AF694981

BEST PRACTICES

Position & Guidance Documents of ASHP

2023–2024 Edition

ashp

The ASHP policies in this book, positions and guidance documents, are intended to foster improvements in pharmacy practice and patient care. The content of individual positions and guidance documents should be assessed in the context of your own health system, its policies and procedures, as well as applicable federal and state laws and regulations.

Guidance documents, in particular, evolve because of advances in technology, new knowledge from research, and lessons from experience. Additionally, medication information is constantly evolving because of ongoing research and clinical experience, and it is often subject to interpretation and unique clinical situations. The American Society of Health-System Pharmacists (ASHP) endeavors to ensure the completeness and timeliness of the information presented. However, the reader is advised that the publisher, contributors, editors, and reviewers make no representations concerning the suitability of the information for any purpose, and are not responsible for the immediate currency of the information, for any errors or omissions, or for any consequences arising from the use of these materials. All decisions made within the context of pharmacy practice should be based on the independent judgment of the practitioner.

ASHP is the collective voice of pharmacists who serve as patient care providers in hospitals, health systems, ambulatory clinics, and other healthcare settings spanning the full spectrum of medication use. The organization's more than 60,000 members include pharmacists, student pharmacists, and pharmacy technicians. For 80 years, ASHP has been at the forefront of efforts to improve medication use and enhance patient safety. For more information about the wide array of ASHP activities and the many ways in which pharmacists advance healthcare, visit ASHP's website, ashp.org, or its consumer website, www.SafeMedication.com.

Editor: Bruce Hawkins

Published by the American Society of Health-System Pharmacists, 4500 East-West Highway, Suite 900, Bethesda, MD 20814.

ASHP® is a service mark of the American Society of Health-System Pharmacists®, Inc.; registered in the U.S. Patent and Trademark Office.

© 2024, American Society of Health-System Pharmacists®, Inc. All rights reserved.

No part of this publication may be reproduced or transmitted in any form or by any means, electronic or mechanical, including photocopying, microfilming, and recording, or by any information storage and retrieval systems, without written permission from the American Society of Health-System Pharmacists®.

ISBN: 978-1-58528-703-1 (paperback)
ISBN: 978-1-58528-704-8 (adobe pdf)
ISBN: 978-1-58528-705-5 (ePub)
DOI: 10.37573/9781585287048

10 9 8 7 6 5 4 3 2

Contents

*Indicates content that has been added or revised since the 2019–2020 edition.

DOI 10.37573/9781585287048.FM

Drug Distribution and Control

*Indicates content that has been added or revised since the 2019–2020 edition.

Ethics

*Indicates content that has been added or revised since the 2019–2020 edition.

*Indicates content that has been added or revised since the 2019–2020 edition.

*Indicates content that has been added or revised since the 2019–2020 edition.

Medication Safety

Medication Therapy and Patient Care

ORGANIZATION AND DELIVERY OF SERVICES

*Indicates content that has been added or revised since the 2019–2020 edition.

*Indicates content that has been added or revised since the 2019–2020 edition.

SPECIFIC PRACTICE AREAS

*Indicates content that has been added or revised since the 2019–2020 edition.

*Indicates content that has been added or revised since the 2019–2020 edition.

Pharmaceutical Industry

DRUG PRODUCTS, LABELING, AND PACKAGING

MARKETING

Pharmacy Management

*Indicates content that has been added or revised since the 2019–2020 edition.

*Indicates content that has been added or revised since the 2019–2020 edition.

Practice Settings

Research

ASHP Therapeutic Position Statements

ASHP Therapeutic Guidelines

*Indicates content that has been added or revised since the 2019–2020 edition.

Page Locator for Guidance Documents by Type and Title

ASHP Statements

DOI 10.37573/9781585287048.FM

ASHP Guidelines

ASHP Report

ASHP Technical Assistance Bulletins

Introduction

ASHP is the largest association of pharmacy professionals in the United States, representing 60,000 pharmacists, student pharmacists, and pharmacy technicians in all patient care settings, including hospitals, ambulatory clinics, and health-system community pharmacies. For over 80 years, ASHP has championed innovation in pharmacy practice, advanced education and professional development, and served as a steadfast advocate for members and patients. In addition, ASHP is the accrediting body for pharmacy residency and technician training programs, and provides comprehensive resources to support pharmacy professionals through every stage of their career.

The Compendium

ASHP, since its founding, has developed official professional policies in the form of policy positions and guidance documents about pharmacy practice, first for hospitals, and then for the continuum of practice settings in integrated health systems. Since 1984, these policies have been compiled annually in this compendium, a compilation of ASHP policy positions, statements, guidelines, technical assistance bulletins, therapeutic position statements, therapeutic guidelines, and selected ASHP-endorsed documents. *Best Practices* reflects the intent of ASHP's professional policies to foster improvements in pharmacy practice and patient care.

The compendium is organized by topic to help readers quickly locate related documents. The table of contents is structured by topic, and under each topic the relevant ASHP policy positions, statements, guidelines, technical assistance bulletins, and endorsed documents are listed. The therapeutic documents are listed by type. Following the table of contents is a page locator for documents by type and title, and the index lists each document, to assist readers who are accustomed to searching for a specific document by its title.

Origins and Purposes of ASHP's Policy Positions and Guidance Documents

Policy positions generally originate with an ASHP council and are approved by the ASHP Board of Directors and ASHP House of Delegates. Some policy positions originate as House of Delegate resolutions. Statements, guidelines, and technical assistance bulletins originate with an ASHP council or commission. Statements are approved by the Board of Directors and the House of Delegates, because of their broad philosophical nature. Other types of documents are approved by the Board of Directors only. Therapeutic position statements and therapeutic guidelines originate with the ASHP Council on Therapeutics and are approved by the Board of Directors.

There is a gradation in detail among the guidance documents. Policy positions are short pronouncements, intended to address professional practice. Often, principles established in policy positions are elaborated on in statements and guidelines. Statements express basic philosophy, guidelines offer programmatic advice, and technical assistance bulletins offer more detailed programmatic advice. Of the two types of therapeutic documents, therapeutic guidelines are thorough discussions of drug use and therapeutic position statements are concise responses to specific therapeutic issues.

The guidance documents of ASHP represent a consensus of professional judgment, expert opinion, and documented evidence. They provide guidance and direction to ASHP members and pharmacy practitioners and to other audiences who affect pharmacy practice. Their use may help to comply with federal and state laws and regulations, to meet accreditation requirements, and to improve pharmacy practice and patient care. They are written to establish reasonable goals, to be progressive and challenging, yet attainable as "best practices" in applicable health-system settings. They generally do not represent minimum levels of practice, unless titled as such, and should not be viewed as ASHP requirements.

The use of ASHP's guidance documents by members and other practitioners is strictly voluntary. Their content should be assessed and adapted based on independent judgment to meet the needs of local health-system settings.

The need for authoritative guidance in pharmacy practice has grown with changes in health care and with the shifting influences from regulatory, accrediting, risk-management, financing, and other bodies. Because of the complex nature of ASHP guidance documents, ASHP does not typically undertake immediate development of new documents or expedited revisions to existing documents in response to environmental changes. Other ASHP activities and services, such as educational sessions at national meetings and *American Journal of Health-System Pharmacy (AJHP)* articles, provide more timely information that may be helpful, until sufficient experience is gained to serve as the basis for a document.

Definitions

The types of guidance documents included in this compendium are defined as follows:

ASHP Policy Position: A pronouncement on an issue related to pharmacy professional practice, as approved by the Board of Directors and House of Delegates.

ASHP Statement: A declaration and explanation of basic philosophy or principle, as approved by the Board of Directors and the House of Delegates.

ASHP Guideline: Advice on the implementation or operation of pharmacy practice programs, as approved by the Board of Directors.

ASHP Technical Assistance Bulletin: Specific, detailed advice on pharmacy programs or functions as developed by an ASHP staff division in consultation with experts, as approved by the Board of Directors.*

ASHP Therapeutic Guideline: Thorough, systematically developed advice for health-care professionals on appropriate use of medications for specific clinical circumstances, as approved by the Board of Directors.

DOI 10.37573/9781585287048.FM

ASHP Therapeutic Position Statement: Concise statements that respond to specific therapeutic issues of concern to health care consumers and pharmacists, as approved by the Board of Directors.

ASHP-Endorsed Document: Professional policy developed by another organization that offers guidance on some aspect of pharmacy practice or medication use, as approved by the Board of Directors.

**The ASHP Board of Directors voted in November 1997 to discontinue the title "Technical Assistance Bulletin" in ASHP guidance documents, assigning the title "Guidelines" in its place. Over time, the title "Guidelines" will replace the title "Technical Assistance Bulletin" on existing documents when they are revised.*

Development of Guidance Documents

The responsible ASHP council or commission recommends the development of a guidance document after considering whether the topic: a) has generated a need among practitioners for authoritative advice; b) has achieved some stability and there is sufficient experience upon which to base a statement or guideline; c) is relevant to the practice of a significant portion of ASHP's members; d) is within the purview of pharmacy practice in health systems; e) is without other sufficient guidance; and f) does not pose significant legal risks to ASHP. Another consideration is whether ASHP leadership believes that there is room for improvements in practice and that an ASHP document would foster that improvement. The Board of Directors must support the recommendations before developmental processes begin.

The processes used to draft and review new or revised documents vary depending on the body responsible for their development and on the type of document. These processes are described below. Once approved, the document draft becomes an official ASHP policy and is published in *AJHP*, added to ASHP's Web site, and incorporated into the next edition of this compendium. Therapeutic documents are reviewed and revised as needed every three years, and policy positions and practice documents every five years.

ASHP Statements and Guidelines

Any of the ASHP policy-recommending bodies (councils and commissions) may initiate and oversee the development of ASHP statements and guidelines; however, most of them are initiated by the Council on Pharmacy Practice. The development of these documents generally includes the following steps:

1. A group of experts on a given topic volunteers to develop a preliminary draft. Drafters are selected based on demonstrated knowledge of the topic and their practice settings. Most often, the drafters are ASHP members.
2. The draft is sent by ASHP to reviewers who have interest and expertise in the given topic. Reviewers consist of members and selected individuals knowledgeable in the content area, representatives of various ASHP bodies, and other professional organizations. A draft of particular interest to ASHP's membership may be published in *AJHP*, posted on ASHP's Web site, or discussed at an open hearing or in a network forum during an ASHP Summer or Midyear Clinical meeting to solicit comments.
3. Based on the comments, a revised draft is submitted to the appropriate ASHP policy-recommending body for action. When the draft meets the established criteria for content and quality, that body recommends that the Board of Directors approve the document.

ASHP Therapeutic Guidelines and Therapeutic Position Statements

The Council on Therapeutics (COT) has responsibility for the development of ASHP therapeutic guidelines and ASHP therapeutic position statements.

Therapeutic Guidelines—The development of these documents generally includes the following steps:

1. When the COT identifies a topic for therapeutic guidelines development, ASHP formally solicits proposals for a contractual arrangement with an individual, group, or organization to draft the guidelines document and coordinate its review. The contractor will work with a panel of 6–10 experts appointed by ASHP who have diverse backgrounds relevant to the topic.
2. A systematic analysis of the literature is performed, and scientific evidence is evaluated based on predetermined criteria. Recommendations in the document are based on scientific evidence or expert consensus. When expert judgment must be used, the document indicates the scientific reasoning that influenced the decision. Scientific evidence takes precedence over expert judgement. Each recommendation is accompanied by projections of the relevant health and cost outcomes that could result.
3. The expert panel and COT review each draft of the guidelines document and provide comments. This process is repeated until the expert panel and COT are satisfied with the content.
4. ASHP solicits multidisciplinary expert input on the draft. Reviewers consist of members and selected individuals knowledgeable in the content area, representatives of various ASHP bodies, and other professional organizations.
5. Once the above processes are completed, COT recommends that the ASHP Board of Directors approve it.

ASHP Therapeutic Position Statements (TPS)—The development of these documents generally includes the following steps:

1. One or more experts on a given topic are assigned to draft the TPS. Drafters are selected based on demonstrated knowledge of the topic and their practice setting. Most often, the drafters are ASHP members.
2. The proposed draft document is reviewed by COT, which may suggest modifications. This process is repeated until COT is satisfied with the content.
3. ASHP solicits multidisciplinary expert input on the draft. Reviewers consist of members and selected individuals knowledgeable in the content area, representatives of various ASHP bodies, and other professional organizations.
4. Once the above processes are completed, COT finalizes the draft and recommends that the ASHP Board of Directors approve it.

Access to ASHP Positions and Guidance Documents

Besides publishing in *AJHP* and this compendium, policy positions and guidance documents are available through ASHP's Web site at www.ashp.org. They are located at the "Policy Positions & Guidelines" heading under "Pharmacy Practice" on the ASHP Web site (https://www.ashp.org/Pharmacy-Practice/Policy-Positions-and-Guidelines), where a chronological compendium of policy positions (*ASHP Policy Positions 1982–2023*) is also available.

Opportunities to Be a Part of Guidance Document Development

ASHP members determine the needs for policy guidance documents. They write and review the drafts. And, as members of policy-recommending bodies, the Board of Directors, and House of Delegates, they approve the documents.

ASHP members are encouraged to take an active role in the development of documents by suggesting topic ideas for new documents or modifications to current ones, volunteering to be drafters or reviewers, and completing survey and evaluation forms. Members may comment on or express their interests in participating in the development of documents by contacting the editor by e-mail at standards@ashp.org.

Mission Statement of the American Society of Health-System Pharmacists (ASHP)

The mission of pharmacists is to help people achieve optimal health outcomes. ASHP helps its members achieve this mission by advocating and supporting the professional practice of pharmacists in hospitals, health systems, ambulatory clinics, and other settings spanning the full spectrum of medication use. ASHP serves its members as their collective voice on issues related to medication use and public health.

Approved by the ASHP Board of Directors, December 6, 2012.

Copyright © 2012, American Society of Health-System Pharmacists. All rights reserved. Contact ASHP for reprint and permissions requests. This content may not be used for commercial purposes without the express written consent of ASHP.

Vision Statement of the American Society of Health-System Pharmacists (ASHP)

ASHP's vision is that medication use will be optimal, safe, and effective for all people all of the time.

Approved by the ASHP Board of Directors, December 6, 2012.

Copyright © 2012, American Society of Health-System Pharmacists. All rights reserved. Contact ASHP for reprint and permissions requests. This content may not be used for commercial purposes without the express written consent of ASHP.

DOI 10.37573/9781585287048.FM

ASHP Policy Positions, Statements, Guidelines, and Technical Assistance Bulletins

DOI 10.37573/9781585287048

Automation and Information Technology

DOI 10.37573/9781585287048

Automation and Information Technology

2303

INTEROPERABILITY OF PATIENT-CARE TECHNOLOGIES

Source: Council on Pharmacy Management

To encourage interdisciplinary development and implementation of standards that foster foundational, structural, semantic, and organizational interoperability of health information technology (HIT); further,

To encourage the integration, consolidation, and harmonization of medication-related databases used in patient-care technologies to reduce the risk that outdated, inaccurate, or conflicting data might be used and to minimize the resources required to maintain such databases; further,

To encourage healthcare organizations to adopt HIT that utilizes industry standards and can access, exchange, integrate, and cooperatively use data within and across organizational, regional, and national boundaries.

This policy supersedes ASHP policy 1302.

Rationale

The interoperability of patient-care technologies should be a standard across any hospital or health system. The development and implementation of standards would promote timely and seamless portability of information and optimize patient-care technologies that utilize medication-related databases. The installation of these technologies will aid pharmacy data, data analytics, and support activities that mitigate medication errors, medication diversion, and other health outcomes. This form of uniformity in information sharing will increase workflow efficiency and reduce delay in duties for pharmacy and other healthcare workers.

Although it is important to recognize the differences among technologies used in patient care, there is a need to have both a standardized format to describe medications as well as means for efficiently managing the medication databases in order to safely populate and update the different technologies that rely on drug information. Coalitions such as the Pharmacy e-Health Information Technology Collaborative are important in providing expertise, organizing and participating in stakeholder events, and advocating for best practices. It may, however, be necessary for other organizations to convene stakeholders to develop standards for the harmonization of medication-related databases.

2304

PATIENT MEDICATION DELIVERY SYSTEMS

Source: Council on Pharmacy Practice

To foster the clinical and technical expertise of the pharmacy workforce in the use of medication delivery systems; further,

To advocate for key decision-making roles for the pharmacy workforce in the selection, implementation, maintenance, and monitoring of medication delivery systems; further,

To urge hospitals and health systems to directly involve departments of pharmacy and interprofessional stakeholders in performing appropriate risk assessments before new medication delivery systems are implemented or existing systems are upgraded; further,

To advocate that medication delivery systems employ patient safety-enhancing capabilities and be interoperable with health information systems; further,

To encourage continuous innovation and improvement in medication delivery system technologies; further,

To foster development of tools and resources to assist the pharmacy workforce in designing and monitoring the use of medication delivery systems.

Rationale

Technological advances in medication delivery systems and administration devices frequently enable improved control of medication administration. Smart infusion pumps are becoming the standard of care for delivering intravenous fluids and medications because they allow for a greater level of control, accuracy, and precision with drug delivery. They are designed to provide users with clinical decision support for programmed doses and infusion rates in order to identify errors before medications or fluids are infused. Smart pump technology and data systems can help improve safety practices by recording and offering reports regarding pump-related errors, alerts, compliance to the institution's drug library, and overrides. ASHP advocates that to enhance patient safety, medication delivery systems interface with information systems, allow interoperability with the electronic health record, and employ dose error reduction software, including but not limited to standardized medication drug libraries with dosing limits, clinical advisories, and other patient safety-enhancing capabilities.

The design, maintenance, monitoring, and continuous quality improvement of medication delivery systems is an interdisciplinary process that requires ongoing collaboration among many disciplines. The pharmacy workforce has an integral role in ensuring the safe and effective management of medication delivery systems, including advising the interprofessional care team on their use. Pharmacists are a resource for education, therapy selection, monitoring, and troubleshooting of smart pump and other drug delivery systems to help improve patient safety and reduce medication errors. In efforts to optimize drug use, pharmacists should participate in organizational and clinical decisions with regard to these systems and devices.

2332

BARCODING OF LOT NUMBER AND EXPIRATION DATE

Source: House of Delegates

To advocate that the Food and Drug Administration and organizations that develop barcode standards require barcodes contain lot number and expiration date on all immediate product packages to enable automated collection and validation of this information during medication preparation, dispensing, and administration processes; further,

To educate regulatory and safety organizations that barcode scanning versus manual logging of lot numbers and expirations is critical for patient safety and preparation sterility and improves data visibility for medication recalls; further,

DOI 10.37573/9781585287048.001

To advocate that state boards of pharmacy, regulatory agencies, and accrediting bodies delay punitive action on rules requiring logging of lot number and expiration dates during sterile product preparation until this information is made available on immediate product barcodes.

Rationale

The current Food and Drug Administration (FDA) barcode rule requires the National Drug Code (NDC), lot number, and expiration date on all saleable medication packages. FDA created an exception for immediate packages, which include unit dose packages and individual vials sold as lots in boxes. More than 90% of products dispensed in a hospital are immediate packages. The FDA exception requires that the barcodes on these immediate packages be linear (1D) barcodes. Due to the technology of 1D barcodes, it is difficult to fit the larger barcode containing additional characters needed to code lot number, expiration date, and NDC on labels of inner packages. As a result, the 1D barcodes required on inner packages only contain the NDC. 2D barcodes require less label space than 1D barcodes, and 2D scanners can read 1D and 2D barcodes. Many products dispensed are saleable packages that only contain 2D barcodes, and 2D barcode readers are significantly less expensive and more reliable than the 1D laser scanners used in the past. Hospitals have responded by widely adopting use of 2D scanners.

A proposed FDA rule will allow but not require 2D barcodes and require only the inclusion of the NDC in the barcode. The FDA states that the reason for these requirements is that the expansion of the NDC to 12 digits will create issues for manufacturers that code a 10-digit NDC number in the barcode and don't have the label space to expand the 1D barcode to 12 digits. The proposed rule will not guarantee that barcodes on inner products contain lot number and expiration date. FDA has stated that they are addressing the immediate package requirements in the revised rule, but this is only true for the NDC 12-character expansion and not for the encoding of lot and expiration date.

Multiple state boards of pharmacy, including California and Texas, require hospitals to log the NDC, lot number, and expiration dates on all intravenous (IV) products that are compounded or repackaged. United States Pharmcopeia (USP) Chapter 797 is adding the same requirements, effective November 1, 2023. The logging of lot numbers and expiration dates is not a second check but an attempt to track medications all the way to the patient in the case of recalls and event reporting. With IV workflow systems and barcodes with lot number and expiration dates, an IV product can be prepared and documented with only two barcode scans. Current linear barcodes require scans of the NDC, multiple mouse clicks, and many keystrokes on a keyboard to enter the data. For example, a two-component IV product with a base solution and one additive was reported to require 22 keystrokes and 2 mouse clicks at a minimum if lot number and expiration date are not in the barcode. In addition, putting a keyboard into the sterile environment or pulling hands in and out of the sterile field threatens sterility. Dispersing this data entry work in the middle of a complicated IV workflow will not only create data entry or transcription errors but will increase the potential for computation errors, as the preparer keys in or handwrites a long series of seemingly random numbers while computing, measuring, and verifying doses.

Software vendors have acknowledged that their systems already have the functionality to capture lot number and expiration dates, if available, through barcode scanning, replacing numerous keystrokes. This functionality has not only been added to IV preparation functions but also to dispensing and medication administration functions as well. In addition, many systems allow barcode scans to be initiated by foot switches, permitting users to avoid touching scanners, therefore minimizing potential impacts on sterility. One vender has reported that they are in the process of adding automatic checks for expired medications and recalled lot numbers during all medication barcode scanning functions throughout the medication-use process. Significant safety improvements and time savings can be realized through automated checking of expiration dates and recalls throughout the medication-use process, including automated dispensing cabinet restocking.

Although state boards of pharmacy and USP are considering and implementing rules to track medications to the patient and validate expiration dates, there is a general lack of understanding how these rules impact IV preparation workflows and corresponding medication safety and sterility of IV preparation. It is important that rulemakers understand these impacts and implement rules to require the inclusion of lot number and expiration date on immediate product barcodes. Healthcare organizations should communicate the need for NDC, lot number, and expiration date on all immediate products, including repackaged products and investigational medications, to the FDA and GS1, the barcode standards organization that defines medication barcode standards, to assure the resulting barcodes meet the needs of health systems.

2204

MOBILE HEALTH TOOLS, CLINICAL APPS, AND ASSOCIATED DEVICES

Source: Council on Pharmacy Management

To advocate that patients, pharmacists, and other healthcare professionals be involved in the selection, approval, and management of patient-centered mobile health tools, clinical software applications ("clinical apps"), and associated devices used by clinicians and patients for patient care; further,

To foster development of tools and resources to assist pharmacists in designing and assessing processes to ensure safe, accurate, supported, and secure use of mobile health tools, clinical apps, and associated devices; further,

To advocate that decisions regarding the selection, approval, and management of mobile health tools, clinical apps, and associated devices consider patient usability, acceptability, and usefulness and should further the goal of delivering safe and effective patient care that optimizes outcomes; further,

To advocate that mobile health tools, clinical apps, and associated devices that contain health information be interoperable and, if applicable, be structured to allow incorporation of health information into the patient's electronic health record and other essential clinical systems to facilitate optimal health outcomes; further,

To advocate that pharmacists be included in regulatory and other evaluation and approval of mobile health tools, clinical apps, and associated devices that involve medications or medication management; further,

To encourage patient education and assessment of competency in the use of mobile health technologies; further,

To enhance patient awareness on how to access and use validated sources of health information integrated with mobile health tools, clinical apps, and associated devices.

This policy supersedes ASHP policy 1708.

Rationale

Digital health technologies, including mobile health (mHealth) applications (apps), hold great potential to improve health and healthcare. There is nearly ubiquitous use of smartphones and an ever-growing and increasingly sophisticated suite of health apps. These apps are providing a wide range of medical functions that span the care continuum from prevention to diagnosis to care management. The adoption of these digital solutions is further amplified by their accessibility, low cost, and personalized features. In addition, their ability to provide practical functions such as health education, tracking of symptoms and side effects, appointment management, and social support make them compelling healthcare tools. With the proliferation of mHealth tools, clinical apps, and associated devices, healthcare organizations need to address the potential barriers and risks of application use. Particular concerns include (1) assessing the quality of mHealth tools, clinical apps, and associated devices; (2) standardizing choices and use across the organization; (3) ensuring the security of data and data storage; and (4) patient usability, acceptability, and usefulness (e.g., generational differences in acceptance of technology). To maximize the effectiveness of mHealth tools, clinical apps, and associated devices, they must be selected, approved, and managed with the goal of improving care and with input from representatives of all affected parties, including patients, physicians, pharmacists, and other healthcare professionals. In addition, their effectiveness is enhanced when they are interoperable (as described in ASHP policy 1302, Interoperability of Patient-Care Technologies) and the data stored within them can be incorporated into the patient's electronic health record (EHR) and other essential clinical systems.

Providers and patients currently have little guidance regarding use of these resources or the management of the data they provide. The Food and Drug Administration and other regulatory agencies are just beginning to determine the scope of their oversight regarding standardized evaluation and validation processes. As medication-use experts, pharmacists can contribute to the regulatory evaluation and approval of mHealth tools, clinical apps, and associated devices that involve medications or medication management. For example, pharmacists can help assess the quality of information presented (e.g., incorrect or incomplete information, variation in content, incorrect or inappropriate response to patient needs) and mitigate inconsistencies with patient education resources provided by an organization (e.g., discharge education). ASHP is committed to fostering development of resources to help pharmacists ensure safe, accurate, supported, and secure use of mHealth tools, clinical apps, and associated devices. Patient engagement strategies include patient education and competency assessment and enhanced patient awareness of how to access and use validated sources of health information integrated with mHealth tools, clinical apps, and associated devices. Product customer assistance teams for mHealth tools, clinical apps, and associated devices should be leveraged to provide direct support to sustain these efforts. Patient engagement with these tools will: (1) increase communication between patient and providers, leading to increased patient satisfaction; (2) enhance sharing of health information using EHRs; and (3) enable patients to have access to their health data, which empowers them with the knowledge of their health conditions and helps them make informed treatment choices.

2246

AUTOVERIFICATION OF MEDICATION ORDERS

Source: Council on Pharmacy Practice

To recognize the importance of pharmacist verification of medication orders, and the important role pharmacists have in developing and implementing systems for autoverification of select medication orders; further,

To recognize that autoverification of select medication orders under institution-guided criteria can help expand access to pharmacist patient care; further,

To discourage implementation of autoverification as a means to reduce pharmacist hours; further,

To promote and disseminate research, standards, and best practices on the safety and appropriateness of autoverification of medication orders; further,

To encourage healthcare organizations to develop policies, procedures, and guidelines to determine which care settings, medications, and patient populations are appropriate candidates for autoverification of select medication orders in order to support the implementation of autoverification models for those circumstances; further,

To advocate for regulations and accreditation standards that permit autoverification of select medication orders in circumstances in which it has proven safe.

Rationale

The purpose of autoverification of medication orders is to improve medication-use safety and quality and more efficiently and effectively utilize pharmacy personnel. When autoverification functionality is used, medications ordered via computerized provider order entry (CPOE) are evaluated against predetermined parameters in electronic health records (EHRs). Orders that fall within set parameters are autoverified and available to be administered; those that fall outside the parameters require review by a pharmacist. Critical values, patient history, and clinical decision support tools are used to create the algorithm that determines whether a medication order is reviewed. The healthcare community has long recognized the importance of pharmacist verification of medication orders, and that role is no less important when developing and implementing systems for autoverification of select medication orders. Recent experience has shown that autoverification of medication orders, when done safely and efficiently, can allow more effective use of pharmacist resources by expanding access to pharmacist patient care.

In the 2016 ASHP survey of health systems, 51.6% of hospitals utilized the autoverification functionality in the CPOE system; this rose to 62.2% utilization by the 2019 survey. Of the health systems surveyed in 2019 that utilized autoverification, 52.9% autoverified in selected areas (e.g., all emergency department orders, perioperative orders); 50.2% identified selected medications for autoverification in specific areas (e.g., pain medications in the emergency department); and 17.1% of hospitals had autoverification for select medications (e.g., flushes, influenza vaccine) throughout the hospital. Between 2016 and 2019, overall use of autoverification and autoverification of select medications throughout the hospital and for select medications in certain areas increased. In contrast, the use of autoverification for all medications in a select area of the hospital decreased from 2016 to 2019.

According to the ASHP survey, the most commonly cited reasons for not implementing autoverification were patient safety concerns (40.4%); "our hospital has not discussed this" (23.2%); and requirements by law, regulation, or accreditors (22.9%). Less common reasons were that EHR software does not have the functionality (6.9%) and EHR limitations on criteria used for autoverification (4.6%). Healthcare professionals have also expressed a concern about medication optimization: medication appropriateness may not be the same as medication optimization. Pharmacy directors have also stated that staffing determinations based on pharmacist workload and other measurable metrics must be carefully considered; autoverification should not be a mechanism for reducing pharmacist hours, which would negate the potential to expand patient care services.

2255

THERAPEUTIC INDICATION FOR PRESCRIBED MEDICATIONS

Source: Council on Therapeutics

To advocate that all healthcare professionals involved in a patient's care have immediate access to the intended therapeutic purpose of prescribed medications in order to ensure safe and effective medication use; further,

To encourage all healthcare settings to optimize the use of clinical decision support systems with indications-based prescribing; further,

To advocate for implementation of a universal, interoperable coding system for labeled therapeutic indications that can be integrated throughout the medication-use process, enabling optimum clinical workflows and decision support functionality; further,

To advocate for federal and state laws and regulations to include diagnosis-based indication(s) on medication order(s) and prescription(s), and to allow the withholding of indication on medication prescription labels when patient privacy risks outweigh benefits.

This policy supersedes ASHP policies 0305 and 2123.

Rationale

The Joint Commission (TJC) *Comprehensive Accreditation Manual for Hospitals* includes standards that specify that healthcare professionals involved in the medication-use process should have access to and use patient and medication information important in the prescribing, dispensing, administration, and monitoring of medications. In addition to its accreditation standards, TJC's 2022 national patient safety goals for hospitals include improved staff communication (getting important test results to the right staff person on time) and safe use of medications (recording and passing along correct information about a patient's medications). It is important to recognize that medication indications are used not only by pharmacists, nurses, and physicians but also other important members of the healthcare team, including but not limited to respiratory therapists, social workers, physical therapists, and others who utilize this information to guide patient care.

The Institute for Safe Medication Practices (ISMP) has offered recommendations, including clearly specified dosage form, drug strength, and complete directions on all prescriptions; indication on all outpatient prescriptions and on inpatient PRN orders; with name pairs known to be problematic, reducing the potential for confusion by writing prescriptions using both the brand and generic names; listing both brand and generic names on medication administration records and automated dispensing cabinet computer screens; and, whenever possible, determining the purpose of the medication before dispensing or administering it.

Several well-known studies have demonstrated reductions in wrong-patient errors and adverse events with the inclusion of indication on the prescription order. In 2010, Equale (*Drug Saf.* 2010;33:559–67) described the accuracy of indication information in electronic health records (EHRs). Galanter (*J Am Med Inform Assoc.* 2013;20:477–81) focused on preventing wrong-patient medication errors with the use of indication-based prescribing. Indication-based alerts resulted in an interception rate of 0.25 interceptions per 1000 alerts. One team of investigators conducted a trial of inpatient indication-based prescribing using computerized provider order entry with drugs commonly used off-label (*Appl Clin Inf.* 2011;2:94–103). Off-label prescription drug use without strong scientific evidence has also been associated with increased rates of adverse drug events (*JAMA Internal Medicine* 2016;176:55–63). The authors suggested that use of and proper documentation of therapeutic indication can help improve surveillance and safety and decrease risk. This additional safety check is critical in limiting errors due to wrong and/or look-alike/sound-alike medications. In addition to error prevention, indication-based prescribing can improve patient engagement, patient education, and provide pharmacists with information that may be necessary for prior authorizations or claim processing. To foster successful implementation of indication-based prescribing in EHRs, several authors have documented the success of starting electronic prescriptions with a problem or indication list first before medications can be selected to reduce time and medication errors while maintaining clinician satisfaction.

In several countries, including Canada and Spain, the EHR includes indication as part of comprehensive documentation. ASHP first developed official policy on the importance of pharmacists' access to indications in 1993. In 1996, the National Coordinating Council for Medication Error Reporting and Prevention recommended including the purpose of medication orders because of concerns about safety, unless considered inappropriate by the prescribers. In 1999, the Institute for Safe Medication Practices recommended including the purpose of prescribing on all written orders. In 2004, the National Association of Boards of Pharmacy (NABP) approved a resolution encouraging national and state medical associations to support legislative and regulatory efforts to require prescribers to include indications for all oral, written, and electronically transmitted prescriptions. In 2012, the United States Pharmacopeia made amendments to the standards for prescription container labeling to include "purpose-for-use" language. In 2015, the National Council of Prescription Drug Plans drafted language to recommend diagnosis and SNOMED indication be sent with any prescription. Despite these recommendations, few states have adopted any laws requiring inclusion of indication on all medication orders or prescriptions.

More recently, ISMP has recommended updating the five "rights" of patient, drug, dose, time, and route to include a sixth "right": the right indication. They cite benefits of indication-based prescribing as (1) helping to prevent errors by narrowing medication choices; (2) empowering and educating patients, which helps increase patient adherence; (3) improving communications among the healthcare team, patients, and families; (4) facilitating medication reconciliation; (5) helping prescribers select the best medications for their patients; and (6) aiding in measuring drug effectiveness and learning from off-label use.

ASHP also has policy on off-label use that encourages the use of the three authoritative drug compendia, peer-reviewed literature, and consultation with experts in research and clinical practice to make specific coverage decisions. ASHP supports informed decision-making that promotes third-party reimbursement for drug products approved by the Food and Drug Administration (FDA) appropriately prescribed for unlabeled uses.

Implementation and use of interoperable clinical decision support systems with indications-based prescribing would be eased by agreement on a universal coding system for labeled therapeutic indications. The FDA, the National Council for Prescription Drug Programs, and other organizations should work collaboratively to select and implement such a system.

Furthermore, ASHP recognizes that there are circumstances in which it would be inappropriate to include diagnosis on a medication order, and encourages such exceptions in federal and state laws and regulations. One clear example of such an exception would be six protected categories of drugs (antidepressants, antipsychotics, anticonvulsants, immunosuppressants for treatment of transplant rejection, antiretrovirals, and antineoplastics), as including these may inadvertently result in breaches in patient privacy.

2147

PHARMACIST'S ROLE IN HEALTHCARE INFORMATION SYSTEMS

Source: Council on Pharmacy Management

To strongly advocate key decision-making roles for pharmacists in the planning, selection, design, implementation, and maintenance of medication-use information systems, electronic health records, computerized provider order entry systems, and e-prescribing systems to balance the security and integrity of data with the ability to facilitate clinical decision support, data analysis, and education of users for the purpose of ensuring the safe and effective use of medications; further,

To advocate for incentives to hospitals and health systems for the adoption of patient-care technologies; further,

To recognize that design, maintenance, and cyber-security of medication-use information systems is an interdisciplinary process that requires ongoing collaboration among many disciplines; further,

To advocate that pharmacists must have accountability for strategic planning and direct operational aspects of the medication-use process, including the successful deployment of medication-use information systems and continuity plans when the systems are unavailable.

This policy supersedes ASHP policies 1211 and 1701.

Rationale

ASHP recognizes that design, maintenance, and cyber-security of healthcare information systems (e.g., medication-use information systems, electronic health records, computerized provider order entry systems, e-prescribing systems) is an interdisciplinary process that requires ongoing collaboration across many disciplines. Maintaining the privacy of health information, in compliance with the Health Insurance Portability and Affordability Act (HIPAA), and ensuring patient safety in the face of cyber-attacks are essential concerns for every healthcare organization. Given the ever-evolving nature of pharmacist patient care, medication use, and health information technology, it is essential pharmacists have key decision-making roles in the planning, selection, design, implementation, and maintenance of such systems in order to help prevent and respond to cyber-attacks. To ensure the safe and effective use of medications, pharmacists must have accountability for strategic planning and direct operational aspects of the medication-use process, including the successful deployment of medication-use-related information systems by assessing vulnerabilities and vendor systems to validate the security and integrity of the data. Increased connectivity with vendor systems creates a mutual need to share access to patient information and other vital data, so risk mitigation must be considered at all points of access. This includes, for example, facilitating clinical decision support by assessing the minimum amount of patient health information vendors require to provide services, data analysis, education of users, and developing and implementing business continuity plans, to include fail-over testing of these plans, for when the systems are unavailable.

2015

NETWORK CONNECTIVITY AND INTEROPERABILITY FOR CONTINUITY OF CARE

Source: Council on Pharmacy Management

To advocate the use of electronic information systems, with appropriate security controls, that enable the integration of patient-specific data that is accessible in all components of a health system; further,

To support the use of technology that allows the transfer of patient information needed for appropriate medication management across the continuum of care; further,

To urge computer software vendors and pharmaceutical suppliers to provide standards for definition, collection, coding, and exchange of clinical data used in the medication-use process; further,

To pursue formal and informal liaisons with appropriate healthcare associations to ensure that the interests of patient care and safety in the medication-use process are fully represented in the standardization, integration, and implementation of electronic information systems; further,

To strongly encourage health-system administrators, regulatory bodies, and other appropriate groups to provide health-system pharmacists with full access to patient-specific clinical data; further,

To advocate that client-vendor agreements include timelines for data destruction; further,

To oppose the selling of data for unauthorized uses; further,

To educate health-system leaders about potential use and misuse of shared data.

This policy supersedes ASHP policy 0507.

Rationale

For the past two decades, the U.S. health system has been racing to take advantage of the potential that digital health information offers for improved patient care. Each institution and practice has invested in information systems that work for its specific situation. These systems were developed by multiple vendors, each with their own proprietary structures and labels. Information was and continues to be found in silos, within health systems, within institutions, even within departments.

In 2004, an executive order created the Office of the National Coordinator for Health Information Technology (ONC). ONC is the primary federal entity charged with coordination of nationwide efforts to implement and advance health information technology and the electronic exchange of health information. The 2009 Health Information Technology for Economic and Clinical Health (HITECH) Act provided the Department of Health and Human Services with additional authority to promote health information technology, including the secure exchange of electronic health information.

As defined by the Healthcare Information and Management Systems Society (HIMSS), interoperability is "the ability of different information systems, devices, or applications to connect, in a coordinated manner, within and across organizational boundaries to access, exchange and cooperatively use data amongst stakeholders, with the goal of optimizing the health of individuals and populations." ONC has developed a roadmap for interoperability and created calls to action for entities with specific roles in our healthcare system (e.g., the Calls to Action for People and Organizations That Deliver Care and Services).

As government agencies, standards-setting organizations, and professional associations work toward interoperability of health information technology, it is important to ensure this includes the ability of healthcare providers and patients to securely access and use health information from different sources and settings relevant to medication use to ensure patient-centered continuity of care.

Along with secure access and sharing of health information, providers and health systems must be cognizant of how a vendor will handle data, how it plans to safeguard data, and whether and how data will be used for secondary purposes (e.g., research, advertising).

ASHP recognizes that continuity of care is a vital requirement in the appropriate use of medications. Pharmacists have responsibility for ensuring continuity of care as patients move from one setting to another (e.g., ambulatory care, inpatient care, community pharmacy, home care). Achieving information systems that have the ability to share relevant patient care data securely across care settings is a critical step in optimizing medication use across care settings.

1529

ONLINE PHARMACY AND INTERNET PRESCRIBING

Source: Council on Pharmacy Practice

To support efforts to regulate prescribing and dispensing of medications via the Internet; further,

To support legislation or regulation that requires online pharmacies to list the states in which the pharmacy and pharmacists are licensed, and, if prescribing services are offered, requires that the sites (1) ensure that a legitimate patient-prescriber relationship exists (consistent with professional practice standards) and (2) list the states in which the prescribers are licensed; further,

To support mandatory accreditation of online pharmacies by the National Association of Boards of Pharmacy Verified Internet Pharmacy Practice Sites or Veterinary-Verified Internet Pharmacy Practice Sites; further,

To support appropriate consumer education about the risks and benefits of using online pharmacies; further,

To support the principle that any medication distribution or drug therapy management system must provide timely access to, and interaction with, appropriate professional pharmacist patient-care services.

This policy was reviewed in 2020 by the Council on Pharmacy Practice and by the Board of Directors and was found to still be appropriate.

Rationale

ASHP's vision to make medication use safe, optimal, and effective includes supporting efforts to protect the public from unscrupulous website operators who illegally provide medications online. Patients are entitled to know whether the healthcare providers prescribing and dispensing their medications are licensed, and in which states they are licensed. ASHP supports legislation and regulations that would require online pharmacies to provide such information. To further guarantee patient safety, ASHP advocates mandatory accreditation of such sites by the National Association of Boards of Pharmacy (NABP) Verified Internet Pharmacy Practice Sites (VIPPS) and Veterinary-Verified Internet Pharmacy Practice Sites (Vet-VIPPS) accreditation programs for online pharmacies to assure the public that the pharmacies are compliant with federal and state regulations and NABP criteria. Education of consumers will be required to ensure that online pharmacies are used wisely, and use of online pharmacies should involve appropriate pharmacist counseling.

1418

RISK ASSESSMENT OF HEALTH INFORMATION TECHNOLOGY

Source: Council on Pharmacy Management

To urge hospitals and health systems to directly involve departments of pharmacy in performing appropriate risk assessment before new health information technology (HIT) is implemented or existing HIT is upgraded, and as part of the continuous evaluation of current HIT performance; further,

To advocate that HIT vendors provide estimates of the resources required to implement and support new HIT; further,

To collaborate with HIT vendors to encourage the development of HIT that improves patient-care outcomes; further,

To advocate for changes in federal law that would recognize HIT vendors' safety accountability.

This policy was reviewed in 2019 by the Council on Pharmacy Management and by the Board of Directors and was found to still be appropriate.

Rationale

The adoption of HIT in hospitals has been increasing at a quickening pace. The ASHP National Survey—2012 reports the adoption of the following: full paperless electronic health record (EHR) (18.6%), computerized provider order entry with clinical decision support (CPOE with CDS) (54.4%), bar-coded medication administration (BCMA) (65.5%), and smart pumps (77%). The adoption of HIT has undoubtedly been spurred by the American Recovery and Reinvestment Act (ARRA) and the Health Information Technology for Economic and Clinical Health Act (HITECH) provisions under Meaningful Use (MU) of the EHR. Hospitals have been incentivized to implement EHRs that meet the MU criteria by increased reimbursement through Medicare and/or Medicaid payments. Due to the strict guidelines and the rush to meet incentive payments, many providers are questioning whether some HIT is being implemented too quickly.

The implementation of HIT within the medication-use process has been proven to prevent and decrease errors, improve quality, and prevent waste. A key premise of the Office of the National Coordinator for Health Information Technology (ONC) report "Health Information Technology Patient Safety Action & Surveillance Plan" (July 2013) is that HIT, when fully integrated into health care delivery organizations, facilitates substantial improvements in health care quality and safety as compared to paper records. As hospitals and providers implement HIT within their institutions and practices, however, they often encounter new types of errors and problems. The medical literature is starting to see reports of these unintended consequences of HIT, so continuous monitoring of these systems is required. It has become increasingly important to properly assess the interface between HIT and users to identify whether any new risk has been introduced to the system and implement HIT appropriately, taking into account medication-use processes and human factors. Critical questions hospitals and health systems face include (1) when do HIT advances exceed the capacity for integration into workflow, (2) when does HIT begin to introduce risk into the medication-use process rather than improve patient safety, and (3) what are the accountabilities of HIT providers, regulators, and providers to ensure the necessary product development and assessments are made before implementation of new HIT.

ASHP advocates that the pharmacy department be part of the implementation team for any medication-related technology within an institution. Technology assessment tools should be applied by pharmacists and others to proactively determine gaps in function prior to implementation, during upgrades, and as part of the continuous evaluation of HIT performance. The use of failure modes effects analysis (FMEA) and other resources should be considered. Risk assessment should also be considered when implementing any new technology to ensure that unintended consequences are minimized.

Regulatory and accreditation organizations include components of risk assessment and quality improvement within their criteria, but hospitals need to incorporate these into their overall plans. Such risk assessments could result in less attention on some HIT implementations. Finally, federal law needs to recognize vendors' accountability for the safety of their products as implemented.

1212

CLINICAL DECISION SUPPORT SYSTEMS

Source: Council on Pharmacy Management

To advocate for the development of clinical decision support (CDS) systems that are proven to improve medication-use outcomes and that include the following capabilities: (1) alerts, notifications, and summary data views provided to the appropriate people at the appropriate times in clinical workflows, based on (a) a rich set of patient-specific data, (b) standardized, evidence-based medication-use best practices, and (c) identifiable patterns in medication-use data in the electronic health record; (2) audit trails of all CDS alerts, notifications, and follow-up activity; (3) structured clinical documentation functionality linked to individual CDS alerts and notifications; and (4) highly accessible and detailed management reporting capabilities that facilitate assessment of the quality and completeness of CDS responses and the effects of CDS on patient outcomes.

This policy was reviewed in 2023 by the Council on Pharmacy Management and by the Board of Directors and was found to still be appropriate.

Rationale

Clinical decision support (CDS) systems provide timely information, usually at the point of care, to help inform decisions about a patient's care. CDS can effectively improve patient outcomes and lead to higher-quality healthcare. CDS systems are now commonly administered through electronic medical records and other computerized clinical workflows, which has been facilitated by increasing global adoption of electronic medical records with advanced capabilities. Despite these advances, there remain unknowns regarding the effect CDS systems have on the providers who use them, patient outcomes, and costs. There have been numerous published examples of CDS system success stories, but notable setbacks have also demonstrated that CDS systems are not without risks. Ongoing advocacy is needed for evidence-based improvements in CDS systems that minimize risk in design, implementation, evaluation, and maintenance; provide actionable data analytics; and support the medication-use process.

1020

ROLE OF PHARMACISTS IN SAFE TECHNOLOGY IMPLEMENTATION

Source: Council on Pharmacy Practice

To affirm the essential role of the pharmacist in the evaluation, implementation, and ongoing assessment of all technology intended to ensure safety, effectiveness, and efficiency of the medication-use process.

This policy was reviewed in 2020 by the Council on Pharmacy Practice and by the Board of Directors and was found to still be appropriate.

Rationale

Effective use of automation and technology solutions improves efficiency, allows more time for direct patient care, and ensures safe medication management. The Joint Commission Sentinel Event Alert published in December 2008 outlined patient safety concerns specific to technology implementation and recommended specific actions to reduce error and patient harm. The Institute for Safe Medication Practices (ISMP) has published related recommendations for specific technologies and noted recently that one drug delivery device was marketed to promote physician autonomy as a benefit of its use.

This policy was reviewed in 2017 by the Council on Public Policy and by the Board of Directors and was found to still be appropriate.

0712

ELECTRONIC HEALTH AND BUSINESS TECHNOLOGY AND SERVICES

Source: Council on Pharmacy Practice

To encourage pharmacists to assume a leadership role in their hospitals and health systems with respect to strategic planning for and implementation of electronic health and business technology and services; further,

To encourage hospital and health-system administrators to provide dedicated resources for pharmacy departments to design, implement, and maintain electronic health and business technology and services; further,

To advocate the inclusion of electronic health technology and telepharmacy issues and applications in college of pharmacy curricula.

This policy was reviewed in 2017 by the Council on Pharmacy Practice and by the Board of Directors and was found to still be appropriate.

0105

COMPUTERIZED PRESCRIBER ORDER ENTRY

Source: Council on Administrative Affairs

To advocate the use of computerized entry of medication orders or prescriptions by the prescriber when (1) it is planned, implemented, and managed with pharmacists' involvement, (2) such orders are part of a single, shared database that is fully integrated with the pharmacy information system and other key information system components, especially the patient's medication administration record, (3) such computerized order entry improves the safety, efficiency, and accuracy of the medication-use process, and (4) it includes provisions for the pharmacist to review and verify the order's appropriateness before medication administration, except in those instances when review would cause a medically unacceptable delay.

This policy was reviewed in 2021 by the Council on Pharmacy Management and by the Board of Directors and was found to still be appropriate.

9813

REGULATION OF AUTOMATED DRUG DISTRIBUTION SYSTEMS

Source: Council on Legal and Public Affairs

To work with the Drug Enforcement Administration and other agencies to seek regulatory and policy changes to accommodate automated drug distribution in health systems.

ASHP Statement on Bar-Code-Enabled Medication Administration Technology

Position

The American Society of Health-System Pharmacists (ASHP) encourages health systems to adopt bar-code-enabled medication administration (BCMA) technology to improve patient safety and the accuracy of medication administration and documentation. To support the goal of having all medications electronically verified before they are administered, BCMA systems should be used in all areas of health systems in which medications are used. Pharmacists must be involved in the interdisciplinary planning, development, implementation, and management of BCMA systems and must ultimately be responsible for developing and maintaining the infrastructure required to ensure BCMA success. Health systems deploying BCMA programs must provide the funding and staffing necessary to permit pharmacists to fulfill this role.

ASHP urges the Food and Drug Administration (FDA) and other regulatory agencies, standard-setting bodies, contracting entities, health systems, and others to mandate that pharmaceutical manufacturers use symbologies that are readily deciphered by commonly used scanning equipment to code for the National Drug Code (NDC), lot number, and expiration date on all unit dose, unit-of-use, and injectable drug packaging. Pharmaceutical manufacturers should also provide all medications used in health systems in unit dose packages. FDA, pharmaceutical manufacturers and packagers, and the manufacturers of BCMA systems should collaborate to minimize or eliminate the causes of false rejection of valid medication doses. Certain characteristics of the current NDC identification system contribute to the burden of implementing BCMA systems, and ASHP urges stakeholders to participate in efforts to develop a system that more reliably identifies the unique drug (or combination of drugs), strength, dosage form, and route of administration.

Although bar-coding systems are currently a widely used point-of-care technology, ASHP recognizes that other types of machine-readable coding (e.g., radio-frequency identification) may evolve. ASHP supports the use of new technologies that are as effective as or improve upon existing systems and believes the principles outlined in this statement apply to such systems. ASHP urges further research on such systems as well as research that will definitively determine the extent to which BCMA systems reduce preventable medication errors and provide a financial return on investment for health systems.

Background

Since the 1980s, health care practitioners and policymakers have recognized the potential benefits of using bar-coding technology in the medication dispensing and administration process.[1–5] Although there is a consensus of professional judgment and expert opinion on the advancement of BCMA technology, more studies are needed to definitively determine the impact of BCMA systems on medication errors and the finances of health systems. ASHP believes that optimally implemented BCMA systems have tremendous potential to improve patient safety. In addition, the reengineering of the medication-use process required to implement a BCMA system can provide opportunities for performance improvement in patient care and clinical documentation.

A 2005 ASHP survey estimated that only 13.2% of hospitals used a BCMA system.[6] Although this percentage is small, it represents an almost 10-fold increase since 2002.[7] The rapid adoption of BCMA systems presents challenges to health systems, and ASHP believes that pharmacists have a crucial role in responding to those challenges.

Role of the Pharmacist

Pharmacists should take the lead in ensuring that the implementation of BCMA systems and the reengineering of the medication-use system address the complexities of the process and that the goal of improving patient safety is achieved. Poor design and inadequate planning can compromise the effectiveness of a BCMA system and may even introduce new sources of error into the medication-use process.[8] Growing experience with BCMA systems has produced a body of knowledge that will aid hospitals and health systems in the adoption of BCMA systems.[9–12]

Pharmacy leadership needs to engage the chief information officer, chief nursing officer, and other key stakeholders in planning for BCMA systems as early as possible. Pharmacists and nurses should be involved with the preinstallation evaluation and selection of the BCMA system. Allowing end users to provide crucial advice about system design will increase acceptance and utility of the system.

Implementation of a BCMA system must be accompanied by the development of policies and procedures that ensure the system's safety. These policies and procedures should be developed by an interdisciplinary team that includes pharmacists.[10] Pharmacists and nurses should be involved with postinstallation evaluation and system improvement.

The role of nurses as end users of this technology should not be underestimated; nursing involvement is essential to successful system implementation and use. Processes for delivery and storage of medications (e.g., in medicine rooms or bedside storage spaces) should be examined by pharmacists and nurses to avoid workarounds or diversion.

Elements of a BCMA System

Although every hospital and health system will need to develop a BCMA system that meets its own needs, the following general principles should guide the implementation and use of such systems.

Use of the BCMA system should be universal within the health system. To the fullest extent feasible, every patient, care provider, and medication should receive a unique identifier, and that identifier should be used not only to verify care prescribed for a patient but also to document every significant step in the medication-use process.

DOI 10.37573/9781585287048.002

A process should be in place to ensure simple, secure, and controllable placement and replacement of a patient identification tag. To ensure that there is only one active wristband per patient, this process should discourage the printing of multiple labels.[12] In addition to appropriate human-readable information, machine-readable patient wristbands should contain information (e.g., a photograph or the patient's medical record number) in order to uniquely identify the patient.

The BCMA system should have a secure user-identification system. Every care provider should be assigned and use a unique identifier. The care provider administering a medication should be able to use the BCMA system to verify that the medication to be administered is appropriate for the patient (i.e., confirming that the five rights of medication administration[13] are met). The BCMA system should document the information in the electronic medication administration record.

The pharmacy must be able to ensure that doses received in patient care areas can be scanned without inappropriate rejection and that those scans reliably indicate whether the medication is appropriate for a particular patient. For the implementation of a BCMA system to succeed, the health system must commit the pharmacy resources necessary to verify that each incoming medication is scannable and that the data encoded within its bar code accurately represent the product.

Every medication possible should be packaged in unit doses, and each unit dose package should be labeled with both human-readable medication identification information and a machine-readable code that includes the medication's unique identifier and, when feasible, its lot number and expiration date. Pharmacy information systems must be able to generate bar codes for multiple-component items. Pharmacy departments must develop a validation process for ensuring that every item has a bar code that can be scanned by all equipment supporting the BCMA system, including pharmacy automation systems, automated medication storage and distribution devices, and nursing BCMA scanning units.

An adequate number of scanners should be provided for each patient care area to facilitate scanning at peak times. Scanners should have the capacity to autodiscriminate the variety of symbologies encountered on pharmaceutical and pharmacy-prepared containers.

Finally, contingency plans should exist to ensure patient safety during system downtime. These policies should require that medications administered during downtime are retrospectively documented electronically in the medical record so that decision-support systems accurately reflect clinical trends associated with the patient, medication administration, and medication effects.

Conclusion

ASHP encourages health systems to adopt BCMA technology, with the goal of having all medications electronically verified before they are administered. Pharmacists must ultimately be responsible for developing and maintaining the infrastructure necessary to ensure BCMA success, and health systems deploying BCMA systems must provide the funding and staffing necessary to permit pharmacists to fulfill this role.

ASHP believes that pharmaceutical manufacturers should be required to place machine-readable coding that includes the NDC, lot number, and expiration date on all unit dose, unit-of-use, and injectable drug packaging, using symbologies that are readily deciphered by commonly used scanning equipment. ASHP also urges further research that will definitively determine the extent to which BCMA systems reduce preventable medication errors or provide a financial return on investment for health systems.

References

1. Hokanson JA, Keith MR, Guernsey BG et al. Potential use of barcodes to implement automated dispensing quality assurance programs. *Hosp Pharm.* 1985; 20:327–37.
2. Nold EG, Williams TC. Barcodes and their potential applications in hospital pharmacy. *Am J Hosp Pharm.* 1985; 42:2722–32.
3. Barry GA, Bass GE, Eddlemon JK et al. Bar-code technology for documenting administration of large-volume intravenous solutions. *Am J Hosp Pharm.* 1989; 46:282–7.
4. Lefkowitz S, Cheiken H, Barhart MR. A trial of the use of bar code technology to restructure a drug distribution and administration system. *Hosp Pharm.* 1991; 26:239–42.
5. Meyer GE, Brandell R, Smith JE et al. Use of bar codes in inpatient drug distribution. *Am J Hosp Pharm.* 1991; 48:953–66.
6. Pedersen CA, Schneider PJ, Scheckelhoff DJ. ASHP national survey of pharmacy practice in hospital settings: dispensing and administration—2005. *Am J Health-Syst Pharm.* 2006; 63:327–45.
7. Pedersen CA, Schneider PJ, Scheckelhoff DJ. ASHP national survey of pharmacy practice in hospital settings: dispensing and administration—2002. *Am J Health-Syst Pharm.* 2003; 60:52–68.
8. Patterson ES, Cook RI, Render ML. Improving patient safety by identifying side effects of introducing bar coding in medication administration. *J Am Med Inform Assoc.* 2002; 9:540–53.
9. Patterson E, Rogers M, Render M. Fifteen best practice recommendations for bar-code medication administration in the Veterans Health Administration. *Joint Comm J Qual Saf.* 2004; 30:355–65.
10. Neuenschwander M, Cohen MR, Vaida AJ et al. Practical guide to bar coding for patient medication safety. *Am J Health-Syst Pharm.* 2003; 60:768–79.
11. ASHP Research and Education Foundation Implementing a bar-coded medication safety program: a pharmacist's toolkit. www.ashpfoundation.org/MainMenuCategories/Education/SpecialPrograms/ImplementingaBarCodedMedSafetyProgram.aspx (accessed 2008 Dec 3).
12. Cummings J, Bush P, Smith D et al. Bar-coding medication administration overview and consensus recommendations. *Am J Health-Syst Pharm.* 2005; 62:2626–9.
13. 10 Golden rules for administering drugs safely. In: McGovern K. Preventing medication errors. Springhouse, PA: Springhouse; 1994:2–3.

Suggested Readings or Other Resources

- ASHP guidelines on preventing medication errors in hospitals. *Am J Hosp Pharm.* 1993; 50:305–14.
- Aspden P, Wolcott J, Bootman JL et al., eds. Preventing medication errors: quality chasm series. Washington, DC: National Academies Press; 2007.
- Cohen MR, ed. Medication errors. Washington, DC: American Pharmaceutical Association; 1999.
- Johnson CL, Carlson RA, Tucker CL et al. Using BCMA software to improve patient safety in Veterans Administration medical centers. *J Healthc Inf Manage.* 2002; 16:46–51.
- Leape LL. Error in medicine. *JAMA.* 1994; 272:1851–7.
- Poon EG, Cina JL, Churchill W et al. Medication dispensing errors and potential adverse drug events before and after implementing bar code technology in the pharmacy. *Ann Intern Med.* 2006; 145:426–34.
- Puckett F. Medication management component of a point of care information system. *Am J Health-Syst Pharm.* 1995; 52:1305–9.

Developed through the ASHP Section of Pharmacy Informatics and Technology and approved by the ASHP Board of Directors on March 7, 2008, and by the ASHP House of Delegates on June 10, 2008. Supersedes ASHP policy position 0308.

Copyright © 2009, American Society of Health-System Pharmacists, Inc. All rights reserved. Contact ASHP for reprint and permissions requests. This content may not be used for commercial purposes without the express written consent of ASHP.

Arash T. Dabestani, Pharm.D., M.H.A. and Alicia B. Perry, Pharm.D., are gratefully acknowledged for drafting versions of this statement.

The bibliographic citation for this document is as follows: American Society of Health-System Pharmacists. ASHP statement on bar-code-enabled medication administration technology. *Am J Health-Syst Pharm.* 2009; 66:588–90.

ASHP Statement on Bar-Code Verification During Inventory, Preparation, and Dispensing of Medications

Position

The American Society of Health-System Pharmacists encourages hospital and health-system pharmacies to incorporate bar-code scanning into inventory management, dose preparation and packaging, and dispensing of medications. The purpose of such scanning is to ensure that drug products distributed, deployed to intermediate storage areas, or used in the preparation of patient doses are the correct products, are in-date, and have not been recalled. Such bar-code scanning should be employed in:

- Stocking of inventory both in the pharmacy and in other locations from which patient medications may be dispensed (e.g., an automated dispensing device).
- Manual packaging of oral solid and liquid medications.
- Compounding, repackaging, and labeling processes (e.g., scanning of source ingredients).
- Retrieving medications from automated dispensing devices.
- Dispensing from the pharmacy to any location.

Prudent use of bar-coding technology in these processes will enhance patient safety and the quality of care by improving the accuracy of core pharmacy functions, closing potential gaps in the bar-code-assisted medication administration (BCMA) process, and allowing better allocation of pharmacists' knowledge and skills.

Background

Discussion of the role of technology in improving medication safety almost universally focuses on BCMA or computerized provider order entry (CPOE), despite evidence of medication errors that neither CPOE nor BCMA could prevent.[1,2] A number of activities in the medication-use process create opportunities for error outside of medication ordering and administration systems, such as:

- Receiving of inventory from suppliers and stocking of inventory locations from which patient medications may be dispensed (e.g., stocking unit-based automated dispensing devices with medications that may not be delivered to the bedside in their original packaging).
- Packaging of medications, which has become more prevalent as BCMA systems are more widely adopted by health systems and manufacturers have discontinued unit dose packaging of medications.
- Manual packaging of liquid medications in ready-to-administer form.
- The compounding of medications.
- The dispensing of patient-specific medications (e.g., 24-hour medication carts, nurse servers).

In addition, for BCMA to function, a vast majority of doses must be accurately bar coded, meaning there must be a highly reliable relationship between the information in the bar code and the contents of the dose. Additionally, the bar code must be readable by commercially-available scanners. Although doses delivered directly from manufacturer-labeled packages generally meet these conditions, there are numerous drug products that may not:

- Commercial products may lack a readily readable bar code, may have an irregular package shape that confounds the ability of scanning equipment to read the bar code, or may have a bar code in a symbology format that cannot be interpreted by the institution's bar-code scanning software.
- Nurse-prepared medications (e.g., insulin doses, heparin boluses, or syringes pre-drawn in the operating room) may be prepared at a location other than the patient's bedside, with the result that there is no labeling of any kind on the dose when it is administered.
- Compounded medications (e.g., sterile preparations) are often labeled by the pharmacy with a bar code that references a prescription or order number that describes the intended contents of the prescribed dose but provides no assurance that the prescribed contents were actually used in the product's preparation.

Benefits of Bar-Code Verification During Inventory, Preparation, and Dispensing

Initial estimates of the contribution of pharmacy dispensing errors to the overall medication errors were quite low.[3] However, recent reports have suggested that adding bar coding to the pharmacy dispensing process can significantly reduce opportunities for medication errors at the bedside and reduce the occurrence of potential adverse drug reactions.[4–6] Incorporating bar-code scanning in inventory management, dose preparation and packaging, and dispensing can improve patient safety in the following ways:

- Scanning during stocking in the pharmacy or patient-care locations (e.g., loading of an automated dispensing device) can help ensure that the product is placed in the correct location.
- Scanning during the retrieval of medications mitigates the hazards of erroneous medication stocking, which is especially important in the case of automated dispensing devices, where there is a potential risk that caregivers will override controls and remove medications for immediate use.
- Scanning of source ingredients during compounding, repackaging, or labeling processes can ensure that labeled doses contain the appropriate ingredients. Additionally, such scanning creates a reliable link between the information in the final package's bar code, its contents, and the National Drug Code (NDC) of the source container, which may be required to satisfy billing requirements (e.g., those of the Centers for Medicare & Medicaid Services).

DOI 10.37573/9781585287048.003

- Scanning on dispensing can help prevent look-alike, sound-alike medication substitution errors that are difficult to visually detect, can identify and remove from distribution drug products whose bar codes are missing or unreadable, and prevent the distribution of expired or recalled products or facilitate retrieval in case of a recall.
- Scanning during any of these activities permits accumulation of an audit trail for each transaction in the inventory, preparation, and dispensing process. This information provides indications of the frequency of error encounter and detection, a record of the amount of time needed to perform selected functions, and evidence of success or failure of manual processes to deliver the correct medication.

Bar-code verification is optimized, and its potential negative impacts on productivity minimized, when the scanning system is configured to use bar codes on bulk packages (e.g., the bar code on an unopened case of unit-dose-packaged tablets) to confirm the contents of each item in the case, especially during batch processes. For patient-specific doses, each individual container used for the dose must be scanned.

The equipment and training costs for a pharmacy-based bar-code scanning implementation is quite small, especially when compared to those of BCMA systems.[7] Pharmacy-based bar-code scanning implementation may be considered a prerequisite for BCMA success, because unreadable bar codes are a significant cause of BCMA implementation failures.[8,9]

Limitations

As with BCMA, adoption of bar code scanning within distribution processes creates the necessity to ensure that the scanning system will recognize and appropriately respond to every bar code it scans. This verification activity is likely to create significant additional work for the pharmacy. Pharmacies planning on implementing such systems must plan for the resources needed to ensure that properly bar-coded products are presented to, and readable by, the scanning system.

In addition, as with other bar-code technology implementations, pharmacy-based bar-code scanning systems will only be beneficial if appropriately deployed. For example, given the need to scan three vials of medication to prepare an IV admixture, such a system cannot distinguish between scanning each vial and scanning the same vial three times, although the latter defeats the purpose of the scanning. Any program of pharmacy-based bar-code scanning should be accompanied by appropriate training, policies, and procedures to promote and optimize safe use of the system, as well as a regular program of auditing to ensure that the program is being properly deployed by staff. Additionally, such programs require hospitals and health systems to compile and maintain a complete database of bar codes in use throughout the institution. The availability of such information in a timely fashion is a well-recognized problem.[10] An incomplete database or the absence of bar codes on drug products can undermine the entire system, as the system cannot properly recognize and evaluate the drug products being scanned. Procedures should address such issues as the expected behavior while scanning occurs, specific prohibited acts, and the penalties associated with known at-risk behavior.[11]

In addition, this statement should not be interpreted to express a preference for bar-code scanning over other forms of automated identification of medications. Currently, bar coding is the least-expensive mechanism to introduce and deploy throughout the medication management cycle.[12] Should other technologies (e.g., radio-frequency identification) demonstrate similar or better capabilities, the principles articulated in this statement will continue to apply.

Validation

As with all such systems, bar coding on dispensing presumes that the scanning software, the scanning hardware, and the associated underlying database are accurate and complete. To ensure accuracy and completeness, organizations using a bar coding process will need to validate both that the software operates as expected and that the underlying database information is correct and reliable. A process will also need to be in place to immediately remediate problems if it is discovered that the hardware, software, or database are not operating properly.

Conclusion

Prudent use of bar-code scanning in inventory management, dose preparation and packaging, and dispensing of medications can enhance patient safety and the quality of care. Such scanning also provides the opportunity to accumulate and use statistics on the pharmacy distributive operation that can direct more appropriate staffing, identify sources of routine error, and generally permit better management of the drug distribution process.

References

1. Wolf R. Preventable medication error responsible for infant deaths. Injury Board.com. Available at: http://dallas.injuryboard.com/medical-malpractice/preventable-medication-error-responsible-for-infant-deaths.aspx?googleid=206592 (accessed 2010 Jan 11).
2. Institute for Safe Medication Practices. Failed check system for chemotherapy leads to pharmacist's no contest plea for involuntary manslaughter. www.ismp.org/Newsletters/acutecare/articles/20090423.asp (accessed 2010 Mar 4).
3. Bates DW, Cullen DJ, Laird N et al. Incidence of adverse drug events and potential adverse drug events. Implications for prevention. ADE Prevention Study Group. *JAMA*. 1995; 274:29–34.
4. Cina J, Fanikos J, Mitton P et al. Medication errors in a pharmacy-based bar-code-repackaging center. *Am J Health-Syst Pharm.* 2006; 63:165–8.
5. Poon EG, Cina JL, Churchill W et al. Medication dispensing errors and potential adverse drug events before and after implementing bar code technology in the pharmacy. *Ann Intern Med.* 2006;145:426–34.
6. Ragan R, Bond J, Major K et al. Improved control of medication use with an integrated bar-code-packaging and distribution system. *Am J Health-Syst Pharm.* 2005; 62:1075–9.
7. Maviglia SM, Yoo JY, Franz C et al. Cost-benefit analysis of a hospital pharmacy bar code solution. *Arch Intern Med.* 2007; 167:788–94.

8. Koppel R, Wetterneck T, Telles JL et al. Workarounds to barcode medication administration systems: their occurrences, causes and threats to patient safety. *J Am Med Inform Assoc.* 2008;15:408–23.
9. Young D. VA pursues bar code quality. *Am J Health-Syst Pharm.* 2004; 61:1312–4.
10. ASHP statement on bar-code-enabled medication administration technology. *Am J Health-Syst Pharm.* 2009; 66:588–90. www.ashp.org/DocLibrary/Best Practices/AutoITStBCMA.aspx. (accessed 2010 Mar 4).
11. ASHP policy position 0910: reporting medication errors. In: Hawkins B, ed. *Best practices for hospital and health-system pharmacy: positions and guidance documents of ASHP.* 2009–2010 ed. Bethesda, MD: American Society of Health-System Pharmacists; 2006:160. www.ashp.org/DocLibrary/BestPractices/MedMisPositions09.aspx (accessed 2010 Mar 08).
12. Cummings J, Bush P, Smith D et al. Bar-coding medication administration: overview and consensus recommendations. *Am J Health-Syst Pharm.* 2005; 62:2626–9.

Suggested Reading

- Bates DW, Cullen JC, Laird N et al. Incidence of adverse drug events and potential adverse drug events. *JAMA.* 1995; 274:29–34.
- Nold EG, Williams TC. Bar codes and their potential applications in hospital pharmacy. *Am J Hosp Pharm.* 1985; 42:2722–32.
- Meyer GE, Brandell R, Smith JE et al. Use of bar codes in inpatient drug distribution. *Am J Hosp Pharm.* 1991; 48:953–66.
- Santell JP, Hicks RW, McMeekin J et al. Medication errors: experience of the United States Pharmacopeia (USP) MEDMARX reporting system. *J Clin Pharmacol.* 2003; 43:760–7.
- Ness JE, Sullivan SD, Stergachis A. Accuracy of technicians and pharmacists in identifying dispensing errors. *Am J Health-Syst Pharm.* 1994; 51:354–7.
- Oswald S, Caldwell R. Dispensing error rate after implementation of an automated pharmacy carousel system. *Am J Health-Syst Pharm.* 2007; 64:1427–31.
- Cina J, Fanikos J, Mitton P et al. Medication errors in a pharmacy-based bar-code-repackaging center. *Am J Health-Syst Pharm.* 2006; 63:165–8.
- Ambrose PJ, Saya FG, Lovett LT et al. Evaluating the accuracy of technicians and pharmacists in checking unit dose medication cassettes. *Am J Health-Syst Pharm.* 2002; 59:1183–8.
- Shane R. Current status of administration of medicines. *Am J Health-Syst Pharm.* 2009; 66:s42–s48.
- Blair R. Medication transformation: pharmacists on the floor. A Midwest healthcare system takes bar code technology to new heights, as part of an enterprise initiative to optimize patient safety. *Health Manag Technol.* 2004; 25:26, 28, 30.
- Nanji KC, Cina J, Patel N et al. Overcoming barriers to the implementation of a pharmacy bar code scanning system for medication dispensing: a case study. *J Am Med Inform Assoc.* 2009; 16:645–50.

Developed through the ASHP Section of Pharmacy Informatics and Technology and approved by the ASHP Board of Directors on April 15, 2010, and by the ASHP House of Delegates on June 6, 2010.

This statement was drafted by the ASHP Section of Pharmacy Informatics and Technology 2009–2010 Section Advisory Group on Pharmacy Operations Automation (Dennis A. Tribble, Pharm.D.; Ron Burnette, B.S.Pharm., M.B.A.; Dawn M. Biller; Leslie Brookins, M.S.; Richard Capps III, Pharm.D.; Marvin H. Choi; Kavish J. Choudhary, Pharm.D., M.S.; Seth Aaron Cohen, Pharm.D.; Thomas W. Cooley M.B.A.; Arash T. Dabestani, Pharm.D., M.H.A., FABC; Charles De la Torre, M.S., MIS; Doina Dumitru, Pharm.D., M.B.A.; Christopher Fortier, B.S.Pharm.; Barbara Giacomelli, Pharm.D., MBA, FASHP; Staci Hermann, M.S., Pharm.D.; Gary L. Johnson, Jr., Pharm.D., M.H.A.; Seth A. Kuiper, Pharm.D.; Denise Mckenzie, B.S.Pharm.; Rhonda B. McManus, Pharm.D.; Eric C. Nemec, II, Pharm.D.; Beth Prier, Pharm.D., M.S.; Brad Rognrud, M.S., R.Ph.; Kevin A. Scheckelhoff, M.B.A.; Paul M. Seelinger, B.S.Pharm.; Suzanne B. Shea, M.B.A.; David A. Tjhio, M.S., Pharm.D.; Christopher J. Urbanski, M.S.; Gwen Volpe, B.S.Pharm.; Rayburn Brian Vrabel, Pharm.D.; and Robynn P. Wolfschlag, M.B.A.).

ASHP gratefully acknowledges the following organizations and individuals for reviewing drafts of this statement (review does not imply endorsement): American Association of Critical Care Nurses (AACCN); American Nurses Association (ANA); Institute for Safe Medication Practices (ISMP); Rhode Island Society of Health System Pharmacists (RISHP); South Carolina Society of Health-System Pharmacists (SCSHP); Wyoming Society of Health-System Pharmacy (WSHP); Linda Annecchini, M.S.; James L. Besier, Ph.D., FASHP; Carol J. Bickford, Ph.D., RN-BC (ANA); Denny C. Briley, Pharm.D.; Mary E. Burkhardt, M.S., FASHP; Richard Capps, Pharm.D.; William W. Churchill, M.S.; Debra Cowan, Pharm.D.; Michele Danish, Pharm.D, FASHP; Brent I. Fox, Pharm.D., Ph.D.; Karl F. Gumpper, BCNSP, BCPS, FASHP; Kathleen M. Gura, Pharm.D., BCNSP, FASHP; J. Chad Hardy, Pharm.D., M.S.; Robi Hellman, RN, MSN, CNS (AACCN); Matthew R. Keith, B.S.Pharm., FASHP; Stan Kent, M.S.; Thomas E. Kirschling, Pharm.D., M.S.; Jim Lile, Pharm.D.; Jeff Little, Pharm.D., M.P.H.; Donald Lynx, M.B.A., FASHP; Leslie R. Mackowiak, M.S.; Linda Gore Martin, Pharm.D., M.B.A., BCPS (WSHP); Denise McKenzie, CPhT; Joel Melroy, Pharm.D., M.S., BCPS (SCSHP); Ian Orensky, Pharm.D., M.S.; Stephanie C. Peshek, Pharm.D., M.B.A., FASHP; Tommie Peterson, B.S.Pharm.; James Ponto, M.S., BCNP, FASHP; Brad Rognrud, M.S.; Martha J. Roberts, Pharm.D. (RISHP); Richard I. Sakai, Pharm.D., FASHP, FCSHP; Ronald Schneider, B.S.Pharm., M.H.A.; Paul Seelinger, B.S.Pharm.; Suzanne Shea, M.B.A.; Armen Simonian, Pharm.D.; Kirby K. Stiening, B.S.Pharm.; George Taniguchi, Pharm.D., M.P.H., M.A.; Greg Teale, Pharm.D.; Jennifer Thomas, Pharm.D.; Melanie J. Townsend, Pharm.D., BCPS; Dennis A. Tribble, Pharm.D.; Chris L. Tucker, B.S.Pharm.; Chris Urbanski, M.S.; Allen J. Vaida, Pharm.D., FASHP (ISMP); Rayburn B. Vrabel, Pharm.D.; Kelley A. Wasicek, B.S.Pharm.; and Jody Jacobson Wedret, FASHP, FCSHP.

Copyright © 2011, American Society of Health-System Pharmacists, Inc. All rights reserved. Contact ASHP for reprint and permissions requests. This content may not be used for commercial purposes without the express written consent of ASHP.

The bibliographic citation for this document is as follows: American Society of Health-System Pharmacists. ASHP statement on bar-code verification during inventory, preparation, and dispensing of medications. *Am J Health-Syst Pharm.* 2011; 68:442–5.

ASHP Statement on the Pharmacist's Role in Clinical Informatics

Position

ASHP believes that pharmacists have the training, knowledge, background, and responsibility to assume a significant role in clinical informatics.

Background

Healthcare organizations continue to invest a significant amount of financial and human resources in health information technology (HIT) initiatives, including advanced clinical systems, electronic health records, business intelligence and analytics tools, and applications that deliver the highest levels of patient safety and value. This growth has not only led to a considerable demand for HIT workers but, more importantly, has identified the need for a work force with training and skills to create a successful and safe interface between HIT and the healthcare delivery system. This work force must understand healthcare, information and communication technology, and the people, processes, and culture of an organization. The intersection of these skills has commonly been described as the discipline of biomedical and health informatics, more recently termed *clinical informatics*.[1] Evidence continues to emerge regarding the value that a well-trained individual in clinical informatics can bring to an organization faced with implementing highly complex and transformative HIT systems.[2,3]

Pharmacy informatics has grown to be an integral discipline within the clinical informatics domain, centered on the effective management and delivery of medication-related data, information, and knowledge across systems that support the medication-use process. Pharmacists' professional identity, education, training, and experience with medication management make them ideal candidates to play a significant role and fill a critical need in pharmacy informatics. Their firm understanding of core pharmacy operations, clinical practice, the medication-use process, standards, and regulations and their long history of utilizing technology to support medication management provide the essential components for effectively transitioning into this role. Despite the growing number of formally trained pharmacy informaticists, the path and skills required for a career in informatics have varied considerably, emphasizing the need to build core competencies and grow the number of available programs.[4–6] The American Board of Medical Specialties (ABMS) recognition of clinical informatics as a physician subspecialty will likely play an important role in evolving pharmacy informatics beyond its current state to one with a clinical edge, centered on analytics and delivering information and knowledge at the point of care. This ABMS decision may also impact the development of a standardized, interprofessional educational road map for individuals seeking a career in pharmacy informatics.[7–9]

Roles and Responsibilities

Pharmacists who practice clinical informatics must collaborate with other healthcare and information technology professionals to promote the safe, efficient, effective, timely, and optimal use of medications. They contribute to the transformation of healthcare by analyzing, designing, implementing, maintaining, and evaluating information and communication systems that improve medication-related outcomes and strengthen the pharmacist–patient relationship. The role of pharmacy informaticists revolves around their knowledge of pharmacy practice, safe medication use, clinical decision-making, and the improvement of medication therapy outcomes, combined with their understanding of the discipline of informatics and HIT systems.[10] Their primary roles and responsibilities must encompass five broadly defined categories:

- Data, information, and knowledge management: managing medication-related information while promoting integration, interoperability, and information exchange.
- Information and knowledge delivery: delivering medication-related information and knowledge throughout the clinical knowledge life cycle, from the point of knowledge generation through cataloging, embedding knowledge into the workflow, and measuring the usage and effectiveness of that knowledge.
- Practice analytics: developing point-of-business analytic solutions for improving decision-making.
- Applied clinical informatics: applying user experiences, research, and theoretical informatics principles to improve clinical practice and usability.
- Leadership and management of change: leading and participating in the procurement, development, implementation, customization, management, evaluation, and continuous improvement of clinical information systems.

Data, Information, and Knowledge Management. Pharmacy informaticists play a key role in maintaining the data, information, and knowledge assets across all systems that support medication management. They are instrumental in ensuring data quality and safety, minimizing data-quality risks, and affirming medication-related data, information, and knowledge management best practices.[10,11] Data quality and information management best practices encompass

- Providing the appropriate level of data governance and stewardship.
- Adopting standard human- and machine-interpretable formats.
- Utilizing controlled terminology for integration and interoperability.
- Ensuring that data are accurate, accessible, complete, consistent, current, timely, precise, at the appropriate level of granularity, reliable, relevant, conforming, and understandable across all data-quality management domains.
- Ensuring the consistent use of maps to internal and external standards and reference data.
- Ensuring that system architecture supports data interchange.
- Ensuring that data, information, and knowledge are audited, measured, and evaluated for effectiveness.

DOI 10.37573/9781585287048.004

- Ensuring that data, information, and knowledge assets are validated, integrated, normalized, consolidated, and routinely optimized.
- Developing infrastructure for knowledge, metadata, and terminology management.
- Ensuring that information is readily and rapidly understood and accessed within the workflow.
- Ensuring that information and knowledge are centrally managed, collaboratively developed, and easily disseminated and maintained.
- Ensuring that information and knowledge are platform independent.
- Developing tools to effectively maintain and manage data, information, and knowledge.

Maintenance roles and responsibilities include

- Corrective maintenance: taking the corrective and educative steps required to correct problems with the utilization of a clinical information system or technology.
- Customized maintenance: modifying features already in production systems that require updating or modification for user needs; customized maintenance is essential in clinical information systems, as healthcare is constantly changing (e.g., new drugs, new treatment guidance, new procedures).
- Enhancement maintenance: improving the performance of applications and people associated with the use of tools.
- Preventive maintenance: taking steps in advance to reduce the risk of a problem, including testing before a new release or system upgrade.[12]

Information and Knowledge Delivery. Healthcare delivery is inherently complex and knowledge dependent, and it is becoming ever more challenging for providers to absorb and assimilate the growing volume and granularity of knowledge needed for safe and effective patient care. The clinical knowledge available is often conflicting, misaligned, and not readily identified or available at the point of care. To serve the needs of any clinical encounter, relevant patient-centered knowledge must be accessible to the person supplying care at the right time in the workflow. Such knowledge can be delivered proactively (before decisions are made), interactively (as decisions are made), or asynchronously or passively as reference information that can be searched online. Pharmacy informatics plays a key role in supporting and overseeing the core processes involving information and knowledge delivery throughout the clinical knowledge life cycle. This role includes knowledge discovery and creation, knowledge application and delivery, and knowledge asset management.

Knowledge Discovery and Creation. As technology-driven transactions for results, ordering, documentation, task completion, communication, and patient monitoring continue to grow, so will the amount of data. Pharmacy informatics plays a key role in analyzing these data for the purposes of understanding performance, evaluating processes, and reporting, predicting, and harvesting new information to create new knowledge for improving outcomes.

Knowledge Application and Delivery. Pharmacy informatics is responsible for leveraging knowledge at the right time and place within a provider's workflow to improve caregiver effectiveness, work satisfaction, patient satisfaction, and the quality of care. Pharmacy informatics must continue to evolve to optimize the use of clinical decision support and develop tools that reduce information overload and provider burden. Pharmacy informatics is responsible for looking beyond the traditional means of delivering knowledge by analyzing process and outcomes data from existing applications to develop and implement new solutions for embedding knowledge into the workflow.[13]

Knowledge Asset Management. Pharmacy informatics must play a significant role in managing and supporting a healthcare system's technology-enabled medication information and knowledge assets. This role would include assisting with authoring, encoding, cataloging, versioning, updating, disseminating, and maintaining an inventory of medication-related information and knowledge. Despite the emergence of commercial content-management systems and groupware, pharmacy informatics must provide the appropriate level of oversight and governance for these activities and play a role in the development of future knowledge asset–management systems that support end-to-end knowledge engineering.

Practice Analytics. The healthcare industry has historically generated large amounts of data driven by financial, regulatory, compliance, and patient care–related activities. These data have primarily been stored in hard copy form, making them difficult to process through traditional database management tools. Paper records have also limited opportunities for the effective exchange of information with other healthcare systems and for providing actionable insight on reducing costs, improving performance, and making decisions. The recent infusion of financial incentives and regulation involving HIT from the American Recovery and Reinvestment Act[14] has fueled the implementation of technologies across the United States, contributing to an exponential growth of available and usable healthcare data. Healthcare organizations are looking for every opportunity to transform and leverage data into information that provides concise, timely, descriptive, predictive, and prescriptive insight into their business and clinical data. Business intelligence (BI) and business analytics (BA) processes and technologies are enabling health systems to improve their performance and maintain their competitive advantage while creating an additional demand for clinical informatics professionals. Pharmacy informatics plays a significant role in all efforts surrounding medication management–related BI and BA activities. Pharmacy informaticists' understanding of basic software and database design, ability to grasp the big picture, and functional knowledge of detail, coupled with their analytical skills, create opportunities to develop evidence-driven answers for practice improvement and performance questions, such as

- How are pharmacists performing in relation to cost, quality, and service?
- How can pharmacists improve performance and safety within and outside of their service lines?
- How can pharmacy practice identify patients who are at risk for readmission?
- How can pharmacy practice identify patients requiring medication therapy management services?[15,16]

Pharmacy informatics roles and responsibilities in BI and BA must include

- Ensuring data are standardized, structured, and modeled to support a data-driven BI and BA culture.
- Creating effective analytics tools that allow for multiple formats and layers of analysis, from summary reports on individual patient encounters to an entire population of patients.
- Developing, maintaining, and ensuring the quality of clinical, operational, and financial dashboards, scorecards, screening tools, and surveillance tools to guide the achievement of treatment and strategic goals.
- Driving analytics to the frontline by creating greater end-user accessibility to BI and BA tools.
- Monitoring the effectiveness of tools and information to deploy or further develop point-of-care or analytical systems.

Applied Clinical Informatics. Pharmacy informatics plays a key role in delivering informatics research principles and best practices to the bedside. Through informal and formal partnerships with the research community, pharmacy informaticists must work collaboratively with members of various disciplines to improve the effectiveness, efficiency, and safety of systems that support medication management. They must actively participate in relevant associations and workgroups in the clinical informatics field to maintain their current skills and play a significant role in the following activities:

- Acquiring professional perspective: understanding and analyzing the history and values of the discipline and its relationship to other fields while demonstrating an ability to read, interpret, and critique the core literature.
- Analyzing problems: analyzing, understanding, abstracting, and modeling a specific biomedical problem in terms of data, information, and knowledge components.
- Producing solutions: troubleshooting and effectively analyzing problems to identify and understand the spectrum of possible solutions and generating designs that capture essential aspects of solutions and their components.
- Articulating the rationale: defending the specific solution and its advantage over competing options.
- Implementing, evaluating, and refining: implementing the solution (including obtaining necessary resources and managing projects), evaluating it, and iteratively improving it.
- Innovating: creating new theories, typologies, frameworks, representations, methods, and processes to address clinical informatics problems.
- Working collaboratively: teaming effectively with partners within and across disciplines.
- Educating, disseminating, and discussing: communicating effectively to students and other audiences in multiple disciplines in persuasive written and oral forms.

Leading and Managing Change. To ensure that HIT systems support safe and effective medication use, pharmacy informaticists are expected to lead as well as manage the risks and changes associated with the development, implementation, safety, and use of systems that support medication management. Their knowledge and skills in comprehending and evaluating organizational culture, managing change, working effectively in interdisciplinary teams, communicating, synthesizing user requirements, and articulating HIT needs within the context of broad strategic goals allow them to play a significant role in

- Leading health-system, professional, industry, regulatory, standards-setting, and governmental organizations to sound conclusions regarding the use of technology in medication management.
- Leading and managing the evaluation and communication of the potential risks of a newly implemented technology and developing plans to mitigate potential hazards.
- Translating user requirements into safe and effective system designs.
- Implementing project management best practices.
- Attaining key leadership roles within the healthcare technology industry, professional practice associations, and healthcare technology organizations.[4,10,11]

Conclusion

As the scope for the development and complexity of systems that support medication management continues to grow, so does the need for individuals to lead, manage, and evaluate them. Pharmacy informaticists are uniquely qualified and possess the necessary skills to fulfill this need. Their knowledge of pharmacy practice and safe medication use, combined with their understanding of informatics concepts, methods, and tools, provides the framework for effectively leading and participating in the procurement, customization, development, implementation, management, evaluation, and continuous improvement of clinical information systems.

References

1. Hersh W, Margolis A, Quiros F, et al. Building a health informatics workforce in developing countries. *Health Aff.* 2010; 29:274–7.
2. Price Water House Cooper Health Research Institute. Needles in a haystack: seeking knowledge with clinical informatics. www.pwc.com/us/en/health-industries/publications/needles-in-a-haystack.jhtml (accessed 2015 Jan 9).
3. Kilbridge PM, Classen DC. The informatics opportunities at the intersection of patient safety and clinical informatics *J Am Med Inform Assoc.* 2008; 15:397–407.
4. American Society of Health-System Pharmacists. ASHP statement on the pharmacist's role in informatics. *Am J Health-Syst Pharm.* 2007; 64:200–3.
5. Tribble DA, Poikonen J, Blair J, et al. Whither pharmacy informatics. *Am J Health-Syst Pharm.* 2009; 66:813–5.
6. HIMSS Pharmacy Informatics. What is pharmacy informatics? www.himss.org/library/pharmacy-informatics (accessed 2015 Jan 9).
7. Dolan PL. Clinical informatics now a subspecialty. www.amednews.com/article/20111010/business/310109962/6/ (accessed 2015 Jan 9).

8. Detmer DE, Lumpkin JR, Williamson JJ. Defining the medical subspecialty of clinical informatics. *J Am Med Inform Assoc.* 2009; 16:167–8.
9. Safran C, Shabot MM, Munger BS, et al. Program requirements for fellowship education in the subspecialty of clinical informatics. *J Am Med Inform Assoc.* 2009; 16:158–66.
10. Fox BI, Thrower MR, Felkey BG. Building core competencies in pharmacy informatics. Washington, DC: American Pharmacists Association; 2010.
11. Gardner RM, Overhage JM, Steen EB, et al. AMIA Board White Paper: core content for the subspecialty of clinical informatics. *J Am Med Inform Assoc.* 2009; 16:153–7.
12. Stratis Health. Health information technology toolkit: ongoing system maintenance, administration, and data quality management. www.stratishealth.org/documents/HITToolkitcoordination/ongoing_system_maintenance.doc (accessed 2015 Jan 9).
13. Sittig DF, Wright A, Simonaitis L, et al. The state of the art in clinical knowledge management: an inventory of tools and techniques. *Int J Med Inform.* 2010; 79:44–57.
14. American Recovery and Reinvestment Act of 2009 (P.L. 111-5, 123 Stat. 115-521). www.gpo.gov/fdsys/pkg/PLAW-111publ5/html/PLAW-111publ5.htm (accessed 2015 Jan 9).
15. Advisory Board Company. Business intelligence and analytics in health care: a primer. www.advisory.com/Research/Health-Care-IT-Advisor/Research-Notes/2011/Business-Intelligence-and-Analytics-in-Health-Care (accessed 2015 Jan 9).
16. Sage Growth Partners. The changing role of health analytics for providers. www.sage-growth.com/index.php/2012/02/the-changing-role-of-analytics-for-health-care-providers/ (accessed 2015 Jan 9).

Developed through the ASHP Section of Pharmacy Informatics and Technology and approved by the ASHP Board of Directors on April 10, 2015, and by the ASHP House of Delegates on June 7, 2015.

Mark Siska, M.B.A./TM, B.S.Pharm., is gratefully acknowledged for drafting this statement.

ASHP gratefully acknowledges Alan Chung, Pharm.D.; Carol Hope, Pharm.D., M.S.ChemEng., M.S.Biosciences; Beth Breeden, D.Ph., M.S., CPHIT, CPEHR; and the 2013–14 and 2014–15 Section of Pharmacy Informatics and Technology Section Advisory Groups on Professional Development for their contributions to this statement.

ASHP also gratefully acknowledges the following organizations and individuals for reviewing draft versions of this document (review does not imply endorsement): American Association of Colleges of Pharmacy (AACP); American Medical Informatics Association Pharmacoinformatics Working Group Leadership (AMIA-PWGL); Kansas Council of Health-System Pharmacists (KCHP); New Hampshire Society of Health-System Pharmacists (NHSHP); Pharmacy HIT Collaborative (PHITC); Ernest R. Anderson Jr., M.S., FASHP; Janinah Barreto, Pharm.D., M.S.; Paul J. Barrett, Pharm.D., M.P.A., BCPS, FASHP; Carol J. Bickford, Ph.D., RN-BC, CPHIMS; Sarah Bledsoe, Pharm.D.; Lynette R. Bradley-Baker, Ph.D. (AACP); Max E. Burchett Jr., Pharm.D.; Gregory Burger, Pharm.D., CPPS (KCHP); Michelle DeLuca Fraley, Pharm.D., RPD; Barbara Giacomelli, Pharm.D., M.B.A., FASHP; Nancy Hope Goodbar, Pharm.D., BCPS; James Hoffman, Pharm.D., M.S.; Joan Kapusnik-Uner, Pharm.D., FASHP; Emily Kirkwold, Pharm.D.; Janet M. Kozakiewiz, M.S., Pharm.D., FASHP; Kabeer Mago, Pharm.D.; Ben McDaniel, Pharm.D.; Karen Michaud, Pharm.D., BCPS; Richard Pacitti, Pharm.D., M.B.A.; Lois F. Parker, B.S.Pharm.; Shea Polk, Pharm.D.; James A. Ponto, M.S., B.S.Pharm., BCNP, FASHP; Jason J. Schafer, Pharm.D., M.P.H., BCPS; Philip J. Schneider, M.S.; Terry L. Seaton, Pharm.D., FCCP, BCPS (AMIA-PWGL); Nancy R. Smestad, M.S., CMI; Shelly Spiro, B.S.Pharm., FASCP (PHITC); Mark St. Cyr, D.Ph., M.P.H.; Craig Stern, Pharm.D., M.B.A.; Tate N. Trujillo, Pharm.D., BCPS, FCCM, FASHP; Elizabeth Wade, Pharm.D., BCPS (NHSHP); Jody Jacobson Wedret, B.S.Pharm., FASHP; and Marc Willner, Pharm.D.

This statement supersedes the ASHP Statement on the Pharmacist's Role in Informatics dated June 27, 2006.

Copyright © 2016, American Society of Health-System Pharmacists, Inc. All rights reserved. Contact ASHP for reprint and permissions requests. This content may not be used for commercial purposes without the express written consent of ASHP.

The bibliographic citation for this document is as follows: American Society of Health-System Pharmacists. ASHP statement on the pharmacist's role in clinical informatics. *Am J Health-Syst Pharm.* 2016; 73:410–3.

ASHP Statement on the Pharmacist's Role with Respect to Drug Delivery Systems and Administration Devices

Technological advances in drug delivery systems and administration devices frequently enable improved control of drug administration. Such advances may offer numerous potential benefits to patients, including improved therapeutic outcomes in disease management, improved patient compliance with drug regimens, and greater efficiency and economy in disease therapy. These advances constitute an important aspect of pharmaceutical knowledge and are routinely incorporated into pharmacy practice as they occur.

A drug delivery system is defined as one in which a drug (one component of the system) is integrated with another chemical, a drug administration device, or a drug administration process to control the rate of drug release, the tissue site of drug release, or both. A drug administration device is an apparatus that is used for introducing a drug to the body or controlling its rate of introduction. Drug delivery systems include (but are not limited to) osmotic pumps, thermal isolation, transdermal patches, lipsomal encapsulation, iontophoresis, phonophoresis, magnetic migration, and implantation. Drug administration devices include (but are not limited to) mechani cal (e.g., balloon-driven), gravity-driven, and electromechanical pumps. Some of the latter are portable, implantable, computer controlled, or patient controlled. Some enable the simultaneous infusion of multiple drugs. Drug administration control devices include plasma concentration monitoring and administration rate monitoring devices, which incorporate computers.

Pharmacists bear a substantial responsibility for ensuring optimal clinical outcomes from drug therapy and are suited by education, training, clinical expertise, and practice activities to assume responsibility for the professional supervision of drug delivery systems and administration devices. As a natural extension of efforts to optimize drug use, pharmacists should participate in organizational and clinical decisions with regard to these systems and devices. Some decisions and activities in which pharmacists should participate follow. Others may be appropriate as well.

1. Research and development of innovative drug delivery systems and administration devices.
2. Evaluation and research to determine the direct and comparative efficacy, safety, and cost-effectiveness of specific drug delivery systems and administration devices.
3. In conjunction with pharmacy and therapeutics committees (or other appropriate medical staff committees), decisions to choose or exclude particular drug delivery systems and administration devices for use in specific organizational settings.
4. Development of organization-specific policies and procedures regarding the acquisition, storage, distribution, use, maintenance, and ongoing product quality control of drug delivery systems and administration devices.
5. Choice of a particular drug delivery system or administration device for use in a specific patient's drug therapy.
6. Direct communication with patients to instruct them in the use of such systems and devices and to gather information necessary to monitor the outcome of their therapy.
7. Monitoring of the ongoing clinical effectiveness and suitability of specific drug delivery systems or administration devices with respect to specific patients and the communication of clinically relevant observations and recommendations to prescribers and other health professionals involved in the patients' care.

Failures or malfunctions of drug administration devices may lead to patient harm. Reports of such problems should be made in accordance with the provisions of the Safe Medical Devices Act of 1990 (PL 101–629).

Recommendations for Additional Reading

- Acevedo ML. Electronic flow control. *NITA*. 1983; 6:105–6.
- Akers MJ. Current problems and innovations in intravenous drug delivery. Considerations in using the i.v. route for drug delivery. *Am J Hosp Pharm*. 1987; 44:2528–30.
- Alexander MR. Current problems and innovations in intravenous drug delivery. Developing and implementing a contract for electronic infusion devices. *Am J Hosp Pharm*. 1987; 44:2553–6.
- Anderson RW, Cohen JE, Cohen MR, et al. Hospital pharmacy symposium on new concepts in parenteral drug delivery. *Hosp Pharm*. 1986; 21:1033–55.
- Baharloo M. Iontophoresis and phonophoresis: a role for the pharmacist. *Hosp Pharm*. 1987; 22:730–1.
- Block LH, Shukla AJ. Drug delivery in the 1990s. *US Pharm*. 1986; 11(Oct):51–6, 58.
- Boothe CD, Talley JR. Mechanical and electronic intravenous infusion devices. Part 1. *Infusion*. 1986; 10:6–8.
- Chandrasekaran SK, Benson H, Urquhart J. Methods to achieve controlled drug delivery, the biomedical engineering approach. In: Robinson JR, ed. Sustained and controlled release drug delivery systems. New York: Marcel Dekker; 1978:557–93.
- Colangelo A. Current problems and innovations in intravenous drug delivery. Drug preparation techniques for i.v. drug delivery systems. *Am J Hosp Pharm*. 1987; 44:2550–3.
- Davis SR. Latest developments in drug delivery systems—abstracts. *Hosp Pharm*. 1987; 22:890–908.
- Goodman MS, Wickham R. Venous access devices: oncology nurse overview. *Hosp Pharm*. 1985; 20:495–511.

DOI 10.37573/9781585287048.005

- Holm A, Campbell N. Role of institutional review boards in facilitating research, marketing of drugs and devices, and protecting human subjects. *Drug Dev Ind Pharm.* 1985; 11:1–12.
- Juliano RL. Drug delivery systems. New York: Oxford University Press; 1980.
- Kelly WN, Christensen LA. Selective patient criteria for the use of electronic infusion devices. *Am J IV Ther Clin Nutr.* 1983; 10(Mar):18, 19, 21, 25, 26, 29.
- Kirschenbaum B, Klein S. Pharmacy-coordinated infusion device evaluation. *Am J Hosp Pharm.* 1984; 41:1181–3.
- Leff RD. Current problems and innovations in intravenous drug delivery. Features of i.v. devices and equipment that affect i.v. drug delivery. *Am J Hosp Pharm.* 1987; 44:2530–3.
- Longer MA, Robinson JR. Sustained-release drug delivery systems. In: Gennaro AR, ed. Remington's pharmaceutical sciences. Easton, PA: Mack Publishing Company; 1985:1644–61.
- McFarlane AE. Role for pharmacists in the provision of medical devices. *Aust J Hosp Pharm.* 1986; 16:78.
- Mutschler E. Now and future of drug delivery systems. *Pharm Tech.* 1983(Suppl); 7:13–5.
- Nahata MC. Current problems and innovations in intravenous drug delivery. Effect of i.v. drug delivery systems on pharmacokinetic monitoring. *Am J Hosp Pharm.* 1987; 44:2538–42.
- Piecoro JJ Jr. Current problems and innovations in intravenous drug delivery. Development of an institutional i.v. drug delivery policy. *Am J Hosp Pharm.* 1987; 44:2557–9.
- Polack AE, Roberts MS. Drug delivery systems. *Med J Aust.* 1986; 144:311–4.
- Rapp RP. Current problems and innovations in intravenous drug delivery. Considering product features and costs in selecting a system for intermittent i.v. drug delivery. *Am J Hosp Pharm.* 1987; 44:2533–8.
- Reilly KM. Current problems and innovations in intravenous drug delivery. Problems in administration techniques and dose measurement that influence accuracy of i.v. drug delivery. *Am J Hosp Pharm.* 1987; 44:2545–50.
- Reiss RE. Volumetric IV pumps. *Pharm Tech.* 1983(Suppl); 7:46–9.
- Self TH, Brooks JB, Lieberman P, et al. The value of demonstration and role of the pharmacist in teaching the correct use of pressurized bronchodilators. *Can Med Assoc J.* 1983; 128:129–31.
- Selton MV. Implantable pumps. *CRC Crit Rev Biomed Eng.* 1987; 14:201–40.
- Smith KL. Developments in drug delivery systems. *Hosp Pharm.* 1987; 22:905–6.
- Talley JR. Mechanical and electronic intravenous infusion devices. Part 2. *Infusion.* 1986; 10:31–4.
- Talley JR. Mechanical and electronic intravenous infusion devices. Part 3. *Infusion.* 1986; 10:58–62.
- Talsma H, Crommelin DJA. Liposomes as drug delivery systems, part I: preparation. *Pharm Tech.* 1992(Oct); 16:98, 100, 102, 104, 106.
- Urquhart J. Implantable pumps in drug delivery. *Pharm Tech.* 1983(Suppl); 7:53–4.
- Zenk KE. Current problems and innovations in intravenous drug delivery. Intravenous drug delivery in infants with limited i.v. access and fluid restriction. *Am J Hosp Pharm.* 1987; 44:2542–5.

This statement was reviewed in 1998 by the Council on Professional Affairs and by the ASHP Board of Directors and was found to still be appropriate.

Approved by the ASHP Board of Directors, November 18, 1992, and the ASHP House of Delegates, June 9, 1993. Revised by the ASHP Council on Professional Affairs. Supersedes a previous version approved by the ASHP House of Delegates on June 5, 1989, and the ASHP Board of Directors on November 16, 1988.

Copyright © 1993, American Society of Hospital Pharmacists, Inc. All rights reserved. Contact ASHP for reprint and permissions requests. This content may not be used for commercial purposes without the express written consent of ASHP.

The bibliographic citation for this document is as follows: American Society of Hospital Pharmacists. ASHP statement on the pharmacist's role with respect to drug delivery systems and administration devices. *Am J Hosp Pharm.* 1993; 50:1724–5.

ASHP Statement on the Pharmacy Technician's Role in Pharmacy Informatics

Position

The American Society of Health-System Pharmacists (ASHP) believes that specially trained pharmacy technicians can assume important supportive roles in pharmacy informatics. These roles include automation and technology systems management, project management, end-user training and education, policy and governance, process improvement, analytics and reporting, and inventory and financial management. Such advanced roles require pharmacy technicians to gain expertise in information technology (IT) systems, including knowledge of interfaces, computer management techniques, trouble shooting and database maintenance.[1,2] This knowledge could be acquired through specialized training or experience in a health science or allied scientific field (e.g., health informatics). With appropriate safeguards and supervision, pharmacy technician informaticists (PTIs) will manage IT processes in health-system pharmacy services, ensuring a safe and efficient medication-use process.

Background

The National Library of Medicine has defined health informatics as "the interdisciplinary study of the design, development, adoption and application of IT-based innovations in healthcare services delivery, management and planning."[3] Health informatics is a discipline at the intersection of information science, healthcare, and computer science that designs and delivers information to improve clinical care, individual and public healthcare, and biomedical research. Health informatics optimizes the usability, acquisition, and processing of health-related information, using resources and tools that span the IT spectrum, from people to processes, from information to knowledge, and from algorithms to data. The broad definition of health informatics and the number of disciplines involved present an opportunity for the growth of subspecialties within the field. One of these subspecialties is pharmacy informatics, which has been defined as "the use and integration of data, information, knowledge, technology, and automation in the medication-use process for the purpose of improving health outcomes."[4] ASHP believes that pharmacists have the unique knowledge, expertise, and responsibility to assume a significant role in health informatics.[4] Similarly, properly trained and qualified pharmacy technicians play a key supporting role in the field of informatics.[5]

The potential for health informatics to improve health outcomes has prompted the healthcare industry, large healthcare purchasers, and state and federal governments to undertake sweeping health information technology (HIT) initiatives. These initiatives have greatly increased the demand for a highly skilled HIT workforce. The United States Bureau of Labor Statistics estimates that 29,000 new medical records and HIT technician jobs will be created between 2019 and 2029.[6] This tremendous increase will affect organizations' ability to recruit and retain the qualified personnel necessary for healthcare operations. Although not all pharmacy technicians are qualified to fill this pressing need, an emerging cadre of specialized PTIs will help fill these important roles. The purpose of this statement is to provide a preliminary description of the potential roles and responsibilities of the PTI in the evolving HIT landscape as well as the knowledge, skills, and abilities required to assume those roles and responsibilities.

Roles and Responsibilities

In general, the PTI is a healthcare professional, working under the supervision of a registered pharmacist, who uses their knowledge to influence and adapt IT systems to improve the effectiveness and efficiency of the health system and the medication-use process. The roles of PTIs vary, depending on the needs of the healthcare institution and the knowledge, skills, and abilities of the individual. PTIs specializing in the management of health-system pharmacy informatics may, for example, perform workflow assessment and optimization in clinical, administrative, educational, or research domains; adapt software controls to existing workflow; implement and follow inventory management best practices; lead and/or coordinate measures to manage budgetary expectations; provide subject-matter expertise for new technology assessment and usability; or serve as a resource for pharmacist informaticists when system updates are needed or problems are identified. Areas of responsibility can also vary considerably and may include automation and technology systems management, project management, end-user training and education, policy and governance, process improvement, analytics and reporting, and inventory and financial management.

Automation and Technology Systems Management. With training and experience in health informatics, the PTI can serve as a knowledgeable expert for placement, configuration, building, monitoring, maintenance, and troubleshooting of automation and technology systems, and provide users and staff with consultative support. They may assist or lead in assessing the functions, benefits, and constraints of technology and automation systems for drug procurement, pharmacy inventory management, prescribing medications, order processing, distribution and dispensing of medications, administering and documenting administration of medications, medication diversion monitoring, and clinical monitoring. Other responsibilities may include consulting, advising, and educating staff on methods and means to optimize automation and technology systems, as well as integration of information and workflow processes to achieve successful adoption and application of new technologies to support healthcare operations and systems.

PTIs provide and analyze relevant technological or administrative data to identify, quantify, and resolve organizational or operational problems. They integrate software applications for technological services by: (1) evaluating the unique needs of the specific services in conjunction with the capabilities of the software and coordinating required modifications; (2) reviewing the effectiveness of the systems

DOI 10.37573/9781585287048.006

and procedures to assure optimum benefit to patient-care activities; (3) determining the cause of and the solution to problems when functionality is compromised; and (4) coordinating with vendor resources to assist in issue resolution under the guidance of a pharmacist informaticist.

PTIs may develop, modify, and test components specific to fields and data that individualize or customize applications to user roles or needs while maintaining integrity among multiple software packages. They may provide for maintenance and updating of site parameters and site-specific files to ensure proper functioning of complex, interrelated, and interdependent software applications, while effectively and efficiently managing multiple competing priorities.

Project Management. PTIs may lead or collaborate with pharmacist informaticists in implementing and managing technology and information systems based on a shared understanding of system requirements, capabilities, and limitations. They may serve as an interdisciplinary team member to complete HIT system initiatives using analytical and evaluative techniques to assess the effectiveness of results and other related programs. For example, they may contribute to planning for acquisition and implementation of a technology or automation system by assisting the pharmacist informaticist in developing a plan for the evaluation of the system; writing a request for proposal (RFP) for a system; assessing responses to the RFP; or developing a plan for implementation, testing, or maintenance of the system. Further, they may participate in the implementation of a technology or automation system by contributing to system installation (including supplemental buildouts), testing, and training of staff for use of the system, as well as maintaining the system according to an established plan. Development of contingency plans for failure or compromise of technology or automation systems may also involve PTIs.

End-User Training and Education. PTIs identify end-user educational requirements and training needs and develop educational programs, instructional materials, and appropriate tools to educate users and support staff at all levels of the organization. Additionally, they may contribute to didactic discussions to pharmacy learners on rotation with the pharmacy informatics team, including but not limited to pharmacy technician students, pharmacy students, and pharmacy residents. PTIs monitor end-user satisfaction to drive enhancements and improve performance. In a supportive role with the pharmacist informaticist, PTIs may work to ensure technological changes are aligned with the organizational needs and participates in process improvement, root cause analysis, and system (re)design teams.

Policy and Governance. PTIs maintain state-of-the-art knowledge of changes in technology, regulatory, and the clinical environment to identify, propose, formulate, and support new or revised major technological policies and directives for automation and systems technology. In collaboration with informaticists, analysts, IT and pharmacy, they may lead or participate in structuring of programmatic and security requirements for data access in IT to ensure that best practices are applied to operational requirements. Finally, they instruct staff members in the proper use of information management tools and security procedures in compliance with policy, regulations, and best practices.

Process Improvement. PTIs maintain ongoing professional, collegial relationships with onsite peers, pharmacist informaticists, technical support staff, administrative staff, and healthcare professionals within the facility and/or health system. They may need to contact clinical subject-matter experts and offsite technical support personnel as needed. External contacts may include contract developers, for whom PTIs can serve as a primary contact and knowledge resource. Additionally, PTIs maintain open communication with end-users and stakeholders to gather feedback on systems and opportunities for improvement, monitor effects of implemented changes, and solicit feedback on proposed changes to perpetuate the continuous improvement cycle.

Analytics and Reporting. Standard reports from clinical and automation systems may be extracted, compiled, and analyzed by PTIs to facilitate organizational and individual decision-making. PTIs may customize reports and provide database management to address organizational needs not addressed through standard reporting tools. PTIs may provide extracted data for clinical research, operational review, or validation of informatics implementations. Reporting may then be incorporated into visual dashboards that managers may review for tracking of operational functions such as completion of medication reconciliations or absent administration documentation for unreconciled dispenses.

PTIs may analyze or interpret data, including evaluation of the validity of measures used to generate outcomes related to patient management systems. PTIs collaborate with pharmacist informaticists to develop recommendations for improving clinical data management methods, follow-up procedures, and timely compliance with regulatory guidelines.

Inventory and Financial Management. PTIs maintain and manage processes that oversee drug shortage mitigation, departmental quality assurance, formulary and inventory management, and various software interfaces (e.g., 340B split billing and management, perpetual inventory systems).

PTIs maintain appropriate charging controls to ensure accurate patient and third-party billing. They may be engaged with pharmaceutical wholesalers and distributors to validate price files in clinical and automation systems, as well as Healthcare Common Procedure Coding System (HCPCS) coding, units, and quantities. Charging and transaction interfaces are also monitored for errors in charge application, quantities, or amounts. This monitoring may include bar coded medication administration (BCMA) monitoring and maintenance.

Knowledge, Skills, and Abilities

Due to their combination of technological knowledge, skills, abilities, experience, and training, PTIs are uniquely qualified to serve in pharmacy informatics. They are required to understand IT systems, including interfaces, computer management techniques, problem resolution, and database maintenance. They must be competent in pharmacy operations, medications, and medical terminologies as well as medication-use workflow processes, including drug procurement, pharmacy inventory, medication ordering, order management, dispensing, drug preparation, distribution, regulatory guidance, and billing systems.

Thorough knowledge of the clinical environment is required, including practices, procedures, policies, strengths, and weaknesses, and effective use of data to track and manage patient care. Knowledge of emerging and state-of-the-art technology, regulations, programs, and processes related to health informatics is necessary for PTIs to propose administrative and clinical policies and directives, instruct practitioners on the changes and application of new policies and directives, and provide leadership on informatics committees or teams.

Practical, in-depth knowledge of automation and software systems that affect clinical practice, as well as knowledge of technologies that may benefit healthcare delivery processes is required. When available, PTIs should pursue and complete training, certification and courses for the specific technology, and employer should provide support if it is used in the facility. PTIs should be able to troubleshoot functionality issues, develop solutions, and ensure quality management of clinical operations.

PTIs should have comprehensive knowledge of the data life cycle, including data design, collection, and management, in order to input, retrieve, analyze, summarize, and present information effectively. The required knowledge base is extensive and includes but is not limited to usability, data standards, data validation, understanding content relationships, data security, and interoperability among systems.

PTIs should understand common network standards, network architectures, the functions and purposes of common hardware components, configurations, and the design of safe technology and automation systems. Additionally, the PTI should possess the database skills to successfully create patient and medication information data sets and successfully construct reports.

The PTI should be skilled in communicating both orally and in a variety of written media for a variety of audiences, from information technology and clinical experts to end-users. As a specialist with training and experience in health informatics, they guide the evolution of automation technology and processes using creative and well-developed interpersonal skills to achieve effective communication with end-users and management.

Conclusion

The ASHP Practice Advancement Initiative provides several recommendations regarding use of technology to ensure medication safety.[5] Meeting these recommendations requires an expansion of pharmacy resources devoted to the implementation and maintenance of HIT operating at the top of their licenses. A trained and educated PTI has unique skill sets that combine technical knowledge with an understanding of medication vocabulary and pharmacy operational workflow. Through these specialized skills, they are able to support and coordinate pharmacy technologies under the direction of the pharmacy department or an accountable pharmacist. The PTI possesses a working knowledge of the technology and automation systems and processes that support the medication-use system and can contribute to ensuring their safety and efficiency.

References

1. American Society of Health-System Pharmacists. ASHP statement on the roles of pharmacy technicians. *Am J Health-Syst Pharm.* 2016;73:928–30. https://www.ashp.org/-/media/assets/policy-guidelines/docs/statements/roles-of-pharmacy-technicians.pdf
2. American Society of Health-System Pharmacists. ASHP policy position 1203, qualifications of pharmacy technicians in advanced roles. Accessed November 1, 2021. https://www.ashp.org/pharmacy-practice/policy-positions-and-guidelines/browse-by-document-type/policy-positions?loginreturnUrl=SSOCheckOnly
3. National Library of Medicine. Health Services Research Information Central: Health Informatics. Accessed December 13, 2021. https://www.nlm.nih.gov/hsrinfo/informatics.html
4. American Society of Health-System Pharmacists. ASHP statement on the pharmacist's role in clinical informatics. *Am J Health-Syst Pharm.* 2016; 73:410–3.
5. American Society of Health-System Pharmacists. ASHP Practice Advancement Initiative 2030. *Am J Health-Syst Pharm.* 2020;77:113–122.
6. US Bureau of Labor Statistics. Occupational outlook handbook: medical records and health information technicians. Accessed November 1, 2021. www.bls.gov/ooh/healthcare/medical-records-and-health-information-technicians.htm

Other Resources

- American Society of Health-System Pharmacists. Pharmacy technician informatics specialist web resource page. Accessed November 1, 2021. https://www.ashp.org/pharmacy-practice/resource-centers/informatics/pharmacy-technician-informatics-specialist
- Nemec II EC, Pawola JA, Shah B. Online resources for informatics education and training. *Am J Health-Syst Pharm.* 2016;73:1131–1134. doi:10.2146/ajhp150659
- Fox BI, Flynn AJ, Fortier CR, et al. Knowledge, skills, and resources for pharmacy informatics education. *Am J Pharm Educ.* 2011; 5:93. doi: 10.5688/ajpe75593
- American Society of Health-System Pharmacists. Pharmacy informatics certificate. Accessed November 1, 2021. https://store.ashp.org/Default.aspx?TabID=251&productId=830829873

Developed through the ASHP Section of Pharmacy Informatics and Technology and approved by the ASHP Board of Directors on November 2, 2021, and by the ASHP House of Delegates on March 25, 2022. This statement supersedes the ASHP Statement on the Pharmacy Technician's Role in Pharmacy Informatics dated June 3, 2013.

ASHP gratefully acknowledges the contributions of authors of the previous version of this statement: Nancy R. Smestad, M.S.; Trinh Le, M.S., FASHP; Adelaide Quansah-Arku, B.S.B.A.; Karl F. Gumpper, BCNSP, BCPS, FASHP; and Andy Laegeler, Pharm.D., M.S.

The authors have declared no potential conflicts of interest.

Bryan Shaw, PharmD, Vizient, Inc., Irving, TX.

Shawn Boland, PharmD, DPLA, MS, CPPS, Meritus Health, Hagerstown, MD.

Danielle Baker, CPhT, Meritus Health, Hagerstown, MD.

Mary Tucker, CPhT, BD (Becton, Dickinson and Company), San Diego, CA.

Cynthia Jeter, CPhT, CPP, BGS, McKesson RxO, Springdale, AR.

Yuqi Zhou, BS, PharmD (candidate), University of Minnesota College of Pharmacy, Minneapolis, MN.

Copyright © 2022, American Society of Health-System Pharmacists, Inc. All rights reserved. Contact ASHP for reprint and permissions requests. This content may not be used for commercial purposes without the express written consent of ASHP.

The bibliographic citation for this document is as follows: American Society of Health-System Pharmacists. ASHP statement on the pharmacy technician's role in pharmacy informatics. *Am J Health-Syst Pharm*. 2022; 79(17):1449–52.

ASHP Statement on Telehealth Pharmacy Practice

Position

ASHP believes appropriately trained and equipped pharmacists can use telehealth to remotely oversee pharmacy operations and provide distributive, clinical, analytical, consultative, and managerial services. ASHP advocates for telehealth utilization in suitable functions of pharmacy operations and patient care to improve patient outcomes, expand access to healthcare, enhance patient safety, achieve effective cost-of-care, and interact with other healthcare team members. ASHP further advocates that boards of pharmacy adopt compatible regulations that enable the use of United States–based telehealth services within and across state lines for appropriate practice settings and that additional research be conducted to establish best practices for telehealth.

Background

Telehealth. Definitions of telehealth vary widely.[1] The Agency for Healthcare Research and Quality has defined telehealth as "the use of information and telecommunications technology in healthcare delivery for a specific patient involving a provider across distance or time."[2] The Health Resources and Services Administration (HRSA) of the US Department of Health and Human Services (HHS) defines telehealth more broadly: "the use of electronic information and telecommunications technologies to support and promote long-distance clinical healthcare, patient and professional health-related education, and public health and health administration. Technologies include videoconferencing, the internet, store-and- forward imaging, streaming media, and landline and wireless communications."[3] The 2020 American Medical Association (AMA) Telehealth Playbook[4] defines telehealth as "a digital health solution that connects the patient and clinician through real-time audio and video technology" and states that telehealth "can be used as an alternative to traditional in-person care delivery and, in certain circumstances, can be used to deliver care such as the diagnosis, consultation, treatment, education, care management, and self-management of patients."

The Centers for Medicare & Medicaid Services (CMS) distinguishes between telehealth and telemedicine, at least as it concerns Medicaid, defining "Telehealth (or Telemonitoring)" as "the use of telecommunications and information technology to provide access to health assessment, diagnosis, intervention, consultation, supervision and information across distance."[5] CMS follows this definition by saying "[t]elehealth includes such technologies as telephones, facsimile machines, electronic mail systems, and remote patient monitoring devices, which are used to collect and transmit patient data for monitoring and interpretation." CMS notes that although such technologies "do not meet the Medicaid definition of telemedicine they are often considered under the broad umbrella of telehealth services" and may nevertheless be covered and reimbursed as part of a Medicaid coverable service.[5] Other authors[6] have also made this distinction, while some organizations do not; the American Academy of Pediatrics states that the terms telemedicine and telehealth "are considered synonymous and are used interchangeably to describe use of electronic information and telecommunications technologies to support clinical healthcare, patient and professional health-related education, public health and health administration."[7]

Just as many definitions of telehealth include a broader scope of virtual healthcare services than does telemedicine, ASHP believes telehealth pharmacy practice is a more appropriate overarching term for the virtual delivery of pharmacists' patient care services than telepharmacy. For the purposes of this document, ASHP defines telehealth pharmacy practice as use of electronic information and telecommunications technology by pharmacists to provide patient care services. This definition reflects the broad spectrum of pharmacy practice. Telehealth patient care services and operations may include, but are not limited to, the following:

- Comprehensive medication management
- Chronic disease state management,
- Medication selection and dispensing
- Sterile and nonsterile compounding verification
- Patient assessment and evaluation
- Adverse drug event detection and monitoring
- Patient counseling
- Medication reconciliation
- Clinical consultation
- Outcomes assessment
- Healthcare data analysis
- Interacting with other healthcare practitioners
- Healthcare personnel supervision
- Provision of drug information
- Oversight of aspects of pharmacy operations

Practice Advancement Initiative 2030 (PAI 2030). The ASHP PAI states that the pharmacy enterprise "must have sufficient resources to develop, implement, and maintain technology-related medication-use safety standards."[8] It further recommends that virtual pharmacy services "should be deployed to optimize operational and clinical services that extend patient care services and enhance continuity of care."[8]

Telehealth Pharmacy Practice Applications

Telehealth pharmacy practice has demonstrated value in a variety of settings for medication selection, order review, and dispensing; intravenous (IV) admixture verification; patient counseling and monitoring; and clinical services.[9] Telehealth pharmacy services have long proven useful in supporting settings that perform medication-use activities when a pharmacist is not physically present or pharmacy resources may be limited, such as at geographically isolated ambulatory clinics and healthcare facilities.[10–13] Telehealth also provides a solution for order review and verification in tertiary medical centers when staffing, particularly in specialty areas such as oncology and pediatrics, is limited (eg, due to attrition or staff turnover), creating a mechanism for health systems to provide enterprise level pharmacy services throughout the

DOI 10.37573/9781585287048.007

system even when not all pharmacies operate 24 hours per day.[14,15] Other facilities may use telehealth services for supplemental workload balancing, which includes network workload balancing and on-call assistance.[14] In addition, telehealth provides a tool for virtual monitoring, assessment, detection, decision-making, and adverse drug event management.[16]

Medication Selection, Order Review, and Dispensing. Telehealth has been used successfully to enable pharmacists to be directly involved in the medication selection process for patients at geographically remote hospitals. Specific tasks may include but are not limited to remote review of new medication orders, entry of orders into the patient's electronic health record, release of medication from an automated dispensing cabinet, and electronic supervision of technicians in the performance of pharmacy operations.[10–13,17–20]

IV Admixture Verification. Although technology systems for remote checking of IV admixture preparation were originally designed to reduce contamination risk by reducing the need for pharmacists to physically enter sterile compounding areas to review and verify finished preparations, these and similar technologies can be used for verification of admixtures at different stages of preparation, across multiple sites, and over long distances.[20,21] The technology also reduces exposure risk by reducing the number of pharmacy personnel and other providers having to handle hazardous medications, such as chemotherapy. Documentation and safety can also be enhanced with these systems, as images capture lot numbers and expiration dates in addition to the step-by-step processes of preparation. Some of these systems perform in-process verification steps (eg, barcode verification of correct product selection, gravimetric verification of additive quantities), which provide additional assurance to the remote pharmacist that the preparation is correct.

Patient Counseling and Monitoring. Pharmacists have been using telecommunications technology to counsel patients about the proper use of their medications for as long as telephone service lines have been available. Early examples of pharmacists employing videoconferencing technology to counsel geographically remote patients include the outreach program by a Federally Qualified Health Center (FQHC) in eastern Washington State[22] and another program in North Dakota.[23] The Indian Health Service has also implemented videoconferencing technology to provide pharmacist services to remote areas of Alaska,[24] and the US Navy has deployed use of this technology worldwide.[25] Other examples include the use of videoconferencing to provide comprehensive medication management,[26] chronic disease state management (eg, diabetes mellitus, chronic obstructive pulmonary disease, congestive heart failure and other cardiovascular conditions, post-MI cardiac rehabilitation, gout),[27–38] specialty pharmacy services (eg, oncology, autoimmune diseases, multiple sclerosis, cystic fibrosis),[39–42] and mental and behavioral health telehealth.[43,44] Implementation of intensive care unit telemedicine services, including telehealth pharmacy practice, led to reduced hospital length of stay, an increase in institutional best practice adherence, and lower rates of preventable complications.[45] Pharmacists are also being encouraged to use mobile applications to communicate with patients to help them manage their diseases and medications.[46,47]

Expanding Pharmacy Services. ASHP supports implementation of telehealth services to "maintain pharmacy operations and pharmacist-led comprehensive medication management that extend patient care services to and enhance continuity of care for rural or medically underserved populations."[48] Telehealth can be used to enable on-site pharmacy activities if the pharmacist is not physically located at the point of pharmacy operation or patient care.

Millions of Americans live in areas, both rural and urban, devoid of pharmacies.[49] Until recently, much of the focus of expanding telehealth pharmacy practice has been on rural areas. According to the 2019 National Pharmacist Workforce Study (NPWS),[50] more licensed pharmacists were unemployed or working outside of pharmacy than in the 2014 NPWS,[51] which suggests there has not been a shortage of pharmacists. However, workforce issues continue to plague rural areas.[52] Between 2003 and 2018, 16% (1,231) of independently-owned rural pharmacies closed.[53] Similarly, 180 rural hospitals closed between 2005 and 2021, causing pharmacists and other professionals to leave rural areas for employment.[54] Telehealth pharmacy services in retail and hospital pharmacy settings can help fill the gap.[55–57] More recently, attention has also turned to the problem of "pharmacy deserts" in urban areas,[58,59] as FQHCs and other healthcare institutions increase utilization of telehealth and explore strategies such as remote dispensing.[60–62]

Federal Regulation. Federal regulation of telehealth has evolved, and CMS has established standards for telehealth.[63] The Health Insurance Portability and Accountability Act64 (HIPAA) and Subtitle D of the Health Information Technology for Economic and Clinical Health (HITECH) Act,[65] which was enacted as part of the American Recovery and Reinvestment Act of 2009,[66] address privacy and security concerns associated with electronic transmission of health information. The Food and Drug Administration (FDA) has jurisdiction over medical software and equipment that may be involved in healthcare, whether online, mobile, or in-house. Pharmacists communicating with a patient via a mobile application should ensure it is compliant with FDA standards.[67]

ASHP advocates for changes in federal (eg, Social Security Act), state, and third-party payment programs to define pharmacists as healthcare providers and provide an infrastructure supporting sustainability of pharmacist-provided patient care services and improved interactions between pharmacists and other healthcare providers that benefit patient care.[68,69] ASHP recognizes that reimbursement for those provider services may be contingent on credentialing by payers and other appropriate bodies. ASHP further encourages health systems to include pharmacists in their credentialing and privileging processes in a manner consistent with other healthcare professionals to assess pharmacists' competence to engage in patient care services, including telehealth pharmacy practice.[70] Provider status and institutional privileging and credentialing processes expand pharmacists' ability to bill for services they are already providing, enhancing the health system's reimbursement for services and facilitating ongoing growth of telehealth pharmacy practice. In addition, the federal government and accrediting bodies should collaboratively establish standards for telehealth pharmacy practice and associated technologies, and incorporate regulatory and reimbursement imperatives to encourage adoption of standards regarding telehealth practice that would foster wider adoption and improve patient care.

State Regulation. The Model State Pharmacy Act and Model Rules of the National Association of Boards of Pharmacy (Model Act), while not a federal standard, provides boards of pharmacy with model language for developing state laws or board rules.[71] The Model Act defines telehealth-related terms and provides requirements for remote pharmacy services. Many states now have specific regulations for telehealth.[72] However, these state laws and regulations demonstrate wide variation in the application and control of telehealth systems.[73] States have variously described telehealth pharmacy practice in terms of remote order management with or without dispensing using automated dispensing cabinets, remote supervision of medication order filling with or without automated medication order dispensing, and inpatient dispensing activities (including IV preparation). When providing pharmacy services across state lines, pharmacists must be aware of the regulations of the state in which the pharmacist is located and the state in which the patient is receiving care.[74] State laws and regulations vary on the definition of telehealth, licensing requirements, education and training for participating pharmacists and technicians, practice setting restrictions, and geographical limitations for the remotely practicing pharmacist. State laws and regulations also vary widely regarding the technology required to implement telehealth. Although most stipulate a camera and some audio exchange between the pharmacy and the remote pharmacist, the specification of the types of technology (video vs still, telephone vs voice over internet protocol [VoIP]) and the types and amounts of transactional information captured vary widely. Some state boards of pharmacy have identified specific training, certification, or experience that pharmacy technicians engaged in telehealth must possess.[75,76]

As use of telehealth expands, state board of pharmacy regulations and state laws regarding its use should evolve while avoiding mandating technologies that could impede future improvements in patient care and the medication-use process. ASHP advocates that federal and state governments adopt laws and regulations that modernize and standardize telehealth practices nationwide and facilitate the use of US-based telehealth services to enhance interprofessional practices. ASHP further advocates that boards of pharmacy and state agencies that regulate pharmacy practice address the following regarding telehealth pharmacy practice:

1. Education and training of participating pharmacists
2. Education, training, certification by the Pharmacy Technician Certification Board, and licensure of participating pharmacy technicians
3. Communication and information systems requirements
4. Remote order entry, prospective order review, verification of the completed medication order before dispensing, and dispensing
5. Direct patient-care services, including comprehensive medication management and medication therapy management services and patient counseling and education
6. Licensure (including reciprocity) of participating pharmacies and pharmacists
7. Service arrangements that cross state borders
8. Service arrangements within the same corporate entity or between different corporate entities
9. Service arrangements for workload relief in the point-of-care pharmacy during peak periods
10. Pharmacist access to all applicable patient information
11. Development and monitoring of patient safety, quality, and outcomes measures[77]

ASHP advocates for interstate pharmacist licensure to expand the mobility of pharmacists, especially during emergencies, and to enhance their ability to practice in multiple states, which is particularly important to telehealth pharmacy practice.[78] The National Association of Boards of Pharmacy's (NABP) Electronic Licensure Transfer Program[79] is a good first step toward true interstate licensure but should be enhanced at the state level to meet the needs presented by the rapid expansion of telehealth pharmacy practice. ASHP supports exploration of licensure models (eg, endorsements, interstate agreements) that would allow pharmacists to provide specific services across state lines and encourages advocacy to implement such models.[78,80]

In addition, some state legislatures have passed laws ensuring that insurance reimbursements for telehealth are the same as for non-telehealth services. Whether these statutes can or will be applied to pharmacy-related telehealth services in those states remains unanswered. Many of the telehealth payment models involving pharmacists have been implemented in managed care organizations that see the value of increasing frequency of visits and follow-up to improve quality of care in chronic disease state management.[81] As payment shifts toward value-based care, insurance payers may be increasingly interested in telehealth models.[82]

Reimbursement for Telehealth Pharmacy Practice Services

ASHP advocates for reimbursement for pharmacists' provision of telehealth pharmacy services commensurate with the complexity and duration of service and consistent with other healthcare providers, to ensure that patients can maintain access to vital services.[83] During the COVID-19 public health emergency, hospitals, health systems, and clinics quickly pivoted to providing patient services via telehealth. CMS, commercial payers, and state policy makers have indicated that they would like to maintain telehealth services after the pandemic. Because pharmacists are not currently recognized as healthcare providers through Medicare Part B, reimbursement for telehealth services has been challenging.[84]

ASHP advocates for full recognition of pharmacists as reimbursable healthcare providers through Medicare, Medicaid, and all health insurance plans.[68] Since this has not yet been fully realized, as an interim step, ASHP supports federal and state legislation and regulation that would provide qualified pharmacists (ie, as determined by the state board of pharmacy or the credentialing board of a qualified healthcare institution) provider status to bill for services rendered through telehealth.[83] ASHP also advocates billing for services using existing billing codes, and expansion of those codes, as the current set is limited and does not capture the full potential of clinical pharmacy services, including services provided via telehealth.[85]

Telehealth Infrastructure

The technology infrastructure required for the implementation and maintenance of telehealth services may be scalable and adjusted to fit the care setting. Two intra-system facilities may already share a network, a pharmacy information system, and possibly an order management system. In this scenario, perhaps the only additional equipment needed is a digital communication system for transmission of any orders not provided via computerized provider order entry (CPOE).

In contrast, the inter-system model provides telehealth services to a facility external to the health system. This could involve a variety of infrastructures; for example, a cloud-based health information exchange (HIE) where all patients and care providers interact through a variety of hardware and software. Additionally, all data may be stored in a relational database or data warehouse.

As more pharmacists are providing telehealth management, it is recommended that organizations investigate the feasibility of integrating telehealth solutions (eg, videoconferencing software, remote monitoring devices) into the electronic health record (EHR). Telehealth EHR integration streamlines workflow, optimizes cognitive workload, minimizes clinician burden, and facilitates documentation.[86,87] In addition, incorporation of decision support tools, machine learning, and internet-of-things technologies will offer greater insights, earlier prediction, and better care by pharmacists to patients and caregivers in a variety of settings, ranging from institutional to home-based care.

With all electronic systems and workflow processes, redundancies and contingency plans must be carefully outlined and readily referenced in organizational policies and procedures to ensure continuity of operations and safety in instances of unplanned events.

Security of Information and Equipment

The security and integrity of patient data is of paramount importance when determining the information technology setup of a telehealth system.[88] Security is vital when accessing and modifying patient records. Adherence to HIPAA[64] and HITECH[65] regulations are important to both the providers of telehealth pharmacy services as well as the entities who receive them. As security continues to be threatened by breaches and ransomware, facilities are tightening their security policies. Telehealth pharmacy providers may notice additional layers of security such as multifactor authentication requirements for access to their network or electronic medical record, as well as shorter workstation session timeouts with inactivity.

Security is important wherever telehealth pharmacy is practiced. It is important to note that some states require that pharmacists work only from licensed pharmacies. This includes home-based practices and corporate environments that may need to be licensed as a professional pharmacy according to state regulations. A professional and secure environment should be provided in every setting. Care should be taken to keep the environment a professional workspace with all necessary references, resources, confidentiality, and data security practices.

Patient-Centric Considerations for the Telehealth Pharmacy Visit

The environment for provision of telehealth services should be evaluated from the patient's point of view. It should provide proper lighting to allow the patient to clearly see the pharmacist's face. Dress and appearance should be consistent with what would be seen within a healthcare facility. Ideally, the camera is at eye level to simulate a true face-to-face interaction. The background should appear professional, be free from clutter and commotion, and provide a sense of privacy. Audio and video quality should be verified with the recipient upon initiation of the visit. The patient should be allowed access to all applicable patient care records during an encounter when possible.[89]

Conclusion

Telehealth is a method used in pharmacy practice in which pharmacists utilize electronic information and telecommunications technology to provide patient care services. Telehealth services that adhere to ASHP practice guidelines allow expanded coverage, improved patient safety, and enhanced communication between patients, healthcare providers, and pharmacists. Variability in laws between states and evolving regulations must be closely monitored when implementing services. ASHP advocates for more research to investigate a refined definition and best practices in the implementation and delivery of telehealth services.[90]

References

1. Skelley JW, Parrott AM, Lassiter J, et al. Establishing the definitions for telehealth. In: DeRemer CE, ed. *Telehealth: Strategies for Establishing Pharmacy Practice Models in Ambulatory Care Settings.* American Society of Health-System Pharmacists; 2022. doi:10.37573/9781585286928.002
2. Totten AM, Womack DM, Eden KB, et al; Pacific Northwest Evidence-based Practice Center. *Telehealth: Mapping the Evidence for Patient Outcomes from Systematic Reviews.* Agency for Healthcare Research and Quality; 2016. Accessed January 13, 2022. https://effectivehealthcare.ahrq.gov/sites/default/files/pdf/telehealth_technicalbrief.pdf
3. Office for the Advancement of Telehealth, Health Resources and Services Administration. Telehealth Programs. Accessed January 13, 2022. https://www.hrsa.gov/rural-health/telehealth
4. American Medical Association. *Telehealth Implementation Playbook.* Revised February 2022. Accessed July 13, 2022. https://www.ama-assn.org/system/files/ama-telehealth-playbook.pdf
5. Centers for Medicare & Medicaid Services. Telemedicine. Medicaid.gov. Accessed January 13, 2022. https://www.medicaid.gov/medicaid/benefits/telemedicine/index.html
6. van Dyk L. A review of telehealth service implementation frameworks. *Int J Environ Res Pub Health.* 2014;11:1279–1298. doi:10.3390/ijerph110201279

7. American Academy of Pediatrics. What is telehealth? Accessed January 13, 2022. https://www.aap.org/en-us/professional-resources/practicetransformation/telehealth/Pages/Whatis-Telehealth.aspx
8. American Society of Health-System Pharmacists. Practice Advancement Initiative (PAI) 2030 recommendations. Accessed January 13, 2022. www.ashp.org/Pharmacy-Practice/PAI/PAI-Recommendations
9. Stratton T. Review of research on telepharmacy. In: *Telemedicine*. SMGroup; May 20, 2016. Accessed July 13, 2022. http://www.smgebooks.com/telemedicine/chapters/TELMED-16-03.pdf
10. Keeys CA, Dandurand K, Harris J, et al. Providing nighttime pharmaceutical services through telepharmacy. *Am J Health-Syst Pharm*. 2002;59:716–721.
11. Boon AD. Telepharmacy at a critical access hospital. *Am J Health-Syst Pharm*. 2007;64:242–244.
12. Peterson CD, Rathke A, Skwiera J, et al. Hospital telepharmacy network: delivering pharmacy services to rural hospitals. *J Pharm Technol*. 2007;23:158–165.
13. Stratton TP, Worley MM, Schmidt M, et al. Implementing after-hours pharmacy coverage for critical access hospitals in northeast Minnesota. *Am J Health-Syst Pharm*. 2008;65:1727–1734.
14. American Society of Health-System Pharmacists. ASHP guidelines on remote medication order processing. *Am J Health-Syst Pharm*. 2010;67:672–677.
15. Amkreutz J, Lenssen R, Marx G, et al. Medication safety in a German telemedicine centre: implementation of a telepharmaceutical expert consultation in addition to existing tele-intensive care unit services. *J Telemed Telecare*. 2020;26(1–2):105–112. doi:10.1177/1357633X18799796.
16. Copeland AC, Foster MC, Muluneh B, et al. The utility of a telemedicine platform to monitor adherence and adverse effects of tyrosine kinase inhibitors. *Leuk Lymphoma*. 2019;60:1842–1844. doi:10.1080/10428194.2018.1551540
17. Casey M, Elias W, Knudson A, et al. Implementation of telepharmacy in rural hospitals: potential for improving medication safety. Upper Midwest Rural Health Research Center; 2008. Accessed March 30, 2016. http://rhrc.umn.edu/wp-content/files_mf/telepharmacy.pdf
18. Mahaney L, Sanborn M, Alexander E. Nontraditional work schedules for pharmacists. *Am J Health-Syst Pharm*. 2008;65:2144–2149.
19. Garrelts JC, Gagnon M, Eisenberg C, et al. Impact of telepharmacy in a multihospital health system. *Am J Health-Syst Pharm*. 2010;67:1456–1456.
20. Wakefield DS, Ward MM, Loes JL, et al. Implementation of a telepharmacy service to provide round-the-clock medication order review by pharmacists. *Am J Health-Syst Pharm*. 2010;67:2052–2057.
21. O'Neal BC, Worden JC, Couldry RJ. Telepharmacy and bar-code technology in an i.v. chemotherapy admixture area. *Am J Health-Syst Pharm*. 2009;66:1211–1217.
22. Clifton GD, Byer H, Heaton K, et al. Provision of pharmacy services to underserved populations via remote dispensing and two-way videoconferencing. *Am J Health-Syst Pharm*. 2003;60:2577–2582.
23. Peterson CD, Scott DM, Rathke A, et al. Establishing a central order entry system for delivering telepharmacy services to remote rural hospitals. *J Pharm Technol*. 2010;26:179–186.
24. Rose JL. Improved and expanded pharmacy care in rural Alaska through telepharmacy and alternative methods demonstration project. *Int J Circumpolar Health*. 2007;66 (suppl 1):14–22.
25. Traynor K. Navy takes telepharmacy worldwide. News. *Am J Health-Syst Pharm*. 2010;67:1134–1136.
26. Badowski ME, Wright EA, Bainbridge J, et al. Implementation and evaluation of comprehensive medication management in telehealth practices. *J Am Coll Clin Pharm*. 2020;3:520–531. Accessed January 13, 2020. https://doi.org/10.1002/jac5.1210
27. Nye AM. A clinical pharmacist in telehealth team care for rural patients with diabetes. *N C Med J*. 2017;78:183–184. doi:10.18043/ncm.78.3.183
28. Maxwell LG, McFarland MS, Baker JW, et al. Evaluation of the impact of a pharmacist-led telehealth clinic on diabetes-related goals of therapy in a veteran population. *Pharmacotherapy*. 2016;36:348–356.
29. Shane-McWhorter L, McAdam-Marx C, Lenert L, et al. Pharmacist-provided diabetes management and education via a telemonitoring program. *J Am Pharm Assoc*. 2015;55:516–526.
30. Shane-McWhorter L, Lenert L, Petersen M, et al. The Utah Remote Monitoring Project: improving healthcare one patient at a time. *Diabetes Technol Ther*. 2014;16:653–660.
31. McFarland M, Davis K, Wallace J, et al. Use of home telehealth monitoring with active medication therapy management by clinical pharmacists in veterans with poorly controlled type 2 diabetes mellitus. *Pharmacotherapy*. 2012;32:420–426.
32. Margolis A, Young H, Lis J, et al. A telepharmacy intervention to improve inhaler adherence in veterans with chronic obstructive pulmonary disease. Letter. *Am J Health-Syst Pharm*. 2013;70:1875–1876.
33. Peeples L. Telepharmacy helps keep HF pts close to heart. *Pharmacy Practice News*. Published November 13, 2018. Accessed January 13, 2022. www.pharmacypracticenews.com/Clinical/Article/11-18/Telepharmacy-Helps-Keep-HF-Pts-Close-to-Heart/53282
34. Coakley C, Hough A, Dwyer D, et al. Clinical video telehealth in a cardiology pharmacotherapy clinic. *Am J Health-Syst Pharm*. 2013;70:1974–1975.
35. Omboni S, Tenti M. Telepharmacy for the management of cardiovascular patients in the community. *Trends Cardiovasc Med*. 2019;29:109–117. doi:10.1016/j.tcm.2018.07.002
36. Aberger EW, Migliozzi D, Follick MJ, et al. Enhancing patient engagement and blood pressure management for renal transplant recipients via home electronic monitoring and web-enabled collaborative care. *Telemed J E Health*. 2014;20:850–854.
37. Peretti A, Amenta F, Tayebati SK, et al. Telerehabilitation: Review of the state-of-the-art and areas of application. *JMIR Rehabil Assist Technol*. 2017;4(2):e7. www.ncbi.nlm.nih.gov/pmc/articles/PMC5544892/ (accessed 13 Jan 2022).

38. Goldfien RD, Ng MS, Yip G, et al. Effectiveness of a pharmacist-based gout care management programme in a large integrated health plan: results from a pilot study. *BMJ Open*. 2014;4:e003627. doi:10.1136/.bmjopen-2013-003627
39. Chen ZJ, Liang WT, Liu Q, et al. Use of a remote oncology pharmacy service platform for patients with cancer during the COVID-19 pandemic: implementation and user acceptance evaluation. *J Med Internet Res*. 2021;23:e24619. doi:10.2196/24619
40. Howren A, Tsao NW, Choi HK, et al. eHealth-supported decentralized multidisciplinary care for gout involving rheumatology, pharmacy, and dietetics: proof-of-concept study. *Clin Rheumatol*. 2020;39:1241–1249. doi:10.1007/s10067-019-04809-6
41. Settle JR, Maloni HW, Bedra M, et al. Monitoring medication adherence in multiple sclerosis using a novel web-based tool: a pilot study. *J Telemed Telecare*. 2016;22:225–233. doi:10.1177/1357633X15597115
42. Muirhead CA, Sanford JN, McCullar BG, et al. One center's guide to outpatient management of pediatric cystic fibrosis acute pulmonary exacerbation. *Clin Med Insights Pediatr*. 2016;10:57–65. doi:10.4137/CMPed.S38336
43. Uscher-Pines L, Thompson J, Taylor P, et al. Where virtual care was already a reality: experiences of a nationwide telehealth service provider during the COVID-19 pandemic. *J Med Internet Res*. 2020;22:e22727. doi:10.2196/22727
44. Nieves JE, Stack KM, Cruz M. Telepharmacy in mental health outpatient case management. *J Pharm Technol*. 2007;23:281–283.
45. Meidl TM, Woller TW, Iglar AM, et al. Implementation of pharmacy services in a telemedicine intensive care unit. *Am J Health-Syst Pharm*. 2008;65:1464–1469.
46. Dayer L, Heldenbrand S, Anderson P, et al. Smartphone medication adherence apps: potential benefits to patients and providers. *J Am Pharm Assoc*. 2013;53:172–181.
47. Holdford DA, Inocencio TJ. Adherence and persistence associated with an appointment-based medication synchronization program. *J Am Pharm Assoc*. 2013;53:576–583.
48. American Society of Health-System Pharmacists. ASHP policy 2029: preserving patient access to pharmacy services by medically underserved populations. In Hawkins B, ed. *Best Practices: Positions and Guidance Documents of ASHP*. 2020–2021 ed. American Society of Health-System Pharmacists; 2021.
49. Telepharm, LLC. State-by-state pharmacy deserts map. Accessed January 13, 2022. https://info.telepharm.com/state-pharmacy-deserts-map
50. Arya V, Bakken BK, Doucette WR, et al. National Pharmacist Workforce Study 2019. Pharmacy Workforce Center, Inc.; January 2020. Accessed January 13, 2022. https://www.aacp.org/sites/default/files/2020-03/2019_NPWS_Final_Report.pdf
51. Gaither CA, Schommer JC, Doucette WR, et al. 2014 National Pharmacist Workforce Survey. Midwest Pharmacy Workforce Research Consortium; 2015. Accessed January 13, 2022. https://www.aacp.org/sites/default/files/finalreportofthenationalpharmacistworkforcestudy2014.pdf
52. Rural Health Information Hub. Rural pharmacy and prescription drugs. Accessed January 13, 2022. https://www.ruralhealthinfo.org/topics/pharmacy-and-prescription-drugs
53. Salako A, Ullrich F, Mueller KJ. Update: independently owned pharmacy closures in rural America, 2003–2018. *Rural Policy Brief*. 2018;2018(2):1–6.
54. Cecil G. Sheps Center for Health Services Research, University of North Carolina at Chapel Hill. Rural hospital closures: 2005-present. https://www.shepscenter.unc.edu/programs-projects/rural-health/rural-hospital-closures/
55. Sarkar R, Metzger B, Sayre H, et al. Telepharmacy and access to pharmaceutical services in rural areas. Marshall Digital Scholar. Published June 1, 2018. Accessed January 13, 2022. https://mds.marshall.edu/mgmt_faculty/218/
56. Pathak S, Haynes M, Qato DM, et al. Telepharmacy and quality of medication use in rural areas, 2013–2019. *Prev Chronic Dis*. 2020;17:E101. doi:10.5888/pcd17.200012
57. Todd K, Ullrich F, Mueller K; RUPRI Center for Rural Health Policy Analysis, University of Iowa College of Public Health Department of Health Management and Policy. Rural pharmacy closures: implications for rural communities. *Rural Policy Brief*. 2013;(2012 5):1–5.
58. Qato DM, Daviglus ML, Wilder J, et al. 'Pharmacy deserts' are prevalent in Chicago's predominantly minority communities, raising medication access concerns. *Health Aff (Millwood)*. 2014;33:1958–1965. doi:10.1377/hlthaff.2013.1397
59. Pednekar P, Peterson A. Mapping pharmacy deserts and determining accessibility to community pharmacy services for elderly enrolled in a state pharmaceutical assistance program. *PLoS One*. 2018;13:e0198173. doi:10.1371/journal.pone.0198173
60. Guadamuz JS, McCormick CD, Choi S, et al. Telepharmacy and medication adherence in urban areas. *J Am Pharm Assoc (2003)*. 2021;61(2):e100–e113. doi:10.1016/j.japh.2020.10.017
61. Lori UP, Bouskill KE, Jessica S, et al. Experiences of Medicaid programs and health centers in implementing telehealth. *Rand Health Q*. 2020;8(4):RR-2564-ASPE.
62. Hudd TR, Tataronis GR. The impact of an urban telepharmacy on patient medication adherence in a Federally Qualified Health Center. *J Pharm Tech*. 2011;27(3):117–122. doi:10.1177/875512251102700304
63. Centers for Medicare & Medicaid Services. Telehealth. Accessed January 13, 2022. https://www.cms.gov/Medicare/Medicare-General-Information/Telehealth
64. Centers for Medicare & Medicaid Services. Privacy and security information. Accessed January 13, 2022. https://www.cms.gov/Regulationsand-Guidance/Administrative-Simplification/HIPAA-ACA/PrivacyandSecurityInformation
65. Department of Health and Human Services. Health information privacy: HITECH Act enforcement interim final rule. Accessed January 13, 2022. http://www.hhs.gov/ocr/privacy/hipaa/administrative/enforcementrule/hitechenforcementifr.html

66. The American Recovery and Reinvestment Act of 2009, Pub L No 111–5 (2009).
67. Food and Drug Administration. Device software functions including mobile medical applications. Accessed January 13, 2022. https://www.fda.gov/medical-devices/digital-health-centerexcellence/device-software-functionsincluding-mobile-medical-applications
68. American Society of Health-System Pharmacists. ASHP policy 1502, pharmacist recognition as a healthcare provider. In: Hawkins B, ed. *Best Practices: Positions and Guidance Documents of ASHP*. 2020–2021 ed. American Society of Health-System Pharmacists; 2021. Accessed January 13, 2022. www.ashp.org/Pharmacy-Practice/Policy-Positions-and-Guidelines/Browse-by-Document-Type/Policy-Positions
69. American Society of Health-System Pharmacists. ASHP policy 1215, pharmacist's role in team-based care. In: Hawkins B, ed. *Best Practices: Positions and Guidance Documents of ASHP*. 2020–2021 ed. American Society of Health-System Pharmacists; 2021. Accessed January 13, 2022. www.ashp.org/Pharmacy-Practice/Policy-Positions-and-Guidelines/Browse-by-Document-Type/Policy-Positions
70. American Society of Health-System Pharmacists. ASHP policy 2011, credentialing and privileging by regulators, payers, and providers of collaborative practice. In: Hawkins B, ed. *Best Practices: Positions and Guidance Documents of ASHP*. 2020–2021 ed. American Society of Health-System Pharmacists; 2021. Accessed January 13, 2022. www.ashp.org/Pharmacy-Practice/Policy-Positions-and-Guidelines/Browse-by-Document-Type/Policy-Positions
71. National Association of Boards of Pharmacy. Model pharmacy act/rules. Accessed January 13, 2022. https://nabp.pharmacy/resources/model-pharmacy-act/
72. National Association of Boards of Pharmacy. Survey of pharmacy law—2020. Accessed January 13, 2022. https://nabp.pharmacy/resources/publications/survey-of-pharmacy-law/
73. Thomas L, Capistrant G. State Telemedicine Gaps Analysis, Physician Practice Standards & Licensure. American Telemedicine Association; 2017. Accessed January 13, 2022. https://utn.org/resources/downloads/50-state-telemedicinegaps-analysis-physician-practicestandards-licensure.pdf
74. Compton-Brown A, Mooradian S. State regulation of telepharmacy. Pharmacy Times. Published March 23, 2016. Accessed January 13, 2022. www.pharmacytimes.com/view/state-regulation-of-telepharmacy
75. National Conference of State Legislatures. State regulation of compounding pharmacies. Accessed January 13, 2022. http://www.ncsl.org/research/health/regulatingcompounding-pharmacies.aspx
76. Casey MM, Sorensen TD, Elias W, et al. Current practices and state regulations regarding telepharmacy in rural hospitals. *Am J Health-Syst Pharm.* 2010;67:1085–1092.
77. American Society of Health-System Pharmacists. ASHP policy 1310: regulation of telepharmacy. In: Hawkins B, ed. *Best Practices: Positions and Guidance Documents of ASHP*. 2020–2021 ed. American Society of Health-System Pharmacists; 2021. Accessed January 13, 2022. www.ashp.org/Pharmacy-Practice/Policy-Positions-and-Guidelines/Browse-by-Document-Type/Policy-Positions
78. American Society of Health-System Pharmacists. ASHP policy 2030, interstate pharmacist licensure. In: Hawkins B, ed. *Best Practices: Positions and Guidance Documents of ASHP*. 2020–2021 ed. American Society of Health-System Pharmacists; 2021. Accessed January 13, 2022. www.ashp.org/Pharmacy-Practice/Policy-Positions-and-Guidelines/Browse-by-Document-Type/Policy-Positions
79. National Association of Boards of Pharmacy. Licensure. Accessed January 13, 2022. https://nabp.pharmacy/programs/licensure/
80. American Society of Health-System Pharmacists. ASHP policy 0909, regulation of interstate pharmacy practice. In: Hawkins B, ed. *Best Practices: Positions and Guidance Documents of ASHP*. 2020–2021 ed. American Society of Health-System Pharmacists; 2021. Accessed January 13, 2022. www.ashp.org/Pharmacy-Practice/Policy-Positions-and-Guidelines/Browse-by-Document-Type/Policy-Positions
81. Longo KG. Telepharmacy business model allows satellite operation and increased patient convenience. Drug Topics. Published November 22, 2018. Accessed January 13, 2022. https://www.drugtopics.com/view/telepharmacy-business-model-allowssatellite-operation-and-increasedpatient-convenience
82. Littauer SL, Dixon DL, Mishra VK, Sisson EM, Salgado TM. Pharmacists providing care in the outpatient setting through telemedicine models: a narrative review. *Pharm Pract.* 2017;15(4):1134. doi:10.18549/PharmPract.2017.04.1134
83. American Society of Health-System Pharmacists. ASHP policy 2141, Pharmacist Engagement in and Payment for Telehealth. In: Hawkins B, ed. *Best Practices: Positions and Guidance Documents of ASHP*. 2020–2021 ed. American Society of Health-System Pharmacists; 2021. Accessed January 13, 2022. www.ashp.org/Pharmacy-Practice/Policy-Positions-and-Guidelines/Browse-by-Document-Type/Policy-Positions
84. Kliethermes MA, Reiter J, Maack B. Foundational elements of billing for telehealth pharmacy practice. In: DeRemer CE, ed. *Telehealth: Strategies for Establishing Pharmacy Practice Models in Ambulatory Care Settings*. American Society of Health-System Pharmacists; 2022. Accessed January 13, 2022. https://doi.org/10.37573/9781585286928.006
85. American Society of Health-System Pharmacists. ASHP policy 1710, revenue cycle compliance and management. In: Hawkins B, ed. *Best Practices: Positions and Guidance Documents of ASHP*. 2020–2021 ed. American Society of Health-System Pharmacists; 2021. Accessed January 13, 2022. www.ashp.org/Pharmacy-Practice/Policy-Positions-and-Guidelines/Browse-by-Document-Type/Policy-Positions
86. American Hospital Association Center for Health Innovation. Telehealth: a path to virtual integrated care. Accessed January 13, 2022. https://www.aha.org/system/files/media/file/2019/02/MarketInsights_TeleHealthReport.pdf

87. Jason C. What are the top telehealth, EHR integrations in healthcare? EHRIntelligence. Published October 9, 2020. Accessed January 13, 2022. https://ehrintelligence.com/news/what-are-the-top-telehealth-ehrintegrations-in-healthcare
88. Hall JL, McGraw D. For telehealth to succeed, privacy and security risks must be identified and addressed. *Health Aff (Millwood).* 2014;33:216–221. doi:10.1377/hlthaff.2013.0997
89. Food and Drug Administration. 21st Century Cures Act. Accessed January 13, 2022. www.fda.gov/regulatoryinformation/selected-amendmentsfdc-act/21st-century-cures-act
90. American Society of Health-System Pharmacists. ASHP policy 2117, education and training in telehealth. In: Hawkins B, ed. *Best Practices: Positions and Guidance Documents of ASHP*. 2020–2021 ed. American Society of Health-System Pharmacists; 2021. Accessed January 13, 2022. www.ashp.org/Pharmacy-Practice/Policy-Positions-and-Guidelines/Browse by Document-Type/Policy-Positions

---

Developed through the ASHP Section of Pharmacy Informatics and Technology and approved by the ASHP Board of Directors on March 14, 2022, and by the ASHP House of Delegates on May 19, 2022. This statement supersedes the ASHP Statement on Telepharmacy dated November 18, 2016.

ASHP gratefully acknowledges the contributions of authors of the previous version of this statement: Emily Alexander, PharmD, BCPS; C. David Butler, PharmD, MBA; Andrea Darr, PharmD, BCPS; Matthew T. Jenkins, PharmD, MS Robert D. Long, BSPharm; Colleen J. Shipman, PharmD, MPH, BCPS; and Timothy P. Stratton, PhD, BCPS, FAPhA. ASHP also gratefully acknowledges the following individuals for reviewing this statement (review does not imply endorsement): Courtney Coffman, PharmD; Mary Ann Kliethermes, PharmD FAPhA, FCIOM; Maritza Lew, PharmD PMP, CPHIMS; Tim Lynch, PharmD, MS, FASHP, FABC, FWSPA; Katie Clark McKinney, PharmD, MS, BCPS, FACHE, FASHP; Dennis Tribble, PharmD, FASHP; and Jody E. Jacobson Wedret, BSPharm, FASHP, FCSHP.

The authors have declared no potential conflicts of interest.

Brendan R. Begnoche, PharmD, Garnet Health Medical Center, Middletown, NY.

C. David Butler, PharmD, MBA, Teradata, Inc. Richmond, VA.

Paige H. Carson, PharmD, BCPS, CDE, CPP, Atrium Health, Charlotte, NC.

Andrea Darr, PharmD, BCPS, AveleCARE, LLC, Sioux Falls, SD.

Matthew T. Jenkins, PharmD, MS, University of Virginia Health System, Charlottesville, VA.

Trinh Le, MS, MBA, FASHP, UNC Health Care, Raleigh, NC.

Robert B. McDaniel, PharmD, CMQ, The University of Texas MD Anderson Cancer Center, Houston, TX.

Hesham Mourad, PharmD, EMBA, BCPS, BCCCP, CPHIMS, Mayo Clinic, Jacksonville, FL.

Colleen J. Shipman, PharmD, MPH, BCPS, Oregon Health and Science University, Portland, OR.

Timothy P. Stratton, PhD, BCPS, FAPhA, University of Minnesota College of Pharmacy, Duluth, Duluth, MN.

Kelvin Tran, PharmD, Houston, TX.

Kong (Kit) Wong, PharmD, BCACP, VA Capitol Health Care Network (VISN 5), Washington, DC.

Copyright © 2022, American Society of Health-System Pharmacists, Inc. All rights reserved. Contact ASHP for reprint and permissions requests. This content may not be used for commercial purposes without the express written consent of ASHP.

The bibliographic citation for this document is as follows: Begnoche BR, Butler CR, Carson PH, et al. ASHP statement on telehealth pharmacy practice. *Am J Health-Syst Pharm.* 2022; 79(19):1728–35.

ASHP Statement on the Use of Artificial Intelligence in Pharmacy

Position

Pharmacists are responsible for determining which aspects of medication use and management are best handled by pharmacists, by artificial intelligence (AI), or by pharmacists who receive advice from AI-based systems. Pharmacists should use scientific approaches to determine the degree to which AI is used to automate specific medication-use tasks. Full automation using AI should be reserved for algorithmic tasks for which it is demonstrated that AI performs as well or better than pharmacists. AI of proven value should be adopted and used so that pharmacists can make better decisions and focus their expertise on solving new and confounding problems for patients, families, and organizations.

Pharmacists are uniquely positioned to be key contributors and domain experts in the advancement of AI in healthcare. Pharmacists should lead the design, implementation, and ongoing evaluation of AI-related applications and technologies that affect medication-use processes and tasks. Pharmacists should define appropriate medication-related use cases for AI-enabled technology and provide foresight for anticipated future applications. It is also important for pharmacists to assist in validating AI for clinical use. At a minimum, AI should be evaluated for accuracy and interpretability. In addition, pharmacists should be prepared to adapt to AI through education and continued engagement.

Background

The US healthcare landscape is rapidly evolving, driven by rising costs, an aging population, and an increased emphasis on personalized medicine. As healthcare becomes increasingly digitized, unprecedented amounts of data offer valuable opportunities to better understand and thus improve patient care and pharmacy practice. The increasing digitization of healthcare data further accelerates the need for increased automation and scalability. Pharmacy must be prepared to embrace and lead efforts in making efficient use of advanced technologies to address all aspects of the quadruple aim (improving access, reducing costs, improving outcomes, and optimizing clinician satisfaction).[1]

AI is the theory and development of computer systems to perform tasks normally requiring human intelligence, such as visual perception, language processing, learning, and problem solving.[2] AI, when deployed optimally, has the ability to "augment human intelligence and improve decision-making and operational processes."[3] As the ASHP Commission on Goals noted at its 2019 meeting, AI capabilities are rapidly evolving within healthcare, with both clinical and operational implications for pharmacy.[4] This technology allows for automation of routine and manual tasks and provides a higher level of clinical decision support for the clinician across every aspect of medication management, including procurement, storage, ordering, verifying, dispensing, administering, and monitoring. As this technology advances, its deployment in the healthcare system has the potential to create new roles for pharmacists and alter the scope of pharmacist care.[5]

ASHP has developed this statement to define the role and position of pharmacists and pharmacy technicians in the advancement of AI in the care of patients. This statement was developed not simply to consider potential applications of AI within the current practice of pharmacy but also to plan for how this technology will need to be developed and implemented in coming years. Although this position is similar to the positions of other health-professional organizations contemplating how AI will drive change in their practices, it is uniquely focused on identifying opportunities specific to the practice of pharmacy. This statement is based on consensus opinion and professional judgment among experts on AI in pharmacy. Pharmacy practice settings impacted by this policy include informatics, acute care, ambulatory, community, education, public health, policy, industry, research, and development.

Responsibilities of Pharmacists in AI

For AI implementation, pharmacists should actively seek to address the following 3 key questions:

1. Which medication- or therapy-related tasks are appropriate for AI to address?
2. How should AI models be evaluated?
3. For each type of use case, which AI learning approach(es) is(are) most appropriate?

As AI methodology and techniques evolve, pharmacists should define appropriate medication-related clinical-use cases for AI-enabled technology based on AI's current capabilities, providing foresight for anticipated future applications. Every health system should include an AI-integration road map as an important part of strategic planning.[4] Any clinical AI platform implemented in the health system related to medication use or monitoring should be validated by a pharmacist prior to implementation and receive continual evaluation by a pharmacist for its contextual accuracy and interpretability. As new techniques and methodologies come into practice, establishing best practices for clinical validation and bias reduction will be a critical component in AI optimization. Pharmacists should develop and maintain clinical validation standards for AI at the local and national levels, outlining the varying levels of required evidence for safety and efficacy before deploying AI-enabled technology.[4] Clinical validation standards should

- Take into account the level of risk involved in the AI activity and its level of autonomy
- Balance stringency with the need for rapid innovation
- Include definitions and requirements for interpretability for any model used in the medication-use process

Impact on Pharmacy. As AI automates routine, manual, and repeatable tasks, pharmacists' time and focus can shift to complex clinical tasks that provide direct, empathetic patient care in a high-touch and humanistic way.[6,7] AI systems have the potential to off-load time-consuming tasks, such as routine monitoring, patient and medication safety surveillance,

DOI 10.37573/9781585287048.008

and data processing. AI technology can run in the background to provide information in a visually digestible and easily interpretable way, at the appropriate time to aid the pharmacist in patient-care decisions.

AI also has the potential to synthesize and become a new source of evidence-based data with which pharmacists will need to be actively engaged. As AI capacity develops further into the diagnostic space, it has the potential to shift healthcare paradigms, with some diagnoses being confirmed independently through AI-enabled devices and applications.[8,9] Eventually, patients may receive continuous diagnostic surveillance. Pharmacy leadership should focus on improving access to care through scalable models centered on AI-enabled diagnostic surveillance and pharmacy medication management, especially for underserved patient populations. Given the novelty of this technology, systems should be designed with a functional level of autonomy that corresponds to the level of trust users can confidently place in the system.[10]

In addition to its impact on care-delivery models, AI is expanding the medication armamentarium. Advances in AI capabilities are enabling the emergence of software platforms designed for patients with chronic disease states to be used with, or in place of, medication therapy.[11] Given the anticipated trend of increasing development and use of digital therapeutics and a blend between chemical, biological, and digital therapies, pharmacists should be involved in the design of AI-enabled digital therapeutics.[12,13] Pharmacists should have access to the summarized data from AI-enabled digital therapeutics for safety and efficacy monitoring. Pharmacy organizations should seek out opportunities to collaborate with other healthcare organizations to be involved in creating guidance and standards on how to incorporate AI-enabled digital therapeutics into patient care.

Informatics

Pursuant to the rigor applied to clinical trial design and the practice of evidence-based medicine, AI models need to be trained, evaluated, corrected, and applied to data that match clinical practice. AI models that run on poorly sourced data, data with disproportionate representation, or correlated data assumed to be causal could unintentionally magnify systemic bias or discrimination.[14–16] In addition, AI models require maintenance and monitoring as clinical practice and data inputs or data distributions change over time. With their background in experimental design, research methodology, and problem solving, pharmacists (especially pharmacists specialized in informatics) have ideal baseline skill sets for AI development and implementation.[17] Pharmacists can further specialize in AI and data science, or develop partnerships with data scientists to develop, test, and validate new AI models related to medication management, and should promote development of interdisciplinary teams or dedicated positions for integrating AI solutions within the health system.

Clinical Applications

Pharmacists should be open and willing to make changes to traditional clinical workflows by leveraging AI and AI-enabled clinical-decision support systems to improve patient care.[18] AI applications are expanding from diagnostics to therapy recommendations. Because medications are a central focus of therapy recommendation models, pharmacists should take a central role in leading the research, development, implementation, and quality improvement of these models. Pharmacy departments should work with healthcare systems to leverage pharmacists and future emerging AI-enabled diagnostic tools and decision support tools to evaluate models, improve care, lower costs, and provide comprehensive medication management for patients.

Pharmacy Operations

From an operational standpoint, AI platforms can be used to tighten inventory management,[19] facilitate product verification, and help pharmacists perform at the top of their skill set. As AI becomes more reliable, standard pharmacy operations will become increasingly automated, allowing pharmacists to focus more on high-value patient-care activities. Rather than merely adopting AI, it is important that pharmacy executives lead the effort to define the future of pharmacy and the role of the pharmacist in an environment where AI is pervasive. As pharmacy departmental leadership looks at operational AI systems to develop and deploy, they should prioritize systems and applications that promote personalized, continuous, and preventive care.[20]

Education and Engagement

Education about and exposure to AI is necessary throughout all domains of pharmacy practice.[1] Pharmacy students should be introduced to the essentials of data science and fundamentals of AI through a health informatics curriculum during their PharmD education. Pharmacists must also be given the opportunity to develop an understanding of AI through continuing education. Data science courses or pharmacy residencies with a focus on AI topics should be made available for pharmacists seeking more hands-on involvement in AI development, governance, and use. As these technologies rapidly evolve, the pharmacy education system must remain agile to ensure our profession is equipped to steward these transformations of care.

Conclusion

Advances in technology through AI stand to substantially change how care is delivered to patients. In all aspects of the medication-use process, there are opportunities to refine and augment existing pharmacy workflows to improve both safety and efficiency. Pharmacists will be necessary in leading innovation on how AI models and technologies are developed, validated, and activated to enact change. Further, pharmacists must be poised to capitalize on the operational gains and enhanced clinical guidance made possible by AI technology to enhance patient care. To carry this out, pharmacy needs to continue to build on education that will enable current and future generations of pharmacists and pharmacy technicians to shape the evolution of AI technology. The scope and impact of changes to come will cross into all aspects of pharmacy practice, requiring continued engagement by all in the field.

References

1. Sikka R, Morath JM, Leape L. The quadruple aim: care, health, cost and meaning in work. *BMJ Qual Saf.* 2015;24(10):608–610.
2. Oxford Dictionaries, English. Definition of artificial intelligence. https://en.oxforddictionaries.com/definition/artificial_intelligence. Accessed September 16, 2019.
3. Hodges BD. Learning from Dorothy Vaughan: artificial intelligence and the health professions. *Med Educ.* 2018;52(1):11–13.
4. Executive summary of the 2019 ASHP commission on goals: impact of artificial intelligence on healthcare and pharmacy practice. *Am J Health-Syst Pharm.* 2019;76(24):2087–2092.
5. Stead WW. Clinical implications and challenges of artificial intelligence and deep learning. *JAMA.* 2018;320(11):1107–1108.
6. Vermeulen LC, Eddington ND, Gourdine MA et al. ASHP foundation pharmacy forecast 2019: strategic planning advice for pharmacy departments in hospitals and health systems. *Am J Health-Syst Pharm.* 2019;76(2):71–100.
7. Israni ST, Verghese A. Humanizing artificial intelligence. *JAMA.* 2019;321(1):29–30.
8. Orihuela Y. Health care in 2030: AI and the shifting role of your pharmacist. Forbes. February 2018. https://www.forbes.com/sites/forbestechcouncil/2018/02/23/health-care-in-2030-ai-and-the-shiftingrole-of-your-pharmacist. Accessed September 16, 2019.
9. Abràmoff MD, Lavin PT, Birch M, Shah N, Folk JC. Pivotal trial of an autonomous AI-based diagnostic system for detection of diabetic retinopathy in primary care offices. *NPJ Digit Med.* 2018;1:39.
10. Proud RW, Hart JJ, Mrozinski RB. Methods for determining the level of autonomy to design into a human spaceflight vehicle: a function specific approach. NASA Technical Reports Server website. https://ntrs.nasa.gov/archive/nasa/casi.ntrs.nasa.gov/20100017272.pdf. Published September 1, 2003. Accessed September 13, 2019.
11. Akili Interactive. Akili achieves primary efficacy endpoint in pediatric ADHD pivotal trial. December 4, 2017. https://www.akiliinteractive.com/news-collection/akili-achieves-primary-efficacyendpoint-in-pediatric-adhd-pivotal-trial. Accessed September 16, 2019.
12. Farr C. Can "digital therapeutics" be as good as drugs? April 7, 2017. MIT Tech Rev. https://www.technologyreview.com/s/604053/can-digitaltherapeutics-be-as-good-as-drugs/. Accessed September 16, 2019.
13. Espie CA, Emsley R, Kyle SD et al. Effect of digital cognitive behavioral therapy for insomnia on health, psychological well-being, and sleep-related quality of life: a randomized clinical trial. *JAMA Psychiatry.* 2019;76(1):21–30.
14. Executive Office of the President. Big Data: A Report on Algorithmic Systems, Opportunity, and Civil Rights; May 2016. https://obamawhitehouse.archives.gov/sites/default/files/microsites/ostp/2016_0504_data_discrimination.pdf. Accessed September 16, 2019.
15. Char DS, Shah NH, Magnus D. Implementing machine learning in health care—addressing ethical challenges. *New Engl J Med.* 2018;378(11):981–983.
16. American Medical Association. Proceedings of the 2018 Annual Meeting of the American Medical Association House of Delegates. https://www.amaassn.org/system/files/2018-10/a18-botreports.pdf. Accessed September 16, 2019.
17. Taulli T. Hiring for the AI (artificial intelligence) revolution—part I. Forbes. January 26, 2019. https://www.forbes.com/sites/tomtaulli/2019/01/26/hiring-for-the-ai-artificial-intelligencerevolution-part-i/. Accessed September 16, 2019.
18. Zhang Y, Trepp R, Wang W, Luna J, Vawdrey DK, Tiase V. Developing and maintaining clinical decision support using clinical knowledge and machine learning: the case of order sets. *J Am Med Inform Assoc.* 2018; 25(11):1547–1551.
19. Pham T, Tran T, Phung D et al. DeepCare: a deep dynamic memory model for predictive medicine. In: Bailey J, ed. *Advances in Knowledge Discovery and Data Mining.* New York, NY: Springer International Publishing; 2016:30–41.
20. Chilcott M. How data analytics and artificial intelligence are changing the pharmaceutical industry. Forbes. May 2018. https://www.forbes.com/sites/forbestechcouncil/2018/05/10/how-dataanalytics-and-artificial-intelligence-arechanging-the-pharmaceutical-industry/. Accessed May 13, 2019.

Suggested Readings and Other Resources

- ASHP Statement on the Pharmacist's Role in Clinical Informatics. *AJHP.* 2016;73(6):410–413.
- American Medical Association. Augmented intelligence in health care policy report. https://www.ama-assn.org/system/files/2019-01/augmented-intelligence-policyreport.pdf. Published January 2019. Accessed August 28, 2020.
- Beam AL, Kohane IS. Big data and machine learning in health care. *JAMA.* 2018;319(13):1317–1318.
- Carroll WM. Artificial Intelligence, nurses and the quadruple aim. *Online J Nurs Inform.* 2018;22(2). https://www.himss.org/library/artificialintelligence-nurses-and-quadrupleaim. Accessed August 28, 2020.
- National Science & Technology Council. The National Artificial Intelligence Research and Development Strategic Plan: 2019 Update; 2019. https://www.nitrd.gov/pubs/National-AI-RD-Strategy-2019.pdf. Accessed August 28, 2020.
- Ng A, Soo K. *Numsense! Data Science for the Layman: No Math Added.* Singapore: Annalyn Ng and Kenneth Soo; 2017.
- Office of the National Coordinator for Health Information Technology. Artificial intelligence for health and health care; 2017. https://www.healthit.gov/sites/default/files/jsr-17-task-002_aiforhealthandhealthcare12122017.pdf. Accessed August 28, 2020.
- American Medical Association. A primer on artificial and augmented intelligence; 2018. https://www.ama-assn.org/system/files/2018-11/a18-clrpdreports.pdf. Accessed August 28, 2020.

- Rajkomar A, Dean J, Kohane I. Machine learning in medicine. *N Engl J Med.* 2019;380(14):1347–1358.
- Savadjiev P, Chong J, Dohan A et al. Demystification of AI-driven medical image interpretation: past, present and future. *Eur Radiol.* 2019;29(3):1616–1624.

Approved by the ASHP Board of Directors on November 19, 2019, and by the ASHP House of Delegates on May 20, 2020. Developed through the ASHP Section of Pharmacy Informatics and Technology

ASHP gratefully acknowledges the following individuals for reviewing the current version of the statement: Allen Flynn, PharmD, PhD; Amey C. Hugg, BSPharm, CPHIMS, FKSHP; Beth Prier, PharmD, MS, CPHIMS; Chris Urbanski, BSPharm, MS, FASHP; Dennis Tribble, Pharm, FASHP; Eric Maroyka, PharmD, BCPS; Jay Dorris, PharmD; Jessica Hill, PharmD, BCPS, BCACP; Katayoon Kathy Ghomeshi, PharmD, MBA, BCPS, CPPS; Kerry Goldrosen, PharmD, BCPS; Maritza Lew, PharmD, CPHIMS, PMP; Seth Hartman, PharmD, MB; and Sylvia Belford, PharmD, MS, CPHIMS, FASHP.

The authors have declared no potential conflicts of interest.

Nick Schutz, PharmD, North Memorial Health, Robbinsdale, MN.

Casey A. Olsen, PharmD, Pharmacy Department, Advocate Aurora Health, Oak Brook, IL.

Andrew J. McLaughlin, PharmD, MBA, Cerner Corporation, Kansas City, MO.

Whitley M. Yi, PharmD, BCPS, Department of Pharmacy, University of North Carolina Medical Center, Chapel Hill, NC.

Scott D. Nelson, PharmD, MS, Vanderbilt University Medical Center, Nashville, TN.

Asha L. Kalichira, PharmD, MS, Enterprise Information Services, CedarsSinai Health System, Los Angeles, CA.

Andrew H. Smith, RPh, MHA, Novant Health, Clinical Informatics, Fort Mill, SC.

Katherine A. Miller, PharmD, MHA, FASHP, The University of Kansas Health System, Kansas City, KS

Trinh Le, MS, RPh, FASHP, Information Services Division, UNC Health, Morrisville, NC.

Bruce W. Chaffee, PharmD, FASHP, Department of Pharmacy Services, Michigan Medicine, Ann Arbor, MI.

CDR Kendra Worthy Woodbury, PharmD, MS, Food and Drug Administration, CDER Office of Translational Sciences, Office of Computational Science, Silver Spring, MD.

Hardik Patel, PharmD, Pharmacy Department, NorthShore University HealthSystem, Evanston, IL.

Copyright © 2020, American Society of Health-System Pharmacists, Inc. All rights reserved. Contact ASHP for reprint and permissions requests. This content may not be used for commercial purposes without the express written consent of ASHP.

The bibliographic citation for this document is as follows: American Society of Health-System Pharmacists. ASHP statement on the use of artificial intelligence in pharmacy. *Am J Health-Syst Pharm.* 2020;77:2015–18.

ASHP Statement on Use of Social Media by Pharmacy Professionals

Position

The American Society of Health-System Pharmacists (ASHP) encourages pharmacy professionals working in hospitals and health systems who use social media to do so in a professional, responsible, and respectful manner. Such use may complement and enhance their relationships with patients, caregivers, other members of the health care team, and the public. To achieve that goal, pharmacy professionals should

- Thoroughly consider the purposes and potential outcomes of participation in social media and develop the strategies and skills required to effectively utilize social media to meet their goals.
- Exercise professional judgment and adhere to professional standards and legal requirements in both private and public social media communications, especially legal and ethical obligations to protect the privacy of personal health information.

Background

The term "social media" may be defined as online tools that allow interaction among individuals. Examples include professional networks such as ASHP Connect, career-building networks such as LinkedIn, and sites such as Facebook and Twitter that are primarily social but which may serve multiple purposes.[1–3] Informational sites regarding medical information that allow for commentary from users and medical professionals (e.g., PharmQD, The Pharmacist Society, Sermo) should also be considered collaborative social media.

Social media have transformed the way people communicate by reducing barriers to the exchange of information, increasing both the amount of communication and the number of people who can participate. Health care organizations (e.g., hospitals, health systems, professional societies, pharmaceutical companies, patient advocacy groups, pharmacy benefit companies) have chosen to use social media for both communication and marketing.

Like other health care professionals, pharmacy professionals have adapted to advancing technology and are using social media to communicate with patients, caregivers, other health care professionals, and the public. Pharmacy professionals (including pharmacy students as professionals in training) should continue to incorporate these new tools into the armamentarium of pharmacy practice and apply them with professional judgment to pursue the goal of helping people make the best use of medications. Social media provide pharmacy professionals with opportunities to educate patients and practitioners, seek advice from and provide advice to colleagues, optimize the medication use of individual patients and populations, promote the role of pharmacists in caring for patients, and engage in debate about issues in health care practice and policy, among other things.[1–5]

Participation in Social Media

Hospitals or health systems that choose to use social media or permit practice-related social media use by staff should have in place policies and procedures that

- Balance the benefits social media provide with the obligations and liabilities they may create.
- Encourage the development and application of best practices by users of social media.

The details of such policies, procedures, and best practices are beyond the scope of this statement, which has as its purpose to briefly outline some of the considerations that should guide pharmacy professionals' participation in social media.

Pharmacy professionals should carefully consider the purposes and potential outcomes of their participation in social media and develop the strategies and skills required to achieve their goals. They need to be aware of and employ best practices when using social media, because health care practitioners, including pharmacy professionals, are held to a higher standard of professionalism within and outside the workplace than members of the public.[6] Pharmacy professionals who participate in social media should strive for a high degree of professionalism in their communications and ensure that patient privacy is not compromised.

Professionalism

ASHP has long advocated for the adoption of high professional aspirations for pharmacy practice. Pharmacists' responsibilities as professionals include "advancing the well-being and dignity of their patients, acting with integrity and conscience, [and] collaborating respectfully with health care colleagues."[7] The following recommendations for the use of social media represent high professional aspirations, and pharmacy professionals are encouraged to exercise their professional judgment in incorporating them into their practices.

Advancing the Well-Being and Dignity of Patients. The following recommendations can help pharmacy professionals who choose to participate in social media advance the well-being and dignity of patients.

1. Medical advice offered through social media should be provided in accordance with the professional standards of pharmacy practice. For example, pharmacy professionals should provide medical advice only with a complete understanding of the patient's medical conditions and only if they accept the associated liabilities, especially those regarding privacy and the requirements of pharmacy practice. Pharmacy professionals should be aware that providing medical advice may create a pharmacist–patient relationship, with all its attendant obligations and liabilities. All online relationships should conform to the ethical boundaries of an appropriate pharmacist–patient relationship.[8]

DOI 10.37573/9781585287048.009

2. Pharmacy professionals should be cognizant of both the benefits and limitations of online communication. Social media may serve especially well as a point of initial contact or as a convenient way to maintain contact between patients and care providers, but professionals must recognize when a patient's health care needs would be better met through other means (e.g., phone consultation, office visit).
3. Pharmacy professionals should view social media as a means to not only provide timely and accurate drug information but also to rebut inaccurate, misleading, or outdated information. While the purpose of specific social media content may not always be apparent, pharmacy professionals need to be aware of and alert to the use of social media for marketing and sales purposes.
4. Complaining about or disparaging patients, even in general terms, does not advance the dignity of patients or the profession. Communications that contain patients' identifying information would violate privacy requirements, which are discussed in more detail below. Pharmacy professionals should keep in mind that simply avoiding the name of a patient may not be sufficient to avoid patient identification.

Acting with Integrity and Conscience. The following recommendations are intended to assist pharmacy professionals to act with integrity and conscience in their use of social media.

1. Pharmacy professionals should carefully distinguish between personal and professional information within social media and make conscientious decisions regarding who will have access to personal or professional information. Although some organizations recommend use of a strictly personal page and a separate, strictly practice-related page,[9] professionals will quickly recognize the difficulty of making such distinctions. The higher standards of conduct expected of professionals, even in personal behavior, apply as well to their participation in social media.[6,10]
2. Pharmacy professionals must be conscious that content posted to social media may have consequences on reputations or careers for years to come, reflect poorly upon the pharmacy profession, or undermine patient confidence in the care provided. Postings on social media should be subject to the same professional standards and ethical considerations as other personal or public interactions.
3. The apparent anonymity provided by social media does not release pharmacy professionals from their ethical obligation to disclose potential conflicts of interest, especially when representing themselves as professionals. Some circumstances may require personal identification or disclosure of potential competing interests.[9]
4. Although all pharmacists should use social media in ways that set positive examples for pharmacy students and residents, preceptors and mentors have a special responsibility to model appropriate practices.[7,11]

Collaborating Respectfully with Health Care Colleagues. Although social media can and should be used to promote healthy debate about health care and pharmacy practice, such debate should be conducted in a respectful manner. Reasoned debate sometimes requires constructive criticism, but pharmacy professionals should not use social media to make ad hominem comments or needlessly denigrate specific care providers, institutions, or professions.

Patient Privacy

Health care professionals have long confronted the challenge of "communicat[ing] freely with each other while maintaining patient confidentiality and privacy."[12] Social media, by their very nature, present new issues of privacy and confidentiality by extending the reach of communications. The following recommendations may help pharmacy professionals protect patient privacy and confidentiality as they navigate this new terrain.

1. Pharmacy professionals should continue to adhere to all laws, regulations, standards, and other mandates intended to protect patient privacy and confidentiality in all environments, including social media.[8]
2. Pharmacy professionals should exercise professional judgment and employ established best practices to ensure compliance with privacy requirements when communicating with patients or about specific patient cases on social media.[9,13,14]
3. Pharmacy professionals should select privacy settings in social media accounts that provide the greatest degree of protection for personal information, keeping in mind that privacy settings are not perfect and that information posted online is likely permanent. Continuous self-monitoring of privacy settings is necessary, as social media sites change privacy policies.[10]

Conclusion

Social media are emerging as important modes of communication and are increasingly being used for personal, professional, and business communication, as well as for patient care. As medical professionals held to high standards of personal, professional, ethical, and moral conduct, pharmacy professionals have a responsibility to use social media appropriately.

References

1. Fox BI, Varadarajan R. Use of Twitter to encourage interaction in a multi-campus pharmacy management course. *Am J Pharm Educ.* 2011; 75(5):88.
2. Estus E. Using Facebook within a geriatric pharmacotherapy course. *Am J Pharm Educ.* 2010; 74(8):145.
3. Cain J, Fox BI. Web 2.0 and pharmacy education. *Am J Pharm Educ.* 2009; 73(7):120.
4. Clauson KA, Seamon MJ, Fox BI. Pharmacists' duty to warn in the age of social media. *Am J Health-Syst Pharm.* 2010; 67:1290–3.
5. Mattingly TJ, Cain J, Fink JL. Pharmacists on Facebook: online social networking and the profession. *J Am Pharm Assoc.* 2010; 50:424–7.
6. Williams J, Field C, James K. The effects of a social media policy on pharmacy students' Facebook security settings. *Am J Pharm Educ.* 2011; 75(9):177.

7. American Society of Health-System Pharmacists. ASHP statement on professionalism. *Am J Health-Syst Pharm.* 2008; 65:172–4.
8. University of California, San Diego. Guidelines and best practices for online social media use by student pharmacists. http://pharmacy.ucsd.edu/current/pdf/Social_Media_Guidelines.pdf (accessed 2012 Feb 1).
9. Ohio State Medical Association. Social networking and the medical practice: guidelines for physicians, office staff, and patients. www.osma.org/files/documents/tools-and-resources/running-a-practice/social-media-policy.pdf (accessed 2012 Feb 1).
10. American Medical Association. AMA policy: professionalism in the use of social media. www.ama-assn.org/ama/pub/meeting/professionalism-social-media.shtml (accessed 2012 Feb 1).
11. Kukreja P, Sheehan AH, Riggins J. Use of social media by pharmacy preceptors. *Am J Pharm Educ.* 2011; 75(9):176.
12. American Society of Health-System Pharmacists. ASHP statement on confidentiality of patient health care information. *Am J Health-Syst Pharm.* 2009; 66:411–2.
13. Dimov V. Case reports and HIPAA rules. http://casesblog.blogspot.com/2005/07/case-reports-and-hipaa-rules.html (accessed 2012 Feb 1).
14. Dimov V. How to write a medical blog and not get fired. http://casesblog.blogspot.com/2008/02/how-to-write-medical-blog-and-not-get.html (accessed 2012 Feb 1).

Developed through the ASHP Pharmacy Student Forum and the ASHP Section of Pharmacy Informatics and Technology and approved by the ASHP Board of Directors on April 13, 2012, and by the ASHP House of Delegates on June 10, 2012.

This statement was drafted by Ashley M. Overy, Pharm.D. The following individuals are also acknowledged for their contributions to this statement: Kevin A. Clauson, Pharm.D.; Brent I. Fox, Pharm.D., Ph.D.; Karl F. Gumpper, BCNSP, BCPS, FASHP; Arpit Mehta, Pharm.D.; and David R. Witmer, Pharm.D. The drafters and contributors have declared no potential conflicts of interest.

ASHP gratefully acknowledges the following individuals and organizations for reviewing drafts of this statement (review does not imply endorsement): Academy of Managed Care Pharmacy (AMCP); Paul Barrett, Pharm.D., M.P.A., BCPS, FASHP; Mark Brueckl, M.B.A. (AMCP); Jeff Cain, Ed.D., M.S.; Michael S. Edwards, Pharm.D., M.B.A., BCOP, FASHP; Erin R. Fox, Pharm.D.; Becky Harvey, Pharm.D.; John Hertig, Pharm.D., M.S.; Justin Julius, Pharm.D.; Nishaminy Kasbekar, Pharm.D., FASHP; Linda McElhiney, Pharm.D., FASHP, FIACP; Sean Mirk, Pharm.D.; John F. Mitchell, Pharm.D., FASHP; David B. Moore, M.P.A., CPh.; Linda A. Nelson, Pharm.D.; Agatha Nolen, Ph.D.; James Ponto, M.S., FASHP; Curt W. Quap, M.S., FASHP; Marcus Ravnan, Pharm.D.; Jamie S. Sinclair, M.S., FASHP; Kelly M. Smith, Pharm.D., BCPS, FASHP, FCCP; and Jody Jacobson Wedret, B.S.Pharm., FASHP, FCSHP.

Copyright © 2012, American Society of Health-System Pharmacists, Inc. All rights reserved. Contact ASHP for reprint and permissions requests. This content may not be used for commercial purposes without the express written consent of ASHP.

The bibliographic citation for this document is as follows: American Society of Health-System Pharmacists. ASHP statement on use of social media by pharmacy professionals. *Am J Health-Syst Pharm.* 2012; 69:2095–7.

ASHP Guidelines on the Design of Database-Driven Clinical Decision Support: Strategic Directions for Drug Database and Electronic Health Records Vendors

ASHP believes that use of clinical decision support (CDS) tools can make patient care more efficient and effective.[1] Currently available pharmacotherapy CDS systems are not as effective as they need to be at helping all practice settings achieve the goal of safe and effective pharmacotherapy. The focus of these guidelines is commercially available pharmacotherapy warning systems such as drug interaction, allergy, and dose monitoring CDS. Pharmacotherapy warning CDS systems are collectively referred to as "database-driven CDS" in these guidelines. Database-driven alert associations are compiled by drug database vendors and are incorporated as alerts into clinical information systems by electronic health record (EHR) vendors. All practice settings are usually limited in their ability to customize the content of messages or severity levels of alerts created by the drug database or EHR vendors. In contrast, free-form, rule-based alerts are created by users based on coded logic rules using information contained in the EHR database. Although free-form, rule-based alerts are an important tool, these guidelines limit their focus to active, interruptive database warnings. These guidelines outline an approach that would provide all practice settings with the power and flexibility to implement database-driven CDS so that it is a useful tool for improving the quality, cost efficiency, and safety of medication use. Adoption of this functionality by all practice settings is of course critical to meeting the goal of delivering improved, patient-centered care. These database-driven CDS rules should be shareable between all practice settings so that each institution can make the customizations needed for its particular circumstances.

Purpose

The purposes of these guidelines are to describe essential functions and capabilities that should be available to reduce alert fatigue, increase user satisfaction, and increase the effectiveness of these CDS systems; and to advocate for collaboration between health information system vendors, drug database vendors, and the end-user community on design and testing of the CDS systems as well as new algorithmic models for pharmacotherapy warnings.

Background

There are two different types of CDS, passive and active, as well as several types of active CDS (**Figure 1**).

1. *Passive CDS.* This type of CDS directs the user toward the most appropriate practices unobtrusively; examples include order sets and limited selections in drop-down lists or check boxes. Passive CDS is derived from population data, or more commonly clinical guidelines, and is therefore not patient-specific by nature. It is left to the patient's healthcare provider to make these patient-specific.
2. *Active CDS.* There are two types of active CDS, interruptive and noninterruptive. Active CDS is patient-specific in that it uses at least two pieces of patient data to trigger an alert (e.g., two interacting drugs, or the patient's age and an ordered dose).

FIGURE 1. Types of clinical decision support (CDS).

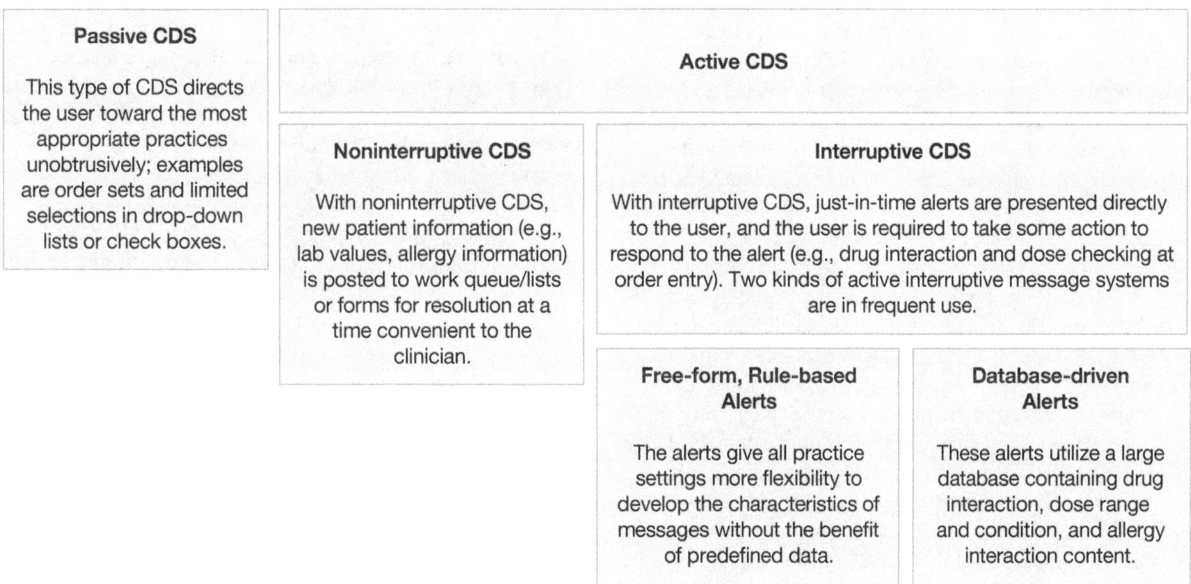

DOI 10.37573/9781585287048.010

a. *Noninterruptive CDS.* With noninterruptive CDS, new patient information (e.g., lab values, allergy information) is posted to work queue/lists or forms for resolution at a time convenient to the clinician.

b. *Interruptive CDS.* With interruptive CDS, just-in-time alerts are presented directly to the user, and the user is required to take some action to respond to the alert (e.g., drug interaction and dose checking at order entry). Two kinds of active interruptive message systems are in frequent use:

   i. *Database-driven alerts.* These alerts utilize a large database containing drug interaction, dose range and condition, and allergy interaction content.

   ii. *Free-form, rule-based alerts.* The alerts give all practice settings more flexibility to develop other decision models and the characteristics of patient-specific messages. Ideally, in the future it will be common for free-form CDS rules to be able to access the content of commercially developed pharmacotherapy CDS databases.

Although database-driven CDS systems have been commercially available for over 30 years, most of these systems have not progressed beyond the use of simple rules for drug–drug, drug–food, and drug–allergy checking. Most provide limited logic to determine a patient's true susceptibility to these drug interactions, and some provide limited drug–disease state screening and age-based dose checking.[2] Most currently available database-driven CDS systems have excellent content and can generally inform the right person; however, they have limited options for format, channel, and right time in workflow. These limitations cause a high incidence of false-positive alerts in computerized prescriber-order-entry and pharmacy information systems, which can in turn decrease users' sensitivity to alerts, also known as "alert fatigue." Alert fatigue is more than just an annoyance; it increases the risk of harm to both patients and providers.[2–4] The lack of clinical usefulness of the majority of drug interaction, drug allergy, and dose monitoring tools has been demonstrated by physician alert override rates that exceeded 90% in some studies.[3–8] The relevance and specificity of CDS tools will be improved, and the value of CDS tools enhanced, when the rate of meaningful warnings is increased and the incidence of clinically irrelevant alerts is reduced. Achieving these goals will require more than the currently available simple logic, especially for dose monitoring and mathematical algorithms. These systems also need broader access to the rich patient data that are now available in the EHR.

The meaningful use requirements of the American Recovery and Reinvestment Act[9] contain explicitly stated objectives for CDS, spurring healthcare facilities to invest in new EHR systems with an increased focus on CDS. Although these systems are the most current ones available, many of them continue to use the same simple logic for database-driven CDS. What is needed is more sophisticated logic, such as statistical methods and branching algorithms to reduce the false-positive and false-negative alerts. The Agency for Healthcare Research and Quality recommends that CDS developers consider the CDS Five Rights model, which states "that we can achieve CDS-supported improvements in desired healthcare outcomes if we communicate:

1. The ***right information:*** evidence-based, suitable to guide action, pertinent to the circumstance
2. To the ***right person:*** considering all members of the care team, including clinicians, patients, and their caretakers
3. In the ***right CDS intervention format:*** such as an alert, order set, or reference information to answer a clinical question
4. Through the ***right channel:*** for example, a clinical information system (CIS) such as an electronic medical record (EMR), personal health record (PHR), or a more general channel such as the Internet or a mobile device
5. At the ***right time in workflow:*** for example, at time of decision/action/need."[10]

The Healthcare Standards Organization Health Level Seven (HL7) and the American National Standards Institute have developed and maintain a standard programming language design for clinical informaticists to build medical logic modules capable of sophisticated clinical logic. There are also many HL7 standards (e.g., Arden Syntax, GELLO, HQMF, Infobutton, DSS) that can assist in this endeavor and offer a mechanism across all practice settings around the world to collaborate on the development of effective database-driven CDS.[11] Use of these standards could improve the ability for users to share logic developed to capitalize on the functionality presented below.

ASHP encourages pharmacists, hospital and health-system administrators, drug database vendors, and EHR system vendors to use the recommendations in these guidelines to increase the usefulness and flexibility of database-driven CDS tools. In essence, the goal of their collaborative efforts should be to provide the flexibility and customization capabilities as are currently available in the free-form rules engines provided by most EHR vendors today. This would allow users to build alerts that have greater specificity and higher positive predictive performance.

Essential CDS Capabilities

The following are essential database-driven CDS capabilities that should be available in all EHR systems for any combination of drug database vendor and EHR vendor used by a hospital or health system. These recommendations are not listed in order of feasibility or priority; all are considered vitally important for the development of more patient appropriate care.

1. The institution should be able to configure and/or customize "drug groups" that can be used in alert triggers or criteria. Drug groups should be defined as lists of individual medication products or generic or therapeutic groupings. Individual medication products should be capable of being included in multiple drug groups, and drug groups should be able to subsume other drug groups. The drug group construct should be an option for using the configuration functionality described below. The drug group must have a free-text comment field of at least 1000 characters to allow the institution to identify the drug group's owner and purpose and to construct a history of changes.

2. Warnings should be available in real time and be capable of being tailored to the specific patient situation using available patient information (e.g., age, gender, weight, laboratory values, radiology procedures, dietary needs, diagnosis, current problem list, location of care delivery) together with information contained in the drug database to construct inclusion and exclusion criteria that make alerts more useful and reduce alert fatigue. The patient information should conform to standard terminology, such as Logical Observation Identifiers Names and Codes (LOINC) for laboratory tests. The drug database vendor should consider developing an external database that translates standard terminologies (e.g., RxNorm, LOINC, Systematized Nomenclature of Medicine, and International Classification of Diseases codes) to an internal dictionary of medical terms used in their knowledge base.
3. Medication-order-specific information (e.g., dosage forms, routes, frequencies, dose, order status, ordering provider) should also be available to be utilized in alert inclusion and exclusion criteria.
4. All practice settings should have the ability to (a) customize how an alert looks (e.g., color, shape, audio, size) to emphasize the criticality or type of warning, and (b) offer response options based on characteristics of the potential harm (e.g., prevalence of problem, extent of risk or severity) (see "Notification System" in **Figure 2**).
5. All practice settings should have the ability to configure the information displayed in the warnings. The CDS rule development language must enable the rule to build patient-specific alert messages during rule execution. The following five basic types of logic must be supported by the rule development tool kit.
    a. *String handling.* This type of logic allows the rule developer to incorporate useful patient- specific suggestions based on patient information. It also allows displaying of useful data such as allergies, relevant medications, and other patient characteristics or data, in the form of text or structured data values, directly into the warning message, so the information contained in the alert can help the clinician determine the best response to the alert.
    b. *Loop functions.* This type of logic allows alert designers to gather or group all related information into a single warning (e.g., sort through lists of patient data to find relevant drug, lab result, or diagnosis). In addition, the loop functions should allow the use of mathematical algorithms (e.g., statistical methods to test trends of data, calculate glomerular filtration rate, or perform patient scoring).
    c. *Math functions.* This type of logic allows an alert to perform calculations and must include logarithmic and other standard mathematical functions. This will be necessary to perform specialized calculations that are available in but not retrievable from the EHR.
    d. *Trends over time.* This type of logic provides the ability to configure alerts based on trends in data over a defined period of time (e.g., decrease in hemoglobin of 2 grams in 2 days, or increase of hemoglobin $A_{1c} > 2.0\%$ in 3 months).
    e. *Conditional statements.* If-then-else statements that direct action based on the result of a Boolean logic statement (AND, OR, NOT). Duration conveniences must allow construction of temporal logic such as:
        1. If age < 6 days then ...
        2. Else if age < 2 years then ...

        In this case, age (a duration) is automatically converted to days and then years.
6. All practice settings should have the ability to configure whether a warning acknowledgment cannot be bypassed (i.e., a "hard stop"), can only be bypassed by documenting a valid reason for bypassing the alert (i.e., a "soft stop"), or can be bypassed without documenting a reason, and whether an additional comment is required by user type and venue (e.g., critical care, ambulatory). If a drop-down menu is utilized, it should specifically relate to the context and content of an alert.
7. Users should be able to take action from the synchronous alert presentation window. Such actions should be specific to the type of alert presented and include at least the following seven choices, by type of user or user category:
    a. Discontinue the conflicting order.
    b. Cancel the order being entered.
    c. Modify the order being entered (e.g., change dose, dosage form, route, frequency, start date, or end date).
    d. Modify the preexisting order (e.g., change dose, dosage form, route, frequency, start date, or end date).
    e. Add monitoring orders (e.g., laboratory tests or other parameters).
    f. Continue with current order as requested.
    g. Suspend the current order (i.e., put it in a held/suspended state).
8. The EHR system should be able to handle logic rules that determine how an alert can be transmitted to the clinician as well as specifying the individuals and/or groups that are to receive the alert. The importance of the alert should also be included in the logic rules for determining who is notified about the alert and how they are notified. The alert notification should be able to be transmitted in any electronic form, depending on the technology available at the institution, including but not limited to the electronic message inbox within the EHR, e-mail (where the alert information is available within the e-mail message), pagers, text message, fax, and printers. Encryption or secured messaging must be utilized to protect patient health information. The alert notification system should include a means of stratifying the alert importance and associating the type of alert notification with the level of the alert (e.g., an alert of moderate importance would be e-mailed to the clinician, whereas a more urgent alert such as a direct allergy match would be sent via text message). This type of stratification would be included in the logic using "if-then" types of statements.

FIGURE 2. Conceptual schematic of a potential new architecture with a clinical rules engine (CRE). Not shown here is the integrated development environment, where the rules are built by a clinician analyst. CPOE = computerized provider order entry, eMAR = electronic medication administration record, MedIA = medication interaction alert (e.g., drug–drug, drug–allergy, dose check, drug–disease).

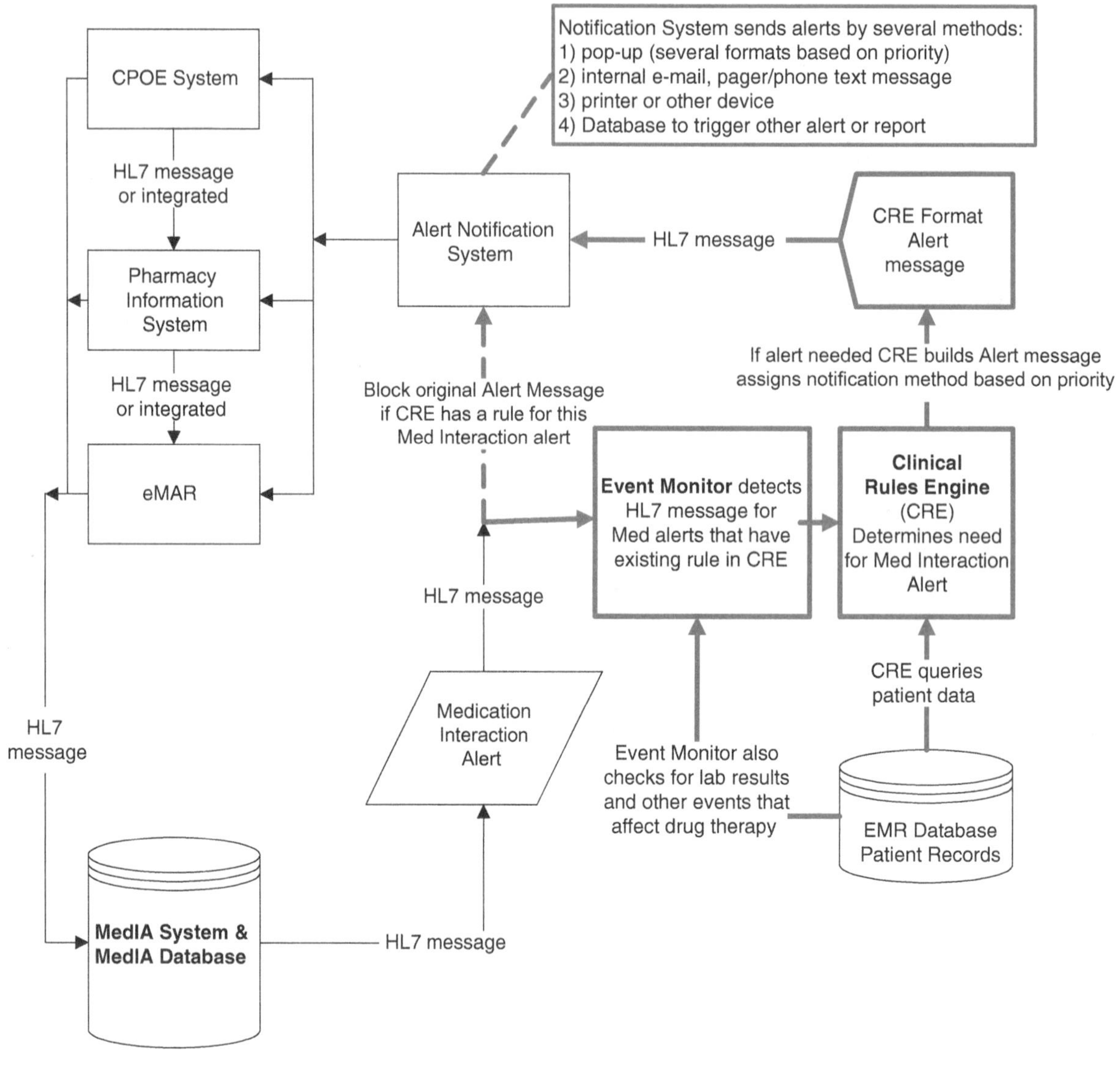

9. The EHR system should provide the capability to allow all practice settings to determine whether end users can customize the conditions under which they must respond to specific alerts within the larger list of alerts assigned to them. Appropriate warnings and audit trails must be in place to support this functionality. Database managers should be able to customize the conditions and options for the user to respond to specific alerts to
   a. "Snooze" the alert: delaying a response to the alert, whether globally or for user-identified individual patients for a predetermined amount of time with the ability to limit how many times an alert may be ignored before an action is required.
   b. Forward the alert: send the alert to an EHR message box with a time constraint based on the follow-up action needed.

10. The alerts system should allow sub-second response times (i.e., the absence of user waiting for system response) for warning notification and filing user response. Although response time is contingent upon a practice setting's hardware configuration, a short response time is essential to winning user acceptance. Reporting or database updates should not impact real-time system performance.

11. All practice settings should have the capability to configure and record (or track) when an alert notification displays, which implies when the checking occurs (e.g., when the medication is first selected, when a portion of the order information is changed, when the order or group of orders is filed). If an alert is overridden but then the triggering order is discontinued within a certain time period of the alert firing, the data should

indicate that the alert had a user response that resulted in discontinuing an order.

12. Clinicians and EHR system managers should have easy access to the supporting data available for each alert viewed in the EHR. Supporting evidence, including citations, should be available as specified in the American Recovery and Reinvestment Act of 2009 Stage 2 meaningful-use requirements.[9] Supporting evidence formats that should be available would include
    a. References that are included with the data imports from the various knowledge databases.
    b. Internal system policies and protocols.
    c. External reference databases or guidelines.

    EHR systems should be able to display these references, the quality of the references, and any other supporting evidence provided by the knowledge vendor. EHRs should allow links to external databases or documentation when deemed appropriate by the institution. These links should allow viewing of more details than what is presented in the initial alert. Supporting information should be easily retrieved by the user as part of the typical workflow. Supporting evidence should be formatted so that it could be presented in either a soft- or hard-alert format.
13. If there is additional information located within the EHR that is relevant to the alert, the EHR should provide a link or other means of easily accessing that content as part of the clinician workflow. Examples would include
    a. Allergy information.
    b. All orders flagged by the alert.
    c. Links to orders needed for entry as determined by the alert (e.g., laboratory test, medication).

    Setting up links for internal or custom external documents via the EHR alert should be a simple process.
14. The EHR system should provide the ability to invoke the database for synchronous and asynchronous checking based on different system transactions (i.e., not only order entry). Examples include laboratory test values filing to the patient chart, entering of patient information (e.g., diagnosis, problem, allergy), medication administration (see "Event Monitor" in Figure 2), or to delay alert notification to allow completion of orders (e.g., for an aminoglycoside order, allowing time for the practitioner to determine whether serum creatinine, drug levels, or a consult has also been ordered).
15. The CDS system must log all alert warnings and user actions taken in response to the alert (i.e., record alert outcomes). Those alert outcomes should include, at a minimum, the following:
    a. User who has received the alert.
    b. Users who have viewed the alert.
    c. Overridden alerts.
    d. Alerts that have occurred and had an action taken on them.
    e. Subsequent actions taken from the synchronous alert or view window.
    f. Current patient data related to the alert.
    g. Communications associated with the alert (e.g., reasons, required responses, comments).
16. All responses entered during the alert session should be available to subsequent users who view either the order or alert via inquiry and as part of subsequent alerts at order verification or other transactions related to the order. The inquiry should provide the ability for a user to check a patient's record for any alerts displayed in the system, including a historical account of all alerts that have displayed for a patient (pertaining to the current or prior inpatient or outpatient visits), including all information mentioned in item 15 above.
17. Data related to user actions in response to alerts and messages must be available within the context of CDS, and standard queries should be available. Data on alerts and responses to those alerts should be exportable to an external database or spreadsheet to support retrospective auditing. Studies are needed to determine if documenting override reasons improves or diminishes alert effectiveness and patient outcomes. Rates of overrides and other simple measures of alert effectiveness can be useful for identifying potential opportunities to improve system performance, but additional studies are needed to document the effect of changes made to CDS alerting rules. The reporting mechanism should facilitate the capture of the chronological history of alerts associated with an order across the multiple users who receive them.
18. Outcome documentation should be consistent across vendor systems so that healthcare organizations can accurately compare and benchmark database-driven CDS outcomes among organizations. To achieve this goal, vendors and CDS researchers may need to establish a consensus database schema for CDS outcomes.
19. The alerts system must facilitate easy identification of any facility-specific custom data that will be affected by modifications that a vendor has made to data or functionality.
20. CDS rules must be easily exportable to a text file. The exported rule must contain rule logic and all documentation contained in the rule. The exported rule does not have to contain external data queries or external destination logic referenced within the rule's logic, as this information is unique to the hospital or health system.
21. The CDS system must allow batch import of CDS rules from standalone files of prespecified types and formats. There must be options to overwrite existing rules and add new rules.
22. The CDS system must allow users to flag alerts for usefulness or intrusiveness so as to give the user a mechanism to provide immediate feedback to the CDS team. This functionality would be an extremely helpful tool to allow for a real-time evaluation tool for CDS, especially when changes are made to a system before the CDS team has a chance to collect and collate data.

Conclusion

Database-driven CDS could have a major impact on the quality, safety, and cost of healthcare. Unfortunately, its potential is largely unfulfilled due to the high number of false-positive warnings produced by most CDS systems. Alert fatigue from these warnings is common among physician and pharmacist users of EHR systems. To realize the promise of CDS, drug database and EHR vendors must work collaboratively to develop CDS systems that offer flexible patient-specific checking, reduce false-positive and false-negative warnings, and provide useful warning information to clinicians. It is of equal importance that all practice settings embrace this new functionality and aggressively use it to improve the specificity and appropriateness of patient care. By giving all practice settings the power to tailor drug database warning systems as they do with their EHR rules engines, the needed specificity to patient factors can be obtained.

References

1. Bates DW, Cohen M, Leape LL, et al. Reducing the frequency of errors in medicine using information technology. *J Am Med Inform Assoc.* 2001; 8:299–308.
2. Kuperman GJ, Reichley RM, Bailey TC. Using commercial knowledge bases for clinical decision support: opportunities, hurdles, and recommendations. *J Am Med Inform Assoc.* 2006; 13:369–71.
3. Kesselheim A, Cresswell K, Phansalkar S, et al. Clinical decision support systems could be modified to reduce "alert fatigue" while still minimizing the risk of litigation. *Health Aff.* 2011; 30:2310–7.
4. Phansalkar S, van der Sijs H, Tucker AD, et al. Drug–drug interactions that should be noninterruptive in order to reduce alert fatigue in electronic health records. *J Am Med Inform Assoc.* 2013; 20:489–93.
5. Lin CP, Payne TH, Nichol WP, et al. Evaluating clinical decision support systems: monitoring CPOE order check override rates in the Department of Veterans Affairs' computerized patient record system. *J Am Med Inform Assoc.* 2008; 15:620–6.
6. Payne TH, Nichol WP, Hoey P, et al. Characteristics and override rates of order checks in a practitioner order entry system. *Proc AMIA Symp.* 2002:602–6.
7. Weingart SN, Toth M, Sands DZ, et al. Physicians' decisions to override computerized drug alerts in primary care. *Arch Intern Med.* 2003; 163:2625–31.
8. Karsh BT. Clinical practice improvement and redesign: how change in workflow can be supported by clinical decision support (June 2009). AHRQ publication no. 09-0054-EF. http://healthit.ahrq.gov/sites/default/files/docs/page/09-0054-EF-Updated_0.pdf (accessed 2014 Sep 26).
9. Centers for Medicare and Medicaid Services. Meaningful use. www.cms.gov/Regulations-and-guidance/Legislation/EHRIncentivePrograms/Meaningful_Use.html (accessed 2014 Sep 26).
10. Agency for Healthcare Research and Quality. Chapter 1: approaching clinical decision support in medication management. Section 2: overview of CDS five rights. Improving medication use and outcomes with clinical decision support: a step-by-step guide. http://healthit.ahrq.gov/ahrq-funded-projects/clinical-decision-support-initiative/chapter-1-approaching-clinical-decision/section-2-overview-cds-five-rights (accessed 2014 Sep 26).
11. Health Level Seven International. HL7 standards—master grid. www.hl7.org/implement/standards/product_matrix.cfm?ref=nav (accessed 2014 Sep 26).

Developed through the ASHP Section of Pharmacy Informatics and Technology Section Advisory Group on Clinical Information Systems. Approved by the ASHP Section of Pharmacy Informatics and Technology Executive Committee on December 6, 2014, and by the ASHP Board of Directors on April 10, 2015.

David Troiano, B.S.Pharm., M.S.I.A., CPPS, is Director of Consulting, Dearborn Advisors, Chicago, IL. Michael A. Jones, Pharm.D., is Informatics Pharmacist for Clinical Decision Support, University of Colorado Hospital, Aurora. Andrew H. Smith, B.S.Pharm., M.H.A., is Pharmacy Clinical Applications Analyst, Novant Health, Winston-Salem, NC. Raymond C. Chan, Pharm.D., is Informatics Residency Coordinator—Information Technology, Sentara HealthCare, Norfolk, VA. Andrew P. Laegeler, M.S., Pharm.D., is Pharmacy Informatics Operations Manager, Harris County Hospital District, Houston, TX. Trinh Le, B.S.Pharm, M.S., FASHP, is Clinical Pharmacy Manager—Informatics, Department of Pharmacy, University of North Carolina Health Care, Chapel Hill. Allen Flynn, Pharm.D., is Solutions Designer, Health Practice Innovators, Ann Arbor, MI. Bruce W. Chaffee, Pharm.D., is Coordinator for Strategic Projects and Adjunct Clinical Associate Professor of Pharmacy, Department of Pharmacy Services, College of Pharmacy, University of Michigan, Ann Arbor.

Copyright © 2015, American Society of Health-System Pharmacists, Inc. All rights reserved. Contact ASHP for reprint and permissions requests. This content may not be used for commercial purposes without the express written consent of ASHP.

The bibliographic citation for this document is as follows: American Society of Health-System Pharmacists. ASHP guidelines on the design of database-driven clinical decision support: strategic directions for drug database and electronic health records vendors. *Am J Health-Syst Pharm.* 2015; 72:1499–505.

ASHP Guidelines on Pharmacy Planning for Implementation of Computerized Provider-Order-Entry Systems in Hospitals and Health Systems

Purpose and Scope

The purpose of these guidelines is to provide guidance to pharmacists in hospitals and health systems on planning for, implementing, and enhancing safe computerized provider-order-entry (CPOE) systems. To date, most CPOE guidelines have concentrated on the functionality required of a CPOE system, despite the fact that most CPOE system implementations occur using commercial systems whose functionality is largely pre-determined. These guidelines are intended to help pharmacy directors, managers, informaticists, and project managers successfully engage in this type of CPOE system implementation. CPOE is commonly part of a larger health information technology (IT) plan or system implementation. Though many health care technologies impact patient care and pharmacy practice, this guideline will focus on CPOE only. This document is the first of a planned series of ASHP guidelines on CPOE and related technologies and addresses the planning phase of a health-system CPOE implementation, primarily focusing on acute care and associated ambulatory care clinics. The guideline will focus on using CPOE in the medication-use process, though it is important to realize that CPOE includes all orders for patient care (laboratory, nursing, respiratory, and others). Topics covered in these guidelines include

- Developing an interdisciplinary planning and implementation team.
- Defining the vision, goals, and objectives of the CPOE system.
- Establishing essential metrics to measure the success of CPOE system implementation.
- Understanding current and future workflow in order to reengineer the medication-use process as part of CPOE system implementation.
- Planning for scope and depth of clinical decision support (CDS).
- Determining the functionality that ensures the safety of the CPOE system.
- Educating and training health care providers to use the CPOE system.

Terms used in these guidelines are defined in the appended glossary. The recommendations presented in these guidelines can be used for strategic planning with the organization's decision-makers, drafting contract provisions, prospectively comparing CPOE systems, and creating an implementation plan. These guidelines should be used in conjunction with other literature on the topic and information from prospective or selected CPOE vendors. Pharmacists should exercise professional judgment in assessing their health system's needs regarding CPOE systems and in adapting these guidelines to meet those needs.

CPOE and the Electronic Health Record

In its 1999 report *To Err is Human*,[1] the Institute of Medicine (IOM) shocked the nation with its estimate of deaths due to medical errors. Two large studies, one conducted in New York[2,3] and the other in Utah and Colorado,[4] revealed adverse events occurring in 2.9% and 3.7% of hospitalizations, respectively. Over half of these adverse events were judged to be preventable. Based on these studies, IOM estimated that 44,000–98,000 Americans die each year due to medical errors in hospitals.[1] Many of these deaths are caused by medication errors or preventable adverse drug events (ADEs).[5,6]

When it was recognized that errors resulting in preventable ADEs involved a wide range of drug classes and most commonly occurred at the prescribing stage,[7] interest in CPOE systems grew. In a second report, *Crossing the Quality Chasm: A New Health System for the 21st Century*,[8] the IOM called for IT, including CPOE, to take a central role in the redesign of the health care system to improve quality, increase efficiency, and reduce errors. In addition to IOM, organizations such as the Leapfrog Group and the National Quality Forum have pushed for hospitals to adopt CPOE.[9,10] The American Recovery and Reinvestment Act of 2009 (Recovery Act) authorizes the Centers for Medicare and Medicaid Services (CMS) to provide reimbursement incentives for eligible professionals and hospitals who are successful in becoming "meaningful users" of certified electronic health record (EHR) technology. This law will likely increase the adoption of CPOE in hospitals and health systems.[11]

CPOE has the potential to affect the ordering of all medications, laboratory tests, medical imaging, nursing orders, and more. Even a basic CPOE system can eliminate illegible and incomplete orders and facilitate efficient order processing through instantaneous transmission of orders to hospital departments such as pharmacy and laboratory. Additionally, CPOE integrated with a pharmacy information system and the electronic medication administration record (eMAR) can nearly eliminate transcription errors, resulting in another potential 6% decrease in ADEs.[7] A homegrown CPOE system has been shown to decrease medication errors by 55–80%.[12,13] There are many reports of improvements in physician practices and patient outcomes with health IT related to ordering,[14–21] but in some reports it is difficult to distinguish whether the benefits were due to CPOE, CDS, the EHR, or a combination of all three. The synergy of the three of these will likely lead to the most significant improvements.[15,16] Although there are many reported benefits to CPOE, there is a growing body of research pointing to new problems introduced by CPOE. These new problems are collectively known as e-iatrogenesis, which is defined as patient harm caused at least in part by the application of health IT.[22] Though the systems themselves may contribute to these problems, design and implementation decisions play a role in the avoidance of these new errors.

DOI 10.37573/9781585287048.011

More recently, attention has focused on the development of an integrated information system to support the coordination and integration of clinical and business processes. The terminology for such information systems is evolving, with *enterprise information system* sometimes used to describe the broader system that integrates clinical and business systems, and *EHR* used to describe the clinical information system, which may include a patient portal or the ability to link to a personal health record (PHR).[23] CPOE must be viewed in the context of the EHR, which would integrate CPOE, CDS, and departmental information systems and make patient-specific clinical information available to providers.

The EHR is a longitudinal electronic record of patient health information generated by one or more encounters in any care delivery setting.[24] It contains medical histories, medication histories, laboratory test results, diagnostic images, clinical documentation, progress notes, narrative summaries (such as operative reports or consultations), and other information related to patient encounters. EHRs provide the ability to manipulate, organize, and present data in ways that are clinically meaningful during the care planning, ordering, and care processes and allow broad clinician access to patient-specific clinical information, which is important to clinical quality and patient safety. When fully deployed within a facility through protected networks, the EHR serves as an information source and platform to coordinate patient care and communicate with the health care team. In addition, codified data can be used to trigger effective CDS as well as to provide data for continuous quality improvement.

For CPOE to be most useful it must be deployed as part of an EHR and not as a stand-alone module. CPOE is the process of health care providers entering orders and related information directly into the EHR. It places the provider at the center of patient care, allowing direct access and secure sharing of health information.

The EHR, including electronic clinician (e.g., physician, pharmacist, nurse) documentation with CPOE and CDS, is important to support the complex effort needed to improve hospital care.[15,16] The integration of CPOE and CDS within an EHR can create a platform upon which to build and improve the delivery of health care today and in the future. Many organizations implement these in a stepwise fashion because of the enormous work effort and the significant workflow changes required. Although there is no single solution that fits every circumstance, the literature offers many examples for others to follow or avoid.[25–28] Regardless of the vendor, organization size, or other factors that could potentially affect success, there are quite a number of implementation decisions that can increase the likelihood of a clinician-accepted CPOE installation that leads to quality and safety improvements.

Planning for the Transition to CPOE

A successful CPOE implementation starts with a well-organized, realistic plan. In planning for the transition to CPOE, initial tasks include assembling an interdisciplinary planning and implementation team; developing a vision, goals, and objectives for the CPOE system; establishing essential baseline and post-go-live metrics; mapping current physician, pharmacist, and nurse workflows as they relate to the medication-use process; defining the desired medication-use process; and planning for CDS. Project management and change management skills are vital for the conversion to CPOE. Because the enormous change in workflow will affect every clinician, standard project management and change management tools, such as a formal project charter, will help keep the implementation on track and manage expectations. Establishing a plan for communication is important from day 1.

Assembling an Interdisciplinary Planning and Implementation Team

The transition to CPOE is an immense cultural change that will affect every member of the health care team. No individual or department will be exempt from the impact of CPOE. Support for the project at the executive level is a prerequisite. Medical and administrative leadership/sponsorship are instrumental in the development of a clear vision for CPOE. An interdisciplinary team approach to planning and implementation is essential for a safe, well- designed, user-friendly, and successful CPOE system.

Physicians must be central players in the decision-making process, as prescriber buy-in and acceptance is crucial to CPOE success. Key departments (such as pharmacy, nursing, laboratory, radiology, admissions, dietary, and respiratory therapy) must dedicate resources and be involved in the initial effort, including workflow/ process analysis and redesign, system analysis, integration between ancillary systems, review of organizational culture, and compliance with regulatory, legal, and reimbursement requirements.

The involvement of pharmacists in the development and implementation of CPOE is essential for several reasons. Pharmacists have the benefit of years of experience with electronic order entry systems. Pharmacists' experience with human factors issues related to the interaction between human and computer is invaluable, even though pharmacy systems may differ from CPOE systems in significant ways. In addition, the medication-order-entry aspect of CPOE systems leads to the most significant increase in patient safety and is likely the most complex part of the system.[21,29–32] The initial decision to purchase a completely integrated CPOE system or develop one that can interface with existing electronic systems (e.g., the pharmacy department's information system) is an important one that would benefit from the pharmacist's perspective. Although the number of successful implementations is increasing on a yearly basis,[33] the complexity of the systems should not be underestimated.

Collaboration among health care staff and the IT department is critical to the selection, implementation, and maintenance of CPOE systems. Although a CPOE system cannot be developed and implemented without IT expertise, the CPOE system is intended to serve the best interests of patients and clinicians. Clinicians and IT staff do not always talk the same language, and differences of opinion are not uncommon. Though difficult at times, these groups must work together for success. IT understands the technical aspects, but physicians, nurses, and pharmacists are best suited to determine how the CPOE system can be implemented to best serve the interests of patients and clinicians.

Recommendations for Team Structure. The organization should carefully consider the structure of the interdisciplinary implementation team, which should include physicians, nurses, pharmacists, IT staff, the chief medical information officer, and staff from all ancillary departments (e.g., laboratory services, respiratory therapy). In addition to front-line practitioners, patient safety and quality improvement staff can help immensely with some of the workflow and design decisions. CPOE systems by definition require ownership by the medical staff. Therefore, prescribers (mainly physicians) must be actively solicited for system requirements and be involved in key decisions. CPOE system design, including the content, the user interface, and the flow of CDS, will be influenced by the vendor's product, but acceptance will ultimately reside with the medical staff.

The team structure for implementing CPOE must take into account the interests and expertise of the following types of individuals:

- *Clinical content experts.* Physicians, pharmacists, mid-level providers, nurses, and practitioners of other disciplines who have clinical knowledge and workflow experience that can help shape the CPOE system to be most useful in the local environment.
- *Medical record content experts.* Health care information management representatives who oversee the legal medical record.
- *Technical experts.* Typically, IT professionals who understand the capabilities of the system, write or configure the software, and test and troubleshoot problems.
- *Front-line users.* Physicians, nurses, pharmacists, and others who care for patients on a regular basis and who will understand the positive and negative implications of each proposal regarding CPOE. CPOE's effects on nurses cannot be overstated. The workflow of incoming information completely changes with the implementation of CPOE. The unit secretary will no longer be the gatekeeper and notifier of new orders. The development of an electronic means to notify nurses of new orders must be considered and incorporated into the nursing workflow to enhance patient care.
- *Project managers.* Individuals responsible for overseeing the completion of project tasks and managing timelines and resources. There may be both a facility project manager and a project manager for the vendor or outside contractor.
- *Workflow analysts.* Team members responsible for analyzing the workflow and processes of patient care, from admission through the entire hospitalization (including transfers, surgeries, and procedures) to discharge.
- *Project sponsors.* Clinician champions and organization leaders who can, with frequent reports from the CPOE team, help overcome the many real and imagined barriers to the CPOE transition and keep the implementation on track.
- *Others.* Ancillary staff whose roles or responsibilities may change with the implementation of CPOE.

Representatives from each of these areas of expertise should work together regularly, in a variety of committees and work group formats. The team should report to a key organizational committee (e.g., the pharmacy and therapeutics [P&T] committee) as well as medical staff or other governance-related bodies. Communication with many formal committees is important as early as possible. The hospital should consider the merits of compensation for time spent away from clinical duties. The health system's existing committee structure may be utilized as oversight authority for CPOE initiatives before, during, and after the system goes live. However, it is highly recommended to create small work groups consisting of physicians, administrators, pharmacists, nurses, and IT personnel to make and approve design decisions and form specific task groups as needed when policy or process issues arise. Quick and timely action will be required during the implementation phase to keep the project moving forward on schedule and in an organized and cohesive manner. This interdisciplinary group should refer matters of policy to existing policy-making committees (e.g., P&T committee, medication safety committee, executive committee, practice guidelines committee, leadership council). The interdisciplinary CPOE committee is not a policymaking committee, but rather a tool to provide structure to existing policies. Some organizations may find it necessary to keep this new formal committee for ongoing oversight of clinical information systems and CDS decision-making.

Pharmacists are needed to provide oversight of medication-use process development. Pharmacist involvement should begin in the initial CPOE planning stages and continue throughout all phases of CPOE development and optimization. The pharmacists that serve on the interdisciplinary team would ideally be relieved of clinical duties to the extent possible in order to commit much of their time to the complex project. Those pharmacists could remain in the pharmacy or be physically relocated to whatever space the interdisciplinary team is allocated. Any pharmacist chosen to serve on the team should be

- A team player
- Well-respected within and outside the pharmacy department
- A good communicator
- Knowledgeable about all facets of the medication-use system, especially the thought process prescribers use to determine a treatment or treatment plan
- Well-versed in the regulatory and legal requirements of medication management
- Current on patient safety initiatives and issues, both external and internal to the health system
- Detail-oriented, with sharp analytical skills
- Open to new ideas
- Very interested in informatics
- Capable of handling stressful situations and limited time lines
- Able to differentiate the requirements of an ordering system from those of a dispensing system and translate those requirements for others

Outside Consultants. External consultants may be used in a variety of roles, including evaluation and vendor selection as well as project management and post- implementation assessments. Use of outside consultants may be warranted if there are insufficient resources, lack of on-site knowledge of the vendor's application, or a desire for a quicker implementation timeline. Consultants add a unique dimension to the team structure in that they have experienced how other hospitals have solved similar problems, can offer a variety of solutions based on their experience from other facilities, and have a network of colleagues they can contact for advice. Having a consultant engaged early in the process can provide continuity to the development and implementation processes.

External consultants should work in conjunction with permanent members of the implementation team. It is important that the permanent members of the team know and understand how the system was designed, how its components fit together, and how each item was built by the consultants. Changes in one part of the system may have intended and unintended downstream effects. Modifications to the system are inevitable, and the on-site team must have the knowledge to understand and execute the necessary future changes. It is detrimental to have this knowledge leave with the consultant when the contract expires. Formal documentation and knowledge transfer meetings should be part of the consultant deliverables.

Allocating Resources. The resources required to manage the transition to a CPOE system will vary, based on a number of factors: the size and complexity of the institution, whether it is an academic or a community setting, types of patients served, current IT infrastructure, the scope of the CPOE project, commitment of implementation project team members, degree of system integration, and other circumstances. There are no general rules about the time, money, or number of employees required for such a transition. Vendors may perform an assessment to help determine the resources that will be required based on the institution's circumstances.

The resources needed should be identified and approved before the project begins, and monitoring of ongoing resource needs and allocation will be necessary. Planning often focuses on capital expenses, underestimating the personnel required to build, test, maintain, improve, and train staff on the use of the system.[29] Having these resources in place is critical to the success of an implementation. During planning and implementation, resource needs may vary, based on project activities. Following implementation, order sets and CDS are integral components of managing care, and the ongoing maintenance to keep the care components current and in line with practice requires ongoing resources. In addition, as the complexity of the system increases with enhancements and user requests, resources needed for ongoing management may increase. Understanding these needs before implementation can help in resource planning.

Developing a Vision for the CPOE System

A vision statement helps describe where the organization wants to be after CPOE implementation and helps define decision-making criteria and the framework for metrics. It is imperative that the CPOE vision align tightly with the vision of the organization as a whole. Large-scale projects should include a clear organizational vision, which might be as simple as increasing patient safety or improving provider access to information. Taking the time to develop these criteria will focus the team throughout the design and implementation processes, help the team communicate the rationale for the necessary change that front-line clinicians will have to make, and lay the groundwork for ongoing measurement.

CPOE is a vital component of the institution's overall patient safety and IT development plans. It is important to establish from the beginning that CPOE is a clinical intervention and not an IT implementation. The implementation team should determine whether there are other issues that may influence CPOE implementation, such as new buildings or other system changes (e.g., pharmacy, bar-coding, or eMAR systems). The team should review and attempt to anticipate trends in regulation or best practices (e.g., from CMS, the Joint Commission, the Institute for Safe Medication Practices, or ASHP) and adopt practices from similar sites that have implemented CPOE. Finally, it should be remembered that CPOE is only one element of the hospital's IT infrastructure. Care should be taken to integrate these disparate systems, with the end result of a complete EHR.

Pharmacy involvement in CPOE development and implementation will be related mainly to medication use within the health system. Pharmacists often have experience with entry of medication orders into a computer system. This experience can be used to help providers adapt to the changes that come with CPOE, but pharmacists should be aware of the differences between ordering medications and verifying and dispensing them. Financial goals, hospital infrastructure, integration, and regulatory compliance also play an important role in the development of a vision for CPOE.

Developing a vision for medication orders in a CPOE system can be divided into three main tasks: defining the goals and objectives for the CPOE system, mapping the current and desired medication-use processes, and determining CPOE system performance requirements to reach those goals. An organization's physicians, nurses, pharmacists, other providers, and administrators can team up to prepare this vision. The vision might include describing how products should be named for easy identification or the configuration of special populations of orders. Consideration should also be given to how medication orders relate to other orders, laboratory test results, allergies, and other clinical information.

Defining Goals and Objectives for the CPOE System

Implementing CPOE is an immense cultural change that involves every part of an organization. After an overarching vision for the components of the CPOE system has been established, the implementation team should reach out to all areas of the institution to develop and explain the goals and objectives of the CPOE system. Widespread understanding and acceptance of these goals and objectives will facilitate development and implementation of the CPOE system. The central goals of a CPOE system typically include improving medication safety and the quality of health care processes.

Medication Safety. Improving the safety of the medication-ordering process should always be in the forefront of any design decision, programming modification, or enhancement to CPOE. The analysis of the existing medication-use process (see "Mapping the Current Medication-use Process" below) should identify any safety deficiencies that can be corrected with CPOE, as well as the strengths of the current processes. The addition of safety features to CPOE will be an ongoing endeavor, as acceptance of the system grows and clinicians realize how the system can improve their practices.

CPOE systems need to be monitored for unexpected safety failures. CPOE can introduce previously unknown safety failures through user interaction with the system, programming changes, or poor system design.[26] To prevent the introduction of new medication errors, careful analysis, review, and testing needs to be conducted with initial implementation and subsequent additions, modifications, and enhancements. Constant surveillance for errors and unanticipated outcomes is an ongoing necessity.[29] This evaluation can also be used to develop the goals and objectives for implementation.

A major impetus behind CPOE is that the deployment of a well-designed CPOE system with effective CDS can reduce medication errors and ADEs. A systematic review of the effects of CPOE with CDS on medication errors and ADEs supports the successful use of CPOE in health care facilities.[18] Many hospitals will implement CPOE to improve patient care, while focusing less on research that explores its impact. Nevertheless, internal systems for tracking medication errors and ADEs should be continually used to assess the impact of CPOE. CPOE could potentially

- Reduce some forms of ADEs or medication errors.
- Qualitatively change some forms of ADEs or medication errors (e.g., an error of omission may become a wrong-time error).
- Introduce new types of ADEs or medication errors (e.g., a physician may select the wrong drug or wrong patient from a list appearing on the computer screen or inappropriately select a default dose).

Quality of Health Care Processes. In addition to improving medication safety, the goals of CPOE implementation may include such things as decreasing drug or laboratory costs, reducing the time required for pharmacist medication order review, improving data collection, or increasing communication among health care team members. If efficiencies from the direct entry of medication orders by the physician result in time savings in the pharmacy, the pharmacy department could potentially direct more pharmacist resources to patient interaction or areas such as pharmacotherapy consultation, pharmacokinetics, anticoagulation monitoring, drug regimen review, antibiotic streamlining, or intravenous-to-oral (i.v.-to-p.o.) conversions. Such goals will be different for every organization, but it is important to establish them during the planning phase of the project. The transition to CPOE represents a major paradigm shift for most organizations. The organized, goal-oriented institution will benefit from creating concise, measurable goals and objectives.[19]

Establishing Baseline Data

In conjunction with the analysis of the current medication-use process, the interdisciplinary team should develop a clear and complete understanding of the institution's current medication safety data (e.g., medication errors, ADEs) as well as the resources devoted to the manual medication order system.[34,35] It is important to track data for at least three months in advance of implementation to assemble adequate baseline data. These data can then be compared with data from the CPOE system at designated intervals. Data should be tracked over time to assess the impact of the CPOE on the medication-use process. This information can help identify workflow bottlenecks or discrepancies in the CPOE system, providing opportunities for improvement. Examples of data that may change with the implementation of CPOE and CDS include errors related to known drug allergies, ADEs related to drug–drug interactions, prescribing errors related to drug dose, and drugs withheld due to contraindications identified via CDS.

Establishing Post-Go-Live Metrics

Implementation metrics can be used to help measure achievement of organizational goals. Comparing baseline and post-go-live measures can identify which areas have improved and which need further review. Metrics are quantitative, measurable parameters, and may include

- Order entry time (e.g., average time it takes a provider to enter an order[36])
- Compliance with established evidence-based order sets
- Number of entered orders
- Missing doses
- Pharmacist interventions related to order entry problems
- Changes to scheduled administration times in the system
- First dose medication administration turnaround time
- Assess possible financial indicators of success
- Frequency of provider contact (e.g., pages for questions or errors on order entry)
- Documented medication errors

When reporting these data, the hospital should be careful not to overstate the impact of the CPOE system on patient outcomes. The measures listed above are process measures, not outcome measures. For example, although the CPOE system may have flagged a patient allergy and prevented administration of the medication, it is possible that even without the CPOE system the pharmacist or nurse would have identified the allergy and intervened before the drug was administered.

It is important to identify and report new errors or ADEs introduced by the CPOE system.[22,25,26,31,37–40] The hospital should actively engage clinicians at all levels in open dialogue and reporting of such issues. These reports should be used to make rapid changes in the design of the system in the spirit of continuous quality improvement.

Describing the Current Medication-Use Process and System Design

To ensure that the integrity, safety, and efficiency of the entire current medication process are maintained, if not enhanced, it is important to perform a complete analysis of the current medication-use process. This analysis should include the interdisciplinary workflows associated with medication use for multiple types of medications. The output can be represented in a variety of ways, including flow charts, narrative scenarios, analyzed issue/problem reports, and comparisons of current practices to known best practices.

The analysis of the current medication-use process should consider a variety of medication order types, based on frequency of use or potential impact on patient safety, in all different process settings (e.g., acute care, critical care, emergency department), procedural areas (e.g., diagnostic imaging), and patient populations (e.g., pediatric, geriatric, adult). The project team should consider a representative group of orders that includes the basic types of orders prescribers typically write. How orders are currently entered into the system may not necessarily be intuitive to a physician. Most importantly, the project team should consider how the prescriber currently orders medications and what would make the most sense to the prescriber when ordering electronically. CPOE systems should be designed from the prescribers' perspective, with an eye on how orders flow over the course of their existence, to encompass all facets of medication use, ensuring the process is complete from medication reconciliation through ordering, renewing, and discontinuing. Complex medication orders and/or protocols may need special attention because of current technology limitations or workflow differences. The types of medication orders that should be reviewed and included in the design, as well as the processes across which they should be considered, are listed in **Figure 1**.

The description of the current medication-use process should be developed from a number of sources: observation, paper order sets, discussion with clinicians, and the knowledge of those who have worked on the organization's previous process-improvement efforts. This process is an opportunity to engage staff pharmacists who service various areas of the organization. Pharmacists often have a broad view of the medication-use process, seeing it from end to end, both receiving orders from physicians and helping address complex administration scheduling issues. The project team should strive to understand the current state of the medication-use process in terms of the components listed in **Table 1**, which also lists the form best used to represent the component.

Developing the Future Medication-Use Process and System Design

Once the current state of the medication-use process is well understood, one or more instances of the future state (depending on the plan for phasing in the CPOE system) can be designed. This future state should be designed to meet or exceed the current levels of service and other important designated metrics and priorities (e.g. patient safety, first-dose delivery time) and address any desired improvements.

The CPOE system should be designed to support the hospital's ideal medication-use process as much as is possible. The system should be configured to support clinicians and promote improved patient care processes, rather than compromising these processes to accommodate system functionality. It will likely be necessary (and desirable) to change many of the key work processes to ensure that benefits (such as improved medication safety) are achieved. A description of the ideal medication-use process is beyond the scope of these guidelines, but key steps in a typical medication-use process are outlined in **Figure 2**.

A successful CPOE design is a combination of process, information systems, and supporting technologies that work together to allow the desired improvements to occur. **Figures 3–6** list some of the process and technology enhancements that should be considered for incorporation into the new process/technology/system design.

The desired benefits of the CPOE implementation should be clearly identified, and the process and system design should make those benefits possible. The design should include the practices, work processes, and

FIGURE 1. Types of medication orders and processes that should be reviewed and included in CPOE design.

Medication Order Types

Oral solids	Medical staff protocols that include medications
Oral liquids	Automated dispensing device overrides
Topicals	Irrigations
High-risk medications (e.g., anticoagulants, heparin, insulin, or potassium chloride)	Immunizations
Compounded medications, such as triple mix or acetazolamide suspension (e.g., oral swish-and swallow or dermatological preparations made in the pharmacy)	Patient-controlled analgesia, including epidural analgesia
Combination products (e.g., hydrocodone-acetaminophen, multi-drug inhalers)	Sliding scale insulin and heparin
Combination doses	Chemotherapy standard and non-standard protocols
Respiratory therapy	Conditional orders
Total parenteral nutrition	Hemodialysis, peritoneal dialysis, and continuous renal replacement solutions
I.V. medications	Investigational medications
Piggy-back i.v.'s	Herbal medications
Continuous infusion medications and titrations	Ophthalmic or otic medications
Flushes	Injectable medications (e.g., i.v. push, i.m.)
	Medications used in operative and procedural areas
	Linked or interdependent orders
	Medications used for diagnostic imaging

Medication Order Processes

Ordering (physician or other clinician)	Medication schedule changes
Electronic signature, signing of verbal orders	Holding orders
Medication reconciliation	Code medications
Preparation and labeling	On-call to operating room or procedures
Medication order review	Future orders
Dispensing and distribution (including interface to automated dispensing devices)	Negative orders (e.g., do not give aspirin)
Administration and documentation	Charging
	Transfer orders

TABLE 1.
Components of the Medication-use Process and Formats Best Suited to Representing Them

Component	Representation
Activities performed	Process flow chart
Strengths and weaknesses of the current process	Text/table
The person(s) performing the activities	Text
The information needed in order to perform the activitiy	Text
The tools and systems used to perform the activity	Flow chart
The outputs of the activity and where they are sent/recorded	Text
The time/effort used to perform the activities'	Text
The barriers, constraints, reductions in efficiency, and limitations on the activity	Text

technological components in an integrated fashion. General process design principles are listed in **Figure 7**.

The future state design should be an interdisciplinary effort that considers the entire medication-use process, even though parts of the process may not change or may not change much with CPOE implementation. It is important to maintain the continuity and integrity of the process by making sure that the design of the component activities is compatible and completely accounts for manual or previously automated processes.

The draft future state design is typically done with a small interdisciplinary group of clinicians (the "core team") who understand the current process and the capabilities and limitations of the CPOE system. This group should consist of clinicians who order (physicians, nurse practitioners, and pharmacists), dispense (pharmacists and pharmacy technicians), and administer (nurses and physicians) medications. This core team should have dedicated time for the project, or at least be relieved of their regular staff schedules for the time spent working on the project. The charge of this group is to weave into the system design the following factors:

- Existing work processes and systems
- Best practices
- New systems, with consideration for their capabilities and limitations
- Physical limitations (e.g., space, facility issues, staffing limitations)
- Political issues (e.g., organizational priorities, limited physician cooperation or interest in CPOE)
- Desired benefits and performance improvements
- Compliance with regulatory, legal, and reimbursement requirements

This redesign typically starts with a high-level process flow diagram that describes the activities performed by each member in the medication-use process, coupled with demonstrations of the system capabilities and flow. Through successive iterations, the workflow and system design is brought into increasing levels of detail and expanded to address the factors listed above.[34] Once the core team is satisfied with the design, practicing clinicians can be brought in to validate and improve the design. The clinicians involved in these process redesign sessions should be experienced and practicing clinicians who understand the current process and will likely find the potential issues with the new processes. These process redesign sessions should be as practically focused as possible and should demonstrate prototypes of orders and output from the system. They should provide a forum to discuss what to do and how it will be done. The redesign will likely take at least three or four sessions to cover the necessary detail of all the affected processes. The information gathered from these sessions can then be used to complete the process and system design and build the policy and procedure and training documents.

Failure Mode and Effects Analysis. A safety analysis of the future state design should be done prior to implementation to identify unintended or unidentified consequences.[41] Failure mode and effects analysis (FMEA) is a useful tool to prospectively evaluate the potential risks associated with the new process and identify inconsistencies or omissions that may have the unwanted effect of increasing risk to patient safety rather than reducing it.[41–44]

Other Design Considerations. It should be determined whether there are required elements at provider order entry in order for the pharmacy to verify orders (e.g., patient allergies, weight). Integrated systems start to break down the silos in which physicians, nurses, and pharmacists sometimes practice. There should be one shared field for allergy and weight documentation, so any expected workflow changes need to be discussed prior to implementation. Though it is the right thing to do, this standardization often uncovers workflow issues that were previously hidden in the paper process. The current process for handling allergy conflicts or drug interactions should be examined and it should be determined how users will handle an alert in a critical or time-dependent area, such as the emergency room. It should also be determined whether there is a need for an additional set of elements for order processing (e.g., laboratory or other results).

Medication Use within the Context of CPOE and the EHR. Whether your organization implements CPOE alone or along with other parts of the EHR (such as the eMAR), other parts of the medication-use process will be affected. To meet the long-term goal of a complete EHR, all medication orders should be included in CPOE. Having disparate ordering systems (i.e., manual and electronic systems) causes confusion, creates additional work for health care professionals, and presents risks to patient safety. The hospital must recognize that CPOE

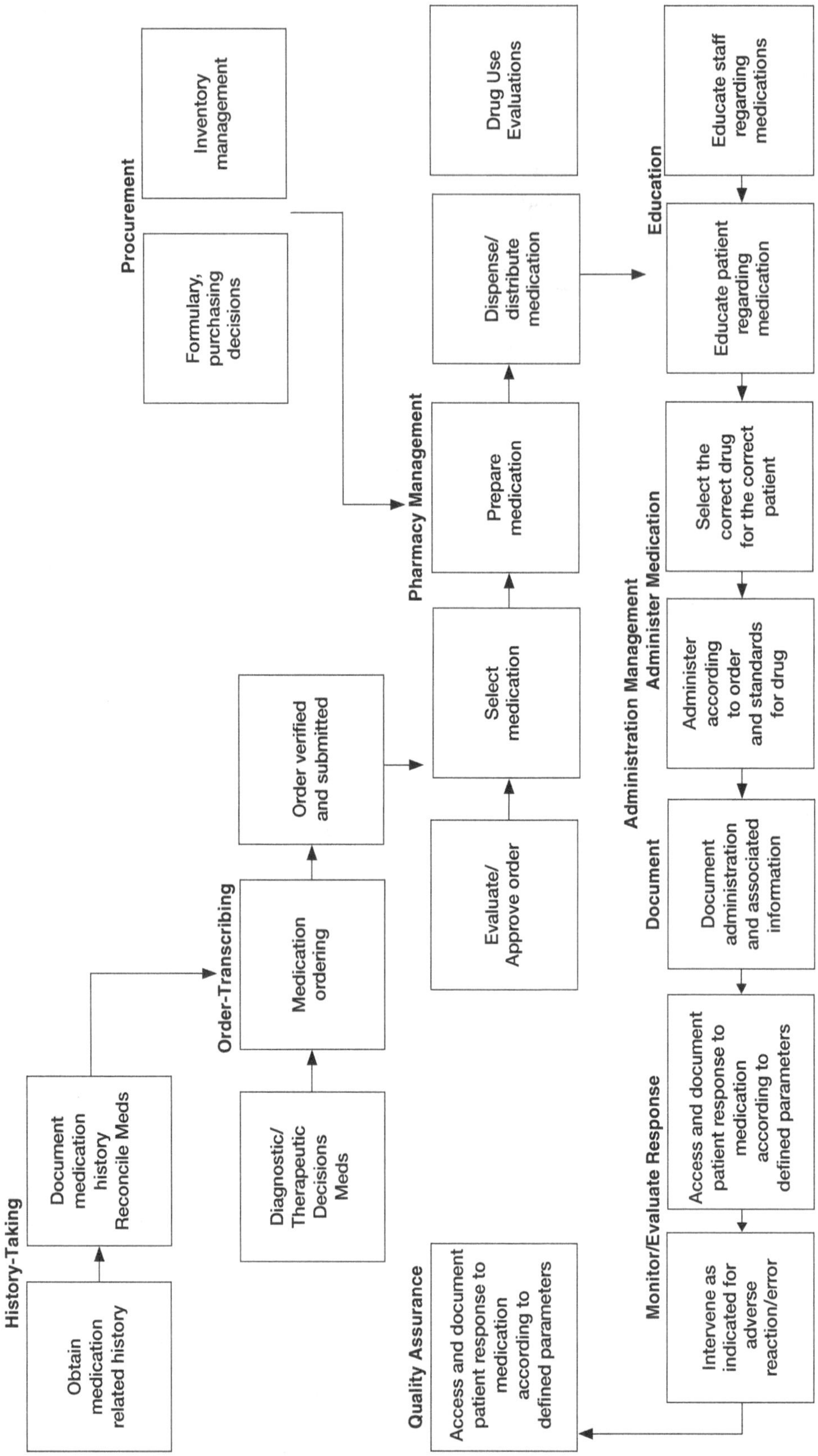

FIGURE 2. Medication-use process model. Reprinted, with permission, from reference 32. Copyright, VHA, Inc. 2001.

FIGURE 3. Potential process and technology interventions in order writing and submission to improve medication safety. Reprinted, with permission, from reference 32. Copyright VHA, Inc. 2001.

Ordering: Order Writing and Submission

Process Interventions

- Establish standards for abbreviations
- Establish policies that do not accept incomplete or vague orders such as "continue previous medications"
- Establish standard protocols for drug dosing and administration
- Develop standard order sets to include drug order, time associated tests, and associated medicines
- Provide routine staff education on common causes of error
- Educate staff on back-up procedures for system down time
- Establish policies for routine review and updating of current orders
- Monitor the bypass of rules and alerts to complete order
- Do not dispense drug prior to written order or verbal order verification unless critical
- Minimize verbal order use

Technology Interventions

- Implement tools to guide the user:
  - Order entry (CPOE) with standard order sets and protocols
  - Mandatory fields to complete an order
  - Rules-based ordering to include dose adjustment, interaction checking, and accompanying orders
- Provide formulary selections
- Provide mobile charting devices to allow for ordering at the point of care
- Adequate back-up procedures for system down
- Updated Mar generated by CPOE or pharmacy sytem on routine basis (minimum every 24 hours)
- Automated reminders or alerts for changes in patient status
- Automated dispensing units do not dispense drug prior to order verification unless a critical medication

FIGURE 4. Potential process and technology interventions in medication history-taking and medication reconciliation to improve medication safety. Reprinted, with permission, from reference 32. Copyright VHA, Inc. 2001.

Medication History-Taking and Medication Reconciliation

Process Interventions

- Establish procedures for obtaining admission history
- Establish minimum data set to include medications, diagnoses, height, weight, and allergies
- Establish accountability for obtaining minimum data set
- Use standardized templates
- Multi-disciplinary clinical documentation
- Instruct patient/family on need to bring all current medications with them, including over-the-counter medications
- Select and identify "record of truth"
- Establish communication links with primary and extended care providers to support transitions in level of care
- Replace free text with checklists when appropriate
- Establish standard abbreviations for medication recording
- Provide wallet cards or other forms to prompt patients to bring complete home medication information

Technology Interventions

- Implement tools to guide the user
- Clinical documentation with templates and checklists
- Prompts for required fields to include minimum data set
- Flags to highlight changes in minimum data set from previous data
- Improve access to patient record through implementation of computer-based patient record/clinical data repository
- Establish communication links with primary and extended care providers to support transitions in level of care
- Provide mobile charting devices to allow for documentation at the point of care
- Structured for computer-based clinical documentation
- Technology adherence to standards

FIGURE 5. Potential process and technology interventions in pharmacy evaluation of orders to improve medication safety. Reprinted, with permission, from reference 32. Copyright VHA, Inc. 2001.

Pharmacy Evaluation of Orders

Process Interventions

- Establish standards for abbreviations
- Establish policies that do not accept incomplete or vague orders such as "continue previous medications"
- Develop standard order sets to include drug order, associated tests and associated medications
- Provide routine staff education on common causes of error
- Do not dispense drug prior to order evaluation unless critical
- Establish procedures for evaluation of orders and when to clarify
- Establish procedures for pharmacy dosing
- Develop procedures for escalating an order that is on hold for clarification

Technology Interventions

- Adequate back-up procedures for system downtime
- Minimize system downtime
- Automated reminders or alerts for patient changes in status
- Pharmacy alerts and reminders based on change in lab value, drug-to-drug interaction, dose-checking, drug-to-diagnosis, drug-to-allergy checking
  - Targeted alerts that vary by individual receiving them to reduce alert fatigue
  - Ability to view online clinical information to include: lab values, clinical documentation and orders
  - Interfaces to auto-populate pharmacy system with ADT, laboratory, clinical documentation
  - Access to drug knowledge base

FIGURE 6. Potential process and technology interventions in administering medications to improve medication safety. Reprinted, with permission, from reference 32. Copyright VHA, Inc. 2001. RFID = radio frequency identification.

Administering Medications	
Process Interventions	**Technology Interventions**
Standardize medication administration times	MAR with time based schedule
Standardize equipment for IV infusion; minimize number of different kinds of devices	Electronic MAR
Provide tools that assist staff in calculating correct rate of infusion	Automated drug distribution carts at the point of care
Stock pre-mixed IV drugs	Smart infusion pumps
Establish standard dose packaging and labeling	Alerts to caregiver to obtain and document clinical information prior to administering a drug
Patients with multiple IV access lines have line clearly marked at distal end	Bar code/RFID administration systems
Distal ports of non-IV tubing incompatible with medication oral syringe	Comprehensive wireless network coverage
Standard protocols for the physical assessment prior to administering a specific drug throughout the hospital	Needleless administration system
	Other medication delivery technologies

FIGURE 7. General CPOE process design principles.

CPOE Process Design Principles
Standardization of order entry and management information and workflows across the organization to the degree possible.
Simplifying processes.
Creating an effective interdisciplinary, team-based approach (i.e., improving communication).
Designing mechanisms for reporting and learning from errors.
Seeking redundancy through use of technology to support clinical decision making.
Avoiding reliance on memory.
Using constraints and forcing functions where appropriate.
Simulating planned and unplanned events for how people interact with each other and technology.
Planning for failure and designing for recovery.
Providing access to a core set of integrated clinical information at the time and point of decision-making.

may increase the amount of time the medical staff spends on prescribing medications, at least in the beginning.[45,46] Therefore, there must be considerable dialogue with the medical staff about their role in the overall medication-use process. It is important that they understand that CPOE is an effective way for them to communicate their orders and improve the timeliness, accuracy, and safety of patient care and that efficiency should improve over time. The hospital should provide incentives for prescribers to utilize the system and disincentives for giving verbal orders or continuing to handwrite orders. To facilitate use of the system, prescribers should have access to the CPOE system from multiple venues, including their offices and homes and via wireless computers. If clinicians have the ability to enter orders from multiple locations such as home or office, a defined process should exist to easily reach the prescriber if there is a problem with the order (e.g., non-formulary, lack of availability).

All new orders should be verified by a pharmacist and reviewed by a nurse, and these actions should be documented in the EHR prior to medication administration. The nurse should work directly in the EHR for all clinical documentation, including medication administration. To comply with the "five rights" of medication administration,[47] a workstation must be available close to the patient's bedside with ready access to that patient's relevant information to facilitate resolution of any questions on the medications that arise. **Figure 8** lists some design considerations for the workgroup as new workflows are designed for different clinical scenarios.

Computers (both wired and wireless) should be available in sufficient quantities so that no clinician has to wait to use one. It is critical that the technologies used for stationary and mobile computing be matched to the anticipated workflow. It is likely that stationary computers, handheld devices (e.g., personal digital assistants), and tablet and cart-mounted computers will all be needed for some part of medication ordering for various users. If they are not part of an integrated system, the CPOE, eMAR, and pharmacy information systems should be available on the same computer to facilitate switching between systems. Any other technologies that are used by providers (e.g., voice recognition) should not only be on the same computer but ideally available from these devices as well. Users should be able to easily switch between different applications if needed, and clinical data should freely flow between applications so that the pharmacist and other providers have real-time access to the same information.

Planning for CDS

CPOE is an important part of an organization's plan for improved safety and quality. The addition of CDS to the EHR and CPOE is essential for the prevention of adverse events and improvement in patient outcomes.[17,20,21] A full discussion of CDS is beyond the scope of this document. ASHP plans to cover the topic in future guidelines. The purpose of this section is to provide an overview of CDS that will allow incorporation of CDS to be addressed in planning.

CDS can be defined as providing the appropriate clinicians with clinical knowledge and/or patient information intelligently filtered and presented at appropriate times to enhance patient care.[48] CDS has many intervention types, including but not limited to the following[49]:

- Documentation forms/templates (structured guidance, required or restricted fields, checklists)
- Relevant data presentation (optimize decision making by ensuring all pertinent data are considered)

FIGURE 8. CPOE design considerations.

Design Considerations
How do orders post to the MAR, and what is the relationship between the MAR and intake/output flowsheets?
Are there other documentation flowsheets that are also used or needed (e.g., patient-controlled anesthesia, continuous renal replacement therapy)?
When do orders need to be approved by pharmacy before a nurse can chart or administer the first dose of the medication?
Can nursing staff easily tell when the order has been verified by pharmacy?
Is there a mechanism to have critically needed orders available on the eMAR before pharmacist review?
What medication information is displayed to the nurse for administration (i.e., both brand and generic names)?
How are orders sorted on the MAR (e.g., are as-needed orders separated from scheduled orders)?
Are administration instructions and notes required (e.g., do not administer oral ciprofloxacin with Maalox)? Will they be supplied from the CPOE system or from the pharmacy system?
Are nondrug items needed on the MAR (e.g., wet to dry dressings)? If so, how will these items be entered (i.e., are these orders that pharmacy must review and approve)? Can some type of treatment administration record be created for these items?
Is there a chart on removal from an automated dispensing cabinet or are auto-charting functions in use?
How will the health system develop a bar-coding system for medication administration?
Override rates of alerts by both pharmacists and providers to better set sensitivities for the warning.
Order verification times by pharmacists to determine turn-around times for different priorities of medication ordering.
Compliance to clinical practice guidelines and order sets.
If integration of the CPOE system is available with automated dispensing devices, then monitoring for overrides would be warranted.
Monitoring free-text orderables in the system, to better address the provider's needs and provide guidance for appropriate formulary build.
Does the software provide the ability to designate a medication and document "First Dose Effectiveness"?
How are enteral nutritional supplements and tube feeding supplements documented, ordered, etc?
Does the software provide "Query Tools"?
Will provider, pharmacist, nursing software "Hand Off" IT tools be needed?
Does the software handle "Look-A-Like, Sound-A-Like" medications and due to this aspect should generate medication nomenclature be utilized exclusively?
Does the software provide the functionality for "after hours" entry and how will the review be completed if pharmacy service is closed?
How will MAR/eMAR handle multi-component medication orders?
How will MAR/eMAR process fractional doses of medication package forms?
How will reporting needs be developed and integrated into the system for users? When?
How are co-signatures or verbal order sign-offs obtained?

- Order/prescription creation facilitators (pick-lists, pre-completed order sentences and order sets)
- Protocol/pathway support (multistep care plans, link to evidence or protocol, pertinent reference information or institution-specific best practice guidance)
- Alerts and reminders (drug–drug interactions, therapeutic duplication, drug–disease, allergy alerts, and others)
- Automated ADE detection based on patient symptoms, labs, diagnostic results, and patient notes

Because CDS has such a broad definition, the line between CDS and CPOE is not always clear. Basic forms of CDS, such as fully defined order sentences and order sets, are an important aspect of CPOE and can decrease errors while enhancing clinician acceptance of the system.[27,28] This type of basic CDS encourages clinicians to make proper choices initially rather than alerting them to potentially problematic choices after the fact and is an essential part of any CPOE implementation.

An organization must recognize that to realize the benefits of CDS, the CPOE system must be accepted by clinicians and used effectively. Poor design or too many alerts could lead to system rejection or, even worse, unanticipated outcomes such as increased errors or adverse events.[25,26,50–53]

Some CDS, including checks for allergies, drug–drug interactions, drug duplications, and dose ranges, are typically delivered via an interruptive alert to the user or displayed as a passive warning on an order entry screen. Such CDS should be considered before CPOE implementation, but designers should keep in mind that a high number of interruptive alerts may cause clinicians to ignore alerts altogether and may even threaten clinician acceptance of CPOE. The way alerts are prioritized and presented to the user may be as important as which alerts are presented. Alerts for very serious clinical situations may be ignored when lost in a sea of less important ones.[54] Some vendor systems allow clients to change severity levels or even disable some alerts in an effort to bring alert interruptions to a better signal-to-noise ratio and thus decrease the potential for alert fatigue, particularly for physician recipients.[50–52] Ideally, there needs to be an alternative mechanism to provide CDS feedback to prescribers that is not intrusive but still allows the prescriber to know that there may be issues with an order. If ignored, these alerts can be acted upon by the pharmacist.

The strategy for prioritization of CDS should be defined as early as possible, and pharmacists should take a leading role in all medication-related CDS. It is likely that organizations will be eager to implement CDS along with CPOE. Pharmacists should ensure that the CPOE system is implemented with basic CDS, such as order sets and sentences, while using appropriate caution when implementing alerts.[27] Although vendor systems are continuously improving and may allow tiering of alerts, there is typically a significant amount of work necessary to vet any changes and carry out the technical work involved in the customization. The combination of pharmacists' clinical knowledge of drugs and their experience with the interruptive alerts that have been present in pharmacy information systems for years provide pharmacists with a unique understanding of the many implications of implementing medication-related CDS. Pharmacists should work with medical leadership, either through the P&T, informatics, or another interdisciplinary committee, to decide how and when medication-related CDS will be added to CPOE. Pharmacists are well positioned to formulate local evidence criteria, collect information on medication therapy outcomes, and to bring together institutional health providers for the purpose of setting priorities and targeted outcomes where select IT interventions are made. The design, implementation, and optimization of CDS is an exciting area of opportunity for pharmacists now and in the years to come.

Elements of a Safe CPOE System

Minimum Features and Functions. The implementation group and key stakeholders should consider what features and functions of the CPOE system are desired both now and in the future. Starting with a pilot group of users allows experience with the system to build and permits users to work through some process issues before system usage is widespread. Any pilot should be brief, with plans for a rollout shortly after addressing the major discoveries. A highly sophisticated system may take so long to develop that interest is lost, or it may be too sophisticated or rigid in its initial application to be well accepted.

An important consideration during CPOE implementation is the determination of which functionalities are required for go-live. CPOE will always be a work in progress, and there will be opportunities for modifications and enhancements. At a minimum, the project team should evaluate all existing manual medication ordering processes, including such complex orders as epidurals, patient-controlled analgesia, weight-based dosing, lab-result-dependent dosing, tapering medication doses, total parenteral nutrition, and chemotherapy, along with critical patient safety functionality driven from known internal or external sentinel events. An agreed-upon list of basic functionality should be established in order to ensure a timely yet successful go-live. If some complex or high-risk medication orders will be left on paper at the initial go-live (e.g., chemotherapy), be sure this is well communicated during training. As well, this principle applies to other identified yet unresolved design topics. The project team will to need re-visit these topics for completion in the post-go-live period.

General Features and Functions. The user interface is often a problematic aspect of CPOE. Users have been reported to enter orders for the wrong patient or to select the wrong item (or wrong feature of an order) unintentionally because they did not use selection lists properly or because it is very easy to select the wrong item from a drop-down list.[38] The CPOE user interface should incorporate appropriate human-factors engineering to avoid risk-prone workflows and controls (e.g., memorized mnemonic codes or function keys, long selection lists) that may produce order-entry errors. The order entry functionality should be independent of patient setting (e.g., inpatient, outpatient), and users should be able to combine data (e.g., order history) from all settings without a need for independent searches or screen selections. The system should include an online help function for system navigation and provide notification if another user modifies the patient record while an order session is ongoing, without losing the session. All displays should contain the patient name, patient location, user name, and function in consistent screen locations. The system should support third-party data entry for prescribers by simultaneous display of the same session in multiple locations and default fields where possible or helpful. The CPOE system should permit user definition of data elements and fields that can be attached to any portion of the database. The system should permit user-friendly, error-free medication order processing by providing the functionalities for the CPOE interface and order processing listed in **Figure 9**.

Levels of Access. The team will need to determine the levels of access or security permitted to staff throughout the hospital. The team may find it easier to begin with the current level of privileges for existing systems.

In general, pharmacists require a high level of access (full access to medication orders, and in some cases the ability place lab orders) because they cover multiple areas; place, alter, or discontinue orders; and may practice under protocols that require monitoring of laboratory test results. There may be different levels of access within the pharmacy department (e.g., actions by a pharmacy student, intern, or resident may need to be reviewed by a senior pharmacist; pharmacy technicians may require different levels of access, depending on duties). Staff may also need off-site or alternative site access.

In addition to pharmacy personnel access, the design team will need to determine levels of access for other staff members. This should include all categories of physicians that practice at the site (e.g., attendings, specialists, consultants, community clinicians with privileges, residents or other trainees, fellows, and medical students). The medical staff office, medical staff executive committees, or P&T committees may be able to make recommendations for appropriate access based on existing policies. Nursing will need to consider similar access issues and ensure compliance with provider practice acts. Ideally, these issues are addressed by existing policies that will only need to be reviewed and implemented. Other ancillary staff will need to be granted access, depending on their need for information and orders that will be built within CPOE and routed to the appropriate department for action.

User Levels and Co-Signatures. The CPOE system should permit restriction of medication orders by user type, individual order, or class of order. Each medication order should indicate the name and user level of the ordering party. The CPOE system should support the entry of unverified orders and the editing and verification of unverified orders, and this function should be role-based and restricted. The system should also support the creation of reminders or inbox messages for orders that require a co-signature. The pending prescriber co-signature name should default into the field from service, team, or coverage schedules, and there should be an option to override the name. The system should provide the ability to require that all orders be countersigned prior to placing a discharge order if the organization wishes to implement this.

Medication Order Status. Considerations regarding medication order status include the following:

- Whether all orders must be reviewed by a pharmacist before they are active or posted to the MAR.
- If the answer to the above question is yes, the process in which the organization will handle urgent medications that are administered before pharmacist review.

FIGURE 9. Functionalities for CPOE interface and order processing.

CPOE Interface

- Multiple active sessions on one display (i.e., ability to put a current order session on hold and review other information, then return to the original work session without losing the work in progress).
- Side-by-side viewing of active order lists and any system-maintained order list (e.g., a standard order set, personal favorites list, or critical path order set).
- Alignment of orders by department while in side-by-side view.
- Switching between applications on the same display without exiting order functions.
- Utilization of all functions via either keyboard or mouse.
- Forward and backward navigation anywhere in the application.
- Access to the Internet from anywhere in the orders application.
- Access from multiple locations (e.g., sign-on, viewing, data entry, and verification at clinical or remote location).
- Order entry with minimal (<3) screen flips and user definition of defaulted fields.

CPOE Medication Order Processing

- Ability to return user to previous screen.
- Online access to error message documentation.
- Hospital-defined error messages.
- Ability to audit and track all errors and alerts.
- Robust search functionality available from all screens.
- Support for coding all diagnoses, tests, and procedures with institutional, departmental, and user-definable subsets of preferred terms (e.g., the appropriate edition of the International Classification of Diseases,[55] SnoMed CT,[56] or others).
- Ability to establish cross-references for tests or procedures, including:
  - Information regarding the name of a procedure or test (i.e., the ability to use alternate names for a procedure).
  - Information regarding indications for, execution of, cost of, and medical literature pertinent to a procedure.
  - Diagnosis codes that can be restricted based on type of exam or test.
  - Diagnosis code restrictions that staff can override by direct entry of the code or access to full table for lookup.
  - Ability to enter a diagnosis code along with reason for exam.
  - Ability to maintain orders online for the duration of the patient stay and to display the status of the orders (e.g., open, in process, completed, scheduled to expire, expired) during order inquiry.
  - Ability to store, display, and print patient test instructions as well as preparation instructions for the order.
- Ability to perform global set-up changes (i.e., changes to a master file table element can be optionally set to automatically populate all relevant items throughout the table).
- Ability to update patient service and physician(s).
- Ability to clearly note, flag and color-code order status.
- Option to have active orders remain visible on the same screen while writing new orders.
- Ability to view all orders, including stopped and interrupted (partially entered) orders.
- Automatic assignment of unique order identification numbers used in mapping to other systems, with the order identification number large enough, or based on an algorithm, so that such numbers are not repeated within 5 years.
- Ability to retain multiple order numbers or other unique identifiers from other systems.
- Option to manually update order status, with the ability to restrict such updates to specific order items or specific users or user classes.
- Ability to create user-defined order status.
- One-step cancel/reorder process.
- Discontinue, discontinue/renew, cancel occurrence, and hold order functions.
- Automatic calculations.
- Option to input order information using free text.
- Ability to search for, track, and audit free text orders.
- Ability to drill down for detail from every screen.
- Ability to drill down to the following during the order entry process:
  - Medication and doses, since initial orders include suspended and discontinued orders.
  - Termination date and time of current orders.
  - Allergies (coded).
  - Patient diagnoses (coded).
  - Demographic information.
  - Visit information (medical).
  - Physicians responsible for the patient (resident, attending, and consultant physicians, at a minimum).
  - Active and completed orders with dates and times.
  - Patient location and service.
- Modules with data specific to clinical specialties, including sets for reporting results, CDS, and order sets.

- Should the CPOE system have some medications on override for urgent use? Are these medications always on override or are there alternative methods for ordering them?
- Does the pharmacy have sufficient staff to deal with the volume of orders? Pharmacy will potentially see all changes, i.v. fluid orders, discontinuation orders, and titration orders. Design considerations will need to address the disposition of the orders prior to implementation.
- If a prescriber enters and then changes an order, how are those two orders reconciled into one order?
- How does the system handle an order by a physician assistant or student that requires a co-signature before becoming active?
- Do hold orders need a defined duration to be accepted? Do these orders automatically discontinue if on hold for a certain amount of time?

Except in urgent situations as described by the Joint Commission,[57] a pharmacist should verify every medication order prior to drug dispensing and administration. Once verified by a pharmacist, the order should populate the pharmacy computer system, generate labels and other items necessary for dispensing, release the drug in the automated dispensing device (if applicable), and populate the eMAR as an active order. The order should be available to the eMAR as soon as it is placed, but it should be clear to the nurse whether the pharmacist has verified the order or not.

Order History. The CPOE system should permit viewing of orders from all previous patient encounters regardless of enterprise location, setting, or patient status. The system should be capable of storing and retrieving previous patient order lists and sorting, reporting, and printing patient order lists by date and date range, setting, patient status (e.g., discharge), service, department, and provider.

The system should allow pharmacists to maintain eMARs and permit online updates, provide online capability to automatically generate a hard copy of eMARs for downtime back-up, provide the ability to display and/or print patient medication profiles or eMARs on demand or at a specified time, and include the ability to have multiple formats that are definable by systems-level staff.

Documentation in the eMAR. The CPOE system should seamlessly build the eMAR from orders in real time. Some institutions may want medication administration time changes to be modifiable from the eMAR, and the eMAR may have a bi-directional interface to the pharmacy information system (if it is not an integrated system). The system should provide the ability to enable bar-code medication documentation. Pharmacist order validation should automatically update the eMAR. The pharmacy and nursing departments should work together to ensure that the eMAR is designed to be readable and user-friendly from the nurse's perspective. Pharmacists and nurses should have the ability to add or delete patient allergies, enter special instructions, change administration times, and place medication orders on or remove them from hold or conditional status. Changes made to administration times in the eMAR should back- populate the CPOE and pharmacy information systems.

Medication Orderable Design and Build Considerations

The design and build of the medication orderables are key tasks in implementing the CPOE system. Care should be taken in designing and building the formulary or formularies, as well as the standard orders and order sets that are built from the formulary. The pharmacy department must have direct involvement in this task.

The CPOE formulary cannot be simply a copy of the pharmacy inventory. Prescribers need to have the orderables constructed to match how they order medications (therapeutic entity), rather than how the pharmacy maintains medication inventory (dosage form/product). In addition, care must be exercised when deciding on the default dose, frequency, and route values for items that will be displayed to the prescriber and in developing the construction of standard orders. Medication errors can result from a hurried prescriber accepting the default that he or she assumes must be correct.[25] The CPOE system should be able to generate formulary lists by generic name, trade name, and dosage form.

The CPOE system should allow routine online updating of the formulary and clinical checks of information without system functionality downtime. The system should provide authorized personnel the ability to maintain and display the formulary with pertinent data (e.g., formulary code, generic name, trade name, national drug code [NDC], or American Hospital Formulary Service [AHFS] number), while limiting access to certain formulary data by role. The CPOE system should include the ability to identify whether an i.v. with a medication additive is to be handled as a large-volume i.v. or as a small-volume i.v. for appropriate handling within the pharmacy department for compounding and dispensing. The system should allow the ability to make changes to the medication identifier (NDC or RxNorm identifier), communicate those changes to other systems, and receive changes from other systems.

Build Considerations

IT analysts design and build the system from documents or order sets reviewed and approved by the multidisciplinary group. Standard IT processes should be followed, beginning with the design phase. Once the design has been approved, IT staff should build the system in a test environment. A test environment protects from mishaps in the live (or "production") environment. It is important for the test environment to match the production environment so that testers get a true feel for how the build will work and interact. IT staff should meet with nursing and pharmacy throughout building and testing phases to resolve any issues that may arise.

After the builder is satisfied that the requested build or order set is complete, the builder should then develop a testing plan. The builder should work through the test plan initially and sign off when the build works as designed.

Next, pharmacy and nursing should perform testing. This testing should involve patient scenarios throughout the patient's visit. Pharmacy is integral to this process and should ensure proper medication management and workflow. When the build passes pharmacy and nursing testing, physicians should review, test, and sign off.

When all aspects have been tested and fixed, and any necessary education is completed, the build may be moved to production. Follow-up is critical to ensure the build meets the needs of providers and is not adversely affecting ancillary staff. A mechanism to report issues quickly must be established, so that the implementation team can investigate and resolve them. The CPOE group should maintain reports of problems and review those lists for recurrent issues. Providing feedback and updates to the persons reporting problems is vital to progression of the project. Clinicians need to know they have been heard and resolution is being sought.

Dependent or Joined Orders. Support for dependent or joined orders is important in the case of i.v. medications and the diluent used for administration, two drugs to be taken together, or a drug and a measurement requirement (e.g., digoxin and pulse rate). The CPOE system needs to make it easy for the prescriber to order these types of formulary items. The system should be flexible enough for the prescriber to select the drug form and size or indicate the diluent for an i.v. piggy-back when ordering if so desired or to allow these choices to be made once the order reaches the pharmacy system.

Order Sets. Requiring providers to use a CPOE system requires a change in workflow, and many fear it may increase the time clinicians spend processing orders.[46] Configuring pre-constructed order sentences and order sets prior to implementing CPOE may increase speed, accuracy, and acceptability of CPOE.[27,28,58] Careful deliberation is needed prior to the creation of CPOE order sets, including consideration of how order sets are currently developed and revised (e.g., by department or by individual practitioners), what the process to propose and review order sets is, and what level of medical oversight is in place for order set development and use. It is also important to understand ordering patterns when developing order sets for use by clinicians. Many organizations use this opportunity to improve and standardize across important aspects of care, such as post-operative nausea and vomiting or pain management, as well as move to evidence-based order sets from their legacy order sets.[28]

The system should permit development of specific admission pathways (e.g., order sets capable of including any type of order and intervention) and integrate with data documented elsewhere in the EHR (e.g., medical histories, medication lists, laboratory results, diagnostic images, clinical documentation, progress notes, narrative summaries [such as operative reports or consultations]). Order set availability should be limitable by user, user role, location, service, or patient status or diagnosis. The system should permit an unlimited number of orders within an order set and an unlimited number of order sets within departments, across departments, and with user-definable time parameters. Order sets can include nursing orders, tests, and medications, and should include appropriate laboratory tests at appropriate intervals to assist in monitoring therapy. Though many systems allow users to create and save their own order sets in a favorites list, this flexibility needs to be weighed against the desire to standardize care by allowing hospital-based order sets only.[28] Discontinuation of an order set should trigger the automatic ability to review, edit, or discontinue all linked orders.

Because the CPOE system may permit initiation of standard order sets with a single action (mouse click, keyboard stroke, etc.), order sets' ease of use may lead to inappropriate or excess medications being ordered. Order sets should be allowed to include linked orders, but orders grouped in a standard order set need not be linked. The institution should decide whether all orders in the set are going to be active once they are signed or if prescribers are required to actively check and click on each medication before signing.

The CPOE system should require designation of an owner (i.e., department, service, person, or role) for each order set. CPOE order sets should be reviewed on a periodic basis for therapy updates. Item and service maintenance should be performed at the departmental level, with updates in item or service definition flagged for review by the owner of the standard order set containing that item or service (i.e., the change triggers a report that the order set requires review). The CPOE system should support restriction of departmental or service standard order set creation or editing by role or individual.

The CPOE system should support standard order set maintenance and review by

- Grouping order sets by department/service
- Dating the creation and review of order sets
- Providing periodic (user-defined intervals or dates, or as-needed) reporting of standard order sets that require review by owner (department, service, person, or role)
- Permitting global changes

Critical Pathways and Protocol Order Sets. Critical pathways and paper-based order sets, a very basic form of CDS already widely used in hospitals, provide a starting point in efforts to standardize care and improve quality and safety through the CPOE system. With the implementation of evidence-based order sets, organizations can provide the prescriber with a direct link to the electronic literature supporting the recommended practice. The work of synthesizing and classifying the available evidence is done by organizations such as the National Guideline Clearinghouse[59] and the Cochrane Database of Systematic Reviews.[60] Organizations may incorporate these guidelines into electronic order sets and critical pathways, in addition to providing the link to give prescribers point-of-care access to the evidence-based literature at the time of order entry.

The CPOE system should support all functions listed under general order sets for critical pathways and protocol order sets. The system should provide a default set of protocols that are available by service and physician and a default set of protocols that are restricted by location. The CPOE system should include an alert system for orders not completed within user-defined time parameters or time parameters required by critical paths or research protocol.

Medication Order Linking. The CPOE system should include the ability to identify orders as linked and sequential or mutually exclusive or time off-set, and to specify intervals, as well as cascade changes in future orders to maintain sequence and timing. It should permit an order stop to automatically bring up any linked orders for re-verification, with the default being to cancel unless re-verified. The system should provide automatic re-sequencing of future orders if any item identified as sequential is moved on the timeline, and it should permit linked orders (i.e., reflexive occurrences that trigger other procedures) that cascade through multiple levels.

Favorites Lists. The CPOE system should permit use of favorites lists by individual user that may include orders for multiple departments (e.g., laboratory, pharmacy, radiology). The system should provide default components of medication prescribing ("Sigs"), such as dose route frequency, and length of order, that are user-definable at the nursing unit level and that have discharge orders or discharge worksheet functionality. The system should provide default Sigs and permit users to save favorite Sigs in user favorites. Users should be able to create favorites lists that include orders from multiple departments on one list. Favorites lists should be fully editable on an ad hoc basis for an active order session, and user-specific favorites lists should be editable by the user. Users should be able to designate any order list as a favorite and may name or rename the list ad hoc (i.e., the save function automatically prompts for name, defaulting to the existing name if available). There should be an option to save an order list as a favorite, either as a new favorite or as a replacement for an existing favorite; that option should be available during any ordering session. Favorites lists should be allowed to contain ordering details that default into the order, and default details should be editable and replaceable during order entry. The CPOE system should support context-specific favorites lists by user, nursing unit, service, and diagnosis, and by combinations of user and diagnosis or by combinations of user, diagnosis, and setting (e.g., outpatient, inpatient). User favorites lists should be copied and shared easily, and the system should allow favorites lists to be built by opening and then editing standard order sets and saving as a favorite. Favorites lists may also include reminders. The system should permit review of favorites lists.

Pharmacy Department Considerations

The ideal CPOE system will have to be integrated with or have a fully functional bi-directional interface with the hospital's pharmacy computer system so that orders entered or modified in one system will populate fields in the other system, avoiding the need for dual order entry. The bi-directional feature of an interface is important because it prevents potentially dangerous discrepancies between data in the pharmacy and EHR systems and removes the transcription step of the medication-use process. In addition, if the distribution and administration components of medication management are not linked, then documentation and billing will not be either, causing more opportunities for error and audit problems.

In their day-to-day interaction with the CPOE system, pharmacists should be working primarily in the pharmacy system, which has all relevant patient information fully integrated with the EHR and CPOE module. The pharmacist's roles include verifying all orders, reviewing and responding to alerts, and clinical monitoring of the patient. The pharmacist should have security privileges to enter and modify orders under protocol (such as formulary or formulation changes).The pharmacist should see all orders within a particular group of orders so that they can see the context in which each individual drug order was prescribed. Additionally, any functionality to help the pharmacist prioritize the review and approval of orders will improve the care of patients.

Pharmacists should receive and work with orders electronically in a queue. Patients with stat orders should appear at the top of the list and be clearly differentiated from less urgent orders. Pharmacists should have the ability to screen their view of orders based on the nursing units they are responsible for on a given shift. At no time should a pharmacist be able to view orders for more than one patient at the same time.

When working with paper orders, pharmacists often gain insight into the medication orders from the context of the surrounding patient care orders. CPOE systems should preserve that context so that pharmacists can view an order in terms of the other therapies, tests, nutrition, and nursing care surrounding it.

Communication Among Departments

The CPOE system should allow for notification of clinicians for pending orders needing signature via e-mail, pager, text message, or inbox message. Pharmacist order notification should be allowed via printout, work queue, e-mail message, system message, or pager. The default method for receiving notification of orders should be definable by the department or service, and the system should support special notification methods for specific services or items different from the departmental or service default, without affecting summary reporting by department. Users should be able to print orders to alternate locations and to send messages, orders, and alerts to additional departments (including information about scheduling and priority of orders) as a single order is being entered or completed. The CPOE system should have an option that order placement generates user-defined worklists. The system should also provide the ability to e-mail patient and preparation instructions and to reference on-call lists.

Education and Training of Health Care Providers

The rate of adoption of the new CPOE system may be directly linked to the extent of training provided to users prior to and during the implementation. One cannot spend too much time training users, as the change the new system entails will be overwhelming. This training can be in the form of formal classroom training, local expert training, or "at-the-elbow" support and training (the type of training typically most welcomed by physicians) during implementation. Organizations may find the most success in using a combination of all three. The more familiar the users are with the system at the time of implementation, the easier the transition will be.

The facility should train and employ a group of prescriber "super users." These users will support the go-live, help the institution refine the CPOE system to be as efficient as possible, and serve as liaisons and CPOE champions to the other members of the medical staff. There should be ongoing, open dialogue with leadership and medical staff members to continually improve the system.

Each training session should be geared toward the type of user, since utilization will differ by clinician type (e.g., physician, respiratory therapist, nurse, pharmacist, laboratory technician). The initial training of users is important, but ongoing training for new users, changes in programming, and functionality require that training be given a high priority after transition to the new system.

Overview of System. The initial introduction to the system should familiarize the user with the layout of the system. It should review toolbars and menus of each application. The first glimpse should include any definitions that are new or to which meanings may be different from the current process.

Accessing Data. This section of training should familiarize the user with the various methods for accessing data. It should provide information on sorting and filtering data. Because access to data will vary based upon the type of user, separating different user types for training purposes at this stage may be beneficial, and this is a good time to discuss security and privileges.

Documenting Information. This section should teach users how to document information pertinent to their practices. These tasks would include adding basic patient information and documentation onto flow sheets, as well as clinical progress notes.

Orders. The training sessions on medication orders will be the most comprehensive. Some users will be limited to ordering tests or procedures specific to their practices. Physicians, nurses, and pharmacists, however, will spend a large percentage of their time in the CPOE system working with orders. Time should be taken to demonstrate each type of order. After the demonstration, users should practice working with all types of orders that they may process in various scenarios. Though documented information may be sparse in test domains, practicing with realistic patient scenarios will provide the best training results and prepare the user for success when using the live CPOE system.

Pilot Project. A pilot with a defined scope is advisable at the beginning of the implementation phase. Organizers should consider the length of the pilot, which patients will be included, what the objectives of the pilot are (i.e., testing system performance, workflow, completeness of ordering), and what happens at the conclusion of the pilot (e.g., more programming, more testing, another pilot, or live rollout). Consideration should be given to type of prescriber/practitioner, order types and number of patient transfers into or out of pilot test area as well as flow of patient information to non-pilot areas. Because user feedback is a valuable objective of the pilot, organizers should develop and use a formal evaluation tool for the pilot clinicians. A time analysis should be performed, comparing how long it takes the pharmacy to process orders with the CPOE system versus their previous workflow. If the time analysis demonstrates a negative impact on workload, the facility may consider making appropriate staffing adjustments. These adjustments will vary, based on the percentage of orders directly entered by the prescriber, and should be continually assessed. True final measurement of process performance capabilities will likely not be realized until implementation processes have been completed and stabilized. A time analysis should also be performed comparing how long it takes CPOE-trained nursing staff to administer and document medications in the CPOE system versus the manual system. This analysis should determine whether time is saved by eliminating manual transcription of orders and manual development and maintenance of MARs. If the time analysis demonstrates a negative impact on workload, the facility should make appropriate staffing adjustments. These adjustments will vary, based on the percentage of orders directly entered by the prescriber, and should be continually assessed.

Conclusion

These guidelines provide guidance to pharmacists in hospitals and health systems on planning for and implementing safe CPOE systems. Pharmacists should utilize their unique knowledge and skills as part of the interdisciplinary CPOE planning and implementation team. Participation by pharmacists is critical in defining the vision, goals, and objectives of the CPOE system; establishing essential metrics to measure the success of CPOE system implementation; re-engineering the medication-use process as part of CPOE system implementation; determining the functionality that ensures the safety of the CPOE system; planning for CDS; and educating and training health care providers to use the CPOE system. Finally, for optimal benefits to patients, organizations should realize that the implementation is merely the beginning and that pharmacists should continue to take a central role in ongoing system optimization and continued CDS implementation.

References

1. Kohn LT, Corrigan JM, Donaldson MS, eds. *To err is human—building a safer health system.* Washington, DC: National Academy Press; 1999.
2. Brennan TA, Leape LL, Laird NM, et al. Incidence of adverse events and negligence in hospitalized patients. Results of the Harvard Medical Practice Study I. *N Engl J Med.* 1991; 324:370–6.
3. Leape LL, Brennan TA, Laird NM, et al. The nature of adverse events in hospitalized patients: Results from the Harvard Medical Practice Study II. *N Engl J Med.* 1991; 324:377–84.
4. Thomas EJ, Studdert DM, Burstin HR, et al. Incidence and types of adverse events and negligent care in Utah and Colorado. *Med Care.* 2000; 38:261–71.
5. Phillips DF, Christenfeld N, Glynn LM. Increase in U.S. medication-error deaths between 1983 and 1993. *Lancet.* 1998; 351:643–4.
6. Bates DW, Spell N, Cullen DJ, et al. The costs of adverse drug events in hospitalized patients. *JAMA.* 1997; 277:307–11.
7. Bates DW, Cullen DJ, Laird N, et al. Incidence of adverse drug events and potential adverse drug events. Implications for prevention. ADE Prevention Study Group. *JAMA.* 1995; 274:29–34.
8. Corrigan JM, Donaldson MD, Kohn LT, et al. Crossing the quality chasm: a new health system for the 21st century. Washington, DC: National Academy Press; 2001.
9. Birkmeyer JD, Dimick JB. The Leapfrog Group's Patient Safety Practices, 2003: The Potential Benefits of Universal Adoption. Leapfrog Group; February 2004. www.leapfroggroup.org/media/file/Leapfrog-Birkmeyer.pdf (accessed 2009 Jan 22).
10. National Quality Forum (NQF). Safe Practices for Better Healthcare-2009 Update: A Consensus Report. Washington, DC: NQF; 2009.

11. American Recovery and Reinvestment Act of 2009 [ARRA] (P.L. 111-5, 123 Stat. 115-521). http://edocket.access.gpo.gov/2010/E9-31217.htm (accessed 2010 May 19).
12. Bates DW, Teich JM, Lee J, et al. The impact of computerized physician order entry on medication error prevention. *J Am Med Inform Assoc.* 1999; 6:313-21.
13. Bates DW, Leape LL, Cullen DJ, et al. Effect of computerized physician order entry and a team intervention on prevention of serious medication errors. *JAMA.* 1998; 280:1311-6.
14. Hunt DL, Haynes RB, Hanna SE, et al. Effects of computer-based clinical decision support systems on physician performance and patient outcomes: a systemic review. *JAMA.* 1998; 289:1330-46.
15. Amarasingham R, Plantinga L, Diener-West M, et al. Clinical information technologies and inpatient outcomes: a multiple hospital study. *Arch Intern Med.* 2009; 169:108-11.
16. Bates DW. The effects of health information technology on inpatient care. *Arch Intern Med.* 2009; 169:105-7.
17. Wolfstadt JI, Gurwitz JH, Field TS, et al. The effect of computerized physician order entry with clinical decisions support on the rates of adverse drug events: a systematic review. *J Gen Intern Med.* 2008; 23:451-8.
18. Ammenwerth E, Schnell-Inderst P, Machan C, et al. The effect of electronic prescribing on medication errors and adverse drug events: a systematic review. *J Am Med Inform Assoc.* 2008; 15: 585-600.
19. Eslami S, de Keizer NF, Abu-Hanna A. The impact of computerized physician medication order entry in hospitalized patients—a systematic review. *Int J Med Informatics.* 2008; 77:365-76.
20. Teich JM, Merchia PR, Schmiz JL, et al. Effects of computerized physician order entry on prescribing practices. *Arch Intern Med.* 2000; 160:2741-7.
21. Chaudry B, Wang J, Wu S, et al. Systematic review: impact of health information technology on quality, efficiency and costs of medical care. *Ann Intern Med.* 2006; 144:E-12-22.
22. Weiner JP, Kfuri T, Chan K, et al. "e-Iatrogenesis": the most critical unintended consequence of CPOE and other HIT. *J Am Med Inform Assoc.* 2007; 14:387-8.
23. Healthcare Information and Management Systems Society (HIMSS) Enterprise Information Systems Steering Committee. Clinical perspectives on enterprise information technology. www.himss.org/content/files/ClinicalPerspectives_whitepaper_052907.pdf (accessed 2009 Aug 26).
24. Healthcare Information and Management Systems Society (HIMSS). Electronic health record. www.himss.org/ASP/topics_ehr.asp (accessed 2009 Aug 26).
25. Koppel R, Metlay JP, Cohen A, et al. Role of computerized physician order entry systems in facilitating medication errors. *JAMA.* 2005; 293:1197-203.
26. Han YY, Carcillo JA, Venkataraman ST, et al. Unexpected increased mortality after implementation of a commercially sold computerized physician order entry system. *Pediatrics.* 2005; 116:1506-12.
27. Kuperman GJ, Bobb AM, Payne TH, et al. Medication-related clinical decision support in computerized provider order entry systems: a review. *J Am Med Inform Assoc.* 2007; 14:29-40.
28. Bobb AM, Payne TH, Gross PA. Viewpoint: controversies surrounding use of order sets for clinical decision support in computerized provider order entry. *J Am Med Inform Assoc.* 2007; 14:41-7.
29. Bates DW. Computerized physician order entry and medication errors: finding a balance. *J Biomed Informatics.* 2005; 38:259-61.
30. Kaushal R, Shojania KG, Bates DW. Effects of computerized physician order entry and clinical decision support systems on medication safety: a systematic review. *Arch Intern Med.* 2003; 163:1409-16.
31. Bobb A, Gleason K, Husch M, et al. The epidemiology of prescribing errors: the potential impact of computerized prescriber order entry. *Arch Intern Med.* 2004; 164:785-92.
32. Kilbridge PM, Classen DC. A process model of inpatient medication management and information technology interventions to improve patient safety. VHA Research Series, vol. 1. Irving, TX: VHA Inc.; 2001.
33. Pedersen CA, Gumpper KF. ASHP national survey on informatics: Assessment of the adoption and use of pharmacy informatics in U.S. hospitals—2007. *Am J Health-Syst Pharm.* 2008; 65:2244-64.
34. Khajouei R, Jaspers MW. The impact of CPOE medication systems' design aspects on usability, workflow and medication orders: a systematic review. *Methods Inf Med.* 2010; 49:3-19.
35. Niazkhani Z, Pirnejad H, Berg M, et al. The impact of computerized provider order entry systems on inpatient clinical workflow: a literature review. *J Am Med Inform Assoc.* 2009; 16:539-49.
36. Wietholter J, Susan Sitterson S, Allison S. Effects of computerized prescriber order entry on pharmacy order-processing time. *Am J Health-Syst Pharm.* 2009; 66:1394-8.
37. Kaushal R, Jha AK, Franz C, et al. Return on investment for a computerized physician order entry system. *J Am Med Inform Assoc.* 2006; 13:261-6.
38. Campbell EM, Sittig DF, Ash JS, et al. Types of unintended consequences related to computerized provider order entry. *J Am Med Inform Assoc.* 2006; 13:547-56.
39. Campbell EM, Guappone KP, Sittig DF. Computerized provider order entry adoption: implications for clinical workflow. *J Gen Intern Med.* 2009; 24:21-6.
40. Singh H, Mani S, Espadas D, et al. Prescription errors and outcomes related to inconsistent information transmitted through computerized order entry: a prospective study. *Arch Intern Med.* 2009; 169:982-9.
41. Bonnabry P, Despont-Gros C, Grauser D, et al. A risk analysis method to evaluate the impact of a computerized provider order entry system on patient safety. *J Am Med Inform Assoc.* 2008; 15:453-60.
42. Kozakiewicz JM, Benis LJ, Fisher SM, et al. Safe chemotherapy administration: using failure mode and effects analysis in computerized prescriber order entry. *Am J Health-Syst Pharm.* 2005; 62:1813-6.
43. Coles G, Fuller B, Nordquist K, et al. Using failure mode effects and criticality analysis for high-risk processes at three community hospitals. *Jt Comm J Qual Patient Saf.* 2005; 31:132-40.

44. Beuscart-Zéphir MC, Pelayo S, Bernonville S. Example of a human factors engineering approach to a medication administration work system: potential impact on patient safety. *Int J Med Inform.* 2010; 79:e43–57.
45. Kuperman GJ, Gibson RF. Computer physician order entry: benefits, costs, and issues. *Ann Intern Med.* 2003; 139:31–9.
46. Bates DW, Boyle DL, Teich JM. Impact of computerized physician order entry on physician time. *Proc Annu Symp Comput Appl Med Care.* 1994:996.
47. McGovern K. 10 Golden rules for administering drugs safely. In: Preventing medication errors. Springhouse, PA: Springhouse; 1994:2–3.
48. Osheroff JA, Pifer EA, Teich JM, et al. Improving outcomes with clinical decision support: an implementer's guide. Chicago: Healthcare Information and Management Systems Society; 2005.
49. Osheroff J, ed. Improving medication use and outcomes with clinical decision support: a step-by-step guide. Chicago: Healthcare Information and Management Systems Society; 2009.
50. Weingart SN, Toth M, Sands DZ, et al. Physicians' decisions to override computerized drug alerts in primary care. *Arch Intern Med.* 2008; 163:2625–31.
51. Igboechi CA, Ng CL, Yang CS, et al. Impact of computerized prescriber order entry on medication errors at an acute tertiary care hospital. *Hosp Pharm.* 2003; 38:227–31.
52. Hsieh TC, Kuperman GJ, Jaggi T, et al. Characteristics and consequences of drug allergy alert overrides in a computerized physician order entry system. *J Am Med Inform Assoc.* 2004; 11:482–91.
53. Nebeker JR, Hoffman JM, Weir CR, et al. High rates of adverse drug events in a highly computerized hospital. *Arch Intern Med.* 2005; 165:1111–6.
54. Paterno MD, Maviglia SM, Gorman PN, et al. Tiering drug-drug interaction alerts by severity increases compliance rates. *J Am Med Inform Assoc.* 2009; 16:40–6.
55. International classification of diseases, ninth revision, clinical modification (ICD-9-CM). www.cdc.gov/nchs/about/otheract/icd9/abticd9.htm (accessed 2009 Jan 27).
56. SnoMed Clinical Terms (SnoMed CT). www.nlm.nih.gov/research/umls/Snomed/snomed_main.html (accessed 2009 Aug 28).
57. Medication Management Standard MM.4.10—preparing and dispensing. In: Comprehensive accreditation manual for hospitals. Oakbrook Terrace, IL: Joint Commission on the Accreditation of Healthcare Organizations: 2006:MM-10.
58. Payne TH, Hoey PJ, Nichol P, et al. Preparation and use of preconstructed orders, order sets, and order menus in a computerized provider order entry system. *J Am Med Inform Assoc.* 2003; 10:322–9.
59. National Guideline Clearinghouse. www.guideline.gov (accessed 2009 Jan 22).
60. Cochrane Database of Systematic Reviews. www.cochrane.co.uk (accessed 2009 Jan 22).

Appendix—Glossary of Terms and Abbreviations

Adverse drug event (ADE): ASHP defines a significant ADE as any unexpected, unintended, undesired, or excessive response to a drug that

1. Requires discontinuing the drug (therapeutic or diagnostic),
2. Requires changing the drug therapy,
3. Requires modifying the dose (except for minor dosage adjustments),
4. Necessitates admission to a hospital,
5. Prolongs stay in a health care facility,
6. Necessitates supportive treatment,
7. Significantly complicates diagnosis,
8. Negatively affects prognosis, or
9. Results in temporary or permanent harm, disability, or death.

Bar-code-assisted medication administration (BCMA): A methodology involving the use of scanners and software to verify all medications electronically before they are administered to patients. These systems may also document the medication in the eMAR.

Clinical decision support (CDS): Clinical decision support systems are interactive computer programs or other tools, which are designed to assist physicians and other health professionals with decision making tasks usually at the point of care.

Computerized provider-order-entry; alternatively, computerized prescriber-order-entry (CPOE): An electronic system that health care professionals can use to enter drug, treatment, and test orders and transmit the orders directly to the department responsible for fulfilling the order.

e-iatrogenesis: Patient harm caused at least in part by the application of health information technology including but not limited to the systems and/or the design and implementation of the system.

Electronic health record (EHR): An electronic record of health-related information on an individual that conforms to nationally recognized interoperability standards and that can be created, managed, and consulted by authorized clinicians and staff across more than one health care organization.

Electronic medication administration record (eMAR): A version of the medication administration record viewable online and not printed.

Electronic medical record (EMR): An electronic record of health-related information on an individual that can be created, gathered, managed, and consulted by authorized clinicians and staff within one health care organization.

Enterprise information system: Broader system that integrates clinical systems such as an EHR and business systems such a scheduling and/or financial systems and quality reporting systems.

Leadership: Within a health-system, leadership may address three leadership groups: The governing body, the chief executive and other senior managers, and the leaders of the licensed independent practitioners.

Legal medical record (LMR): The legal health record is the documentation of health care services provided to an individual during any aspect of health care delivery in any type of health care organization. It is consumer or patient-centric. The legal health record contains individually identifiable data, stored on any medium, and collected and directly used in documenting health care or health status.

National drug code (NDC): A universal 11-digit product identifier used in the United States for drugs intended for human use. The Drug Listing Act of 1972 requires registered drug establishments to provide the Food and Drug Administration (FDA) with a current list of all drugs manufactured, prepared, propagated, compounded, or processed by it for commercial distribution.

Orderable: An authoritative direction or instruction from a prescriber to perform a task (e.g., a radiology test or administer a medication or treatment).

Medication administration record (MAR): Medication administration record usually handwritten or printed from an electronic pharmacy information system.

Personal health record (PHR): An electronic record of health-related information on an individual that conforms to nationally recognized interoperability standards and that can be drawn from multiple sources while being managed, shared, and controlled by the individual.

RxNorm: RxNorm is a standardized nomenclature for clinical drugs and drug delivery devices and is produced by the National Library of Medicine.

Sponsorship: An identified executive or clinical leader who assumes responsibility for another person or a group during a period of project planning implementation follow-up.

Systematized nomenclature of medicine (SNOMed): A multiaxial, hierarchical classification system. As in any such system, a disease may be located in a body organ, which results in a code in a topography axis and may lead to morphological alterations represented by a morphology code.

Workflow: The flow or progress of work done by a company, industry, department, or person.

Developed through the ASHP Section of Pharmacy Informatics and Technology and approved by the ASHP Board of Directors on September 24, 2010.

A work group of the ASHP Section of Pharmacy Informatics and Technology Section Advisory Group on Clinical Information Systems is gratefully acknowledged for developing these guidelines: Anne M. Bobb, B.S.Pharm.; Jennifer Boehne, Pharm.D.; W. Lynn Ethridge, Pharm.D.; J. Chad Hardy, Pharm.D., M.S.; Randy Herring, B.S.Pharm.; Richard S. Jacobs, Pharm.D.; Michael A. Jones, Pharm.D.; Timothy W. Lynch, Pharm.D., M.S.; Leslie R. Mackowiak, M.S.; Tommy J. Mannino, B.S.; Jayson J. Przybyla, Pharm.D.; Brendan J. Reichert, M.S.; Ranee M. Runnebaum, Pharm.D.; Nancy R. Smestad, M.S.; David L. Troiano, M.B.A., MSIA; Laura L. Tyndall, Pharm.D.; and Lori Wright, Pharm.D.

ASHP also gratefully acknowledges the contributions of the following people: Bruce W. Chaffee, Pharm.D.; Toby Clark, M.Sc., FASHP; Kate Farthing, Pharm.D., BCPS; Burt W. Finkelstein, Pharm.D.; William L. Fritz, M.S., FASHP; Kimberly A. Galt, Pharm.D., FASHP; Barry R. Goldspiel, Pharm.D., FASHP; Frances M. Jordan, M.B.A., FASHP; Renee B. Marino, Pharm.D.; Kevin C. Marvin, M.S., FASHP; Steven Meisel, Pharm.D.; Alicia S. Miller, M.S.; Sandi Mitchell, M.S.I.S., FASHP; Kuldip R. Patel, Pharm.D.; Alicia B. Perry, Pharm.D.; John Poikonen, Pharm.D.; Mark H. Siska, B.S.Pharm.; and Mary Windle, Pharm.D.

ASHP also acknowledges the following organizations and individuals for reviewing drafts of these guidelines (review does not imply endorsement): American Academy of Family Physicians (AAFP); American Association of Critical Care Nurses (AACCN); American Health Information Management Association (AHIMA); American Hospital Association (AHA); California Society of Health-System Pharmacists (CSHP); Healthcare Information and Management Systems Society (HIMSS); Jeanine (Porter) Abrons, Pharm.D., M.S.; Christel Anderson (HIMSS); Dan Buffington; Peggy Brashear, B.S.Pharm.; Tim R. Brown, Pharm.D., FASHP; Dominick A. Caselnova III, M.H.A.; Thomas W. Cooley, M.B.A.; Debby Cowan, Pharm.D.; Michele Danish, Pharm.D., FASHP; Neil Davis; Charlie De la Torre; Robert DeChristoforo, M.S., FASHP; Jean Douglas, Pharm.D.; Brent R. Ekins, Pharm.D., DABA; Elizabeth Fang, Pharm.D.; Tim Lanese, M.B.A., FASHP, CPHIMS; Lisa Gunther Lum, Pharm.D., FASHP, FCSHP; Robi Hellman, RN, MSN, CNS (AACCN); James M. Hoffman, Pharm.D., M.S., BCPS; Carol J. Hope, Pharm.D., M.S.; Amey Hugg; Joan E. Kapusnik-Uner, Pharm.D., FCSHP; Linda L. Kloss, RHIA, FAHIMA (AHIMA); Ronald E. Lay, M.S.; Jeff Little, Pharm.D.; Bob Lobo, Pharm.D.; LTC Eric M. Maroyka, Pharm.D., BCPS; Greg Matsuura, Pharm.D., BCPS; Patrick J. McDonnell, Pharm.D.; Michael McGregory, Pharm.D., M.B.A., BCPS; Robert Moore, B.S.Pharm., BCPS; Susan J. Morikawa, Pharm.D., BCPS; Kevin Olsen, RN, BSN; Peg Panella-Spangler M.S.; Christine Pavlak, M.H.A., FASHP; Stephanie C. Peshek, Pharm.D., FASHP; Tommie Peterson; Minh James Pham, Pharm.D.; James A. Ponto, M.S., BCNP, FASHP; Donald W. Rucker, M.D.; Richard Sakai; Kevin Scheckelhoff; Thomas R. Schafer, Pharm.D., BCPS; Terry Seaton, Pharm.D.; Suzanne Shea; Pamela Shellner, M.A., RN (AACCN); Clyde Spence, Pharm.D., M.B.A.; Richard L. Stambaugh, Pharm.D., M.S., BCPS; Craig S. Stern, Pharm.D., M.B.A.; Scott H. Takahashi, Pharm.D., FCSHP (CSHP); Dennis A. Tribble, Pharm.D.; Jody Jacobson Wedret, FASHP, FCSHP; Rich Umbdenstock (AHA); Ray Vrabel, Pharm.D.; Steven E. Waldren, M.D., M.S. (AAFP); Eric Weber; Barbara White, M.S., PMP, FASHP.

Copyright © 2011, American Society of Health-System Pharmacists, Inc. All rights reserved. Contact ASHP for reprint and permissions requests. This content may not be used for commercial purposes without the express written consent of ASHP.

The bibliographic citation for this document is as follows: American Society of Health-System Pharmacists. ASHP guidelines on pharmacy planning for implementation of computerized provider- order-entry systems in hospitals and health systems. *Am J Health-Syst Pharm.* 2011; 68:e9–31.

ASHP Guidelines on Remote Medication Order Processing

Purpose

Because of the complexity of the care that pharmacists provide patients, the American Society of Health-System Pharmacists (ASHP) advocates that patients have 24-hour access to the pharmacist responsible for their care and that the pharmacist be physically accessible to the patient when feasible. ASHP recognizes that such access is not always possible and encourages the development of remotely delivered pharmacist care as a supplement to onsite care.

Medication order review is one aspect of pharmacist patient care. All health-system pharmacies have an obligation to provide a review of medication orders that ensures safe medication use.[1] When onsite pharmacist review is not available, health systems may determine that remote pharmacist review of medication orders is a suitable alternative. The purpose of these guidelines is to describe the policies and procedures that must be in place to safely employ remote medication order processing (RMOP). Health-system policies and procedures regarding RMOP should address quality assurance and safety; access to drug information and hospital policy resources; training and orientation; minimum technical standards and specifications; confidentiality, privacy, and security; regulatory and accreditation standards; and communication and problem resolution. These guidelines also describe some general considerations for RMOP implementation, and **Appendix A** provides a checklist for assessing implementation readiness. **Appendix B** contains an outline of a model agreement for RMOP. A glossary of terms used in these guidelines appears in **Appendix C**.

Because of the rapid pace of change, differences in practice settings and RMOP models, and the complexities of health care organizational arrangements, aspects of these guidelines may not be applicable to all settings. These guidelines are not intended to describe best practices for the operational relationships between satellite and central pharmacies in acute care settings. Readers should also note that these guidelines do not attempt to address all aspects of remotely delivered pharmacist care and should interpret them as limited to the subject of RMOP. These guidelines address remote order verification only when medication order fulfillment occurs through automated medication storage and distribution devices. Remote end verification of the dispensed drug product (e.g., visual approval of the drug product by video camera or other means) is beyond the scope of these guidelines. Health-system administrators and pharmacy managers should therefore exercise their professional judgment in assessing and adapting these guidelines to meet the needs of their particular settings and to comply with the health care organization's policies and procedures.

Models of RMOP Services

The technologies used in RMOP are relatively new and rapidly changing, so different methods for RMOP have evolved, and further evolution should be encouraged. At least two models of RMOP are currently in use: contracted services and supplemental workload balancing, which includes network workload balancing and on-call assistance. Each of these models has unique characteristics that must be considered in planning for its use.

Contracted Services. In this model, a hospital pharmacy that is not continuously open contracts with a larger hospital or a service to provide RMOP when its pharmacy is closed. This model is typically applied when a hospital without 24-hour pharmacy services has sufficient automated dispensing cabinet capacity that RMOP allows nursing staff to keep functioning without having a pharmacist present,[2] although some institutions have developed models for remote verification by pharmacists of dispensing performed by pharmacy technicians at the client site.[3]

Supplemental Workload Balancing. Similar to the model described above, in this case a health system with a number of hospitals relies on the ones that have a 24-hour pharmacy department or on a service to provide RMOP for hospitals whose pharmacies are closed or that experience unanticipated peaks in order processing workload. For example, in an on-call model, a staff pharmacist from the client site or a contracted service is placed on call to help with managing workload. This pharmacist works remotely (sometimes from a home office, where allowed by state regulation) to help the client's pharmacy department manage unanticipated peaks in order processing workload (often on the second or third shift). In this model, the remote pharmacist is responsible for medication order entry and/or review, and medication order fulfillment occurs through the client-site pharmacy.

Quality Assurance and Safety

Medication-use management and safety in the RMOP environment require special efforts in the coordination of quality-assurance, quality-improvement, and patient safety practices between the client site and the remote site. Differences in local practice standards and organizational cultures, combined with unique human factors issues, have the potential to magnify the risk of errors. Quality, safety, and risk management strategies should be jointly examined and agreed on and should address the procedures and communication pathways unique to RMOP systems. These include critical workflow steps and handoffs involved in medication ordering, review, and verification; communication among prescriber, pharmacist, and nurse; and assessing the patient's response to drug therapy and achieving desired therapeutic outcomes.

Review of the Patient's Profile. The remote pharmacist must be able to review the patient's profile for

- Medication history and medication reconciliation reports
- Diagnosis
- Allergies and prior adverse drug reactions
- Height, weight, age (measured versus estimated), and sex
- Pregnancy status for women of childbearing potential

DOI 10.37573/9781585287048.012

- Duplications of drug therapies
- Potential drug interactions
- Pertinent laboratory data
- Other information as needed

Clarification of Medication Orders. The remote pharmacist must have a process by which he or she can clarify the medication order with the prescriber. The remote pharmacist must alert other health care providers caring for the patient (e.g., the client nursing and pharmacy staff) of the need for additional review and clarification. There must be a mechanism for the remote pharmacist to readily communicate by phone or leave a note in the patient profile for other health care providers, including the client site pharmacy staff, to clarify the order or otherwise respond within an appropriate period of time. The remote pharmacy must have a mechanism for timely follow-up on medication orders that are pending clarification.

Quality-Assurance and Medication Error Reporting Systems. The remote pharmacy must participate in the client site's quality-assurance and medication error reporting systems. These systems should include the collection and reporting of medication errors and process variances as described below:

- The medication error reporting system should include potential adverse events that reach the patient (with or without harm) and potential adverse events that are intercepted before reaching the patient.
- Medication error reports related to RMOP procedures and communications should be tracked by outcome, type, cause, severity, preventability, and source.
- Corrective action plans should be directed toward the system failures that contributed to or caused the error, variance, or adverse event.
- Policies and procedures should ensure that quality-assurance data and medication error reports are jointly reviewed in a timely manner by pharmacy leadership and safety officers (if applicable) at both the client and remote sites and that relevant information is shared with relevant frontline practitioners at both sites, including remote pharmacists and client-site nursing and pharmacy staff.

The quality-assurance program should include indicators that measure important aspects of RMOP, including measures of (1) timeliness (e.g., elapsed time to receive and verify an order), (2) system performance (e.g., percentage of time information technology systems are not available for RMOP), (3) compliance with contractual requirements, (4) employee satisfaction at the client and remote sites, and (5) unanticipated problems (e.g., breaks in privacy standards, communication and handoff problems).

Handoff Communication. The remote site should have a documented process for handoff communication that meets the requirements of Joint Commission National Patient Safety Goals.[4]

Access to Drug Information and Hospital Policy Resources

Drug Information Resources. Drug information resources are essential tools for health care organizations. Drug information resources, specific to the needs and scope of patients served, are essential for practicing evidence-based medicine in a safe and efficient manner. In health care systems that use RMOP procedures, each institution needs point-of-care access to internal and external drug information systems. Internal drug information resources include the client's formulary, laboratory reference values, newsletters, and drug-use guidelines based on local standards. External drug information resources include commercially available electronic and print media that organize information into full-text and bibliographic retrieval systems.

Drug information resources available in the remote pharmacy should at a minimum meet the state board of pharmacy requirements for both the client and remote pharmacy sites and include the current edition of a drug information reference (hard copy or electronic). Other reference material (hard copy or electronic media) should be available, depending on the scope of care being provided. Recommended clinical and drug information reference materials available in the remote pharmacy include

- Two sources of pediatric dosing information (ideally, one of which is the same resource used by clinicians in the remote pharmacy)
- Internet access to online drug information resources, including the Food and Drug Administration
- Drug compatibility and drug interaction resources
- Poison information and poison control resources (at a minimum, the telephone number for a certified poison control center)
- Drug information center contact number

Drug information requirements, resources, and staff competencies in the use of drug information systems should be reviewed at least annually to ensure that patient care needs are met.

Hospital Policy and Procedures. The minimum information on client site hospital policies and procedures that the remote pharmacist should have available is

- Client site's pharmacy department's policies and procedures
- Client site's formulary
- Client site's relevant nursing department policies and procedures
- Standard medication administration times
- Standard drip concentrations or drug protocols
- High-risk policies including the "Do Not Use" abbreviations list
- Drug-specific clinical guidelines
- Restrictions by indication or prescriber
- Chemotherapy protocols, pain protocols, and anticoagulation protocols
- Standing or protocol orders
- Pre- and postoperative antibiotic selection and administration protocols, and other protocols as determined
- Therapeutic interchange list
- Client's policies and procedures for processing nonformulary medication orders
- Client's policies and procedures for handling a clinical message order to alert nursing staff and pharmacy department of the need to address an issue at a future time

- Client's pharmacokinetic and renal dosing policies along with written medical staff approval to write orders in the patient's chart if required to comply with these policies

The remote site must have a procedure that ensures the timely and complete communication of changes in client site hospital policies and procedures, including changes to formularies and medication protocols.

Training and Orientation

Pharmacists, through training and orientation, are competent to review and enter medication orders written by prescribers into a computerized database to maintain a complete patient profile. This patient profile can be used by nurses and other providers to access medications appropriate for their patients. This training and orientation are critical for pharmacists to accurately document and transcribe the appropriate information to maintain an accurate and up-to-date profile. Requirements for training and orientation include the following:

- All education and orientation are documented in a permanent record maintained in the pharmacy department of the remote site (if applicable) and shared with client sites or in the pharmacy department of the client site, as appropriate.
- All pharmacy personnel accessing the pharmacy information system are tested for competency prior to use of the system and annually thereafter.
- When upgrades or significant changes are made to the client site's computer system, the client site will communicate to the remote site the need for follow-up training.
- When significant changes are made to the client site's clinical policies or procedures, the client site will communicate to the remote site the need for follow-up training.
- The client and the remote site must have a process for documenting the remote pharmacist's competencies. If the remote site is responsible for the documentation of those competencies, the client and the remote site must have a system for reporting those competencies to the client.

Minimum Technical Standards and Specifications

The client and the remote site must ensure that the following minimum technical standards and specifications are met:

- The remote site must have access to the client's network or Internet, phone, and scan or fax access to the client.
- The remote site must have the ability to access the client facility via the client's Internet solution or via the client's computer network.
- The remote site must, to the extent possible, have redundant systems in place to ensure RMOP service availability (e.g., computer network and Internet connectivity, other information systems used to facilitate RMOP).
- The remote site must have the ability to operate remotely the client's order transmittal system.
- The systems used by the remote pharmacist to view the patient orders and other medical information must comply with the technical standards set by the Health Insurance Portability and Accountability Act of 1996 and ensure technical and physical safeguarding of patient health care information.

Confidentiality, Privacy, and Security

To ensure the confidentiality, privacy, and security of patient health care information, the following conditions must be met:

- Remote pharmacists must adhere to the client's confidentiality policy.
- The remote site, if a business entity, must have a signed business associate agreement with the client.
- The client must provide individual pharmacist-specific access to the client's hospital computer system.

Regulatory Considerations

State regulation of RMOP varies considerably. The client and the remote site should jointly analyze state regulations governing pharmacy practice at both sites to determine and meet applicable requirements. This analysis should be repeated on a routine basis, as regulations may change. To ensure regulatory compliance, at a minimum the following should be verified and approved by the client and the remote site before implementing RMOP:

- Remote site's approval to operate by the client's state board of pharmacy, if required.
- The policy and procedure manual for the RMOP operation, including but not limited to procedures for handling computer system or connectivity downtime, issue escalation, annual competency renewal verification, and communication between the client site and remote site personnel.
- Copies of all licensure required by the states in which the client and the remote site are located (some states require remote pharmacists to have a consultant license in addition to a state pharmacist license for each hospital for which the pharmacist performs RMOP services).
- Copies of any hospital job-specific competency requirements for pharmacy personnel.

Communication and Problem Resolution

To ensure the safety of the RMOP service, the client and the remote site must establish effective communication channels between personnel at the two sites. Communication among prescriber, pharmacist, and nurse will be critical to assessing the patient's response to drug therapy and achieving desired therapeutic outcomes. The remote pharmacist must have the ability to immediately contact the prescriber or client site's nursing staff to discuss any concerns identified during review of the patient's information. The client must provide its nursing supervisor with a 24-hour telephone number to contact the remote site or remote pharmacist and encourage nurses to communicate with the remote pharmacist. In the event the nursing supervisor is unable to resolve a problem or concern, the client pharmacist on call is available for consultation and problem resolution if the problem cannot wait until the client pharmacist is on duty again. Patient profile information, including laboratory results, should be communicated to the remote site electronically; oral communication of laboratory results should be limited to exceptional circumstances, and such oral communications should be documented in the patient medical record as soon as possible. Downtime procedures should provide mechanisms for direct communication among the remote pharmacist, nurses, and the prescriber.

Considerations for Implementation

The success of RMOP implementation will depend on a host of specific factors. Below are some considerations that are generally applicable. Appendix A provides a brief checklist for implementation readiness.

- Terms of the contract or agreement should allow flexibility for the number of orders processed, since estimates prior to "go-live" may be inaccurate.
- Early and frequent communication between the client site and the remote site, especially in the first few weeks after go-live, is critical to the success of the implementation and ongoing operation.
- After-hours technical support at both the remote site and the client site will be essential to the success of the implementation and ongoing operation. Plan for information technology support in advance of go-live.
- Education will be required for all nurses at the client site, not just those whose shifts coincide with RMOP coverage. In particular, changes to the client site's override processes will need to be planned in collaboration with nurses.
- The client should implement a mechanism for communication between the remote site and nursing via the electronic medication administration record (eMAR) system. For example, if the remote pharmacist reviews the patient's home medication reconciliation list and identifies items not stocked by the pharmacy, it would be helpful to have a drug dictionary item (e.g., "Pharmacy Note to Nurse") whereby the remote pharmacist can make an entry in the eMAR that informs nurses that the remote pharmacist has reviewed the order but that some action at the client site is required.

Conclusion

ASHP believes that patients should have 24-hour access to the pharmacist responsible for their care and that the pharmacist should be physically accessible to the patient when feasible. Because 24-hour pharmacy services are not achievable in all circumstances, health systems may employ remote pharmacist review and processing of medication orders. The purpose of these guidelines is to describe the policies and procedures that must be in place to safely employ RMOP. Health-system policies and procedures regarding RMOP should address quality assurance and safety; access to drug information and hospital policy resources; training and orientation; minimum technical standards and specifications; confidentiality, privacy, and security; regulatory and accreditation standards; and communication and problem resolution. Given the rapid pace of change in technology, differences in practice settings and RMOP models, and the complexities of health care organizational arrangements, health-system administrators and pharmacy managers should exercise their professional judgment in assessing and adapting these guidelines to their particular settings.

References

1. The Joint Commission. Elements of performance for medication management standard 4.10 (preparing and dispensing). Comprehensive accreditation manual for hospitals. Oakbrook Terrace, IL: The Joint Commission; 2007:MM-10.
2. Stratton TP, Worley MW, Schmidt M, et al. Implementing after-hours pharmacy coverage for critical access hospitals in northeast Minnesota. *Am J Health-Syst Pharm.* 2008; 65:1727–34.
3. Clifton GD, Byer H, Heaton K, et al. Provision of pharmacy services to underserved populations via remote dispensing and two-way videoconferencing. *Am J Health-Syst Pharm.* 2003; 60:2577–82.
4. The Joint Commission. 2009 National Patient Safety Goals: hospital program. www.jointcommission.org/PatientSafety/NationalPatientSafetyGoals/09_hap_npsgs.htm. (accessed 2009 Dec 28).

Appendix A—Checklist/Assessment for Implementation Readiness

1. All automation has been tested and is functional, including
   a. Communication of medication orders (fax machines or scanners)
   b. Computer systems maintaining patient profiles
   c. Connectivity to automated medication dispensing cabinets
   d. Electronic reference resources
   e. Remote connectivity
2. All personnel training for remote site and client site is completed and documented:
   a. Computer systems
   b. Clinical guidelines
   c. Client site pharmacy policies and procedures related to review, authorization, and entry of medication orders
   d. Communication procedures
3. Pre-go-live test of mock patients and scenarios has been performed for
   a. Fax/scan orders
   b. Admission, transfer, and discharge of patient
   c. Medication order entry
   d. Communication procedures
4. System downtime protocols have been well communicated to all applicable personnel at both the remote site and client site (e.g., pharmacy, nursing, information technology, and administrative personnel)
5. Go-live date and service level expectations have been well communicated to all applicable personnel at both the remote site and client site
6. Communication process that includes quality reporting, system changes/availability, and policy and procedure updates as well as shift change communication has been agreed on, established, and well communicated to all applicable personnel at both the remote site and client site

Appendix B—Outline for Model Agreement Between Remote Site and Client

The agreements between a remote site and the client must be approved by both contract office and risk management in both facilities (if applicable). The agreement should include

1. Services to be provided, including the roles of both parties:
    a. Hours of service
    b. Technology requirements
    c. Order processing services
    d. All clinical services provided
    e. Management services
    f. Quality measures
    g. Other services (e.g., vacation, emergency, or other hours of coverage)
    h. Qualification of pharmacy and pharmacists
    i. Security of information
    j. Limitations
    k. Access to records, including information required to review patient profiles
2. Terms and renewal of the agreement
3. Mutual indemnification and insurance
4. Termination of the agreement, including changes in laws or regulations
5. Confidentiality, including requirements set by the Health Insurance Portability and Accountability Act of 1996
6. Limitations of liability
7. No exclusion from federal health care programs
8. Dispute resolution
9. Fees and payment terms:
    a. Hourly rates
    b. Per-order rates
    c. Order volume
    d. Overpayment and underpayment exposure
    e. Penalty charges
    f. Addition of new services
10. Miscellaneous issues, including
    a. Independent contractors
    b. Notices
    c. Compliance with the terms
    d. Rights of the parties
    e. Conflict of laws
    f. Compliance with laws, regulations, guidelines, and accrediting body standards (e.g., Joint Commission)

Appendix C—Glossary

Terms used to describe remote medication order processing (RMOP) practices are evolving and vary considerably. Readers should be alert to these inconsistencies and exercise caution in interpreting the literature. The following terms are used in these guidelines:

Client: The health care organization receiving the RMOP service.

Client site: The site receiving the RMOP service (the site where the patient is receiving care).

RMOP: Medication order processing provided by a remote pharmacist; this term includes remote order entry and remote order review.

Remote pharmacist: A licensed pharmacist processing the medication order from the remote site.

Remote site: The site that is electronically linked to the client site via a computer system and/or a video or auditory communication system approved by the appropriate state board(s) of pharmacy. The remote site may be a licensed pharmacy or other location permitted by the appropriate state board(s) of pharmacy.

Developed through the ASHP Council on Pharmacy Management and approved by the ASHP Board of Directors on September 25, 2009.

ASHP gratefully acknowledges the expert panel that authored these guidelines. At the time of writing, members of the expert panel held the following positions. Bruce Thompson, M.S., was Director of Pharmacy Services, Hennepin County Medical Center, Minneapolis, MN; Greg Conrad was Director, Pharmacy, Willamette Falls Hospital, Oregon City, OR; Michael O. Gum was Pharmacy Director, Presbyterian Hospital, Charlotte, NC; John M. Kessler, Pharm.D., BCPS, was Founder and Chief Clinical Officer, SecondStory Health LLC, Carrboro, NC; Tim Larson was Pharmacy Director, Cardinal Rxe-source Center–Chicago region, Westmont, IL; Dallas Moore, M.S., was Pharmacy Director, American Fork Hospital–Intermountain Healthcare, American Fork, UT; Kelly Morrison was Director of Sales & Marketing, Rxe-source, Cardinal Health, Houston, TX; and Mickey Price was Vice President, Rxe-source, Cardinal Health, Dublin, OH.

The contributions of Stephen R. Novak, M.P.A., FASHP, to these guidelines are gratefully acknowledged. At the time of his contribution, Mr. Novak was Director, Pharmacy Services, Pardee Hospital, Hendersonville, NC. ASHP also acknowledges the following organizations and individuals for reviewing drafts of these guidelines (review does not imply endorsement): Accreditation Council for Pharmacy Education (ACPE); Healthcare Information and Management Systems Society (HIMSS) Pharmacy Informatics Task Force; Emily Alexander, Pharm.D., BCPS; David B. Archer, D.Ph.; David Aresco, B.S.Pharm., FASCP; John A. Armitstead, M.S., FASHP; Darrel W. Box, M.H.A.; Michael Brown, Pharm.D.; Kimberly K. Daugherty, Pharm.D., BCPS; Doug DeJong, M.B.A., FASHP; Mike Dudzik, M.H.A.; Francis J. Dunn, Jr., B.S.Pharm.; Jeanne Ezell, M.S., FASHP; Kelly Guhr, Pharm.D., BCPS; George Hill, M.B.A.; Linda Horton, Pharm.D.; Jody Jacobson Wedret, FASHP, FCSHP; Ken Kester, Pharm.D., J.D.; Patricia Kienle, M.P.A., FASHP; Nancy Konieczny, M.B.A.; Donald H. Lynx, M.B.A., FASHP; Lynnae M. Mahaney, M.B.A.; Peter G. Mayberry; Roland Patry, Dr.P.H., FASHP; James A. Ponto, M.S., BCNP, FASHP; Cliff Richards, Pharm.D.; Mike Rouse, B.Pharm.(Hons), M.P.S. (ACPE); Terry Seaton, Pharm.D., FCCP, BCPS; Timothy P. Stratton, Ph.D., BCPS, FAPHA; Basil J. Thoppil, M.Sc., Pharm.D.; and Dennis A. Tribble, Pharm.D.

Copyright © 2010, American Society of Health-System Pharmacists, Inc. All rights reserved. Contact ASHP for reprint and permissions requests. This content may not be used for commercial purposes without the express written consent of ASHP.

The bibliographic citation for this document is as follows: American Society of Health-System Pharmacists. ASHP guidelines on remote medication order processing. *Am J Health-Syst Pharm.* 2010; 67:672–7.

ASHP Guidelines on the Safe Use of Automated Compounding Devices for the Preparation of Parenteral Nutrition Admixtures

Purpose

Automated compounding devices (ACDs) are frequently used by pharmacists for the extemporaneous preparation of parenteral nutrition (PN) admixtures. This continuing shift from manual compounding procedures comes as a result of significant advances in automated technology, as well as in response to changing healthcare demands to provide admixture compounding in a safer, more efficient, and more accurate manner. As of 2019, approximately 29% of hospitals in the United States use ACDs. Larger teaching facilities are more likely to implement ACDs, with approximately 58% of hospitals with 400 beds or greater having an ACD in their workflow.[1] Compounders are also used for other types of intravenous (IV) admixtures and in other settings, including home care and long-term care facilities; therefore, the overall magnitude of their use is substantial. As with other automated systems or devices, the benefits can be realized only when the technology is used appropriately. Significant patient harm may occur when safety and quality assurance measures are overlooked or circumvented.[2]

The purpose of these guidelines is to outline key issues that should be considered to safely and cost-effectively incorporate this technology into the pharmacy operations of healthcare organizations. The guidelines focus on PN admixtures, but the recommendations may also be applicable to the use of compounders for other types of IV admixtures. The term "healthcare organization" is used throughout the guidelines as a general descriptor and is intended to be inclusive of any practice setting or type of facility in which compounders are used. These guidelines should be used in conjunction with the ASHP Guidelines on Compounding Sterile Preparations[3]; the American Society for Parenteral and Enteral Nutrition (ASPEN) Standards of Practice for Nutrition Support Pharmacists[4]; the ASPEN, Academy of Nutrition and Dietetics, and ASHP consensus statement on optimizing the electronic health record (EHR) in the parenteral nutrition workflow[5]; and device manufacturers' instruction manuals and training materials. The recommendations in these guidelines represent a consensus of professional judgment, expert opinion, and documented evidence. They are written to establish reasonable goals and to be progressive and challenging yet attainable as best practices in applicable settings. They do not represent minimum levels of practice, and pharmacy professionals are encouraged to exercise their professional judgment in assessing their organization's needs for ACDs and in adapting these guidelines to meet those needs.

Background

The act of extemporaneously compounding any parenteral formulation is complex and not without inherent risks; therefore, compounding tasks are best performed by personnel most qualified to do so. An incompatible, unstable, or contaminated IV infusion may induce significant patient morbidity and even mortality.[2] Pharmacists are specifically educated and legally responsible for performing these tasks safely. Pharmacists are also responsible for training other personnel to perform relatively simple tasks with the least risk possible.

The extemporaneous preparation of multi-additive products, such as PN admixture compounding, should be performed under the direct supervision of a pharmacist and in the appropriate environment according to United States Pharmacopeia (USP) standards and regulatory guidelines.[6] The historical method of compounding these multicomponent admixtures has been to manually use gravity-driven transfers for large-volume additives, such as amino acids, dextrose, lipids, and sterile water. Small-volume additives, such as electrolytes, trace minerals, multivitamins, and drugs, have often been added manually and separately with a syringe. Thus, this compounding method is limited by the visual inspection of volumes transferred between stock containers, as well as by the precision of the calibrations marked on the stock containers or transfer devices.

The manual method of PN admixture compounding is labor-intensive and requires multiple manipulations of infusion containers, sets, syringes, needles, and other equipment, which can lead to extrinsic contamination of the final admixture with sterile and/or nonsterile contaminants. A sterile contaminant can be particulate matter from elastomeric vial enclosures (needle cores), and nonsterile contaminants can be bacteria and other infectious materials. Minimizing the number of extemporaneous manipulations of the parenteral infusion containers and supplies improves compounding efficiency and reduces the risk of extrinsic contamination and associated sequelae.[7]

Technology utilization as an alternative approach to PN admixture compounding has led to potentially improved compounding accuracy with the use of fluid pump technology and software that controls the compounder pump. Fluid can be delivered from the source container to the final container using either a volumetric or a gravimetric fluid pumping system. Volumetric systems transfer a specified volume of fluid from a source container to a final container via a rotary peristaltic pump. The tubing is stretched around a rotor and, as the rotor turns, the solution is pulled from the source container and pushed toward the final container. Measurements are based on the theory that each rotor movement advances a constant amount of fluid through the system. The total volume delivered is calculated by the volume pulled into the tubing by each rotor movement multiplied by the number of movements. These systems usually incorporate a final check of the actual total bag weight by comparing it with a calculated expected weight.

In gravimetric systems, measurement of fluid volume delivered from the source container to the final container is

DOI 10.37573/9781585287048.013

performed by weighing the fluid transferred and dividing the weight by the solution's known specific gravity, thereby converting weight to volume. Two types of gravimetric pumps are available, additive and subtractive; additive pumps are the most common. With an additive pump, a single load cell is positioned to measure each fluid as it is delivered to the final container. With a subtractive pump, load cells are positioned beneath the source containers to measure each fluid as it is being pumped from its source container. Weight is determined by subtracting the post-transfer weight from the pre-transfer weight of the container for each source solution. When all transfers are completed, the system compares the actual total bag weight with a calculated expected weight.

Compared with manual methods, the software application available with ACDs leads to improved compounding accuracy, enforcement of proper compounding sequence, and a reduction in opportunities for human touch contamination. However, preparing PN admixtures with an ACD is not an error-free process. Previous literature has reported higher error rates with manual compounding than with ACDs.[8,9] Organizations may improve the safety of using PN compounding systems by requiring that all doses being compounded pass through an order entry/clinical decision support system and by ensuring that those systems' clinical decision support features are properly enabled and configured.[10]

Justification for the Use of ACDs

When is it appropriate to use compounders, and how will decisions affect others within and outside the pharmacy department? It is incumbent upon the pharmacist to ensure that the department is fully knowledgeable about the operation of the compounder and that a minimum acceptable standard of pharmacy practice is met. First, internal decisions need to be made to justify the expenses associated with this technology. Second, policies and procedures should be in place to assess workflow, establish training programs, and standardize compounder use in the specific pharmacy practice setting. Third, changing current compounder contracts may result in more cost than the savings that might appear in the new contracts. Specifically, the initial incorporation of an automated compounder into daily pharmacy practice is a labor-intensive effort, and such transitions can be disruptive and can even increase the risk of errors, particularly during staff orientation to new devices. Such changes must be carefully reviewed and, if they are determined to be worthwhile, a well-coordinated transition plan should be devised in advance. Whether transition costs (including the potential for unused sets and supplies) can be deferred to the new contract is another factor for consideration.

The principal emphasis associated with using ACDs in healthcare organizations should be improving patient care and enhancing mixed PN prepared in the pharmacy while maintaining efficiency and cost-effectiveness. "Cost-effectiveness" is a relative term with respect to personnel, as the labor saved is often redirected to other aspects of pharmacist care that could also improve patient safety. Time that was previously spent on operations associated with PN admixture compounding can now be aimed at other issues, such as optimization of drug and nutritional therapies, reorganization of product utilization, quality assurance programs, and augmentation of other core pharmacy services.

Specific points related to cost justification of ACDs may include the following:

1. Enhanced efficiency and worker safety during the PN compounding process and patient safety with parenteral use.
2. Reduction in labor associated with manually compounded PN admixtures. Assessment of the overall labor and material costs associated with the current manual compounding methods should include hidden costs, such as pharmacists' time to perform calculations, quality assurance checks, and compounder set-up, as well as staff training (initial and ongoing).
3. Reduction in waste through more efficient use of base solutions and additives. Inventory can often be reduced by consolidating source solutions to a few high-concentration, large-volume additives.

In some cases, in which the cost of implementing automated compounding technology in one facility is prohibitive, healthcare organizations have opted to explore regional compounding centers or outsourcing to contractors.

Performance Requirements and Responsibilities

Use of automated devices for compounding PN admixtures should be clearly defined by the healthcare organization and the manufacturer. This definition should include the ongoing responsibilities of the pharmacy department and those of the manufacturer during and after implementation of the compounder in the pharmacy practice setting.

Three areas need to be clearly defined before choosing an automated compounding system: (1) the system's performance requirements, (2) the manufacturer's responsibilities, and (3) the pharmacy department's responsibilities. Performance requirements of the automated compounding system should ensure the following at a minimum:

1. The compounder exceeds the level of accuracy achieved with manual compounding. The ACD should be accurate to within 5% of the amount programmed, with verification of the amount pumped versus the programmed amount for each ingredient.
2. The ACD has inherent safeguards (e.g., barcode technology), including the ability to detect inadvertent source-solution mix-ups; the ability to detect situations that could result in inaccurate deliveries, such as occluded transfer-set tubing and empty source containers; and the ability to keep incompatible source solutions separate.
3. The automated compounding software alerts the user when formulation issues arise.
4. The automated compounding software meets ASPEN standards for PN label formats.[10]
5. The automated compounding software assists the pharmacist in producing physicochemically compatible PN formulations.
6. The automated compounding software provides useful clinical information.
7. The automated compounding software interfaces with the existing EHR wherever possible to allow orders transfer from the EHR to the compounder after pharmacist verification to help in optimizing patient care and avoiding therapeutic duplications.

The contractual agreement with the manufacturer should provide continuous support of the compounder and software, including information and software updates, problem solving, and emergency coverage. The Food and Drug Administration (FDA) considers all ACDs class II devices,[11] and as such they must comply with federal regulations. The manufacturer's responsibilities are as follows:

1. The manufacturer should ensure compliance with all FDA requirements for medical devices.
2. The manufacturer should provide support for the compounder and its software throughout the life of the contract.
3. The manufacturer should routinely provide the latest version of the compounder software in a timely manner.
4. The manufacturer should ensure adequate availability of compounding supplies.
5. The manufacturer should provide detailed information and instructions on the appropriate use of the compounder and its software. References should be provided when appropriate.
6. The manufacturer should comply with FDA requirements for reporting adverse events.

Within the pharmacy department, specific policies and procedures should be developed to address responsibilities for compounder operations and maintenance, staff training, and monitoring compounder performance at all times. Before selecting and implementing an automated compounder, the pharmacy department should do the following:

1. Define and agree on automated compounding system needs and performance requirements.
2. Develop an implementation team with a lead person.
3. Develop a set of policies and procedures.
4. Develop a well-defined plan for backup and downtime procedures.

Control of the ACDs in Daily Operations

The pharmacy department is responsible for the use, maintenance, and performance of the ACD, including decisions about who has access to the compounder and its operations. Specific consideration should be given to the following:

1. Only designated pharmacy department personnel should have access to the compounder and its software. The level of access should correspond to the level of authority and expertise of the personnel.
2. Before being granted access to a compounder, pharmacy personnel should pass established competency standard testing.
3. Access to and use of the compounder by pharmacy support personnel (e.g., pharmacy technicians, students, other designated support staff) should be directly supervised by an authorized pharmacist.
4. The additive configuration or sequence of the compounder for compounding PN admixtures should not be altered from the established format without the authorization of a designated pharmacist.
5. Unless allowed per approved facility specific policy, the compounder should not be used for any purpose other than PN admixture compounding without authorization from a designated pharmacist. If the compounder is used for other extemporaneous drug preparation, this should be done separately from the schedule for PN admixtures. The use of the compounder in this manner will likely require the use of new compounding sets and admixture configurations.
6. Operation of the compounder should follow manufacturer recommendation (e.g., tubing changes).
7. With the current prevalence of medication shortages, pharmacist review and verification should be required for any changes to individual product ingredients (needed to reflect availability, shortages, and conservation, among other variables) and to prevent ordering of unavailable products.
8. Only the core equipment needed should be in the hood when compounding, and unnecessary items should not be kept or stored in the hood (e.g., extra labels and needles).
9. If the ACD will be used for multiple patient populations (e.g., adults and pediatrics), an authorized pharmacist should ensure the formula templates are clearly marked to avoid compounding errors, such as using incorrect ingredient concentrations.

Safety and Efficacy Features

The complexity of ACD functions makes it imperative that the pharmacy department develop a specific plan for ensuring safe and efficacious use at all times. The safety and efficacy features should outline the core principles necessary for carrying out the complex tasks of PN compounding. The plan should identify the minimum standards that are routinely assessed through an established monitoring and surveillance program. ACDs on the market differ in hardware design, mechanisms of fluid transfer, and software applications. Consequently, sterility and quality assurance testing procedures and measures are also different, including routine assessments of accuracy in the delivery of correct amounts of nutrients. Consideration should be given to the following in accordance with the device manufacturer's specific instructions:

1. Establishing minimum competency standards for all personnel who have access to and operate the compounder. Competency standards should ensure that the compounder user has sufficient expertise to identify errors that may inadvertently bypass quality assurance systems. For all personnel operating the compounder, the competency standards should be reviewed and validated on a routine basis to ensure compliance with federal and local regulation along with sterile compounding standards (e.g., USP general chapter 79712).
2. Establishing specific procedures for the operation of the compounder that standardize its use, irrespective of the individual operator. Changes in compounder operations should occur only when authorized and should be communicated to all staff involved in compounding.
3. Including sterility and quality assurance measures that meet USP general chapter 797 sterile compounding standards to avoid extrinsic contamination and ensure accurate delivery of PN additives.[12]
4. Ensuring that compounder tubing changes occur at appropriate specified time intervals in accordance with the manufacturer's recommendations.

5. Devising methods for assessing and calibrating the accuracy of the compounder in delivering precise levels of substrates and additives in accordance with the manufacturer's recommendations.
6. Developing a plan on how to utilize reports included within the automated compounding in documenting daily activities.
7. Developing a contingency plan and a readily available backup system or method for providing uninterrupted PN therapy to patients in the event of compounder failure.
8. Ensuring that adequate amounts of solutions and supplies for automated compounding are on hand.

Quality Assurance Monitoring and Documentation

ACDs are intended to provide a higher margin of accuracy and to streamline the labor-intensive tasks associated with the manual extemporaneous preparation of large-volume, multi-additive PN admixtures and other admixtures. The compounders are not designed to replace oversight functions, which require the expertise of a pharmacist.

The pharmacy department may work with other departments to assess the compounder's performance if such expertise is not available within the pharmacy department. For example, portions of PN admixtures may be sent to the healthcare organization's laboratory to determine dextrose content. However, laboratory methods are usually designed for biological rather than pharmaceutical systems and should be validated to meet USP requirements for the components being tested. If outside departments participate in the quality assurance program, their methods should be appropriately validated in accordance with USP specifications and the results documented within the pharmacy department records on the compounder's performance.

The pharmacy department should develop a monitoring and surveillance plan with output reports that encompasses the principles outlined under the section on safety and efficacy features. The plan should detail specific policies and procedures that will ensure the continuing operation of the ACD at optimum performance levels at all times. The data generated by the monitoring procedures should be reported to the pharmacy director and other appropriate oversight personnel and kept as a permanent record of the compounder's operations. These reports should be regularly reviewed in the assessment of trends and other long-term measures of performance. Specific consideration should be given to the following:

1. Establishing performance standards and continuous quality assurance measures for assessing the compounder's performance and product quality during setup and in process (during compounding) and end-process testing.
2. Establishing quality assurance testing of user-defined software variables validating that the correct responses to user commands occur.
3. Validating all quality assurance testing before implementation.
4. Establishing a minimum performance standard for each quality assurance test (e.g., deviations in the accuracy of delivering a single additive cannot exceed a predetermined percentage error without immediate corrective actions).
5. Documenting all quality assurance data daily. A comprehensive review of the data and documentation of performance trends should be performed at scheduled intervals as necessitated by aseptic conditions. The compounder should have scheduled, routine cleaning and maintenance according to the manufacturer's recommendations to ensure proper operation.
6. The availability of readily accessible reports from the compounding device is a feature that should be considered when selecting a device.

Storage, Inventory, and Medication Shortages

The pharmacy department is responsible for housing the ACD, related disposable supplies, and admixture ingredients. Other departments, such as materials management or supply chain, may order and store additional supplies for the compounder yet defer to the pharmacy for the selection of the components necessary for proper compounder operation. Specific consideration should be given to the following:

1. Maintaining an adequate inventory of supplies necessary for compounder operation and patient needs.
2. Procuring large-volume PN components (amino acids, dextrose, and lipids) that have adequate physicochemical data that ensure the stability, compatibility, and safety of the final formulations commensurate with the data for single-source products.
3. Any proposed substitute products should be assessed for compatibility and approved by designated pharmacy personnel qualified to do so and possibly by the pharmacy and therapeutics committee if clinical issues are identified.
4. If a healthcare organization's contract requires a change in the brand of parenteral products, designated pharmacy personnel should verify that the new products are compatible. If a new product is approved, designated pharmacy personnel should verify that the new product is compatible, add it to the compounder formulary, and revise the admixture requirements and instructions relevant to the compounder's operations. In addition, EHR updates need to happen in the same time to make the transition seamless.

Hospitals and medical facilities across the nation are dealing with shortages of medications and supplies daily. The reasons behind drug shortages are varied and complex. According to the FDA, the leading causes of drug shortages are manufacturing problems, delays in manufacturing or shipping, and lack of availability of the active pharmaceutical ingredient.[13] Specific consideration concerning drug shortages should be given to the following:

1. Changes made in the EHR in response to a drug shortage should be associated with matching changes to the PN components within the ACDs. This is imperative to avoid patient harm in the midst of an urgent response to a critical medication shortage.
2. Having multiple concentrations of a specific medication loaded in an automated dispensing cabinet carries a risk of infusing the wrong concentration; proper use of barcode technology and other safeguards built within the ACDs minimize that risk.

Education and Training

PN is a complex therapeutic modality reflected in complex prescriptions with dozens of ingredients, each with clinical rationales, dosing implications, and interaction potential. As such, the pharmacist reviewing the PN order should demonstrate competency to optimize the delivery of safe and effective therapy. In addition, the pharmacist and/or the pharmacy technician preparing or directly supervising the preparation of the PN should demonstrate competency to prepare an appropriate and safe admixture for each patient. Institutions should implement policies and procedures addressing determination of competent PN order review and preparation. Competence should be assessed initially and on an annual basis at a minimum. Any identified medication errors related to PN order review or preparation will necessitate more frequent competency assessment in addition to a systematic review of the PN use process.[14] Specific consideration should be given to ensuring the following:

1. Pharmacy administration determines the individuals who will be responsible for education and training in the use of the compounders.
2. All education and training are documented in a permanent record maintained in the pharmacy department and in personnel files.
3. All pharmacy personnel using or supervising compounder operations are tested at regular intervals to ensure that individuals meet the department's minimum competency standards.
4. Retraining, competency assessment, and appropriate documentation accompany upgrades and new versions of the compounder to ensure the continued proficiency of personnel, safety of compounder operations, and adequacy of oversight.

Device Variability

ACDs are marketed by several manufacturers. Even though there are similarities among compounders, there may be significant differences in the design, accuracy, operation, maintenance, software, and manufacturing support, among other things. The safe operation and supervision of any given compounder depend on adherence to the manufacturer's specific instructions and continuous quality assurance monitoring of compounder performance. The safe and efficient operation of an automated compounding system depends on defined responsibilities for the pharmacy and manufacturer, as well as on strict adherence to policies, procedures, and quality assurance programs.

Conclusion

ACDs are frequently used for extemporaneous preparation of PN admixtures to provide admixture compounding in a safer, more efficient, and more accurate manner. As with other automated systems or devices, benefits can be realized only when the technology is used appropriately, and significant patient harm may occur when safety and quality assurance measures are overlooked or circumvented. These guidelines outline key issues that should be considered to safely and cost-effectively incorporate this technology into the pharmacy operations of healthcare organizations. Pharmacy professionals are encouraged to exercise their professional judgment in assessing their organization's needs for ACDs and in adapting these guidelines to meet those needs.

References

1. Automated Compounding Devices. Pharmacy Purchasing & Products. Published 2019. Accessed July 28, 2021. https://www.pppmag.com/article/2431
2. Food and Drug Administration. Safety alert: hazards of precipitation associated with parenteral nutrition. *Am J Hosp Pharm.* 1994;51:1427–1428.
3. American Society of Health-System Pharmacists. ASHP guidelines on compounding sterile preparations. *Am J Health-Syst Pharm.* 2014;71:145–166. doi:10.2146/sp140001
4. Tucker A, Ybarra J, Bingham A, et al. American Society for Parenteral and Enteral Nutrition (A.S.P.E.N.) standards of practice for nutrition support pharmacists. *Nutr Clin Pract.* 2015;30:139–146. doi:10.1177/0884533614550318
5. Vanek VW, Ayers P, Kraft M, et al. A call to action for optimizing the electronic health record in the parenteral nutrition workflow. *Am J Health-Syst Pharm.* 2018;75:1400–1420. doi:10.2146/ajhp180276
6. American Society of Hospital Pharmacists. ASHP technical assistance bulletin on quality assurance for pharmacy-prepared sterile products. *Am J Hosp Pharm.* 1993;50:2386–2398.
7. McClendon RR. A comparative evaluation of methods used to compound parenteral nutrition solutions. *Nutr Support Serv.* 1983;3:46–49.
8. Eckel SF, Higgins JP, Hess E, et al. Multicenter study to evaluate the benefits of technology-assisted workflow on i.v. room efficiency, costs, and safety. *Am J Health-Syst Pharm.* 2019;76: 895–901. doi:10.1093/ajhp/zxz080
9. Lin AC, Deng Y, Thaibah H, et al. The impact of using an intravenous workflow management system (IVWMS) on cost and patient safety. *Int J Med Inform.* 2018;115:73–79.
10. Ayers P, Adams S, Boullata J, et al. American Society for Parenteral and Enteral Nutrition. A.S.P.E.N. parenteral nutrition safety consensus recommendations. *JPEN J Parenter Enteral Nutr.* 2014;38(3):296–333. doi:10.1177/0148607113511992.
11. Trautman KA. *The FDA and Worldwide Quality System Requirements Guidebook for Medical Devices.* ASQ Quality Press; 1997.
12. United States Pharmacopeial Convention. General chapter <797> pharmaceutical compounding—sterile preparations. Accessed July 28, 2021. https://www.usp.org/compounding/general-chapter-797
13. Fox ER, Sweet BV, Jensen V. Drug shortages: a complex health care crisis. *Mayo Clinic Proc.* 2014.89(3):361–373.
14. Boullata JI, Holcombe B, Sacks G, et al; Parenteral Nutrition Safety Committee, American Society for Parenteral and Enteral Nutrition. Standardized competencies for parenteral nutrition order review and parenteral nutrition preparation, including compounding: the ASPEN model. *Nutr Clin Pract.* 2016;31(4):548–555. doi:10.1177/0884533616653833

Developed through the ASHP Section of Pharmacy Informatics and Technology and approved by the ASHP Board of Directors on September 3, 2021. These guidelines supersede the ASHP Guidelines on the Safe Use of Automated Compounding Devices for the Preparation of Parenteral Nutrition Admixtures dated April 27, 2000.

ASHP gratefully acknowledges the contributions of authors of the previous version of these guidelines: David F. Driscoll, PhD; Katherine Giampietro, MHA; and Michael D. Sanborn, MS, FASHP, FACHE.

The authors have declared no potential conflicts of interest.

Benjamin Iredell, PharmD, MBA, BCPS, Cedars-Sinai Medical Center, Los Angeles, CA.

Hesham Mourad, PharmD, BCPS, BCCCP, CPHIMS, Mayo Clinic, Jacksonville, FL.

Nancy A. Nickman, PhD, RPh, University of Utah College of Pharmacy, Salt Lake City, UT, and University of Utah Health, Salt Lake City, UT.

Hao Dieu, PharmD, Kaiser Permanente, Walnut Creek, CA.

Gary Austin, PharmD, BCPS, BD, Detroit, MI.

Rani Goradia, PharmD, Marshfield Clinic Health System, Woodbury, MN.

Joseph Scott Wade, PharmD, WVU Medicine, Morgantown, WV.

Justin Goette, PharmD, Lexington Medical Center, West Columbia, SC.

Tanya O. Ezekiel, PharmD, BCPS, Prisma Health, Columbia, SC.

Brendan R. Begnoche, PharmD, Nuvance Health, Danbury, CT.

Andrew Liu, PharmD, CPHIMS, Nordic Consulting, Chicago, IL.

Stacey English, PharmD, MHCI, Children's Hospital of the King's Daughters, Norfolk, VA.

Copyright © 2022, American Society of Health-System Pharmacists, Inc. All rights reserved. Contact ASHP for reprint and permissions requests. This content may not be used for commercial purposes without the express written consent of ASHP.

The bibliographic citation for this document is as follows: American Society of Health-System Pharmacists. ASHP guidelines on the safe use of automated compounding devices for the preparation of parenteral nutrition admixtures. *Am J Health-Syst Pharm.* 2022; 79:730–5.

ASHP Guidelines on the Safe Use of Automated Dispensing Cabinets

Automated dispensing cabinet (ADC) technology is used to improve patient care, enhance the efficiency and accuracy of medication dispensing in the medication-use system, support medication storage and security, and provide evaluation of ADC-user interactions. ADC use has become widespread in healthcare institutions, with 93% of hospitals using ADCs in their medication-use systems,[1] and 70.2% using ADCs as a primary method of maintenance dose distribution.[2]

Implementation steps and objectives to support an ADC system include the following:

- Software and hardware technology for optimal operations are available and supported by knowledgeable staff
- ADC maintenance is supported with adequate personnel, minimum downtime, and analytical reporting for ordering and restocking
- Staff education and competency on ADC operation are supported at a high level
- Interfaces to other technologies supporting medication use (eg, intravenous [IV] infusion systems) are created to enable efficient workflows and enhanced medication diversion detection
- Interoperability is established with the electronic health record (EHR) and related systems
- Safe and secure operation is ensured with real-time reporting functionality of medication diversion
- Mechanical operation and inventory management capabilities exist to allow efficient, accurate, and optimized availability of medication
- Employment of other technology is used, eg, barcode scanning, biometric identification, special storage and alerting features
- ADCs in procedural and non-acute extended patient care areas (eg, long-term care, ambulatory clinics) have the same standard of medication control as traditional patient care areas
- These guidelines address components of ADC technology implementation and important detailed steps to meet and maintain basic ADC requirements.

Background

Appropriate, accurate, and timely distribution of medications to patients is a well-established responsibility of pharmacists. Use of ADCs has become the standard of care for the medication-use process in healthcare systems.[2] ASHP supports use of ADCs, because they are essential to provide quality patient care, secure storage of medications, and ensure viability of the medication-use process in healthcare organizations.

These ASHP guidelines reflect the evolving and increased use of ADCs to improve patient safety and allow secure access to a broad selection of medications. Consideration of the use of ADCs must include serious evaluation of existing and potential opportunities for error and the implementation of mitigating strategies to minimize or prevent such errors. Pharmacists have a professional responsibility to ensure that appropriate policies, procedures, and quality assurance programs are in place to address the safety, accuracy, security, and patient confidentiality of automated pharmacy systems, including ADCs.[3]

Requirements

ADCs must provide accurate and controlled storage, dispensing, and monitoring of medications while providing medications in an efficient and safe manner. The ability of ADCs to accomplish these requirements has improved since their introduction in the late 1980s, leading to the technology becoming the primary means of medication distribution.[1,2] To be successful at implementing and sustaining ADC benefits, an organization must ensure that the ADC will help optimize the medication-use process and meet financial, operational, and clinical goals of the organization.

Information Technology Infrastructure

Technical infrastructure that will best support the system and allow for smooth operation and future growth is of utmost importance. Infrastructure requirements include servers, interfaces, upgrades, integration with other systems, and security. It is essential to ensure that both physical and personnel infrastructure necessary to maintain the system are in place.

Servers. Servers are typically client-hosted but are becoming increasingly cloud-based as health systems move away from owning and maintaining their own servers.[4] Regardless of the hosting approach, servers should be readily available and highly reliable to minimize workflow interruptions. Servers must be adequately sized to store both formulary and user information, as well as transactional information for analytics and reporting, and should be scalable to allow for future growth. Consideration should also be given to minimizing the amount of redundant software maintenance (eg, formulary maintenance). Depending on an organization's size, an ADC server might be a single standalone server. Larger organizations and integrated delivery networks (IDNs) may employ integrated servers that work together but physically separate different data components into separate servers. Options for server redundancy to offer protection and limit interruptions in the event of unplanned downtime must also be considered. A range of options are available, from data refreshes every few hours to more frequent data refreshes that support minimal losses in the event of unplanned downtime.

Partnering with the information technology (IT) department is essential for proper server maintenance, such as operating system patches and security software to protect against viruses and malware, as well as the integrity of frequent data backups. Maintenance may be supplied internally by the system for virtual machines or by the vendor (more

DOI 10.37573/9781585287048.014

commonly for standalone servers). In either case, IT should be engaged to assist and help coordinate proper server security. Finally, an organizational downtime and recovery policy and procedure should be developed and implemented to minimize disruptions in patient care.

Interfaces. With the growth of large healthcare IDNs and proliferation of multiple electronic clinical applications used within healthcare systems, ADC vendors have moved toward integrated platforms that simplify and standardize system maintenance. The ADC system must work seamlessly with other clinical systems, which include at a minimum EHRs, pharmacy information systems (PISs), and admission/discharge/transfer systems. Each of these other systems serve as the source of primary data for the formulary, barcodes, patient information, medication profile, and medication orders. The ADC provides source information for other clinical systems through interfaces based on Health Level Seven International (HL7) standards. Affected clinical systems include inventory information for the PIS, dispense information for billing systems (for organizations that charge on dispense), usage information for inventory management systems, and user information for a domain management system. Finally, many systems also use interface engines to streamline system connectivity, especially when multiple systems come from the same vendor.

During the build phase of ADC system implementation, all interfaces must be thoroughly tested to ensure that both accurate and current information is transmitted into the ADC system. In addition to the ADC vendor, the organization and EHR vendor play important roles in successful implementation and maintenance of the ADC system. Both the ADC and EHR vendors have test plans for the implementation process, which should be used in conjunction with the organization's testing plan, and all will be incorporated to create successful interfaces. If there is a change in EHR or ADC vendor, new interfaces and a retrievable archive of dispense data for reference purposes needs to be created.

System Integration. In addition to foundational clinical systems described above, integration of several optional systems with the ADC system must be completed if they are used. Other dispensing devices, such as central pharmacy robotics, or ADC replenishment may require connectivity. Pharmacy inventory management systems used to manage a perpetual inventory based on all pick and restock transactions within the pharmacy must also be considered. These systems may utilize dispensing robotics and can also be used for both central fill within a hospital or across a healthcare system. Finally, many healthcare organizations also use a controlled substances (CS) system that provides secure storage for CS and integrates with the ADC system to provide secure CS dispensing.

Database management within the ADC system involves maintenance of information integral to ADC workflow, including ADC formularies, barcodes, users, user roles, rules, and alerts. In multihospital IDNs, these databases are typically shared between all sites to streamline support processes and allow for sharing of ADC formulary, barcodes, and user role information. There are scenarios in which IDNs are required to maintain separate databases at each facility (eg, separate PIS and/or different ADC version), but typically the goal is to get all facilities on a single database.

Upgrades. ADC upgrades involve updating hardware and/or software. While hardware upgrades are not uncommon, timely software upgrades may coincide to prolong the life of cabinets. These efforts may allow for core hardware to remain in place (sometimes with an option of swapping drawer types or configurations within the drawers) while any major software updates occur. There may also be the option of keeping the cabinet intact while changing the computer system that drives the cabinets. This model allows for new functionality and changes to the user interface while minimizing costs by allowing the healthcare organization to continue using existing hardware. Upgrades will also involve updates to the operating system, which can include security patches and necessary hardware changes.

Safe and Secure Operation

Topics to be considered to ensure safe and secure operation of ADCs include but are not limited to access control, medication stocking and dispensing, the override function, return and waste of medications, emergency access, ADC placement, and alerts.

Access Control. Safe and secure operation of ADCs starts with well-defined processes for granting and maintaining user access. Current technology allows for centralized user management through the IT or pharmacy department. A domain management system allows for centralized control of access to multiple applications, while the user can utilize the same credentials for each application. For ADC systems, the domain management system must allow for immediate suspension of access if an employee is suspended, terminated, or under investigation.

The ADC should also have a mechanism to lock accounts of inactive users who have not been successfully authenticated within a facility-defined time period. The organization's ADC access policy should address privileges of all clinical team members who administer or manage medications, including learners. A single ADC system often supports multiple facilities within an IDN and should use the same user templates and policy to create standardization throughout the organization.

Biometric identification may be available for an ADC system. Staff should be required to use biometrics, and if a particular individual's biometrics are unable to be consistently recognized, the use of user ID and password or an alternative workflow recognized by regulatory bodies and organizational policy should be followed. Use of biometric ID data must meet individual state requirements for security and user consent.

Medication Stocking and Dispensing. Organizations should establish processes for loading and withdrawal of medications from the ADC by the pharmacy, including how and when medications are supplied to the ADC and authorized personnel. The layout and type of storage areas within the ADC can ensure the correct medication, dose, and dosage form are being refilled or withdrawn. When medications are refilled, barcode technology should be consistently used to ensure medication is placed in the correct storage area. ADCs can be configured so that personnel refilling an ADC are required to scan both the medication and the storage area to minimize the number of ADC fill errors.

The barcode database is a critical component to ensure safe ADC use when stocking, removing, and returning medications to the ADC. The pharmacy department should establish procedures for addition and maintenance of barcodes in the database. Only appropriately trained and credentialed staff members should add barcodes to the drug dictionary. Typically, one credentialed pharmacy staff member adds the barcode and a pharmacist verifies the barcode, or the barcode is otherwise as allowed by state regulations.

All medications dispensed from the pharmacy should have a barcode. Although most medications have a barcode incorporated by the manufacturer, pharmacy is responsible for adding barcodes for compounded or repackaged items and those items with unusable barcodes. Supplemental barcode labeling may be provided by special equipment or under contract with a wholesaler or other specialty company.

Barcode technology should be used when a practitioner removes medication from an ADC for administration. Risk avoidance should be weighed carefully against the time requirement for a practitioner to scan on removal. Organizations utilizing barcode-assisted medication administration (BCMA) technology reduce risk of error. If the ADC is configured with drawers that limit access to a medication and barcode scanning is required for adding medications to the device, the risk of a wrong medication being dispensed is greatly reduced. When a practitioner is returning a medication to the ADC, barcode scanning should be used to verify the medication and storage location.

ADC systems may allow remote queuing of medication withdrawals. The process allows a practitioner to select patient medications for withdrawal while away from the ADC by completing the process through HER integration or a Web-based portal. When medications are in the queue, the practitioner can access them at the ADC. Remote access to the ADC should be considered a tool to decrease wait times and allow optimization of workflow. Nurses may also witness and document waste of medications via the EHR or Web portal, rather than at the ADC. Organizations should evaluate processes for workflow benefits and compliance with laws and regulations.

ADCs can be configured as either open-access or restricted devices. Restricted machines only allow access to medications via a verified medication order or defined automatic override list. In open-access devices, individuals administering medications have unrestricted access to all medications in the machine. The Institute for Safe Medication Practices (ISMP) does not recommend the use of open-access devices.[5] Open-access devices should be limited to areas where pharmacists are unable to review medication orders (eg, ambulatory, radiology, and operative areas), due to standards and regulations that require prospective review of medication orders by pharmacists. Restricted devices have been successfully deployed in the emergency department (ED), where historically open-access devices have been used. As more pharmacists begin to review ED orders, ADCs should be converted to restricted status to limit opportunity for error. Successful conversion of an ED -based ADC to restricted access can be accomplished by partnering with ED personnel to develop appropriate turnaround times, override lists, and autoverification algorithms.[6]

Override Function. If a medication stored in a restricted ADC is needed but there is not an active order on the patient profile, permission to override may be allowed, although this practice is discouraged. Medications can have access grouped by practitioner type, specialty, or location to ensure they are unit-specific and available only for emergency needs or approved protocols.[5] A list of override medications should be defined by the organization's pharmacy oversight committee, typically the pharmacy and therapeutics committee. Guidance for developing this list is available both from ASHP7 and ISMP.[8] A policy should be developed to define the criteria by which a medication can be added to the override list and the frequency with which the list shall be reviewed. Development of this list requires weighing risk versus benefit (ie, potentially delayed patient care against the reduced risk achieved by pharmacist review of the medication order).

The reason for an override must be documented when withdrawing a medication so that data can be standardized for later analysis. A second individual should be required to verify the correct patient, medication, dosage form, dose, strength, route, frequency, duration of therapy, and indication upon override removal of medications included in a list of high-alert medications or from certain ADCs.[7] ADCs should be configured to require entering a minimum number of letter characters (ISMP[8] recommends using at least 5 letters) during a medication search to decrease the likelihood of similar medication names appearing on the screen. The number and types of overrides should be regularly reviewed for process improvement and identification of safety issues.

Return and Waste of Medications. Organizations must develop policies and standard procedures that follow federal and state laws for medications returned or wasted using an ADC. The ADC can be configured to require documentation of the reason for wasting a medication. Standardized responses for medication waste documentation should be developed to support data analysis and process improvement. When returning unopened medication, the ADC can be configured to return it only to the original storage area or to a separate returned medication space, and barcode scanning should be employed to ensure the medication is returned to the proper location.

Emergency Access. ADCs rely on electrical power and are typically equipped with a battery backup. However, procedures are necessary to outline processes for dispensing medications in the event of an extended power loss.

ADC Placement. The number of devices to deploy and placement are important decisions. Several factors impact the number of ADCs in patient care areas, including number of beds, patient acuity, floor plan, budget, medication distribution model, and other institution-specific issues. Pharmacy and nursing distribution experiences and vendor recommendations will drive an appropriate ADC ratio for each care area. ADCs should be located in areas that are well illuminated and ventilated, central to patient care areas, connected to the hospital network and systems, supplied with emergency power, and have efficient caregiver workspace with a quiet zone designation.

ADC size is also a factor in determining placement. Time-motion studies may be done to determine ideal locations. State laws and regulations may require ADCs to be placed in a secured and/or locked area.

Alerts. ADC systems allow for passive or active messaging and alerts to guide clinical decision-making. Alerts should be standardized and approved across an IDN using a governing body and developed with consideration for alert fatigue. The process for developing new alerts should include stakeholders from those who will receive the alert and consideration of other safety measures already in place for a particular medication. For example, alerting should only provide information that is relevant at the time of administration if the alert appears on withdrawal of a medication from the ADC. Metrics on alert overrides should be consistently and periodically evaluated, including metrics per individual and rationales, and the governing body should consider the effectiveness of each alert.[9] Consider the Five Rights of Clinical Decision Support[10] when developing and maintaining alerts.

Configuration and Inventory Selection

Configuration of ADCs can be highly customized, depending on device design and organizational preference. Cabinets may be configured with drawers, towers, or a combination of both, in various sizes. Options may include return bins, integrated locks on refrigeration units, or other customizations. Frame selection and configuration are driven by several factors, including the organization's distribution model, space available for equipment, number and type of medications to be stored, control level requirements, and the care role of the user. Within each device, the number of storage locations may vary and include open or lidded pockets with features that guide users to specific medications or allow ease of reconfiguration.

Safe Configuration Considerations. Safety is the primary concern when determining medication configuration within the ADC. Restricting access to medications through appropriate configuration reduces the potential for inadvertently selecting the wrong medication. ADCs should be configured to prevent clinically inappropriate medications from being loaded into specific cabinets without prior approval (eg, enabling ADC features to prevent adult-sized medications from being loaded in ADCs for pediatric and neonatal use). Storage of high-alert medications, reversal agents, medications with common look-alike/sound-alike (LASA) names and packaging, and agents prone to diversion within a matrix drawer or tower is inappropriate.[5] Each medication and strength should be loaded in an individual, locked ADC compartment that opens only when the specific medication is requested. If neuromuscular blocking agents (NMBAs) must be stored in ADCs (in a critical care, ED, or perioperative setting), organizations should standardize storage practices by keeping NMBAs in lock-lidded pockets with a prominently displayed auxiliary label on the pocket that states: "WARNING: CAUSES RESPIRATORY ARREST—PATIENT MUST BE VENTILATED."[5,11-13] Organizations should also consider using an interactive alert that requires users to enter or select clinically relevant information for removal of the NMBA (eg, purpose for removal, patient ventilation status).[11,13] Interactive alerts can also be used to warn staff when removing other high-alert medications and are customizable. LASA or high-alert medications, and medications with multiple strengths, should be positioned throughout the ADC, rather than near one another, to minimize incorrect restocking or retrieval. Access to refrigerated medications should be monitored through the ADC system whenever possible and may be accomplished via an integrated refrigerator or ADC-connected lock that provides simple access to information and temperature monitoring. Secure refrigeration bins should be utilized for types of medications that require refrigerated storage. Items with a limited beyond-use date (BUD) outside of refrigeration should be labeled with the appropriate BUD and stored in a drawer away from the computer/monitor or any warm or heated sections of the cabinet.

To address staff safety, frequently dispensed medications should be positioned in an area of the ADC that is ergonomically friendly for both pharmacy and nursing staff. For example, placement of frequently used medications toward the bottom of the ADC should be avoided to reduce the need for bending or stooping to retrieve or restock.

Inventory Selection Considerations. The pharmacy department, as part of an interdisciplinary committee that provides medication safety oversight,[5] should develop criteria for determining medications and quantities that will be stored under different levels of access control in specific configurations of drawers, bins, pockets, or other compartments. Criteria should be determined based on the organization's medication distribution model, needs, and acuity of patients and should address all elements listed in **Box 1**. Medication storage practices should be routinely reviewed and adjusted based on prescribing patterns, utilization, and specific unit needs. When possible, a small number of ADC pockets should be kept unassigned in the event they are needed for a patient-supplied medication or other unique situation.

Monitoring, Reporting, and Surveillance

Topics to be addressed regarding monitoring, reporting, and surveillance include but are not limited to inventory counts; discrepancy management; diversion surveillance, monitoring, and detection; and medication dispense transaction reconciliation.

Inventory Counts. Because ADCs have become a common source of diversion, CS should only be stored in secured pockets (individually locked-lidded), and strict attention should be paid to ADC CS inventory counts. Par levels should be kept to quantities that facilitate ease of counting to increase inventory accuracy. Pocket settings should include blind counts, which require the user to count the remaining number of items in the pocket and enter this information into the ADC to complete the transaction.[14,15] Blind counts alone will not guarantee that inventories stay accurate; regular cycle counts of pockets must be included in written policies and documented accordingly when completed. Based on a case study by Blackmere et al,[16] it may be most productive for nursing to perform a weekly count only of CS accessed since the last inventory 3 weeks out of every month and then complete a full inventory of CS once a month. Cycle counts should be intermittently observed to prevent blind count work-arounds. Removal or unloading of CS that are not frequently used will decrease CS inventory time, decrease risk of delays in detecting diversion of low- or no-use CS, and make a valuable internal footprint available.

BOX 1. Inventory Selection Criteria

Frequency and appropriateness of individual medication use

Identification of medications considered to be inappropriate for inclusion in ADCs, such as products with short expiration dates, with special preparation or storage requirements, that present cross-contamination risks, or are hazardous

Party responsible for medication safety oversight and administrative control of medication availability in the ADC, such as the pharmacy and therapeutics committee[5]

Specification of the individual(s) responsible for adding, modifying, or reviewing formulary items on a regular and ongoing basis to ensure they correctly display and interface map with other devices or applications

Tall-man lettering, standardized concentration displays, and form designations as examples of many items that improve safety in use

Procedures to prevent and minimize the incorrect return of medications directly to the ADC by nursing staff to decrease the potential for error

Procedures for keeping policies, procedures, and education current

Policies addressing medication integrity, including:

- The importance of accuracy and integrity of product labels
- How to handle medications that are removed from an ADC but not used
- How to account for medication waste
- Checking products for expiration and BUDs
- Identification and follow-up on tampered products
- Product storage
- Procedures for delivering medications to patient care units and individual patients

Controls that ensure accurate restocking of ADCs, such as:

- Steps to ensure the ADC system permits use of barcoding to restock correct medication in correct drawer, bin, or pocket
- Access controls on drawers, bins, and pockets, including software restrictions and use of location lights and/or locking bin or pocket systems that support safe access
- Process redundancies to ensure correct restocking
- Standardization of restocking procedures to limit process variation

Abbreviations: ADC, automated dispensing cabinet; BUD, beyond-use date.

CS waste creates a significant opportunity for diversion. Witness or second nurse electronic identification via biometric signatures should be required for items wasted and items returned to the ADC return bin (direct return to a pocket should not be allowed). Organizational policy should require that the second authorized user either witness the waste or return the CS to the ADC return bin prior to signing as a witness.[4,14] In the event waste is returned to the pharmacy for testing, procedures should be in place to maintain proper chain of custody during the return process. Implementation of a mechanical or chemical CS waste disposal system that deactivates and renders CS irretrievable may help standardize the waste disposal practice.[17] Policies and procedures should include how waste is managed outside of the ADC to minimize the potential for diversion.

Discrepancy Management. Discrepancies between actual inventory count and recorded count occur frequently enough that constant vigilance to notification and swift reconciliation are required to minimize loss, identify process improvements, and adhere to state and federal regulations with respect to CS losses. ISMP[5] and the California Hospital Association Medication Safety Committee (CHAMSC)[15] recommend discrepancies be resolved upon discovery, no later than end of shift. Further, CHAMSC advises that discrepancies not resolved by end of shift be jointly reviewed by pharmacy and patient care leadership, with resolution within 24 hours.[15] The ASHP Guidelines on Preventing Diversion of Controlled Substances provide additional recommendations on discrepancy management.[14]

Diversion Surveillance, Monitoring, and Detection. Every facility or institution that manages CS is at risk for diversion. Those reporting little or no drug diversion are likely not providing adequate oversight and surveillance.[18] As part of a CS diversion prevention plan, institutions should form a diversion response team and establish routine diversion surveillance processes that will proactively monitor staff involved in CS ordering, inventory, dispensing, administration, and documentation activities.[14] Staff members involved in diversion surveillance should receive training to understand ADC user patterns that may indicate diversion.

Because manual data and report review are tedious and time consuming, diversion detection software options should be evaluated and employed to facilitate the review process.[17] Installing security cameras in medication rooms that provide a bird's-eye view of ADC activity has also become a common practice in many institutions. It is important to work closely with the organization's security and human resources departments to review state laws and labor contracts that might constrain the use of such surveillance, as well as determine the organization's policies and procedures regarding security footage review.

Medication Dispense Transaction Reconciliation. Medication dispensing from ADCs consists of many individual transactions, which may include order, dispense, administration, waste, return, and cancel transactions. ADC reports, as described by New and Overmire,[18] should be reviewed at least monthly by the diversion surveillance team or as defined by the organization. Diversion monitoring and surveillance procedures should include a comparison of ADC dispense transactions with the medication administration record to identify unusual or unreconciled activity to determine whether there are gaps in practice competencies or potential diversion. Dispense transactions can be considered reconciled when matched to a prescriber's order and the dose dispensed is equal to the dose charted as administered plus any amount of drug documented as wasted or returned. These transactions should be reconciled in a timely manner during the normal course of a clinician's work shift.

Dispense event review can be a tedious and resource-intensive process. Organizations should support CS administration practices that minimize the risk of diversion, such as the following:

- Time lapse between CS retrieval from storage area and the time of administration and documentation, waste, and return is appropriate.
- Dose dispensed is package-size equivalent to, or closest available to, the dose to be administered.[14]
- Only healthcare providers operating within the scope of their practice may dispense and administer CS.
- CS are removed from the ADC for one patient at a time.
- The person dispensing CS from the ADC is also the person who administers and documents the medications outside of acceptable emergency situations.
- CS drawn into a syringe is labeled per institutional policy.[15]

Maintenance and Monitoring

ADCs require ongoing maintenance and monitoring to ensure operational safety and efficiency. Additionally, policies and procedures related to access, proper use, daily tasks, and ongoing maintenance are necessary to ensure the system is being used appropriately and maintained for optimal performance and inventory savings.

Access Monitoring. The process of credentialing ADC users ensures correct access levels and privileges for end-users, which allows complete tracking of any user transactions related to system security. Pharmacy and nursing employees perform many basic tasks as they interact with the ADC. In addition to keeping the system running efficiently, certain tasks must be performed on daily, weekly, monthly, 90-day/quarterly, semiannual, or annual schedules, depending on the organization's goals, time, and availability of resources. Some organizations choose to use basic reports for task management, while others invest in comprehensive analytical platforms to streamline the task management process and to provide additional insight into ADC use. Regardless of the approach, a list of basic pharmacy and nursing tasks can be found in **Table 1**.

Maintenance and Optimization. ADCs require hardware maintenance, as well as software updates, upgrades, and optimization. In some cases, vendors may be contractually obligated to provide preventive maintenance to manage ADC issues (full hard drive files, equipment failures, operating system patches, and antivirus software updates). It is important to install the latest operating system, software, and malware updates. Upgrades should be completed in a timely manner and remain a top priority for the health system IT department to ensure efficient use of the ADCs.

It is important to have a maintenance checklist that includes the following:

- Determination of optimization processes and frequencies
- Volume and type of inventory in each device
- Optimal par levels based on usage
- Stock out analysis
- Barcode and alert maintenance
- Override list monitoring and associated reconciliation policies
- Test system maintenance
- Cleaning and infection control measures[19]
- Spare parts inventory
- Software and hardware updates

Monitoring the existing fleet of ADCs in relation to changing patient care needs and medication-use process demands will facilitate future equipment planning. Existing nursing units may require additional ADCs, new nursing units may need new ADCs, and older cabinets may need to be replaced. Enhancements and new products are released periodically.

TABLE 1.
Employee ADC Interaction Tasks

Pharmacy Staff	Nursing Staff and Other Clinicians
Restocking/stock outs	
Patient-specific medication stock and removal	Removing, returning, and/or wasting medications
Expired medication removal	
Returned medication maintenance	
Recalled medications status	
Discrepancy resolution	Discrepancy resolution
CS monitoring	CS monitoring (eg, counting)
Patient-specific medication maintenance	
System integrity (eg, are any cabinets malfunctioning?)	
Inventory optimization	Inventory optimization

CS, controlled substances.

Keeping up-to-date with existing systems and competitive systems will help users make informed decisions on what is needed for a particular facility or institution.

Education and Training

Education and training are important and necessary with any automated system implementation or upgrade and standard components of a robust and complete project plan. Adequate lead time must be planned for development of educational materials and scheduling of training sessions prior to system go-live dates. Attention should be given to development of training materials and sessions that meet the needs of varying user types and roles, as well as workflow differences between patient care areas. Education should include not only technical skills but also the theory and policies supporting proper use (eg, the reasoning behind not overriding).

Vendors should provide standard training support for new implementations and significant upgrades. Health systems should designate personnel that can train new and existing employees on an ongoing basis. Training strategies should include scheduled classroom training sessions as well as self-guided online training courses provided through either a vendor website or the organization's intranet. Hands-on classroom sessions should be highly encouraged, if not mandatory. Because there will always be exceptions, flexibility to accommodate ad hoc training sessions and online courses should be used to fill training gaps to ensure 100% education coverage. For example, online access to full training manuals might be preferable to printing a copy for each individual trainee. Pocket-sized guides or similar education aids may be helpful for users to reference until familiar with normal daily usage. The project manager or designated hospital resource should assemble the training plan to determine which roles need training and at what level, and to ensure accurate training documentation of all staff members.

An adequate number of certified trainers should be available to cover the various roles and staff members who need training. Certain staff members may be identified as super-users who need to be properly trained and/or certified to provide education to any end user, regardless of role. Super-users can also provide support to certified trainers when there are large numbers of staff to be trained. Super-users should be familiar with the environment and staff they will train, and may also serve as added support staff during implementations. Night and weekend shift staff might need extra training and support.

Once initial ADC implementation and training is completed, it is important to plan for ongoing training for new and existing team members. Succession planning and cross-training for key members (such as administrators and super-users) of the ADC team as they move to new roles or leave the organization should also be anticipated. Live or self-guided training courses, manuals, best practices, quick guides, on-screen help, and posted 1-800 help desk numbers are important tools to provide immediate support and keep users' skills up to date. It is helpful to provide the centralized help desk with a decision tree to triage calls and determine what can be quickly resolved by the help desk and where to direct other issues.

Competency of users should be assessed annually or as defined by the organization's policies and procedures, especially when ADC software upgrades include new features. Sites may consider permanently installing a training ADC for testing and training.

Health systems may change ADC vendors, and the above recommendations can be used to guide education and training. User experience will change with a new vendor, including computer screens, medication compartments and drawers, and procedures. Workflows between vendors can vary greatly, and an additional step of mapping workflow changes from vendor to vendor will be needed to ensure staff understands the current state and future state.

Perioperative ADC Use

Use of ADCs in perioperative areas is expanding due to the need for health systems to obtain better inventory control, improve efficiency, and improve accountability for non-controlled and controlled drugs specifically stored and administered in the perioperative area.[20] There are typically two ADC choices to consider for these specialized areas: standard ADCs that are adapted to perioperative use, or anesthesia ADCs, which take the form of an automated cart and are typically used in surgical suites and procedural rooms.

A key point to consider when expanding an ADC medication distribution system into the perioperative area is determining which users will be using the ADC. A user's role will determine their ADC access and privileges in the perioperative area. Frequently, standard ADCs are in core operative areas near operating room (OR) suites for use by nurses or surgeons. In the perioperative area, diverse levels of staff may need access (eg, anesthesiologists, anesthesia techs, nurses, and nurse anesthetists). A licensed healthcare provider will be independently ordering, removing, and administering medications. Perioperative nurses are most likely removing medications from the ADC based on surgery-specific preference documents. Standard ADCs used in the perioperative area are generally open-access machines that store many medications needed for surgeries taking place in OR suites. These can be used as added storage for anesthesia-specific medications that are either too large to fit in anesthesia-specific machines or are critical and could be quickly accessed if out of stock in anesthesia machines.

Anesthesia ADCs specifically for use by anesthesia, surgical, and procedural staff vary in functionality when compared to standard ADCs. These specialized ADCs have improvements in workflow, CS accountability, and access to critical medications as primary features and are visually quite different from their standard ADC counterparts. Commonly, anesthesia ADCs contain high-alert medications, and care needs to be taken in how these medications are stored in ADCs, including proximity to other LASA medications, use of alerts, use of locked compartments, and creation of surgery-specific virtual kits to help ensure appropriate selection of medications.[4,5,12] High-alert medications such as NMBAs require special attention to selection requirements.[4,5,11,13]

Advantages to implementing more specialized anesthesia ADCs in the perioperative area include increased medication security, added inventory visibility (particularly useful during medication shortage situations), and speeding up provider access to medications during surgical procedures. Operational challenges include ensuring provider buy-in with the correct process of removal to ensure accurate administration documentation, inventory counts, and standardizing medication and supply layout between anesthesia ADCs. Anesthesia ADCs also have the capability to interface with external or embedded products that allow providers to comply more easily with The Joint Commission and American Society of Anesthesiologists syringe labeling requirements.[21,22] Anesthesia ADCs may assist in providing accurate medication administration charging if the appropriate ADC and EHR interfaces have been developed and integrated. Some limitations to implementing anesthesia ADCs include challenges with restocking based on availability of the OR suite, and discrepancies between physical and electronic inventory levels.

Many anesthesia ADCs are equipped with features to allow flexibility around use. Helpful mobility features include wireless access, wheels, and a backup uninterrupted power source in cases of power loss. These features allow for repositioning based on case-type for rooms where space is tight and bed orientation is critical. With increased mobility, the security of the anesthesia ADC needs to be considered to ensure no devices are taken out of an OR suite inappropriately.

ADC settings and configurations. Perioperative ADCs have different configuration requirements unique to the areas they serve. An appropriate timeout interval is important in all locations of perioperative ADCs to ensure users have prompt access when needed but that limits are in place to prevent unrestricted access while keeping accurate user documentation. In the OR suite, the timeout interval could be configured to be longer than the interval on the nursing floors due to the need for ongoing access throughout an OR case. Review of settings to limit access to CS without reverification of user identity is important to ensure ongoing accountability and security. Patient lists in perioperative areas need to be configured to ensure prompt access to patients and limit creation of temporary patient records. Some considerations when setting patient lists include configuration of patient location in the EHR, access to patients in the perioperative ADC following discharge for case reconciliation, and the need to have access to all patients admitted. Broader access creates greater need for safeguards to ensure quicker detection of inappropriate access. Like use of system-level kits for a standardized patient treatment protocol in non-OR areas, access to appropriate medications for specific treatment protocols and surgery cases can similarly be facilitated through creation and management of medication kits in perioperative care areas. Prompt access to emergency medications must also be granted. Due to the fast pace of perioperative areas, secure storage and dispensing of CS may best be accomplished by placing CS into single-use pockets. Then, if a provider requests one vial of a CS, they get access to only one vial. This limitation helps ensure CS counts remain correct, prevents discrepancies, and enables quick access to CS for anesthesia providers. There may also be requests to stock items other than medications in the ADC. Ordering, stocking, and replenishment of such items should be discussed with end-users to ensure adequate systems are in place to replenish supplies promptly and clearly designate who is responsible for ongoing management.

Processes for medication returns to the ADC must be discussed with the perioperative department to ensure that processes match workflow and prevent restocking issues. One option for returning medications recommended by ISMP[5] includes returning unused medications to a one-way return bin. When making determinations on preferred workflow, the size of the return bin, expected volume of medications returned to the bin, and processes needed to clear the bin need to be determined. The return bin can securely store CS waste after the provider has electronically wasted leftover medications at the ADC if the decision is made to have pharmacy manage all physical waste. Safeguards also need to be in place to ensure chain of custody for all CS and to ensure that CS waste placed in return bins is trackable and secure throughout the reconciliation process. Depending on the EHR and anesthesia ADC vendors, there may be some available interfacing capabilities that allow transaction information to flow from the ADC to the EHR, including removals, returns, and waste transactions. Select EHRs also have the capability for a CS reconciliation report at the end of an OR case that alerts the provider to any CS discrepancies. This capability also helps keep accurate CS accountability. When implementing anesthesia ADCs, the organization will need to make a policy decision on how to handle partially administered CS (eg, return all partially administered doses to pharmacy for reconciliation versus allowing providers to waste with a witness).

ADC Use Outside the Hospital

Use of ADCs is expanding from hospital to off-site, non-acute areas, such as long-term care facilities, hospice, skilled nursing homes, ambulatory care clinics, rehabilitation facilities, standalone surgery centers, freestanding emergency rooms, and veterinary hospitals. Inclusion of ADCs in non-acute areas has been facilitated by the ability to collect, control, and maintain all transaction information and accurately track medication movement in and out of the system for the enhanced security, accuracy, and accountability of medications. In addition to "starter doses" of medications, ADCs can store emergency kits and supply continuous dosing of CS when appropriately registered.[23] Sites may be miles from the pharmacy that monitors them. The implementation of an ADC in a non-acute setting is impacted by the same considerations given to implementation in acute care locations, but further considerations include those outlined in **Box 2**.[24]

Switching ADC Systems

Hospital systems may replace ADC systems entirely. Regardless of whether upgrades occurred over time, new versions of ADCs that provide previously unused or unavailable options may be available. Processes should be mapped to minimize potential for error and test for accuracy as if it were a new system. The swap of an ADC system should be treated like a new installation, with appropriate training to ensure safety, accuracy, and efficiency in the medication-use process.

Mechanisms should be in place to determine quality of installation (done completely and correctly), operation of the system (as installed it, fits the needs of the organization and contractual specifications), and processes (good fit for workflows within the organization and supported by laws, regulations, policies and procedures).

BOX 2. ADC Implementation and Considerations for Off-Site Use

Cost justification

- Ability to decrease inventory through better management
- Cost of monthly lease and service agreement
- Regulatory/licensing requirements
- Ownership of the device
- DEA licensure requirements (ie, how medications are transferred and tracked from pharmacy to the nonacute area)
- Creation and management of override lists for access to medications prior to order verification
- Adherence to regulations around use of ADCs in nonacute areas

Operations

- Requesting restocking of medications
- Servicing and maintenance of the ADC
- Refilling the ADC, pharmacy vs nonpharmacy staff
- User access and management
  - May require new roles that did not have access historically
  - New or updated privileges may be required
- Type of access to ADC (restricted or open)
  - If restricted, will medications require pharmacy verification prior to removal?
  - If open access, what is process for order review, including steps to take in the event of a delay or an error?
- Policy and procedures for access to medications during system malfunction or electrical outage

Security

- Securing medications during transport to be tamper evident?
- Safety of staff during transport
- Physically security of the ADC
- Video surveillance

Accountability

- Responsibility for reconciliation
- Responsibility for electronic surveillance of activity at the ADC
- Monitoring activity on the ADC if located in care areas that are closed nights or weekends, or temporarily have no patients
- Responsibility for temperature monitoring and response to alerts

System design and interoperability

- Address differences in EMR vendors between organizations and nonacute areas
- Reconcile differences in formularies among organizations' off-site area(s) and hospital
- Access to system software to make changes to settings and build

DEA, Drug Enforcement Administration; ADC, automated dispensing cabinet.

Regulations

Pharmacy personnel must be familiar with state and federal laws concerning ADC use, report diversion where required, and stay up-to-date with changes. At present, most ADCs are not regulated as medical devices, so organizations are responsible for ensuring that vendors are responsive to patient safety or diversion issues, as they are not required to be reported to the Food and Drug Administration (FDA). However, some anesthesia ADCs are regulated by the FDA and do require safety reporting. ADC use is part of an integrated approach in the medication-use process and rarely operates in isolation. With technological advancements, interoperability with other systems such as smart pumps and EHRs, and the hacking potential with any connected device, these systems may be considered medical devices by the FDA in the future. Until then, it is imperative that organizations take appropriate steps to report issues that may impact diversion or patient safety to vendors and appropriate agencies to ensure appropriate evaluation and timely resolution.

Future Considerations

Organizations should communicate suggestions that would improve the interoperability, safety, and efficiency of ADCs and enhance the medication-use process to ADC vendors. In addition, vendors should have a method of documenting and deploying best ideas and practices, as well as innovating with safe and efficient methods of medication distribution that align with customer objectives and state and federal laws.

ADCs are abundant in hospitals, store and distribute medications as a primary tool in the medication-use cycle, and are becoming progressively more interoperable with other hospital systems and devices. As a result, ADCs need to continually evolve with technology improvements, workflow enhancements, and proactive monitoring, which can help organizations keep medication distribution systems safe for patients, efficient for providers, and in compliance with state, federal, and Drug Enforcement Administration requirements.

References

1. Halvorson RM. State of pharmacy automation 2019. *Pharmacy Purchasing and Products*. 2019;16:50, 52–53.
2. Schneider PJ, Pedersen CA, Scheckelhoff DJ. ASHP national survey of pharmacy practice in hospital settings: dispensing and administration—2017. *Am J Health-System Pharm*. 2018;75:1203–1226.
3. ASHP statement on the pharmacist's responsibility for distribution and control of drug products. In: Hawkins BH, ed. *ASHP Best Practices 2020–21*. American Society of Health-System Pharmacists; 2021. Accessed May 1, 2021. https://www.ashp.org/-/media/assets/policy-guidelines/docs/statements/pharmacists-responsibilitydistribution-control-drug-products.ashx
4. Cloud Standards Customer Council 2017. Impact of cloud computing on healthcare version 2.0. Accessed May 6, 2021. https://www.omg.org/cloud/deliverables/CSCC-Impact-of-Cloud-Computing-on-Healthcare.pdf
5. Institute for Safe Medication Practices. Guidelines for safe use of automated dispensing cabinets. Published February 7, 2019. Accessed May 6, 2021. https://www.ismp.org/resources/guidelines-safe-use-automateddispensing-cabinets
6. Ortman MJ, Johnson EG, Jarrell DH, et al. ASHP Guidelines on Emergency Medicine Pharmacist Services. *Am J Health-Syst Pharm*. 2021;78:261–275. doi. org/10.1093/ajhp/zxaa378
7. ASHP Section of Inpatient Care Practitioners. Practice resource for automated dispensing cabinet overrides. Accessed May 2, 2021. www.ashp.org/-/media/assets/pharmacy-practice/resource-centers/patient-safety/patient-safety-practiceresource-for-automated-dispensingcabinet-overrides.ashx
8. Institute for Safe Medication Practices. ISMP guidelines for safe electronic communication of medication information. Published January 16, 2019. Accessed May 6, 2021. https://www.ismp.org/node/1322
9. Partnership for Health IT Patient Safety. Safe practices to reduce CPOE alert fatigue through monitoring, analysis, and optimization. Published 2021. Accessed May 1, 2021. https://d84vr99712pyz.cloudfront.net/p/pdf/hit-partnership/partnership_whitepaper_alertfatigue_final.pdf
10. Osheroff JA, Teich JM, Levick D, et al. *Improving Outcomes with Clinical Decision Support: An Implementer's Guide*, 2nd ed. Taylor & Francis; 2012.
11. Institute for Safe Medication Practices. Paralyzed by mistakes - reassess the safety of neuromuscular blockers in your facility. Published June 16, 2016. Accessed May 6, 2021. https://www.ismp.org/resources/paralyzed-mistakes-reassess-safetyneuromuscular-blockers-your-facility
12. Institute for Safe Medication Practices. ISMP targeted medication safety best practices for hospitals. Published February 21, 2020. Accessed May 6, 2021. https://www.ismp.org/guidelines/best-practices-hospitals
13. Institute for Safe Medication Practices. Safety enhancements every hospital must consider in wake of another tragic neuromuscular blocker event. Published February 17, 2019. Accessed May 6, 2021. https://www.ismp.org/resources/safety-enhancements-everyhospital-must-consider-wake-anothertragic-neuromuscular
14. Brummond PW, Chen DF, Churchill WW, et al. ASHP guidelines on preventing diversion of controlled substances. *Am J Health-System Pharm*. 2017;74:325–348.
15. California Hospital Association Medication Safety Committee. Reducing controlled substances diversion in hospitals. Published May 2013. Accessed May 6, 2021. https://www.chpso.org/sites/main/files/fileattachments/controlled_substance_diversion.pdf
16. Blackmere J, Crowson K, Danley B, et al. Determining the most efficient controlled substance inventory practice that minimizes discrepancies and maximizes security. Accessed May 6, 2021. https://www.bd.com/documents/case-studies/medication-supply-management/DI_Managing-Controlled-Substances_CS_EN.pdf
17. Belisle C. Establishing a controlled substance compliance program. *Pharmacy Purchasing and Products*. 2017;14:2–5.
18. New K, Overmire L. Utilize ADC transaction data to detect diversion. *Pharmacy Purchasing and Products*. 2017;14:10–17.
19. Institute for Safe Medication Practices. Considerations for automated dispensing cabinets (ADC) usage during COVID-19. Published April 16, 2020. Accessed May 6, 2021. www.ismp.org/resources/considerationsautomated-dispensing-cabinets-adcusage-during-covid-19
20. Bickham P, Golembiewski J, Meyer T, et al. ASHP guidelines on perioperative pharmacy services. *Am J Health-Syst Pharm*. 2019;76:903–920.
21. The Joint Commission. National Patient Safety Goals effective January 2019: Hospital Accreditation Program. Accessed May 6, 2021. https://www.jointcommission.org/-/media/tjc/documents/standards/national-patientsafety-goals/historical/npsg_chapter_hap_jan2019.pdf
22. American Society of Anesthesiologists. Statement on labeling of pharmaceuticals for use in anesthesiology. Amended December 13, 2020. Accessed May 6, 2021. https://www.asahq.org/standards-and-guidelines/statementon-labeling-of-pharmaceuticals-foruse-in-anesthesiology

23. Drug Enforcement Administration, United States Department of Justice. Preventing the accumulation of surplus controlled substances at long term care facilities (final rule). 70 Fed. Reg. 25462. Published May 13, 2005. Accessed May 6, 2021. **https://www.govinfo.gov/content/pkg/FR-2005-05-13/pdf/05-9538.pdf**
24. White L. Key success factors in the implementation of an automated dispensing system in a community pharmacy. *Int J Healthcare Tech Mgmt.* 2009;10(6):393–407.

Developed through the ASHP Section of Pharmacy Informatics and Technology and approved by the ASHP Board of Directors on May 20, 2021. These guidelines supersede the ASHP Guidelines on the Safe Use of Automated Dispensing Devices dated July 21, 2009.

ASHP gratefully acknowledges the following organizations and individuals for reviewing these guidelines (review does not imply endorsement): Allina Health (AH), American Society of Consultant Pharmacists ASCP), Institute for Healthcare Improvement (IHI), Institute for Safe Medication Practices (ISMP), Omnicell, University of Kentucky Healthcare (UKH), Carol J. Bickford, PhD, RN-BC, CPHIMS, FAMIA, FHIMSS, FAAN; Sarah Bledsoe, PharmD, CPHIMS; Arnold E. Clayman, PD, FASCP (ASCP); Monica L. Commins, PharmD; Michael Dejos, PharmD, BCPS, LSSBB; Michael Dickens, RPh; Mary Durham, PharmD, MS, BCPS; Frank Federico, RPh (IHI); Jenni Fors, PharmD, BCPS; Roy Guharoy, PharmD, MBA, FCCP, FASHP; Karl Gumpper, MSMI, RPh, CPHIMS, FASHP; Jessica Hill, PharmD, BCPS, BCACP; Matthew J. Hoover, PharmD, MS, BCCCP; Amey Hugg, BSPharm, CPHIMS, FKSHP; Christi Jen, PharmD, BCPS; Matthew Kelm, PharmD, MHA; Patricia C. Kienle, RPh, MPA, FASHP; Darla Klementz, PharmD; Eric C. Kutscher, PharmD, MBA, FASHP; Stephen M. LaHaye, PharmD, BCPS; Chung-Shien Lee, PharmD, BCPS, BCOP; Maritza Lew, BS, PharmD, CPHIMS, PMP; Patrick J. McDonnell, PharmD, FASHP; Kathryn Clark McKinney, PharmD, MS, BCPS, FACHE, FASHP; Scott D. Nelson, PharmD, MS; David Ngo, PharmD, BCPS; James R Rinehart, RPh, MS, FASHP; Ashley Schaber, PharmD, BCPS, NCPS, MPH; Erin K. Scott, RPh; Devlin V Smith, PharmD (UKH); Robert L. Stein, PharmD, JD; James G. Stevenson, PharmD, FASHP, FFIP (Omnicell); Rebecca A. Taylor, PharmD, MBA, FASHP; Dennis Tribble, PharmD, FASHP; Alan Vaida, PharmD, FASHP (ISMP); Tyler Vest, PharmD, MS, BCPS; Geralyn Waters, PharmD, BCPS; Jody Jacobson Wedret, RPh, FASHP, FCSHP; Michelle Dusing Wiest, PharmD, BCPS, FASHP; and Matt Wolf, PharmD, MBA, BCPS (AH).

The authors have declared no potential conflicts of interest.

Ryan Cello, PharmD, UC Davis Health, Sacramento, CA.

Matthew Conley, PharmD, BCPS, AdventHealth-Central Florida Division, Orlando, FL.

Thomas Cooley, BS Pharm, MBA, Brigham and Women's Hospital, Boston, MA.

Charlie De la Torre, BS Pharm, MS, BayCare Health System, Clearwater, FL.

Mitchell Dorn, PharmD, MS, The Ohio State University Wexner Medical Center, Columbus, OH.

Darren S. Ferer, RPh, CPHIMS, Kaleida Health, Buffalo, NY.

Nancy A. Nickman, BS Pharm, MS, PhD, University of Utah Health, Salt Lake City, UT, and College of Pharmacy, University of Utah, Salt Lake City, UT.

David Tjhio, PharmD, Becton Dickinson, Inc., San Diego, CA.

Chris Urbanski, BS Pharm, MS, FASHP, Becton Dickinson, Inc., San Diego, CA.

Gwen Volpe, RPh, Lean Six Sigma Black Belt, FASHP, Fresenius Kabi USA, LLC, Lake Zurich, IL.

Copyright © 2022, American Society of Health-System Pharmacists, Inc. All rights reserved. Contact ASHP for reprint and permissions requests. This content may not be used for commercial purposes without the express written consent of ASHP.

The bibliographic citation for this document is as follows: American Society of Health-System Pharmacists. ASHP guidelines on the safe use of automated dispensing cabinets. *Am J Health-Syst Pharm.* 2022; 79:e71–e82.

Drug Distribution and Control

DOI 10.37573/9781585287048

Drug Distribution and Control

2222

PHARMACIST'S ROLE IN MEDICATION PROCUREMENT, DISTRIBUTION, SURVEILLANCE, AND CONTROL

Source: Council on Pharmacy Practice

To affirm the pharmacist's expertise, responsibility, and oversight in the procurement, distribution, surveillance, and control of all medications used within health systems and affiliated services; further,

To assert that the pharmacy leader retains the authority to determine the safe and reliable sourcing of medications; further,

To assert that the pharmacy workforce is responsible for the coordination of medication-related care, including optimizing access, ensuring judicious stewardship of resources, and providing intended high-quality clinical care; further,

To encourage payers, manufacturers, wholesalers, accreditation bodies, and governmental entities to enhance patient safety by supporting the health-system pharmacy workforce's role in medication procurement, distribution, surveillance, and control.

This policy supersedes ASHP policy 0232.

Rationale

Pharmacists are accountable for ensuring that medications will be optimally used in the care setting in which they work. (For the purposes of this policy, "medications" include those used by inpatients and outpatients, large- and small-volume injectables, radiopharmaceuticals, diagnostic agents including radiopaque contrast media, anesthetic gases, bloodfraction drugs, dialysis fluids, respiratory therapy drugs, biotechnologically produced drugs, investigational drugs, drug samples, drugs brought to the setting by patients or family, and other chemicals and biological substances administered to patients to evoke or enhance pharmacologic responses.) The pharmacist and pharmacy workforce, as part of their leadership over all aspects of the medication-use process, are responsible for medication procurement, distribution, surveillance and control. One of the central roles of the pharmacist and pharmacy workforce in hospitals, health systems, and affiliated services is to oversee and assume accountability for these responsibilities while also supporting patient access to medications and engaging in clinical services to optimize medication use. While recognizing the stakeholders that influence medication procurement, distribution, surveillance, and control such as payers, manufacturers, wholesalers, accreditation bodies, and governmental entities, pharmacists require the autonomy to make decisions related to these aspects for their institutions and affiliated service provision.

2145

REDUCTION OF UNUSED PRESCRIPTION DRUG PRODUCTS

Source: Council on Pharmacy Practice

To recognize that unused prescription drug products contribute to drug misuse, abuse, and diversion; further,

To advocate for staffing, research, education, and best practices to ensure appropriate quantities of prescription drug products are prescribed, reconciled, and dispensed; further,

To advocate that the pharmacy workforce take a leadership role in reducing excess quantities of unused prescription drug products, including the provision of patient and caregiver education, raising public awareness, and supporting and integrating medication take-back programs.

This policy supersedes ASHP policy 1702.

Rationale

According to the Centers for Disease Control and Prevention (CDC), almost 5% of the U.S. population over 12 years old used prescription pain relievers for nonmedical reasons in 2010, resulting in 15,000 overdose deaths. A major source of diversion is unused prescription drug products, such as those left over after a patient has gained relief from temporary pain. Although prescribers and other healthcare providers have long been aware of the dangers of unused prescription drug products, incentives for overprescribing remain. The desire to minimize office visits, concern about undertreatment of pain, and prohibitions against partial fills and refills of controlled substances contribute to overprescribing. In addition to the risk of misuse, abuse, and diversion, research reveals that as many as 10 million prescriptions go unused every year, resulting in up to $5 billion in wasted medication (Lenzer J. *BMJ* 2014; 349:g7677). There is clearly a need for concentrated effort to minimize medication waste from unused prescription drug products.

ASHP recognizes the need for research on best practices to ensure appropriate quantities of drug products are prescribed, reconciled, and dispensed, which will include study of the effectiveness of partial fills or refills of prescription drug products, among other solutions. ASHP has concerns about quantity and duration limits, because rigid restrictions on treatment options may result in adverse patient outcomes.

Appropriate community return and disposal of excess prescription drug products reduce diversion, accidental poisoning risk, and environmental harm. ASHP advocates for pharmacist pharmacy workforce leadership in reducing excess quantities of unused prescription drug products through appropriate pain management practices and development and implementation of prescription drug product return and disposal programs.

2042

CONTROLLED SUBSTANCES DIVERSION PREVENTION

Source: Council on Pharmacy Management

To enhance awareness by the pharmacy workforce, other healthcare workers, and the public of the potential threats to the public and patient care and safety presented by diversion of controlled substances; further,

To encourage healthcare organizations to develop controlled substances diversion prevention programs (CSDPPs) and supporting policies that delineate the core administrative elements and system- and provider-level controls needed to

DOI 10.37573/9781585287048.015

deter diversion of controlled substances at all stages of medication use; further,

To encourage healthcare organizations to address in their CSDPPs the roles, responsibilities, and oversight of all workers who may have access to controlled substances to ensure compliance with applicable laws and scopes of practice; further,

To encourage healthcare organizations to ensure that all healthcare workers are appropriately screened for substance abuse prior to initial employment and that surveillance, auditing, and monitoring are conducted on an ongoing basis to support a safe patient-care environment, protect co-workers, and discourage controlled substances diversion; further,

To advocate that pharmacists take principal roles in collaborative, interdisciplinary efforts by organizations of healthcare professionals, patient advocacy organizations, and regulatory authorities to develop and promote best practices for preventing drug diversion and appropriately using controlled substances to optimize and ensure patient access and therapeutic outcomes; further,

To advocate that the Drug Enforcement Administration and other regulatory authorities interpret and enforce laws, rules, and regulations to support patient access to appropriate therapies, minimize burdens on pharmacy practice, and provide reasonable safeguards against fraud, misuse, abuse, and diversion of controlled substances.

This policy supersedes ASHP policies 1614 and 1709.

Rationale

Pharmacy managers and pharmacists-in-charge have increasing responsibility for ensuring controlled substance management and storage across large healthcare organizations. This responsibility has increased as acquisition of physician office practices, clinics, and other non-hospital business units continue.

According to the Drug Enforcement Administration (DEA) *2019 National Drug Threat Assessment Summary*, controlled substances are responsible for the most drug-involved overdose deaths and are the second most commonly abused substances in the United States. Traffickers continue to manufacture and distribute counterfeit controlled substances, often containing fentanyl and other opioids, along with nonopioid illicit drugs in attempts to expand their customer base and increase profits.

All pharmacies and healthcare organizations that handle controlled substances are required to have storage and distribution systems in place that prevent diversion. Due to the numerous medication access points embedded within hospital distribution systems, diversion can be difficult to detect. Overall, diversion incidents continue to decline; however, controlled substances lost in transit or diverted by medical professionals remain a prevalent threat across the U.S. that can lead to patient harm. Drug addiction among healthcare workers is well documented. One survey suggested that nurses who reported a perception of easier availability of controlled substances were almost twice as likely as others to divert and use a controlled substance. In another survey published in *AJHP*, 19% of pharmacists reported use of a controlled substance without a prescription during the preceding 12 months. Even the most conservative estimates are that 8–12% of physicians will develop a substance abuse problem at some point during their career, although the exact rate of substance abuse among physicians is uncertain.

To ensure compliance with applicable laws and scopes of practice, ASHP advocates that healthcare organizations develop controlled substances diversion prevention programs and policies to describe the roles, responsibilities, and oversight of all personnel who have access to controlled substances throughout the organization. The ASHP Guidelines on Preventing Diversion of Controlled Substances offer detailed suggestions on implementation guidance for pharmacists to employ proactive measures and mitigate diversion in their institutions and communities. ASHP also supports pre-employment screening and ongoing surveillance, auditing, and monitoring of all healthcare workers to reduce the risk of controlled substances diversion.

Healthcare institutions face many challenges in managing controlled substances. New laws and regulations, including DEA quotas and controlled substances monitoring requirements at community outpatient dispensing facilities, are meant to decrease diversion and illegal activity but are also impacting patients and pharmacists. In addition, the DEA has allowed hospitals and clinics with an onsite pharmacy and status as an authorized collector to maintain collection receptacles onsite and administer mail-back programs for controlled substances, adding another layer of complexity to controlled substance disposal. Pharmacists in healthcare organizations are required to meet standards and comply with laws and regulations from a variety of sources, including the DEA, The Joint Commission, Det Norske Veritas, other accreditation organizations, and state and federal governments. The ASHP Statement on the Pharmacist's Role in Substance Abuse Prevention, Education, and Assistance offers detailed suggestions for pharmacists in addressing substance abuse in their institutions and communities.

0303

PHARMACY DRUG THEFT

Source: House of Delegates Resolution

To support the development of policies and guidelines for health-system pharmacists designed to deter drug product theft and thereby enhance both the integrity of the drug distribution chain and the safety of the workplace; further,

To encourage the development of systems that limit the diversion and abuse potential of medications, including high-cost drugs and controlled substances, and thereby reduce the likelihood that these products will be targets of theft.

This policy was reviewed in 2019 by the Council on Pharmacy Management and by the Board of Directors and was found to still be appropriate.

9903

OPTIMIZING THE MEDICATION-USE PROCESS

Source: Council on Administrative Affairs

To urge health-system pharmacists to assume leadership, responsibility, and accountability for the quality, effectiveness, and efficiency of the entire medication-use process (including prescribing, dispensing, administration, monitoring, and education) across the continuum of care; further,

To urge health-system pharmacists to work in collaboration with patients, prescribers, nurses, and other health care providers in improving the medication-use process.

This policy was reviewed in 2019 by the Council on Pharmacy Management and by the Board of Directors and was found to still be appropriate.

ASHP Guidelines on Preventing Diversion of Controlled Substances

Purpose

Controlled substances (CS) diversion in health systems can lead to serious patient safety issues, harm to the diverter, and significant liability risk to the organization. Diversion puts patients at risk of harm, directly or indirectly, including inadequate relief of pain, inaccurate documentation of their care in the medical record, exposure to infectious diseases from contaminated needles and drugs, and impaired healthcare worker (HCW) performance.[1,2] In addition to patient harm, there are regulatory and legal risks to the organization, including fraudulent billing and liability for resulting damages, and decreased community confidence in the healthcare system. These guidelines provide a detailed and comprehensive framework to support organizations in developing their CS diversion prevention program (CSDPP) in order to protect patients, HCWs, the organization, and the community at-large. Ultimately, each organization is responsible for developing a CSDPP that complies with applicable federal and state laws and regulations, but also one that applies technology and diligent surveillance to routinely review process compliance and effectiveness, strengthen controls, and seek to proactively prevent or detect diversion.[3,4]

Although rarely discussed openly, diversion of CS is common, and serious events have highlighted the prevalence of this issue and its implications. It is estimated that 10–15% of HCWs misuse alcohol or drugs at some point in their careers, which is similar to the general population.[5] HCW may also divert for sale or for use by someone else. With the role HCWs have in taking care of patients and the accessibility of CS in their work environment, organizations must routinely evaluate their employees, systems, and patient care environments for opportunities to prevent diversion.[6,7] It is imperative that healthcare organizations develop CSDPPs that include support systems for the workforce (eg, employee assistance programs, professional monitoring programs), methods to monitor the effectiveness of diversion prevention efforts, and patient safety considerations. Education on the signs and symptoms of impaired HCWs—supported by rigorous monitoring and surveillance, human resources management, awareness of state and national diversion reporting requirements, and substance abuse treatment programs—is paramount for healthcare organizations. In addition, healthcare organizations are not immune to the larger societal issues associated with substance abuse, including the recent exponential rise in accidental overdoses, and should therefore ensure that there are systems in place to positively influence procurement and storage, prescribing, preparation and dispensing, administration, and proper disposal and wasting of CS.[8–15]

There are many points in the medication management process where diversion may occur (**Figure 1**). CSDPPs that build in tight control through process checks and balances, diligent surveillance, and prompt interventions are required to prevent, promptly identify, and investigate suspected diversion. Such programs require proactive surveillance and a rapid response by key stakeholders, using established processes and time frames as defined by the organization. Clear policies, procedures, and lines of accountability must be in place for conducting such investigations, reporting findings, and implementing corrective action plans in a timely and thorough manner. The purpose of these guidelines is to provide guidance to health systems on planning for and implementing best practices when establishing a comprehensive CSDPP. Making a comprehensive CSDPP a strategic priority will require engaged leadership oversight that promotes a culture of organizational awareness and transparency, implements and evaluates the effectiveness of systems and processes, and works toward continuous improvement. The guidelines provide recommendations on developing CS diversion prevention strategies and a framework for integrating those strategies into a comprehensive organizational program that ensures consistent implementation across the organization, regardless of setting. The recommendations outline a collaborative, interdisciplinary approach to and accountability for CS diversion prevention and response within the organization. Some topics outlined in these guidelines are the subjects of other ASHP Best Practices documents, which should be referred to for additional information and guidance. Pharmacy leadership and other key stakeholders within healthcare organizations should use their professional judgment when determining applicability to their own needs and circumstances.

Scope

These guidelines address all settings in which health-system pharmacies typically have responsibility for purchasing, procuring, distributing, wasting, and disposing of CS, including, but not limited to, acute care settings, outpatient and community pharmacies, organization-owned clinics, long-term care facilities, physician practices, and free-standing emergency rooms and ambulatory surgery centers. The broad range of CS diversion prevention strategies recommended in this document supports a culture of safety for patients and HCWs and defines how to address impaired HCWs. To encourage dissemination and adoption of these strategies and recommendations, **Appendix A** defines terms used in this document and in diversion prevention generally. **Appendix B** provides additional guidance regarding implementation strategies, examples of best practices, and key action steps described within the guidelines that can assist in self-assessment. Some of these approaches are relatively straightforward and can be implemented within the pharmacy. Other approaches are more complex and require collaboration throughout the organization and, in some cases, with vendors. Successful diversion prevention requires systematic attention to and integration of both types of approaches. When selecting and implementing these strategies, it is essential that the organization remain mindful of patient safety and the quality of patient care; patients must still be ensured access to timely care and effective pain management.

DOI 10.37573/9781585287048.016

FIGURE 1. Examples of common risk points and methods of diversion. CS = controlled substances, DEA = Drug Enforcement Administration, ADC = automated dispensing cabinet.

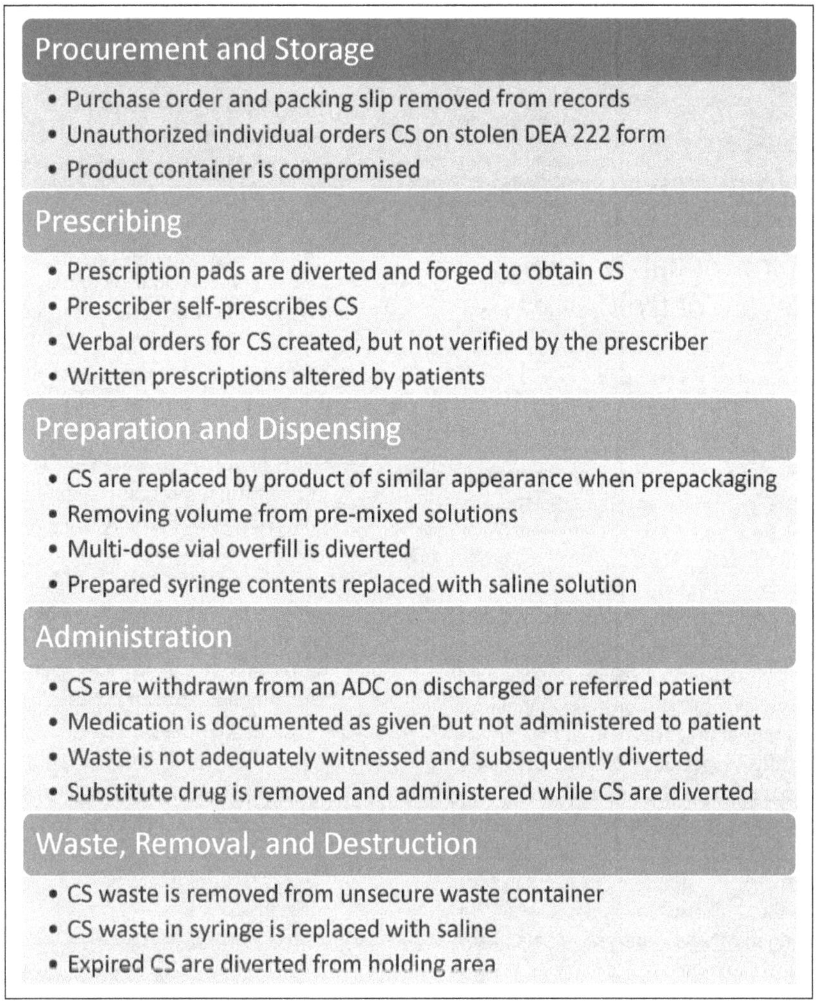

Core Elements of a CSDPP

A comprehensive CSDPP includes core administrative elements (eg, legal and regulatory requirements, organization oversight and accountability), system-level controls (eg, human resources management, automation and technology, monitoring and surveillance, and investigation and reporting), and individual-level controls (eg, chain of custody; storage and security; internal pharmacy controls; prescribing and administration; returns, waste, and disposal) (**Figure 2**). This framework is driven by key principles that include a collaborative approach, setting clear lines of accountability and responsibility, implementation of standard processes, and a culture of continuous readiness and quality improvement. When an organization has locations with multiple Drug Enforcement Administration (DEA) licenses, all organizational policies and procedures related to the CSDPP should be applied consistently.

Legal and Regulatory Requirements

The movement and transfer of CS, from procurement and storage to prescribing, dispensing, administration, waste, and disposal, is highly regulated by federal and state laws and regulations as well as compliance standards (eg, those of accrediting organizations and the Centers for Medicare & Medicaid Services). These requirements must serve as the foundation for the organization's policies and procedures.[6,7,16,17] Whether implemented manually or through the use of technology, policies and procedures must reflect current legal and regulatory requirements, including, but not limited to, those pertaining to records retention and forms completion; DEA registration and power-of-attorney designations; procurement and accounting of inventory, including biennial inventory; security and storage; prescription authentication and reporting (eg, prescription monitoring programs); surveillance, investigation and reporting of CS diversion or loss; authorization to access CS (ie, to procure, prescribe, handle, transport, dispense, or administer); and documentation of waste and transfer. When applicable, the CSDPP integrates requirements of state-level CSDPPs and procedures, such as those required by professional licensure boards.

Billing and Fraud Implications. CS diversion also has billing fraud implications. When there are diversions with known documentation or processes that have impacted the integrity of the billing process, additional actions may be required. Organizations, with input from pharmacy, should take the

FIGURE 2. Controlled substances diversion prevention program.

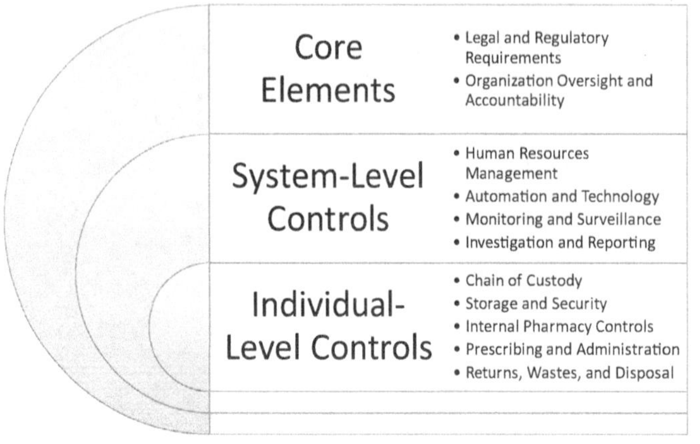

initiative to self-monitor practices to prevent, identify, and correct potential fraud, waste, or abuse in collaboration with relevant departments (eg, corporate compliance, finance, and internal audit).[18]

DEA Registrations. The organization should be aware of applicable DEA registrations under its control and appoint a registrant who will be accountable for enforcement of requirements. Registrations and powers of attorney issued by a DEA registrant should be current and re-evaluated on a regular basis (ie, at least annually). There should be procedures in place for reporting suspected or known diversion to DEA and other required local authorities, with the designated person submitting reports in accordance with requirements. Local DEA and law enforcement may vary in their requirements and preferences for how and when to report suspected diversion or theft. Furthermore, states vary in their requirements for who may handle and transport CS, for licensure and registration of providers, and for provider assistance programs. Those responsible for their CSDPP should be familiar with local and state requirements and work collaboratively to minimize risk to the organization and ensure public safety. Organizations should ensure completeness and integrity of required documentation, required elements in manual and electronic forms of documentation (ie, procurement and disposition records and inventories), surveillance findings and actions, discrepancy investigations, and reports to DEA and other authorities; such documentation should be readily retrievable for the minimum timeframe established by law and as required by the organization.

Patient's Own Medications, Medical Cannabis, Marijuana, and Illicit Substances. Healthcare organizations should develop procedures for the disposition of patients' CS, medical cannabis, marijuana, and illicit substances brought into a facility.[19] Policies and procedures should address notification of the local authorities and referral to substance abuse programs when patients bring illicit substances into the organization, as required by law.[20] Pharmacy leaders, representatives of other affected HCWs, and the security department should work closely with the organization's legal counsel to interpret and weigh legal, regulatory, and accreditation requirements regarding these substances, as well as the rights of individual patients, in developing the organization's policies. It should be noted that, especially in the case of medical cannabis and marijuana, possession and prescription laws vary from state to state.

Organization Oversight and Accountability

It is imperative that organizations establish a CSDPP that discourages diversion and strengthens accountability, rapidly identifies suspected diversion and responds to known or suspected diversion incidents, and continually seeks to improve controls. Strong organization oversight with broad HCW participation and a clear accountability structure provides a framework for a capable program.

Organizations should support the CSDPP by providing adequate resources, including human resources, facility controls, and technology. The pharmacy executive, whose central role is responsibility for the organization's medication use system, will be an essential resource for a successful CSDPP. Key elements for organization oversight and accountability include the following (see Appendix B for additional guidance):

- The organization establishes an interdisciplinary CS management program in compliance with statutory and regulatory requirements and with systems that discourage diversion and enhance accountability. Established policies and procedures address all points of access, reflect a segregation of duties where there are overlapping processes for diversion risk, and ensure that the chain of custody and individual accountability are maintained, documented and verifiable at all times.
- CS-related policies are reviewed at regular intervals and when there is a notable change in the organization's circumstances or structure (eg, additional campuses, departments, or service lines) to ensure that they are current, meet applicable practice standards, reflect best practices when possible, and are consistent across the organization.
- HCWs authorized to access or handle CS are trained and competent in established policies, procedures, and regulatory requirements.
- As part of its CSDPP, an organization defines a structure that identifies and supports specific organization accountabilities with respect to oversight and implementation of the program.
- The organization establishes an interdisciplinary CSDPP committee to provide leadership and direction for developing policies and procedures and for overseeing the CSDPP. The CSDPP committee is proactive in its prevention efforts and addresses prevention control, diversion detection, incident investigation, reporting procedures, and quality improvement activities.
- The CSDPP committee is led by a designated diversion officer who coordinates all aspects of the program. The functions of this committee are integrated with existing compliance management programs, and the committee reports at least quarterly directly to the senior leadership of the organization.
- Committee members are identified and have clear roles with defined expectations. Suggested committee membership includes staff from the following departments: medicine, anesthesia, pharmacy, nursing, security, human resources, compliance, risk management, administration, legal, media/communications, information technology, and Employee Health. Pharmacy must have a leadership role on the CSDPP committee.

- A diversion response team should be established to respond immediately to suspected incidents and report findings to the CSDPP. Stakeholder notifications should be tiered and based on the stage and findings of the investigation.

Human Resources Management

It is important that healthcare organizations approach CS diversion prevention with the same diligence they would apply to any potential compromise to patient safety and create a culture of awareness that supports an effective organization-wide CSDPP. A comprehensive human resources approach to support the CSDPP should at a minimum include (1) a written employee and provider substance abuse policy and procedures; (2) an HCW education and awareness program; (3) a supervisor training program; (4) an employee and provider assistance program; (5) peer support and systems (eg, pharmacist recovery networks); (6) requirements for drug testing, including a for-cause policy for drug and blood-borne pathogen testing; (7) return-to-work policies for HCWs[21]; and (8) sanctions for performance and diversion violations. Pharmacists should participate in or contribute to the development of substance abuse prevention and assistance programs within healthcare organizations.[22]

First and foremost, organizations must implement policies to protect patients from potential harm related to substance abuse and diversion and have a process to remove an HCW suspected of being impaired from delivering patient care and to prevent further access to CS either pending investigation or after a confirmed diversion or policy breach. Organization policies should ensure compliance with federal and state laws regarding referral to local law enforcement and applicable licensing boards. The organization's senior leadership should determine the repercussions or sanctions for confirmed thefts or diversion, and should ensure that those repercussions or sanctions are consistently applied across all locations and disciplines. HCW sanctions should take into account whether the HCW is supporting his or her own substance use disorder (or that of an associate) or there has been theft of CS for sale and financial gain. The organization's substance abuse policy should address circumstances in which an HCW is diverting to support a substance use disorder. Such diversion should be referred to applicable licensing boards, and the HCW should be referred to a substance abuse program. The substance abuse policy should also address actions to take when a person separates from the employer during the course of an investigation or does not comply with substance abuse program or other requirements, and includes guidance on when the organization should inform local authorities and the relevant licensing board.

There are signs that signal possible CS diversion, and all HCWs need to understand their role in recognizing diversion. The organization's senior leadership should communicate the expectation that HCWs speak up when they become aware of or suspect an issue related to CS diversion and should ensure that HCWs will be protected from retaliation if they report a suspected issue related to CS diversion. The organization should therefore establish and communicate ways for HCWs to speak up anonymously (eg, compliance hotline, paper or electronic submission), preferably to a neutral party. The organization should treat such information as confidential and take all reasonable steps to protect the confidentiality of the information and the identity of the HCW furnishing the information.

All HCWs should receive initial orientation and annual education in diversion prevention and substance abuse and diversion awareness (signs and behavior patterns and symptoms of impairment) and reporting options. Initial education and at least annual competency assessment on medication diversion and CS policies and procedures should be required before granting, or continuing to grant, an HCW authorization to access CS. HCWs should be made aware that random compliance checks will occur and that HCWs will be held accountable for complete compliance with policies, laws, and record-keeping requirements. Furthermore, the employer should inform HCWs that they have the responsibility to report suspected drug diversion and that the employer will treat such information as confidential.[16] The organization should emphasize the importance of reporting the signs of a potentially impaired HCW or suspected CS diversion and the potential impact on patient care, including ramifications for failure to report. Managers should also receive training about signs, symptoms, and behavior alerts; what to do when they suspect an HCW is impaired; managing an HCW in recovery; and their responsibilities should they become aware of a known or suspected diversion.

The organization should establish a process to support recovery for HCWs who are diverting CS for an active substance abuse problem (ie, an employee assistance program process, which may include mandatory program referral, reporting to the relevant state board or professional assistance program, and a contract for the HCW's return to work). Drug testing for cause should be permitted, and, as required for investigations or by licensing boards or other employment contracts, organizations should implement standardized and reliable testing and validation for drug screening. The organization should have policies to address the assessment of an HCW's ability to return to patient care when there has been a for-cause investigation. Furthermore, the organization should have a policy that addresses how to handle situations when there may be an additional impact on patient care, such as an infection control risk, and should address requirements for further testing (eg, human immunodeficiency virus, hepatitis C).

If HCW services are contracted, agreements should ensure that all contracted HCWs receive education regarding CS and that the contracted company will immediately notify the organization if there is disciplinary action against an HCW or if an HCW is removed because of an impairment issue. Furthermore, for contracted HCWs, the contract should define or otherwise provide clear processes and accountability for monitoring, investigating, and reporting suspected diversion, and there should be transparency with regard to sanctions, external reporting, and remediation.

Organizations will need to establish policies and procedures to manage situations and offer staff support (eg, bereavement support, employee assistance programs) when diversion results in an HCW overdose or death in the workplace. These situations will require all of the investigation and discovery aspects of any suspected diversion, but will also require that determinations be made regarding which authorities need to be immediately contacted, whether evidence will need to be quarantined, and whether and how the chain of custody will be documented. See Appendix B for additional guidance.

Automation and Technology

Automated dispensing technology, including automated dispensing cabinets (ADCs), prepackaging devices, and diversion monitoring software have been developed to assist with the management of CS, including inventory control; documentation of removal, administration, and waste; billing; chain of custody tracking; and auditing.[23] The use of ADCs has become the standard of care for the medication-use process in healthcare systems because they are essential to provide quality patient care, provide secure yet accessible storage of medications, and ensure viability of the medication-use process in healthcare organizations.[23] Automated dispensing and surveillance solutions that support adequate control, surveillance, and auditing processes should be implemented, at minimum, in high-risk areas. For example, areas commonly considered to be high risk include the main pharmacy CS vault, anesthesia and procedural areas, emergency departments, surgery centers, and remote locations. Despite their perceived ease of implementation and use, automated dispensing and surveillance technologies still require diligence in the development of meaningful and readily retrievable reports, investigation of trends and variances, and review of the impact of changes in the automation technology. Pharmacists and other stakeholders in the organization should only engage with vendors who will work collaboratively to develop adequate implementation testing, HCW training, and maintenance and upgrade plans for their technology solutions. Key elements of automation and technology to support a CSDPP include the following (see Appendix B for additional guidance):

- An interdisciplinary team that includes pharmacy representation participates in the selection and implementation of all medication-related automated systems (eg, surveillance software) and technology (eg, ADCs, syringe and infusion pumps, security devices) to ensure they support diversion control, surveillance, and auditing of CS and meet legal, regulatory, and functionality requirements. Pharmacy has an integral role in the selection and implementation process. Any changes or upgrades to existing technology are reviewed by key stakeholders, including pharmacy, to assess the impact on systems of control, surveillance, and auditing, and the changes are tested and vetted to ensure that implementation meets legal, regulatory, and functionality requirements. A report of this assessment and any gaps identified with the new system/upgrade and a plan for remedy are documented in a formal report and reviewed by the CSDPP committee before implementation.
- CS management automation and technology vendors collaborate with healthcare organizations to provide adequate solutions that support control, surveillance, and auditing functions that address the entire chain of custody, up to and including administration to the patient, and have the ability to track waste, identify discrepancies, and pull data from technology systems into actionable reports, including, but not limited to, trending of information that supports diversion surveillance.
- Technology solutions facilitate and clearly document chain of custody points, wherever possible.
- Storage and access to CS within ADCs is limited to unit-of-use, when possible, and access is restricted to one drug and strength at a time (ie, matrix drawers should not be used).
- Records generated from technology solutions are readily retrievable and contain information required to conduct investigations and fulfill investigator requests. Reporting capability is tested to ensure that data within reports are complete, accurate, and integrated into actionable reports that are readily retrievable.
- Integrated technology solutions (eg, diversion monitoring software, ADC medical record integration, and barcode verification) are utilized for dispensing, monitoring, reporting, and surveillance.
- All HCWs are adequately trained regarding their roles and responsibilities in the use of automation and technology, including surveillance capabilities, and their competency is assessed. Competency is assessed when an HCW assumes a new position, annually, or when there is a relevant change to existing technology.
- A pharmacist is designated to oversee ADCs, including selection, maintenance, and inventory management, and to ensure that procedures are in place to limit access to CS in ADCs by minimizing the number of authorized individuals with access, as well as the ability to immediately add or rescind access privileges.
- Policies and procedures that address access, security, documentation, recovery, and post-event reconciliation are established in the event of automation downtime or system failure.

Monitoring and Surveillance

The organization, through its CSDPP committee, should define, review, and audit relevant data that could indicate potential CS diversion and ensure that trends and variances are acted on in a timely manner and that corrective action plans are implemented (**Figure 3**). All variances should signal an opportunity for improvement and require investigation. CS monitoring and surveillance rely on the availability and use of data and information, including timely access

FIGURE 3. Monitoring and Surveillance Cycle.

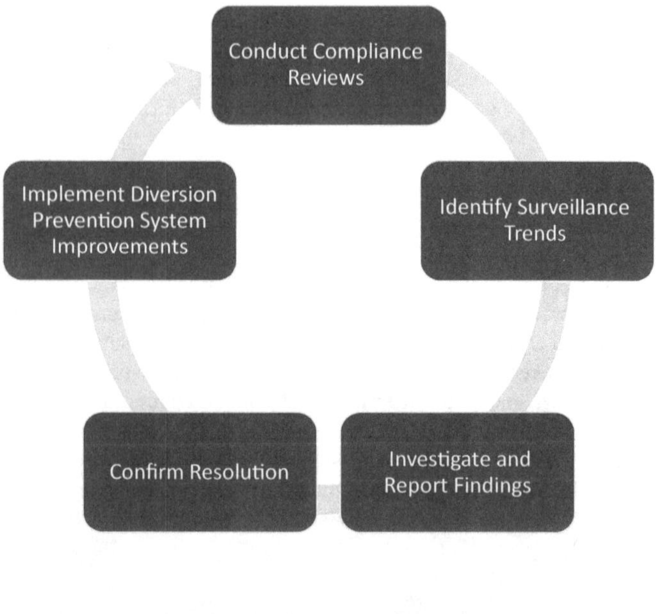

to actionable reports that support an effective surveillance and detection system. Furthermore, the CSDPP should assess the comprehensiveness and level of documentation and response to suspected diversion events and compliance with established policies and procedures. Automated systems and diversion monitoring software are recommended to support efficient surveillance, particularly for high-risk or high-volume locations. The CSDPP committee, with input from the designated diversion officer, designated pharmacist representative, and pharmacy compliance team (if applicable), should oversee the organization's monitoring and surveillance efforts, including identifying required and routine compliance reviews, determining surveillance metrics for trend reports, assigning responsibility for and frequency of review, providing facility oversight, and conducting established audits of facility-based diversion monitoring and documentation of suspected diversion events. The organization, through the CSDPP committee, should establish and review, at least annually, surveillance requirements, including the definition of monitoring and surveillance measures, thresholds of variance that require action, reporting frequency, and surveillance procedures. The organization, through the CSDPP committee, should ensure that all elements are implemented, conducted in a timely manner, investigated, and reported as required. Core program elements and controls (Figure 2) should be regularly audited for compliance on a scheduled basis (eg, at least annually). The CSDPP committee should provide facility oversight to ensure that established audits for facility-based diversion monitoring are conducted and documented. The use of diversion monitoring software with advanced analytics capability to support monitoring and surveillance activities is strongly recommended.

Surveillance. Surveillance processes should be interdisciplinary and touch all aspects of the CS management system, from purchasing, inventory management, preparation, administration, waste, and disposal, to documentation through expired product management. Key process indicators (KPIs) should be established, reviewed, and revised at least annually. (See **Table 1** for example KPIs). CS auditing should be performed on a regularly scheduled basis, as determined by processes in a particular area, such as anesthesia, patient care units, special procedure areas, ambulatory care areas, and the pharmacy, focusing on identified risk points (Figure 1) and previous events. Self-audits should be conducted within areas as well as regularly scheduled audits by individuals external to the area being audited. The organization should periodically audit compliance with all diversion controls, including human resources requirements for individuals authorized to handle CS (eg, completion of required background checks, documentation of training and competency requirements for authorized HCWs, compliance with licensure board reporting, testing for fitness for duty, random drug-testing requirements, and compliance with rehabilitation program requirements). Important examples of recommended surveillance practices include the following (see Appendix B for additional guidance):

- The healthcare organization assigns a pharmacist, with adequate support staff and dedicated time for surveillance monitoring, who is accountable for optimizing the implementation and functionality of ADCs and diversion monitoring software reporting capabilities. Other disciplines (eg, nursing, quality assurance, anesthesia providers) are actively involved in surveillance monitoring and audits and assist with evaluation of trends and incident investigation.
- Processes for procurement surveillance are followed by all areas that purchase CS under their own DEA license (eg, research areas). For all purchases, authorization (eg, power of attorney) is verified. The healthcare organization reviews purchase history through regularly scheduled audits to identify potential diversion through variations or changes in volume or pattern. CS purchase invoices are compared with CS orders and receipt into the pharmacy's perpetual inventory. Because the invoice–receipt pair may be removed with CS diversion, invoices also are reconciled to statements or wholesale purchase history reports to detect missing invoices. A process is in place to identify unusual peaks in quantity or frequency of CS purchased and to conduct periodic reviews of the quantity of CS removals from the main inventory to patient care areas compared with actual documentation and/or patient care charges.
- Verification of a perpetual inventory should be conducted on a regular basis with the frequency consistent with the controls to limit the time frame for discovery. It is important to identify inventory discrepancies in a timely manner so the reason for the discrepancy can be more easily investigated. CS managed through ADCs have ADC counts verified (by blind count) each time a CS drawer is accessed. Unless verified by blind count, CS in ADCs are inventoried weekly. CS storage areas outside ADCs are inventoried at each shift change by two authorized HCWs. CS inventory in the pharmacy CS vault is counted at least monthly. A biennial physical inventory of all CS is completed and documented per DEA requirements (or per state requirements, whichever is the more strict interpretation).
- Movement of CS throughout the organization is traced, and all transactions are reconciled (eg, reports match CS vault transactions with receipt into the ADC and/or paper inventory record with nurse signature of receipt).
- Prescribing practices and prescribing trends are evaluated, and significant variation from peers should be reviewed.
- ADC reports are reviewed at least monthly by pharmacy and patient care managers as defined by the organization, and the results of the review and any actions are documented. Reports compare ADC activity with medication administration records. Patient response to medication (ie, pain management) is also evaluated against medication administration records, documentation of response, and patient interview. The medication record is reviewed for the amount and quantity administered and compared with what other HCWs administer on subsequent shifts (when there is no change in patient condition).
- Nursing management integrates routine auditing and surveillance activities into core daily, weekly, or monthly responsibilities, including staff education regarding signs of diversion, symptoms of substance abuse, and diversion-reporting procedures; review of nursing removal, return, overrides, and wasting records; development, implementation, and monitoring of procedures for witnessing CS-related transactions;

TABLE 1.
Examples of Surveillance Key Process Indicators

Diversion Risk Point	Key Process Indicators
Procurement and inventory	Random inventory audits (to ensure the perpetual inventory count is correct) Inventory adjustment reasons and user Destocks Inventory statistics (amount dispensed, top movers, top issued medications, etc) Missing medication alerts
Preparation and dispensing	Overrides Quantity purchased vs. dispensed Discrepancies/time (day, month, etc) Discrepancy resolution by user Types of medications with top discrepancies Will-call audits (community-based prescriptions) Destock transactions Dispenses "off the clock" Dispensing consistent with pain scales Destock and null transactions Suspicious order monitoring Post-case reconciling Time between event and detection Time between event and resolution Dispenses post discharge or transfer from unit Temporary patient additions
Prescribing	Verify active prescriber DEA license Only authorized prescribers are ordering CS (audit) Review and trend CS verbal orders that have not been cosigned Prescribing patterns trends compared to peers Suspicious order monitoring
Administration	Overrides User unlinked orders in relation to overrides Cancelation patterns/null transactions Returns Sole user (dispense, waste, return or issue) Out of area/unit dispensing/global list transactions Anesthesia post case reconciliation Anomalous user activity checks Gaps in documentation Delays in administration Delays in documentation Verbal read back or no cosign by location
Waste and removal	Waste patterns Waste witness patterns Time to document waste Delayed waste documentation from time of administration High waste products High waste procedures Full waste transactions
Overall process integrity	Post-case reconciliation Tracer audits (from the last biennial to a random day) Control substance safety reporting Submission information for DEA 106 reports State control substance filings Outstanding discrepancies Time to resolve discrepancies DEA/significant loss reports Expired CS trends

Abbreviations: CS, controlled substances; DEA, Drug Enforcement Administration.

and investigation and reporting of suspected diversion in accordance with organization procedures.

- Nursing management conducts random patient interviews to verify that patients received the CS and had the expected therapeutic response (eg, that the medication adequately controlled pain) and also compares responses to nursing patient assessment notes and medication administration records. Inconsistencies found on patient interview or multiple patients experiencing lack of medication efficacy may point to diversion at the time of administration. When possible, medication administration is integrated with clinical assessment in the electronic medication record. Incidents in which patient response is not as expected and all nurses are experiencing similar lack of medication efficacy are reported to the pharmacy for further investigation of product integrity; there are case reports of prepackaged CS containing the wrong medication, and these circumstances could signal a medication error.
- A process is in place to resolve CS discrepancies and specify the time in which discrepancies must be resolved. It is recommended that CS discrepancies be reported to the supervisor in charge and resolved as soon as possible upon discovery, preferably no later than the end of the work shift, and that discrepancies deemed to be resolved are reviewed by the supervisor to ensure the legitimacy of the resolution. Discrepancies that cannot be resolved ("unresolvable discrepancies") are reported immediately to pharmacy and are jointly reviewed by pharmacy and patient care leadership, with resolution within 24–72 hours.
- Pharmacy is immediately notified of and supports the reconciliation investigation when an unresolvable discrepancy is discovered, and a pharmacist is responsible for overseeing the investigation of the discrepancy, even when a technician assists with these duties.
- Provider transactions are reviewed for poor documentation patterns (eg, failure to document, corrections in the pharmacy CS vault or ADCs), and trends of users and cosigners are tracked. A trend of poor documentation practices by HCWs is reviewed for possible diversion.
- Pharmacy, in collaboration with nursing supervision, reconciles all CS orders against administration records, at minimum, in high-risk areas, by comparing the amount dispensed with the amount documented as administered and the amount documented as wasted. This reconciliation may occur through surveillance analytics technology. Random, monthly audits may be conducted in areas that are not high-risk or supported by surveillance analytics.
- The organization identifies specific high-risk CS medications that are randomly assayed, and procedures include random testing of waste from all high-risk or high-volume areas (eg, pharmacy sterile products preparation, surgery and anesthesia areas), as permitted by and in accordance with state and federal rules and regulations.

High-Risk Areas. The organization should identify high-risk areas (eg, surgery, anesthesia, intensive care units, sterile compounding areas, emergency departments) and include an assessment of risk for diversion (eg, known diversion points), ease of detection (eg, high-volume locations, level of oversight and controls, state of awareness of patients), and probability of harm (eg, potential to impact the quality of care). Automation and technology should be utilized in all high-risk areas to facilitate security controls and optimization of automated monitoring and surveillance technology. High-risk areas should be defined by the organization but include areas where the same provider is prescribing, obtaining, preparing, and administering the medication, such as surgery centers, operating rooms, and procedural and anesthesia areas. High-risk areas are also locations where high volumes of CS are ordered, prescribed, stored, prepared, and dispensed within the same location. The main pharmacy is considered a high-risk area.

Anesthesia and operating rooms are high-risk areas for which organizations should consider additional controls. Documentation of doses administered in the health record should be routinely reconciled with documentation of doses dispensed, waste, and return quantities as well as prescribed doses. The pharmacist should be responsible for all drugs and CS dispensed and distributed in these settings. Pharmacy technicians, under the supervision of the pharmacist, could be assigned many of the responsibilities for these daily activities as permitted by state and federal law. If there is a satellite pharmacy, minimal drug stock should be kept in each surgical suite, and additional drug inventory should be maintained within a pharmacy location to the extent possible. Satellite pharmacies supporting surgery and procedural areas should be staffed whenever the areas providing surgery and administering anesthesia are normally staffed. If the satellite pharmacy is not open 24 hours a day, it may be necessary to establish an after-hours drug supply. The pharmacy and anesthesiology departments should collaborate to decide the drugs and quantities required for this supply, including an assessment of the smallest appropriate dose and packaging, and the accountability system to be used. Supply levels should be checked, reconciled, and replenished daily. Dedicated pharmacy resources within the perioperative area allow for more active and timely monitoring of CS utilization and identification of possible diversion. Systems to track drugs used, adjust par levels as needed, and monitor drug expiration dates should be devised. The ASHP Guidelines on Perioperative Pharmacy Services provide specific guidance on best practices unique to CS management for these patient care areas and services.[24]

Investigation and Reporting of Suspected Diversion

It is imperative that there is a detailed and thorough approach to investigating and reporting suspected diversion. Incomplete investigations and follow-up can have serious patient care, legal, personal reputation, and compliance implications. Any unresolvable discrepancy should be considered a possible diversion and escalated to an investigation, with notifications to occur as defined in the organization's CSDPP. Processes should be in place to trigger an immediate investigation, the appropriate internal and external communications, and the completion of required reporting. Although the supervisor in the area where diversion is suspected will assist in conducting the investigation, those external to the area should be involved to ensure that biases do not influence the investigation. The pharmacy director or his or her designee and diversion officer (if different) should be notified immediately of any suspected diversion within the organization and participate in all active investigations. Investigation and reporting procedures should include the following (see Appendix B for additional guidance):

- Guidance is provided by the CSDPP with regard to the review process, including who will coordinate the investigation, appropriate team members, leadership and organization legal counsel notification, documentation of the investigation, and coordination of internal and external reporting.
- Investigations are conducted as thoroughly and completely as possible; at a minimum, reporting occurs when it is determined that the discrepancy is unresolved or that there has been a known theft or diversion. As the investigation proceeds, there is an escalation and broadening of notifications specified in the policies and procedures defined by the CSDPP.
- Investigations involving contracted HCWs are conducted in collaboration with the contracted entity and with full transparency.
- If the organization becomes aware of an arrest of an HCW for illicit use of CS, the organization immediately conducts an investigation of the HCW's transactions to assess whether diversion has occurred. The organization assesses whether to suspend, transfer, or terminate the HCW or take other action (eg, remove access to CS) or impose other sanctions against the HCW. The organization immediately removes access privileges to CS if diversion is suspected until the investigation is completed and a determination of diversion or other risks to patient care is made.
- The organization establishes guidelines for engaging external entities, such as DEA, licensure boards, laboratories (for testing), and local law enforcement. Guidance is provided with regard to review processes to determine who is required to be notified, when to notify, who is responsible for contacting the agency, and other circumstances for the notification. The organization fulfills reporting requirements for diversion or other unaccountable loss of CS in accordance with laws and regulations.
- The organization defines, in accordance with the law, when a DEA Form 106 should be completed for discrepancies that remain ultimately unresolved. There are clear responsibilities for completion of DEA Form 106 for a theft or significant loss, who is to be notified, and when. Even if the loss cannot be quantified due to the nature of the diversion method, DEA must still be notified.

Quality Improvement. For significant diversions, a quality-improvement review should be initiated by the CSDPP committee, including a root cause analysis and recommendations to prevent future occurrences. Representatives from the area where there is a suspected diversion should be engaged in the investigation and refinement of prevention strategies. Furthermore, the CSDPP should coordinate a proactive diversion risk review, such as by conducting a failure modes and effects analysis of processes, particularly when there are drug shortages, new drug products and dosage forms are approved, new technology or technology upgrades are implemented, and new drug delivery systems are implemented. Results of the risk review should be used to make system improvements as part of the organization's performance-improvement activities.

Communications. The organization should have a clearly defined, full-disclosure policy and process to communicate to patients and families who are affected by CS diversion. The organization should also have guidelines for engaging the media and managing external public relations upon conclusion of the investigation. Policies and processes should specify when to notify the media, what internal communications are required, and who is responsible for contacting the media representative and approving media communications. External communications need to also consider and protect HCW privacy and confidentiality.

Chain of Custody

Effective diversion control systems depend on implementing retrievable evidence that the chain of custody is maintained at all times and at all points when the transfer of CS occurs between individuals, whether within or external to the pharmacy (eg, courier transport to other facilities, use of pneumatic tube systems, transfer to emergency medical service providers, collection receptacle inventory, or transfer from contract pharmacy services). Chain-of-custody controls depend on the ability to reliably audit the trail of transfer. Every point along the chain of custody should be identified and reviewed to detect and address any gaps. The organization should establish and enforce a policy stating that HCWs with access to CS may not delegate their access to another HCW in a way that will alter the audit trail for the chain of custody (eg, not sharing electronic medical record, ADC, or pharmacy door passcodes; not providing key access and entry to unauthorized HCWs); utilizing biometric identification whenever possible prevents this type of circumvention. The delivery of CS to a storage location without witness and receipt confirmation by another authorized HCW may not meet the intent of the chain of custody requirement. In addition, controls should be built in when transfer is made via transport mechanisms (eg, a pneumatic tube system) to ensure that the CS is received and verified as received by an identifiable, authorized individual.

Measures should be in place to ensure the integrity and security of CS, the chain of custody, and the safety of personnel transporting CS. Secure, lockable, and tamper-evident delivery containers (eg, carts, trays, or boxes) should be used to transport CS. The packaging should not reveal the contents during transport (eg, an opaque container). Contents should be blind counted and documented upon receipt. Locking mechanisms, when used, should be tamper-resistant and traceable (eg, plastic tie locks with unique, verifiable, numerical identifier). The chain of custody must also apply to laboratory services (internal or external) used to analyze syringes or other products as part of an investigation or random assay process.

In circumstances in which CS prescriptions or drugs are dispensed directly to patients (eg, in emergency departments, discharge prescriptions, and home infusion), procedures must ensure that the chain of custody is maintained and documented.

If CS are provided to emergency medical services (eg, ambulance services), the organization should ensure that procedures are in place that comply with local, state, and federal requirements and ensure that the chain of custody is maintained and the disposition of CS is documented and retrievable. See Appendix B for additional guidance.

Storage and Security

Storage and security of CS require a coordinated approach that includes facility controls (eg, camera surveillance), physical access controls (eg, locks or biometric access technology), and frequent inventory checks and surveillance to allow discrepancies to be discovered in a timely manner. Key elements of CS storage and security include the following (see Appendix B for additional guidance):

- CS are stored in a locked and secured location (eg, ADC, safe, locked cabinet/ drawer) at all times unless in the direct physical control of an authorized individual. When implementing or assessing facility and physical access controls, the security and safety of HCWs are taken into consideration.
- Storing CS in transportable lock boxes or "fanny packs" is avoided. If used, such lock boxes or packs follow the same requirements for storage, security, and chain-of-custody controls as other inventory. Unattended and transportable lock boxes are not considered secure and are stored in a locked area accessible only to authorized personnel when not in use or otherwise unattended. Lock-out times for electronic locks on carts (eg, medication or anesthesia carts) containing CS are limited to the narrowest window of time that is appropriate for the particular setting.
- There is a defined process to ensure that only authorized individuals have access to CS. Access to CS storage areas is minimized and limited to authorized personnel. There is a complete assessment of all HCWs with access privileges to ensure that only those permitted to access have access (ie, currently employed, temporary employees, or licensed independent practitioners with privileges), and removal of access privileges occurs immediately upon separation.
- There are policies and procedures regarding CS access, including restrictions through assignment, key controls, and the use of passwords. Access permissions should be monitored at least every 6 months and revised when appropriate (eg, separation or job change). For ADCs, biometric identification with a user ID is preferred over passwords. CS cabinets and carts that are not ADCs are secured with an electronic lock that requires a user-specific biometric identification, code, or badge swipe. Access is recorded and retrievable for surveillance.
- Where keys are used (eg, lock boxes, refrigerated storage boxes, and infusion pumps), they are unique to the device, when possible, and there is a procedure to track keys and their chain of custody, secure keys after hours, replace lost keys, and change locks if keys are lost.
- Any HCW authorized to have access to or prescribe CS will be able to provide appropriate photo identification upon request.
- Camera surveillance should be considered (1) in locations where there is high risk for diversion (eg, main pharmacy vault, packaging areas, community pharmacy), (2) in locations where electronic or biometric access is not available, (3) in remote locations; and used to assist with an active diversion investigation. Video should be retained and retrievable for a timeframe sufficient to allow for adequate incident investigation. It is important to work closely with the organization's security and human resources departments to review state laws and labor contracts that might constrain the use of such surveillance, as well as determine the organization's policies and procedures regarding security footage review.
- ADC technology should be utilized in high-volume CS areas, including the pharmacy, anesthesia and surgery locations, high-volume clinics, and outpatient procedure areas.
- When delivering CS to an ADC, restocking an ADC, or pulling returns from the return bin, there should be a witness or other verification process (as previously described in the Monitoring and Surveillance section).
- Controls are in place to monitor pharmacy inventories for discrepancies. In areas outside of the pharmacy, at least one of those conducting the inventory is licensed. Within pharmacy areas with ADC vault management, CS are manually inventoried by two rotating, licensed, or otherwise authorized pharmacy personnel (eg, pharmacy technicians) monthly. For high-volume or high-risk areas, more frequent verification audits are considered to prevent or minimize inventory count discrepancies and minimize the time window for discovery of the discrepancy. For pharmacies without ADC vault management, a physical inventory is conducted at least once per month but preferably weekly. At least one of those conducting the inventory is a licensed pharmacist. The inventory count includes expired or otherwise unusable CS awaiting disposal or transfer to a reverse distributor.
- CS counts managed by ADCs or done manually are verified by a blind count each time a CS drawer, pocket, cabinet, or refrigerator is accessed, except when unit-of-use dispensing technology is deployed.
- Inventory verification is conducted for CS managed by ADCs by two authorized HCWs if a blind count has not been performed within one week. CS not managed through ADCs are manually inventoried by two authorized HCWs at the beginning and end of every shift when the area is open for services.
- Patient-specific CS infusions are contained in a secured lock box utilizing no-port tubing unless under constant surveillance. Keys and access to these controls are limited and tracked as with any keys and lock boxes.
- Documents used to procure or prescribe CS (eg, DEA Form 222, blank prescriptions, security printer paper) are secured and monitored with the same diligence as CS to prevent theft or loss.

CS Brought into the Hospital by Patients

Procedures are established that address special circumstances to ensure controls are in place to secure CS and prevent diversion of CS brought into the organization by patients. Patients should be encouraged to return their own medications to home via a household member or authorized agent when possible. Alternatively, patients or their authorized agent may be provided with an envelope to mail prescriptions to their home or directed to a collection receptacle for disposal. Organizations should, in collaboration with local and state authorities, consider providing a public collection (or "take-back") receptacle for disposal of CS by patients or their agent.

CS should only be allowed when they are to be administered to the patient pursuant to a medication order, on behalf of the patient, and with their consent. These medications should be inventoried and stored in a secure location. When a patient is not able to maintain security of their own medications due to loss of competence or death, or when medications are abandoned, documentation of the patient's home medications, quantity inventoried, and signatures of two verifying HCWs should be recorded in the medical record upon receipt of the medications, and arrangements made as soon as possible for appropriate disposition. The organization should define the period of time to be considered abandonment, and in such instances, should dispose of the medications as allowed by law or contact their local DEA Diversion Field Office for guidance on proper disposal procedures. CS should be stored in a secure location until disposition and chain of custody documented (eg, the patient or patient's authorized agent should sign that he or she has received the medication and its quantity.) When patients bring illicit substances into the organization, procedures should address notification of the local authorities as required by law.[19,20]

Internal Pharmacy Controls

Internal pharmacy controls include controls related to procurement, preparation, and dispensing of CS. These processes typically apply only to pharmacy locations. Diversion can occur at various points within these processes, and it is important to apply key principles to effectively minimize opportunities for diversion. Key principles include limiting the number of people authorized to order CS, creating separation of duties and rotation of HCWs through various responsibilities within the process, and observing for variation in processes. It is recommended that these processes be audited by external (to the pharmacy) review at least biannually. Examples of recommended procurement, preparation, and dispensing controls follow; see Appendix B for additional guidance.

Procurement Controls

- All CS are procured from the pharmacy. If other departments or individuals are authorized to procure CS, there are checks and balances established to ensure the same policies and procedures are consistently followed throughout the organization.
- There are purchasing safeguards in place that prohibit ordering of CS by those not authorized by the organization. CS may only be ordered by authorized individuals (DEA registrant and for Schedule II CS, those with power of attorney granted).
- An electronic CS ordering system (CSOS) is utilized, eliminating or minimizing use of paper DEA Form 222s.
- When paper DEA Form 222s are used, those forms are locked in a secure location, recorded on a perpetual inventory log, and accessible only to those authorized to procure CS. CSOS order files are backed up to an organization-based system to ensure that archived files are readily retrievable by designated personnel.
- Separation of duties exists between the ordering and receipt of CS. Two authorized individuals count and check in CS received and confirm that the order, invoice, and product-received documentation match. At least one of the receivers is licensed. The process is overseen by a licensed pharmacist.
- There is a process to investigate and remedy discrepancies when CS are received in the pharmacy from the wholesaler or other distributor.
- There are processes to track, reconcile, and audit CS products where preparation is outsourced to and received from a third party.
- Procedures exist that ensure the chain of custody is maintained for interorganization transfer or transport of CS (eg, from a central distribution hub).
- Procedures define the controls and required documentation when CS are transferred between pharmacies.
- All CS procurement paperwork is reviewed for completion and filed according to applicable laws and regulations. Procedures are in place for patient care areas of the organization that are considered under common control that support the pharmacist-in-charge to provide oversight and authority to ensure proper procurement controls are being utilized.

Preparation and Dispensing Controls

- A perpetual inventory is maintained, and a blind-count process is used when adding or removing CS from a pharmacy inventory location.
- Access to inventory is limited, with controls to identify who accessed the inventory, when the inventory was accessed, and what changes were made to the inventory; access controls provide a readily retrievable audit trail.
- To minimize diversion through drug product alteration or tampering, drug products are inspected for alteration or tampering, and any potential discrepancy is investigated for possible diversion.
- To minimize diversion during repackaging, CS are purchased and dispensed in unit dose packaging whenever possible. Diversion controls are in place when CS are repackaged, and repackaged products are routinely inspected to ensure product integrity.
- Delivery and restocking of CS in patient care and procedural areas require an auditable verification of delivery and receipt.
- Returns from the patient care and procedural areas (eg, emptying a return bin) have an auditable verification of return. Returns are inspected for integrity.

Prescribing and Administration

CS may only be ordered by prescribers who are licensed in accordance with the DEA and authorized to prescribe CS. When possible and permitted or required by law, CS orders and prescriptions are generated and transmitted by electronic systems with controlled access, except in emergency situations. When written prescriptions are used, there are controls in place to track and secure these prescriptions and paper used to print prescriptions (see the Storage and Security section). Order sets and guidelines that include CS should be evaluated in accordance with organizational guidelines, are supported by clinical evidence, and align with the lowest unit-of-use products to minimize waste. Guidelines, restrictions, and diversion controls should not delay patient treatment or compromise patient needs. Key elements of prescribing and administration diversion controls include the following (see Appendix B for additional guidance):

- A valid order from an authorized prescriber exists for all CS administered, and the number of CS allowed via ADC override status is minimized.
- There is a process to identify and verify authorized prescribers within either an electronic or a manual ordering system. There is also a process to identify and verify authorized prescribers and prescriptions written by medical residents or other providers who are authorized to prescribe CS under the organization's DEA registration (eg, use of a suffix).
- Pharmacists clarify orders for which the prescriber or order is questionable with regard to prescriber identity or other legitimacy of the prescription or order. Pharmacists and prescribers query the prescription drug monitoring program (PDMP) to assist with prescription initiation and dispensing, respectively, when necessary or required by law.
- Active prescriptions and orders for CS are reevaluated regularly, and CS orders are reordered per the organization's policies when a patient transfers to a different level of care. The medical staff, in coordination and consultation with pharmacy, determines and establishes an automatic stop-order system for CS when there is not a specific time or number of doses prescribed.
- CS are retrieved from the storage location and administered to patients by a licensed provider within his or her scope of practice, and such administration is documented in the medical record. When administration is scheduled "as needed," the administration can be correlated to the patient assessment (eg, established pain assessment criteria).
- Access to medications for a particular patient is suspended immediately at discharge.
- CS are retrieved from inventory by the authorized HCW responsible for administering the medication to the patient and as close to the time of administration as possible, as defined by organization and appropriate to the care setting. Procedures for exceptions in emergency situations or settings are defined, and these exceptions are reviewed for appropriateness. The CS retrieved for a patient is the package size equivalent to, or the closest available to, the dose to be administered.
- CS packaging (eg, vials, prefilled syringe systems, unit dose packages of oral dosage forms) is inspected for integrity when being inventoried, before dispensing, and upon administration.
- Generally, outside of pharmacy compounding areas and in patient care areas, CS are not drawn up into syringes in advance, and sequential dosing is avoided, recognizing that these processes may be necessary in some procedural areas. Specifically, single-dose syringes and vials are not used to deliver multiple doses. The syringes prepared in these procedural areas are labeled as required by approved procedures and kept under the direct control of the person preparing the syringes until administration. When sequential doses are required from a single syringe (eg, during procedures), there is a method in place to track the doses ordered versus those administered.
- Policies and procedures address the documentation of CS issued but unused, and there is a process to return the unused CS to inventory. Returns should be placed in a one-way, secure return bin and not returned to the original pocket in the ADC. These products should not be restocked until inspected for tampering.

Returns, Waste, and Disposal

Policies and procedures should define how waste will be accounted for, tracked, and disposed of to prevent unauthorized access. To minimize waste, when possible, CS are stocked in ready-to-use form (eg, avoiding the use of multidose vials or oral liquids) and in the lowest commercially available units for doses frequently prescribed for patients. Waste may include products prepared for administration but not administered to the patient (eg, when a provider discontinues an order or a patient refuses administration), or drug product remaining after a partial dose is removed from its packaged unit (eg, oral liquids or vial). Waste may also include overfill in vials and drug product remaining in transdermal delivery systems. The organization's waste handling practices should maintain chain of custody to minimize the risk for CS diversion. CS should be wasted immediately or as close to the time of administration as possible.

The wasting of all CS requires an independent witness and documentation; at least one, but preferably both, of the witnesses should be licensed. Procedures should define what constitutes complete and timely documentation of waste. An individual witnessing CS wasting should verify the product label, that the volume or amount being wasted matches the documentation, that the drug product being wasted physically matches the drug product in the documentation, and that the wasting occurs per policy for safe disposal and in a manner that makes the CS non-retrievable (as defined by the DEA).[16] The entire process of drawing up and wasting before administration should be witnessed so the individual verifying can be certain that the actual CS is being wasted and not a substituted or adulterated product. Approved methods and secure containers for returns, wastes, and disposal of CS are as defined in federal, state, county, and municipal laws and regulations. Key elements of returning, wasting, and disposing of CS include (see Appendix B for additional guidance):

- All issued but unused CS that may be potentially reusable are returned to the pharmacy or to a designated, secure return location. All returns to the pharmacy and when using a reverse distributor require that the chain of custody be maintained and that witness of transfer is documented.
- In patient care areas where waste is documented through the ADC, the waste is documented by the person who retrieved and administered the medication and, to the extent possible, in the same device from which the medication was removed.
- In patient care areas, unless selected for random assay (see the Monitoring and Surveillance section), unusable CS products, including patient-specific partially used preparations, are immediately wasted and witnessed by authorized individuals per specific organization procedures.

- Procedures are established that ensure the chain of custody is maintained when waste is transferred to the pharmacy for conducting random assays.
- Partially used preparations or containers are not returned to the pharmacy for disposal, except for purposes of random assay. The act of wasting and the documentation of CS waste are completed by the same HCW who accesses and administers the medication, when feasible. Examples of cases in which this may not be feasible include wasting a CS infusion, patient-controlled analgesia cartridge, or multiday patch. Within the pharmacy, CS waste from compounded sterile preparations is documented with a cosignature and randomly assayed at least quarterly.
- CS overfill is considered an unusable product and is wasted and documented according to established procedures.
- For defined high-risk areas (eg, surgical, anesthesia, procedural, high volume) and/or specific high-risk CS medications (eg, fentanyl), waste is witnessed and reconciled with the medication administration record by an authorized HCW. Dispense transactions can be considered reconciled when matched to a prescriber's order and the dose dispensed is equal to the dose charted as administered plus any amount of drug documented as wasted or returned.
- Approved methods for wasting CS are defined in policies and procedures and comply with universal precautions and organization waste disposal requirements.
- CS product are secured to prevent tampering or made otherwise non-retrievable (eg, use of deactivating, deterring, and solidifying agents.)
- Expired CS are clearly identified as such and stored in a separate, secured location from other medications, and inventory is monitored until return via a reverse distributor or destruction and disposal in accordance with legal requirements. Before final transfer to a reverse distributor, DEA Form 222 is audited against amounts transferred. Expired or otherwise unusable CS are not retained or stored in the pharmacy for long periods of time, and the frequency of returns ensures that inventory is not allowed to accumulate. Returns or destruction occurs at least quarterly.

Community and Mail Delivery Pharmacies

Over 30% of hospitals and health systems operate community pharmacies.[25] It is important to consider and address controls unique to these operations. Organizations should include their community pharmacies within the scope of their CSDPP oversight and proactively seek to improve controls. Community pharmacies may require additional registration, certification, or record-keeping (eg, drug collection receptacle site registration or compliance with the Combat Methamphetamine Epidemic Act of 2005) related to CS.[26] Community pharmacies within health systems should be aware that they are at risk for both internal and external theft and diversion, and CS diversion management controls need to consider public access and the possibility of diversion from fraudulent prescriptions.

Security measures and other physical controls, such as camera surveillance throughout the pharmacy, are imperative in this setting to deter and monitor for suspected theft and provide an avenue for discrepancies to be resolved in a timely manner. Badge reader or biometric access should be required for access to all areas where CS are stored. These systems provide physical access control, limit access to appropriate personnel, and create a perpetual log of HCWs who have accessed the storage area or cabinet. To deter theft, bulk containers of Schedule III, IV, and V CS should be dispersed among non-CS inventory, where permitted by law. Schedule II CS requiring refrigeration should be stored among other refrigerated medications, preferably in a locked compartment.

Inventory adjustments to CS medications pose a significant internal diversion risk. Depending on who within the pharmacy has security access to perform CS inventory adjustments, community pharmacies should consider having auditing systems in place to track and validate inventory adjustments performed by staff. Audits should also be routinely conducted to ensure CS purchases are reconciled with quantity dispensed and on-hand inventory to identify discrepancies in inventory and dispensing trends. In addition to CS inventory adjustments, CS prescriptions awaiting delivery or pick-up ("will call" area), and canceled prescriptions are significant internal diversion risks. Controls such as tamper-resistant packaging should be used when possible and procedures implemented to ensure chain of custody is maintained when dispensing or delivering CS to the patient (as with a meds-to-beds program). Community pharmacies should develop policies and procedures for an accounting of will-call and canceled prescriptions and consider developing reports or tracking methods to identify any CS medications that have not been picked up from will-call within a specific period of time (eg, 10 days) or have been canceled and returned to stock. Furthermore, organizations should consider interfacing their point-of-sale system with their prescription management software and develop a report to reconcile processed prescriptions with prescriptions in will-call and sold.

Fraudulent prescriptions also pose a significant risk for diversion in the CS supply chain. Community pharmacies should utilize a variety of diversion prevention and monitoring tools when reviewing CS prescriptions, including internal pharmacy documentation and dispensing records, third-party utilization reviews, and PDMP databases, if applicable. Prior to dispensing, prescriptions should be reviewed for patient prescriber red flags (eg, concomitant opioid/benzodiazepines prescribed, high daily doses, cash-only claims, and "doctor shopping"). Investigation and resolution of red flags to determine the legitimacy of a prescription should be documented and retrievable. Red flag trends noted with prescribers or patients should also be monitored for trends that indicate prescriptions may not be for a legitimate medical purpose.

Community pharmacies should attempt to receive electronic CS prescriptions when possible. If hard-copy prescriptions are accepted, community pharmacies should develop a system to document which employee received the CS prescription at prescription intake and validate that it was not introduced into the pharmacy dispensing system for fraudulent purposes. The same system should be utilized to document which HCW processed the CS prescription. Finally, the CS prescriptions should be filed sequentially, and community pharmacies should consider developing a system to audit hardcopy prescriptions for documentation of chain of custody from employee to patient, such as signature of receipt.

There should be a complete and accurate written or electronic perpetual inventory record for the receipt (CSOS and DEA Form 222) and disposition of all Schedule II medications, filed in sequential order. The perpetual inventory should be updated each time a Schedule II CS medication is received and should be verified by two employees, one of whom is a licensed provider. Furthermore, the same sign-off process in the perpetual inventory log should occur with each fill of a Schedule II CS. When possible, community pharmacies should utilize labels from the prescription management software to record the quantity filled in the perpetual inventory log. Community pharmacies should also consider implementing a system for monitoring partial fills of Schedule II CS, as this is a risk for diversion. Schedule II CS medications should be audited each month to ensure correct counts and that the perpetual log has been signed off by two authorized HCWs. All records, including but not limited to prescriptions, DEA Form 222s, CSOS receiving documents, perpetual inventory logs, and discrepancy reports, should be kept for a specified time as determined by the organization and relevant regulations. When discrepancies are identified, their investigation and resolution should be evaluated by a third party, such as the CSDPP, internal or external auditing personnel. Key elements of community-based pharmacy management of CS include (see Appendix B for additional guidance):

- During nonbusiness hours, CS are stored in an area secured by a physical barrier with security access controls (which may include a locked room within a secured facility) that can only be accessed when authorized pharmacy personnel are present.
- The organization has systems in place for documentation and monitoring of CS inventory adjustments made by pharmacy employees, CS prescriptions cancelled and returned to stock, and CS prescriptions left at will-call (eg, prescriptions remaining 10 days after being filled).
- CS safety controls (eg, bar code verification, weight checks, drug photo identification labels) should be considered when implementing automated dispensing technology. When automated checks are not available for dispensing, the quantity dispensed is verified and documented with a second authorized person.
- Diversion prevention and monitoring tools are utilized as appropriate to determine the legitimacy of CS prescriptions, including PDMP reporting and checks, in accordance with state requirements.
- Chain of custody and security is maintained when holding prescriptions in the will-call area and when delivering medications to patients, such as with a "meds-to-beds" prescription delivery service, for example, by use of tamper-evident security bags.
- The pharmacy's point-of-sale system is interfaced with prescription management software and has reports designed to identify discrepancies.
- For mail returns, documentation, chain of custody, inventory, and security controls are ensured from the point it is received until it is wasted or re-shipped.
- CS purchases are compared and reconciled with dispensing and on-hand inventory at least monthly.

Special Considerations

Although it is impossible to predict all scenarios, and procedures may need to be customized for unique circumstances and settings, these guidelines present core principles applicable to all settings, and exceptions should be minimized. Examples of areas where special considerations may apply include both high- and low-volume areas, such as organization-owned physician practices, research areas, off-campus clinics, rehabilitation facilities, alternate sites of care (eg, home infusion services, virtual hospitals), and free-standing emergency rooms and surgery centers. Organizations or other regulatory agencies may elect to designate a non-scheduled medication (eg, growth hormone, gabapentin, PDE-5 inhibitors, types of insulin, propofol) as a locally controlled item based on what is determined to be at "high risk" for diversion. In these circumstances, the same principles described in these guidelines may be applied.

Conclusion

Healthcare organizations should develop a framework for integrating CS diversion prevention strategies into a comprehensive CSDPP. With engaged leadership and interprofessional collaboration, organizations can foster a culture of organizational and individual awareness and accountability for CS diversion prevention and response.

References

1. Schaefer MK, Perz JF. Outbreaks of infections associated with drug diversion by US healthcare personnel. *Mayo Clin Proc.* 2014;89:878–887.
2. Berge KH, Dillon KR, Sikkink KM, et al. Diversion of drugs within healthcare facilities, a multiple-victim crime: patterns of diversion, scope, consequences, detection, and prevention. *Mayo Clin Proc.* 2012;87:674–682.
3. Minnesota Department of Health and Minnesota Hospital Association. Road map to controlled substance diversion prevention 2.0. Published 2015. Accessed June 7, 2022. https://www.health.state.mn.us/facilities/patientsafety/drugdiversion/docs/divroadmap041812.pdf
4. California Hospital Association Medication Safety Collaborative Committee. Reducing controlled substances diversion in hospitals. Accessed June 7, 2022. https://www.chpso.org/sites/main/files/file-attachments/controlled_substance_diversion.pdf?1368720872
5. Baldisserri MR. Impaired healthcare professional. *Crit Care Med.* 2007;35(suppl):S106–116.
6. The Joint Commission. MM.08.01.01: the organization evaluates the effectiveness of its medication management system. In: *Comprehensive Accreditation Manual for Hospitals 2019.* Joint Commission Resources; 2019.
7. Centers for Medicare & Medicaid Services. Conditions of participation for hospitals, §482.11, compliance with federal, state, and local laws. Accessed June 7, 2022. http://cms.hhs.gov/Regulations-and-Guidance/Guidance/Manuals/downloads/som107ap_a_hospitals.pdf

8. Mattson CL, Tanz LJ, Quinn K, et al. Trends and geographic patterns in drug and synthetic opioid overdose deaths—United States, 2013–2019. *MMWR Morb Mortal Wkly Rep.* 2021;70:202–207.
9. Siegel J, O'Neal B. Prevention of controlled substance diversion—scope, strategy, and tactics. Code N: multidisciplinary approach to proactive drug diversion prevention. *Hosp Pharm.* 2007;42:244–248.
10. O'Neal B, Bass K, Siegel J. Prevention of controlled substance diversion—scope, strategy, and tactics. Diversion in the operating room. *Hosp Pharm.* 2007;42:359–363.
11. Siegel J, Wierwille C, O'Neal B. Prevention of controlled substance diversion—scope, strategy, and tactics. The investigative process. *Hosp Pharm.* 2007;42:466–469.
12. O'Neal B, Siegel J. Prevention of controlled substance diversion—scope, strategy, and tactics. Use of diversion detection software. *Hosp Pharm.* 2007;42:564–572.
13. Siegel J, O'Neal B. Prevention of controlled substance diversion—scope, strategy, and tactics. Code N: the intervention process. *Hosp Pharm.* 2007;42:653–6.
14. O'Neal B, Siegel J. Prevention of controlled substance diversion—scope, strategy, and tactics. Diversion in the pharmacy. *Hosp Pharm.* 2007;42:145–148.
15. Martin ES, Dzierba SH, Jones DM. Preventing large-scale controlled substance diversion from within the pharmacy. *Hosp Pharm.* 2013;48:406–412.
16. Code of Federal Regulations, Title 21 Food and Drugs, Chapter II, Drug Enforcement Administration, Department of Justice. Accessed June 7, 2022. https://www.ecfr.gov/current/title-21/chapter-II
17. Office of Diversion Control, Drug Enforcement Administration. *Pharmacist's Manual: An Informational Outline of the Controlled Substances Act.* Published October 8, 2020. Accessed June 7, 2022. https://www.deadiversion.usdoj.gov/GDP/(DEA-DC-046R1)(EO-DEA154R1)_Pharmacist's_Manual_DEA.pdf
18. Centers for Medicare & Medicaid Services. Pharmacy self-auditing. Control practices to improve Medicaid program integrity and quality patient care—booklet 2: controlled substances. Published December 2015. Accessed June 7, 2022. https://www.cms.gov/Medicare-Medicaid-Coordination/Fraud-Prevention/Medicaid-Integrity-Education/Downloads/pharmacy-selfaudit-booklet2-control-substances.pdf
19. American Society of Health-System Pharmacists. ASHP policy position 1522: disposition of illicit substances. Accessed June 7, 2022. https://www.ashp.org/-/media/assets/policy-guidelines/docs/browse-by-document-type-policy-positions-1982-2022-with-rationales-pdf.pdf
20. American Society of Health-System Pharmacists. Frequently asked questions: DEA rule on disposal of controlled substances (DEA-316). Updated October 20, 2014. Accessed June 7, 2022. https://www.ashp.org/-/media/assets/advocacy-issues/docs/ashp-frequently-asked-questions-dea-proposed-rule-on-the-disposal-of-controlled-substances-dea-316.ashx?la=en&hash=E037298EACE95084EA0B64BAE3E75BFC59F94833
21. Missouri Bureau of Narcotics and Dangerous Drugs. Drug diversion in hospitals: a guide to preventing and investigating diversion issues. Published August 2016. Accessed June 7, 2022. http://health.mo.gov/safety/bndd/doc/drugdiversion.doc
22. American Society of Health-System Pharmacists. ASHP statement on the pharmacist's role in substance abuse prevention, education, and assistance. *Am J Health-Syst Pharm.* 2016;73:e267-e270. https://www.ashp.org/-/media/assets/policy-guidelines/docs/statements/pharmacists-role-substance-abuse-prevention-education-assistance.pdf
23. Cello R, Conley M, Cooley T, et al. ASHP guidelines on the safe use of automated dispensing cabinets. *Am J Health-Syst Pharm* 2022;79:e71-e82. Accessed June 7, 2022. https://www.ashp.org/-/media/assets/policy-guidelines/docs/guidelines/safe-use-of-automated-dispensing-devices.ashx
24. Bickham P, Golembiewski J, Meyer T, et al. ASHP guidelines on perioperative pharmacy services. *Am J Health-Syst Pharm.* 2019;76:903–920. doi:10.1093/ajhp/zxz073
25. Pedersen CA, Schneider PJ, Scheckelhoff DJ. ASHP national survey of pharmacy practice in hospital settings: monitoring and patient education—2015. *Am J Health-Syst Pharm.* 2016;73:1307–1330.
26. Drug Enforcement Administration. CMEA (Combat Methamphetamine Epidemic Act of 2005). Accessed June 7, 2022. https://www.deadiversion.usdoj.gov/meth/cma2005.htm

Appendix A—Definitions of Terms Related to Diversion Prevention

All terms used in these guidelines have the definition set forth in Title 21 United States Code Controlled Substances Act (CSA) (Section 102 of the Act [21 USC 802]) or part 1300 of Title 21 Code of Federal Regulations, except where noted.

Administer: Defined in the CSA [CSA §102(2); 21 USC 802(2)] (2), the term refers to the direct application of a controlled substance to the body of a patient or research subject by (a) an individual practitioner (or, in his presence, by his authorized agent), or (b) the patient or research subject at the direction and in the presence of the individual practitioner, whether such application be by injection, inhalation, ingestion, or any other means.

Advanced analytics: Advanced analytics capability is the application of machine learning and artificial intelligence technology solutions to assist with efficient data interpretation and analysis, with tools such as dashboards, identification of trends and insights.

Audit trail: Defined in the DEA regulations [21 CFR 1300.03] but not in the CSA, the term refers to a record showing who has accessed an information technology application and what operations the user performed during a given period.

Automated dispensing system: Defined in DEA regulations [21 CFR 1304.02(g)] but not in the CSA, the term refers to a mechanical system that performs operations or activities, other than compounding or administration, relative to the storage, packaging, counting, labeling, and dispensing of medications and which collects, controls, and maintains all transaction information.

Automated dispensing cabinet: Computer-controlled, decentralized medication-dispensing system designed for use in healthcare facilities allowing for computer-controlled storage and dispensing of drugs and devices to licensed health care professionals near the point of care.

Biometric: Defined in DEA regulations [21 CFR 1300.03] but not in the CSA, the term refers to authentication based on measurement of the individual's physical features or repeatable actions where those features or actions are both distinctive to the individual and measurable.

Blind count: A physical inventory taken by personnel who perform a hands-on count of inventory without access to the quantities currently shown on electronic or other inventory systems. Blind counts are used to assess the integrity of the automated inventory systems. (Source: www.businessdictionary.com/definition/blind-count.html)

Deliver: Defined in the CSA [CSA §102(10); 21 USC 802(10)], the term refers to the actual, constructive, or attempted transfer of a controlled substance or a listed chemical, whether or not there exists an agency relationship.

Dispense: Defined in the CSA [CSA §102(10); 21 USC 802(10)] but not in DEA regulations, the term means to deliver a controlled substance to an ultimate user or research subject by, or pursuant to the lawful order of, an individual practitioner, including the prescribing and administering of a controlled substance and the packaging, labeling, or compounding necessary to prepare the substance for delivery. Additionally, the term *dispenser*, as defined in the CSA [CSA §102(10); 21 USC 802(10)] and DEA regulations [21 CFR 1304.02(c)], means an individual practitioner, institutional individual practitioner, pharmacy, or pharmacist who dispenses a controlled substance.

Distribute: Defined in the CSA [CSA §102(10); 21 USC 802(10)] but not in DEA regulations, the term means to deliver (other than by administering or dispensing) a controlled substance or a listed chemical. The term *distributor* means a person who so delivers a controlled substance or a listed chemical.

Diversion: The term includes any unaccountable loss, theft, use for unintended purposes, or tampering of a drug. For purposes of these guidelines, *drug diversion* is a medical and legal concept involving the transfer of any legally prescribed drug from the individual for whom it was prescribed to another person for any illicit use, including any deviation that removes a prescription drug from its intended path from the manufacturer to the intended patient.

Healthcare worker: Refers to an employee, individual practitioner, or contracted worker who provides services within an organization and who has access to controlled substances.

Inventory: Defined in DEA regulations [21 CFR 1304.11], controlled substances inventory "on hand" includes CS in the possession of or under the control of the registrant, including substances returned by a customer, ordered by a customer but not yet invoiced, stored in a warehouse on behalf of the registrant, and substances in the possession of employees of the registrant and intended for distribution as complimentary samples. Unusable CS being held for return or destruction are considered as part of inventory.

Individual practitioner: Defined in the CSA [CSA §102(20); 21 USC 802(20)] but not in DEA regulations, the term refers to a physician, dentist, veterinarian, scientific investigator, pharmacy, organization, or other person licensed, registered, or otherwise permitted, by the United States or the jurisdiction in which the individual practitioner practices or does research, to distribute, dispense, conduct research with respect to, administer, or use in teaching or chemical analysis, a controlled substance in the course of professional practice or research.

Long-term care facility: Defined in DEA regulations [21 CFR 1306.02(e)] but not in the CSA, the term refers to a nursing home or a retirement care, mental care, or other facility or institution that provides extended healthcare to resident patients.

Password: Defined in DEA regulations [21 CFR 1300.03] but not in the CSA, the term refers to a secret code, typically a character string (letters, numbers, and other symbols), that a person memorizes and uses to authenticate his identity.

Pharmacist: Defined in DEA regulations [21 CFR 1304.02(g)] but not in the CSA, the term refers to any individual licensed by a state to dispense controlled substances and also includes any other person (eg, pharmacist intern) authorized by a state to dispense controlled substances under the supervision of a pharmacist licensed by that state.

Prescription: Defined in DEA regulations [21 CFR 1300.01(b)] but not in the CSA, the term refers to an order for medication which is dispensed to or for an ultimate user but does not include an order for medication which is dispensed for immediate administration to the ultimate user (eg, an order to dispense a drug to a bed patient for immediate administration in a hospital is not a prescription).

Readily retrievable: Defined in DEA regulations [21 CFR 1304.02(h)] but not in the CSA, the term means that certain records are kept by automatic data-processing systems or other electronic or mechanized recordkeeping systems in such a manner that they can be separated out from all other records in a reasonable time and/or records are kept on which certain items are asterisked, redlined, or in some other manner visually identifiable apart from other items appearing on the records.

Reverse distributor: Defined in DEA regulations [21 CFR 1306.02(e)] but not in the CSA. The term *reverse distribute* means to acquire controlled substances from another registrant or law enforcement agent for the purpose of (a) return to the registered manufacturer or another registrant authorized by the manufacturer to accept returns on the manufacturer's behalf or (b) destruction. A *reverse distributor* is a person registered with the DEA as a reverse distributor.

Significant loss: A significant diversion is any unaccountable loss of a controlled substance. Some states and local authorities may have specific requirements for what is considered significant. Organizations should formally define what is considered a significant loss and ensure consistent application to investigations and reporting requirements. In its 1971 regulation, 21 CFR 1301.74(c), DEA provided the following list of factors to consider when making determinations about whether losses are significant:

- The actual quantity of controlled substances lost in relation to the type of business,
- The specific controlled substances lost,
- Whether the loss of the controlled substances can be associated with access to those controlled substances by specific individuals, or whether the loss can be attributed to unique activities that may take place involving the controlled substances,
- A pattern of losses over a specific time period, whether the losses appear to be random, and the results of efforts taken to resolve the losses, and, if known,
- Whether the specific controlled substances are likely candidates for diversion, and
- Local trends and other indicators of the diversion potential of the missing controlled substance.

Waste: A quantity of controlled substance that has not been used and is unable to be used (eg, single-use vial, discontinued intravenous infusion) after being removed from inventory in order to fill a medication order or prescription.

Appendix B—Controlled Substances Diversion Prevention Program Self-Assessment Guide[a,b]

Organization Oversight and Accountability

- The organization establishes a controlled substances (CS) diversion prevention program (CSDPP).
- The organization establishes an interdisciplinary CSDPP committee to provide leadership and direction for developing policies and procedures for overseeing the CSDPP. A pharmacy representative has a leadership role on the CSDPP committee, and there is a designated diversion officer who coordinates activities of the CSDPP. The diversion officer should have a license and a college degree in pharmacy or nursing, with at least 5 years of healthcare experience; ideally, the diversion officer would be a licensed pharmacist with 10 years or more of experience as a staff or managerial pharmacist and an advanced management degree (eg, MHA or MBA). The diversion officer should have a thorough understanding of medication management systems and technologies (eg, ADCs, medication carts, repackaging systems); CS surveillance and management systems and techniques; federal and state regulatory compliance requirements; and auditing techniques. The diversion officer should be familiar with operations of the pharmacy department (eg, ordering, receiving, storage, preparation, distribution, administration, returns, wasting) as well as other pertinent areas (perioperative, anesthesia, procedure, clinic, research, and community pharmacy areas). The diversion officer should be able to lead the complex investigatory processes of an interdisciplinary team, which will require strong analytical and communication skills, attention to detail, organization, ability to work independently and collaboratively, and a commitment to healthcare ethics and confidentiality. The Diversion Officer should have formal training in the processes of conducting a drug diversion investigation and process improvement techniques, including conducting root cause analyses, and, if performing interviews or interrogation, in those techniques as well. The diversion officer should have the ability to work with local, state, and federal law enforcement organizations during criminal investigations, as well as with state licensing agencies and national accrediting organizations. The diversion officer should have the ability to work with the organization's human resources department and hospital leadership to develop strong policies to protect HCWs and mitigate HCW diversion risks. Familiarity with the causes, symptoms, recognition, and treatment of substance use disorder and human behavioral assessment is desirable, as is a passion for patient safety and protecting the organization from diversion. Diversion officers should be familiar with national, state, and local drug abuse and diversion trends. They should be involved with national, state, and local organizations and efforts to help raise awareness of drug diversion, and attend local, state, and national diversion meetings.
- The CSDPP committee
  - Includes representatives from, but not limited to, the following departments: medical staff, anesthesia, pharmacy, nursing, security, human resources, compliance, risk management, administration, legal, communications, information technology, and Employee Health.
  - Ad hoc members such as infection control, infectious diseases, or media/public relations may be added depending on the circumstances of the diversion.
  - Establishes a charter that includes membership composition, roles and responsibilities, reporting structure, and meeting frequency.
  - Is proactive in its prevention efforts and actively addresses prevention control, diversion detection, incident investigation, and reporting procedures (eg, minutes that document monitoring trend reports, quality-improvement efforts and outcomes of those efforts, compliance with existing procedures, and reviews of internal and external audits and action plans).
- The functions of the CSDPP committee are integrated with existing compliance management programs, and the committee reports at least quarterly directly to the senior leadership of the organization.
- A diversion response team that can rapidly and effectively respond to suspected incidents is established, with notifications tiered based on the stage of investigation.
- The diversion response team members conduct diversion risk rounds.[c] Diversion risk rounds involve observation of areas where controlled medications are received, stored, or utilized, as well as interaction with staff and patients in these locations. The objectives are to assess security, monitor compliance with regulations and institutional policy, and initiate process improvement where warranted.

- Established policies and procedures reflect federal, state, and local regulatory requirements.
- Policies and procedures build in closed-loop chain of custody with individual accountability that is readily auditable.
- CS diversion incidents are collated, reviewed, and analyzed to identify further opportunities for improvement in existing systems.
- Surveillance data are trended and shared with the CSDPP committee to review on at least a quarterly basis. Trended information is acted upon, corrective actions are implemented, and resolution of the identified issue is verified.
- The CSDPP conducts failure modes and effects analysis to identify potential points of risk and prevention strategies.[d]
- The CSDPP ensures that policies and procedure reflect a segregation of duties where there is overlapping processes for diversion risk.
- The organization identifies high-risk areas where CS diversion could occur and implements specialized controls and more focused surveillance for these areas when warranted.
- Drug Enforcement Administration (DEA) licenses and other relevant registrations are current, and power-of-attorney designees are reevaluated at least annually.
- The organization collaborates and cooperates with key external stakeholders, including local DEA officials, local law enforcement, wholesalers, technology vendors, state licensure boards, and contract pharmacy services.

Human Resources Management (Staff Education, Expectations, Culture, Support)

- The organization implements a process to remove a healthcare worker (HCW) suspected of being impaired from delivering patient care and to prevent further access to CS either pending investigation or after a confirmed diversion or policy breach.
- The organization has a clearly defined full disclosure policy and process to communicate to patients and families that are affected by CS diversion.
- The organization conducts pre-employment background checks for HCWs who have access to CS in the course of their job responsibilities.
- When HCWs with access to CS are suspended, terminated, or otherwise separated, the pharmacy and designated system administrator are notified immediately so access to CS can be removed promptly, within a time frame defined by the organization.
- Known diverters who are licensed or registered are reported to the appropriate licensing or registration board as required by state law.
- A comprehensive human resources and occupational health approach to support the CSDPP at a minimum consists of (a) a written employee and provider substance abuse policy; (b) an HCW education and awareness program; (c) a supervisor training program; (d) an employee and provider assistance program; (e) peer support and systems (eg, pharmacist recovery network); (f) requirements for drug testing, including a for-cause policy for drug testing; (g) return-to-work policies for HCWs; and (h) sanctions for performance and diversion violations.
- The CSDPP ensures that training of all staff with access to CS is mandatory and occurs annually and when there is a significant change in policies or procedures.
- Pharmacists participate in or contribute to the development of substance abuse prevention and assistance programs within the organization.
- The organization's senior leadership emphasizes the importance of reporting signs of a potentially impaired HCW or suspected CS diversion and its potential impact on patient care, including ramifications for failure to report; communicates the expectation that staff speak up when they become aware of or suspect an issue related to CS diversion; and ensures and communicates that staff will be protected from retaliation if they report a suspected CS diversion or impaired HCW.
- The organization establishes and communicates ways for staff to speak up anonymously (eg, telephone hotline, paper or electronic submission) and posts signs explaining how to report suspected diversion near every CS point of access.
- All HCWs receive annual education in diversion prevention and substance abuse and diversion awareness (signs and behavior patterns and symptoms of impairment) and reporting; and managers receive training in signs, symptoms, and behavior alerts, what to do when they suspect an HCW may be impaired, and managing HCWs in recovery.
- The organization establishes a process to support recovery and peer assistance programs for those who have diverted for an active substance abuse problem.
- Drug testing for cause is permitted, and, as required by licensing boards or other employment contracts, organizations implement reliable testing and validation for drug screening.
- Human Resources (or Employee Health, if they are the individual responsible for drug testing) should be informed of the suspected drug(s) involved to ensure the appropriate test panel is used so a drug test does not result in a false negative.
- The organization establishes behavioral standards and norms among all HCWs that discourage the abuse of CS.
- An ongoing CS diversion education program is in place to promote the safe handling of CS and awareness of medication diversion. Education on medication diversion and CS policies and procedures is required before authorizing HCW access to CS.
- The organization develops and enforces sanctions for CSDPP policy and procedure violations.
- If provider services are contracted, contracts provide that all contracted workers receive education regarding CS and that the contracted company notifies the organization immediately if there is disciplinary action against an HCW or if an HCW is removed because of an impairment issue.

Automation and Technology

- ADCs are implemented, at minimum, in all high-risk locations (eg, surgery or anesthesia areas, central pharmacy).
- An interdisciplinary team that includes pharmacy representation participates in the selection and implementation of all medication-related automated systems (eg, surveillance software) and technology (eg, ADCs, syringe and infusion pumps, security devices) to ensure they support CS diversion control, surveillance, and auditing and meet legal, regulatory, and functionality requirements.
- Pharmacy representatives have an integral role in the selection and implementation of all medication-related automated systems and technology.
- The organization works proactively with vendors to ensure there is adequate training and implementation testing before installing or upgrading new technology equipment or software.
- Changes in or upgrades to existing technology are reviewed by key stakeholders, including pharmacy representatives, to assess potential impacts on systems of CS control, surveillance, and auditing, and changes or upgrades are tested and vetted to ensure implementation meets legal, regulatory, and functionality requirements.
- Records generated from technology solutions are readily retrievable and contain information required to conduct investigations and fulfill investigator requests.
- Reporting capability is tested to ensure that records with complete and accurate information are readily retrievable.
- Surveillance reports generated from automated technology solutions are produced on a scheduled basis, as determined by the CSDPP, and include but are not limited to discrepancies, overrides, user metrics, and inventory reports (see Monitoring and Surveillance section).
- Staff is adequately trained regarding their roles and responsibilities in the use of automation and technology, and competency is assessed when an HCW is on boarded to a new position or responsibilities, annually thereafter, and when there is a relevant change to existing technology.
- Access to CS in ADCs is limited to authorized individuals, and there is a process in place to immediately add or rescind access privileges (eg, suspected diverters can be removed immediately, other users [e.g., terminated HCWs] removed within 24 hours, and temporary HCWs added as necessary).
- Administrative privileges that allow staff to add, delete, or change access permissions for ADC users are limited to as few individuals as possible, and a record of all actions is maintained.
- Policies and procedures specify that ADC overrides should be limited only to clearly defined situations. The amount of CS available for dispensing via ADC override functionality is minimized, and the process is directed by a comprehensive policy and review process that includes ensuring use is clinically appropriate, a valid order exists, and there is appropriate documentation in the medical record.
- The pharmacy department is the party responsible for authorizing access to CS and for adding and removing users to ADCs. If this authority is delegated to informatics or security personnel, the pharmacy department should still maintain responsibility to oversee the process and ensure that established procedures are followed. The activities of those with access to system administration functionality should be reviewed at least annually by a neutral party.
- Controls are in place to limit lock-out access times, and this access discontinued as soon as possible when patients are transferred or discharged.
- ADC or electronic vault downtime procedures are defined to maintain control, documentation, and accountability of CS. Considerations for downtime procedures include but are not limited to backup surveillance (eg, cameras); storage, access, and security controls; information management (eg, PDMP and decision support alerts, interface functionality); and recovery.
- ADC admission, transfer, and discharge patient profile information is managed in a timely manner.

Monitoring and Surveillance

- The CSDPP committee identifies surveillance reports (eg, discrepancy and user transactions), metrics, responsibility for conducting reviews, timeframe for resolution, and frequency of reviews (see Table 1 for example KPIs).
- The organization, through the CSDPP committee, establishes surveillance requirements, including defining monitoring and surveillance measures, thresholds of variance that require action, reporting frequency, and surveillance procedures, and ensures that all elements are implemented, conducted in a timely manner, investigated, and reported as required.
- The CSDPP committee provides facility oversight to ensure that established audits for facility-based diversion monitoring are conducted and documented.
- There is a process defining the escalation of discrepancies that cannot be resolved ("unresolvable discrepancies") or CS policy and procedure violations that include the director of pharmacy or designated pharmacy manager and other hospital leadership, including the chief executive officer, as appropriate.
- Surveillance processes are interdisciplinary and touch all aspects of the CS management system, from purchasing to waste and disposal.
- Self-audits are conducted within areas as well as regularly scheduled audits by individuals external to the area being audited.
- The organization periodically audits human resources requirements for individuals authorized to handle CS, including
    - Completion of required background checks.
    - Documentation of training and competency requirements for authorized staff.
    - Compliance with random drug testing requirements.
    - Compliance with licensure board reporting and rehabilitation program requirements.

- Drug purchase history is monitored through regularly scheduled audits to identify diversion through variations or changes in volume or pattern.
  - CS purchase invoices are compared to CS purchase orders and receipt into the pharmacy's perpetual inventory.
  - Invoices are reconciled to statements or wholesale purchase history reports to detect missing invoices.
  - A process is in place to identify unusual peaks in quantity or frequency of CS purchases (eg, quarterly review of purchases over the prior 12- 24 months).
  - Wholesaler is able to flag unusual peaks in quantity or frequency of CS purchased.
- A perpetual inventory of all CS is maintained and verified on a scheduled basis, consistent with the control system used (eg, inventory managed with ADCs with closed compartments and unit-of-use access limitations versus manual inventory).
  - CS counts from ADCs are verified (blind count) each time a CS drawer is accessed, and a complete inventory for CS in ADCs is conducted weekly by two authorized HCWs. The inventory count is not required for drugs accessed and verified during that week.
  - Deliveries, replenishment, and stocking of CS in patient care areas will be done by authorized pharmacy personnel and require an auditable verification of delivery and receipt.
  - CS inventory in the pharmacy CS vault is counted at least monthly.
  - Outside pharmacy areas, CS storage areas in which CS are not managed through ADCs are inventoried at each shift change by two authorized HCWs.
  - A biennial physical inventory of all CS is completed and documented per DEA requirements (or per state requirements, whichever is the stricter interpretation).
- ADC reports are routinely monitored to ensure overrides occur only as permitted by policies and procedures. ADC override reports are reviewed daily to ensure an order exists during the time the medication was accessed from the ADC, and corresponding documentation is in the medication administration record (MAR).
- Reports match CS vault transactions with receipt into ADC and/or paper inventory record with signature of receipt.
- Diversion monitoring software is implemented to support surveillance activities.
- A person is dedicated to surveillance monitoring and is accountable for optimizing implementation and functionality of diversion monitoring software. Other disciplines (eg, nursing quality, anesthesia providers) are actively involved in surveillance audits and assist with evaluation of trends and incident investigation.
- Reports that monitor CS use in patient care areas are reviewed at least monthly by pharmacy and patient care managers as defined by the organization. The organization has a process to generate CS trend data and reports:
  - Tracking and trending of patient care usage.
  - Reports compare ADC activity with the prescriber order and MAR.
  - The MAR is reviewed for amount and quantity administered compared to what other caregivers administer on subsequent shifts (without patient change in condition).
  - ADC CS activity is compared to peers with similar staffing responsibilities and appointments.
  - Transaction activity (eg, inventory abnormalities, removal of quantities greater than prescribed dose, cancellations, returns, and waste) is compared with peers.
  - The MAR is reviewed for transactions that occur abnormally (eg, after a patient is discharged or transferred to another unit.)
- Prescribing practices are reviewed for unusual trends or patterns, such as variance in prescribing compared to peers.
- Patient response to medication (eg, pain management) is also evaluated against medication administration, documentation of response, and patient interview.
- Nursing management conducts random patient interviews to verify that patients received pain medication and that the medication adequately controlled pain and also compares responses to nursing patient assessment notes and MAR.
- Nursing management integrates routine auditing and surveillance activities into core daily, weekly, or monthly responsibilities, including staff education regarding signs of diversion, symptoms of substance abuse, and diversion reporting procedures; review of nursing removal, return, and wasting records; development, implementation, and monitoring of procedures for witnessing CS-related transactions; and investigation and reporting of suspected diversion in accordance with organization procedures.
- CS storage inventory transactions are routinely compared with the MAR (eg, anesthesia record, sedation record, electronic MAR) to ensure appropriate documentation of administration and waste.
- Anesthesia CS audits are performed on a regularly scheduled basis, as determined by the process for managing CS for anesthesia, identified risk points, and previous events.
- CS discrepancies are reported to the supervisor in charge, who reviews and attempts to resolve the discrepancy no later than the end of the work shift. Discrepancies that cannot be resolved (unresolvable discrepancies) are reported immediately to the pharmacy department and are jointly reviewed by pharmacy and patient care leadership, with resolution within 24–72 hours.
- The supervising or other designated pharmacist is notified of unresolvable discrepancies in ADCs and supports the reconciliation investigation; a pharmacist has responsibility for investigating the discrepancy, even when a pharmacy technician assists with these duties.

- A trend of poor documentation practices by an HCW is reviewed by his or her immediate supervisor (eg, nursing or pharmacy manager, department chair) for possible diversion.
- There is a procedure for random assay testing of waste from all high-risk, high-volume areas, including areas for pharmacy sterile products preparation, anesthesia administration, and surgery.
- CS dispensed in high-risk settings (eg, for operating room cases or procedures) are reconciled by pharmacy against what CS were documented as administered or wasted.

Investigation and Reporting of Suspected Diversion

- The organization creates and implements a standard process to investigate discrepancies that are not resolved (unresolvable discrepancies) or other discovered or suspected diversions.
- Any unresolvable discrepancy is considered a possible diversion and escalated to investigation, and notifications occur as defined by the CSDPP.
- A process is in place to report and respond to suspected diversions and prompt an immediate investigation:
    - There is a way to report (anonymously, if desired) a suspected CS diversion 24 hours-per-day/7 days-per-week (eg, pager, phone, or other emergency alert notification system).
    - An interdisciplinary drug diversion response team is in place to provide consultation, direction, and oversight for suspected diversion incidents.
    - Designated team members external to the area under investigation are also involved to ensure the impartiality of the investigation of incident.
    - A standardized process exists for interviewing suspected CS diverters.
    - Guidelines are in place for the handling of suspected impaired HCWs and drug testing, including guidance when for-cause testing may be initiated.
- A defined process is in place for the internal and external reporting of medication diversion incidents.
- The pharmacy director or his or her designee and diversion officer (if different) are notified immediately of any suspected diversion within the organization, participate in all active investigations regarding CS diversion, and are informed of the outcomes of all investigations.
- There are guidelines for determining whether a CS loss is considered significant, which include factors such as
    - Quantity of CS lost in relation to the type of business.
    - The specific type(s) of CS lost.
    - Whether the loss can be associated to access by specific individuals or can be attributed to unique activities.
    - A pattern of losses over a specific time period, whether the losses appear to be random, and the results of efforts taken to resolve the losses.
    - Whether the specific CS are likely candidates for diversion.
    - Local trends and other indicators of the diversion potential.
- There are guidelines for engaging others internal to the organization, such as the risk management, legal, and human resources departments, as well as leadership levels of medical staff and administration. Guidelines specify who will coordinate the investigation, including communications to appropriate team members, conducting the investigation, and coordinating internal and external reporting.
- If the organization becomes aware of an arrest of an HCW for illicit use of CS, the organization immediately conducts an investigation of the HCW's transactions to assess whether diversion has occurred. The organization assesses whether to suspend, transfer, terminate, or take other action (eg, remove access to CS) or other sanctions against the HCW. The organization immediately removes access privileges to CS if diversion is suspected, until the investigation is complete and a determination of diversion or other risks to patient care is made.
- The organization establishes guidelines for engaging external entities, such as DEA, licensure boards, laboratories (for testing), and local law enforcement. Guidelines specify who is required to be notified, when notifications take place, who is responsible for contacting the agency/designated representative, and the time frame and circumstances for notification.
- The organization fulfills all reporting requirements for diversion or other unaccountable loss of CS in accordance with laws and regulations.
    - Investigations are conducted as thoroughly and completely as possible; reporting occurs when it is determined that the discrepancy is unresolved or that there has been a known theft or diversion
    - Organizational policy defines when a DEA Form 106 should be completed with discrepancies that remain ultimately unresolved. There are clear responsibilities for completion of a DEA Form 106 for a theft or significant loss, who within the organization is to be notified, and when.

Quality improvement

- For significant diversions, a quality-improvement review is initiated, including a root cause analysis and recommendations to prevent future occurrences.
- Representative(s) from the area where there is a suspected diversion are engaged in the investigation and refinement of prevention strategies.
- Proactive, systemic analyses of CS processes are conducted, such as a failure mode and effects analysis, to identify risk points and take action to improve diversion prevention practices.

Communications

- Organizational guidelines specify how to respond to media inquiries, when to notify the media, what internal communications are required, and who is responsible for approving media communications and contacting the media representative.

Chain of Custody

- Authorized HCWs verify dispensing and receipt of CS and are secured immediately. In areas without ADC storage, the HCW delivering and the HCW receiving CS both cosign documentation of receipt.

- When using an ADC for dispensing and storage of CS, transactions should be tracked and reconciled electronically.
- Sending CS via a pneumatic tube system is not recommended; if employed, delivery requires a secure transaction function (eg, not a generic passcode when CS is received in a patient care area).
- Persons transporting CS (eg, couriers) are trained and competent in relevant organizational policies and procedures.
- When using a courier for CS transport, procedures and documentation are in place to ensure receipt of CS at the final destination. CS delivery to areas with ADCs requires co-signature for delivery and return.
- Hand-offs during a patient procedure are generally avoided, but in the event a hand-off is unavoidable, such as during an active surgical case (eg, prepared case trays, break coverage, or change of shift), there are procedures to document the chain of custody and document provider transfer of CS.
- Secure, lockable, and tamper-evident delivery containers (eg, carts, trays, boxes, prescription bags) are used to deliver CS. Packaging does not make the contents apparent (eg, opaque containers).
- When used, tamper-resistant or tamper-evident mechanism on transport containers should be traceable (eg, plastic tie locks with a unique numerical identifier).
- There is a process to ensure that chain of custody is maintained when transferring CS to a laboratory service (internal or external) analyzing products as part of an investigation or random assay process.
- Dispensing a prescription for CS to patients from patient care areas, such as the emergency department, is not recommended; if such dispensing occurs, chain of custody is documented from the provider to the patient.
- The organization establishes a procedure for transfer of CS to emergency medical services that complies with federal, state, and local requirements.
- When discharging and transporting patients to another location outside of the licensed organization, it is recommended, when clinically feasible, to discontinue CS infusions and provide incremental dosing during transport, then re-start upon arrival at the new facility or arrange for continuity of therapy when the patient is received for transport.

Storage and Security (Facilities, Requirements, Inventory Management)

- CS are securely stored in a locked location (ie, ADC, safe, locked cabinet/drawer, refrigerator) accessible only to authorized individuals at all times unless in the direct physical control of an authorized individual. CS not under the direct physical control of an authorized individual are stored in an area allowing direct observation at all times and where distractions are minimized.
    - Environmental services and other support staff should not have access to central CS storage locations when unattended (eg, after hours).
    - When used, lock boxes are stored in a secure location when left unattended.
    - Codes for electronic or keypad locks on cabinets or carts are not set at the manufacturer's default code and are protected with a strong code (eg, not "1-2-3-4").
    - Lock-out times for electronic locks on carts (eg, medication carts, anesthesia carts) containing CS are limited to the narrowest window of time appropriate for the particular setting.
    - There is a procedure to track keys, secure keys after hours, replace lost keys, and change locks, and there is evidence of compliance with those procedures.
    - Storage of CS in patient care area refrigerators is minimized and access limited to authorized HCWs. CS stored in compartments or boxes within refrigerators are secured and key access limited. For example, keys may be kept in a dedicated single-access pocket in the ADC that opens when the CS is selected from the patient profile and returned to the pocket after removing the CS.
    - Storage areas, including medication rooms, have a window to allow visibility within the area. Backpacks, purses, and bags are not allowed in these areas. Camera surveillance is present in primary CS pharmacy storage and preparation areas (eg, CS vault).
- Access to CS storage areas is minimized and limited to authorized staff.
    - When key lock security is used, chain of custody is maintained for keys, and there is a process to secure keys after hours in locations not in continuous operation.
    - There are policies and procedures regarding CS access, including restrictions through assignment, key controls, use of passwords, and schedule for changing lock codes (where there is not biometric or card reader access).
    - At least every 6 months there is a complete assessment of all staff with access privileges to ensure that only those permitted access have access (eg, authorized HCWs, temporary employees, independent practitioners with privileges). Inactive users (eg, those who have not accessed the system within a specified period of time) have their access suspended or removed.
    - Removal of access occurs immediately when HCWs are terminated. For auditing purposes, staff termination reports (date and time) are reconciled against date and time of documented removal of access.
    - Patient-specific CS infusions are contained in a secured, locked box utilizing no-port tubing unless under constant surveillance. Keys and access to these controls are limited and tracked.
- CS storage locations are reviewed by security personnel to evaluate the potential need for enhanced physical security controls (eg, glass break alarms, door sweeps, cameras, and door contact detectors). Panic buttons should be considered as part of the overall security system and should be accessible to staff in the main storage location (eg, main pharmacy, vault) and public-facing locations (eg, community pharmacies).

- The central pharmacy vault is considered a high-risk location and should be supported by automated dispensing technology.
- Within pharmacy areas with ADC vault management, CS inventory verification counts are conducted by two rotating, licensed, or otherwise authorized pharmacy providers monthly. For pharmacies without ADC technology vault management, a physical inventory is conducted at least once per month, preferably weekly.
  - Inventory count includes expired and otherwise unusable CS awaiting disposal or transfer to reverse distributor.
  - CS counts done via ADCs and manual systems are verified by a blind count each time a CS location (eg, drawer, pocket, and refrigerator) is accessed.
- ADC technology is utilized in areas with a high volume of CS use, including the pharmacy, anesthesia and surgery areas, high-volume clinics, and outpatient procedure areas.
- User identification and biometric authentication are used rather than passwords. When biometric authentication is not available, password security on ADCs follows institutional policy and standards and includes requirements for password complexity and frequent changes. Organizations should develop countermeasures when biometrics authentication technology is available, but an HCW is not able to use biometrics.
- For manual access to CS, signature and initial logs recording receipt and disposition are maintained as appropriate. Any HCW receiving, transferring, or dispensing CS will be able to provide photo identification upon request.
- Camera surveillance is considered for high-risk locations (eg, receiving areas, central pharmacy vault location, and approved waste receptacles), remote areas, areas where electronic or biometric access are not available, distribution locations (eg, public access or other exchange locations), and when for-cause surveillance is required to support an investigation.
- Procedures are implemented to secure storage of DEA forms, and access to forms is limited to authorized individuals.
  - There are procedures and documentation (eg, a log book) for tracking the receipt and filling of DEA Form 222.
  - Blank DEA Form 222s are listed consecutively on a log documenting the disposition of each form.
  - The DEA Form 222 log is stored separately from unused DEA forms.
  - DEA Form 222s are not pre-signed.
- Procedures are implemented to secure prescription pads and paper, and access is limited to authorized individuals.
  - Prescription blanks and paper for printing prescriptions are dispensed per patient rather than the entire prescription pad.
  - There is a method (eg, numbering system) to allow for tracking of individual prescriptions.
- Organizations consider providing, in collaboration with local and state authorities, a public collection ("take-back") receptacle or kiosk for disposal of CS by patients. Pharmacists should ensure the security of the receptacle (eg, bolting to floor and surveillance) and ensure witnessed removal and that the chain of custody is maintained. Other measures for returns control should be considered, such as recording package weight and inspecting for shipping package integrity until transfer or disposition.
- Procedures are established that ensure controls are in place to secure CS and prevent diversion in the rare cases in which CS is brought into the organization by patients.
  - Patient's own CS should only be administered to the patient pursuant to an authorized prescriber's order. Documentation of patient's own CS, quantity inventoried, and signatures of two verifying HCWs should be recorded in the medical record.
  - Patient's own medications may be mailed home, returned home by a designated agent of the patient, or disposed of by the patient in a collection receptacle.
  - When there is a physician order to use the patient's own CS, the patient's CS are secured and tracked via a perpetual inventory record, and any remaining doses are the responsibility of the patient to take home or dispose of in a collection receptacle upon discharge.
  - CS that cannot be returned to home, are unable to be secured by the patient, or are abandoned by the patient are inventoried and stored securely per organization policies until disposition can be arranged. The chain of custody is always maintained (eg, the patient or patient's representative signs that he or she has received the CS, noting the quantity and signature of receipt).
  - If patients bring illicit substances into the organization, procedures address notification of the local DEA office and law enforcement, as required by law, and as advised by those authorities.

Internal Pharmacy Controls

Procurement controls

- All CS are procured by the pharmacy. If other departments or individuals are authorized to procure CS, there are checks and balances established to ensure the same policies and procedures are consistently followed throughout the organization.
- The number of people authorized to order CS is limited to individuals authorized and defined by policy.
- Ordering is integrated into automated inventory tracking systems when possible, based on usage or established par levels, and need for adjustments is monitored. There is a process in place to monitor for a wide variation (eg, increase) in ordering quantities, frequency of ordering, or unusual products ordered (eg, bulk bottles when unit-dose is usually stocked).
- Electronic CS ordering system (CSOS) is used and CSOS order files are backed up to an organization-based system to ensure that archived files are readily retrievable by designated personnel.

- If DEA Form 222s are used, they are secured, and the DEA Form 222 accountability and control log includes
  - DEA order form number
  - Date the form was received from the DEA
  - Date the form was issued for use
  - The company the form was issued to
  - The initials (if the organization uses a signature/initial log) or signature of user
- Separation of duties exists between the ordering and receipt of CS.
  - Upon receipt, two authorized individuals conduct a visual inspection for package integrity, count, sign (two signatures), and date (packing slip) and confirm that what is received matches what was ordered and invoiced (purchase order and invoice).
  - A pharmacist reconciles CS received against what is indicated on the delivery ticket or invoice and documents receipt as required; the documents will be signed or initialed and dated. CS purchase invoices are compared to CS orders and receipt into the pharmacy's perpetual inventory. Since the invoice–receipt pair may both be removed with CS diversion, invoices also are reconciled to statements or wholesale purchase history reports to detect missing invoices. Staff should be cross-trained and rotated through functions related to procurement and prepackaging.
  - All drug invoices should indicate the total number of pages in the invoice. The pharmacist in charge or delegate must verify that drugs detailed in all the pages of an invoice are being received.
  - Automated vault technology is utilized in the central pharmacy main storage location, and receipts reports are reconciled with delivery ticket and invoice.
  - If the HCW who provides the second count at check-in is not a pharmacy employee (eg, at a small organization where only one pharmacy employee is available), the designated HCWs receive appropriate training.
  - CSOS orders are acknowledged as received within 7 days of receiving the order.
  - CS inventory levels are routinely reviewed, and orders are based on usage to minimize excess stock.
- There are processes to track and reconcile CS products when preparation is outsourced to a third-party vendor.
- There are procedures for interorganization transfer and transport of CS, including distribution from or to a central distribution hub within an organization.
- There are procedures for transfer of CS between pharmacies.
- The organization establishes a policy that discrepancies in the procurement process will be documented and brought to the attention of the director of pharmacy or designated pharmacy manager immediately.

Preparation and dispensing controls

- A perpetual inventory is maintained and a blind count process is used when adding or removing CS from a pharmacy inventory location.
- Access to CS inventory is limited, with controls to identify who accessed the inventory, when the inventory was accessed, and what changes were made to the inventory.
- Effective access controls are in place to ensure the integrity of the inventory and provide for accurate, timely surveillance.
- To minimize opportunities for CS diversion during repackaging, CS are purchased and dispensed in unit dose packaging whenever possible, and when repackaging is required, it is configured to minimize waste. There are diversion controls in place when CS are repackaged by pharmacy personnel, including separation of duties and chain of custody controls.
- ADC technology is utilized in patient care areas for the distribution and accountability of CS.
- In patient care areas, ADC-managed CS counts are verified by a blind count each time a CS drawer/pocket/cabinet is accessed (unless unit-of-use dispensing technology is employed).
- In patient care areas, CS managed through ADCs are manually inventoried by two authorized HCWs if a blind count has not been performed within one week.
- In patient care areas, CS not managed through ADCs are manually inventoried by blind count by two authorized HCWs every shift. The perpetual inventory log includes the drug product, quantity, date, and signatures of those conducting the inventory.
- CS managed through ADCs are stored in a location with single pocket or unit of use access when possible.
- Barcode-scanning is utilized when replenishing ADCs.
- When dispensing, removal from the pharmacy inventory is matched to the refill transaction on the patient care unit to validate that CS reach their destination.
- CS returned from nursing units to the return bin of the ADC or to the pharmacy are matched to the CS received by the pharmacy and documented in the perpetual inventory or a return to active inventory transaction on the ADC.
- Returns from the patient care and procedural areas (eg, emptying a return bin) have an auditable verification of return. Returns are inspected for integrity.

Prescribing and Administration

- A valid order from a licensed, authorized prescriber exists for all CS administered, and the number of CS allowed via ADC override status is minimized.
- There is a process to identify and verify authorized prescribers within either an electronic or manual ordering system. There is also a process to identify and verify authorized prescribers and prescriptions written by medical residents or other providers who are authorized to prescribe CS under the organization's DEA registration (eg, use of a suffix).
- CS prescriptions and orders are periodically audited to ensure they are only initiated by authorized prescribers.
- Pharmacists clarify any orders for which prescriber identity is uncertain or other factors create doubt about the legitimacy of the prescription or order.
- Oral orders for CS entered into the medical record are reviewed for appropriateness and accuracy by the ordering prescriber before cosigning orders.

- Oral orders that have not been cosigned are reviewed and trended.
- The use of range orders for CS is prohibited.
- Prescriptions or orders for CS are reevaluated regularly (eg, through use of automatic stop reminders, by discontinuing and reordering CS per organizational policy when patients transfer to a different level of care). Medical staff, in coordination and consultation with the pharmacy department, develops and implements an automatic stop-order system for CS when there is not a specific time or number of doses prescribed.
- Organization policy prohibits authorized prescribers prescribing for themselves or an immediate family member.
- The organization assesses lock-out times for ADCs and duration for temporary access, including appropriate number and units of ADCs for which each HCW is granted access.
- CS are retrieved from inventory for one patient at a time, and as close to the time of administration as possible, as defined by organization and appropriate to the care setting. CS retrieved for a patient is the package size equivalent to, or closest available to, the dose to be administered.
- When being administered to a patient, CS infusions are secured in locked infusion pumps.
- All CS drawn up into syringes, if not immediately administered, are labeled per organizational policy, and the initials of the HCW who drew up the drug are written on the label. Syringes are kept under the direct control of the person preparing the syringes until administration to the patient, and the initials on prepared syringes are verified immediately before administration to ensure that the syringe has not been switched. Generally, only single doses are drawn up into a syringe. When sequential doses are required from a single syringe, there is a method to track the dose ordered versus the dose administered.
- In areas in which CS are not managed through ADCs, CS disposition and administration records are accurate and include the following information:
  - Date and time administered
  - Medication name
  - Medication strength
  - Dosage form
  - Dose administered
  - Signature of the HCW who administered the dose
  - Amount wasted (if applicable), with cosignature
  - Proof of count verification per shift
  - Signature of HCW who transferred the balance forward when transcribing to a new record

Returns, Waste, and Disposal

- CS are stocked in as ready-to-use form as possible (eg, avoiding the use of multidose vials or oral liquids) and in the lowest commercially available units frequently prescribed to patients. Inventory and practice is routinely evaluated for opportunities to reduce the need to waste.
- Procedures require that CS be wasted immediately or as close to the time of administration as possible; there is an established timeframe allowed per policy.
- The wasting of all CS requires an independent witness and documentation, except in situations in which waste is being returned to the pharmacy for assay and wasting.
- CS waste receptacles are installed adjacent and in line of sight to the ADC console for witnessing and documenting waste.
- An individual witnessing CS wasting verifies that the volume and amount being wasted match the documentation and physically watches the medication being wasted per policy for safe disposal and in a manner that the CS is not retrievable.
- There is a procedure for wasting fentanyl transdermal patches according to Food and Drug Administration or state-specific guidelines in a manner that renders the fentanyl non-retrievable or otherwise deactivated before disposal.
- Pharmaceutical waste containers render CS unrecoverable, non-retrievable, and unusable. Containers and their keys are secured, and a process for waste removal and disposal that ensures that chain-of-custody controls are maintained is implemented.
- Potentially reusable products issued from ADCs are returned to a secure, one-way, return bin or pocket and not to the original ADC pocket, and these returns are witnessed and have an auditable verification of return. Returns are inspected for integrity.
- Empty CS containers are discarded in limited-access waste containers that render the waste non-retrievable and waste procedures comply with organizational procedures for waste management.
- Expired or otherwise unusable CS are clearly identified as such and stored in a location separate from other medications. They are properly accounted for with a perpetual inventory list that is regularly verified, as is other CS inventory within the pharmacy, and the inventory is monitored until return via reverse distributor or destruction and disposal in accordance with legal requirements. The frequency of returns and destruction ensures that inventory is not allowed to accumulate, but returns and destruction are done at least quarterly.
- Documentation is provided by the reverse distributor, is verified, and corresponds with the pharmacy perpetual inventory record of expired and unusable CS before the drugs leave the pharmacy.
- DEA registrant or his or her designee assists with all phases of transfer of CS to a reverse distributor or hazardous waste disposal company.
- Items returned via reverse distribution are reconciled with the reverse distribution log of CS.
- If the inventory quantities are double-counted separately by the reverse distributor, these recorded quantities should be reviewed and reconciled with the pharmacy inventory list before the medications leave the pharmacy.

Community and Mail Order Pharmacies

- There are physical access controls, such as secured storage cabinets only accessible by badge or biometric access, to limit and track access by personnel.
- The organization considers placing cameras and panic buttons in high-risk areas such as CS storage areas,

dispensing areas, verification areas, will-call, and drug take-back receptacles.

- The organization has security measures in place (eg, cameras) to monitor theft and provide an avenue for discrepancies to be resolved in a timely manner.
- The organization ensures that required registration and documentation is completed and current for special programs (eg, drug collection receptacle site registration, compliance with the Combat Methamphetamine Epidemic Act of 2005 [CMEA]).
- The pharmacy has developed a report or auditing process to compare CS purchases with utilization to identify discrepancies and trends.
- The pharmacy has a system for processing hard-copy CS prescriptions that provides documentation of the chain of custody and files CS prescriptions sequentially.
- The pharmacy has a system in place to audit documentation of the chain of custody, including dispensing to the patient or their authorized representative. The pharmacy maintains a perpetual inventory of Schedule II CS that is maintained and audited at least monthly.
- The pharmacy utilizes labels from prescription management software in the perpetual inventory log to identify the quantity of Schedule II CS filled.
- The pharmacy has established procedures for managing and documenting partial fills of CS.
- Pharmacy collection receptacle sites meet appropriate DEA registration requirements.
- The pharmacy complies with the CMEA requirements, including sales tracking, training, and self-certification.

---

[a]This implementation guidance includes recommendations reprinted with permission from the following: Minnesota Hospital Association's Road Map to Controlled Substance Diversion Prevention 2.0; 2015, The California Hospital Association Medication Safety Collaborative Committee's Reducing Controlled Substances Diversion in Hospitals (https://www.chpso.org/sites/main/files/file-attachments/controlled_substance_diversion.pdf?1368720872), and Berge KH, Dillon KR, Sikkink KM, et al. Diversion of drugs within health care facilities, a multiple-victim crime: patterns of diversion, scope, consequences, detection, and prevention. *Mayo Clin Proc.* 2012; 87:674–82.

[b]This implementation guidance does not include all legal requirements and is intended to enhance diversion prevention controls in the health-system setting and should complement policies and procedures required by state, federal, and local authorities as well as accreditation agencies.

[c]New K. Diversion risk rounds: a reality check on your drug-handling policies (2015). http://www.diversionspecialists.com/wp-content/uploads/Diversion-Risk-Rounds-A-Reality-Check-on-Your-Drug-Handling-Policies.pdf (accessed 2021 Sept 20).

[d]Nolan K, Zullo AR, Bosco E, et al. Controlled substance diversion in health systems: A failure modes and effects analysis for prevention. *Am J Health-Syst Pharm.* 2019;76:1158–64.

Developed through the ASHP Council on Pharmacy Management by an expert panel of ASHP members and approved by the ASHP Board of Directors on July 28, 2022. These guidelines supersede a previous version dated October 28, 2016.

ASHP gratefully acknowledges the authors of the previous version of these guidelines: Philip W. Brummond, PharmD, MS; David F. Chen, MBA; William W. Churchill, MS, FMSHP; John S. Clark, PharmD, MS, BCPS, FASHP; Kevin R. Dillon, PharmD, MPH; Doina Dumitru, PharmD, MBA, FASHP; Lynn Eschenbacher, PharmD, MBA, FASHP; Toni Fera, PharmD; Christopher R. Fortier, PharmD, FASHP; Kristine K. Gullickson, PharmD, FASHP; Kristen Jurakovich; Stan Kent, MS, FASHP; Jennifer Keonavong, PharmD, BCPS; Christine Marchese, PharmD; Tricia Meyer, PharmD, MS; Lee B. Murdaugh, PhD; Richard K. Ogden Jr., PharmD, MBA, BCPS; Brian C. O'Neal, PharmD, MS, FASHP; Steve Rough, MS, FASHP; and Rafael Saenz, PharmD, MS, FASHP; Jacob S. Smith, PharmD, MBA.

ASHP also gratefully acknowledges the following organizations and individuals for reviewing these guidelines (review does not imply endorsement): Atrium Health Wake Forest Baptist (AHWFB); California Society of Health-System Pharmacists (CSHP); Federal Bureau of Prisons (BOP); Mercy Hospitals and Health Care (MHHC); National Association of Boards of Pharmacy (NABP); Society of Hospital Medicine (SHM); The Johns Hopkins Hospital (JHH); THRIV Coalition for IV Accuracy; University of North Carolina (UNC) Health; Daniel T. Abazia, PharmD, BCPS, CPPS; Amisha Arya, PharmD, BCSCP, CJCP; Tegan J. Buckley, PharmD, BCPS, BCGP; Greg Burger, MS, RPh; Maureen Burger, MSN, RN, CPHQ, FACHE; Lemrey "Al" Carter, MS, PharmD, RPh (NABP); Carl Coats, PharmD, MHA, BCPS; Thomas Cooley, RPh, BS, MBA; Angela Covington, PharmD, MBA, BCPS; Loriann De Martini, PharmD, MPH, BCGP (CSHP); Doina Dumitru, PharmD, MBA, FASHP; Agnes Ann Feemster, PharmD, BCPS (JHH); Evan Frasure, PharmD, BCPS; Jenna Goldstein, MS (SHM); Kim Harris, RPh (MHHC); John Hertig, PharmD, MS, CPPS, FASHP; Amey C. Hugg, BS Pharm, CPHIMS, FKSHP; Alifiya F. Hyderi, PharmD, BCPS; Terri Jorgenson, RPh, BCPS; Bonnie Levin, PharmD, MBA, FASHP; CAPT Michael Long, RPh, MPH (BOP); Pashmina Malik, PharmD, MPH; Eric Maroyka, PharmD, BCPS; Nisha Mathew, PharmD BCPS CPh; JoAnne Myhre, CPhT, FMSHP, BA; Danielle Neal, PharmD, MBA, BCPS, DPLA (AHWFB); Mark Neuenschwander, BA (THRIV); Sheetal Patel-House, PharmD, MS, MBA (UNC); Barbara Petroff, MS, RPh, FASHP, FNHIA, BCSCP; Mary Petrovskis, PharmD, MS, BCPS; Carol A. Purcell, MSN, RN, CNML; Beth Weisz Riead, PharmD, MHA; James Rinehart, RPh, MS, FASHP; Samantha Roberts, PharmD, MBA; Dennis Tribble, PharmD, FASHP; Tyler A. Vest, PharmD, MS, BCPS, BCSCP; Elizabeth Wade, PharmD, BCPS, FASHP; and Amy Young, PharmD.

The authors and contributors have declared no potential conflicts of interest.

John Clark, PharmD, MS, BCPS, FASHP; University of Michigan Health and University of Michigan College of Pharmacy, Ann Arbor, MI.

Toni Fera, BS Pharm, PharmD; Independent Healthcare Consultant, Pittsburgh, PA.

Christopher Fortier, PharmD, FASHP; Massachusetts General Hospital, Boston, MA.

Kristine Gullickson, PharmD, MBA, FASHP, FMSHP; Allina Health Abbott Northwestern Hospital, Minneapolis, MN.

Amanda Hays, PharmD, MHA, BCPS, CPHQ, DPLA, FASHP; Becton, Dickinson and Company, San Diego, CA.

Lee Murdaugh, BS Pharm, PhD; Cardinal Health, Dublin, OH.

Ricky Ogden, Jr., PharmD, MBA, BCPS, FACHE; Children's Mercy Kansas City, Kansas City, MO.

Brian O'Neal, PharmD, MS, FASHP; Children's Mercy Kansas City, Kansas City, MO.

Jordan Rush, PharmD, MS; UNC Health, Chapel Hill, NC.

Tyler Vest, PharmD, MS, BCPS, BCSCP; Duke University Hospital, Durham, NC.

Copyright © 2022, American Society of Health-System Pharmacists, Inc. All rights reserved. Contact ASHP for reprint and permissions requests. This content may not be used for commercial purposes without the express written consent of ASHP.

The bibliographic citation for this document is as follows: American Society of Health-System Pharmacists. ASHP guidelines on preventing diversion of controlled substances. *Am J Health-Syst Pharm.* 2022; 79(24):2279–2306.

ASHP Guidelines on Managing Drug Product Shortages

Purpose

Drug product shortages can adversely affect drug therapy, compromise or delay medical procedures, result in medication errors, and cause patient harm.[1-38] In addition to these potential problems, healthcare professionals are also increasingly concerned about the tremendous resources required to address shortages, estimated at $209 million in 2013 for the purchase of more-expensive substitutes alone, which excludes other significant costs (e.g., drugs purchased "off contract," therapeutic alternatives, added labor).[39,40] Drug product shortages adversely affect healthcare organization finances by increasing the cost of delivering patient care, largely through the personnel costs required to manage the multiple pharmacy automation systems and electronic medical record changes that must be adjusted in the face of a drug shortage.[40] In addition, shortages create high levels of frustration and stress for everyone involved, including purchasing agents, pharmacists, pharmacy technicians, nurses, physicians, and patients.[15,41,42] Pharmacy leaders need to educate all members of the healthcare team as well as organizational leadership about the complex and challenging nature of the drug shortage problem as well as what is being done to manage shortages.

Managing drug product shortages is particularly complex for practitioners in hospitals and other acute care settings because these facilities routinely treat patients with acute or emergent conditions, use a significant number of medically necessary or single-source products, and use high-cost new drugs and technologies. These healthcare providers are challenged during drug product shortages to ensure the provision of seamless, safe, and therapeutically equivalent drug therapy, preferably at comparable costs. The pharmacy department must take a leadership role in efforts to develop and implement appropriate strategies and processes for informing practitioners of shortages and ensuring the safe and effective use of therapeutic alternatives. Strategic planning is required for managing drug product shortages, just as it is for disasters such as major weather events or mass casualty incidents.[43] The purpose of these guidelines is to provide a framework for healthcare teams in patient care settings that can be used to develop policies and procedures that minimize the effects of drug shortages on quality of care. These guidelines are focused on minimizing the impact on patient care because it is impossible for healthcare organizations to prevent drug shortages from happening. Although drug shortages are a symptom of broader problems in the U.S. drug product marketplace, these issues are beyond the scope of this document.[44-47]

Patient Safety

Drug shortages are a cause of significant patient safety concerns. Medication errors are more likely to occur (1) when a pharmacy alters how a product is ordered, prepared, or dispensed or (2) when prescribing practices change to less-familiar alternative agents, especially agents that are less efficacious, have a worse adverse-effect profile, or require an unusual or difficult dosing regimen. Best practices for managing drug shortages must first consider the potential impact on patient safety. Data documenting patient harm due to drug shortages are limited to case reports and survey data. The Institute for Safe Medication Practices (ISMP) is the leading source of aggregate data.[13,15,16] A medication-error reporting and review system is an essential component of a medication safety system. Errors and near misses should be reported internally and externally, and analyzed.[48,49]

Factors That Contribute to Drug Product Shortages

For the purpose of these guidelines, a drug product shortage is defined as a supply issue that affects how the pharmacy prepares or dispenses a drug product or influences patient care when prescribers must use an alternative agent. Shortages can be the result of 1 or a combination of factors throughout the supply chain. The supply chain includes producers of raw materials, manufacturers, regulators, wholesalers/distributors, prime vendors, group purchasing organizations, healthcare organizations, and the patient. Factors that contribute to drug product shortages include the unique market for drug products, manufacturing and quality problems, production delays and lack of manufacturing capacity, manufacturer business decisions, shortages of active pharmaceutical ingredients (APIs) or raw materials, restricted distribution and allocation of drug products, and inventory practices.

Unique Market for Drug Products. Drug products are a unique commodity because they do not follow the fundamental economic laws of supply and demand. A first-line agent remains a first-line agent, regardless of price. Unlike other markets, consumers (i.e., patients) have little or no control over prescription product selection in healthcare organizations. In addition, because there is no required disclosure of information regarding manufacturers or manufacturing sites, purchasers of drug products are unable to make educated purchasing decisions based on the quality of a supplier. Purchasers of drug products are unable to make selections based on the quality of a supplier because there is no required transparency regarding the manufacturer or manufacturing site of a drug product.[50]

Manufacturing and Quality Problems. The majority of drug shortages are caused by a production delay due to a failure of quality management at the final product's manufacturing site.[51] For example, the most recent data available show that 46.6–55.1% of sterile injectable anti-infective and cardiovascular drug shortages from 2012 through 2014 were from manufacturing plants that received a warning letter from the Food and Drug Administration (FDA) for failure to comply with manufacturing standards.[44] Quality is not rewarded in the drug product marketplace, because manufacturing is not transparent. The current pass-fail system of FDA approval provides no opportunity for purchasers to favor companies

DOI 10.37573/9781585287048.017

with higher manufacturing standards over companies with lower standards.[51] Although FDA has plans to require manufacturers to provide quality metrics, such as batch failure rates or the number of complaints, neither FDA nor purchasers of drug products have any method to review even these simple metrics.[52] FDA has focused its responsibility for quality on the Office of Pharmaceutical Quality, whose mission is to ensure that quality medications are available for the American public.[53]

Production Delays and Lack of Capacity. Manufacturing capacity issues or delays were the cause of 30% of drug product shortages from 2011 through 2013.[54] Many production delays actually stem from quality problems that delay production for a single manufacturer, and other manufacturers do not have the capacity to make up for the difference. Generic drug products are particularly susceptible to shortages because, unlike branded products, redundancy is typically not built into the production process. Generic products are typically manufactured on lines that prepare multiple products. An additional manufacturing line is generally not available as a contingency for generic products.[55] These types of shortages frequently occur with generic injectable agents, as tight profit margins and the complexities of production limit the number of manufacturers and lead to high market shares; in many cases, a single manufacturer may have over 50% of the market share for specific therapeutic categories.[51] A small number of manufacturers (fewer than 7) comprise the vast majority of all injectable drug products,[51] and more than one third of injectable drug products are produced by just 1 or 2 manufacturers.[51,55]

Manufacturer Business Decisions. Manufacturers' business decisions are based on a variety of factors, including availability of generic products, market size, patent expiration, drug approval status, regulatory compliance requirements, and anticipated clinical demand. Frequently, the decision to manufacture a new product forces production tradeoffs because many generic manufacturers function at full capacity.[51,56]

Shortages of APIs or Raw Materials. Shortages of APIs or raw materials are rare but can result in drug product shortages.[51,55] An API shortage can be particularly disruptive if there is only 1 supplier; however, manufacturers' sources of API are considered proprietary and are rarely publicly disclosed.

Restricted Distribution and Allocation of Drug Products. Most healthcare organizations obtain the majority of their drug products through wholesale distributors. Restricted distribution methods that bypass the normal supply chain can also contribute to shortages. Manufacturers may limit the availability of and access to specific drug products to selected pharmacies, clinicians, and patients complying with manufacturer agreements based on market approval requirements and/or postmarketing surveillance. A manufacturer can also place restrictions on the availability of products by requiring healthcare organizations to order directly from the manufacturer or through a specialty distributor to receive an allocation.

Inventory Practices. Inventory reductions permitted by advanced communication and transportation efficiencies within the supply chain may amplify the effects of a shortage on healthcare organizations. Most manufacturers, distribution centers, and healthcare organizations use just-in-time inventory management to reduce the cost of inventory on hand, increase inventory turns, minimize expenses, and optimize cash flow. This strategy is recognized as sound business management but allows unexpected shortages at any stage in the supply chain to significantly impact purchasers and patients. Some manufacturers and distributors use inventory management strategies that minimize end-of-quarter or end-of-year product inventories or limit shipment based on yearly quotas.[57] Poor ordering practices, stockpiling before announced price increases, hoarding caused by rumors of an impending shortage, and unexpected delivery delays may also affect inventory levels in individual healthcare organizations. Hospitals in rural areas face additional inventory challenges caused by distant distribution centers and the inability to easily borrow an item from a nearby hospital. Drug product shortages may also occur when hospitals in an area disproportionately use the same wholesaler. Some shortages are wholesaler dependent, as shortages of drugs can occur when contracts with suppliers are delayed.

Planning for Drug Product Shortages

The pharmacy department can lead effective drug shortage management by ensuring that its organization has the necessary infrastructure and a well-defined management strategy in place before a shortage occurs. To effectively respond to drug product shortages, several essential elements of infrastructure must be in place before a shortage occurs: a drug shortage team, a resource allocation committee, and established processes for approving alternative therapies and addressing ethical considerations.

Drug Product Shortage Team. The first step is to identify an interdisciplinary team of key staff who can make decisions and access information. The drug product shortage team needs to understand the organization's processes for change and how to expedite results. At a minimum, the drug product shortage team should be able to identify persons responsible for the following activities: data gathering and monitoring; purchasing alternatives; changing storage, preparation, and dispensing procedures; deciding to conserve or ration; implementing technology changes; and communications. The drug shortage team should develop a list of ad hoc stakeholders to consult for specific shortages. A specific point person should be designated to lead drug shortage efforts, but no single person can manage all drug shortage planning and response activities alone.

Resource Allocation Committee. Although consideration of the ethical implications of drug shortages may be discussed within the organization's existing committee structure (e.g., the ethics committee), a resource allocation committee should be formed to directly oversee the allocation of scarce resources such as drug products. The resource allocation committee should include, at a minimum, representatives from the departments of pharmacy, nursing, social work, and medicine; a patient representative; and a representative from the organization's ethics committee.[58] When a drug shortage affects a specific therapeutic area, other departments or disciplines may need to be represented, and a clinician with expertise in that area should provide representation on the committee. Committee members should be identified in advance and be available to assume membership on the committee when the need arises.[58,59] All members of the committee should disclose any bias or potential conflicts of interest in advance if possible.[60]

The committee should carefully determine appropriate patient characteristics and clinical evidence for prioritization and rationing of medications.[58,59,61,62] Because drug shortages will evolve, ethics protocols should allow for feedback and amendment.[62] Standardizing the ethics framework in advance avoids the need for bedside decisions and allows clinicians to contemplate complexities and appropriate rationales before difficult choices need to be made.[60,62,63] Protocols should also address how to manage the distress clinicians can experience when making such difficult decisions.[60]

Interruption of clinical trials is another potential consequence of drug shortages that has potential ethical implications. Organizations must ensure that study sponsors and principal investigators are aware of drug shortages that may affect clinical trials. Healthcare organizations should appropriately allocate remaining medications, halt trial enrollment, or continue patients on the standard-of-care treatment only as necessary until the drug shortage has resolved.[58]

Process for Approving Alternative Therapies. A formal process for identifying and approving therapeutic alternatives for the healthcare organization should be established. The healthcare organization's decision-making process about alternative agents should involve timely collaboration among representatives of medicine, nursing, pharmacy, and other affected disciplines, and those decisions should be approved by the appropriate medical committees as promptly as possible. Organizations should follow the same steps and processes used in changing any drug product in their system to ensure that key steps in managing automation and technology are not missed.

Process for Addressing Ethical Considerations. As drug shortages have become more common, healthcare organizations and providers have become more adept at identifying and utilizing therapeutic alternatives. Nevertheless, situations arise in which it is difficult to simply substitute an alternative agent, if available at all.[58] Drug shortages have become a barrier to clinicians providing the most appropriate and evidence-based care to patients and may create mistrust between patients and providers.[64,65] The appropriate management of drug shortages requires carefully balancing what is good for an individual and what is good for a group of individuals or society.[60,61]

As the number of drug shortages has grown, several ethical frameworks for appropriately rationing these resources have been proposed.[58,60,66] One method that reflects the fundamental healthcare principles of justice, beneficence, and nonmaleficence is an adaptation of Daniels and Sabin's[67] "accountability for reasonableness," amended by several authors to address drug shortages.[58,60,61] Because there isn't 1 ethical framework to provide complete guidance for all drug shortage dilemmas, the framework should be adapted by organizations to address their particular circumstances.[63] The main principles of this method are as follows:

- *Transparency:* details of the process are made public and available for scrutiny.
- *Relevance:* a neutral observer would be able to apply the process to a broad range of differing situations.
- *Appeals and revision:* those who feel wronged by the process have a way to appeal and have the original decision reversed if appropriate.
- *Enforcement:* the process is mandatory, and its results are required to be applied.
- *Fairness:* the process is to be applied to all, regardless of the type of patient or prominence of clinician treating that particular patient.[58,60,66]

Just as the therapeutic management of drug shortages requires healthcare organizations to prospectively institute guidelines or restrictions, ethical procedures and protocols should be developed and put into place before the need for them arises.[65] Variations in these protocols may be necessary for different classes and uses of drugs; the rationing of anti-infectives and oncological agents, for example, is quite different.[59–61,66]

Responding to Drug Product Shortages

The identification of a shortage initiates a cascade of events surrounding drug procurement and therapeutic decision-making (**Figure 1**). When a shortage is identified, the drug product shortage team should conduct an operational and therapeutic assessment to evaluate its potential impact. A shortage impact analysis based on the 2 assessments and an evaluation of procedural and financial implications should be used to assess the potential impact on patient care. The drug shortages team should use that impact analysis to develop a final action plan for approval and implementation. An institution's success in responding to shortages is typically dependent on how well the system can change drug products in their system under nonshortage conditions.

Operational Assessment

The operational assessment should be performed by the point person or that person's designee, working with others as necessary. The assessment validates the details of the shortage, estimates the supply of the drug product in shortage available on hand and from alternative sources, evaluates past usage, and estimates the supply of alternative therapies.

Details and Duration of Shortage. The pharmacy team can contact product manufacturers, distributors, FDA, the Centers for Disease Control and Prevention (CDC), and other sources to determine the cause of the shortage and its expected timing and duration. This information may already be available on the ASHP Drug Shortage Resource Center website (www.ashp.org/Drug-Shortages) or the FDA Drug Shortages website (www.fda.gov/Drugs/DrugSafety/DrugShortages). If it is not, visitors to the sites should report the shortage online. Predictions of when the product will be available help the healthcare organization develop its short- and long-term strategies. Because the status of a shortage can change quickly, follow-up communications with manufacturers may be required to obtain updates on previous estimates of product availability.

Inventory on Hand. Once a shortage is identified, pharmacy staff should assess the inventory on hand and estimate the time period it will cover. Available inventory includes all supplies of the drug product within the healthcare organization, including the pharmacies, inpatient units, ambulatory

FIGURE 1. Process for decision-making in the management of drug product shortages.

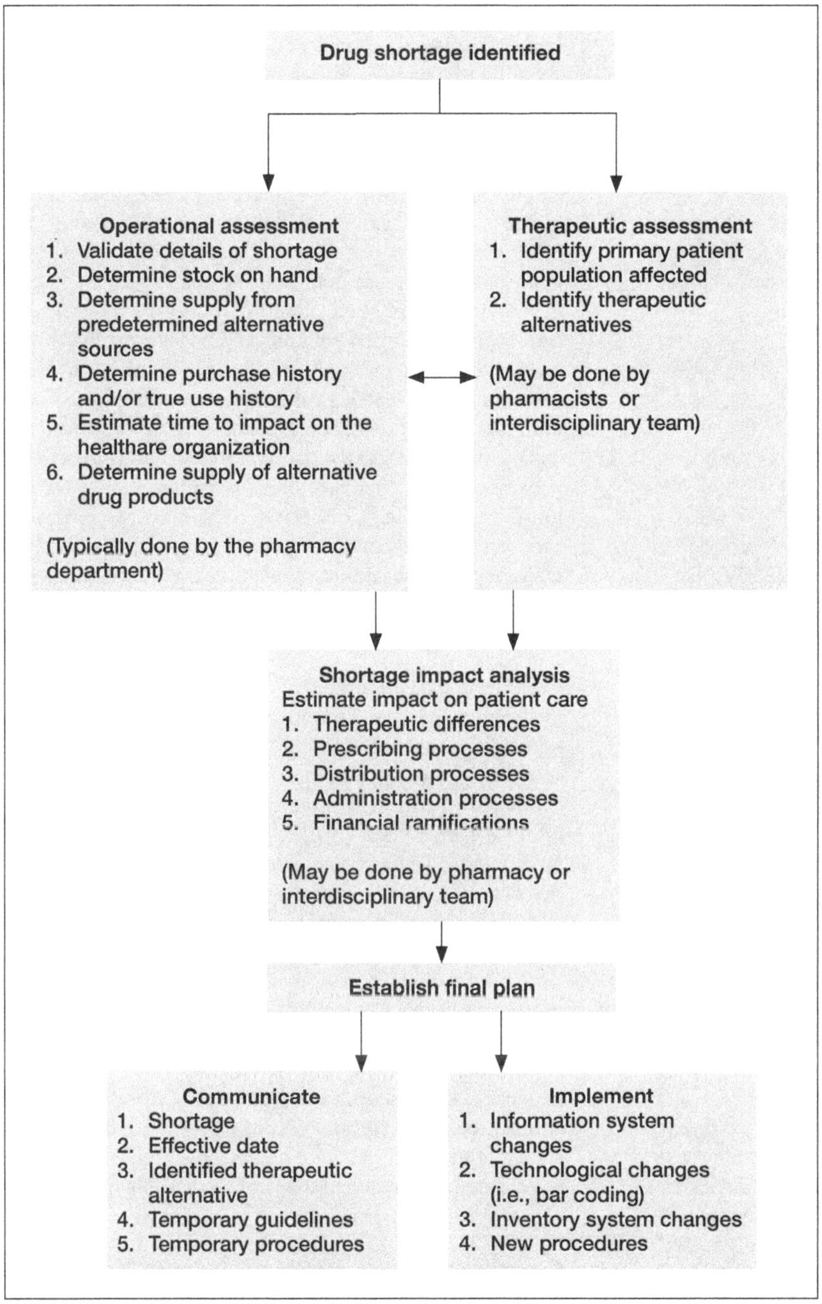

care clinics, automated medication storage and distribution devices, floor stock, code carts, and prepared trays. The pharmacy should estimate how long the healthcare organization can endure a shortage based on available quantities and historical usage, converting inventory counts of alternative drug products into common measurement units (e.g., common dose, days of therapy) to augment estimates of use.

Therapeutic Assessment

The therapeutic assessment can be performed by the point person, that person's designee, or other members of the drug shortage team as necessary. The assessment identifies the primary patient populations affected and identifies therapeutic alternatives.

Patient Prioritization. When a limited supply of a drug remains available and alternatives for specific patient groups are undesirable, a healthcare organization may prioritize use of the drug for specific patient groups. National organizations (e.g., CDC or an organization of healthcare specialists) may provide guidance on patient prioritization. Medication-use evaluation data on prescribing and utilization trends, if available for the drug in question, may be useful in developing prioritization criteria to guide appropriate drug use. Additional criteria, such as therapeutic use (curative versus palliative), may also be helpful in guiding appropriate use of the drug. Such criteria are particularly helpful in dealing with long-term shortages. To restrict product use for select patients or services in the healthcare organization, criteria should be developed by an interprofessional team. An ethical framework for allocating particularly scarce or lifesaving products is essential as is evidence-based decision making with regard to alternatives.[58,63]

Therapeutic Alternatives. Therapeutic alternatives should be inventoried and availability assessed to ensure adequate supplies to meet new demand. In many cases, supplies of the best alternative agent may be affected by the response to the shortage. If therapeutic alternatives are not on the formulary or not currently stocked in the system, there should be a process to expedite adding the new product to all systems (e.g., the electronic health record [EHR], smart pump libraries, automated dispensing cabinets [ADCs]). If a compounded medication is an appropriate alternative, organizations must decide whether resources are available to compound inhouse or if the best solution is to purchase the compounded medication from an FDA-registered outsourcing facility.

Shortage Impact Analysis

A shortage impact analysis evaluates all factors relevant to the shortage (e.g., duration, current and available inventory, medical necessity, affected patient populations, alternative therapies) to determine the shortage's potential impact on patient care and costs. Such analyses should include a threat analysis for severe shortages to determine whether surgeries or other treatments must be canceled. Healthcare organizations should develop a mitigation strategy for patients whose treatments are no longer available. This strategy may include sending patients to another facility that has the drug in stock or developing a process to postpone elective surgeries. Shortages affect safe medication practices throughout the medication distribution and administration process within a healthcare organization. When considering alternative dosage forms or therapies, pharmacists must consider changes in look-alike/sound-alike procedures, barcoding, distribution paths, and the impact on automation, contract compliance, and final product preparation.[68] Healthcare organizations should evaluate the time required to implement any changes into electronic systems. The extent to which a healthcare organization will be affected by a given shortage depends on the severity of the shortage's impacts; the organization's scope, level of services, and service population; and the organization's agility in switching drug products given the constraints of information system changes (e.g., EHR, smart pump libraries, ADCs).

Financial Ramifications. Drug shortages result in increased costs due to a variety of causes: the higher cost of off-contract purchases of drug products or more-expensive alternative agents and the increased personnel costs to develop plans, relocate or compound drug products, and make changes to the EHR and other information systems. Healthcare organizations should make every effort to track all drug and personnel costs related to shortages as well as lost revenue from canceled treatments or surgeries. An accounting of these costs is helpful when explaining budget variance or proposing plans for additional staff or funds.

Final Action Plan

The healthcare organization should develop a final action plan prior to sending a comprehensive communication about the shortage. The final action plan can be used to double-check all elements of the management plan. The plan should state whether a conservation approach will be used to conserve remaining supplies or smaller future allocations or if the shortage will require use of an alternative agent. Examples of management and conservation strategies include par adjustments, centralization of inventory (e.g., removing from ADCs and floor stock), repackaging into smaller dosage units, extending beyond-use dating (when approved by FDA and manufacturer or verified through *United States Pharmacopeia* chapter 797-compliant process), i.v.-to-p.o. conversion, discontinuing nonessential therapy, limiting use of product to uses supported by evidence, and using a different strength or size of product. In some cases, a combination of these actions will be necessary for optimal clinical efficacy. For shortages that require canceled surgeries or treatments, the rationing plan for remaining supplies should be included. The organization should coordinate a specific time for making changes in information systems (e.g., EHR, smart pump libraries, ADCs, and other databases) and ensure that sufficient staff are available to re-enter orders, move stock between ADCs, or take other follow-up actions. Finally, it is essential that everyone understand their roles and the timing required for effective implementation as well as the dynamic nature of drug shortages that may require revisions to the plan.

Communication

Clear communication with all affected clinicians about the status of a shortage is vital. Administrators should also be included in communications, particularly if the shortage may result in canceled surgeries or treatments or significantly increased costs. Multiple communication methods are better than a single strategy. The EHR can also play a communication role to provide prescribers information at the time of medication order. The shortage management team should understand each member's role and share information quickly, efficiently, and in a timely manner. Information should be shared prospectively about both anticipated and confirmed shortages to allow appropriate preparation. Communication within the pharmacy department should include all staff members, including pharmacy technicians. Pharmacists who specialize in a specific clinical area (e.g., intensive care, transplantation) can be especially helpful in relaying information about shortages to their healthcare colleagues during rounds. All pharmacy shifts should receive the same message, and the communication methods should be adapted to the organization's culture, using multiple methods whenever possible (standing meetings, texts, emails, intranet, blogs). Communications to affected prescribers and other healthcare providers should include those in training (e.g., students and residents). Some healthcare organizations may designate a specific department to manage communications; others may find that a collaborative strategy involving various organizational departments and committees works best.

Disclosure to Patients. Healthcare organizations should establish policies and protocols regarding the disclosure of drug shortage information to patients and the extent of such disclosures.[59,65] Patients or family members should be counseled when a drug product shortage will delay or compromise care, especially when patients have been stabilized on the drug product and alternatives may be less effective.[58,63,69,70] Disclosure may vary depending on the type of clinical situation. In an emergent situation, decisions about disclosure need to balance transparency and other critical factors involved in providing care. In the case of an elective procedure, it must be decided how patients will be provided an understanding of the potential risks from less efficacious drugs or those with more adverse effects.[65] When the patient's need for a drug will recur, communications should address, before drug initiation, the possibility that the full course of treatment may not be available. Concerns that the full course of the regimen may not be available may warrant consideration of alternatives.

Communication with Media. Media outlets may be interested in reporting on severe shortages; working with the media can highlight the impact that drug shortages have on patient care. Organizations and individuals should work with their public affairs officers before speaking to the media and should keep in mind that updates may be necessary, especially when a shortage resolves. For all communications, it is important to balance timeliness and completeness and to be transparent about how decisions to ration are made and whether there is a method for appeals or exceptions.

Inventory System Changes

Stockpiling Restraint. Inventory management is a challenge in the face of a shortage. Stockpiling (hoarding) and speculative purchasing in advance of an anticipated shortage can exacerbate the shortage, disrupt efficient distribution, and divert supplies away from healthcare organizations with patients in need.[71] Healthcare organizations should refrain from stockpiling drugs anticipated to go into shortage as well as alternatives. Stockpiling causes 2 distinct problems: (1) stockpiling can cause artificial shortages when healthcare organizations drain the supply chain and demand exceeds manufacturing capacity, and (2) stockpiled inventory is costly and may not be absorbed by normal usage if shortages do not occur as anticipated.

Speculative purchasing in response to a potential shortage has drawbacks as well, depending on the likely cause of the shortage and where it might occur in the supply chain. Problems may arise that appear to pose a shortage threat but never reach end users, because the supply chain, from raw material to finished product, may contain several months' supply; that long lead time allows corrections that avert the shortage. Finally, during shortages, manufacturers and distributors often allocate product on the basis of past usage, so an initial stockpile order generally has no impact on increasing an allocation.

Purchasing from Outside Pharmacies and Inhouse Compounding. Healthcare organizations must establish clear guidelines for dealing with situations in which a product is available only from a compounding source or nontraditional source or when a critical drug is not available at all. Each healthcare organization must determine its philosophies on purchasing drugs from the gray market or compounding pharmacies and on inhouse compounding. These decisions should be made before the pressure and emotion of a specific shortage occur. Each option and its potential effect on patient risk should be evaluated. Nontraditional drug product sources (e.g., secondary wholesalers) have extremely limited supplies, and the quality of these products may be questionable, as the provenance of the medication may be unknown. Pedigree requirements of the Drug Supply Chain Security Act may alleviate these concerns as they are implemented.[72] Products from compounding pharmacies may also present risks to patients (e.g., inefficacy, adulteration, lack of sterility); tragically, several deaths have been associated with improperly sterilized compounded products. Healthcare organizations may choose to compound products if they can meet the necessary guidelines; however, obtaining raw materials may be difficult in some cases.

Conclusion

Drug product supply issues are a frequent problem affecting healthcare organizations. Organizations can mitigate the effects of shortages by establishing an infrastructure for dealing with shortages before they occur. Although it is impractical to prepare for every potential shortage, proper planning can reduce adverse effects on patient care and healthcare organization costs and prevent problems from escalating into crises. The keys to success will undoubtedly be found in the effectiveness of information gathering; teamwork to assess options; ability to rapidly make changes in information systems; and communication with providers, patients, and administrators.

References

1. Storey MA, Weber RJ, Besco K et al. Evaluation of parenteral nutrition errors in an era of drug shortages. *Nutr Clin Pract.* 2015; 31:211–7.
2. American Society of Anesthesiologists. 2012 ASA drug shortage survey results. www.asahq.org/advocacy/fda-and-washington-alerts/washington-alerts/2012/04/2012-asa-drug-shortage-survey-results (accessed 2018 Jul 10).
3. Norton SA, Soghier L, Hatfield J et al. Zinc deficiency dermatitis in cholestatic extremely premature infants after a nationwide shortage of injectable zinc—Washington, DC, December 2012. *MMWR.* 2013; 62:136–7. [Erratum, *MMWR.* 2013; 62:196.]
4. De Oliveira GS Jr, McCarthy RJ. Drug shortages in perioperative medicine: past, present, or future? *Anesth Analg.* 2015; 121:259–61.
5. De Oliveira GS Jr, Theilken LS, McCarthy RJ. Shortage of perioperative drugs: implications for anesthesia practice and patient safety. *Anesth Analg.* 2011; 113:1429–35.
6. Salazar EG, Bernhardt MB, Li Y et al. The impact of chemotherapy shortages on COG and local clinical trials: a report from the Children's Oncology Group. *Pediatr Blood Cancer.* 2015; 62:940–4.
7. Emanuel EJ, Shuman K, Chinn D et al. Impact of oncology drug shortages. http://ascopubs.org/doi/abs/10.1200/jco.2013.31.18_suppl.cra6510 (accessed 2018 Jul 10).
8. Goldsack JC, Reilly C, Bush C et al. Impact of shortages of injectable oncology drugs on patient care. *Am J Health-Syst Pharm.* 2014; 71:571–8.
9. Goozner M. Drug shortages delay cancer clinical trials. *J Natl Cancer Inst.* 2012; 104:891–2.
10. Griffith MM, Gross AE, Sutton SH et al. The impact of anti-infective drug shortages on hospitals in the United States: trends and causes. *Clin Infect Dis.* 2012; 54:684–91.
11. Griffith MM, Pentoney Z, Scheetz MH. Antimicrobial drug shortages: a crisis amidst the epidemic and the need for antimicrobial stewardship efforts to lessen the effects. *Pharmacotherapy.* 2012; 32:665–7.
12. Hanson C, Thoene M, Wagner J et al. Parenteral nutrition additive shortages: the short-term, long-term and potential epigenetic implications in premature and hospitalized infants. *Nutrients.* 2012; 4:1977–88.
13. Institute for Safe Medication Practices. Drug shortages threaten patient safety (July 29, 2010). www.ismp.org/resources/drug-shortages-threaten-patient-safety (accessed 2018 Jul 10).
14. Institute for Safe Medication Practices. Drug shortages continue to compromise patient care (January 11, 2018). www.ismp.org/resources/drug-shortages-continue-compromise-patient-care (accessed 2018 Jul 19).
15. Institute for Safe Medication Practices. Drug shortages: National survey reveals high level of frustration, low level of safety (September 23, 2010). www.ismp.org/resources/special-issue-drug-shortages-national-survey-reveals-high-level-frustration-low-level (accessed 2018 Jul 10).

16. Institute for Safe Medication Practices. A shortage of everything except errors: Harm associated with drug shortages (April 19, 2012). www.ismp.org/resources/shortage-everything-except-errors-harm-associated-drug-shortages (accessed 2018 Jul 10).
17. Kosarek L, Hart SR, Schultz L et al. Increase in venous complications associated with etomidate use during a propofol shortage: an example of clinically important adverse effects related to drug substitution. *Ochsner J.* 2011; 11:143–6.
18. Krisl JC, Fortier CR, Taber DJ. Disruptions in the supply of medications used in transplantation: implications and management strategies for the transplant clinician. *Am J Transplant.* 2013; 13:20–30.
19. Mazer-Amirshahi M, Hawley KL, Zocchi M et al. Drug shortages: implications for medical toxicology. *Clin Toxicol.* 2015; 53:519–24.
20. Mazer-Amirshahi M, Pourmand A, Singer S et al. Critical drug shortages: implications for emergency medicine. *Acad Emerg Med.* 2014; 21:704–11.
21. McBride A, Holle LM, Westendorf C et al. National survey on the effect of oncology drug shortages on cancer care. *Am J Health-Syst Pharm.* 2013; 70:609–17.
22. McHugh SM, Ibinson JW. Anesthesiology in the era of drug shortages: use of a succinylcholine infusion for a laparoscopic sigmoid colectomy due to a shortage of neostigmine. *J Clinical Anesth.* 2013; 25:79–81.
23. McLaughlin M, Kotis D, Thomson K et al. Effects on patient care caused by drug shortages: a survey. *J Manag Care Pharm.* 2013; 19:783–8.
24. Metzger ML, Billett A, Link MP. The impact of drug shortages on children with cancer—the example of mechlorethamine. *N Engl J Med.* 2012; 367:2461–3.
25. Mirtallo JM, Holcombe B, Kochevar M et al. Parenteral nutrition product shortages: the A.S.P.E.N. strategy. *Nutr Clin Pract.* 2012; 27:385–91.
26. Moffett BS, Mossad EB. Drug shortages: implications on pediatric anesthesia practice and management resources. *J Clinical Anesth.* 2012; 24:677–9.
27. Mruk AL, Record KE. Antimicrobial options in the treatment of adult staphylococcal bone and joint infections in an era of drug shortages. *Orthopedics.* 2012; 35:401–7.
28. Neavyn MJ, Boyer EW, Bird SB et al. Sodium acetate as a replacement for sodium bicarbonate in medical toxicology: a review. *J Med Toxicol.* 2013; 9:250–4.
29. Nickel RS, Keller F, Bergsagel J et al. Mitoxantrone as a substitute for daunorubicin during induction in newly diagnosed lymphoblastic leukemia and lymphoma. *Pediatr Blood Cancer.* 2014; 61:810–4.
30. Osterholm MT. Shortage of antimicrobials wider, more severe than thought. *Clin Infect Dis.* 2000; 30:preceding table of contents.
31. Paparella SF. Drug shortages in the emergency department: managing a threat to patient safety. *J Emerg Nurs.* 2012; 38:466–9.
32. Plogsted S, Adams SC, Allen K et al. Parenteral nutrition electrolyte and mineral product shortage considerations. *Nutr Clin Pract.* 2016; 31:132–4.
33. Reed BN, Fox ER, Konig M et al. The impact of drug shortages on patients with cardiovascular disease: causes, consequences, and a call to action. *Am Heart J.* 2016; 175:130–41.
34. Pluss-Suard C, Pannatier A, Ruffieux C et al. Changes in the use of broad-spectrum antibiotics after cefepime shortage: a time series analysis. *Antimicrob Agents Chemother.* 2012; 56:989–94.
35. Pramyothin P, Kim DW, Young LS et al. Anemia and leukopenia in a long-term parenteral nutrition patient during a shortage of parenteral trace element products in the United States. *J Parenter Enteral Nutr.* 2013; 37:425–9.
36. Printz C. Medication shortages threaten cancer care: the oncology community and the FDA tackle ongoing drug shortage problem. *Cancer.* 2012; 118:289–91.
37. Quadri F, Mazer-Amirshahi M, Fox ER et al. Antibacterial drug shortages from 2001 to 2013: implications for clinical practice. *Clin Infect Dis.* 2015; 60:1737–42.
38. Ralls MW, Blackwood RA, Arnold MA et al. Drug shortage-associated increase in catheter-related blood stream infection in children. *Pediatrics.* 2012; 130:e1369–73.
39. Premier. Drug shortages 2014: a Premier healthcare alliance update. www.premierinc.com/wpdm-package/drug-shortages-press-resources/?wpdmdl=3325&ind=nrBpFZ99rM8HAsnKDI-C46IHzLP3L6LkqYBuEezDWgmFszq2_ILP3v9-dnfv6lcPOkesuoDBg4sWvLrBf6XRPA (accessed 2018 Jul 19).
40. Kaakeh R, Sweet BV, Reilly C et al. Impact of drug shortages on U.S. health systems. *Am J Health-Syst Pharm.* 2011; 68:1811–9.
41. Institute for Safe Medication Practices. Part I of our national survey on drug shortages reveals high level of frustration, low regard for safety. *ISMP Medication Safety Alert!* March 21, 2001.
42. Thompson CA. Pharmacist converted frustration about drug shortages into action. *Am J Health-Syst Pharm.* 2012; 69:182–4.
43. Hick JL, Hanfling D, Courtney B et al. Rationing salt water—disaster planning and daily care delivery. *N Engl J Med.* 2014; 370:1573–6.
44. U.S. Government Accountability Office. Drug shortages: certain factors are strongly associated with this persistent public health challenge (GAO-16-595, July 2016). www.gao.gov/assets/680/678281.pdf (accessed 2018 Jan 18).
45. American Society of Health-System Pharmacists. 2014 Drug Shortages Summit. www.ashp.org/-/media/assets/drug-shortages/docs/drug-resources-2014-drug-shortages-summit.ashx (accessed 2018 Jan 18).
46. American Society of Health-System Pharmacists. 2013 Drug Shortages Summit: evaluating long-term solutions. www.ashp.org/-/media/assets/drug-shortages/docs/drug-resources-2013-drug-shortages-summit.ashx (accessed 2018 Jan 18).
47. American Society of Health-System Pharmacists. 2010 Drug Shortages Summit summary report. www.ashp.org/-/media/assets/drug-shortages/docs/drug-resources-2010-drug-shortages-summit.ashx (accessed 2018 Jan 18).

48. American Society of Health-System Pharmacists. ASHP statement on reporting medical errors. *Am J Health-Syst Pharm.* 2000; 57:1531–2.
49. American Society of Health-System Pharmacists. ASHP guidelines on preventing medication errors in hospitals. *Am J Health-Syst Pharm.* 2018; 75:In Press.
50. Fox ER, Tyler LS. Call to action: finding solutions for the drug shortage crisis in the United States. *Clin Pharmacol Ther.* 2013; 93:145–7.
51. Woodcock J, Wosinska M. Economic and technological drivers of generic sterile injectable drug shortages. *Clin Pharmacol Ther.* 2013; 93:170–6.
52. Food and Drug Administration. Submission of quality metrics data: guidance for industry (draft guidance, November 2016). www.fda.gov/ucm/groups/fdagov-public/@fdagov-drugs-gen/documents/document/ucm455957.pdf (accessed 2018 Jul 19).
53. Food and Drug Administration. Office of Pharmaceutical Quality homepage. www.fda.gov/AboutFDA/CentersOffices/OfficeofMedicalProductsandTobacco/CDER/ucm418347.htm (accessed 2016 Jul 22).
54. U.S. Government Accountability Office. Drug shortages: public health threat continues, despite efforts to help ensure product availability (GAO-14-194, February 2014). www.gao.gov/assets/670/660785.pdf (accessed 2018 Feb 14).
55. Fox ER, Sweet BV, Jensen V. Drug shortages: a complex health care crisis. *Mayo Clin Proc.* 2014; 89:361–73.
56. Office of the Assistant Secretary for Planning and Evaluation. Economic analysis of the causes of drug shortages (October 28, 2011). https://aspe.hhs.gov/sites/default/files/pdf/108986/ib.pdf (accessed 2016 Jul 22).
57. Jensen V, Rappaport BA. The reality of drug shortages—the case of the injectable agent propofol. *N Engl J Med.* 2010; 363:806–7.
58. Rosoff PM. Unpredictable drug shortages: an ethical framework for short-term rationing in hospitals. *Am J Bioethics.* 2012; 12:1–9.
59. Griffith MM, Patel JA, Sutton SH et al. Prospective approach to managing antimicrobial drug shortages. *Infect Control Hosp Epidemiol.* 2012; 33:745–52.
60. Jagsi R, Spence R, Rathmell WK et al. Ethical considerations for the clinical oncologist in an era of oncology drug shortages. *Oncologist.* 2014; 19:186–92.
61. Beck JC, Smith LD, Gordon BG et al. An ethical framework for responding to drug shortages in pediatric oncology. *Pediatr Blood Cancer.* 2015; 62:931–4.
62. Flynn J, Chubbs K, Gladney-Martin S et al. Triage in times of drug shortage. *Healthc Manage Forum.* 2015; 28:202–5.
63. Unguru Y, Fernandez CV, Bernhardt B et al. An ethical framework for allocating scarce life-saving chemotherapy and supportive care drugs for childhood cancer. *J Natl Cancer Inst.* 2016; 108:djv392.
64. Lipworth W, Kerridge I. Why drug shortages are an ethical issue. *Australas Med J.* 2013; 6:556–9.
65. Char DS, Magnus D.Ethics of disclosure regarding drug shortages that affect patient care. *Anesth Analg.* 2015; 121:262–3.
66. Valgus J, Singer EA, Berry SR et al. Ethical challenges: managing oncology drug shortages. *J Oncol Pract.* 2013; 9:e21–3.
67. Accountability for reasonableness. In: Daniels N, Sabin JE. Setting limits fairly: Can we learn to share medical resources? New York: Oxford Univ. Press; 2002:43–66.
68. Pick AM, Massoomi F, Neff WJ et al. A safety assessment tool for formulary candidates. *Am J Health-Syst Pharm.* 2006; 63:1269–72.
69. Hsia IK, Dexter F, Logvinov I et al. Survey of the national drug shortage effect on anesthesia and patient safety: a patient perspective. *Anesth Analg.* 2015; 121:502–6.
70. Rosoff PM, Patel KR, Scates A et al. Coping with critical drug shortages: an ethical approach for allocating scarce resources in hospitals. *Arch Intern Med.* 2012; 172:1494–9.
71. Myers CE. Artificial shortages of drug supplies. *Am J Health-Syst Pharm.* 1999; 56:727.
72. Food and Drug Administration. Key provisions of the Drug Supply Chain Security Act. www.fda.gov/Drugs/DrugSafety/DrugIntegrityandSupplyChainSecurity/DrugSupplyChainSecurityAct/ucm565168.htm (accessed 2018 Jan 18).

Developed through the ASHP Council on Pharmacy Management and approved by the ASHP Board of Directors on June 19, 2018. These guidelines supersede the ASHP Guidelines on Managing Drug Product Shortages dated January 15, 2009.

ASHP gratefully acknowledges the contributions made to previous versions of these guidelines by Annette Birt, M.B.A., M.P.H.; Ken B. James, Pharm.D.; Heather Kokko, Pharm.D.; Sandra Salverson, Pharm.D., BCPS; and Donna L. Soflin, B.S.Pharm.

ASHP gratefully acknowledges the following organizations and individuals for reviewing these guidelines (review does not imply endorsement): American Association of Pharmacy Technicians; American Pharmacists Association; Canadian Pharmacists Association; Idaho Society of Health-System Pharmacists; Ellena Anagnostis, M.S., Pharm.D., BCPS; Jason Babby, Pharm.D.,BCPS; Bona E. Benjamin, B.S.Pharm.; Kate Bidwell, Pharm.D., BCPS; Jennifer L. Brandt, Pharm.D., FASHP; Ryan Burke, Pharm.D.; John S. Clark, Pharm.D., M.S., BCPS; Shelita Dattani, Bsc.Phm., Pharm.D.; Michael D. Dickens, Pharm.D.; Elizabeth Duncan, Pharm.D.; Ashley Duty, Pharm.D., M.S.; Katie Gauen, Pharm.D.; Anne Gonzales-Luna, Pharm.D.; Stephen M. LaHaye, Pharm.D., BCPS; Molly Billstein Leber, Pharm.D., BCPS, FASP; Jim Lile, Pharm.D., FASHP; Charles E. "Kurt" Mahan, Pharm.D., Ph.C.; Susan Mankad, Pharm.D.; Michelle McCarthy, Pharm.D., FASHP; Brenna Mehta, Pharm.D.; Cristian Merchan, Pharm.D., BCCCP; Kathleen Morneau, Pharm.D., BCPS; Judy Neville; Robert S. Oakley, FASHP; Lois F. Parker, B.S.Pharm., FASHP; Stacey Pattie, Pharm.D., BCPS; Stephanie Peshek, FASHP; James Ponto, M.S., BCNP, FASHP; Emily Prabhu, Pharm.D., BCPS; Ed C. Rainville, Pharm.M.S.; James R. Rinehart, M.S., FASHP; Catherine L. Shely, Pharm.D.; Elizabeth Snipes, Pharm.D.; Christopher Snyder, Pharm.D.; Ami Vyas, Ph.D., M.B.A., M.S.; Geralyn Waters, Pharm.D.; Roger Woolf, Pharm.D.; and Amy M. Young, Pharm.D.

Dr. Fox is a member of the *AJHP* Editorial Board. The authors have declared no other potential conflicts of interest.

Erin R. Fox, Pharm.D., BCPS, FASHP, Senior Director of Drug Information and Support Services, University of Utah Health, and Adjunct Associate Professor, University of Utah College of Pharmacy, Salt Lake City, UT.

Milena M. McLaughlin, Pharm.D., M.Sc., BCPS-AQ ID, AAHIVP, Associate Professor, Department of Pharmacy Practice, Midwestern University, Chicago College of Pharmacy, Downers Grove, IL and HIV/ID Clinical Pharmacist, Department of Pharmacy, Northwestern Memorial Hospital, Chicago, IL.

Copyright © 2018, American Society of Health-System Pharmacists, Inc. All rights reserved. Contact ASHP for reprint and permissions requests. This content may not be used for commercial purposes without the express written consent of ASHP.

The bibliographic citation for this document is as follows: American Society of Health-System Pharmacists. ASHP guidelines on managing drug product shortages. *Am J Health-Syst Pharm.* 2018; 75:1742–50.

ASHP Guidelines for Selecting Pharmaceutical Manufacturers and Suppliers

Pharmacists are responsible for selecting, from hundreds of manufacturers and suppliers of drugs, those that will enable them to fulfill an important obligation: ensuring that patients receive pharmaceuticals and related supplies of the highest quality and at the lowest cost. These guidelines are offered as an aid to the pharmacist in achieving this goal.

Obligations of the Supplier

Pharmacists may purchase with confidence the products of those suppliers meeting the criteria presented here. Other factors such as credit policies, delivery times, and the breadth of a supplier's product line also must be considered when selecting a supplier.

Technical Considerations

1. On request of the pharmacist, the supplier should furnish
   a. Analytical control data.
   b. Sterility testing data.
   c. Bioavailability data.
   d. Bioequivalency data.
   e. Descriptions of testing procedures for raw materials and finished products.
   f. Any other information that may be indicative of the quality of a given finished drug product.

   Testing data developed by independent laboratories should be identified by the supplier. All information should be supplied at no charge.
2. There should be no history of recurring product recalls indicative of deficient quality control procedures.
3. The supplier should permit visits (during normal business hours) by the pharmacist to inspect its manufacturing and control procedures.
4. All drug products should conform to the requirements of *The United States Pharmacopeia—The National Formulary (USP—NF)* (the most recent edition) unless otherwise specified by the pharmacist. Items not recognized by *USP—NF* should meet the specifications set forth by the pharmacist.
5. To the extent possible, all products should be available in single unit or unit dose packages. These packages should conform to the "ASHP Technical Assistance Bulletin on Single Unit and Unit Dose Packages of Drugs."[1]
6. The name and address of the manufacturer of the final dosage form and the packager or distributor should be present on the product labeling.
7. Expiration dates should be clearly indicated on the package label and, unless stability properties warrant otherwise, should occur in January or July.
8. Therapeutic, biopharmaceutic, and toxicologic information should be available to the pharmacist on request. Toxicity information should be available around the clock.
9. Patient/staff educational materials that are important for proper use of the product should be routinely available.
10. On request, the supplier should furnish proof of any claims made with respect to the efficacy, safety, and superiority of its products.
11. On request, the supplier should furnish, at no charge, a reasonable quantity of its products to enable the pharmacist to evaluate the products' physical traits, including pharmaceutical elegance (appearance and absence of physical deterioration or flaws), packaging, and labeling.

Distribution Policies

1. Whenever possible, delivery of a drug product should be confined to a single lot number.
2. Unless otherwise specified or required by stability considerations, not less than a 12-month interval between a product's time of delivery and its expiration date should be present.
3. The supplier should accept for full credit (based on purchase price), without prior authorization, any unopened packages of goods returned within 12 months of the expiration date. Credits should be in cash or applied to the institution's account.
4. The supplier should ship all goods in a timely manner, freight prepaid, and enclose a packing list with each shipment. All items "out of stock" should be noted, and the anticipated availability of the item should be clearly indicated. There should be no extensive recurrence of back orders.
5. The supplier should warrant title to commodities supplied, warrant them to be free from defects and imperfections and fit for any rational use of the product, and indemnify and hold the purchaser harmless against any and all suits, claims, and expenses, includ-ing attorneys' fees, damages, and injuries or any claims by third parties relating to the products.

Marketing and Sales Policies

1. The supplier should not, without written consent, use the pharmacist's or his or her organization's name in any advertising or other promotional materials or activities.
2. The supplier should honor formulary decisions made by the organization's pharmacy and therapeutics committee, and the supplier's sales representatives should comply with the organization's regulations governing their activities.
3. The supplier should not offer cash, equipment, or merchandise to the organization or its staff as an inducement to purchase its products.
4. Discounts should be in cash or cash credit, not merchandise, and should be clearly indicated on invoices and bills rather than consisting of end-of-year rebates or similar discount practices.

DOI 10.37573/9781585287048.018

5. In entering into a contract to supply goods, the supplier should guarantee to furnish, at the price specified, any minimum amount of products so stated. If the supplier is unable to meet the supply commitment, the supplier should reimburse the organization for any excess costs incurred in obtaining the product from other sources. If, during the life of the contract, a price reduction occurs, the lower price should prevail.
6. All parties to the bidding process should respect the integrity of the process and the contracts awarded thereby.

Responsibilities of the Purchaser

It may be desirable to purchase drugs or other commodities on a competitive bid basis. The pharmacist should ensure that competitive bidding procedures conform to the guidelines below:

1. Invitations to bid should be mailed to the suppliers' home offices with copies to their local representatives (if any), unless suppliers specify otherwise.
2. Potential bidders should be given no less than 3 weeks to submit a bid.
3. The opening date for bids should be specified and honored by the purchaser.
4. The language of the invitation to bid should be clear and should indicate the person (and organization address and telephone number) the bidder should contact in the event of questions or problems. Specifications should be complete with respect to products, packagings, and quantities desired.
5. If bidding forms are used, they should contain adequate space for the bidder to enter the information requested.
6. The winning bidder should be notified in writing. Unsuccessful bidders may be informed of who won the award at what price, if they so request.
7. The quantities specified in the invitation to bid should be a reasonable estimate of requirements.
8. If the invitation to bid is offered on behalf of a group of purchasers, the individual members of the group should not engage in bidding procedures of their own and should purchase the goods in question from the winning bidder.

Reference

1. American Society of Hospital Pharmacists. ASHP technical assistance bulletin on single unit and unit dose packages of drugs. *Am J Hosp Pharm.* 1985; 42:378–9.

Approved by the ASHP Board of Directors, November 14, 1990. Revised by the ASHP Council on Professional Affairs. Supersedes previous versions approved November 17–18, 1983, and September 22, 1989.

Copyright © 1991, American Society of Hospital Pharmacists, Inc. All rights reserved. Contact ASHP for reprint and permissions requests. This content may not be used for commercial purposes without the express written consent of ASHP.

The bibliographic citation for this document is as follows: American Society of Hospital Pharmacists. ASHP guidelines for selecting pharmaceutical manufacturers and suppliers. *Am J Hosp Pharm.* 1991; 48:523–4.

Preparation and Handling

2139

SAFE AND EFFECTIVE EXTEMPORANEOUS COMPOUNDING

Source: Council on Pharmacy Practice

To affirm that extemporaneous compounding of medications, when done to meet immediate or anticipatory patient needs, is part of the practice of pharmacy and is not manufacturing; further,

To support the principle that medications should not be extemporaneously compounded when drug products are commercially and readily available in the form necessary to meet patient needs; further,

To encourage the pharmacy workforce members who compound medications to use only drug substances that have been manufactured in Food and Drug Administration-registered facilities and that meet official United States Pharmacopeia (USP) compendial requirements, where those exist; further,

To advocate that all compounding activities meet applicable USP standards and federal and state regulations; further,

To support the principle that the pharmacy workforce be adequately trained and have sufficient facilities and equipment that meet technical and professional standards to ensure the quality of compounded medications; further,

To encourage USP to develop drug monographs for commonly compounded preparations; further,

To educate prescribers and other healthcare professionals about the potential risks associated with the use of extemporaneously compounded preparations.

This policy supersedes ASHP policy 0616.

Rationale

The practice of compounding has evolved along with the profession of pharmacy and it remains an essential component of patient care and pharmacy practice. With advances in pharmaceutical manufacturing, the need for preparation of individualized medications based on a prescription or medication order has decreased but not disappeared. Extemporaneous compounding of medications, when done to meet immediate or anticipatory patient needs, will likely always be an essential part of the practice of pharmacy, and cannot be replaced by any manufacturing model currently envisioned. Commercially and readily available drug products in the form necessary to meet patient needs should always be preferred to extemporaneously compounded alternatives. When extemporaneous compounding is required, it should meet strict requirements to protect patients from receiving substandard or poor-quality medications that pose a safety risk to their health and well-being. In particular, extemporaneously compounded sterile preparations must ensure highest quality. Extemporaneous compounding should be performed only using drug substances that have been manufactured in Food and Drug Administration-registered facilities and that meet official United States Pharmacopeia (USP) compendial requirements. Such compounding should only be performed by adequately trained pharmacists and pharmacy technicians, in facilities and with equipment that meet technical and professional standards to ensure the quality and integrity of the compounded medication, and in accordance with USP standards and other applicable federal and state regulations. To facilitate such a high level of compounding, USP should develop drug monographs for commonly compounded preparations. ASHP and its members have always devoted a great deal of effort to promoting safe extemporaneous compounding, through education of pharmacists and pharmacy technicians, publication of best practices, and advocacy, recognizing the inherent risks of any such endeavor. Pharmacists and pharmacy technicians have a responsibility to safely prepare and distribute compounded medications to meet the unique and customized therapeutic needs of their patients, and ASHP and pharmacists therefore have a responsibility to educate prescribers and other healthcare professionals about the potential risks associated with the use of extemporaneously compounded preparations.

2024

SAFETY AND EFFICACY OF COMPOUNDED TOPICAL FORMULATIONS

Source: Council on Therapeutics

To encourage pharmacists to take a leadership role in developing processes that would ensure quality, safety, and effectiveness of compounded topical formulations; further,

To advocate that ASHP expand its repository of evidence-based formulations that could serve as a resource for compounding topical formulations; further,

To advocate that public and private payers and healthcare providers collaborate to create standardized and efficient methods for authorizing payment for medically necessary compounded topical formulations; further,

To encourage hospitals and health systems to develop policies and procedures to guide clinicians in making informed decisions regarding the prescribing and use of compounded topical formulations; further,

To encourage pharmacists to take a leadership role in developing and providing education on the safety and efficacy of compounded topical formulations to providers and consumers.

Rationale

Compounded topical formulations are meant to be customized for individuals whose needs cannot be met by commercially available drugs. Unlike the drugs made by conventional manufacturers that require Food and Drug Administration (FDA) approval, compounded drugs such as various topical formulations are not evaluated by the FDA for safety, effectiveness, or quality, and many are exempt from the new-drug approval process, current good manufacturing practice, and other FDA requirements. In addition, quality standards for compounded drugs are generally lower than those for FDA-approved drugs; therefore, compounded drugs can pose increased safety risks (e.g., being contaminated or having the wrong potency) or lack efficacy.

Because some drugs do have FDA approval for topical application, clinicians and patients may not be aware of potential safety risks or potential lack of effectiveness associated with certain ingredients and combinations of ingredients in compounded topical pain creams. When these

DOI 10.37573/9781585287048.019

agents are compounded, at least one of the ingredients is an active ingredient in an FDA-approved topical pain cream (e.g., lidocaine), while the remaining ingredients may be active ingredients in drugs approved by the FDA for non-topical administration to treat non-pain-related indications (e.g., antidepressants, anticonvulsants, antivirals, narcotics). In addition, the literature supporting the use of the additional agents outside their normal vehicle of administration is often not well designed or sufficiently powered to demonstrate efficacy. A study published by the U.S. Department of Defense found that these combination-compounded pain creams were no better than placebo creams and, given their higher costs, which had escalated to a cost of $6 million per day, should no longer be used.

Issues of fraud are also well known with compounded topical formulations. In August 2018, the Department of Health and Human Services Office of Inspector General (OIG) found that from 2006 to 2015, spending for these drugs increased 625%, and spending for compounded topical drugs—such as creams, gels, and ointments—grew at an even faster pace. Medicare Part D sponsors cover these drugs under certain circumstances. The OIG also found that Part D spending for compounded topical drugs increased 2353% from 2010 to 2016, rising from $13.2 million to $323.5 million. Much of this growth occurred from 2014 to 2016, when spending increased by more than $200 million and raised concerns that the drugs that were billed to Part D were not always dispensed or medically necessary. Upon investigation, the OIG found that many of the parties charging Part D were located in a handful of cities, with thousands of prescriptions written by a single provider and filled by a limited number of pharmacies. This led HHS to conclude that the prescribers may not have had legitimate doctor-patient relationships with the beneficiaries.

Given these challenges, pharmacists will need to assume a leadership role in developing processes to ensure the quality, safety, and effectiveness of compounded topical formulations, including developing and providing education on compounded topical formulations for providers and consumers, and expanding the ASHP repository of evidence-based formulations. Public and private payers and healthcare providers will need to collaborate to create standardized and efficient methods for authorizing payment for medically necessary compounded topical formulations, and hospitals and health systems will need to develop policies and procedures to guide clinicians in making informed decisions regarding prescribing and use of compounded topical formulations.

1903

COMPOUNDED STERILE PREPARATION VERIFICATION

Source: Council on Pharmacy Practice

To advocate that health systems adopt automation and information technology to facilitate in-process and final verification of compounded sterile preparations (CSPs) to ensure CSP quality; further,

To advocate that, until such time as automation or technology can be implemented, independent in-process and final verification of CSPs be performed; further,

To oppose the use of the syringe pull-back method or other proxy methods of CSP verification.

This policy supersedes ASHP policy 1617.

Rationale

Adoption of automation and information technology for preparing and dispensing compounded sterile preparations (CSPs) is increasing but not evenly distributed among healthcare organizations. A 2017 ASHP survey showed that 64% of hospitals did not use any technology for sterile product preparation activities. Only 26.9% of health systems surveyed employed barcode verification in their IV medication preparation and verification process. The survey found that 12.8% of all health systems surveyed used drug workflow software to manage IV drug preparation, verification, and dispensing. There are many reasons for these disparate rates of adoption. Each institution has a different break-even point of investment versus return, and challenges of implementation can be daunting. Some organizations have implemented automated compounding technology only to withdraw it later. These technologies may slow the preparation and verification process; however, the enhanced safety outweighs losses in operational efficiency.

Information technology and automation, including robotics, can be used to improve the safety of CSP compounding. Although IV workflow technologies continue to be developed and improved, the majority of pharmacy departments continue to compound manually without the assistance of barcode or other technologies. Health systems have been slow to adopt IV workflow technology, with only 27% of respondents to the 2017 survey indicating their departments use barcode scanning to verify the ingredients in CSPs. If automated procedures are not employed, there are only two methods of in-process or final verification: real-time, direct, and independent visualization, or retroactive, proxy verification (e.g., the syringe pull-back method). The dangers of the syringe pull-back method have been well demonstrated, and the 2016 Institute for Safe Medication Practices (ISMP) Guidelines for Safe Preparation of Compounded Sterile Preparations discourage its use.

1813

USE OF CLOSED-SYSTEM TRANSFER DEVICES TO REDUCE DRUG WASTE

Source: Council on Pharmacy Practice

To recognize that a growing body of evidence supports the ability of specific closed-system transfer devices (CSTDs) to maintain sterility beyond the in-use time currently recommended by United States Pharmacopeia Chapter 797, when those CSTDs are used with aseptic technique and following current sterile compounding standards; further,

To foster additional research on and develop standards and best practices for use of CSTDs for drug vial optimization; further,

To educate healthcare professionals, especially pharmacists and pharmacy technicians, about standards and best practices for use of CSTDs in drug vial optimization.

This policy was reviewed in 2023 by the Council on Pharmacy Practice and by the Board of Directors and was found to still be appropriate.

Rationale

A 2016 study estimated that the U.S. may spend close to $2 billion on oncology drug products that are discarded because they come in vials in which the volume of drug product exceeds what is needed for most doses. Considerable savings are gained when the leftover contents of those vials are used. One practice that has shown promise in optimizing use of leftover drug product is the use of closed-system transfer devices (CSTDs) to facilitate the transfer of drug product from one reservoir to another. CSTDs prevent the release of hazardous drugs during compounding and administration and have primarily been used throughout the medication-use process to minimize healthcare workers' exposure to hazardous drugs. Some CSTDs use a mechanical barrier that can also prevent the ingress of environmental contaminants, which has prompted study of their ability to safely prolong the sterility of drug product in vials. A growing number of studies have been generating data that indicate specific CSTDs have the possibility of maintaining sterility and extending in-use time when used under sterile conditions defined by United States Pharmacopeia Chapter 797. Although some CSTDs have an FDA-approved indication for use to prevent microbial ingress with studied dwell times of up to 168 hours when maintained in an ISO Class 5 environment using proper aseptic technique, they do not have an explicit indication for extending the in-use time of drug products. Until the data from the studies can be validated and applied, standard-setting entities and regulators will not permit this practice. ASHP therefore advocates that the existing evidence that supports the ability of properly used CSTDs to maintain sterility and extend in-use times be recognized, and encourages research and development of guidance by standard-setting entities and regulators regarding safe use of CSTDs for drug vial optimization.

0903

PHARMACEUTICAL WASTE

Source: Council on Pharmacy Practice

To collaborate with regulatory bodies and appropriate organizations to develop standards for the disposal of pharmaceutical hazardous waste as defined in the Resource Conservation and Recovery Act (RCRA), for the purpose of simplifying the disposal of these substances by health systems; further,

To encourage pharmaceutical manufacturers and the Environmental Protection Agency (EPA) to provide guidance and assistance to hospitals and health systems in proper pharmaceutical waste disposal and destruction efforts; further,

To advocate that EPA update the list of hazardous substances under RCRA and establish a process for maintaining a current list; further,

To urge federal, state, and local governments to harmonize regulations regarding disposal of hazardous pharmaceutical waste; further,

To advocate that the Food and Drug Administration standardize labeling of drug products with information relating to appropriate disposal; further,

To promote awareness within hospitals and health systems of pharmaceutical waste regulations; further,

To encourage research on the environmental and public health impacts of drug products and metabolites excreted in human waste; further,

To encourage pharmaceutical manufacturers to streamline packaging of drug products to reduce waste materials.

This policy was reviewed in 2019 by the Council on Pharmacy Practice and by the Board of Directors and was found to still be appropriate.

0614

SAFE DISPOSAL OF PATIENTS' HOME MEDICATIONS

Source: Council on Professional Affairs

To minimize the patient safety consequences and public health impact of inappropriate disposal of patients' home medications by working collaboratively with other interested organizations to (1) develop models for patient-oriented medication disposal programs that will minimize accidental poisoning, drug diversion, and potential environmental impact, (2) advocate that the pharmaceutical industry and regulatory bodies support the development and implementation of such models, and (3) educate health professionals, regulatory bodies, and the public regarding safe disposal of unused home medications.

This policy was reviewed in 2021 by the Council on Pharmacy Practice and by the Board of Directors and was found to still be appropriate.

ASHP Guidelines on Compounding Sterile Preparations

Purpose

The compounding of medications is a fundamental part of pharmacy practice. All compounding personnel, mainly pharmacists and pharmacy technicians, are responsible for compounding and dispensing sterile products and preparations of correct ingredient identity, purity (freedom from physical contaminants, such as precipitates,[1] and chemical contaminants), strength (including stability[2] and compatibility), and sterility and for dispensing them in appropriate containers that are labeled accurately and appropriately for the end user. In contemporary health care organizations, patients receive compounded sterile preparations (CSPs) that are stored for extended periods before use. It has long been recognized that extended storage of CSPs may allow for the growth of a pathological bioburden of microorganisms[3] and that patient morbidity and mortality can result from contaminated or incorrectly compounded sterile preparations.[4–9] When quality monitoring is inadequate, personnel responsible for sterile compounding may not know that inaccurate or contaminated products are dispensed.[10–13]

These guidelines are intended to help compounding personnel prepare CSPs of high quality and reduce the potential for harm to patients and consequences for compounding personnel. The recommendations in these guidelines are based on published data, when available; on expert opinion and procedures used in similar industries; and on applicable regulations and standards. These guidelines are a revision of the 2000 *ASHP Guidelines on Quality Assurance of Pharmacy-Prepared Sterile Products*,[14] with the goals of providing more current recommendations and harmonizing the ASHP guidelines with *United States Pharmacopeia* (*USP*) chapter 797, Pharmaceutical Compounding—Sterile Preparations.[15] To help achieve that harmonization, these guidelines employ the definitions and terminology of *USP* chapter 797 rather than those of the previous guidelines.

Many health care settings also use CSPs prepared by compounding pharmacies. Although these guidelines may be useful in assessing the quality of CSPs prepared by compounding pharmacies, more information on the topic of outsourcing sterile compounding services is available in the *ASHP Guidelines on Outsourcing Sterile Compounding Services*.[16]

Finally, while these guidelines are generally applicable to all personnel who prepare CSPs and all facilities in which CSPs are prepared, pharmacists and other health care professionals responsible for the preparation, selection, and use of CSPs are urged to use professional judgment in interpreting and applying these guidelines to their specific circumstances. Users of these guidelines are cautioned that the information provided is current as of publication and are urged to consult current editions of original sources (e.g., laws, regulations, and applicable standards, including USP compendial standards) to ensure patient safety as well as legal and regulatory compliance.

Legal and Regulatory Considerations

Significant legal and regulatory changes have taken place since publication of the previous ASHP guidelines (**Figure 1**).

At the time of its publication, section 503A of the U.S. Food and Drug Administration Modernization Act (FDAMA) served to define the limits of legitimate compounding.[18] When section 503A of FDAMA was ruled unconstitutional in 2001, the delineation between compounding and manufacturing reverted to earlier regulations based on the Federal Food, Drug, and Cosmetics Act.[19] Under those regulations, compounding is considered part of the practice of pharmacy and in most states, is governed by state law and regulation. Manufacturing is regulated by the federal government through the auspices of the Food and Drug Administration (FDA). In most cases, extemporaneously compounded preparations must be prepared pursuant to a prescriber's prescription for a specific patient. Some states have specific regulations dealing with CSPs for office use. Some pharmacies whose primary purpose is preparing CSPs for hospitals and other facilities may be registered with the FDA as manufacturers and must adhere to federal good manufacturing practices. Some state boards of pharmacy permit one pharmacy to compound for another pharmacy under central fill regulations. Most pharmacies compound only pursuant to a prescriber's prescription and follow state regulations regarding compounding.

On January 1, 2004, *USP* chapter 797, Pharmaceutical Compounding—Sterile Preparations,[15] became official, replacing *USP* chapter 1206, Sterile Drug Products for Home Use.[20] The change from a chapter numbered above 1000 to a chapter below 1000 marked a change from an advisory standard to an enforceable one. *USP* chapter 797 has since been revised.[15] Some state regulations require full compliance with *USP* chapter 797, some have indirect references to the chapter, some do not mention the chapter, and some have additional regulations.[21] The National Association of Boards of Pharmacy supports the incorporation of compounding regulations into state pharmacy practice legislation by including such wording in the association's Model Rules and Model State Pharmacy Act.[22] State boards of pharmacy should be consulted to determine the current status of sterile compounding regulations, as there are significant differences in regulation among states.

Accreditation Considerations

The Centers for Medicare and Medicaid Services (CMS) Hospital Conditions of Participation and Interpretive Guidelines, the Joint Commission, the American Osteopathic Association's Healthcare Facilities Accreditation Program, and DNV Healthcare's National Integrated Accreditation for Healthcare Organizations all include statements concerning safe practices for storage and preparation of sterile compounds.[23–26] Clinics, long-term care facilities, home care organizations, rehabilitation facilities, and physician offices (all of which come under the purview of *USP* chapter 797[15])

DOI 10.37573/9781585287048.020

FIGURE 1. Evolution of Sterile Compounding Standards, 1970—2010. Adapted from *The ASHP Discussion Guide on USP Chapter <797> for Compounding Sterile Preparations.*[17] NCCLVP, National Coordinating Committee on Large Volume Parenterals; CSPs, compounded sterile preparations; USP, United State Pharmacopeia; TAB, technical assistance bulleting; FDAMA, Food and Drug Administration Modernization Act; PCAB, Pharmacy Compounding Accreditation Board.

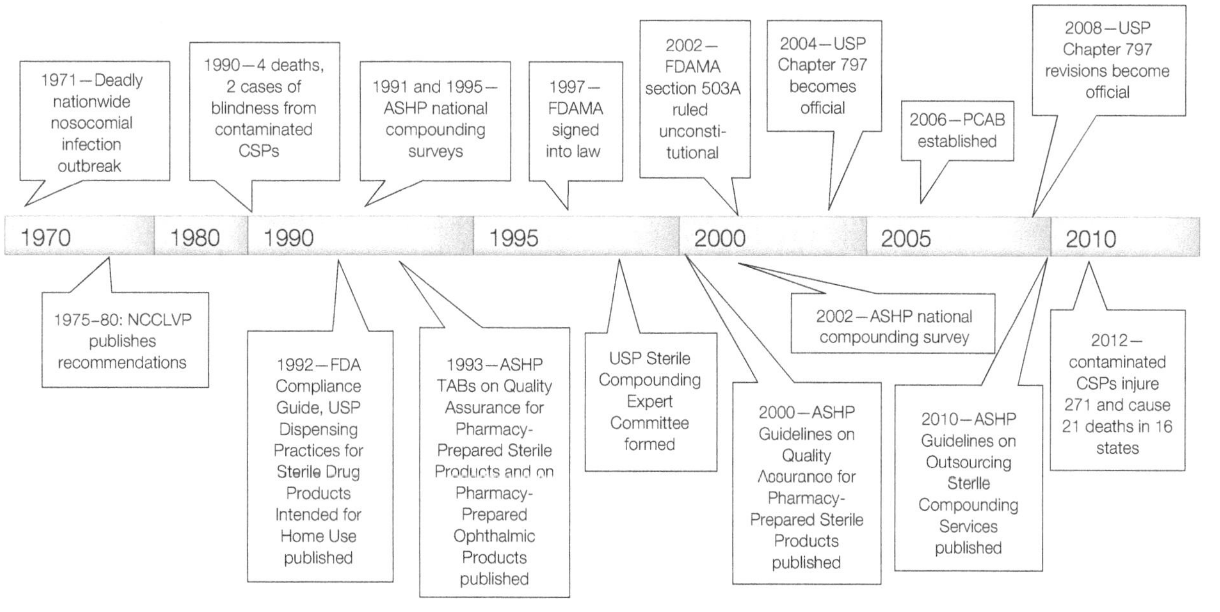

may all be subject to specific additional governance of sterile compounding practices, depending on the agencies regulating or accrediting the facility. In addition, organizations preparing hazardous drugs[27,28] should comply with National Institute for Occupational Safety and Health (NIOSH) recommendations to ensure that compounding personnel are operating in a safe environment.[29,30]

Other Compounding-Related Guidelines

ASHP provides several guidelines for safe compounding practices[28,31,32] and a discussion guide on *USP* chapter 797[17] and has recognized *USP* chapter 797 as a relevant practice standard in the *ASHP Guidelines: Minimum Standard for Pharmacies in Hospitals.*[33] Other professional organizations also provide guidance on specific aspects of compounding. Standards for prescribing, preparation, administration, and monitoring of parenteral nutrition are available through the American Society for Parenteral and Enteral Nutrition.[34,35] The Institute for Safe Medication Practices provides recommendations for preventing medication errors, including those involving CSPs.[36,37] The Infusion Nurses Society offers standards, professional development, and resources for all aspects of infusion care.[38] The Controlled Environment Testing Association (CETA) provides numerous CETA Application Guides (CAGs) for the proper use, cleaning, and certification of primary engineering controls (PECs) and buffer areas (generally referred to as "cleanrooms").[39-45] *Guidelines for Hand Hygiene in Healthcare Settings,*[46] *Guidelines for Prevention of Intravascular Catheter-Related Infections,*[47] *Guidelines for Environmental Infection Control in Healthcare Facilities,*[48] and *Protect Patients Against Preventable Harm from Improper Use of Single-dose/Single-use Vials,*[49] all from the Centers for Disease Control and Prevention (CDC), serve as the backbone for most infection prevention practices in the United States. Safe infusion, injection, and medication vial practices have been addressed by CMS[50] and the Association for Professionals in Infection Control and Epidemiology,[51] and the Association of peri-Operative Registered Nurses has recommended practices for medication safety in perioperative settings.[52]

Physical Facilities and Equipment

Design and Functionality Requirements

Facility requirements are intended to establish a safe environment for compounding CSPs. The International Organization for Standardization (ISO) air cleanliness classification of the compounding environment is a critical measure that is affected by facility design.

Primary Engineering Controls (PECs). A PEC is a device or room that provides an ISO Class 5 environment for compounding CSPs. PECs all rely on a special type of high-efficiency particle air (HEPA) filter that is ≥99.99% efficient in removing particles as small as 0.3 microns in size (the most penetrating particle size [MPPS], which refers to the largest-sized particle that may escape the filter, although particles of all sizes may be captured). The unidirectional (horizontal or vertical) HEPA-filtered air must provide sufficient velocity to sweep particles away from the direct compounding area and maintain unidirectional flow during preparation of CSPs. (More information about HEPA filtration and first-air concepts can be found in the ASHP publications *Compounding Sterile Preparations,*[53] *Basics of Aseptic Compounding Technique,*[54] *Getting Started in Aseptic Compounding,*[55] and *Compounding Sterile Preparations: ASHP Video Guide to USP*.[56])

PEC devices include laminar airflow workbenches (LAFWs), biological safety cabinets (BSCs), compounding aseptic isolators (CAIs), and compounding aseptic containment isolators (CACIs) (**Table 1**). Properly designed,

TABLE 1.
Primary Engineering Controls (PECs)

PEC Device	Used to Prepare Non-Hazardous CSPs	Used to Prepare Hazardous CSPs
Conventional	Laminar airflow workbench (LAFW)	Class II Biological safety cabinet (BSC)
Isolators	Compounding aseptic isolator (CAI)	Compounding aseptic containment isolator (CACI)

unidirectional airflow CAIs function in a similar manner as LAFWs, but the direct compounding area does not interact with room air because it is within a closed system, with the air sweeping particles away from the compounding site. Smoke tests of PECs assist a facility in verifying unidirectional airflow and lack of turbulence and reverse flows.

CAIs or CACIs located outside of an ISO Class 7 environment must be coupled with documentation from the manufacturer that the device will meet or exceed *USP* chapter 797 standards under these conditions and be dynamically tested on site to USP 797 and CETA requirements. If the CACI used for hazardous drug preparation is located outside the buffer area (see **Architecture**, below), it must be located in a segregated and dedicated area that maintains at least 0.01-inch water column negative pressure and maintains, at a minimum, 12 air changes per hour (ACPH).

Architecture. The sterile compounding area includes a well-lit buffer area and ante area (both are secondary engineering controls) and an area for storage of sterile products and supplies. A buffer area (or "cleanroom") is defined as an area where a PEC is located and where activities such as preparation, compounding, and staging of CSPs occur. This area should provide adequate space for the PEC and may include a limited amount of shelving and/or carts for staging of compounding (not for storing stock). An ante area provides space for hand washing, garbing, and product decontamination; it also serves as a way to further segregate the buffer area from other, less-clean areas of the facility. Water sources, such as sinks or floor drains, are not permitted in the buffer area and should not be immediately adjacent to segregated compounding areas outside of a buffer area. A storage area outside the buffer and ante areas should provide adequate space for placement of sterile products and supplies.

The sterile compounding area (ante and buffer areas) may be constructed of either hard- or soft-walled enclosures, with the zones being delineated by open or closed architecture. Closed architecture is formed by walls and doors between the buffer and ante areas and is required for high-risk compounding (**Table 2**).

Open architecture has openings between the buffer and ante areas and relies on a defined airflow velocity to divide the two areas, which are marked by a line of demarcation; this type of facility may only be utilized for low- and medium-risk compounding. Demarcation lines should be indicated by colored tiles or other elements integrated into the flooring pattern but may be as simple as marking on the floor.

Facilities for preparation of radiopharmaceuticals have some different requirements. Refer to *USP* chapter 797[15] and other relevant standards for specifics.

TABLE 2.
Facilities Features Required for Specific Types of Compounding (Data from *USP* Chapter 797[15] Except as Noted)

	Low-Risk with ≤12-hour BUD (Non-Hazardous)	Low-Risk (Non-Hazardous)	Medium-Risk (Non-Hazardous)	High-Risk (Non-Hazardous)	Hazardous Drugs
Architectural Style[a]	Segregated	Open or closed	Open or closed	Closed	Closed
Buffer zone ISO classification	N/A	ISO Class 7 or better	ISO Class 7 or better	ISO Class 7 or better	ISO Class 7 or better
Ante area ISO classification	N/A	ISO Class 8 (ISO Class 7 if opens into negative pressure area) or better	ISO Class 8 (ISO Class 7 if opens into negative pressure area) or better	ISO Class 8 (ISO Class 7 if opens into a negative pressure area) or better	ISO Class 7 or better
Minimum air exchanges for buffer area[b]	N/A	30	30	30	30
Minimum air exchanges for ante area[c]	N/A	20 if ISO 8; 30 if ISO 7	20 if ISO 8; 30 if ISO 7	20 if ISO 8; 30 if ISO 7	30
Pressure	N/A	Positive	Positive	Positive	Negative

[a]Architectural style ("open" and "closed") is not defined in *USP* chapter 797, but the concept of physical separation of ante areas and buffer rooms is described in the chapter. For the purposes of these guidelines, "closed architecture" indicates that the buffer and ante areas are separated by a door (i.e., are physically separate rooms) and maintain a pressure differential of no less than 0.02-inch water column positive pressure. "Open architecture" indicates that the buffer and ante areas are in one room, not separated by a door (i.e., not physically separated). Displacement airflow is used to separate open architecture spaces, with at least 40 feet per minute of airflow across the entire plane of the opening. A segregated compounding area contains a PEC within a restricted space.

[b]If an ISO Class 5 recirculating device is in place, a minimum of 15 air changes per hour (ACPH) is sufficient if the ACPH is 30 between the device and the area supply HEPA filters.

[c]*USP* chapter 797 does not address the air changes in ISO Class 8 ante areas. The FDA Aseptic Processing Guide57 recommends a minimum of 20 ACPH to maintain ISO 8. However, this is a minimum value intended for industry. Since ante areas for CSPs include ungowned personnel and other activities, a minimum of 30 ACPH is best practice for ISO Class 8 ante areas and required for ISO 7 ante areas.

Facilities without *USP* chapter 797-compliant ante areas and buffer areas may prepare low-risk, non-hazardous CSPs in a PEC within a segregated compounding area. A segregated compounding area is an unclassified space (i.e., an area with no specific ISO classification) and does not include ante or buffer areas. It is required to be separated from activities that are not essential to the preparation of CSPs; not be located adjacent to food preparation sites, warehouses, or construction sites; and not have unsealed windows or doors that connect to the outdoors or high-traffic areas.[15] This architecture type is most often seen in satellite pharmacies, small hospitals, procedural areas, or clinics. The beyond-use dating for sterile preparations compounded in a segregated compounding area cannot exceed 12 hours (see **Expiration and Beyond-Use Dating**).

Buffer Areas

Air Supply. A buffer area differs from an ordinary ventilated room by having the following:

- Increased air supply.
- HEPA filtration (the filtered air should be introduced at the ceiling, with returns mounted low on the walls; ceiling-mounted returns should not be used) including a terminal air filter (a filter at the end of the heating, ventilation, and air conditioning [HVAC] ducting).
- Room pressurization.
- A perforated plate or swirl supply air diffuser (if an air diffuser is necessary); high-induction supply air diffusers should not be used in buffer areas.

Structural components must be coupled with HEPA filtration and air exchanges in order to provide a complete buffer area environment and proper ISO classifications. Buffer areas must meet or exceed ISO Class 7 air cleanliness standards. Ante areas must at least meet ISO Class 8 standards; ante areas opening into a negative pressure preparation area must meet ISO Class 7 standards. The number of ACPH is based upon air/room pressure, velocity or air handler capacity, HEPA flow restriction, duct size, the amount of processing completed on a daily basis, and temperature. ACPH must occur at a minimum of 30 times per hour in buffer and ante areas, but may need to be increased in high-traffic/high-volume areas in order to maintain the room's specified ISO classification (Table 2) under dynamic conditions. Facilities may incorporate the contribution of up to 15 air changes per hour from a LAFW in the total air changes per hours in a nonhazardous buffer area. By design, these devices filter room air as it passes through the HEPA filter.

Airflow within the room should be as steady as possible, having as few interruptions as possible. Within the PEC, it must be unidirectional,[39] with as few interruptions in steady airflow as possible. PEC placement within the room should be well designed, with PECs placed where they are least affected by opened doors, HVAC systems, or personnel traffic. For non-hazardous preparations, positive pressure is required between rooms physically divided by walls or doors (closed architecture style) and should be maintained at a minimum of positive 0.02 inch water column. If a room does not have physical barriers (i.e., has an open architecture style) and relies on a line of demarcation, the displacement airflow concept requiring air velocity of 40 feet per minute (0.2 meter per second) from the buffer area across the entire plane of line of demarcation into the ante area is required. Open architecture is not permitted in areas used for high-risk preparations.

When designing buffer areas, facilities must consider workflow patterns, such as how personnel performing double-checks will affect air quality. If supervisory personnel are not located in the buffer area, movement in and out of the buffer area is likely to increase airflow interruption. Communication devices should be used to minimize traffic between areas, and cameras may be installed to supplement supervision of staff or check compounding accuracy, if permitted by state regulations.

Surfaces. Surfaces of any kind in the buffer area and ante area must be smooth, impervious, and easy to clean, with no cracks or crevices that could trap dust or contaminants. All materials used in the facilities must be non-shedding. Walls and ceilings must be made of either hard plastic or epoxy-painted gypsum board. If ceiling tiles are used, they must be coated with hard polymer and caulked both around the perimeter and around each tile. Ceiling lights must be smooth, mounted flush, and sealed. Floors should be made of wide, heavy-duty sheet vinyl, rubber, or epoxy that is coved around the corners and rolled up onto the walls. Paint must be an epoxy, acrylic, or other non-porous sealant type.

Work surfaces should preferably be stainless steel, but at a minimum are required to be non-porous and easily sanitized. Carts and shelves, ideally made of stainless steel wire, nonporous plastic, or rustproof metal, should be easy to move and clean, if necessary. Office equipment (e.g., computers and components [including washable keyboard and mouse], telephones, printers) placed in the buffer area must be easily cleanable and placed in such a manner that they have no material impact on the ISO air cleanliness classification of the area.

Renovations

To meet requirements for sterile compounding, many facilities choose to renovate existing space rather than construct new facilities. Whether designing a new area or retrofitting one, the specific types (e.g., hazardous or nonhazardous) and risk levels of CSPs that will be prepared in the area should guide the facility design and construction. A plan for how operations will continue without interruption should be devised prior to construction.

Power and Other Utility Interruptions

The facility's emergency management plan should include steps to meet patient-care needs during time of utility interruptions, including the need for CSPs. In some cases, immediate-use procedures may be safely implemented to meet some needs. Methods to identify and safely meet interim compounding needs or address patient-care needs with noncompounded alternatives should be developed, put into standard operating procedures (SOPs), inserviced to staff, and tested as part of the organization's emergency planning process.

Pharmacy Compounding Devices

Pharmacy compounding devices are utilized to increase efficiency while decreasing the potential for human error. Devices that do not create their own ISO Class 5 environment must be located within an ISO Class 5 PEC and adhere to applicable standards for accuracy and precision. All compounding devices must be monitored and validated for accuracy consistent with device manufacturer specifications.

Automated Compounding Devices (ACDs) are utilized to accurately combine multiple drugs and solutions into a single delivery container. These devices are most commonly used for parenteral nutrition preparation, but may be used for cardioplegia solutions, continuous renal replacement therapy, or other complex processes. *ASHP Guidelines on the Safe Use of Automated Compounding Devices for the Preparation of Parenteral Nutrition Admixtures*[32] should be consulted for further details on utilizing ACDs. Accuracy and precision testing for ACDs is required by *USP* chapter 797[15] and incorporate gravimetric, volumetric, and chemical analyses. These analyses, as determined by facility protocol, must be monitored and recorded on a daily basis, with evaluation for outliers occurring at least weekly.

Repeater pumps are devices used to pump a preset volume of fluid in a consistent and reproducible manner. They must be calibrated according to manufacturer specifications, which may depend on the volume and frequency of use.

Robotic systems automate the compounding and labeling of parenteral doses in syringes and bags using an enclosed chamber that must create an ISO Class 5 air cleanliness environment or better.

The proper use of ACDs, repeater pumps, robotic systems, and other compounding equipment used in the preparation of CSPs remains the responsibility of the pharmacist.

Cleaning and Disinfecting

Cleaning with a germicidal detergent and water will remove visible solids or soiling before disinfecting. Disinfecting removes microbial contamination. It is critical that an appropriate germicidal detergent and water be used to clean all surfaces of the buffer and ante areas in addition to all of the PECs. Great care must be exercised to avoid getting the HEPA filters wet during cleaning. Cleaning with a germicidal detergent will leave a residue that needs to be removed from work surfaces (e.g., counter and PEC surfaces). This residue is best removed by using sterile 70% isopropyl alcohol (IPA).

Appendix II of *USP* chapter 797[15] provides information on types of products that can be used for cleaning and disinfecting the ante and buffer areas, including floors, walls, and ceilings. Choice of cleaning and disinfection products should be approved by the organization's appropriate authority (e.g., the Infection Control Committee).

Policies and procedures must be developed to ensure consistent practices, including dilution of cleaning products. **Table 3** describes the minimum frequency for cleaning surfaces used to compound low- and medium-risk CSPs in the sterile compounding area.

TABLE 3.
Minimum Frequency for Cleaning of Specific Sites (Reprinted with Permission from *USP* Chapter 797[15])

Site	Minimum Frequency
ISO Class 5 PEC	Beginning of each shift Before each batch Every 30 minutes when compounding After spills When surface contamination is known or suspected
Counters and easily cleanable work surfaces	Daily
Floors	Daily
Walls	Monthly
Ceilings	Monthly
Storage shelving	Monthly

Environmental Monitoring

Environmental monitoring and related documentation must be completed on a routine basis to ensure adequate environmental and personnel controls are in place to prevent contamination of CSPs. Ensuring a safe compounding environment requires viable and nonviable airborne particle testing, pressure differential or displacement airflow measurement, temperature monitoring, and surface disinfection sampling and assessment. Nonviable particles are particles that do not contain a living organism, such as particles shed from paper or dust. Viable particles are living organisms, such as bacteria or fungal spores, that require nonviable particles to travel. Monitoring of humidity,[39,44] sound,[39] and lighting[39] may also be considered by facilities to enhance the environmental monitoring program.

Each element of the monitoring program must be included in a sampling plan with sample locations, methods of collection, sampling frequency, and other specifics depending on the type of monitoring being performed. The environmental monitoring sampling frequency must occur at a minimum as listed below, with possible additional times based on the type of testing:

- At the commissioning and certification of new facilities and equipment.
- Every six months during routine re-certification of equipment and facilities.
- After any facility or equipment maintenance, including construction or remodeling of adjacent departments or work on shared air handlers.
- At any point when problems are identified with products, preparations, or employee technique or if a CSP is suspected to be the source of a patient infection.

Records of data collected through the monitoring program must be maintained as part of the overall quality assurance program of the facility. The data should be reviewed by management personnel or their designees and by the facility's Infection Control Committee to ensure that the findings of the reports are addressed. **Table 4** provides an overview of environmental monitoring requirements.

Temperature Monitoring. Any controlled temperature area used for compounding sterile preparations or for storage of sterile products or CSPs must be monitored at least once daily and results documented in a log. The facilities should maintain a comfortable room temperature (20 °C [68 °F] or cooler) for properly garbed compounding personnel. If facilities use continuous temperature recording devices, they must be monitored and documented once daily to ensure they are functioning properly. Controlled temperature ranges are listed in **Table 5**.

Pressure Differential or Air Displacement. Since positive- and/or negative-pressure rooms are required for sterile compounding, the appropriate differential pressure or air

TABLE 4.
Environmental Monitoring Requirements (Adapted from *USP* Chapter 797[15])

Parameter	Monitored By	Frequency
Temperature	Compounding personnel or facilities management staff (if electronic monitoring is centralized)	Documented daily (at a minimum)
Pressure differential or velocity across line of demarcation	Compounding personnel	Documented each shift (preferably), daily (at a minimum)
	Qualified certifier	At least every 6 months
Nonviable particles	Qualified certifier	At least every 6 months
Surface sampling	Compounding or laboratory personnel	Periodically, as defined by compounding and infection control personnel, at least every 6 months or after significant changes in procedures or cleaning practices
Electronic device sample of viable particles	Compounding personnel or qualified certifier	At least every 6 months

TABLE 5.
Controlled Temperatures (Data from *USP* General Notices and Requirements[58])

Storage Condition	Centigrade	Fahrenheit
Room temperature	20 to 25 °C	68 to 77 °F
Cold temperature (refrigerated)	2 to 8 °C	36 to 46 °F
Freezer (frozen)	−25 to −10 °C	−13 to 14 °F

displacement velocities must be maintained. If closed architecture is used, a pressure differential between general, ante, and buffer areas must be monitored. A facility with open architecture design must monitor the differential airflow across the opening between ante and buffer areas.

A pressure gauge or velocity meter must be in place to monitor airflow between relevant areas. Pressure between ISO Class 7 positive-pressure areas and the general area must be at least 5 Pa (0.02-inch water column). Negative pressure areas should have no less than 2.5 Pa (0.01-inch water column) negative pressure to adjacent positive pressure. A monitored pressure indicator must be installed to ensure proper pressurization. If differential airflow is used as a measure, the velocity must be at least 0.2 meter per second (40 feet per minute).

Results of pressure differential and/or velocity of air displacement must be reviewed and documented each shift (at least daily) or by a continuous device with alarms.

Nonviable Airborne Particle Testing Program. Determination of the ISO classification of an area or device is dependent on nonviable particle testing ("certification"), which must be completed by qualified personnel complying with the Certification Guide for Sterile Compounding Facilities (CAG-003-2006).[39] PECs such as LAFWs, BSCs, CAIs, and CACIs must be certified every 6 months and whenever the device is relocated or serviced. Both primary (LAFWs, BSCs, CAIs, and CACIs) and secondary engineering controls (buffer areas and ante areas) must be checked for total particle counts every 6 months according to the manufacturer's specifications or CETA recommendation and when a device or room is relocated or altered. Thresholds for each ISO class are presented in **Table 6**.

Viable Airborne Particle Testing Program. Classified space (PECs and buffer and ante areas) must undergo routine viable particle testing. The testing plan should include the required sample locations, method of collection, frequency, the volume of air to be tested, and the time of day testing will occur. Testing must occur every 6 months in all compounding areas (PECs, buffer areas, ante areas, and areas adjacent to segregated compounding areas) as part of the overall compounding recertification process. The method of testing must be impaction via an electronic air sampling device, as settling plates alone are not considered an acceptable method.

Sampling plans should be detailed and include all high-traffic locations within the compounding area and any sites prone to contamination. Turbulence caused by airflow disruption, such as within an ISO Class 5 LAFW or doorways, should be included in the testing plan, along with areas where garbing, cleaning, labeling, and staging occur. In segregated compounding areas, sampling should include locations within the ISO Class 5 PEC and other areas in close proximity to the PEC.

Viable particle testing must be performed using a general microbiological growth medium, such as sterile nutrient agar. In facilities that compound high-risk preparations,

TABLE 6.
Particle Limits for Sterile Compounding Areas (Adapted from *USP* Chapter 797[15])

	Primary Engineering Controls (LAFW, BSC, CAI, CACI)	Buffer Area and Ante-Area Opening into a Negative Pressure Room	Ante-Area Opening Only into a Positive Pressure Room
ISO Class	5	7	8
Limit on number of ≥ 0.5 micron particles/m^3 of air	3,520	352,000	3,520,000

testing must also be done with a medium that supports fungal growth, such as malt extract. The growth medium should be incubated (outside of the sterile preparation area) according to the manufacturer's recommendations.

Sample data must be reviewed as a means of evaluating control of the compounding environment. Results above recommended action levels (see **Table 7**) should prompt reevaluation of work practices, cleaning procedures, and HEPA filtration. Any microbial growth that results from viable environment sampling must be identified to the genus level by microbiology personnel. If any highly pathogenic organisms (e.g., gram-negative rods or yeasts) are identified, infection control specialists should immediately be consulted to assist in formulating a response to the situation.

Surface Disinfection Sampling and Assessment. Touch contamination originating from contaminated work surfaces must be minimized and prevented if possible. Surface sampling provides facilities with a snapshot of the effectiveness of their disinfection procedures (including technique and cleaning products) and must be part of the overall quality assurance plan. Using a sterile nutrient agar contact plate for flat surfaces or swabs for equipment and other non-flat surfaces, sampling must be performed in all ISO classified areas on a periodic basis, at a minimum, every 6 months or when significant procedural or cleaning changes are implemented. A specific plan detailing the location of each sample must be devised so that the same locations are repeated with each testing session. Contact plates require pressing a plate directly to the surface being tested, while swabbing requires swabbing an area, submersing the swab in the correct amount of diluent, and then swabbing onto or into a sterile nutrient agar surface. Agar plates will leave a residue on contact surfaces that must be cleaned with sterile water and disinfected with sterile 70% IPA.

Results must be reported in colony-forming units (CFUs) per plate. Reevaluation of work practices and cleaning procedures should occur if the CFU count exceeds the suggested action levels (**Table 8**). Investigation into the source of contamination should be undertaken, the sources eliminated, and the area cleaned and re-sampled.

Environmental monitoring and quality assurance programs and documentation may be completed by a limited number of personnel in any given facility, but the actions of all compounding personnel may affect these two critical elements of compliance. All compounding personnel should be familiar with all facility policies and procedures specific to CSPs, even if the procedures are not typically their responsibility.

TABLE 7.
Viable Environmental Monitoring Recommended Action Levels for Microbial Contamination (Adapted from *USP* Chapter 797[15])

ISO Classification	Recommended Action Levels for Microbial Contamination (CFUs/m^3)[a]
5	1[b]
7	10
8 or above	100

[a]CFUs/m^3, colony-forming units per cubic meter.

[b]Samples from ISO Class 5 environments should normally yield no microbiological contaminants.

Expiration and Beyond-Use Dating

A manufacturer's expiration date is the date assigned pursuant to manufacturer testing. The drug product is guaranteed by the manufacturer to be safe and effective up to the listed date when products are stored as described in the product labeling.

A beyond-use date (BUD) is the date or time after which administration of a CSP shall not be initiated. As described in previous ASHP guidelines[14] and in *USP* chapter 797,[15] the BUD is determined from the date or time the preparation is compounded, its chemical stability, and the sterility limits described later in these guidelines. Both the stability of the components and the sterility limits described above must be taken into consideration when determining BUDs, and the BUD must be the shorter of the sterility dating or chemical stability dating. Information regarding stability dating procedures and defaults can be found in *USP* chapter 795, Pharmaceutical Compounding—Non-Sterile Preparations,[59] and other published literature sources.[60,61]

Processes such as thin-layer chromatography (TLC) and high-performance liquid chromatographic (HPLC) assays are the most reliable means of determining the stability of a product and should be used in place of theoretical predictions of stability when published literature is not available. The use of commercial reference laboratories that offer qualitative and quantitative testing may serve as a key resource for end-product testing.

Risk Level Classification

In these guidelines, as in previous ASHP guidelines[14] and *USP* chapter 797,[15] CSPs are stratified by potential risk of microbial contamination into three primary categories: low-,

TABLE 8.
Recommended Action Levels for Personnel Testing (Adapted from *USP* Chapter 797[15])

	PEC	Buffer Area	Ante Area
Viable airborne particle testing action levels for contamination (CFUs per cubic meter [1000 L] of air per plate)	>1	>10	>100
Surface sample contamination (CFUs per plate)	>3	>5	>100
Glove fingertip sampling	>3	N/A	N/A

[a]CFUs = colony-forming units.

medium-, and high-risk CSPs, with an additional category for CSPs intended for immediate use[15] and a sub-category for low-risk CSPs intended for use within 12 hours.[15] The potential risk is based on the danger of exposing multiple patients to microbial bioburden and based on microbial growth factors influenced by product storage time, temperature and product ability to support microbial growth, surface and time exposure of critical sites, and microbial bioburden in the environment. Compounding personnel must determine the appropriate risk level and the appropriate BUD for use based upon chemical stability and the potential for microbial, physical, or chemical contamination during compounding. In making a risk-level determination, compounding personnel must evaluate where the preparation is being made, the number of components or the number of aseptic breaches needed to compound the preparation, and the complexity of the compounding process. When circumstances make risk-level assignment unclear, guidelines for the more stringent risk level should prevail. For examples and a comparison of the risk levels, requirements, and BUDs to be used in risk-level determination, see **Table 9**.

TABLE 9.
CSP Risk Levels and Beyond-Use Dates (BUDs) (Adapted from *USP* Chapter 797[15])[a]

Risk Category	Compounding Location	Garbing Required	Aseptic Technique Required	Examples	BUDs of CSP Stored at Room Temperature	Refrigerated	Frozen (≤ 10 °C)
Low-risk	ISO Class 5 PEC, ISO Class 7 buffer area, ISO Class 8[b] ante area	Yes	Yes	Reconstitution of a single-dose vial, single preparation of a small volume parenteral, single large volume IV replacement fluids with no more than 3 components	48 hours	14 days	45 days
Low-risk with < 12-hour BUD	ISO Class 5 PEC segregated from other operations	Yes	Yes	Same as low-risk examples, non-hazardous preparations only	12 hours	12 hours	N/A
Medium-risk	ISO Class 5 PEC, ISO Class 7 buffer area, ISO Class 8[b] ante area	Yes	Yes	Batched syringes, total parenteral nutrition, ophthalmic preparations made from sterile products, pooled admixtures, batch-compounded preparations without bateriostatic additives, preparations made using automated compounders or other automated devices, elastomeric pumps	30 hours	9 days	45 days
High-risk	ISO Class 5 PEC, ISO Class 7 buffer area, ISO Class 7 ante area	Yes	Yes	CSPs prepared from bulk, nonsterile components or in final containers which are not sterile; preparations that must be terminally sterilized before administration	24 hours	3 days	45 days
Immediate-use	Medication preparation areas should be clean, uncluttered, and functionally separate[c]	No	Yes	Emergent use preparations such as epidurals prepared by anesthesia for immediate injection or infusion, diagnostics, any non-hazardous preparations that might cause harm due to delays in administration	1 hour	N/A	N/A

[a]ISO = International Organization for Standardization, PEC = primary engineering control, IV = intravenous.

[b]Ante area must be ISO 7 if it opens into a negative pressure buffer area.

[c]*Source*: The Joint Commission. MM.05.01.07, EP2.[24]

Low-Risk CSPs

This category encompasses simple admixtures involving closed-system transfer, measuring, and mixing of three or fewer commercially manufactured sterile products (including the infusion solution). Low-risk compounding conditions must include all of the following:

- CSPs are compounded using aseptic technique within an ISO Class 5 PEC (e.g., LAFW, BSC, CAI, or CACI) that is located within an ISO Class 7 buffer area with an ISO Class 8 ante area.
- Each container, including the final container, may not be entered more than twice to prepare the CSP.
- Compounding is limited to aseptic manipulations of disinfected containers using sterile needles and syringes.

Low-Risk CSPs for Use Within 12 Hours. Under limited circumstances, sterile compounding may occur in a segregated compounding area (such as a satellite pharmacy or dedicated sterile compounding space) in which the ISO Class 5 PEC is not located within an ISO Class 7 buffer area. A segregated compounding area is a designated space, either a demarcated area or room, in which compounding is restricted to preparing low-risk, nonhazardous CSPs with a beyond-use time of no more than 12 hours from the time of preparation. All other requirements for low-risk CSPs must be followed, with the exception that the ISO Class 5 PEC is not required to be located within an ISO Class 7 buffer area. The PEC must be separate from other operations, including sinks and other water sources or drains, and away from unsealed windows or doors that connect to high traffic areas, construction, warehouses, or food preparation areas. Distinct labeling for conveying short BUDs should be considered.

Medium-Risk CSPs

This category encompasses preparations requiring more complex compounding processes, including:

- Multiple doses of sterile products combined or pooled to prepare a product that will be administered either to multiple patients (i.e., batching of syringes or large volumes), or one patient on multiple occasions (e.g., preparation for use over several days).[49]
- More than three commercially available sterile products are used to produce the compound.
- More complex compounding processes (e.g., total parenteral nutrition).

All requirements for low-risk compounding regarding location and aseptic technique must be followed.

High-Risk CSPs

High-risk CSPs are those

- Prepared from nonsterile ingredients, including manufactured products not intended for sterile routes of administration.
- Compounded using a nonsterile device prior to terminal sterilization.
- Containing nonsterile water that are stored for more than 6 hours before sterilization.
- Exposed to conditions worse than ISO Class 5 air quality for longer than 1 hour, if they contain or are compounded from sterile contents of commercially manufactured products or CSPs without antimicrobial preservatives.
- Containing bulk ingredients whose chemical purity and content strength are not verified by labeling and documentation from suppliers or by direct determination.
- Prepared by compounding personnel who are improperly garbed or gloved.

Presterilization procedures for high-risk level CSPs, such as weighing and mixing, shall be completed in no worse than an ISO Class 8 environment.

CSPs in this category must be terminally sterilized before administration to patients. Terminal sterilization is defined by the FDA as the application of a lethal process (e.g., steam under pressure or autoclaving) to sealed containers for the purpose of achieving a sterility assurance level of less than 10^{-6} or a probability of 1 nonsterile unit per 1 million sterilized units.[57] For CSPs that are heat-labile and cannot be processed as above, sterilization using an alternative method, such as a sterilizing grade 0.22 micron filter, must be done. Filtration only achieves a sterility assurance level of 10^{-3}, which is only 1 nonsterile unit per one thousand filtrated units. All filters used to sterilize CSPs must undergo filter integrity (bubble-point) testing.

Immediate-Use CSPs

The immediate-use category should be reserved for emergent use or situations in which adhering to low-risk compounding procedures would add additional risk due to delays in patient care. Examples of such situations may include cardiopulmonary resuscitation, diagnostic procedures, or short-stability medications that must be prepared immediately before administration outside health care facilities (e.g., in home infusion or emergency care at the accident site or in an ambulance). Immediate-use CSPs do not need to be compounded in an ISO Class 5 environment and garbing and gowning are not required, as long as all of the following criteria are met:

- Hand hygiene per CDC recommendations.[46]
- Aseptic technique is followed.
- No hazardous drugs are used.
- Only simple transfer of no more than three sterile, nonhazardous drugs in the manufacturer's original containers are involved in the compounding, and no more than two entries into any one container occur.
- No more than 1 hour elapses from the time compounding commences to the time administration to the patient begins (although best practice dictates that there are no intervening steps between compounding and administration).
- No batching or storage of CSPs occurs.
- The preparation is labeled with patient identification, names and amounts of all ingredients, name or initials of preparer, and exact 1-hour BUD and time.

If CSPs prepared for immediate use are not administered within 1 hour, they must be properly discarded. All medications must be labeled to meet regulatory and accreditation standards and in accordance with facility policy.

Point-of-Care Activation Systems

Point-of-care (POC) activation systems (i.e., vial/bag systems) create a physical barrier between components (fluid and medication) that can be activated to allow the components to mix. These devices are designed to create a closed system by which the end user activates the components just prior to the administration of the medication. BUDs for these products are based on the individual manufacturer's recommendations for labeling and dating. **Table 10** provides a summary of manufacturer-recommended BUDs for POC systems at time of publication. To decrease potential for contamination and errors, POC systems that will be attached and stored for longer than 1 hour prior to activation should be assembled (but not activated) by pharmacy staff within an ISO Class 5 environment. Activation of the devices should be completed at the point of care just prior to administration.

Ampuls, Single-Dose, and Multiple-Dose Containers

Ampuls may not be reused or saved at any time during the compounding process. To minimize particulate contamination, 5 micron filter straws or filter needles must be used when withdrawing contents of ampuls. Refer to the drug labeling for manufacturer's recommendations concerning filtration.

The environmental conditions in which drug vials are entered determine the BUD for the CSP. Single-dose vials are intended to be used to prepare single doses; however, in times of critical need, contents from unopened single-dose/single-use vials may be repackaged for multiple patients.[49] This repackaging should only be performed by qualified health care personnel in accordance with the procedures described in these guidelines and in *USP* chapter 797.[15]

Pharmacy bulk packages (PBPs), a type of vial containing many single doses,[65] must be considered a single-dose vial for purposes of determining BUDs. Manufacturer's information for each PBP contains recommended BUDs, which are usually between 4 and 8 hours.

Multiple-dose vials may be reused or saved up to the manufacturer's recommended BUD, if they are not opened in a direct patient-care area and if facility policy does not require a shorter period.[66] If there is no manufacturer recommendation, multiple-dose vials may be reused or saved up to a maximum of 28 days or for a shorter period dictated by facility policy. **Table 11** illustrates the dating for these products based on environmental conditions.

The person who first punctures a multiple-dose container intended for re-use must note the BUD and other information required by facility policy (e.g., his or her initials) on the vial or attached label. A label indicating "use by" clarifies that the date is the BUD rather than the opening date. If a vial lacks a BUD, it should not be used and should be properly discarded.

Batch Compounding and Sterility Testing

Use of CSPs stored for extended periods of time is guided by the chemical stability of components and the sterility limits of the CSP defined above. If medium-risk batches are prepared and assigned a BUD within those limits, no sterility testing

TABLE 10.
Beyond-Use Date (BUD) at Room Temperature for Point-of-Care Activated Devices Assembled in ISO Class 5 Environment[a]

Device	Company	BUD[b]	Applicable Products
ADD-Vantage[62]	Hospira	30 days from date diluent removed from overwrap	
Mini Bag Plus[63]	Baxter	15 days from date diluent removed from overwrap	50 and 100 mL bags
Mini-Bag Plus[63]	Baxter	30 days from date diluent removed from overwrap	100 mL containers docked with the following drugs: cefazolin 1 g, cefuroxime (Zinacef) 750 mg, ceftriaxone (Rocephin) 1 g, aztreonam (Azactam) 1 g, piperacillin and tazobactam (Zosyn) 3.375 g
addEASE[64]	B. Braun	70 days	When connected to 50 mL and 100 mL bags
		56 days	When connected to Excel 250 mL bags

[a]Information is current as of January 2011. The manufacturer's package insert should always be checked for the most current recommendation for dating.

[b]BUD for assembled but not activated system.

TABLE 11.
Beyond-Use Dates for Ampuls, Single-Dose, and Multiple-Dose Containers (Adapted from *USP* Chapter 797[15])

Container	Opened and Maintained within an ISO Class 5 Environment	Opened Outside an ISO Class 5 Environment or Taken from ISO Class 5 Conditions to Less Clean Air
Ampuls	One time use; cannot be stored	One time use; cannot be stored
Single-dose vials	One time use, cannot be stored; contents of unopened vial may be repackaged in times of critical need[49]	One time use; cannot be stored
Pharmacy bulk packages	6 hours[a]	Not intended for use outside ISO 5 environment
Multiple-dose vials	28 days[a]	28 days[a]

[a]Unless otherwise specified by manufacturer.

is required. However, if those limits are exceeded, each batch must be tested for sterility according to the requirements of *USP* chapter 71.[67]

Facilities that wish to store CSPs for periods longer than those described above must complete sterility testing for each batch to determine the extended BUD. Each batch of any risk-level CSP intended for storage outside the limits described above must be tested for sterility, according to the requirements of *USP* chapter 71, *Sterility Tests*.[67] The results must be evaluated along with stability data to establish the extended BUD. The policies and procedures of the individual facility must outline the processes used to determine extended BUDs.

Batches of high-risk CSPs prepared as multiple-dose vials intended for administration to multiple patients, batches of high-risk CSPs exposed for more than 12 hours to temperatures of 2 to 8 °C (36 to 46 °F) or for more than 6 hours to temperatures above 8 °C (46 °F) before sterilization, or batches of more than 25 identical, single-dose, high-risk CSPs must undergo sterilization and microbial and bacterial endotoxin (pyrogen) testing prior to dispensing or administration. Sterility testing, as outlined in *USP* chapter 71, must be completed prior to dispensing or administration.[67] *USP* Membrane Filtration, *USP* Direct Inoculation of the Culture Medium, or another testing method that produces verification results statistically comparable with those methods may be utilized.[67]

If sterility testing results are not received prior to dispensing, procedures must be in place for daily observation of the sterility test specimens, immediate recall of dispensed CSPs, and notification of patients and their physicians if microbial or fungal growth is observed. An investigation into the root cause of contamination must occur if sterility testing is positive.

All high-risk CSPs prepared in batches of more than 25 units, with the exception of inhalation or ophthalmic preparations, must be tested to ensure that they do not contain excessive bacterial endotoxins, as described in *USP* chapter 85, Bacterial Endotoxins Test,[68] and *USP* chapter 151, Pyrogen Test.[69] Endotoxin limits (reported in *USP* endotoxin units/hour/kg or units/hour/m^2), if established, are included in the official monograph for the product or may be found in other formula sources. If specific endotoxin limits are not available, default guidance can be found in *USP* chapter 85.[68]

For high-risk preparations, batches of 25 or fewer CSPs do not require sterility testing.[15] However, facilities should consider sterility testing of such CSPs as part of their quality assurance plans to ensure that proper procedures are being followed.

Outsourced CSPs

Outsourcing the preparation of CSPs to pharmacies that specialize in sterile compounding provides an option for facilities that cannot or do not wish to prepare all or some types of CSPs (e.g., radiopharmaceuticals, high-risk CSPs, parenteral nutrition) in their own facility. Facilities considering outsourcing compounding should consult the *ASHP Guidelines on Outsourcing Sterile Compounding Services*.[16] The decision to use CSPs prepared by outside compounding pharmacies should be reviewed and approved by hospital leadership,[23,70] and such use should only occur in accordance with written policies and procedures.

Administration of CSPs

USP chapter 797 does not include any specifications for administration or timing during this crucial period of the drug delivery cycle. CDC provides the most comprehensive guidance regarding administration of intravenous medications, including administration times, frequency of infusion set changes, use of filters, and prevention of catheter-related infections.[38,47]

Personnel

Personnel Responsibilities

The term *compounding personnel* refers to any individual involved in compounding sterile preparations, regardless of profession. Compounding personnel are responsible for ensuring that CSPs are accurately identified, measured, diluted, and mixed and are correctly purified, sterilized, packaged, sealed, labeled, stored, dispensed, distributed, and disposed of if not used. Emphasis should be on the need to maintain quality standards for the control of processes, components, and environments and for the skill and knowledge of personnel who prepare CSPs.

Accurate identification and inspection of quality and purity of non-sterile chemicals or non-sterile ingredients are necessary for the integrity of the finished preparations. Upon arrival from the manufacturer and subsequently after opening, bulk packages should be inspected for breaks in the package or closure integrity and for proper appearance, color, odor, and texture.

If nonsterile ingredients are not official *USP* or *National Formulary* products, compounding personnel must require a Certificate of Analysis from the manufacturer to accompany the products.[59] Once a product is received from the manufacturer, the date of receipt must be clearly marked on each package. If a manufacturer's expiration date is not provided, chemicals should be given a three-year BUD from the time of opening unless inspection or testing deems the product within drug monograph specification (if available) to be used for a longer time.[59]

Compounding personnel must have an understanding of how combining different agents in a preparation may affect bioavailability, compatibility (visual and chemical), pH, and concentration effects. Factors that influence stability (e.g., temperature, pH, sorption, photolysis, and chemical degradation) must be carefully evaluated and supported by references or appropriate testing.

Compounding personnel must understand and demonstrate competency in aseptic technique and for the products and systems used in CSP preparation, such as needles, syringes, administration sets, fluid containers, and compounding devices. Aseptic principles and techniques are explained in depth in *Compounding Sterile Preparations*[53] and demonstrated in *Basics of Aseptic Compounding Technique*,[54] *Getting Started in Aseptic Compounding*,[55] and *Compounding Sterile Preparations: ASHP's Video Guide to Chapter* .[56] Personnel must understand the types of PECs, HEPA filtration, and airflow concepts that are critical to sterile compounding.

Policies should be developed in conjunction with employee health or infection control personnel to set thresholds for health status fitness for compounding personnel. Compounding personnel with weeping sores, rashes, conjunctivitis, or respiratory infections must not participate in compounding processes until these conditions resolve.

Hygiene and Garbing. Proper preparation for sterile, nonhazardous drug compounding must include effective hand hygiene and garbing procedures. To minimize the number of particles introduced into the sterile compounding area and to minimize the risk of bacteria, all outer jackets and sweaters, visible jewelry, and cosmetics must be removed prior to initiating the handwashing and garbing processes. Personal electronic devices (e.g., cell phones, MP3 players) and any associated attachments must be removed prior to hand hygiene and garbing and should not be used within the sterile compounding area.

Hand hygiene must be performed prior to and after gowning and includes:

- Washing hands, under the fingernails, wrists, and up to the elbow for 30 seconds with a facility-approved agent.
- Drying hands and arms with nonshedding disposable towels or an electronic hand dryer.
- Sanitizing hands with application of a waterless, alcohol-based hand rub (ABHR) with persistent activity prior to donning sterile gloves.

Garbing occurs in the ante area and should be sequenced as follows (from "dirtiest" to "cleanest"):

- Don shoe covers, hair and beard covers, and a mask.
- Perform hand hygiene.
- Don gown, fastened securely at the neck and wrists.
- Sanitize hands using an ABHR and allow hands to dry.
- Enter the buffer area (if facility layout dictates, this step may occur after the following two steps).
- Don sterile powder-free gloves.
- Sanitize the gloves with application of 70% sterile IPA and allow gloves to dry.

Studies support the use of sterile rather than nonsterile gloves in the reduction of initial bioburden.[71] Furthermore, nonsterile gloves run the risk of cross-contamination from hands touching multiple gloves as they are removed from a stock box or container. Gloves must be inspected by personnel on a routine basis during the compounding process to check for tears or holes. The gloves should be disinfected with sterile 70% IPA throughout the compounding process and each time contaminated items are touched.

When high-risk compounding operations prior to terminal sterilization occur, personnel must glove and garb as stated above.

When exiting the compounding area during a work shift, gowns that are not soiled may be removed and retained in the ante area and re-worn during the same work shift. All other garb, including gloves, must be removed and replaced, and proper hand hygiene must be completed before re-entering the compounding area. When CAIs are utilized, compounding personnel must glove and garb as above, unless the manufacturer of the isolator provides written documentation based on environmental testing that any or all of the components of personnel hygiene and garbing are not required based on the PECs of the facility where the device is located.

Proper garb should always be used with CACIs, because personnel will be handling hazardous materials. Vials may be contaminated, even upon delivery,[72–74] and the garb is needed to protect compounding personnel from unexpected drug residue and from inadvertent spills.

Compounding Areas. Compounding personnel must understand the purposes of and relationships between ante, buffer, segregated, and storage areas. A systematic process of entering and exiting the various areas is necessary to minimize contamination. Food, drinks, and gum are prohibited in all of these areas. Since shedding from paper and labels provides a source of nonviable particles, only paper products essential to the compounding process should be allowed in the buffer area. Corrugated cardboard packaging must be eliminated from buffer areas and should be eliminated from ante areas, with all products and components such as needles, syringes, and tubing removed from their outer cardboard packaging and decontaminated by wiping the individual packages (if not in an overwrap) with a suitable disinfectant (e.g.,70% IPA) prior to entering the buffer area.

When used for sterile compounding, items in plastic or foil overwrap should remain in the overwrap until introduced into the ISO Class 5 PEC, at which point they should be opened immediately before placing in the PEC and the overwrap immediately discarded.[75] Items stored in the buffer area but not in an overwrap must be decontaminated again prior to entering the PEC, as items may be stored in a buffer area for an extended period of time and may become contaminated by dust or other particles.

Packaging and Labeling

Packaging and subsequent labeling are critical to patient safety. Packaging must be appropriate to preserve both sterility and stability until the BUD. Proper labeling requires an understanding of compounding risk levels and how to determine BUDs based on both stability and sterility.

Labels for single compounded preparations must, at a minimum, include the following:

- Names of active ingredients
- Amounts or concentrations of active ingredients
- BUD and time
- Storage requirements
- Identification of responsible compounding personnel

Labels for batch-prepared CSPs must also include:

- Control or lot number
- Appropriate auxiliary labeling (including precautions)
- Device-specific instructions (when appropriate)

Federal and state regulations and accreditation requirements may necessitate additional label information before the CSP is dispensed to a specific patient.

Verification of compounding accuracy and sterility incorporates physical inspection, ensuring compounding accuracy processes are in place, and (when applicable) sterility and endotoxin testing. Finished preparation evaluation is the responsibility of compounding personnel and should be performed during the compounding process and when the preparation leaves the storage area. Visual inspection should assess particulate matter, coring, cloudiness, leaks, and container and closure integrity.

Compounding accuracy checks must comply with federal and state dispensing regulations and include accuracy of the product or preparation and the labeling. Prescription orders, compounding procedures, records, and materials used to prepare the compounds should be evaluated. A process should be implemented to confirm that the compounding process and end-preparation testing are properly done. Checking procedures should follow facility policy and procedures and may be accomplished via cameras or other devices, by video recordings, or by keeping the used additive containers and syringes with the final product until checked. The check ideally should be performed by someone other than the compounder to decrease confirmation bias. Accuracy can be further verified by weighing when applicable and practical. When using an ACD, specific gravity values must be independently confirmed after being entered to ensure proper volumes are delivered during the compounding process.

Storage of CSPs

Temperatures of areas used for storage on patient-care and procedural units, including room temperature and in refrigerators, freezers, and warmers, must be monitored and recorded daily. On at least a monthly basis, compounding personnel or designated pharmacy personnel should evaluate storage areas for appropriate secure conditions, separation of drugs and food, and proper use and disposal of single- and multiple-dose vials.

Control and Oversight of IV Solutions

Some facilities delegate storage and distribution of parenteral solutions to materials management. Since the products are prescription drugs, the pharmacy must maintain oversight, including selection of appropriate products, package sizes, and forms; safe and secure storage; and temperature control. IV solutions that contain medications (e.g., potassium chloride, heparin, dopamine, dextran, mannitol) or high-risk agents (e.g., sterile water, sodium chloride greater than 0.9%, and parenteral nutrition components) should be stored in and distributed by the pharmacy.

Transporting CSPs

All personnel involved in the handling, transport, or storage of CSPs, whether they are compounding personnel or not, must be properly trained to complete these tasks, and the performance of all personnel, including contractors, must be monitored for compliance with facility policies. Transportation methods for CSPs should be evaluated, as some forms of transportation, such as pneumatic tube systems, may adversely affect stability or integrity. Pneumatic tube delivery may require additional padding around containers to ensure that heat and light exposure and impact are minimized. Some preparations may degrade if shaken, and therefore personnel, including pharmacy and nursing personnel, should be aware of which preparations may not be delivered via a pneumatic tube device.

Hazardous drug transport must incorporate measures to maintain CSP integrity while minimizing the risk of drug residue exposure to patients, personnel, and the environment. These preparations should always be delivered in a bag to prevent leakage or accidental exposure during transport, and they should not be delivered using a pneumatic tube device due to the risk of contamination to the environment if breakage occurs. Cleaning protocols for pneumatic tube systems are inadequate for hazardous drug contamination throughout the system.

Transport may occur outside of the compounding facility to other facilities or directly to patients. In these situations, compounding personnel must ensure physical integrity, sterility, and stability are maintained during transit. Proper packaging must be chosen to prevent contamination, leaks, damage, and temperature variations and to protect the end recipients and transporting personnel from harm. Handling and exposure instructions should be legibly displayed on the outside of shipping containers. BUDs, storage instructions, and disposal instructions for out-of-date preparations must be available to recipients, and recipients must be able to properly store CSPs (e.g., in a refrigerator or freezer, if necessary).

Redispensing CSPs

If facility policy allows redispensing of CSPs, the process must only be done by compounding personnel to ensure continued sterility, purity, and stability. Facilities must determine how to track original preparation and thaw dates (if applicable) and be able to detect product tampering. There must be policies and procedures in place to provide assurance of proper storage conditions for each product or preparation (e.g., refrigeration, protection from light, package integrity) before redispensing. CSPs must not be redispensed if package integrity has been compromised, including temperature variations.

Personnel Responsibilities for Handling, Preparation, and Disposal of Cytotoxic and Other Hazardous Agents

The Occupational Safety and Health Administration (OSHA) requires that employers and employees be made aware of the hazards of all chemicals used in the workplace, including drugs.[76] Compounding personnel of reproductive capability shall confirm in writing that they understand the risks of handling hazardous drugs.[15] Personnel at high risk of exposure to hazardous drugs should be enrolled in a medical surveillance program. In many larger facilities, the employee's health department will determine who should be enrolled. Specific guidance about surveillance for health care workers exposed to hazardous drugs is available from NIOSH,[77] as is a list of drugs NIOSH considers hazardous.[27] The risks of occupational exposure to hazardous drugs and their potential effects on compounding personnel should be conveyed to employees during employee orientation and in an ongoing manner through continuing education and monitoring at least annually. Training and competency programs should be provided in addition to competencies for compounding of non-hazardous sterile drugs, with details of differentiating the garbing, storage, preparation, and disposal procedures for hazardous drugs. *USP* chapter 797 requires that training, at a minimum, include:

- Safe aseptic manipulation practices.
- Negative pressure techniques when compounding.
- Proper utilization of a BSC or CACI.
- Correct use of closed-system transfer devices (CSTDs), if used.

- Containment, cleanup, and disposal procedures for breakages and spills.
- Treatment of personnel contact and inhalation exposure.[15]

OSHA requires more general training on chemical label elements and safety data sheet (SDS) format.[76] When training or evaluating competency, facilities may choose products to objectively evaluate hazardous drug compounding technique. These products utilize dyes or fluorescence to determine personnel technique and assess for spills or hazardous drug exposures.

Definitions of hazardous drugs and proper handling of hazardous drugs, including receiving, distribution, stocking, inventorying, preparation, transport, and disposal, are all concepts discussed in detail in the *ASHP Guidelines on Handling Hazardous Drugs*.[28]

Personnel Responsibilities for Specialty Preparations

Specialty preparations (e.g., allergen extracts, radiopharmaceuticals, and evolving technology and therapeutics such as biologics and nanotechnology) provide specific treatments for patients and require specialized procedures to be followed. Although compounding of intradermal or subcutaneous injections of allergen extracts would ideally occur under conditions for similar risk-level CSPs, they may not necessarily be subject to the same personnel, environmental, and storage requirements as for other CSPs of a similar risk level, as long as the following criteria outlined by *USP* chapter 797,[15] in conjunction with the American Academy of Otolaryngic Allergy and the Joint Council of Allergy, Asthma and Immunology,[78] are met:

- Compounding process involves simple transfer using sterile components and allergen products.
- All allergen extracts contain effective preservatives to prevent microbial growth.
- All hand hygiene, garbing, and gloving procedures for low-risk compounding, with the exception of donning shoe covers, must be followed.
- Ampul necks and vial stoppers are disinfected by wiping with sufficient amounts of sterile 70% IPA to ensure that the critical sites remain wet for 10 seconds and are allowed to dry.
- Direct contact contamination of critical sites is minimized by utilizing aseptic compounding.
- Multiple-dose vials are labeled with the name of one patient and a BUD and storage temperature range based on manufacturer recommendations or published literature. Single-dose extracts are not to be stored for subsequent use after entry.

Nuclear pharmacies are regulated by the Nuclear Regulatory Commission as well as other applicable pharmacy laws and regulations. *USP* chapter 823, Radiopharmaceuticals for Positron Emission Tomography,[79] provides the standards for production facilities. Once the components for use in positron emission tomography are released as finished preparations, handling, manipulation, and use are considered compounding by *USP* chapter 797[15] and for the purposes of these guidelines. Low-risk-level radiopharmaceuticals are those compounded from sterile components with a volume of less than 100 mL for a single-dose injection or no more than 30 mL taken from a multiple-dose container.[15] These radiopharmaceutical preparations must be compounded in an ISO Class 5 PEC within an ISO Class 8 environment.

Non-radiopharmaceuticals compounded in nuclear pharmacies must be compounded under full USP 797 compliant conditions. The radiopharmaceutical exemption in USP chapter 797[15] does not apply to non-radiopharmaceuticals.

The concept of limiting radiation exposure to a level that is as low as reasonably achievable (ALARA) must be adhered to for handling, compounding, and visual inspection of products. Technetium-99m/molybdenum-99 generator system operations and storage must occur within an ISO Class 8 environment and must further comply with all manufacturer's recommendations and federal and state regulations. Manufacturer's guidelines for BUDs should be followed for radiopharmaceutical multiple-dose vials that are compounded with technetium-99m and exposed to ISO Class 5 conditions with no direct contact contamination.

Personnel Compounding Competency

Touch contamination remains the primary cause of microbial contamination in sterile compounding.[71,80] For this reason, personnel training and assessment of competency are of utmost importance to ensure the lowest possible risk for contamination due to human error. For low- and medium-risk operations, training and competency assessment are required initially upon hire or upon transfer to compounding responsibilities, and again at least every 12 months for all staff involved in the compounding of sterile products. High-risk operations require more frequent assessments, and staff must be evaluated upon hire or transfer and again at least every six months.

As part of the training competency assessment, a written test that evaluates knowledge about proper compounding SOPs, aseptic technique, cleaning and garbing, environmental monitoring, calculations, risk levels and BUDs, and quality assurance principles must be successfully completed. Thresholds for passing the written examination should be set by the facility. While written tests assess knowledge, hands-on observation of daily duties assesses for proper technique. Personnel should be able to demonstrate at least the following in a hands-on, witnessed assessment, as applicable to their compounding responsibilities:

- Proper hand hygiene technique (see Appendix III of *USP* chapter 797[15] for a sample assessment form).
- Proper gloving and garbing technique, including successful glove fingertip test (see Appendix III of *USP* chapter 797[15] for a sample assessment form).
- Proper aseptic technique, including successful media-fill test (see Appendix IV of *USP* chapter 797[15] for a sample assessment form).
- Proper cleaning and disinfecting procedures, including successful surface sampling test (see Appendix V of *USP* chapter 797[15] for a sample assessment form and Appendix II for information about cleaning products).
- Competency in the compounding of hazardous drugs.
- Competency in the compounding of allergen extracts.
- Competency in the compounding of radiopharmaceuticals.

- Competency in the use of sterile devices, such as filter needles, injection port adapters, sterile fluid transfer devices, and CSTDs.
- Competency in the use of pharmacy compounding devices.
- Ability to fill pump reservoirs.
- Competency to perform end-product testing and sterilization.

USP chapter 797[15] requires specific assessments to be completed using sterile nutrient agar growth media to test for potential contamination. Personnel-specific examples of this type of testing include media-fill testing of aseptic technique and glove fingertip testing of compounding personnel.

Media-Fill Testing

As described in *USP* chapter 797, the media-fill component of personnel assessment provides an objective evaluation of aseptic technique.[15] Media-fill tests should be customized to mimic the most challenging preparations compounded by personnel on a regular basis in a specific facility. Testing should occur at least every 12 months for personnel who compound low- and medium-risk preparations, while testing at least every 6 months is required for personnel involved in compounding high-risk preparations. The actual testing should take place under conditions that reflect realistic workflow, such as the end of a shift, to simulate a worst-case scenario environment for compounding sterile preparations. Once started, the test should be completed without interruption. Fluid culture media are available commercially for low- and medium-risk evaluations. High-risk assessments may utilize nonsterile nutrient medium in a powder form, which may be diluted and sterilized by filter methods. Finished tests should be incubated per manufacturer's recommendations. If incubators are in the pharmacy, they must be placed outside the sterile compounding area. Ideally, the facility's microbiology services should incubate and read the tests, providing an independent evaluation by qualified individuals. Turbidity in the culture media signifies failure of the media-fill testing and requires retesting of compounding personnel. Personnel who fail these tests will require retraining and may not compound sterile preparations until tests have been repeated with successful results.

Glove Fingertip Testing

Three sets of glove fingertip evaluations must be completed with no growth prior to personnel being allowed to compound sterile preparations. This initial testing involves compounding personnel completing all necessary hand hygiene and garbing procedures (with the exception of applying sterile 70% IPA to gloves). Immediately upon completion of these procedures, the glove fingertip and thumb samples from each hand are placed on sterile nutrient agar plates. The samples should be incubated (such as by the facility's microbiology personnel) according to manufacturer standards. This test must be successfully completed three times initially, then at least every 12 months. Personnel compounding high-risk products must successfully complete the test at least every 6 months. Suggested thresholds for contamination limits can be found in Table 6. Patterns of failures (personnel, media, or facility) must be evaluated as part of the facility's quality assurance plan. Qualified microbiology personnel and the facility's infection control practitioner should be consulted.

Growth Media Requirements

Sterile nutrient agar for media-fill testing, plates for fingertip testing, and surface testing materials are available from multiple vendors. *USP* chapters 797 and 1116 provide specifications and requirements.[15,81] The media-fill testing growth media and viable airborne particle plates should utilize a Soybean-Casein Digest medium, which may also be sold as Tryptic Soy Agar/Broth. The agar plates for glove fingertip testing and surface testing should utilize general nutrient agar with neutralizing agents such as lecithin and polysorbate 80.

SOP Development

SOPs are documents containing detailed, step-by-step instructions on how to perform a task or procedure so that all personnel consistently perform the task or procedure in the same manner. SOPs are part of a good quality assurance program within the pharmacy. They provide assurance that:

- Equipment and facilities are properly maintained in good working order.
- Personnel are properly educated, trained, and evaluated.
- Supplies are received, stored, and disposed of properly and meet compendial standards.
- All tasks and procedures are performed uniformly and documented.

There are several components that should be included in an SOP:

- *Title*—should clearly identify the task.
- *SOP number*—an internal department number assigned by the organization to identify it.
- *Author(s)*—the name of the person or persons who write the SOP so that problems and revisions can be addressed.
- *Date effective*—date when the SOP is implemented into the compounding routine.
- *Authorization signature*—person or committee that approves the SOP.
- *Responsibility*—person- or persons-in-charge who are responsible for making sure that the SOP is performed properly.
- *Purpose of the procedure*—brief explanation of why the SOP is necessary or being implemented.
- *Equipment and supplies required*—list of equipment and supplies needed to perform the SOP.
- *Procedure*—detailed step-by-step explanation that can be easily followed by different individuals with the same results. The instructions should be concise to minimize any required interpretation.
- *References*—references should be listed to support the implementation and use of the SOP.
- *Documentation form*—easily accessible written record or log that demonstrates that the SOP is being performed routinely and properly.
- *Revision*—documentation of the date that an SOP has been reviewed and the name of the reviewer.

USP chapter 797[15] lists and recommends SOPs and should be reviewed to guide the pharmacy department in developing, writing, and implementing SOPs. There should be SOPs written to address tasks or procedures in the following general categories:

- *Personnel*—training, education, skills, competency evaluations, and responsibilities.
- *Facilities*—access, cleaning, maintenance, use, monitoring, and testing.
- *Equipment*—calibration, maintenance, cleaning, certification, verification, and use.
- *Supplies*—ordering, storing, certification, inspection, and disposal.
- *Compounding procedures*—preparation of various sterile compounded medications (e.g., batches, total parenteral nutrition, hazardous drugs, epidural, patient-controlled analgesia, or ophthalmics), formulas, assigning BUDs, handling, and packaging.
- *Safety*—injuries, hazardous spills, and accidental exposures.
- *Quality assurance*—inspection of CSPs, testing of CSPs, BUDs, delivery, and storage of final CSPs, patient monitoring, adverse event reporting, and personnel and environmental monitoring.
- *Administration*—record keeping and management.

All significant procedures performed in a pharmacy should be covered by SOPs and documentation. These procedures should be routinely reviewed and modified for improvements at least annually.

Quality Assurance Program

The purpose of a quality assurance program is to provide a mechanism for monitoring, evaluating, correcting, and improving activities and processes. A quality assurance program should review and analyze objective data and use these data to develop action plans. Facilities should actively work to correct problems detected and improve activities and processes as needed. Any plan designed to correct problems should include follow up parameters to make certain actions were taken and were effective.

Activities and processes that are identified based on their high frequency, high risk, or problem-prone nature should have specific monitoring and evaluation criteria assigned for objective and measurable assessment. The quality assurance program should encompass any and all activities that are included in previous sections of this document as elements which should be assessed and documented. This includes, but is not limited to:

- Personnel training and assessment
- Environmental monitoring
- Equipment calibration and maintenance

Specific quality assurance measures, pursuant to each risk level compounded in a facility, include routine cleaning and disinfection and air quality testing, visual confirmation of proper garbing procedures, review of all orders and preparations to ensure accuracy of compounded products, and visual inspection of final CSPs to confirm the absence of particulate matter or leakage.

A critical part of any quality assurance program is proper documentation, corrective action, and follow-up. Institutions must determine how results will be reported and evaluated, including development of action limits and thresholds. Thresholds and follow-up mechanisms must be in place prior to initiating a quality assurance program or immediately after collecting initial benchmark data. Responsible persons for completing these tasks should be identified and trained, if necessary, in the proper execution of the quality assurance plan. Results of monitoring and measurements should be reported within and outside of the department responsible for compounding practices to committees such as Infection Control and Quality Improvement.

If corrective action is needed, the problem should be resolved as soon as possible. Assessment of problems with compounding errors, evident contamination during preparation, quarantine, or patterns of personnel or environmental monitoring outside the established parameters require formal follow-up. A root cause analysis, including participation by other facility experts such as infection control personnel, should be completed.[82] For situations needing more time for corrective measures, an action plan should be developed and followed. Indicators and effectiveness of the quality assurance program should be reassessed annually.

New technologies, procedures, and policies should be incorporated on an as-needed basis. A failure mode and effects analysis of new techniques can serve as a valuable proactive assessment of the ease and value prior to introduction into the compounding process.[83]

References

1. Hasegawa GR. Caring about stability and compatibility. *Am J Hosp Pharm.* 1994; 51:1533–4. [editorial]
2. Stability considerations in dispensing practice (general information chapter 1191). In: The United States pharmacopeia, 34th rev., and The national formulary, 29th ed. Rockville, MD: The United States Pharmacopeial Convention; 2011:742–5.
3. Guynn JB Jr, Poretz DM, Duma RJ. Growth of various bacteria in a variety of intravenous fluids. *Am J Hosp Pharm.* 1973; 30:321–5.
4. Selenic D, Dodson DR, Jensen B, et al. *Enterobacter cloacae* bloodstream infection in pediatric patients traced to a hospital pharmacy. *Am J Health-Syst Pharm.* 2003; 60:1440–6.
5. Hughes CF, Grant AF, Lick BD, et al. Cardioplegic solution: a contamination crisis. *J Thorac Cardiovasc Surg.* 1986; 91:296–302.
6. Dugleaux G, Coutour XL, Hecquard C, et al. Septicemia caused by contaminated parenteral nutrition pouches: the refrigerator as an unusual cause. *J Parenter Enteral Nutr.* 1991; 15:474–5.
7. Sachs GS. Microbial contamination of parenteral nutrition—How could it happen? *J Parenter Enteral Nutr.* 2011; 35:432.
8. Traynor K. Meningitis outbreak challenges hospital pharmacies. *Am J Health-Syst Pharm.* 2012; 69:2024–6.
9. Pierce LR, Gaines A, Varricchio R, et al. Hemolysis and renal failure associated with use of sterile water for injection to dilute 25% human albumin solution. *Am J Health-Syst Pharm.* 1998; 55:1057,1062,1070.
10. Flynn EA, Pearson RE, Barker KN. Observational study of accuracy in compounding i.v. admixtures at five hospitals. *Am J Health-Syst Pharm.* 1997; 54:904–12.

11. Morris AM, Schneider PJ, Pedersen CA, et al. National survey of quality assurance activities for pharmacy-compounded sterile preparations. *Am J Health-Syst Pharm.* 2003; 60:2567–76.
12. Santell JP, Kamalich RF. National survey of quality assurance activities for pharmacy-prepared sterile products in hospitals and home infusion facilities—1995. *Am J Health-Syst Pharm.* 1996; 53:2591–605.
13. Kastango ES, Douglass K. Improving the management, operations and cost effectiveness of sterile-product compounding. *Int J Pharm Compd.* 1999; 3:253–8.
14. American Society of Health-System Pharmacists. ASHP Guidelines on Quality Assurance for Pharmacy-Prepared Sterile Products. *Am J Health-Syst Pharm.* 2000; 57:1150–69.
15. Pharmaceutical compounding—sterile preparations (general information chapter 797). In: The United States Pharmacopeia, 36th rev., and the National Formulary, 31 ed. Rockville, MD: The United States Pharmacopeial Convention; 2013: 361–98.
16. American Society of Health-System Pharmacists. ASHP guidelines on outsourcing sterile compounding services. *Am J Health-Syst Pharm.* 2010; 67:757–65.
17. ASHP Discussion Guide on USP Chapter ; 2008. www.ashp.org/s_ashp/docs/files/DiscGuide797-2008.pdf (accessed 2012 Dec 28).
18. Food and Drug Administration Modernization Act of 1997, Pub. L. No. 105-115, 111 Stat. 2296. www.fda.gov/RegulatoryInformation/Legislation/FederalFoodDrugandCosmeticActFDCAct/SignificantAmendmentstotheFDCAct/FDAMA/default.htm (accessed 2012 Dec 28).
19. Office of Regulatory Policy and Office of Compliance, Center for Drug Evaluation and Research (CDER), Food and Drug Administration. Guidance for FDA staff and industry. Compliance policy guides manual. Sec. 460.200. Pharmacy compounding. www.fda.gov/ICECI/ComplianceManuals/CompliancePolicyGuidanceManual/ucm074398.htm (accessed 2012 Dec 28).
20. Sterile drug products for home use (general information chapter 1206). In: The United States pharmacopeia, 23rd rev., and The national formulary, 19th ed. Rockville, MD: The United State Pharmacopeial Convention; 1995:2130–43.
21. Douglas K, Kastango E, Cantor P. State regulations impact USP compliance. *Pharm Purch Prod.* 2012; 9:S18–S21.
22. National Association of Boards of Pharmacy. Model State Pharmacy Act and Model Rules of the National Association of Boards of Pharmacy. www.nabp.net/publications/model-act/ (accessed 2012 Dec 28).
23. CMS Hospital Conditions of Participation and Interpretative Guidelines, Centers for Medicare and Medicaid Services (CMS), Department of Health and Human Services. *State Operations Manual Appendix A—Survey Protocol, Regulations and Interpretive Guidelines for Hospitals*, Rev 78 (12-22-11). Washington, DC: Government Printing Office; 2011. www.cms.gov/Regulations-and-Guidance/Guidance/Manuals/downloads/som107ap_a_hospitals.pdf (accessed 2012 Dec 28).
24. Comprehensive accreditation manual for hospitals: the official handbook. Oakbrook Terrace, IL: The Joint Commission; 2012.
25. American Osteopathic Association. Healthcare Facilities Accreditation Program, 2009 Accreditation Requirements for Healthcare Facilities; 2009.
26. DNV Healthcare. National Integrated Accreditation for Healthcare Organizations (NIAHO), Interpretive Guidelines and Surveyor Guidance, Revision 10; 2012.
27. National Institute for Occupational Safety and Health [NIOSH]. NIOSH List of Antineoplastic and Other Hazardous Drugs in Healthcare Settings 2012. www.cdc.gov/niosh/docs/2012-150/ (accessed 2012 Dec 28).
28. American Society of Health-System Pharmacists. ASHP guidelines on handling hazardous drugs. *Am J Health-Syst Pharm.* 2006; 63:1172–93.
29. National Institute for Occupational Safety and Health [NIOSH]. NIOSH alert: preventing occupational exposure to antineoplastic and other hazardous drugs in health care settings; 2004. www.cdc.gov/niosh/docs/2004-165/#g (accessed 2012 Dec 28).
30. National Institute for Occupational Safety and Health [NIOSH]. Personal protective equipment for health care workers who work with hazardous drugs (NIOSH document 2009-16). www.cdc.gov/niosh/docs/wp-solutions/2009-106/ (accessed 2012 Dec 20).
31. American Society of Hospital Pharmacists. ASHP technical assistance bulletin on pharmacy-prepared ophthalmic products. *Am J Hosp Pharm.* 1993; 50:1462–3.
32. American Society of Health-System Pharmacists. ASHP guidelines on the safe use of automated compounding devices for the preparation of parenteral nutrition admixtures. *Am J Health-Syst Pharm.* 2000; 57:1343–8.
33. American Society of Health-System Pharmacists. ASHP guidelines: minimum standard for pharmacies in hospitals. *Am J Health-Syst Pharm.* 2013; 70:1619–30.
34. ASPEN Task Force for the Revision of Safe Practices for Parenteral Nutrition: Mirtallo J, Canada T, Johnson D, et al. Safe Practices for Parenteral Nutrition. *J Parenter Enteral Nutr.* 2004; 28(6):S39–S70.
35. Bankhead R, Boullata J, Brantley S, et al. Enteral nutrition practice recommendations. *J Parenter Enteral Nutr.* 2009; 33:122–67.
36. Institute for Safe Medication Practices [ISMP]. 2004 ISMP medication safety self assessment for hospitals. Huntington Valley, PA: ISMP; 2004. www.ismp.org/selfassessments/Hospital/2004Hospsm.pdf (accessed 2012 Dec 28).
37. Institute for Safe Medication Practices [ISMP]. Proceedings from the ISMP Sterile Preparation Compounding Safety Summit: Guidelines for SAFE Preparation of Sterile Compounds; 2012. www.ismp.org/tools/guidelines/IVSummit/IVCGuidelines.pdf (accessed 2012 Dec 28).
38. Infusion Nurses Society. Infusion nursing standards of practice. *J Infus Nurs.* 2011; 34(1S):S1–S110.
39. Controlled Environment Testing Association [CETA]. CETA certification guide for sterile compounding facilities (CAG-003-2006) (revised January 31, 2012).

www.cetainternational.org/reference/CAG-003-2006v11.pdf (accessed 2012 Dec 28).

40. Controlled Environment Testing Association [CETA]. Servicing hazardous drug compounding primary engineering controls (CAG-005-2007). www.cetainternational.org/reference/CAG005-v15.pdf (accessed 2012 Dec 28).
41. Controlled Environment Testing Association [CETA]. Application guide for the use of surface decontaminants in biosafety cabinets (CAG-004-2007). www.cetainternational.org/reference/CAG0042007i.pdf (accessed 2012 Dec 28).
42. Controlled Environment Testing Association [CETA]. Compounding isolator testing guide (CAG-002-2006) (revised December 2008). www.cetainternational.org/reference/CETACompoundingIsolatorTesting Guide2006.pdf (accessed 2012 Dec 28).
43. Controlled Environment Testing Association [CETA]. Application guide for the use of compounding isolators in compounding sterile preparations in healthcare facilities (CAG-001-2005) (revised December 2008). www.cetainternational.org/reference/Applications GuideBarrierIsolator-CAG-001-2005.pdf (accessed 2012 Dec 28).
44. Controlled Environment Testing Association [CETA]. CETA Certification Matrix for Sterile Compounding Facilities (CAG-008-2010) (updated January 2012). www.cetainternational.org/reference/CAG-008-2010v2.pdf (accessed 2012 Dec 20).
45. Controlled Environment Testing Association [CETA]. CETA Certification Application Guide USP Viable Environmental Sampling & Gowning Evaluation (CAG-009-2011v3). www.cetainternational.org/reference/CAG-009v3.pdf (accessed 2012 Dec 28).
46. Centers for Disease Control and Prevention [CDC]. Guidelines for hand hygiene in healthcare settings. *MMWR* 2002; 51(RR16):1–45. www.cdc.gov/mmwr/preview/mmwrhtml/rr5116a1.htm (accessed 2012 Dec 28).
47. O'Grady NP, Alexander M, Burns LA, et al. 2011 Guidelines for the Prevention of Intravascular Catheter-Related Infections. Centers for Disease Control and Prevention, 2012. www.cdc.gov/hicpac/pdf/guidelines/bsi-guidelines-2011.pdf (accessed 2012 Dec 28).
48. Centers for Disease Control and Prevention [CDC]. Guidelines for Environmental Infection Control in Healthcare Facilities. *MMWR.* 2003; 52(RR10):1–42. www.cdc.gov/mmwr/preview/mmwrhtml/rr5210a1.htm (accessed 2012 Dec 28).
49. Centers for Disease Control and Prevention, National Center for Emerging and Zoonotic Infectious Diseases (NCEZID), Division of Healthcare Quality Promotion (DHQP). Protect Patients Against Preventable Harm from Improper Use of Single-Dose/Single-Use Vials. www.cdc.gov/injectionsafety/CDCposition-SingleUseVial.html (accessed 2012 Dec 28).
50. Centers for Medicare & Medicaid Services [CMS]. Single use of single dose/single use medications to prevent healthcare-associated infections. www.cms.gov/Medicare/Provider-Enrollment-and-Certification/SurveyCertificationGenInfo/Policy-and-Memos-to-States-and-Regions-Items/Survey-and-Cert-Letter-12-35.html (accessed 2012 Dec 28).
51. Dolan SA, Felizardo G, Barnes S, et al. APIC position paper: Safe injection, infusion, and medication vial practices in health care. *Am J Infect Control.* 2010; 38:167–72.
52. Chapter 17. Recommended Practices for Medication Safety. In: Conner R, Blanchard J, Burlingame B, et al. (eds). Perioperative Standards and Recommended Practices. Denver, CO: Association of periOperative Registered Nurses (AORN); 2012:251–300.
53. Buchanan EC, Schneider PJ. Compounding sterile preparations, 3rd ed. Bethesda, MD: American Society of Health-System Pharmacists; 2009.
54. American Society of Health-System Pharmacists [ASHP]. Basics of aseptic compounding technique. Bethesda, MD: ASHP; 2006.
55. Davis K, Sparks J. Getting started in aseptic compounding. Bethesda, MD: American Society of Health-System Pharmacists; 2008.
56. Kienle PC. Compounding sterile preparations: ASHP video guide to chapter . Bethesda, MD: American Society of Health-System Pharmacists; 2009.
57. U.S. Department of Health and Human Services, Food and Drug Administration, Office of Regulatory Affairs. Guidance for industry: sterile drug products produced by aseptic processing—current good manu facturing practice. September 2004. www.fda.gov/downloads/Drugs/GuidanceComplianceRegulatory Information/Guidances/UCM070342.pdf (accessed 2012 Dec 28).
58. General notices and requirements. In: The United States pharmacopeia, 34th rev., and The national formulary, 29th ed. Rockville, MD: The United States Pharmacopeial Convention; 2011:11–12.
59. Pharmaceutical compounding—nonsterile preparations (general information chapter 795). In: The United States pharmacopeia, 34th rev., and The national formulary, 29th ed. Rockville, MD: The United States Pharmacopeial Convention; 2011:330–6.
60. Trissel LA. Handbook on injectable drugs. 17th ed. Bethesda, MD: American Society of Health-System Pharmacists; 2013.
61. Bing CD, Nowobilski-Vasilios A. Extended stability for parenteral drugs. 5th ed. Bethesda, MD: American Society of Health-System Pharmacists; 2013:321.
62. Personal communication from Hospira. December 16, 2008.
63. Personal communication from Baxter. December 18, 2008.
64. Personal communication from B. Braun. December 26, 2008.
65. Injections (general information chapter 1). In: The United States pharmacopeia, 34th rev., and The national formulary, 29th ed. Rockville, MD: The United States Pharmacopeial Convention; 2011:33–8.

66. Centers for Disease Control and Prevention, National Center for Emerging and Zoonotic Infectious Diseases (NCEZID), Division of Healthcare Quality Promotion (DHQP). Safe Injection Practices to Prevent Transmission of Infections to Patients. www.cdc.gov/injectionsafety/IP07_standardPrecaution.html (accessed 2013 Jan 30).
67. Sterility tests (general information chapter 71). In: The United States pharmacopeia, 34th rev., and The national formulary, 29th ed. Rockville, MD: The United States Pharmacopeial Convention; 2011:65–70.
68. Bacterial endotoxins test (general information chapter 85). In: The United States pharmacopeia, 34th rev., and The national formulary, 29th ed. Rockville, MD: The United States Pharmacopeial Convention; 2011: 78–82.
69. Pyrogen test (general information chapter 151). In: The United States pharmacopeia, 34th rev., and The national formulary, 29th ed. Rockville, MD: The United States Pharmacopeial Convention; 2011:115–7.
70. Oversight of Care, Treatment, and Services Provided through Contractual Agreement (Standard LD.04.03.09). Comprehensive accreditation manual for hospitals: the official handbook. Oakbrook Terrace, IL: The Joint Commission; 2012.
71. Trissel LA, Gentempo JA, Saenz LM, et al. Effect of two work practice changes on the microbial contamination rates of pharmacy-compounded sterile preparations. *Am J Health-Syst Pharm.* 2007; 64:837–41.
72. Sessink PJ, Boer KA, Scheefhals AP, et al. Occupational exposure to antineoplastic agents at several departments in a hospital: environmental contamination and excretion of cyclophosphamide and ifosfamide in urine of exposed workers. *Int Arch Occup Environ Health.* 1992; 64:105–12.
73. Kiffmeyer TK, Ing KG, Schoppe G. External contamination of cytotoxic drug packing: safe handling and cleaning procedures. *J Oncol Pharm Pract.* 2000; 6:13.
74. Connor TH, Sessink PJ, Harrison BR et al. Surface contamination of chemotherapy drug vials and evaluation of new vial-cleaning techniques: results of three studies. *Am J Health-Syst Pharm.* 2005; 62:475–84.
75. Kastango ES, Wagner JT, Kastango KB, et al. Generation of particulate matter during handling of needle and syringe packaging. *Am J Health-Syst Pharm.* 2008; 65:1443–50.
76. OSHA Hazard Communication Standard (revised 2012). www.osha.gov/dsg/hazcom/index.html. (accessed 2012 Dec 28).
77. National Institute for Occupational Safety and Health [NIOSH]. Medical surveillance for healthcare workers exposed to hazardous drugs. NIOSH Publication No. 2013-103; November 2012. www.cdc.gov/niosh/docs/wp-solutions/2013-103/ (accessed 2012 Dec 28).
78. Joint Council of Allergy, Asthma, and Immunology. Allergen Immunotherapy Extract Preparation Guidelines. www.jcaai.org/file_depot/0-10000000/20000-30000/27387/folder/62846/Allergen_Extract_Preparation_Guidelines.pdf (accessed 2012 Dec 28).
79. Radiopharmaceuticals for positron emission tomography—compounding (general information chapter 823). In: The United States pharmacopeia, 34th rev., and The national formulary, 29th ed. Rockville, MD: The United States Pharmacopeial Convention, 2011:385–9.
80. Thomas M, Sanborn MD, Couldry R. I.V. admixture contamination rates: Traditional practice site versus a class 1000 cleanroom. *Am J Health-Syst Pharm.* 2005; 62:2386–92.
81. Microbiological evaluation of clean rooms and other controlled environments (general information chapter 1116). In: The United States pharmacopeia, 34th rev., and The national formulary, 29th ed. Rockville, MD: The United States Pharmacopeial Convention; 2011: 633–41.
82. Agency for Healthcare Research and Quality Patient Safety Network (AHRQ PSNet). Patient safety primer: root cause analysis. www.psnet.ahrq.gov/primer.aspx?primerID=10 (accessed 2012 Dec 28).
83. DeRosier J, Stalhandske E, Bagian JP, et al. Using health care failure mode and effects analysis: the VA National Center for Patient Safety's prospective risk analysis system. *Jt Comm J Qual Improv.* 2002; 28: 248–67.

Approved by the ASHP Board of Directors on June 2, 2013. Developed through the ASHP Council on Pharmacy Practice. These guidelines supersede the ASHP Guidelines on Quality Assurance for Pharmacy-Prepared Sterile Products dated April 27, 2000.

Patricia C. Kienle, M.P.A., FASHP, is gratefully acknowledged for leading the development of and drafting substantial portions of these guidelines. Linda F. McElhiney, Pharm.D.; Richard B. Osteen, D.Ph.; Ed Troell, M.B.A.; Fred Massoomi, Pharm.D., FASHP; Kathleen Sheehy, M.B.A.; and Angela T. Cassano, Pharm.D., BCPS, are also gratefully acknowledged for their contributions to these guidelines.

ASHP gratefully acknowledges the following individuals for reviewing these guidelines (review does not imply endorsement): Caryn D. Bing, M.S., FASHP; E. Clyde Buchanan, M.S., FASHP; Ryan A. Forrey, Pharm.D., M.S.; Eric S. Kastango, M.B.A., FASHP; Lee B. Murdaugh, Ph.D.; Daryl McCollum, Pharm.D.; Luci A. Power, M.S.; Philip J. Schneider, M.S., FASHP; and James T. Wagner.

Copyright © 2014, American Society of Health-System Pharmacists, Inc. All rights reserved. Contact ASHP for reprint and permissions requests. This content may not be used for commercial purposes without the express written consent of ASHP.

The bibliographic citation for this document is as follows: American Society of Health-System Pharmacists. ASHP guidelines on compounding sterile preparations. *Am J Health-Syst Pharm.* 2014; 71:145–66.

ASHP Guidelines on Handling Hazardous Drugs

ASHP published its first guidance on hazardous drugs (HDs) in 1983 as part of the 1983–84 ASHP Practice Spotlight: Safe Handling of Cytotoxic Drugs.[1,2] This was followed by technical assistance bulletins in 1985 and 1990 and the ASHP Guidelines on Handling Hazardous Drugs in 2006.[3–5] The 2006 guidelines were created to harmonize with the National Institute for Occupational Safety and Health (NIOSH) Alert: Preventing Occupational Exposure to Antineoplastic and Other Hazardous Drugs in Health Care Settings issued in 2004.[6] The ASHP 2006 HD guidelines were current to 2005.

In 2007, the United States Pharmacopeial Convention revised *United States Pharmacopeia (USP)* chapter 797 (Pharmaceutical Compounding—Sterile Preparations)[7] to harmonize with the NIOSH 2004 Alert. It became effective May 1, 2008, establishing many of the NIOSH recommenda tions as enforceable requirements. On February 1, 2016, *USP* published a new general chapter, chapter 800, Hazardous Drugs—Handling in Healthcare Settings.[8] Unlike the other publications regarding HDs noted above, *USP* chapter 800 is not a guidance document but an enforceable standard, containing both best practice recommendations and mandates for reducing the occupational exposure of healthcare workers who handle nonsterile and sterile HDs. The standards set by *USP* chapter 800 are applicable in all settings in which HDs are compounded and administered and where healthcare workers may come into contact with HD residue, not just hospitals and clinics.

With the increasing number of publications on this topic, the inclusion of older material in these guidelines has been limited to landmark or other crucial studies. The ASHP 1990 technical assistance bulletin and 2006 guidelines provide historic overviews of this topic. Sections of *USP* chapter 800 are discussed in this document, but the ASHP Guidelines on Handling Hazardous Drugs are not intended to modify, interpret, or be a substitute for the provisions of *USP* chapter 800. These updated guidelines include information from the literature, NIOSH, and *USP* and are current to October 2017.

Purpose

Significant advances in the awareness of safe handling of HDs have been made since the previous version of these guidelines was published in 2006. NIOSH has created a topics page to maintain a bibliography of NIOSH HD documents, publications on occupational exposure to antineoplastic and other HDs, and research on safe handling drawn from the published literature.[9] After more than 30 years of published guidance, international research indicates that occupational exposure to HDs continues, negative reproductive outcomes continue, and barriers to adherence to safe handling guidance remain. The purposes of these updated guidelines are to (1) inform readers about new and continuing concerns for healthcare workers handling HDs and (2) provide information on recommendations and requirements, including those regarding controls and equipment that have been developed since the publication of the 2006 ASHP guidelines.

Because newer studies have shown that contamination is widespread in healthcare settings and that more workers than previously thought are exposed, these guidelines should be implemented wherever HDs are received, stored, prepared, transported, administered, or disposed.[8–11]

Comprehensive reviews of the literature covering anecdotal and case reports of surface contamination, worker exposure, and risk assessment are available from NIOSH,[6,9,12] the Occupational Safety and Health Administration (OSHA),[13,14] and individual authors.[15–20] The primary goal of this document is to provide recommendations for the safe handling of HDs. These guidelines represent the research and recommendations of many groups and individuals who have worked tirelessly over decades to reduce the potential harmful effects of HDs on healthcare workers. The research available to date, as well as the opinions of thought leaders in this area, is reflected in the guidelines. Where possible, recommendations are evidence based. In the absence of published data, professional judgment, experience, and common sense have been used.

Background

Healthcare workers may be exposed to HDs at many points during manufacture, distribution, receipt, storage, transport, compounding, and administration, as well as during waste handling and care of treated patients.[6] All workers involved in these activities, as well as in equipment maintenance and repair, have the potential for contact with uncontained drug. One study of worker contact with surfaces contaminated with HDs identified a number of job categories not traditionally expected to be exposed.[11] Unit clerks, transport workers, ward aides, dietitians, and oncologists were observed touching contaminated surfaces. A follow-up study documented cyclophosphamide in the urine of these workers, concluding that workers in the drug administration setting, even those who were not responsible for administering the drugs to patients (i.e., volunteers, oncologists, ward aides, and dietitians), had the largest proportion of samples exceeding the limit of detection (LOD) for cyclophosphamide.[21] These results suggest that it is reasonable to expand the list of potentially exposed workers. Recent studies have also begun to examine the impact on families and caregivers of home treatments with HDs[22–24]; however, the scope of these guidelines is limited to workers in healthcare settings.

Exposure to HDs in the workplace has been associated with acute and short-term reactions as well as long-term effects. Anecdotal and case reports in the literature range from skin-related and ocular effects to flu-like symptoms and headache.[6,17] Reproductive studies on healthcare workers have shown an increase in fetal abnormalities, fetal loss, and fertility impairment resulting from occupational exposure to these potent drugs.[25–28] An extensive study published in 2012 documented increased spontaneous abortions in nurses exposed to HDs in the workplace.[26] An increase in learning disabilities among offspring as a result of occupational exposure to these potent drugs has also been reported.[27]

Antineoplastic drugs and immunosuppressants are some of the types of drugs included on lists of known or suspected human carcinogens by the National Toxicology Program[29] and the International Agency for Research on

DOI 10.37573/9781585287048.021

Cancer.[30] Although the increased incidence of cancers for occupationally exposed groups has been investigated, with varying results,[31–34] 2 related studies described evidence of drug uptake (drug being incorporated into workers' bodies) and chromosomal changes in oncology workers exposed to workplaces contaminated with HD residue.[35,36] The DNA of exposed workers showed a statistically significant increase in the frequency of damage to chromosome 5 or 7 and an increase in frequency of damage to chromosome 5 alone. As signature lesions in chromosomes 5, 7, and 11 have been shown to be associated with chemotherapy treatment-related myelodysplastic syndrome and acute myeloid leukemia, these results provide additional evidence of harmful effects from occupational exposure to HDs.[37,38] These conclusions are bolstered by recent meta-analyses of comet assay, micronuclei and chromosomal aberration data in healthcare workers that have shown increases in chromosomal damage in workers exposed to antineoplastic drugs.[39–41]

Continuing Exposure. Before the publication of the 2004 NIOSH Alert, a 1999 study done in 3 cancer treatment centers in the United States and 3 in Canada provided strong evidence of surface contamination with antineoplastic HDs in compounding and infusion areas.[42] Measurable amounts of cyclophosphamide, ifosfamide, and fluorouracil were detected in 75% of the pharmacy wipe samples and 65% of the infusion area wipe samples. The levels of contamination were higher in the pharmacy areas than in the drug infusion areas. The number of positive wipe sampling results was related to the amount of drug prepared and administered.

A NIOSH-sponsored study of 3 university-based U.S. cancer centers published in 2010 reexamined HD contamination and other risk points from the 1999 study.[10,42] The 2010 study measured surface contamination of at least 1 of the 5 drugs (cyclophosphamide, ifosfamide, fluorouracil, paclitaxel, and cytarabine) in 75% of the pharmacy wipe samples and 43% of the infusion wipe samples. The study confirmed that HD contamination is generally widespread, even with engineering controls such as class II biological-safety cabinets (BSCs); that pharmacy areas have more contaminated surfaces; and that the contamination is in higher concentrations than in nursing areas. Most importantly, this study confirmed that there had been little progress in reducing HD contamination in similar healthcare settings in the United States in the 10 years between the studies.

A series of multisite studies on HD contamination was published by a research team in British Columbia.[11,21,43] Through interviews and observations, 11 job categories with the potential for HD exposure by dermal contact with potentially contaminated surfaces were identified within 6 medical sites.[11] In addition to those workers traditionally thought to be exposed, workers who had possible dermal contact with HDs included receiving staff, unit clerks, ward aides, and even volunteers. In investigating contaminated surfaces, the researchers noted that although the BSC had the highest frequency of contact in the compounding area, the pen inside the BSC and the isopropyl alcohol spray bottle were frequently touched.[11] I.V. pumps, countertops, and waste containers were the most contacted surfaces in the infusion areas. The team collected surface wipe samples at the participating sites, using cyclophosphamide as the marker drug.[11] Of the 275 surface samples collected, 35% were above the LOD. As in the 2010 U.S. study,[10] the pharmacy compounding areas had the majority of contaminated wipes (47 of 85) and the highest concentration of drug.[11] Additional surface wipe sampling done at the same 6 medical sites[43] produced a total of 438 samples from 55 categories of surfaces in 5 drug handling stages (delivery, preparation, transport, administration, and waste), with 159 (36%) having concentrations above the LOD. The most-contaminated surfaces by stage were the drug delivery elevator button, drug preparation pen (possibly from the BSC), transport bin for drug pickup, drug administration i.v. pump, and waste elevator button.[43] In the original study,[11] the BSC was noted to be the most frequently touched item in the drug preparation area; however, the pen used in the BSC was the most contaminated. Other items such as a marker and tweezers kept in the BSC were also heavily contaminated, probably resulting in glove contamination during each contact. While routine cleaning of the BSC surface was reported, miscellaneous items, such as the pen, were probably not included in that cleaning. Measurable HD contamination on elevator buttons is concerning for workers, and visitors may also be exposed to this risk.

In addition, this research team sought to determine whether healthcare workers from the earlier studies were at risk of cyclophosphamide uptake through dermal contact with contaminated surfaces or by other means.[21] Participants identified from the prior studies as potentially exposed agreed to provide urine samples to quantify the urine concentration of nonmetabolized cyclophosphamide. Cyclophosphamide levels greater than the LOD were found in 55% of urine samples.[21] Participants from departments where drug preparation and drug administration do not occur (i.e., shipping/receiving, transport, nutrition, and materials management) had the highest average urinary concentration levels of cyclophosphamide.[21] When the results were stratified by job title, unit clerks had the highest average urinary cyclophosphamide concentration. The authors identified 2 factors associated with cyclophosphamide uptake: (1) whether a worker had a duty to handle antineoplastic HDs and (2) whether a worker received training on safe drug handling, and concluded that interventions to minimize this risk should be more broadly applied.

A review of studies of healthcare worker exposure to antineoplastic HDs published in the United States, Canada, and Europe after publication of the 2004 NIOSH HD Alert revealed no decrease in contamination.[44] In addition, separating the publications by origin, the review found that only 9 of 71 such studies were done by U.S. researchers, and most of those were sponsored by medical device manufacturers. U.S. critics of HD safe handling guidance often note the lack of evidence of exposure as well as the recommendations to mitigate it. The exceptionally small number of U.S. studies found in this literature review may indicate a basic lack of interest in conducting such research in the United States.

Routes of Exposure. Numerous studies have shown the presence of HDs in the urine of healthcare workers.[10,21,45–47] In a review of 20 studies from 1992 to 2011 examining biomarkers of exposure in healthcare workers handling antineoplastic HDs, 17 studies found drug in workers' urine.[19] One of the studies in that review described no response in 50 subjects, but the study did note that all subjects demonstrated postshift exposure to platinum.[47] A study by Wick et al.,[46] which was not included in the review, demonstrated that 6 of 8 participants' 24-hour urine samples had cyclophosphamide and ifosfamide levels above the LOD. Hon et al.[21] collected 201 urine samples from 103 subjects, including those in job categories with low expectation of exposure; 55% had levels exceeding the LOD for cyclophosphamide, with unit clerks having the highest average level.

HDs may enter the body through inhalation, dermal absorption, accidental injection, ingestion of contaminated foodstuffs, or mouth contact with contaminated hands. Inhalation was previously suspected as the primary route of exposure, but 1 or more of these routes might be responsible for workers' exposure. More recent studies, especially those looking at healthcare workers not directly involved with HD compounding and administration, support the theory that dermal contact with contaminated surfaces is the primary route of exposure.[18,19,21,48–50]

An alternative to dermal absorption, where HDs penetrate unprotected skin after contact with contaminated surfaces, is that surface contamination transferred to hands may be ingested via the hand-to-mouth route.[51,52] Researchers have examined hand sampling as a measure of exposure.[51] Using a technique of wipe sampling, similar to that done for work surfaces, healthcare workers' hands may be swabbed to check for HD contamination.[51] One study of workers at 6 sites analyzed a total of 225 wipe samples, 20% of which were above the LOD for cyclophosphamide.[52] Contaminated hands may transfer HD residue to other surfaces and other workers as well as contribute to hand-to-mouth transfer. Hand sampling may offer an alternative to surface sampling in monitoring HD contamination and exposure.

Hazard Assessment. The risk to workers from handling HDs is the result of a combination of the inherent toxicity of the drugs and the extent to which workers are exposed to the drugs in the course of their daily job activities. Both hazard identification (the qualitative evaluation of the toxicity of a given drug) and an exposure assessment (the amount of worker contact with the drug) are required to complete a hazard assessment. As the hazard assessment is specific to the safety program and safety equipment is in place at a work site, a formal hazard assessment may not be available for most practitioners. An alternative is a performance-based, observational approach. Observation of current work practices, equipment, and the physical layout of work areas where HDs are handled at any given site will serve as an initial assessment of appropriate and inappropriate practices.[6]

NIOSH defines a risk assessment as characterization of potentially adverse health effects from human exposure to environmental and occupational hazards. Risk assessment can be divided into 5 major steps: hazard identification, dose–response assessment, exposure assessment, risk characterization, and risk communication.[4]

USP chapter 800 introduced the term *assessment of risk*, which allows an entity to perform an evaluation of risk to determine alternative containment strategies and/or work practices to those described in *USP* chapter 800 for some dosage forms of HDs that may not pose a significant risk of direct occupational exposure.[8] An assessment of risk may only be used for drugs on the NIOSH list that are neither HD active pharmaceutical ingredients (APIs) nor antineoplastics requiring HD manipulation. According to *USP* chapter 800, the assessment of risk must, at a minimum, consider the type of HD, the dosage form, the risk of exposure, the packaging involved, and how the drug will be manipulated.

If an assessment of risk is performed, the entity must document the alternative containment strategies and/or work practices specific to the drugs and dosage forms so as to minimize healthcare workers' exposure. The assessment of risk must be reviewed and documented at least every 12 months. An assessment of risk should not be confused with a *risk assessment*, as the hazard identification step is not done by the entity. *USP* chapter 800 describes the requirements and restrictions of an assessment of risk.[8]

Definition of HDs

The 1990 ASHP technical assistance bulletin proposed criteria to determine which drugs should be considered hazardous and handled within an established safety program.[4] The technical assistance bulletin's definition of HDs was revised by the NIOSH Working Group on Hazardous Drugs for the 2004 alert.[6] These definitions are compared in **Table 1**. For purposes of these guidelines, the definition from the 2004 NIOSH Alert is used (**Appendix A**).

NIOSH. The NIOSH 2004 HD Alert contained an appendix of HD lists compiled from information provided by 4 organizations that had generated lists of HDs for their respective institutions, as well as a list from the Pharmaceutical Research and Manufacturers of America.[6] NIOSH adopted a mechanism both to review its HD criteria and to update its HD list every 2 years by reviewing the existing drugs on the HD list and examining newly approved drugs, and drugs with new Food and Drug Administration (FDA) warnings against the NIOSH HD criteria. The review process for the addition of the new listings is described in the *Federal Register*.[53]

From 2004 through 2012, NIOSH recommended that standard precautions or universal precautions be taken in handling HDs. In 2014, with the addition of many nonantineoplastic drugs and drugs in tablet and/or capsule form to the list, NIOSH noted that no single approach could cover the diverse potential occupational exposures to the drugs.[54] This change required the development of a new format for the 2014 NIOSH list of HDs, which for the first time divided HDs into 3 groups:

- **Group 1:** antineoplastic drugs (AHFS Classification 10:00) [ASHP/AHFS DI 2013]. Many of these drugs may also pose a reproductive risk for susceptible populations.
- **Group 2:** nonantineoplastic drugs that meet 1 or more of the NIOSH criteria for an HD. Some of these drugs may also pose a reproductive risk for susceptible populations.
- **Group 3:** drugs that primarily pose a reproductive risk to men and women who are actively trying to conceive and women who are pregnant or breast-feeding (some of these drugs may be present in breast milk).

The 2016 NIOSH HD list retains this 3-group format.[55] The most current NIOSH list of HDs, along with other NIOSH HD documents, may be found on the NIOSH Hazardous Drug Exposures in Healthcare Topics Page.[56]

USP Chapter 800. In 2016, *USP* chapter 800 adopted the NIOSH HD list as the list of antineoplastic and other HDs that an organization wishing to comply with *USP* chapter 800

TABLE 1.

Comparison of NIOSH and ASHP Definitions of Hazardous Drugs

NIOSH[6]	ASHP[4]
Carcinogenicity	Carcinogenicity in animal models, in the patient population, or in both as reported by the International Agency for Research on Cancer
Teratogenicity or developmental toxicity[a]	Teratogenicity in animal studies or in treated patients
Reproductive toxicity[a]	Fertility impairment in animal studies or in treated patients
Organ toxicity at low doses[a]	Evidence of serious organ or other toxicity at low doses in animal models or in treated patients
Genotoxicity[b]	Genotoxicity (i.e., mutagenicity and clastogenicity in short-term test systems)
Structure and toxicity profile of new drugs that mimic existing drugs determined hazardous by the above criteria	. . .

[a]The National Institute for Occupational Safety and Health (NIOSH) definition contains the following explanation: "All drugs have toxic side effects, but some exhibit toxicity at low doses. The level of toxicity reflects a continuum from relatively nontoxic to production of toxic effects in patients at low doses (for example, a few milligrams or less). For example, a daily therapeutic dose of 10 mg/day or a dose of 1 mg/kg/day in laboratory animals that produces serious organ toxicity, developmental toxicity, or reproductive toxicity has been used by the pharmaceutical industry to develop occupational exposure limits (OELs) of less than 10 micrograms/meter^3 after applying appropriate uncertainty factors [Sargent and Kirk 1988; Nauman and Sargent 1997; Sargent et al. 2002]. OELs in this range are typically established for potent or toxic drugs in the pharmaceutical industry. Under all circumstances, an evaluation of all available data should be conducted to protect health care workers."[6]

[b]The NIOSH definition contains the following explanation: "In evaluating mutagenicity for potentially hazardous drugs, responses from multiple test systems are needed before precautions can be required for handling such agents. The EPA evaluations include the type of cells affected and in vitro versus in vivo testing [51 Fed. Reg. 34006-34012 (1986)]."[6]

must begin with.[8] This list may be modified to include only the drugs that they handle and must be reviewed at least every 12 months. The list must be dynamic: whenever a new agent or dosage form is used by the organization, it should be reviewed against the list. The NIOSH HD criteria must be used to identify HDs that enter the market after the most recent version of the NIOSH HD list and to assess any investigational drugs used by the organization.

OSHA. The OSHA Hazard Communication Standard (HCS) was updated in 2012 to align with the United Nations Globally Harmonized System of Classification and Labeling of Chemicals.[57] The revised HCS defines a hazardous chemical as any chemical that is classified as a physical or health hazard, simple asphyxiant, combustible dust, pyrophoric gas, or hazard not otherwise classified.[58] It further defines a health hazard as a chemical that is classified as posing 1 of the following hazardous effects: acute toxicity (any route of exposure), skin corrosion or irritation, serious eye damage or irritation, respiratory or skin sensitization, germ cell mutagenicity, carcinogenicity, reproductive toxicity, specific target organ toxicity (single or repeated exposure), or aspiration hazard. The criteria for determining whether a chemical is classified as a health hazard are detailed in Appendix A to §1910.1200—Health Hazard Criteria.[59] In addition, the HCS requires that drugs that pose a health hazard (with the limited exception of those in solid, final forms for direct administration to the patient, such as tablets or pills) be included on lists of hazardous chemicals to which employees are exposed. As a federal standard, the HCS is the definitive document establishing compliance with all phases of this right-to-know legislation, including the definition of *hazardous* and the requirements for the Safety Data Sheet (SDS). In addition, the HCS requires that the hazards of all chemicals produced or imported into a workplace are classified and that information concerning the classified hazards is transmitted to employers and employees.[57]

A list of HDs in use in the facility is required by the OSHA HCS and by *USP* chapter 800.[8,57] The Joint Commission, in Elements of Performance for Medication Management (MM).01.01.03, requires that hospitals identify in writing their high-alert and hazardous medications.[60]

HDs as Sterile Preparations

Many HDs are designed for parenteral administration, requiring aseptic reconstitution or dilution to yield a final sterile preparation. As such, the compounding of these products is regulated as sterile pharmaceutical compounding by *USP* chapter 797.[7] The intent of *USP* chapter 797 is to protect patients from improperly compounded sterile preparations (CSPs) by regulating facilities, equipment, and work practices to ensure the sterility of extemporaneously CSPs. *USP* chapter 797 addresses not only the sterility of a preparation but also the accuracy of its composition. Because many HDs are very potent, there is little margin for error in compounding.

HDs, as CSPs, are regulated by both *USP* chapters 797 and 800 for compounding environments.[7,8] The compounding of nonsterile HDs must meet the criteria in *USP* chapter 795, Pharmaceutical Compounding—Nonsterile Preparations,[61] as well as *USP* chapter 800.[8] With the adoption of *USP* chapter 800, the HD section will be removed from *USP* chapter 797.

USP chapter 800 has changed the requirements for HD handling, storage, and compounding environments to emphasize containment, including the containment primary engineering control (C-PEC), the device in which compounding takes place, and the containment secondary engineering control (C-SEC), the room in which the C-PEC is placed.[8] Major revisions in engineering controls adopted by *USP* chapter 800 include a requirement that certain areas be under negative pressure relative to surrounding areas to contain HDs and minimize the risk of exposure.[8]

External ventilation (i.e., exhausting to the outside) is advocated to achieve negative pressure. Because HDs are also compounded in areas adjacent to patients and family members (e.g., in chemotherapy infusion centers), inappropriate environmental containment puts them and healthcare workers at risk.[8]

Recommendations

The recommendations below stem from the dedicated and thoughtful efforts of numerous groups and individuals over many years. Where possible, the recommendations are evidence based. In the absence of published data, the professional judgment and opinions of thought leaders have been relied upon. In this document, the term *must* is used to denote a requirement of generally applicable laws, regulations, or practice standards; the term *should* indicates a generally accepted recommendation that is not drawn from an authoritative reference. Healthcare professionals are encouraged to rely on their professional judgment, experience, and common sense in applying these recommendations to their unique circumstances, as no set of guidelines on this topic can address all the needs of every healthcare facility.

Safety Program

Policies and procedures for the safe handling of HDs must be in place for all situations in which these drugs are used throughout a facility. A comprehensive safety program must be developed that deals with all aspects of the safe handling of HDs. This program must be a collaborative effort, with input from all affected departments, such as pharmacy, nursing, medical staff, environmental services, transportation, maintenance, employee health, risk management, industrial hygiene, clinical laboratories, and safety. New research indicates that HD contamination is more widespread than generally believed and that worker exposure extends beyond the primarily accepted occupations.[11,21] It is important to make all affected workers aware of the potential risks and to train them in appropriate safety precautions.[62]

Per *USP* chapter 800, each facility handling HDs must have a designated person who is qualified and trained to be responsible for developing and implementing appropriate procedures; overseeing entity compliance with this chapter and other applicable laws, regulations, and standards; ensuring competency of personnel; and ensuring environmental control of the storage and compounding areas.[8]

As many HDs are also hazards that are identified in the revised HCS, the requirements of the HCS must also be met.[57] A fundamental element of this safety program is the SDS, formerly the Material Safety Data Sheet, mandated by the HCS.[63] Employers are required to have an SDS available for all hazardous agents, including HDs, in the workplace. A comprehensive safety program must include a process for monitoring and updating the SDS database. When an HD is purchased for the first time, an SDS must be received from the manufacturer or distributor. The SDS should define the appropriate handling precautions, including protective equipment, controls, and spill management associated with the drug. SDS collections are available online through the specific manufacturer or through safety-information services. In the event an online service is used, a proper contingency plan must be in place to access this vital information in the event of a system failure.

Drugs that have been identified as requiring safe handling precautions should be clearly labeled at all times during their transport, storage, and use. The HCS requires a list of hazardous chemicals be present in the workplace as part of the written hazard communication program.[64] The HCS applies to all workers, including those handling HDs at the manufacturer and distributor levels. Employers are required to develop and implement employee training programs regarding workplace hazards and protective measures.[64]

USP chapter 800 requires that all personnel who handle HDs are responsible for understanding the fundamental practices and precautions and for continually evaluating these procedures and the quality of final HDs to prevent harm to patients, minimize exposure to personnel, and minimize contamination of the work and patient-care environment.[8]

The HCS and *USP* chapter 800 require employee training to the tasks they will perform as part of the safety program.[8,57] Personnel competency must be demonstrated every 12 months and documented.[8]

The outsides of the vials of many commercial HDs are contaminated when the vials are received in the pharmacy.[50,65–68] In 1 study, the contamination extended to the inside of the packing cartons and onto the package inserts placed around the vial within the carton.[68] This study found cyclophosphamide contamination on 100% of the cyclophosphamide vials, the outside outer packaging, and the inside outer packaging that were sampled.[68] Package leaflets (inserts) were also sampled, with 90–100% of samples found to be above the LOD. In addition, the researchers sampled primary packaging containing tablets (blister packages) of 50-mg cyclophosphamide tablets. Cyclophosphamide was quantified in all wipe samples from the tablet blister packages.[68]

Such contamination on packaging presents an exposure risk to anyone opening drug cartons or handling the vials, including workers receiving open or broken shipping cartons or selecting vials to be repackaged at a distribution point (e.g., a worker at the drug wholesaler selecting HDs for shipping containers, a pharmacy worker dividing an HD in a multidose container for repackaging into single-dose containers). These activities present risks, especially for workers who too often receive inadequate safety training.[62] Environmental services staff and patient care assistants who handle drug waste and patient waste are also at risk and are not always included in the safe handling training required by safety programs. Safety programs must identify and include all workers who may be at risk of exposure.[11,43,62]

New packaging techniques for HD vials include a film wrapper on the vials and reinforcement of the bottom of the vials with a plastic disk. Studies of specialty packaging methods have shown that these resist breakage and that the wrapper is less contaminated than detected in previous studies of the glass of the vial itself.[67,69] The packaging (cartons, vials, ampules) of HDs should be properly labeled by the manufacturer or distributor with a distinctive identifier that notifies personnel receiving them to don appropriate personal protective equipment (PPE) during their handling. Sealing these drugs in plastic bags at the distributor level provides an additional level of safety for workers who are required to unpack cartons. *USP* chapter 800 requires policies and procedures and standard operating procedures (SOPs) for labeling, packaging, and transport of HDs.[8] It should be noted that *USP* chapter 800 does not apply to manufacturers or distributors. Distributors may provide special packaging and labeling if requested by their customers.

Labeling, Packaging, Storing, and Transport of HDs from Point of Receipt

The safety program should address the entire lifecycle of HD handling, including receipt, storage, and transportation. Drug packages, bins, shelves, and storage areas for HDs must bear distinctive labels identifying those drugs as requiring special handling precautions.

Receipt of HDs. According to *USP* chapter 800, HDs listed as antineoplastic HDs on the current NIOSH HD list[55,56] and all HD APIs must be unpacked in areas that are neutral/normal or negative pressure relative to the surrounding areas.[8] HDs must not be removed from their external shipping containers in sterile compounding areas or in any area that is under positive pressure to the surrounding areas.[8] During receipt of HDs, visual examination of cartons for outward signs of damage or breakage is an important initial step in the receiving process. Policies and procedures must be in place for handling damaged cartons or containers of HDs (e.g., returning the damaged goods to the distributor using appropriate containment techniques).[8] These procedures should include the use of PPE, which must be supplied by the employer. HD spill kits must be available in the receiving area.[8] The spill kit should contain complete PPE, including a NIOSH-certified respirator, in the event no ventilation protection is available where damaged HD containers are handled.[8,70,71] As required by OSHA, a complete respiratory program, including proper training and fit-testing, must be completed by all staff required to use respirators.[70] Surgical masks do not provide adequate protection from the harmful effects of these drugs.

USP chapter 800 contains a table listing the summary of requirements for receiving and handling damaged HD shipping containers.[8] *USP* chapter 800 prefers that damaged shipping containers be transported to a C-PEC designated for nonsterile compounding before opening.[8]

Storing HDs. Segregation of HD inventory from other drug inventory improves control and reduces the number of staff members potentially exposed to the danger.[5] *USP* chapter 800 requires that HDs listed as antineoplastic HDs on the current NIOSH HD list[55,56] that require manipulation (more than counting or repackaging of final dosage forms) and HD APIs be stored separately from non-HDs.[8] HDs should be stored so as to prevent contamination and personnel exposure. These HDs must be stored in areas with sufficient external exhaust ventilation (i.e., negative-pressure rooms) having at least 12 air changes per hour (ACPH).[8] The non-antineoplastic, reproductive risk–only, and final HD dosage forms of antineoplastic HDs, as contained on the current NIOSH HD list,[55,56] may be stored with other inventory per *USP* chapter 800 if the facility's assessment of risk and policy allow it.[8]

HDs placed in inventory should be protected from potential breakage by storage in bins that have high fronts and on shelves that have guards to prevent accidental falling.[5] *USP* chapter 800 notes that HDs must be stored to prevent spillage or breakage if the container falls.[8] Special care must also be taken to secure shelves and other storage containers in the event of earthquakes or other natural disasters as appropriate. The bins must also be appropriately sized to properly contain all stock. Care should be taken to separate HD inventory to reduce potential drug errors (e.g., pulling a look-alike vial from an adjacent drug bin). To reduce transfer of HD residue from vials and cartons, all staff members must wear gloves tested to ASTM D6978 for resistance to chemotherapy (i.e., chemotherapy gloves). NIOSH notes that single chemotherapy gloves are sufficient in receiving, unpacking, and placing HDs into storage, unless there is a spill.[55] Because many studies have shown that HD residue on the drug vial itself is routine and that contamination has been reported in significant amounts,[65–69] staff should consider wearing double chemotherapy gloves when receiving, unpacking, stocking, and inventorying these drugs and selecting HD packages for further handling.[5,20] Per NIOSH 2016 recommendations, a gown and respiratory protection should also be used when spills or leaks are of concern (e.g., if a carton appears damaged) during HD receiving, unpacking, and storage activities.[55]

Transport of HDs. All transport of HD packages must be done in a manner to reduce environmental contamination in the event of accidental dropping.[5] HD packages must be placed in sealed containers and labeled with a unique identifier. Carts or other transport devices must be designed with guards to protect against falling and breakage. All individuals transporting HDs must have safety training that includes spill control and have spill kits immediately accessible.[5,57] Staff handling HDs or cleaning areas where HDs are stored or handled must be trained to recognize the unique identifying labels used to distinguish these drugs and areas.[57] Warning labels and signs must be clear to non-English readers. All personnel who work with or around HDs must be trained to appropriately perform their jobs using the established precautions and required PPE.[57]

Environment

It has long been shown that HD contamination is widespread in healthcare settings, even when primary compounding controls are in place.[6,10,11,21,42–46] *USP* chapter 800 focuses on containment of HD contamination, which is illustrated in the new terminology of ventilation controls.[8] Many prior recommendations for controlled, ventilated areas for storage and handling HDs will become mandates when *USP* chapter 800 becomes effective.[8] Similar to NIOSH and ASHP recommendations, *USP* chapter 800 requires that HDs be handled within a program that promotes patient safety, worker safety, and environmental protection.[5,6,8] Facilities must identify all areas where HDs are stored or handled.[5,6,8] As staff members in some jobs may not be proficient in English, using signs with verbal and pictorial warnings is preferred.[57] HDs should be handled in restricted areas where access is limited to authorized personnel trained in handling requirements. Break rooms and refreshment areas for staff, patients, visitors, and others should be located away from areas of potential HD contamination to reduce unnecessary exposure to staff, visitors, and others. *USP* chapter 800 requires that specific areas are designated for defined HD tasks, including receipt and unpacking, storing HDs, and compounding nonsterile and sterile HD preparations.[8] *USP* chapter 800 also requires that certain HD areas have negative pressure from surrounding areas to contain HDs and minimize risk of exposure.[8]

Compounding. Only individuals trained in the compounding of HDs should do so.[5,6,8] HDs should be compounded in a controlled area where access is limited to authorized personnel trained in handling requirements.[5,6] Sterile and nonsterile HDs must be compounded in environments that have a negative pressure to all adjacent areas.[8] Positive-pressure environments for HD compounding must not be used because of the potential spread of airborne contamination from contaminated packaging, poor handling technique, and spills.[5] Ventilation controls for sterile and nonsterile compounding are covered in the Ventilated Engineering Controls section below.

Administration. Only individuals trained in the administration of HDs should do so.[5,6,8] Nurses who administer HDs and care for patients receiving chemotherapy should meet the requirements of the Oncology Nursing Society (ONS) position statement on administration.[72] During administration, access to the administration area should be limited to patients receiving therapy and essential personnel. Eating, drinking, applying makeup, and the presence of foodstuffs should be avoided in patient care areas while HDs are administered. For inpatient therapy, where lengthy administration techniques may be required, hanging or removing HDs should be scheduled to reduce exposure of family members and ancillary staff and to avoid the potential contamination of dietary trays and personnel.

Because much of the compounding and administration of HDs throughout the United States are done in outpatient or clinic settings with patients and their family members near the compounding area, care must be taken to minimize environmental contamination and to maximize the effectiveness of cleaning (decontamination) activities. The design of such areas must include surfaces that are readily cleaned and decontaminated. Upholstered and carpeted surfaces should be avoided, as they are not readily cleaned. Several studies have shown floor contamination and the ineffectiveness of cleaning practices on both floors and surfaces.[10,36,37,40,73,74]

HDs may also be administered in nontraditional locations, such as the operating room, which presents challenges in training of personnel and in proper containment of the drugs and drug residue. Intracavitary administration of HDs (e.g., into the bladder, peritoneal cavity, or chest cavity) frequently requires equipment for which locking connections may not be available. Inhalation of some HDs to treat certain diseases also has the potential for significant worker exposure as well as environmental contamination, as closed-system administration is problematic. All staff members who handle HDs should receive safety training that includes recognition of HDs and appropriate spill response. HD spill kits, containment bags, and disposal containers must be available in all areas where HDs are handled.

Ventilated Engineering Controls

Engineering controls protect workers by removing hazardous conditions or by placing a barrier between the worker and the hazard. To safely handle HDs, ventilated engineering controls are required for primary and secondary containment of sterile and nonsterile forms of these drugs. For compounding sterile preparations, *USP* chapter 797 designated primary engineering controls, buffer areas, and clean rooms as ventilated engineering controls that provided appropriate air quality.[7] *USP* chapter 800 applies to both sterile and nonsterile compounding of HDs and has modified *USP* chapter 797 terminology to emphasize the key requirement in handling HDs, which is containment.[8] *USP* chapter 800 divides ventilated engineering controls for containment as C-PEC, used for the actual compounding, and C-SEC, in which the C-PEC is placed.[8] These guidelines only present a summary of *USP* chapters 797 and 800 and are not meant to interpret the standards and best practices described in those documents.

C-PECs

A C-PEC is defined in *USP* chapter 800 as a ventilated device designed and operated to minimize worker and environmental exposures to HDs.[8] A C-PEC functions by controlling emissions of airborne contaminants through the following[8]:

- The full or partial enclosure of a potential contaminant source.
- The use of airflow capture velocities to trap and remove airborne contaminants near their point of generation.
- The use of air pressure relationships that define the direction of airflow into the cabinet.
- The use of high-efficiency particulate air (HEPA) filtration on all potentially contaminated exhaust streams.

The C-PEC required is dictated by the type of compounding being performed, as well as other factors.

Nonsterile Compounding. For nonsterile HD compounding, a C-PEC that provides personnel and environmental protection, such as a class I BSC or containment ventilated enclosure (CVE), must be used. A C-PEC for nonsterile use does not require unidirectional airflow because the critical environment does not need to be International Organization for Standardization classified.[8] A class II BSC or a compounding aseptic containment isolator (CACI) may be used if it is dedicated to nonsterile compounding. The C-PECs used for manipulation of nonsterile HDs must either be externally vented (preferred) or have HEPA filters in series as a containment system to exhaust into the work area.[8] HEPA filters do not trap vapors and should not be used for handling vaporous HDs, either as nonsterile APIs or in other nonsterile forms.[6,75] *USP* chapter 800 allows a C-PEC that is usually used for sterile compounding (e.g., class II BSC or CACI, as defined by *USP* chapter 797, as revised in 2008) to be used for occasional nonsterile HD compounding if it is decontaminated, cleaned, and disinfected before resuming sterile compounding in that C-PEC.[8] As cleaning and decontaminating a C-PEC has not been shown to be very effective, this is not a preferred option.[73,74,76,77] The C-PEC used for nonsterile compounding must be placed in a C-SEC that has at least 12 ACPH, is externally vented, and is at negative pressure relative to adjacent areas.[8]

Sterile Compounding. To compound sterile HDs, as with any sterile compounding, the standards in *USP* chapter 797 must be followed.[7] Sterile HDs must be compounded in a

C-PEC that provides ISO class 5 or better air quality and unidirectional airflow. A class II or class III BSC or a CACI is an appropriate ventilated engineering control for compounding sterile HDs.[8] C-PECs for sterile compounding must be located in a C-SEC that is either an ISO class 7 buffer room with an ISO class 7 anteroom (preferred) or an unclassified containment segregated compounding area (C-SCA).[8] *USP* chapter 800 requires C-PECs used for compounding of sterile HDs to be externally vented to the outside.[8]

Class II BSCs. Class II BSCs have been used to provide product, personnel, and environmental protection while compounding sterile HDs for over 3 decades. As specific and sensitive analytic methods have been developed to measure representative or marker HDs, studies have shown continuing HD contamination on surfaces in HD work areas and detected HDs in the urine of healthcare workers exposed to these drugs while compounding in a class II BSC.[10,16,42,46] The exact cause of contamination has yet to be determined, but it is probably a combination of issues. Studies have shown that (1) there is contamination on the outside of vials received from manufacturers and distributors,[65–69] (2) work practices required to maximize the effectiveness of the class II BSC are neglected or not taught,[78,79] and (3) the potential vaporization of HD solutions may reduce the effectiveness of the HEPA filter in providing containment.[75,80] Studies of surface contamination have discovered deposits of HDs on the floor in front of the class II BSC, indicating that drug may have escaped through the open front of the BSC onto contaminated gloves or the final product, or into the air.[10,42,46] Workers must understand that the class II BSC does not prevent the generation of contamination within the cabinet and that the effectiveness of such cabinets in containing HD contamination depends on operators' use of proper technique and strict adherence to policies and procedures.

Class II BSCs types A2, B1, and B2 are acceptable under *USP* chapter 800 for compounding sterile HDs.[8] *USP* chapter 800 notes that the type A2 cabinet, which recirculates a portion of the HD-contaminated air through HEPA filters while exhausting the remainder to the outside, can be reliably integrated with ventilation systems and accommodates the pressurization requirements of *USP* chapter 800 for the C-SEC. Class II type B2 BSCs exhaust all air from the cabinet through an outside ventilation system, recirculating none of the HD-contaminated air within the cabinet.[81] *USP* chapter 800 notes that these are typically reserved for use with volatile components. Class II type A1 BSCs are not appropriate for HDs, as they are not designed for integration with an outside ventilation system to exhaust to the outside.[81] Class II type A2 and B1 BSCs recirculate a portion of the contaminated air but are designed to connect to an outside ventilation system and exhaust the predominant amount.[81] A new class II BSC, the type C1, is currently available but is not certified by NSF International (NSF).[82,83] The class II type C1 cabinet is a recirculating cabinet with outside exhaust capabilities. It may be useful in handling HDs, but additional testing and validation are needed to document this.

Most class II BSCs recirculate contaminated air within the cabinet through HEPA filters, which may not trap all HDs, allowing them to pass into the HEPA-filtered air.[75,80,83] The class II BSC is designed with air plenums that are unreachable for surface decontamination; the plenum under the work tray collects room dirt and debris that mix with HD residue when the cabinet is operational.[4] Drafts, supply-air louvers, and other laminar airflow equipment placed adjacent to the class II BSC can interfere with the containment properties of the inflow air barrier, resulting in contamination of the work environment.[81,84] Additional information on classes and types of BSCs is available through the Centers for Disease Control and Prevention (CDC).[81] More information on the design and use of class II BSCs is available from NSF/American National Standards Institute (ANSI) standard 49.[83] Recommendations for use of class II BSCs are listed in **Appendix B**.

Alternatives to Class II BSCs. *USP* chapter 800 identifies the class III BSC and the CACI as acceptable ventilated engineering controls for compounding sterile HDs. These offer alternatives to the open-front class II BSC.[8]

Class III BSC. By definition, a class III BSC is a totally enclosed, ventilated cabinet of leak-tight construction.[81] Operations in the cabinet are conducted through fixed-glove access. The cabinet is maintained under negative air pressure. Supply air is drawn into the cabinet through HEPA filters. The exhaust air is treated by double HEPA filtration or by HEPA filtration and incineration. Class III cabinets are not exhausted through the general exhaust system. The class III BSC is designed for use with highly toxic or infectious material. Because of the costs of purchasing and operating a class III BSC, it is not commonly used for extemporaneous compounding of sterile preparations.[5]

CACI. A CACI is a form of compounding isolator specifically designed for compounding pharmaceutical ingredients or preparations that provides worker protection from exposure to undesirable levels of airborne drug throughout the compounding and material transfer processes and provides an aseptic environment with unidirectional airflow for compounding sterile preparations.[7,8] Air exchange with the surrounding environment should not occur unless the air is first passed through a microbial retentive filter (HEPA minimum) system capable of containing airborne concentrations of the physical size and state of the drug being compounded. Where volatile HDs are prepared, the exhaust air from the compounding isolator should be appropriately removed by properly designed building ventilation.[7,8]

Unlike class II BSCs, which have a standard to which they are designed and validated,[83] there have been few performance measures for the compounding isolator. *USP* chapter 797 created performance criteria for the CACI, including unidirectional airflow,[7] and the Controlled Environment Testing Association has established several performance guides, testing requirements, and servicing instructions that may be used with CACIs to ensure their effectiveness for the compounding of HDs.[85–88]

For compounding sterile preparations, the filtered air and airflow must achieve an ISO class 5 environment within the CACI.[7,89] The totally enclosed design may reduce the escape of contamination during the compounding process, and the CACI may be less sensitive to drafts and other laminar airflow equipment. Issues unique to CACIs include pressure changes when accessing the fixed-glove assembly, pressure changes in the main chamber when accessing the antechamber (compounding isolator pass-through), and ergonomic considerations associated with a fixed-glove assembly. Compounding isolators must be continuously monitored for leaks in the gloves and the fixed-glove assembly. Glove changes must be done routinely, and facilities must have policies for the frequency of such changes. As in all sterile HD compounding, the glove closest to the sterile preparation must be sterile.

CACIs, like class II BSCs, do not prevent the generation of contamination within the cabinet workspace, and their effectiveness in containing contamination depends on proper technique.[41,90,91] The potential for the spread of HD contamination from the antechamber and main chamber of the CACI to the workroom may be reduced by surface decontamination, but no wipe-down procedures have been studied. Surface decontamination may be more readily conducted in CACIs than in class II BSCs; however, opening the front of the CACI to improve access may allow surface contamination to escape the enclosure. Cleaning the enclosure through the glove ports generally requires tools and may be difficult for some operators. (See the Decontamination, Deactivation, and Cleaning section below for more information.)

Recirculating CACIs depend on high-efficiency (HEPA or ultra-low penetrating air) filters. These filters may not sufficiently remove volatile HD contamination from the airflow. CACIs that discharge air into the workroom, even through high-efficiency filters, present exposure concerns similar to those of unvented class II BSCs. If there is a possibility that the HDs handled in them may vaporize, they will not be contained in a filter. *USP* chapter 800 requires outside exhaust.[8] CACIs used for compounding HDs should be at negative pressure or use a pressurized airlock to the surrounding areas to improve containment. Some compounding isolators rely on a low-particulate environment rather than laminar airflow technology to protect the sterility of the preparations and are not recommended for compounding sterile hazardous preparations.[8] Recommendations for use of class III BSCs and CACIs are summarized in **Appendix C**.

C-SECs

USP chapter 800 requires that C-PECs used to compound sterile and nonsterile HDs be located in a C-SEC, which may be either an ISO class 7 buffer room with an ISO class 7 anteroom (preferred) or an unclassified C-SCA.[8] The C-SEC must be vented to the outside, be physically separated from non-HD preparation areas, have appropriate ACPH, and be at negative pressure to all adjacent areas. If the negative pressure in the C-SEC is supplied either all or in part by the C-PEC, the C-PEC must operate continuously.[8] The C-PEC must also operate continuously if used for sterile compounding.[8] The allowance for HD compounding in a C-SCA is new, as this was not allowed in *USP* chapter 797 and will be allowed only after *USP* chapter 800 takes effect.[7,8] The beyond-use date of all CSPs compounded in a C-SCA, however, must be limited as described in *USP* chapter 797.[7,8]

Containment Supplemental Engineering Controls

USP chapter 800 describes a third level of control, a containment supplemental engineering control, which provides adjunct controls to offer an additional level of protection during compounding or administration of HDs.[8]

The device most frequently discussed in this category is the closed-system drug-transfer device (CSTD). The NIOSH definition of a CSTD, adopted by *USP* chapter 800, is a drug transfer device that mechanically prohibits the transfer of environmental contaminants into the system and the escape of HD or vapor concentrations outside the system.[6,8] The continued discovery of HD contamination in compounding and administration areas, despite adherence to HD safe handling guidelines, has generated an interest in CSTDs, especially for administration areas where C-PECs are not available during HD administration. The initial CSTD, developed in Europe, was tested in 1996–97 during compounding and administration by 3 nurses for 1 year in an outpatient setting. Compared to surface contamination of similar work areas reported in the literature, the closed system was more effective than the BSC in reducing contamination during preparation.[92]

In originally defining the CSTD in 2004, NIOSH did not specify design or performance criteria for what constitutes an effective CSTD.[6] A number of devices marketed as CSTDs have appeared since 2004. These devices are designated by FDA as class II medical devices, not requiring premarket approval.[93] The FDA 510(k) process does not establish independent performance standards for devices submitted as "substantially equivalent" nor does it test or approve these devices. Based on a successful review of the manufacturer's 510(k) submission, FDA clears the new device for sale in the United States [93] Many devices marketed for i.v. compounding or administration have been cleared by the FDA 510(k) process under various product codes. Many of the devices marketed and used for HD compounding are not CSTDs by definition and may not be appropriate for HD use. FDA created a product code, ONB, specifically for a closed antineoplastic and HD reconstitution and transfer system.[94] Although applications under this code are not independently tested by FDA, the application process is more stringent for the manufacturer and the code specifically addresses antineoplastics and HDs. Products that are marketed as CSTDs but have not been cleared by FDA under the product code ONB should not be considered CSTDs.

Although some CSTDs have been shown in peer-reviewed studies to limit the potential of generating aerosols and reduce HD contamination in the workplace, not all marketed CSTDs have been studied, and no surrogate or marker HD has been shown to be superior in measuring CSTD effectiveness or has been universally adopted for that purpose. The NIOSH topics page includes an expanded bibliography of publications related to CSTDs.[95] In the absence of a performance standard, NIOSH is attempting to develop protocols to test the containment performance of both the physical barrier type of CSTD and CSTDs designed to operate using air-cleaning technologies.[96,97] Difficulties encountered in this attempt include the selection of surrogates to represent HDs and the method to capture and analyze the surrogates. The NIOSH protocols are a positive step in evaluating these devices. As other products become available, they should meet the definition of CSTDs established by NIOSH[6] and should be required to demonstrate their effectiveness in independent studies.[8] CSTDs (or any other ancillary devices) are not a substitute for using a ventilated cabinet.[6,8]

The use of ventilated engineering controls during the compounding of HDs provides protection for the worker as well as the sterile preparation. During the administration of HDs, there are no similar controls available. For these reasons, *USP* chapter 800 has determined that CSTDs should be used when compounding HDs and that CSTDs must be used when administering antineoplastic HDs when the dosage form allows and the device is physically or chemically compatible with the HD to be used.[8]

USP chapter 800 notes that there is no certainty that all CSTDs will perform adequately, and, without a standard for evaluating CSTD containment, users will have to rely on independent, peer-reviewed studies and demonstrated contamination reduction to evaluate performance claims.[8]

PPE

PPE provides worker protection to reduce exposure to HD aerosols and residues. However, in the hierarchy of controls, PPE is the least-effective measure for protecting workers.[98] Additional PPE may be required to handle the HDs outside of a C-PEC, such as treating a patient or cleaning a spill. The NIOSH list of antineoplastic and other HDs provides general guidance on PPE for possible scenarios that may be encountered in healthcare settings.[12] NIOSH has also created a Workplace Solution on PPE containing detailed recommendations with references.[99] Disposable PPE must not be reused. Reusable PPE, such as a face shield or cartridge respirator, must be decontaminated and cleaned after use. *USP* chapter 800 has an extensive discussion of PPE and its appropriate use but requires that the entity develop SOPs for PPE based on its own safety plan and assessment of risk.[8] The following summary of PPE use is not designed to replace or interpret the best practice mandates of *USP*.[7,8]

Removal of PPE. PPE used to compound HDs, dispose of HDs, and clean up an HD spill should be considered contaminated with HD residue. PPE used to administer HDs, perform patient care, or discard patient waste should be considered contaminated with HD residue and potentially contaminated with infectious material. Removal of PPE must be done cautiously to avoid transferring contamination to skin, the environment, or other surfaces that may be touched with uncovered skin. Wearing double gloves provides an additional barrier to possible contamination transfer as the hands are covered until the last item of PPE is removed. After any handling of HDs, the outer gloves should be removed 1 at a time with the contaminated glove fingers touching only the outer surface of the other glove, never the inner surface. The first glove should be removed and then turned inside out. Still wearing the inner, clean glove, personnel should place the fingers underneath the wrist of the second, outer glove and roll the glove down, turning it carefully inside out to avoid touching the outside. The face shield, if worn, should be removed next, while avoiding contact with the front. Personnel should then remove the gown, using care to avoid transfer of contamination to clothes and skin. They should then turn the gown inside out, fold it tightly, and discard it as trace waste. Other PPE (e.g., hair coverings, facemask, shoe coverings) should then be carefully removed, from least contaminated to most contaminated. The inner gloves should be removed last and discarded in the HD disposal container. Hands should be washed with soap and water.

Gloves. Gloves are essential when handling HDs. Glove use has been more clearly described by *USP* and NIOSH as the definition of HDs has expanded to include nonantineoplastic HDs and reproductive risk–only HDs and the catalog of formulations of HDs similarly enlarged to encompass APIs used in compounding, final dosage forms of compounded HD preparations, and manufactured HD products.[8,55]

Although double gloving is required by *USP* chapter 800 in only select circumstances,[8] wearing 2 pairs of gloves allows removal of the outer glove while the skin of the hand and wrist is still covered. Changing the outer glove while retaining the inner glove during any HD handling is a work practice that provides added protection against skin contact with HDs. Many studies have shown that areas where HDs are handled have significant surface contamination and workers are at risk of absorbing HDs through uncovered skin any time they come into contact with this contamination.[10,11,21,43,46] A single, thicker glove, tested as a chemotherapy glove, may provide the same protection as 2 pairs of chemotherapy gloves against permeation during compounding and administration, but it does not provide the protection of never having exposed skin in a contaminated area. Double gloving and good work practices provide better protection. Facilities writing policies and procedures, especially detailing work practices, should consider requiring wearing double chemotherapy gloves when receiving and stocking HDs, selecting HD packages for further handling, handling drug waste and patient waste, cleaning spills, performing routine cleaning with detergents and disinfectants, and any situation in which an exposed hand or wrist may create a risk of touch contamination with HD residue on surfaces. NIOSH allows single gloves for receiving, unpacking, and placing HDs in storage.[55] Because broken cartons and containers of HDs represent a major risk of worker exposure while receiving and unpacking, any package that does not appear intact should be handled with 2 pairs of chemotherapy gloves. Workers should visually examine the shipping container or tote for damage, as described in *USP* chapter 800, and then determine the appropriate PPE.[8] NIOSH also allows single gloves for handling intact, unit-dose oral agents when no cutting or crushing is required.[55] NIOSH recommends double gloves for spill control and for cleaning and disposal of HD waste and patient waste.[55] *USP* chapter 800 and Table 5 of the current NIOSH HD list should be consulted for specific information about glove use.[8,55]

ASTM International has developed testing standards for assessing the resistance of medical gloves to permeation by chemotherapy drugs, ASTM D6978-05 (2013).[100] This standard tests gloves for resistance to permeation to a group of HDs selected for characteristics of toxicity, diluent, and ability to permeate standard gloving material, among others. Gloves are not tested for all known HDs because of the cost and lack of assays for many drugs, so these drugs act as markers for permeability. Gloves passing this ASTM standard may be labeled as "chemotherapy gloves." ASTM F739-12e1 (2012) is also a permeation standard, but it is specific neither to gloves nor to chemotherapy drugs and should not be used to test chemotherapy gloves.[100–102] The performance requirement of ASTM F739-12e1 is only one tenth that of ASTM D6978-05, and ASTM F739-12e1 is performed at room temperature rather than body temperature, which results in less drug permeation being measured and less-protective gloves to be marketed as chemotherapy gloves.[100–102] Staff purchasing gloves and staff using them for handling HDs must verify that the gloves are tested against ASTM D6978. *USP* chapter 800 requires that chemotherapy gloves must meet ASTM D6978.[8]

Many guidance documents have recommended gloves both for sterile compounding and for any handling of HDs be powder-free to avoid powder particulates from contaminating sterile processing areas and to prevent absorption of HD contaminants, which may increase the potential for dermal contact.[5] This issue was resolved when FDA issued a ban on powdered gloves effective January 18, 2017.[103] FDA states that the use of powder on medical gloves presents numerous risks to patients and healthcare workers, including inflammation, granulomas, and respiratory allergic reactions.[103]

As latex sensitivity is a concern to healthcare workers and patients, gloves made of nitrile and neoprene have been tested against different HDs, with nitrile demonstrating a high resistance to permeation by multiple HDs.[104–106] In a review of glove standards and studies done in the European Union and United States, Landeck et al.[107] determined that for gloves used for extended exposure to HDs, double gloving, the use of thicker gloves, and frequent glove changes increased worker protection. They recommend regular glove changes every 15–20 minutes with constant exposure to chemotherapy drugs.[107]

USP chapter 800 requires that gloves selected for use with HDs must meet ASTM D6978-05 (or its successor) and requires that 2 pairs of chemotherapy gloves are used for compounding sterile and nonsterile HDs. For sterile compounding, the outermost glove must be sterile.[7,8] During sterile compounding in a class II BSC, 2 pairs of ASTM D6978-approved gloves are required, with the outermost pair being sterile. During sterile compounding in a class III BSC and a CACI, both of which are equipped with attached gloves or gauntlets, the gauntlet, sleeve and fixed-glove assembly must be cleaned and disinfected before sterile compounding using an appropriate cleaner and disinfectant applied with a sterile wiper. The fixed glove, if disposable, must be changed before compounding and sanitized per the manufacturer's instructions. A pair of sterile ASTM D6978-approved gloves must be placed in the pass-through and brought into the C-PEC work area and donned over the glove connected to the gauntlet or over the fixed-glove assembly. The outermost glove must be sterile. Supplies of sterile ASTM D6978-approved gloves must be kept near the C-PEC to allow changing of the outermost glove as needed.

USP chapter 800 notes that chemotherapy gloves should be worn for handling all HDs, including nonantineoplastic HDs and for reproductive risk–only HDs, and that 2 pairs of chemotherapy gloves are required for administering antineoplastic HDs.[8] Gloves should be inspected for visible defects before donning. When double gloves are worn with a gown, the inner glove should be placed underneath the gown cuff and the outer glove over the gown cuff. There should be no skin exposed at the wrist.

Based on the ASTM D6978 permeability testing, the maximum recommended wear time for gloves is 30 minutes. Certain drugs may permeate more quickly (e.g., carmustine, thiotepa).[100] When handling these drugs, gloves should be changed according to the permeation time listed on the glove packaging. Gloves should be removed immediately if torn, punctured, or knowingly contaminated. The same wear-time restrictions apply to the outermost glove in the class III BSC or CACI.

When compounding in a class II BSC, gloves (at minimum the outermost gloves) must be changed whenever it is necessary to exit and reenter the BSC. Gloves worn during the administration of HDs must be removed at the completion of administration, if gloves are visibly damaged or contaminated, and before leaving the administration area to prevent the spread of HD residue to other areas. For the aseptic protection of sterile preparations, the outermost sterile gloves must be sanitized with an appropriate disinfectant (e.g., sterile isopropyl alcohol 70%) by wiping with a sterile wiper saturated with the disinfectant when reentering the BSC. Personnel should never spray anything on contaminated gloves or any other potentially contaminated surface, as this may generate aerosols and spread HD contamination.[108]

When removing HD gloves, the contaminated glove fingers must only touch the outer surface of the glove, never the inner surface. If the innermost glove becomes contaminated, both pairs of gloves must be changed. Both the innermost and outermost gloves should be considered contaminated, and glove surfaces must never contact the skin or any surface that may be touched by the unprotected skin of others. HD contamination may be distributed to other surfaces during compounding, other handling, or glove removal and may be a source of surface contamination and subsequent dermal absorption of HDs by workers not actively involved in the compounding, administration, or other tasks involving HDs or who are not wearing PPE.[11,21,109] Gloves used to compound HDs in the class II BSC should be placed in a sealable plastic bag for containment within the C-PEC before disposal as contaminated waste. The outermost glove attached to the class III BSC or CACI fixed glove or gauntlet must be removed from the assembly and placed in a sealable plastic bag for containment within the C-PEC before disposal as contaminated waste. During compounding, HD contamination may be transferred to the gloves or gauntlets and then transferred to the surfaces of all items within the C-PEC. Fixed-glove and gauntlet surfaces must be cleaned after HD compounding to avoid the potential spread and cross-contamination of HD residue to other surfaces. All final preparations must be surface decontaminated while wearing ASTM D6978-approved gloves to avoid spreading contamination, and the clean inner glove must be used to apply labels.

Proper hand hygiene must be practiced before donning and after removing any PPE. Hands should be cleaned with soap and water after PPE is removed. Sanitizing gels should not be used until hands are thoroughly cleaned of HD residue, as rubbing gels into hands may increase the dermal absorption of any HD residue.[110]

Recommendations for use of gloves are summarized in **Appendix D**.

Gowns. Gowns are worn during the compounding of HD preparations to protect the preparation from the worker, the worker from the preparation, or both.[5] Any sterile compounding requires PPE to protect the aseptic compounding environment from the biological contamination that is presented by the worker. The requirements of both *USP* chapters 797 and 800 must be met for sterile compounding.[7,8] *USP* chapter 800 requires gowns; head, hair, and shoe covers; and 2 pairs of chemotherapy gloves for compounding sterile and nonsterile HDs.[8] HD compounding in an enclosed environment, such as a class III BSC or a CACI, has not been exempted from the gowning requirement. *USP* chapter 800 further requires that gowns that show resistance to permeability by HDs be worn when administering injectable antineoplastic HDs. Additional policies for gowns, as for other PPE, must be established by the entity and delineated in the procedures.

The selection of gowning materials depends on the goal of the process. Personal protective gowns are recommended during the handling of HD preparations to protect the worker from inadvertent exposure to extraneous drug particles on surfaces or generated during the compounding process and leakage of any liquid forms of HDs. HD gowns must be disposable and shown to resist HD permeability. Disposable gowns made of polyethylene-coated polypropylene (e.g., spunbond/meltblown/spunbond) provide better protection than uncoated gowns.[5,8] Basic characteristics for HD gowns include that they close in the back with no open front, have long sleeves with tight-fitting elastic or knit cuffs to fit over gloves, and have no seams or closures to allow powder or liquid HD residue to pass through.[5,8] Washable garments (e.g., laboratory coats, scrubs, cloth gowns) absorb fluids and provide no barrier against HD absorption and permeation.[5,8] To avoid spreading contamination, potentially contaminated clothing must never be taken home.[8]

There is no specific standard for gowns or gowning materials to be tested for permeation by HDs. ASTM F739-12e1 is a test method for permeation by liquids and gases through protective clothing materials under conditions of continuous contact, but it does not specify drugs or concentrations to be tested and has no performance standard for an acceptable resistance to HD permeation.[101] Some gowns are tested using the ASTM F739 parameters and the chemotherapy drugs and concentrations from D6978.[100] This practice has not been studied for effectiveness or safety. HD gowns should be coated and labeled as impervious per manufacturer testing.

Gowns should be changed per the manufacturer's recommendations. If there is no specific information, coated gowns should be changed every 2–3 hours.[5,8] Gowns must be changed immediately after a spill or splash. Contamination of gowns during glove changes must be a consideration. If the inner pair of gloves requires changing, a gown change may be needed. Gowns worn as barrier protection in the handling of HDs must never be worn outside the immediate handling areas. Gowns worn during administration should be changed when leaving the patient care area and immediately if contaminated. Gowns should be removed carefully and properly disposed of as trace-contaminated waste to avoid becoming a source of contamination to other staff and the environment.[5,6] Gowns used for cleaning or spill management may be more heavily contaminated. These gowns should be contained in sealable bags and discarded as bulk hazardous waste.

Researchers have looked at gown contamination with fluorescent scans, high-performance liquid chromatography, and tandem mass spectrometry.[111,112] In 1 study, researchers scanned nurses and pharmacists wearing gowns during the compounding and administration of HDs.[111] Of a total of 18 contamination spots detected, 5 were present on the gowns of nurses after drug administration. No spots were discovered on the gowns of pharmacists after compounding. In contrast, researchers using a more sensitive assay placed pads in various body locations, both over and under the gowns used by the subjects during compounding and administration of cyclophosphamide and ifosfamide.[112] Workers wore short-sleeved nursing uniforms, disposable or cotton gowns, and vinyl or latex gloves. More contamination was found during compounding than administration. Contamination found on the pads placed on the arms of preparers was consistent with the design and typical work practices used in a class II BSC, where the hands and arms are extended into the contaminated work area of the cabinet. Remarkably, 1 preparer had contamination on the back of the gown, possibly indicating touch contamination with the class II BSC during removal of the final product. Pads were used in 2 additional studies to assess HD contamination on the workers' bodies.[113,114] Pads placed on the arms and chest of workers involved in compounding and administration showed evidence of touch contamination with HD residue on the studied areas. Without protective gowns, the HD residue may have contaminated skin or worker clothing, resulting in drug uptake or transfer.

Recommendations for the use of gowns are summarized in **Appendix E**.

Eye and Face Protection. Many HDs are irritating to the eyes and mucous membranes. Appropriate eye and face protection must be worn when there is a risk of spills or splashes, when HD waste materials are handled, or when working outside of a C-PEC (e.g., administration in the surgical suite, working at or above eye level, cleaning a spill). Face shields should be used in combination with goggles to provide a full range of protection against splashes to the face and eyes. Although face shields provide improved skin protection, face shields alone do not deliver full eye and face protection.[8,99] Goggles must be used when eye protection is required.[8] Eyeglasses alone or safety glasses with side shields do not sufficiently protect the eyes from splashes and therefore are not suitable when handling HDs. A full-face piece respirator provides complete eye and face protection.[8]

Respirator Protection. Staff unpacking HDs that are not contained in plastic should wear an elastomeric half-mask with a multigas cartridge and P100 particulate filter.[8] All workers who may use a respirator must be fit-tested by a certified fit tester and instructed on the use of the appropriate respirator according to the OSHA Respiratory Protection Standard.[70,71] A respirator of the correct size and suitable to the aerosol size, physical state (i.e., particulate or vapor), and concentration of the airborne drug must be available at all times. Surgical masks do not provide respiratory protection and therefore should on no occasion be used when respiratory protection is required for HDs.[6,8] N95 respirators offer no protection against gases and vapors and negligible protection against direct liquid splashes.[71] A surgical N95 respirator provides the respiratory protection of an N95 respirator and, like a surgical mask, provides a barrier to splashes, droplets, and sprays around the nose and mouth.[8]

Shoe and Hair Coverings. Shoe and hair coverings must be worn throughout the sterile compounding process to minimize particulate contamination of the critical work zone and the preparation.[7] With the potential for HD contamination on the floor in the compounding and administration areas, donning of 2 pairs of shoe coverings, as the contamination-control mechanism, must occur. Contaminated shoe covers must never be worn outside of the immediate HD area to avoid spreading contamination.[8] The outer shoe covers must be removed with gloved hands when exiting the compounding area. Gloves are required, and care must be taken, when removing hair or shoe covers, to prevent contamination from spreading to uncontaminated areas. Hair and shoe coverings used in the HD handling areas must be contained, along with used gloves, and discarded as trace contaminated waste in the appropriate waste receptacle. Shoe coverings that are overtly contaminated, as in spill cleanup, should be disposed of as hazardous waste.

Work Practices

Compounding Sterile HDs. Work practices for the compounding of sterile HDs differ somewhat with the use of a specific C-PEC. Good organizational skills are essential to minimize contamination and maximize productivity. All activities not requiring a critical environment (e.g., checking labels, performing calculations) should be completed before accessing the C-PEC. All items needed for compounding must be gathered before beginning work to eliminate the need to exit the C-PEC once compounding has begun. Two pairs of ASTM D6978-approved gloves should be worn to gather HD vials, due to the frequent findings of HD residue on vials, and 1 or 2 pairs of ASTM D6978-approved gloves may be worn to gather other supplies. All areas where HDs are received, stored, handled, and wasted have been shown to be contaminated with HD residue. Prudent practice is to wear 2 pairs of gloves.[6,8,10,11,20,21,43] After tasks are completed, these gloves should be carefully removed and discarded as contaminated waste. Fresh ASTM D6978-approved gloves must be donned before aseptic manipulation. For the compounding of sterile HDs, the ASTM D6978-approved glove closest to the sterile preparation must be sterile.

Only supplies and drugs essential to compounding the dose or batch should be placed in the work area of the C-PEC. C-PECs should not be crowded to avoid unnecessary HD contamination and disrupting airflow. Luer-Lok connections on syringes and on all compounding and ancillary devices must be used whenever possible for manipulating HDs, as they are less likely to separate during compounding and administration.

Spiking an i.v. set into a solution containing HDs or priming an i.v. set with HD solution in an uncontrolled environment must be avoided. One recommendation is to attach and prime the appropriate i.v. set to the final container in the C-PEC before adding the HD. CSTDs should achieve a dry connection between the administration set and the HD's final container. This connection allows the container to be spiked with a secondary i.v. set and the set to be primed by backflow from a primary non-HD solution. This process may be done outside the C-PEC, reducing the potential for surface contamination of the i.v. set during the compounding process. Only CSTDs that have been tested to achieve a dry connection may be considered for use with this technique. Personnel should avoid placing the i.v. set on the surface of the C-PEC during compounding to reduce the transfer of HD residue from the surface of the C-PEC to the surface of the i.v. set. Care must also be taken to avoid contaminating the tubing with HD residue from the surface of the gloves. A new i.v. set must be used with each dose of HD. Once attached, the i.v. set must never be removed from an HD dose, thereby preventing the residual fluid in the bag, bottle, or tubing from leaking and contaminating personnel and the environment.

In order to avoid inadvertent contamination of the outer surface of the bag by transfer of HD residue, transport bags must never be placed in the C-PEC work area during compounding. Final HD preparations must be surface decontaminated after compounding is complete. In any type of C-PEC, clean ASTM D6978-approved gloves must be worn when labeling and placing the final HD preparation into the transport bag. Handling final preparations and transport bags with gloves contaminated with HD residue will result in the transfer of the contamination to other workers. Personnel should don clean ASTM D6978-approved gloves whenever there is a doubt as to the cleanliness of the inner or outer gloves.

Working in Any C-PEC. With or without ancillary devices (e.g., CSTDs), none of the available ventilated engineering controls can provide 100% protection for the worker. Personnel must recognize the limitations of the equipment and address them through appropriate work practices.[4,5] PPE use with C-PECs is addressed by *USP*[8] and NIOSH[55] (see also the PPE section above). The effectiveness of C-PECs in containing HD contamination depends on proper technique.[47] HD contamination from the work area of the CACI (e.g., on the surfaces of the final preparation) may be brought into the antechamber or airlocks of the CACI and ultimately into the workroom environment. Surface decontamination of the preparation before removal from the CACI's main chamber should reduce the HD contamination that could be transferred to the workroom, but no wipe-down procedures for final preparations have been studied. Surface contamination may be removed by using isopropyl alcohol, sterile water, peroxide, or sodium hypochlorite solutions on disposable pads and wiping the surface of the final preparation, provided the packaging is not permeable to the solution and the labels remain legible and intact.

Recommendations for working in C-PECs are summarized in **Appendix F**.

Class II BSCs. Class II BSCs use unidirectional, vertical-flow, HEPA-filtered air (ISO class 5) as their controlled aseptic environment. Before beginning an operation in a class II BSC, personnel should follow the hand-washing and PPE requirements of *USP* chapters 797 and 800.[7,8] For cleaning the class II BSC, nonsterile ASTM D6978-approved gloves are appropriate. Sterile ASTM D6978-approved gloves must be available near the class II BSC to allow changes of gloves during sterile HD compounding. The class II BSC work surface should be cleaned of surface contamination with detergent, sodium hypochlorite, and neutralizer or an independently tested alternative cleaner. Between cleanings, the compounding surface must be disinfected with sterile 70% isopropyl alcohol applied with a sterile wiper, never using a spray. For the class II BSC, the front shield must be lowered to the proper level to protect the face and eyes. The operator should be seated so that his or her shoulders are at the level of the bottom of the front shield. All drugs and supplies needed to aseptically compound a dose or batch should be gathered and disinfected with sterile 70% isopropyl alcohol before being placed in the direct compounding area (DCA) of the C-PEC. Exiting and reentering the work area should be avoided. Being careful not to place any sterile objects below them, i.v. bags and bottles may be hung from the bar. All items must be placed well within the class II BSC, away from the unfiltered air at the front barrier. By design, the intended work zone within the class II BSC is the area between the front and rear air grilles. The containment characteristics of the class II BSC are dependent on the airflow through both the front and back grilles; these grilles should never be obstructed. Due to the design of the class II BSC, the quality of HEPA-filtered air is lowest at the sides of the work zone, so manipulations should be performed at least 6 inches away from each sidewall in the horizontal plane. A small waste-sharps container may be placed along the sidewall toward the back of the BSC. Per *USP* chapter 800, a plastic-backed preparation mat should be placed on the work surface of a C-PEC before compounding HDs.[8] One study has suggested that a plastic-backed absorbent preparation pad in a class II BSC may interfere with airflow,[112] but another study determined that use of a flat firm pad that did not block the grilles of the cabinet had no effect on airflow.[115] The use of a large pad that might block the front or rear grilles must be avoided. In addition, because a pad may absorb small spills, it may become a source of HD contamination for anything placed upon it. Preparation pads are not readily decontaminated and must be replaced and discarded after preparation of each batch and frequently during compounding. The mat should be changed immediately if a spill occurs.[8] Equipment for HD compounding must be dedicated. Work practices for sterile compounding of HDs must adhere to *USP* chapters 797 and 800.[7,8] More information on the design and use of class II BSCs is available from the CDC[81] and NSF/ANSI Standard 49-2016.[83]

Class III BSCs and CACIs. At least 1 pair of ASTM D6978-approved gloves should be worn to prepare for work in a class III BSC or a CACI. Using 2 pairs of gloves allows changing only the outer pair while handling vials and supplies. Wearing gloves, workers must gather all drugs and supplies needed to aseptically compound an HD dose or batch, sanitize them, and ready them for placement into the antechamber of the compounding isolator. Supplies and drugs in the antechamber are disinfected with sterile 70% isopropyl alcohol when taken into the main chamber (the DCA) of the compounding isolator, where the drug and supplies are used to compound the dose. The contaminated supplies are removed using the closed trash system of the compounding isolator, if so equipped, or sealed into a transport bag and removed via the antechamber for disposal as contaminated waste. The dose is then labeled and placed into a sealable bag for transport in the antechamber. The transport bag is never placed in the DCA of the compounding isolator to avoid contaminating the outer surface.

For sterile compounding, the gloves closest to the sterile preparation must also be sterile.[7,8] Sterile gloves must be placed into the antechamber to be transferred into the DCA. Additional work practices may include cleaning off the gloves or gauntlets and final preparation after initial compounding and before handling the label and sealable transport bag. Care must be taken when transferring products out of the antechamber and disposing of waste through the antechamber or trash chute to avoid accidental contamination.

Aseptic Technique. Stringent aseptic technique, described by Wilson and Solimando[116] in 1981, remains the foundation of any procedure involving the use of needles and syringes in manipulating sterile dosage forms. This technique, when performed in conjunction with negative-pressure technique, minimizes the escape of drug from vials and ampules. Needleless devices have been developed to reduce the risk of blood-borne pathogen exposure through needle sticks. None of these devices has been tested for reduction of HD contamination, and the appropriateness of these devices in the safe handling of HDs has not been determined. CSTDs have been developed to reduce the release of HD residue during compounding, but not all HDs or all types of sterile compounding are compatible with CSTDs. Stringent aseptic technique using needles and syringes is a necessary skill, especially for those occasions when no ancillary device is available or appropriate.

In reconstituting HDs in vials, it is critical to avoid pressurizing the contents of the vial. Pressurization may cause the drug to spray out around the needle or through a needle hole or a loose seal, aerosolizing the HD into the work zone. Pressurization can be avoided by creating a slight negative pressure in the vial. Too much negative pressure, however, can cause leakage from the needle when it is withdrawn from the vial. The safe handling of HD solutions in vials or ampules requires the use of a syringe that is no more than three-fourths full when filled with the solution, which minimizes the risk of the plunger separating from the syringe barrel.[116] For reconstitution, once the diluent is drawn up, the needle is carefully inserted into the upright HD vial stopper, being careful not to core the stopper. The syringe plunger is then pulled back (to create a slight negative pressure inside the vial), so that air is drawn into the syringe. Small amounts of diluent should be transferred slowly into the HD vial as equal volumes of air are removed. The needle should be kept in the vial, and the contents should be swirled carefully until dissolved. For a liquid HD, the vial is kept upright while a syringe and needle are prepared. A slightly smaller amount of air than the amount of the required HD dose is drawn into the syringe. The needle is inserted into the vial stopper, being careful not to core the stopper, and the vial is inverted with the syringe and needle inserted. The proper amount of drug solution should be gradually withdrawn while equal volumes of air are exchanged for solution. The exact volume needed must be measured while the needle is in the vial, and any excess drug should remain in the vial. With the vial in the upright position, the plunger should be drawn back past the original starting point to again induce a slight negative pressure before removing the needle. The needle hub should be clear of drug solution before the needle is removed.

If an HD is transferred to an i.v. bag, care must be taken to puncture only the septum of the injection port and avoid puncturing the sides of the port or bag. After the drug solution is injected into the i.v. bag, the i.v. port, container, and set (if attached by pharmacy in the C-PEC) should be surface decontaminated. Wearing clean gloves (or the inner glove), personnel should label the final preparation, including an auxiliary warning, and cover the injection port with a protective seal. The final container should be placed into a sealable bag to contain any possible leakage.[4]

To withdraw HDs from an ampule, the neck or top portion should be gently tapped.[116] After the neck is wiped with sterile 70% isopropyl alcohol, a 5-µm filter needle or straw should be attached to a syringe that is large enough that it will not be more than three-fourths full when holding the drug. The fluid should then be drawn through the filter needle or straw and cleared from the needle and hub. After this, the needle or straw is exchanged for a needle of similar gauge and length; any air and excess drug should be ejected into a sterile vial (leaving the desired volume in the syringe); aerosolization should be avoided. The drug may then be transferred to an i.v. bag or bottle. If the dose is to be dispensed in the syringe, the plunger should be drawn back to clear fluid from the needle and hub. The needle should be replaced with a locking cap, and the syringe should be surface decontaminated and labeled.

Training and Demonstration of Competence. The OSHA HCS and *USP* chapter 800 require employee training for the tasks that will be performed as part of the safety program.[8,57] The HCS details the requirements for worker information and training in paragraph H of the HCS regulation.[57] In the 2008 revision of *USP* chapter 797, which includes HDs, the training requirements note that compounding personnel of reproductive capability must confirm in writing that they understand the risks of handling HDs.[7] This requirement is also in *USP* chapter 800.[8] ONS provides an excellent example of a worker agreement to handle HDs in the 3rd edition of *Safe Handling of Hazardous Drugs*.[110]

Personnel must be trained before handling HDs as part of their job responsibilities.[8,57] Staff handling HDs must demonstrate competency before commencing responsibilities and at least every 12 months thereafter.[8] All staff who will be compounding HDs must be trained in the stringent aseptic and negative-pressure techniques necessary for working with sterile HDs as well as all primary, secondary, and supplementary engineering controls.[8] Once trained, staff must demonstrate competence by an objective method, and competency must be reassessed on a regular basis.[117] Additional training should be carried out whenever new equipment or procedures are put in place. All training and competency testing must be clearly documented as part of the worker's safety record.[8,57]

Compounding and Handling of Nonsterile HD Dosage Forms. Nonsterile compounding of HD dosage forms must adhere to *USP* chapter 795 and *USP* chapter 800.[8,61] Best practices and mandates for other activities involved in handling of nonsterile HD forms (e.g., tablets, oral liquids) are provided in *USP* chapter 800.[8] Guidance for PPE when handling nonsterile HD dosage forms is available from NIOSH.[55]

Although nonsterile dosage forms of HDs contain varying proportions of drug to nondrug (nonhazardous) components, there is the potential for personnel exposure to and environmental contamination with the hazardous components if HDs are handled (e.g., packaged) by pharmacy staff. Most HDs are not available in liquid formulations; however, such formulations are often prescribed for small children and adults with feeding tubes. Recipes for extemporaneously compounded oral liquids may start with the parenteral form or an API, or they may require that tablets be crushed or capsules opened. Tablet trituration has been shown to cause fine dust formation and local environmental contamination.[118] Healthcare personnel should avoid manipulating HDs (e.g., crushing tablets, opening capsules) if possible. Liquid formulations are preferred if solid oral dosage forms are not appropriate for the patient. If HD dosage forms do require manipulation such as crushing tablets or opening capsules for a single dose, personnel must don appropriate PPE and use a plastic pouch to contain any dust or particles generated.

USP chapter 800 requires that compounding of nonsterile HDs be performed in a C-PEC that provides environmental and personnel protection. A class I BSC or CVE is acceptable equipment for this task. A CACI or a class II BSC may also be used if it is dedicated to nonsterile compounding. *USP* chapter 800 allows a C-PEC used for sterile HD compounding to be used for nonsterile HD compounding, provided that the C-PEC is decontaminated, cleaned, and disinfected before resuming sterile compounding in that same device. As noted above, cleaning and decontaminating a C-PEC has not been shown to be very effective, making this an undesirable solution.[73,74,76,77]

Nonsterile HD dosage forms, like oral HD capsules or tablets, vary in their risk of causing occupational exposure. The level of risk, however, depends on the tasks required to prepare and dispense the doses. Manual counting of solid medications may be problematic if, for example, repeated handling of a large container of tablets has created a loose powder or residue of tablet dust. Exposure to the dust or residue may present a risk of powder inhalation or skin contact. *USP* chapter 800 notes that an assessment of risk should be conducted to determine the appropriate containment strategies for the HD tasks required of the worker.[8]

There are risks associated with automatic pill counters, especially high-speed delivery devices. One study studied a number of drugs dispensed in this manner and found measurable drug dust concentrations in the air surrounding such devices.[119] Pill dust was generated in a variety of worker-related tasks, such as emptying and refilling the drugs in the device canisters.[119] Cleaning the device or the canisters using compressed air produced the highest amount of contamination in the air. The researchers found that workers directly involved with the automatic pill counters and those who hand-filled prescriptions were exposed to higher air concentrations of tablet fillers, like lactose, than workers who did other jobs such as administrative or office work.[119] In studies of surface contamination with sterile HDs, measurable drug levels have been found in workers, most likely due to contact of uncovered skin with drug-contaminated surfaces.[21,46] Drug residue generated in any task may be found on work surfaces and result in a potential occupational exposure. Work practices and cleaning procedures must be in place to at least reduce this exposure. Procedures for nonsterile HD compounding and other handling, as well as the appropriate use of equipment (C-PECs and other devices) for this purpose, must be developed to avoid the release of aerosolized powder or liquid into the environment during manipulation of HDs.

Recommendations for preparation and handling of nonsterile HD dosage forms are summarized in **Appendix G.**

Decontamination, Deactivation, Cleaning, and Disinfection. All guidelines agree that decontamination of areas where HDs are stored, compounded, administered, wasted, or otherwise handled is critical to reduce the levels of HD residue on various surfaces.[5,6,8,110,120] All areas where HDs are handled and all reusable equipment and devices must be decontaminated. Decontamination occurs by inactivating, neutralizing, or physically removing HD residue from nondisposable surfaces (e.g., stainless steel C-PECs) and transferring it to absorbent, disposable materials (e.g., wipes, pads, towels) appropriate to the area being cleaned. The decontaminating, deactivating, cleaning, and disinfecting agents selected must be appropriate for the type of HD contaminants, location, and surfaces to be cleaned. Consult manufacturer or supplier information for compatibility with cleaning agents used.[8] Agents used for decontamination, deactivation, and cleaning should be applied through the use of wipes wetted with appropriate solution and not delivered as a spray to avoid aerosolizing and/or spreading HD residue.

Cleaning processes must be validated for solutions and methods by surface wipe sampling of HDs that have appropriate assays.[73,74,76,77,121–124] In addition, sterile compounding (ISO 5) areas and devices must be subsequently disinfected.[7,8] Appropriate preparation of materials used in compounding before introduction into the C-PEC, including spraying (for non-HD-contaminated supplies) or wiping with sterile 70% isopropyl alcohol or appropriate disinfectant, is also necessary for sterile compounding.[7]

All personnel who perform decontamination, deactivation, cleaning, and disinfection activities must be trained in appropriate procedures to protect themselves and the environment from contamination.[7,8] Proper PPE must be worn when performing these tasks (see the PPE section above). All disposable materials must be discarded to meet state and federal Environmental Protection Agency (EPA) regulations and the entity's policies.[8]

Decontamination, deactivation, and cleaning. Decontamination may be defined as cleaning or deactivating. Deactivating an HD is preferred, but no single process has been found to deactivate all currently available HDs from different surface materials.[76,77,121] A 2013 study created terms to clarify the types of HD decontaminants tested on glass and stainless steel as elimination type (cleaners) and degradation type (deactivators).[76] Elimination-type solutions dissolve chemical products on surfaces, and degradation-type solutions react with the chemical structure of HD compounds, leading to their degradation and formation of noncytotoxic compounds. Elimination-type detergents, solutions, solvents, and surfactants and degradation-type cleaners were applied to stainless steel and glass surfaces that were contaminated with 10 HDs and removed.[76] Wipe samples were collected from the surfaces and analyzed for HD residue. All tested decontamination agents reduced the HD residue on the surfaces, but none totally removed it. Sodium hypochlorite was found to be very effective but damaged the stainless steel (no neutralizer was used in this study). Solutions containing anionic surfactants were very effective cleaners and had a high safety ratio but did not deactivate any HD. A second research team used similar solutions on gemcitabine and fluorouracil and found that these cleaning procedures were able to reduce HD contamination but did not completely eliminate it.[124] These researchers concluded that it might be more effective to adapt cleaning procedures to the variety of drug compounds and surface types rather than continue with a singular approach.[124]

The 2 studies also examined removing HD contamination from glass surfaces.[76,124] The cleaning agents and application methods may be useful in decontaminating HD vials before placing them into the C-PEC. The outer surface of HD vials has been shown to be contaminated with HD residue.[65–69] The amount of HD contamination placed into the C-PEC may be reduced by surface decontamination (i.e., wiping down) the HD vials. Care must be taken to avoid damaging the information on the vial label.

In a 2015 study, 70% isopropyl alcohol was compared to sodium dodecyl sulfate in 20% isopropyl alcohol for the routine decontamination of 10 antineoplastic agents from the surfaces of U.K.-designed BSCs.[77] This study concluded that 70% isopropyl alcohol was only 49% efficient at achieving decontamination for the 10 antineoplastic agents tested. The sodium dodecyl sulfate–20% isopropyl alcohol solution averaged 82% overall; however, vincristine and epirubicin demonstrated cleaning efficacies lower than 20% to both tested solutions. Therefore, the use of alcohol for disinfecting stainless steel surfaces may result in the spread of contamination rather than any actual cleaning.[77] Additional considerations with sodium dodecyl sulfate–isopropyl alcohol 20% include whether a rinse is needed with sodium dodecyl sulfate and that 20% isopropyl alcohol is insufficient as a disinfectant, requiring additional application of an effective disinfecting solution.

Decontamination of C-PECs should be conducted per manufacturer recommendations. The SDS for many HDs recommends sodium hypochlorite solution as an appropriate deactivating agent.[125,126] Researchers have shown that strong oxidizing agents, such as sodium hypochlorite, are effective deactivators of many HDs.[125] There are commercially available products that provide a system for decontamination and deactivation using sodium hypochlorite, detergent, and thiosulfate to neutralize the hypochlorite and deactivate other HDs.[73] Other nonchlorine bleach commercial disinfectant and sporicidal cleaners may provide appropriate decontamination from HDs.[127,128] Although it is not possible to perform analysis for all of the HDs, a selection of different chemical HDs with different diluents may provide sufficient markers of the type of contaminants on a given surface. The manufacturer of the deactivating cleaner should provide independent laboratory analysis and documentation of effective cleaning. A decontamination (cleaning/deactivating) process should include 1 or more cleaning or deactivating agents and the method used to apply it and the use of a neutralizer or rinse step, if needed. The entire process should be validated by wipe sampling the various surfaces to determine whether the HD has been removed. As there are many types of chemical HDs, analysis of a number of them, preferably various types, would be needed to validate a given process.

A ventilated cabinet that runs continuously should be cleaned before the day's operations begin and at regular intervals or when the day's work is completed. *USP* chapter 800 further states that the work surface of the C-PEC must be decontaminated between the compounding of different HDs.[8] The C-PEC must be decontaminated at least daily (when used), anytime a spill occurs, before and after certification, anytime power interruption occurs, and if the ventilation device is moved.[8] Ventilated C-PECs (i.e., class II and III BSCs and some CACIs) have air plenums that handle contaminated air. These plenums are designed for fumigation of the contamination from biological agents traditionally handled in the BSCs. The plenums are not designed for surface decontamination of drug or nonbiological residue, and many of the contaminated surfaces (plenums) cannot be reached for surface cleaning.[4,5,81] The area under the C-PEC work tray should be cleaned at least monthly to reduce the contamination level in the BSCs and CACIs where appropriate.[4]

Disinfection. The selection and use of disinfectants in healthcare facilities are guided by several properties, such as microbicidal activity, inactivation by organic matter, residue, and shelf life. Many disinfectants registered by EPA are 1-step disinfectants, formulated to be effective in the presence of light-to-moderate soiling without a precleaning step. However, when the surface to be disinfected has heavy soiling, a cleaning step is recommended before the application of the disinfectant. Trained compounding personnel are responsible for developing, implementing, and practicing the procedures for cleaning and disinfecting the DCAs written in the SOPs.[7] A 2013 study demonstrated the importance of SOPs by demonstrating that the efficacy of chemical decontamination of HD work surfaces depends not only on the cleaning solution used but also on the cleaning protocol.[122] It is necessary to adapt the protocol to the surface to clean, and it must be standardized and validated.[124] Cleaning and disinfecting agents are to be used with careful consideration of compatibilities, effectiveness, and inappropriate or toxic residues.[7]

Administration of HDs. Studies of infusion areas where HDs are administered have demonstrated significant HD surface contamination, which creates exposure risks for nurses, other workers, patients, and visitors to these areas.[10,11,21,46,129] A 2017 study[129] that measured surface contamination directly related to the administration of HDs found the incidence and amount of contamination from marker drugs cyclophosphamide and fluorouracil were higher than previously reported in studies that examined overall contamination in the infusion area.[10,42] Practices for administration of HDs must protect patients, workers, and the environment.[6,8,110,120] The need for more protection in the infusion area is addressed in *USP* chapter 800, which provides direction on improved practices, including the required use of a CSTD for administration of antineoplastic HDs when the dosage form allows.[8]

Policies and procedures governing the administration of HDs must be jointly developed by nursing and pharmacy for the mutual safety of healthcare workers. These policies should supplement policies designed to protect patient safety during administration of all drugs. All policies affecting multiple departments must be developed with input from managers and workers from the affected areas. Extensive nursing guidelines for the safe and appropriate administration of HDs have been developed by ONS[110,120] and *USP*.[8] Guidance on best practices for HD administration may also be found on the OSHA safety and health topics page on HDs.[13,14]

Recommendations for reducing exposure to HDs during administration in all practice settings are listed in **Appendix H**.

Spill Management. Policies and procedures must be developed to attempt to prevent spills and govern the cleanup of HD spills. Written procedures must specify who is responsible for spill management and must address the size and scope of the spill. Spills must be contained and cleaned up immediately by trained workers.

Spill kits containing all of the materials needed to clean up spills of HDs should be assembled or purchased (**Appendix I**). These kits should be readily available in all areas where HDs are routinely handled. A spill kit should accompany delivery of injectable HDs to patient care areas even though they are transported in a sealable plastic bag or container. If HDs are being prepared or administered in a nontraditional area (e.g., home setting, operating room, procedure area, radiology or unusual patient care area), a spill kit and respirator must be obtained by the drug handler. Signs must be available to warn of restricted access to the spill area.[8]

Only trained workers with appropriate PPE and respirators should attempt to manage an HD spill. All workers who may be required to clean up a spill of HDs must receive proper training in spill management and in the use of PPE and NIOSH-certified respirators.[70,71] Policies and procedures should describe how to establish access to workers trained to the OSHA Hazardous Waste Operations and Emergency Response Standard who may provide spill management in the event of a large spill.[130]

The circumstances and handling of spills should be documented. Staff and nonemployees exposed to an HD spill should also complete an incident report or exposure form and report to the designated emergency service for initial evaluation.

All spill cleanup materials, including PPE used for spill management, must be disposed of as hazardous waste in accordance with EPA Resource Conservation and Recovery Act (RCRA) regulations.[131,132] Spill cleanup materials must not be discarded as chemotherapy waste or biohazard waste. Additional information on spill control practices is available on the OSHA Safety and Health Topics page.[13,14]

Recommendations for spill cleanup procedure are summarized in **Appendix J**.

Worker Contamination. Procedures must be in place to address worker contamination, and protocols for medical attention must be developed before the occurrence of any such incident. OSHA requires suitable facilities for quick drenching or flushing of the eyes and body where workers may be exposed to injurious corrosive materials.[133] Limitations on having running water and drains in HD compounding areas conflict with these requirements. An alternative is to have a portable emergency eyewash station or emergency kits containing isotonic eyewash supplies and soap immediately available in areas where HDs are handled. Workers who are contaminated during the spill or spill cleanup or who have direct skin or eye contact with HDs require immediate treatment. OSHA-recommended steps for treatment are outlined in **Appendix K**.[133] Additional information on personnel contamination is available on the OSHA Safety and Health Topics page.[13,14]

Hazardous Waste Containment and Disposal

In 1976, the RCRA was enacted to provide a mechanism for tracking hazardous waste from its generation to disposal.[134] Regulations promulgated under the RCRA are enforced by EPA and apply to pharmaceuticals and chemicals discarded by pharmacies, hospitals, clinics, and other commercial entities. The RCRA outlines 4 characteristics of hazardous waste (D codes)[135] and contains lists of agents that are to be considered hazardous waste when they are discarded (P and U codes).[132] Any discarded drug that is on 1 of the lists (a "listed" waste) or meets 1 of the criteria (a "characteristic" waste) is considered hazardous waste. EPA has provided some relief for pharmaceuticals over the years by excluding epinephrine salts and weak medicinal nitroglycerin from the list, though epinephrine base and other forms of nitroglycerin are still listed.[136] Not all states have adopted these exemptions, so state hazardous waste regulations and interpretations should be consulted. In addition to a few others, the listed drugs include warfarin, nicotine, dalfampridine (4-aminopyridine), and physostigmine, as well as 7 current chemotherapy drugs: arsenic trioxide, chlorambucil, cyclophosphamide, daunomycin, melphalan, mitomycin C, and streptozocin.[137] They require handling, containment, and disposal as RCRA hazardous waste.

Every state except Iowa and Alaska is authorized to implement its own hazardous waste program, and these programs may be more stringent than EPA. State and local regulations must be considered when establishing a hazardous waste and HD disposal policy for a given institution.[138]

The RCRA allows for the exemption of empty containers from hazardous waste regulations. Empty containers are defined as those that have held U-listed or characteristic wastes and from which all wastes have been removed that can be removed using the practices commonly employed to remove materials from that type of container and no more than 3% by weight of the total capacity of the container remains in the container.[139] Disposal guidelines developed by the National Institutes of Health (NIH) and published in 1984 coined the term "trace-contaminated" waste using the 3% rule.[140] Note that a container that has held an acute hazardous waste listed in §261.33(e), such as arsenic trioxide, is not considered empty by the 3% rule[141] and that spill residues from cleanup of hazardous agents are considered hazardous waste.[132]

It is important that distinctions be drawn between HDs from an OSHA (HCS) and NIOSH employee exposure perspective and hazardous waste from an EPA perspective. *USP* chapter 800 uses *antineoplastic hazardous drugs* to refer to those HDs generally used as chemotherapy in oncology treatment.[8] For example, antineoplastic drugs listed in table 1, group 1, of the NIOSH 2016 HD list[55] are both employee hazards and hazardous to the environment based on their acknowledged toxicity. EPA hazardous waste regulations have not kept up with drug development, with over 100 chemotherapy drugs not listed by EPA.[142] The recommendation, therefore, is to manage all antineoplastic drugs as hazardous waste through a permitted hazardous waste treatment, storage, and disposal facility. Assuming that an organization is no longer disposing of any waste drugs by discarding them down the sewer drain, those listed in table 2, group 2, and table 3, group 3, of the NIOSH HD list[55] could be managed as nonhazardous pharmaceutical waste through incineration at a permitted regulated medical waste or waste-to-energy facility. To emphasize the difference between HDs and hazardous waste, the term *chemotherapy* will be used to denote antineoplastic HDs. The healthcare organization always has the option to manage all NIOSH HDs as hazardous waste, of course, if sorting is problematic. It is important to review state regulations for stricter definitions of hazardous waste; in Minnesota, for example, these drugs must be managed as hazardous waste.[143]

Trace-Contaminated Chemotherapy Drug Waste. By the NIH definition of trace chemotherapy waste,[140] "RCRA-empty" containers, needles, syringes, trace-contaminated gowns, gloves, pads, and empty i.v. sets may be collected and incinerated at a regulated medical waste incinerator. Sharps used in the preparation of chemotherapy should not be placed in red sharps containers, since sharps are most frequently disinfected by autoclaving or microwaving, not by incineration, and pose a risk of aerosolization to waste-handling employees.

Bulk Chemotherapy and RCRA Drug Waste. Although the terminology is not official, the terms *bulk chemotherapy* and *RCRA drug waste* have been used to differentiate containers that have held either (1) RCRA-listed or characteristic hazardous waste or (2) any chemotherapy drugs that are not RCRA empty or any materials from chemotherapy or hazardous waste drug spill cleanups. These wastes should be managed as hazardous waste.

Dual Infectious–Hazardous Waste. If a situation arises where a syringe with a needle containing a listed chemotherapy drug cannot be used, it should be managed as a dual waste. A black needle box labeled for both hazardous and biohazardous wastes should be used for containment. The contract with the hazardous waste disposal company should have this waste stream listed on the waste profile. The cost of this waste stream is typically higher than others, so it should be used only when needed.

Once hazardous waste has been identified, it must be collected, stored, and transported according to specific EPA and Department of Transportation (DOT) requirements.[134,144] Properly labeled, leakproof, and spill-proof containers of nonreactive plastic are required for areas where hazardous waste is generated. DOT packing group II containers are required for transportation.[145] Needles, scalpels, and waste contaminated with blood or other body fluids must not be mixed with hazardous waste.

Only individuals who meet OSHA-mandated hazardous waste awareness training may transport the hazardous waste containers from satellite accumulation areas in the pharmacy and nursing units to the storage accumulation sites.[146,147] Hazardous waste must be properly manifested and transported by a federally permitted hazardous waste transporter to a federally permitted hazardous waste storage, treatment, and disposal facility.[131] A licensed contractor may be hired to manage the hazardous waste program. The waste generator, however, may be held liable for mismanagement of hazardous waste. Investigation of a contractor, including verification of possession and type of license, should be completed and documented before a contractor is engaged.

In addition to determining what types of containers and what methods of sorting an organization will implement to properly manage both OSHA and EPA HD wastes, it is important to understand how generating hazardous waste impacts an organization as a whole. Additional departments need to be involved, such as laboratory and maintenance, which may also generate other types of RCRA hazardous wastes. EPA defines waste generation status by the total amount of hazardous waste generated per calendar month.[148] Small- and large-quantity generators are determined by the amount of P-, U-, and D-listed wastes that are discarded on a monthly basis. The Hazardous Waste Generator Improvements Rule took effect federally on May 30, 2017.[148] States had until July 1, 2018, to adopt it or have until July 1, 2019, if legislation is required.[148] The rule changes the name of "conditionally exempt small quantity generators" to "very small quantity generators" (VSQGs). Waste management requirements are more stringent for large-quantity generators than for small-quantity generators (SQGs) and VSQGs.[149] The removal of epinephrine salts and medicinal nitroglycerin from the P-list is a tremendous benefit to healthcare facilities, since only 1 kg (2.2 lb) of P-listed waste per calendar month causes the organization to become a large-quantity generator.

In the past, healthcare facilities had to count the weight of the containers that held P-listed waste toward their generator status. In a 2011 memo, EPA provided additional options, including counting only the residue of the waste.[149] Since most of the P-listed waste containers are warfarin stock bottles, warfarin unit-dose blister packs, or nicotine wrappers, hospitals can use the residue calculation in the memo to document that their P-listed waste does not exceed 1 kg in a calendar month or 1 kg of stored P-listed waste. This practice may enable the facility to remain a VSQG or SQG, depending on the volume of other hazardous waste generated. If an organization is documenting P-listed residues only and total hazardous waste generation per month (not just pharmacy waste) is below 100 kg, it is a VSQG; if the total is 100–1,000 kg, it is an SQG. Again, some states have not accepted this option, so state regulations must be consulted.

On September 25, 2015, EPA published its Proposed Rule: Management Standards for Hazardous Waste Pharmaceuticals.[150] When the final version of the rule is published, it will be important for organizations to review and modify their programs accordingly, as the proposed rule contained very significant hazardous pharmaceutical waste management changes, many of them beneficial to healthcare facilities.

Medical Screening and Surveillance and Alternative Duty

Many drugs described in this document as hazardous are acutely toxic or are known or suspected human carcinogens; many more cause adverse reproductive outcomes.[55] Decades of literature show that HD contamination in the healthcare work environment is absorbed into healthcare workers.[6,9–12,15,19] Marker HDs have been measured in the urine of workers who routinely handle HDs during the course of patient care.[10,21,46,48,49] HD levels have also been found in the urine of workers not directly responsible for HD compounding or administration.[21] This continued worker exposure has prompted many groups to advocate that healthcare workers tasked with handling HDs be identified and enrolled in medical screening programs before job placement and periodically during employment and that they be maintained in a systematic medical surveillance program.[6,13,14,27,110,120]

Medical screening and surveillance should be part of the comprehensive safety program for controlling workplace exposure to HDs, which must include engineering controls, training, work practices, and PPE. Such safety programs must be able to identify potentially exposed workers and those who might be at higher risk of adverse health effects due to this exposure. Guidance on medical surveillance programs is available from *USP*,[8] OSHA,[14] and NIOSH.[151]

Because reproductive risks have been associated with exposure to HDs, alternative duty (work assignments that do not involve handling HDs) should be offered to individuals who are pregnant, breast-feeding, or attempting to conceive or father a child.[14,28] Employees' physicians should be involved in making these determinations. Guidance on alternative duty is available from NIOSH.[28]

All workers who handle HDs should be routinely monitored in a medical surveillance program.[6,8,14,28,110] Medical surveillance involves the collection and interpretation of data for the purpose of detecting changes in the health status of working populations. Medical surveillance programs involve assessment and documentation of symptom complaints, physical findings, and laboratory values (such as a blood count) to determine whether there is a deviation from the expected norms. NIOSH encourages employees who handle HDs to participate in medical surveillance programs that are provided in the workplace.[6] Limited resources may preclude the implementation of a comprehensive medical surveillance program for healthcare workers who are exposed to HDs. Workers handling HDs are encouraged to inform their personal healthcare providers of their occupation and possible HD exposure when obtaining routine medical care.[6]

Robotics

Robotics may be defined as mechanical devices that perform programmed, complex, and repetitive manipulations that mimic human behavior without continuous input from an operator. Robotic i.v. automation presents an opportunity for improving safety and efficiency in the compounding process by increasing accuracy and consistency for patients and reducing HD direct exposure for compounding staff.[152] There are currently a number of robots and automated devices that are marketed for sterile HDs, and manufacturers should provide evidence-based data to support the use of any of these devices in compounding sterile HD doses to provide patient safety and worker safety. There may also be legal requirements when using these devices in a pharmacy licensed through a state board of pharmacy, and these devices must also meet provisions of *USP* chapter 797 when used for sterile compounding.[7,153]

Studies have examined the accuracy of robotic devices compounding HDs for patient safety but did not include environmental contamination or worker safety considerations.[154,155] Limited studies have been published examining the ability for robotics to reduce HD surface contamination during sterile compounding or to impact the safety of healthcare workers interacting with the robot during HD compounding. One study reported on observed work practices where the robot was found to produce a significant reduction in the number of potentially harmful staff safety events during compounding; however, no marker of exposure of staff was used during the study and neither robot cleaning nor waste disposal tasks were addressed.[156]

Environmental contamination has been evaluated by wipe sampling for cyclophosphamide during robotic compounding by different manufacturers' robots. In the first study, cyclophosphamide was measured on work surfaces, in air samples, and in urine samples of workers.[157] Wipe samples of the subjects' hands were also collected. Cyclophosphamide was detected on most surfaces inside the robot in small amounts, and the outer glove had the most contamination. The vials and ports of the i.v. bags where cyclophosphamide was injected had higher and more consistent contamination. No cyclophosphamide was detected on the personal air samplers or in the 14 urine samples of the 2 technicians.

Although the contamination detected in the robot was low, the study identified work practices that needed improvement, such as cleaning HD vials before placing them into the robot, which may have resulted in cyclophosphamide transfer to gloves and final products.

In a second study, wipe samples were used to compare measured cyclophosphamide surface contamination in a BSC and robot after similar compounding over a 4-day period.[158] The detection rate for cyclophosphamide contamination was 70% of surface samples in the BSC versus 15% using the robot. Overall, cyclophosphamide contamination was quite low for both settings compared to that found in the literature.

These studies demonstrate that robotic HD compounders are dependent on work practices surrounding the actual compounding to achieve the lowest levels of contamination and the best protection for workers and the environment. Additional research is needed to evaluate the place of robotic HD compounders in patient and worker safety. Information about robotics in sterile compounding is available from ASHP.[159]

Environment Sampling for HDs

Surface wipe sampling of healthcare settings for HD contamination is advocated as a means of environmental quality and control.[6,8] Surface wipe sampling should be done routinely, first to determine a benchmark of contamination and then to monitor the effectiveness of safe handling programs. As no acceptable levels of HD surface contamination have been determined by any regulatory agency, surface wipe sampling should determine an operational baseline of at least several marker HDs from which a facility action level may be determined. Surface wipe sampling provides a way to determine the efficacy of HD handling equipment, ancillary devices, work practices, cleaning methods, and disposal and is currently the method of choice to determine surface contamination of the workplace with these drugs.[160] Wipe sampling should also be done if a lapse in the safe handling program occurs, which may result in an excursion beyond a predetermined action level of HD surface contamination.[6,8,161,162]

Since it has been postulated that dermal uptake is the most likely route of occupational exposure to most HDs in healthcare settings, especially low-molecular-weight antineoplastic drugs, surface wipe sampling is a useful tool to evaluate contamination of the healthcare facility with HDs.[48,79] Wipe-sampling methodology can be used for most classes of drugs. Published studies have focused on several sentinel antineoplastic drugs, most commonly cyclophosphamide, ifosfamide, fluorouracil, methotrexate, and doxorubicin, though others are reported in the literature.[9] As analytic methods become more sophisticated, more drugs can be analyzed simultaneously.

No standards exist for acceptable or allowable surface concentrations for HDs in the healthcare setting. Surface contamination levels for cyclophosphamide in early studies led *USP* to describe a 1-ng/cm^2 action level for cyclophosphamide, above which drug uptake was believed to occur. More recent studies looking at a large number of samples done with standardized sampling and assay techniques have proposed hygienic guidance values for surface wipe sampling that are based on reporting 50th and 75th percentiles[161] or 90th percentiles[108,162] of samples. Hygienic guidance values are not based on endpoints of either HD uptake by workers or any measurable health effect. The Monitoring-Effect Study of Wipe Sampling in Pharmacies (MEWIP) method conducted in 130 German pharmacies looked at surface contamination with cyclophosphamide, docetaxel, etoposide, fluorouracil, gemcitabine, ifosfamide, methotrexate, and paclitaxel.[108] Based on the 90th percentile of the contamination values, they recommend a substance-independent performance-based guidance value of 0.1 ng/cm^2 as the action level.[108] This is significantly more stringent than *USP*'s observation.[8] Kibby[163] conducted a review of studies with concurrent surface wipe-sampling and urine monitoring for sentinel HDs and noted that no statistically significant correlation was found between the 2 types of studies. He further noted that none of the reviewed studies found detectable HDs in the urine for median surface levels below 0.01 ng/cm^2. This value, as the others, is not based on endpoints of any measurable health effect.

Guidance values and action levels are dependent on the methods used for wipe sampling and analytic assays, which have varied greatly in studies.[9] The basic methodology that should be common to all protocols for wipe sampling was reviewed by Connor et al.[160] They stressed that proper validation of the sampling method is critical to obtaining reproducible results and being able to compare results across studies. *USP* notes there are currently no certifying agencies for vendors of wipe sample kits.[8] Therefore, individuals purchasing or specifying the selection of a kit must be responsible for verifying its effectiveness. Factors to consider when selecting a wipe-sampling kit or a laboratory to perform the analysis include validated sampling and analytic methods, extraction efficiency of drug from surface material, recovery of drug from sampling material, LOD, limit of quantification, and the qualifications and certifications of the laboratory.[160]

No regulations or standards exist for allowable or acceptable HD surface concentrations in healthcare settings, and many questions remain about the potential health risks associated with exposure to existing levels of environmental surface contamination. However, prudent practice dictates that levels of HD surface contamination should be reduced to as low as reasonably achievable.[15,110]

Conclusion

These guidelines represent the recommendations of many groups and individuals who have worked diligently over decades to reduce the potential of harmful effects on healthcare workers exposed to HDs. No set of guidelines on this topic, however comprehensive, can address all the needs of every healthcare facility. Healthcare professionals are encouraged to rely on their professional judgment, experience, and common sense in applying these recommendations to their unique circumstances and to take into account evolving federal, state, and local regulations, as well as the requirements of appropriate accrediting institutions. As additional research is needed in this area, healthcare workers must act as their own advocates and encourage studies that look at adverse health outcomes as well as practice standards that improve worker safety.

References

1. Stolar MH, Power LA, Viele CS. Recommendations for handling cytotoxic drugs in hospitals. *Am J Hosp Pharm.* 1983; 40:1163–71.
2. Stolar MH, Power LA. The 1983–84 ASHP practice spotlight: safe handling of cytotoxic drugs. *Am J Hosp Pharm.* 1983; 40:1161.
3. American Society of Hospital Pharmacists. ASHP technical assistance bulletin on handling cytotoxic drugs in hospitals. *Am J Hosp Pharm.* 1985; 42:131–7.
4. American Society of Hospital Pharmacists. ASHP technical assistance bulletin on handling cytotoxic and hazardous drugs. *Am J Hosp Pharm.* 1990; 47:1033–49.
5. American Society of Health-System Pharmacists. ASHP guidelines on handling hazardous drugs. *Am J Health-Syst Pharm.* 2006; 63:1172–93.
6. National Institute for Occupational Safety and Health. NIOSH alert: preventing occupational exposure to antineoplastic and other hazardous drugs in health care settings. www.cdc.gov/niosh/docs/2004-165/ (accessed 2018 Feb 28).
7. Pharmaceutical compounding—sterile preparations (general information chapter 797). In: The United States pharmacopeia, 39th rev., and The national formulary, 34th ed. Rockville, MD: United States Pharmacopeial Convention; 2016:626–70.
8. Hazardous drugs—handling in healthcare settings (general information chapter 800). In: The United States Pharmacopeia, 39th rev., and The national formulary, 34th ed. First supplement. Rockville, MD: United States Pharmacopeial Convention; 2016.
9. National Institute for Occupational Safety and Health. Safety and health topics: hazardous drug exposures in healthcare: antineoplastic agents. www.cdc.gov/niosh/topics/hazdrug/antineoplastic.html (accessed 2018 Feb 28).
10. Connor TH, DeBord G, Pretty JR et al. Evaluation of antineoplastic drug exposure of health care workers at three university-based US cancer centers. *J Occup Environ Med.* 2010; 52:1019–27.
11. Hon CY, Teschke K, Chua P et al. Occupational exposure to antineoplastic drugs: identification of job categories potentially exposed throughout the hospital medication system. *Saf Health Work.* 2011; 2:273–81.
12. National Institute for Occupational Safety and Health. Safety and health topics: occupational exposure to antineoplastic agents and other hazardous drugs: effects of occupational exposure. www.cdc.gov/niosh/topics/hazdrug/effects.html (accessed 2018 Feb 28).
13. Occupational Safety and Health Administration. Safety and health topics. Hazardous drugs. www.osha.gov/SLTC/hazardousdrugs/index.html (accessed 2018 Feb 28).
14. Occupational Safety and Health Administration. Controlling occupational exposure to hazardous drugs. www.osha.gov/SLTC/hazardousdrugs/controlling_occex_hazardousdrugs.html (accessed 2018 Feb 28).
15. Baker ES, Connor TH. Monitoring occupational exposure to cancer chemotherapy drugs. *Am J Health-Syst Pharm.* 1996; 53:2713–23.
16. Sessink PJ, Bos RP. Drugs hazardous to healthcare workers: evaluation of methods for monitoring occupational exposure to cytostatic drugs. *Drug Saf.* 1999; 20:347–59.
17. Harrison BR. Risks of handling cytotoxic drugs. In: Perry MC, ed. The chemotherapy source book. 3rd ed. Philadelphia: Lippincott, Williams and Wilkins; 2001:566–82.
18. Connor TH, McDiarmid MA. Preventing occupational exposures to antineoplastic drugs in health care settings. *CA Cancer J Clin.* 2006; 56:354–65.
19. Suspiro A, Prista J. Biomarkers of occupational exposure to anticancer agents: a minireview. *Toxicol Lett.* 2011; 207:42–52.
20. Power LA, Coyne JW. Hazardous drugs as compounded sterile preparations. In: Buchanan EC, Schneider PJ, Forrey RA, eds. Compounding sterile preparations. 4th ed. Bethesda, MD: American Society of Health-System Pharmacists; 2017:171–202.
21. Hon CY, Teschke K, Shen H et al. Antineoplastic drug contamination in the urine of Canadian healthcare workers. *Int Arch Occup Environ Health.* 2015; 88:933–41.
22. Yuki M, Sekine S, Takase K et al. Exposure of family members to antineoplastic drugs via excreta of treated cancer patients. *J Oncol Pharm Pract.* 2013; 19:208–17.
23. Yuki M, Takase K, Sekine S et al. Evaluation of surface contamination with cyclophosphamide in the home setting of outpatients on cancer chemotherapy. *J Nurs Educ Pract.* 2014; 4:16–23.
24. Yuki M, Ishida T, Sekine S. Secondary exposure of family members to cyclophosphamide after chemotherapy of outpatients with cancer: a pilot study. *Oncol Nurs Forum.* 2015; 42:665–71.
25. Ratner PA, Spinelli JJ, Beking K et al. Cancer incidence and adverse pregnancy outcome in registered nurses potentially exposed to antineoplastic drugs. *BMC Nurs.* 2010; 9:15.
26. Lawson CC, Rocheleau CM, Whelan EA et al. Occupational exposures among nurses and risk of spontaneous abortions. *Am J Obstet Gynecol.* 2012; 206:327.e1–8.
27. Martin S. Chemotherapy handling and effects among nurses and their offspring. *Oncol Nurs Forum.* 2005; 32:425.
28. Connor TH, Lawson CC, Polovich M et al. Current intelligence bulletin XX: reproductive risks associated with hazardous drug exposures in healthcare workers: recommendations for reducing exposures. www.cdc.gov/niosh/docket/archive/pdfs/NIOSH-279/CIBXX-reporRisk-279.pdf (accessed 2018 Feb 28).
29. National Toxicology Program. Report on carcinogens, 14th ed. https://ntp.niehs.nih.gov/pubhealth/roc/index-1.html (accessed 2018 Feb 28).
30. International Agency for Research on Cancer. IARC monographs on the evaluation of carcinogenic risks to humans (2012). Pharmaceuticals. Volume 100A. http://monographs.iarc.fr/ENG/Monographs/vol100A/index.php (accessed 2018 Feb 28).
31. Skov T, Lynge E, Maarup B et al. Risks for physicians handling antineoplastic drugs. *Lancet.* 1990; 336:1446.

32. Skov T, Maarup B, Olsen J et al. Leukaemia and reproductive outcome among nurses handling antineoplastic drugs. *Br J Ind Med.* 1992; 49:855–61.
33. Gunnarsdottir HK, Aspelund T, Karlsson T et al. Occupational risk factors for breast cancer among nurses. *Int J Occup Environ Health.* 1997; 3:254–8.
34. Fransman W, Kager H, Meijster T et al. Leukemia from dermal exposure to cyclophosphamide among nurses in the Netherlands: quantitative assessment of the risk. *Ann Occup Hyg.* 2014; 58:271–82.
35. McDiarmid MA, Oliver MS, Roth TS et al. Chromosome 5 and 7 abnormalities in oncology personnel handling anticancer drugs. *J Occup Environ Med.* 2010; 52:1028–34.
36. McDiarmid MA, Rogers B, Oliver MS. Chromosomal effects of non-alkylating drug exposure in oncology personnel. *Environ Mol Mutagen.* 2014; 55:369–74.
37. Pedersen-Bjergaard J, Christiansen DH, Andersen MK et al. Causality of myelodysplasia and acute myeloid leukemia and their genetic abnormalities [review]. *Leukemia.* 2002; 16:2177–84.
38. Pedersen-Bjergaard J, Andersen MK, Christiansen DH et al. Genetic pathways in therapy-related myelodysplasia and acute myeloid leukemia. *Blood.* 2002; 99:1909–12.
39. Sakhvidi MJ, Hajaghazadeh M, Mostaghaci M et al. Applicability of the comet assay in evaluation of DNA damage in healthcare providers' working with antineoplastic drugs: a systematic review and meta-analysis. *Int J Occup Environ Health.* 2016; 22:52–67.
40. Villarini M, Gianfredi V, Levorato S et al. Occupational exposure to cytostatic/antineoplastic drugs and cytogenetic damage measured using the lymphocyte cytokinesis-block micronucleus assay: a systematic review of the literature and meta-analysis. *Mutat Res/Rev Mutat Res.* 2016; 770:35–45.
41. Roussel C, Witt KL, Shaw PB et al. Meta-analysis of chromosomal aberrations as a biomarker of exposure in healthcare workers occupationally exposed to antineoplastic drugs. *Mutat Res/Rev Mutat Res.* In press.
42. Connor TH, Anderson RW, Sessink PJ et al. Surface contamination with antineoplastic agents in six cancer treatment centers in Canada and the United States. *Am J Health-Syst Pharm.* 1999; 56:1427–32.
43. Hon CY, Teschke K, Chu W et al. Antineoplastic drug contamination of surfaces throughout the hospital medication system in Canadian hospitals. *J Occup Environ Hyg.* 2013; 10:374–83.
44. Hon CY, Barzan C, Astrakianakis G. Identification of knowledge gaps regarding healthcare workers' exposure to antineoplastic drugs: review of literature, North America versus Europe. *Saf Health Work.* 2014; 5:169–74.
45. Pethran A, Schierl R, Hauff K et al. Uptake of antineoplastic agents in pharmacy and hospital personnel. Part I: monitoring of urinary concentrations. *Int Arch Occup Environ Health.* 2003; 76:5–10.
46. Wick C, Slawson MH, Jorgenson JA et al. Using a closed-system protective device to reduce personnel exposure to antineoplastic agents. *Am J Health-Syst Pharm.* 2003; 60:2314–20.
47. Mason HJ, Blair S, Sams C et al. Exposure to antineoplastic drugs in two UK hospital pharmacy units. *Ann Occup Hyg.* 2005; 49:603–10.
48. Fransman W, Roeleveld N, Peelen S et al. Nurses with dermal exposure to antineoplastic drugs: reproductive outcomes. *Epidemiology.* 2007; 18:112–9.
49. Sottani C, Porro B, Cornelli M et al. An analysis to study trends in occupational exposure to antineoplastic drugs among health care workers. *J Chromatog B.* 2010; 878:2593–605.
50. Hama K, Fukushima K, Hirabatake M et al. Verification of surface contamination of Japanese cyclophosphamide vials and an example of exposure by handling. *J Oncol Pharm Pract.* 2011; 18:201–6.
51. Hon CY, Astrakianakis G, Danyluk Q et al. Pilot evaluation of dermal contamination by antineoplastic drugs among hospital pharmacy personnel. *Can J Hosp Pharm.* 2011; 64:327–32.
52. Hon CY, Teschke K, Demers PA et al. Antineoplastic drug contamination on the hands of employees working throughout the hospital medication system. *Ann Occup Hyg.* 2014; 58:761–70.
53. Centers for Disease Control and Prevention. NIOSH list of antineoplastic and other hazardous drugs in healthcare settings 2014: proposed additions and deletions to the NIOSH hazardous drug list. Docket number: CDC-2013-0007; NIOSH-233. www.cdc.gov/niosh/docket/review/docket233/pdf/CDC-2013-0007.pdf (accessed 2018 Feb 28).
54. National Institute for Occupational Safety and Health. NIOSH list of antineoplastic and other hazardous drugs in healthcare settings, 2014. www.cdc.gov/niosh/docs/2014-138/default.html (accessed 2018 Feb 28).
55. National Institute for Occupational Safety and Health. NIOSH list of antineoplastic and other hazardous drugs in healthcare settings, 2016. www.cdc.gov/niosh/docs/2016-161/default.html (accessed 2018 Feb 28).
56. National Institute for Occupational Safety and Health. Workplace safety and health topics: hazardous drug exposures in health care. www.cdc.gov/niosh/topics/hazdrug/ (accessed 2018 Feb 28).
57. Occupational Safety and Health Administration. Hazard communication standard. 29 C.F.R. 1910.1200. www.osha.gov/pls/oshaweb/owadisp.show_document?p_table=STANDARDS&p_id=10099 (accessed 2018 Feb 28).
58. Occupational Safety and Health Administration. Hazard communication standard. 29 C.F.R. 1910.1200(c). Definitions. www.osha.gov/pls/oshaweb/owadisp.show_document?p_table=STANDARDS&p_id=10099 (accessed 2017 Mar 30).
59. Occupational Safety and Health Administration. Hazard communication standard. 29 C.F.R. 1910.1200. Appendix A. Health hazard criteria (mandatory). www.osha.gov/pls/oshaweb/owadisp.show_document?p_table=STANDARDS&p_id=10100 (accessed 2018 Feb 28).
60. Joint Commission. Medication management standard MM.01.01.03: the hospital safely manages high-alert and hazardous medications. In: Elements of performance for medication management. Comprehensive

accreditation manual for hospitals: the official handbook. Oakbrook Terrace, IL: Joint Commission Resources; 2016.

61. Pharmaceutical compounding—nonsterile preparations (general information chapter 795). In: The United States pharmacopeia, 40th rev., and The national formulary, 35th ed. Second supplement. Rockville, MD: United States Pharmacopeial Convention; 2017:675–83.
62. Hon CY, Teschke K, Shen H. Healthcare workers' knowledge, perceptions and behaviors regarding antineoplastic drugs: survey from British Columbia, Canada. *J Occup Environ Hyg.* 2015; 12:669–77.
63. Occupational Safety and Health Administration. Hazard communication standard. 29 C.F.R. 1910.1200. Appendix D. Safety data sheets (mandatory). www.osha.gov/pls/oshaweb/owadisp.show_document?p_table=STANDARDS&p_id=10103 (accessed 2018 Feb 28).
64. Occupational Safety and Health Administration. Hazard communication standard. 29 C.F.R. 1910.1200(a)(2). www.osha.gov/pls/oshaweb/owadisp.show_document?p_table=STANDARDS&p_id=10099 (accessed 2018 Feb 28).
65. Connor TH, Sessink PJ, Harrison BR et al. Surface contamination of chemotherapy drug vials and evaluation of new vial-cleaning techniques: results of three studies. *Am J Health-Syst Pharm.* 2005; 62:475–84.
66. Touzin K, Bussieres JF, Langlois E et al. Cyclophosphamide contamination observed on the external surfaces of drug vials and the efficacy of cleaning on vial contamination. *Ann Occup Hyg.* 2008; 52:765–71.
67. Power LA, Sessink PJ, Gesy K et al. Hazardous drug residue on exterior vial surfaces: evaluation of a commercial manufacturing process. *Hosp Pharm.* 2014; 49:355–62.
68. Hedmer M, Georgiadi A, Rämme Bremberg E et al. Surface contamination of cyclophosphamide packaging and surface contamination with antineoplastic drugs in a hospital pharmacy in Sweden. *Ann Occup Hyg.* 2005; 49:629–37.
69. Schierl R, Herwig A, Pfaller A et al. Surface contamination of antineoplastic drug vials: comparison of unprotected and protected vials. *Am J Health-Syst Pharm.* 2010; 67:428–29.
70. Occupational Safety and Health Administration. Respiratory protection standard. 29 C.F.R. 1910.134. www.osha.gov/SLTC/respiratoryprotection/standards.html (accessed 2018 Feb 28).
71. National Institute for Occupational Safety and Health. Respirators. www.cdc.gov/niosh/topics/respirators/ (accessed 2018 Feb 28).
72. Oncology Nursing Society. ONS position statement: education of the nurse who administers and cares for the individual receiving chemotherapy, targeted therapy, and immunotherapy. www.ons.org/advocacy-policy/positions/education/chemotherapy-biotherapy (accessed 2018 Feb 28).
73. Touzin K, Bussières JF, Langlois É et al. Pilot study comparing the efficacy of two cleaning techniques in reducing environmental contamination with cyclophosphamide. *Ann Occup Hyg.* 2010; 54:351–9.
74. Chu WC, Hon CY, Danyluk Q et al. Pilot assessment of the antineoplastic drug contamination levels in British Columbia hospitals pre- and post-cleaning. *J Oncol Pharm Pract.* 2012; 18:46–51.
75. Larson RR, Khazaeli MB, Dillon HK. A new monitoring method using solid sorbent media for evaluation of airborne cyclophosphamide and other antineoplastic agents. *Appl Occup Environ Hyg.* 2003; 18:120–31.
76. Lamerie TQ, Nussbaumer S, Décaudin B et al. Evaluation of decontamination efficiency of cleaning solutions on stainless steel and glass surfaces contaminated by 10 antineoplastic agents. *Ann Occup Hyg.* 2013; 57:456–69.
77. Anastasi M, Rudaz S, Lamerie TQ et al. Efficacy of two cleaning solutions for the decontamination of 10 antineoplastic agents in the biosafety cabinets of a hospital pharmacy. *Ann Occup Hyg.* 2015; 59:895–908.
78. Sessink PJ, Wittenhorst BC, Anzion RB et al. Exposure of pharmacy technicians to antineoplastic agents: reevaluation after additional protective measures. *Arch Environ Health.* 1997; 52:240–4.
79. Kromhout H, Hoek F, Uitterhoeve R et al. Postulating a dermal pathway for exposure to antineoplastic drugs among hospital workers: applying a conceptual model to the results of three workplace surveys. *Ann Occup Hyg.* 2000; 44:551–60.
80. Kiffmeyer TK, Kube C, Opiolka S et al. Vapor pressures, evaporation behavior and airborne concentrations of hazardous drugs: implications for occupational safety. *Pharm J.* 2002; 268:331–7.
81. Centers for Disease Control and Prevention. Biosafety in microbiological and biomedical laboratories, 5th ed. Appendix A—primary containment for biohazards: selection, installation and use of biological safety cabinets. www.cdc.gov/biosafety/publications/bmbl5/ (accessed 2018 Feb 28).
82. Labconco. Product information: class II, type C1 biosafety cabinets. www.labconco.com/category/class-ii-type-c1 (accessed 2018 Feb 28).
83. NSF International Standard/American National Standard. NSF/ANSI 49–2016 Annex E. Biosafety cabinetry: design, construction, performance, and field certification. www.nsf.org/newsroom_pdf/NSF_49-2016_Annex_E.pdf (accessed 2018 Feb 28).
84. Clark RP, Goff MR. The potassium iodide method for determining protection factors in open-fronted microbiological safety cabinets. *J Appl Bacteriol.* 1981; 51:439–60.
85. CAG-001-2005: applications guide for the use of compounding isolators in compounding sterile preparations in healthcare facilities. Raleigh, NC: Controlled Environment Testing Association; 2005 (revised 2008).
86. CAG-002-2006: compounding isolator testing guide. Raleigh, NC: Controlled Environment Testing Association; 2006 (revised 2008).
87. CAG-004-2007: application guide for the use of surface decontaminants in biosafety cabinets. Raleigh, NC: Controlled Environment Testing Association; 2007 (revised 2008).
88. CAG-005-2007: CETA servicing hazardous drug compounding primary engineering controls. Raleigh, NC: Controlled Environment Testing Association; 2007.

89. Standard 14644-1. Cleanrooms and associated environments—part 1: classification of air cleanliness by particle concentration. 2nd ed. Geneva: International Organization for Standardization; 2015.
90. Crauste-Manciet S, Sessink PJ, Ferrari S et al. Environmental contamination with cytotoxic drugs in healthcare using positive air pressure isolators. *Ann Occup Hyg.* 2005; 49:619–28.
91. Kopp B, Crauste-Manciet S, Guibert A et al. Environmental and biological monitoring of platinum-containing drugs in two hospital pharmacies using positive air pressure isolators. *Ann Occup Hyg.* 2013; 57:374–83.
92. Sessink PJ, Rolf ME, Ryden NS. Evaluation of the PhaSeal hazardous drug containment system. *Hosp Pharm.* 1999; 34:1311–7.
93. Food and Drug Administration Center for Devices and Radiological Health. Premarket notification (510k) process. www.fda.gov/medicaldevices/device regulationandguidance/howtomarketyourdevice/premarketsubmissions/premarketnotification510k/default.htm (accessed 2018 Feb 28).
94. Food and Drug Administration Center for Devices and Radiological Health. Product code classification database. Product code ONB. www.accessdata.fda.gov/scripts/cdrh/cfdocs/cfPCD/classification.cfm?ID=ONB (accessed 2018 Feb 28).
95. National Institute for Occupational Safety and Health. Safety and health topics: hazardous drug exposures in healthcare. Environmental sampling, decontamination, protective equipment, robotics, closed system transfer devices, and work practice. Closed system drug-transfer devices (CSTDs) and similar devices. www.cdc.gov/niosh/topics/hazdrug/sampling.html (accessed 2018 Feb 28).
96. National Institute for Occupational Safety and Health. A vapor containment performance protocol for closed system transfer devices used during pharmacy compounding and administration of hazardous drugs. www.cdc.gov/niosh/docket/review/docket288/pdfs/a-vapor-containment-performance-protocol-for-closed-system-transfer-devices.pdf (accessed 2018 Feb 28).
97. National Institute for Occupational Safety and Health. A performance test protocol for closed system transfer devices used during pharmacy compounding and administration of hazardous drugs. www.cdc.gov/niosh/docket/review/docket288a/pdfs/aperformancetestprotocolforclosedsystemtransferdevices.pdf (accessed 2018 Feb 28).
98. National Institute for Occupational Safety and Health. Workplace safety and health topics: hierarchy of controls. www.cdc.gov/niosh/topics/hierarchy/ (accessed 2018 Feb 28).
99. National Institute for Occupational Safety and Health. Personal protective equipment for health care workers who work with hazardous drugs. DHHS (NIOSH) publication no. 2009-106 (2008). www.cdc.gov/niosh/docs/wp-solutions/2009-106/ (accessed 2018 Feb 28).
100. ASTM D6978-05: standard practice for assessment of resistance of medical gloves to permeation by chemotherapy drugs. West Conshohocken, PA: ASTM International; 2013.
101. ASTM F739-12e1: standard test method for permeation of liquids and gases through protective clothing materials under conditions of continuous contact. West Conshohocken, PA: ASTM International; 2012.
102. Connor TH, Power LA, Massoomi F et al. Are gloves and gowns safe for handling chemotherapy? *Pharm Purch Prod.* 2015. www.pppmag.com/download.php?file=documents/V12N1/pdfs/ppp_1501_ppe.pdf (accessed 2018 Feb 28).
103. Food and Drug Administration. Banned devices; powdered surgeon's gloves, powdered patient examination gloves, and absorbable powder for lubricating a surgeon's glove (effective January 18, 2017). www.federalregister.gov/documents/2016/12/19/2016- 30382/banned-devices-powdered-surgeons-gloves-powdered-patient-examination-gloves-and-absorbable-powder (accessed 2018 Feb 28).
104. Wallemacq PE, Capron A, Vanbinst R et al. Permeability of 13 different gloves to 13 cytotoxic agents under controlled dynamic conditions. *Am J Health-Syst Pharm.* 2006; 63:547–56.
105. Dolezalova L, Odraska P, Gorna L et al. [Evaporation of selected cytotoxic drugs and permeation of protective gloves—research into the occupational risks of health care personnel handling hazardous cytotoxic drugs (CYTO project).] *Klin Onkol.* 2009; 22:218–22. In Czech.
106. Capron A, Destree J, Jacobs P et al. Permeability of gloves to selected chemotherapeutic agents after treatment with alcohol or isopropyl alcohol. *Am J Health-Syst Pharm.* 2012; 69:1665–70.
107. Landeck L, Gonzalez E, Koch OM. Handling chemotherapy drugs—do medical gloves really protect? *Int J Cancer.* 2015; 137:1800–5.
108. Kiffmeyer T, Tuerk J, Hahn M et al. Application and assessment of a regular environmental monitoring of the antineoplastic drug contamination level in pharmacies—the MEWIP project. *Ann Occup Hyg.* 2013; 57:444–55.
109. Hon CY, Abusitta D. Causes of health care workers' exposure to antineoplastic drugs: an exploratory study. *Can J Hosp Pharm.* 2016; 69:216–23.
110. Polovich M, Olsen M. Safe handling of hazardous drugs. 3rd ed. Pittsburgh: Oncology Nursing Society; 2017.
111. Labuhn K, Valanis B, Schoeny R et al. Nurses' and pharmacists' exposure to antineoplastic drugs: findings from industrial hygiene scans and urine mutagenicity tests. *Cancer Nurs.* 1998; 21:79–89.
112. Minoia C, Turci R, Sottani C et al. Application of high performance liquid chromatography/tandem mass spectrometry in the environmental and biological monitoring of health care personnel occupationally exposed to cyclophosphamide and ifosfamide. *Rapid Commun Mass Spectrom.* 1998; 12:1485–93.
113. Turci R, Minoia C, Sottani C et al. Occupational exposure to antineoplastic drugs in seven Italian hospitals: the effect of quality assurance and adherence to guidelines. *J Oncol Pharm Pract.* 2011; 17:320–32.

114. Sottani C, Porro B, Imbriani M et al. Occupational exposure to antineoplastic drugs in four Italian health care settings. *Toxicol Lett.* 2012; 213:107–15.
115. NuAire. Containment capabilities of a class II, type A2 BSC using a chemo pad on the work surface. Technical bulletin GTB0131. www.nuaire.com/media/wysiwyg/bulletins-general/biological-safety-cabinets/GTB0131%20Containment%20Capabilities%20of%20a%20%20Class%20II,%20Type%20A2%20Biosafety%20Cabinet%20using%20Chemo%20Pad%20on%20the%20Worksurface.pdf (accessed 2018 Feb 28).
116. Wilson JP, Solimando DA. Aseptic technique as a safety precaution in the preparation of antineoplastic agents. *Hosp Pharm.* 1981; 15:575–81.
117. Harrison BR, Godefroid RJ, Kavanaugh EA. Quality assurance testing of staff pharmacists handling cytotoxic agents. *Am J Health-Syst Pharm.* 1996; 53:402–7.
118. Shahsavarani S, Godefroid RJ, Harrison BR. Evaluation of occupational exposure to tablet trituration dust. Paper presented at ASHP Midyear Clinical Meeting. Atlanta, GA; 1993 Dec 6.
119. Fent K, Mueller C. Pharmaceutical dust exposure at pharmacies using automatic dispensing machines: a preliminary study. *J Occup Environ Hyg.* 2014; 11:695–705.
120. Polovich M, Olsen M, LeFebvre K. Chemotherapy and biotherapy guidelines and recommendations for practice. Pittsburgh: Oncology Nursing Society; 2014.
121. Roberts S, Khammo N, McDonnell G et al. Studies on the decontamination of surfaces exposed to cytotoxic drugs in chemotherapy workstations. *J Oncol Pharm Pract.* 2006; 12:95–104.
122. Lé LM, Jolivot PA, Sadou-Yaye H et al. Effectiveness of cleaning of workplace cytotoxic surface. *Int Arch Occup Environ Health.* 2013; 86:333–41.
123. Hon CY, Chua PP, Danyluk Q et al. Examining factors that influence the effectiveness of cleaning antineoplastic drugs from drug preparation surfaces: a pilot study. *J Oncol Pharm Pract.* 2014; 20:210–6.
124. Bohlandt A, Groeneveld S, Fischer E et al. Cleaning efficiencies of three cleaning agents on four different surfaces after contamination by gemcitabine and 5-fluorouracil. *J Occup Environ Hyg.* 2015; 12:384–92.
125. Johnson EG, Janosik JE. Manufacturers' recommendations for handling spilled antineoplastic agents. *Am J Hosp Pharm.* 1989; 46:318–9.
126. Gonzalez R, Massoomi F. Manufacturers' recommendations for handling spilled hazardous drugs. *Am J Health-Syst Pharm.* 2010; 67:1985–6.
127. Contec Healthcare. PeridoxRTU sporicidal disinfectant for decontaminating hazardous drugs. www.contechealthcare.com/files/documents/HCA001_Peridox_HazardousDrugs.pdf (accessed 2018 Feb 28).
128. Contec Healthcare. Peridox RTU. Hazardous drug cleaning removal test report. www.contechealthcare.com/files/documents/Peridox_RTU_Hazardous-Drug-Cleaning-Removal-Test-Summary.pdf (accessed 2018 Feb 28).
129. Bartel SB, Tyler TG, Power LA. Multicenter evaluation of a new closed system drug-transfer device in reducing surface contamination by antineoplastic hazardous drugs. *Am J Health-Syst Pharm.* 2018; 75:199–211.
130. Occupational Safety and Health Administration. OSHA standards. Hazardous waste operations and emergency response. 29 C.F.R. 1910.120. www.osha.gov/pls/oshaweb/owadisp.show_document?p_table=STANDARDS&p_id=9765 (accessed 2018 Feb 28).
131. U.S. Environmental Protection Agency. Protection of environment. Hazardous waste management system: general. 40 C.F.R. 260. www.ecfr.gov/cgi-bin/text-idx? &node=pt40.28.260&rgn=div5 (accessed 2018 Feb 28).
132. U.S. Environmental Protection Agency. Discarded commercial chemical products, off-specification species, container residues, and spill residues thereof. 40 C.F.R. 261.33. www.ecfr.gov/cgi-bin/text-idx?node=se40.26.261_133 (accessed 2018 Feb 28).
133. Occupational Safety and Health Administration. OSHA standards. Medical and first aid. 29 C.F.R. 1910.151(c). www.osha.gov/pls/oshaweb/owadisp.show_document?p_table=STANDARDS&p_id=9806 (accessed 2018 Feb 28).
134. Resource Conservation and Recovery Act of 1976. U.S. Code Title 42. Chapter 82, solid waste disposal. www.gpo.gov/fdsys/pkg/USCODE-2011-title42/html/USCODE-2011-title42-chap82.htm (accessed 2018 Feb 28).
135. U.S. Environmental Protection Agency. Characteristics of hazardous waste. 40 C.F.R. 261.20–24. www.ecfr.gov/cgi-bin/text-idx?&node=pt40.28.261&rgn=div5#sp40.28.261.c (accessed 2018 Feb 28).
136. U.S. Environmental Protection Agency. Memorandum excluding epinephrine salts. http://yosemite.epa.gov/osw/rcra.nsf/ea6e50dc6214725285256bf00063269d/9c30209e1466f980852579ea0067cd97!OpenDocument (accessed 2018 Feb 28).
137. U.S. Environmental Protection Agency. Hazardous waste. Defining hazardous waste: listed, characteristic and mixed radiological wastes. www.epa.gov/hw/defining-hazardous-waste-listed-characteristic-and-mixed-radiological-wastes#PandU (accessed 2018 Feb 28).
138. U.S. Environmental Protection Agency. State authorization under the Resource Conservation and Recovery Act (RCRA). www.epa.gov/rcra/state-authorization-under-resource-conservation-and-recovery-act-rcra (accessed 2018 Feb 28).
139. U.S. Environmental Protection Agency. Residues of hazardous waste in empty containers. 40 C.F.R. 261.7. www.ecfr.gov/cgi-bin/retrieveECFR? &n=pt40.28.261&r=PART&ty=HTML#se40.28.261_17 (accessed 2018 Feb 28).
140. Vaccari PL, Tonat K, DeChristoforo R et al. Disposal of antineoplastic wastes at the National Institutes of Health. *Am J Hosp Pharm.* 1984; 41:87–93.
141. U.S. Environmental Protection Agency. Residues of hazardous waste in empty containers—definition of "empty." 40 C.F.R. 261.7(b)(1)-(3). www.ecfr.gov/cgi-bin/retrieveECFR? &n=pt40.28.261&r=PART&ty=HTML#se40.28.261_17 (accessed 2018 Feb 27).

142. U.S. Environmental Protection Agency Office of Inspector General. Report: EPA inaction in identifying hazardous waste pharmaceuticals may result in unsafe disposal. www.epa.gov/office-inspector-general/report-epa-inaction-identifying-hazardous-waste-pharmaceuticals-may-result (accessed 2018 Feb 28).
143. Minnesota Pollution Control Agency. Alternate method to evaluate pharmaceutical waste for the lethality characteristic. March 2015. www.pca.state.mn.us/sites/default/files/w-hw4-45b.pdf (accessed 2018 Feb 28).
144. Pipeline and Hazardous Materials Safety Administration. Hazardous materials table, special provisions, hazardous materials communications. 49 C.F.R. 172.1-172.123. www.ecfr.gov/cgi-bin/retrieveECFR?&n=pt49.2.172&r=PART&ty=HTML (accessed 2018 Feb 28).
145. Federal Motor Carrier Safety Administration. How to comply with federal hazardous materials regulations. www.fmcsa.dot.gov/regulations/hazardous-materials/how-comply-federal-hazardous-materials-regulations (accessed 2018 Feb 28).
146. Occupational Safety and Health Administration. OSHA standards. Hazardous waste operations and emergency response. Initial training. 29 C.F.R. 1910.120(e)(3)(i). www.ecfr.gov/cgi-bin/text-idx?&node=se29.5.1910_1120&rgn=div8 (accessed 2018 Feb 28).
147. Occupational Safety and Health Administration. OSHA standards. Hazardous waste operations and emergency response. Emergency response to hazardous substances releases. 29 C.F.R. 1910.120(q)(1-6). www.ecfr.gov/cgi-bin/text-idx?&node=se29.5.1910_1120&rgn=div8 (accessed 2018 Feb 28).
148. U.S. Environmental Protection Agency. Hazardous waste generator regulatory summary. www.epa.gov/hwgenerators/hazardous-waste-generator-regulatory-summary (accessed 2018 Feb 28).
149. U.S. Environmental Protection Agency. Memo: containers that once held P-listed pharmaceuticals (November 4, 2011). https://yosemite.epa.gov/osw/rcra.nsf/0/57B21F2FE33735128525795F00610F0F/$file/14827.pdf (accessed 2018 Feb 28).
150. U.S. Environmental Protection Agency. Proposed rule: management standards for hazardous waste pharmaceuticals (September 25, 2015). www.epa.gov/hwgenerators/proposed-rule-management-standards-hazardous-waste-pharmaceuticals (accessed 2018 Feb 28).
151. National Institute for Occupational Safety and Health. Medical surveillance for healthcare workers exposed to hazardous drugs. DHHS (NIOSH) publication no. 2013–103 (2012). www.cdc.gov/niosh/docs/wp-solutions/2013-103/ (accessed 2018 Feb 28).
152. Fox BI, Felkey BG. Automated intravenous preparation: robots for the pharmacy. *Hosp Pharm.* 2009; 44:255–6,264.
153. Volpe G, Cohen S, Capps RC et al. Robotics in acute care hospitals. *Am J Health-Syst Pharm.* 2012; 69:1601–3.
154. Yaniv AW, Knoer SJ. Implementation of an i.v.-compounding robot in a hospital-based cancer center pharmacy. *Am J Health-Syst Pharm.* 2013; 70:2030–7.
155. Masini C, Nanni O, Antaridi S et al. Automated preparation of chemotherapy: quality improvement and economic sustainability. *Am J Health-Syst Pharm.* 2014; 71:579–85.
156. Seger AC, Churchill WW, Keohane CA et al. Impact of robotic antineoplastic preparation on safety, workflow, and costs. *J Oncol Pract.* 2012; 8:344–9.
157. Sessink PJ, Leclercq GM, Wouters DM et al. Environmental contamination, product contamination and workers exposure using a robotic system for antineoplastic drug preparation. *J Oncol Pharm Pract.* 2015; 21:118–27.
158. Schierl R, Masini C, Groeneveld S et al. Environmental contamination by cyclophosphamide preparation: comparison of conventional manual production in biological safety cabinet and robot-assisted production by APOTECAchemo. *J Oncol Pharm Pract.* 2016; 22:37–45.
159. Erickson BA, Boyce CA. Sterile compounding technology. In: Buchanan EC, Schneider PJ, Forrey RA, eds. Compounding sterile preparations, 4th ed. Bethesda, MD: American Society of Health-System Pharmacists; 2017:363–407.
160. Connor TH, Zock MD, Snow AH. Surface wipe sampling for antineoplastic (chemotherapy) and other hazardous drug residue in healthcare settings: methodology and recommendations. *J Occup Environ Hyg.* 2016; 13:658–67.
161. Schierl R, Bohlandt A, Nowak D. Guidance values for surface monitoring of antineoplastic drugs in German pharmacies. *Ann Occup Hyg.* 2009; 53:1–9.
162. Hedmer M, Wohlfart G. Hygienic guidance values for wipe sampling of antineoplastic drugs in Swedish hospitals. *J Environ Monit.* 2012; 14:1968–75.
163. Kibby T. A review of surface wipe sampling compared to biologic monitoring for occupational exposure to antineoplastic drugs. *J Occup Environ Hyg.* 2017; 14:159–74.

Appendix A—Glossary

Active pharmaceutical ingredient (API): Any substance or mixture of substances intended to be used in the compounding of a drug preparation, thereby becoming the active ingredient in that preparation and furnishing pharmacologic activity or other direct effect in the diagnosis, cure, mitigation, treatment, or prevention of disease in humans and animals or affecting the structure and function of the body.[8]

Alternative duty: Performance of other tasks that do not include the direct handling of HDs.[8]

Antechamber: Chamber in a compounding isolator that leads to the main compounding chamber. The antechamber is used to load supplies and drugs into the isolator and unload final preparations and waste.

Anteroom: An ISO class 7 or cleaner room where personnel hand hygiene, garbing procedures, and other activities that generate high particulate levels are performed. The anteroom is the transition room between the unclassified area of the facility and the buffer room.[8]

Antineoplastic drug: A chemotherapeutic agent that controls or kills cancer cells. Drugs used in the treatment of cancer are cytotoxic but are generally more damaging to dividing cells than to resting cells.[6]

Aseptic: Free of living pathogenic organisms or infected materials.[6]

Assessment of risk: Evaluation of risk to determine alternative containment strategies and/or work practices.

Beyond-use date (BUD): The date or time beyond which a compounded preparation cannot be used and must be discarded (see *USP* chapters 795 and 797).[7,61] The date or time is determined from the date or time when the preparation was compounded.

Biological safety cabinet (BSC): BSCs or biosafety cabinets are used as the primary means of containment for working safely with infectious microorganisms. Biosafety cabinets are designed to prevent biological exposure to personnel and the environment and may also protect experimental material from being contaminated when appropriate practices and procedures are followed. Class II BSCs have been adopted for use in compounding HDs as they protect the product, the worker, and the environment. Descriptions of the various classes and types of BSCs may be found in the CDC Biosafety in Microbiological and Biomedical Laboratories, 5th ed., Appendix A.[81]

Buffer room: A type of C-SEC under negative pressure that meets ISO class 7 or better air quality where the C-PEC that generates and maintains an ISO class 5 environment is physically located. Activities that occur in this area are limited to the preparation and staging of components and supplies used when compounding HDs.[8]

Chemotherapy drug: A chemical agent used to treat diseases. The term usually refers to a drug used to treat cancer.[6]

Chemotherapy glove: A medical glove that meets the ASTM Standard Practice for Assessment of Resistance of Medical Gloves to Permeation by Chemotherapy Drugs (D6978) or its successor.[8]

Chemotherapy waste: Discarded items such as gowns, gloves, masks, i.v. tubing, empty bags, empty drug vials, needles, and syringes used while preparing and administering antineoplastic agents.[6]

Classified space: An area that maintains an air cleanliness classification based on ISO.[8]

Cleaning: The process of removing soil (e.g., organic and inorganic material) from objects and surfaces, normally accomplished by manually or mechanically using water with detergents or enzymatic products.[8]

Closed system: A device that does not exchange unfiltered air or contaminants with the adjacent environment.[6]

Closed-system drug-transfer device (CSTD): A drug-transfer device that mechanically prohibits the transfer of environmental contaminants into the system and the escape of HD or vapor concentrations outside the system.[6]

Compounded preparation: A nonsterile or sterile drug or nutrient preparation that is compounded in a licensed pharmacy or other healthcare-related facility in response to or anticipation of a prescription or a medication order from a licensed prescriber.[8]

Compounding aseptic containment isolator (CACI): A specific type of compounding aseptic isolator (CAI) that is designed for the compounding of sterile HDs. The CACI is designed to provide worker protection from exposure to undesirable levels of airborne drugs throughout the compounding and material transfer processes and to provide an aseptic environment with unidirectional airflow for compounding sterile preparations.[8]

Compounding aseptic isolator (CAI): An isolator specifically designed for compounding sterile, nonhazardous pharmaceutical ingredients or preparations. The CAI is designed to maintain an aseptic compounding environment throughout the compounding and material transfer processes.[8]

Compounding personnel: Individuals who participate in the compounding process.[8]

Containment primary engineering control (C-PEC): A ventilated device designed and operated to minimize worker and environmental exposures to HDs by controlling emissions of airborne contaminants through the following:

- The full or partial enclosure of a potential contaminant source,
- The use of airflow capture velocities to trap and remove airborne contaminants near their point of generation,
- The use of air pressure relationships that define the direction of airflow into the cabinet, and
- The use of HEPA filtration on all potentially contaminated exhaust streams.[8]

Containment secondary engineering control (C-SEC): The room with fixed walls in which the C-PEC is placed. It incorporates specific design and operational parameters required to contain the potential hazard within the compounding room.[8]

Containment segregated compounding area (C-SCA): A type of C-SEC with nominal requirements for airflow and room pressurization as they pertain to HD compounding.[8]

Containment ventilated enclosure (CVE): A full or partial enclosure that uses ventilation principles to capture, contain, and remove airborne contaminants through HEPA filtration and prevent their release into the work environment.[8]

Cytotoxic: A pharmacologic compound that is detrimental or destructive to cells within the body.[6]

Deactivation: Treating a chemical agent (such as an HD) with another chemical, heat, ultraviolet light, or another agent to create a less hazardous agent.[6]

Decontamination: Inactivation, neutralization, or removal of toxic agents, usually by chemical means.[6] Surface decontamination may be accomplished by the transfer of HD contamination from the surface of a nondisposable item to disposable ones (e.g., wipes, gauze, towels).

Direct compounding area (DCA): A critical area within an ISO class 5 primary engineering control where critical sites are exposed to unidirectional HEPA-filtered air, also known as first air.[7]

Disinfecting: Removal of viable organism from surfaces using 70% isopropyl alcohol or other appropriate disinfectant before compounding of sterile HDs.

Don: To put on PPE.[8]

Engineering controls: Devices designed to eliminate or reduce worker exposures to chemical, biological, radiological, ergonomic, or physical hazards. Examples include laboratory fume hoods, glove bags, retracting syringe needles, sound-dampening materials to reduce noise levels, safety interlocks, and radiation shielding.[6]

Environmental Protection Agency (EPA)-registered disinfectant: Antimicrobial products registered with EPA for healthcare use against pathogens specified in the product labeling.[8]

Externally vented: Exhausted to the outside.[8]

Final dosage form: Any form of a medication that requires no further manipulation before administration.[8]

Genotoxic: Capable of damaging DNA and leading to mutations.[6]

Globally Harmonized System of Classification and Labeling of Chemicals: A system for standardizing and harmonizing the classification and labeling of chemicals.[8]

Goggles: Tight-fitting eye protection that completely covers the eyes, eye sockets, and facial area that immediately surrounds the eyes. Goggles provide protection from impact, dust, and splashes. Some goggles fit over corrective lenses.[8]

Hazardous drug (HD): Any drug identified by at least 1 of the following 6 criteria: carcinogenicity, teratogenicity or developmental toxicity, reproductive toxicity in humans, organ toxicity at low doses in humans or animals, genotoxicity, and new drugs that mimic existing HDs in structure or toxicity.[6]

Hazardous waste: Any waste that is an RCRA-listed hazardous waste (40 C.F.R. 261.30-261.33) or that meets an RCRA characteristic of ignitability, corrosivity, reactivity, or toxicity as defined in 40 C.F.R. 261.21-.24.[6]

Healthcare settings: All hospitals, medical clinics, outpatient facilities, physicians' offices, retail pharmacies, and similar facilities dedicated to the care of patients.[6]

Healthcare workers: All workers who are involved in the care of patients. These include pharmacists, pharmacy technicians, nurses (registered nurses, licensed practical nurses, nurses' aides, etc.), physicians, home healthcare workers, and environmental services workers (housekeeping, laundry, and waste disposal).[6]

High-efficiency particulate air (HEPA) filter: Filter rated 99.97% efficient in capturing particles 0.3 µm in diameter.[6]

Horizontal-laminar-airflow hood (horizontal-laminar airflow clean bench): A device that protects the work product and the work area by supplying HEPA-filtered air to the rear of the cabinet and producing a horizontal flow across the work area and out toward the worker.[6]

Laboratory coat: A disposable or reusable open-front coat, usually made of cloth or other permeable material.[6]

Mutagenic: Capable of increasing the spontaneous mutation rate by causing changes in DNA.[6]

Negative-pressure room: A room that is maintained at a lower pressure than the adjacent areas; therefore, the net flow of air is into the room.[8]

Pass-through: An enclosure with interlocking doors that is positioned between 2 spaces for the purpose of reducing particulate transfer while moving materials from 1 space to another. A pass-through serving negative-pressure rooms needs to be equipped with sealed doors.[8] (Note: A pass-through located before the main chamber of a compounding isolator is an antechamber.)

Personal protective equipment (PPE): Items such as gloves, gowns, respirators, goggles, and face shields that protect individual workers from hazardous physical or chemical exposures.[6]

Positive-pressure room: A room that is maintained at a higher pressure than the adjacent areas; therefore, the net flow of air is out of the room.[8]

Repackaging: The act of removing a product from its original primary container and placing it into another primary container, usually of smaller size.[8]

Respirator: A type of PPE that prevents harmful materials from entering the respiratory system, usually by filtering hazardous agents from workplace air. A surgical mask does not offer respiratory protection.[6]

Risk assessment: Characterization of potentially adverse health effects from human exposure to environmental or occupational hazards. Risk assessment can be divided into 5 major steps: hazard identification, dose–response assessment, exposure assessment, risk characterization, and risk communication.[6]

Safety data sheet (SDS): An informational document that provides written or printed material concerning a hazardous chemical (previously known as a Material Safety Data Sheet). The SDS is prepared in accordance with the HCS.[8]

Spill kit: A container of supplies, warning signage, and related materials used to contain the spill of an HD.[8]

Standard operating procedure (SOP): Written procedures describing operations, testing, sampling, interpretation of results, and corrective actions that relate to the operations that are taking place.[8]

Supplemental engineering control: An adjunct control (e.g., a CSTD) that may be used concurrently with primary and secondary engineering controls. Supplemental engineering controls offer additional levels of protection and may facilitate enhanced occupational protection, especially when handling HDs outside of primary and secondary engineering controls (e.g., during administration).[8]

Surface decontamination: Transfer of HD contamination from the surface of nondisposable items to disposable ones (e.g., wipes, gauze, towels). No procedures have been studied for surface decontamination of HD-contaminated surfaces. The use of gauze moistened with 70% isopropyl alcohol, sterile water, peroxide, or sodium hypochlorite solutions may be effective. The disposable item, once contaminated, must be contained and discarded as hazardous waste.

Unclassified space: A space not required to meet any air cleanliness classification based on ISO.[8]

Ventilated cabinet: A type of engineering control designed for purposes of worker protection (as used in these guidelines). These devices are designed to minimize worker exposures by controlling emissions of airborne contaminants through (1) the full or partial enclosure of a potential contaminant source, (2) the use of airflow capture velocities to capture and remove airborne contaminants near their point of generation, and (3) the use of air pressure relationships that define the direction of airflow into the cabinet. Examples of ventilated cabinets include BSCs, containment isolators, and laboratory fume hoods.[6]

Appendix B—Recommendations for Use of Class II BSCs

1. Use of a class II BSC must be accompanied by a stringent program of work practices, including training, demonstrated competence, contamination reduction, and decontamination when used for compounding sterile and nonsterile HDs.
2. The class II BSC has an 8–10 inch opening in the front where drugs and supplies are placed into the cabinet and whereby the compounder accesses the cabinet. Studies show that this opening is a source of HD contamination transfer to the environment. Care must be taken to restrict unnecessary movements in and out of the cabinet.
3. A class II BSC used for sterile HD compounding must provide ISO class 5 or better air quality and unidirectional airflow and be externally vented.
4. A class II BSC used for nonsterile compounding must meet the *USP* chapter 800 requirements for all C-PECs.[8] It must be externally vented (preferred) or have redundant HEPA filters in series as an exhaust. Class I BSCs and CVEs are also acceptable C-PECs for nonsterile compounding.
5. The class II BSC (as for all C-PECs) must be located in an externally vented, physically separate, negative pressure C-SEC with appropriate ACPH to be used for compounding sterile and nonsterile HDs.
6. The C-SEC may be either an ISO class 7 buffer room with an ISO class 7 anteroom (preferred) or an unclassified containment segregated compounding area (C-SCA).
7. Class II BSCs (as for all C-PECs) used in a facility that compounds both sterile and nonsterile HDs must be placed in separate rooms unless all the *USP* chapter 800 requirements for placement in the same room are met.
8. The class II BSC (as for all C-PECs) must run continuously if it supplies some or all of the negative pressure in the C-SEC or if it is used to compound sterile HDs.
9. A plastic-backed preparation mat that does not interfere with airflow to the front or back air grilles should be placed on the work surface of the class II BSC. The mat must be changed routinely in batch compounding and immediately if a spill occurs.
10. Appropriate chemotherapy PPE must be worn when compounding or cleaning a class II BSC. For sterile compounding, PPE must be donned per *USP* chapter 797 instructions.[7]
11. The class II BSC must be decontaminated and disinfected before sterile compounding of HDs and routinely during batch compounding.
12. For sterile compounding, reduce the bioburden in the class II BSC by wiping down supplies with an appropriate disinfectant before placing them in the cabinet.
13. Reduce the HD contamination burden in the class II BSC by wiping down HD vials with a decontaminant such as 0.5% sodium hypochlorite wipers[76] and then with a disinfectant such as sterile 70% isopropyl alcohol before placing them in the cabinet.
14. Consider using an FDA ONB-cleared CSTD while compounding HDs in a class II BSC. Studies document a decrease in drug contaminants inside a class II BSC when some such devices are used.[6,8]
15. Contain supply and drug waste in the class II BSC in an appropriate waste bag or hard plastic container. Do not discard waste during operations in the class II BSC, as entering and exiting the cabinet are significant sources of HD contamination transfer.
16. Once HD compounding is complete, wipe down the dose(s), then label and transfer to clean transport bags, wearing noncontaminated gloves.
17. Decontaminate the class II BSC after completing HD compounding.
18. Remove PPE according to SOPs and policies and procedures and discard in an appropriate waste container.
19. Wash hands thoroughly with soap and water.

Appendix C—Recommendations for Use of Class III BSCs and CACIs

1. Use of a class III BSC or CACI must be accompanied by a stringent program of work practices, including training, demonstrated competence, contamination reduction, and decontamination when used for compounding sterile and nonsterile HDs.
2. A class III BSC or CACI used for sterile HD compounding must provide ISO cclass 5 or better air quality and unidirectional airflow in the main work chamber and be externally vented.
3. A class III BSC or CACI must achieve containment at all times during the operation of the cabinet and during the transfer process from the antechamber (compounding isolator pass-through) to the main work chamber and in reverse.
4. A class III BSC or CACI used for nonsterile compounding must meet the *USP* chapter 800 requirements for all C-PECs.[8] It must be externally vented (preferred) or have redundant HEPA filters in series as an exhaust.
5. The class III BSC or CACI (as for all C-PECs) must be located in an externally vented, physically separate, negative-pressure C-SEC with appropriate ACPH to be used for compounding sterile and nonsterile HDs.
6. The C-SEC may be either an ISO class 7 buffer room with an ISO class 7 anteroom (preferred) or an unclassified C-SCA.
7. Class III BSCs or CACIs (as for all C-PECs) used in a facility that compounds both sterile and nonsterile HDs must be placed in separate rooms unless all the *USP* chapter 800 requirements for placement in the same room are met.
8. The class III BSC or CACI (as for all C-PECs) must run continuously if it supplies some or all of the negative pressure in the C-SEC or if it is used to compound sterile HDs.
9. A plastic-backed preparation mat that does not interfere with airflow through the cabinet may be placed on the work surface of the class III BSC or CACI. The mat must be changed routinely during compounding and immediately if a spill occurs.

10. A class III BSC and CACI have sleeves and a fixed glove assembly or a gauntlet to access the main work chamber in the cabinet. Always inspect the condition of the sleeves and gauntlet as well as disposable gloves to ensure they are intact and not damaged. The sleeves and/or gauntlet must be decontaminated before and after HD compounding and disinfected before sterile compounding.
11. The decontamination and disinfecting process must be done in such a manner that surface contamination is contained in both the main chamber and antechamber (compounding isolator pass-through).
12. Gloves or gauntlets must not be replaced before completing appropriate decontamination and disinfecting of the cabinet. Use the device manufacturer's recommendations for changing gloves without breaking the HD containment.
13. Sterile gloves must be donned over the gauntlet or fixed glove before compounding sterile HDs (see glove section for additional details). In a negative pressure cabinet, the additional glove may require being taped to the fixed glove to avoid risking it being dislodged.
14. Appropriate chemotherapy PPE must be worn when compounding or cleaning a class III BSC or CACI. There is no exemption from the requirement for wearing a chemotherapy gown when compounding in a class III BSC or CACI. For sterile compounding, don PPE per *USP* chapter 797 instructions.[7] Sterile gloves tested to ASTM Standard D-6978 for chemotherapy gloves must be available near the cabinet to allow placement of the gloves into the antechamber to affix to the fixed glove assembly.
15. The class III BSC or CACI must be decontaminated and disinfected before sterile compounding of HDs and routinely during batch compounding.
16. For sterile compounding, reduce the bio-burden in the class III BSC or CACI by wiping down supplies with an appropriate disinfectant before placing them in the cabinet antechamber.
17. Reduce the HD contamination burden in the class III BSC or CACI by wiping down HD vials with a decontaminant such as 0.5% sodium hypochlorite wipers[76] and then with a disinfectant such as sterile 70% isopropyl alcohol before placing them in the cabinet antechamber.
18. Consider using an FDA ONB-cleared CSTD while compounding HDs in a class III BSC or CACI. Studies document a decrease in drug contaminants inside a C-PEC when some such devices are used.[6,8]
19. Once HD compounding is complete, wipe down the outer glove and the dose(s), then label and transfer to the antechamber. Final doses should be placed in clean transport bags in the antechamber by someone wearing clean, tested chemotherapy gloves.
20. Contain supply and drug waste in the class III BSC or CACI in an appropriate waste bag or hard plastic container. Remove and contain the outer glove with other HD waste. Transfer the contained waste into the antechamber for removal and disposal. Alternatively, use the waste containers attached to the cabinet, if available.
21. Decontaminate the class III BSC or CACI after completing HD compounding.
22. Remove PPE according to SOPs and policies and procedures and discard in appropriate waste container.
23. Wash hands thoroughly with soap and water.

Appendix D—Recommendations for Use of Gloves

1. Two pairs of ASTM D6978-tested gloves are required for compounding sterile and nonsterile HDs, for the administration of HDs, and for cleanup of HD spills.
2. Chemotherapy gloves should be worn for handling all HDs, including nonantineoplastics, and for reproductive risk–only HDs.
3. Double gloves should be worn during any handling of HD shipping cartons or drug vials and handling of HD waste or waste from patients recently treated with HDs.
4. Select powder-free, high-quality gloves made of latex, nitrile, polyurethane, neoprene, or other materials that meet ASTM D6978 for chemotherapy gloves.
5. Inspect gloves for visible defects.
6. For sterile HD compounding, the outer glove must be sterile.
7. Sanitize gloves with sterile 70% isopropyl alcohol or other appropriate disinfectant before performing any aseptic compounding activity. Wipe gloves using a saturated wipe; never spray.
8. Change gloves every 30 minutes during compounding or immediately when damaged or contaminated, unless otherwise recommended by the manufacturer's documentation.
9. Remove outer gloves after wiping down final preparation but before labeling or removing the preparation from the C-PEC.
10. Outer gloves must be placed in a containment bag while in the C-PEC.
11. In a C-PEC with fixed gloves and sleeves, these must be surface cleaned after compounding is completed to avoid spreading HD contamination to other surfaces.
12. Clean gloves (e.g., the clean inner gloves) should be used to surface decontaminate the final preparation, place the label onto the final preparation, and place the preparation into the antechamber and transport bag.
13. Wear fresh gloves to complete the final check, place preparation into a clean transport bag, and remove the bag from the antechamber.
14. Remove gloves with care to avoid contamination. Specific procedures for removal must be established and followed.
15. Outer gloves should be removed and contained inside the C-PEC.
16. Change gloves after administering an HD dose or when leaving the immediate administration area.
17. Dispose of contaminated gloves as contaminated waste.
18. Wash hands with soap and water after removing gloves.

Appendix E—Recommendations for Use of Gowns

1. Gowns should be worn during compounding, during administration, when handling waste from patients recently treated with HDs, and when cleaning up spills of HDs.
2. Select disposable gowns of material tested to be protective against the HDs to be used.
3. Gowns must be changed per the manufacturer's information for permeation of the gown. If no permeation information is available for the gowns used, change them every 2–3 hours or immediately after a spill or splash.
4. Remove gowns with care to avoid spreading contamination. Specific procedures for removal must be established and followed.[7,8]
5. To avoid spreading HD contamination and exposing other healthcare workers, gowns worn in HD handling areas must not be worn to other areas.
6. Dispose of gowns immediately upon removal.
7. Contain and dispose of contaminated gowns as trace chemotherapy waste.
8. Wash hands after removing and disposing of gowns.

Appendix F—Recommendations for Working in Any C-PEC

1. The C-PEC must be appropriately vented to the outside. Check all gauges and alarms before using a C-PEC for compounding HDs.
2. Select the appropriate C-PEC for the type of HD compounding (sterile or nonsterile).
3. PPE appropriate to the C-PEC must be worn when compounding HDs in a C-PEC.
4. The use of a C-PEC must be accompanied by a stringent program of work practices, including operator training and demonstrated competence, contamination reduction, and decontamination.
5. Decontaminate the C-PEC before beginning HD compounding at the beginning of the day and per the established decontamination schedule. If rinsing is required, use sterile water for irrigation to remove the cleaning agent.
6. Disinfect the C-PEC with sterile 70% isopropyl alcohol before beginning sterile HD compounding and routinely during batch compounding. Use sterile wipers to apply the disinfectant. Do not spray anything into a C-PEC used for HD compounding to avoid aerosolizing or transferring HD residue.
7. Do not place unnecessary items in the work area of the C-PEC, where HD contamination from compounding may settle on them.
8. Do not crowd the C-PEC.
9. Gather all needed supplies before beginning compounding. Avoid exiting and reentering the work area of the C-PEC.
10. A plastic-backed preparation mat that does not interfere with airflow through the C-PEC may be placed on the work surface of the direct compounding area. The mat must be changed routinely during compounding and immediately if a spill occurs.
11. Appropriate handling of the preparation in the C-PEC, including wiping with sterile 70% isopropyl alcohol or another appropriate disinfectant, is necessary for sterile compounding.
12. Reduce the HD contamination burden in the C-PEC by wiping down HD vials before placing them in the C-PEC.
13. To avoid inadvertent contamination of the outside surface, transport bags must never be placed in the C-PEC work area during compounding.
14. Final preparations should be surface decontaminated within the C-PEC and placed into the transport bags, wearing clean gloves, taking care not to contaminate the outside of the transport bag.
15. Decontaminate the work surface of the C-PEC before and after compounding per the manufacturer's recommendations or with detergent, sodium hypochlorite solution, and neutralizer, or another tested decontaminating cleaner.
16. Decontaminate all surfaces of the C-PEC at the end of the batch, day, or shift, as appropriate to the workflow according to facility policy. Typically, a C-PEC in use 24 hours a day would require decontamination 2 or 3 times daily. Disinfect the C-PEC before compounding a dose or batch of sterile HDs with sterile 70% isopropyl alcohol.
17. Wipe down the outside of the class II BSC front opening and the floor in front of the BSC with detergent, sodium hypochlorite solution, and neutralizer, or another tested decontaminating cleaner, at least daily.
18. Wipe down the inside and outside of the antechamber door of the class III BSC or CACI at least daily and the handle of the antechamber frequently with detergent, sodium hypochlorite solution, and neutralizer, or another tested decontaminating cleaner.
19. Seal and then decontaminate surfaces of waste and sharps containers before removing from the C-PEC.

Appendix G—Recommendations for Compounding and Handling Nonsterile HD Dosage Forms

1. HDs should be labeled or otherwise identified as such to prevent improper handling.
2. Tablet and capsule forms of HDs should not be placed in automated counting machines, which subject them to stress and may introduce powdered contaminants into the work area.
3. During routine handling of nonsterile HDs and contaminated equipment, workers should wear 2 pairs of gloves that meet ASTM D6978 requirements.[100]
4. Counting and pouring of HDs should be done carefully, and clean equipment should be dedicated for use with these drugs.
5. Contaminated equipment should be cleaned initially with gauze saturated with sterile water; further cleaned with detergent, sodium hypochlorite solution,

and neutralizer; and then rinsed. The gauze and rinse should be contained and disposed of as contaminated waste.

6. Crushing tablets or opening capsules should be avoided; liquid formulations should be used whenever possible.
7. During the compounding of HDs (e.g., crushing, dissolving, or preparing a solution or an ointment), workers should wear nonpermeable gowns and double gloves. Compounding should take place in a ventilated cabinet.
8. Compounding nonsterile forms of HDs in equipment designated for sterile products must be undertaken with care. Appropriate containment, deactivation, and disinfection techniques must be utilized.
9. HDs should be dispensed in the final dose and form whenever possible. Unit-of-use containers for oral liquids have not been tested for containment properties. Most exhibit some spillage during preparation or use. Caution must be exercised when using these devices.
10. Bulk containers of liquid HDs, as well as specially packaged commercial HDs, must be handled carefully to avoid spills. These containers should be dispensed and maintained in sealable plastic bags to contain any inadvertent contamination.
11. Disposal of unused or unusable noninjectable dosage forms of HDs should be performed in the same manner as for hazardous injectable dosage forms and waste.

Appendix H—Recommendations for Reducing Exposure to HDs During Administration in All Practice Settings[110,120]

Intravenous Administration

1. Only trained and certified staff may administer HDs.
2. Appropriate PPE must be worn when administering HDs.[8,55]
3. The use of gloves, gown, and face shield (as needed for splashing) is required.
4. Gloves for handling HDs must be tested to and meet ASTM D6978 for chemotherapy gloves.[8,100]
5. Two pairs of tested chemotherapy gloves are required for administering injectable antineoplastic HDs.[8]
6. Gather all necessary equipment and supplies, including PPE.
7. CSTDs are required when the dosage form allows.
8. Use needleless systems whenever possible.
9. Use Luer-Lok fittings for all needleless systems, syringes, needles, ancillary devices, infusion tubing, and pumps. If a CSTD cannot be used, position gauze pads to catch leaks from needleless and other devices that may leak at connection points.
10. Designate a workplace for handling HDs.
11. Have a spill kit and HD waste container readily available.
12. Procedure for gowning and gloving: Wash hands, don first pair of gloves, don gown and face shield, and then don second pair of gloves. Gloves should extend beyond the elastic or knit cuff of the gown. Double gloving requires 1 glove to be worn under the cuff of the gown and the second glove over the cuff.
13. Always work below eye level.
14. Visually examine HD dose while it is still contained in the transport bag.
15. If HD dose appears intact, remove it from the transport bag while wearing gloves.
16. Place a plastic-backed absorbent pad under the administration site to absorb leaks and prevent drug contact with the patient's skin.
17. If priming occurs at the administration site, prime i.v. tubing with an i.v. solution that does not contain HDs or prime using the backflow method.
18. Use the transport bag as a containment bag for HD containers and i.v. sets and all materials contaminated with HDs.
19. Discard HD i.v. containers with the administration sets attached; do not remove the set.
20. Wash surfaces that come into contact with HDs with detergent, sodium hypochlorite solution, and neutralizer, if appropriate.
21. Wearing gloves, contain and dispose of materials contaminated with HDs.
22. To remove PPE, carefully begin with outer gloves. Still wearing the inner gloves, remove remaining PPE from least to most contaminated and discard as trace waste.
23. HD waste containers must be sufficiently large to hold all discarded material, including PPE.
24. Do not push or force materials contaminated with HDs into the waste container.
25. Carefully remove, contain, and discard gloves.
26. Wash hands thoroughly after removing gloves.

Intramuscular or Subcutaneous Administration

1. The use of double gloves and gown is required.
2. Gather all necessary equipment and supplies, including PPE.
3. Use Luer-Lok safety needles or retracting needles or shields.
4. Syringes should have Luer-Lok connections and be less than three-fourths full.
5. Designate a workplace for handling HDs.
6. Have a spill kit and HD waste container readily available.
7. Procedure for gloving: wash hands and then don double gloves (1 pair under gown, 1 over).
8. Always work below eye level.
9. Visually examine HD dose while still contained in transport bag.
10. If HD dose appears intact, remove it from the transport bag.
11. Remove the syringe cap and connect appropriate safety needle.
12. Do not expel air from syringe or prime the safety needle.
13. After administration, discard HD syringes (with the safety needle attached) directly into an HD waste container.

14. Wearing gloves, contain and dispose of materials contaminated with HDs.
15. Do not push or force materials contaminated with HDs into the HD waste container.
16. Carefully remove, contain, and discard gloves.
17. Wash hands thoroughly after removing gloves.

Oral Administration

1. Double gloves are required, as is a face shield if there is a potential for spraying, aerosolization, or splashing.
2. Workers should be aware that tablets or capsules may be coated with a dust of residual HD that could be inhaled, absorbed through the skin, ingested, or spread to other locations and that liquid formulations may be aerosolized or spilled.
3. No crushing or compounding of oral HDs may be done in an unprotected environment.
4. Gather all necessary equipment and supplies, including PPE.
5. Designate a workplace for handling HDs.
6. Have a spill kit and HD waste container readily available.
7. Procedure for gloving: wash hands and don double gloves.
8. Always work below eye level.
9. Visually examine HD dose while it is still contained in transport bag.
10. If HD dose appears intact, remove it from the transport bag.
11. Place a plastic-backed absorbent pad on the work area, if necessary, to contain any spills.
12. After administration, wearing double gloves, contain and dispose of materials contaminated with HDs into the HD waste container.
13. Do not push or force materials contaminated with HDs into the HD waste container.
14. Carefully remove, contain, and discard gloves.
15. Wash hands thoroughly after removing gloves.

Appendix I—Recommended Contents of HD Spill Kit

1. Sufficient supplies to absorb a spill of about 1,000 mL (volume of 1 i.v. bag or bottle).
2. Appropriate PPE to protect the worker during cleanup, including 2 pairs of disposable gloves (1 outer pair of heavy utility gloves and 1 pair of inner gloves tested to ASTM D6978).
3. Disposable HD-resistant gown or coverall tested against HD permeability.
4. Disposable HD-resistant shoe covers.
5. Chemical splash goggles.
6. Protective face shield to be used with goggles (for full range of splash protection).
7. NIOSH-approved disposable respirator.[a]
8. Absorbent, plastic-backed sheets or spill pads.
9. Disposable toweling.
10. At least 2 sealable, thick plastic hazardous waste disposal bags (prelabeled with an appropriate warning label).
11. One disposable scoop for collecting glass fragments.
12. One puncture-resistant container for glass fragments.
13. An approved cartridge respirator for use with contents of spill kit.[a]

[a]Respirators may only be used by workers who have been trained and fit-tested to the appropriate respirator.

Appendix J—Recommendations for Spill Cleanup Procedure

General

1. Assess the size and scope of the spill. Call for trained help, if necessary.
2. Spills that cannot be contained by 2 spill kits may require outside assistance.
3. Post signs to limit access to spill area.
4. Obtain spill kit and respirator.
5. Don appropriate PPE, including inner and outer gloves and respirator.
6. Once fully garbed, contain spill using spill kit.
7. Carefully remove any broken glass fragments and place them in a puncture-resistant container.
8. Absorb liquids with spill pads.
9. Absorb powder with damp disposable pads or soft toweling.
10. Spill cleanup should proceed progressively from areas of lesser to greater contamination.
11. Completely remove and place all contaminated material in the disposal bags.
12. Rinse the area with water and then clean with detergent, sodium hypochlorite solution, and neutralizer or other validated decontamination solution.
13. Rinse the area several times and place all materials used for containment and cleanup in disposal bags. Seal bags and place them in the appropriate final container for disposal as RCRA hazardous waste.
14. Carefully remove all PPE using the inner gloves. Place all disposable PPE into disposal bags. Seal bags and place them into the hazardous waste container (not trace-contaminated waste).
15. Remove inner gloves; contain in a small, sealable bag; and then place into the appropriate final container for disposal as hazardous waste.
16. Wash hands thoroughly with soap and water.
17. Once a spill has been initially decontaminated, have the area cleaned by housekeeping, janitorial staff, or environmental services.

Spills in a C-PEC

1. Spills occurring in a C-PEC should be cleaned up immediately.
2. Obtain a spill kit if the volume of the spill exceeds 30 mL or the contents of 1 drug vial or ampule.
3. Utility gloves (from spill kit) should be worn to remove broken glass in the C-PEC. Take care not to damage the sleeve or fixed-glove assembly in the class III BSC or CACI.

4. Place glass fragments in the puncture-resistant HD waste container located in the C-PEC.
5. Thoroughly clean and decontaminate the C-PEC.
6. Clean and decontaminate the drain spillage trough located under the class II BSC or similarly equipped class III BSC or CACI.
7. If the spill results in liquid being introduced onto the HEPA filter or if powdered aerosol contaminates the "clean side" of the HEPA filter, use of the C-PEC should be suspended until the equipment has been decontaminated and the HEPA filter replaced.

Appendix K—OSHA-Recommended Steps for Immediate Treatment of Workers with Direct Skin or Eye Contact with HDs[133]

1. Call for help, if needed.
2. Immediately remove contaminated clothing.
3. Flood affected eye with water or isotonic eyewash for at least 15 minutes.
4. Clean affected skin with soap (not a disinfectant cleanser) and water; rinse thoroughly.
5. Obtain medical attention.
6. Document exposure in employee's medical record and medical surveillance log.
7. Supplies for emergency treatment (e.g., soap, eyewash, sterile saline for irrigation) should be immediately located in any area where HDs are stored, compounded, or administered.

Developed through the ASHP Council on Pharmacy Practice and approved by the ASHP Board of Directors on July 30, 2018.

Luci A. Power, M.S., Power Enterprises, San Francisco, CA.

Joseph W. Coyne, B.Pharm., Coyne Consulting, Mundelein, IL.

The contributions of Charlotte Smith, B.S.Pharm., M.S., and Wendy M. Wong, Pharm.D., BCOP, to these guidelines are acknowledged. ASHP also acknowledges the following individuals for their contributions to previous versions of these guidelines: CAPT (ret.) Joseph H. Deffenbaugh Jr., M.P.H.; CDR Bruce R. Harrison, M.S., BCOP; Dayna McCauley, Pharm.D., BCOP; Melissa A. McDiarmid, M.D., M.P.H.; and CAPT Kenneth R. Mead, Ph.D., PE.

ASHP gratefully acknowledges the following individuals for reviewing the current version of the guidelines (review does not imply endorsement): Thomas H. Connor, Ph.D.; Ryan Forrey, Pharm.D., M.S., FASHP; Patricia C. Kienle, B.S.Pharm., M.P.A., FASHP; and Martha Polovich, Ph.D., RN, AOCN.

The authors have declared no potential conflicts of interest.

These guidelines supersede the ASHP guidelines on handling hazardous drugs dated January 12, 2006 (*Am J Health-Syst Pharm.* 2006; 63:1172–93).

Copyright © 2018, American Society of Health-System Pharmacists, Inc. All rights reserved. Contact ASHP for reprint and permissions requests. This content may not be used for commercial purposes without the express written consent of ASHP.

The bibliographic citation for this document is as follows: American Society of Health-System Pharmacists. ASHP guidelines on handling hazardous drugs. *Am J Health-Syst Pharm.* 2018; 75:1996–2031.

ASHP Technical Assistance Bulletin on Compounding Nonsterile Products in Pharmacies

Introduction

Pharmacists are the only health care providers formally trained in the art and science of compounding medications.[1,2] Therefore pharmacists are expected, by the medical community and the public, to possess the knowledge and skills necessary to compound extemporaneous preparations. Pharmacists have a responsibility to provide compounding services for patients with unique drug product needs.

This Technical Assistance Bulletin is intended to assist pharmacists in the extemporaneous compounding of nonsterile drug products for individual patients. Included in this document is information on facilities and equipment, ingredient selection, training, documentation and record keeping, stability and beyond-use dating, packaging and labeling, and limited batch compounding. This document is not intended for manufacturers or licensed repackagers.

Facilities and Equipment

Facilities. It is not necessary that compounding activities be located in a separate facility; however, the compounding area should be located sufficiently away from routine dispensing and counseling functions and high traffic areas. The area should be isolated from potential interruptions, chemical contaminants, and sources of dust and particulate matter. To minimize chemical contaminants, the immediate area and work counter should be free of previously used drugs and chemicals. To minimize dust and particulate matter, cartons and boxes should not be stored or opened in the compounding area. The compounding area should not contain dust-collecting overhangs (e.g., ceiling utility pipes, hanging light fixtures) and ledges (e.g., windowsills). Additionally, at least one sink should be located in or near the compounding area for hand washing before compounding operations. Proper temperature and humidity control within the compounding area or facility is desirable.

Work areas should be well lighted, and work surfaces should be level and clean. The work surface should be smooth, impervious, free of cracks and crevices (preferably seamless), and nonshedding. Surfaces should be cleaned at both the beginning and the end of each distinct compounding operation with an appropriate cleaner or solvent. The entire compounding facility should be cleaned daily or weekly (as needed) but not during the actual process of compounding.

Equipment. The equipment needed to compound a drug product depends upon the particular dosage form requested. Although boards of pharmacy publish lists of required equipment and accessories, these lists are not intended to limit the equipment available to pharmacists for compounding.[2] Equipment should be maintained in good working order. Pharmacists are responsible for obtaining the required equipment and accessories and ensuring that equipment is properly maintained and maintenance is documented.

Weighing Equipment. In addition to a torsion balance, pharmacists who routinely compound may need to use a top-loading electronic balance that has a capacity of at least 300 g, a sensitivity of ±1 mg (or 0.1 mg), and 1-mg, 100-mg, 1-g, and 100-g weights for checking. Balances should be maintained in areas of low humidity and should be stored on flat, nonvibrating surfaces away from drafts. At least annually, the performance of balances should be checked according to the guidelines found in *Remington's Pharmaceutical Sciences*,3 *USP XXII NF XVII: The United States Pharmacopeia–The National Formulary (USP–NF)*,4 or *USP DI Volume III: Approved Drug Products and Legal Requirements*[5] or the instructions of the balance manufacturer. Performance should be documented.

Weights should be stored in rigid, compartmentalized boxes and handled with metal, plastic, or plastic-tipped forceps—not fingers—to avoid scratching or soiling. Since most Class III prescription balances are only accurate to ±5 or 10 mg, Class P weights may be used for compounding purposes.[4] The *USP–NF* recommends that the class of weights used be chosen to limit the error to 0.1%. In practical terms this means that Class P weights can be used for weighing quantities greater than 100 mg.

The minimum weighable quantity must be determined for any balance being used for compounding. To avoid errors of 5% or more on a Class III balance with a sensitivity requirement of 6 mg, quantities of less than 120 mg of any substance should not be weighed. Smaller quantities may be weighed on more sensitive balances. If an amount is needed that is less than the minimum weighable quantity determined for a balance, an aliquot method of measurement should be used.

Measuring Equipment. The pharmacist should use judgment in selecting measuring equipment. The recommendations given in the *USP–NF* General Information section on volumetric apparatus should be followed. For maximum accuracy in measuring liquids, a pharmacist should select a graduate with a capacity equal to or slightly larger than the volume to be measured. The general rule is to measure no less than 20% of the capacity of a graduate. Calibrated syringes of the appropriate size may be preferred over graduated cylinders for measuring viscous liquids such as glycerin or mineral oil, since these liquids drain slowly and incompletely from graduated cylinders. Viscous liquids may also be weighed if this is more convenient, provided that the appropriate conversions from volume to weight are made by using the specific gravity of the liquid. Thick, opaque liquids should be weighed. For example, if a formulation specifies 1.5 mL of a liquid, it is better to use a 3-mL syringe with appropriate graduations to measure 1.5 mL than to use a 10-mL graduated cylinder, since quantities of less than 2.0 mL cannot be accurately measured in a 10-mL graduate. Also, if an opaque, viscous chemical, such as Coal Tar, USP, must be measured, it is more accurate to weigh the substance than to try to read a meniscus on a graduated cylinder or a fill line on a syringe.

DOI 10.37573/9781585287048.022

For volumes smaller than 1 mL, micropipettes are recommended, in sizes to cover the range of volumes measured. Two or three variable pipettes can usually cover the range from about 50 μL to 1 mL.

Although conical graduates are convenient for mixing solutions, the error in reading the bottom of the meniscus increases as the sides flare toward the top of the graduate. Therefore, for accurate measurements, cylindrical graduates are preferred. Conical graduates having a capacity of less than 25 mL should not be used in prescription compounding.[4]

Compounding Equipment. Pharmacists need at least two types of mortars and pestles—one glass and one Wedgwood or porcelain. The sizes of each will depend on the drug products being compounded. Glass mortars should be used for liquid preparations (solutions and suspensions) and for mixing chemicals that stain or are oily. Generally, glass mortars should be used for antineoplastic agents. Because of their rough surface, Wedgwood mortars are preferred for reducing the size of dry crystals and hard powder particles and for preparing emulsions. Porcelain mortars have a smoother surface than Wedgwood mortars and are ideal for blending powders and pulverizing soft aggregates or crystals. When Wedgwood mortars are used for small amounts of crystals or powders, the inside surface may first be lightly dusted with lactose to fill any crevices in which the crystals or powders might lodge. If the contact surfaces of the mortar and pestle become smooth with use, rubbing them with a small amount of sand or emery powder may adequately roughen them. Over extended use, a pestle and a mortar become shaped to each other's curvature. Thus, to ensure maximum contact between the surface of the head of each pestle and the interior of its corresponding mortar, pestles and mortars should not be interchanged.[3]

The compounding area should be stocked with appropriate supplies. Although supply selection depends on the types of products compounded, all areas should have weighing papers, weighing cups, or both to protect balance pans and spatulas. Glassine weighing papers (as opposed to bond weighing paper) should be used for products such as ointments, creams, and some dry chemicals. Disposable weighing dishes should also be stocked for substances like Coal Tar, USP.

Each compounding area should have stainless steel and plastic spatulas for mixing ointments and creams and handling dry chemicals. The pharmacist should exercise judgment in selecting the size and type of spatula. Small spatula blades (6 inches long or less) are preferred for handling dry chemicals, but larger spatula blades (>6 inches) are preferred for large amounts of ointments or creams and for preparing compactible powder blends for capsules. Plastic spatulas should be used for chemicals that may react with stainless steel blades. A variety of spatulas should be stocked in the compounding area, including 4-, 6-, and 8-inch stainless steel spatulas (one each) and 4- and 6-inch plastic spatulas (one each). Imprinted spatulas should not be used in compounding, since the imprinted ink on the spatula blade may contaminate the product.

The compounding area should contain an ointment slab, pill tile, or parchment ointment pad. Although parchment ointment pads are convenient and reduce cleanup time, parchment paper cannot be used for the preparation of creams because it will absorb water. Therefore, an ointment slab or pill tile is necessary. If suppositories are compounded, appropriate suppository molds, either reusable or disposable, should be available.

Other useful equipment and supplies may include funnels, filter paper, beakers, glass stirring rods, a source of heat (hot plate or microwave oven), a refrigerator, and a freezer—in some cases, an ultrafreezer capable of maintaining temperatures as low as −80 °C.

Ingredients

Ideally, only USP or NF chemicals manufactured by FDA-inspected manufacturers should be used for compounding. Although chemicals labeled USP or NF meet *USP–NF* standards for strength, quality, and purity for human drug products, the facilities in which the chemicals were manufactured may not meet FDA Good Manufacturing Practice (GMP) standards. In the event that a needed chemical is not available from an FDA-inspected facility, the pharmacist should, by next best preference, obtain a USP or NF product. If that is not available, the pharmacist should use professional judgment and may have to obtain the highest-grade chemical possible. Chemical grades that may be considered in this situation are ACS grade (meeting or exceeding specifications listed for reagent chemicals by the American Chemical Society) and FCC grade (meeting or exceeding requirements defined by the Food Chemicals Codex). Additional professional judgment is especially necessary in cases of chemical substances that have not been approved for *any* medical use. Particularly in these cases, but also in others as needed, the pharmacist, prescriber, and patient should be well informed of the risks involved.

Selection of ingredients may also depend on the dosage form to be compounded. In most cases, the prescriber specifies a particular dosage form, such as a topical ointment, oral solution or rectal suppository. Sometimes, however, the prescriber relies on the pharmacist to decide on an appropriate form. Irrespective of how the drug order is written, the pharmacist should evaluate the appropriateness of ingredients and the drug delivery system recommended. Factors to consider in selecting the dosage form include (1) physical and chemical characteristics of the active ingredient, (2) possible routes of administration that will produce the desired therapeutic effect (e.g., oral or topical), (3) patient characteristics (e.g., age, level of consciousness, ability to swallow a solid dosage form), (4) specific characteristics of the disease being treated, (5) comfort for the patient, and (6) ease or convenience of administration.

In checking the physical form of each ingredient, the pharmacist should not confuse drug substances that are available in more than one form. For example, coal tar is available as Coal Tar, USP, or Coal Tar Topical Solution, USP; phenol is available as Liquified Phenol, USP, or Phenol, USP; sulfur is available as Precipitated Sulfur, USP, or Sublimed Sulfur, USP. If ingredients are liquids, the pharmacist should consider compounding liquid dosage forms such as solutions, syrups, or elixirs for the final product. If ingredients are crystals or powders and the final dosage form is intended to be a dry dosage form, options such as divided powders (powder papers) or capsules should be considered. If ingredients are both liquids and dry forms, liquid formulations such as solutions, suspensions, elixirs, syrups, and emulsions should be considered.

Care must be exercised when using commercial drug products as a source of active ingredients. For example, extended-release or delayed-release products should not be crushed. Also, since chemicals such as preservatives and excipients in commercial products may affect the overall stability and bioavailability of the compounded product, their presence should not be ignored. Information on preservatives and excipients in specific commercial products can be found in package inserts and also in the dosage form section of selected product monographs in *USP DI Volume I.*[6]

If an injectable drug product is a possible source of active ingredient, the pharmacist should check the salt form of the injectable product to make sure it is the same salt form ordered. If it is necessary to use a different salt because of physical or chemical compatibility considerations or product availability, the pharmacist should consult with the prescriber. Some injectable products contain active constituents in the form of prodrugs that may not be active when administered by other routes. For example, if an injectable solution is a possible source of active ingredient for an oral product, the pharmacist must consider the stability of the drug in gastric fluids, the first-pass effect, and palatability. Also, if injectable powders for reconstitution are used, expiration dating may have to be quite short.

Storage

All chemicals and drug products must be stored according to *USP–NF* and manufacturer specifications. Most chemicals and drug products marketed for compounding use are packaged by the manufacturer in tight, light-resistant containers. Chemicals intended for compounding should be purchased in small quantities and stored in the manufacturer's original container, which is labeled with product and storage information. This practice fosters the use of fresh chemicals and ensures that the manufacturer's label remains with the lot of chemical on hand. Certificates of purity for chemical ingredients should be filed for a period of time no less than the state's time requirement for retention of dispensing records.

The manufacturer's label instructions for storage should be followed explicitly to ensure the integrity of chemicals and drug products and to protect employees. Most chemicals and commercial drug products may be stored at controlled room temperature, between 15 and 30 °C (59 and 86 °F); however, the pharmacist should always check the manufacturer's label for any special storage requirements. Storage information provided for specific commercial drug products in *USP DI Volume I* and on product labels follows the definitions for storage temperatures found in the General Notices and Requirements section of *USP–NF.* An acceptable refrigerator maintains temperatures between 2 and 8 °C (36 and 46 °F); an acceptable freezer maintains temperatures between −20 and −10°C (− 4 to +14 °F)

To protect pharmacy employees and property, hazardous products such as acetone and flexible collodion must be stored appropriately. Safety storage cabinets in various sizes are available from laboratory suppliers.

Personnel

Compounding personnel include pharmacists and supportive personnel engaged in any aspect of the compounding procedures.

Training. The pharmacist—who is responsible for ensuring that the best technical knowledge and skill, most careful and accurate procedures, and prudent professional judgment are consistently applied in the compounding of pharmaceuticals—must supervise all compounding activities and ensure that supportive personnel are adequately trained to perform assigned functions. Both pharmacists and the compounding personnel they supervise should participate in programs designed to enhance and maintain competence in compounding. Training programs should include instruction in the following areas:

- Proper use of compounding equipment such as balances and measuring devices—including guidelines for selecting proper measuring devices, limitations of weighing equipment and measuring apparatus, and the importance of accuracy in measuring.
- Pharmaceutical techniques needed for preparing compounded dosage forms (e.g., levigation, trituration, methods to increase dissolution, geometric dilution).
- Properties of dosage forms (see Pharmaceutical Dosage Forms in *USP–NF*) to be compounded and related factors such as stability, storage considerations, and handling procedures.
- Literature in which information on stability, solubility, and related material can be found (see suggested references at the end of this document).
- Handling of nonhazardous and hazardous materials in the work area, including protective measures for avoiding exposure, emergency procedures to follow in the event of exposure, and the location of Material Safety Data Sheets (MSDSs) in the facility.[7–10]
- Use and interpretation of chemical and pharmaceutical symbols and abbreviations in medication orders and in product formulation directions.
- Pharmaceutical calculations.

Procedures should be established to verify the ability of staff to meet established competencies. These procedures may include observation, written tests, or quality control testing of finished products.

Attire. Personnel engaged in compounding should wear clean clothing appropriate for the duties they perform. Protective apparel, such as head, face hand, and arm coverings, should be worn as necessary to preclude contamination of products and to protect workers.

Generally, a clean laboratory jacket is considered appropriate attire for most personnel performing nonsterile compounding activities. Personnel involved in compounding hazardous materials should wear safety goggles, gloves, a mask or respirator, double gowns, and foot covers as required, depending on the substance being handled. To avoid microbial contamination of compounded drug products, written policies should be established that address appropriate precautions to be observed if an employee has an open lesion or an illness. Depending on the situation, an affected employee may be required to wear special protective apparel, such as a mask or gloves, or may be directed to avoid all contact with compounding procedures.

Reference Materials

Pharmacists and supportive personnel must have ready access to reference materials on all aspects of compounding (see suggested references at the end of this document). Earlier editions of some references, such as *Remington's Pharmaceutical Sciences,* provide more comprehensive compounding information than do the later editions. Information on compounding extemporaneous dosage forms from commercially available products can sometimes be obtained from the product's FDA-approved labeling (package insert), the manufacturer, a local pharmacy college, or a drug information center. It is essential that the stability and proper storage conditions for extemporaneous products be thoroughly researched. Therefore, the availability of adequate references and appropriate training in the use of the references is important.

Documentation and Record Keeping

Each step of the compounding process should be documented. Pharmacists should maintain at least four sets of records in the compounding area: (1) compounding formulas and procedures, (2) a log of all compounded items, including batch records and sample batch labels (see section on packaging and labeling), (3) equipment-maintenance records, including documentation of checks of balances, refrigerators, and freezers, and (4) a record of ingredients purchased, including certificates of purity for chemicals (see section on ingredient selection) and MSDSs.

Compounding procedures should be documented in enough detail that preparations can be replicated and the history of each ingredient can be traced. Documentation should include a record of who prepared the product (if the compounder is not a pharmacist, the supervising pharmacist should also sign the compounding record); all names, lot numbers, and quantities of ingredients used; the order of mixing, including any interim procedures used (such as preparing a solution and using an aliquot); the assigned beyond-use date; and any special storage requirements (see section on stability and expiration dating). Compounding formulas and procedures should be written in a typeface that can be read easily. If formulas originate from published articles, copies of the articles should be attached to or filed with the written procedures.

Equipment maintenance and calibrations should be documented and the record maintained in an equipment-maintenance record file. Refrigerator and freezer thermometers should be checked and documented routinely, as should alarm systems indicating that temperatures are outside of acceptable limits.

Follow-up contact with patients who have received extemporaneously compounded products is recommended to ascertain that the product is physically stable and that no adverse effects have occurred from use of the product. Documentation of the contact and the findings is recommended.

Stability, Expiration, and Beyond-Use Dating

The *USP–NF*[4] defines stability as the extent to which a dosage form retains, within specified limits and throughout its period of storage and use, the same properties and characteristics that it possessed at the time of its preparation. The *USP–NF* lists the following five types of stability:

- Chemical
- Physical
- Microbiological
- Therapeutic
- Toxicological

Factors affecting stability include the properties of each ingredient, whether therapeutically active or inactive. Environmental factors such as temperature, radiation, light, humidity, and air can also affect stability. Similarly, such factors as particle size, pH, the properties of water and other solvents employed, the nature of the container, and the presence of other substances resulting from contamination or from the intentional mixing of products can influence stability.[4]

Since compounded drug products are intended for consumption immediately or storage for a very limited time, stability evaluation and expiration dating are different for these products than for manufactured drug products. According to criteria for assigning dating in the *USP–NF*[4] General Notices and Requirements section and the Code of Federal Regulations,[11] the pharmacist labeling extemporaneously compounded drug products should be concerned with the beyond-use date as used by *USP–NF* or the expiration date as used by the Code of Federal Regulations. For uniformity, the term *beyond-use date* will be used in the remainder of this bulletin. The beyond-use date is defined as that date after which a dispensed product should no longer be used by a patient.

Determination of the period during which a compounded product may be usable after dispensing should be based on available stability information and reasonable patient needs with respect to the intended drug therapy. When a commercial drug product is used as a source of active ingredient, its expiration date can often be used as a factor in determining a beyond-use date. For stability or expiration information on commercial drug products, the pharmacist can refer to *USP DI Volume I.*[6] If no information is available, the manufacturer should be contacted. When the active ingredient is a USP or NF product, the pharmacist may be able to use the expiration dating of similar commercial products for guidance in assigning a beyond-use date. In addition, the pharmacist can often refer to published literature to obtain stability data on the same active ingredient under varying conditions and in different formulations.[12]

The pharmacist must assess the potential for instability that may result from the new environment for the active ingredients—from the combination of ingredients and the packaging materials. According to *USP–NF*,[4] hydrolysis, oxidation-reduction, and photolysis are the most common chemical reactions that cause instability. When the possibility of such reactions exists, the pharmacist should seek additional stability data or consider other approaches. These could, in extreme cases, include the preparation and dispensing of more than one compounded drug product or the use of alternative methods of dosing. For some drugs, the latter methods might include, for example, crushing a tablet or emptying the contents of a hard gelatin capsule into an appropriate food substance at each dosing time.

In assigning a beyond-use date for compounded drug products, the pharmacist should use all available stability information, plus education and experience in deciding how factors affecting product stability should be weighted. In the absence of stability data to the contrary or any indication of a stability problem, the following general criteria for assigning maximum beyond-use dates are recommended. It must be emphasized that these are *general* criteria. Professional judgment as discussed elsewhere in this section must be used in deciding when these general criteria may not be appropriate.

- When a manufactured final-dosage-form product is used as a source of active ingredient, use no more than 25% of the manufacturer's remaining expiration dating or six months, whichever is less.
- When a USP or NF chemical not from a manufactured final-dosage-form product is used, use no more than six months.
- In other cases, use the intended period of therapy or no more than 30 days, whichever is less.

All compounded products should be observed for signs of instability. Observations should be performed during preparation of the drug product and any storage period that may occur before the compounded drug product is dispensed. A list of observable indications of instability for solid, liquid, and semisolid dosage forms appears in *USP–NF*.

Packaging and Labeling

The packaging of extemporaneously compounded products for ambulatory patients should comply with regulations pertaining to the Poison Prevention Packaging Act of 1970. These regulations can be found in *USP–NF*.[4]

Containers for compounded products should be appropriate for the dosage form compounded. For example, to minimize administration errors, oral liquids should never be packaged in syringes intended to be used for injection.

The drug product container should not interact physically or chemically with the product so as to alter the strength, quality, or purity of the compounded product. Glass and plastic are commonly used in containers for compounded products. To ensure container inertness, visibility, strength, rigidity, moisture protection, ease of reclosure, and economy of packaging, glass containers have been the most widely used for compounded products.[3] Amber glass and some plastic containers may be used to protect light-sensitive products from degradation; however, glass that transmits ultraviolet or violet light rays (this includes green, blue, and clear ["flint"] glass) should not be used to protect light-sensitive products.

The use of plastic containers for compounded products has increased because plastic is less expensive and lighter in weight than glass. Since compounded products are intended for immediate use, most capsules, ointments, and creams should be stable in high-density plastic vials or ointment jars. Only plastic containers meeting *USP–NF* standards should be used.[4] Reclosable plastic bags may be acceptable for selected divided powders that are intended to be used within a short period of time.

Each compounded product should be appropriately labeled according to state and federal regulations. Labels should include the generic or chemical name of active ingredients, strength or quantity, pharmacy lot number, beyond-use date, and any special storage requirements. If a commercial product has been used as a source of drug, the generic name of the product should be used on the label. The trade name should not be used because, once the commercial drug product has been altered, it no longer exists as the approved commercial product. Listing the names and quantities of inactive ingredients on labels is also encouraged. The coining of short names for convenience (e.g., "Johnson's solution") is strongly discouraged; these names provide no assistance to others who may need to identify ingredients (e.g., in emergency circumstances).

Capsules should be labeled with the quantity (micrograms or milligrams) of active ingredient(s) per capsule. Oral liquids should be labeled with the strength or concentration per dose (e.g., 125 mg/5 mL or 10 meq/15 mL). If the quantity of an active ingredient is a whole number, the number should not be typed with a decimal point followed by a zero. For example, the strength of a capsule containing 25 mg of active ingredient should be labeled as 25 mg and not 25.0 mg. In cases where the dosage strength is less than a whole number, a zero should precede the decimal point (e.g., 0.25 μg).[3]

In expressing salt forms of chemicals on a label, it is permissible to use atomic abbreviations. For example, HCl may be used for hydrochloride, HBr for hydrobromide, Na for sodium, and K for potassium.

Vehicles should also be stated on labels, especially if similar products are prepared with different vehicles. For example, if a pharmacist prepares two potassium syrups, one using Syrup, USP, as the vehicle and one using a sugar-free syrup as the vehicle, the name of the vehicle should be included on the labels.

Liquids and semisolid concentrations may be expressed in terms of percentages. When the term "percent" or the symbol "%" is used without qualification for solids and semisolids, percent refers to weight in weight; for solutions or suspensions, percent refers to weight in volume; for solutions of liquids in liquids, percent refers to volume in volume.[4]

Labels for compounded products that are prepared in batches should include a pharmacy-assigned lot number. Assignment of a pharmacy lot number must enable the history of the compounded product to be traced, including the person compounding the product and the product's formula, ingredients, and procedures. Being able to trace the history of a batch is essential in cases of a drug product recall or withdrawal.

In the preparation of labels for batches of compounded products, all extra labels should be destroyed, since pharmacy lot numbers change with each batch. If computers, memory typewriters, or label machines are used to print batch labels, care must be taken to ensure that the memory and printing mechanism have been cleared and the correct information is programmed before any additional labels are made. It is a good practice to run a blank label between each batch of labels to ensure that the memory has been erased or cleared. To document the information printed on each set of labels, a sample label printed for the batch should be attached to the compounded-product log. If labels are sequentially prepared for different drug products, procedures should exist to minimize the risk of mislabeling the compounded products. These procedures should ensure, for example, that labels for one drug product are physically well separated from labels for any other drug product.

Auxiliary labels are convenient for conveying special storage or use information. Auxiliary labels should be attached conspicuously to containers, if possible. If the container is too small for both a general label and an auxiliary label, special storage and use instructions should appear on the label in a format that will emphasize the instructions.

Limited Batch Compounding

The purpose of extemporaneously compounding products is to provide individualized drug therapy for a particular patient. When a pharmacist is repeatedly asked to prepare identical compounded products, it may be reasonable and more efficient for the pharmacist to prepare small batches of the compounded product.

Batch sizes should be consistent with the volume of drug orders or prescriptions the pharmacist receives for the compounded product and the stability of the compounded product. The pharmacist should use judgment in deciding reasonable batch sizes. Product assays should be performed by a chemical analysis laboratory on a regular basis to ensure product consistency among various lots, product uniformity, and stability. Analyses should be repeated every time an ingredient (active or inert) or procedure is changed. Documentation of assay findings should be filed for a period no less than the state's time requirement for the retention of dispensing records.

General Compounding Considerations

To provide the patient with the most stable drug product, the pharmacist should take the following steps upon receiving a prescription order that requires compounding.

First, the pharmacist should determine if a similar commercial product is available. A pharmacist can refer to various reference texts to check the availability of identical or similar products. Package inserts from commercially available products also contain information on inactive ingredients that can be compared with the requested formulation. If there is a commercially manufactured identical product, the local availability of the product should be determined.

When a similar product is commercially available, the pharmacist should determine which ingredients are different from the requested formulation to decide whether or not the commercial product can be used. At this stage, the pharmacist should seek answers to the following questions:

- Are all of the ingredients appropriate for the condition being treated?
- Are the concentrations of the ingredients in the drug order reasonable?
- Are the physical, chemical, and therapeutic properties of the individual ingredients consistent with the expected properties of the ordered drug product?

If the answers to these questions are positive, the pharmacist should consult the prescriber about the possibility of dispensing the commercial product. (In some states, pharmacists may not be required to obtain permission from the prescriber to dispense a commercial product if the formulation is identical to the drug order.) Dispensing a commercial product is preferable to extemporaneously compounding a drug product because commercial products carry the manufacturer's guarantee of labeled potency and stability.

If there is not a commercial product available with the same or similar formulation, the pharmacist should consider asking the prescriber the following questions:

- What is the purpose of the order? There may be another way to achieve the purpose without compounding a product.
- Where did the formula originate (article, meeting, colleague)?
- How will the drug product be used?
- Does the patient have other conditions that must be considered?
- For how long will the drug product be used?

If possible, the pharmacist should obtain a copy of the original formula to determine the extent to which the formulation has been tested for stability. When documentation is not available, the pharmacist should review the ingredients for appropriateness and reasonable concentrations.

For drug products that must be compounded, the pharmacist should closely observe the compounded drug product for any signs of instability. Such observations should be performed during preparation of the drug product and during any storage period that may occur before the compounded drug product is dispensed.

If specific packaging information is not available, a light-resistant, tight container, such as an amber vial or bottle, should be used to maximize stability (see section on packaging and labeling).

The pharmacist should label the compounded drug product, including an appropriate beyond-use date and storage instructions for the patient.

Specific Compounding Considerations

Accepted, proven compounding procedures for products including solutions, suspensions, creams, ointments, capsules, suppositories, troches, emulsions, and powders may be found in reference sources or the pharmacy literature. For additional information, pharmacists should check references cited in this document or consult colleagues or colleges of pharmacy with known expertise in compounding.

Glossary

For the purposes of this document, the following terms are used with the meanings shown.

Active ingredient: Any chemical that is intended to furnish pharmacologic activity in the diagnosis, cure, mitigation, treatment, or prevention of disease or to affect the structure or function of the body of man or other animals.[4]

Batch: Multiple containers of a drug product or other material with uniform character and quality, within specified limits, that are prepared in anticipation of prescription drug orders based on routine, regularly observed prescribing patterns.

Cold: Any temperature not exceeding 8 °C (46 °F).[4]

Commercially available product: Any drug product manufactured by a producer registered with the Department of Health and Human Services as a pharmaceutical manufacturer.

Compounding: The mixing of substances to prepare a drug product.

Container: A device that holds a drug product and is or may be in direct contact with the product.[3]

Cool: Any temperature between 8 and 15 °C (46 and 59 °F).[4]

Drug product: A finished dosage form that contains an active drug ingredient usually, but not necessarily (in the case of a placebo), in combination with inactive ingredients.[4]

Extemporaneous: Impromptu; prepared without a standard formula from an official compendium; prepared as required for a specific patient.

Inactive ingredient: Any chemical other than the active ingredients in a drug product.[4]

Manufacturer: Anyone registered with the Department of Health and Human Services as a producer of drug products.[14]

Sensitivity requirements: The maximal load that will cause one subdivision of change on the index plate in the position of rest of the indicator of the balance.[4]

Stability: The chemical and physical integrity of a drug product over time.[4]

Trituration: The reducing of substances to fine particles by rubbing them in a mortar with a pestle.[3]

Warm: Any temperature between 30 and 40 °C (86 and 104 °F).[4]

Suggested References

Product Availability

American Drug Index
Drug Facts & Comparisons
Physicians' Desk Reference
The Extra Pharmacopoeia (Martindale)
CHEMSOURCES
AHFS Drug Information

Compounding Techniques

Compounding Companion PC-Based Software
King's *Dispensing of Medications*
Remington's Pharmaceutical Sciences
Contemporary Compounding column in *U.S. Pharmacist*

Pharmaceutical Calculations

Stoklosa and Ansel's *Pharmaceutical Calculations*
Math—Use It or Lose It column in *Hospital Pharmacy*
Calculations in Pharmacy column in *U.S. Pharmacist*

Drug Stability and Compatibility

American Journal of Hospital Pharmacy
ASHP's *Handbook on Extemporaneous Formulations*
ASHP's *Handbook on Injectable Drugs*
International Pharmaceutical Abstracts
Journal of the Parenteral Drug Association (now *Journal of Pharmaceutical Science and Technology*)
Canadian Society of Hospital Pharmacists *Extemporaneous Oral Liquid Dosage Preparations*
Pediatric Drug Formulations
Physicians' Desk Reference
Contemporary Compounding column in *U.S. Pharmacist*
AHFS Drug Information
The Merck Index

References

1. Pancorbo SA, Campagna KD, Devenport JK, et al. Task force report of competency statements for pharmacy practice. *Am J Pharm Educ.* 1987; 51:196–206.
2. Allen LV Jr. Establishing and marketing your extemporaneous compounding service. *US Pharm.* 1990; 15(Dec):74–7.
3. Remington's pharmaceutical sciences. 18th ed. Gennaro AR, ed. Easton, PA: Mack Publishing; 1990; 1630–1, 1658, 1660.
4. The United States Pharmacopeia, 22nd rev., and The National Formulary, 17th ed. Rockville, MD: The United States Pharmacopeial Convention; 1989.
5. USP DI Volume III: Approved drug products and legal requirements. 14th ed. Rockville, MD: The United States Pharmacopeial Convention; 1994.
6. USP DI Volume I: Drug information for the health care professional. 14th ed. Rockville, MD: The United States Pharmacopeial Convention; 1994.
7. 29 §C.F.R. 1910. 1200(1990).
8. ASHP technical assistance bulletin on handling cytotoxic and hazardous drugs. *Am J Hosp Pharm.* 1990; 47:1033–49.
9. Feinberg JL. Complying with OSHA's Hazard Communication Standard. *Consult Pharm.* 1991; 6:444, 446, 448.
10. Myers CE. Applicability of OSHA Hazard Communication Standard to drug products. *Am J Hosp Pharm.* 1990; 47:1960–1.
11. 21 C.F.R. §211.137.
12. Connors KA, Amidon GL, Stella VJ. Chemical stability of pharmaceuticals: a handbook for pharmacists. 2nd ed. New York: Wiley; 1986.
13. American Society of Hospital Pharmacists. ASHP guidelines on preventing medication errors in hospitals. *Am J Hosp Pharm.* 1993; 50:305–14.
14. Fitzgerald WL Jr. The legal authority to compound in pharmacy practice. *Tenn Pharm.* 1990; 26(Mar):21–2.

Approved by the ASHP Board of Directors, April 27, 1994. Developed by the Council on Professional Affairs.

Copyright © 1994, American Society of Hospital Pharmacists, Inc. All rights reserved. Contact ASHP for reprint and permissions requests. This content may not be used for commercial purposes without the express written consent of ASHP.

The bibliographic citation for this document is as follows: American Society of Hospital Pharmacists. ASHP technical assistance bulletin on compounding nonsterile products in pharmacies. *Am J Hosp Pharm.* 1994; 51:1441–8.

Distribution

2022

DISPENSING BY NONPHARMACISTS AND NONPRESCRIBERS

Source: Council on Public Policy

To reaffirm the position that to ensure optimal patient outcomes all medication dispensing functions must be performed by, or under the supervision of, a pharmacist; further,

To reaffirm the position that any relationships that are established between a pharmacist and other individuals in order to carry out the dispensing function should preserve the role of the pharmacist in (a) maintaining appropriate patient safety, (b) complying with regulatory and legal requirements, and (c) providing individualized patient care; further,

To advocate that all medication dispensing, regardless of setting, be held to the same regulatory standards that apply to dispensing by a pharmacist; further,

To urge pharmacists to assume a leadership role in medication dispensing in all settings to ensure adherence to best practices.

This policy supersedes ASHP policy 0010.

Rationale

The Council recognizes the reality of limited pharmacist availability and lack of comprehensive pharmacy services in many settings, including public health clinics, rural and urban outreach clinics, and hospital emergency departments. However, the Council believes that responsibility and services of pharmacists are critical to safe medication use and that all dispensing, regardless of setting, should meet the same standards that apply to pharmacies and pharmacists. The Council believes that the current *ASHP Minimum Standard for Pharmaceutical Services in Ambulatory Care* is explicit and pertinent to the practice of dispensing by nonpharmacists and nonprescribers. The Council also noted that this type of drug delivery and dispensing arrangement does not constitute collaborative drug therapy management as defined in ASHP policy 9903.

1913

PHARMACEUTICAL DISTRIBUTION SYSTEMS

Source: Council on Pharmacy Management

To support drug distribution business models that meet the requirements of hospitals and health systems with respect to availability and timely delivery of products, minimizing short-term outages and long-term product shortages, managing and responding to product recalls, fostering product-handling and transaction efficiency, preserving the integrity of products as they move through the supply chain, and maintaining affordable service costs; further,

To oppose manufacturers, distributors, and wholesalers restricting or making availability of drug products contingent on how those products are used; further,

To encourage selection of a wholesale distributor that (1) purchases products only from a manufacturer before distribution to the purchasing end user; (2) is licensed in the state where it is conducting business; (3) complies with the requirements of the Drug Supply Chain Security Act; (4) is accredited under the National Association of Boards of Pharmacy Verified-Accredited Wholesale Distributors program; and (5) uses information systems that are interoperable with common types of pharmacy systems.

This policy supersedes ASHP policy 1707.

Rationale

Wholesalers and distributors have traditionally contracted with hospitals and health systems for basic drug product distribution and other services. Many wholesalers have made a large portion of their revenue through speculative buying and other business practices that are no longer desirable because of requirements for pedigrees, the risk of buying counterfeit or adulterated products, demands by manufacturers to limit product transactions, and the need to manage drug recalls. These changes, plus the vast diversification of many wholesaler distributors, have resulted in new business models that will affect how hospitals acquire and manage pharmaceuticals. These changing models for distribution may result in higher costs for hospitals and health systems, as current wholesaler distribution systems have become very efficient.

Additionally, some wholesalers have required that pharmacies ensure certain drugs are not used or sold for use for particular purposes, and there are concerns that this practice could grow. ASHP supports wholesaler and distribution business models that meet the requirements of hospitals and health systems, which includes the ability for pharmacies to obtain drug products for established patient care uses without restriction.

ASHP supports using strict vendor vetting policies to prevent sales from nonreputable or gray market vendors. Vendors should purchase products only from a manufacturer, not a secondary source; should be licensed in the state in which it operates; comply with the requirements of the Drug Supply Chain Security Act; be accredited under the National Association of Boards of Pharmacy *Verified-Accredited Wholesale Distributors (VAWD) program*; and use information systems that are interoperable with common types of pharmacy systems. VAWD accreditation requires a rigorous criteria compliance review to ensure that a wholesale distribution facility operates legitimately, is licensed in good standing, and employs security and best practices for safe prescription drug distribution from manufacturers to pharmacies. As of 2018, 23 states had recognized VAWD accreditation.

0310

TECHNICIAN-CHECKING-TECHNICIAN PROGRAMS

Source: Council on Administrative Affairs

To advocate technician-checking-technician programs (with appropriate quality control measures) in order to permit redirection of pharmacist resources to patient care activities; further,

To advocate state board of pharmacy approval of these programs.

This policy was reviewed in 2023 by the Council on Pharmacy Management and by the Board of Directors and was found to still be appropriate.

DOI 10.37573/9781585287048.023

Rationale

Technician-checking-technician (tech-check-tech) programs create advanced roles for certified pharmacy technicians with appropriate training and education. These programs allow pharmacists' time to be redirected to additional clinical and cognitive functions, such as drug therapy management activities. Tech-check-tech programs, with appropriate quality control, are an acceptable alternative to pharmacists checking unit dose medication carts. Many state boards of pharmacy still require that pharmacists perform this activity and will consider exceptions to this requirement only upon specific request. Not all states allow technicians to perform final checks or allow them to do so only after obtaining a variance from the Board in limited situations. In 2022, 17 states allowed tech-check-tech programs with varying degrees of oversight (NABP 2022 Survey of Pharmacy Law, p. 60).

ASHP Statement on Pharmacist's Responsibility for Distribution and Control of Drug Products

A fundamental purpose of pharmaceutical services in any setting is to ensure the safe and appropriate use of drug products and drug-related devices. Fulfillment of this responsibility is enhanced through the pharmacist's involvement in all aspects of the use of drugs.[1]

This involvement should include decisions and actions with respect to the evaluation, procurement, storage, distribution, and administration of all drug products. The pharmacist is responsible for development, in consultation with appropriate other professionals, departments, and interdisciplinary committees in the setting, of all drug-use control policies. The pharmacist should be directly responsible for the control and distribution of all stocks of drugs.

The Federal Food, Drug, and Cosmetic Act defines the term *drug* as "(A) articles recognized in the official United States Pharmacopeia, official Homeopathic Pharmacopeia of the United States, or official National Formulary, or any supplement to any of them; and (B) articles intended for use in the diagnosis, cure, mitigation, treatment, or prevention of disease in man or other animals; and (C) articles (other than food) intended to affect the structure or any function of the body of man or other animals; and (D) articles intended for use as a component of any article specified in clauses (A), (B), or (C) of this paragraph; but does not include devices or their components, parts, or accessories."[2]

For purposes of this document, drugs include those used by inpatients and outpatients, large- and small-volume injections, radiopharmaceuticals, diagnostic agents including radiopaque contrast media, anesthetic gases, blood-fraction drugs, dialysis fluids, respiratory therapy drugs, biotechnologically produced drugs, investigational drugs, drug samples, drugs brought to the setting by patients or family, and other chemicals and biological substances administered to patients to evoke or enhance pharmacologic responses.

The pharmacist's responsibility for drug-use control extends throughout the setting served. This purview extends to all pharmacy satellite locations (inpatient and outpatient, including those serving the general public), emergency rooms, surgical and labor and delivery suites (and related areas such as recovery rooms), anesthesiology, nuclear medicine, radiology, dialysis areas, ambulatory care clinics and treatment (including surgery) areas, respiratory therapy areas, central sterile supply centers, blood banks, intensive care areas, cardiac catheterization suites, research areas, and all other areas in which drugs are handled and used. The pharmacist should be responsible for drug-use policies and routine inspection of all drug stocks, even if direct custody and distribution are not possible.

The pharmacist also has an advocacy responsibility with respect to decisions and policies about the use of drug-related devices as they affect drug therapy. As appropriate, the pharmacist may also be assigned direct responsibility for control and distribution of drug-related devices.[3] Drug-related devices include electromechanical pumps, devices for administration of injectable drugs, devices for monitoring plasma drug concentration, and devices for monitoring drug administration rate.

DOI 10.37573/9781585287048.024

References

1. American Society of Hospital Pharmacists. ASHP guidelines: minimum standard for pharmacies in institutions. *Am J Hosp Pharm*. 1985; 42:372–5.
2. 21 U.S.C. §321 (g) (1).
3. American Society of Hospital Pharmacists. ASHP statement on the pharmacist's role with respect to drug delivery systems and administration devices. *Am J Hosp Pharm*. 1989; 46:802–4.

This statement was reviewed in 2005 by the Council on Professional Affairs and by the Board of Directors and was found to still be appropriate.

Approved by the ASHP Board of Directors, November 16, 1994, and by the ASHP House of Delegates, June 5, 1995. Revised by the ASHP Council on Professional Affairs. Supersedes a previous version dated June 3, 1992.

Copyright © 1996, American Society of Health-System Pharmacists, Inc. All rights reserved. Contact ASHP for reprint and permissions requests. This content may not be used for commercial purposes without the express written consent of ASHP.

The bibliographic citation for this document is as follows: ASHP statement on the pharmacist's responsibility for distribution and control of drug products. In: *Practice Standards of ASHP 1996–97*. Deffenbaugh JH, ed. Bethesda, MD: American Society of Health-System Pharmacists; 1996.

ASHP Statement on Unit Dose Drug Distribution

The unit dose system of medication distribution is a pharmacy-coordinated method of dispensing and controlling medications in organized health-care settings.

The unit dose system may differ in form, depending on the specific needs of the organization. However, the following distinctive elements are basic to all unit dose systems: medications are contained in single unit packages; they are dispensed in as ready-to-administer form as possible; and for most medications, not more than a 24-hour supply[a] of doses is delivered to or available at the patient-care area at any time.[1,2]

Numerous studies concerning unit dose drug distribution systems have been published over the past several decades. These studies indicate categorically that unit dose systems, with respect to other drug distribution methods, are (1) safer for the patient, (2) more efficient and economical for the organization, and (3) a more effective method of utilizing professional resources.

More specifically, the inherent advantages of unit dose systems over alternative distribution procedures are

1. A reduction in the incidence of medication errors.
2. A decrease in the total cost of medication-related activities.
3. A more efficient usage of pharmacy and nursing personnel, allowing for more direct patient-care involvement by pharmacists and nurses.
4. Improved overall drug control and drug use monitoring.
5. More accurate patient billings for drugs.
6. The elimination or minimization of drug credits.
7. Greater control by the pharmacist over pharmacy workload patterns and staff scheduling.
8. A reduction in the size of drug inventories located in patient-care areas.
9. Greater adaptability to computerized and automated procedures.

In view of these demonstrated benefits, the American Society of Hospital Pharmacists considers the unit dose system to be an essential part of drug distribution and control in organized health-care settings in which drug therapy is an integral component of health-care delivery.

References

1. Summerfield MR. Unit dose primer. Bethesda, MD: American Society of Hospital Pharmacists; 1983.
2. American Society of Hospital Pharmacists. ASHP technical assistance bulletin on hospital drug distribution and control. *Am J Hosp Pharm.* 1980; 37:1097–1103.

DOI 10.37573/9781585287048.025

[a]In long-term care facilities, a larger supply of medication (e.g., 48 or 72 hours) may be acceptable.

Approved by the ASHP Board of Directors, November 16, 1988, and by the ASHP House of Delegates, June 5, 1989. Supersedes previous versions approved by the House of Delegates on June 8, 1981, and by the Board of Directors on April 19, 1975, and November 13–14, 1980.

Copyright © 1989, American Society of Hospital Pharmacists, Inc. All rights reserved. Contact ASHP for reprint and permissions requests. This content may not be used for commercial purposes without the express written consent of ASHP.

The bibliographic citation for this document is as follows: American Society of Hospital Pharmacists. ASHP statement on unit dose drug distribution. *Am J Hosp Pharm.* 1989; 46:2346.

ASHP Technical Assistance Bulletin on Hospital Drug Distribution and Control

Drug control (of which drug distribution is an important part) is among the pharmacist's most important responsibilities. Therefore, adequate methods to assure that these responsibilities are met must be developed and implemented. These guidelines will assist the pharmacist in preparing drug control procedures for all medication-related activities. The guidelines are based on the premise that the pharmacy is responsible for the procurement, distribution, and control of *all* drugs used within the institution. In a sense, the entire hospital is the pharmacy, and the pharmacy service is simply a functional service extending throughout the institution's physical and organizational structures.

It should be noted that, although this document is directed toward hospitals, much of it is relevant to other types of health-care facilities.

Pharmacy Policies, Procedures, and Communications

Policy and Procedure Manuals.[1] The effectiveness of the drug control system depends on adherence to policies (broad, general statements of philosophy) and procedures (detailed guidelines for implementing policy). The importance of an up-to-date policy and procedure manual for drug control cannot be overestimated. All pharmacy staff must be familiar with the manual; it is an important part of orientation for new staff and crucial to the pharmacy's internal communication mechanism. In addition, preparing written policies and procedures requires a thorough analysis of control operations; this review might go undone otherwise.

Drug control begins with the setting of policy. The authority to enforce drug control policy and procedures must come from the administration of the institution, with the endorsement of the medical staff, via the pharmacy and therapeutics (P&T) committee and/or other appropriate committee(s). Because the drug control system interfaces with numerous departments and professions, the P&T committee should be the focal point for communications relating to drug control in the institution. The pharmacist, with the cooperation of the P&T committee, should develop media such as newsletters, bulletins, and seminars to communicate with persons functioning within the framework of the control system.

Inservice Training and Education. Intra- and interdepartmental education and training programs are important to the effective implementation of policies and procedures and the institution's drug control system in general. They are part of effective communication and help establish and maintain professional relationships among the pharmacy staff and between it and other hospital departments. Drug control policies and procedures should be included in the pharmacy's educational programs.

Standards, Laws, and Regulations

The pharmacist must be aware of and comply with the laws, regulations, and standards governing the profession. Many of these standards and regulations deal with aspects of drug control. Among the agencies and organizations affecting institutional pharmacy practice are those described below.

Regulatory Agencies and Organizations. The U.S. government, through its Food and Drug Administration (FDA), is responsible for implementing and enforcing the federal Food, Drug, and Cosmetic Act. The FDA is responsible for the control and prevention of misbranding and of adulteration of food, drugs, and cosmetics moving in interstate commerce. The FDA also sets label requirements for food, drugs, and cosmetics; sets standards for investigational drug studies and for marketing of new drug products; and compiles data on adverse drug reactions.

The U.S. Department of the Treasury influences pharmacy operation by regulating the use of tax-free alcohol through the Bureau of Alcohol, Tobacco and Firearms. The U.S. Department of Justice affects pharmacy practice through its Drug Enforcement Agency (DEA) by enforcing the Controlled Substances Act of 1970 and other federal laws and regulations for controlled drugs.

Another federal agency, the Health Care Financing Administration, has established Conditions of Participation for hospitals and skilled nursing facilities to assist these institutions to qualify for reimbursement under the health insurance program for the aged (Medicare) and for Medicaid.

The state board of pharmacy is the agency of state government responsible for regulating pharmacy practice within the state. Practitioners, institutions, and community pharmacies must obtain licenses from the board to practice pharmacy or provide pharmacy services in the state. State boards of pharmacy promulgate numerous regulations pertaining to drug dispensing and control. (In some states, the state board of health licenses the hospital pharmacy separately or through a license that includes all departments of the hospital.)

Standards and guidelines for pharmaceutical services have been established by the Joint Commission on Accreditation of Hospitals (JCAH)[2] and the American Society of Hospital Pharmacists (ASHP)[3]. The United States Pharmacopeial Convention also promulgates certain pharmacy practice procedures as well as official standards for drugs and drug testing. Professional practice guidelines and standards generally do not have the force of law but rather are intended to assist pharmacists in achieving the highest level of practice. They may, however, be employed in legal proceedings as evidence of what constitutes acceptable practice as determined by the profession itself.

In some instances, both federal and state laws may deal with a specific activity; in such cases, the more stringent law will apply.

DOI 10.37573/9781585287048.026

The Medication System

Procurement: Drug Selection, Purchasing Authority, Responsibility, and Control.[4–6] The selection of pharmaceuticals is a basic and extremely important professional function of the hospital pharmacist who is charged with making decisions regarding products, quantities, product specifications, and sources of supply. It is the pharmacist's obligation to establish and maintain standards assuring the quality, proper storage, control, and safe use of all pharmaceuticals and related supplies (e.g., fluid administration sets); this responsibility must not be delegated to another individual. Although the actual purchasing of drugs and supplies may be performed by a nonpharmacist, the setting of quality standards and specifications requires professional knowledge and judgment and must be performed only by the pharmacist.

Economic and therapeutic considerations make it necessary for hospitals to have a well-controlled, continuously updated formulary. It is the pharmacist's responsibility to develop and maintain adequate product specifications to aid in the purchase of drugs and related supplies under the formulary system. The *USP–NF* is a good base for drug product specifications; there also should be criteria to evaluate the acceptability of manufacturers and distributors. In establishing the formulary, the P&T committee recommends guidelines for drug selection. However, when his knowledge indicates, the pharmacist must have the authority to reject a particular drug product or supplier.

Although the pharmacist has the authority to select a brand or source of supply, he must make economic considerations subordinate to those of quality. Competitive bid purchasing is an important method for achieving a proper balance between quality and cost when two or more acceptable suppliers market a particular product meeting the pharmacist's specifications. In selecting a vendor, the pharmacist must consider price, terms, shipping times, dependability, quality of service, returned goods policy, and packaging; however, prime importance always must be placed on drug quality and the manufacturer's reputation. It should be noted that the pharmacist is responsible for the quality of all drugs dispensed by the pharmacy.

Records. The pharmacist must establish and maintain adequate recordkeeping systems. Various records must be retained (and be retrievable) by the pharmacy because of governmental regulations; some are advisable for legal protection, others are needed for JCAH accreditation, and still others are necessary for sound management (evaluation of productivity, workloads, and expenses and assessment of departmental growth and progress) of the pharmacy department. Records must be retained for at least the length of time prescribed by law (where such requirements apply).

It is important that the pharmacist study federal, state, and local laws to become familiar with their requirements for permits, tax stamps, storage of alcohol and controlled substances, records, and reports.

Among the records needed in the drug distribution and control system are

- Controlled substances inventory and dispensing records.
- Records of medication orders and their processing.
- Manufacturing and packaging production records.
- Pharmacy workload records.
- Purchase and inventory records.
- Records of equipment maintenance.
- Records of results and actions taken in quality-assurance and drug audit programs.

Receiving Drugs. Receiving control should be under the auspices of a responsible individual, and the pharmacist must ensure that records and forms provide proper control upon receipt of drugs. Complete accountability from purchase order initiation to drug administration must be provided.

Personnel involved in the purchase, receipt, and control of drugs should be well trained in their responsibilities and duties and must understand the serious nature of drugs. All nonprofessional personnel employed by the pharmacy should be selected and supervised by the pharmacist.

Delivery of drugs directly to the pharmacy or other pharmacy receiving area is highly desirable; it should be considered mandatory for controlled drugs. Orders for controlled substances must be checked against the official order blank (when applicable) and against hospital purchase order forms. All drugs should be placed into stock promptly upon receipt, and controlled substances must be directly transferred to safes or other secure areas.

Drug Storage and Inventory Control. Storage is an important aspect of the total drug control system. Proper environmental control (i.e., proper temperature, light, humidity, conditions of sanitation, ventilation, and segregation) must be maintained wherever drugs and supplies are stored in the institution. Storage areas must be secure; fixtures and equipment used to store drugs should be constructed so that drugs are accessible only to designated and authorized personnel. Such personnel must be carefully selected and supervised. Safety also is an important factor, and proper consideration should be given to the safe storage of poisons and flammable compounds. Externals should be stored separately from internal medications. Medications stored in a refrigerator containing items other than drugs should be kept in a secured, separate compartment.

Proper control is important wherever medications are kept, whether in general storage in the institution or the pharmacy or patient-care areas (including satellite pharmacies, nursing units, clinics, emergency rooms, operating rooms, recovery rooms, and treatment rooms). Expiration dates of perishable drugs must be considered in all of these locations, and stock must be rotated as required. A method to detect and properly dispose of outdated, deteriorated, recalled, or obsolete drugs and supplies should be established. This should include monthly audits of all medication storage areas in the institution. (The results of these audits should be documented in writing.)

Since the pharmacist must justify and account for the expenditure of pharmacy funds, he must maintain an adequate inventory management system. Such a system should enable the pharmacist to analyze and interpret prescribing trends and their economic impacts and appropriately minimize inventory levels. It is essential that a system to indicate subminimum inventory levels be developed to avoid "outages," along with procedures to procure emergency supplies of drugs when necessary.

In-House Manufacturing, Bulk Compounding, Packaging, and Labeling.[7,8] As with commercially marketed drug products, those produced by the pharmacy must be accurate in identity, strength, purity, and quality. Therefore, there must be adequate process and finished product controls for all manufacturing/bulk compounding and packaging operations. Written master formulas and batch records (including product test results) must be maintained. All technical personnel must be adequately trained and supervised.

Packaging and labeling operations must have controls sufficient to prevent product/package/label mixups. A lot number to identify each finished product with its production and control history must be assigned to each batch.

The Good Manufacturing Practices of the FDA is a useful model for developing a comprehensive control system.

The pharmacist is encouraged to prepare those drug dosage forms, strengths, and packagings that are needed for optimal drug therapy but that are commercially unavailable. Adequate attention must be given to the stability, palatability, packaging, and labeling requirements of these products.

Medication Distribution (Unit Dose System).[9–11] Medication distribution is the responsibility of the pharmacy. The pharmacist, with the assistance of the P&T committee and the department of nursing, must develop comprehensive policies and procedures that provide for the safe distribution of all medications and related supplies to inpatients and outpatients.

For reasons of safety and economy, the preferred method to distribute drugs in institutions is the *unit dose* system. Although the unit dose system may differ in form depending on the specific needs, resources, and characteristics of each institution, four elements are common to all: (1) medications are contained in, and administered from, single unit or unit dose packages; (2) medications are dispensed in ready-to-administer form to the extent possible; (3) for most medications, not more than a 24-hour supply of doses is provided to or available at the patient-care area at any time; and (4) a patient medication profile is concurrently maintained in the pharmacy for each patient. Floor stocks of drugs are minimized and limited to drugs for emergency use and routinely used "safe" items such as mouthwash and antiseptic solutions.

(1) Physician's drug order: writing the order. Medications should be given (with certain specified exceptions) only on the *written* order of a qualified physician or other authorized prescriber. Allowable exceptions to this rule (i.e., telephone or verbal orders) should be put in written form immediately and the prescriber should countersign the nurse's or pharmacist's signed record of these orders within 48 (preferably 24) hours. Only a pharmacist or registered nurse should accept such orders. Provision should be made to place physician's orders in the patient's chart, and a method for sending this information to the pharmacy should be developed.

Prescribers should specify the date and time medication orders are written.

Medication orders should be written legibly in ink and should include

- Patient's name and location (unless clearly indicated on the order sheet)
- Name (generic) of medication
- Dosage expressed in the metric system, except in instances where dosage must be expressed otherwise (i.e., units, etc.)
- Frequency of administration
- Route of administration
- Signature of the physician
- Date and hour the order was written

Any abbreviations used in medication orders should be agreed to and jointly adopted by the medical, nursing, pharmacy, and medical records staff of the institution.

Any questions arising from a medication order, including the interpretation of an illegible order, should be referred to the ordering physician by the pharmacist. It is desirable for the pharmacist to make (appropriate) entries in the patient's medical chart pertinent to the patient's drug therapy. (Proper authorization for this must be obtained.[12]) Also, a duplicate record of the entry can be maintained in the pharmacy profile.

In computerized patient data systems, each prescriber should be assigned a unique identifier; this number should be included in all medication orders. Unauthorized personnel should not be able to gain access to the system.

(2) Physician's drug order: medication order sheets. The pharmacist (except in emergency situations) must receive the physician's original order or a direct copy of the order before the drug is dispensed. This permits the pharmacist to resolve questions or problems with drug orders before the drug is dispensed and administered. It also eliminates errors which may arise when drug orders are transcribed onto another form for use by the pharmacy. Several methods by which the pharmacy may receive physicians' original orders or direct copies are

1. Self-copying order forms. The physician's order form is designed to make a direct copy (carbon or NCR) which is sent to the pharmacy. This method provides the pharmacist with a duplicate copy of the order and does not require special equipment. There are two basic formats:
   a. Orders for medications included among treatment orders. Use of this form allows the physician to continue writing his orders on the chart as he has been accustomed in the past, leaving all other details to hospital personnel.
   b. Medication orders separated from other treatment orders on the order form. The separation of drug orders makes it easier for the pharmacist to review the order sheet.
2. Electromechanical. Copying machines or similar devices may be used to produce an exact copy of the physician's order. Provision should be made to transmit physicians' orders to the pharmacy in the event of mechanical failure.
3. Computerized. Computer systems, in which the physician enters orders into a computer which then stores and prints out the orders in the pharmacy or elsewhere, are used in some institutions. Any such system should provide for the pharmacist's verification of any drug orders entered into the system by anyone other than an authorized prescriber.

(3) Physician's drug order: time limits and changes. Medication orders should be reviewed automatically when the patient goes to the delivery room, operating room, or a different service. In addition, a method to protect patients from indefinite, open-ended drug orders must be provided. This

may be accomplished through one or more of the following: (1) routine monitoring of patients' drug therapy by a pharmacist; (2) drug class-specific, automatic stop-order policies covering those drug orders not specifying a number of doses or duration of therapy; and (3) automatic cancellation of all drug orders after a predetermined (by the P&T committee) time interval unless rewritten by the prescriber. Whatever the method used, it must protect the patient, as well as provide for a timely notification to the prescriber that the order will be stopped *before* such action takes place.

(4) Physician's drug order: receipt of order and drug profiles. A pharmacist must review and interpret every medication order and resolve any problems or uncertainties with it before the drug is entered into the dispensing system. This means that he must be satisfied that each questionable medication order is, in fact, acceptable. This may occur through study of the patient's medical record, research of the professional literature, or discussion with the prescriber or other medical, nursing, or pharmacy staff. Procedures to handle a drug order the pharmacist still believes is unacceptable (e.g., very high dose or a use beyond that contained in the package insert) should be prepared (and reviewed by the hospital's legal counsel). In general, the physician must be able to support the use of the drug in these situations. It is generally advisable for the pharmacist to document actions (e.g., verbal notice to the physician that a less toxic drug was available and should be used) relative to a questionable medication order on the pharmacy's patient medication profile form or other pharmacy document (not in the medical record).

Once the order has been approved, it is entered into the *patient's medication profile.* A medication profile must be maintained in the pharmacy for all inpatients and those outpatients routinely receiving care at the institution. (Note: Equivalent records also should be available at the patient-care unit.) This essential item, which is continuously updated, may be a written copy or computer maintained. It serves two purposes. First, it enables the pharmacist to become familiar with the patient's total drug regimen, enabling him to detect quickly potential interactions, unintended dosage changes, drug duplications and overlapping therapies, and drugs contraindicated because of patient allergies or other reasons. Second, it is required in unit dose systems in order for the individual medication doses to be scheduled, prepared, distributed, and administered on a timely basis. The profile information must be reviewed by the pharmacist *before* dispensing the patient's drug(s). (It also may be useful in retrospective review of drug use.)

Patient profile information should include

- Patient's full name, date hospitalized, age, sex, weight, hospital I.D. number, and provisional diagnosis or reason for admission (the format for this information will vary from one hospital to another).
- Laboratory test results.
- Other medical data relevant to the patient's drug therapy (e.g., information from drug history interviews).
- Sensitivities, allergies, and other significant contra-indications.
- Drug products dispensed, dates of original orders, strengths, dosage forms, quantities, dosage frequency or directions, and automatic stop dates.
- Intravenous therapy data (this information may be kept on a separate profile form, but there should be a method for the pharmacist to review both concomitantly).
- Blood products administered.
- Pharmacist's or technician's initials.
- Number of doses or amounts dispensed.
- Items relevant or related to the patient's drug therapy (e.g., blood products) not provided by the pharmacy.

(5) Physician's drug order: records. Appropriate records of each medication order and its processing in the pharmacy must be maintained. Such records must be retained in accordance with applicable state laws and regulations. Any changes or clarifications in the order should be written in the chart. The signature(s) or initials of the person(s) verifying the transcription of medication orders into the medication profile should be noted. A way should be provided to determine, for all doses dispensed, who prepared the dose, its date of dispensing, the source of the drug, and the person who checked it. Other information, such as the time of receipt of the order and management data (number of orders per patient day and the like) should be kept as desired. Medication profiles also may be useful for retrospective drug use review studies.

(6) Physician's drug order: special orders.[5,6,13,14] Special orders (i.e., "stat" and emergency orders and those for nonformulary drugs, investigational drugs, restricted use drugs, or controlled substances) should be processed according to specific written procedures meeting all applicable regulations and requirements.

(7) Physician's drug order: other considerations. The pharmacy, nursing, and medical staffs, through the P&T committee, should develop a schedule of standard drug administration times. The nurse should notify the pharmacist whenever it is necessary to deviate from the standard medication schedule.

A mechanism to continually inform the pharmacy of patient admissions, discharges, and transfers should be established.

(8) Intravenous admixture services.[15] The preparation of sterile products (e.g., intravenous admixtures, "piggybacks," and irrigations) is an important part of the drug control system. The pharmacy is responsible for assuring that all such products used in the institution are (1) therapeutically and pharmaceutically appropriate (i.e., are rational and free of incompatibilities or similar problems) to the patient; (2) free from microbial and pyrogenic contaminants; (3) free from unacceptable levels of particulate and other toxic contaminants; (4) correctly prepared (i.e., contain the correct amounts of the correct drugs); and (5) properly labeled, stored, and distributed. Centralizing all sterile compounding procedures within the pharmacy department is the best way to achieve these goals.

Parenteral admixtures and related solutions are subject to the same considerations presented in the preceding sections on "physician's drug order." However, their special characteristics (e.g., complex preparation or need for sterility assurance) also mandate certain additional requirements concerning their preparation, labeling, handling, and quality control. These are described in Reference 15.

It is important that the pharmacy is notified of any problems that arise within the institution pertaining to the use of intravenous drugs and fluids (infections, phlebitis, and product defects).

(9) Medication containers, labeling, and dispensing: stock containers. The pharmacist is responsible for labeling medication containers. Medication labels should be typed or machine printed. Labeling with pen or pencil and the use of adhesive tape or china marking pencils should be prohibited. A label should not be superimposed on another label. The label should be legible and free from erasures and strikeovers. It should be firmly affixed to the container. The labels for stock containers should be protected from chemical action or abrasion and bear the name, address, and telephone number of the hospital. Medication containers and labels should not be altered by anyone other than pharmacy personnel. Prescription labels should not be distributed outside the pharmacy. Accessory labels and statements (shake well, may not be refilled, and the like) should be used as required. Any container to be used outside the institution should bear its name, address, and phone number.

Important labeling considerations are

1. The metric system should be given prominence on all labels when both metric and apothecary measurement units are given.
2. The names of all therapeutically active ingredients should be indicated in compound mixtures.
3. Labels for medications should indicate the amount of drug or drugs in each dosage unit (e.g., per 5 mL and per capsule).
4. rugs and chemicals in forms intended for dilution or reconstitution should carry appropriate directions.
5. he expiration date of the contents, as well as proper storage conditions, should be clearly indicated.
6. The acceptable route(s) of administration should be indicated for parenteral medications.
7. Labels for large volume sterile solutions should permit visual inspection of the container contents.
8. Numbers, letters, coined names, unofficial synonyms, and abbreviations should not be used to identify medications, with the exception of approved letter or number codes for investigational drugs (or drugs being used in blinded clinical studies).
9. Containers presenting difficulty in labeling, such as small tubes, should be labeled with no less than the prescription serial number, name of drug, strength, and name of the patient. The container should then be placed in a larger carton bearing a label with all necessary information.
10. The label should conform to all applicable federal, state, and local laws and regulations.
11. Medication labels of stock containers and repackaged or prepackaged drugs should carry codes to identify the source and lot number of medication.
12. Nonproprietary name(s) should be given prominence over proprietary names.
13. Amount dispensed (e.g., number of tablets) should be indicated.
14. Drug strengths, volumes, and amounts should be given as recommended in References 11 and 16.

(10) Medication containers, labeling, and dispensing: inpatient medications.[11,16] Drug products should be as ready for administration to the patient as the current status of pharmaceutical technology permits. Inpatient medication containers and packages should conform to applicable *USP* requirements and the guidelines in References 11 and 16.

Inpatient self-care and "discharge" medications should be labeled as outpatient prescriptions (see below).

(11) Medication containers, labeling, and dispensing: outpatient medications.[17] Outpatient medications must be labeled in accordance with state board of pharmacy and federal regulations. As noted, medications given to patients as "discharge medication" must be labeled in the pharmacy (not by nursing personnel) as outpatient prescriptions.

The source of the medication and initials of the dispenser should be noted on the prescription form at the time of dispensing. If feasible, the lot number also should be recorded.

An identifying check system to ensure proper identification of outpatients should be established.

Outpatient prescriptions should be packaged in accordance with the provisions of the Poison Prevention Packaging Act of 1970 and any regulations thereunder. They must also meet any applicable requirements of the *USP.*

Any special instructions to or procedures required of the patient relative to the drug's preparation, storage, and administration should be either a part of the label or accompany the medication container received by the patient. Counseling of the patient sufficient to ensure understanding and compliance (to the extent possible) with his medication regimen must be conducted. Nonprescription drugs, if used in the institution, should be labeled as any other medication.

(12) Delivery of medications. Couriers used to deliver medications should be reliable and carefully chosen.

Pneumatic tubes, dumbwaiters, medication carts, and the like should protect drug products from breakage and theft. In those institutions having automatic delivery equipment, such as a pneumatic tube system, provision must be made for an alternative delivery method in case of breakdown.

All parts of the transportation system must protect medications from pilferage. Locks and other security devices should be used where necessary. Procedures for the orderly transfer of medications to the nurse should be instituted; i.e., drug carts or pneumatic tube carriers should not arrive at the patient-care area without the nurse or her designee acknowledging their arrival.

Medications must always be properly secured. Storage areas and equipment should meet the requirements presented in other sections of these guidelines.

(13) Administration of medications. The institution should develop detailed written procedures governing medication administration. In doing so, the following guidelines should be considered:

1. All medications should be administered by appropriately trained and authorized personnel in accordance with the laws, regulations, and institutional policies governing drug administration. It is particularly important that there are written policies and procedures defining responsibility for starting parenteral infusions, administering all intravenous medications, and adding medications to flowing parenteral fluids. Procedures for drug administration by respiratory therapists and during emergency situations also should be established.

Exceptions to any of these policies should be provided in writing.

2. All medications should be administered directly from the medication cart (or equivalent) at the patient's room. The use of unit dose packaged drugs eliminates the need for medication cups and cards (and their associated trays), and they should not be used. A medication should not be removed from the unit dose package until it is to be administered.
3. Medications prepared for administration but not used must be returned to the pharmacy.
4. Medications should be given as near the specified time as possible.
5. The patient for whom the medication is intended should be positively identified by checking the patient's identification band or hospital number or by other means as specified by hospital policy.
6. The person administering the medication should stay with the patient until the dose has been taken. Exceptions to this rule are specific medications which may be left at the patient's bedside upon the physician's written order for self-administration.
7. Parenteral medications that are not to be mixed together in a syringe should be given in different injection sites on the patient or separately injected into the administration site of the administration set of a compatible intravenous fluid.
8. The pharmacy should receive copies of all medication error reports or other medication-related incidents.
9. A system to assure that patients permitted to self-medicate do so correctly should be established.

(14) Return of unused medication. All medications that have not been administered to the patient must remain in the medication cart and be returned to the pharmacy. Only those medications returned in unopened sealed packages may be reissued. Medications returned by outpatients should not be reused. Procedures for crediting and returning drugs to stock should be instituted. A mechanism to reconcile doses not given with nursing and pharmacy records should be provided.

(15) Recording of medication administration. All administered, refused, or omitted medication doses should be recorded in the patient's medical record according to an established procedure. Disposition of doses should occur immediately after administering medications to each patient and before proceeding to the next patient. Information to be recorded should include the drug name, dose and route of administration, date and time of administration, and initials of the person administering the dose.

Drug Samples and Medical Sales Representatives.[18] The use of drug samples within the institution is strongly discouraged and should be eliminated to the extent possible. They should never be used for inpatients (unless, for some reason, no other source of supply is available to the pharmacy). Any samples used must be controlled and dispensed through the pharmacy.

Written regulations governing the activities of medical sales representatives within the institution should be established. Sales representatives should receive a copy of these rules and their activities should be monitored.

Investigational Drugs.[13] Policies and procedures governing the use and control of investigational drugs within the institution are necessary. Detailed procedural guidelines are given in Reference 13.

Radiopharmaceuticals. The basic principles of compounding, packaging, sterilizing, testing, and controlling drugs in institutions apply to radiopharmaceuticals. Therefore, even if the pharmacy department is not directly involved with the preparation and dispensing of these agents, the pharmacist must ensure that their use conforms to the drug control principles set forth in this document.

"Bring-In" Medications. The use of a patient's own medications within the hospital should be avoided to the extent possible. They should be used only if the drugs are not obtainable by the pharmacy. If they are used, the physician must write an appropriate order in the patient's medical chart. The drugs should be sent to the pharmacy for verification of their identity; if not identifiable, they must not be used. They should be dispensed as part of the unit dose system, not separate from it.

Drug Control in Operating and Recovery Rooms.[19] The institution's drug control system must extend to its operating room complex. The pharmacist should ensure that all drugs used within this area are properly ordered, stored, prepared, and accounted for.

Emergency Medication Supplies. A policy to supply emergency drugs when the pharmacist is off the premises or when there is insufficient time to get to the pharmacy should exist. Emergency drugs should be limited in number to include only those whose prompt use and immediate availability are generally regarded by physicians as essential in the proper treatment of sudden and unforeseen patient emergencies. The emergency drug supply should not be a source for normal "stat" or "p.r.n." drug orders. The medications included should be primarily for the treatment of cardiac arrest, circulatory collapse, allergic reactions, convulsions, and bronchospasm. The P&T committee should specify the drugs and supplies to be included in emergency stocks.

Emergency drug supplies should be inspected by pharmacy personnel on a routine basis to determine if contents have become outdated and are maintained at adequate levels. Emergency kits should have a seal which visually indicates when they have been opened. The expiration date of the kit should be clearly indicated.

Pharmacy Service When the Pharmacy Is Closed. Hospitals provide services to patients 24 hours a day. Pharmaceutical services are an integral part of the total care provided by the hospital, and the services of a pharmacist should be available at all times. Where around the clock operation of the pharmacy is not feasible, a pharmacist should be available on an "on call" basis. The use of "night cabinets" and drug dispensing by nonpharmacists should be minimized and eliminated wherever possible.

Drugs must not be dispensed to outpatients or hospital staff by anyone other than a pharmacist while the pharmacy is open. If it is necessary for nurses to obtain drugs when the pharmacy is closed and the pharmacist is unavailable, written procedures covering this practice should be developed. They generally should provide for a limited supply of the drugs most commonly needed in these situations; the drugs should be in proper single dose packages and a log should be kept of all doses removed. This log must contain the date and time the drugs were removed, a complete description of the drug product(s), name of the (authorized) nurse involved, and the patient's name.

Drugs should not be dispensed to emergency room patients by nonpharmacist personnel if the pharmacy is open. When no pharmacist is available, emergency room patients should receive drugs packaged, to the extent possible, in single unit packages; no more than a day's supply of doses should be dispensed. The use of an emergency room "formulary" is recommended.[20]

Adverse Drug Reactions. The medical, nursing, and pharmacy staffs must always be alert to the potential for, or presence of, adverse drug reactions. A written procedure to record clinically significant adverse drug reactions should be established. They should be reported to the FDA, the involved drug manufacturer, and the institution's P&T committee (or its equivalent). Adverse drug reaction reports should contain

- Patient's age, sex, and race.
- Description of the drug reaction and the suspected cause.
- Name of drug(s) suspected of causing the reaction.
- Administration route and dose.
- Name(s) of other drugs received by patient.
- Treatment of the reaction, if any.

These reports, along with other significant reports from the literature, should be reviewed and evaluated by the P&T committee. Steps necessary to minimize the incidence of adverse drug reactions in the facility should be taken.

Medication Errors. If a medication error is detected, the patient's physician must be informed immediately. A written report should be prepared describing any medication errors of clinical import observed in the prescribing, dispensing, or administration of a medication. This report, in accordance with hospital policy, should be prepared and sent to the appropriate hospital officials (including the pharmacy) within 24 hours.

These reports should be analyzed, and any necessary action taken, to minimize the possibility of recurrence of such errors. Properly utilized, these incident reports will help to assure optimum drug use control. Medication error reports should be reviewed periodically by the P&T committee. (It should be kept in mind that, in the absence of an organized, independent error detection system, most medication errors will go unnoticed.)

The following definitions of medication errors are suggested. A *medication error* is broadly defined as a dose of medication that deviates from the physician's order as written in the patient's chart or from standard hospital policy and procedures. Except for errors of omission, the medication dose must actually reach the patient; i.e., a wrong dose that is detected and corrected before administration to the patient is not a medication error. Prescribing errors (e.g., therapeutically inappropriate drugs or doses) are excluded from this definition.

Following are the nine categories of medication errors:

1. *Omission error:* the failure to administer an ordered dose. However, if the patient refuses to take the medication, no error has occurred. Likewise, if the dose is not administered because of recognized contraindications, no error has occurred.
2. *Unauthorized drug error:* administration to the patient of a medication dose not authorized for the patient. This category includes a dose given to the wrong patient, duplicate doses, administration of an unordered drug, and a dose given outside a stated set of clinical parameters (e.g., medication order to administer only if the patient's blood pressure falls below a predetermined level).
3. *Wrong dose error:* any dose that is the wrong number of preformed units (e.g., tablets) or any dose above or below the ordered dose by a predetermined amount (e.g., 20%). In the case of ointments, topical solutions, and sprays, an error occurs only if the medication order expresses the dosage quantitatively, e.g., 1 inch of ointment or two 1-second sprays.
4. *Wrong route error:* administration of a drug by a route other than that ordered by the physician. Also included are doses given via the correct route but at the wrong site (e.g., left eye instead of right).
5. *Wrong rate error:* administration of a drug at the wrong rate, the correct rate being that given in the physician's order or as established by hospital policy.
6. *Wrong dosage form error:* administration of a drug by the correct route but in a different dosage form than that specified or implied by the physician. Example of this error type include use of an ophthalmic ointment when a solution was ordered. Purposeful alteration (e.g., crushing of a tablet) or substitution (e.g., substituting liquid for a tablet) of an oral dosage form to facilitate administration is generally not an error.
7. *Wrong time error:* administration of a dose of drug greater than ± X hours from its scheduled administration time, X being as set by hospital policy.
8. *Wrong preparation of a dose:* incorrect preparation of the medication dose. Examples are incorrect dilution or reconstitution, not shaking a suspension, using an expired drug, not keeping a light-sensitive drug protected from light, and mixing drugs that are physically/chemically incompatible.
9. *Incorrect administration technique:* situations when the drug is given via the correct route, site, and so forth, but improper technique is used. Examples are not using Z-track injection technique when indicated for a drug, incorrect instillation of an ophthalmic ointment, and incorrect use of an administration device.

Special Considerations Contributing to Drug Control

Pharmacy Personnel and Management.[21–24] Adequate numbers of competent personnel and a well-managed pharmacy are the keys to an effective drug control system. References 21–24 provide guidance on the competencies required of the pharmacy staff and on administrative requirements of a well-run pharmacy department.

Assuring Rational Drug Therapy: Clinical Services.[21,25] Maximizing rational drug use is an important part of the drug control system. Although all pharmacy services contribute to this goal in a sense, the provision of drug information to the institution's patients and staff and the pharmacy's clinical services are those that most directly contribute to rational drug therapy. They are, in fact, institutional pharmacists' most important contributions to patient care.

Facilities. Space and equipment requirements relative to drug storage have been discussed previously. In addition to these considerations, space and equipment must be sufficient to provide for safe and efficient drug preparation and distribution, patient education and consultation, drug information services, and proper management of the department.

Hospital Committees Important to Drug Control.[26,27] Several hospital committees deal with matters of drug control, and the pharmacist must actively participate in their activities. Among these committees (whose names may vary among institutions) are the P&T committee, infection control committee, use review committee, product evaluation committee, patient care committee, and the committee for protection of human subjects. Of particular importance to the drug control system are the formulary and drug use review (DUR) functions of the P&T committee (although DUR in many institutions may be under a use review or quality-assurance committee).

Drug Use Review.[28] Review of how drugs are prescribed and used is an important part of institutional quality-assurance and drug control systems. DUR programs may be performed retrospectively or, preferably, concurrently or prospectively. They may utilize patient outcomes or therapeutic processes as the basis for judgments about the appropriateness of drug prescribing and use. Depending on the review methodology, the pharmacist should be involved in

1. Preparing, in cooperation with the medical staff, drug use criteria and standards.
2. Obtaining quantitative data on drug use, i.e., information on the amounts and types of drugs used, prescribing patterns by medical service, type of patient, and so forth. These data will be useful in setting priorities for the review program. They also may serve as a measure of the effectiveness of DUR programs, assist in analyzing nosocomial infection and culture and sensitivity data, and help in preparing drug budgets.
3. Reviewing medication orders against the drug use criteria and standards.
4. Consulting with prescribers concerning the results of 3 above.
5. Participating in the followup activities of the review program, i.e., educational programs directed at prescribers, development of recommendations for the formulary, and changes in drug control procedures in response to the results of the review process.

It should be noted that the overall DUR program is a joint responsibility of the pharmacy and the organized medical staff; it is not unilaterally a pharmacy or medical staff function.

Quality Assurance for Pharmaceutical Services.[29] To ensure that the drug control system is functioning as intended, there should be a formalized method to (1) set precise objectives (in terms of outcome and process criteria and standards) for the system; (2) measure and verify the degree of compliance with these standards, i.e., the extent to which the objectives have been realized; and (3) eliminate any noncompliance situations. Such a *quality-assurance program* will be distinct from, though related to, the DUR activities of the department.

Drug Recalls. A written procedure to handle drug product recalls should be developed. Any such system should have the following elements:

1. Whenever feasible, notation of the drug manufacturer's name and drug lot number should appear on outpatient prescriptions, inpatient drug orders or profiles, packaging control records, and stock requisitions and their associated labels.
2. Review of these documents (prescriptions, drug orders, and so forth) to determine the recipients (patients and nursing stations) of the recalled lots. Optimally, this would be done by automated means.
3. In the case of product recalls of substantial clinical significance, a notice should go to the recipients that they have a recalled product. The course of action they should take should be included. In the case of outpatients, caution should be exercised not to cause undue alarm. The uninterrupted therapy of the patients must be assured; i.e., replacement of the recalled drugs generally will be required. The hospital's administration and nursing and medical staffs should be informed of any recalls having significant therapeutic implications. Some situations also may require notifying the physicians of patients receiving drugs that have been recalled.
4. Personal inspection of all patient-care areas should be made to determine if recalled products are present.
5. Quarantine of all recalled products obtained (marked "Quarantined—Do Not Use") until they are picked up by or returned to the manufacturer.
6. Maintenance of a written log of all recalls, the actions taken, and their results.

Computerization.[30] Many information handling tasks in the drug control system (e.g., collecting, recording, storing, retrieving, summarizing, transmitting, and displaying drug use information) may be done more efficiently by computers than by manual systems. Before the drug control system can be computerized, however, a comprehensive, thorough study of the existing manual system must be conducted. This study should identify the data flow within the system and define the functions to be done and their interrelationships. This information is then used as the basis to design or prospectively evaluate a computer system; any other considerations, such as those of the hospital accounting department, are subordinate.

The computer system must include adequate safeguards to maintain the confidentiality of patient records.

A backup system must be available to continue the computerized functions during equipment failure. All transactions occurring while the computer system is inoperable should be entered into the system as soon as possible.

Data on controlled substances must be readily retrievable in written form from the system.

Defective Drug Products, Equipment, and Supplies. The pharmacist should be notified of any defective drug products (or related supplies and equipment) encountered by the nursing or medical staffs. All drug product defects should be reported to the USP–FDA–ASHP Drug Product Defect Reporting Program.

Disposal of Hazardous Substances. Hazardous substances (e.g., toxic or flammable solvents and carcinogenic agents) must be disposed of properly in accordance with the requirements of the Environmental Protection Agency or other applicable regulations. The substances should not be poured indiscriminately down the drain or mixed in with the usual trash.

Unreconstituted vials or ampuls and unopened bottles of oral medications supplied by the National Cancer Institute (NCI) should be returned to the NCI's contract storage and distribution facility.

Other intact products should be returned to the original source for disposition.

Units of anticancer drugs no longer intact, such as reconstituted vials, opened ampuls, and bottles of oral medications, and any equipment (e.g., needles and syringes) used in their preparation require a degree of caution greater than with less toxic compounds to safeguard personnel from accidental exposure. The National Institutes of Health recommends that all such materials be segregated for special destruction procedures. The items should be kept in special containers marked *"Danger—Chemical Carcinogens."* Needles and syringes first should be rendered unusable and then placed in specially marked plastic bags. Care should be taken to prevent penetration and leakage of the bags. Excess liquids should be placed in sealed containers; the original vial is satisfactory. Disposal of all of the above materials should be by incineration to destroy organic material.

Alternate disposal for BCG vaccine products has been recommended by the Bureau of Biologics (BOB). The BOB suggests that all containers and equipment used with BCG vaccines be sterilized prior to disposal. Autoclaving at 121 °C for 30 minutes will sterilize the equipment.

At all steps in the handling of anticancer drugs and other hazardous substances, care should be taken to safeguard professional and support services personnel from accidental exposure to these agents.

References

1. Ginnow WK, King CM Jr. Revision and reorganization of a hospital pharmacy policy and procedure manual. *Am J Hosp Pharm.* 1978; 35:698–704.
2. Accreditation manual for hospitals 1980. Chicago: Joint Commission on Accreditation of Hospitals; 1979.
3. Publications, reprints and services. Washington, DC: American Society of Hospital Pharmacists; current edition.
4. American Society of Hospital Pharmacists. ASHP guidelines for selecting pharmaceutical manufacturers and distributors. *Am J Hosp Pharm.* 1976; 33:645–6.
5. American Society of Hospital Pharmacists. ASHP guidelines for hospital formularies. *Am J Hosp Pharm.* 1978; 35:326–8.
6. American Society of Hospital Pharmacists. ASHP statement of guiding principles on the operation of the hospital formulary system. *Am J Hosp Pharm.* 1964; 21:40–1.
7. American Society of Hospital Pharmacists. ASHP guidelines for repackaging oral solids and liquids in single unit and unit dose packages. *Am J Hosp Pharm.* 1979; 36:223–4.
8. 21 CFR Parts 210 and 211. Current good manufacturing practices in manufacturing, processing, packing or holding of drugs. April 1979.
9. Sourcebook on unit dose drug distribution systems. Washington, DC: American Society of Hospital Pharmacists; 1978.
10. American Society of Hospital Pharmacists. ASHP statement on unit dose drug distribution. *Am J Hosp Pharm.* 1975; 32:835.
11. American Society of Hospital Pharmacists. ASHP guidelines for single unit and unit dose packages of drugs. *Am J Hosp Pharm.* 1977; 34:613–4.
12. American Society of Hospital Pharmacists. ASHP guidelines for obtaining authorization for pharmacists' notations in the patient medical record. *Am J Hosp Pharm.* 1979; 36:222–3.
13. American Society of Hospital Pharmacists. ASHP guidelines for the use of investigational drugs in institutions. *Am J Hosp Pharm.* 1979; 36:221–2.
14. American Society of Hospital Pharmacists. ASHP guidelines for institutional use of controlled substances. *Am J Hosp Pharm.* 1974; 31:582–8.
15. Recommendations of the National Coordinating Committee on Large Volume Parenterals. Washington, DC: American Society of Hospital Pharmacists; 1980.
16. National Coordinating Committee on Large Volume Parenterals. Recommendations for the labeling of large volume parenterals. *Am J Hosp Pharm.* 1978; 35:49–51.
17. American Society of Hospital Pharmacists. ASHP guidelines on pharmacist-conducted patient counseling. *Am J Hosp Pharm.* 1976; 33:644–5.
18. Lipman AG, Mullen HF. Quality control of medical service representative activities in the hospital. *Am J Hosp Pharm.* 1974; 31:167–70.
19. Evans DM, Guenther AM, Keith TD, et al. Pharmacy practice in an operating room complex. *Am J Hosp Pharm.* 1979; 36:1342–7.
20. Mar DD, Hanan ZI, LaFontaine R. Improved emergency room medication distribution. *Am J Hosp Pharm.* 1978; 35:70–3.
21. American Society of Hospital Pharmacists. ASHP minimum standard for pharmacies in institutions. *Am J Hosp Pharm.* 1977; 34:1356–8.
22. American Society of Hospital Pharmacists. ASHP guidelines on the competencies required in institutional pharmacy practice. *Am J Hosp Pharm.* 1975; 32:917–9.

23. American Society of Hospital Pharmacists. ASHP training guidelines for hospital pharmacy supportive personnel. *Am J Hosp Pharm.* 1976; 33:646–8.
24. American Society of Hospital Pharmacists. ASHP competency standard for pharmacy supportive personnel in organized health care settings. *Am J Hosp Pharm.* 1978; 35:449–51.
25. American Society of Hospital Pharmacists. ASHP statement on clinical functions in institutional pharmacy practice. *Am J Hosp Pharm.* 1978; 35:813.
26. American Society of Hospital Pharmacists. ASHP statement on the pharmacy and therapeutics committee. *Am J Hosp Pharm.* 1978; 35:813–4.
27. American Society of Hospital Pharmacists. ASHP statement on the hospital pharmacist's role in infection control. *Am J Hosp Pharm.* 1978; 35:814–5.
28. Antibiotic use review and infection control: evaluating drug use through patient care audit. Chicago: InterQual, Inc.; 1978.
29. Model quality assurance program for hospital pharmacies, revised. Washington, DC: American Society of Hospital Pharmacists; 1980.
30. Sourcebook on computers in pharmacy. Washington, DC: American Society of Hospitals Pharmacists; 1978.

Developed by the ASHP Council on Professional Affairs. Approved by the ASHP Board of Directors, March 20, 1980. Revised November 1981.

This document contains numerous references to various official ASHP documents and other publications. Inclusion of the latter does not constitute endorsement of their content by the Society; they are, however, considered to be useful elaborations on certain subjects contained herein. To avoid redundancy with other ASHP documents, relevant references are cited in many sections of these guidelines. Most may be obtained from ASHP through its publications catalog.

Copyright © 1980, American Society of Hospital Pharmacists, Inc. All rights reserved. Contact ASHP for reprint and permissions requests. This content may not be used for commercial purposes without the express written consent of ASHP.

The bibliographic citation for this document is as follows: American Society of Hospital Pharmacists. ASHP technical assistance bulletin on hospital drug distribution and control. *Am J Hosp Pharm.* 1980; 37:1097–103.

ASHP Technical Assistance Bulletin on Repackaging Oral Solids and Liquids in Single Unit and Unit Dose Packages

To maximize the benefits of a unit dose drug distribution system, all drugs must be packaged in single unit or unit dose packages.[a] However, not all drugs are commercially available in single unit (or unit dose) packages. Therefore, the institutional pharmacist must often repackage drugs obtained in bulk containers (e.g., bottles of 500 tablets) into single unit packages so that they may be used in a unit dose system.

Certain precautions must be taken if the quality of drugs repackaged by the pharmacist is to be maintained. The guidelines presented herein will assist the pharmacist in developing procedures for repackaging drugs in a safe and acceptable manner:

1. The packaging operation should be isolated, to the extent possible, from other pharmacy activities.
2. Only one drug product at a time should be repackaged in a specific work area. No drug products other than the one being repackaged should be present in the immediate packaging area. Also, no labels other than those for the product being repackaged should be present in the area.
3. Upon completion of the packaging run, all unused stocks of drugs and all finished packages should be removed from the packaging area. The packaging machinery and related equipment should then be completely emptied, cleaned, and inspected before commencing the next packaging operation.
4. All unused labels (if separate labels are used) should be removed from the immediate packaging area. The operator should verify that none remains in the packaging machine(s). If labels are prepared as part of the packaging operation, the label plate (or analogous part of the printing apparatus) should be removed or adjusted to "blank" upon completion of the run. This will help assure that the correct label is printed during any subsequent run. There should be a procedure to reconcile the number of packages produced with the number of labels used (if any) and destroyed (if any) and the number of units or volume of drug set forth to be packaged.
5. Before beginning a packaging run, an organoleptic evaluation (color, odor, appearance, and markings) of the drug product being repackaged should be made. The bulk container should also be examined for evidence of water damage, contamination, or other deleterious effects.
6. All packaging equipment and systems should be operated and used in accordance with the manufacturer's or other established instructions. There should be valid justification and authorization by the supervisor for any deviation from those instructions on the part of the operator.
7. The pharmacist should obtain data on the characteristics of all packaging materials used. This information should include data on the chemical composition, light transmission, moisture permeability, size, thickness (alone or in laminate), recommended sealing temperature, and storage requirements.
8. Unit dose packages and labels should, to the extent possible, comply with the "ASHP Guidelines for Single Unit and Unit Dose Packages of Drugs."[1]
9. Whenever feasible, a responsible individual, other than the packaging operator, should verify that (a) the packaging system (drug, materials, and machines) is set up correctly and (b) all procedures have been performed properly. Ultimate responsibility for all packaging operations rests with the pharmacist.
10. Control records of all packaging runs must be kept. These records should include the following information: (1) complete description of the product, i.e., name, strength, dosage form, route of administration, etc.; (2) the product's manufacturer or supplier; (3) control number; (4) the pharmacy's control number if different from the manufacturer's; (5) expiration dates of the original container and the repackaged product; (6) number of units packaged and the date(s) they were packaged; (7) initials of the operator and checker (if any); (8) a sample of the label and, if feasible, a sample of the finished package, which should not be discarded until after the expiration date and which should be examined periodically for signs of deterioration; and (9) description (including lot number) of the packaging materials and equipment used.
11. It is the responsibility of the pharmacist to determine the expiration date to be placed on the package, taking into account the nature of the drug repackaged, the characteristics of the package, and the storage conditions to which the drug may be subjected. This date must not be beyond that of the original package.[b]
12. All drugs should be packaged and stored in a temperature- and humidity-controlled environment to minimize degradation caused by heat and moisture. A relative humidity of 75% at 23 °C should not be exceeded. Packaging materials should be stored in accordance with the manufacturer's instructions and any applicable regulations.
13. Written procedures (both general and product specific) governing repackaging operations should be prepared and updated as required. Any deviation from these procedures should be noted and explained on the control record. Operators must understand the procedures (and operation of all packaging equipment) before commencing the run.
14. Applicable FDA and USP requirements concerning the type of package required for specific drug products must be followed.
15. Drugs and chemicals with high vapor pressures should be stored separately from other products to minimize cross contamination.

DOI 10.37573/9781585287048.027

References

1. American Society of Hospital Pharmacists. ASHP guidelines for single unit and unit dose packages of drugs. *Am J Hosp Pharm.* 1977; 34:613–4.
2. Stolar MH. Expiration dates of repackaged drug products. *Am J Hosp Pharm.* 1979; 36:170. Editorial.

---

[a]A *single unit* package is one which contains one discrete pharmaceutical dosage form, e.g., one tablet or one 5-mL volume of liquid. A *unit dose* package is one which contains the particular dose of drug ordered for the patient. A *single unit* package is a *unit dose (or single dose)* package if it contains that particular dose of drug ordered for the patient.

[b]For specific recommendations on expiration date policy, see Reference 2.

Revised by the ASHP Board of Directors, November 16–17, 1978.

Developed originally by a joint working group of the American Society of Hospital Pharmacists and the American Society of Consultant Pharmacists and representatives of the drug packaging industry. The original document subsequently was approved officially by the Boards of Directors of ASHP and ASCP. FDA reviewed the original document and commended ASHP and ASCP for developing the guidelines.

Copyright © 1983, American Society of Hospital Pharmacists, Inc., and American Society of Consultant Pharmacists. All rights reserved. Contact ASHP for reprint and permissions requests. This content may not be used for commercial purposes without the express written consent of ASHP.

The bibliographic citation for this document is as follows: American Society of Hospital Pharmacists. ASHP technical assistance bulletin on repackaging oral solids and liquids in single unit and unit dose packages. *Am J Hosp Pharm.* 1983; 40:451–2.

ASHP Technical Assistance Bulletin on Single Unit and Unit Dose Packages of Drugs

Drug packages must fulfill four basic functions:

1. Identify their contents completely and precisely.
2. Protect their contents from deleterious environmental effects (e.g., photodecomposition).
3. Protect their contents from deterioration due to handling (e.g., breakage and contamination).
4. Permit their contents to be used quickly, easily, and safely.

Modern drug distribution systems use single unit packages to a great extent and, in fact, such packages are central to the operation of unit dose systems, intravenous admixture services, and other important aspects of pharmacy practice. These guidelines have been prepared to assist pharmaceutical manufacturers and pharmacists in the development and production of single unit and unit dose packages, the use of which has been shown to have substantial benefits.

A *single unit* package is one that contains one discrete pharmaceutical dosage form, i.e., one tablet, one 2-mL volume of liquid, one 2-g mass of ointment, etc. A *unit dose* package is one that contains the particular dose of the drug ordered for the patient. A single unit package is also a *unit dose* or *single dose* package if it contains the particular dose of the drug ordered for the patient. A unit dose package could, for example, contain two tablets of a drug product.

General Considerations

Packaging Materials. Packaging materials (and the package itself) must possess the physical characteristics required to protect the contents from (as required) light, moisture, temperature, air, and handling. The material should not deteriorate during the shelf life of the contents. Packages should be of lightweight, nonbulky materials that do not produce toxic fumes when incinerated. Materials that may be recycled or are biodegradable, or both, are to be preferred over those that are not. Packaging materials should not absorb, adsorb, or otherwise deleteriously affect their contents. Information should be available to practitioners indicating the stability and compatibility of drugs with various packaging materials.

Shape and Form. Packages should be constructed so that they do not deteriorate with normal handling. They should be easy to open and use, and their use should require little or no special training or experience. Unless the package contains a drug to be added to a parenteral fluid or otherwise used in compounding a finished dosage form, it should allow the contents to be administered directly to the patient (or IPPB apparatus or fluid administration set) without any need for repackaging into another container or device (except for ampuls).

Label Copy. Current federal labeling requirements must be adhered to, with attention also given to the items at right. The desired copy and format are as follows:

Nonproprietary Name
(and proprietary name if to be shown)
Dosage Form (if special or other than oral)
Strength
Strength of Dose and Total Contents Delivered
(e.g., number of tablets and their total dose)
Special Notes (e.g., refrigerate)
Expiration Date
Control Number

1. *Nonproprietary and proprietary names.* The nonproprietary name and the strength should be the most prominent part of the package label. It is not necessary to include the proprietary name, if any, on the package. The name of the manufacturer or distributor should appear on the package. In addition, the name of the manufacturer of the finished dosage form should be included in the product labeling. The style of type should be chosen to provide maximum legibility, contrast, and permanence.
2. *Dosage form.* Special characteristics of the dosage form should be a part of the label, e.g., extended release. Packages should be labeled as to the route of administration if other than oral, e.g., topical use. In a package containing an injection, the acceptable injectable route(s) of administration should be stated on both outer and inner packages, i.e., both on the syringe unit and carton (if any).
3. *Strength.* Strength should be stated in accordance with terminology in the *American Hospital Formulary Service.* The metric system should be used, with dosage forms formulated to provide the rounded-off figures in the *USP* table of approximate equivalents and expressed in the smallest whole number. Micrograms should be used through 999, then milligrams through 999, then grams. Thus, 300 mg, *not* 5 gr, nor 325 mg, nor 0.3 g; 60 mg, *not* 1 gr, nor 0.06 g, nor 64.5 mg, nor 65 mg; 400 mcg, *not* 1/150 gr, nor 0.4 mg, nor 0.0004 g; mL (milliliters) should be used instead of cc (cubic centimeters).
4. *Strength of dose and total contents delivered.* The total contents and total dose of the package should be indicated. Thus, a unit dose package containing a 600-mg dose as two 300-mg tablets should be labeled "600 mg (as two 300-mg tablets)." Likewise, a 500-mg dose of a drug in a liquid containing 100 mg/mL should be labeled "Delivers 500 mg (as 5 mL of 100 mg/mL)."
5. *Special notes.* Special notes such as conditions of storage (e.g., refrigerate), preparation (e.g., shake well or moisten), and administration (e.g., not to be chewed) that are not obvious from the dosage form designation are to be included on the label.
6. *Expiration date.* The expiration date should be prominently visible on the package. If the contents must be reconstituted prior to use, the shelf life of the final product should be indicated. Unless stability data warrant otherwise, expiration dates should fall during January and July to simplify recall procedures.

DOI 10.37573/9781585287048.028

7. *Control number (lot number).* The control number should appear on the package.

Product Identification Codes. The use of product identification codes, appearing directly on the dosage form, is encouraged.

Evidence of Entry. The package should be so designed that it is evident, when the package is still intact, that it has never been entered or opened.

Specific Considerations

Oral Solids

1. *Blister package.* A blister package should
   a. Have an opaque and nonreflective backing (flat upper surface of package) for printing.
   b. Have a blister (dome or bubble) of a transparent material that is, preferably, flat bottomed.
   c. Be easily peelable.
   d. If it contains a controlled substance, be numbered sequentially for accountability purposes.
2. *Pouch package.* A pouch package should
   a. Have one side opaque and nonreflective for printing.
   b. Be easily deliverable, i.e., large tablets in large pouches, small tablets in small pouches.
   c. Tear from any point or from multiple locations.
   d. If it contains a controlled substance, be numbered sequentially for accountability purposes.
3. The packages should be such that contents can be delivered directly to the patient's mouth or hand.

Oral Liquids

1. The packages should be filled to deliver the labeled contents. It is recognized that overfilling will be necessary, depending on the shape of the container, the container material, and the formulation of the dosage form.
2. The label should state the contents as follows: Delivers ____mg (or g or mcg) in ____mL.
3. If reconstitution is required, the amount of vehicle to be added should be indicated. These directions may take the form of "fill to mark on container" in lieu of stating a specific volume.
4. Syringe-type containers for oral administration should not accept a needle and should be labeled "For Oral Use Only."
5. Containers should be designed to permit administration of contents directly from the package.

Injectables

1. The device should be appropriately calibrated in milliliters and scaled from the tip to the fill line. Calibrated space may be built into the device to permit addition of other drugs. The label should state the contents as follows: Delivers ____mg (or g or mcg) in ____mL.
2. An appropriate size needle may be an integral part of the device. The needle sheath should not be the plunger. The plunger should be mechanically stable in the barrel of the syringe.
3. The device should be of such a design that it is patient ready and assembly instructions are not necessary.
4. The sheath protecting the needle should be a nonpenetrable, preferably rigid material, to protect personnel from injury. The size of the needle should be indicated.
5. The device should be of such a design that easy and visible aspiration is possible. It should be as compact as possible and of such a size that it can be easily handled.

Parenteral Solutions and Additives

1. The approximate pH and osmolarity of parenteral solutions should be stated on the label. The amount of overfill also should be noted. Electrolyte solutions should be labeled in both mEq (or millimole) and mg concentrations. Solutions commonly labeled in terms of percent concentration, e.g., dextrose, should also be labeled in w/v terms.
2. Parenteral fluid container labels should be readable when hanging and when upright or in the normal manipulative position.
3. Drugs to be mixed with parenteral infusion solutions should be packaged into convenient sizes that minimize the need for solution transfers and other manipulations.
4. Partially filled piggyback-type containers should
   a. Be recappable with a tamperproof closure.
   b. Have a hanger.
   c. Have volume markings.
   d. Be designed to minimize the potential for contamination during use.
   e. Contain a partial vacuum for ease of reconstitution.
5. If an administration set is included with the container, it should be compatible with all large volume parenteral delivery systems.

Other Dosage Forms—Ophthalmics, Suppositories, Ointments, etc. Dosage forms other than those specifically discussed above should be adequately labeled to indicate their use and route of administration and should adhere to the above and other required package labeling and design criteria.

Approved by the ASHP Board of Directors, November 14–15, 1984. Revised by the ASHP Council on Clinical Affairs. Supersedes the previous version, which was approved on March 31–April 1, 1977.

Copyright © 1985, American Society of Hospital Pharmacists, Inc. All rights reserved. Contact ASHP for reprint and permissions requests. This content may not be used for commercial purposes without the express written consent of ASHP.

The bibliographic citation for this document is as follows: American Society of Hospital Pharmacists. ASHP technical assistance bulletin on single unit and unit dose packages of drugs. *Am J Hosp Pharm.* 1985; 42:378–9.

Education and Training

DOI 10.37573/9781585287048

Education and Training

2301

EDUCATION AND TRAINING IN DIGITAL HEALTH

Source: Council on Education and Workforce Development

To acknowledge that digital health is a growing modality that supports the pharmacy workforce in providing patient care; further,

To support training and education for the pharmacy workforce in innovative models that support digital health services; further,

To advocate for involvement of the pharmacy workforce in research on digital health services and outcomes.

Rationale

Continuous development of digital health technology is rapidly redefining the provision of healthcare. Digital health is a broad, multi-faceted term used to describe a wide category of practices, products, and processes. The U.S Food and Drug Administration has stated that "the broad scope of digital health includes categories such as mobile health (mHealth), health information technology (IT), wearable devices, telehealth and telemedicine, and personalized medicine."

To ensure that pharmacists are involved in the care of patients using digital health technologies, training and education must be developed that supports the pharmacy workforce. The interoperability and integration of digital health technologies into electronic health records is crucial. Research supporting digital health technologies for improved patient outcomes, while maintaining security and improving interoperability with electronic health records, is needed to foster continued development of these technologies and applications.

2329

WELL-BEING AND RESILIENCE OF THE PHARMACY WORKFORCE

Source: Council on Education and Workforce Development

To affirm that occupational burnout adversely affects an individual's well-being and healthcare outcomes; further,

To acknowledge that the healthcare workforce encounters unique stressors throughout their education, training, and careers that contribute to occupational burnout; further,

To declare that healthcare workforce well-being and resilience requires shared responsibility among healthcare team members and between individuals and organizations; further,

To provide resources to empower individuals and institutions to embrace well-being and resilience as a priority supported by organizational culture; further,

To promote that pharmacy leadership collaborate with their institutions to assess the well-being and resilience of the pharmacy workforce and identify effective prevention and intervention strategies; further,

To encourage hospitals and health systems to invest in the development and assessment of interprofessional programs that prevent occupational burnout while supporting well-being, and to support nonpunitive participation in these programs.

This policy supersedes ASHP policy 1825.

DOI 10.37573/9781585287048.029

Rationale

Clinician burnout can have serious, wide-ranging consequences on individual clinicians and learners, health care organizations, and patient care. Occupational burnout is a syndrome characterized by a high degree of emotional exhaustion, high depersonalization (e.g., cynicism), and a low sense of personal accomplishment from work due to both internal and external factors. The results follow a 2018 study in the *American Journal of Health-System Pharmacy* (*AJHP*) that found 53 percent of health-system pharmacists self-reported a high degree of burnout caused by increasing stresses and demands. Occupational burnout affects today's pharmacy workforce at unprecedented rates. At the individual level, pharmacy staff burnout can result in medication errors and increased patient harm. At the hospital or healthcare system level, the consequences of occupational burnout include disengagement, loss of productivity, and employee turnover, which can lead to inefficiency and financial problems for healthcare organizations. Stress in our clinical learning environment can affect all healthcare learners, with negative outcomes ranging from poor well-being to substance abuse to depression, even suicide. A 2017 *AJHP* article reported that pharmacy residents working more than 60 hours per week reported high levels of stress, depression, and hostility.

ASHP joined the National Academy of Medicine (NAM) Action Collaborative on Clinician Well-Being and Resilience in 2017. The goals of the Collaborative are to:

1. Raise the visibility of clinician anxiety, burnout, depression, stress, and suicide.
2. Improve baseline understanding of challenges to clinician well-being.
3. Advance evidence-based, multidisciplinary solutions to improve patient care by caring for the caregiver.

The NAM Action Collaborative Conceptual Model depicts both individual and external factors affecting well-being and resilience and indicates that it requires a combined effort from the individual and the system to address and prevent occupational burnout.

Studies suggest that burnout is a problem of the entire healthcare organization as well as individual clinicians, so maintaining clinician well-being and resilience requires a combined effort by the individuals and their employers. To be successful, interventional programs must promote prevention, recognition, and treatment of burnout, and healthcare organizations must foster a culture that supports not just nonpunitive participation in these interprofessional programs but a sense of personal empowerment for developing and maintaining resilience. A healthcare organization with a resilient workforce will provide the best healthcare outcomes.

Supporting the well-being of the pharmacy workforce requires sustained attention and action at organizational, state, and national levels, as well as investment in research and information sharing to advance evidence-based solutions. A pharmacy workforce with the ability to thrive during adversity—a resilient workforce—is essential to combat burnout and support higher-quality care, increased patient safety, and improved patient satisfaction.

2201

STATE-SPECIFIC REQUIREMENTS FOR PHARMACIST AND PHARMACY TECHNICIAN CONTINUING EDUCATION

Source: Council on Education and Workforce Development

To advocate for the standardization of state pharmacist and pharmacy technician continuing education requirements; further,

To advocate that state boards of pharmacy adopt continuing professional development as the preferred model to maintain competence.

This policy supersedes ASHP policy 1111.

Rationale

All 50 states require continuing education for pharmacists as a means of maintaining their competence, and many states have similar requirements for pharmacy technicians. State requirements for continuing education differ, in numbers of hours and the time frame within which they must be collected and reported, for example. Some state boards of pharmacy have established specific educational requirements for individual topic areas they concluded should be mandatory. These initially included topics such as state-specific pharmacy law and human immunodeficiency virus and acquired immune deficiency syndrome, but more recently, states have included requirements for education on topics such as medication and patient safety, pain and palliative care, patient management, and administration of injectables. Some states also specify the number of hours that must be obtained by "live" presentation rather than home-study courses. As more states develop unique requirements, many pharmacists who are licensed in multiple states are finding it difficult to meet the unique requirements of each individual state.

Pharmacy technician license and continuing education requirements vary widely by state, depending on whether the state requires national certification through the Pharmacy Technician Certification Board (PTCB), completion of a state board-approved or accredited pharmacy technician training program, on-the-job training, or some other measure of competence. To maintain PTCB certification, pharmacy technicians must complete specific continuing education requirements including law, patient safety, or sterile compounding, depending on their level of certification.

For over a decade, ASHP has encouraged individuals, healthcare organizations, and states to embrace continuing professional development (CPD) as a means of maintaining and demonstrating competence. CPD involves personal self-appraisal, educational plan development, plan implementation, documentation, and evaluation, and has been endorsed by the Accreditation Council for Pharmacy Education and other pharmacy organizations for use by pharmacists and pharmacy technicians. Broader adoption of CPD into state CE requirements would facilitate its use and improve pharmacy practice.

2203

PRECEPTOR SKILLS AND ABILITIES

Source: Council on Education and Workforce Development

To collaborate with pharmacy organizations and colleges of pharmacy on the development of standards to enhance the quality of experiential education and pharmacy residency precepting; further,

To provide tools, education, and other resources to develop and evaluate preceptor skills.

This policy supersedes ASHP policy 1201.

Rationale

The quality and effectiveness of the pharmacy workforce can be positively influenced by the quality of pharmacy preceptors. Growth in the number and size of colleges of pharmacy has increased demand for teaching sites and for qualified preceptors to provide experiential training and residency rotations at those sites. Although nearly all colleges of pharmacy endeavor to provide robust preceptor training, efforts to develop preceptors may be inconsistent or ineffective due to resource constraints. In addition to improved training of preceptors, the profession needs a mechanism for evaluating the skills of preceptors and educators.

2216

CAREER COUNSELING

Source: Council on Education and Workforce Development

To advocate that structured student-centered career counseling begin early and continue throughout college of pharmacy curricula; further,

To urge pharmacists to partner with colleges of pharmacy for participation in structured and unstructured student-centered career counseling; further,

To encourage colleges of pharmacy to provide professional development opportunities for faculty and other pharmacy professionals to promote equitable and inclusive student-centered career counseling approaches; further,

To urge colleges of pharmacy to develop an assessment process to evaluate the equity and inclusivity of their career counseling.

This policy supersedes ASHP policy 8507.

Rationale

To ensure students are exposed to the increasing diversity of postgraduate opportunities and ensure their success in obtaining those opportunities, a structured student-centered career counseling approach must be taken. ACPE Standards 14.4 (Advising) and 19.5 (Faculty/Staff Development) address career counseling but fail to address current concerns about equity and inclusivity in career counseling. Promoting a more equitable and inclusive student-centered career counseling approach will ideally result in a more diverse pharmacy workforce that is nimble and able to provide patient care services in more underserved communities and nontraditional care settings.

2230

ADVANCING DIVERSITY, EQUITY, AND INCLUSION IN EDUCATION AND TRAINING

Source: Council on Education and Workforce Development

To advocate that health systems and organizations cultivate training and education partnerships that advance diversity, equity, and inclusion; further,

To advocate that all members of the pharmacy workforce actively participate in the equitable training and education of people from marginalized populations.

Rationale

People from marginalized populations, including Black, Indigenous, and People of Color (BIPOC) and others, can experience disparities when receiving or accessing healthcare. Implicit biases exist against underrepresented minorities among many healthcare providers, which can perpetuate medication nonadherence, decrease trust in healthcare, and ultimately increase morbidity and mortality (Hall WJ, Chapman MV, Lee KM, et al. Implicit racial/ethnic bias among health care professionals and its influence on health care outcomes: a systematic review. *Am J Public Health.* 2015; 105:e60-e76).

ASHP created the Task Force on Racial Diversity, Equity, and Inclusion in June 2020. One of its three focus areas was education and training, which resulted in two key recommendations (13 and 16). The first of these recommendations encourages hospitals and health systems to include statements and/or integrate expectations into their departments' planning and operations for the equitable training of underrepresented minorities. Further, the Task Force recommended hospitals and health systems partner with knowledgeable organizations to help educate and train the pharmacy workforce on how to support future underrepresented minority pharmacy workforce members (e.g., training on implicit bias, cultural competency, and fostering an inclusive climate)(Report of the ASHP Task Force on Racial Diversity, Equity, and Inclusion. *Am J Health-Syst Pharm.* 2021; 78:903–906). Organizations are encouraged to partner with their respective offices of diversity, equity, and inclusion (DEI) as well as local or national organizations to support these education and training efforts (e.g., National Association for Equity, Diversity, and Inclusion [NAEDI] and Government Alliance on Race and Equity [GARE]). By advancing DEI in the education and training of the pharmacy workforce, all members of the pharmacy workforce can positively impact patient care.

2231

CULTURAL COMPETENCY

Source: Council on Education and Workforce Development

To foster the ongoing development of cultural humility and competency within the pharmacy workforce; further,

To educate the pharmacy workforce to interact with patients and caregivers in a manner that demonstrates respect for and responsiveness to personal and social identities; further,

To educate healthcare providers on the importance of providing culturally congruent care to achieve quality care and patient engagement.

This policy supersedes ASHP policy 1613.

Rationale

The United States is rapidly becoming a more diverse nation. Culture influences a patient's belief and behavior toward health and illness. Cultural humility and competence can significantly affect clinical outcomes. Research has shown that overlooking cultural beliefs may lead to negative health consequences. According to the National Center for Cultural Competency, there are numerous examples of benefits derived from the impact of cultural competence on quality and effectiveness of care in relation to health outcomes and well-being. Further, pharmacists can contribute to providing "culturally congruent care," which can be described as "a process of effective interaction between the provider and client levels" of healthcare that encourages provider cultural competence while recognizing that "[p]atients and families bring their own values, perceptions, and expectations to healthcare encounters which also influence the creation or destruction of cultural congruence." The Report of the ASHP Ad Hoc Committee on Ethnic Diversity and Cultural Competence and the ASHP Statement on Racial and Ethnic Disparities in Health Care support ways to raise awareness of the importance of cultural competence in the provision of patient care so that optimal therapeutic outcomes are achieved in diverse populations.

When considering holistic approaches to patient care, clinicians should recognize and respond effectively to all personal and social identities, including but not limited to the categories of sexual identity and gender expression, age, national origin, socioeconomic origin, ethnicity, culture, gender, race, religion or spirituality, and physical, sensory, or mental disability. Spiritually congruent care may be expressed in prayer requests, in clinician-chaplain collaborations, and through health care organizations' religious accommodations for patients and staff. Numerous publications have outlined the role of spirituality in overall health, longevity, and quality of life, especially for patients with severe illness. The pharmacy workforce should be educated on the importance of individual patient spirituality and its impact on health and on ways to facilitate patient access to spiritual care services.

2104

FOSTERING LEADERSHIP DEVELOPMENT

Source: Council on Education and Workforce Development

To work with healthcare organization leadership to foster opportunities, allocate time, and provide resources for members of the pharmacy workforce to move into leadership roles; further,

To encourage leaders to seek out and mentor members of the pharmacy workforce in developing administrative, managerial, and leadership skills; further,

To encourage members of the pharmacy workforce to obtain the skills necessary to pursue administrative, managerial, and leadership roles; further,

To encourage colleges of pharmacy and ASHP state affiliates to collaborate in fostering student leadership skills through development of co-curricular leadership opportunities, leadership conferences, and other leadership promotion programs; further,

To reaffirm that residency programs should develop leadership skills through mentoring, training, and leadership opportunities; further,

To foster leadership skills for members of the pharmacy workforce, including skills for pharmacists to use on a daily basis in their roles as leaders in patient care.

This policy supersedes ASHP policy 1611.

Rationale

In their 2013 report, Is there still a pharmacy leadership crisis? A seven-year follow-up assessment (*Am J Health-Syst Pharm.* 2013; 70:443–7), White and Enright anticipated a high rate in turnover of pharmacy directors and middle managers over the coming decade. Healthcare organizations must address this ongoing challenge if there are to be a sufficient number of new directors and managers to fill those positions. Factors that may contribute to a shortage of potential new leaders and managers include:

- New graduates frequently accept clinical positions or positions in drug distribution. After a few years, they may have a desire to assume managerial positions in health-system pharmacies, but training programs may not be convenient for them, and they may not have the resources to obtain training.
- Health-system pharmacy management positions do not turnover often. Prospective managers view those positions as unavailable for the near future, so there is little incentive to obtain training to be ready to move into those positions.
- Job satisfaction among pharmacy managers appears low to prospective managers.
- Frequent turnover in organizational administrative positions (above pharmacy) is frustrating to pharmacy directors, because they continually need to inform new administrators about the organization's medication-use strengths and weaknesses and the pharmacy department's roles, strategic plans, and priorities for sustaining quality and making improvements. In those turnover circumstances, diligently achieved pharmacy service improvements can sometimes be eroded and reversed. The ensuing frustration can induce pharmacy directors to depart voluntarily from management positions and make those positions unattractive to others.
- Flattening of organizational structures in healthcare organizations has eliminated numerous managerial positions in pharmacies, leaving fewer pharmacists to serve as mentors for prospective managers. Without positive role models, it is difficult for pharmacists to gain good management experience.
- Pharmacy management positions that combine clinical and management responsibilities sometimes allow little time for clinical work.
- Many pharmacists, even those in managerial positions, have no training in personnel administration. Skills such as conflict resolution and negotiation are rarely taught in pharmacy curricula but are very important in leadership positions.
- In some healthcare organizations, managers receive raises predicated on overall organizational or departmental performance. However, the compensation of some staff may be based on individual performance. These differing bases can lead to instances in which the compensation of those supervised is higher than that of their managers. When that occurs, it can be a disincentive to individuals considering management positions.

Leadership and managerial potential in today's student pharmacists, pharmacy technicians, and new graduates is as high as it has ever been, but more effort is needed to nurture that potential and develop leadership and management skills in practice. Colleges of pharmacy, state associations, residency programs, pharmacy technician training programs, and practitioners themselves need to foster the development of leadership and management skills.

ASHP can help foster leadership competencies at all levels of practice through actions such as providing education about leadership and management roles, developing web-based resources, and facilitating networking among leaders, managers, and those aspiring to such roles. Leadership continues to be a critical area for development, as leadership is a necessary competency in the provision of patient care. There are multiple avenues available to pharmacists for leadership development and ASHP should take the lead in fostering this effort.

2105

INTERPROFESSIONAL EDUCATION AND TRAINING

Source: Council on Education and Workforce Development

To advocate for interprofessional education as a component of didactic and experiential education in pharmacy workforce education and training programs; further,

To support interprofessional education, mentorship, and professional development for healthcare professionals and learners; further,

To urge collaboration with other healthcare professionals and executives in the development of education and training models for interprofessional, team-based, patient-centered care; further,

To foster documentation and dissemination of outcomes achieved as a result of interprofessional education of healthcare professionals.

This policy supersedes ASHP policy 1612.

Rationale

Pharmacist involvement in team-based patient care improves medication-use safety and quality and reduces healthcare costs. For patient-care teams to be effective, they must possess unique skills that facilitate effective team-based interactions. Some pharmacists are exposed to team-based care models through interprofessional education and interaction with students of other disciplines when they are student pharmacists. Some colleges of pharmacy have very effective interprofessional didactic courses that include medical, pharmacy, nursing, and other healthcare professional students. Additionally, most experiential rotations involve interaction with other members of the healthcare team and help students of all disciplines learn about the expertise of other team members. However, not all colleges and schools are effective in providing interprofessional education that facilitates team-based patient care. The reasons vary, but may include differences in teaching philosophies or a lack of access to other health professional schools at the university or campus.

The Hospital Care Collaborative (HCC) has described common principles for team-based care. The HCC principles recognize the knowledge, talent, and professionalism of all team members and support role delineation, collaboration, communication, and the accountability of individual team members and the entire team. The HCC principles note that collaboration of the healthcare team can lead to improved systems and processes that provide care more efficiently and result in better patient outcomes. The HCC states that current undergraduate and postgraduate professional education of team members is inadequate to promote true team functions.

ASHP believes that interprofessional education is important not only for student pharmacists but also throughout one's professional career. Similarly, it is important for other professionals on the team so that collaboration and synergistic relationships can develop. Failure to establish these collaborative working relationships early in one's career can result in poor interactions in years to come. A positive working relationship, including interprofessional mentorship, with physicians and nurses is productive, while a bad working relationship can be counterproductive and devastating to all parties, including patients.

2106

PHARMACY EDUCATION AND TRAINING MODELS

Source: Council on Education and Workforce Development

To promote pharmacy education and training models that: (1) provide experiential and residency training in interprofessional patient care; (2) use the knowledge, skills, and abilities of students and residents in providing direct patient care; and (3) promote use of innovative and contemporary learning models; further,

To encourage the collaboration between colleges of pharmacy and residency programs with accreditation agencies on innovative education and training models; further,

To support the assessment and dissemination of the impact of these pharmacy education and training models on the quality of learner experiences and patient care outcomes.

This policy supersedes ASHP policy 1829.

Rationale

Pharmacy training models are continuously evolving. The ideal training model includes characteristics such as flexibility to be useful in all patient care settings, providing patient care through an interprofessional team, and allowing team members to practice at the top of their licenses. Many healthcare organizations are successfully employing innovative and contemporary training models. One such model is the layered learning approach to residency and student pharmacist training, in which a pharmacist oversees multiple residents, student pharmacists, and sometimes generalist pharmacists. Each member of this pharmacy team is integrated into a patient care team, with specific roles and responsibilities, but each also has accountability to the supervising pharmacist. The layered learning model may be more practical in larger institutions, however, because they have more staff, residents, and student pharmacists than smaller hospitals. ASHP recognizes that it is important to individualize the training program to the practice site and its corresponding practice model, and supports the assessment of the impact of these pharmacy training models on the quality of learner experiences and patient care outcomes.

2107

PHARMACY INTERNSHIPS

Source: Council on Education and Workforce Development

To encourage state boards of pharmacy to adopt the standardized pharmacy internship hour requirements recommended in the National Association of Board of Pharmacy Model Rules for Pharmacy Interns; further,

To support structured requirements, goals, and objectives for pharmacy internship experiences, in alignment with requirements for introductory and advanced pharmacy practice experiences; further,

To promote new staffing models that offer expanded roles for pharmacy interns, providing work experiences that build upon their knowledge and help them develop as future pharmacists.

This policy supersedes ASHP policy 1110.

Rationale

State boards of pharmacy vary with respect to the pharmacy internship requirement. Some state boards of pharmacy allow internship hour requirements to be completed as part of the pharmacy curriculum. Other state boards of pharmacy require students to complete internship hours outside of the pharmacy curriculum.

Inconsistencies in internship requirements among states have had significant implications for pharmacy residents. Pharmacy graduates from a state with minimal internship requirements may relocate to a state post-graduation for employment with stringent internship requirements, sometimes delaying their eligibility for licensure until they can complete internship requirements. Greater standardization would prevent these issues as new graduates relocate to other states.

The National Association of Boards of Pharmacy Model Rules for Pharmacy Interns requirements coincide with the ACPE Accreditation Standards and Guidelines. In the rule, boards of pharmacy are strongly encouraged to utilize these Accreditation Standards and Guidelines as a basis for the establishment and revision of board standards for pharmacy practice experiences.

2027

RESIDENCY TRAINING FOR PHARMACISTS WHO PROVIDE DIRECT PATIENT CARE

Source: Council on Education and Workforce Development

To recognize that optimal direct patient care by a pharmacist requires the development of clinical judgment, which can be acquired only through experience and reflection on that experience; further,

Pharmacists who provide direct patient care should have completed an ASHP-accredited residency or have attained comparable skills through practice experience; further,

To support the position that the completion of an ASHP-accredited postgraduate-year-one residency be required for all new college or school of pharmacy graduates who will be providing direct patient care.

This policy supersedes ASHP policies 0701 and 0005.

Rationale

Pharmacists who engage in direct patient care can improve patient outcomes and significantly decrease the overall costs of the healthcare system. Completion of a postgraduate pharmacy residency enables a pharmacist to maximize the provision of these direct patient care services. The use of well-trained pharmacy technicians and technological advances will minimize pharmacists' dispensing roles. Based on the assumption that in the next 20–30 years most pharmacists will be providing direct patient care, it is incumbent upon the pharmacy profession to ensure that pharmacists are in a position to make the most effective interventions when selecting, modifying, and monitoring patients' drug therapy regimens.

Pharmacy students who graduate meet the minimum competency requirements based on pharmacy licensing examinations; however, pharmacists who have completed a residency are better equipped to provide direct patient care due to advanced training based on repetitive practice, preceptor guidance, and the additional interdisciplinary training they receive. This direction is consistent with ASHP's Long-Range Vision for the Pharmacy Workforce in Hospitals and Health Systems.

Similar to the medical model in which medical school graduates complete a residency that allows for the standardization of physician training and the attainment of an appropriate level of competency, the profession of pharmacy would benefit from a similar standardization of training. The value of pharmacy residency programs has been demonstrated over time and has stimulated a significant increase in accredited residency programs as well as employer demand for residency-trained pharmacists. An increasing number of pharmacy graduates are completing one or two years of residency training after graduating in order to bolster their clinical skills and develop clinical judgement, which is acquired only through experience and reflection on that experience.

The number of available residencies in the U.S. is now at nearly 2600 programs. The growth in the number of pharmacy school graduates has begun to plateau while PGY1 residency positions has grown 11% in the last three years.

1911

PHARMACY EXPERTISE IN STERILE COMPOUNDING

Source: Council on Education and Workforce Development

To support colleges of pharmacy in providing sterile compounding and aseptic technique instruction in didactic and experiential curricula that reflect the needs of the workforce; further,

To promote the use of sterile compounding training programs to foster an increase in the number of pharmacists and pharmacy technicians with sterile compounding expertise; further,

To advocate that pharmacists and pharmacy technicians who work in sterile compounding attain compounded sterile preparations advanced certifications.

This policy supersedes ASHP policy 0915.

Rationale

ASHP distinguishes between two needs related to pharmacy expertise in sterile compounding: a need for new pharmacy graduates to possess baseline training and knowledge of sterile compounding, and the need for pharmacists with an advanced body of knowledge on sterile compounding, especially in pharmacy departments where complex compounded sterile preparations (CSPs) are compounded.

Although there is a clear need for students to have a basic understanding of sterile compounding upon graduation, education in colleges of pharmacy on sterile compounding varies. Sterile compounding and aseptic technique instruction are important areas of pharmacy practice to incorporate in the didactic curriculum and during experiential education.

The complexity of intravenous therapy, the risk of errors or patient harm, and new biologic therapies all demand a higher level of expertise in sterile compounding in the pharmacy, however. United States Pharmacopeia Chapter 797 and other efforts have increased the focus on the quality of CSP compounding and have prompted organizations to improve staff training, facilities, and procedures. In such an environment, there is a clear need for pharmacists whose education, training, and experience in sterile compounding provide expertise rather than baseline knowledge. To demonstrate competency, pharmacy technicians should attain PTCB's advanced Compounded Sterile Preparation Technician (CSPT) certification, and pharmacists, the Board of Pharmacy Specialties (BPS) Compounded Sterile Preparations Pharmacy (BCSCP) certification.

1912

PHARMACY TECHNICIAN TRAINING AND CERTIFICATION

Source: Council on Education and Workforce Development

To advocate for adoption of a national standard for accreditation of pharmacy technician education and training programs; further,

To advocate that a pharmacy technician education and training program accredited by ASHP and the Accreditation Council for Pharmacy Education (ACPE) be required for all new pharmacy technicians by the year 2022; further,

To advocate that all pharmacy technicians be required to obtain and maintain Pharmacy Technician Certification Board certification; further,

To foster expansion of ASHP/ACPE-accredited pharmacy technician education and training programs.

This policy supersedes ASHP policy 1609.

Rationale

In January 2017, the Pharmacy Technician Certification Board (PTCB) suspended the condition that by 2020 the completion of an accredited technician education and training program would be required to be eligible for the PTCB certification exam. There is no indication that PTCB will reinstate that requirement; however, ASHP supports completion of an education and training program accredited by ASHP and the Accreditation Council for Pharmacy Education (ACPE) as well as PTCB certification for all pharmacy technicians. Although education requirements have been added by PTCB to take the certification exam starting in 2020, completion of an accredited education and training program is only one pathway for eligibility for the exam; PTCB also recognizes equivalent work experience. If an applicant has completed an unaccredited program, there is a required attestation for the content of that program.

In 2018, ASHP and ACPE developed revised national standards that serve as a guide for the development of ASHP/ACPE-accredited pharmacy technician education and training programs. These standards serve as the criteria for the evaluation of new and established pharmacy technician training programs and will help ensure that pharmacy technicians possess the knowledge, skills, and abilities necessary for their critical role on the healthcare team. A number of environmental factors, including changes in state laws allowing for expanded roles, responsibilities, and authority for pharmacy technicians, prompted the reassessment of the standards, which were last revised in 2015. ASHP supports more uniform state statutes and regulations regarding pharmacy technicians. The anticipated increase in demand for enrollment in ASHP/ACPE-accredited training programs will require an expansion of the number and distribution of such programs, including innovative education and training formats.

The target date of 2022 was included to provide a goal for requiring that all new pharmacy technicians in hospitals and health systems complete a pharmacy technician education and training program accredited by ASHP and ACPE. The date is in line with the initiatives and timeline of the Stakeholder Advisory Committee (the Committee). This Committee continues to advance the recommendations of the Pharmacy Technician Stakeholder Consensus Conference (Toward uniform standards for pharmacy technicians: Summary of the 2017 Pharmacy Technician Stakeholder Consensus Conference), the national consensus conference that engaged all sectors of pharmacy to define basic knowledge, skills, and abilities of pharmacy technicians, to promote and define advanced competencies, and to promote national definitions and regulation of pharmacy technicians. The Committee uses the recommendations and consensus statements to guide their work. Two of these statements are as follows:

2.1 The profession of pharmacy should move urgently towards the development and adoption of national standards for pharmacy technician education.

2.2 The profession of pharmacy should set a target for implementation of the national standard for pharmacy technician education at 3 to 5 years after adoption of the standard.

The accreditation standard for the education and training of pharmacy technicians was revised and approved by both the ASHP and ACPE Boards in June of 2018. Consistent with recommendation 2.2, 2022 is a reasonable target to require accredited training for new pharmacy technicians as it is four years from the time the new standard was developed. The new standard was developed based on a job analysis of more than 44,000 pharmacy technicians in the U.S. The group developing the standard included educators; representatives from community, hospital, and chain pharmacy practice; and members of the Pharmacy Technician Accreditation Commission. More than 500 public comments were received and evaluated for inclusion in the revised standard before it was sent to the Boards of ASHP and ACPE for approval. The revised standard is divided into entry level and advanced, as recommended at the Pharmacy Technician Stakeholder Consensus Conference. This differentiation allows practice settings to have different education and training requirements based on the needs of the position. Additionally, boards of pharmacy can develop requirements based on entry-level competencies as a minimum standard and the advanced level can be an added credential that can be pursued based on employer requirements.

The Committee is currently working with the National Association of Boards of Pharmacy (NABP) to modify the Model State Pharmacy Act and Model Rules of the National Association of Boards of Pharmacy. At the NABP national meeting in May 2019, a resolution was passed to convene a task force of stakeholders to evaluate and make recommendations to NABP regarding the education requirements, practice responsibilities, and competence assessments for pharmacy technicians. Additionally, work is being done at the state level with individual boards of pharmacy to evaluate requirements for accredited education and training for new pharmacy technicians.

This activity follows consensus statement 5.2: The level of urgency for achieving state-to-state consistency in regulation of pharmacy technicians' scope of practice, education, certification, and licensure or regulation is high.

At the state level, advocacy will include several specific issues for boards of pharmacy to include as they consider regulations for technicians:

- There should be clear distinctions between pharmacy technicians and student pharmacists. Technician requirements should not be applied to student pharmacists.
- There should be a provision for a "technician in training" that would allow a technician who is enrolled in an accredited education and training program to be eligible to work in a pharmacy as long they complete the program in some prescribed amount of time (e.g., 12–18 months).

1917

PHARMACY TECHNICIAN STUDENT DRUG TESTING

Source: Pharmacy Technician Forum

To advocate for the use of pre-enrollment, random, and for-cause drug testing as a mandatory component throughout any accredited or unaccredited pharmacy technician training program and practice experience, based on defined criteria with appropriate testing validation procedures; further,

To encourage pharmacy technician training programs to develop policies and processes to identify impaired individuals; further,

To encourage pharmacy technician training programs to facilitate access to and promote programs for treatment and to support recovery; further,

To encourage pharmacy technician training programs to use validated testing panels that have demonstrated effectiveness detecting commonly misused, abused, or illegally used substances.

Rationale

Pharmacy technicians are essential members of the healthcare team and help ensure the health, safety, and welfare of patients. They have access to controlled substances and confidential information, and operate in settings that require the exercise of good judgment and ethical behavior. In addition, some state boards of pharmacy have reported that drug-abusing and -diverting persons are enrolling in pharmacy technician training programs to access drugs during experiential training and employment. Thus, an assessment of a pharmacy technician student's possible impairment, which could diminish his or her capacity to function in such a setting, is imperative to promote the highest level of integrity in healthcare services.

ASHP recognizes that drug testing pharmacy technician students, whose responsibilities may bring them into contact with controlled substances, is an essential element of diversion prevention programs. Pre-enrollment, random, and for-cause drug testing should be performed based on defined criteria, with appropriate testing validation procedures, and have demonstrated effectiveness detecting commonly abused or illegally used substances.

1918

MINIMUM EDUCATIONAL QUALIFICATION STANDARDS FOR PHARMACISTS

Source: House of Delegates Resolution

To support minimum educational qualification standards for pharmacists to practice pharmacy that are consistent with the licensing standards of state boards of pharmacy; further,

To oppose the basic education requirement within the Office of Personnel Management Classification & Qualifications—General Schedule Qualification Standards—Pharmacy Series, 0660, requiring a Doctor of Pharmacy or Doctor of Philosophy degree as the minimum qualification to practice pharmacy.

Rationale

In September 2017, the U.S. Office of Personnel Management (OPM) issued a new qualification standard for pharmacists, GS-0660. The new standard lists the basic educational requirement for pharmacists as a Doctor of Pharmacy (Pharm.D.) or Doctor of Philosophy (Ph.D.) degree. To set this requirement, OPM must have determined that pharmacy cannot be performed by persons without one of these degrees, because Title 5 U.S.C. 3308 permits the establishment of minimum educational requirements only when OPM has determined that the work cannot be performed by persons who do not possess the prescribed minimum education.

All 50 states currently allow pharmacists with a bachelor's degree in pharmacy (B.S.Pharm.) to obtain licensure and practice pharmacy, which indicates that all state legislatures or regulators have concluded that pharmacists with a B.S.Pharm. degree can practice pharmacy safely and effectively. In the U.S., the B.S.Pharm. degree was awarded until 2005; in 2006, the Pharm.D. degree became the only entry-level degree awarded. A 2014 survey of the pharmacy workforce found that only 40% of pharmacists had earned a Pharm.D. The minimum educational requirements set by OPM would automatically disqualify 60% of pharmacists from entering the federal government workforce, an inequitable practice not seen outside the federal sector. The OPM minimum educational requirement also creates a monumental challenge to building and maintaining the pharmacist workforce the Department of Defense needs to support U.S. warfighting efforts and take care of veterans. ASHP recognizes that pharmacists must possess the education, training, and experience required to effectively, efficiently, and responsibly fulfill their roles. Further, ASHP supports licensure by a state board of pharmacy as the minimum requirement for pharmacy practice in its Minimum Standard for Pharmacies in Hospitals.

1826

STUDENT PHARMACIST DRUG TESTING

Source: Council on Education and Workforce Development

To advocate for the use of pre-enrollment, random, and for-cause drug testing throughout pharmacy education and pharmacy practice experiences, based on defined criteria with appropriate testing validation procedures; further,

To encourage colleges of pharmacy to develop policies and processes to identify impaired individuals; further,

To encourage colleges of pharmacy to facilitate access to and promote programs for treatment and to support recovery; further,

To encourage colleges of pharmacy to use validated testing panels that have demonstrated effectiveness detecting commonly misused, abused, or illegally used substances.

This policy was reviewed in 2023 by the Council on Education and Workforce Development and by the Board of Directors and was found to still be appropriate.

Rationale

The Mental Health Parity Act of 1996 stipulated that large group health plans cannot impose annual or lifetime dollar limits on mental health benefits that are less favorable than those imposed on medical or surgical benefits. Therefore, health insurers and group health plans are required to provide the same level of benefits for mental health and/or substance use treatment and services that they do for medical or surgical care. The Affordable Care Act (ACA) later amended this law to also include individual health plans. The ACA also embraces substance use disorders as one of the ten elements of essential health benefits.

Most colleges of pharmacy require students to be enrolled in health insurance and therefore should receive similar benefits for mental health and substance use services and treatment. Despite regulation of opioid prescriptions, opioid-related overdoses are at an all-time high. Research indicates that the best help for someone with a substance use problem or disorder is early interventions. With the growth of substance use disorder clinics and increasing coverage from insurance, recovery is now an obtainable outcome. Efficacy of treatment and rehabilitation as well as the accessibility of such programs further supports the importance of colleges of pharmacy facilitating access to students seeking services or treatment for substance use problems or disorders.

In addition, drug testing should be supported by an addiction recovery program, as outlined in the ASHP Statement on the Pharmacist's Role in Substance Abuse Prevention, Education, and Assistance.

1827

COLLABORATION ON EXPERIENTIAL EDUCATION

Source: Council on Education and Workforce Development

To encourage practitioner contributions to pharmacy education; further,

To encourage pharmacists and pharmacy leaders to recognize their professional responsibility to contribute to the development of new pharmacy practitioners; further,

To promote collaboration of experiential teaching sites with the colleges of pharmacy (nationally or regionally), for the purpose of fostering preceptor development, standardization of experiential rotation schedule dates and evaluation tools, and other related matters; further,

To encourage colleges of pharmacy and health systems to define and develop collaborative organizational relationships that support patient care and advance the missions of both institutions in a mutually beneficial manner.

This policy supersedes ASHP policies 0315 and 0804.

This policy was reviewed in 2023 by the Council on Education and Workforce Development and by the Board of Directors and was found to still be appropriate.

Rationale

As stated in the ASHP Statement on Professionalism, one of the fundamental services of a professional is recruiting, nurturing, and securing new practitioners to that profession's ideals and mission. Because the principles of institutional pharmacy practice are not emphasized in typical pharmacy curricula, professional socialization is especially important for pharmacists who practice in those settings. The experiential education experience of student pharmacists is a partnership between colleges of pharmacy and the experiential teaching sites. Collaboration between the colleges of pharmacy and experiential training sites on preceptor development, standardized rotation schedule dates, evaluation tools, and other materials helps to assure the best possible experience for student pharmacists, preceptors, and the experiential education site. In addition, collaboration allows both entities to fulfill their missions by participating in mutually beneficial activities, improving patient outcomes, and helping students and their institutions achieve educational and research objectives.

1706

ASHP GUIDELINES, STATEMENTS, AND PROFESSIONAL POLICIES AS AN INTEGRAL PART OF THE EDUCATIONAL PROCESS

Source: Council on Education and Workforce Development

To encourage all educators of the pharmacy workforce to use ASHP statements, guidelines, and professional policies as an integral part of education and training.

This policy was reviewed in 2022 by the Council on Education and Workforce Development and by the Board of Directors and was found to still be appropriate.

Rationale

ASHP members create professional policy that reflect best practices and influence the future direction of the profession and patient care. ASHP's professional policies contain varying levels of detail, but all contain guiding principles for the profession. The use of professional policy should be incorporated into all forms of professional education, including pharmacy and technician students, residents, and practitioners and widely used across the pharmacy profession.

1317

EDUCATION AND TRAINING IN HEALTH CARE INFORMATICS

Source: Council on Education and Workforce Development

To recognize the significant and vast impacts of health-system information systems, automation, and technology changes on safe and effective use of medications; further,

To foster, promote, and lead the development of and participation in formal health care informatics educational programs for pharmacists, pharmacy technicians, and student pharmacists.

Rationale

With growing use of automation and technology, there is a growing need for informatics-trained pharmacists and pharmacy technicians, yet there are few training programs or residencies. This shortage of trained individuals has led to on-the-job training and potentially less-than-optimal implementation of new information systems and technology. New educational programs, or adaptation of existing ones, would help ease this lack of trained individuals and lead to better technology outcomes. To most effectively accomplish this goal, ASHP must lead the development of such programs and encourage participation by pharmacists, pharmacy students, and pharmacy technicians.

This policy was reviewed in 2023 by the Council on Education and Workforce Development and by the Board of Directors and was found to still be appropriate.

1203

QUALIFICATIONS OF PHARMACY TECHNICIANS IN ADVANCED ROLES

Source: Council on Education and Workforce Development

To recognize that highly trained and skilled pharmacy technicians working in advanced roles regularly perform complex and critical medication-use procedures, and that a safe and effective medication-use process depends significantly on the skills, knowledge, and competency of those pharmacy technicians to perform those tasks; further,

To reaffirm that all pharmacy technicians should complete an ASHP-accredited training program, be certified by the Pharmacy Technician Certification Board, and be licensed by state boards of pharmacy; further,

To advocate that beyond those requirements pharmacy technicians working in advanced roles should have additional training and should demonstrate ongoing competencies specific to the tasks to be performed; further,

To advocate that expansion of pharmacy technician duties into expanded, advanced roles should include consideration of potential risk to patients and that ongoing quality assurance metrics should be established to assure patient safety.

This policy was reviewed in 2022 by the Council on Education and Workforce Development and by the Board of Directors and was found to still be appropriate.

Rationale

A growing number of hospitals utilize pharmacy technicians in advanced or specialized roles beyond those traditionally filled by technicians: medication preparation, distribution, and purchasing. These advanced or specialized roles include performing medication reconciliation, collecting laboratory data, and managing automation and technology, among others. While there has been a good deal of discussion about minimum standards for education and training of pharmacy technicians in general, there has been little discussion about technicians in these specialized roles. These advanced roles will require different skills and competencies, and pharmacy technicians will require additional, task-specific training and should demonstrate competency before being allowed to perform such tasks. Hospitals and health systems will need to consider the potential risk to patients of expanding the roles of pharmacy technicians and establish quality assurance metrics to assure patient safety.

1108

QUALITY OF PHARMACY EDUCATION AND EXPANSION OF COLLEGES OF PHARMACY

Source: Council on Education and Workforce Development

To support the Accreditation Council for Pharmacy Education's continuing role of promulgating accreditation standards and guidelines and engaging in sound accreditation processes to ensure quality in the education provided by colleges of pharmacy; further,

To acknowledge that, in addition to a robust curriculum, access to quality experiential educational sites and the availability of qualified faculty (including preceptors and specialty-trained clinical faculty) are essential determinants of the ability to expand enrollment in existing or additional colleges of pharmacy; further,

To oppose expansion of enrollment in existing or new colleges of pharmacy unless well-designed projections demonstrate that such enrollment increases are necessary to maintain a viable pharmacist workforce.

This policy was reviewed in 2021 by the Council on Education and Workforce Development and by the Board of Directors and was found to still be appropriate.

Rationale

The growth in the number and capacity of colleges of pharmacy in recent years has been remarkable. Ten years ago, when there was a severe pharmacist shortage, new colleges were welcomed to help meet the anticipated needs of the pharmacy workforce. The pharmacist shortage has now abated, but new colleges continue to be established and capacity of existing colleges expanded. This growth, along with other factors, has led to considerable difficulty for colleges of pharmacy in locating experienced faculty. There are also growing concerns about the limited number of quality experiential education sites and how future demands for training will be met. These two factors alone have raised worries about the quality of education and the readiness of new pharmacy graduates. High quality can be ensured through the existing mechanism of Accreditation Council for Pharmacy Education (ACPE) accreditation, regardless of the number of colleges and the number of students. However, this assumes rigid enforcement of ACPE's accreditation standards and guidelines, the availability of qualified faculty and preceptors, and an adequate capacity in practice to provide the necessary experiential education.

The Council discussed the mismatch between pharmacy workforce supply and demand. Demand far exceeded supply in 2000, but growth in colleges and other factors now have supply exceeding demand. The Council discussed how there could be better planning to avoid these situations, both of which are costly to the health care system and present risks to quality and patient care. It was suggested that well-designed workforce projections might be useful in determining the need for new or expanded educational capacity.

1109

RESIDENCY EQUIVALENCY

Source: Council on Education and Workforce Development

To acknowledge the distinct role of ASHP-accredited residency training in preparing pharmacists to be direct patient-care providers; further,

To recognize the importance of clinical experience in developing practitioner expertise; further,

To affirm that there are no objective means to convert or express clinical experience as equivalent to or a substitute for the successful completion of an ASHP-accredited residency.

This policy was reviewed in 2021 by the Council on Education and Workforce Development and by the Board of Directors and was found to still be appropriate.

Rationale

ASHP's position on the need for residency-trained pharmacists is well established and described in the *ASHP Long-Range Vision for the Pharmacy Workforce in Hospitals and Health Systems*. It has been suggested that a way to achieve the goal of having all pharmacists in direct patient-care roles be residency trained would be to establish a process for reviewing a "portfolio" against pre-established criteria to grant a "residency equivalency." The Council, Board, and House concluded that both residency training and experience are important and valuable, but different, and that it would not be appropriate to create a process that attempts to convert one into the other. The intent of the goal of having all new college of pharmacy graduates who provide direct patient care residency trained by 2020 is to enhance the skills of those practitioners, and the creation of a residency equivalency process might dilute the value of that residency training and undermine achievement of the goal.

The Council, Board, and House also discussed the process used by ASHP to waive the requirement for a postgraduate year one (PGY1) residency for experienced practitioners who wish to enter a postgraduate year two (PGY2) residency directly. While this process does consider total experience in granting the waiver, and may seem to contradict the recommended policy, the applicant still completes a residency, ultimately gaining those experiences unique to residency training.

1112

INNOVATIVE RESIDENCY MODELS

Source: Council on Education and Workforce Development

To support the development of innovative residency models that meet ASHP accreditation requirements.

This policy was reviewed in 2021 by the Council on Education and Workforce Development and by the Board of Directors and was found to still be appropriate.

Rationale

A growing number of residency programs have developed residency positions that are "nontraditional," in that they do not occur in a contiguous 12-month period beginning in July and finishing the following June. Some of these innovative programs schedule the participant for one month as a resident, followed by two months as staff, with this cycle repeated over a three-year period. This allows some individuals, usually experienced individuals already on staff at the institution, to complete a residency while maintaining a more consistent work schedule and lifestyle. Some other settings have adopted a model geared toward new graduates, alternating months between residency rotation and staffing.

The concept of innovative, nontraditional residencies allows another way for established pharmacists to obtain a pharmacy residency when a conventional 12-month contiguous program is not possible. The Council, Board, and House expressed support for this model as long as ASHP accreditation standards and residency goals and objectives are utilized as they would be in a conventional program.

1008

EMPLOYMENT CLASSIFICATION AND DUTY HOURS OF PHARMACY RESIDENTS

Source: Council on Public Policy

To advocate that pharmacy residents should be classified as exempt employees; further,

To advocate that pharmacy residents be subject to duty hour limits (similar to resident physicians) with respect to all clinical and academic activities during their training program in accordance with the Accreditation Council on Graduate Medical Education (ACGME) standards and ASHP accreditation standards for pharmacy residency programs.

This policy was reviewed in 2020 by the Council on Public Policy and by the Board of Directors and was found to still be appropriate.

Rationale

In some states, pharmacy residents are classified as nonexempt employees (eligible for overtime pay) in accordance with guidance from state employment offices. ASHP believes that there is an important job classification distinction between pharmacists employed by a hospital or health system and pharmacy residents who are part of an organization's residency program. Specifically, pharmacy residents are in an organized, directed, and accredited postgraduate training program that builds upon knowledge, skills, attitudes, and abilities gained from an accredited professional pharmacy-degree program. Pharmacy residents receive a salary and are subject to the same duty hours as physicians. Classifying pharmacy residents as non-exempt employees is overly burdensome and counterproductive to the residency experience and the objectives of the training program. Moreover, such misclassification could inhibit the development of an important component of the pharmacy workforce at a time of increased demand for pharmacist services as health care reform is implemented.

0913

PHARMACY STUDENT EXPERIENCES IN MEDICALLY UNDERSERVED AREAS

Source: Council on Education and Workforce Development

To encourage colleges of pharmacy to require student learning experiences in traditionally medically underserved areas and with diverse patient populations.

This policy was reviewed in 2019 by the Council on Education and Workforce Development and by the Board of Directors and was found to still be appropriate.

Rationale

Numerous reports demonstrate how pharmacy students and practice sites benefit from experiential rotations in rural and urban settings, especially in settings or areas classified as medically underserved. Students learn about the cultural, financial, language, and other challenges encountered in these settings, and these skills are often invaluable when they enter practice. In addition, a student's exposure to a new practice area may result in more interest in such sites and provide career choices that might otherwise not have been considered.

ASHP does not support mandating rotations in these settings, since there are many ways to provide the interaction, and there are concerns about how colleges could develop an infrastructure for providing these experiences. The challenges of finding good teaching sites in these settings are formidable and include a limited number of sites, a lack of qualified preceptors, and geographic distances from the college that result in housing needs.

The Accreditation Council for Pharmacy Education currently requires colleges of pharmacy to ensure that graduates can provide patient-centered care that addresses cultural diversity. Although experiential rotations may be the most common way for students to be exposed to diverse patient populations, there are many other creative ways in which this goal is being accomplished. Some colleges, for example, require students to perform service learning projects with a focus on underserved populations.

0916

CONTINUING PROFESSIONAL DEVELOPMENT

Source: Council on Education and Workforce Development

To endorse and promote the concept of continuing professional development (CPD), which involves personal self-appraisal, educational plan development, plan implementation, documentation, and evaluation; further,

To continue the development of a variety of mechanisms and tools that pharmacists can use to assess their CPD needs; further,

To encourage individual pharmacists to embrace CPD as a means of maintaining their own professional competence; further,

To encourage pharmacy managers to promote CPD as the model for ensuring the competence of their staff; further,

To collaborate with other pharmacy organizations, state boards of pharmacy, accrediting bodies, and regulatory bodies in the development of effective methods for implementing CPD; further,

To strongly support objective assessment of the impact of CPD on pharmacist competence; further,

To endorse the efforts of colleges of pharmacy and ASHP-accredited pharmacy residency programs to teach the principles, concepts, and skills of CPD.

This policy was reviewed in 2019 by the Council on Education and Workforce Development and by the Board of Directors and was found to still be appropriate.

Rationale

Maintaining competence throughout one's career is part of a professional's obligation. Traditionally, this has been done through continuing education (CE) activities, but CE has several shortcomings. There is often no mechanism to ensure that CE is effective, since most CE activities have no summative evaluation component. (Summative evaluation takes place at the completion of a program to determine whether goals and objectives have been met.) In addition, CE programs are not usually curricular, are not always competency-directed, and tend to be content-oriented rather than skill-based. There is little evidence that CE changes practice or has an impact on patient outcomes.

Continuing professional development (CPD) is a model that addresses many of the shortcomings of the CE model. CPD differs from CE in that it is ongoing and includes the entire scope of an individual's practice, it is often undertaken in partnership with the professional's employer, it is practitioner-centered and self-directed, and it is intended to be outcomes-oriented. Many pharmacy professionals already assume responsibility for their professional growth and development by reflecting on their practice, recognizing needs, and seeking educational opportunities and activities that will meet those needs. Even when these activities are not documented or reported, this process incorporates many of the principles of CPD.

CPD is a cyclical, five-step process that begins with a self-appraisal by the individual professional to determine educational needs and progresses through the development of a personal plan to meet those needs, an action phase in which the professional participates in the activities identified in the personal plan, a documentation component in which the professional keeps records of all CPD activities in which he or she participates, and an evaluation phase to determine whether the CPD needs were met, if practice has been improved, if patients have benefited, and if learning was or was not accomplished (and why). This step then feeds back into the self-appraisal stage and the cycle continues.

In the self-appraisal phase, identification of CPD needs may be accomplished through personal assessment, performance review by a manager or supervisor, an audit exercise undertaken with other professionals, or as a requirement of a professional organization or regulatory body. There are a variety of mechanisms that pharmacists can use to self-assess their CPD needs. Self-assessment is not a skill most professionals learn during their professional education and training, however. For CPD to be effective, professionals must learn this skill before entering the CPD cycle, in colleges of pharmacy and residency programs.

In the next phase, the personal plan, the professional identifies resources and actions to meet the identified CPD needs. Activities may be informal, such as study clubs, observation of a colleague's practice, and conversations with colleagues, or they may be more formal, such as CE workshops, short courses, seminars, self study programs, or graduate-level course work.

Whether formal or informal, managed CPD requires the documentation of participation in these activities. This documentation becomes the foundation of the professional's CPD portfolio. Documentation of participation in formal activities is usually given by the provider, but more informal and self-directed activities, such as observation of a colleague's practice, require the individual to establish a format for documentation in the portfolio.

In the final phase, which feeds back into self-appraisal, the professional self-evaluates, is evaluated by a manager or supervisor, enlists the aid of peers, or is evaluated by an external (e.g., regulatory) body. It is important in this phase to determine whether learning was or was not accomplished (and if not, why not) and to feed this back into the ongoing CPD cycle.

0917

PHARMACY RESIDENCY TRAINING

Source: Council on Education and Workforce Development

To continue efforts to increase the number of ASHP-accredited pharmacy residency training programs and positions available.

This policy was reviewed in 2019 by the Council on Education and Workforce Development and by the Board of Directors and was found to still be appropriate.

Rationale

ASHP is committed to achieving the goal that by the year 2020 all new college of pharmacy graduates who will be providing direct patient care will be required to complete an ASHP-accredited postgraduate-year-one residency (see ASHP policy 2027). To accomplish this goal, ASHP will need to increase the number of ASHP-accredited pharmacy residency training programs and positions.

0704

RESIDENCY PROGRAMS

Source: Council on Education and Workforce Development

To strongly advocate that all pharmacy residency programs become ASHP-accredited as a means of ensuring and conveying program quality.

This policy was reviewed in 2022 by the Council on Education and Workforce Development and by the Board of Directors and was found to still be appropriate.

0510

COMMUNICATION AMONG HEALTH-SYSTEM PHARMACY PRACTITIONERS, PATIENTS, AND OTHER HEALTH CARE PROVIDERS

Source: Council on Educational Affairs

To foster effective communication (with appropriate attention to patients' levels of general and health literacy) among health-system pharmacy practitioners, patients, and other health care providers; further,

To develop programs to enable pharmacy students, residents, and health-system pharmacy practitioners to self-assess their levels of health literacy and general communication skills; further,

To develop methods with which pharmacy students, residents, and health-system pharmacy practitioners can assess the level of general and health literacy of patients; further,

To disseminate information about resources for students, residents, and health-system pharmacy practitioners to use in working with patients and others having specific communication needs.

This policy was reviewed in 2020 by the Council on Education and Workforce Development and by the Board of Directors and was found to still be appropriate.

0325

PUBLIC FUNDING FOR PHARMACY RESIDENCY TRAINING

Source: Council on Legal and Public Affairs

To support legislation and regulation that ensures public funding for accredited pharmacy residency programs consistent with the needs of the public and the profession; further,

To oppose legislation or regulation involving reimbursement levels for graduate medical education that adversely affects pharmacy residencies at a rate disproportionate to other residency programs.

This policy was reviewed in 2018 by the Council on Public Policy and by the Board of Directors and was found to still be appropriate.

ASHP Statement on Precepting as a Professional Obligation

Position

The American Society of Health-System Pharmacists (ASHP) believes that all pharmacists have a professional obligation to give back to the profession through involvement in the precepting process of students and postgraduate trainees. ASHP encourages pharmacy practice leaders, practitioners, postgraduate trainees, and faculty members to embrace the responsibility to be involved in the precepting process in an effort to advance pharmacy practice and improve patient care. To this end, ASHP urges all pharmacists and healthcare institutions to accept this responsibility and commit time and resources to the precepting process and the development of precepting skills.

ASHP encourages pharmacy practice leaders to create a culture of teaching and learning, integrate precepting as a practice philosophy, support an organizational commitment to well-being, and facilitate the integration of learners into patient care services and scholarly work. Pharmacy leaders and administrators, colleges of pharmacy, faculty, and current preceptors have a responsibility to foster and support the evidence-based development of the precepting skills of all pharmacy practitioners and postgraduate trainees, facilitate the development of practice models that provide regular opportunities to precept learners, encourage all pharmacists to be involved in the precepting process, and support the assessment of training programs' outcomes.

Background

Upon graduation, all pharmacists pledge to use their knowledge, skills, experiences, and values to train the next generation by taking the Oath of a Pharmacist.[1] The apprenticeship model of "see one, do one, teach one" is grounded in centuries of tradition across many healthcare disciplines. Current apprenticeship models, such as the Cognitive Apprenticeship Model, encourage the development of observable skills and critical thinking skills that are fundamental to contemporary practice.[2] The evolution of the current pharmacy education system and apprenticeship models requires preceptor supervision during experiential learning and postgraduate training.

Precepting consists of providing a learner with practical experiences in a practice setting in which they can develop and apply principles of pharmacy practice. The precepting process begins within the college of pharmacy curricula and co-curricula and extends through advanced pharmacy practice experiences (APPEs) and postgraduate trainee experiences. Throughout this prolonged process, preceptors serve vital roles by providing instruction, mentorship, coaching, facilitation, assessment, and feedback to learners. The precepting process teaches more than clinical skills by promoting skill development in professionalism, communication, teamwork, interprofessional collaboration, leadership, time management, and professional values as well as facilitating professional identity formation (PIF).[3] Involvement in the precepting process and experiential learning consists of more than serving as the primary preceptor on rotations and may extend to opportunities such as team precepting, shadowing experiences, speaking engagements, providing feedback to learners, facilitating topic discussions, learner mentoring, learner supervision, and more.

Experiential learning is fundamental to the application of knowledge and skills gained during didactic curricula.[3,4] To determine if students are practice ready, colleges of pharmacy utilize entrustable professional activities (EPAs), which are workplace tasks or responsibilities students are entrusted to perform in the experiential setting with direct or distant supervision.[5] Evaluation of entrustability levels of EPAs requires input from preceptors to assign a degree of trust in student competence. While mastery of EPAs requires the learner to gain foundational knowledge, skills, and attitudes in didactic curricula, these activities cannot be adequately replicated in the classroom; therefore, they should be fully elucidated and evaluated in the experiential setting.[4] Likewise, postgraduate programs require qualified preceptors to provide appropriate training, supervision, and guidance to all postgraduate trainees as they progress toward competence using the postgraduate trainee program's defined assessment scale.[6]

Preceptors are necessary to ensure learners attain the desired level of competency for practice; however, a dearth of preceptors has been a long-standing problem. Experiential site and preceptor capacity are frequent concerns of experiential education directors.[7] There are several contributing factors to this persistent preceptor shortage. First, colleges of pharmacy must adhere to the Accreditation Council for Pharmacy Education (ACPE) accreditation standards, which require enough preceptors to deliver and evaluate students in the experiential setting.[8] Between 2000 to 2020, there was a greater than 70% increase in the number of colleges of pharmacy, and since 2013, there has been a 65% increase in postgraduate training programs.[9] Furthermore, preceptors of postgraduate trainees require advanced training and/or experience to meet postgraduate training standards.[6] These requirements and expansion of programs may limit the number of experiential sites or individuals available to precept at any given time, which may worsen if all pharmacists do not accept precepting as a professional responsibility.

Another contributing factor to these shortages may be pharmacist burnout. Burnout is increasingly associated with work-related stressors, resulting in decreased clinician job satisfaction, productivity, interprofessional teamwork, and mental health. Increasing concerns about the personal ability to effectively balance patient care, administrative, teaching, and other roles may negatively influence pharmacists' interest in precepting. The consequences of burnout to patient care reinforce the need of colleges of pharmacy and healthcare institutions to systematically commit to the well-being of all pharmacy practitioners, pharmacy technicians, and learners.

Within the challenges of our ever-evolving healthcare and educational systems, high-quality preceptors are needed now more than ever. Their contributions continue the rich tradition of pharmacists as one of the most trusted healthcare professionals and bring value to healthcare institutions, learners, and patients.

DOI 10.37573/9781585287048.030

Value of Precepting

The amount of literature demonstrating mutual benefit for learners, preceptors, healthcare institutions, and patients is vast.[3,10] Ultimately, a synergistic relationship among stakeholders can improve patient care by aligning the goals of colleges of pharmacy, learners, preceptors, and healthcare institutions and embracing precepting as a practice philosophy.[11] Additionally, when learners are used as pharmacist extenders, clinical productivity increases, personal and professional growth ensues, and institutional metrics improve.[3,10]

Value to Learners. Preceptors are often one of the most influential teachers learners encounter as part of their training. They significantly influence learners' PIF through instructing, modeling, coaching, and facilitating as learners internalize and demonstrate the values and behaviors of pharmacists in practice. Preceptors' provision of feedback on learners' performance and their intraprofessional and interprofessional interactions are instrumental in learners' professional socialization and identity development. Preceptors also significantly impact learners' career choices and trajectories, personal and professional development, involvement in professional advocacy, and participation in scholarly activities.[3] Learners also benefit from collaborating with various professionals in their interprofessional practice experiences.

Value to Preceptors. There is tangible value for preceptors who incorporate students and postgraduate trainees into experiential learning opportunities. Incorporation of learners as pharmacist extenders helps preceptors expand their clinical services to patients and allows them to accommodate more learners, particularly when the Layered Learning Practice Model (LLPM) is used. The LLPM is the teaching approach in which seasoned clinical preceptors supervise learners' clinical and precepting experience and train postgraduate trainees to precept students.[12] Learners may also serve as productive members of the LLPM. In addition to gaining supervised autonomy, learners develop foundational precepting skills by participating in near peer teaching as appropriate for their development. This model utilizes a team approach so that pharmacists, postgraduate trainees, students, and technicians within larger healthcare teams maximize and extend the reach of pharmacy services.

Incorporating learners also allows preceptors to increase scholarly activities. Preceptors have ample opportunities to collaborate with learners for presenting and publishing abstracts, posters, and manuscripts.[3] These partnerships can help advance preceptors' research goals while developing learners' scholarly skills. Preceptors can leverage journal clubs or presentations on upcoming literature or clinical topics to maintain an updated knowledge base. Precepting is a professionally rewarding opportunity to influence future pharmacy clinicians and leave an enduring legacy on the future of the profession.[3]

Value to Healthcare Institutions and Patients. Abundant literature documents the benefits of learners to healthcare institutions. Utilization of learners at healthcare institutions improves institutional metrics by expanding pharmacy services and advancing research agendas and dissemination rates.[10,13] For example, literature has shown tangible benefits of learners when they participate in taking medication histories, optimizing transitions of care, performing discharge counseling, practicing medication therapy management, and administering vaccinations.[10] Involvement of learners in these activities has been associated with the prevention of errors, decreases in medication costs, increased patient interventions and encounters, and decreased pharmacist-to-patient ratios.[10,14] Finally, trainees often apply for positions within their training institution, creating a pipeline of future employees.

Responsibilities of Stakeholders

Positively impacting patient care is the shared vision of learners, preceptors, healthcare institutions, colleges of pharmacy, and professional organizations, and preceptors are necessary to achieve that vision.[11] Preceptors provide an invaluable aspect of pharmacy education as they empower learners to independently apply their knowledge and skills in real-world situations. Colleges of pharmacy uphold the responsibility to prepare APPE-ready students by adhering to ACPE standards regarding experiential learning, and postgraduate training programs uphold the responsibility to ensure postgraduate trainees are practice or advanced practice ready. Practitioners involved in the precepting process play an integral role in determining these outcomes for learners. When experiential learning is thoughtfully designed, students, postgraduate trainees, preceptors, healthcare institutions, and ultimately patients benefit.[3,15]

Preceptors have diverse learning needs and preferences, and healthcare institutions vary in development resources available to preceptors. Preceptor development is instrumental in supporting the design of experiential learning and preparing preceptors for teaching and mentoring within the precepting process. To improve preceptor efficiency and maximize learning, development regarding in-the-moment experiential teaching is crucial, and additional training and sharing best practices in leveraging learners to help meet institutional goals should be a priority. It is imperative that professional organizations, colleges of pharmacy, and healthcare institutions collaborate to provide evidence-based preceptor development resources in a variety of media and formats and promote an inclusive and equitable culture of teaching and learning. As such, the continual professional development of preceptors is a shared responsibility among these entities.

Responsibilities of Professional Organizations

Professional organizations play a pivotal role in the development of precepting standards and preceptor development resources. ASHP and ACPE provide guidance on the standards and requirements for preceptor training and development.[6,8] Professional organizations should collaborate with preceptors, healthcare institutions, and colleges of pharmacy to provide practical and contemporary preceptor development resources and programming to meet the standards. These organizations are equipped to spotlight best teaching practices and practice models of their diverse members.[16] Professional organizations are also positioned to advocate for the importance of precepting and preceptor development to pharmacists and healthcare institutions.

Responsibilities of Colleges of Pharmacy and Postgraduate Training Programs

In addition to providing preceptor development resources to meet individual and group preceptor development needs, colleges of pharmacy and postgraduate training programs can assist in the creation, research, and dissemination of best practices in precepting and innovative practice models to spur the development of others.[11] Colleges of pharmacy and postgraduate training programs also aid in the development of preceptors and healthcare institutions through sharing de-identified aggregate feedback from learners, quality assurance programs, and in the acknowledgment of quality precepting through recognition programs.[16]

Responsibilities of Healthcare Institutions

It is critical to the training of the next generation of pharmacists that healthcare institutions embrace the responsibility to support preceptor development and to develop precepting as a practice philosophy within their institutions. Practice and research models that integrate learners and leverage them to extend pharmacy services should be encouraged and highlighted. Particular importance should be placed on the well-being of busy preceptors who are balancing clinical, professional, and precepting responsibilities. While preceptors continue to adapt to newer educational models that discourage long didactic sessions, preceptors need time for the precepting process. Protected time may be necessary for planning practice experiences, orienting learners, reviewing expectations, discussing learner background and goals, completing and delivering feedback and evaluations, reviewing learner's work, and providing teaching pearls from learning activities. Although this time may vary based on the specific site and infrastructure in place, leadership discussions with precepting teams can help determine what type of support is needed and foster collaborative solutions.

Additionally, this responsibility includes providing financial support to attend preceptor development offerings, protected time to be involved in the precepting process and attend training and development programs, access to development resources, and an organizational commitment to employee well-being. The expectation of precepting as a practice philosophy should be included in role descriptions, performance appraisals, and career ladders to encourage and recognize effective precepting. Examples of competency areas on performance appraisals include commitment to precepting, advocacy for the profession, communication and collaboration, qualities of the learning environment, use of teaching and learning strategies that develop clinical reasoning and other skills, feedback and assessment practices of learners, content expertise, contribution in the area precepted, and ongoing professional engagement.[6,17,18] These competencies may also serve as a framework for self- and peer assessment that are essential to professional development as well as guide preceptor development plans.[17,18,19,20]

Responsibilities of Preceptors

Preceptors should approach precepting with a commitment to lifelong learning and continual personal and professional growth. Strategies to implement this philosophy include continuing professional development (CPD) and the self-directed assessment seeking (SDAS) approaches. In CPD, learning needs are identified through self-assessment and reflection; specific, measurable, achievable, relevant, time-bound (SMART) goals are developed to meet learning needs; the effectiveness of the plan is assessed; and learning is applied to teaching practices.[19,20] Recognizing the limitations of self-assessment alone, the SDAS performance improvement process involves seeking feedback and assessment from external sources such as peers and learners, self-reflecting to identify areas of strength and growth, and developing a plan for improvement.[21] Development plans may include preceptor development offered through written, online, on-demand, live, and other resources. The Habits of Preceptors Rubric is an example of a criterion-referenced tool to support preceptors engaged in self-directed assessment to guide CPD.[22] Preceptors may also create a teaching or precepting philosophy to guide their work. Postgraduate trainees and students also have important roles in preceptor development through provision of constructive and professional feedback on learning experiences and precepting practices. Preceptors should create an environment and foster dialogue that encourages and welcomes feedback from learners throughout a rotation. In addition, colleges of pharmacy and postgraduate trainee programs should train learners to provide constructive, meaningful feedback for learning experiences and preceptors.

Incorporating Precepting into Practice

Serving as a liaison between classroom education and practical application, preceptors are role models for the practice of pharmacy and share the art of the profession with learners. Preceptors are vital to modeling professionalism, communication, and application of skills and knowledge when they advise, mentor, and provide feedback during thoughtfully designed experiential learning. Additionally, throughout postgraduate training, it is imperative that trainees not only learn to precept effectively, but also to employ those skills by becoming preceptors themselves following completion of postgraduate training. All pharmacists with practice experience, including those with and without postgraduate training, have a responsibility to be involved in the precepting process.

Preceptors have a responsibility to be involved not only in training learners, but also in the continuous quality improvement process of the training. Both colleges of pharmacy and postgraduate trainee programs have set standards for continuous quality improvement. ACPE 2016 Standard 20 requires that colleges of pharmacy solicit preceptors for continuous quality improvement of educational programs, especially in experiential learning, and ASHP standards require that preceptors provide input related to continuous improvement and formal postgraduate trainee program evaluation.[6,8] These efforts ensure that experiential learning for both students and postgraduate trainees remain parallel with contemporary practice. Preceptors and learners are vital to these quality improvement processes to ensure patient care and outcomes and institutional metrics are optimized.

Finally, preceptors are encouraged to publish examples of the value of precepting as a practice philosophy, the value of learners as pharmacist extenders, and the impact of learners on patient outcomes through scholarly work. As precepting is incorporated into daily practice, this scholarly work reflects contemporary practice, documents value to other healthcare institutions, provides a framework for the development of effective precepting, and encourages other healthcare institutions to embrace precepting as a professional responsibility. Disseminating both positive and negative outcomes as scholarly work is vital to optimizing outcomes for all stakeholders, most importantly patients.

Conclusion

ASHP believes involvement in the precepting process of learners is the professional responsibility of all pharmacy practice leaders, pharmacists, postgraduate trainees, and faculty to advance pharmacy practice and improve patient outcomes. All pharmacy stakeholders play a vital role in embracing precepting as a practice philosophy and supporting a culture of teaching and learning in the experiential setting. Professional organizations, pharmacy leaders and administrators, colleges of pharmacy, and healthcare institutions should support pharmacists, postgraduate trainees, and pharmacy technicians in developing and utilizing precepting skills, provide resources for formal precepting training and development, and promote learner and preceptor well-being.

References

1. American Association of Colleges of Pharmacy. Oath of a Pharmacist. https://www.aacp.org/sites/default/files/2021-12/oath-of-a-pharmacist-pdf-2021.pdf (accessed December 15, 2022).
2. Lyons K, McLaughlin JE, Khanova J et al. Cognitive apprenticeship in health sciences education: a qualitative review. *Adv in Health Sci Educ.* 2017; 22:723–739.
3. DeRemer CB, Gant KO, Ordonez ND et al. Precepting fundamentals. In: *Preceptor's Handbook for Pharmacists*, 4th ed. Bethesda, MD: American Society of Health-System Pharmacists; 2020:1–26.
4. Persky AM, Fuller KA, Cate OT. True entrustment decisions regarding entrustable professional activities happens in the workplace, not in the classroom setting. *Am J Pharm Educ.* 2021; 85:Article 8356.
5. American Association of Colleges of Pharmacy. Curriculum Outcomes and Entrustable Professional Activities (COEPA) 2022. Patient Care Provider Domains and Example Supporting Tasks. https://www.aacp.org/sites/default/files/2022-11/coepa-document-final.pdf (accessed December 15, 2022).
6. American Society of Health-System Pharmacists. ASHP Accreditation Standard for Postgraduate Residency Programs. https://www.ashp.org/-/media/assets/professional-development/residencies/docs/examples/ASHP-Accreditation-Standard-for-Postgraduate-Residency-Programs-effective-July-2023.pdf (accessed December 15, 2022).
7. Danielson J, Craddick K, Eccles D et al. A qualitative analysis of common concerns about challenges facing pharmacy experiential programs. *Am J Pharm Educ.* 2015; 79(1):Article 06.
8. Accreditation Council for Pharmacy Education. Accreditation Standards and Key Elements for the Professional Program in Pharmacy Leading the Doctor of Pharmacy Degree. Standards 2016. https://www.acpe-accredit.org/pdf/Standards2016FINAL.pdf (accessed December 15, 2022).
9. American Society of Health-System Pharmacists. ASHP Match Statistics. Natmatch.com. https://natmatch.com/ashprmp/stats.html (accessed December 15, 2022).
10. Mersfelder TL, Bouthilier MJ. Value of the student pharmacist to experiential practice sites: a review of the literature. *Ann Pharmacother.* 2012; 46:541–8.
11. Taylor CT, Adams AJ, Albert EL et al. AACP Reports. Report of the 2014–2015 Professional Affairs Standing Committee: producing practice-ready pharmacy graduates in an era of value-based health care. *Am J Pharm Educ.* 2015;79: Article s12.
12. Pinelli NR, Eckel SF, Vu MB et al. The layered learning practice model: Lessons learned from implementation. *Am J Health-Syst Pharm.* 2016; 73:2077–82.
13. Slack MK, Martin JM, Islam S. A systematic review of extramural presentations and publications from pharmacy student research programs. *Am J Pharm Educ.* 2016; 80:Article 100.
14. Delgado O, Kernan WP, Knoer SJ. Advancing the pharmacy practice model in a community teaching hospital by expanding student rotations. *Am J Health-Syst Pharm.* 2014; 71:1871–6.
15. Soric MM, GLowczewski JE, Lerman RM. Economic and patient satisfaction outcomes of a layered learning model in a small community hospital. *Am J Health-Syst Pharm.* 2016; 73(7): 456–462.
16. Worrall CL, Chaira DS, Aistropeb EA et al. AACP Reports. Priming the preceptor pipeline: Collaboration, resources, and recognition: The Report of the 2015–2016 Professional Affairs Standing Committee. *Am J Pharm Educ.* 2016; 80: Article S19.
17. Walter S, Mulherin K, Cox CD. A preceptor competency framework for pharmacists. Part 2 of a 3-part series. *Curr Pharm Teach Learning.* 2018;10:402–410.
18. Larson S, Davis LE, Stevens AM et al. Development of a tool to assess and advance the effectiveness of preceptors: the habits of preceptors rubric. *Am J Health-Syst Pharm.* 2019; 76:1762–9.
19. Accreditation Council for Pharmacy Education. Accreditation Council for Pharmacy Education Guidance on Continuing Professional Development (CPD) for the Profession of Pharmacy. https://www.acpe-accredit.org/pdf/CPDGuidance%20ProfessionPharmacyJan2015.pdf (accessed December 15, 2022).
20. Tofade T, Kim J, Lebovitz L et al. Introduction of a continuing professional development tool for preceptors: lessons learned. *J Pharm Pract.* 2015; 28:212–219.
21. Eva KW, Regehr G. "I'll never play professional football" and other fallacies of self- assessment. *J Contin Educ Health Prof.* 2008; 28:14–19.
22. Davis LE, Pogge EK, Larson S, Storjohann T, Early N. Evaluating the change in preceptor habits while enrolled in a teaching and learning curriculum using the habits of preceptors rubric. *J Am Coll Clin Pharm.* 2021; 4:137–146.

Additional Information

This statement was developed through the ASHP Section of Pharmacy Educators and was appproved by the ASHP Board of Directors on December 16, 2022, and by the ASHP House of Delegates on June 11, 2023.

Acknowledgments

ASHP gratefully acknowledges the following organizations and individuals for reviewing this statement (review does not imply endorsement): American Association of Colleges of Pharmacy (AACP); Kelly Bach, PharmD, BCPS, BCCCP, BCGP; Jaclyn Boyle, PharmD, MS, MBA, BCACP; Lynette Bradley-Baker (AACP), PhD, CAE, RPh; Aaron Burton, PharmD, MBA, BCPS; Angela Chu, PharmD, BCPS; Michelle Chu, PharmD, BCACP, APh; Mary Petrea Cober, PharmD, BCNSP, BCPPS, FASPEN; Justin W. Cole, PharmD, BCPS; Janet Cooley, PharmD, BCACP; Jeffrey Cook, PharmD, MS, MBA, CHFP; Kate Cozart, MEd, PharmD, BCPS, BCGP, BCACP; Julie Dagam, PharmD, BCPS, FASHP, FPSW; Vi Doan, PharmD, BCOP; Collins Enwerem; Judy Huang, PhD, PharmD, BCPS, AAHIVP; Indrani Kar, PharmD, DPLA; Allison R. King, PharmD, FASHP; Denise Kolanczyk, PharmD, BCPS; Trisha LaPointe, PharmD, BCPS, FASHP; Suzanne Larson, PharmD; Brody Maack, PharmD, BCACP, CTTS; Nancy C. MacDonald, PharmD, BCPS, FASHP; Jessica Merlo, PharmD, BCACP; Rachel Meyers, PharmD; Hesham Mourad, PharmD, EMBA, BCPS, BCCCP, CPHIMS; Marianne Pop, PharmD, MPH, BCPS; Marjorie Shaw Phillips, MSPharm, RPh, FASHP, CIP; Joshua Raub, PharmD, BCPS; Anthony Scott, PharmD, MBA; Susan Skledar, RPh, MPH, FASHP; Winter Smith, PharmD, BCPS; Mate Soric, PharmD, BCPS, FCCP; Alexandria Stringberg, PharmD, BCPS; Emmeline Tran, PharmD, BCPS; Michelle Turner, PharmD, BCPS, BCIDP; Marnie Wickizer, PharmD; Jordan L Wulz, PharmD, MPH, BC-ADM; and David Zimmerman, PharmD, BCCCP.

Authors

Jennifer N. Wisniewski, PharmD, BCPA, Assistant Professor, Medical University of South Carolina College of Pharmacy, Charleston, SC

Charlene R. Williams, PharmD, BCACP, CDCES, Director of Preceptor Development and Clinical Assistant Professor, University of North Carolina Eshelman School of Pharmacy, Asheville, NC

Dana G. Carroll, PharmD, BCPS, BCGP, CDCES, Clinical Professor, Auburn University Harrison School of Pharmacy, Tuscaloosa, AL

Lisa M. Richter, PharmD, BCPS, BCCCP, FASHP, Director of Experiential Outreach and Assessment and Associate Professor of Practice, North Dakota State University School of Pharmacy, Fargo, ND

Sarah Eudaley, PharmD, BCPS, Assistant Professor and Department of Clinical Pharmacy and Translational Science, The University of Tennessee Health Science Center, Memphis, TN

Kazuhiko Kido, PharmD, MS, BCPS, BCCP, Clinical Associate Professor, West Virginia University Health Sciences Directory, Morgantown, WV

Disclosures

The authors have declared no potential conflicts of interest.

Copyright © 2023, American Society of Health-System Pharmacists, Inc. All rights reserved.

Note: This statement had not been published in the *American Journal of Health-System Pharmacy (AJHP)* when *Best Practices for Hospital & Health-System Pharmacy 2023-2024* went to press. Some minor editorial difference may exist between this document and the official one that will eventually appear in *AJHP* and subsequent editions of this publication.

Definitions of Pharmacy Residencies and Fellowships

Pharmacy residencies (originally termed "internships") began in the early 1930s, primarily for the purpose of training pharmacists for the management of pharmacy services in hospitals. The first nonacademic residency program is believed to have been conducted by Harvey A. K. Whitney at the University of Michigan Hospital.[1] Approximately 10 years later, the first residency program combined with formal graduate studies was created.[2] Developments in these programs eventually led the American Society of Hospital Pharmacists to establish, in 1948, standards for pharmacy internships in hospitals.[3] Those standards defined an internship as "a period of organized training in an accredited hospital pharmacy under the direction and supervision of personnel qualified to offer such training."

Two types of internships were recognized, nonacademic and academic. The nonacademic internship consisted of a period of training in a hospital pharmacy. The academic internship consisted of training in a hospital pharmacy and study in an accredited graduate school associated with a college of pharmacy and leading to a Master of Science degree.

In 1962, following several revisions in the standards, ASHP established an accreditation process and accreditation standards for residencies in hospital pharmacy.[4,5] In this action, the term "internship" was replaced by "residency." A residency was defined as "a postgraduate program of organized training . . ." (and further detailed within the various standards). In 1985, the concept that a resident's training should be *directed* was incorporated into the definition.[6–9] It was also acknowledged that a residency is practice oriented and that it is possible for a residency to focus on a defined (specialized) area.

During the early 1970s, numerous residencies developed in *clinical* practice, leading to the establishment, in 1980, of accreditation standards for clinical pharmacy and specialized residency training.[10,11] In 1986, the American Pharmaceutical Association published a compilation of programmatic essentials for community pharmacy residencies.[12] In that same year, the American College of Apothecaries published specific guidelines for the accreditation of community pharmacy residencies.[13]

Paralleling these developments and fostered by a growing sophistication and clinical thrust in institutional pharmacy practice, postgraduate research-oriented programs (generally termed "fellowships") developed in the 1970s. These programs were conducted primarily in colleges of pharmacy and in academically based health centers to educate and train individuals to conduct pharmacy research. A 1981 survey of fellowship programs reported the existence of 58 fellowships in 19 topic areas.[14] Two-thirds of these fellowships had existed for 3 years or less. The oldest program had existed for less than 9 years. The ASHP Research and Education Foundation initiated clinical fellowships in 1978 and defined a pharmacy fellowship as "a directed, but highly individualized program [that] emphasizes research. The focus of a pharmacy fellowship is to develop the participant's (the fellow's) ability to conduct research in his or her area of specialization."[15,16]

ASHP publishes an annual directory of ASHP-accredited residency programs. In 1985, there were 184 accredited programs.[17] The American College of Clinical Pharmacy publishes an annual listing of residencies and fellowships conducted by its members. In 1985, ACCP reported the availability of 51 such residencies and 83 such fellowships.[18] Another source reported 115 known fellowships in 1986.[19] In that year, there were 12 clinical fellowships sponsored by the ASHP Research and Education Foundation in nine areas of specialization.

By 1986, a lack of conformity had arisen in the use of the terms "residency" and "fellowship," and considerable potential existed for program applicants to be misinformed or misled regarding program purposes and content. In 1986, at the recommendation of the ASHP Commission on Credentialing, ASHP invited six other national pharmacy organizations to discuss the issue and develop consensus definitions for the terms. The definitions and interpretations that follow resulted from that conference. These definitions and interpretations are viewed as accurate for current residencies and fellowships yet sufficiently broad and flexible to allow the development of new types of programs. Education, practice, and research developments may generate changes in residencies and fellowships and ultimately stimulate revisions in the definitions and interpretations.

Residency

Definition. A pharmacy residency is an organized, directed, postgraduate training program in a defined area of phamacy practice.

Interpretation. Residencies exist primarily to train pharmacists in professional practice and management activities. Residencies provide experience in integrating pharmacy services with the comprehensive needs of individual practice settings and provide indepth experiences leading to advanced practice skills and knowledge. Residencies foster an ability to conceptualize new and improved pharmacy services. Within a given residency program, there is considerable consistency in content for each resident. In addition, accreditation standards and program guidelines produced by national pharmacy associations provide considerable program content detail and foster consistency among programs.

A residency is typically 12 months or longer in duration, and the resident's practice experiences are closely directed and evaluated by a qualified practitioner–preceptor. A residency may occur at any career point following an entry-level degree in pharmacy. Individuals planning practice-oriented careers are encouraged to complete all formal academic education before entry into a residency.

Fellowship

Definition. A pharmacy fellowship is a directed, highly individualized, postgraduate program designed to prepare the participant to become an independent researcher.

Interpretation. Fellowships exist primarily to develop competency in the scientific research process, including conceptualizing, planning, conducting, and reporting research. Under

DOI 10.37573/9781585287048.031

the close direction and instruction of a qualified researcher-preceptor, the participant (the fellow) receives a highly individualized learning experience that utilizes research interests and knowledge needs as a focus for his or her education and training. A fellowship graduate should be capable of conducting collaborative research or functioning as a principal investigator.

Fellowships are typically offered through colleges of pharmacy, academic health centers, or specialized health-care institutions. Fellowships are usually offered for predetermined, finite periods of time, often exceeding 12 or even 24 months. Individuals planning research-oriented careers should expect to complete formal education in research design and statistics either before or during a fellowship. A fellowship candidate is expected to possess basic practice skills relevant to the knowledge area of the fellowship. Such skills may be obtained through practice experience or through an appropriate residency and should be maintained during the program.

References

1. Niemeyer G. Ten years of the American Society of Hospital Pharmacists, 1942–1952: education and training. *Bull Am Soc Hosp Pharm.* 1952; 9:363–75.
2. American Society of Hospital Pharmacists. Approval program for internships in hospital pharmacy. *Bull Am Soc Hosp Pharm.* 1955; 12:309–13.
3. American Society of Hospital Pharmacists. Standards for internships in hospital pharmacies. *Bull Am Soc Hosp Pharm.* 1948; 5:233–4.
4. American Society of Hospital Pharmacists. Minimum standard for pharmacy internship in hospitals. *Bull Am Soc Hosp Pharm.* 1955; 12:288–90.
5. American Society of Hospital Pharmacists. Accreditation standard for residency in hospital pharmacy. *Am J Hosp Pharm.* 1963; 20:378–80.
6. American Society of Hospital Pharmacists. Accreditation standard for pharmacy residency in a hospital. *Am J Hosp Pharm.* 1971; 28:189–90.
7. American Society of Hospital Pharmacists. Accreditation standard for pharmacy residency in a hospital. *Am J Hosp Pharm.* 1973; 30:1129.
8. American Society of Hospital Pharmacists. ASHP accreditation standard for pharmacy residency in a hospital (with guide to interpretation). *Am J Hosp Pharm.* 1979; 36:74–80.
9. American Society of Hospital Pharmacists. ASHP accreditation standard for hospital pharmacy training (with guide to interpretation). *Am J Hosp Pharm.* 1985; 42:2008–18.
10. American Society of Hospital Pharmacists. ASHP accreditation standard for residency training in clinical pharmacy (with guide to interpretation). *Am J Hosp Pharm.* 1980; 37:1223–8.
11. American Society of Hospital Pharmacists. ASHP accreditation standard for specialized residency training (with guide to interpretation). *Am J Hosp Pharm.* 1980; 37:1229–32.
12. American Pharmaceutical Association, Academy of Pharmacy Practice. APhA community pharmacy residency program: programmatic essentials. *Am Pharm.* 1986; NS26:35–43.
13. American College of Apothecaries. Guidelines for accreditation of community pharmacy residencies. Memphis, TN: American College of Apothecaries; 1986.
14. Kaul AF, Powell SH, Cyr DA. Postgraduate pharmacy fellowships. *Drug Intell Clin Pharm.* 1981; 15:981–5.
15. ASHP Commission on Credentialing. Statement of definition of pharmacy fellowships and residency. Bethesda, MD: American Society of Hospital Pharmacists; 1981.
16. McConnell W. Fellowship program in critical care pharmacy. In: Majerus TC, Dasta JF, eds. Practice of critical care pharmacy. Rockville, MD: Aspen Systems; 1985:59–68.
17. American Society of Hospital Pharmacists. Residency directory. Accredited pharmacy residency programs and programs participating in the 1986 ASHP resident matching program. Bethesda, MD: American Society of Hospital Pharmacists; 1985.
18. American College of Clinical Pharmacy. Residency and fellowship programs offered by members of the American College of Clinical Pharmacy, 1986–87. Kansas City, MO: American College of Clinical Pharmacy; 1986.
19. Kaul AF, Janosik JE, Powell SH. Postgraduate pharmacy fellowships (1985–86). *Drug Intell Clin Pharm.* 1986; 20:203–8.

Developed by an ad hoc consortium made up of representatives from the American Association of Colleges of Pharmacy (AACP), the American College of Apothecaries (ACA), the American College of Clinical Pharmacy (ACCP), the American Pharmaceutical Association (APhA), the American Society of Consultant Pharmacists (ASCP), the American Society of Hospital Pharmacists (ASHP), and the National Association of Retail Druggists (NARD); the consortium was convened by ASHP and met on August 4, 1986. Approved by the ASHP Board of Directors, November 20, 1986, and subsequently approved by ACCP, APhA, ASCP, ACA, and AACP.

Copyright © 1987, American Society of Hospital Pharmacists, Inc. All rights reserved. Contact ASHP for reprint and permissions requests. This content may not be used for commercial purposes without the express written consent of ASHP.

The bibliographic citation for this document is as follows: American Society of Hospital Pharmacists. Definitions of pharmacy residencies and fellowships. *Am J Hosp Pharm.* 1987; 44:1142–4.

Ethics

DOI 10.37573/9781585287048

Ethics

2320

PHARMACOEQUITY

Source: Council on Pharmacy Practice

To raise awareness that disparities in clinical practice negatively impact healthcare outcomes and compromise pharmacoequity; further,

To recognize the impact of social determinants of health on pharmacoequity and patient outcomes; further,

To advocate for drug availability, drug pricing structures, pricing transparency, and insurance coverage determinations that promote pharmacoequity; further,

To advocate that the pharmacy workforce identify and address risks and vulnerabilities to pharmacoequity as part of comprehensive medication management services; further,

To advocate for resources, including technology, that improve access to care for marginalized and underserved populations where pharmacy access is limited; further,

To encourage the pharmacy workforce to identify and mitigate biases in healthcare decision-making that compromise pharmacoequity.

Rationale

Pharmacoequity aims to ensure that all individuals regardless of race and ethnicity, socioeconomic status, or availability of resources, have access to the highest quality medications required to manage their health needs. Barriers contributing to the lack of pharmacoequity include decreased access to care, increased costs of care, and differences in care based on provider bias (Essien UR, Dusetzina SB, Gellad WF. A policy prescription for reducing health disparities—achieving Pharmacoequity. *JAMA*. 2021;326(18):1793. doi:10.1001/jama.2021.17764). These barriers have helped raise awareness of the ABCs of solutions for promoting pharmacoequity: access, bias, and costs.

Decreased access to care may be due to insufficient prescription drug coverage or residing in a pharmacy desert. The current trends in the price of prescription drugs, combined with lack of insurance or underinsurance, results in lower use of prescribed medications and nonadherence. Pharmacists can help build culturally competent structures to reduce racial and ethnic disparities in healthcare through various means, including promoting a more diverse work force, increasing awareness of disparities, promoting culturally competent care and services, researching and implementing best practices for providing culturally competent care, and ensuring effective communication with patients and among providers (ASHP Statement on Racial and Ethnic Disparities in Health Care, *Am J Health-Syst Pharm.* 2008; 65:728–33, doi.org/10.2146/ajhp070398).

Ensuring that all individuals regardless of race and ethnicity, socioeconomic status, or availability of resources have access to the highest quality medications required to meet their needs will require a multifaceted approach. Promotion of culturally competent structures through increased awareness of disparities and diversification of the workforce, in addition to improving medication affordability and pharmacy access, are all steps needed to attain pharmacoequity.

2036

RACIAL AND DISCRIMINATORY INEQUITIES

Source: House of Delegates

To acknowledge that racism, discrimination, and inequities exist in healthcare and society; further,

To assert that racism, or any form of discrimination or injustice, has no value in society and cannot be tolerated; further,

To fervently commit to creating a just and inclusive healthcare system and society.

Rationale

ASHP and its members have long been committed to eliminating racial and ethnic disparities in healthcare and recognize the need to further strengthen that commitment following the recent killings of George Floyd, Ahmaud Arbery, and Breonna Taylor. ASHP has pledged to take actionable steps through the creation of a Board of Directors–appointed Task Force on Racial Diversity, Equity, and Inclusion. The Task Force is charged with taking inventory of ASHP's efforts in the areas of racial diversity, equity, and inclusion as they relate to issues facing Black Americans, and for making related recommendations on new or enhanced efforts ASHP may undertake. ASHP further seeks to help eliminate racism, discrimination, and inequities that impact other minority and underrepresented populations and to help improve diversity, equity, and inclusion in healthcare and society.

1704

MEDICAL AID IN DYING

Source: Board of Directors

To affirm that a pharmacist's decision to participate or decline to participate in medical aid in dying for competent, terminally ill patients, where legal, is one of individual conscience; further,

To reaffirm that pharmacists have a right to participate or decline to participate in medical aid in dying without retribution; further,

To take a stance of studied neutrality on legislation that would permit medical aid in dying for competent, terminally ill patients.

This policy was reviewed in 2022 by the Council on Pharmacy Practice and by the Board of Directors and was found to still be appropriate.

Rationale

Medical aid in dying (also called physician-assisted dying, physician-assisted suicide, physician aid in dying, physician-assisted death, hastened death, medically assisted dying, and death with dignity) has been legal in some areas of the U.S. since Oregon passed its Death with Dignity Law in 1995. By 2016, one sixth of U.S. citizens lived in a jurisdiction in which medical aid in dying was available, and more states were contemplating legislation to legalize it. Experience in Oregon and elsewhere demonstrates that pharmacists in those jurisdictions may be confronted with the difficult ethical question of whether to participate in medical aid in dying.

DOI 10.37573/9781585287048.032

For purposes of this policy position, ASHP adapts a common definition of medical aid in dying: the practice in which a physician provides a prescription for a lethal dose of medication to a terminally ill, competent patient at the patient's request that the patient can self-administer at a time of his or her choosing to end his or her life. ASHP notes that many of the terms commonly used to describe this practice ignore the patient care and dispensing roles of pharmacists as well as the roles of other healthcare professionals, such as hospice nurses, in providing care for patients requesting medical aid in dying. ASHP recognizes the utility of a term such as "medical aid in dying" that addresses the roles of all healthcare providers involved in or affected by the practice but acknowledges the term's ambiguity regarding self-administration of the lethal dose. ASHP therefore explicitly distinguishes medical aid in dying from all forms of euthanasia, which is not the subject of this policy.

ASHP takes a position of studied neutrality on whether pharmacists should participate in medical aid in dying. Studied neutrality has been defined as "the careful or premeditated practice of being neutral in a dispute" and has as it goals "to foster a respectful culture among people of diverse views and to guide action that does not afford material advantage to a [particular] group." (Johnstone M-J. Organization Position Statements and the Stance of "Studied Neutrality" on Euthanasia in Palliative Care. *J Pain Symp Manag.* 2012; 44:896–907.) ASHP respects the diversity of views of its members and other pharmacists on medical aid in dying and adopts a position of studied neutrality to promote patient autonomy and access to care and to protect pharmacists' professional integrity and comity.

The Code of Ethics for Pharmacists states that "a pharmacist promises to help individuals achieve optimum benefit from their medications [and] to be committed to their welfare" and that "a pharmacist promotes the right of self-determination and recognizes individual self-worth by encouraging patients to participate in decisions about their health." In pharmacist decision-making about participation in medical aid in dying, those principles may clash. Self-determination dictates that patients should be free to exercise their ethical and legal right to choose or decline any legally available treatment. Many healthcare professionals, and their organizations (including the American Medical Association, the American College of Physicians, and the American Nurses Association), question whether death is ever an acceptable therapeutic goal. Others (including the American Academy of Hospice and Palliative Medicine and the American Psychological Association) acknowledge in their statements of neutrality that society may determine that medical aid in dying falls within a spectrum of treatments and withholding of treatments that has as its goal the relief of suffering through a compassionately hastened death, even while recognizing the risks of such a practice.

Pharmacists, like other healthcare professionals, have a right to examine and act on the moral and ethical issues involved in providing care to patients. ASHP policy position 0610, Pharmacist's Right of Conscience and Patient's Right of Access to Therapy, outlines the rights and responsibilities of pharmacists and other pharmacy employees who decline to participate in therapies that they find morally, religiously, or ethically troubling, including the right to reasonable accommodation of their right to conscience in a nonpunitive manner. Procedures should be in place to ensure that healthcare organizations can provide mission-compatible care to patients, and that healthcare providers practicing there are not a barrier to the organization's ability to provide that care. In adopting its position of studied neutrality on pharmacist involvement in medical aid in dying, ASHP recognizes that adopting a position in favor of participation would infringe on the moral and ethical prerogatives of pharmacists. ASHP similarly recognizes that a stance against participation would make the same infringement and in addition present the risk of legal or professional sanction for pharmacists who participate in medical aid in dying where it is legal.

ASHP also takes a position of studied neutrality on whether medical aid in dying should be legally permitted for competent, terminally ill patients. ASHP recognizes that society may interpret the principle of patient autonomy to include the right to therapies that some may find morally, religiously, or ethically troubling, including medical aid in dying. Recognizing as well the role of healthcare professionals as guardians against practices that would undermine patient autonomy, ASHP advocates that, when permitted, medical aid in dying only be available to competent, terminally ill patients who freely and knowledgeably make that choice.

ASHP joins other healthcare professional organizations in noting that medical aid in dying is inextricably linked with hospice, palliative, and other end-of-life care. ASHP will therefore continue to advocate that patients receive appropriate pharmacist care at the end of life, including pain management (ASHP policy 1722), support in dying (ASHP policy 0307), and hospice and palliative care.

1531

PHARMACIST ROLE IN CAPITAL PUNISHMENT

Source: Council on Pharmacy Practice

To acknowledge that an individual's opinion about capital punishment is a personal moral decision; further,

To oppose pharmacist participation in capital punishment; further,

To reaffirm that pharmacists have a right to decline to participate in capital punishment without retribution.

This policy was reviewed in 2020 by the Council on Pharmacy Practice and by the Board of Directors and was found to still be appropriate.

Rationale

Since 1977, when Oklahoma became the first state to adopt execution by lethal injection, many healthcare professional organizations have adopted policies opposing participation by members of their respective professions in capital punishment. The American Medical Association (AMA), the American Nurses Association (ANA), and the American Pharmacists Association (APhA) are among these groups; however, a wide variety of organizations have spoken out on the issue. The consistent theme of the opposition of those organizations is that the intentional infliction of death is contrary to the mission of healthcare and therefore unethical. ASHP's previous policy on pharmacist participation in capital punishment, which was adopted in 1984 and has been reaffirmed several times since, emphasized the pharmacist right to conscience when deciding whether to participate in capital punishment.

The role of pharmacists in execution by lethal injection changed substantially after Hospira relocated its thiopental sodium manufacturing to Italy in 2011. The European Union bans the export of thiopental sodium to countries where it may be used in executions, including the U.S. The ban resulted in severe shortages of the drug, which was the cornerstone of the three-drug cocktail used in lethal injections. (At least nine drug manufacturers have followed suit in prohibiting use of their products for lethal injection.) States responded by substituting compounded anesthetic preparations or instituting other drug protocols, which came under criticism after several executions in which prisoners appeared to suffer despite being medicated. These developments increased the role of pharmacists in preparing and/or compounding drugs for execution by lethal injection, which in turn increased the scrutiny of that role both inside and outside the profession.

That increased scrutiny comes at a time when pharmacists are rapidly expanding their roles on the patient care team and are being recognized as patient care providers. This proposed policy developed by the ASHP Council on Pharmacy Practice recognizes that one's beliefs about capital punishment are a personal, individual decision but opposes pharmacist participation in capital punishment because it is contrary to their role as healthcare providers. Given the ethical questions about pharmacist participation in capital punishment, pharmacists should not be punished for their refusal to participate.

1403

PHARMACIST'S ROLE ON ETHICS COMMITTEES

Source: Council on Pharmacy Practice

To advocate that pharmacists should be included as members of hospital and health-system ethics committees; further,

To encourage pharmacists to actively seek ethics consultations as appropriate; further,

To encourage pharmacists serving on ethics committees to seek advanced training in health care ethics.

This policy was reviewed in 2019 by the Council on Pharmacy Practice and by the Board of Directors and was found to still be appropriate.

Rationale

Many hospitals have a committee or other process by which they consider ethical decisions related to patient care. Many issues that face these committees involve medications, yet often pharmacists do not serve on the committee or are not directly involved in the decision-making process. The number of ethical issues involving medications is expected to increase, given many new and unique drug products coming into the market. Pharmacist involvement would better inform these committees and consultations. To effectively contribute to decision-making on ethics, pharmacists will require advanced education on the subject.

1116

ETHICAL USE OF PLACEBOS IN CLINICAL PRACTICE

Source: Council on Pharmacy Practice

To affirm that the use of placebos in clinical practice is ethically acceptable only when patients have been informed of and agree to such use as a component of treatment; further,

To encourage hospitals and health systems to develop policies and procedures to guide clinicians in making informed decisions regarding the use of placebos; further,

To oppose the use of pharmacologically active substances or medications as placebos.

This policy was reviewed in 2021 by the Council on Pharmacy Practice and by the Board of Directors and was found to still be appropriate.

Rationale

The Council reviewed previous action on ASHP policy 0517, the American Medical Association (AMA) *Opinion on Placebo Use in Clinical Practice*, and the *ASHP Guidelines on Clinical Drug Research*, which state in part:

> The principal investigator or designee is responsible for obtaining informed consent from each subject who is eligible for participation in the study (i.e., meets inclusion and exclusion criteria). The informed consent process shall conform to current federal and state regulations. IRB approval of the consent form (and assent form for minors) is required. Review by legal counsel may be desirable.

After comparing use of placebos for research to prescribing for clinical use, the Council agreed with the stance expressed by AMA, i.e., patients should be informed of and agree to use of a placebo as a therapeutic intervention. The Council believed that the informed consent process should be reserved for research and medical interventions, where a consent contract and oral explanation of the patient's rights are required. In addition, the Council expressed concern that advocating informed consent could lead to a mistaken assumption that clinical use of placebos requires the review and approval of an institutional review board.

The Council disputed the AMA definition of a placebo as "a substance provided to a patient that the physician believes has no specific pharmacological effect upon the condition being treated," however, and recommended that a placebo should be defined as an inert substance. The Board and the House concurred. Research on placebos found differing definitions of the term but did not provide an established or official definition. The Council concluded that the current policy lacks clarity in that it addresses an undefined term. The Council requested that ASHP identify the appropriate standards-setting or regulatory body to provide this definition or determine whether ASHP should establish a definition for the purpose of its policy.

The Council noted a number of other unresolved issues that require further exploration and action by ASHP. These include research for definitive guidance on the ethics of clinical placebo use, potential ethical dilemmas for pharmacists, and compliance with professional standards and regulatory requirements for reviewing placebo orders for appropriateness, labeling placebo prescriptions, and counseling patients. The Council suggested a comprehensive review by a bioethicist be published in AJHP.

0610

PHARMACIST'S RIGHT OF CONSCIENCE AND PATIENT'S RIGHT OF ACCESS TO THERAPY

Source: Council on Legal and Public Affairs

To recognize the right of pharmacists, as health care providers, and other pharmacy employees to decline to participate in therapies they consider to be morally, religiously, or ethically troubling; further,

To support the proactive establishment of timely and convenient systems by pharmacists and their employers that protect the patient's right to obtain legally prescribed and medically indicated treatments while reasonably accommodating in a nonpunitive manner the right of conscience; further,

To support the principle that a pharmacist exercising the right of conscience must be respectful of, and serve the legitimate health care needs and desires of, the patient, and shall provide a referral without any actions to persuade, coerce, or otherwise impose on the patient the pharmacist's values, beliefs, or objections.

This policy was reviewed in 2021 by the Council on Pharmacy Practice and by the Board of Directors and was found to still be appropriate.

Rationale

ASHP affirms pharmacists' right to decline to participate in therapies they consider to be morally, religiously, or ethically troubling but recognizes that a right of conscience must balance a pharmacist's deeply held beliefs with his or her professional duty and the patient's right to access legally prescribed and medically indicated treatments. To achieve this balance, systems to protect the patient's right to timely access to therapy should be developed in advance of the presentation of a prescription to a pharmacist or other employee who might exercise the right of conscience. The right of conscience therefore creates an affirmative responsibility on the part of the pharmacist to proactively notify his or her employer about therapies of concern. In addition, a pharmacist exercising the right of conscience must respect and serve the legitimate healthcare needs and desires of the patient and must provide a referral without any actions to persuade, coerce, or otherwise impose on the patient the pharmacist's values, beliefs, or objections. For the purposes of this policy, "referral" is defined in a manner similar to that used by the American Academy of Family Physicians (Consultations, Referrals, and Transfers of Care; 2012 COD): a referral is a request from one pharmacist to another to assume responsibility for management of one or more of a patient's specified problems, for a specified period of time, until the problem(s)' resolution, or on an ongoing basis, and represents a temporary or partial transfer of care to another pharmacist for a particular condition. When conscience requires a pharmacist also to decline to refer the patient to a specific provider who can provide the legally prescribed and medically indicated treatment, the pharmacist should offer impartial guidance to patients about how to inform themselves regarding access to the therapy. The National Catholic Bioethics Center suggests that healthcare providers declining to refer may assist patients with accomplishing a transfer of care to another provider or institution of the patient's choosing by providing a general list of other providers or institutions based on geographic vicinity or area of specialty, so long as the list is not developed based on the criterion of whether the providers are known or believed to offer the therapy in question. Institutions should have processes in place to ensure that the transfer of care process does not interfere with the patient's right to obtain legally prescribed and medically indicated treatments. Any accommodations made on the basis of a pharmacist's decision to exercise the right of conscience should be nonpunitive.

0013

PATIENT'S RIGHT TO CHOOSE

Source: Council on Legal and Public Affairs

To support the right of the patient or his or her representative as allowed under state law to develop, implement, and make informed decisions regarding his or her plan of care; further,

To acknowledge that the patient's rights include being informed of his or her health status, being involved in care planning and treatment, and being able to request or refuse treatment; further,

To support the right of the patient in accord with state laws to (a) formulate advance directives and (b) have health care practitioners who comply with those directives.

This policy was reviewed in 2015 by the Council on Public Policy and by the Board of Directors and was found to still be appropriate.

ASHP Statement on Leadership as a Professional Obligation

Position

The American Society of Health-System Pharmacists (ASHP) believes that the pharmacy workforce has a professional obligation to serve as leaders in the safe and effective use of medications. These leaders have an obligation to encourage pharmacy practitioners, administrators, faculty members, preceptors, technicians, and learners to advance patient care and strengthen the pharmacy profession by embracing the responsibility to exert leadership within their practices and across their organizations. ASHP urges the pharmacy workforce to accept this responsibility, actively seek the development of leadership skills, and exercise leadership when working with others within and outside of the profession.

ASHP encourages colleges of pharmacy, pharmacy technician training programs, and employers to grow the pipeline for developing a diverse group of future leaders by extending beyond management coursework and integrating education on leadership as a practice philosophy throughout the training and curriculum. The pharmacy workforce shares the responsibility to mentor pharmacy students, pharmacy residents, pharmacists, pharmacy technicians, and non-pharmacist support staff. Pharmacy workforce members in formal leadership roles have a specific responsibility to: 1) foster the development of leadership skills among others within the workforce; 2) facilitate the development of practice models that provide regular opportunities to exercise leadership; 3) encourage others to exercise leadership in practice; and 4) build relationships across the organization to serve as the voice of pharmacy and safe medication use. ASHP also encourages hospital and health-system executives to support the development of leadership skills of all healthcare professionals.

Leadership in Practice

The ASHP Statement on Professionalism includes leadership ("influenc[ing] others with unquestionable integrity") as a professional responsibility shared by individuals and the institutions where they work.[1] The ASHP Statement on the Roles and Responsibilities of the Pharmacy Executive explains the formal leadership roles of the pharmacy executive, including the responsibility to successfully build and manage relationships with diverse groups to ensure pharmacy is involved with strategic planning and decision making processes.[2] As both of those statements highlight, the pharmacy workforce also has the professional obligation to serve as leaders in the safe and effective use of medications.

Definitions of leadership commonly focus on working toward goals and exerting influence.[3] For example, Nahata[4] stated that leadership "is about a vision, direction, strategies, motivating, and inspiring." The focus on goals and influence guides understanding of the inherent requirement for leadership in pharmacy. The success of current pharmacy practice models and the successful implementation of future models rest on the ability of members of the profession to influence others. In the complex and evolving healthcare environment, leadership from the pharmacy workforce is required to promote and advance the profession and our care for patients. Thus, leadership is not an option—it is a professional obligation.

The most successful organizations facilitate the inclusive development of routine leadership roles and encourage participation in those roles. The frontline pharmacy workforce must exhibit themselves as leaders each time they step into the workplace. The practice of effectively influencing the behavior of physicians, pharmacists, nurses, pharmacy technicians, learners, support staff, and other healthcare team members to optimize medication safety and patient outcomes constitutes successful leadership. Such leadership often requires pharmacy team members to work across interprofessional teams to optimize patient safety and medication use. Innovative practice models can support the development of both clinical and leadership skills. ASHP encourages development and implementation of these types of practice models.

Each pharmacy workforce member's personal and professional experiences affect how they approach the patients and decisions that come before them. The diversity of their perspectives and lived experiences fosters decision-making that better reflects the whole population, resulting in better, richer analyses as clinicians and healthcare leaders. When pharmacy leadership includes all voices and perspectives, practicing members of the team and members of the public are more likely to trust theirs will be heard. The ASHP Task Force on Racial Diversity, Equity, and Inclusion has put forth recommendations to promote this aspect of leadership.[5]

The obligation to develop a pharmacy workforce prepared for professional leadership requires colleges of pharmacy, pharmacy technician training programs, and employers to adopt the training of leadership and its values. Currently, leadership training is inconsistently present in both academic and practice settings. White's survey[6] as well as the report of the American Association of Colleges of Pharmacy Argus Commission[7] support the need for formalized training programs to cultivate the required leadership training among learners. To cultivate high-quality candidates to fill the pharmacy leadership gap, the report also recommends expansion of didactic leadership training, distance learning programs, the use of social media for networking and mentorship, and an increased focus on the full spectrum of leadership. All members of the pharmacy workforce should take personal responsibility for leadership of the medication-use process and for mentorship of learners, pharmacy technicians, and other colleagues. Although it is not the exclusive responsibility of formal pharmacy leaders such as pharmacy directors and managers, formal leaders must foster and support diverse leadership among the members of a pharmacy team.

The pharmacy workforce also has an obligation to exert leadership and participate in shaping the future of the profession.[8] Participation in professional societies such as ASHP and ASHP state affiliates provides opportunities to shape the future of the profession and affords excellent opportunities

DOI 10.37573/9781585287048.033

for the development of leadership skills. Professional organizations such as ASHP and ASHP state affiliates also have an obligation to encourage the development of leadership skills and support their development among their memberships.

Conclusion

Leadership is a professional obligation of all members of the pharmacy workforce and not the exclusive responsibility of those who hold formal leadership roles or titles. All members of the pharmacy workforce should accept the obligation to develop and exert leadership skills to ensure the safe and effective use of medications. Colleges of pharmacy, pharmacy technician training schools, professional organizations, and employers should encourage the development of these skills among learners and practitioners and should provide both formal training and opportunities for all team members to develop leadership capability and capacity.

References

1. American Society of Health-System Pharmacists. ASHP statement on professionalism. *Am J Health-Syst Pharm.* 2022; 79:1612–1616.
2. American Society of Health-System Pharmacists. ASHP statement on the roles and responsibilities of the pharmacy executive. *Am J Health-Syst Pharm.* 2021; 79:497–499.
3. Holdford DA. Leadership theories and their lessons for pharmacists. *Am J Health-Syst Pharm.* 2003; 60:1780–1786.
4. Nahata MC. Balancing leadership and management. *Am J Pharm Educ.* 2001; 65:295–296.
5. American Society of Health-System Pharmacists. Report of the ASHP Task Force on Racial Diversity, Equity, and Inclusion. *Am J Health-Syst Pharm.* 2021; 78:903–906. doi.org/10.1093/ajhp/zxab078
6. White SJ. Will there be a pharmacy leadership crisis? An ASHP Foundation Scholar-in-Residence report. *Am J Health-Syst Pharm.* 2005; 62:845–55.
7. Kerr RA, Beck DE, Doss J et al. Building a sustainable system of leadership development for pharmacy: report of the 2008–09 Argus Commission. *Am J Pharm Educ.* 2009; 73(suppl):S5.
8. ASHP Practice Advancement Initiative 2030: New recommendations for advancing pharmacy practice in health systems. *Am J Health-Syst Pharm.* 2020; 77:113–121.

Additional Resources

American Society of Health-System Pharmacists. ASHP statement on advocacy as a professional obligation. *Am J Health-Syst Pharm.* 2019; 76:251–4.

American Society of Health-System Pharmacists. Section of Pharmacy Practice Leaders. https://www.ashp.org/pharmacy-practice-leadership

American Society of Health-System Pharmacists. Leadership Resource Center. https://www.ashp.org/pharmacy-practice/resource-centers/leadership

ASHP Foundation Pharmacy Leadership Academy.® https://www.ashpfoundation.org/leadership-development/pharmacy-leadership-academy

American Society of Health-System Pharmacists. Pharmacy Leadership Certificate: Management Basics. https://elearning.ashp.org/products/10194/pharmacy-leadership-management-basics-certificate

ASHP Practitioner Recognition Program. https://www.ashp.org/about-ashp/awards/board-of-directors-awards/ashp-fellows

The American Society of Health-System Pharmacists accredits pharmacy residency training programs in the following topic areas:

- Community-Based Pharmacy Administration and Leadership
- Corporate Pharmacy Administration and Leadership
- Health System Pharmacy Administration and Leadership
- Pharmacy Administration and Leadership with Masters (Community; Health-System; Specialty)
- Specialty Pharmacy Administration and Leadership

Additional Information

Developed through the ASHP Council on Pharmacy Management and approved by the ASHP Board of Directors on February 28, 2023, and by the ASHP House of Delegates on May 18, 2023. This statement supersedes the ASHP Statement on Leadership as a Professional Obligation dated June 12, 2011.

Acknowledgments

The contributions of Ashley Mains Espinosa, PharmD, MS, CPHIMS, FASHP, and David R. Witmer, PharmD, to the previous version of this statement are gratefully acknowledged.

Authors

Ashley Mains Espinosa, PharmD, MS, CPHIMS, FASHP, DocStation, Denver, CO

Arpit Mehta, PharmD, MPH, MHA, Allegheny Health Network, Pittsburgh, PA

Tara Behring Vlasimsky, PharmD, BCACP, BCPS, FASHP, Intermountain Health, Denver, CO

Disclosures

The authors have declared no potential conflicts of interest.

Copyright © 2023, American Society of Health-System Pharmacists, Inc. All rights reserved.

Note: This statement had not been published in the *American Journal of Health-System Pharmacy (AJHP)* when *Best Practices for Hospital & Health-System Pharmacy 2023-2024* went to press. Some minor editorial difference may exist between this document and the official one that will eventually appear in *AJHP* and subsequent editions of this publication.

ASHP Statement on Pharmacist's Decision-making on Assisted Suicide

Preamble

Consistent with the intent of the Code of Ethics for Pharmacists "to state publicly the principles that form the fundamental basis of the roles and responsibilities of pharmacists," the American Society of Health-System Pharmacists issues this Statement on Pharmacist Decision-making on Assisted Suicide. The practice of providing competent patients with pharmaceutical means of ending their lives raises issues of professional obligations to patients and to other professionals involved in patient care. We affirm the ASHP policy (9802) that supports the right of a pharmacist to participate or not in morally, religiously, or ethically troubling therapies.

This Statement establishes a framework for pharmacist participation in the legal and ethical debate about the appropriate care of patients at the end of life. This Statement will help pharmacists resolve the growing questions about the ethical obligations of health care professionals to provide care and alleviate suffering. It is hoped that this framework and its use by pharmacists will virtually eliminate a patient's request for assisted suicide.

When asked to evaluate and comment on legislative, regulatory, or judicial actions or on organizational policies of health systems regarding pharmaceutical care, pharmacists should use the principles expressed in this Statement in developing their responses.

Guiding Principles

Professional Tradition. The basic tenet of the profession is to provide care and affirm life. The pharmacy profession is founded on a tradition of patient trust. The trust developed between each patient and members of the health care team makes it important for each professional to examine the moral and ethical issues of patients' requests for assistance in dying. Pharmacists should serve as advocates for the patient throughout the continuum of care.

Respect for Patients. *Patient autonomy.* Pharmacists should ensure the rights of competent patients to know about all legally available treatment options while communicating to patients and their caregivers (including family members if appropriate) the overall duty of health care professionals to preserve life.

Confidentiality. Pharmacists should maintain the confidentiality of all patient information, regardless of whether they agree with the values underlying the patient's choice of treatment or decision to forgo any particular treatment.

Decision-making. Patients' ability to exercise their ethical and legal right to choose or decline treatment is dependent upon pharmacists informing patients and their health care providers about the nature of pharmaceutical options. Those options are constantly changing, given the dynamic aspect of the pharmaceutical marketplace and the evolving nature of hospice care and available palliative treatments.

Health Care Systems. *Collaboration.* Collaboration among members of the health care team must occur at both the patient care and the public policy levels. It is the pharmacist's responsibility to educate members of the health care team about the pharmacotherapeutic options available in treating the patient's condition. Health care team members include the patient, members of the patient's family, and caregivers.

Confidentiality. The patient's right of confidentiality and right to determine his or her therapy, including end-of-life decisions, shall be respected, included, and considered in the decision process in health care systems. Pharmacists should maintain the confidentiality of all patient information, regardless of whether they agree with the values underlying the patient's choice of treatment or decision to forgo any particular treatment.

Covenant with society. Health care is delivered in a system in which each profession makes a contribution on the patient's behalf. An act in one part of the system has consequences in other parts of that system. Each profession has a covenant with society, founded on a relationship of trust with the patient. The trust developed between each patient and members of the health care team makes it important for each professional to examine the moral and ethical issues of patients' requests for assistance in dying.

Barriers to care. Health care professionals must address the following barriers to adequate end-of-life care:

1. Inadequate knowledge and use of pain- and symptom-management therapies.
2. The paucity of published data related to the ingestion of lethal drugs and the outcomes thereof.
3. Insufficient education of health care professionals about end-of-life and palliative care issues.
4. Inadequate recognition that end-of-life care is the responsibility of the entire health care team.
5. Legal and regulatory issues that deter appropriate provision of pain and symptom management.

Professional Obligations. *Conscientious objection.* Pharmacists must retain their right to participate or not in morally, religiously, or ethically troubling therapies. Procedures should be in place to ensure that employers are able to provide care to the patient and provide adequate services to the patient and caregiver. The employer has specific responsibilities, and the employee cannot be a barrier to the employer's ability to fulfill those obligations. Employers must reasonably accommodate the employee pharmacist's right to not participate in morally, religiously, or ethically troubling therapies.

Obligation to the patient. Pharmacists should support appropriate drug therapy to ensure that palliative care and aggressive pain management are available for all patients in need. Pharmacists, as part of their professional responsibility, must offer to provide counseling services to the patient and caregivers and be prepared to provide pharmaceutical care to the patient until the end of life.

Obligation to team members. The pharmacist, as a member of a health care team responsible for the care of a patient, is accountable for providing the team members with detailed information concerning efficacious use of pharmaceutical and other therapies available that may affect the options open to the patient.

DOI 10.37573/9781585287048.034

As active members of an interdisciplinary team caring for patients, pharmacists must be central participants in all decisions relating to medication management of the patient. Pharmacists should respect the opinions and specific areas of expertise of the other members of the health care team.

Pharmacist education. Pharmacists are often inadequately trained in the care of dying patients. Therefore, pharmacists' education at all levels (undergraduate, graduate, continuing education) should be sensitive to these issues and offer the development of skills and knowledge concerning care of the dying. Pharmacists should make a personal, professional commitment to learn more about end-of-life care.

Recommended Readings

Supreme Court Decisions

1. *Washington v. Glucksberg,* decided June 26, 1997.
2. *Vacco v. Quill,* decided June 26, 1977.
3. Angell M. The Supreme Court and physician-assisted suicide—the ultimate right. *N Engl J Med.* 1997; 336: 50–3.
4. Annas GJ. The bell tolls for a constitutional right to physician-assisted suicide. *N Engl J Med.* 1997; 337:1098–103.
5. Burt RA. The Supreme Court speaks: not assisted suicide but a constitutional right to palliative care. *N Engl J Med.* 1997; 337:1234–6.
6. Gostin LO. Deciding life and death in the courtroom: from *Quinlan to Cruzan, Glucksberg,* and *Vacco*—a brief history and analysis of constitutional protection of the "right to die" *JAMA* 1997; 278:1523–8.
7. Orentlicher D. The Supreme Court and physician-assisted suicide: rejecting assisted suicide but embracing euthanasia. *N Engl J Med.* 1997; 337:1236–9.
8. Palmer LI. Institutional analysis and physicians' rights after *Vacco v. Quill, Cornell J Law Public Policy.* 1998; 7:415–30.

Professional Organization Position Statements/Policies

1. American Bar Association house of delegates. Report of action taken at 1997 annual meeting.
2. American Pharmaceutical Association. Code of Ethics for Pharmacists.
3. American Pain Society. Treatment of pain at the end of life.
4. National League for Nursing. Life-terminating choices: a framework for nursing decision-making.
5. American Medical Association Policy on Physician-Assisted Suicide, 1996.
6. American Nurses Association. Position statement on assisted suicide.
7. American Geriatrics Society. Position statement on the care of dying patients.
8. National Hospice Organization.

Assisted Suicide

1. Dixon KM, Kier KL. Longing for mercy, requesting death: pharmaceutical care and pharmaceutically assisted death. *Am J Health-Syst Pharm.* 1998; 55:578–85.
2. Hamerly JP. Views on assisted suicide: perspectives of the AMA and the NHO. *Am J Health-Syst Pharm.* 1998; 55:543–7.
3. Lee BC. Views on assisted suicide: the aid-in-dying perspective. *Am J Health-Syst Pharm.* 1998; 55: 547–50.
4. Meier DE, Emmons CA, Wallenstein S et al. A national survey of physician-assisted suicide and euthanasia in the United States. *N Engl J Med.* 1998; 338: 1193–201.
5. Mullan K, Allen WL, Brushwood DB. Conscientious objection to assisted death: can pharmacy address this in a systematic fashion? *Ann Pharmacother.* 1996; 30:1185–91.
6. Rupp MT. Issues for pharmacists in assisted patient death. In: Battin MP, Lipman AG, eds. Drug use in assisted suicide and euthanasia. Binghamton, NY: Haworth; 1996.
7. Rupp MT. Physician-assisted suicide and the issues it raises for pharmacists. *Am J Health-syst Pharm.* 1995; 52:1455–60.
8. Rupp MT, Isenhower HL. Pharmacists' attitudes toward physician-assisted suicide. *Am J Hosp Pharm.* 1994; 51:69–74.
9. Stein GC. Assisted suicide: an issue for pharmacists. *Am J Health-Syst Pharm.* 1998; 55:539. Editorial.
10. Van der Maas PJ, van der Wal G, Haverkate I et al. Euthanasia, physician-assisted suicide, and other medical practices involving the end of life in the Netherlands, 1990–1995. *N Engl J Med.* 1996; 335:1699–705.
11. Van der Wal G, van der Maas PJ, Bosma JM et al. Evaluation of the notification procedure for physician-assisted death in the Netherlands. *N Engl J Med.* 1996; 335:1706–11.
12. Vaux KL. Views on assisted suicide: an ethicist's perspective. *Am J Health-Syst Pharm.* 1998; 55:551–3.

End-of-Life Care

1. Foley KM. Competent care for the dying instead of physician-assisted suicide. *N Engl J Med.* 1997; 336:54–8.
2. Quill TE, Lo B, Brock DW. Palliative options of last resort: a comparison of voluntarily stopping eating and drinking, terminal seda-tion, physician-assisted suicide, and voluntary active euthanasia. *JAMA.* 1997; 278:2099–104.
3. Suicide prevention: efforts to increase research and education in palliative care. Washington, DC: General Accounting Office, 1998 Apr; report HEHS-98-128.

Miscellaneous

1. Board of Directors report on the Council on Legal and Public Affairs, ASHP House of Delegates Session—1994.
2. Board of Directors report on the Council on Professional Affairs, ASHP House of Delegates Session—1998.
3. Board of Directors report on the Council on Legal and Public Affairs, ASHP House of Delegates Session—1998.

4. Statement of Attorney General Reno on Oregon's Death with Dignity Act. June 5, 1998.
5. Schnabel J, Schnabel G. Pharmacy information. In: Haley K, Lee M, eds. The Oregon Death With Dignity Act: A Guidebook for Health Care Providers. Portland: Oregon Health Sciences University, Center for Ethics in Health Care; 1998 Mar.

This statement was reviewed in 2013 by the Council on Pharmacy Practice and by the Board of Directors and was found to still be appropriate.

Approved by the ASHP Board of Directors, April 21, 1999, and by the ASHP House of Delegates, June 7, 1999. Developed by the Council on Legal and Professional Affairs.

Copyright © 1999, American Society of Health-System Pharmacists, Inc. All rights reserved. Contact ASHP for reprint and permissions requests. This content may not be used for commercial purposes without the express written consent of ASHP.

The bibliographic citation for this document is as follows: American Society of Health-System Pharmacists. ASHP statement on pharmacist's decision-making on assisted suicide. *Am J Health-Syst. Pharm.* 1999; 56:1661–4.

ASHP Statement on Professionalism

Position

Professionalism, achieved by consistent demonstration of core values and guiding principles to obtain desired health and wellness outcomes, must be embodied by the pharmacy workforce. The pharmacy workforce engaged in ASHP includes pharmacists, pharmacy residents, pharmacy interns, and pharmacy technicians and may include other nonpharmacist support staff (eg, data scientists, inventory specialists, department business managers) in acute and ambulatory care settings. The pharmacy workforce must fulfill the responsibilities that stem from their profession's guiding principles and professional oath. Among those responsibilities are advancing the well-being and dignity of patients, acting with high personal standards of integrity and competence, using shared decision-making among healthcare providers to improve patient engagement and empowerment, and seeking justice in the stewardship of healthcare resources. ASHP urges the pharmacy workforce to dedicate themselves to practice with compassion and respect for patients, caregivers, and colleagues. The pharmacy workforce should commit to serving humanity, creating an equitable and inclusive healthcare system and society, resolving conflicts in a professional manner, pursuing continuous professional development and leadership development, and engaging in professional associations and advocacy, as well as further developing analytical thinking and ethical reasoning, effective interpersonal skills, and personal well-being and resilience. All forms of discrimination (eg, on the basis of race, color, sex, national origin, religion, sexual orientation/identity, age, disability), harassment (including sexual harassment), and malicious behaviors such as bullying, intimidation, or exploitation go against the core beliefs of the profession. ASHP encourages the pharmacy workforce to advance patient care and strengthen the pharmacy profession by promoting and modeling professionalism in everyday practice across diverse settings, roles (eg, administrators, preceptors), and institutions. Pharmacists must provide person centered care through medication optimization, considering effectiveness, safety, costs, and each patient's specific factors and individual needs. The pharmacy workforce should partner with interprofessional healthcare teams across the continuum of care to improve access to high-quality healthcare and comprehensive medication management services for the communities in which they work and reside. ASHP encourages the pharmacy workforce to serve as role models (eg, mentors, advisors) to student pharmacists, residents, technicians, and colleagues in a manner that promotes the adoption of high professional aspirations for pharmacy practice and personal standards of integrity and competence. Organizations should nurture professionalism, communicate with transparency, deliver high-quality patient care by ensuring staff competency and expertise, and ensure patient safety in collaboration with the broader healthcare community.

Background

Instilling professionalism and fostering professional identity formation are continued areas of focus for the pharmacy workforce, as roles and practice models have evolved.[1,2] According to the Interprofessional Professionalism Collaborative (IPC), interprofessional professionalism is defined as "consistent demonstration of core values evidenced by professionals working together, aspiring to, and wisely applying principles of altruism and caring, excellence, ethics, respect, communication, and accountability to achieve optimal health and wellness in individuals and communities."[3]

Pharmacy is not the only profession fostering professionalism among its members. Professional associations from the American College of Physicians–American Society of Internal Medicine to the American College of Dentistry have convened task forces, developed white papers and charters, and initiated programs to increase the professionalism of their members.[4–10] The IPC that defined interprofessional professionalism represents 12 health professions' programs and one medical education assessment organization.[3]

Professionalism warrants continued emphasis because changes in healthcare delivery and society have the potential to erode the professional standards of healthcare providers.[4] Among the changes confronting the pharmacy profession are momentum to eliminate racial and ethnic disparities in healthcare and foster diversity, equity, and inclusion in healthcare and society[11]; expansion of the pharmacist's role in patient care[1]; and technology-driven changes in pharmacy's core responsibilities and communications.[1] With increased social media use blurring public and private personas, there is a need for professionalism in all forms of communication, which includes e-professionalism, or "the attitudes and behaviors reflecting traditional professionalism paradigms that are manifested through digital media."[12,13] Direct communication should be used to resolve perceived conflicts that may challenge the pharmacy workforce's ability to serve patients, teams, and the profession. As changes mount, it is in the best interest of our profession and the public we serve to reaffirm our foundational principles. The pharmacy workforce must therefore define for ourselves the principles that will guide us in our unique practice settings.

Guiding Principles and Responsibilities for the Pharmacy Workforce

The use of the term "profession" to describe a group of individuals pursuing an occupation or career is based on the idea that these individuals profess a common purpose.[14] The common purpose for pharmacists and pharmacy technicians surrounding the provision of patient care is eloquently stated in the Oath of a Pharmacist,[15] Code of Ethics for Pharmacists,[16] and Pharmacy Technician Code of Ethics.[17]

Professing these principles creates responsibilities for the pharmacy workforce. Foremost among these responsibilities is the obligation to place the well-being of patients at the center of pharmacy practice. Among the responsibilities

DOI 10.37573/9781585287048.035

listed in the codes of ethics, there is a clear foundation of principles that establish trust, including acting with honesty and integrity at all times and respecting the values and abilities of all colleagues and healthcare providers. There must be zero tolerance in the pharmacy profession for discrimination (eg, on the basis of race, color, sex, national origin, religion, sexual orientation/identity, age, disability), harassment (including sexual harassment), and malicious behaviors such as bullying, intimidation, and exploitation.[18,19]

Many of the other guiding principles flow from the pharmacy workforce's covenantal relationship with a patient. To provide the best possible patient care, the pharmacy workforce must dedicate themselves to maintaining professional competence through lifelong learning and self-assessment. Professional education and advancing standards of practice can only be achieved through a profession's collective efforts; the pharmacy workforce therefore commits themselves to serve not only their patients, but also their profession. Finally, the pharmacy workforce commits themselves to improving healthcare institutions not simply for the well-being of individual patients, but for the benefit of society as a whole.

Incorporating Professionalism into Practice

ASHP encourages the pharmacy workforce and institutions to incorporate into their practices the guiding principles set forth in the Oath of a Pharmacist and codes of ethics,[15–17] as well as other professional characteristics (**Figures 1 and 2**).[8–10]

Practicing and aspiring members of the pharmacy workforce should develop a personal plan for continuing professional development, encourage their colleagues to do the same, and share the results. Professional development should be viewed as an opportunity to enhance one's practice and contribute to the advancement of the pharmacy profession, rather than an obligation to be fulfilled in the most expedient manner.

One fundamental tenet of a professional is recruiting, nurturing, and shaping new practitioners to that profession's ideals and mission.[20] In fact, professional identity formation or internalizing a profession's core values and beliefs can be a means to professionalization.[2,21] Pharmacy workforce curricula should address professional identity formation and professional behaviors. Additionally, the pharmacy workforce needs to prevent "inconsistent socialization," through which the principles of professionalism instilled in students and trainees are undermined by a lack of professionalism in the role models they encounter when they enter practice.[22] Pharmacy departments can avoid inconsistent socialization by promoting a culture of professionalism in the workplace through personnel recruitment and evaluation systems that emphasize professional development.[22] Regardless of the level of support they receive, however, the pharmacy workforce must commit themselves fully to their mentorship responsibilities.

ASHP urges the pharmacy workforce to serve as mentors to students, trainees, and colleagues in a manner that fosters the adoption of high professional aspirations for pharmacy practice, high personal standards of integrity and competence, a commitment to serve humanity, habits of analytical thinking and ethical reasoning, and a commitment to lifelong learning. Practice sites should designate preceptors, implement preceptor training programs, encourage preceptor adherence to the highest professional standards, solicit student and resident feedback on preceptorship, and reward high-performing preceptors.[7] Institutions should also explore ways to promote mentorship relationships among staff as well as continuous open feedback and self-reflection. ASHP encourages the pharmacy workforce, particularly new practitioners, to actively seek mentors.

To make practice sites more conducive to professional behavior, institutions can develop personnel recruitment, orientation, and evaluation systems that encourage continuing professional development and promote well-being.[23] Additionally, the pharmacy workforce can advance the cause of professionalism in healthcare by reinvigorating the mission development processes of their institutions, encouraging those institutions to revise their mission statements to describe how they will address such ethical issues as the treatment of patients, employees, and staff; institutions' responsibilities to their communities, to other institutions, and to their own futures; the need to honor founding traditions and sustaining principles; and the complex interactions of legal and ethical responsibilities and their obligations to meet legislatively and socially defined needs.[24]

In 1976, Anderson called on hospital pharmacists to "create a code that reflects our relationships with all of the different people and conditions under which we practice."[20] The time has come for the pharmacy workforce to join forces with other healthcare providers and patients to engage what has been called "the new authorities of healthcare" to attain the kind of healthcare system our patients deserve and our society demands.[24]

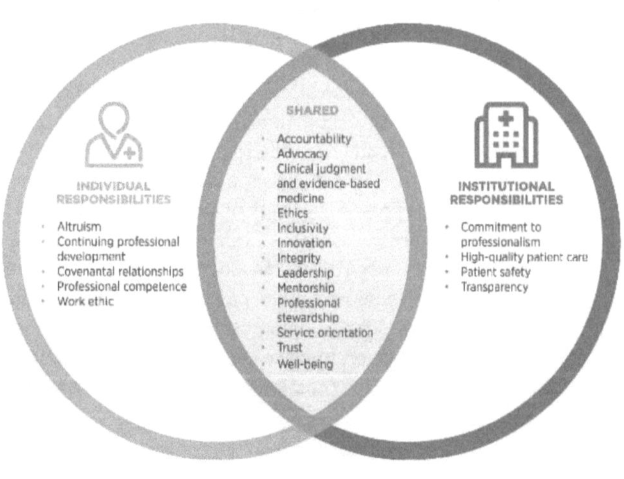

FIGURE 1. Individual, shared, and institutional professionalism responsibilities.

Conclusion

The pharmacy profession's guiding principles are described in the Oath of a Pharmacist,[15] Code of Ethics for Pharmacists,[16] and the Pharmacy Technician Code of Ethics.[17] As healthcare and society evolve, the pharmacy workforce must reaffirm the responsibilities that stem from their profession's guiding principles.

FIGURE 2. Description of individual, shared, and institutional professionalism responsibilities.

INDIVIDUAL RESPONSIBILITIES

- **Altruism:** Embrace selfless concern for the well-being of others
- **Continuing professional development:** Commit to continuing professional development to enhance one's professional practice
- **Covenantal relationships:** Value the patient-provider relationship
- **Professional competence:** Maintain knowledge, skills, and abilities
- **Work ethic:** Approach tasks with discipline, diligence, and hard work

SHARED RESPONSIBILITIES

- **Accountability:** Accept responsibility in accordance with the professional values
- **Advocacy:** Champion advocacy and professional advancement for safe and effective patient care
- **Clinical judgment and evidence-based medicine:** Incorporate clinical judgement and evidence-based medicine into therapeutic decision-making
- **Ethics:** Act in a manner guided by conscience
- **Inclusivity:** Promote a just health care system that values diversity, equity, and inclusion
- **Innovation:** Advance the profession through transformational practices
- **Integrity:** Exhibit high personal standards
- **Leadership:** Influence others with unquestionable integrity
- **Mentorship:** Serve as a professional role model
- **Professional stewardship:** Nurture the profession and pharmacy workforce
- **Service orientation:** Meet the needs of others
- **Trust:** Cultivate with honesty, consistency, and competency
- **Well-being:** Promote a culture of wellness

INSTITUTIONAL RESPONSIBILITIES

- **Commitment to professionalism:** Commit to professionalism as a core organizational value
- **High-quality patient care:** Commit to safe and effective, equitable patient care
- **Patient safety:** Ensure fail-safe medication use
- **Transparency:** Communicate with a culture of clarity and trust

References

1. ASHP Practice Advancement Initiative 2030: new recommendations for advancing pharmacy practice in health systems. *Am J Health-Syst Pharm.* 2020;77(2):113–121. doi:10.1093/ajhp/zxz271
2. ASHP policy 2129, professional identity formation. In: Hawkins B, ed. *Best Practices: Positions and Guidance Documents of ASHP.* 2020–2021 ed. American Society of Health-System Pharmacists; 2021. Accessed August 19, 2021. http://www.ashp.org/Pharmacy-Practice/Policy-Positions-and-Guidelines/Browse-by-Document-Type/Policy-Positions
3. Frost JS, Hammer DP, Nunez LM, et al. The intersection of professionalism and interprofessional care: development and initial testing of the interprofessional professionalism assessment (IPA). *J Interprof Care.* 2019;33(1):102–115.
4. ABIM Foundation, ACP–ASIM Foundation, and European Federation of Internal Medicine. Medical professionalism in the new millennium: a physician charter. *Ann Intern Med.* 2002;136:243–246.
5. Yeager AL. Dental ethics for the 21st century: learning from the Charter on Medical Professionalism. *J Am Coll Dent.* 2002;69:53–60.

6. Popp RL, Smith SC Jr. Cardiovascular professionalism and ethics in the modern era. *J Am Coll Cardiol.* 2004;44:1722–1723.
7. American Society of Health-System Pharmacists. 2001 ASHP Leadership Conference on Pharmacy Practice Management executive summary. From management to leadership: the building blocks of professionalism. *Am J Health-Syst Pharm.* 2002;59:661–665.
8. American Pharmaceutical Association Academy of Students of Pharmacy—American Association of Colleges of Pharmacy Council of Deans Task Force on Professionalism. White paper on pharmacy student professionalism. *J Am Pharm Assoc.* 2000;40:96–102.
9. Popovich NG, Hammer DP, Hansen DJ, et al. Report of the AACP Professionalism Task Force, May 2011. *Am J Pharm Educ.* 2011;75(10):S4.
10. American College of Clinical Pharmacy. Tenets of professionalism. Commentary. *Pharmacotherapy.* 2009;29(6):757–759.
11. Report of the ASHP Task Force on Racial Diversity, Equity, and Inclusion. Published January 2021. Accessed August 19, 2021. https://www.ashp.org/-/media/assets/about-ashp/docs/DEI-Task-Force-Recommendations.ashx
12. Cain J, Romanelli F. E-professionalism: a new paradigm for a digital age. *Curr Pharm Teach Learn.* 2009;1:66–70.
13. Chisholm-Burns MA, Spivey CA, Jaeger MC, et al. Development of an instrument to measure pharmacy student attitudes toward social media professionalism. *Am J Pharm Educ.* 2017;81(4):65.
14. Knowlton CH, Penna RP. *Pharmaceutical Care.* 2nd ed. American Society of Health-System Pharmacists; 2003:4.
15. Oath of a Pharmacist. Developed by the American Pharmaceutical Association Academy of Students of Pharmacy/American Association of Colleges of Pharmacy Council of Deans (APhA-ASP/AACP-COD) Task Force on Professionalism, June 26, 1994. Revised November 2021. Accessed August 19, 2021. https://www.pharmacist.com/About/Oath-of-a-Pharmacist
16. Code of ethics for pharmacists. In: Hawkins B, ed. *Best Practices: Positions and Guidance Documents of ASHP.* 2020–2021 ed. American Society of Health-System Pharmacists; 2021. Accessed August 19, 2021. www.ashp.org/Pharmacy-Practice/Policy-Positions-and-Guidelines/Browse-by-Document-Type/Policy-Positions
17. American Association of Pharmacy Technicians. Pharmacy technician code of ethics. Published January 1996. Accessed August 19, 2021. https://www.pharmacytechnician.com/pharmacy-technician-code-of-ethics/
18. ASHP policy 2131, zero tolerance of harassment, discrimination, and malicious behaviors. In: Hawkins B, ed. *Best Practices: Positions and Guidance Documents of ASHP.* 2020–2021 ed. American Society of Health-System Pharmacists; 2021. Accessed August 19, 2021. www.ashp.org/Pharmacy-Practice/Policy-Positions-and-Guidelines/Browse-by-Document-Type/Policy-Positions
19. Bissell BD, Johnston JP, Smith RR, et al. Gender inequity and sexual harassment in the pharmacy profession: Evidence and call to action. *Am J Health-Syst Pharm.* 2021;78:2059–2076.
20. Anderson RD. 1976 Harvey A.K. Whitney lecture: the peril of deprofessionalization. *Am J Hosp Pharm.* 1977;34:133–139. Reprinted in *Am J Health-Syst Pharm.* 2004;61:2373–2379.
21. Mylrea MF, Gupta TS, Glass BD. Professionalization in pharmacy education as a matter of identity. *Am J Pharm Educ.* 2015;79(9):142.
22. Manasse HR Jr, Stewart JE, Hall RH. Inconsistent socialization in pharmacy—a pattern in need of change. *J Am Pharm Assoc.* 1975;15:616–621, 658.
23. Hammer DP, Berger BA, Beardsley RS, et al. Student professionalism. *Am J Pharm Educ.* 2003;63:1–29.
24. Reiser SJ, Banner RS. The Charter on Medical Professionalism and the limits of medical power. *Ann Intern Med.* 2003;138:844–846.

Developed through the ASHP Council on Education and Workforce Development and approved by the ASHP Board of Directors on January 20, 2022, and by the ASHP House of Delegates on March 25, 2022. This statement supersedes a previous version dated June 26, 2007.

The authors have declared no potential conflicts of interest.

Angela L. Bingham, PharmD, BCPS, BCNSP, BCCCP, FASPEN, FCCP, FASHP, Philadelphia College of Pharmacy, Philadelphia, PA.

Seena L. Haines, PharmD, BCACP, CHWC, FAPhA, FCCP, FASHP, FNAP, RYT 500, University of Mississippi Medical Center, Jackson, MS, and University of Mississippi School of Pharmacy, Jackson, MS.

Jenna Summerlin, PharmD, Johns Hopkins All Children's Hospital, St. Petersburg, FL.

Carol Heunisch, PharmD, BCPS, BCCP, NorthShore University HealthSystem, Skokie, IL.

Copyright © 2022, American Society of Health-System Pharmacists, Inc. All rights reserved. Contact ASHP for reprint and permissions requests. This content may not be used for commercial purposes without the express written consent of ASHP.

The bibliographic citation for this document is as follows: Bingham AL, Haines SL, Summerlin J, Heunisch C. ASHP statement on professionalism. *Am J Health-Syst Pharm.* 2022; 79(18):1612–1616.

ASHP Guidelines on Pharmacists' Relationships with Industry

In the practice of their profession, pharmacists should be guided only by the consideration of patient care. Pharmacists should neither accept nor retain anything of value that has the potential to affect materially their ability to exercise judgments solely in the interests of patients. A useful criterion in determining acceptable activities and relationships is this: Would the pharmacist be willing to have these relationships generally known? Notwithstanding this responsibility, pharmacists may benefit from guidance in their relationships with industry. To this end, the following suggestions are offered.

Gifts and Hospitality

Gifts, hospitality, or subsidies offered to pharmacists by industry should not be accepted if acceptance might influence, or appear to others to influence, the objectivity of clinical judgment or drug product selection and procurement.

Continuing Education

Providers of continuing education that accept industry funding for programs should develop and enforce policies to maintain complete control of program content.

Subsidies to underwrite the costs of continuing-education conferences, professional meetings, or staff development programs can contribute to the improvement of patient care and are permissible. Payments to defray the costs of a conference should not be accepted directly or indirectly from industry by pharmacists attending the conference or program. Contributions to special or educational funds for staff development are permissible as long as the selection of staff members who will receive the funds is made by the department of pharmacy.

It is appropriate for faculty at conferences or meetings to accept reasonable honoraria and reimbursement for reasonable travel, lodging, and meal expenses. However, direct subsidies from industry should not be accepted to pay the costs of travel, lodging, or other personal expenses of pharmacists attending conferences or meetings, nor should subsidies be accepted to compensate for the pharmacists' time.

Scholarships or other special funds to permit pharmacy students, residents, and fellows to attend carefully selected educational conferences may be permissible as long as the selection of students, residents, or fellows who will receive the funds is made by the academic or training institution.

Consultants and Advisory Arrangements

Consultants who provide genuine services for industry may receive reasonable compensation and accept reimbursement for travel, lodging, and meal expenses. Token consulting or advisory arrangements cannot be used to justify compensating pharmacists for their time, travel, lodging, and other out-of-pocket expenses.

Clinical Research

Pharmacists who participate in practice-based research of pharmaceuticals, devices, or other programs should conduct their activities in accord with basic precepts of accepted scientific methodology. Practice-based drug studies that are, in effect, promotional schemes to entice the use of a product or program are unacceptable.

Disclosure of Information

To avoid conflicts of interest or appearances of impropriety, pharmacists should disclose consultant or speaker arrangements or substantial personal financial holdings with companies under consideration for formulary inclusion or related decisions. To inform audiences fully, speakers and authors should disclose, when pertinent, consultant or speaker and research funding arrangements with companies.

Additional Issues

The advice in this document is noninclusive and is not intended to limit the legitimate exchange of prudent scientific information.

This guideline was reviewed in 2001 by the Council on Legal and Public Affairs and by the ASHP Board of Directors and was found to still be appropriate.

Approved by the ASHP Board of Directors, November 20, 1991. Developed by the ASHP Council on Legal and Public Affairs.

The language used in many of the guidance issues contained in this document was adapted, with permission, from documents developed by the American Medical Association (*JAMA*. 1991; 265:501) and the American College of Physicians (*Ann Intern Med.* 1990; 112:624–6).

Copyright © 1992, American Society of Hospital Pharmacists, Inc. All rights reserved. Contact ASHP for reprint and permissions requests. This content may not be used for commercial purposes without the express written consent of ASHP.

The bibliographic citation for this document is as follows: American Society of Hospital Pharmacists. ASHP guidelines on pharmacists' relationships with industry. *Am J Hosp Pharm.* 1992; 49:154.

DOI 10.37573/9781585287048.036

Code of Ethics for Pharmacists

Preamble

Pharmacists are health professionals who assist individuals in making the best use of medications. This Code, prepared and supported by pharmacists, is intended to state publicly the principles that form the fundamental basis of the roles and responsibilities of pharmacists. These principles, based on moral obligations and virtues, are established to guide pharmacists in relationships with patients, health professionals, and society.

Principles

I. ***A pharmacist respects the covenantal relationship between the patient and pharmacist.***

Interpretation: Considering the patient-pharmacist relationship as a covenant means that a pharmacist has moral obligations in response to the gift of trust received from society. In return for this gift, a pharmacist promises to help individuals achieve optimum benefit from their medications, to be committed to their welfare, and to maintain their trust.

II. ***A pharmacist promotes the good of every patient in a caring, compassionate, and confidential manner.***

Interpretation: A pharmacist places concern for the well-being of the patient at the center of professional practice. In doing so, a pharmacist considers needs stated by the patient as well as those defined by health science. A pharmacist is dedicated to protecting the dignity of the patient. With a caring attitude and a compassionate spirit, a pharmacist focuses on serving the patient in a private and confidential manner.

III. ***A pharmacist respects the autonomy and dignity of each patient.***

Interpretation: A pharmacist promotes the right of self-determination and recognizes individual self-worth by encouraging patients to participate in decisions about their health. A pharmacist communicates with patients in terms that are understandable. In all cases, a pharmacist respects personal and cultural differences among patients.

IV. ***A pharmacist acts with honesty and integrity in professional relationships.***

Interpretation: A pharmacist has a duty to tell the truth and to act with conviction of conscience. A pharmacist avoids discriminatory practices, behavior or work conditions that impair professional judgment, and actions that compromise dedication to the best interests of patients.

V. ***A pharmacist maintains professional competence.***

Interpretation: A pharmacist has a duty to maintain knowledge and abilities as new medications, devices, and technologies become available and as health information advances.

VI. ***A pharmacist respects the values and abilities of colleagues and other health professionals.***

Interpretation: When appropriate, a pharmacist asks for the consultation of colleagues or other health professionals or refers the patient. A pharmacist acknowledges that colleagues and other health professionals may differ in the beliefs and values they apply to the care of the patient.

VII. ***A pharmacist serves individual, community, and societal needs.***

Interpretation: The primary obligation of a pharmacist is to individual patients. However, the obligations of a pharmacist may at times extend beyond the individual to the community and society. In these situations, the pharmacist recognizes the responsibilities that accompany these obligations and acts accordingly.

VIII. ***A pharmacist seeks justice in the distribution of health resources.***

Interpretation: When health resources are allocated, a pharmacist is fair and equitable, balancing the needs of patients and society.

The endorsement of this document was reviewed in 2017 by the Council on Pharmacy Practice and by the Board of Directors and was found to still be appropriate.

Copyright © 1994, American Society of Health-System Pharmacists, Inc. All rights reserved. Contact ASHP for reprint and permissions requests. This content may not be used for commercial purposes without the express written consent of ASHP.

Endorsed by the American Society of Health-System Pharmacists House of Delegates on June 3, 1996 (ASHP Policy 9607). Proceedings of the 47th annual session of the ASHP House of Delegates. *Am J Health-Syst Pharm.* 1996; 53:1805. ASHP Reports.

DOI 10.37573/9781585287048.037

Formulary Management

(Medication-Use Policy Development)

DOI 10.37573/9781585287048

Formulary Management

2308

PHARMACOGENOMICS

Source: Council on Therapeutics

To advocate that pharmacists take a leadership role in pharmacogenomics-related patient testing, based on current or anticipated medication therapy; further,

To advocate for the inclusion of pharmacogenomic test results in medical and pharmacy records in a format that clearly states the implications of the results for drug therapy and facilitates availability of the genetic information throughout the continuum of care and over a patient's lifetime; further,

To encourage health systems to support an interprofessional, evidenced-based effort to implement appropriate pharmacogenomics services and to identify and determine appropriate dissemination of actionable information to appropriate healthcare providers for review; further,

To encourage pharmacists to educate prescribers and patients about the use of pharmacogenomic tests and their appropriate application to drug therapy management; further,

To advocate that all health insurance policies provide coverage for pharmacogenomic testing to optimize patient care; further,

To advocate that drug product manufacturers and researchers conduct and report outcomes of pharmacogenomic research to facilitate safe and effective use of medications; further,

To encourage research into the economic and clinical impact of preemptive pharmacogenomic testing; further,

To encourage pharmacy workforce education on the use of pharmacogenomics and its application to therapeutic decision-making.

This policy supersedes ASHP policy 2113.

Rationale

Clinical pharmacogenomics is the practice of using genetic information to guide optimal drug selection and drug dosing for patients to maximize therapeutic effects, improve outcomes, and minimize toxicity. Currently, pharmacogenomic testing is used for specific drug-gene pairs in patients currently taking a medication associated with a gene or prior to initiating therapy. Pharmacists are especially prepared to take a leadership role in selecting appropriate tests as they have an understanding of pharmacokinetic and pharmacodynamics properties of drugs in specific diseases and patient populations.

Over the past 10 years, the Clinical Pharmacogenetics Implementation Consortium (CPIC) has published over 23 guidelines that cover 19 genes and 46 drugs across several therapeutic areas as well as resources to facilitate the implementation of pharmacogenomics into routine clinical practice and the electronic health record. These guidelines include indications for which drugs and genes are most likely to be clinically useful based on current evidence. However, barriers such as prioritizing testing, interpretation for actionable results, incorporation of genomic data into the electronic health record, and reimbursement remain. Furthermore, there is also the challenge of how to ensure that the results of pharmacogenomic tests stay with the patient throughout their health journey. Implementation of pharmacogenomic testing has the potential to improve patient care by decreasing failed treatment attempts due to medication ineffectiveness or adverse effects and by increasing effectiveness of improperly dosed medications.

The advent of widely available pharmacogenomic tests, many of which are also marketed to the public, introduces another layer of complexity. The Food and Drug Administration (FDA) has alerted patients and healthcare providers that claims for many genetic tests to predict a patient's response to specific medications have not been reviewed by the FDA and may not have the scientific or clinical evidence to support their use. Changing drug treatment based on the results from such a test could lead to inappropriate treatment decisions and potentially serious health consequences for the patient. It is imperative to identify clinically significant drug-gene pairs, as these may prevent adverse events, and such identification should be performed preemptively, as with DPYD genotyping prior to starting patients on fluoropyrimidines. There may also be a role for the FDA to provide incentives for manufacturers to conduct pharmacogenomic testing to optimize drug-gene patient paring.

Another barrier that many providers and patients encounter is insurance coverage of pharmacogenomic testing. A 2019 JAPhA article found that coverage and payments of pharmacogenomics varied by the company and gene-drug pairs and remain suboptimal. The article found that, of gene-drug indication group (GDIG), 50% were mentioned in policies but were covered less than 20% of the time. When mentioned in a policy, 7 GDIGs were uniformly covered, and 11 GDIGs were uniformly not covered. Overall, insurance companies covered approximately 40% of GDIGs mentioned in their policies. Additionally, preemptive pharmacogenomics suffers from a lack of economic and outcomes data supporting its more widespread adoption into practice. Such data would provide impetus for reimbursement from third-party payers. The number of genes tested in preemptive testing is typically greater than for reactive testing, meaning the number of actionable pharmacotherapeutic interventions made will increase. To ensure a sustainable preemptive pharmacogenomic testing system, clinical decision support is crucial for the implementation of evidence-based treatment decisions because it will become less feasible for a clinician specializing in pharmacogenomics to provide a recommendation for each pharmacogenomically actionable medication.

Furthermore, the ASHP Statement on the Pharmacist's Role in Clinical Pharmacogenomics states that pharmacogenomics has an essential place in pharmacy education because pharmacists should be educated to be able to recommend pharmacogenomic testing for drug and dosage selection; design patient-specific drug and dose regimens based on the patient's pharmacogenomic profile and other pertinent information; educate patients, pharmacists, and other healthcare professionals about pharmacogenomic principles and appropriate indications for clinical pharmacogenomic testing; and communicate pharmacogenomic-specific drug therapy recommendations to the healthcare team.

DOI 10.37573/9781585287048.038

2016

MEDICATION FORMULARY SYSTEM MANAGEMENT

Source: Council on Pharmacy Management

To declare that decisions on the management of a medication formulary system, including criteria for use, (1) should be based on clinical, ethical, legal, social, philosophical, quality-of-life, safety, comparative effectiveness, and pharmacoeconomic factors that result in optimal patient care; (2) must include the active and direct involvement of physicians, pharmacists, and other appropriate healthcare professionals; and (3) should not be based solely on economic factors; further,

To support the concept of a standardized medication formulary system among components of integrated health systems when standardization leads to improved patient outcomes; further,

To oppose independent payer-directed formulary decisions that would increase the complexity of the medication-use system.

This policy supersedes ASHP policies 9601 and 1805.

Rationale

A formulary is a continually updated list of medications and related information, representing the clinical judgment of pharmacists, physicians, and other experts in the diagnosis and treatment of disease and promotion of health. A formulary includes, but is not limited to, a list of medications, standardized medication concentrations, and medication associated products or devices, medication-use policies, important ancillary drug information, decision-support tools, and organizational guidelines. The multiplicity of medications available, the complexities surrounding their safe and effective use, and differences in their relative value make it necessary for healthcare organizations to have medication-use policies that promote rational, evidence-based, clinically appropriate, safe, and cost-effective medication therapy. The formulary system is the ongoing process through which a healthcare organization establishes policies on the use of drugs, therapies, and drug-related products and identifies those that are most medically appropriate and cost-effective to best serve the health interests of a given patient population.

As described in more detail in the ASHP Statement on the Pharmacy and Therapeutics Committee and the Formulary System, a fundamental characteristic of the formulary system is that all decisions are made based on factors that result in optimal patient care, include the involvement of appropriate healthcare professionals, and are not based solely on economic factors.

Formulary management techniques may differ under an integrated or network system versus an individual healthcare entity. Standardized drug formularies within integrated health systems increase coordination complexity, but help drive standardized medication use processes across sites of care.

Additionally, insurance coverage of medications should not interfere with the safe and effective provision of care. For example, some hospitals are currently being forced to administer a specific payer-preferred biosimilar drug to a covered patient, which requires hospitals to stock a different product for each payer and then ensure the correct one is dispensed. This costly and resource-intensive practice also has medication safety implications and negatively affects supply chain efficiency. Biosimilar drugs are considered to be therapeutically equivalent, but the current Food and Drug Administration (FDA) approval process does not include a determination of interchangeability between reference and biosimilar products. Because the substitution of a biosimilar for a reference product is a decision outside the FDA regulatory process, it is therefore a matter of state pharmacy law. The obligation to have a specific payer-preferred biosimilar results in hospitals and health systems devoting significant resources to procure, store, label, and dispense payer-preferred biosimilars. This duplication adds complexity to the medication-use process, and as more biosimilars become available, the potential for harmful medication errors will increase. The use of biosimilars was a key cost-reduction concept in the Affordable Care Act. However, in May 2018, the price linkage cost-reduction concept within Medicare Part B was rescinded. Going forward, reimbursement will be based on the specific biosimilar product pricing. The full impact of this change for individual healthcare organizations will depend on patient and payer mix. Biosimilars that are priced at a lower acquisition cost compared to the innovator product are likely to stagnate or lose market share due to a low reimbursement margin. As a result, pricing of biosimilars may increase to make the reimbursement margin competitive with the innovator product, leaving healthcare organizations in search of other cost reduction opportunities.

1802

GENE THERAPY

Source: Council on Pharmacy Management

To assert that health-system decisions on the selection, use, and management of gene therapy agents should be managed as part of the medication formulary system in that (1) decisions are based on clinical, ethical, legal, social, philosophical, quality-of-life, safety, comparative effectiveness , and pharmacoeconomic factors that result in optimal patient care; and (2) such decisions must include the active and direct involvement of physicians, pharmacists, and other appropriate healthcare professionals; further,

To advocate that gene therapy be documented in the permanent patient health record; further,

To advocate that documentation of gene therapy in the permanent patient health record accommodate documentation by all healthcare team members, including pharmacists.

This policy supersedes ASHP policy 0103.

This policy was reviewed in 2023 by the Council on Pharmacy Management and by the Board of Directors and was found to still be appropriate.

Rationale

Gene therapy is an emerging area of medicine, and pharmacists should take a leadership role in managing these therapies and associated devices under the medication formulary systems in their institutions.

As described in more detail in the ASHP Guidelines on the Pharmacy and Therapeutics Committee and the Formulary System, a fundamental characteristic of the formulary system is that all decisions are made based on factors that result in optimal patient care, include the involvement of appropriate healthcare professionals, and are not based solely on economic factors. Pharmacy should be integral in the development of procedures regarding storage, prescribing, dosing, preparation, labeling, dispensing, transport, and other challenges with clinical decision support tools when working with this medication class. It is important that gene therapy be documented in the permanent patient health record to ensure accurate and complete documentation of the care provided to patients and to validate the impact of therapies on patient outcomes and that all healthcare providers involved in providing gene therapy, including pharmacists, be able to document the patient care provided. This includes the ability for the pharmacist to verify the gene therapy product when use of free text entry or volumetric dosages with drug-specific protocols are utilized, to ensure the accuracy of the dose, product, and labeling.

1820

MEDICAL DEVICES

Source: Council on Public Policy

To advocate that the Food and Drug Administration (FDA) and manufacturers of drug preparation, drug distribution, and drug administration devices and associated new technologies ensure transparency, clarity, and evidence be provided on the intended use of devices and technologies in all phases of the medication-use process; further,

To advocate that the FDA and device manufacturers ensure compatibility between the intended use of any device and the drugs to be used with that device.

This policy supersedes ASHP policy 9106.

This policy was reviewed in 2023 by the Council on Public Policy and by the Board of Directors and was found to still be appropriate.

Rationale

The lines between devices, drugs, and technology are blurring as new and innovative technologies combine drugs and devices. Because drugs and medical devices undergo different approval processes, it is important that compatibility between the intended use of any device and the drugs to be used with that device be ensured during the approval process so that unintended and possibly detrimental consequences do not occur. In addition, clinicians require information about the intended use of devices in all phases of the medication-use process in order to make the best-informed decisions about patient care.

0817

GENERIC SUBSTITUTION OF NARROW THERAPEUTIC INDEX DRUGS

Source: Council on Therapeutics

To support the current processes used by the Food and Drug Administration (FDA) to determine bioequivalence of generic drug products, including those with a narrow therapeutic index, and to recognize the authority of the FDA to decide if additional studies are necessary to determine equivalence; further,

To oppose a blanket restriction on generic substitution for any medication or medication class without evidence from well-designed, independent studies that demonstrate inferior efficacy or safety of the generic drug product.

This policy was reviewed in 2020 by the Council on Therapeutics and by the Board of Directors and was found to still be appropriate.

8708

THERAPEUTIC INTERCHANGE

Source: Council on Legal and Public Affairs

To support the concept of therapeutic interchange of various drug products by pharmacists under arrangements where pharmacists and authorized prescribers interrelate on behalf of patient care.

This policy was reviewed in 2019 by the Council on Pharmacy Practice and by the Board of Directors and was found to still be appropriate.

ASHP Statement on the Use of Medications for Unlabeled Uses

The freedom and responsibility to make drug therapy decisions that are consistent with patient-care needs is a fundamental precept supported by ASHP. This activity is a professional duty of pharmacists not limited by language in Food and Drug Administration (FDA)-approved product labeling.

The prescribing, dispensing, and administration of FDA-approved drugs for uses, treatment regimens, or patient populations that are not reflected in FDA-approved product labeling often represent a therapeutic approach that has been extensively studied and reported in medical literature. Such uses are *not* indicative of inappropriate usage. Health-care professionals should appreciate the critical need for freedom in making drug therapy decisions and understand the implications of unlabeled uses. ASHP supports third-party reimbursement for FDA-approved drug products appropriately prescribed for unlabeled uses.

Definition of Unlabeled Use

The FDA approves drug products for marketing in the United States. Such a product approved for marketing is often termed an "FDA-approved drug." FDA also approves each drug product's labeling (container label, package insert, and certain advertising); the term "FDA-approved labeling" applies here. Drug uses that are not included in the indications or dosage regimens listed in the FDA-approved labeling are defined as "unlabeled uses." For purposes of this document, unlabeled use includes the use of a drug product in (1) doses, (2) patient populations, (3) indications, or (4) routes of administration that are not reflected in FDA-approved product labeling.

It is important to recognize that FDA cannot approve or disapprove physician prescribing practices of legally marketed drugs. FDA does regulate what manufacturers may recommend about uses in their products' labeling and what manufacturers can include in advertising and promotion.

The sometimes-used term "unapproved use" is a misnomer, implying that FDA regulates prescribing and dispensing activities. This term should be avoided.[1] Other terminology that is sometimes used to describe unlabeled use includes "off-label use," "out-of-label use," and "usage outside of labeling."

According to FDA, unlabeled use encompasses a range of situations that extend from inadequate to carefully conceived investigations, from hazardous to salutary uses, and from infrequent to widespread medical practice. Accepted medical practice often involves drug use that is not reflected in FDA-approved drug-product labeling.[2]

Health-Care Issues Related to Unlabeled Use

Access to Drug Therapies. The prescribing and dispensing of drugs for unlabeled uses are increasing.[3,4] In many clinical situations, unlabeled use represents the most appropriate therapy for patients. Failure to recognize this or, more importantly, regarding such use as "unapproved" or "experimental" may restrict access to necessary drug therapies.

Lack of Practice Standards. Well-defined medical practice standards that differentiate between experimental therapies and established practice will probably always be somewhat lacking, owing to the advancement of medical science and the dynamic nature of medical practice. Standards of practice for certain drug therapies, particularly biotechnologically produced drugs, cancer chemotherapy, and AIDS treatments, are continually evolving. The dynamic nature of these drug therapies makes it difficult for professional societies to review scientific data expediently and to develop standards that remain absolutely current.

Failure of Package Insert and FDA-Approved Labeling to Reflect Current Practice. For FDA-approved product labeling to be modified, scientific data must be submitted by a product's manufacturer to FDA to support any additional indication(s) and dosage regimen(s). Once they are submitted, FDA must review the data and make a decision to permit alteration of the package insert.

Knowing that unlabeled uses are permitted, and knowing that the accumulation and submission of scientific data to FDA to modify labeling is a time-consuming and often expensive process, some pharmaceutical manufacturers elect not to pursue labeling changes. Therefore, a product's labeling sometimes fails to represent the most current therapeutic information for a drug, and situations naturally occur when it is appropriate to prescribe drugs for unlabeled uses.

Pharmacist's Role

ASHP believes that pharmacists in organized health-care settings bear a significant responsibility for ensuring optimal outcomes from all drug therapy. With respect to unlabeled uses, the role of the pharmacist should be to

1. Fulfill the roles of patient advocate and drug information specialist.
2. Develop policies and procedures for evaluating drug orders (prescriptions) and dispensing drugs for unlabeled uses in their own work settings. Such policies and procedures might address the documentation of scientific support, adherence to accepted medical practice standards, or a description of medical necessity.
3. Develop proactive approaches to promote informed decisionmaking by third-party payers for health-care services.

Role of Drug Information Compendia

The Medicare Catastrophic Coverage Act of 1988 (now repealed) included the statements that "in carrying out the legislation, the Secretary [of Health and Human Services] shall establish standards for drug coverage. In establishing such standards, which are based on accepted medical practice, the Secretary shall incorporate standards from such current authoritative compendia as the Secretary may select."[5] Specific compendia recommended were the *AHFS Drug Information, AMA Drug Evaluations,* and *USP Dispensing*

DOI 10.37573/9781585287048.039

Information, Volume I. Despite the repeal of the Act, some third-party payers have adopted guidelines that endorse these three compendia as authoritative information sources with respect to unlabeled uses for drug products.

Positions on Unlabeled Use

FDA Position. A statement entitled "Use of Approved Drugs for Unlabeled Indications" was published in the *FDA Drug Bulletin* in April 1982 to address the issues of appropriateness and legality of prescribing approved drugs for uses not included in FDA's approved labeling. This statement included the following:

> The Food, Drug and Cosmetic Act does not limit the manner in which a physician may use an approved drug. Once a product has been approved for marketing, a physician may prescribe it for uses or in treatment regimens or patient populations that are not included in approved labeling. Such "unapproved" or, more precisely, "unlabeled" uses may be appropriate and rational in certain circumstances, and may, in fact, reflect approaches to drug therapy that have been extensively reported in medical literature.[1]

Other Organizations. Other organizations that have published positions on the issue of unlabeled uses of drug products are the Health Care Financing Administration (HCFA),[6] the Blue Cross and Blue Shield Association of America (BC/BS),[7] and the Health Insurance Association of America (HIAA).[8]

The American Medical Association, American Society of Clinical Oncology, Association of American Cancer Institutes, Association of Community Cancer Centers, Candlelighters Childhood Cancer Foundation, Memorial Sloan Kettering Cancer Center, National Cancer Institute, and the National Institute of Allergy and Infectious Diseases jointly developed a consensus statement and recommendations regarding use and reimbursement of unlabeled uses of drug products.[9]

These statements are consistent with the ASHP position.

Reimbursement Issues

As a cost-containment measure, most third-party payers exclude coverage for experimental therapies. Drug therapy coverage decisions are complicated, because often it is difficult to differentiate among an accepted standard of practice, an evolving standard of practice, and investigational therapies. Data demonstrating medical necessity and improved patient outcome are often difficult to retrieve. Consequently, insurance carriers and managed care providers have sometimes elected to cover only those indications included in FDA-approved drug-product labeling and have frequently denied coverage for unlabeled uses of drug products.

ASHP believes that such coverage denials restrict patients from receiving medically necessary therapies that represent the best available treatment options. A growing number of insurance carriers are following the BC/BS and HIAA guidelines that encourage the use of the three authoritative drug compendia, peer-reviewed literature, and consultation with experts in research and clinical practice to make specific coverage decisions. ASHP supports informed decisionmaking that promotes third-party reimbursement for FDA-approved drug products appropriately prescribed for unlabeled uses.

References

1. Use of approved drugs for unlabeled indications. *FDA Drug Bull.* 1982; 12:4–5.
2. Nightingale SL. Use of drugs for unlabeled indications. *FDA Q Rep.* 1986(Sep); 269.
3. Mortenson LE. Audit indicates many uses of combination therapy are unlabeled. *J Cancer Program Manage.* 1988; 3:21–5.
4. Off-label drugs: initial results of a national survey. Washington, DC: U.S. General Accounting Office. 1991:1–27.
5. PL 100-360, 1988.
6. Health Care Financing Administration. Medicare carriers' manual. Section 2050.5. Washington, DC: U.S. Department of Health and Human Services; 1987 Aug.
7. Statement on coverage recommendation for FDA-approved drugs. Chicago: Blue Cross and Blue Shield Association; 1989 Oct 25.
8. Statement of the Health Insurance Association of America (HIAA) on coverage for unapproved drugs and drug-related costs. Presented to the National Committee to Review Current Procedures for Approval of New Drugs for Cancer and AIDS. 1989 Oct 25.
9. Cancer economics. *Cancer Lett.* 1989; Suppl(Jun):2–3.

Approved by the ASHP Board of Directors, November 20, 1991, and by the ASHP House of Delegates, June 1, 1992. Developed by the Council on Professional Affairs.

Copyright © 1992, American Society of Hospital Pharmacists, Inc. All rights reserved. Contact ASHP for reprint and permissions requests. This content may not be used for commercial purposes without the express written consent of ASHP.

The bibliographic citation for this document is as follows: American Society of Hospital Pharmacists. ASHP statement on the use of medications for unlabeled uses. *Am J Hosp Pharm.* 1992; 49:2006–8.

ASHP Guidelines on Medication-Use Evaluation

Purpose

These guidelines describe essential elements of the medication-use evaluation (MUE) process for healthcare organizations. These elements include the goals and objectives of a MUE, performance improvement methods, a description of indicators suggesting the need for an MUE, how to prioritize and select medications and processes for evaluation, typical steps in the process, the roles and responsibilities of the interdisciplinary team, common problems and pitfalls, and useful resources.

Goals, Objectives, and Definitions of MUE

MUE is a systematic and interdisciplinary performance improvement method with an overarching goal of optimizing patient outcomes via ongoing evaluation and improvement of medication utilization.[1] Various terms have been employed to describe programs intended to achieve this goal; in addition to MUE, *drug use evaluation* (DUE) and *drug utilization review* (DUR) have also been used.[1-3] Although these terms are sometimes used interchangeably, MUE may be differentiated in that it emphasizes improving patient outcomes and quality of life through assessment of clinical outcomes via a multidisciplinary approach whereas DUE and DUR generally refer to an ongoing, systematic, criteria-based, drug- or disease-specific assessment that ensures appropriate medication utilization at the individual patient level.[3] Historically, the American Society of Health-System Pharmacists (ASHP) has considered MUE to encompass DUE in its broadest application,[1] so these guidelines continue to use MUE as a preferred term.

When developing a MUE, clinicians should also take into consideration its focus. For example, a MUE may focus on patient-centered therapeutic outcomes (e.g., clinical events, quality of life) or on process elements related to appropriate medication usage (e.g., prescribing, dispensing). In this way, an initial MUE may identify suboptimal therapeutic outcomes experienced by patients, which may trigger a separate MUE focused on aspects of the medication use process and vice-versa. Specific objectives, examples of MUE designs, and their foci (i.e., therapeutic or process outcomes) are presented in **Table 1**.

Performance Improvement Framework

Healthcare organizations routinely use performance improvement methods to improve safety, efficacy, quality, and efficiency in patient care. Many accreditation bodies, such as the Joint Commission, require annual reviews of a hospital formulary along with other quality and safety improvement strategies that would benefit from such a framework. These methods may be applied in the setting of MUE, which can be considered one component of a performance improvement program. One performance improvement framework that aligns with the MUE process is FOCUS-PDCA (**Figure 1**).[4] These steps include:

- Find the process to be targeted for improvement
- Organize the team that knows the process
- Clarify current knowledge of the process
- Understand causes of process variation
- Select process improvement
- Plan: develop a solution
- Do: implement improvements
- Check: evaluate the results
- Act: determine what changes are needed moving forward and implement those changes.

The steps in the FOCUS-PDCA model may need to be repeated in an ongoing, systematic manner.

Indicators Suggesting a Need for an MUE

The occurrence of certain events in a stage of the medication-use process may indicate opportunities to improve medication use and justify undertaking an MUE (**Table 2**).[1,5] Generally, these events may represent trends or deviations in medication use within a health system, availability or discontinuation of drugs, or new knowledge regarding drug therapy.

Prioritizing Medications and Medication-Use Processes for Evaluation

The indicators described above may reveal specific medications or medication-use processes that should be evaluated in an MUE. The following partial list of characteristics may help prioritize the selection of a particular medication or medication-use process, based on its magnitude or severity of effect on patients or the medication-use system (other characteristics will likely emerge with the introduction of new medications and technologies):

- The medication is known or suspected to cause adverse events or is used in the treatment of patients who may be at high risk for adverse events.
- The medication interacts with another medication, food, or diagnostic procedure in a way that presents a significant health risk.
- The medication or process affects a large number of patients, or the medication is frequently prescribed.
- The medication or process is a critical component of care for a specific disease, condition, or procedure.
- The medication is potentially toxic or causes discomfort at normal doses.
- The medication is most effective when used in a specific way.
- The medication is under consideration for formulary retention, addition, or deletion.
- The medication has been the subject of a Food and Drug Administration (FDA) recall, safety alert, or market withdrawal.
- The medication has not been approved by the FDA.
- The medication has not been evaluated in a high-risk population (pregnant females, pediatric patients, obese patients, etc.).

DOI 10.37573/9781585287048.040

TABLE 1.
Common MUE Objectives, MUE Examples, and Type of Outcome (Therapeutic or Process)

Objective	MUE Example	Therapeutic or Process Outcome
Promoting optimal medication therapy	Compare efficacy before and after introduction of a biosimilar therapeutic substitution policy	Therapeutic
	Evaluate the frequency of patients who qualified for, but did not receive, an approved therapeutic substitution	Process
Improve patient safety	Evaluate the incidence of major bleeding in patients treated with thrombolytic therapy	Therapeutic
	Evaluate the frequency of use of thrombolytic therapy in inappropriate candidates	Process
Standardize to reduce unnecessary variation	Compare rates of adverse events in patients receiving standard vs highly concentrated vasopressor infusions	Therapeutic
	Evaluate the prescribing frequency of concentrations outside of the standard concentration policy for vasopressors	Process
Optimize drug therapy	Determine the time in therapeutic range for patients treated with a medication requiring pharmacokinetic therapeutic drug monitoring	Therapeutic
	Evaluate the frequency of appropriate dose changes when an interacting medication is introduced	Process
Assess value of innovative practices	Compare the rates of blood pressure control in a physician- vs pharmacist-managed hypertension service	Therapeutic
	Evaluate the frequency of physician referral to a pharmacist-led hypertension management service	Process
Meet quality or regulatory standards	Determine the percentage of patients with heart failure readmitted after discharge	Therapeutic
	Determine the percentage of patients receiving required medication discharge education	Process
Minimize costs	Compare infection cure rates before versus after involvement of an antimicrobial stewardship pharmacist	Therapeutic
	Compare costs of antimicrobial therapy before versus after involvement of an antimicrobial stewardship pharmacist	Process

Abbreviation: MUE, medication-use evaluation.

- The medication or process is one for which its use would have a negative effect or no therapeutic impact on patient outcomes.
- The process is an innovative or newly initiated practice and its effects on patient care are unknown.
- Use of the medication or medication process is considered expensive and the cost benefit is unknown.
- To determine if clinicians are complying with medication formulary restrictions or facility guidelines for use.
- To evaluate pharmacist-directed collaborative practices, such as dosing protocols or algorithms (pharmacy per protocol or pharmacy to dose) to verify appropriate action steps.
- Analytic tools (e.g., failure mode and effects analysis, risk priority numbers, cause and effect diagrams, control chart) or scoring systems (e.g., harm criteria) suggest the need for intervention.

Steps of the MUE Process Using FOCUS-PDCA

While the specific approach varies with the practice setting and patient population being served, many steps common to MUE fall within the FOCUS-PDCA model framework for process improvement mentioned earlier (Figure 1). However, the following common steps often occur in an ongoing MUE process.

1. Find the process to target for improvement:
   - Establish the need for the MUE (see Table 2 for indicators of need for MUE).
2. Organize the team:
   - Establish organizational authority for the MUE process and engage subject matter experts and representative stakeholders:
     - Inform healthcare professionals (and others as necessary) in the practice setting(s) about the objectives and expected benefits of the MUE process.
     - Set priorities for in-depth analysis of important aspects of medication use.
     - Educate healthcare professionals involved with the MUE on the guidelines, treatment protocols, and standards of care.
     - Establish mechanisms for timely communication among healthcare professionals.
   - Decide on the team for the MUE:
     - Core teams tend to include pharmacists, pharmacy residents, student pharmacists, pharmacy technicians, and key stakeholders such as nurses, physicians, and other allied health professionals.

FIGURE 1. Components of the FOCUS-PDCA process improvement model applied to medication-use evaluation.

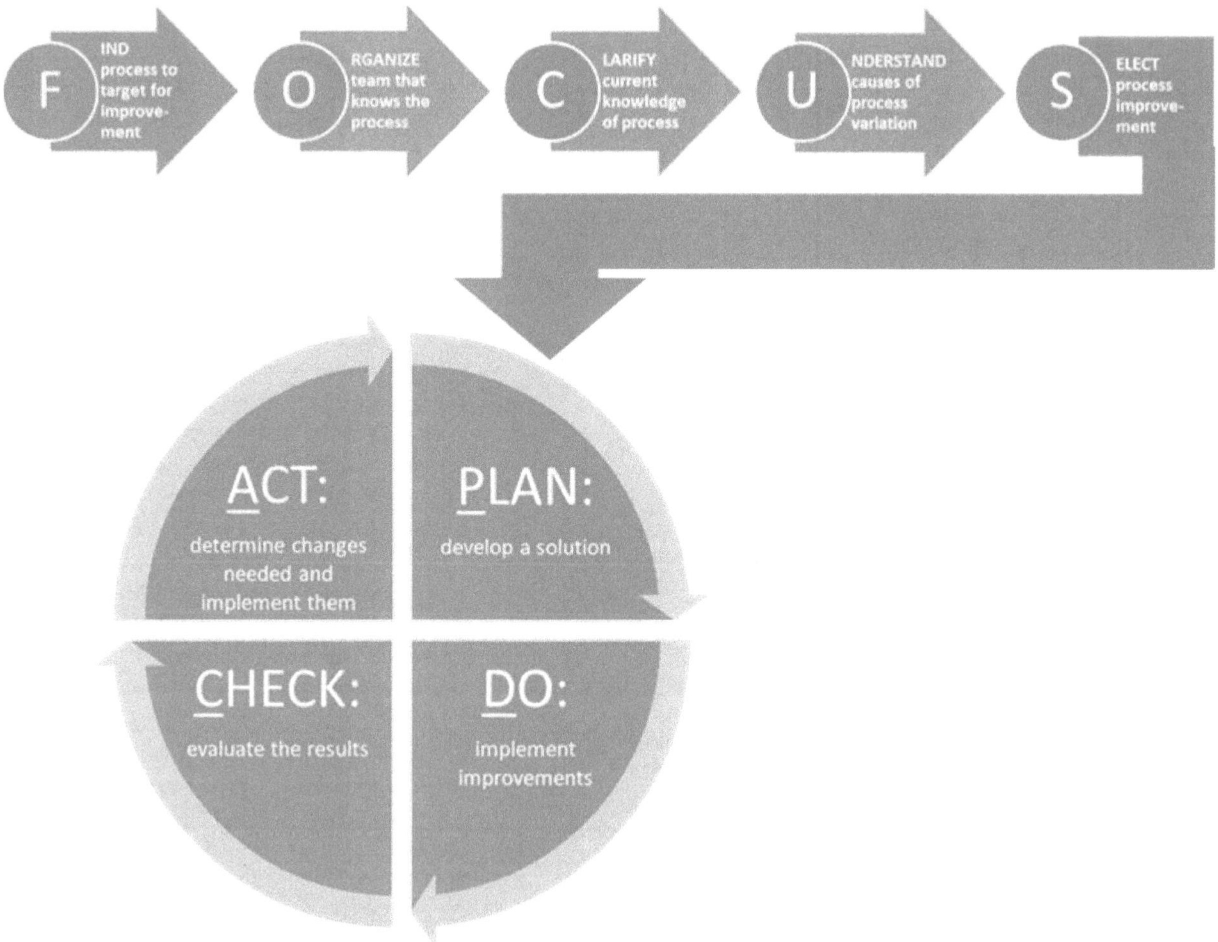

TABLE 2.
Indicators of Need for Medication-Use Evaluation at Different Steps in Medication-Use Process[a]

Step	Indicator
Prescribing	• Market entry or withdrawal of approved drug products • Regulatory actions such as drug recalls, market withdrawals, or safety alerts • Publication of guidelines or high-impact studies that may change treatment patterns • New organizational interventions to improve medication therapy, such as changes to protocols or formularies • Changes in use of, or requests for, nonformulary medications • Changes to pharmacy clinical services to improve medication therapy • Introduction of or changes in quality indicators, such as those published by the Centers for Medicare & Medicaid Services, or other regulatory or accrediting bodies
Dispensing	• Signs of process failures, such as wasted medication or delayed medication delivery • Incorrect medication preparation • Dosing that requires clinician preparation or compounding • Ensuring compliance with regulatory requirements (eg, United States Pharmacopeia chapters 795, 797, 800)
Administration	• Medication misadventures related to medication delivery systems • Multiple medication concentrations, units of measure, or infusion rates
Monitoring	• Adverse events, including medication errors, preventable adverse drug reactions, and toxicity • Signs of treatment failures, such as unexpected readmissions and bacterial resistance to anti-infective therapy • Patient dissatisfaction or deterioration in quality of life attributable to drug therapy
Systems management and control	• Procurement requirements, specialty pharmacy requirements, risk evaluation and mitigation strategies (REMS) programs, restricted distribution channels, or other access challenges • Drug shortages requiring replacement or therapeutic substitution • Diversion of controlled substances • Lack of standardization or confusion within the medication-use process • Changes in contracts, cost, or spending on drugs • Organizational priorities such as budget constraints or cost-saving initiatives

[a]This table does not provide an exhaustive list of characteristics.

  - Consider engaging experts in informatics, data analytics, performance improvement and/or biostatistics whenever possible.
- ▸ Provide training to the staff involved with the MUE.

3. Clarify current knowledge:
   - ▸ Build MUE criteria using the above guidelines, treatment protocols, and standards of care in the medication-use process.
   - ▸ Identify the key question to answer, measurable objectives, and the timeline for the MUE. Objectives must be measurable, relevant, and easy to obtain/collect. See Table 1 for details.
   - ▸ Design MUE by deciding on methodology and selecting sample population, sample size, and inclusion and exclusion criteria.
   - ▸ Create a data collection plan. Include a data dictionary to standardize definitions for collected variables and sources utilized for collection:
     - Generate reports from the electronic medical record (EMR) whenever possible in order to limit manual chart abstraction.
     - Determine sample size and variables to collect. Estimate the potential time required for manual chart reviews and the ideal number of team members. Any set sample size should represent a larger group of population.
     - Establish thresholds for evaluating achievement of targeted measures by using past performance and/or utilization reports or published benchmarks, if available.
     - Conduct data collection and schedule intermittent progress evaluations as needed, depending on project timeline. Look for outlying data (e.g., 80 lbs accidentally entered instead of 80 kg for 55 year-old, 6-foot, healthy male).
   - ▸ Analyze data using appropriate statistical tests:
     - Descriptive statistics are appropriate for many MUEs (e.g., measures of central tendency, measures of variability, percentage of patients meeting a certain outcome). If there are 2 or more distinct groups within the analysis, inferential statistics may also be considered.
   - ▸ Document results and compare them to your anticipated outcomes.
   - ▸ Share MUE results using appropriate text and visuals (e.g., figures, tables) with the MUE team and key stakeholders.
4. Understand the causes of process variation:
   - ▸ If outcomes do not meet desired thresholds, conduct root cause analyses to determine the source of the problem.
   - ▸ Consider using tools that assist in identifying variation in the process (e.g., Five Whys).[6]
   - ▸ Punitive reactions to quality concerns are often counterproductive. It is important to communicate and commend positive achievements as well.
5. Select process improvement:
   - ▸ Brainstorm and engage key stakeholders to develop ideas that would address the root cause of the process variation:
     - Whenever possible, solutions that "hardwire" workflows and those that do not rely on someone to remember to do something during particular circumstances are preferred.
     - Ensure the selected solution aligns with the department and organization's goals, adds value, and is both technically and financially feasible.
     - Consider using a tool such as the "FACES"[7] tool to evaluate and prioritize recommendations:
       - ▸ Feasibility: How easily and quickly can the change be made?
       - ▸ Acceptability: How willing are those impacted to make the change?
       - ▸ Cost/Benefit: How much does the cost outweigh the benefit?
       - ▸ Effectiveness: How effectively will this change solve the problem?
       - ▸ Sustainability: How will the change last over time?
6. Plan:
   - ▸ Create a plan to specify what actions will be taken, how it will be done, who is responsible for each task, and what the desired timeline will be.
   - ▸ Establish a plan for data collection and measuring success once the solution is implemented. Success should be assessed in terms of improved healthcare outcomes, which may include but is not limited to morbidity, mortality, adverse events, quality of life, healthcare resource utilization, and cost savings.
7. Do:
   - ▸ Implement the identified solution(s).
8. Check:
   - ▸ Complete follow-up data collection on the new process following implementation of corrective actions.
   - ▸ Obtain feedback from the MUE team and other disciplines regarding lessons learned in order to brainstorm solutions to overcome obstacles, challenges, and inefficiencies of MUE methods.
9. Act:
   - ▸ Take steps necessary to maintain the improvement. If the identified solution was piloted, develop a plan to roll out the optimized solution to the entire process.
   - ▸ When sustained reproducible improvement is seen, revise criteria, guidelines, treatment protocols, standards of care policies, or point-of-care tools in the EMR (e.g., hard stops, automatic conversions) when indicated.
   - ▸ Communicate findings of the MUE and the newly implemented processes to affected parties (e.g., newsletters, seminars).

- Consider publishing MUE results (e.g., poster, manuscript) outside of the institution if appropriate. Although MUEs are within the scope of operational activities, this type of quality assurance or quality improvement (QA/QI) work does not preclude publication. It is important that MUE results be accurately presented either as research or non-research, depending on whether it was designed to contribute to generalizable knowledge, which would then fall within the realm of research.[8] Most peer-reviewed journals do require, at minimum, a statement regarding review and/or exemption by a human subjects protection committee or institutional review board. Local governing groups should be consulted for external publication and presentation requirements.

Roles and Responsibilities in the MUE Process

The roles of pharmacists and other healthcare professionals in MUE may vary according to practice setting, organizational goals, and available resources. The organizational body (e.g., quality management or QI committee, pharmacy and therapeutics committee) responsible for the MUE process should have, at a minimum, a prescriber (most commonly a physician), pharmacist, nurse, and an administrator or health-system representative. Pharmacist extenders, including pharmacy technicians, student pharmacists, and pharmacy residents should also participate in conducting MUEs in facilities and healthcare systems where allowed. Other healthcare professionals and subject matter experts should contribute their unique perspectives when the evaluation and improvement processes address their areas of expertise and responsibility. Ad hoc committees or temporary working groups, which include at a minimum a pharmacist as the MUE lead and subject matter expert(s), can be assigned to develop MUEs for specific QI efforts. Best practices should be established in settings whenever possible to enhance the structure around how MUE committees conduct, report, implement, and complete evaluations. In addition, systematic evaluations should be conducted when possible to assess the attributes of the interdisciplinary team in regard to subject matter expertise, leadership in the program or healthcare system, and overall ability to implement and sustain the MUE findings. In settings in which only a small number of healthcare professionals are available (e.g., some community hospitals, rural hospitals, or clinics), extensive MUEs conducted by a large interdisciplinary team may not be an option. In such instances, the pharmacist at the smaller facility may be responsible for the design, conduct, analysis, and reporting of an MUE. Implementation of findings from the MUE may require assistance from the hospital administration in such facilities.

QI programs with a high degree of interdisciplinary participation provide an optimal mechanism to conduct MUEs. Although other disciplines should be encouraged to assist in development of MUEs, pharmacists, by virtue of their expertise and mission to ensure appropriate medication use, remain the primary healthcare professional responsible for the development and coordination of MUEs. Pharmacists should continue to exert leadership and work collaboratively with other members of the healthcare team in the ongoing MUE process. The responsibilities of pharmacists (with the assistance of pharmacist extenders such as pharmacy technicians, student pharmacists, and pharmacy residents) in the MUE process should include:

- Developing an operational plan for MUE programs and processes that is consistent with the health system's overall goals and resource capabilities.
- Working collaboratively with prescribers, subject matter expert(s), and others to develop criteria for specific medications and to design effective medication-use processes and assessments.
- Ensuring optimal input from subject matter expert(s) and interdisciplinary groups in the design of the MUE efforts, when possible.
- Reviewing individual medication utilization against medication-use criteria and consulting with prescribers and others in the process as needed.
- Collecting, analyzing, and evaluating patient-specific data to identify, resolve, and prevent medication-related problems, enhance medication effectiveness, and improve patient outcomes.
- Ensuring the integrity of the collected data.
- Interpreting and reporting MUE findings, as well as recommending and facilitating changes in medication-use processes.
- Providing information and education based on MUE findings.
- Assisting in implementation of optimal findings in the facility or healthcare system.
- Evaluating the outcomes of implemented MUE findings when appropriate and assessing the effect on the facility or healthcare system.
- Ensuring that systems are in place to sustain the implemented MUE findings in the facility or healthcare system whenever possible.
- Ensuring that MUEs emphasize QI versus research.

Common Problems and Pitfalls

Common problems and pitfalls to avoid in performing MUE activities are presented in **Table 3**. These pitfalls often involve lack of interdisciplinary involvement, including authoritative medical staff; poor documentation and communication of the MUE process; and inadequate education of affected staff regarding outcomes of the MUE and improvements to the medication-use system.

Conclusion

These guidelines describe essential elements of the MUE process for healthcare organizations. MUE is an ongoing, systematic, and interdisciplinary performance improvement method that has an overarching goal of optimizing patient outcomes through evaluation and improvement of medication-use processes. MUE may be considered one component of a performance improvement program, and its steps may be described using the FOCUS-PDCA model framework. The occurrence of certain events in a stage of the medication-use process may indicate opportunities to improve medication use and justify undertaking an MUE, and the characteristics provided may help prioritize

TABLE 3.
Problems, Pitfalls, and Barriers to Completing a Successful Medication-Use Evaluation

Category	Explanation
Lack of authority	An MUE process that does not involve the medical staff is likely to be ineffective. Authoritative medical staff support and formal organizational recognition of the MUE process are necessary to support changes and incorporate best practices.
Lack of organization, structure, or leadership	Without a clear definition of the roles, responsibilities, and accountabilities of individuals involved to complete tasks and reach milestones, an MUE process may not succeed.
Poor communication	Everyone included in the MUE process should understand its importance to the health system, its goals, and its procedures. The pharmacist should manage the MUE process and have the responsibility and authority to ensure timely communication among all professionals involved in the MUE process. Criteria for medication use should be communicated to all affected professionals prior to the evaluation of care. MUE activity should be a standing agenda item for appropriate quality-of-care committees responsible for aspects of medication use.
Poor documentation	MUE activities should be well documented, including summaries of MUE actions with respect to individual medication orders and the findings and conclusions from collective evaluations. Documentation should address recommendations made and follow-up actions.
Lack of involvement	The MUE process is not a one-person task, nor is it the responsibility of a single department or professional group. Medication-use criteria should be developed through an interdisciplinary consensus process. Lack of administrative support can severely limit the effectiveness of MUE. The benefits of MUE should be conveyed in terms of improving patient outcomes and minimizing health-system costs.
Data integrity	Data collection efforts are often interdisciplinary and can involve student pharmacists, pharmacy interns, pharmacy residents, and others. Data are often found in different medical record locations and can be interpreted differently, often resulting in discrepancies. Teams should agree on sources and interpretation before data collection begins.
Lack of follow-through	A one-time study or evaluation independent of the overall MUE process will have limited success in improving patient outcomes. The effectiveness of initial actions must be assessed and the action plan adjusted if necessary. It is important not to lose sight of the improvement goals.
Evaluation methodology that impedes patient care	Data collection should not consume so much time that patient care activities suffer. Interventions that can improve care for an individual patient should not be withheld because of the sampling technique or evaluation methodology.
Lack of scope	Consider inclusion of unique or under-represented populations (e.g., neonates, pediatric patients, pregnant women, etc.) in project scope.
Lack of readily retrievable data	Collaboration with analytics or information solutions teams should occur to ensure the majority of discrete data fields are generated through reporting mechanisms.
Lack of hard-wired corrective actions	When sub-optimal processes are uncovered, corrective actions should be hard-wired (e.g., forcing functions in the electronic health record) whenever possible. Remedies relying on education and provider memory are often ineffective in promoting lasting change.
Lack of education	If results from a MUE are not disseminated through the education of appropriate staff, a change in process or patient care will not occur.

Abbreviation: MUE, medication-use evaluation.

the selection of a particular medication or medication-use process for MUE. The success of an MUE process should be assessed in terms of improved patient outcomes, one of which may be lower cost. Interdisciplinary participation is crucial to successful MUEs. Although other disciplines should be encouraged to participate in MUEs, pharmacists remain the primary healthcare professionals responsible for the development and coordination of MUEs due to their expertise and mission to ensure appropriate medication use.

References

1. Phillips MS, Gayman JE, Todd MW. ASHP guidelines on medication-use evaluation. *Am J Health-Syst Pharm.* 1996; 53:1953–1955.
2. Academy of Managed Care Pharmacy. Drug utilization review. https://www.amcp.org/about/managed-care-pharmacy-101/concepts-managed-care-pharmacy/drug-utilization-review. Published July 18, 2019. Accessed January 27, 2020.
3. World Health Organization. *Drug and Therapeutics Committees—A Practical Guide.* http://apps.who.int/medicinedocs/en/d/Js4882e/8.5.html. Accessed January 27, 2020.
4. Agency for Healthcare Research and Quality. Health literacy universal precautions toolkit, 2nd ed. Plan-do-study-act (PDSA) directions and examples. https://www.ahrq.gov/professionals/quality-patient-safety/quality-resources/tools/literacy-toolkit/healthlittoolkit2-tool2b.html. Published February 2015. Accessed January 27, 2020.
5. Thomas JK, Nau DP. Quality improvement and the medication use system. In: Malone PM, Malone MJ, Park SK, eds. *Drug Information: A Guide for Pharmacists.* 6th ed. New York, NY: McGraw-Hill; 2018.

6. Institute for Healthcare Improvement. 5 Whys: Finding the Root Cause. www.ihi.org/resources/Pages/Tools/5-Whys-Finding-the-Root-Cause.aspx. Accessed January 27, 2020.
7. O'Connor PE, Cohn JV. *Human Performance Enhancement in High-Risk Environments: Insights, Developments, and Future Directions from Military Research*. Santa Barbara, CA: ABC-CLIO; 2010:200.
8. U.S. Department of Veterans Affairs. Office of Research & Development program guide: 1200.21. VHA operations activities that may constitute research. October 28, 2011. https://www.research.va.gov/resources/policies/ProgramGuide-1200-21-VHA-Operations-Activities.pdf. Published January 19, 2019. Accessed January 27, 2020.

Resources

Resources that may be helpful in the design and implementation of MUEs include the following.

- Veterans Affairs Center for Medication Safety. VA Medication use evaluation (MUE) toolkit. https://www.pbm.va.gov/PBM/vacenterformedicationsafety/tools/MUEToolkit.pdf. Updated July 2012. Accessed January 27, 2020
- World Health Organization. Introduction to drug utilization research. http://apps.who.int/medicinedocs/en/d/Js4876e/4.6.html. Published 2003. Accessed January 27, 2020.
- Academy of Managed Care Pharmacy. Drug utilization review. https://www.amcp.org/about/managed-care-pharmacy-101/concepts-managed-care-pharmacy/drug-utilization-review. Published July 18, 2019. Accessed January 27, 2020.
- Institute for Healthcare Improvement. Science of improvement: testing changes. http://www.ihi.org/resources/Pages/HowtoImprove/ScienceofImprovementTestingChanges.aspx. Accessed January 27, 2020.
- Fanikos J, Jenkins KL, Piazza G, Connors J, Goldhaber SJ. Medication use evaluation: pharmacist rubric for performance improvement. *Pharmacotherapy*. 2014;34(Suppl 1):5S-13S.
- Thomas JK, Nau DP. Quality improvement and the medication use system. In: Malone PM, Malone MJ, Park SK, eds. *Drug Information: A Guide for Pharmacists*. 6th edition. New York, NY: McGraw-Hill; 2018.
- Anderson KC, Brown C. Medication use policy and performance assessment. In: Gabay M, ed. *The Clinical Practice of Drug Information*. 1st ed. Burlington, MA: Jones & Bartlett; 2016.
- Faley B, Fanikos J. Best practices for medication utilization evaluations in postsurgical pain management. *Curr Emerg Hosp Med Rep*. 2017;5(1):33–40.

Developed through the ASHP Council on Pharmacy Practice and approved by the ASHP Board of Directors on May 15, 2020. These guidelines supersede the ASHP Guidelines on Medication-Use Evaluation dated April 24, 1996.

ASHP gratefully acknowledges the following organizations and individuals for reviewing these guidelines (review does not imply endorsement): American Pharmacists Association (APhA); Institute for Healthcare Improvement (IHI); Maryland Society of Health-System Pharmacy (MSHP) Legislative Committee; Thomas S. Achey, Pharm.D., MS, BCPS; Nicole Acquisto, Pharm.D., FCCP, BCCCP; Tyler B. Clay, Pharm.D.; Michael C. Dejos, Pharm.D., BCPS, LSSBB, DPLA; Frank Federico, R.Ph. (IHI); Paul Fina, Pharm.D., BCACP; Katie Foster, M.S., Pharm.D., FCCM; Rena Gosser, Pharm.D., BCPS; Kathleen M. Gura, Pharm.D., BCNSP, FASHP; Charzetta H. James, Pharm.D., M.B.A., M.H.A., FACHE, CPH, PRS; Isha John, Pharm.D., M.B.A. (APhA); Indrani Kar, Pharm.D.; Nicole Kiehle, Pharm.D., BCPS (MSHP); Patrick M. Malone, Pharm.D., FASHP; Kathryn Clark McKinney, Pharm.D., M.S., BCPS, FACHE, FASHP; Valerie Dee Nolt, Pharm.D., BCPPS; Maryann Oertel, Pharm.D., BCPS; Preetham Talari, M.D., FACP, SFHM; Philip Trapskin, Pharm.D., BCPS; Tyler A. Vest, Pharm.D., M.S., BCPS; and Jody Jacobson Wedret, R.Ph., FASHP, FCSHP.

John Fanikos declares having served as the lead investigator for the RE-VECTO surveillance study (for which Boehringer Ingelheim provided research support) and as a consultant to Portola and Ipsen.

Janna Afanasjeva, Pharm.D., BCPS, Clinical Assistant Professor, University of Illinois at Chicago.

Muriel Burk, Pharm.D., Clinical Pharmacist Specialist, Veterans Affairs (VA) Center for Medication Safety—Pharmacy Benefit Management (PBM) Services, Hines, IL.

Francesca (Fran) Cunningham, Pharm.D., Director, Veterans Affairs (VA) Center for Medication Safety, Associate Chief Consultant, Pharmacy Benefits Management (PBM) Services, Hines, IL.

John Fanikos, B.S.Pharm., M.B.A., Executive Director of Pharmacy Services, Brigham and Women's Hospital, Adjunct Professor of Clinical Pharmacy, Massachusetts College of Pharmacy and Health Sciences, Boston, MA.

Michael Gabay, Pharm.D., J.D., BCPS, Clinical Associate Professor, Pharmacy Practice, University of Illinois at Chicago.

Genevieve (Jeni) Hayes, Pharm.D., M.S.Pharm., BCPS, Clinical Specialist—Outcomes Management, Medication Safety, Use & Policy, MUSC Health, Charleston, SC.

Patricia L. Masters, Pharm.D., BCPS, Clinical Pharmacy Coordinator, Mount Auburn Hospital, Cambridge, MA.

Ryan Rodriguez, Pharm.D., BCPS, Clinical Assistant Professor, University of Illinois at Chicago.

Mark J. Sinnett, Pharm.D., FASHP, Director, Clinical and Educational Services, Department of Pharmacy, Montefiore Medical Center, Bronx, NY.

Copyright © 2021, American Society of Health-System Pharmacists, Inc. All rights reserved. Contact ASHP for reprint and permissions requests. This content may not be used for commercial purposes without the express written consent of ASHP.

The bibliographic citation for this document is as follows: American Society of Health-System Pharmacists. ASHP guidelines on medication-use evaluation. *Am J Health-Syst Pharm*. 2021;78:168–75.

ASHP Guidelines on the Pharmacy and Therapeutics Committee and the Formulary System

Purpose

These guidelines outline important considerations and recommend processes for formulary system management within the context of a hospital or health system. Pharmacist responsibilities and roles in managing the formulary system in partnership with other healthcare professionals are embedded throughout. These guidelines also provide assistance to pharmacists in the organization and operation of the pharmacy and therapeutics (P&T) committee or equivalent body, evaluation of medications for formularies and consideration of rational use of medications, and development and implementation of strategies to optimize medication use through the formulary system. A glossary of terms is provided in **Appendix A**.

Formulary and Formulary System

A *formulary* is a continually updated list of available medications and related information, representing the clinical judgment, resulting from a review of the clinical evidence, of physicians, pharmacists, and other clinicians in the diagnosis, prophylaxis, or treatment of disease and promotion of health. A formulary includes, but is not limited to, a list of medications and medication-associated products or devices, medication-use policies, important ancillary drug information, decision-support tools, and organizational guidelines. A formulary system is the ongoing process through which a healthcare organization establishes policies regarding the use of drugs, therapies, and drug-related products, including medication delivery devices, and identifies those that are most medically appropriate, safe, and cost-effective to best serve the health interests of a given patient population.[1] Formulary systems are used in many different settings, including hospitals, acute care facilities, home care settings, and long-term-care facilities, as well as by payers such as Medicare, Medicaid, insurance companies, and managed care organizations. Many organizations have policy statements on the use of formularies.[2–8] These guidelines focus on the use of formulary systems in hospitals and health systems, in both inpatient and outpatient settings.

Evolution of Formularies

Formulary systems have evolved over time. Early formularies began as rudimentary drug lists developed by the military as early as the Revolutionary War and came into more widespread use during the 1950s.[9] Pharmacists, in conjunction with their organizations, developed policies to dispense generic equivalent drugs when a specific brand-name drug was prescribed. In the late 1950s, the ASHP minimum standard for pharmacies in hospitals called for the implementation of a formulary system.[10]

During the 1960s, the concept of a hospital formulary continued to grow. Hospitals developed policies that authorized pharmacists to make generic interchanges in an institutional formulary system based on prior consent from physicians.[11] ASHP and the American Hospital Association (AHA) issued joint statements on the legality of formularies.[12,13] The American Medical Association (AMA) and the American Pharmaceutical (later Pharmacists) Association (APhA) subsequently joined with ASHP and AHA to revise the statements.[14] In 1965, two significant events occurred: (1) Medicare listed formularies as a reimbursement eligibility requirement15 and (2) the Joint Commission on the Accreditation of Hospitals (now known as the Joint Commission) included an active P&T committee in its accreditation requirements.[16] Even with these actions, formularies were typically no more than lists of drugs stocked by the pharmacy.

By the 1980s, literature describing the clinical and economic value of well-designed formularies emerged. Evidence from the hospital setting was published first, soon followed by evidence from the ambulatory care environment.[11] This literature led to more widespread acceptance of formularies by providers, payers, and industry.[5,17]

Today, formulary systems are considered an essential tool for healthcare organizations to foster interprofessional efforts to promote the rational use of medications. Formularies have grown from simple drug lists to comprehensive systems of medication-use policies intended to ensure safe, appropriate, and cost-effective use of pharmaceuticals in patient care.[18]

P&T Committee

The P&T committee is generally the medical staff committee responsible for managing the formulary system. The P&T committee provides an evaluative, educational, and advisory service to the medical staff and organizational administration in all matters pertaining to the use of available medications. The P&T committee should be responsible for overseeing policies and procedures related to all aspects of medication use within an institution.

The P&T committee's organization and authority should be outlined in the organization's medical staff bylaws, medical staff rules and regulations, and other organizational policies, as appropriate. The description of organization and authority becomes even more important as healthcare facilities merge into larger health systems.

Typically, P&T committee member appointments and voting rights are made based on guidance from the medical staff and other affected stakeholders. Voting members may include facility medical staff, other prescribers, pharmacists, nurses, and administrators, and are a representative sample of the organization. If the scope of the P&T committee includes a health system, site representation needs to be addressed to ensure equitable input and voting authority from each facility. Additional supporting P&T committee members may include quality improvement managers, medication safety leaders, informaticists, other healthcare professionals and staff who participate in the medication-use process, and patient and family engagement advisors.

DOI 10.37573/9781585287048.041

The P&T committee should have the following administrative components in place to maximize meeting effectiveness:

- Charter
- Role of the P&T secretary and/or formulary manager
- Committee and subcommittee(s) responsibility and scope
- Process to track attendance
- Definition of quorum
- Process to allow (or disallow) delegation of vote
- Process to appeal committee decisions
- Defined term limits for members
- Process for identifying, disclosing, addressing, and reporting conflicts of interest (COI)
- Policy and procedures
- Approach to voting, including roll call votes to ensure transparency
- Scope of committee responsibility (e.g., specific site or entire system; inpatient or outpatient sites; drugs, devices, and biologics)
- Process for managing minutes, agendas, record keeping, and communication of decisions made

Other responsibilities of the P&T committee include medication-use evaluation (MUE), adverse drug event monitoring and reporting, medication error prevention, medication safety, and development of clinical care plans and medication management initiatives (e.g., delegation and practice protocols, restrictions, guidelines and clinical pathways). Information about these activities is available in ASHP guidelines on the topics.[19–22]

Oversight of a formulary system and the capacity to make appropriate formulary decisions requires consideration of patient care factors and a thorough, unbiased review of the biomedical literature. Voting members should be required to provide COI statements to avoid actual or perceived interference with evidence-based decisions.[23] Some healthcare organizations exclude healthcare professionals with COIs from P&T committee membership, whereas others allow participation in committee discussions but prohibit voting on particular items. Practitioners requesting additions or changes to the formulary should also be required to disclose financial relationships with pharmaceutical companies, payers and insurance companies, and other potential COIs to the P&T committee. Management of COI should be specified in organizational policies and procedures.

Managing the Formulary System

Health systems should develop, maintain, and implement a formulary management process. This evidence-based process should not be based solely on economic factors. The formulary system should have aspects of financial stewardship incorporated and be standardized within integrated health systems when standardization leads to improved patient outcomes, safety, and cost effectiveness. Decisions on the management of a formulary system should be founded on the evidence-based clinical, ethical, legal, social, logistical, philosophical, quality-of-life, safety, and economic factors that result in optimal patient care.[24–26] The process must include the active and direct involvement of physicians, pharmacists, and other appropriate healthcare professionals, as well representatives with expertise in finance, law, and informatics.

Management of a formulary system is a significant component of a healthcare organization's ongoing medication-use policy development process. A comprehensive, well-maintained formulary is tailored to the organization's patient care needs, policy framework, and medication-use systems while ensuring alignment with medication management standards of accrediting organizations.[27] A well-managed formulary system ensures a close relationship among the organization's medication-use policies, the therapies offered by the organization, and the medications routinely stocked in the pharmacy. A formulary also identifies those medications that are most medically appropriate and cost-effective to best serve the health interests of the health system's patient population. The P&T committee should review all medications (see Appendix A) used in the health system. These may include alternative remedies (herbals and supplements), nonprescription drugs, blood derivatives, contrast media, and other diagnostic and treatment agents.[27]

Institutional policies may need to be created for P&T committee evaluation of agents not approved by the FDA (e.g., herbal supplements).

The formulary system should review and approve all policies related to the medication-use process; all medication-use policies, regardless of their origination, should flow through the P&T committee. The organization's medical staff leadership (i.e., the body to which the P&T committee reports) should complete the final policy approval. Policy review and revision should occur as new information becomes available and at regularly established intervals (e.g., annually). The organization should have medication-use policies that address the following:

- How medications are requested for addition to or deletion from the formulary
- How medications are reviewed for addition to or deletion from the formulary, including who performs the reviews
- How and when drug class reviews are conducted
- The process for developing, implementing, and monitoring medication-use guidelines
- Methods and policies for ensuring the safe procurement, prescribing, distribution, administration, and monitoring of medications
- Methods for selection of suitable manufacturers for specific medications (i.e., the pharmacy department is responsible for specifications for the quality, quantity, and source of supply of all medications, chemicals, biologicals, and pharmaceutical preparations used in the diagnosis and treatment of patients)[28]
- The process for using nonformulary agents within the hospital and health system
- The process for managing radiopharmaceuticals
- The process for managing drug product shortages
- The process for developing an organization or health system-specific MUE plan
- Policies regarding specific medication-use processes (e.g., procurement, prescribing, distribution, administration, monitoring, automation, and technology)

- The process for disseminating medication-use policies and how users will be educated regarding the process
- Process for accountability over medication delivery devices (e.g., infusion pumps, dose error reduction software, intranasal atomizers)
- Consideration of medication access through prior authorization processes and patient assistance programs
- Implementation of P&T committee decisions into the electronic health record (EHR)

A formal process to review medication-use policies should be in place. This process may include the use of expert panels or subcommittees of the P&T committee. Expert panels or subcommittees should serve in an advisory role to the P&T committee, and their membership should include recognized experts in their areas of practice. The P&T committee may also find subcommittees that address specific therapeutic areas to be beneficial (e.g., pediatrics, antimicrobial, oncology therapy, cardiovascular, adverse drug reaction, pharmacogenomics, or biotechnology subcommittees). Panels and subcommittees are helpful in applying clinical study results to specific patient populations and developing recommended strategies for the safe and effective use of medications. Subcommittee and panel members can help educate groups of clinicians, who ultimately drive prescribing behaviors, about significant formulary changes. User groups, representing those primarily affected by the policy, may also be helpful.

The P&T committee should have formal interactions (i.e., communication lines) with other committees whose functions may affect the medication-use process. These committees would include those responsible for developing tools to facilitate medication use (e.g., forms or order set review committee, computerized provider order entry committee), those concerned with safety or performance improvement (e.g., quality improvement or patient safety committees), those involved in developing patient care policies (e.g., medical and nursing committees), those involved with investigational medications (e.g., investigational review boards), and other committees whose actions may affect medication use (e.g., nutrition, equipment and supply, and finance committees or patient and family engagement advisors). Recommendations from other committees, subcommittees of P&T, expert panels, and others should be submitted to the P&T committee for review. P&T committee decisions on recommendations should be communicated to the recommending group in a timely fashion.

Finally, the role of pharmaceutical company representatives and medical science liaisons in a healthcare organization should be carefully considered. Organizational guidelines should define appropriate relationships and interactions with such individuals. At a minimum, these guidelines should address the provision of pharmaceutical samples, indirect or direct funding support, and educational programming regarding formulary and nonformulary medications. Applications for formulary additions should be initiated and completed independently by the requesting healthcare provider and not by an industry representative or vendor. Refer to ASHP's Guidelines on Pharmacists' Relationships with Industry for more information on appropriate interactions with industry.[29]

Evaluating Medications for Inclusion in the Formulary

The P&T committee should use a structured, evidence-based process in the evaluation of medications for formulary consideration. The P&T committee should be provided with information that reflects a thorough, accurate, and unbiased review and analysis of the evidence available in the scientific literature. The evaluation process should encourage objective consideration of clinical and care delivery information, facilitate communication, foster positive patient outcomes, and support safe and effective medication ordering, dispensing, administration, and monitoring. Decisions made by the P&T committee should support improved patient care outcomes across the continuum of care, including considerations regarding patient access to medications upon discharge.

Evidence-Based Evaluation. Evidence-based medicine is a systematic approach to the evaluation of biomedical literature and application to clinical practice and should be applied to formulary decision-making for medication product selection.[25] Evidence-based decision-making standardizes and improves the quality of patient care and promotes cost-effective prescribing.[25,26] To practice evidence-based medicine, practitioners must be proficient in retrieving, evaluating, and applying the biomedical literature to clinical practice. Inclusion of a medication on a health system's formulary or the adoption of a medication-use guideline should reflect an evidence-based evaluation. Evidence-based decision-making incorporates the systematic approach to reviewing, evaluating, and applying the biomedical literature to guide formulary decisions. Various types and strengths of evidence (e.g., randomized clinical trials, meta-analyses, case reports, association consensus statements) may be useful in the decision-making process. Although different types of evidence are available for application, those with stronger evidence should be used to drive formulary decisions (e.g., meta-analyses, randomized controlled trials). Other types of evidence have a role in the decision-making process, however, and may be appropriate when stronger evidence is not available. Observational studies (i.e., case–control and cohort studies), case reports, and consensus opinions may be valuable even when stronger evidence is available. Some organizations find it useful to grade evidence when evaluating formulary requests; several tools are available for this purpose.[30–34]

Published evidence and expert opinion are not the only resources available to aid in the formulary decision-making process. Internal data and prescribing and outcomes information may be helpful in formulary decision-making. When published data are not available, it may be appropriate to incorporate expert opinion into the review process. Experts in practice areas sometimes have access to unpublished data or reports that may offer insight into difficult formulary decisions.

The formulary decision-making process should be guided by an independent review of evidence published in the biomedical literature, application of expert opinion, and use of internal data and benchmarking programs (see **Appendix B** for a description of the four major types of reviews used in such evaluations). If a P&T committee uses medication dossiers prepared by a pharmaceutical manufacturer, it should do so with the utmost caution, since the objectivity of these documents may be challenged.

Information used in the formulary decision-making process should be provided to the P&T committee in a written document with a standard format (e.g., a drug monograph, drug review, drug-evaluation document).[35] All information provided in the drug-evaluation document should be referenced to the evidence or identified as a conclusion supported by evidence. Any areas of consensus recommendations or opinion should be clearly identified.

Formulary status recommendations (e.g., from drug information services or expert groups) may be included in the drug-evaluation document. Recommendations should consider the formulary status (addition or rejection) of a medication, as well as the need for restrictions, educational efforts, or policies and procedures to ensure safe and appropriate use within the health system.

Pharmacoeconomic Assessments. Rigorous pharmacoeconomic evaluations can and should be conducted in some cases when reviewing new medications. These evaluations should explicitly state the perspective of the analysis (e.g., patient, healthcare provider, payer) and should include consideration of all costs and consequences relevant to that perspective. When new medications being considered are found to be therapeutically equivalent to existing alternatives (i.e., having equivalent efficacy and safety), then the cost-minimization approach is appropriate. In these circumstances, it is important to consider costs associated with the medication and non-medication-related costs (e.g., costs of administration, monitoring, prolonged hospital stay, operational costs, and laboratory test monitoring; costs to patients and providers).

While cost-effectiveness analysis (evaluating the incremental difference in investment necessary to produce an incremental difference in clinical outcome) is another potentially useful analytic approach, it is not often used for formulary decision-making because of its complexity and need for strong evidence or data. The academic value of this approach lies in its ability to show how little (or how much) must be spent to achieve a particular margin of clinical advantage when comparing an alternative that is more expensive but safer or more efficacious. No standards currently exist to determine what cost is reasonable for a given improvement in outcome; however, it is unreasonable to recommend alternatives of lower quality simply to achieve cost savings. This approach can be used to demonstrate how a decrease in clinical outcomes associated with the use of a less expensive agent can be offset by investing the savings achieved in other interventions that produce even greater total benefits. When evaluating cost-effectiveness, it is important to consider the site of care for administration of the drug.

Cost-utility evaluations (evaluating the incremental difference in investment necessary to produce an incremental difference in quality-of-life-adjusted clinical outcome [e.g., incremental cost per quality-adjusted life-years gained for one medication vs another]) may also be beneficial by serving to reflect patient preference in formulary decision-making. However, the same concerns related to the use of cost-effectiveness evaluations apply to this approach.[36–38]

Decision analysis models incorporating local data can be employed when published pharmacoeconomic data are limited or unavailable. Probabilities for each outcome can be extracted from the published literature or drawn from local data sources, which would provide a more relevant local perspective on outcomes. Costs associated with medications and outcomes should reflect those of the healthcare system.

Pharmacoeconomic analyses published in the medical literature or provided in the manufacturer's formulary dossier should be analyzed carefully before being included as part of the review process. Particular attention should be paid to the assumptions made in these studies. In many situations, assumptions made to simplify economic studies are not valid in particular institutions. Institution-specific costs are often different from the costs used in published studies, and local data should be used when incorporating their results into medication reviews.[39,40]

Even if a formal pharmacoeconomic evaluation is not included in a drug review document, a financial evaluation must be conducted, including consideration of site of care, non-medication-related costs, and financial consequences to the pharmacy and to the organization as a whole.

Formulary Exceptions. Exclusion of a medication from a formulary may affect coverage of and access to the medication. In a closed formulary system, for example, only medications listed on the formulary are covered under the patient's drug benefit. Regardless of health-system setting, the formulary system should include an exception process that provides prescribers and patients with timely access to medications that are not on the formulary but are medically necessary for the care of the patient. The underlying principle for such a process is that unique patient needs may not be satisfied by use of the formulary medications. The formulary exception process should generate information on nonformulary medication use that will enable the P&T committee to evaluate trends in such use. Criteria for approval of nonformulary medications should be developed (e.g., allergy to or therapeutic failure of formulary alternative, condition not treatable by formulary medications) and guidelines for use should be considered for nonformulary medications if they carry patient safety risks, have a risk evaluation and mitigation strategy (REMS), are expensive, and require complicated preparation.

Subformularies. Depending on state regulations, subformularies may be developed and maintained, using the same evidence-based process, to provide lists of appropriate and approved medications for furnishing by nonphysician providers or to specific patient subsets, such as Medicare patients. Health systems must follow specific rules and regulations provided under the U.S. Medicare Modernization Act of 2003 in their evaluation and inclusion of medications in a Medicare formulary for those medications to be covered.[41]

Strategies for Managing Medication Use

Common strategies for managing medication use via the formulary include use of generic drugs, biosimilars, and specialty medications; therapeutic interchange; guided-use policies, clinical practice guidelines; and MUE.

Generic Drugs. Optimizing the number of medication entities and products available from the pharmacy can produce substantial patient care and financial benefits. These benefits are greatly increased through the use of generic equivalents (drugs considered bioequivalent by FDA [i.e., AB-rated drug products[42]]). The use of generic equivalents is encouraged in order to provide the best possible care at an affordable cost. Use of generic drugs that have been deemed bioequivalent by FDA does not require review or approval by the P&T committee, although a review of all new generic medications for key safety issues (e.g., look-alike, sound-alike concerns) should be conducted to prevent medication errors when possible. For some drug categories, such as those with a narrow therapeutic range, a more thorough evaluation of the bioequivalency data and approval of experts or the P&T committee should be considered before implementing a generic substitution.

The P&T committee should establish policies and procedures governing the dispensing of generic equivalents when branded products are ordered. These policies and procedures should include the following points:

- The pharmacist is responsible for selecting from available generic equivalents those drugs to be dispensed pursuant to a prescriber's order for a particular medication.
- The prescriber has the option, at the time of prescribing, to specify the brand or supplier of the drug to be dispensed for that particular medication order if considered clinically justified.
- The prescriber's decision should be based on pharmacologic or therapeutic considerations (or both) relative to that patient.

Biosimilars. A biosimilar is a biological product that is highly similar to and has no clinically meaningful differences from an existing FDA-approved reference product.[43] Several entities have been approved as biosimilars by the FDA, and inclusion of these products on formulary should be considered as a strategy for management of the medication-use system. Biosimilars are not generically equivalent to the reference product, so the P&T committee should be involved in the decision to include these products on formulary. The implications for patients must also be considered, including legal and regulatory restrictions, coverage and reimbursement models by payers, differences in clinical indications or activity between the reference product and the biosimilar, and contractual obligations.

There are several considerations when evaluating biosimilars. When there are multiple biosimilars available for the same reference product, a close review of indications for each of the biosimilars should occur, as the indications that each biosimilar has may differ compared to each other and the reference product. The FDA can deem a biosimilar as interchangeable, however, even if a product does not have this status noted in its labelling. Available switching data should be reviewed closely to determine whether patients currently receiving treatment with the reference product can be switched to the biosimilar. In instances in which the FDA has determined a biosimilar product to be interchangeable, state regulations should be reviewed to determine actions required by the pharmacist when dispensing a biosimilar with an interchangeable status. In instances in which an institution may elect to have both a reference product and a biosimilar on formulary, careful attention should be paid to how these are built in the EHR to ensure the appropriate product is utilized.

Therapeutic Interchange. Therapeutic interchange is the authorized exchange of therapeutic alternatives in accordance with previously established and approved written guidelines, policies, or protocols within a formulary system.[1,44] Drugs appropriate for therapeutic interchange are drug products with different chemical structures that are expected to have similar therapeutic effects and safety profiles when administered to patients in therapeutically equivalent doses. Therapeutic interchange provides pharmacists with the authorization to use a formulary therapeutic alternative in place of a nonformulary medication or a nonpreferred formulary medication without having to contact the prescriber. Ideally, therapeutic interchanges are built into the EHR to allow for seamless substitution of formulary products. A process should be established for when the prescriber wishes to opt out of the interchange. Adequate educational initiatives should be undertaken to ensure that everyone affected (prescribers, patients, pharmacists, nurses, and other healthcare professionals) is notified of the therapeutic interchange.

Guided-Use Strategies. Medications may be added to the formulary with additional processes in place to guide the use of the medications to improve therapeutic outcomes, prevent adverse events, or reduce costs. All guidelines for use for both on- and off-label indications should be developed using evidence-based decisions, based on the current medical literature.[45] Examples of strategies to help guide the use of medications may include the following.

Established-use criteria. Patients must meet the established criteria before the medication is dispensed. A process should be developed to cover situations in which the patient does not meet the established criteria, but the medication is nevertheless determined to be medically necessary. This strategy may also be useful when medications are in short supply.

Restricting drug use by specialty service. A specific service must approve the use of the drug before dispensing. This strategy can be used when inappropriate use or severe adverse effects may occur, and it can also be employed for antimicrobial agents when inappropriate use or overuse can result in resistant organisms and pose a danger to the general patient population or the public. Alternatively, ordering of a specific medication may be limited to a specific group of prescribers (e.g., restricting use of chemotherapy agents to oncologists).

Designating medications for use in specific areas. Such policies can be helpful when administration of a medication requires special equipment or staff with particular skills to use the medication safely (e.g., limiting neuromuscular blockers to operating rooms and critical care areas). Approval of medical director (or designee) before drug use. This strategy is particularly appropriate when the P&T committee has reviewed a high-cost medication and determined that the drug has little or no role in the care of patients at that organization but a prescriber would like to use the medication on a nonformulary basis. This strategy may also be used as an approval pathway for medications requested for use outside of established criteria outlined in the formulary.

Clinical Practice Guidelines. Clinical practice guidelines are developed and disseminated by national and international organizations, but they can also be developed locally.

Whether the medication formulary is a reflection of existing clinical practice guidelines in a particular organization or vice versa, it is critical that the guidelines and formulary are consistent. If a specific medication is recommended by a clinical practice guideline, it should in the majority of cases be on the formulary. As formulary changes are made, agents may need to be removed from or replaced in existing guidelines. Guidelines should avoid recommending use of nonformulary medications, and they can be useful in discouraging nonformulary medication use and guiding the appropriate use of formulary products when necessary.

Guidelines are frequently developed to address complex or particularly expensive medication therapies. However, complicated specialty therapies that will affect the care of very few patients may not justify the time and resources necessary to develop and maintain a guideline. Guidelines may be medication specific or disease oriented and may overlap in their scope of coverage.

The development of a clinical practice guideline should begin with the synthesis of all available biomedical evidence addressing the guideline topic. In many cases, guidelines from other organizations, both national and local, can be used as a starting point for development. The subsequent consensus process, eliciting feedback and input from local stakeholders, is critical. Data from the organization should be used to make informed decisions during the consensus process. After the consensus process is completed, the guideline should be reviewed and approved by the P&T committee.

The dissemination and implementation of guidelines in the practice environment must also be carefully executed. Communication about the availability of guidelines is necessary. Guidelines should be readily available through existing health-system platforms. If feasible, it is recommended to build the guidelines into the computerized provider order entry system (e.g., through order set creation) to facilitate the appropriate care of the patient. Every guideline should include a time frame for future review and revision.

If utilization of a medication is being requested outside established health-system guidelines for appropriate use, scientific evidence to support safety and efficacy should be provided and reviewed to substantiate the request.

Specialty Medications. P&T committees should be involved in the organization's approach to managing specialty medications to ensure the pharmacy has the ability to provide medications in a timely manner, to support patient access to medications, and provide continuity of care. ASHP has resources to aid in specialty pharmacy management, including the ASHP Specialty Pharmacy Resource Guide.[46] This guide provides guidance on dispensing the medication directly to the site of care for patient administration (white bagging) or to the patient, who then carries it to the site of care for administration (brown bagging). Another strategy to consider in management of specialty pharmaceuticals is clear bagging. Clear bagging is the delivery of a patient-specific specialty pharmaceutical directly from a health system's specialty pharmacy directly to the health-system site of service, where it is then administered.[47]

MUE Process. MUE is a quality-improvement activity, but it can also be considered a formulary system management technique. MUEs have traditionally involved evaluating evidence-based criteria to determine the health system's compliance with established standards. Interventions could then be used to improve any aspect of the medication-use process based on MUE data analyses.

MUE can be simply informative (collecting data to guide decision-making) or used to measure the effect of interventions, such as the addition of a new agent to the formulary or the implementation of a new medication-use policy. While MUE often focuses on problem-prone, high-risk, or high-cost medications, MUE can be used to examine any aspect of medication use that is problematic to the institution conducting the evaluation. Medications recently added to the formulary should be evaluated, especially if there is the potential for inappropriate use or adverse effects. This review should occur 6–12 months after their addition to the formulary. High-cost, high-use, or problem-prone medications and outcomes of specific disease states are also good candidates for evaluation.

A systematic plan to monitor, evaluate, and improve medication use should be established within the organization.[19] Such a plan is an accreditation requirement for many organizations (e.g., Joint Commission[27]). The P&T committee, or its equivalent, should be involved in the MUE process. Refer to ASHP's Guidelines on Medication-Use Evaluation for more detailed information conducting an MUE.[19]

Incorporating Patient Safety Issues in the Decision-Making Process

The P&T committee should systematically address medication and patient safety issues as part of its deliberations. The P&T committee should ensure that medication-use policies adequately address potential risk and safety issues. Hospital or health-system medication-event data, including near misses, should consistently be reviewed by the P&T committee, along with recommendations to prevent future events. The P&T committee should also review available information on medication or patient safety events reported by other organizations to identify ways to prevent medication events and disseminate the information to healthcare providers and, when appropriate, patients.

When evaluating a medication for inclusion on the formulary, the P&T committee and its supporting subcommittees or panels should consider adverse effects, preparation issues, sound-alike or look-alike potential, practitioner safety, and dosing or administration issues. If a product has a REMS program, the requirements of this program should be carefully reviewed to ensure the institution can meet the requirements. When implementing formulary decisions for medications that have REMS, there should be processes in place to ensure compliance both during implementation and on an ongoing basis. Proactive assessments should be conducted to identify potential safety concerns posed by use of the medication, and proposed strategies to mitigate those risks should be implemented by the P&T committee. In addition, quality improvement projects to improve the safety of specific medications or to evaluate the processes involved should be conducted and reviewed by the P&T committee. The P&T committee should champion evidence-based fail-safe techniques (e.g., bar-coding) to prevent medication events.

Resources that provide information on medication or patient safety events include the Institute for Safe Medication Practices (www.ismp.org) and Medwatch. The Joint

Commission, Institute for Healthcare Improvement, and National Center on Patient Safety provide information about conducting and examples of failure mode and effects analysis (FMEA) projects on their websites (www.jointcommission.org/, www.ihi.org/, and www.patientsafety.va.gov).

Implementation of Formulary Decisions into the EHR

Use of the EHR to implement, guide, and evaluate decisions made by the P&T committee is essential. EHR technology functionality should be maximized to support drug policy and formulary management decisions. The EHR should provide guidance on dosing, monitoring, and restrictions/limitations at the point of prescription and verification. A standard process, including established expectations for timeliness, should be developed to consistently and efficiently implement these decisions into the EHR. Multi-hospital systems and integrated delivery networks that share the same HER platform and formulary review process should centralize the coordination of implementation.[48] EHR implementation efforts should be coordinated with operational changes and education requirements identified in the decision-making process. Finally, resources and personnel available to support implementation into the EHR should interface with the P&T committee to ensure understanding and shared expectations of the EHR technology functionality. In addition, key content experts charged with evaluating and proposing drug policy and formulary management decisions should collaborate with informatics personnel on the design and validation of EHR content.

Drug Product Shortages

Health systems frequently need to address drug product shortages. Drug product shortages disrupt patient care and impact all aspects of the medication-use system, including purchasing, storage, automation systems, the EHR, preparation, administration, monitoring, and education.

During a drug product shortage, the P&T committee plays an important role. The P&T committee needs to develop strategies to address shortages in a timely manner, including designating appropriate therapeutic alternatives, identifying strategies for mitigating use of available drug product, and establishing use restrictions. All of these strategies should be developed based on available literature and best practices. Therapeutic interchange can be useful in dealing with critical drug product shortages. The P&T committee should work collaboratively with other committees and departments, such as specific medical departments, nursing, and risk management (when necessary) to develop effective management plans for addressing shortages. Given the dynamic nature of drug shortages, it is not always possible to obtain approval from P&T committee members prior to implementation of strategies if there is a need for urgent changes. To make sure the P&T committee is aware of all changes related to drug shortages, organizations should include a drug shortage update as a regular agenda item for the P&T committee. Communication with patients and staff is crucial to effectively manage shortages.

Effective integration of these strategies into the EHR is key to successful implementation of a drug shortage plan. Various strategies exist for communication in the EHR, including placing electronic alerts on medications, blocking the ordering of medications on shortage, and facilitating the build of new medication records or order sets to guide use of alternative agents during the time of the shortage.

More information about managing drug product shortages can be found in the ASHP Guidelines on Managing Drug Product Shortages.[49]

Implementing Medication-Use Policies

Various tools can be used to implement medication-use policies. The policy should be integrated directly into the therapeutic decision-making processes that guide the use of a medication during order entry or incorporated into diagnosis-specific electronic treatment plan. Other specific ways of communicating information about a medication-use policy may include the use of

- Inservice education
- Facility-approved social media
- Grand rounds
- Communication between pharmacists and prescribers
- Staff meetings
- E-mail
- Electronic newsletters
- Prescriber detailing
- Pharmacy or institutional websites

Outcome-driven projects may be beneficial in illustrating the value of a new medication-use policy and support further expansion.

Reimbursement Strategies and Considerations

New payment models require that P&T committee members are astute in their understanding of the hospital and health system's payment policies and reimbursement strategies related to medications. A balanced approach to managing a hybrid reimbursement structure between traditional fee-for-service models and emerging value-based contracts will be required. Financing and reimbursement for medications is complex; hospitals and health systems can no longer exclusively focus on manufacturing contracts, wholesaler agreements, and inpatient reimbursement. Large health systems and integrated systems must consider implications of medication reimbursement by Medicare, Medicaid, commercial, and private payers. If applicable, 340B policies must also be considered. Prior to approval of high-cost drugs, in collaboration with the finance department, there should be a benefits investigation conducted, factoring in local payer mix, plans for financial monitoring, and payer negotiations. The organization should have a defined process and responsible department for validating reimbursement of therapy and financial outcomes over time. Factors include site of care decisions in determining where a medication will be administered. Each organization should have policies on the use of medications not directly procured by the hospital pharmacy. For example, some specialty medication payer agreements circumvent traditional buy-and-bill dispensing channels and instead use white or brown bagging strategies.[47] Furthermore, patient access to medications upon discharge or during transitions of care between care settings needs to be evaluated, and systems need to be in place to ensure continuity of medication use and to decrease the potential to prolong length of stay due to medications initiated during an inpatient stay that may be restricted elsewhere.

Conclusion

A formulary system is the multidisciplinary, evidence-based process employed by an organization to select and use medications that offer the best therapeutic outcomes while minimizing potential risks and costs for patients. Organizations should employ the MUE process to continually improve how medications are used within the organization at all steps in the medication-use process. Medication use is an inherently complex process that requires constant evaluation. Organizations need to implement all necessary tools and processes to meet the goals of safe and effective medication use. Professionals involved in the medication-use process need to know and understand how the organization's medication-use policies and processes can be incorporated into their daily work to ensure medications are used appropriately and safely. Technology offers many opportunities to make those processes more effective and efficient. Communicating the actions related to medication use is a constant challenge that organizations need to address.

References

1. Principles of a sound drug formulary system. In: Hawkins B, ed. *Best Practices for Hospital and Health-System Pharmacy: Positions and Guidance Documents of ASHP*. American Society of Health-System Pharmacists; 2018:233–236.
2. American Heart Association. American Heart Association policy statement on drug formularies. Published 2018. Accessed October 14, 2020. https://www.heart.org/-/media/files/about-us/policy-research/prevention-nutrition/drug-formulary-statement-2018.pdf
3. American College of Physicians. Position paper: therapeutic substitution and formulary systems. Published 1990. Accessed October 14, 2020. https://www.acponline.org/acp_policy/policies/therapeutic_substitution_formulary_systems_1990.pdf
4. Laing R, Tisocki K. How to develop a national formulary based on the WHO model formulary. Published 2004. Accessed October 14, 2020. http://archives.who.int/EMLib/docs/National_MF_Manual2004-8.pdf
5. American Medical Association. Policy H-125.991: drug formularies and therapeutic interchange. Accessed October 14, 2020. https://policysearch.ama-assn.org/policyfinder/detail/formulary?uri=%2FAMADoc%2FHOD.xml-0-227.xml
6. American Medical Association. Policy H-285.965: managed care cost containment involving prescription drugs. Accessed October 14, 2020. https://policysearch.ama-assn.org/policyfinder/detail/drug%20formularies%20?uri=%2FAMADoc%2FHOD.xml-0-2089.xml
7. Academy of Managed Care Pharmacy. AMCP format for formulary submissions. Accessed June 3, 2019. http://www.amcp.org/practice-resources/amcp-format-formulary-submissions/
8. American Academy of Family Physicians. Patient-centered formularies. Accessed October 14, 2020. https://www.aafp.org/about/policies/all/patient-formularies.html
9. Balu S, O'Connor P, Vogenberg FR. Contemporary issues affecting P&T committees. Part 1: The evolution. *P&T.* 2004;29:709–711.
10. American Society of Hospital Pharmacists. Minimum standard for pharmacies in hospitals. *Am J Hosp Pharm*. 1958; 15:992–994.
11. May JR. Formulary systems. In: DiPiro JT, ed. *Encyclopedia of Clinical Pharmacy*. Marcel Dekker; 2002.
12. Willcox AM. The legal basis of the formulary system. *Am J Hosp Pharm*. 1960; 17:603–608.
13. American Society of Hospital Pharmacists, American Hospital Association. Statement of guiding principles on the operation of hospital formularies. *Am J Hosp Pharm*. 1960; 17:609–610.
14. American Society of Hospital Pharmacists, American Hospital Association, American Pharmaceutical Association, et al. Statement of guiding principles on the operation of hospital formularies. *Am J Hosp Pharm.* 1964; 21:40–41.
15. Social Security Administration. Conditions of participation for hospitals. *Am J Hosp Pharm*. 1966; 23:179–180.
16. Lammy PP, Flack HL. Pharmacy and therapeutics committee, consent, and the hospital formulary. *Am J Hosp Pharm*. 1966; 23:662–672.
17. American Medical Association. AMA policy on drug formularies and therapeutic interchange in inpatient and ambulatory patient care settings. *Am J Hosp Pharm*. 1994; 51:1808–1810.
18. Heindel GA, McIntyre CM. Contemporary challenges and novel strategies for health-system formulary management. *Am J Health-Syst Pharm*. 2018; 75:556–560.
19. American Society of Health-System Pharmacists. ASHP guidelines on medication-use evaluation. Published 2020. Accessed October 14, 2020. https://www.ashp.org/-/media/assets/policy-guidelines/docs/guidelines/medication-use-evaluationcurrent.ashx
20. American Society of Health-System Pharmacists. ASHP guidelines on adverse drug reaction monitoring and reporting. *Am J Health-Syst Pharm*. 1995; 52:417–419.
21. American Society of Health-System Pharmacists. ASHP guidelines on preventing medication errors in hospitals. *Am J Health-Syst Pharm*. 2018; 75:1493–1517. Accessed October 14, 2020. https://www.ashp.org/-/media/assets/policyguidelines/docs/guidelines/preventing-medicationerrors-hospitals.ashx
22. American Society of Health-System Pharmacists. ASHP guidelines on the pharmacist's role in the development, implementation, and assessment of critical pathways. *Am J Health-Syst Pharm*. 2004; 61:939–945.
23. Brennan TA, Rothman DJ, Blank L, et al. Health industry practices that create conflicts of interest: a policy proposal for academic medical centers. *JAMA*. 2006; 295:429–433.

24. Nair KV, Ascione FJ. Evaluation of P&T committee performance: an exploratory study. *Formulary.* 2001; 36:136–146.
25. Nakahiro S. Contemporary issues in formulary management. In: Millares M, ed. *Applied Drug Information: Strategies for Information Management.* Applied Therapeutics Inc.; 1998:8.1–8.43.
26. Nakahiro RK, Ho SS, Okamoto MP. Concepts of pharmacoeconomics. In: Millares M, ed. *Applied Drug Information: Strategies for Information Management.* Applied Therapeutics Inc.; 1998:7.1–7.37.
27. The Joint Commission. *Comprehensive Accreditation Manual for Hospitals.* The Joint Commission; April 2018.
28. ASHP guidelines for selecting pharmaceutical manufacturers and suppliers. *Am J Hosp Pharm.* 1991; 48:523–524.
29. American Society of Hospital Pharmacists. ASHP guidelines on pharmacists' relationships with industry. *Am J Hosp Pharm.* 1992; 49:154.
30. Briss PA, Zaza S, Pappaioanou M, et al. Developing an evidence-based guide to community preventive services—methods. *Am J Prev Med.* 2000; 18(suppl 1): 35–43.
31. Atkins D, Best D, Briss PA, et al. Grading quality of evidence and strength of recommendations. *BMJ.* 2004; 328:1490–1498.
32. Guyatt G, Gutterman D, Baumann MH, et al. Grading strength of evidence of recommendations and quality of evidence in clinical guidelines: report from an American College of Chest Physicians task force. *Chest.* 2006; 129:174–181.
33. Harbour R, Miller J. A new system for grading recommendations in evidence based guidelines. *BMJ.* 2001; 323:334–336.
34. Corman SL, Skledar SJ, Culley CM. Evaluation of conflicting literature and application to formulary decisions. *Am J Health-Syst Pharm.* 2007; 64:182–185.
35. Sterné SC, Uchida KM, Iteen SA. Improving the presentation of drug information to pharmacy and therapeutics committees for formulary decisions. *Am J Health-Syst Pharm.* 1996; 53:1162–1164.
36. Reeder CE. Overview of pharmacoeconomics and pharmaceutical outcomes evaluations. *Am J Health Syst Pharm.* 1995; 52(19)(suppl 4):S5–S8.
37. Drummond MF, Sculpher MJ, Torrance GW, et al. *Methods for the Economic Evaluation of Health Care Programmes.* 3rd ed. Oxford University Press; 2005:137–189.
38. Gold MR, Siegel JE, Russell LB, et al., eds. *Cost-Effectiveness in Health and Medicine.* Oxford University Press; 1996:176–213.
39. Sanchez LA. Applied pharmacoeconomics: evaluation and use of pharmacoeconomic data from the literature. *Am J Health-Syst Pharm.* 1999; 56:1630–1638.
40. Ofman JJ, Sullivan SD, Neumann PJ, et al. Examining the value and quality of health economic analyses: implications of utilizing the QHES. *J Manag Care Pharm.* 2003; 9:53–61.
41. U.S. Medicare Prescription Drug, Improvement, and Modernization Act of 2003. Pub. L. No. 108-173.
42. Food and Drug Administration. Approved Drug Products with Therapeutic Equivalence Evaluations (Orange Book). www.fda.gov/cder/ob/. Accessed October 14, 2020.
43. Food and Drug Administration. Biosimilars. Accessed October 14, 2020. https://www.fda.gov/drugs/therapeutic-biologicsapplications-bla/biosimilars
44. Gray T, Bertch K, Galt K, et al. Guidelines for therapeutic interchange—2004. *Pharmacotherapy.* 2005; 25:1666–1680. Accessed October 4, 2020. https://www.accp.com/docs/positions/guidelines/Pharm2511_ACCP-TherapIntchg.pdf
45. American Society of Hospital Pharmacists. ASHP statement on the use of medications for unlabeled uses. *Am J Hosp Pharm.* 1992; 49:2006–2008.
46. American Society of Hospital Pharmacists. ASHP Specialty Pharmacy Resource Guide. Accessed October 14, 2020. https://www.ashp.org/-/media/assets/pharmacy-practice/resource-centers/specialty-pharmacy/specialtypharmacy-resource-guide.ashx
47. McCain J. Part I: distribution models for biologics and other specialty pharmaceutical products. *Biotechnol Healthc.* 2012; 9:8–13.
48. Knoer SJ, Riffle AR. Multihospital health systems: seize the opportunity. *Am J Health-Syst Pharm.* 2018; 75(7):423–429.
49. ASHP guidelines on managing drug product shortages. *Am J Health-Syst Pharm.* 2018; 75:1742–1750. Accessed October 14, 2020. https://www.ashp.org/-/media/assets/policy-guidelines/docs/guidelines/managing-drug-product-shortages.ashx
50. Jamison DT, Breman JG, Measham AR, et al., eds. *Priorities in Health. Chapter 3: Cost-Effectiveness Analysis.* International Bank for Reconstruction and Development/World Bank; 2006.
51. Robinson R. Cost-utility analysis. *BMJ.* 1993; 307(6908):859–862. doi: 10.1136/bmj.307.6908.859
52. Centers for Medicare & Medicaid Services. Electronic health records. Accessed October 14, 2020. https://www.cms.gov/Medicare/EHealth/HealthRecords/index.html

Appendix A—Glossary of Terms

Cost-effectiveness analysis: A method for assessing the gains in health relative to the costs of different health interventions.[50]

Cost utility analysis: A comparison of the costs of different procedures with their outcomes measured in "utility based" units—that is, units that relate to a person's level of well-being and most often expressed as quality adjusted life year(s).[51]

Electronic health record: A digital version of a patient's medical history that is maintained by the provider over time, and may include all of the key administrative clinical data relevant to that person's care under a particular provider, including demographics, progress notes, problems, medications, vital signs, past medical history, immunizations, laboratory data, and radiology reports.[52]

Formulary: A continually updated list of medications and related information, representing the clinical judgment of physicians, pharmacists, and other experts in the diagnosis, prophylaxis, or treatment of disease and promotion of health.

Formulary system: An ongoing process whereby a healthcare organization, through its physicians, pharmacist, and other healthcare professionals, establishes policies on the use of drug products and therapies and identifies drug products and therapies that are the most medically appropriate and cost-effective to best serve the health interests of a given patient population.[1]

Generic substitution: The substitution of drug products that contain the same active ingredient or ingredients and are chemically identical in strength, concentration, dosage form, and route of administration to the drug product prescribed.[1]

Medication: Any prescription medications, sample medications, herbal remedies, vitamins, nutraceuticals, vaccines, or over-the-counter drugs; diagnostic and contrast agents used on or administered to persons to diagnose, treat, or prevent disease or other abnormal conditions; radioactive medications, respiratory therapy treatments, parenteral nutrition, blood derivatives, and intravenous solutions (plain, with electrolytes and/or drugs); and any product designated by the Food and Drug Administration (FDA) as a drug. This definition of medication does not include enteral nutrition solutions (which are considered food products), oxygen, and other medical gases.[27]

Medication-use evaluation: A systematic and interdisciplinary performance improvement method with an overarching goal of optimizing patient outcomes via ongoing evaluation and improvement of medication utilization.[19]

Pharmacy and therapeutics (P&T) committee: An advisory committee that is responsible for developing, managing, updating, and administering a formulary system. Institutions may refer to this committee by a different name.[1]

Therapeutic alternatives: Drug products with different chemical structures but of the same pharmacologic or therapeutic class and usually have similar therapeutic effects and adverse-reaction profiles when administered to patients in therapeutically equivalent doses.[1]

Therapeutic interchange: Authorized exchange of therapeutic alternatives in accordance with previously established and approved written guidelines or protocols within a formulary system.[1,44]

Therapeutic substitution: The act of dispensing a therapeutic alternative for the drug product prescribed without prior authorization of the prescriber. This is an illegal act because only the prescriber may authorize an exchange of therapeutic alternatives.[1]

Appendix B—Drug Evaluation Process

There are four major types of drug reviews: new drug monographs, reevaluations of previous formulary decisions, therapeutic class reviews, and expedited reviews of newly approved medications. Because of the expertise and training of pharmacists (drug information specialists in particular), pharmacists should play an integral part in the preparation and presentation of the drug review document to the P&T committee.

New Drug Monographs. When the Food and Drug Administration (FDA) approves a new drug for marketing that is relevant to the health system, a drug monograph should be prepared for formulary consideration by the P&T committee.

New chemical entities warrant a thorough evaluation and a written drug monograph. A short (e.g., one-page) summary could be provided along with the full monograph.[35] Some organizations use an executive summary format. A new drug that is significantly similar to other available therapeutic alternatives may be presented in a more abbreviated manner (e.g., an abbreviated monograph) provided that the P&T committee or experts agree that the drug is therapeutically equivalent to agents already available on the formulary.

Addenda to Original Monographs Used to Reevaluate Previous Formulary Decisions. Formulary decisions may need to be reassessed based on relevant new information or in light of newly marketed drugs or dosage forms. New data on safety, efficacy, stability, methods of administration, cost, or pharmacoeconomics may warrant a reevaluation of the drug or dosage strengths or formulations stocked by the health system. An addendum to the original monograph summarizing the new information should be developed for evaluation by the P&T committee. The P&T committee may want to establish reassessment dates at the time of formulary review so that the committee can reassess the effect of a formulary decision on quality or cost of care.

Therapeutic Class Reviews. Review of an entire therapeutic class of drugs should be performed at regular intervals, which may be determined by the P&T committee or influenced by regulatory agencies. A therapeutic class review should include all formulary and nonformulary medications within the class and may include institutional utilization or outcomes data and newly published information. Therapeutic class reviews may lead to formulary removal of therapeutically equivalent drugs or a change in restriction or guideline status for a drug.

Expedited Reviews. A process should be available for the P&T committee to conduct an expedited review of a new drug, new indication for a drug, or reevaluation of a previous formulary decision. Criteria should be in place to describe when an expedited review is warranted. For example, approval of a new chemical entity for a disease with no therapeutic alternative may warrant an expedited review to ensure availability of the drug for patients who need it. Likewise, a significant new safety concern may warrant an expedited review for addition of restrictions or removal from the formulary.

Developed through the ASHP Council on Pharmacy Practice and approved by the ASHP Board of Directors on November 16, 2020. These guidelines supersede the ASHP Guidelines on the Pharmacy and Therapeutics Committee and the Formulary System dated January 28, 2008, and the ASHP Statement on the Pharmacy and Therapeutics Committee and the Formulary System dated June 10, 2008.

ASHP gratefully acknowledges the following organizations and individuals for reviewing these guidelines (review does not imply endorsement): American Pharmacists Association (APhA); Maryland Society of Health System Pharmacists (MSHP); Thomas S. Achey, Pharm.D., M.S., BCPS; Ryan C. Costantino, Pharm.D., M.A., BCPS, BCGP; Katie Foster, Pharm.D., M.S., FCCM; Rena Gosser,

Pharm.D., BCPS; Kathleen M. Gura, Pharm.D., BCNSP, FASHP; Charzetta H. James, Pharm.D., CPh., M.B.A., M.H.A., FACHE, PRS; Isha John, Pharm.D., M.B.A. (APhA); Indrani Kar, Pharm.D.; Nicole Kiehle, Pharm.D., BCPS (MSHP); Eric C. Kutscher, Pharm.D., MBA, FASHP; Patrick M. Malone, Pharm.D., FASHP; Nancy MacDonald, Pharm.D., BCPS, FASHP; Kathryn Clark McKinney, Pharm.D., M.S., BCPS, FACHE, FASHP; Valerie Dee Nolt, Pharm.D., BCPPS; James Ponto, M.S., BCNP, FASHP; Preetham Talari, M.D., FACP, SFHM; Philip J. Trapskin, Pharm.D., BCPS; Tyler A. Vest, Pharm.D., M.S., BCPS; Geralyn Waters, Pharm.D., BCPS; Jody Jacobson Wedret, R.Ph., FASHP, FCSHP.

ASHP also gratefully acknowledges the contributions of authors of previous versions of these guidelines: Linda S. Tyler, Pharm.D., FASHP; Mirta Millares, Pharm.D., FCSHP, FASHP; Andrew L. Wilson, Pharm.D., FASHP; Lee C. Vermeulen, Jr., B.S.Pharm., M.S.; J. Russell (Rusty) May, Pharm.D., FASHP; Michael A. Valentino, R.Ph., MHSA; and Sabrina W. Cole, Pharm.D.

The authors have declared no potential conflicts of interest.

Christy Ciccarello, PharmD, MHA, Vice President, Clinical Pharmacy Services, Novant Health, Winston-Salem, NC.

Molly Billstein Leber, PharmD, BCPS, FASHP, Associate Director, Drug Use Policy and Formulary Management, Yale New Haven Health System, New Haven, CT.

Mandy C. Leonard, PharmD, BCPS, System Director, Drug Use Policy and Formulary Management, Department of Pharmacy, Cleveland Clinic, Cleveland, OH.

Todd Nesbit, PharmD, MBA, FASHP, Director of Pharmacy Patient Care Services, The Johns Hopkins Health System, Baltimore, MD.

Mary G. Petrovskis, PharmD, BCPS, PGY2 Health-System Pharmacy Administration Resident, University of North Carolina Medical Center, Chapel Hill, NC.

Emily Pherson, PharmD, BCPS, Assistant Director, Medication Use Policy & Clinical Informatics, The Johns Hopkins Health System, Baltimore, MD.

Heidi A. Pillen, PharmD, FASHP, Director of Pharmacy, Clinical Services & Medication Use Policy, Beaumont Health, Southfield, MI.

Celia Proctor, PharmD, MBA, Assistant Director, System Formulary Management & Integration, The Johns Hopkins Health System, Baltimore, MD.

Jennifer Reddan, PharmD, FASHP, Pharmacy Executive Director, Excelerate, Vizient, Irving, TX.

Copyright © 2021, American Society of Health-System Pharmacists, Inc. All rights reserved. Contact ASHP for reprint and permissions requests. This content may not be used for commercial purposes without the express written consent of ASHP.

The bibliographic citation for this document is as follows: American Society of Health-System Pharmacists. ASHP guidelines on the pharmacy and therapeutics committee and the formulary system. *Am J Health-Syst Pharm*. 2021;78:907–18.

Principles of a Sound Drug Formulary System

These principles have been endorsed by the following organizations:

- Academy of Managed Care Pharmacy
- Alliance of Community Health Plans
- American Medical Association
- American Society of Health-System Pharmacists
- Department of Veterans Affairs, Pharmacy Benefits Management Strategic Healthcare Group
- National Business Coalition on Health
- U.S. Pharmacopeia

Preamble

A coalition of national organizations representing health care professionals, government, and business leaders formed a working group (see **Appendix III**) to develop a set of principles specifying the essential components that contribute to a sound drug formulary system. The Coalition was formed in September 1999 in response to the widespread use of drug formularies in both inpatient and outpatient settings and the lack of understanding about formularies among the public. Also, proposed federal legislation that would provide a prescription drug benefit for Medicare beneficiaries has brought increased attention to the appropriate role and management of drug formulary systems within drug benefit programs.

The formulary system, when properly designed and implemented, can promote rational, clinically appropriate, safe, and cost-effective drug therapy. The Coalition has enumerated these principles, however, because it recognizes that patient care may be compromised if a formulary system is not optimally developed, organized, and administered. This document contains "Guiding Principles" that the Coalition believes must be present for a drug formulary system to appropriately serve the patients it covers. The absence of one or more of these "Guiding Principles" should be cause for careful scrutiny of a formulary system. A glossary (see **Appendix I**) and bibliography (see **Appendix II**) are included with the "Guiding Principles" to clarify terminology and to provide additional resources, respectively.

The Coalition believes that the presence of consensus-based Formulary System Principles can assist decision-makers who must balance the health care quality and cost equation. Further, the Guiding Principles will be a valuable educational tool for national, state, and local public policy makers, health care system administrators, purchasers and third-party payers, practitioners, and consumers and patient advocates. These parties all have an interest in designing formulary systems that ensure patients have access to rational, clinically appropriate, safe, and cost-effective therapy and which supports an affordable and sustainable drug benefit program.

Definitions

Drug Formulary System. An ongoing process whereby a health care organization, through its physicians, pharmacists, and other health care professionals, establishes policies on the use of drug products and therapies, and identifies drug products and therapies that are the most medically appropriate and cost-effective to best serve the health interests of a given patient population.

Drug Formulary. A continually updated list of medications and related information, representing the clinical judgement of physicians, pharmacists, and other experts in the diagnosis and/or treatment of disease and promotion of health.

Guiding Principles

Formulary system decisions are based on scientific and economic considerations that achieve appropriate, safe, and cost-effective drug therapy.

- Clinical decisions are based on the strength of scientific evidence and standards of practice that include, but are not limited, to the following:
  - Assessing peer-reviewed medical literature, including randomized clinical trials (especially drug comparison studies), pharmacoeconomic studies, and outcomes research data.
  - Employing published practice guidelines, developed by an acceptable evidence-based process.
  - Comparing the efficacy as well as the type and frequency of side effects and potential drug interactions among alternative drug products.
  - Assessing the likely impact of a drug product on patient compliance when compared to alternative products.
  - Basing formulary system decisions on a thorough evaluation of the benefits, risks, and potential outcomes for patients; risks encompass adverse drug events (adverse drug reactions and medication errors, such as those caused by confusing product names or labels).
- Economic considerations include, but are not limited, to the following:
  - Basing formulary system decisions on cost factors only after the safety, efficacy, and therapeutic need have been established.
  - Evaluating drug products and therapies in terms of their impact on total health care costs.
  - Permitting financial incentives only when they promote cost management as part of the delivery of quality medical care. Financial incentives or pressures on practitioners that may interfere with the delivery of medically necessary care are unacceptable.

The formulary system encompasses drug selection, drug utilization review, and other tools to foster best practices in prescribing, dispensing, administration, and monitoring of outcomes.

- The formulary system:
  - Provides drug product selection and formulary maintenance (see above).
  - Provides drug use evaluation (also called drug utilization review) to enhance quality of care for patients by assuring appropriate drug therapy.

DOI 10.37573/9781585287048.042

- Provides for the periodic evaluation and analysis of treatment protocols and procedures to ensure that they are up-to-date and are consistent with optimum therapeutics.
- Provides for the monitoring, reporting, and analysis of adverse results of drug therapy (e.g., adverse drug reactions, medication errors) to continuously improve the quality of care.

The Pharmacy and Therapeutics (P&T) Committee, or equivalent body, comprised of actively practicing physicians, pharmacists, and other health care professionals, is the mechanism for administering the formulary system, which includes developing and maintaining the formulary and establishing and implementing policies on the use of drug products.

- The Pharmacy and Therapeutics Committee:
  - Objectively appraises, evaluates, and selects drugs for the formulary.
  - Meets as frequently as is necessary to review and update the appropriateness of the formulary system in light of new drugs and new indications, uses, or warnings affecting existing drugs.
  - Establishes policies and procedures to educate and inform health care providers about drug products, usage, and committee decisions.
  - Oversees quality improvement programs that employ drug use evaluation.
  - Implements generic substitution and therapeutic interchange programs that authorize exchange of therapeutic alternatives based upon written guidelines or protocols within a formulary system. (Note: Therapeutic substitution, the dispensing of therapeutic alternates without the prescriber's approval, is illegal and should not be allowed—see Glossary.)
  - Develops protocols and procedures for the use of and access to non-formulary drug products.

Physicians, pharmacists, and other health care professionals provide oversight of the formulary system.

- Health care organization policies should ensure appropriate oversight of the P&T Committee and its decisions by the medical staff or equivalent body.

The formulary system must have its own policies, or adhere to other organizational policies, that address conflicts of interest and disclosure by P&T committee members.

- Formulary system policies should:
  - Require P&T committee members to reveal, by signing a conflict of interest statement, economic and other relationships with pharmaceutical entities that could influence Committee decisions.
  - Exclude product sponsor representatives from P&T committee membership and from attending P&T committee meetings.
  - Require P&T committee members to adhere to the formulary system's policy on disclosure and participation in discussion as it relates to conflict of interest.

The formulary system should include educational programs for payers, practitioners, and patients concerning their roles and responsibilities.

- The formulary system should:
  - Inform physicians, pharmacists, other health care professionals, patients, and payers about the factors that affect formulary system decisions, including cost containment measures; the procedures for obtaining non-formulary drugs; and the importance of formulary compliance to improving quality of care and restraining health care costs.
  - Proactively inform practitioners about changes to the formulary or to other pharmaceutical management procedures.
  - Provide patient education programs that explain how formulary decisions are made and the roles and responsibilities of the patient, especially the importance of patient compliance with drug therapy to assure the success of that therapy.
  - Disclose the existence of formularies and have copies of the formulary readily available and accessible.
  - Provide rationale for specific formulary decisions when requested.

The formulary system should include a well-defined process for the physician or other prescriber to use a non-formulary drug when medically indicated.

- The formulary system should:
  - Enable individual patient needs to be met with non-formulary drug products when demonstrated to be clinically justified by the physician or other prescriber.
  - Institute an efficient process for the timely procurement of non-formulary drug products and impose minimal administrative burdens.
  - Provide access to a formal appeal process if a request for a non-formulary drug is denied.
  - Include policies that state that practitioners should not be penalized for prescribing non-formulary drug products that are medically necessary.

Appendix I—Glossary

Drug formulary system: An ongoing process whereby a health care organization, through its physicians, pharmacists, and other health care professionals, establishes policies on the use of drug products and therapies, and identifies drug products and therapies that are the most medically appropriate and cost effective to best serve the health interests of a given patient population.

Drug formulary: A continually updated list of medications and related information, representing the clinical judgement of physicians, pharmacists, and other experts in the diagnosis and/or treatment of disease and promotion of health.

Pharmacy & therapeutics (P&T) committee: An advisory committee that is responsible for developing, managing, updating, and administering the drug formulary system.

Generic substitution: The substitution of drug products that contain the same active ingredient(s) and are chemically identical in strength, concentration, dosage form, and route of administration to the drug product prescribed.

Therapeutic alternates: Drug products with different chemical structures but which are of the same pharmacological and/or therapeutic class, and usually can be expected to have similar therapeutic effects and adverse reaction profiles when administered to patients in therapeutically equivalent doses.

Therapeutic interchange: Authorized exchange of therapeutic alternates in accordance with previously established and approved written guidelines or protocols within a formulary system.

Therapeutic substitution: The act of dispensing a therapeutic alternate for the drug product prescribed without prior authorization of the prescriber. This is an illegal act because only the prescriber may authorize an exchange of therapeutic alternates.

Drug utilization review (drug use review, DUR, and drug use evaluation): Process used to assess the appropriateness of drug therapy by engaging in the evaluation of data on drug use in a given health care environment against predetermined criteria and standards.

Appendix II—Bibliography

1. Academy of Managed Care Pharmacy, Concepts in Managed Care Pharmacy Series—Formulary Management (Alexandria, VA: 1998).
2. American Medical Association. Board of Trustees Report PPP, Principles of Drug Utilization Review. In, American Medical Association House of Delegates Proceedings, 140th Annual Meeting. Chicago: American Medical Association; June 1991; 225–7.
3. American Medical Association. Board of Trustees Report 45, Drug Formularies and Therapeutic Interchange. In, American Medical Association House of Delegates Proceedings, 47th Interim Meeting. New Orleans: American Medical Association; December 1993; 155–8.
4. American Medical Association. Council on Ethical and Judicial Affairs Report 2, Managed Care Cost Containment Involving Prescription Drugs. In, American Medical Association House of Delegates Proceedings, 144th Annual Meeting. Chicago: American Medical Association; June 1995; 207–13.
5. American Medical Association. Board of Trustees Report 9, Pharmaceutical Benefits Management Companies. In, American Medical Association House of Delegates Proceedings, 51st Interim Meeting. Dallas: American Medical Association; December 1997; 33–44.
6. American Society of Consultant Pharmacists. Guidelines for the Development of Formulary Systems in Nursing Facilities; July 1996.
7. American Society of Hospital Pharmacists. ASHP Statement on the Formulary System. *Am J Hosp Pharm.* 1983; 40:1384–5.
8. American Society of Hospital Pharmacists. ASHP Guidelines on Formulary System Management. *Am J Hosp Pharm.* 1992; 49:648–52.
9. American Society of Hospital Pharmacists. ASHP Statement on the Pharmacy and Therapeutics Committee. *Am J Hosp Pharm.* 1992; 49:2008–9.
10. American Society of Health-System Pharmacists. ASHP Guidelines on Medication-Use Evaluation. *Am J Health-syst Pharm.* 1996; 53:1953–5.
11. American Society of Hospital Pharmacists. ASHP Technical Assistance Bulletin on Drug Formularies. *Am J Hosp Pharm.* 1991; 48:791–3.
12. American Society of Hospital Pharmacists. ASHP Technical Assistance Bulletin on the Evaluation of Drugs for Formularies. *Am J Hosp Pharm.* 1988; 45:386–7.
13. Covington TR and Thornton JL. The formulary system: A cornerstone of drug benefit management, in A Pharmacist's Guide to Principles and Practices of Managed Care Pharmacy. Ito S and Blackburn S, eds. Foundation for Managed Care Pharmacy, Alexandria VA. 1995:35–49.
14. Dillon MJ. Drug Formulary Management, in Managed Care Pharmacy Practice. Navarro RP ed. Aspen Publishers, Inc., Gaithersburg, MD. 1999:145–65.
15. Hejna CS and Shepherd MD. Pharmacy and therapeutics committee and formulary development, in A Pharmacist's Guide to Principles and Practices of Managed Care Pharmacy. Ito S and Blackburn S, eds. Foundation for Managed Care Pharmacy, Alexandria VA. 1995:27–34.
16. National Committee for Quality Assurance. UM 10 procedures for pharmaceutical management. 2000 Standards for Accreditation of MCOs. 1999:58–60.
17. National Committee for Quality Assurance. UM 10 procedures for pharmaceutical management. 2000 Surveyor Guidelines for the Accreditation of MCOs. 1999:173–82.
18. PCMA Response to American Medical Association Report, I-97, "Pharmaceutical Benefits Management Companies." September 1998.
19. Rucker TD and Schiff GD. Drug formularies: myths-information. *Medical Care.* 1990; 28:928–42. Reprinted in *Hospital Pharmacy,* 1991; 26:507–14.

Appendix III—Coalition Working Group

Academy of Managed Care Pharmacy
Judith A. Cahill, C.E.B.S., Executive Director
Richard Fry, Senior Director, Pharmacy Affairs

American Medical Association
Joseph W. Cranston, Ph.D., Director-Science, Research and Technology

American Society of Health-System Pharmacists
William A. Zellmer, M.P.H., Deputy Executive Vice President

Department of Veterans Affairs
John E. Ogden, Director, Pharmacy Services
Michael A. Valentino, Associate Chief Consultant for Pharmacy Benefits Management

National Business Coalition on Health
Catherine Kunkle, Vice President

U.S. Pharmacopeia
Jacqueline L. Eng, Senior Vice President, Program Development
Keith W. Johnson, Vice President and Director, New and Off-Label Uses
Thomas R. Fulda, Program Director, Drug Utilization Review Programs
Nancy B. Mabie, Assistant Director, Pharmacy Affairs

Observer
AARP
David Gross, Senior Policy Advisor, Public Policy Institute

Public Comment Requested

To ensure that knowledgeable and interested parties beyond the Coalition Working Group had an opportunity to contribute to the Principles development process, a preliminary set of principles was distributed for public comment to 50-plus organizations in February 2000. Comments received were thoroughly reviewed and considered by the Coalition Working Group.

These principles were endorsed by the ASHP Board of Directors on June 4, 2000.

The endorsement of this document was reviewed in 2011 by the Council on Pharmacy Practice and by the Board of Directors and was found to still be appropriate.

Government, Law, and Regulation

DOI 10.37573/9781585287048

Government, Law, and Regulation

2306

SUPPORT FOR FDA EXPANDED ACCESS (COMPASSIONATE USE) PROGRAM

Source: Council on Public Policy

To advocate that the Food and Drug Administration (FDA) Expanded Access (Compassionate Use) Program be the primary mechanism for patient access to drugs for which an investigational new drug application (IND) has been filed, in order to preserve the integrity of the drug approval process and assure patient safety; further,

To advocate for broader patient access to such drugs under the FDA Expanded Access Program; further,

To advocate that IND applicants expedite review and release of drugs for patients who qualify for the program; further,

To advocate that the drug therapy be recommended by a physician and reviewed and monitored by a pharmacist to assure safe patient care; further,

To advocate for the patient's right to be informed of the potential benefits and risks via an informed consent process, and the responsibility of an institutional review board to review and approve the informed consent and the drug therapy protocol; further,

To support the use of the Right-to-Try pathway in instances in which all other options have been exhausted, provided there is (1) a robust informed consent process, and (2) institutional and clinical oversight by a physician and a pharmacist.

This policy supersedes ASHP policy 1508.

Rationale

Patient access to drugs for which an investigational new drug application (IND) has been filed is made available on a limited basis to individual patients under a compassionate-use program regulated by the FDA. With information about clinical trials and drugs under development readily available to patients, there is an increased demand for access to these therapies. In addition, three states have passed laws to permit patients who have exhausted approved drugs and treatment to have access to these potentially lifesaving drugs. Other states may follow suit in the future, and the FDA has begun to respond to this growing patient demand by streamlining its application process for individual patient expanded access. In order to respond to state legislative proposals, ASHP advocates preserving the integrity of drug development through strengthening the evidence-based clinical trial process and expanded patient access.

In 2018, Congress passed Right-to-Try legislation, which, per FDA, "is one pathway for patients diagnosed with life-threatening diseases or conditions who have exhausted all approved treatment options and are unable to participate in a clinical trial to access certain drugs that have not been approved by the Food and Drug Administration (FDA)." The program functions outside of FDA control, with patients and their physicians coordinating directly with manufacturers for access to investigational new drugs. ASHP advocates that the FDA's Compassionate Use Program remain the primary access point for investigational new drugs, but supports the use of Right-to-Try for patients who have exhausted all other options. Furthermore, ASHP advocates for additional patient safety requirements related to informed consent and clinician monitoring for patients accessing investigational new drugs through the Right-to-Try pathway.

DOI 10.37573/9781585287048.043

2307

BIOSIMILAR MEDICATIONS

Source: Council on Public Policy

To encourage the development of safe and effective biosimilar medications in order to make such medications more affordable and accessible; further,

To encourage research on the safety, effectiveness, and interchangeability of biosimilar medications; further,

To support legislation and regulation to allow Food and Drug Administration (FDA) approval of biosimilar medications that are also determined by the FDA to be interchangeable and therefore supports substitution for the reference product without the intervention of the prescriber; further,

To oppose the implementation of any state laws restricting biosimilar interchangeability; further,

To oppose any state legislation that would require a pharmacist to notify a prescriber when a biosimilar deemed to be interchangeable by the FDA is dispensed; further,

To require postmarketing surveillance for all biosimilar medications to ensure their continued safety, effectiveness, purity, quality, identity, and strength; further,

To advocate for adequate reimbursement for biosimilar medications that are approved by the FDA; further,

To promote and develop education of pharmacists, providers, and patients about biosimilar medications and their appropriate use within hospitals and health systems; further,

To advocate for patient, prescriber, and pharmacist choice in selecting the most clinically appropriate and cost-effective therapy.

This policy supersedes ASHP policy 1816.

Rationale

A provision in the Patient Protection and Affordable Care Act created a new pathway for the FDA to approve biosimilar products. The FDA approved its first biosimilar application in March 2015 for filgrastim-sndz, and others (e.g., adalimumab-adbm, adalimumab-atto, bevacizumab-awwb, etanercept-szzs, infliximab-abda, infliximab-dyyb) have followed. The FDA defines a biosimilar drug as "a biologic that is highly similar to and has no clinically meaningful differences from another biologic that is already approved by the FDA (known as the reference product)." During the FDA approval process, a new biosimilar undergoes tests to assess structural and functional components as well as limited preclinical and clinical studies. In order for a biosimilar to be considered interchangeable with its reference product, the FDA requires the manufacturer to additionally show that their biosimilar produces the same clinical result and switching to their biosimilar does not result in any additional risks or diminished efficacy. This typically requires additional trials, which are time consuming and costly. As of 2022, there are over 30 biosimilars approved, not all of which are commercially available, but only a select few have qualified as interchangeable due to these extensive regulatory processes.

At the state level, legislation has been proposed and enacted requiring patient and/or prescriber notification that a biosimilar medication has been interchanged. It is important to note that pharmacists cannot substitute a biosimilar medication unless the FDA has deemed that biosimilar to be interchangeable. As of 2019, 46 states and Puerto Rico have passed biosimilar substitution laws. In some states the prescriber/patient notification is similar to what is required for generic substitution, but in others it goes further. For example, Georgia's biosimilar law requires the pharmacist to notify the prescriber within 48 hours of dispensing the medication (excluding weekends and holidays).

Despite the lack of interchangeable biosimilars, insurance companies have started requiring use of "preferred" biosimilars, leading to issues when attempting to maintain reasonable hospital formularies, patients being required to switch between biosimilar products for nonmedical reasons, and increased burden on the dispensing process when pharmacists have to contact the prescriber with every required biosimilar switch. Therefore, while health systems appear to acquire the biosimilars at lower costs, most are forced to maintain extensive formularies with all of the biosimilars in order to provide the payers preferred biosimilar for a patient. Additionally, this requirement extends into logistical burdens associated with storing, handling, and dispensing multiple similar products and increases the potential for medication errors. Due to lack of interchangeable biosimilars and payers requiring certain biosimilars to be used, a pharmacist is required to contact a prescriber each time a biosimilar needs to be changed. This interrupts workflows and prolongs the process of the patient receiving the drug. Inadvertently dispensing the wrong product to a patient may actually lead to higher cost to the patient if their payer will not cover the dispensed product. Initially identifying which product is covered for a patient, in addition to maintaining documentation about which product is needed for future dispenses, is a time-consuming task on an already strained healthcare system.

ASHP recognizes FDA's authority to determine biosimilar interchangeability, and in cases in which biosimilar products are deemed interchangeable, supports substitution for the reference product without the intervention of the prescriber. Further, ASHP opposes the implementation of any state laws regarding biosimilar interchangeability prior to finalization of FDA guidance and opposes any state legislation that would require a pharmacist to notify a prescriber when a biosimilar deemed to be interchangeable by the FDA is dispensed. FDA's determination of interchangeability should be all that is needed in order to substitute the biosimilar with the reference product. Although FDA guidances are distinct from FDA regulations, they often have profound impacts on healthcare decisions and delivery, so ASHP encourages the FDA to include healthcare practitioners in their development.

ASHP recognizes that postmarketing surveillance and pharmacist evaluation as part of the formulary system before biosimilar use are required to guarantee safe use of biosimilar medications. ASHP also advocates for adequate reimbursement for biosimilars approved by the FDA. This includes opposing payer ability to dictate preferred biosimilars. ASHP encourages payers to work with health systems to align their preferred biosimilar products and for payers to cover multiple biosimilars in order to allow health systems to maintain cost-effective formularies.

2317

EMERGENCY MEDICAL KITS

Source: Council on Pharmacy Practice

To recognize the importance of standardized and readily accessible emergency medical kits (EMKs) in locations with inconsistent emergency medical services; further,

To advocate for the inclusion of pharmacist expertise in policy and regulations for the interprofessional decisions related to the contents, storage, and maintenance of medications in EMKs; further,

To collaborate with other professions and stakeholders to standardize the contents of and locations for EMKs, and to develop guidelines and standardized training for proper use of EMK contents by designated personnel employed in those settings.

Rationale

A social media movement called attention to the lack of standardization in emergency medical kits (EMKs) during an in-flight medical emergency. U.S. CFR 121.803—Emergency Medical Equipment—requires certain medications and supplies for flights in case of medical emergencies but does not require the stocking of naloxone for reversing opioid overdoses or epinephrine auto-injectors for ease of administration, among many other medications and supplies. Many locations with inconsistent access to emergency medical services, such as airplanes, contain a stock of emergency supplies and medications that are not standardized and may not be adequate to manage some emergencies. In 2019, the Aerospace Medical Association Air Transport Medicine Committee sent recommendations to the Federal Aviation Administration regarding the contents of emergency medical kits, including recommendations to add naloxone and an epinephrine auto-injector (EpiPen).

The World Health Organization (WHO) has developed standardized health kits of medicines and medical supplies to meet different health needs in humanitarian emergencies and disasters. These kits are developed to provide reliable and affordable medicines and supplies quickly to those in need. The kits are used by United Nations agencies, nongovernmental organizations, and national governments. The contents of these kits are based primarily on the WHO's Essential Medicines list and guidelines on treatment of specific medical conditions. The contents of the kits are frequently reviewed and updated to adapt to changing needs based on experience in emergency situations. However, the WHO List of Essential Medicines does not specify an auto-injector for use in anaphylaxis.

There is growing concern regarding the need to standardize requirements set by a governing body to ensure that EMKs contain appropriate medications and supplies that are easy to use in an emergency, have been audited to ensure they contain the required items, have been stored appropriately, and do not contain expired products. Standardization of EMK contents would simplify training requirements for those using the kits, which should include what products are contained within the EMKs, how to use them (when appropriate), and when to provide the kits in the case of an emergency. Finally, it is critical to collect and track incident and outcomes data to promote improvement in emergency response, and pharmacist involvement in the interprofessional evaluation of that data is essential.

2322

AVAILABILITY AND USE OF FENTANYL TEST STRIPS

Source: Council on Therapeutics

To affirm that fentanyl test strips (FTS) have a place in harm reduction strategies for people who use drugs; further,

To support legislation that declassifies FTS as drug paraphernalia; further,

To promote public availability of and access to FTS, including zero-cost options; further,

To support the pharmacy workforce in their roles as essential members of the healthcare team in educating the public and healthcare providers about the role of FTS in public health efforts.

Rationale

In April 2021 the National Center for Health Statistics reported that in the past 12-month period there were over 100,000 drug overdose deaths in the United States, with fentanyl responsible for over two thirds of those deaths. Fentanyl, a synthetic opioid, is 50 to 100 times more potent than morphine, and therefore the risk of overdose is higher than with other opioids, particularly when the person consuming the fentanyl is not aware of its presence or has not developed a tolerance to it.

Studies have shown that fentanyl test strips (FTS) are used by people who use drugs (PWUD) to check their drugs for the presence of fentanyl and mitigate overdose risk by making informed decisions about their safety when consuming. The findings of a 2018 study suggest that the distribution and use of rapid fentanyl test strips are a feasible and PWUD-accepted harm reduction tool to detect the presence of fentanyl in illicit drugs. As a result, as part of the effort to reduce overdoses and promote harm reduction, state and county health departments and community organizations across the United States have started to distribute FTS as a low-barrier, inexpensive drug-checking strategy. Through the SUPPORT Act, the Centers for Disease Control and Prevention, the U.S. Department of Health and Human Services, and the Substance Abuse and Mental Health Services Administration are permitted to provide funding to be used to purchase FTS as a part of harm reduction efforts.

Currently, a little more than half the states in the U.S. have laws that declassify FTS as drug paraphernalia. Laws in the remaining states that designate FTS as drug paraphernalia may prevent states and organizations from applying for those grants or using their own funds to purchase FTS. Although many states have legislation in the works to remove this barrier, some states are reluctant to make this change, due to the perception that the use of FTS as quality control devices could encourage PWUD to seek out a stronger high rather than reduce the use of fentanyl, reinforcing risky behavior.

The pharmacy workforce is well equipped to meet the needs of PWUD and the use of FTS. For example, in June of 2022, the Illinois General Assembly passed H.B. 4556, which expands the ability of pharmacists and other healthcare professionals to distribute FTS. The Ohio State University School of Pharmacy offers a naloxone and FTS training and distribution event as an effort to reduce harm, to meet patients where they are, and to provide services along a continuum of care. Legislation and programs like these demonstrate the value of the pharmacy workforce and should be expanded throughout the United States.

2323

DEA SCHEDULING OF CONTROLLED SUBSTANCES

Source: Council on Therapeutics

To advocate that the Drug Enforcement Administration (DEA) establish clear, measurable criteria and a transparent process for scheduling determinations; further,

To urge the DEA to use such a process to re-evaluate existing schedules for all substances regulated under the Controlled Substances Act to ensure consistency and incorporate current science-based evidence concerning scheduling criteria; further,

To advocate that the U.S. Congress, with input from stakeholders, enact clear definitions of the terms *potential for abuse*, *currently accepted medical use*, and *accepted safety for use* in the Controlled Substances Act; further,

To advocate for monitoring of the impact of DEA scheduling of products under the Controlled Substances Act and other abuse-prevention efforts (e.g., prescription drug monitoring programs) on patient access to therapy and on healthcare provider workload; further,

To advocate for the elimination of federal and state laws that create barriers to research on therapeutic use of Schedule I substances.

This policy supersedes ASHP policy 1315.

Rationale

Since its passage in 1970, the Controlled Substances Act (CSA) has served as the foundation of modern drug control policy by regulating the manufacture, importation, possession, use, and distribution of certain substances. The CSA lists eight factors to be considered by the Drug Enforcement Administration (DEA) when deciding if a molecular entity should be scheduled: (1) the potential for abuse; (2) scientific evidence of its pharmacological effect; (3) state of current scientific knowledge regarding the substance; (4) history and current pattern of abuse; (5) scope, duration, and significance of abuse; (6) risk to public health; (7) its psychic or physiological dependence liability; and (8) whether the substance is an immediate precursor of a substance already controlled. The CSA then specifies that the three criteria used to determine the schedule of a substance include (1) its potential for abuse, (2) whether it has a medical use, and (3) its safety and risk of dependence. Several limitations of the aforementioned factors and criteria are worth noting. First, the eight factors are redundant and lack clarity. Second, the CSA does not specify the relationship between the eight factors and the three criteria for scheduling, and the DEA has not yet clarified this matter.

Additionally, the CSA does not explicitly define the terms *potential for abuse* or *accepted medical use*, giving the DEA much discretion to apply the scheduling criteria. The DEA has maintained broad discretion when scheduling substances according to their abuse potential, through court rulings that have upheld the DEA's comparison of the substance in question to already-scheduled substances. The DEA has formally defined the term *currently accepted medical use* in response to repeated litigation regarding the classification of Schedule I substances. The criteria under this definition include:

(1) the drug's chemistry must be known and reproducible; (2) adequate safety studies; (3) adequate and well-controlled studies proving efficacy; (4) the drug must be accepted by qualified experts; and (5) the scientific evidence must be widely available.

The lack of regulatory clarity of the CSA has led to a complicated process and inconsistent scheduling of substances. The language of the CSA implies that for a substance to be placed into a particular schedule, it must fulfill all three criteria. It is entirely possible, however, for one substance to fail to meet all three criteria of one schedule. Nonetheless, the DEA maintains that all scheduled substances without an accepted medical use must be classified as Schedule I, illustrating the conflicting scheduling practices used.

Furthermore, the existing schedules do not take into account evolving evidence about the abuse potential of these drugs. For example, gabapentin and pregabalin are structural analogues of gamma-aminobutyric acid, with pregabalin being classified as Schedule V under the CSA. Gabapentin, however, remains federally uncontrolled. An increase in its abuse has led some states to classify this medication as a Schedule V substance and/or mandate prescription reporting.

Finally, the CSA also places many restrictions on medical research into Schedule I substances, creating barriers that hinder the discovery of their potential therapeutic uses. Therefore, ASHP first recommends that the U.S. Congress use its legislative authority to define, with the input of stakeholders, the aforementioned terms in the CSA to provide a statutory basis for regulatory decision-making that will simplify the scheduling process. ASHP also advocates that the DEA establish clear, measurable criteria, to the extent possible for this complex subject, and a transparent process for scheduling determinations. Further, the DEA is encouraged to use those criteria to re-evaluate current schedule assignments for all controlled substances based on recent evidence. Finally, federal and state legislators are urged to eliminate laws that create barriers to research on Schedule I substances.

2325

NONPRESCRIPTION AVAILABILITY OF SELF-ADMINISTERED INFLUENZA ANTIVIRALS

Source: Council on Therapeutics

To support a behind-the-counter practice model that expands access to self-administered influenza antivirals.

This policy supersedes ASHP policy 2116.

Rationale

Oseltamivir (Tamiflu), zanamivir (Relenza), and baloxavir (Xofluza) are self-administered drugs used for the treatment and chemoprophylaxis of influenza. ASHP supports the availability of self-administered influenza antivirals via a behind-the-counter practice model. Use of this practice model, which has already been adopted for medications such as pseudoephedrine and emergency contraception, would facilitate appropriate use of those antivirals and provide patients with an opportunity to receive assessment and professional consultation from a pharmacist.

There are several perceived advantages and disadvantages of the nonprescription designation for self-administered influenza antivirals. Potential benefits include quicker and improved access for patients, public health value by reducing exposure of sick individuals at provider visits, unlikely development of antiviral resistance (based on currently available data), and experience with oseltamivir as a nonprescription medication in New Zealand since 2007. Potential concerns include stockpiling, shortages, questionable effectiveness, adverse effects, potential reduction of influenza vaccination rates because of perceived antiviral availability, dosing considerations (e.g., renal function, pediatric weight-based dosing), costs, reimbursement for clinical services provided by pharmacists (e.g., point-of-care influenza testing, questionnaire screening tool for oseltamivir dispensing), blunting of other more severe underlying conditions without a provider visit, and overextension of pharmacist responsibilities and duties. Furthermore, potential public health benefits and risks of expanded access must also be considered. With availability over or behind the counter, patients may bypass visiting their primary care providers to obtain antivirals, and pharmacists will therefore need to assume an active role in promoting public health by reporting positive cases to local health departments, should rapid testing and reporting be a requirement of dispensing.

Given the interest in expanding patient access to self-administered influenza antivirals, ASHP advocates that any reclassification should not result in increased costs to patients or pharmacies. Modifications to national, regional, and local drug coverage decisions are needed to ensure that payer policies do not unintentionally restrict or prevent access. In addition, the reclassification will likely result in an increased workload and potential liability associated with pharmacist provision of this care, which includes patient screening (and point-of-care testing, if applicable), patient education, dosing, counseling, and documentation of the care provided in the pharmacy and medical record. ASHP policy 2020, Care-Commensurate Reimbursement, states that pharmacists should be compensated for these kinds of clinical and patient care services.

2326

OVER-THE-COUNTER AVAILABILITY OF HORMONAL CONTRACEPTIVES

Source: Council on Therapeutics

To advocate that hormonal contraceptives be available over the counter (OTC) without age restriction only under conditions that ensure safe use, including the availability of pharmacist consultation to ensure appropriate self-screening and product selection, and that maintain patient confidentiality; further,

To encourage the Food and Drug Administration to require manufacturers to include all patients of childbearing age, including adolescents, in studies to determine the safety and effectiveness of OTC hormonal contraceptives; further,

To advocate that all insurers and manufacturers maintain coverage and limits on out-of-pocket expenditure so that patient access is not compromised.

This policy supersedes ASHP policy 1410.

Rationale

There have been repeated calls to make hormonal contraceptive products more widely available, with the intent of expanding access to women's reproductive health therapies and reducing unintended pregnancies. The American College of Obstetricians and Gynecologists (ACOG) advocates over-the-counter (OTC) access to hormonal contraception, including oral contraceptive pills, the contraceptive patch, contraceptive vaginal rings, and depot medroxyprogesterone acetate injections, without age restrictions. The American Medical Association (AMA), and the American Academy of Family Physicians (AAFP) support OTC access to oral contraceptives. ASHP agrees with ACOG and AMA that there is no clinical justification to restrict access to hormonal contraceptives by adolescents past menarche.

As with other OTC medications, there is recognition that both progestin-only and combined oral contraceptive use carries a very small amount of risk of adverse events and should be determined to be safe and effective for self-use. Progestin-only hormonal methods are generally safe and carry no or minimal risk of venous thromboembolism (VTE), and the VTE risk with combined oral contraceptive use is small compared with the increased risk of VTE during pregnancy and the postpartum period. ASHP advocates that OTC hormonal contraceptives should therefore be available where a patient has access to a pharmacist. Patient self-screening and product selection would be improved through pharmacist-provided consultation that assists patients in identifying absolute and relative contraindications (e.g., hypertension, heart or kidney disease), assessing other patient-specific factors (e.g., adherence practices), and determining when to recommend a referral to seek a higher level of care through the use of counseling and clinical decision-making tools. This process would guide the determination of which contraceptive product would be most safe and effective for an individual patient. ASHP does not believe that the current model for behind-the-counter access to some drug products (e.g., pseudoephedrine, emergency contraception) is appropriate for hormonal contraceptives because such a model would place the pharmacist in a gatekeeping rather than the clinical role that is necessary to ensure safe and effective use of these therapies.

Manufacturers will need to submit a supplemental new drug application for conversion from prescription to OTC status, including post-marketing surveillance reports and studies of consumer behaviors. It is critical that adolescents be included in these studies to assess their label comprehension, aptitude to self-select, and ability to effectively use the OTC hormonal contraceptives.

Given the intent to expand access to these therapies, ASHP advocates along with ACOG and AAFP that the proposed reclassification to OTC should not result in increased costs to patients and should include full insurance coverage without cost sharing. Modifications to national, regional, and local drug coverage decisions may be needed to ensure that payer policies do not unintentionally restrict or prevent access to OTC oral contraceptives.

2330

PHARMACIST PRESCRIBING AUTHORITY FOR ANTIRETROVIRAL THERAPY FOR THE PREVENTION OF HIV/AIDS

Source: Council on Therapeutics

To affirm that drug products for pre-exposure prophylaxis (PrEP) and post-exposure prophylaxis (PEP) for human immunodeficiency virus (HIV) infection prevention should be provided to individuals in a manner that ensures safe and appropriate use; further,

To oppose reclassification of currently available drugs used for PrEP and PEP to nonprescription status; further,

To advocate for legislation and regulation that expands pharmacist scope of practice to encompass initiation of PrEP and PEP therapy; further,

To advocate that the therapies and associated care for PrEP and PEP are available to patients with zero cost-sharing; further,

To support establishment of specific and structured criteria to guide comprehensive pharmacist interventions related to PrEP and PEP; further,

To support the research, education, and training of the pharmacy workforce on the therapeutic, psychosocial, and operationalization considerations of pharmacist-provided PrEP and PEP therapy; further,

To support educating the public regarding the public health benefits of PrEP and PEP.

Rationale

Increasing access to pre-exposure prophylaxis (PrEP) and post-exposure prophylaxis (PEP) for human immunodeficiency virus (HIV) infection prevention is a public health priority. The *Ending the HIV Epidemic in the U.S.* initiative (https://www.hiv.gov/federal-response/ending-the-hiv-epidemic/overview/), for example, includes expanded access to PrEP and PEP in its whole-of-society plan coordinated among agencies across the U.S. Department of Health and Human Services to end the HIV epidemic in the United States by 2030. Despite the increase in the availability of antiretroviral therapies for such prophylaxis, much of the patient population that would benefit from access, particularly those in the black, indigenous, and people of color communities, has been limited by stigma and other barriers, including a requirement for a prescription in many parts of the U.S. One of those barriers to access is that many states do not provide pharmacists independent authority to order and initiate PrEP and PEP therapy. Given the time-sensitive nature of these therapies, patients and their partners would benefit from being able to access them at community pharmacies. Those forced to seek medications through a physician's office or other site of care may struggle to find a timely appointment, especially if they do not have an established primary care provider. In contrast to physicians, community pharmacists are often available without an appointment and pose a potential solution to expanding access to therapy. Through policy, education, and infrastructure changes, pharmacists can be an alternate source for PrEP, expanding availability and further reducing HIV transmission.

ASHP advocates expanding pharmacists' scope of practice to include initiation of PrEP and PEP therapy, including associated screening, testing, monitoring, referrals, product selection, and counseling, as well as the establishment of specific and structured criteria for prescribing, dosing, and dispensing of PrEP and PEP by pharmacists. As one example, California Bill 159, approved in October 2019, authorizes pharmacists who undergo a board-approved training program to supply PrEP and PEP every two years, with a 60-day supply cap and certain conditions under which the therapies can be prescribed. In addition, insurance companies are not allowed to require prior authorization for these drug products. The goal of this law is to get patients on PrEP and then direct them to a prescriber for further care management. Other states, including New York, Colorado, Missouri, and

New Hampshire, are exploring similar programs. As these practices and programs vary from state to state, ASHP also recommends structured criteria be set that optimizes patient care and access to these drug products.

Expanding collaborative practice, in which pharmacists are permitted under an agreement with a prescriber to prescribe a defined list of medications along with associated monitoring, provides an effective way to advance the scope of pharmacy practice nationwide. A Seattle pharmacy operationalized such a program by forming a clinic in which pharmacists perform a history, risk assessment, lab testing, and education before dispensing PrEP. Implementation of a standing order for pharmacists to furnish PrEP for their patients may provide longitudinal benefit, and infrastructure for pharmacists to bill for these services, as well as the facilities to see patients, must accompany such policy changes. To ensure that patients who present for HIV prophylaxis receive comprehensive care, pharmacists should be allowed to order tests for other sexually transmitted infections at the patient's request when possible, as some community pharmacies and other sites of care may not have the ability to provide certain tests onsite.

ASHP opposes reclassification of currently available drugs used for PrEP and PEP (tenofovir and emtricitabine) to nonprescription status, because existing models for nonprescription dispensing do not provide the safeguards required to ensure safe and effective use.

Other barriers to access include a lack of insurance coverage and high out-of-pocket costs, insurers' refusal to cover brand medications when necessary, and insurers failing to cover all formulations, including pediatric formulations. Modifications to national, regional, and local drug coverage decisions are needed to ensure that payer policies do not unintentionally restrict or prevent access. To promote the broadest possible access, ASHP advocates that PrEP and PEP be available to patients with zero cost-sharing, regardless of income or insurance coverage.

Pharmacist initiation of PrEP and PEP therapies will likely result in an increased workload and potential liability associated with provision of this care, which includes patient screening (including point-of-care testing, if applicable), patient education, dosing, counseling, and documentation of the care provided in the pharmacy and medical record. ASHP policy 2020, Care-Commensurate Reimbursement, states that pharmacists should be compensated for these kinds of clinical and patient care services.

A survey of community pharmacists revealed that education and training are needed to advance pharmacy practice in PrEP and PEP therapy. Training in necessary laboratory testing, trauma-informed care, destigmatizaton, and appropriate follow-up should be done to ensure an adequate knowledge base for pharmacists unfamiliar with the procedures. Finally, ASHP supports public education regarding the public health benefits of PrEP and PEP therapy.

2239

DRUG PRICING PROPOSALS

Source: Council on Public Policy

To advocate for drug pricing and transparency mechanisms that ensure patient access to affordable medications, preserve existing clinical services and patient safety standards, and do not increase the complexity of the medication-use system.

Rationale

As drug prices have continued to climb, policymakers have proposed numerous solutions. While each proposal will need to be evaluated on its merits, it is critical that, at a minimum, policy solutions promote transparency, protect patient access to medications, and limit or reduce patient out-of-pocket costs. However, drug pricing solutions should not threaten programs that support expanded patient services (e.g., the 340B Drug Pricing Program), create patient safety risks (e.g., certain drug importation proposals), or add to the administrative or practice burden of healthcare providers.

2101

DIRECT-TO-CONSUMER CLINICAL GENETIC TESTS

Source: Council on Therapeutics

To support research to validate and standardize genetic markers used in direct-to-consumer clinical genetic tests and guide the application of test results to clinical practice; further,

To encourage the Food and Drug Administration (FDA) to continue to regulate direct-to-consumer clinical genetic tests as medical devices and work with the National Institutes of Health to evaluate and approve direct-to-consumer clinical genetic tests; further,

To advocate that direct-to-consumer clinical genetic tests be provided to consumers through the services of appropriate healthcare professionals who order tests from laboratories certified under the Clinical Laboratories Improvement Amendments of 1988 (CLIA); further,

To support FDA policies and procedures regarding advertising of direct-to-consumer clinical genetic tests, including the following requirements: (1) the relationship between the genetic marker and the disease or condition being assessed is clearly presented, (2) the benefits and risks of testing are discussed, and (3) such advertising is provided in an understandable format, at a level of health literacy that allows the intended audience to make informed decisions, and includes a description of the established patient-healthcare provider relationship as a critical source for information about the test and interpretation of test results; further,

To encourage health systems to create policies and procedures addressing direct-to-consumer genetic testing results as it relates to confirmatory testing, integration of genomic information into the healthcare record, genetic counseling, and clinical decision-making; further,

To encourage pharmacists to educate consumers and clinicians on the potential risks and benefits of direct-to-consumer clinical genetic tests for disease diagnosis and decisions involving drug therapy management.

This policy supersedes ASHP policy 1103.

Rationale

Since 2018, the FDA has implemented multiple processes, procedures, and guidance documents surrounding in vitro diagnostics (IVDs), also referred to as direct-to-consumer (DTC) testing. The FDA now reviews DTC tests for moderate- to high-risk medical purposes, to determine the validity of the test claims. The FDA review consists of assessing for analytical validity, clinical validity, and claims made by the company marketing the test about how well it works. Additionally, the FDA reviews descriptive information about the test for accuracy and for an appropriate level of health literacy.

The FDA now regulates DTC tests as medical devices. The specific regulatory requirements depend on the risk classification of the individual IVD. The FDA has been proactive about streamlining the regulation of DTC tests, as well as determining appropriate use by a consumer without the involvement of a healthcare provider.

In October 2018 and April 2019, the FDA issued a safety communication to alert the public to concerns regarding pharmacogenetic tests with unapproved claims to predict an individual's response to a specific therapeutic drug, where these claims may not supported by clinical evidence. Warning letters were sent by the FDA to select companies. Patients and providers were advised the FDA has not evaluated genetic tests, which make claims regarding the effects of a specific medication.

As consumer use of DTC testing continues to be prevalent, it is critical healthcare systems develop policies and best practices related to the utilization of data patients may present to their healthcare teams. Providers should be aware for most medications the relationship between genetic variations and a medication's effects has not been established. If a patient provides a test report from a genetic DTC test claiming to predict a person's response to a specific medication, the healthcare team should seek information in the FDA-approved drug label regarding whether genetic information should be used for determining therapeutic treatment. Confirmatory testing should be ordered by the healthcare team from a CLIA-certified laboratory.

2111

PHARMACIST INVOLVEMENT IN THE STRATEGIC NATIONAL STOCKPILE

Source: Council on Public Policy

To advocate for the inclusion of pharmacist expertise in the development and maintenance of the Strategic National Stockpile (SNS); further,

To advocate for transparency and improvement of SNS processes, including standardization of the request process and enhanced periodic review of SNS contents; further,

To advocate that pharmacists lead distribution of medications and related supplies requested from the SNS.

Rationale

The depletion of the Strategic National Stockpile (SNS) during the COVID-19 pandemic presents an opportunity to significantly improve SNS operations. Pharmacists should be engaged in determining which medications and supplies are included in the SNS, as well as how to maintain quality and ensure the stock remains up to date.

At the outset of the pandemic, hospitals and health systems struggled to make requests to the SNS for both medications and supplies. Because there was a not a clear mechanism for making requests, with the process varying among states, even sharing tips and best practices between providers was not always helpful. The SNS should increase transparency regarding stock and should implement a single consistent process for making requests. Providers should not have to devote huge amounts of time to making SNS requests in the midst of an emergency—and there should be a mechanism for quickly checking on the status of SNS requests to avoid additional wasted time.

Finally, to streamline processes, the SNS should have a standard distribution logistics process for medications and related supplies centered on pharmacists. Ensuring that pharmacists receive distributions of medications and related supplies will allow them time to prepare storage space (e.g., freezer space for remdesivir) and ensure proper storage and handling of products.

2112

MEDICATION PRICE-GOUGING LAWS

Source: Council on Public Policy

To advocate for price-gouging laws that include medications.

This policy supersedes ASHP policy 1622.

Rationale

Price gouging, whether due to shortages or other causes, can result in trafficking in counterfeit and diverted products through gray-market distributors, which can ultimately result in adverse patient outcomes and increased healthcare costs. Strategies, including specific legislation with stiff penalties for price gouging on medications, are needed to deter these activities. Thirty-one states currently have pricegouging laws that prohibit price markups on life-sustaining products (e.g., food, water, fuel), usually during a time of disaster, natural or otherwise. ASHP advocates for laws that specifically address price gouging on medications at any time, rather than predicating action on a triggering event, such as a disaster or shortage.

2114

FDA REQUIREMENT FOR DOSE-RESPONSE INFORMATION

Source: Council on Therapeutics

To advocate that the Food and Drug Administration require drug product manufacturers to (1) identify average dose-response curves for desirable and undesirable effects, and make this information available to healthcare providers; and (2) publish dose-response information, to the extent possible, on factors that lead to differences in pharmacokinetics and pharmacodynamics among individuals; further,

To encourage drug product manufacturers to conduct studies on and publicly report minimum effective dose data.

This policy supersedes ASHP policy 0602.

Rationale

Knowledge of the relationships among dose, drug concentration in blood, and clinical response (effectiveness and undesirable effects) is important for the safe and effective use of drugs. This information can help identify an appropriate starting dose, titration of dosing, and identification of doses that would produce unacceptable side effects or be unlikely to provide added benefit. Important to this understanding is the analysis of the dose–response relationship, particularly with drug levels above the ED50, the dose that provides approximately 50% of the maximum possible drug effect, as efficacy increases only slightly, while adverse effects increase.

Manufacturer dose-finding studies sometimes provide a dose estimate and the range of a drug's population ED50, but this information appears to have little bearing on prescribing. Many are either not aware of this measurement or do not consult the information after the drug is marketed with recommended dosage guidelines. Often overlooked is the variation in individual ED50 depending on body size, pharmacokinetics, and pharmacodynamics. This variation in ED50 may cause the effective dose to be lower in many patients compared with participants in clinical trials. It is important to note that the ED50 also can alert a clinician to the likely useful and safe dose range and should be more widely available. ED50 should be an important variable in drug approval, marketing, and, most importantly, prescribing. Furthermore, numerous observational studies have shown that providers often prescribe increasingly higher levels of treatment, often without clear clinical indication for such high doses. As such, the FDA recommends that dose-response assessment should be an integral part of drug development, including minimum effective doses.

2115

MEDICAL CANNABIS

Source: Council on Therapeutics

To recognize that there is limited evidence to support safe and effective use of medical cannabis; further,

To encourage research that quantifies the therapeutically active components and defines the effectiveness, safety, and clinical uses of medical cannabis; further,

To recognize that there is not a standardized product subject to the same regulations as a prescription drug product, and to advocate for the development of processes that would ensure standardized formulations that would ensure consistent potency and quality of medical cannabis; further,

To advocate for the alignment of federal and state laws to eliminate barriers to research on and therapeutic use of medical cannabis, including review of medical cannabis's status as a Schedule I controlled substance, and its potential for reclassification; further,

To encourage healthcare organizations to develop policies and procedures regarding the handling of medical cannabis consistent with applicable laws, regulations, and accreditation standards; further,

To promote the documentation of medical cannabis use and indication in the electronic health record; further,

To encourage education that prepares pharmacists as part of an interprofessional team to educate patients, caregivers, healthcare providers, and healthcare administrators about therapeutic and legal aspects of medical cannabis use.

This policy supersedes ASHP policy 1101.

Rationale

To date, 33 states and the District of Columbia, Guam, and Puerto Rico have enacted workable medical cannabis laws that provide, or will provide, meaningful access to medical cannabis for qualifying patients. Healthcare providers in those jurisdictions, including pharmacists, are grappling with the challenges presented by medical use of medical cannabis (defined for purposes of this policy as whole or parts of the natural marijuana plant and therapeutic products derived therefrom). ASHP recognizes that there is some evidence supporting the effectiveness of medical cannabis to treat or ameliorate symptoms of disease. The extent and quality of this evidence is limited, however, and even less is known about the safety of medical cannabis, especially related to its long-term use. Well-designed research is necessary to further define the therapeutic uses of medical cannabis, including determination of its therapeutically active components; clinical indications and contraindications; precautions; dosing; routes of administration; adverse effects; drug-drug, drug-disease, and drug-laboratory interactions; and effectiveness compared to existing therapies.

Current inconsistencies in product formulation, potency, and quality are also a hindrance to developing a strong evidence base. Standardizing these factors, to the extent possible, will help ensure the quality and reliability of research results. ASHP encourages efforts by the United States Pharmacopeia to develop quality standards for medical cannabis. Federal legislation and regulation, including marijuana's classification as a Schedule I substance under the Controlled Substances Act, remains a barrier to the necessary research, and ASHP advocates that federal and state laws and regulations be aligned to remove or minimize these barriers.

Conflicting federal and state laws also create confusion about research on and use of medical cannabis, as federal law precludes procurement, storage, preparation, or distribution of medical cannabis by pharmacies or healthcare facilities registered with the Drug Enforcement Administration. Given the complexity of the issues involved, ASHP encourages healthcare organizations to develop policies and procedures regarding medical cannabis to conduct research and provide patient care that is consistent with applicable laws, regulations, and accreditation standards. Recreational or medical use of cannabis should be documented in the patient medical record. ASHP recognizes the need for pharmacists and other healthcare providers to provide education about the unique therapeutic and legal issues created by research on and use of medical cannabis

2118

SUPPLY CHAIN RESILIENCE DURING DISASTERS AND PUBLIC HEALTH EMERGENCIES

Source: Council on Pharmacy Management

To support building an enhanced and resilient hospital and health-system supply chain that is lean and economical during normal operations yet nimble enough to support patient care needs during large surges in demand for pharmaceuticals and medical supplies; further,

To advocate for ongoing federal evaluation of a national hazard vulnerability assessment to determine how pandemics and disasters present risks to healthcare and public health critical infrastructure; further,

To advocate for the development of critical pharmaceutical and medical supply requirement listings based on a national hazard vulnerability assessment to guide the composition of government and distributor-managed emergency stockpiles; further,

To urge Congress and state legislatures to direct medical supply and pharmaceutical distributors to manage both private sector-owned" medical materiel (just-in-time for normal operations) and government-owned/distributor-managed emergency stockpiles (just-in-case for emergencies) that can flow into the private sector supply chain when release of government-owned materiel during public health emergencies, disasters, or contingencies is authorized.

Rationale

Hospitals and health systems experience supply chain challenges for patient care during routine operations, and these challenges can be exacerbated by public health emergencies and disasters. Aspects of the novel coronavirus disease 2019 (COVID-19) pandemic that have required nimbleness in thinking and action are the transformation of organizational governance and the need for speed in decision-making. The COVID-19 pandemic has dramatically changed inventory management and supply chain practices.

Many pre-existing factors contributed to the supply chain crises triggered by COVID-19, including but not limited to overextended supply lines, lean manufacturing, and outsourcing, which have been especially unfavorable for hospitals and health systems running just-in-time (JIT) inventory replenishment. Designed to use capital more efficiently, JIT replenishment relies on highly accurate demand forecasting and tight coordination with suppliers. When there is a sudden increase in demand, from a larger number of buyers trying to purchase the same products at the same time or from the typical number of buyers trying to make larger purchases, the thin supply chains that support JIT inventories can't respond quickly enough, creating long-term backorders at the local, regional, and national levels. An alternative just-in-case (JIC) inventory strategy would maintain extensive inventories to reduce backorder risks in the face of supply and demand uncertainties, but at the cost of forcing organizations to tie up capital in inventory.

During the COVID-19 pandemic, hospital and health-system governance structures had to quickly pivot to accommodate shifts in unexpected operational, clinical, and financial challenges. Organizations quickly embraced the "new normal" of supply chain management conundrums (e.g., shortages of personal protective equipment and critical drug, minimizing drug waste), controversial drug therapy considerations for pharmacy and therapeutics committees, and provisioning planning for alternate care sites (e.g., field hospitals). To prepare the healthcare system to endure the stresses on critical infrastructure caused by future public health emergencies or disasters, a shift toward a hybrid supply chain model needs serious consideration, to reap the benefits of both models and build resiliency into supply chains. Such a system would use information from a national hazard vulnerability assessment to guide the composition of emergency stockpiles of critical pharmaceuticals and medical supplies and require private-sector distributors of those products to manage the supply chains for those stockpiles when they are released during public health emergencies or disasters in addition to their normal operations.

2141

PHARMACIST ENGAGEMENT IN AND PAYMENT FOR TELEHEALTH

Source: Council on Public Policy

To advocate for pharmacists' provision of telehealth services in all sites of care; further,

To advocate that reimbursement for pharmacists' provision of telehealth services be commensurate with the complexity and duration of service and consistent with other healthcare providers.

Rationale

During the COVID-19 public health emergency, hospitals, health systems, and clinics quickly pivoted to providing patient services via telehealth. The Centers for Medicare & Medicaid Services, commercial payers, and state policymakers have indicated that they would like to maintain telehealth services post-pandemic. Because pharmacists are not Medicare-eligible, it has been a struggle to ensure that they can be reimbursed for services provided via telehealth. In particular, it is vital that services be reimbursed at a level commensurate with the complexity and duration of the service and consistent with other healthcare providers, to ensure that patients can maintain access to services.

2142

PHARMACY SERVICES IN A STATE OF EMERGENCY

Source: Council on Public Policy

To advocate that states grant temporary licensure, registration, or any other necessary state-mandated credentials to eligible pharmacies and members of the pharmacy workforce during states of emergency; further,

To encourage expedient licensure or registration for eligible members of the pharmacy workforce during states of emergency; further,

To advocate that state and federal regulatory agencies allow for flexibilities necessary to provide patient care during a declared state of emergency.

Rationale

During the COVID-19 pandemic, both state and federal policymakers scrambled to provide the regulatory flexibility necessary to allow patients to access pharmacist services. Although states are generally willing to be flexible about dispensing during a public health emergency, pharmacy services themselves are not subject to the same degree of flexibility. Specifically, pharmacists, more so than other clinicians, struggled to get temporary licensure across state lines, and pharmacy technicians experienced similar challenges in states that require registration. The lack of access to temporary licensure and registration impeded the ability of pharmacists and pharmacy technicians to move to areas of great need or to volunteer in states with patient surges. Further, pharmacy services require flexibility, particularly around inventory control and the ability to reallocate product and the ability to quickly establish alternate sites of care. During the COVID-19 public health emergency, remdesivir was allocated to the states, and then the state retained full control over distribution, which resulted in situations in which hospitals could not transfer product across state lines to other hospitals, even to related entities, that needed the product more.

2144

AGRICULTURAL USE OF HORMONE AND PROHORMONE THERAPY

Source: Council on Therapeutics

To advocate that the Food and Drug Administration (FDA) and United States Department of Agriculture (USDA) reevaluate the agricultural use of hormone and prohormone therapies for purposes of animal growth promotion based on evidence demonstrating potential adverse effects on human health; further,

To advocate that the FDA and USDA eliminate approval for nontherapeutic uses in agricultural animals of hormone and prohormone therapies that are known to cause adverse effects on human health; further,

To encourage efforts to eliminate the nontherapeutic agricultural uses of hormone and prohormone therapies previously approved by the FDA and USDA; further,

To support the therapeutic use of hormone and prohormone therapies in animals only under the supervision of a veterinarian; further,

To encourage additional research on hormone and prohormone therapies to better define the public health impact of these therapies for agricultural purposes.

This policy supersedes ASHP policy 1102.

Rationale

Natural (e.g., estradiol, progesterone, testosterone) and synthetic (trenbolone, zeranol, melengestrol) hormones are commonly used for growth promotion in beef cattle raised in the United States. While the European Union has banned the use of these substances for growth promotion based on safety concerns, the USDA and FDA have long supported use of these substances based on studies conducted in the 1970s. Of note, a 2002 statement from the FDA stated that the use of hormones for agricultural purposes was safe. However, more recent research has raised new concerns about potential harm to human health, including epidemiological studies demonstrating increased rates of breast cancer in women, testicular cancer and decreased fertility in men, and hormone-related developmental issues in infants and children.

Hormone therapies for agricultural therapies should be re-examined based on this new evidence and because technology for measuring exposure to hormone substances has improved since the initial decision by the USDA and FDA. In addition, research to examine the public health impact of agricultural uses of hormone and prohormone therapies needs to be encouraged.

2004

EVALUATION OF ABUSE-DETERRENT DRUG MECHANISMS

Source: Council on Therapeutics

To encourage manufacturers to develop safe and efficacious abuse-deterrent formulations for drugs known to be abused and misused; further,

To promote research on the efficacy of abuse-deterrent mechanisms in preventing prescription drug abuse, and to support the reporting and dissemination of this information; further,

To advocate for legislation that would limit out-of-pocket expenditures for such formulations.

This policy supersedes ASHP policy 1512.

Rationale

The abuse of certain classes of prescription drugs, including narcotics and stimulants, has had a large impact on public health. One way the Food and Drug Administration (FDA) has sought to curb this activity is through the use of abuse-deterrent formulations (ADFs). ADFs are formulations that permit treatment of a patient's medical condition but reduce the likelihood of diversion, misuse, and abuse, and related adverse outcomes through various mechanisms, such as hindering the extraction of active ingredients, limiting their bioavailability, preventing administration through alternative routes, or making abuse of the manipulated product less attractive or rewarding.

The FDA has been taking steps to incentivize and support the development of opioid formulations with progressively better abuse-deterrent properties. These steps include working with individual sponsors on promising abuse-deterrent technologies, developing appropriate testing methodologies for both innovator and generic products, and publishing guidance on the development and labeling of abuse-deterrent opioids.

Despite these efforts, prescription stimulants used to treat attention deficit hyperactivity disorder have become drugs of choice for young adults, with as many as 20% of college students using such drugs for nonmedical purposes. According to a 2011 study, benzodiazepines were involved in 30.6% of prescription drug-related overdose deaths. However, to date, the FDA has not provided guidance on ADFs for any controlled substance other than opioids.

Despite the groundswell of support for abuse-deterrent opioid formulations, there is not strong evidence that such formulations deter abuse. One study of 232,874 patients across 437 facilities found an increase in abuse prevalence of all opioids after introduction of an abuse-deterrent formulation. That study showed little success in deterring abuse, finding instead that patients had switched to alternative drugs. There may also be unintended consequences of preferring abuse-deterrent formulations to regular formulations, such as increased costs borne by patients who legitimately need the drugs.

There also is a need to demonstrate that these formulations are truly abuse deterrent as well. In April 2015, the FDA published an industry guidance document on *Abuse-Deterrent Opioids—Evaluation and Labeling*. The document explains the FDA's "current thinking about the studies that should be conducted to demonstrate a given formulation has abuse-deterrent properties."

Addressing the growing rate of prescription drug abuse will require a multifaceted strategy; no one tactic will solve the problem. While ASHP supports measures such as abuse deterrent formulations and rescheduling to prevent abuse, more research is necessary to determine which tactics are the most effective at deterring abuse.

2005

QUALITY CONSUMER MEDICATION INFORMATION

Source: Council on Therapeutics

To support efforts by the Food and Drug Administration (FDA) and other stakeholders to improve the quality, consistency, accessibility, targeting, and simplicity of consumer medication information (CMI); further,

To encourage the FDA to work in collaboration with patient advocates and other stakeholders to create evidence-based models and standards, including establishment of a universal literacy level and standardized, patient-focused templates, for CMI; further,

To advocate that research be conducted to validate these models in actual-use studies in pertinent patient populations; further,

To advocate that FDA explore alternative models of CMI content development and maintenance that will ensure the highest level of accuracy, consistency, and currency, and conforms with health literacy requirements; further,

To advocate that the FDA engage a single third-party author to provide editorial control of a highly structured, publicly and easily accessible central repository of CMI in a format that is suitable for ready export; further,

To advocate for laws and regulations that would require all dispensers of medications to comply with FDA-established standards for unalterable content, format, and distribution of CMI.

This policy supersedes ASHP policy 1513.

Rationale

ASHP supports the intent of efforts to improve the quality, consistency, and simplicity of consumer medication information (CMI). The Food and Drug Administration (FDA) defines CMI (previously called patient medication information, or PMI) as "written information about prescription drugs developed by organizations or individuals other than a drug's manufacturer that is intended for distribution to consumers at the time of drug dispensing." CMI is not reviewed or approved by the FDA or a drug's manufacturer.

In the 1970s, the FDA began evaluating the usefulness of patient labeling, and in 1996, *Public Law 104–180* defined PMI "usefulness" as being "scientifically accurate, unbiased in content and tone, sufficiently specific and comprehensive, presented in an understandable and legible format that is readily comprehensible to consumers, timely and up-to-date, enables the consumer to use the medicine properly and appropriately, receive the maximum benefit, and avoid harm." In 2002, the National Association of Boards of Pharmacy conducted a study on the usefulness of PMI and found that 89% of patients in the study received some form of written PMI but that only about 50% of the PMI met the definition of usefulness.

In 2006, the FDA published *guidance* on useful written CMI. However, because CMI improvement efforts were largely based on consensus of expert opinion, rather than quantitative and well-documented evidence, and because subsequent studies were conducted using expert-based focus groups and other study designs that do not reflect typical patients and under flawed methodology, ASHP encourages the development of evidence-based models for CMI that are designed to support desired outcomes (e.g., better medication use, improved patient safety). In addition, research to validate the effectiveness of any new CMI models under real-use conditions by actual patients, including establishment of a universal literacy level for CMI, should be encouraged. Evidence to establish the essential CMI content needed for the safe and effective use of medications by patients remains to be determined.

Although drug information publishers have made significant progress in improving the quality of CMI, this content is often truncated or provided in illegible formats to accommodate size restrictions or marketing information on patient drug information leaflets that are stapled to prescription packaging.

Because of the FDA's long history of failure to ensure the consistency, currency, and accuracy of the professional labeling on which CMI would be based; the potential for inclusion of biased or promotional information; and the resulting patient confusion and possible harm, ASHP strongly opposes any proposal for manufacturer-authored CMI that would not be subject to FDA review. Approximately 85% of professional labeling has not been reviewed or updated since 1992 to reflect FDA's current standard for the Physician Labeling Rule (PLR) format. In addition, numerous inconsistencies and inaccuracies in such labeling continue. Given these limitations, the majority of information on which CMI would be based under such a regime would not be likely to "enhance the safe and effective use of prescription drug products and in turn reduce the number of adverse reactions resulting from medication errors due to misunderstood or incorrectly applied drug information," which is the main goal of the FDA requirements.

ASHP further advocates that state legislatures and regulatory agencies require that all dispensers distribute CMI according to FDA-established standards and be held accountable if CMI content or format is modified in a manner that results in nonconformance to the standards.

Creation and maintenance of CMI by a single third-party author (subject to FDA-contracted standards and quality assurance metrics) would provide clear, concise, unbiased, evidence-based CMI that is both timely and consistent for the same drug and for relevant information within the same drug class. Such coordination of the medication information database would allow for consistency in style and content, as well as more frequently updated content.

Due to the evolution of how information is consumed and accessed and in light of the 2009 *Health Information Technology for Economic and Clinical Health (HITECH) Act*, ASHP also advocates that CMI also be consumable across multiple platforms, including electronic platforms, as more individuals use online medical records to better manage their health and healthcare needs. The Department of Health and Human Services has reported a steady increase in the proportion of individuals who reported having been offered access to their online medical record, with approximately three-quarters of individuals reporting having access to a current list of medications within their online medical record.

2007

USE OF SURROGATE ENDPOINTS FOR FDA APPROVAL OF DRUG USES

Source: Council on Therapeutics

To support efforts by the Food and Drug Administration (FDA) and other stakeholders to qualify the appropriateness of surrogate endpoints; further,

To support the continued use of qualified surrogate endpoints by the FDA as a mechanism to evaluate the effectiveness and safety of new drugs and new indications for existing therapies, when measurement of definitive clinical outcomes is not feasible; further,

To advocate that the FDA consistently enforce existing requirements that drug product manufacturers complete postmarketing studies for drugs approved based on qualified surrogate endpoints in order to confirm that the expected improvement in outcomes occurs, and to require that these studies be completed in a timely manner.

This policy supersedes ASHP policy 1011.

Rationale

Expedited approval programs provided by the FDA have resulted in substantial public health benefits, as illustrated by the use of surrogate endpoints to approve therapies for HIV and AIDS in the 1990s. The FDA provides four mechanisms to expedite the development and review process for drugs: fast track designation, breakthrough therapy designation, accelerated approval, and priority review designation. The structure and requirements for each of these mechanisms differs as described in a *2013 draft guidance for industry*. However, to qualify for any of these programs, a drug must (1) address an unmet medical need, (2) provide benefit over available drug treatments, and (3) be used in the treatment of a serious or life-threatening condition. Further, the FDA guidance states that these programs are "intended to help ensure that therapies for serious conditions are approved and available to patients as soon as it can be concluded that the therapies' benefits justify their risks." Processes used to ensure a favorable risk–benefit profile include, but are not limited to, requirements for postmarketing studies to evaluate safety and effectiveness of the drug as used in real-world scenarios. However, the accelerated approval program is the only program that includes postmarketing studies as a requirement of the program. The FDA has discretion to require additional studies on a case-by-case basis for drug products approved via the other expedited mechanisms. Despite these safeguards, some features of these programs (e.g., smaller clinical trials, alternate trial designs, or limited-duration trials) can result in increased patient risk because less is known about a drug's side effect profile and efficacy due to limited patient exposure. In addition, as with all drugs, safety assessments benefit from use of the drug in post-approval patient populations, which better reflect real-world use than the controlled environment of a clinical trial.

Because these drugs represent medical advances, their post-approval use can be extensive. Further, off-label use of these drug products, like all therapies, is common. Unfortunately, prescribers and other clinicians are frequently unaware that an expedited pathway was utilized and that evidence limitations exist. This scenario raises significant concerns about whether there is sufficient clinician awareness to ensure appropriate use of drugs approved via these pathways. Therefore, ASHP proposes unique labeling requirements that would increase awareness through use of a logo or other mechanism that would be used on an interim basis to inform clinicians about data limitations and provide guidance on appropriate use. This labeling would describe appropriate patient populations and monitoring parameters. Similar labeling requirements have been proposed for a new pathway being considered for the development of antibiotics used to treat life-threatening infections. ASHP supports the approach, but recommends that the increased labeling requirements be discontinued once the drug product manufacturer and FDA agree that sufficient data is available to support safe and effective use, or after the drug manufacturer completes any required postmarketing study commitments.

Given data limitations associated with approval of these therapies, ASHP advocates that the FDA be extremely diligent in ensuring that postmarketing commitments are met. Further, the FDA should use its existing authority as described under 21 CFR 314 subpart H and 21 CFR 601 subpart E if timelines or expectations for these commitments are not satisfactory. This authority allows the FDA to take legal action through penalties that include requiring labeling changes or rescinding marketing approval.

Finally, ASHP believes that there is a need for research to determine whether these expedited pathways are achieving the desired benefits, which include decreasing the time and costs associated with drug product development, lowering overall healthcare costs, and increasing patient access to safe and effective drug therapies.

2012

IMPORTATION OF DRUG PRODUCTS

Source: Council on Public Policy

To oppose wholesale importation of drug products as a method to lower drug costs.

This policy supersedes ASHP policy 0413.

Rationale

Recent efforts to rein in drug pricing have centered on proposals to allow the wholesale importation of drugs (meaning importation of drugs by healthcare providers and distributors on a larger scale, rather than by individuals on a small scale) from foreign countries (e.g., Canada) as a means to reduce patient costs. Although states (e.g., Florida and Colorado) have passed wholesale importation laws, those laws cannot take effect until the state has crafted an importation plan, the Food and Drug Administration (FDA) has signed off on it, and the Department of Health & Human Services (HHS) Secretary has made the required certification to Congress.

Current law allows wholesale importation only in very limited circumstances (i.e., shortages) and requires the HHS Secretary to certify to Congress that allowing importation of drugs will not put public health and safety at risk and that it will result in significant savings. No Secretary has ever been able to make such a certification.

ASHP believes that wholesale importation of drugs cannot be accomplished while: (1) maintaining the integrity of the pharmaceutical supply chain and avoiding the introduction of counterfeit products into the U.S.; (2) providing for continued patient access to pharmacist review of all medications and preserving the patient-pharmacist-prescriber relationship; and (3) providing adequate patient counseling and education, particularly to patients taking multiple high-risk medications. Further, wholesale importation is unlikely to result in significant cost savings and reduces focus on drug pricing solutions that can reduce prices over the long term.

Nothing in this policy should be construed to oppose personal importation of drugs, or importation of drugs and related medical devices to alleviate a drug shortage when such importation is overseen by the FDA.

2013

PUBLIC QUALITY STANDARDS FOR BIOLOGIC PRODUCTS

Source: Council on Public Policy

To oppose federal or state legislation that would remove the requirement for biologic products to adhere to public quality standards; further,

To review and evaluate current public standards to ensure that they are relevant and appropriate to biologic products.

Rationale

ASHP has long recognized that application of quality standards (e.g., United States Pharmacopeia monographs or other applicable guidance) helps guarantee safe use of drugs. ASHP joined virtually all national pharmacy groups, including more than 30 state pharmacy associations, in opposing Congressional efforts to *eliminate monographs for biologic medications* in the 115th and 116th Congresses. The *FDA advocates voluntary standards* for biologic products on the basis of reduced costs and improved access, but the agency does not provide data to justify that stance. The arguments against requiring monographs center on their potential use as a barrier to competition, because manufacturers could incorporate patentable characteristics relevant to the product's safety and efficacy. However, removing monographs for one class of drugs could open the door to removal of standards for other drug classes and to laxer safety standards generally. There is evidence that the monographs do not dampen innovation, as new products continue to enter the market.

2019

ACCESS TO AFFORDABLE HEALTHCARE

Source: Council on Public Policy

To advocate for access to affordable healthcare for all, including coverage of medications and related pharmacist patient care services; further,

To advocate that the full range of available methods be used to (1) ensure the provision of appropriate, safe, and cost-effective healthcare services; (2) optimize treatment outcomes; (3) minimize overall costs without compromising quality; and (4) ensure patient choice of healthcare providers, including pharmacy services; further,

To advocate that healthcare payers seek to optimize continuity of care in their design of benefit plans.

This policy supersedes ASHP policy 1001.

Rationale

This policy expresses ASHP's stance on access to healthcare in the United States. The policy emanated from ASHP policies dealing with affordability and accessibility of pharmaceuticals. ASHP believes that it is important to address the larger issue of healthcare access, particularly due to the impact of the cost of medications on the nation's overall healthcare budget as well as pharmacy budgets in hospitals and health systems. Healthcare should be affordable, but also sufficient to ensure patient access to services.

2021

FUNDING, EXPERTISE, AND OVERSIGHT OF STATE BOARDS OF PHARMACY

Source: Council on Public Policy

To advocate appropriate oversight of pharmacy practice and the pharmaceutical supply chain through coordination and cooperation of state boards of pharmacy and other state and federal agencies whose mission it is to protect the public health; further,

To advocate representation on state boards of pharmacy and related agencies by pharmacists and pharmacy technicians; further,

To advocate that hospitals and health systems are adequately represented on state boards of pharmacy; further,

To advocate for dedicated funds for the exclusive use by state boards of pharmacy and related agencies including funding for the training of state board of pharmacy inspectors and the implementation of adequate inspection schedules to ensure the effective oversight and regulation of pharmacy practice, the integrity of the pharmaceutical supply chain, and protection of the public; further,

To advocate that inspections be performed only by individuals with demonstrated competency in the applicable area of practice.

This policy supersedes ASHP policy 1507.

Rationale

In recent years, the regulatory scope of boards of pharmacy has grown to address new and expanded scopes of practice and healthcare while fulfilling their mission of protecting the public health. In addition, coordination with federal agencies (e.g., Food and Drug Administration, Drug Enforcement Administration) and related state agencies add to the complexity of a state board's mission. With this expanded scope and mission comes the need for additional resources, both financial and human. Specific knowledge acquired by pharmacists and pharmacy technicians is essential to the safe regulation of practice. Thus, inspectors need to have demonstrated competency in the applicable area of practice in order to assure the health and safety of the public.

2023

NEW CATEGORIES OF LICENSED PHARMACY PERSONNEL

Source: Council on Public Policy

To oppose the creation of new categories of licensed pharmacy personnel.

Rationale

State efforts to introduce a "pharmacist assistant" category conflict with longstanding ASHP efforts to support the professional growth of licensed or registered pharmacy technicians. Pursuant to these state proposals, pharmacists could delegate a number of activities that fall under the purview of their practice to the pharmacist assistant, such as receiving telephone calls, prescriptions, tech-check-tech, etc. In effect, this would create another midlevel provider in the pharmacy. Not only would this create confusion regarding terminology and job roles, it would undermine ASHP's work to professionalize the technician role. The policy should not be read as impeding the use of current licensed personnel, including technicians and students.

2025

POSTMARKETING STUDIES

Source: Council on Therapeutics

To advocate that Congress grant the Food and Drug Administration (FDA) authority to require the manufacturer of an approved drug product or licensed biologic product to conduct postmarketing studies on the safety of the product when the agency deems it to be in the public interest and to require additional labeling or withdrawal of the product on the basis of a review of postmarketing studies; further,

To advocate that Congress provide adequate funding to FDA and other agencies to fulfill this expanded mission related to postmarketing surveillance and studies; further,

To advocate that such studies compare a particular approved drug product or licensed biologic product with (as appropriate) other approved drug products, licensed biologic products, medical devices, or procedures used to treat specific diseases; further,

To advocate expansion of studies of approved drug products or licensed biologic products to improve safety and therapeutic outcomes and promote cost-effective use; further,

To encourage impartial public-private partnerships or private-sector entities to also conduct such studies.

This policy supersedes ASHP policies 1004 and 0515.

Rationale

Pharmacists, other members of the healthcare team, patients, and private and public payers need objective, authoritative, and reliable evidence to make the best treatment decisions. Since the passage of the Medicare Prescription Drug, Improvement and Modernization Act of 2003, the Agency for Healthcare Research and Quality (AHRQ) has been tasked with studying the outcomes, comparative clinical effectiveness, and appropriateness of healthcare items and services. For such research to contribute to the practice of evidence-based patient care, good clinical decision-making, and rational drug use, AHRQ must evaluate devices, invasive procedures, and prescription and nonprescription medications, including both labeled and unlabeled uses of prescription drugs. Since prescription drugs represent a significant and growing portion of healthcare costs, the need for such research is increasingly important. Although impartial private sector entities can supplement the research efforts of government agencies such as AHRQ, only the federal government has the ability to support such independent research, provide oversight to safeguard the integrity of the research process, and disseminate the findings.

Furthermore, to ensure safety, the Food and Drug Administration (FDA) has several requirements for manufacturers and programs in place to monitor postmarket adverse events. These requirements and programs include the Division of Medication Error Prevention and Analysis, which is responsible for monitoring and preventing medication errors related to the naming, labeling, packaging, and design for CDER-regulated drugs and therapeutic biological products; the Risk Evaluation and Mitigation Strategy (REMS) program, which is designed to help reduce the occurrence and severity of certain serious risks; by informing and supporting the execution of the safe use conditions described in the medication's FDA-approved prescribing information; the Safe Use Initiative, a program that aims to reduce preventable harm by identifying specific, preventable medication risks and developing, implementing, and evaluating cross-sector interventions with partners who are committed to safe medication use. Other programs include the FDA Adverse Event Reporting System (FAERS), which is a database that contains adverse event reports, medication error reports, and product quality complaints resulting in adverse events that were submitted to FDA, and MedWatch, the FDA Safety Information and Adverse Event Reporting Program, which permits voluntary reporting by consumers and healthcare professionals and mandatory reporting for regulated industry and user facilities. Additionally, the FDA requires that adverse drug events (ADEs) must be reported in accordance with the requirements of 21 CFR 310.305 and 314.80, which require three types of ADE reports: (1) 15-day reports of serious, unlabeled events; (2) 15-day narrative increased frequency reports of serious, labeled events; and (3) periodic reports.

2026

GABAPENTIN AS A CONTROLLED SUBSTANCE

Source: Council on Therapeutics

To advocate that the Drug Enforcement Administration classify gabapentin as a Schedule V substance due to its potential for abuse and patient harm.

Rationale

Gabapentin is a structural analog of gamma-aminobutyric acid that is approved by the Food and Drug Administration (FDA) for post-herpetic neuralgia and as an adjunctive therapy for partial seizures. Gabapentin has been identified as an opportunistic drug of abuse which, when used in conjunction with other medications, particularly opioids, may result in serious adverse events such as respiratory depression and even death. Gabapentin is used due to its low cost, classification as a noncontrolled substance, and increasing rates of on- and off-label prescribing attributable to clinicians' desire for an alternative to opioids for pain management. In the U.S., gabapentin is and remains a noncontrolled substance at the federal level despite evidence suggestive of diversion and abuse with opioids. Most recently, several states have made an effort to combat the diversion and abuse of gabapentin by examining various regulatory approaches, such as reclassification of gabapentin as a controlled substance or mandating the reporting of the prescribing and/or dispensing of gabapentin to a state-level prescription drug monitoring programs (PDMPs). As recently as April 2019, the United Kingdom reclassified gabapentin as a Class C controlled substance, which required similar dispensing and monitoring as controlled substances in the U.S., due to the increase in abuse they have seen in this drug.

As defined by the Drug Enforcement Administration (DEA), Schedule V controlled substances "are defined as drugs with lower potential for abuse than Schedule IV" substances. Schedule IV substances "are defined as drugs with a low potential for abuse and low risk of dependence." Recent data from multiple sources have shown a significant increase in gabapentin misuse, abuse, and diversion over the past 10 years, and one study found that 22% of a sample of 162 opioid-dependent patients had a prescription for gabapentin, of which 40% indicated they used more than prescribed to augment and enhance their opioid experiences.

The criteria used by DEA to determine whether to control or reschedule a drug include (a) the drug's actual or relative potential for abuse; (b) scientific evidence of its pharmacological effect, if known; (c) the state of current scientific knowledge regarding the abuse of the drug or other substance; (d) its history or current pattern of abuse; (e) the scope, duration, and significance of abuse; (f) what, if any, risk there is to public health; (g) its psychic or physiological dependence liability; and (e) whether the substance is a precursor of a substance already controlled under the law.

Based on an assessment using these criteria, gabapentin is similar to other controlled substances found in Schedule V and should therefore be assigned to Schedule V. Because some states have already taken steps to reschedule gabapentin as Schedule V or have added it to their PDMPs, the DEA should take steps to change the schedule status of gabapentin to ensure continuity of care and monitoring.

While it is difficult to predict the impact rescheduling may have on abuse, the current extent of abuse is likely exacerbated by easy access to and excessive supply of these therapies. However, the potential public health benefit of rescheduling must be weighed against concerns about restricting patients' access to treatment and increasing administrative and other burdens on pharmacists and other clinicians. The proposed change to a more restrictive schedule would require stricter recordkeeping and security processes, which could in turn make providers reluctant to prescribe these therapies for patients who need pain management. In balancing these concerns, it should be noted that increased control of drugs with abuse potential is in the best interests of patients and public health. DEA and other stakeholders should monitor the impact of this scheduling change on patient access and practice, as well as monitor the impact of other strategies that have been implemented to minimize the abuse and diversion of these therapies.

2030

INTERSTATE PHARMACIST LICENSURE

Source: Council on Pharmacy Management

To advocate for interstate pharmacist licensure to expand the mobility of pharmacists and their ability to practice.

Rationale

Rapid changes in technology have increasingly allowed healthcare to be delivered at a distance, and the growth of health systems and the consolidation and closing of hospitals in rural areas have created a demand for practitioner mobility across state lines. The century-old state-by-state licensure model of pharmacy has not kept pace with these changes, creating barriers to care. The nursing profession has addressed this challenge by creating the *enhanced Nurse Licensure Compact (NLC)*. Under the NLC, registered nurses and licensed practical/vocational nurses who meet uniform standards are granted one multistate license that provides the privilege to practice in their home state and any other NLC state. This licensing model protects the interests of the state in ensuring the qualifications of its healthcare providers while fostering provider mobility and distance healthcare, increasing access to care. This licensing model has demonstrated its value by growing to include 25 states over 20 years. In addition, the NLC reduces the cost and administrative burden of licensure to both healthcare organizations and providers.

2037

SUPPORT OF THE WORLD HEALTH ORGANIZATION

Source: House of Delegates

To strongly support the mission and work of the World Health Organization in its role in public health preparedness, prevention, and control to improve the health and well-being of people globally.

Rationale

In an age of global travel between and among countries, the efforts to prevent, control, treat, and eradicate diseases and conditions that decrease health and well-being of all peoples are critical to all countries, independent of factors such as income and education. Addressing new vectors of disease transmission and behavioral conditions related to lifestyles and environmental conditions continue to provide challenges that need to be addressed. Agencies such as the World Health Organization that provide evidence-based warnings, guidelines, education, research, and advocacy, and that collect data to help countries prepare their public health infrastructure, are critical in providing all peoples with the tools and resources needed to address critical health issues globally.

2040

PREMARKETING COMPARATIVE CLINICAL STUDIES

Source: Council on Therapeutics

To advocate that Congress grant the Food and Drug Administration (FDA) authority to require premarketing comparative clinical trials when appropriate alternative agent(s) exist on the market, to elucidate the new agent's role and place in therapy for the proposed indication; further,

To recommend that drug manufacturers include a summary of premarketing comparative study results in official product labeling, when available; further,

To advocate that Congress provide adequate funding to FDA and other agencies to support the additional tasks required by such premarketing comparative studies.

This policy supersedes ASHP policy 1506.

Rationale

In the past, new drugs were approved in the United States without a requirement to demonstrate efficacy or safety. Today, the FDA reviews new drug applications focusing on 3 major categories: the safety and efficacy of the drug for the proposed indication(s), appropriateness of the manufacturing process to ensure drug identity, potency, and purity, and proposed drug label information. Randomized controlled trials are the study design of choice to demonstrate the efficacy and safety of a new drug. Today, there is no requirement by the FDA that drug manufacturers conduct premarketing comparative studies due to a lack of legislation providing this express authority. A drug may be approved based on comparison to placebo alone, even if there are comparable treatment options available on the market. Demonstrated efficacy in placebo-controlled trials may overestimate the benefit of the drug and inadvertently lead prescribers to utilize a less effective drug, increases the risk for safety events and delayed time to care goals, and increased cost of care. Comparative clinical studies, when done in advance of approval consideration, may provide clinicians with critical information to stratify which patient populations are most appropriate candidates for a new drug in relation to therapeutic options already on the market.

Recently, the FDA has approved more drugs via expedited approval pathways, creating reliance on postmarketing studies to provide clarity on the role of the therapy in care, as well as for identification of undesirable treatment related effects. While postmarketing data is valuable, it is critical that potential efficacy and safety concerns be identified prior to drug approval where reasonable and applicable. Premarketing trials may not reveal all risks related to a drug, especially those in which the drug is used off label, represent adverse events that may take multiple years to emerge, or other adverse events that are relatively rare. Postmarketing studies provide the best opportunity to identify such events. The FDA should be granted the authority to require premarketing comparative clinical studies when appropriate, taking into account the potential impact of such therapies on patient care and timing to avoid approval delay when necessary in order to ensure expedited availability for indications of unmet need. To ensure that the information in premarketing studies is of high integrity, consensus-driven, evidenced-based, and improves healthcare delivery and outcomes, the FDA could include the input of organizations such as the Pharmacy Quality Alliance and Patient-Centered Outcomes Research Institute. Funding to allow for this expanded scope should be provided to support timely review and consideration of premarketing studies.

2043

DRUG PRODUCT SUPPLY CHAIN INTEGRITY

Source: Council on Pharmacy Management

To encourage the Food and Drug Administration (FDA) and relevant state authorities to take the steps necessary to ensure that (1) all drug products entering the supply chain are thoroughly inspected and tested to establish that they have not been adulterated or misbranded and (2) patients will not receive improperly labeled and packaged, deteriorated, outdated, counterfeit, adulterated, or unapproved drug products; further,

To encourage FDA and relevant state authorities to develop and implement regulations to (1) restrict or prohibit licensed drug distributors (drug wholesalers, repackagers, and manufacturers) from purchasing legend drugs from unlicensed entities and (2) ensure accurate documentation at any point in the distribution chain of the original source of drug products and chain of custody from the manufacturer to the pharmacy; further,

To advocate for the establishment of meaningful penalties for companies that violate current good manufacturing practices (cGMPs) intended to ensure the quality, identity, strength, and purity of their marketed drug product(s) and raw materials; further,

To advocate for improved transparency so that drug product labeling includes a readily available means to retrieve the name and location of the facility that manufactured the specific lot of the product and the country of origin of the active pharmaceutical ingredient; further,

To advocate that this readily retrievable manufacturing information be available prospectively to aid purchasers in determining the quality of a drug product and its raw materials; further,

To foster increased pharmacist and public awareness of drug product supply chain integrity; further,

To urge Congress and state legislatures to provide adequate funding, or authority to impose user fees, to accomplish these objectives.

This policy supersedes ASHP policy 1602.

Rationale

The aspect of drug product selection that is not transparent from the labeling is its quality. This information needs to be readily available so those who make the purchasing decision on behalf of hospitals and health systems can factor quality into the decision. Aspects of manufacture that affect quality include the production and compliance history of a manufacturer, the specific name and location of the manufacturing plant, and the source of raw materials, including active pharmaceutical ingredients. This information has been useful in responding to a recall, but it is also important as part of the procurement process. The FDA's Strategic Plan for Preventing and Mitigating Drug Shortages recommends that purchasers of medications consider quality as a component of the purchasing decision. FDA publishes some quality information about manufacturers; however, in subcontracting and licensing situations, it is not always known who the actual manufacturer is, which specific plant location produced the product, and the country of origin of the active pharmaceutical ingredient.

Hospitals and health-system pharmacy leaders have years of experience in managing the demands and challenges of ensuring that drug supply chain safety and integrity is at the highest level possible. Unfortunately, there are many forces in the marketplace that seek to divert and introduce illicit products into the supply chain.

ASHP has supported efforts to improve the integrity of the drug product supply chain, which has included advocacy on track-and-trace legislation, collaboration with the United States Pharmacopeia (USP) in its efforts on supply chain integrity, leadership in dealing with the various issues arising from drug shortages, and a voice for patients and pharmacists on needed change (regulatory and practice-based) with pharmacy's trading partners to enable pharmacists to secure legitimate drug products.

On November 27, 2013, the Drug Quality and Security Act (DQSA) was signed into law. Title II of the DQSA, the Drug Supply Chain Security Act (DSCSA) sets forth new definitions and requirements related to drug product tracing. The DSCSA outlines critical steps to build an electronic, interoperable system by November 27, 2023, which will identify and trace certain prescription drug products as they are distributed in the United States. Implementation of this new electronic, interoperable system, over a 10-year period, will enhance FDA's ability to help protect U.S. consumers by improving detection and removal of potentially dangerous products from the pharmaceutical distribution supply chain.

1904

NOTIFICATION OF DRUG PRODUCT PRICE INCREASES

Source: Council on Public Policy

To advocate for manufacturers to provide notice and justification to the public and healthcare providers in advance of drug price increases; further,

To advocate for transparency in drug product pricing decisions.

Rationale

Many factors contribute to high drug product costs, and addressing the problem is made difficult by lack of knowledge about the marketplace for those products. For example, rebates negotiated by pharmacy benefit managers (PBMs) and discounts to other buyers make it difficult to determine the actual price of a drug product. ASHP advocates for more publicly accessible information on drug product pricing, such as an annual report on increases in drug product prices. Such information would provide patients and their healthcare providers with the information needed to make drug product purchasing choices. The purpose of this policy is to advocate for laws and regulations that would require drug product manufacturers to publicly report price increases in advance and provide justification for those increases, as well as to advocate for transparency regarding drug product pricing decisions. The policy is intended to increase public knowledge concerning pricing decisions made by different parties in the drug product supply chain (e.g., manufacturers, distributors, PBMs, group purchasing organizations) ho may influence drug product prices.

1905

MITIGATING DRUG PRODUCT SHORTAGES

Source: Council on Public Policy

To advocate for ongoing federal evaluation of how drug product shortages present risks to national security and public health; further,

To advocate that drug product manufacturers be required to disclose manufacturing sites and sources of active pharmaceutical ingredients (APIs) to facilitate such a risk assessment; further,

To recommend that the Food and Drug Administration (FDA) require drug product manufacturers to have contingency plans for maintaining drug supplies; further,

To advocate that drug product manufacturers be required to provide a specific reason for a shortage and an estimated timeline for resolution in their Food and Drug Administration Safety and Innovation Act notifications to FDA; further,

To advocate that FDA be required to publicly provide quality ratings for 503B outsourcing facilities preparing copies of drug products under the exemption for products on FDA's shortage list; further,

To advocate that the Federal Trade Commission be required to evaluate the potential for drug product supply chain interruptions when considering manufacturer consolidations.

Rationale

In November 2017, ASHP convened a *meeting of healthcare professional organizations* to review and identify new opportunities to address the ongoing supply chain and patient care challenges associated with drug product shortages. Participants at the meeting examined how the 2012 FDA Safety and Innovation Act (FDASIA) has impacted drug product shortages and made recommendations to prevent and mitigate future shortages. One of those recommendations was that the federal government undertake an evaluation of the risks drug product shortages could present to national security. Such an evaluation would need to consider the risks posed by sourcing of APIs and excipients, as well as by the location of manufacturing sites.

FDA's *Strategic Plan for Preventing and Mitigating Drug Shortages* recommends that drug product purchasers consider quality in making purchasing decisions. Information that purchasers would find helpful in prospectively assessing drug product quality includes the production and compliance history of a manufacturer, the specific name and location of the manufacturing plant, and the source of raw materials. Because approximately 80 percent of APIs used in U.S. drug product manufacturing comes from foreign sources, FDA has limited ability to inspect and certify that those APIs are unadulterated. In addition, although FDA publishes some quality information about manufacturers, it is sometimes difficult to know who the actual manufacturer is and which specific plant location produced the product, because drug companies may rely on contract manufacturers to produce drug products through licensing agreements. Requiring manufacturers to disclose that information publicly would allow for improved evaluation of a manufacturer's integrity and alignment with current good manufacturing processes. Detailed knowledge of manufacturing sites would also allow the government and healthcare systems to plan for or avoid disruptions to the supply chain like those that followed Hurricanes Irma and Maria in 2017, when supplies of 40 critical pharmaceutical products went into shortage, in part because of disruption to the large number of pharmaceutical manufacturing facilities in Puerto Rico. Lack of information about such disruptions can also lead to hoarding, which exacerbates an existing shortage. To avoid similar disruptions, FDA should require manufacturers to have contingency plans for maintaining drug product supplies during events that could disrupt production, such as natural and manmade disasters (e.g., hurricanes, cyberattacks, electricity failures, shipping disruptions).

FDASIA requires that drug product manufacturers submit a notification of a production disruption to FDA. Manufacturers should also be required to provide in these notices a specific reason for the shortage and an estimated timeline for resolution. This information would be helpful not only to those affected but also in the federal evaluation of the risks posed by drug product shortages. Healthcare providers addressing drug product shortages also need information to evaluate the quality of copies of drug products produced by 503B outsourcing facilities under the exemption for products on FDA's shortage list. Congress should require FDA to publicly provide quality ratings for those manufacturers.

Finally, to avoid future drug product shortages, the Federal Trade Commission should be required to evaluate the potential for drug product supply chain interruptions when considering manufacturer consolidations.

1906

EMERGENCY SUPPLIES OF DRUG PRODUCTS

Source: Council on Public Policy

To advocate for states to allow any pharmacist, during a declared emergency, to dispense without a prescription an emergency supply of a drug product in quantities that meet the needs of patients.

Rationale

Many states allow pharmacists to provide emergency supplies of prescription drug products during or in the immediate aftermath of a declared emergency. States such as Florida allow this practice for up to 72 hours after an emergency has been declared (i.e., a patient can obtain a 72-hour supply during an emergency or disaster). However, the long duration of events like hurricanes demonstrates the need to expand the 72-hour window. Hurricanes, for example, typically generate an emergency declaration prior to the storm, and the impact can last until days after the storm, when flood waters crest. Several states, including California and Texas, allow pharmacists to adequately provide prescription drug products, excluding controlled substances, during disasters, emergencies, or catastrophic events. In California, pharmacists are empowered to use their professional judgment when determining the appropriate quantity of an emergency fill. In these situations, patients without a prescription may use an empty pill bottle or other documentation to demonstrate their need for a drug product. In addition, states sometimes require appropriate follow-up by the pharmacist with the patient's prescriber and supporting documentation of the provision of care under an emergency declaration. American Medical Association policy H-120.933, Emergency Prescription Drug Refills, calls for emergency refills beyond the 72-hour period, excluding controlled substances.

1908

340B DRUG PRICING PROGRAM SUSTAINABILITY

Source: Council on Public Policy

To affirm the intent of the federal drug pricing program (the "340B program") to stretch scarce federal resources as far as possible, reaching more eligible patients and providing more comprehensive services; further,

To advocate for continued access to the 340B program in accordance with the intent of the program; further,

To advocate that reimbursement and contracting policies promote 340B program stability and to oppose reimbursement and savings reductions to covered entities; further,

To advocate for clarification and simplification of the 340B program and any future federal discount drug pricing programs with respect to program definitions, eligibility, and compliance measures to ensure the integrity of the program; further,

To encourage 340B participants to provide appropriate stewardship of the 340B program; further,

To educate pharmacy leaders and health-system administrators about the internal partnerships and accountabilities and the patient-care benefits of program participation; further,

To educate health-system administrators, risk managers, and pharmacists about the resources required to support 340B program compliance and documentation; further,

To encourage communication and education concerning the value of the 340B program; further,

To advocate that the Health Resources & Services Administration Office of Pharmacy Affairs have sufficient regulatory authority to enforce compliance for all stakeholders with the 340B program.

This policy supersedes ASHP policy 1817.

Rationale

Statutory and other policy changes to the federal drug pricing ("340B") program over the years have spurred an increase in the number of hospitals and other eligible entities that participate. Since the program's inception, the number of 340B-eligible and participating hospitals has continued to grow. In response, policymakers and other stakeholders have raised questions over how the discounts are used by covered entities and what value the program brings to their respective communities. Congress has held hearings, and bills have been introduced to reform the program. Among the items Congress is considering are transparency, increasing authority of the Health Resources & Services Administration (HRSA) to oversee the program, reimbursement cuts imposed under Medicare Part B on 340B drugs, and examining policy that passes the discount along to the patient.

Expansion of Medicaid eligibility in 2014 (through provisions in the Affordable Care Act) allowed additional hospitals to participate in the program, further driving scrutiny and questions from policymakers and stakeholders. In response to policymaker and stakeholder concerns, ASHP recognizes the important intent and role of the 340B program and stresses the need for its continued sustainability. These developments demonstrate the need for pharmacy leaders to engage in a strategic response to this compliance environment.

The original intent of the 340B program was "to enable these entities to stretch scarce federal resources as far as possible, reaching more eligible patients and providing more comprehensive services." (H.R. Rept. 102-384, pt. 2, at 12 [1992]). ASHP emphasizes the need for clarification and simplification (to the extent possible) of the program in order to enable compliance and maintain program integrity. Further, there is a need for communication and collaboration with public and private payers to ensure optimization of benefits from the 340B program and related contract and reimbursement policies.

1909

PHARMACIST AUTHORITY TO PROVIDE MEDICATION-ASSISTED TREATMENT

Source: Council on Public Policy

To advocate for the role of the pharmacist in medication-assisted treatment (MAT) for opioid use disorder, including patient assessment, education, prescribing, and monitoring of pharmacologic therapies; further,

To pursue the development of federal and state laws and regulations that recognize pharmacists as providers of MAT for opioid use disorder; further,

To foster additional research on clinical outcomes of pharmacist-driven MAT; further,

To advocate for the removal of barriers for all providers to be able to provide MAT to patients.

Rationale

An estimated 2.5 million Americans suffer from opioid use disorder. In 2017, the President's Commission on Combating Drug Addiction and the Opioid Crisis recommended that the U.S. increase screenings and treatment for opioid use disorder. Many pharmacists have the skills to provide direct care to patients with opioid addiction or assist other healthcare providers in caring for these patients. Although some states allow pharmacists to prescribe controlled substances under collaborative practice agreements, pharmacists are not eligible to obtain a waiver under the Drug Addiction Treatment Act of 2000 to prescribe buprenorphine or other drugs for opioid use disorder. Having such prescribing authority would allow pharmacists to fully exercise their expertise and expand the pool of MAT providers. ASHP advocates the removal of barriers for all providers to be able to provide MAT to patients and encourages additional research on the clinical outcomes of pharmacist-driven MAT.

1922

ANTIMICROBIAL USE IN AGRICULTURE

Source: Council on Therapeutics

To advocate that the Food and Drug Administration (FDA) eliminate future approval of antimicrobials for nontherapeutic uses in agricultural animals that represent a safety risk by contributing to antimicrobial resistance; further,

To encourage efforts to phase out and eliminate the nontherapeutic uses of antimicrobials previously approved by the FDA; further,

To support the therapeutic use of antimicrobials in animals only under the supervision of a veterinarian; further,

To encourage the agricultural industry to report to the appropriate regulatory bodies the specific antimicrobials used, the purpose or indication for their use, and the settings in which they are used; further,

To encourage the FDA, Centers for Disease Control and Prevention, and other stakeholders to monitor and limit, when effective alternatives are available, the therapeutic use of antimicrobials that are essential to the treatment of critically ill human patients; further,

To advocate for the inclusion of pharmacists in antimicrobial surveillance and related public health efforts based on pharmacists' knowledge of antimicrobial drug products and antimicrobial resistance.

This policy supersedes ASHP policy 1009.

Rationale

The use of antibiotics in animal agriculture represents the majority of antibiotic use worldwide and poses significant public health risks. Approximately 80% of antibiotic consumption in the U.S. is dedicated to agricultural purposes. Despite warnings and risks, antibiotics are still excessively used for growth promotion, feed efficiency, and disease prevention in animal agriculture.

ASHP supports the public health approach to antimicrobial use in agricultural animals outlined in the July 2010 FDA *testimony* to Congress. The goal of this approach is to minimize the development of antimicrobial resistance, preserving the effectiveness of antimicrobial therapies that are critical in human medicine. According to the FDA, an enhanced action plan would seek to phase out the use of antimicrobials for nontherapeutic purposes (e.g., animal growth promotion, food efficiency) by eliminating future approvals for new nontherapeutic indications. ASHP also supports the FDA's request for increased statutory authority that would facilitate removal of previously approved nontherapeutic uses of antimicrobials. This two-pronged approach is critical to preserving the effectiveness of existing antimicrobials as well as those in development. ASHP opposes nontherapeutic uses but supports animal use of antimicrobials for therapeutic purposes (e.g., treatment of disease or prevention of disease in animals within a population that has documented disease) when this use occurs under the supervision of a veterinarian. Reporting of the specific antimicrobials used, the purpose or indication for their use, and the settings in which they are used would support achievement of the FDA's action plan. In addition, ASHP advocates that FDA approval and subsequent use of antimicrobials should take into consideration the public health impact of the drugs' use. Pharmacists' knowledge of antimicrobial drugs and antimicrobial resistance will be critical to these efforts, including the identification of antimicrobial classes for which animal treatment use should be minimized in order to retain the effectiveness of these drugs for the treatment of critically ill human patients.

1803

CONFIDENCE IN THE U.S. DRUG APPROVAL AND REGULATORY PROCESS

Source: Council on Public Policy

To support and foster legislative and regulatory initiatives designed to improve public and professional confidence in the drug approval and regulatory process in which all relevant data are subject to public scrutiny.

This policy supersedes ASHP policy 9010.

This policy was reviewed in 2023 by the Council on Public Policy and by the Board of Directors and was found to still be appropriate.

Rationale

Patients, healthcare providers, and private and public payers need objective, authoritative, and reliable evidence about drugs in order to make the best treatment decisions. The basis of the trust in the Food and Drug Administration (FDA) drug approval and regulatory process is public scrutiny of the data used in its decision-making. As medication experts, pharmacists play a critical role in educating the public and other clinicians regarding the drug approval process. This education includes helping to explain FDA decision-making related to medications in order to maintain both public trust in FDA and clinician acceptance of FDA's drug approval processes. ASHP supports efforts to improve public and professional confidence in the FDA's drug approval and regulatory process by expanding public access to relevant data used in FDA decision-making.

1815

IMPACT OF DRUG LITIGATION ADS ON PATIENT CARE

Source: Council on Public Policy

To oppose drug litigation advertisements that do not provide a clear and conspicuous warning that patients should not modify or discontinue drug therapy without seeking the advice of their healthcare provider.

This policy was reviewed in 2023 by the Council on Public Policy and by the Board of Directors and was found to still be appropriate.

Rationale

Many law firms use advertising as a means to generate clients for future litigation, including litigation regarding drugs. These advertisements can generate unnecessary fear for patients taking those drugs and may lead them to modify or discontinue medically necessary therapies. Abruptly discontinuing a drug without consulting a healthcare provider can lead to failed therapy and other adverse effects (e.g., some drugs require a tapered withdrawal to be safely discontinued, and patients on multiple medications may require new dosing or drug interaction assessments). Other than truth-in-advertising laws, there is currently no oversight of these advertisements and no requirement to warn patients about the potential harmful effects of discontinuing their drugs. ASHP agrees with the *American Medical Association* that such ads should be required to have clear and conspicuous warnings that direct patients to speak with their healthcare providers before modifying or discontinuing any drug therapy.

1818

FEDERAL QUALITY RATING PROGRAM FOR PHARMACEUTICAL MANUFACTURERS

Source: Council on Public Policy

To advocate that the Food and Drug Administration (FDA) assign quality ratings to pharmaceutical manufacturers based on the quality of their manufacturing processes, sourcing of active pharmaceutical ingredients and excipients, selection of contract manufacturers, and business continuity plans; further,

To advocate that the FDA consider offering incentives for manufacturers to participate in the program.

This policy was reviewed in 2023 by the Council on Public Policy and by the Board of Directors and was found to still be appropriate.

Rationale

Shortages of critical drug products in hospitals and health systems continue to pose a significant threat to public health, and pharmacists and other clinicians are often challenged with locating supplies of life-saving or life-sustaining drug products at a moment's notice and with very few options to choose from. While the number of new shortages has fallen considerably since 2011, a number of drug products remain in short supply. Drug product shortages are often caused by a manufacturing problem (e.g., contamination) that halts production until the problem is resolved. To address the issue of quality in drug product manufacturing, the FDA has proposed the creation of a manufacturing quality initiative that would highlight companies that employ the best quality manufacturing processes by establishing a rating system that would assign a rating to companies based on their level of quality in the manufacturing process. This rating system could be made public to enable prospective customers to see which companies employ the best quality practices. Further, the rating system could serve as a basis for FDA to offer incentives to companies who consistently rate higher than competitors.

1819

INTRAVENOUS FLUID MANUFACTURING FACILITIES AS CRITICAL PUBLIC HEALTH INFRASTRUCTURE

Source: Council on Public Policy

To advocate that federal and state governments recognize intravenous fluid and associated supply manufacturing facilities as critical public health infrastructure.

This policy was reviewed in 2023 by the Council on Public Policy and by the Board of Directors and was found to still be appropriate.

Rationale

In the wake of hurricane Maria's impact on Puerto Rico in 2017, there has been rising interest in examining drug shortages from a national security perspective. The vulnerability of drug manufacturing on the island of Puerto Rico underscored a need to more closely evaluate the potential impacts of natural disasters on drug manufacturing and the production of critical pharmaceutical supplies. The Department of Homeland Security's list of key infrastructure includes public health infrastructure. ASHP advocates that public health infrastructure be defined to include manufacturing sites of intravenous fluids and associated supplies (i.e., components needed to administer intravenous fluids), and that those sites be afforded the same protections as other critical infrastructure. Such protections should include an evaluation of manufacturing vulnerabilities such as geographic location, vulnerability of surrounding infrastructure such as roads or ports, and whether the company has developed business continuity plans or redundancies in manufacturing. Entities deemed critical public health infrastructure should be required to make necessary changes to ensure that manufacturing is not at risk for a supply disruption.

1713

PARTIAL FILLING OF SCHEDULE II PRESCRIPTIONS

Source: Council on Public Policy

To advocate that state legislatures and boards of pharmacy create consistent laws and rules to allow partial filling of Schedule II drugs; further,

To advocate that public and private entities construct criteria for partial filling to minimize the additional burden on patients, pharmacists, and healthcare organizations; further,

To advocate that pharmacists educate prescribers and patients about options for filling prescriptions for Schedule II drugs, including the risks of overprescribing, while recognizing the patient or caregiver's rights to make their own care and management decisions.

This policy was reviewed in 2022 by the Council on Public Policy and by the Board of Directors and was found to still be appropriate.

Rationale

The issue of opioid abuse and addiction has been at the forefront of federal and state activity. Increasing addiction rates of patients taking powerful opioids have spurred calls for action to help address this growing problem. The issue has become national in scope and has generated discussion among policymakers and healthcare practitioners alike. In mid-2016, Congress passed the *Comprehensive Addiction and Recovery Act of 2016*, legislation aimed at curbing opioid abuse and enhancing access to addiction treatment. States have been considering their own legislative initiatives to address what is increasingly described as an epidemic.

One solution proposed by policymakers is to allow pharmacists to dispense only a portion of the quantity of a Schedule II drug prescribed (e.g., 7 days of the prescribed quantity of the drug rather than an entire 30-day supply).

Such "partial filling" of Schedule II drug prescriptions reduces the potential of opioid addiction for the patient and the risk of diversion for others. Federal law has been changed to permit partial filling of Schedule II drugs, and Massachusetts and Maine have passed laws to allow for partial filling of Schedule II drugs. ASHP advocates that other state legislatures and boards of pharmacy amend pharmacy practice acts and rules to allow for partial filling of Schedule II drugs, and that such laws and rules be made consistent across states. However, ASHP has concerns about quantity and duration limits applied across the board and not on an as-needed basis (e.g., for oncology and palliative care patients). ASHP believes that each patient must be evaluated individually and that polices that allow for partial filling are not indiscriminately applied as an across-the-board mandatory rule. ASHP encourages public and private payers to recognize the additional burden placed on patients and pharmacies by partial filling and to minimize these burdens when possible, including providing appropriate reimbursement for pharmacist activities. ASHP encourages pharmacists to serve as patient advocates by educating prescribers and patients about options for filling prescriptions for Schedule II drugs.

1715

COLLABORATIVE PRACTICE

Source: Council on Public Policy

To pursue the development of federal and state laws and regulations that authorize pharmacists as providers within collaborative practice; further,

To advocate expansion of federal and state laws and regulations that optimize pharmacists' ability to provide the full range of professional services within their scope of expertise; further,

To advocate for federal and state laws and regulations that would allow pharmacists to prescribe and transmit prescriptions electronically; further,

To acknowledge that as part of these advanced collaborative practices, pharmacists, as active members in team-based care, must be responsible and accountable for medication-related outcomes; further,

To support affiliated state societies in their pursuit of state-level regulations allowing collaborative practice for pharmacists.

This policy was reviewed in 2022 by the Council on Public Policy and by the Board of Directors and was found to still be appropriate.

Rationale

Although many states permit pharmacists to serve as providers in collaborative practice, there is great variability in the authority granted to pharmacists. ASHP supports collaborative practice and advocates its expansion to all states, in a variety of diverse practice settings, and at the highest level of pharmacy practice. As new pharmacy practice models emerge, collaborative practice should be a part of those innovations. One of the common barriers to the highest level of collaborative practice is the prohibition of pharmacists transmitting prescriptions electronically. The expansion of collaborative practice, including electronic transmission of prescriptions, will aid in moving the profession forward to the highest level of team-based practice and will enable pharmacists to practice at the top of their licenses, accountable to the patient and the team for medication-related outcomes.

Further, expansion of these team-based models will require both federal and state reimbursement models sufficient to support the practice, including advancement of state-level pay parity acts that ensure payment for pharmacists at least equivalent to that of other providers.

1716

GREATER COMPETITION AMONG GENERIC AND BIOSIMILAR MANUFACTURERS

Source: Council on Public Policy

To advocate for legislation and regulations that promote greater competition among generic and biosimilar pharmaceutical manufacturers.

This policy was reviewed in 2022 by the Council on Public Policy and by the Board of Directors and was found to still be appropriate.

Rationale

A healthy market for generic drug products and biosimilars increases patient access to drugs and lowers drug costs. ASHP recognizes several threats to the health of that market and advocates legislative and regulatory solutions: speeding FDA approval of generic drug applications, especially for lifesaving drugs; reducing drug monopolies by incentivizing competition for additional market entrants; targeting exclusivity protections to truly innovative products; and curbing abuse of risk evaluation and mitigation strategies (REMS) and misuse of FDA's citizen petition process. In 2015, the FDA faced a backlog of nearly 4,000 generic drug applications, with the approval process taking three years or more. ASHP advocates that the FDA be provided the resources needed to evaluate and approve generic drug applications in a safe and timely manner. ASHP also advocates government and market incentives to increase competition for expensive drugs where no competitors exist and encourage additional market entrants. ASHP has long recognized that agreements between generic and brand-name manufacturers when a product's market exclusivity is about to expire have the effect of delaying the marketing of competitor products and limiting patient access to affordable generic drugs. ASHP advocates for legislative and regulatory solutions to limit such agreements, as well as solutions to prevent brand-name manufacturers from extending market exclusivity and preventing market entry by generics by slightly altering the formulation of a product. ASHP further advocates legislation that would prevent frivolous patent infringement litigation by brand-name manufacturers, which is reported to have been initiated with the sole intent to extend market exclusivity. Another solution advocated by ASHP is curbing misuse of REMS, which are reported to have been used to prevent generic manufacturers from accessing drug products. In addition, ASHP advocates for more consumer-accessible information on drug prices and rebates, including an annual report on increases in drug prices, which would provide patients and their healthcare providers with the information they need to make drug purchasing choices. Finally, ASHP encourages appropriate federal review of anticompetitive practices by pharmaceutical manufacturers.

1621

TIMELY BOARD OF PHARMACY LICENSING

Source: Council on Public Policy

To advocate that the National Association of Boards of Pharmacy (NABP) collaborate with boards of pharmacy to streamline the licensure process through standardization and improve the timeliness of application approval; further,

To advocate that NABP collaborate with boards of pharmacy and third-party vendors to streamline the licensure transfer or reciprocity process; further,

To advocate that boards of pharmacy grant licensed pharmacists in good standing temporary licensure, permitting them to engage in practice, while their application for licensure transfer or reciprocity is being processed.

This policy was reviewed in 2021 by the Council on Public Policy and by the Board of Directors and was found to still be appropriate.

Rationale

Pharmacists sometimes face challenges from delays in obtaining licensure by transfer or reciprocity when moving their practice from one jurisdiction to another. Such delay may be due to the need for boards to review pharmacists' licensure records in all jurisdictions in which they are licensed, administer a state pharmacy law exam, complete a criminal background check, and, in some cases, schedule an interview with the board. To address these challenges, boards of pharmacy should allow pharmacists in good standing to immediately practice in a different jurisdiction when they change employment or enter a residency program. Granting pharmacists a temporary license for a period of up to six months while the board completes its review would help meet workforce demands while continuing to safeguard the public health. In some cases, pharmacists who are unable to obtain a license in a timely manner are unable to fully use the skills in which they have been trained. Without a license, the pharmacist may temporarily have to function as a technician or perform other tasks. For pharmacists participating in residency programs outside their jurisdiction of licensure, several months of their residency program can elapse before they receive licensure transfer or reciprocity. Upon completion of a yearlong residency program, many residents move to another jurisdiction to practice and have to start the transfer or reciprocity process again.

Members in several states have reported that in recent years boards of pharmacy have been slow to issue pharmacy licenses. This delay is especially problematic for pharmacy residents from another jurisdiction who rely on boards to grant them a license prior to performing in a clinical capacity. Given that the licensing period can take several months, this delay has presented a problem for pharmacy residents who have a limited timeframe to successfully complete their duties, typically one year. In some cases, state boards are urging residents to obtain a pharmacy technician license; however, this is inappropriate given the expertise and education residents have and the level of practice they're expected to engage in. Given its national scope, NABP is well-positioned to explore a broad solution to this problem rather than the current, incremental, state-by-state approach.

1501

PHARMACIST PARTICIPATION IN HEALTH POLICY DEVELOPMENT

Source: Council on Public Policy

To advocate that pharmacists participate with policymakers and stakeholders in the development of health-related policies at the national, state, and community levels; further,

To develop tools and resources to assist pharmacists in fully participating in health policy development at all levels.

Rationale

Health policy developed at the federal, state, and local levels increasingly impacts medication use, particularly as payment and delivery models require the interprofessional healthcare team to collaboratively deliver care to meet quality and outcomes measures. The perspective of pharmacists practicing in hospital and ambulatory care settings is essential to the development of health policy. At the federal level, policy development includes drug development, distribution, and control; coverage for medication therapy; interoperability of health information; and all aspects of patient safety. Those federal issues also exist at the state and local level, but also include the full range of scope of practice issues.

The absence of hospital and ambulatory care pharmacist input into health policy development leads to suboptimal public policy, inefficient use of resources (public and private), and the potential for suboptimal patient care at the individual patient level and with specific patient populations. Furthermore, poorly developed public policy results in pharmacists being unable to practice at the top of their licenses.

This policy was reviewed in 2020 by the Council on Public Policy and by the Board of Directors and was found to still be appropriate.

1502

PHARMACIST RECOGNITION AS A HEALTHCARE PROVIDER

Source: Council on Public Policy

To advocate for changes in federal (e.g., Social Security Act), state, and third-party payment programs to define pharmacists as healthcare providers; further,

To affirm that pharmacists, as medication-use experts, provide safe, accessible, high-quality care that is cost effective, resulting in improved patient outcomes; further,

To recognize that pharmacists, as healthcare providers, improve access to patient care and bridge existing gaps in healthcare; further,

To collaborate with key stakeholders to describe the covered direct patient-care services provided by pharmacists; further,

To advocate for sustainable compensation and standardized billing processes used by payers for pharmacist services by all available payment programs.

This policy was reviewed in 2020 by the Council on Public Policy and by the Board of Directors and was found to still be appropriate.

Rationale

Recognition of pharmacists as healthcare providers is emerging and being codified in state law as well as in current federal legislative proposals (e.g., H.R. 592, S. 314). In some cases this recognition also includes specified compensation through existing payment mechanisms (e.g., federal Medicare Part B or state Medicaid programs). With recognition, pharmacists should be sustainably compensated for their patient-care services by all public and private payers using standardized billing processes.

1405

AUTOMATIC STOP ORDERS

Source: Council on Pharmacy Practice

To advocate that the Centers for Medicare & Medicaid Services (1) remove the requirement in the Hospital Conditions of Participation that all medication orders automatically stop after an arbitrarily assigned period to include other options to protect patients from indefinite, open-ended medication orders, and (2) revise the remainder of the medication management regulations and interpretive guidelines to be consistent with this practice; further,

To affirm that the requirement for automatic stop orders for all medications is a potential source of medication errors and patient harm; further,

To encourage pharmacists to participate in interprofessional efforts to establish standardized methods to assure appropriate duration of therapy.

This policy was reviewed in 2019 by the Council on Therapeutics and by the Board of Directors and was found to still be appropriate.

Rationale

Automatic stop orders on medications are intended to safeguard patients against unnecessary or prolonged drug therapy, yet they also have been shown to cause medication errors when critical therapy is inadvertently and arbitrarily discontinued. The Centers for Medicare & Medicaid Services Hospital Conditions of Participation (CMS COP) continue to require automatic stop orders for all medications, not accounting for shorter lengths of stay and other means of reviewing drug therapy for appropriateness. The CMS COP should be revised to reflect better, more effective approaches to re-evaluating the appropriateness of medications.

1406

FEDERAL AND STATE REGULATION OF COMPOUNDING

Source: Council on Public Policy

To advocate that the applicable compendial standards of the United States Pharmacopeia be included in state and federal laws and regulations that govern compounding by any health professional; further,

To advocate for mandatory state registration of compounding facilities (e.g., pharmacies, physician offices, clinics, ambulatory surgery centers) that provide products for specific patient prescriptions or in anticipation of specific patient prescriptions or medication orders; further,

To advocate for mandatory Food and Drug Administration registration and current good manufacturing practices requirements for outsourcing facilities that compound and sell products without patient-specific prescriptions across state lines; further,

To advocate for improved patient safety and care through education of regulatory inspectors, increased frequency and improved effectiveness of compliance inspections, and enhancing interagency communications; further,

To advocate that state and federal agencies develop standardized definitions and nomenclature relating to sterile and nonsterile compounding, including but not limited to definitions of compounding, manufacturing, repackaging, and relabeling.

This policy was reviewed in 2019 by the Council on Public Policy and by the Board of Directors and was found to still be appropriate.

Rationale

The practice of compounding has evolved along with the profession of pharmacy. With the advancement of pharmaceutical manufacturing, the preparation of individualized medications based on a prescription or medication order has also evolved. In particular, sterile preparation and related best practices (e.g., ASHP guidelines) and standards of practice (relevant USP chapters) have also evolved. However, cases of contamination, adulteration, and misbranding have persisted, culminating in the meningitis tragedy caused by contaminated sterile preparations compounded by the New England Compounding Center (NECC). That contamination resulted in 64 deaths and over 700 patient cases, as reported by the Centers for Disease Control and Prevention.

The NECC case highlighted the need for accountability and clear regulatory jurisdiction between state boards of pharmacy and the federal Food and Drug Administration. Since 1997, there has been discussion and debate over the proper oversight of compounding. The NECC case demonstrated the real and potential national public health threat posed by the lack of oversight of the practice of compounding. This threat is particularly acute when high-risk sterile products are prepared in large quantities and sold across state lines without adherence to either relevant USP chapters or Food and Drug Administration (FDA) current good manufacturing practices (cGMPs). Over the past 16 years, a series of court decisions in various federal circuits has resulted in a patchwork application of Section 503A of the Federal Food Drug and Cosmetic Act. In addition, a new type of supplier of sterile compounded preparations has emerged to fill a critical need for high-risk sterile preparations for hospitals and health systems. Those health systems are often unable to make the capital and/or human resource investments to prepare these high-risk preparations and seek to use outside suppliers to meet their patients' needs. In 2013, Congress passed H.R. 3204, the Drug Quality and Security Act (DQSA) and President Obama signed it into law (P.L. 113-54) on November 27, 2013. Prior to the passage of the DQSA, these outside suppliers operated as licensed pharmacies and in some cases also registered as drug establishments with the FDA. However, the authority for FDA to inspect and enforce either cGMPs or USP standards was unclear. DQSA is designed to provide that clarity as well as delineate the accountability between the FDA and state boards.

ASHP advocates federal oversight of certain entities that compound and engage in interstate commerce to address the wider public health threat when these preparations can potentially be distributed nationwide. ASHP continues to call for state regulation of compounding by health professionals (including pharmacists, physicians, and nurses) that would require meeting the applicable USP standards. ASHP believes that federally registered compounding facilities should be required to meet applicable cGMPs and that state-registered facilities engaged in "traditional compounding" (i.e., compounding for specific patient prescriptions or in anticipation of specific patient prescriptions or medication orders) be required to meet applicable USP standards. ASHP also advocates for inspection by the relevant regulatory body, training of inspectors, and enhanced communication among federal and state regulatory authorities. Finally, ASHP calls for standard definitions and nomenclature for certain terms that may have different definitions within federal law and regulation and between federal and state law and regulation (FDA, Drug Enforcement Administration [DEA], pharmacy practice act and regulation).

1408

STATE PRESCRIPTION DRUG MONITORING PROGRAMS

Source: Council on Public Policy

To advocate for mandatory, uniform prescription drug monitoring programs that collect real-time, relevant, and standard information from all dispensing outpatient entities about controlled substances and monitored prescriptions; further,

To advocate that the design of these programs should balance the need for appropriate therapeutic management with safeguards against fraud, misuse, abuse, and diversion; further,

To advocate that such programs be structured as part of electronic health records and exchanges to allow prescribers, pharmacists, and other practitioners to proactively monitor data for appropriate assessment; further,

To advocate for full interstate integration to allow for access by prescribers, pharmacists, and other qualified designees across state lines; further,

To advocate for federal and state funding to establish and administer these programs; further,

To promote research, education, and implementation of best practices in prescription drug monitoring programs.

This policy was reviewed in 2019 by the Council on Public Policy and by the Board of Directors and was found to still be appropriate.

Rationale

ASHP recognizes the important contributions to public health made by state prescription drug monitoring programs (PDMPs). To be effective, these programs need to be mandatory; must collect standardized, relevant, and real-time information for analysis and comparison among states; and need to be universal. Some PDMPs do not update information in real time. When updating lags reporting by days (or even weeks), program effectiveness is compromised. Moreover, relevant information is sometimes not required, and not all dispensing sites are required to participate, which impacts the ability of practitioners to make relevant clinical decisions. PDMPs need to be fully integrated across state lines so information from other jurisdictions is available to practitioners and prescribers to assist them in balancing the goals of discouraging prescription drug abuse while providing appropriate therapeutic management. It is also important to ensure the integration and interoperability of these programs with the evolving use of electronic health records and information exchanges so that prescription monitoring programs can be an educational tool for prescribers and practitioners. Finally, adequate state and federal funding is essential to sustain the viability of these programs and to encourage research, education, and implementation of best practices in PDMPs. Such research and education would serve to raise awareness about how to best address the growing public health issue of prescription drug abuse and misuse.

1411

EXPEDITED PATHWAYS FOR FDA DRUG APPROVAL

Source: Council on Therapeutics

To support the use of expedited pathways for Food and Drug Administration (FDA) approval of new drugs that expand access to innovative therapies while protecting patient safety; further,

To advocate for the development of unique labeling requirements that would be used on an interim basis to identify products approved by these pathways in order to increase awareness of data limitations and guide clinician use of these drugs until additional evidence becomes available; further,

To advocate that the FDA be diligent in enforcing postmarketing commitments for drug products approved via expedited pathways, including utilizing its existing authority to enforce penalties when these requirements are not met; further,

To encourage research to evaluate the impact of expedited pathways on drug product development and patient care, including drug development timelines and costs, overall health care costs, patient access to care, and the effectiveness and safety of these therapies.

This policy was reviewed in 2020 by the Council on Public Policy and by the Board of Directors and was found to still be appropriate.

Rationale

Expedited approval programs provided by the FDA have resulted in substantial public health benefits as illustrated by the use of surrogate endpoints to approve therapies for HIV and AIDS in the 1990s. The FDA provides four mechanisms to expedite the development and review process for drugs: fast track designation, breakthrough therapy designation, accelerated approval, and priority review designation. The structure and requirements for each of these mechanisms differs as described in a *2013 draft guidance for industry*. However, to qualify for any of these programs a drug must (1) address an unmet medical need, (2) provide benefit over available drug treatments, and (3) be used in the treatment of a serious or life-threatening condition. Further, the FDA guidance states that these programs are "intended to help ensure that therapies for serious conditions are approved and available to patients as soon as it can be concluded that the therapies' benefits justify their risks." Processes used to ensure a favorable risk–benefit profile include, but are not limited to, requirements for postmarketing studies to evaluate safety and effectiveness of the drug as used in real-world scenarios. However, the accelerated approval program is the only program that includes postmarketing studies as a requirement of the program. The FDA has discretion to require additional studies on a case-by-case basis for drug products approved via the other expedited mechanisms. Despite these safeguards, some features of these programs (e.g., smaller clinical trials, alternate trial designs, or limited-duration trials) can result in increased patient risk because less is known about a drug's side effect profile and efficacy due to limited patient exposure. In addition, as with all drugs, safety assessments benefit from use of the drug in post-approval patient populations, which better reflect real-world use as compared to the controlled environment of a clinical trial.

Because these drugs represent medical advances, their post-approval use can be extensive. Further, off-label use of these drug products, like all therapies, is common. However, prescribers and other clinicians are frequently unaware that an expedited pathway was utilized and that evidence limitations exist. This scenario raises significant concerns about whether there is sufficient clinician awareness to ensure appropriate use of drugs approved via these pathways. Therefore, ASHP proposes unique labeling requirements that would increase awareness through use of a logo or other mechanism that would be used on an interim basis to inform clinicians about data limitations and provide guidance on appropriate use. This labeling would describe appropriate patient populations and monitoring parameters. Similar labeling requirements have been proposed for a new pathway being considered for the development of antibiotics used to treat life-threatening infections. ASHP supports the approach, but recommends that the increased labeling requirements be discontinued once the drug product manufacturer and FDA agree that sufficient data is available to support safe and effective use, or after the drug manufacturer completes any required postmarketing study commitments.

Given data limitations associated with approval of these therapies, ASHP advocates that the FDA be extremely diligent in ensuring that postmarketing commitments are met. Further, the FDA should use its existing authority as described under 21 CFR 314 subpart H and 21 CFR 601 subpart E if timelines or expectations for these commitments are not satisfactory. This authority allows the FDA to take legal action through penalties that include requiring labeling changes or rescinding marketing approval.

Finally, ASHP believes that there is a need for research to determine whether these expedited pathways are achieving the desired benefits, which include decreasing the time and costs associated with drug product development, lowering overall health care costs, and increasing patient access to safe and effective drug therapies.

1412

FDA OVERSIGHT OF LABORATORY-DEVELOPED TESTS

Source: Council on Therapeutics

To advocate that the Food and Drug Administration be granted increased authority to regulate laboratory-developed tests as medical devices, including tests used for pharmacogenetic testing; further,

To support development of a risk-based framework for regulatory oversight of laboratory-developed tests that promotes innovation while providing a mechanism to ensure that test results are reliable, reproducible, and clinically relevant; further,

To encourage expanded availability of commercially marketed pharmacogenetic tests that would be available for use by laboratory and health care professionals to guide drug therapy.

This policy was reviewed in 2023 by the Council on Public Policy and by the Board of Directors and was found to still be appropriate.

Rationale

The use of in vitro pharmacogenetic tests has become increasingly common as efforts continue to achieve the promise of personalized medicine. However, the current system of regulatory oversight of these and other laboratory tests used to guide drug therapy is complex and inconsistent. Some laboratory tests (e.g., companion diagnostics devices) receive premarket review and approval by the Food and Drug Administration (FDA) when the test is either developed in tandem with drug development or following the drug's approval. Other tests, commonly called laboratory-developed tests (LDTs), are proprietary tests that are developed and validated for use at specific laboratory facilities. These tests do not undergo premarket review and approval by the FDA. LDTs currently fall under a mixed system of oversight by the FDA and Centers for Medicare & Medicaid Services (CMS), which regulates these tests based on facilities' compliance to the Clinical Laboratory Improvement Amendments (CLIA). CLIA compliance serves as the primary mechanism for oversight, as the FDA has traditionally practiced discretionary authority, meaning that only a few of the most complex tests are scrutinized by that agency. While an LDT is monitored for validity and reliability at the laboratory where it is conducted, results may not be reproducible if the test is conducted at a different laboratory site. This variability complicates the interpretation and application of this information in patient care. Therefore, ASHP advocates for the FDA to have increased authority to regulate these LDTs as medical devices to ensure that results are reliable, reproducible, and clinically relevant to patient care.

Development of a risk-based framework represents the ideal model to provide sufficient oversight while creating conditions that support continued innovation in this field. Further, the development of nationally validated and marketed tests that are available for use by laboratory and health care professionals is desirable. ASHP believes that this scenario would provide the most assurance to pharmacists and other health care professionals that the results of these tests are reliable, reproducible, and clinically relevant to patient care.

1310

REGULATION OF TELEPHARMACY SERVICES

Source: Council on Public Policy

To advocate that state governments adopt laws and regulations that standardize telepharmacy practices across state lines and facilitate the use of United States-based telepharmacy services; further,

To advocate that boards of pharmacy and state agencies that regulate pharmacy practice include the following in regulations for telepharmacy services: (1) education and training of participating pharmacists; (2) education, training, certification by the Pharmacy Technician Certification Board, and licensure of participating pharmacy technicians; (3) communication and information systems requirements; (4) remote order entry, prospective order review, verification of the completed medication order before dispensing, and dispensing; (5) direct patient-care services, including medication therapy management services and patient counseling and education; (6) licensure (including reciprocity) of participating pharmacies and pharmacists; (7) service arrangements that cross state borders; (8) service arrangements within the same corporate entity or between different corporate entities; (9) service arrangements for workload relief in the point-of-care pharmacy during peak periods; (10) pharmacist access to all applicable patient information; and (11) development and monitoring of patient safety, quality, and outcomes measures; further,

To identify additional legal and professional issues in the provision of telepharmacy services to and from sites located outside the United States.

This policy was reviewed in 2023 by the Council on Public Policy and by the Board of Directors and was found to still be appropriate.

Rationale

In light of continuing advances in technology, there is an increasingly urgent need for state board of pharmacy regulation of the provision of pharmacist care services from off-site locations through electronic technology, which is often referred to, especially in regulation, as *telepharmacy*. In the ASHP Statement on Telehealth Pharmacy Practice, ASHP explains why it prefers the term *telehealth pharmacy practice* to describe both the provision of team-based patient care and oversight of aspects of pharmacy operations (e.g., remote dispensing, order verification, supervision of staff) by pharmacists using electronic information and telecommunications technology.

It is important to acknowledge the regulatory purview of state boards of pharmacy regarding the use of telepharmacy and recognize that the intent of such regulations should be to balance protection of the public health with the increased patient access to the patient care services of pharmacists provided by telepharmacy. Although such regulations should allow for various arrangements across state borders and within or between health systems, they all need to address a number of common concerns.

ASHP advocates that the provision of medication therapy management and other direct patient care services be addressed in any regulation of telepharmacy services and that patient safety, quality, and outcomes measures for these services be developed and monitored. Further, ASHP urges state governments to harmonize the practice of pharmacy across state lines and to require that pharmacy technicians providing telepharmacy services be certified by the Pharmacy Technician Certification Board and licensed by the state board of pharmacy. Finally, ASHP recognizes the need to continue efforts to identify additional legal and professional issues in the provision of international telepharmacy services.

1311

REGULATION OF CENTRALIZED ORDER FULFILLMENT

Source: Council on Public Policy

To advocate changes in federal and state laws, regulations, and policies to permit centralized medication order fulfillment within health care facilities under common ownership.

This policy was reviewed in 2023 by the Council on Public Policy and by the Board of Directors and was found to still be appropriate.

Rationale

Health systems use centralized facilities to provide a range of medications in order to improve efficiency, decrease redundancy, optimize preparation expertise, and decrease overhead and inventory costs. Importantly, health systems use centralized facilities to provide medications that are in short supply or are difficult to compound safely.

The Drug Enforcement Administration prohibits central repackaging and distribution of controlled substances to other facilities that are part of the same health system. Moreover, health systems with facilities in multiple states find additional requirements in each state by boards of pharmacy and other state regulators when providing medications across state borders from a centralized facility.

ASHP recognizes the importance of maintaining practice standards and related safeguards to assure patient safety. In fact, health systems use centralized facilities in order to have the most-qualified personnel prepare these medications in the safest facility. Regulatory changes are needed at the state and federal level to optimally use centralized facilities that are under the common ownership and therefore quality control of the health system.

1216

PHARMACY TECHNICIANS

Source: Council on Public Policy

To advocate that pharmacy move toward the following model with respect to the evolving pharmacy technician workforce as the optimal approach to protecting public health and safety: (1) development and adoption of uniform state laws and regulations regarding pharmacy technicians, (2) mandatory completion of an ASHP-accredited program of education and training as a prerequisite to pharmacy technician certification, (3) mandatory certification by the Pharmacy Technician Certification Board as a prerequisite to licensure by the state board of pharmacy, and (4) licensure of pharmacy technicians by state boards of pharmacy granting the technician permission to engage in the full scope of responsibilities authorized by the state; further,

To advocate, with respect to certification, as an interim measure until the optimal model is fully implemented, that individuals be required either (1) to have completed an ASHP-accredited program of education and training or (2) to have at least one year of full-time equivalent experience as pharmacy technicians before they are eligible to become certified; further,

To advocate that all pharmacy functions be performed under the general supervision of a licensed pharmacist and that licensed pharmacists and technicians be held accountable for the quality of pharmacy services provided.

(*Note:* Licensure is the process by which an agency of government grants permission to an individual to engage in a given occupation upon finding that the applicant has attained the minimal degree of competency necessary to ensure that the public health, safety, and welfare will be reasonably well protected. Certification is the process by which a nongovernmental agency or association grants recognition to an individual who has met certain predetermined qualifications specified by that agency or association.)

This policy was reviewed in 2022 by the Council on Public Policy and by the Board of Directors and was found to still be appropriate.

Rationale

Licensure is the process by which an agency of government grants permission to an individual to engage in a given occupation upon finding that the applicant has attained the minimal degree of competency necessary to ensure that the public health, safety, and welfare will be reasonably well protected. Certification is the process by which a nongovernmental agency or association grants recognition to an individual who has met certain predetermined qualifications specified by that agency or association.

Recommendation D8 of the 2010 *Pharmacy Practice Model Initiative Summit* and subsequent discussion by the ASHP Board of Directors called for licensure of pharmacy technicians. Subsequent ASHP initiatives, including the Pharmacy Advancement Initiatives 2030, support licensure and certification of pharmacy technicians.

Optimal use of pharmacy technicians will enable pharmacists to devote more time to drug therapy management. Uniformity among state laws is essential to achieve the preferred vision for practice. Moreover, requiring licensure rather than registration will enable state boards to require competency, impose disciplinary sanctions, and hold technicians accountable for their actions.

The process proposed for pharmacy technicians to achieve licensure follows the same steps outlined in ASHP policy 0815: education and training, followed by examination and certification, as prerequisites to licensure. The movement to technician licensure was essential to assure the public that the medication-use system includes individuals competent to assist pharmacists to provide and manage their medication regimens. Licensure will provide state boards with the tools necessary to provide that assurance to the public.

1219

STABLE FUNDING FOR HRSA OFFICE OF PHARMACY AFFAIRS

Source: Council on Public Policy

To advocate for a sustainable level of funding, including appropriations, sufficient to support the public health mission of the Health Resources and Services Administration (HRSA) Office of Pharmacy Affairs; further,

To support initiatives of the Office of Pharmacy Affairs, including the 340B Drug Pricing Program and innovative pharmacy service models in HRSA-funded programs; further,

To encourage research on the potential impact of any proposed fees or alternative funding sources for the Office of Pharmacy Affairs.

This policy was reviewed in 2022 by the Council on Public Policy and by the Board of Directors and was found to still be appropriate.

Rationale

The Office of Pharmacy Affairs (OPA) currently relies on general funding from its parent agency, HRSA, and not a line-item annual appropriation to administer the 340B Drug Discount Program. The OPA and HRSA have sought funding to establish a cost recovery (user fee) program to administer the program. The initial fee would be 0.1 percent of the total 340B drug purchases paid by participating covered entities. HRSA and OPA contend that the cost recovery fee will create a sustainable funding source to meet the demands of the existing and projected growth of the 340B program, the changing marketplace, and new statutory program requirements.

There is a need for stable and sustainable funding for the OPA. A variety of funding sources should be considered, perhaps involving entities that do not participate in the 340B program. Any user fee program should include an annual review of the percentage used to determine the annual fee charged to participating entities. In addition, OPA should not be solely dependent on user fees for its program administration; some level of congressional appropriations would serve as an important safeguard against such a dependency.

1223

GLOBALIZATION OF CLINICAL TRIALS

Source: Council on Therapeutics

To encourage the Food and Drug Administration (FDA) to use its existing authority to increase monitoring and inspection of foreign clinical trials to ensure the integrity and quality of those studies; further,

To advocate that the FDA expand its oversight of clinical trials conducted abroad by continuing to pursue innovative strategies, such as increased collaboration with foreign regulatory agencies and changes in domestic regulatory processes that support timely submission of foreign clinical trial information; further,

To encourage the FDA to establish a standardized electronic format and reporting standards that would be required for submission of data from foreign clinical trials; further,

To support the ethical treatment of patients in foreign clinical trials in accordance with international standards designed to protect human subjects; further,

To encourage public and private research to study the impact of the globalization of clinical trials on patient care.

This policy was reviewed in 2022 by the Council on Therapeutics and by the Board of Directors and was found to still be appropriate.

Rationale

More than 80% of marketing applications for drugs approved in fiscal year 2008 were supported by data from foreign clinical trials, and more than 50% were based on data from trials that were conducted entirely outside of the United States. This trend toward the globalization of clinical trials is expected to continue because of potential benefits to drug manufacturers (e.g., decreased costs, availability of treatment-naïve patients). ASHP is concerned that limited experience with clinical trials in some countries could affect data integrity and questioned whether results from foreign clinical trials could always be generalized to patients in the United States because of differences in genetics and cultural factors (e.g., diet, use of supplements). Existing FDA authority allows for oversight of foreign clinical trials, including a requirement for mandatory reporting. However, according to the 2010 Office of Inspector General (OIG) report, *Challenges to FDA's Ability to Monitor and Inspect Foreign Clinical Trials*, only 0.7 percent of foreign trial investigators were inspected in FY 2008 (compared to 1.9% of investigators in the United States). The FDA should increase oversight of foreign clinical trials given the potential for inconsistencies in protocol implementation and concerns about the availability and integrity of data noted in the OIG report. Development of innovative approaches to expand oversight given limited FDA resources is also encouraged. ASHP supports a recent *FDA agreement with the European Medicines Agency* to share information from inspections conducted by that agency and encourages the FDA to establish this type of agreement with other countries, including those whose experience with clinical trials is limited. The FDA should also explore regulatory changes that would support more timely submission of foreign clinical trial information. This recommendation is based on concern that some aspects of current regulations may encourage drug manufacturers to favor foreign clinical trials. For example, submission of an investigational new drug (IND) application triggers FDA oversight, including required submission of clinical trial protocols. Timely submission of an IND is necessary for studies conducted within the United States because it provides an exemption from interstate commerce laws, which is needed to conduct clinical trials. However, interstate commerce laws do not apply abroad. Therefore, there is no requirement or incentive for manufacturers to submit study protocols for foreign trials if they are conducted prior to the IND submission. However, results from those trials are sometimes used to support marketing applications for drug approval. While the FDA can review protocol and data from these studies retrospectively, data omissions and other factors limit the effectiveness of this approach. Earlier submission of this information would enhance the effectiveness of FDA's oversight. Standardization and electronic submission of data from foreign clinical trials should also be encouraged, given the OIG finding that data from these trials was sometimes not available to FDA reviewers. Ethical concerns associated with foreign clinical trials, including documented lapses in informed consent, support the need for improved adherence to ethical standards for conducting clinical research, such as those described in the *International Conference on Harmonization Tripartite Guideline for Good Clinical Practice*, the *Declaration of Helsinki*, and other international guidelines. Finally, the FDA and private entities are encouraged to study the potential patient care impact of the globalization of clinical trials to determine whether there is an impact even when studies are conducted appropriately.

1121

POISON CONTROL CENTER FUNDING

Source: Council on Public Policy

To advocate that poison control centers be considered an essential emergency service; further,

To advocate for new and stable funding mechanisms for poison control centers to continue to provide these essential and valuable services; further,

To support the integration and coordination of poison control center services where appropriate.

This policy was reviewed in 2021 by the Council on Public Policy and by the Board of Directors and was found to still be appropriate.

Rationale

The Council reviewed recent trends by state governments to reduce or eliminate funding for poison control centers and concluded that ASHP policy was needed. The Board and House concurred. The Council, Board, and House agreed with observations by the American College of Emergency Physicians in its June 2010 task force report that the centers are an essential emergency service and part of the infrastructure for an all-hazards emergency preparedness system, including pandemic and bioterrorism response. The Council noted that studies have shown a positive financial benefit provided by the centers; a 2004 report by the Institute of Medicine (IOM) cited a $6.50 cost savings for every dollar invested in poison control centers.

The Council suggested that recent cuts in funding by state governments (e.g., California) as well as proposals to eliminate poison control centers in some states (e.g., New Jersey) demonstrate a need to develop new and stable funding, and the Board and House agreed. The Council further noted that the IOM report concluded that poison control centers should be better integrated and coordinated, and the Board and House agreed that such integration and coordination should be supported where appropriate.

1002

RISK EVALUATION AND MITIGATION STRATEGIES

Source: Council on Public Policy

To advocate for research on the impact of the Food and Drug Administration's Risk Evaluation and Mitigation Strategies (REMS) on patient safety, cost effectiveness, and pharmacy workflow; further,

To advocate pharmacist involvement in the development and implementation of REMS; further,

To urge computer software vendors to assist pharmacists in the identification of and compliance with REMS; further,

To advocate that any REMS that include constraint on traditional drug distribution systems be consistent with ASHP policy on restricted drug distribution.

This policy was reviewed in 2015 by the Council on Public Policy and by the Board of Directors and was found to still be appropriate.

Rationale

Risk Evaluation and Mitigation Strategies (REMS) are part of new authority granted to the Food and Drug Administration (FDA) to ensure that a drug's benefits outweigh its risks. An increasing number of drug products require REMS in order to be marketed, and some REMS require Medication Guides as well as other "elements to assure safe use." These elements beyond a Medication Guide have included prescriber and pharmacist training, patient registry, and additional patient monitoring. ASHP believes that more research should be conducted by either the FDA or drug manufacturers to determine the effectiveness of and need for REMS.

Health-system pharmacists have encountered problems with REMS that were developed without input from health-system pharmacy. Pharmacist input in the development of REMS is essential to avoid unnecessary barriers to patients and burdensome interruptions to pharmacy workflow that could impact patient care and safety.

Drug information and knowledge vendors providing information technology and decision support systems will need to include gateways to specific information about REMS so that pharmacists and other health professionals have access to information about all REMS-required products and the specific requirements for a particular REMS that includes elements to assure safe use.

Finally, REMS that include constraints on traditional drug distribution systems should be consistent with existing ASHP policy on restricted drug distribution.

1003

FDA AUTHORITY ON RECALLS

Source: Council on Public Policy

To strongly encourage the Food and Drug Administration (FDA) to develop a standard recall notification process and European Medicines Agency to share information from inspections conducted by that agency and encourages the FDA to establish this type of format to be used by all manufacturers to facilitate the timely removal of recalled drugs; further,

To advocate that such notification should (1) come from a single source, (2) clearly identify the recalled product, (3) explain why the product is being recalled, (4) provide a way to report having the recalled product, (5) give instructions on what to do with the recalled product, and (6) be provided concurrently to all entities in the supply chain; further,

To advocate that the FDA be given the authority to order mandatory recalls of medications; further,

To urge the FDA to require drug manufacturers and the computer software industry to provide bar codes and data fields for lot number, expiration date, and other necessary and appropriate information on all medication packaging, including unit dose, unit-of-use, and injectable drug packaging, in order to facilitate compliance with recalls or withdrawals and to prevent the administration of recalled products to patients; further,

To urge the FDA to encourage postmarketing reporting of adverse events and product quality issues to enhance the recall system.

This policy was reviewed in 2020 by the Council on Public Policy and by the Board of Directors and was found to still be appropriate.

Rationale

A recall is a manufacturer or distributor's voluntary removal or correction of a marketed product. The Food and Drug Administration (FDA) may request a recall in "urgent situations." For each recall, the manufacturer or distributor develops a recall strategy based upon guidance from the FDA; there is no standard format for recall notices, and communication timelines, format, content, and distribution vary.

Managing product recalls within hospitals and health systems is a complex process. Past recall events have highlighted the complexity of the process and demonstrate the need for improvements to ensure that recalled product can be removed effectively and efficiently to protect patients from inadvertent administration. During the 2008 recall of heparin, for example, 94 hospitals were found to have recalled product remaining on their shelves. Further evaluation of how the recall was implemented revealed flaws in the system. Some pharmacy departments reported that they never received the recall notice; in other cases, recalled product was shipped to the pharmacy after the hospital had completed its review of supplies and quarantined all recalled product.

The FDA must have the authority to clearly communicate with stakeholders about recalls of marketed products. Inconsistent, unclear, and confusing information has been communicated during past recalls. A standardized recall notification process and format would enable practitioners and others in the drug distribution chain to readily identify and respond to a recall. Such a notification process should contain the following elements: a single source to designate a point of contact and control communication, clear identification of the recalled product to assist in removing the product from stock, an explanation of why the product is being recalled in order to understand the nature of the recall and communicate with patients and other stakeholders, a feedback mechanism (a reporting loop) so manufacturers and the FDA know where recalled product is located, instructions on how to return or dispose of the recalled product, and concurrent notification of all entities in the supply chain.

ASHP advocates that the FDA be given the authority to order a mandatory recall of a product to avoid the miscommunication that has occurred in past voluntary recalls. In addition, ASHP has long encouraged the FDA to require that lot number, expiration date, and other necessary information be provided electronically (e.g., by bar code or radio frequency identification) as part of the manufacturer's information on all unit dose, unit-of-use, and injectable drug packaging.

Finally, postmarketing reporting of adverse events and product quality issues must be encouraged. Voluntary reporting will provide information for FDA to analyze to determine with the manufacturer the correct course of action.

1007

REGULATION OF HOME MEDICAL EQUIPMENT MEDICATION PRODUCTS AND DEVICES

Source: Council on Public Policy

To advocate for consistent regulatory oversight of all home medical equipment, with the goals of continuity of care, patient safety, and appropriate pharmacist involvement whenever equipment is used for medication administration; further,

To monitor the impact of the Centers for Medicare & Medicaid Services quality standards on the accreditation of suppliers of medication-related durable medical equipment and supplies.

This policy was reviewed in 2020 by the Council on Public Policy and by the Board of Directors and was found to still be appropriate.

Rationale

Federal and state regulation of home medical equipment (HME) and durable medical equipment (DME) suppliers creates a gap in pharmacist review and input in medication-related aspects of the services these suppliers provide to patients, particularly when a patient is discharged from the hospital to the home. The Centers for Medicare & Medicaid Services (CMS) provides conditions of participation for home health services, and states may regulate HME and DME suppliers, home health agencies, and suppliers of medical gases. Furthermore, CMS has proposed surety bond requirements for pharmacies that are also DME suppliers. The Council recommended and the Board and House agreed that ASHP should advocate for consistent regulatory oversight of these medication-related aspects so that this medication-use process ensures patient safety, improves continuity of care, and guarantees appropriate pharmacist involvement.

0909

REGULATION OF INTERSTATE PHARMACY PRACTICE

Source: Council on Public Policy

To advocate that state governments, including legislatures and boards of pharmacy, adopt laws and regulations that harmonize the practice of pharmacy across state lines in order to provide a consistent, transparent, safe, and accountable framework for pharmacy practice.

This policy was reviewed in 2019 by the Council on Public Policy and by the Board of Directors and was found to still be appropriate.

Rationale

With the emergence of new technology, state borders are becoming more artificial and coordination between states is increasingly needed. To achieve the highest level of patient safety possible, state regulatory bodies need to work closely together to provide a consistent and transparent regulatory framework for pharmacy practice. Dialogue between the National Association of Boards of Pharmacy and individual state boards can help harmonize the practice of pharmacy across state lines by producing model language that can be adopted by individual states.

0811

REGULATION OF DIETARY SUPPLEMENTS

Source: Council on Public Policy

To advocate that Congress grant authority to the Food and Drug Administration (FDA) to (1) require that dietary supplements undergo FDA approval for evidence of safety and efficacy; (2) mandate FDA-approved dietary supplement labeling that includes disclosure of excipients; (3) mandate FDA-approved patient information materials that describe safe use in a clear, standardized format, including the potential for interaction with medications and cautions for special populations; and (4) establish and maintain an adverse-event reporting system specifically for dietary supplements, and require dietary supplement manufacturers to report suspected adverse reactions to the FDA; further,

To oppose direct-to-consumer advertising of dietary supplements unless the following criteria are met: (1) federal laws are amended to include all the requirements described above to ensure that dietary supplements are safe and effective; (2) evidence-based information regarding safety and efficacy is provided in a format that allows for informed decision-making by the consumer; (3) the advertising includes a recommendation to consult with a health care professional before initiating use; (4) any known warnings or precautions regarding dietary supplement–medication interactions or dietary supplement–disease interactions are provided as part of the advertising; and (5) the advertising is educational in nature and includes pharmacists as a source of information.

(*Note:* Dietary supplement as used in this policy is defined by the Dietary Supplement Health and Education Act of 1994, as amended; 21 U.S.C. 321.)

This policy was reviewed in 2023 by the Council on Public Policy and by the Board of Directors and was found to still be appropriate.

Rationale

Under the Dietary Supplement Health and Education Act of 1994 (DSHEA), manufacturers are prohibited from marketing adulterated or misbranded products, and the Food and Drug Administration (FDA) has authority to take action if adulterated or misbranded dietary supplements reach the market. To ensure a safe market for dietary supplements, the FDA needs the authority to require manufacturers to conduct safety and efficacy testing for dietary supplements, provide labeling and information about the content of the product and its safe use, and report suspected adverse reactions to FDA.

In 2007, the FDA announced final regulations requiring current Good Manufacturing Practices (GMPs) for dietary supplements that include testing ingredients and the final product. While the FDA does require all manufacturers to adhere to GMPs, not all supplement manufacturers are GMP certified.

Under the current regulatory and legislative regime, direct-to-consumer advertising of dietary supplements should not occur unless specified criteria are met. Dietary supplement advertising should be strictly regulated by the FDA and the Federal Trade Commission (FTC) to ensure it is truthful and substantiated. The FDA and FTC have published guidance for industry concerning dietary supplement claims. The FDA is primarily responsible for claims on product labeling, while FTC has primary responsibility for claims in advertising, including print and broadcast ads, infomercials, catalogs, and similar direct marketing materials.

0813

MEDICARE PRESCRIPTION DRUG BENEFIT

Source: Council on Public Policy

To strongly advocate a fully funded prescription drug program for eligible Medicare beneficiaries that maintains continuity of care and ensures the best use of medications; further,

To advocate that essential requirements in the program include (1) appropriate product reimbursement; (2) affordability for patients, including elimination of coverage gaps; (3) payment for indirect costs and practice expenses related to the provision of pharmacist services, based on a study of those costs; (4) appropriate coverage and payment for patient care services provided by pharmacists; (5) open access to the pharmacy provider of the patient's choice; (6) formularies with sufficient flexibility to allow access to medically necessary drugs; and (7) well-publicized, unbiased resources to assist beneficiaries in enrolling in the most appropriate plan for their medication needs.

(*Note:* Fully funded means the federal government will make adequate funds available to fully cover the Medicare program's share of prescription drug program costs; eligible means the federal government may establish criteria by which Medicare beneficiaries qualify for the prescription drug program.)

This policy was reviewed in 2020 by the Council on Public Policy and by the Board of Directors and was found to still be appropriate.

0719

FDA AUTHORITY TO PROHIBIT REUSE OF BRAND NAMES

Source: Council on Public Policy

To advocate for Food and Drug Administration authority to prohibit reuse of brand names of prescription and nonprescription drugs when any active component of the product is changed or after any other changes are made in the product that may affect its safe use.

Rationale

To avoid patient safety risks and provider error, FDA should not reuse brand names for drugs. In particular, recent examples of the reuse of product names or minor changes to product names in the nonprescription category (e.g., Zantac 360, Dramamine Drug-Free) have resulted in patient and provider confusion.

This policy was reviewed in 2022 by the Council on Public Policy and by the Board of Directors and was found to still be appropriate.

0516

MANDATORY REGISTRY OF CLINICAL TRIALS

Source: Council on Legal and Public Affairs

To advocate disclosure of the most complete information on the safety and efficacy of drug products; further,

To advocate that the Department of Health and Human Services establish a mandatory registry for all Phase II, III, and IV clinical trials that are conducted on drugs intended for use in the United States; further,

To advocate that each clinical trial have a unique identifier; further,

To advocate that all data from registered clinical trials be posted electronically with unrestricted access, and that such posting occur (1) after Food and Drug Administration approval of the related new product but before marketing begins and (2) as soon as possible for trials completed after initial marketing.

This policy was reviewed in 2023 by the Council on Public Policy and by the Board of Directors and was found to still be appropriate.

Rationale

Incomplete disclosure of data on the safety and efficacy of drug products from clinical trials has negatively impacted patient safety and pharmacy practice. For example, in 2004 unpublished data and results regarding the efficacy and safety of antidepressants in pediatric patients prompted a national analysis of the potential effects of suppressing negative findings in clinical trials. That experience demonstrated that positive and negative data and results should be made available to healthcare providers so they can make the best decisions about medications for their patients.

In 2016, the Department of Health and Human Services issued a final rule that specifies requirements for registering certain clinical trials and submitting summary results information to ClinicalTrials.gov. The rule expands the legal requirements for submitting registration and results information for clinical trials involving U.S. Food and Drug Administration-regulated drug, biological and device products. Similarly, the National Institutes of Health has issued a complementary policy for registering and submitting summary results information to ClinicalTrials.gov for all NIH-funded trials, including those not subject to the final rule. Requirements under the final rule apply to most interventional studies of drug, biological, and device products that are regulated by the FDA.

0413

IMPORTATION OF PHARMACEUTICALS

Source: Council on Legal and Public Affairs

To advocate for the continuation and application of laws and regulations enforced by the Food and Drug Administration and state boards of pharmacy with respect to the importation of pharmaceuticals in order to (1) maintain the integrity of the pharmaceutical supply chain and avoid the introduction of counterfeit products into the United States; (2) provide for continued patient access to pharmacist review of all medications and preserve the patient-pharmacist-prescriber relationship; and (3) provide adequate patient counseling and education, particularly to patients taking multiple high-risk medications; further,

To urge the FDA and state boards of pharmacy to vigorously enforce federal and state laws in relation to importation of pharmaceuticals by individuals, distributors (including wholesalers), and pharmacies that bypass a safe and secure regulatory framework.

This policy was reviewed in 2015 by the Council on Public Policy and by the Board of Directors and was found to still be appropriate.

0012

FDA'S PUBLIC HEALTH MISSION

Source: Council on Legal and Public Affairs

To support the Food and Drug Administration's public health mission of ensuring the safety and effectiveness of drugs, biologics, and medical devices through risk assessment, appropriate product approval, labeling approval, manufacturing oversight, and consultation with health professionals, while deferring to state regulation and professional self-regulation on matters related to the use of drugs, biologics, and medical devices; further,

To support the allocation of sufficient federal resources to allow FDA to meet its defined public health mission; further,

To support the appointment of practicing pharmacists to FDA advisory committees as one mechanism of ensuring that decisions made by the agency incorporate the unique knowledge of the profession of pharmacy for the further benefit of the patient; further,

To support an ongoing dialogue between FDA and ASHP for the purpose of exploring ways to advocate the best use of FDA-regulated products by consumers and health care professionals.

This policy was reviewed in 2020 by the Council on Public Policy and by the Board of Directors and was found to still be appropriate.

ASHP Statement on Advocacy as a Professional Obligation

Position

ASHP believes that all pharmacists have a professional obligation to advocate on behalf of patients and the profession. Pharmacists should stay informed of issues that affect medication-related outcomes and advocate on behalf of patients, the profession, and the public. These issues may include legal, regulatory, financial, and other health policy issues, and this obligation extends beyond the individual practice site to their broader communities. ASHP recognizes that to fulfill this obligation, training and education is needed. ASHP urges all pharmacists to accept this responsibility and to be advocates both within and outside the profession, in the community, and in society as a whole to strengthen the care of our patients.

Role of Professional Organizations in Promoting Advocacy

Advocacy can be defined as an activity by an individual or group to plead a case, support a cause, or to recommend a course of action related to patient-care, political, economic, social, or institutional issues. When attempting to define the advocacy responsibilities for pharmacy, it is instructive to examine the guidance from other healthcare professional organizations regarding advocacy.

One role professional organizations play is to help define the moral and ethical responsibilities of the profession. The American Medical Association (AMA) and the American Nurses Association (ANA) articulate how the members of those professions should be involved in advocacy efforts.

The AMA Code of Medical Ethics states that "physicians, individually and collectively through their professional organizations and institutions, should participate in the political process as advocates for patients (or support those who do) so as to diminish financial obstacles to access health care" and that "the medical profession must work to ensure that societal decisions about the distribution of health resources safeguard the interests of all patients and promote access to health services."[1]

These statements emphasize several responsibilities for the physician outside care for individual patients. Physicians are explicitly urged to participate in the political process as advocates and to make sure societal decisions are in the interest of all patients. Simply providing excellent patient care to patients within the physician's practice is not enough to meet the physician's ethical obligations.

The ANA Code of Ethics with Interpretive Statements Provision 8 states that "[t]he nurse collaborates with other health professionals and the public to protect human rights, promote health diplomacy, and reduce health disparities," which is further elaborated in Interpretive Statement 8.2 to mean that "[n]urses must lead collaborative partnerships to develop effective public health legislation, policies, projects and programs that promote and restore health, prevent illness, and alleviate suffering."[2] Provision 9 emphasizes the important role of nursing professional organizations in advocacy: "The profession of nursing, collectively through its professional organizations, must . . . integrate principles of social justice into nursing and health policy."[2] One prominent nurse advocate has described advocacy as "the cornerstone of nursing—nurses advocate for patients, causes, and the profession. Our advocacy, motivated by moral and ethical principles, seeks to influence policies by pleading or arguing within political, economic, and social systems, and also institutions, for an idea or cause that can lead to decisions in resource allocation that promote nurses, nursing, and all of healthcare."[3]

Advocacy as a Professional Obligation

Current ASHP policies encourage pharmacists to serve as advocates for their patients and the profession. For example, ASHP Policy 1114, Pharmacist Accountability for Patient Outcomes, states in part that ASHP and pharmacists should "promote pharmacist accountability as a fundamental component of pharmacy practice to other healthcare professionals, standards-setting and regulatory organizations, and patients."[4] The ASHP Statement on Leadership as a Professional Obligation notes that "the practice of effectively influencing the behavior of physicians, nurses, pharmacy technicians, interns, support staff, and others to optimize medication safety and patient outcomes constitutes successful leadership."[5] ASHP Policy Position 1501, Pharmacist Participation in Health Policy Development, clearly articulates the role pharmacists should play in developing health policy: "To advocate that pharmacists participate with policymakers and stakeholders in the development of health-related policies at the national, state, and community levels. . . ."[4] The ASHP Statement on the Role of Health-System Pharmacists in Public Health states that "health-system pharmacists should be involved in public health policy decision-making and in the planning, development, and implementation of public health efforts. Health-system pharmacists can improve public health by . . . advocating for sound legislation, regulations, and public policy regarding disease prevention and management; and engaging in public health research."[6]

ASHP not only encourages pharmacists to participate in advocacy efforts but believes that pharmacists have a professional and moral obligation to do so. That obligation stems from the covenantal relationship between the pharmacist and their communities described in the profession's shared Code of Ethics of the Pharmacist and the *Oath of a Pharmacist*. The Code of Ethics of a Pharmacist states that "[a] pharmacist serves individual, community, and societal needs" and "seeks justice in the distribution of health resources."[7] While the Code makes clear that the primary obligation of a pharmacist is to individual patients, the pharmacist's responsibility extends at times beyond the individual to the community and society. The specific instance provided in the language of the Code is the distribution of health resources, in which pharmacists are called upon to seek a just distribution. The *Oath of a Pharmacist*,

DOI 10.37573/9781585287048.044

which graduating student pharmacists across the country swear to, reads in part:

- I will consider the welfare of humanity and relief of suffering my primary concerns.
- I will embrace and advocate changes that improve patient care.[8]

The pharmacist's advocacy responsibilities are also evident in ASHP Vision and Mission statements. The ASHP Vision is "that medication use will be optimal, safe, and effective for all people all of the time," and the ASHP Mission states in part that "ASHP serves its members as their collective voice on issues related to medication use and public health."[9] The broad purview of these statements is reinforced by the ASHP Statement on Professionalism, which implores pharmacists to "commit themselves to improving healthcare institutions not simply for the well-being of individual patients but for the benefit of society as a whole" and "to join forces with other healthcare providers and patients . . . to attain the kind of healthcare system our patients deserve and our society demands."[10]

These professionwide and ASHP policies, like those of our professional counterparts in medicine and nursing, are a clear statement of the professional obligation members of the profession have to involve themselves in the policy-making process to advocate for the needs of patients, the profession, and the public, both within and outside healthcare settings.

Preparing Pharmacist Advocates

Pharmacy education at several different levels includes recommendations that learners develop advocacy skills. The Accreditation Council for Pharmacy Education (ACPE) Accreditation Standards and Key Elements for the Professional Program in Pharmacy Leading to the Doctor of Pharmacy Degree (Standards 2016) include the following learning expectations for professional communications and public health, respectively:

- Analysis and practice of verbal, non-verbal, and written communication strategies that promote effective interpersonal dialog and understanding to advance specific patient care, education, advocacy, and/or interprofessional collaboration goals.
- Exploration of population health management strategies, national and community-based public health programs, and implementation of activities that advance public health and wellness.[11]

These expectations demonstrate that pharmacy students will be taught strategies to be successful advocates for a range of topics, including population health management strategies.

This approach to teaching pharmacy students about population health strategies and other means of advancing public health suggests that pharmacists, as well as students, should begin to think not only about their obligations to individual patients but also to how they might use their training to impact the health of communities or society as a whole. There is a push for more of this type of training for pharmacy students. In 2016, the American Association of Colleges of Pharmacy (AACP) published Public Health and the CAPE 2013 Educational Outcomes: Inclusion, Pedagogical Considerations and Assessment. This paper provides guidance to the pharmacy profession on using the Center for the Advancement of Pharmacy Education (CAPE) 2013 outcomes to incorporate public health within college of pharmacy curricula and in co-curricular programs/activities and delineates public health-related course objectives for both didactic and experiential courses. Two of the recommended competency areas for integration of public health into didactic Pharm.D. curricula are:

- Process of health policy-making (e.g., local, state, federal government).
- Methods for participation in the policy process (e.g., advocacy, advisory processes, opportunities, and strategies to impact policy and public health problems).[12]

Pharmacy residency training also incorporates advocacy. The Required Competency Areas, Goals, and Objectives for Postgraduate Year One (PGY1) Pharmacy Residencies states that one of the criteria for demonstrating "personal, interpersonal, and teamwork skills critical for effective leadership" is that a resident "effectively expresses benefits of personal profession-wide leadership and advocacy."[13]

Conclusion

ASHP believes pharmacists have a moral and ethical professional obligation to advocate for "changes that improve patient care"[8] as well as "justice in the distribution of health resources."[7] Specific ASHP policies on various aspects of healthcare, population health, and public health stem from this general obligation. To meet this professional obligation, pharmacist advocates will need appropriate training and education.

References

1. American Medical Association. AMA Code of Medical Ethics opinion 11.1.4 ((b) and (c)). https://www.ama-assn.org/delivering-care/financial-barriers-health-care-access (accessed 2019 Jan 4).
2. American Nurses Association. ANA Code of Ethics with Interpretive Statements. http://nursingworld.org/DocumentVault/Ethics-1/Code-of-Ethics-for-Nurses.html (accessed 2019 Jan 4).
3. Matthews J. Role of professional organizations in advocating for the nursing profession. *OJIN* 17; 2012: Manuscript 3. http://ojin.nursingworld.org/MainMenuCategories/ANAMarketplace/ANAPeriodicals/OJIN/TableofContents/Vol-17-2012/No1-Jan-2012/Professional-Organizations-and-Advocating.html (accessed 2019 Jan 4).
4. American Society of Health-System Pharmacists. ASHP policy position 1501, pharmacist participation in health policy development; 2005. In: ASHP policy positions 1982–2017. https://www.ashp.org/-/media/assets/policy-guidelines/docs/browse-by-document-type-policy-positions-1982-2018-with-rationales-pdf.ashx? (accessed 2019 Jan 4).
5. American Society of Health-System Pharmacists. ASHP statement on leadership as a professional obligation (2011). https://www.ashp.org/-/media/assets/policy-guidelines/docs/statements/leadership-as-professional-obligation.ashx (accessed 2019 Jan 4).
6. American Society of Health-System Pharmacists [ASHP]. ASHP statement on the role of health-system Ppharmacists in public health (2011). https://www.ashp.org/-/media/assets/policy-guidelines/docs/statements/role-of-health-system-pharmacists-in-public-health.ashx (accessed 2019 Jan 4).

7. American Pharmacists Association. Code of Ethics for Pharmacists (1994, reviewed 2017). https://www.ashp.org/-/media/assets/policy-guidelines/docs/endorsed-documents/code-of-ethics-for-pharmacists.ashx (accessed 2019 Jan 4).
8. American Pharmacists Association. Oath of a pharmacist (revised 2007). http://www.pharmacist.com/oath-pharmacist (accessed 2019 Jan 4).
9. American Society of Health-System Pharmacists. About ASHP. https://www.ashp.org/About-ASHP/What-We-Do (accessed 2019 Jan 4).
10. American Society of Health-System Pharmacists. ASHP statement on professionalism (2008). https://www.ashp.org/-/media/assets/policy-guidelines/docs/statements/professionalism.ashx (accessed 2019 Jan 4).
11. Accreditation Council for Pharmacy Education. Accreditation standards and key elements for the professional program in pharmacy leading to the doctor of pharmacy degree (Standards 2016) https://www.acpe-accredit.org/pdf/Standards2016FINAL.pdf (accessed 2019 Jan 4).
12. Covvey JR, Conry JM, Bullock KC et al. Public Health and the CAPE 2013. Educational outcomes: inclusion, pedagogical considerations and assessment. https://www.aacp.org/sites/default/files/2017-10/PublicHealthSIGCAPEpaper.pdf (accessed 2019 Jan 4).
13. American Society of Health-System Pharmacists. Required competency areas, goals, and objectives for postgraduate year one (PGY1) pharmacy residencies (2015). https://www.ashp.org/-/media/assets/professional-development/residencies/docs/required-competency-areas-goals-objectives (accessed 2019 Jan 4).

Approved by the ASHP Board of Directors on January 19, 2018, and by the ASHP House of Delegates on June 3, 2018. Developed through the ASHP Council on Public Policy.

Jeff Little, Pharm.D., M.P.H., BCPS, FACHE, Saint Luke's Hospital Director of Pharmacy, Kansas City, MO.

Melissa Ortega, Pharm.D., M.S., Tufts Medical Center, Boston, MA.

Michael Powell, M.S.Pharm., FASHP, Optics Performance, LLC, Minden, IA.

Mark Hamm, Pharm.D., M.B.A, BCPS, Director Oncology Services, Advocate Aurora Health, Milwaukee, WI.

The authors have declared no potential conflicts of interest.

Copyright © 2019, American Society of Health-System Pharmacists, Inc. All rights reserved. Contact ASHP for reprint and permissions requests. This content may not be used for commercial purposes without the express written consent of ASHP.

The bibliographic citation for this document is as follows: American Society of Health-System Pharmacists. ASHP statement on advocacy as a professional obligation. *Am J Health-Syst Pharm.* 2019; 76:251–4.

Medication Safety

DOI 10.37573/9781585287048

Medication Safety

2318

RAISING AWARENESS OF THE RISKS ASSOCIATED WITH THE MISUSE OF MEDICATIONS

Source: Council on Pharmacy Practice

To support the pharmacy workforce in outreach efforts to provide education to authorities, patients, and the community on the risks associated with use of medications for nonmedical purposes or from nonmedical sources.

Rationale

Misuse of medications involves the use of prescription and over-the-counter medications in ways that are not prescribed or directed. The use of medications for nonmedical purposes is also a category of misuse. Misuse may lead to serious consequences, such as emergency department visits, hospitalization, and death. While most of the evidence regarding medication misuse is related to opioids, central nervous system depressants, and stimulants, misuse of any medication may result in patient harm. As such, efforts to raise awareness of the risks of misusing any medication needs to be prioritized, in addition to specific medications and medication classes. Pharmacists, as medication experts, can identify red flags and patterns of medication misuse and support community outreach efforts to help patients understand the risks associated with the misuse of medications.

2241

HUMAN USE OF VETERINARY PHARMACEUTICALS

Source: Council on Therapeutics

To oppose human use of pharmaceuticals approved only for veterinary use; further,

To support use of veterinary pharmaceuticals only under the supervision of a licensed veterinarian in compliance with the Animal Medicinal Drug Use Clarification Act of 1994; further,

To encourage state and federal regulatory bodies as well as other stakeholders to monitor the misuse of veterinary pharmaceuticals and, when appropriate, limit the public availability of those pharmaceuticals; further,

To educate healthcare professionals and the public about the adverse effects of human consumption of veterinary pharmaceuticals; further,

To encourage research, monitoring, and reporting on the adverse effects of human consumption of veterinary pharmaceuticals to define the public health impact of and to quantify the strain these agents place on the healthcare system.

Rationale

Medications that are formulated for veterinary use are often supplied at higher concentrations, contain compounds not safe for human use, and require specialized knowledge to administer. The prevalence of drug misuse in the veterinary setting is not well documented, but surveys of veterinarians by the Idaho Board of Veterinary Medicine, Colorado Veterinarians, and Veterinary Hospitals in Pennsylvania found that they suspect 23% of animal owners misuse veterinary medicines on themselves, their children, or friends, and that the most-documented misused drugs are opioids, benzodiazepines, and ketamine. These findings are concerning because animals often require a more potent dose of controlled substances, which can be appealing for individuals with substance use disorders, and medications are often dispensed directly to the animal owner, bypassing pharmacists, who are critical players in prescription drug misuse risk mitigation.

In the United States, licensed veterinarians can prescribe, administer, carry, stock, and dispense medications, including veterinary-only drugs, drug compounds, and FDA-approved over-the-counter veterinary drugs. These drugs are typically veterinary formulations that are not tested for human safety or approved for human use, and the Animal Medicinal Drug Use Clarification Act of 1994 (AMDUCA) permits veterinarians to prescribe those drugs in an "extralabel" manner. Under AMDUCA regulations, "extralabel use" means the actual or intended use of a drug, by or on the order of a veterinarian, in a manner that is not in accordance with approved labeling (similar to off-label use in human medicine). Any deviation from labeled use, by veterinarians or lay persons, is an illegal use unless it meets all the requirements of FDA's extralabel drug-use rules. Deviations from the label include use in a species or production class not on the label and use of a different route of administration.

More recently, the COVID-19 pandemic has exacerbated human consumption of veterinary compounds, as some medications being studied for efficacy against the virus produce promising or equivocal preliminary results that are seized upon by the public and some prescribers, leading to inappropriate prescribing. For example, ASHP, APhA, and AMA have called for an immediate end to the prescribing, dispensing, and use of ivermectin for treatment of COVID-19 outside of a clinical trial. Due to the response of the medical community, many physicians and pharmacies are not writing or filling prescriptions for this medication, driving patients to purchase the animal formulation of ivermectin for human consumption. Earlier in the pandemic, a patient in Arizona consumed chloroquine phosphate meant for fish as a treatment for COVID-19 and died. The FDA, aware of the misuse of chloroquine products, issued a cautionary letter to stakeholders and worked with online marketplaces to remove the products from the market.

Finally, some veterinary compounds produce mild to life-threatening human adverse effects upon accidental or intentional exposure or ingestion. Patients exposed to or ingesting these products present to the emergency department with symptoms that range from bronchospasm, central nervous system stimulation, and miscarriage to sudden death, which demonstrates the need for timely reporting of abuses, misuses, or accidental exposures of these agents.

2132

STANDARDIZING AND MINIMIZING THE USE OF ABBREVIATIONS

Source: Council on Pharmacy Management

To support efforts to standardize and minimize the use of abbreviations in healthcare; further,

DOI 10.37573/9781585287048.045

To oppose use of abbreviations when communicating with patients to enhance transparency and understanding; further,

To encourage education of healthcare professionals and learners on standardizing and minimizing the use of abbreviations across all patient care settings.

This policy supersedes ASHP policy 0604.

Rationale

Although there are anecdotal examples of medical abbreviations causing harm to patients, there is little good clinical evidence to demonstrate that medical abbreviation use is dangerous or is causing problems in the delivery of care. Nevertheless, minimizing or even eliminating the use of medical abbreviations in healthcare has been encouraged for decades. The Institute of Safe Medication Practices regularly receives reports of errors, some of which have resulted in adverse events, due to misinterpretation of medical abbreviations. The Joint Commission has regularly issued updates and guidance on the safe use of medical abbreviations and has also published a short list of dangerous medical abbreviations and dose expressions that should never be used. However, despite many key organizations discouraging the use of medical abbreviations, they continue to be used at an alarming rate. Such use can place new practitioners at great risk when they have to interpret the abbreviations, as the new practitioner may have limited knowledge about what the abbreviations mean. Use of abbreviations should be minimized, and when abbreviation use cannot be avoided, they should be standardized to ensure accurate interpretation. In addition, use of abbreviations when communicating with patients should be avoided to enhance transparency and patients' understanding of their treatment.

2044

DRUG NAMES, LABELING, AND PACKAGING ASSOCIATED WITH MEDICATION ERRORS

Source: Council on Pharmacy Practice

To urge drug manufacturers, drug packagers and repackagers, outsourcing pharmacies, and the Food and Drug Administration to involve patients, practicing pharmacists, nurses, and physicians in decisions about drug names, labeling, and packaging to help eliminate (a) look-alike and sound-alike drug names, and (b) labeling and packaging characteristics that contribute to medication errors; further,

To inform pharmacists and others, as appropriate, about specific drug names, labeling, and packaging that have documented association with medication errors.

This policy supersedes ASHP policy 0020.

Rationale

Confusion caused by drug product names, labeling, and packaging has been associated with medication errors. Despite laws, regulations, and standards that seek to address these areas, safety concerns still exist. For example, the Institute for Safe Medication Practices lists errors and hazards due to look-alike labeling of manufacturer's products third and unsafe labeling of prefilled syringes and infusions by 503B compounders eighth among the top ten medication errors and hazards. ASHP advocates involving representatives of those who use the products—patients, practicing pharmacists, nurses, and physicians—in the decision-making process regarding drug names, labeling, and packaging to provide advice on how to avoid confusion and prevent medication errors. In furtherance of our mission to support pharmacists in helping people achieve optimal health outcomes, ASHP will continue to inform pharmacists, other healthcare providers, government agencies, and the public about specific drug names, labeling, and packaging associated with medication errors.

1505

STATUTORY PROTECTION FOR MEDICATION-ERROR REPORTING

Source: Council on Public Policy

To collaborate with other healthcare providers, professions, and stakeholders to advocate and support state and federal legislative and regulatory initiatives that provide liability protection for the reporting of actual and potential medication errors by individuals and healthcare providers; further,

To provide education on the role that patient safety organizations play in liability protection.

This policy was reviewed in 2020 by the Council on Public Policy and by the Board of Directors and was found to still be appropriate.

Rationale

Medication-error reporting at the state and federal level has been shown to improve medication-use systems and aid in conducting a root cause analysis of a medication error. Liability protection for such reporting at the federal level is necessary to achieve this analysis and improve patient safety. Pharmacists need to be aware of legal protection for error reporting under the federal Patient Safety and Quality Improvement Act of 2005. The Act set up a network of federally sanctioned Patient Safety Organizations (PSOs) that provide protection for healthcare providers, including pharmacy personnel. A PSO is prohibited from identifying individuals or organizations that report and the information used for educational purposes must be de-identified, including contextually as necessary. The Act overrides state protections and supports the collaboration sought among providers who report and work with a PSO.

1524

SUPPORT FOR SECOND VICTIMS

Source: Council on Pharmacy Practice

To acknowledge that the patient is the primary victim in any medical error, unanticipated adverse patient event, or patient-related injury; further,

To acknowledge that involvement by healthcare personnel in such events may cause them to become second victims; further,

To recognize that a just culture and a healthy culture of safety embrace a support system for second victims; further,

To encourage healthcare organizations to establish programs to support second victims; further,

To educate healthcare professionals (including those in training), health organization administrators, and regulatory agencies about the second-victim effect and available resources.

This policy was reviewed in 2020 by the Council on Pharmacy Practice and by the Board of Directors and was found to still be appropriate.

Rationale

The University of Missouri Health System has defined second victims as "healthcare providers who are involved in an unanticipated adverse patient event, in a medical error and/or a patient-related injury and become victimized in the sense that the provider is traumatized by the event." Frequently, these individuals feel personally responsible for the patient outcome. Many feel as though they have failed the patient, second guessing their clinical skills and knowledge base. Individuals involved in a serious adverse patient event may experience the symptoms of post-traumatic stress disorder and may require support to successfully manage the experience.

Healthcare organizations have emphasized establishing a just culture environment to encourage individuals to speak up when they are aware of medication errors. Studies have indicated that many second victims did not feel they received organizational support after these events, however. The Joint Commission, the Institute for Healthcare Improvement, the Institute for Safe Medication Practices (ISMP), and others have advocated for support systems for second victims. The Joint Commission Leadership Standards state that leaders will "make support systems available for staff that have been involved in an adverse or sentinel event."

Healthcare organizations will have to tailor these support system to their needs. Such support systems may, for example, be tiered, with the first tier being unit or department support; the second tier, trained peer support, including patient-safety and risk-management staff; and the third tier, professional counseling support, such as employee assistance programs or social workers. Education of staff on resources available to support the second victim is critical to avoiding adverse impact on the second victim.

1530

STANDARDIZATION OF SMALL-BORE CONNECTORS TO AVOID WRONG-ROUTE ERRORS

Source: Council on Pharmacy Practice

To support the use of medication administration device connectors and fittings that are designed to prevent misconnections and wrong-route errors; further,

To encourage healthcare organizations to prepare for safe transition to use of medication delivery device connectors and adapters that meet International Organization for Standardization standards; further,

To identify and promote the implementation of best practices for preventing wrong-route errors.

This policy was reviewed in 2020 by the Council on Pharmacy Practice and by the Board of Directors and was found to still be appropriate.

Rationale

Interconnectivity among drug delivery devices and their fittings is a significant and preventable cause of serious or fatal wrong-route errors. Connector and tubing design unique to the route of administration that cannot be linked to a device used for a different route is the strongest type of control for these errors.

An international joint working group composed of the International Organization for Standardization (ISO), Association for the Advancement of Medical Instrumentation (AAMI), FDA, manufacturers, clinicians, and other regulators recently initiated development of new ISO connector standards for medical devices for intravascular/hypodermic, limb cuff, enteral, neuraxial, and breathing systems/pressurized medical gas applications. Urethral standards are also planned, but not yet initiated. The new ISO standards are voluntary and intended to facilitate global standardization of medical devices. The FDA has announced that it will only approve or clear an enteral device with a new small-bore connector if it meets the ISO standard or equivalent alternative method. (Small-bore [less than 8.5 mm diameter] connectors are used to link or join devices, accessories, and components for intravascular/hypodermic, neuraxial [epidural, intrathecal, spinal], urinary, enteral, and breathing system/medical gas delivery of medications.) Subsequently, the first ISO standard for enteral device connectors (ANSI/AAMI/ISO 80369-1) has been adopted industrywide. New connectors will be phased in, beginning fourth quarter 2014. The Joint Commission recently published Sentinel Event Alert #53, *Managing risk and transition during transition to new ISO tubing connector standards.* The alert provides suggested actions from the 2014 Get Connected campaign provided by the Global Enteral Device Supplier Association (GEDSA), as well as updates to the recommendations from the 2006 Sentinel Event Alert #36 on tubing misconnections.

In addition, the following statements were issued from the 2008 Global Conference on the Future of Hospital Pharmacy in Basel, Switzerland:

> Pharmacists should ensure that strategies and policies are implemented to prevent wrong route errors, including, for example, labeling of intravenous tubing near insertion site to prevent misconnections, and use of enteral feeding catheters that cannot be connected with intravenous or other parenteral lines.

Oral syringes that are distinctly different from hypodermic syringes should be used to prevent injection of enteral or oral medicines, especially in pediatric patients.

1115

JUST CULTURE

Source: Council on Pharmacy Practice

To recognize that the principles of just culture promote an environment in health care organizations in which safety is valued, reporting of safety risks is encouraged, and a fair process is used to hold staff and leaders accountable; further,

To encourage hospitals and health systems to include just culture as a component in organizational safety culture surveys and quality improvement initiatives.

This policy was reviewed in 2020 by the Council on Pharmacy Practice and by the Board of Directors and was found to still be appropriate.

Rationale

The Council, Board, and House agreed that a specific ASHP policy supporting just culture principles should be developed, and that education on the topic should be an important focus for ASHP. In developing the policy, the Council reviewed principles and methods established by David Marx, a systems safety engineer and just culture educator, and noted the following (Marx, D. *Whack-a-Mole: The Price We Pay for Expecting Perfection.* Plano, TX: By Your Side Studios; 2009):

- The notion that humans can perform perfectly if they are well trained and continuously vigilant is unrealistic. Humans will never be perfect.
- Safe environments anticipate human error and systems are designed accordingly. However, systems will never be perfect.

- Individuals are accountable for behavioral choices that lead to error and leaders are accountable for establishing environments that encourage reporting of unsafe conditions and adverse events.
- Behaviors that cause or may cause errors are addressed regardless of whether harm occurs.
- Individual culpability for adverse events is assessed using a decision algorithm that defines attributes of behaviors and systems and can be summarized as follows:
    1. **Human error:** inadvertent; a mistake; doing other than what should have been done.

       Origin: System design, processes, procedures, training.

       Manage by: correcting system, supporting employee.
    2. **At-risk behavior:** behavioral choice that increases risk where risk is not recognized or is mistakenly believed to be justified.

       Origin: System inefficiencies, such as steps that create rework, are burdensome, or seem irrelevant to outcome. The system incentivizes workarounds and shortcuts that are unsafe.

       Manage by: Improving procedures or processes to remove incentives and reward safe behaviors.
    3. **Reckless behavior:** choosing to behave in a manner that places others at substantial and unjustifiable risk knowing that harmful outcome is likely but indifferent to it.

       Origin: the individual.

       Manage by: remedial action, punitive action.
    4. **Negligence:** determined by using the substitution test, i.e., would another individual in the same work area with comparable experience and qualifications have behaved any differently?

The Council identified significant advantages to this approach, one of the most important being that it encourages reporting of adverse events and provides essential information for improving systems and processes of care. In addition, holding individuals accountable by using criteria to distinguish between behaviors that do or do not merit punishment was perceived to be the fairer approach than a strictly punitive or strictly blame-free approach. Another positive attribute of just culture is that behaviors associated with error are handled with the appropriate responses regardless of whether harm resulted. By focusing on behaviors rather than outcomes, potential errors are averted, safe behaviors are encouraged, and at-risk or reckless behavior is not tolerated.

The Council recognized that while the just culture approach has been accepted by safety leaders, implementation is challenging for a number of reasons. The goals of just culture—to sustain a nonpunitive reporting and learning environment, yet hold individuals accountable for their behavior—seem contradictory. Methods for differentiating behaviors for which to hold an individual accountable tend to use subjective, rather than objective, criteria, and may lead to misinterpretation. Maintaining the just culture approach is particularly challenging under the pressure of media coverage and legal liability when a patient is harmed or dies from an error. The belief that individual practitioners are solely responsible for their errors continues to predominate in the health care professions.

The Council noted that decision-making tools and education are available to support implementation of a just culture. They suggested that ASHP consider providing education and practical tools for implementing fair processes for holding individuals and leadership accountable for medication safety. Council members also characterized just culture as a component of the larger issue of culture of safety and proposed that assessment of just culture as part of assessing general safety culture should be included in ASHP's national survey.

1021

JUST CULTURE AND REPORTING MEDICATION ERRORS

Source: Council on Pharmacy Practice

To encourage pharmacists to exert leadership in establishing a just culture in their workplaces and a nonpunitive systems approach to addressing medication errors while supporting a nonthreatening reporting environment to encourage pharmacy staff and others to report actual and potential medication errors in a timely manner; further,

To provide leadership in supporting a single, comprehensive, hospital- or health-system-specific medication error reporting program that (1) fosters a confidential, nonthreatening, and nonpunitive environment for the submission of medication error reports; (2) receives and analyzes these confidential reports to identify system-based causes of medication errors or potential errors; and (3) recommends and disseminates error prevention strategies; further,

To provide leadership in encouraging the participation of all stakeholders in the reporting of medication errors to this program.

(*Note:* A just culture is one that has a clear and transparent process for evaluating errors and separating events arising from flawed system design or inadvertent human error from those caused by reckless behavior, defined as a behavioral choice to consciously disregard what is known to be a substantial or unjustifiable risk.)

This policy was reviewed in 2020 by the Council on Pharmacy Practice and by the Board of Directors and was found to still be appropriate.

Rationale

"Just culture" is an approach to medical error management that recognizes individual accountability for behavioral choices that compromise safety. The concept of "just culture" was first introduced by Sidney Dekker, a pilot and systems engineer, who recommended a different approach to the view that management of medical error should take a strict systems approach with a "no blame" attitude regarding individual accountability. David Marx, a lawyer and engineer, added additional background and recommendations, including criteria for determining whether error is "human" (i.e., inadvertent and unintended) or the result of behavioral choices that introduce risk.

"Just culture" differs from the "no blame" approach in two ways: (1) intentional actions that introduce risk or lead to error are acknowledged, and (2) an algorithm or criteria are used to determine the type of corrective action that should be taken (e.g., coaching or disciplinary action). "Just culture" has come to be accepted over the "no blame" approach because it allows the safety and health care community to address what Dekker and Marx characterize as at-risk and reckless behavior as causes of error.

ASHP Statement on Reporting Medical Errors

Position

The incidence of death and serious harm caused by mistakes and accidents in health care is unacceptable.[1] This serious public health problem merits top-priority national attention. Addressing this issue will require major reforms and sizable investment of resources throughout the health care system, including the medication use process, which is a particular focus of the American Society of Health-System Pharmacists (ASHP).

ASHP believes that the following steps should be taken as part of a comprehensive national solution to the problem: (1) The establishment of a standardized, uniform nationwide system (with the characteristics noted below) of mandatory reporting of adverse medical events that cause death or serious harm, (2) continued development and strengthening of systems for voluntary reporting of medical errors, and (3) strengthening efforts to implement process changes that reduce the risk of future errors and improve patient care.

The fundamental purpose of reporting systems for medical errors is to learn how to improve the health care delivery process to prevent these errors. Reporting of medical errors must become culturally accepted throughout health care. A major investment of resources will be required in the health care system to apply the lessons derived from the reporting of medical errors. Marshaling those resources is an urgent issue for the governing boards of health care institutions, health care administrators, health professionals, purchasers of health care (including federal and state governments), third party payers, public policy makers, credentialing organizations, the legal profession, and consumers.

Requirements

The primary goal of *mandatory reporting* of adverse medical events that cause death or serious harm should be to foster accountability for health care delivery process changes to prevent errors or adverse medical events. If a patient dies or is seriously harmed because of a mistake or accident in the health care system, the practitioner or institution responsible for the patient's care should report the incident to a designated state health body. Further, states should be obligated to share information based on these reports promptly with a national coordinating body and with national programs that are designed to improve the quality and enhance the safety of patient care.

ASHP's support of a mandatory reporting system is contingent upon the system having the following characteristics:

1. An overall focus on improving the processes used in health care, with the proper application of technical expertise to analyze and learn from reports.
2. Legal protection of confidentiality of patients, health care workers, and the information submitted to the extent feasible while preserving the interest of public accountability.
3. Nonpunitive in the sense that the submission of a report, per se, does not engender a penalty on the reporting institution or practitioner or others involved in the incident.
4. A definition of "serious harm" that concentrates on long-term or irreversible patient harm, so as not to overburden the reporting system.
5. National coordination and strong federal efforts to ensure compliance with standardized methods of reporting, analysis, and follow up, that emphasize process improvement and avoid a culture of blame.
6. Adequate resources devoted to report analysis, timely dissemination of advisories based on report analysis, and development of appropriate quality improvement efforts.
7. Periodic assessment of the system to ensure that it is meeting its intent and not having serious undesired consequences.

Experience associated with current mandatory state reporting of adverse medical events and mandatory public health reporting of certain infectious diseases should be assessed, and the best practices of such programs should be applied to the new system of mandatory reporting of adverse medical events that cause death or serious harm.

The primary goals of *voluntary reporting* of medical errors should be quality improvement and enhancement of patient safety. Reports by frontline practitioners of errors and "near misses" are a strength of such programs when report analysis and communication lead to prevention of similar occurrences. The public interest will be served if protection is granted to individuals who submit reports to voluntary reporting programs. The Medication Errors Reporting Program operated by the United States Pharmacopeia in cooperation with the Institute for Safe Medication Practices is an important initiative that merits strengthening; this program may be a model for voluntary reporting of other types of medical error.

Reference

1. Institute of Medicine Division of Health Care Services Committee on Quality of Health Care in America. To err is human: building a safer health system. Washington, DC: National Academy Press; 1999.

This statement was reviewed in 2005 by the Council on Professional Affairs and by the Board of Directors and was found to still be appropriate.

Approved by the ASHP House of Delegates, June 5, 2000.

Copyright © 2000, American Society of Health-System Pharmacists, Inc. All rights reserved. Contact ASHP for reprint and permissions requests. This content may not be used for commercial purposes without the express written consent of ASHP.

The bibliographic citation for this document is as follows: American Society of Health-System Pharmacists. ASHP statement on reporting medical errors. *Am J Health-Syst Pharm.* 2000; 57:1531–2.

DOI 10.37573/9781585287048.046

ASHP Statement on the Role of the Medication Safety Leader

Position

The American Society of Health-System Pharmacists (ASHP) believes that medication safety is a fundamental responsibility of all members of the profession of pharmacy. For a medication safety program to succeed, however, it is essential that there be an innovative leader to set a vision and direction, identify opportunities to improve the medication-use system, and lead implementation of error-prevention strategies. The medication safety leader's role includes responsibility for leadership, medication safety expertise, influencing practice change, research, and education. ASHP believes that because of their training, knowledge of the medication-use process, skills, and abilities, pharmacists are uniquely qualified to fill the roles and meet the responsibilities of the medication safety leader in hospitals and health systems.

Background

Hospital and health-system pharmacists have improved pharmacy systems over the past 60 years to reduce the risk that medications could harm patients. Medication safety was at the heart of such historic innovations in pharmacy services as unit-dose systems, decentralized clinical pharmacy services, and intravenous admixture services. The crucial leadership role of pharmacists in medication safety has been summarized as follows:

> Pharmacy leadership is the core of a successful medication safety program. Pharmacy leaders can play an enormously important role in performance improvement. They can be part of the senior leadership team's DNA because their impact and view go far beyond the walls of the pharmacy. . . . Pharmacists can play an important role as leaders to reduce patient safety risks, optimize the safe function of medication management systems, and align pharmacy services with national initiatives that measure and reward quality performance.[1]

The landmark Institute of Medicine (IOM) report *To Err Is Human: Building a Safer Health System*[2] generated major patient safety initiatives by government agencies, regulatory and accrediting bodies, professional and organizational associations, and health care organizations. The Joint Commission National Patient Safety Goals (NPSGs)[3] are an example of a response to the original IOM report. The Practice Advancement Initiative (PAI)[4] and the National Quality Forum (NQF) Safe Practice 18: Pharmacist Leadership Structures and Systems[5] incorporate medication safety principles to ensure optimal patient safety and outcomes.

The medication safety leader (also referred to as a medication safety officer, medication safety manager, or medication safety coordinator, among other titles) is a clinical practitioner designated by an organization to serve as the authoritative expert in safe medication use. Traditionally, the medication safety leader has been a clinical pharmacist or manager within the department of pharmacy, although the position is sometimes filled by a nurse or physician. The medication safety leader may report to the organization's pharmacy, risk-management, or quality departments, or to senior administration. The medication safety leader should be positioned on the organizational chart where it will best enhance his or her "ability to affect change and advocate that the position remains targeted on medication safety."[6] Medication safety leadership may encompass a single hospital or a group of organizations (e.g., spanning a health system or at a corporate level of a larger organization). Regardless of organization size, it is critical that the fundamentals of medication safety are the central component of the medication safety leader's job function. Although medication safety leaders may have other responsibilities in smaller institutions, medication safety should remain their core responsibility, and they must be strategically positioned and empowered to lead efforts to reduce the risks of medication use.

The characteristics of a medication safety leader include

1. A strong understanding of the facility's internal systems and processes developed through firsthand experience, observations, medication-use evaluations, interviews, and data analysis for the spectrum of patient populations treated in their organization (e.g., pediatric, geriatric, cardiac, oncology).
2. Clinical expertise and a broad understanding of health care systems and processes to facilitate accurate interpretation of clinical events.
3. Knowledge of and experience with all aspects of the medication-use system, including procurement, prescribing, transcribing, preparation, distribution, administration, documentation, and monitoring.
4. Strong analytical skills and an understanding of statistics, population data, and the concepts of risk and prioritization.
5. Knowledge of performance-improvement methodology and tools, including root cause analysis (RCA), failure mode and effects analysis (FMEA), cause-and-effect diagramming, process-flow mapping, and methods for monitoring projects and measuring the progress of performance-improvement initiatives.
6. Post-graduate specialized training (e.g., medication safety residency or fellowship) or three or more years of health-system practice experience.
7. Demonstrated leadership skills.
8. Excellent small- and large-group presentation skills.
9. Excellent oral communication skills, especially the ability to communicate to all types of health care providers as individuals as well as in small and large groups.
10. Excellent writing and editing skills.
11. Strong personal belief that resolving the problem of medication errors is a systems issue and not an individual health care provider issue.
12. Ability to function proactively rather than reactively.
13. Strong personal belief in the concept of a "just culture"[7] that enhances transparency, opens participation

DOI 10.37573/9781585287048.047

to all health care professionals, and fosters a "lessons learned" environment in an organization's medication error reporting system.

14. Understanding of concepts and application of safety principles, continuous quality improvement, and human factors engineering.
15. Appropriate assertiveness.
16. A passion for medication safety and improving patient outcomes.
17. Proven success in working with interdisciplinary teams and engaging diverse groups.
18. Strong personal belief in engaging patients as part of the health care team.
19. Eagerness to learn from events outside one's own facility (e.g., through external sources of information) to apply learning about what went wrong in order to identify and remedy possible system weaknesses to prevent patient harm.

The scope of a medication safety leader's responsibilities reaches into every corner of the health care system and encompasses many roles, such as educator, preceptor, mentor, detective, compliance officer, risk manager, engineer, accountant, statistician, computer analyst, and counselor. A typical day may include attending safety rounds, precepting pharmacy students and residents, writing policies, reviewing adverse drug events and medication error reports,[8] developing error-prevention strategies, leading process-improvement teams, implementing action items, reviewing smart pump libraries, ensuring safe use of automated medication dispensing systems, assessing the safety of replacement drug products during drug shortages, orienting new professional staff, designing and optimizing the medication reconciliation process, conducting tracers to ensure compliance with accreditation standards (e.g., Joint Commission medication management standards and NPSGs), working with practitioners to resolve acute events, attending medical staff meetings, and educating staff and leaders across the system on the culture of safety. Most medication safety leaders quickly find themselves involved in many projects and committees as well as serving as the contact person when nursing, pharmacy, or medical staff have questions or problems. The medication safety leader needs a solid understanding of patient safety principles and must have the ability to prioritize work activities to have a positive impact on the safety of patient care. The medication safety leader should strive to acquire additional skills crucial to success, such as presentation and communication skills, as well as expertise in process-improvement methodologies such as Six Sigma and Lean. Formalized training in medication safety can be achieved through residency, fellowship, and certificate programs and other methods of continuing education. ASHP supports the expansion of pharmacy education and postgraduate residency training to include an emphasis on medication safety.[9]

Responsibilities of Medication Safety Leaders

Medication safety leaders must collaborate with all types of health care professionals, support staff, and management and consider all components of the medication-use process in all settings of healthcare (e.g., inpatient, clinic, community pharmacies, drug distribution centers) in order to improve medication safety. The medication safety leader's role includes responsibility for leadership, medication safety expertise, influencing practice change, research, and education.

Leadership. To provide leadership, the medication safety leader will

1. Develop a vision of an ideal safe medication-use system for the organization.
2. Oversee the planning, creation, review, and refinement of a medication safety plan.
3. Proactively develop and lead implementation of error-prevention strategies based on practice standards, best practice guidelines (or recommendations), literature review, external error reports, medication safety tools, and analysis of the organization's medication safety data.
4. Ensure medication management and patient safety are core components of overall organization quality and outcomes initiatives.
5. Participate in the planning, design, and implementation of the organization's medication-use technology and automation systems.
6. Build a culture of safety through "lesson learned" education and communication across the entire organization.
7. Oversee processes to collect information on the organization's medication errors and system failures to ensure that they are captured and barriers to reporting are addressed.
8. Ensure compliance with state and federal regulatory and legal requirements relating to medication safety and assist in the accreditation process by ensuring that the organization's medication-use processes meet applicable medication management standards and NPSGs.
9. Support the development and implementation of a second victim/care-for-the-caregiver program.

Medication Safety Expertise. In the role of medication safety expert, the medication safety leader will

1. Serve as an authoritative resource on medication safety for the organization.
2. Contribute the medication safety perspective for technology initiatives.
3. Contribute the medication safety perspective to internal and external emergency-preparedness planning.
4. Serve as an internal consultant to investigate medication safety events or issues and develop recommendations for action.
5. Serve as the chair of the medication safety committee, whose duties may include setting the agenda, reviewing general and specific error reports, and examining the progress of projects and initiatives assigned to the medication safety team.
6. Be knowledgeable in the application and use of a variety of quality-improvement methodologies and tools (e.g., FOCUS-PDCA or Lean methodologies, RCA, FMEA).
7. Collect, review, and analyze the organization's medication-use process, medication errors, adverse drug reactions, and continuous quality-improvement data (e.g., markers of adverse drug events, smart pump event data,

triggers and surveillance information, automated dispensing system and bedside bar-code scanning reports) and use appropriate data analysis techniques to identify needed improvements and develop high-leverage error-reduction strategies.

8. Predict and prepare to manage medication safety issues caused by potential or actual drug product shortages and the use of replacement drug products.
9. Maintain knowledge of trends and developments in the patient safety field through continuous professional development: reading articles, journals, and related material; attending appropriate seminars, conferences, or educational programs; and using information from the Institute for Safe Medication Practices (ISMP) National Medication Error Reporting Program, the Food and Drug Administration (FDA) MedWatch program, and similar programs.
10. Participate at local and national levels in patient safety and medication safety organizations and initiatives. Medication safety leaders are also encouraged to seek and share best practices with other regional safety leaders and practice sites.

Influencing Practice Change. To influence practice change, the medication safety leader will

1. Collaborate with other departments (e.g., pharmacy, risk management, patient safety), hospital or health-system senior leadership, frontline staff, and nursing and medical staff leadership to identify and prioritize safety issues and develop risk-reduction strategies using the methods listed above to identify opportunities to improve medication safety.
2. Manage changes in the medication-use system to enhance medication safety, ensure that appropriate measures are taken to address and resolve medication safety issues, and see that hospital staff and faculty are supported in providing safe care for patients.
3. Work closely with others (e.g., the patient safety officer) to integrate medication safety into the overall strategic plan for patient safety and coordinate medication safety initiatives with organizational patient safety initiatives.
4. Participate in or lead multidisciplinary hospital and health-system committees concerned with medication errors, adverse drug events and reactions, near misses, policy review, safe medication use, new product review, and patient safety to identify risk points and prioritize system improvements to reduce the potential for medication error and patient harm.
5. Consult with and advise specific clinical teams and the hospital and health system generally on opportunities and strategies to improve patient care.
6. Encourage organization wide medication error reporting through an established and accepted error reporting system that utilizes appropriate error detection methods (e.g., trigger tools) and through other appropriate avenues such as the pharmacy and therapeutics committee, medication safety committee, and patient safety committee.
7. Develop effective methods for spreading best medication-use practices throughout the organization.
8. Use continuous quality-improvement principles to assess and report on the status of efforts to improve medication safety.
9. Periodically review and update clinical decision-support tools to alert staff to high-risk situations and educate staff as needed.

Research and Education. To further research and education regarding medication safety, the medication safety leader will

1. Design and assist in the implementation of education and orientation programs in safe medication use, including
2. Development of competency assessment for
    - Staff tasks related to medication safety (e.g., use of smart pumps and automated medication dispensing systems);
    - Education of health care providers, other pertinent staff, and (as possible) patients to ensure they are competent in safe medication-use practices; and
    - Provision of effective ongoing programs and presentations related to safe medication use to diverse audiences (e.g., nursing, pharmacy, respiratory care, and medical staff).
3. Share information about actual or potential medication errors or harm with safety organizations such as ISMP, FDA, drug or product manufacturers, and state error reporting programs.
4. Conduct medication-use safety research through well-designed, externally validated studies and implement evidence-based practices for medication safety.
5. Contribute to the literature on medication safety.
6. Provide medication safety education to pharmacy colleagues, students, and residents, as well as other health care professionals.
7. Integrate medication safety into orientation and training for all health care providers who participate in the medication-use process.

Conclusion

ASHP believes that pharmacists, as experts on medication use, are uniquely qualified to serve as medication safety leaders. Medication safety leaders articulate the vision and direction for improving the safety of the medication-use system to prevent patient harm. The medication safety leader's role includes responsibility for leadership through direction and prioritization, medication safety expertise, influencing practice change, research, and education. Through analysis of the organization's medication safety data and literature review, the medication safety leader will lead development and implementation of proactive error-prevention strategies and build a culture of safety across the organization.

References

1. Burgess LH, Cohen MR, Denham CR. A new leadership role for pharmacists: a prescription for change. *J Patient Saf.* 2010; 6:31–7.
2. Kohn LT, Corrigan JM, Donaldson MS, eds. To err is human: building a safer health system. Washington, DC: National Academy Press; 1999.

3. The Joint Commission. Facts about the National Patient Safety goals. https://www.jointcommission.org/facts_about_the_national_patient_safety_goals/ (accessed 2019 March 7).
4. The consensus of the Pharmacy Practice Model Summit. *Am J Health-Syst Pharm.* 2011; 68:1148–52.
5. National Quality Forum. Safe practices for better healthcare 2009 update: a consensus report. https://www.qualityforum.org/Publications/2009/03/Safe_Practices_for_Better_Healthcare%E2%80%932009_Update.aspx (accessed 2019 March 7).
6. Institute for Safe Medication Practices. The Case for Medication Safety Officers (MSO): A White Paper (Aug 2018). https://www.ismp.org/resources/white-paper-case-medication-safety-officers-mso (accessed 2019 June 8).
7. Marx D. Patient safety and the "just culture": a primer for health care executives. New York: Columbia University Press; 2001.
8. National Coordinating Council for Medication Error Reporting and Prevention. Contemporary view of medication-related harm: a new paradigm. 2015. http://www.nccmerp.org/sites/default/files/nccmerp_fact_sheet_2015-02-v91.pdf (accessed 2019 March 7).
9. American Society of Health-System Pharmacists. Required educational outcomes, goals, and objectives for postgraduate year two (PGY2) pharmacy residencies in medication-use safety. https://www.ashp.org/-/media/assets/professional-development/residencies/docs/pgy2-medication-use-safety.ashx?la=en&hash=642AFA9DCC931BE72EF8877DCD1AC5095D286B60 (accessed 2019 March 7).

Suggested Readings

- Larson CM, Saine D. Medication safety officer's handbook. Bethesda, MD: American Society of Health-System Pharmacists; 2013.
- Cohen MR, ed. Medication errors. Washington, DC: American Pharmacists Association; 2007.
- Manasse HR, Thompson KK, eds. Medication safety: a guide for health care facilities. Bethesda, MD: American Society of Health-System Pharmacists; 2005.
- Hepler CD, Segal R. Preventing medication errors and improving drug therapy outcomes: a management systems approach. Boca Raton, FL: CRC Press; 2003.
- Joint Commission Resources. Medication use: a systems approach to reducing errors, 2nd ed. Oakbrook Terrace, IL: Joint Commission Resources; 2008.
- Committee on Quality of Health Care in America, Institute of Medicine. Crossing the quality chasm: a new health system for the 21st century. Washington, DC: National Academy Press; 2001.
- Committee on Data Standards for Patient Safety, Institute of Medicine. Patient safety: achieving a new standard for care. Washington, DC: National Academy Press; 2004.
- Committee on the Work Environment for Nurses and Patient Safety, Board on Health Care Services, Institute of Medicine. Page A, ed. Keeping patients safe: transforming the work environment of nurses. Washington, DC: National Academy Press; 2004.
- Committee on Identifying and Preventing Medication Errors, Board on Health Care Services, Institute of Medicine. Aspden P, Wolcott JA, Bootman JL, et al., eds. Preventing medication errors. Washington, DC: National Academy Press; 2007.
- National Patient Safety Foundation. Free from harm: accelerating patient safety improvement fifteen years after to err is human. 2015. http://www.npsf.org/?page=freefromharm (accessed 2019 March 7).
- Vaida AJ, Lamis RL, Kenward K, Cohen MR. Assessing the state of safe medication practices using the ISMP medication safety self-assessment for hospitals: 2000 and 2011. *Jt Comm J Qual Patient Saf.* 2014 Feb;40(2):51–67. https://www.ncbi.nlm.nih.gov/pubmed/?term=24716328 (accessed 2019 March 7).
- Chassin MR, Loeb JM. High-reliability health care: getting there from here. The Joint Commission. 2013. https://www.jointcommission.org/assets/1/6/Chassin_and_Loeb_0913_final.pdf
- Hertig J, Hultgren K, Weber R. Using contemporary leadership skills in medication safety programs. Hospital Pharmacy [serial online]. April 2016;51(4): 338–344. https://www.ncbi.nlm.nih.gov/pubmed/27303083 (accessed 2019 March 7).
- American Hospital Association, Health Research & Education Trust, and the Institute for Safe Medication Practices. Pathways for Medication Safety: Leading a Strategic Planning Effort. 2002. http://www.ismp.org/tools/PathwaySection1.pdf (accessed 2019 March7).
- American Hospital Association, Health Research & Education Trust, and the Institute for Safe Medication Practices. Pathways for medication safety: looking collectively at risk. 2002. http://www.ismp.org/tools/PathwaySection2.pdf (accessed 2019 March 7).

Web Resources

www.ashp.org
www.ismp.org
www.safemedication.com
www.medsafetyofficer.org
www.asmso.org
www.ahrq.gov
www.fda.gov/cder/drugSafety.htm
www.ihi.org
www.jointcommission.org/standards_information/npsgs.aspx
www.leapfroggroup.org
www.qualityforum.org
www.nccmerp.org
www.usp.org
www.patientsafety.gov
www.npsf.org

Approved by the ASHP Board of Directors on February 13, 2019, and by the ASHP House of Delegates on June 11, 2019. Developed through the ASHP Section of Inpatient Care Practitioners Section Advisory Group on Medication Safety.

This statement was drafted by Stacy L. Carson, Pharm.D., BCPS, FISMP; Sophia Chhay, Pharm.D.; Michael Dejos, Pharm.D.; Michael O'Connor, Pharm.D., M.S.; and Krystal Moorman, Pharm.D., BCPS; the drafters declared no potential conflicts of interest.

Copyright © 2019, American Society of Health-System Pharmacists, Inc. All rights reserved. Contact ASHP for reprint and permissions requests. This content may not be used for commercial purposes without the express written consent of ASHP.

The bibliographic citation for this document is as follows: American Society of Health-System Pharmacists. ASHP statement on the role of the medication safety leader. *Am J Health-Syst Pharm.* 2019; 77:308–12.

ASHP Guidelines on Adverse Drug Reaction Monitoring and Reporting

Purpose

Pharmacists have the knowledge and expertise needed to develop and organize comprehensive programs that monitor, report, and evaluate adverse drug reactions (ADRs) in health systems. ADR monitoring and reporting programs (hereinafter, "ADR programs") encourage surveillance, facilitate documentation, promote reporting, provide mechanisms for monitoring the safety of drug use, and stimulate the education of healthcare professionals.

The purpose of this document is to provide updated guidance for organizations initiating an ADR program or seeking to improve an existing program. The following topics are covered: common definitions, recommended program features, program goals, and the pharmacist's role in the development of a comprehensive program. The recommendations in these guidelines represent a consensus of documented evidence, expert opinion, and professional judgment. They are written to establish reasonable goals that are progressive and challenging yet attainable as best practices in applicable settings. Pharmacy professionals are encouraged to exercise their professional judgment in assessing and adapting these recommendations to meet the specific needs of their healthcare organizations.

Definitions

The relationship between medication errors, adverse drug events, and adverse drug reactions is described in **Figure 1**. Standardized use of these terms and definitions is recommended in order to focus attention on efforts needed to address ADRs.

Adverse drug event (ADE): harm resulting from medical intervention involving a drug.[1–4]

- Adverse drug events may be preventable (ie, medication errors) or nonpreventable (ie, adverse drug reactions).
- All ADEs are associated with harm.

Harm: impairment of the physical, emotional, or psychological function or structure of the body and pain or injury resulting therefrom.[3]

Adverse drug reaction (ADR): a nonpreventable adverse drug event occurring with usual use of medication.[2,3,5,6]

- ADRs are not associated with medication errors.
- Multiple organizations have defined ADRs; the above definition is a simplified version derived from these multiples sources in an effort to standardize and simply.[2,3,5]
- Side effect is a popular term typically used to describe ADRs that are known to occur with a medication with varying degrees of associated harm.
- Drug withdrawal, drug-abuse syndromes, accidental poisoning, and drug-overdose complications should not be defined as ADRs.

FIGURE 1. Relationship between medication errors and adverse drug events. Adapted from reference 3 and from Morimoto T, Gandhi TK, Seger AC, et al. Adverse drug events and medication errors: detection and classification methods. *Qual Saf Health Care* 2004;13:306–314.

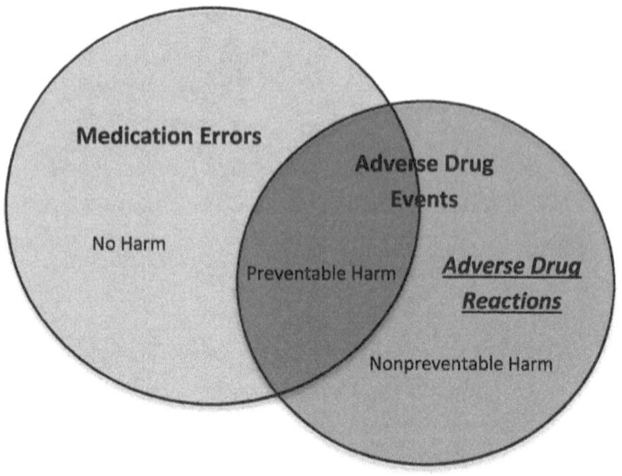

Allergic ADR: an ADR that results from an immunologic hypersensitivity.

Idiosyncratic ADR: an ADR that is peculiar to the individual.

Trigger tool: Chart review, via automated or manual processes, to detect "triggers" that may be representative of an ADE or ADR.[7] The trigger is investigated to determine whether an ADE occurred (eg, if an INR of >7 is the trigger, the chart is then reviewed to determine if warfarin is the cause).

Trigger medications: Medications commonly used to treat ADRs, such as antidotes, reversal agents, steroids, or antihistamines.[7] Administration of a trigger medication does not always indicate that patient harm occurred.

High-alert medications: drugs that bear a heightened risk of causing significant patient harm when they are used in error.[8]

Natural language processing: computer software analysis of text contained in the electronic health record (EHR).[9]

Goals of an ADR Program

The primary goal of an ADR program should be to raise awareness of the risks associated with ADRs, identify ADRs that have occurred, and reduce their risk of associated harm. An ongoing ADR program can provide benefits to the organization, patients, pharmacists, and other healthcare professionals, including (but not limited to) the following:

1. Improving patient care and decreasing length of stay by ensuring safer use of drugs and appropriate follow-up.
2. Educating healthcare professionals and patients about drug effects and increasing their level of awareness regarding ADRs.

DOI 10.37573/9781585287048.048

3. Providing an indirect measure of the quality of drug therapy through identification of potential ADRs and anticipatory surveillance for high-risk drugs or high-risk patients.
4. Complementing organizational risk-management activities and efforts to minimize liability.
5. Assessing the safety of drug therapies.
6. Providing quality-assurance screening to identify opportunities for medication-use evaluation or other performance improvement initiatives.
7. Characterizing ADR incidence. (ASHP does not suggest that there is a predictable rate of incidence or severity of ADRs. The number and severity of ADRs in a given organization or setting would vary with the organization's size, type, patient mix, drugs used, modalities utilized to assess risk and patient harm, the ADR definition used, and ease of reporting.)

ADR Program Features

A comprehensive ADR program should be an integral part of an organization's overall drug-use system and should include the following features (**Figure 2**):

1. A surveillance system that spans the course of the medication-use process, including:
   a. A prospective surveillance system for high-risk drugs or patients at high risk for ADRs, which includes ongoing review of the medical literature, proactive communication to practitioners to increase awareness, and mitigation of potential harm.
   b. An ongoing and concurrent (during drug therapy) surveillance system based on the reporting of suspected ADRs by pharmacists, physicians, nurses, other caregivers, and patients.[10]
   c. A retrospective surveillance system to identify ADRs. This surveillance would include identifying orders for the use of trigger medications that are used to treat common ADRs (eg, orders for immediate doses of antihistamines, epinephrine, or corticosteroids), abrupt discontinuation or decreases in dosage of a drug, patient clinical assessment, or stat orders for laboratory assessment of therapeutic drug levels.[11–13]
   d. Tools such as event monitoring, clinical decision support, and natural language processing can be used to detect certain types of ADRs in clinical databases.[14,15]
2. Date of onset, a description of each suspected ADR, reaction type, and the outcomes from the event should be accurately documented in the patient's medical record. Some EHRs do not readily distinguish between an allergy and significant ADR without additional investigation into the record by the clinician.[14,15] ADR monitoring and reporting programs should ensure timely and appropriate information is provided to clinicians.

FIGURE 2. Features and process of a comprehensive adverse drug reaction (ADR) monitoring and reporting program. Med Safety indicates Medication Safety Committee (or similar organization); P&T, Pharmacy and therapeutics committee (or similar organization).

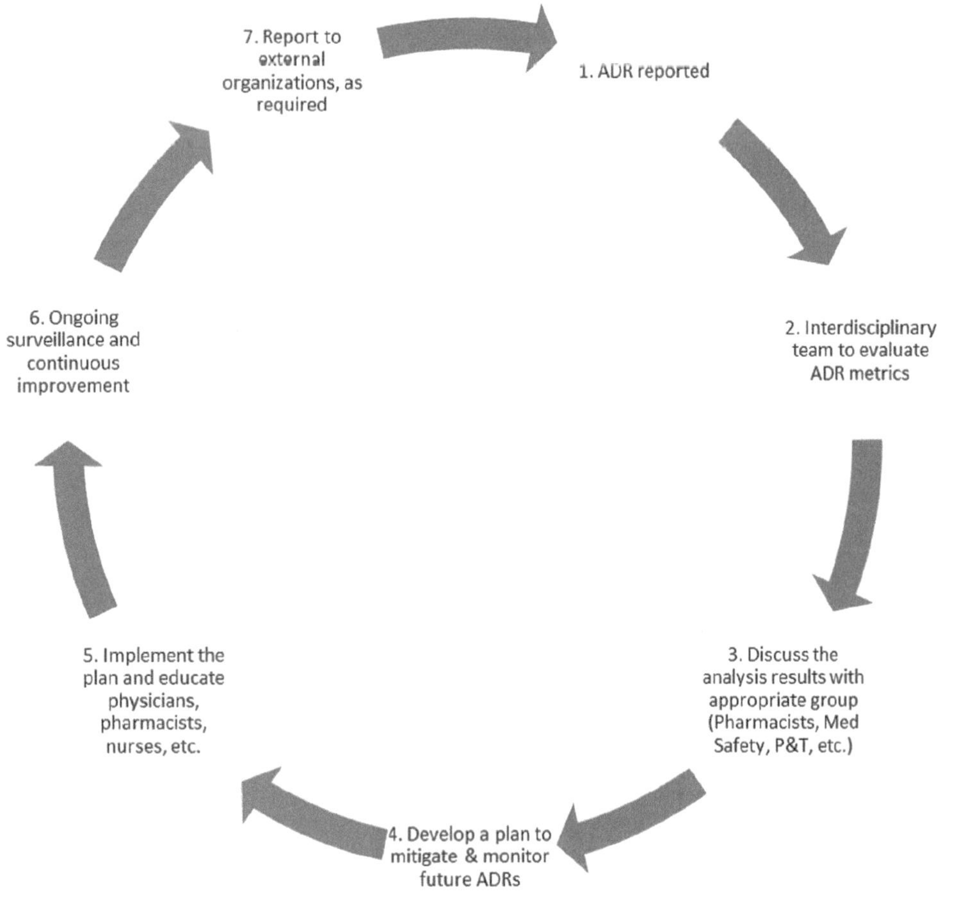

3. Healthcare professionals, patients, or patient representatives should be notified following institutional policy and procedures regarding suspected ADRs.
4. Information regarding suspected ADRs should be reported to the pharmacy department for complete data collection and analysis, including the patient's name, the patient's medical and medication history, a description of the suspected ADR, the temporal sequence of the event, any remedial treatment required, and patient outcomes.[10]
5. High-risk patients should be identified and monitored.
   a. High-risk patients include but are not limited to pediatric patients, geriatric patients, patients with organ failure (eg, hepatic or renal failure), and patients receiving antineoplastics.[11]
6. High-risk drugs should be identified based on prescribing patterns and institutional utilization, and their use should be routinely monitored because they can also be a source of ADRs. Examples of drugs that may be considered as high-risk include but are not limited to aminoglycosides, amphotericin, antineoplastics, corticosteroids, digoxin, anticoagulants, insulin, lidocaine, phenytoin, thrombolytic agents, and opioids.[8,11]
7. The cause(s) of each suspected ADR should be evaluated on the basis of the patient's medical and medication history, the circumstances of the ADR, the results of dechallenge and rechallenge (if any), alternative etiologies, and a literature review.
8. A method for assigning the probability of a reported or suspected ADR should be developed to categorize each ADR. Many algorithms to assist in assessment of the cause of the ADR have been developed. Commonly used algorithms include the Naranjo algorithm, the WHO causality tool, and the Liverpool ADR causality tool; however, there are many others that pharmacists may find useful.[5,16–23] Subjective questions and the professional judgment of a pharmacist can be used as additional tools to determine the probability of an ADR. Questions might include the following:
   a. Was there a temporal relationship between the onset of drug therapy and the adverse reaction?
   b. Was there a dechallenge (ie, did the signs and symptoms of the adverse reaction subside when the drug was withdrawn)?
   c. Can signs and symptoms of the adverse reaction be explained by the patient's disease state?
   d. Were there any laboratory tests that provide evidence for the reaction being an ADR?
   e. What was the patient's previous general experience with the drug?
   f. Was there a rechallenge (ie, did symptoms return when the drug was readministered)?
9. A method for ranking ADRs by severity should be established. A commonly used scale ranks severity into 7 categories according to clinical consequence, including resultant harm and intensity of medical intervention required.[24] The National Cancer Institute Common Terminology Criteria for Adverse Events is a standardized system to quantify or grade the severity of adverse medication reactions.[25] The National Coordinating Council for Medication Error Reporting and Prevention (NCC MERP) also provides a classification that can assist in coding ADEs; it considers factors such as whether an error reached the patient and whether the patient was harmed and to what degree.[26] The NCC MERP classification index included in the document was developed to categorize harm for medication errors. Despite being designed for medication errors, many commercial and governmental reporting programs have adopted the NCC MERP Index and applied it to all event types, including ADRs.
10. Serious or unexpected ADRs should be reported to a medication manufacturer and/or the FDA in accordance with state reporting requirements (Figure 2).
    a. Sequester as much evidence and clinical information as possible prior to reporting.
    b. FDA offers 2 reporting tools, MedWatch[27] and the Vaccine Adverse Event Reporting System (VAERS),[28] which should be used to report events and allow for tracking of national safety signals.
11. ADR reports should be reviewed and evaluated by a designated interdisciplinary committee (eg, medication safety committee, pharmacy and therapeutics committee).
    a. In settings where it is possible, a pharmacy-coordinated ADR team or committee, consisting of but not limited to a physician, nurse, quality improvement leader, an administrator, a pharmacist, and an informaticist (preferably a pharmacy informaticist) is recommended.[29–31]
    b. The interdisciplinary committee should be charged with adopting a definition for the organization, promoting awareness of the consequences of ADRs, establishing mechanisms for identifying and reporting ADRs, reviewing ADR patterns or trends, and developing preventive and corrective interventions.
12. ADR report information and trending should be disseminated to healthcare professional staff members for educational purposes, while maintaining confidentiality. Suggested topics for medical staff education include recognition of ADRs and appropriate and effective care for patients who experience ADRs. Educational programs can be provided in various formats, such as competencies, morning report/safety huddle discussions, newsletters, grand rounds presentations, algorithms for treatment, and interdisciplinary reviews of medication-use evaluations.
13. Findings from an ADR program should be incorporated into the organization's ongoing quality improvement activities. The process should include the following actions:
    a. Case-specific feedback to all appropriate healthcare staff, patients, and caregivers.
    b. Continuous monitoring for trends, clusters, or significant individual ADRs, both internally and externally (eg, manufacturers, state boards, FDA, Institute for Safe Medication Practices).
       i. Internal data can be trended by patient demographics (eg, gender and age), patient care area, involved drug(s) and drug class, reaction type, and severity level. Data can be

reported via descriptive analysis or as a trend (**Figures 3-5** provide examples). This information should be used by the interdisciplinary committee to decide further action, training, or system improvement, as appropriate. The FDA Adverse Event Reporting System (FAERS) can be utilized for trending external data through its public dashboard.[32]

c. Educational efforts to interdisciplinary team for detection, prevention, and reporting of ADRs.

d. Evaluation of prescribing patterns, patient monitoring practices, patient outcomes, and the ADR program's effect on overall and individual patient outcomes.

14. Technology allowing sharing of ADR information, standardization and simplification of reporting, and automated access to external reporting databases such as MedWatch and VAERS is not widely available. Adoption of these features should be considered by the ADR program as they become available.

Role of the Pharmacist in ADR Monitoring and Reporting

Pharmacists are a vital link between the patient and the health system before and during the course of drug therapy.[33,34] Pharmacists are uniquely qualified to provide valuable information on drug products, can play an important role in monitoring adverse events, and help design and implement system improvements related to ADRs in their health systems.[35,36]

Pharmacists should obtain formal endorsement or approval of such programs through appropriate committees (eg, a pharmacy and therapeutics committee and the executive committee of the medical staff) and the organization's administration. In applicable settings, input into the design of the program should be obtained from the medical staff, nursing staff, quality improvement staff, the medical records department, and risk managers.[19,37-39]

The pharmacist should facilitate the following activities:

1. Analysis of each reported ADR.

2. Identification of drugs and patients at high risk for being involved in ADRs.

3. The development of scope, policies and procedures for the ADR-monitoring and reporting program.

4. A description of the responsibilities and interactions of pharmacists, physicians, nurses, risk managers, and other health professionals in the ADR program.

5. Use of the ADR program for educational purposes.

6. Development, maintenance, and routine evaluation of ADR records within the organization, including the use of standardized reporting rate and incidence of onsite ADRs occurrence.

7. The organizational dissemination and use of information obtained through the ADR program.

8. Facilitating the reporting of serious or unexpected ADRs, as outlined in program features section 2, and publication and presentation of important ADRs to the medical community.

Conclusion

Pharmacists are uniquely positioned to assist in the coordination of an ADR program. Programs should focus on surveillance, complete documentation within medical records, reporting to and review by an interdisciplinary committee, and education to achieve an overall goal of reducing the risk and severity of ADRs within an organization. All pharmacists should understand their role in recognizing, evaluating, reporting, and educating both patients and providers on ADRs.

FIGURE 3. Adverse drug reaction (ADR) trending by involved drug using Pareto principle. In the example, Drug A was the top reported medication involved in ADR events, a trend that can be used as a signal to warrant additional investigation.

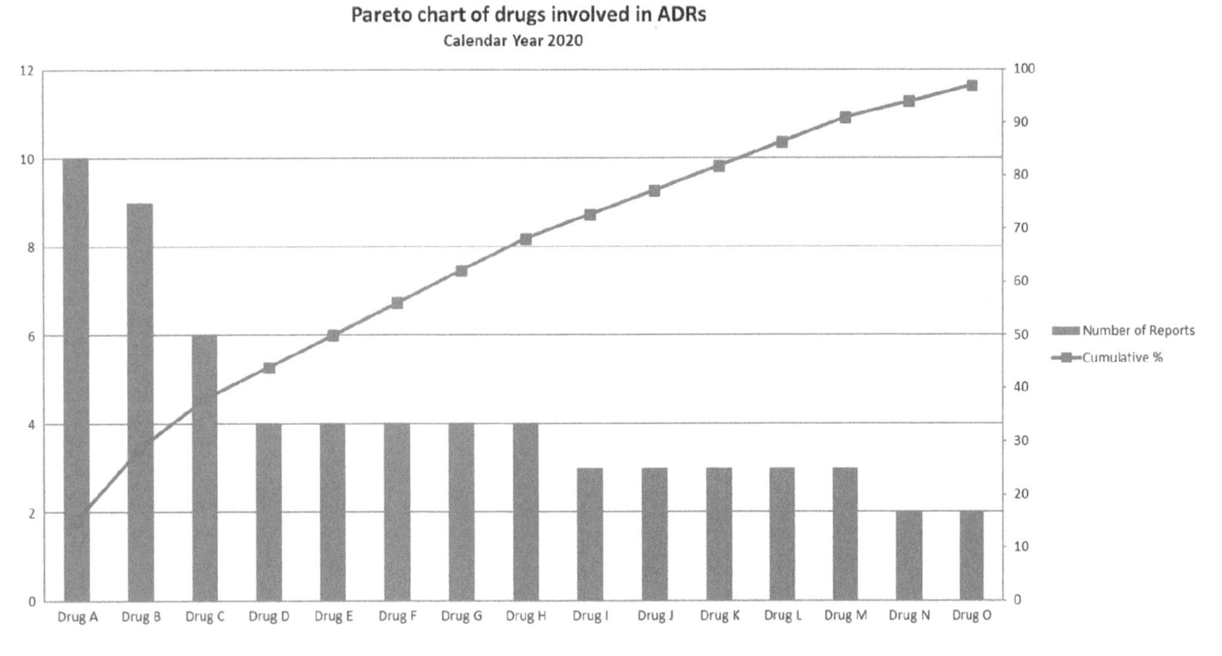

FIGURE 4. Example of monthly adverse drug reaction (ADR) event trending of the top reported medication identified in Figure 3. In the example, shortness of breath (SOB) ADR events involving Drug A were captured on a monthly basis and the event rate compared with the hospital's ADR average (green line) and reported SOB events resulting from the use of Drug A in clinical trials (red line). Based on the trends noted, an intervention was made in August to premedicate patients, and this milestone is depicted on the graph.

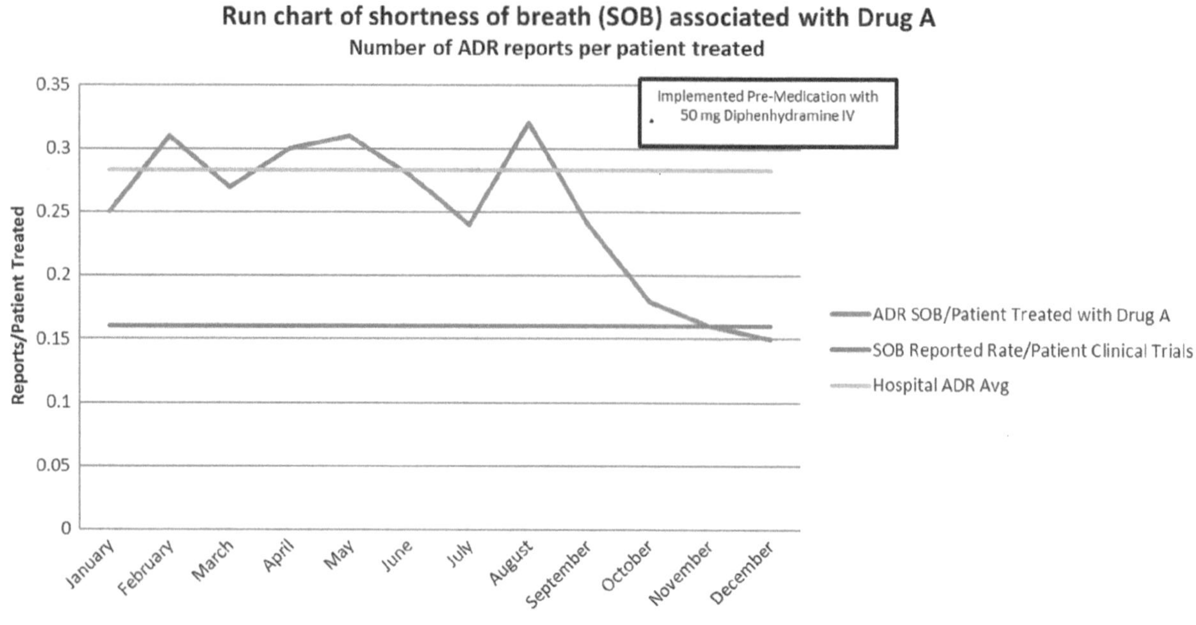

FIGURE 5. Example of organization of data on reported adverse drug reaction events by involved drug class in a pie chart.

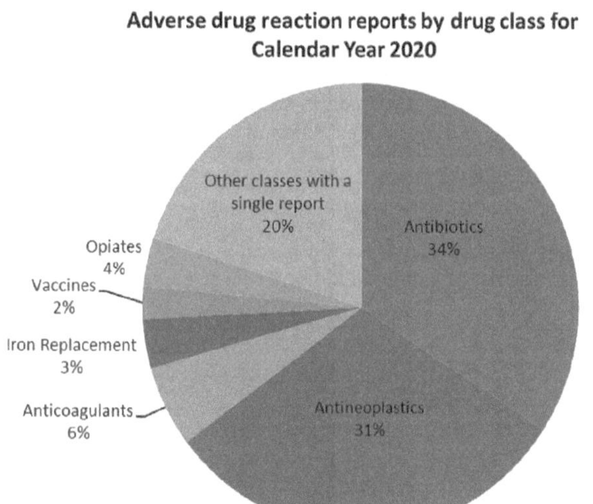

References

1. US Food and Drug Administration. What is a serious adverse event? Accessed January 21, 2021. https://www.fda.gov/safety/reporting-serious-problems-fda/what-serious-adverse-event
2. Requirements for adverse reaction reporting. World Health Organization; 1975.
3. National Coordinating Council for Medication Error Reporting and Prevention. Contemporary view of medication-related harm. A new paradigm. Accessed January 21, 2021. https://www.nccmerp.org/sites/default/files/nccmerp_fact_sheet_2015-02-v91.pdf
4. Kohn LT, Corrigan JM, Donaldson MS. Institute of Medicine. *To Err Is Human: Building a Safer Health System*. National Academy Press; 2000.
5. Karch FE, Lasagna L. Adverse drug reactions. A critical review. *JAMA*. 1975;234(12):1236–41.
6. Edwards IR, Aronson JK. Adverse drug reactions: definitions, diagnosis, and management. *Lancet*. 2000; 356:1255–9. doi:10.1016/S0140-6736(00)02799-9
7. Griffin FA, Resar RK. *IHI Global Trigger Tool for Measuring Adverse Events (Second Edition)*. IHI Innovation Series white paper. Institute for Healthcare Improvement; 2009. Accessed January 21, 2021. http://www.ihi.org/resources/Pages/IHIWhitePapers/IHIGlobalTriggerToolWhitePaper.aspx
8. Institute for Safe Medication Practices. High-alert medications in acute care settings. Published August 23, 2018. Accessed January 21, 2021. https://www.ismp.org/recommendations/high-alert-medications-acute-list
9. Ross MK, Wei W, Ohno-Machado L. "Big data" and the electronic health record. *Med Inform*. 2014;9:97–104.
10. Prosser TR, Kamysz PL. Multidisciplinary adverse drug reaction surveillance program. *Am J Hosp Pharm*. 1990;47:1334–1339.
11. Koch K. Adverse drug reactions. In: Brown T, ed. *Handbook of Institutional Pharmacy Practice*. 4th ed. American Society of Hospital Pharmacists; 2006.
12. Koch KE. Use of standardized screening procedures to identify adverse drug reactions. *Am J Hosp Pharm*. 1990;47:1314–1320.
13. Classen DC, Pestotnik SL, Evans RS, et al. Computerized surveillance of adverse drug events in hospital patients. *JAMA*. 1991;266:2847–2851.
14. Bates DW, Evans RS, Murff H, et al. Detecting adverse events using information technology. *J Am Med Inform Assoc*. 2003;10:115–128.

15. Emmendorfer T, Glassman PA, Moore V, et al. Monitoring adverse drug reactions across a nationwide health care system using information technology. *Am J Health-Syst Pharm.* 2012;69:321–328.
16. Naranjo CA, Busto U, Sellers EM, et al. A method for estimating the probability of adverse drug reactions. *Clin Pharmacol Ther.* 1981;30:239–245.
17. Gallagher RM, Kirkham JJ, Mason JR, et al. Development and inter-rater reliability of the Liverpool adverse drug reaction causality assessment tool. *PLoS One.* 2011;6(12):e28096. doi:10.1371/journal.pone.0028096
18. Jones JK. Adverse drug reactions in the community health setting: approaches to recognizing, counseling, and reporting. *Fam Community Heal.* 1982;5:58–67.
19. Karch FE, Lasagna L. Toward the operational identification of adverse drug reactions. *Clin Pharmacol Ther.* 1977;21:247–254.
20. Kramer MS, Leventhal JM, Hutchinson TA, et al. An algorithm for the operational assessment of adverse drug reactions: I. Background, description, and instructions for use. *JAMA.* 1979;242:623–632.
21. Koh Y, Yap C, Li S. A quantitative approach of using genetic algorithm in designing a probability scoring system of an adverse drug reaction assessment system. *Int J Med Inform.* 2008;77:421–430.
22. Bégaud B, Evreux J, Jouglard J, et al. Imputation of the unexpected or toxic effects of drugs. Actualisation of the methods used in France. *Therapie.* 1985;40:111–118.
23. World Health Organization, Centre UM. The use of the WHO-UMC system for standardised case causality assessment. Published 2014. Accessed January 21, 2021. https://www.who.int/medicines/areas/quality_safety/safety_efficacy/WHOcausality_assessment.pdf
24. Hartwig SC, Siegel J, Schneider PJ. Preventability and severity assessment in reporting adverse drug reactions. *Am J Health-Syst Pharm.* 1992;49:2229–2232.
25. National Cancer Institute. Common Terminology Criteria for Adverse Events (CTCAE) v.5. Accessed January 21, 2021. https://ctep.cancer.gov/protocolDevelopment/electronic_applications/docs/CTCAE_v5_Quick_Reference_5x7.pdf
26. Hartwig S, Denger S, Schneider P. Severity-indexed, incident report-based medication error-reporting program. *Am J Health-Syst Pharm.* 1991;48:2611–2616.
27. US Food and Drug Administration. Medwatch Safety Program. Accessed January 21, 2021. www.fda.gov/safety/medwatch/
28. US Food and Drug Administration. Vaccine Adverse Event Reporting System. Accessed January 21, 2021. https://www.fda.gov/vaccines-bloodbiologics/vaccine-adverse-events/vaers-overview
29. Keith MR, Bellanger-McCleery RA, Fuchs JE Jr. Multidisciplinary program for detecting and evaluating adverse drug reactions. *Am J Hosp Pharm.* 1989;46:1809–1812.
30. Kimelblatt BJ, Young SH, Heywood PM, et al. Improved reporting of adverse drug reactions. *Am J Hosp Pharm.* 1988;45:1086–1089.
31. Nelson R, Shane R. Developing an adverse drug reaction reporting program. *Am J Hosp Pharm.* 1983;40:445–446.
32. US Food and Drug Administration. FDA Adverse Event Reporting System (FAERS) Public Dashboard. Accessed January 21, 2021. https://www.fda.gov/Drugs/GuidanceComplianceRegulatoryInformation/Surveillance/AdverseDrugEffects/ucm070093.htm
33. van Grootheest K, Olsson S, Couper M, et al. Pharmacists' role in reporting adverse drug reactions in an international perspective. *Pharmacoepidemiol Drug Saf.* 2004;13:457–464.
34. Green CF, Mottram DR, Raval D, et al. Community pharmacists' attitudes to adverse drug reaction reporting. *Int J Pharm Pract.* 1999;7:92–99.
35. Emerson A, Martin RM, Tomlin M, et al. Prospective cohort study of adverse events monitored by hospital pharmacists. Hospital Adverse Event Monitoring Study (HAEMS) Group. *Pharmacoepidemiol Drug Saf.* 2001;10:95–103.
36. Forster AJ, Halil RB, Tierney MG. Pharmacist surveillance of adverse drug events. *Am J Health-Syst Pharm.* 2004;61:1466–1472.
37. Swanson KM, Landry JP, Anderson RP. Pharmacy coordinated, multidisciplinary adverse drug reaction program. *Top Hosp Pharm Manage.* 1992;12:49–59.
38. Flowers P, Dzierba S, Baker O. A continuous quality improvement team approach to adverse drug reaction reporting. *Top Hosp Pharm Manage.* 1992;12:60–67.
39. Guharoy S. A pharmacy-coordinated, multidisciplinary approach for successful implementation of an adverse drug reaction reporting program. *Top Hosp Pharm Manage.* 1992;12:68–74.

Developed through the ASHP Section of Inpatient Care Practitioners and approved by the ASHP Board of Directors on May 20, 2021. These guidelines supersede the ASHP Guidelines on Adverse Drug Reaction Monitoring and Reporting dated November 16, 1994.

ASHP gratefully acknowledges the following organizations and individuals for reviewing these guidelines (review does not imply endorsement): American Association of Critical-Care Nurses (AACN); Institute for Healthcare Improvement (IHI); Institute for Safe Medication Practices (ISMP); Maryland Society of Health-System Pharmacy (MSHP); Sandra Leigh Bardas, BSPharm, RPh, FCSHP; James L. Besier, PhD, MS, BSPharm, FASHP; Carol J. Bickford, PhD, RN-BC, CPHIMS, FAMIA, FHIMSS, FAAN; John Bowman, MS, BCPS, FASHP; Jamie N. Brown, PharmD, BCPS, BCACP; Kavish Choudhary, PharmD, MS; Michael R. Cohen, RPh, MS, ScD (hon), DPS (hon), FASHP (ISMP); Michael C. Dejos, PharmD, BCPS, LSSBB, DPLA; Frank Federico, RPh (IHI); Katayoon Kathy Ghomeshi, PharmD, MBA, BCPS, CPPS; Jennifer Howard, PharmD; Anna Hu, PharmD; Melissa Jones, PhD (AACN); Thomas Kaye, RPh, MBA, FASHP; Nicole Kiehle, PharmD, BCPS (MSHP); Eric C. Kutscher, PharmD, MBA, FASHP; Mark A. Malesker, PharmD, FCCP, FCCP, FCCM, FASHP, BCPS; Patrick M. Malone, PharmD, FASHP; Linda Gore Martin, PharmD, MBA, FASHP; Robert B. McDaniel, PharmD, BCPS; Charles D. Ponte, BPharm, PharmD, FAADE, FAPhA, FASHP, FCCP, FNAP; James Ponto, MS, FASHP; Robert L. Poole, PharmD, FPPAG, FCSHP, FASHP; James R. Rinehart, RPh, MS, FASHP; Richard I. Sakai, PharmD, FASHP, FCSHP; Adam Servi, PharmD, RPh, BCPS; Karen W. Smollen, PharmD; Kristin A. Tuiskula, PharmD; Geralyn Waters, PharmD, BCPS; and Debbie Wu, PharmD. ASHP also gratefully acknowledges the contributions of authors of previous versions of these guidelines: Philip E. Johnston, PharmD, Charles P. Coe, BSPharm, and Karen E. Koch, PharmD.

The authors have declared no potential conflicts of interest.

Lynne M. Lee, PharmD, Greene, NY.

Delia Charest Carias, PharmD, BCPS, DPLA, St. Jude Children's Research Hospital, Memphis, TN.

Rena Gosser, PharmD, BCPS, UW Medicine – Harborview Medical Center, Seattle, WA.

Ambra Hannah, PharmD, BCPS, Wellstar Health System, Marietta, GA.

Sarah Stephens, PharmD, BCPS, CPPS, Kaweah Delta Health Care District, Visalia, CA.

William A. Templeman, PharmD, Kaiser Riverside, Riverside, CA.

Copyright © 2022, American Society of Health-System Pharmacists, Inc. All rights reserved. Contact ASHP for reprint and permissions requests. This content may not be used for commercial purposes without the express written consent of ASHP.

The bibliographic citation for this document is as follows: American Society of Health-System Pharmacists. ASHP guidelines on adverse drug reaction monitoring and reporting. *Am J Health-Syst Pharm.* 2022;79:e83–89.

ASHP Guidelines on Preventing Medication Errors in Hospitals

Purpose

The goal of medication therapy is the achievement of defined therapeutic outcomes that improve a patient's quality of life while minimizing patient risk.[1] There are inherent risks, both known and unknown, associated with the use of medications (prescription and nonprescription). This document addresses medication errors, defined as any preventable event that may cause or lead to inappropriate medication use or patient harm while the medication is in the control of the healthcare professional, patient, or consumer. Such events may be related to professional practice, healthcare products, procedures, and systems, including prescribing, order communication, product labeling, packaging, and nomenclature, compounding, dispensing, distribution, administration, education, monitoring, and use.[2]

The landmark Institute of Medicine (IOM) report *To Err Is Human: Building a Safer Health System,* published in 1999, increased the national focus on improvements and the prevention of errors in patient safety.[3] This report drew attention to the significant problem of medical errors in the healthcare system, one type of which is medication errors. Other reports published after 1999 have drawn attention to patient safety improvement efforts, including 5-, 10-, and 15-year updates after *To Err Is Human,*[4–6] as well as the 2007 release of IOM's *Preventing Medication Errors: Quality Chasm Series.*[7] While the original IOM report increased awareness of the significant risk of medical errors, the pace of change is slow, and there is more work to be completed.[6]

The outcomes or clinical significance of many medication errors may be minimal, with few or no consequences that adversely affect a patient. In addition, numerous medication errors go unrecognized and are not detected or reported. Tragically, however, some medication errors result in serious patient morbidity or mortality.[8] Thus, medication errors (including close calls) must not be taken lightly, and risk-reduction strategies and systems should be established to prevent or mitigate patient harm from medication errors.

Reason[9] stated that humans are imperfect, and errors should be expected. A system-based approach should be undertaken at institutions to prevent future errors; this approach strives to change worker conditions and build defenses, barriers, and safeguards to prevent errors from occurring or mitigate the harm if errors do occur.[9] Blaming healthcare workers involved in errors or passively encouraging them to be more careful will not prevent errors since it does not change the underlying conditions that contributed to the error.

The pharmacist should participate in multidisciplinary committees of the organization and take an active role in the evaluation and monitoring of the medication-use process throughout the hospital or healthcare system to examine and improve systems to ensure that medication processes are safe. Furthermore, health-system pharmacists have the responsibility and expertise to lead collaborative, multidisciplinary efforts to prevent medication-related problems that can result in patient harm.[10]

The purpose of these guidelines is to provide the pharmacists with practical recommendations and best practices for preventing and mitigating patient harm from medication errors in the health-system setting. These guidelines are primarily intended to apply to the acute care setting because of the special collaborative processes established in this setting (i.e., formulary system, pharmacy and therapeutics committee, widespread use of automation and electronic health records [EHRs], and opportunity for increased interaction among healthcare providers). However, many of the ideas and principles in these guidelines may be applicable to practice settings outside of the acute care setting, especially in health systems.

Medication errors can occur at any point of the medication-use system.[7] For the purposes of these guidelines, the medication-use system is defined in **Figure 1**.

Planning for Safe Medication Practices

Safe medication practices begin with placing medication safety as anorganizational and departmental priority, and implementing a system that will support these practices. The organization must have a comprehensive program that includes a medication safety leader, key elements in place to provide the structure for safe medication practices, and a successful strategic plan.[10] Key supporting elements include a culture of safety built on principles of just culture that is supported at all levels of the organization (from the C-suite to the frontline), an event-reporting system, an interdisciplinary medication safety team, a continuous improvement philosophy regarding evaluation of errors and harm, and strong designs that assess and reduce the risk of errors. If any of these are not well developed, the organization should address them through the planning process in order to meet the continuing goal of ensuring patient safety.

A culture of patient safety, based on the principles of just culture, provides a solid foundation for safe and effective systems and teamwork. In a just culture, safety is valued, reporting of safety risks is encouraged without penalization, and the staff, leadership, and board of trustees are held accountable using a clear and transparent process that evaluates the errors.[8] The evaluation process separates events arising from a flawed system design or inadvertent human error from behavioral choices that compromise safety[11]; there may be consequences when unjustifiable risk is knowingly taken by an individual.[10] A just culture environment should also include a support system for second victims. Second victims are defined as healthcare providers who are involved in an unanticipated adverse patient event, a medical error, or a patient-related injury and become victimized in the sense that the provider is traumatized by the event.[12,13] Programs should be established to support the second victims and to educate healthcare professionals about the second-victim effect.[14]

A system for reporting and reviewing errors is an essential component of a medication safety system; the goal is to enhance patient safety and prevent patient harm. Errors and close calls should be reported and analyzed (e.g., root cause

DOI 10.37573/9781585287048.049

FIGURE 1. This diagram is a modification of the Joint Commission's medication management system, with the addition of 2 steps: patient admission and discharge. These steps were added to appropriately encompass issues that arise during admission and discharge (e.g., medication history and reconciliation errors, patient education barriers).

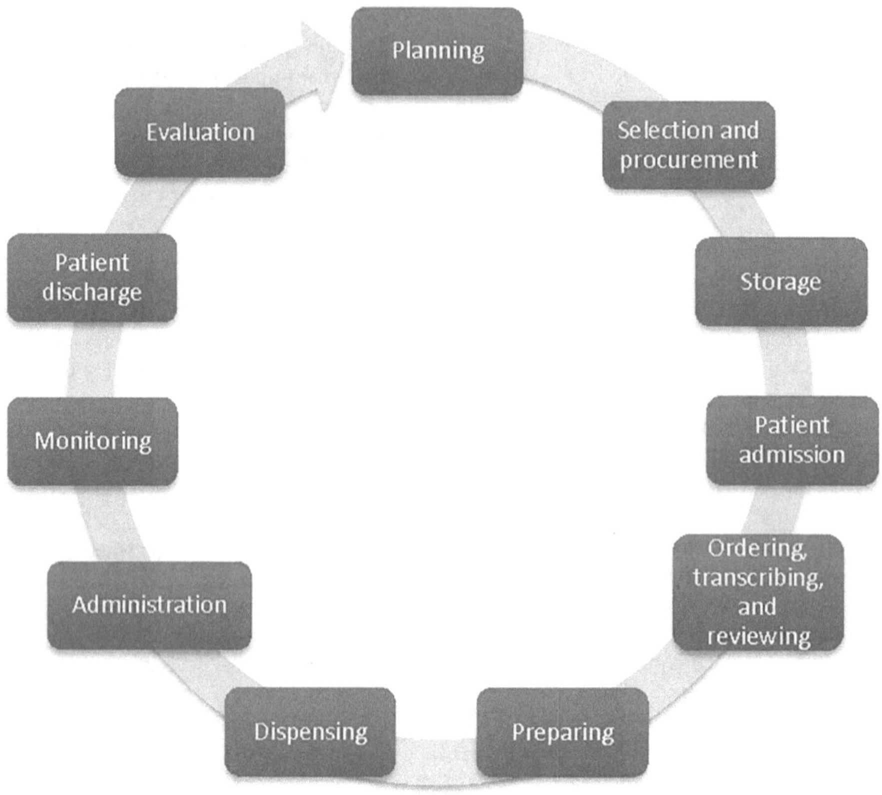

analysis [RCA]) to identify the causes and develop measures to prevent similar occurrences.[5,15,16] Other event detection methods, such as trigger tools, chart review, data from technology, and direct observation, should be considered to complement error-reporting efforts. There are a number of commercially available software systems for online reporting and analysis of medication errors.

A multidisciplinary medication safety team provides a collaborative and systematic approach to addressing medication safety issues and problems as well as proactively assessing risk.[17] In order to ensure overall success, a medication safety leader, preferably a pharmacist, should lead the medication safety efforts throughout the organization. The "ASHP Statement: Role of the Medication Safety Leader" is an important guide.[11] A pharmacist position dedicated to medication safety should be developed to ensure that pharmacists are key safety leaders in the organization.

Lastly, the organization must evaluate and adopt technologies that will help reduce the risk of medication errors and help prevent patient harm.[18,19] Pharmacists must be involved in technology decisions to ensure the safety and effectiveness of technology that impacts the medication-use process.[20] The application of individual technologies will be discussed in subsequent sections.

Risk Assessment. The process of completing a medication safety self-assessment will help a health-system organization identify medication safety risks within its system so that it can prioritize and plan for improvements. Proactive risk assessment tools, such as assessments available from the Institute for Safe Medication Practices (ISMP) (www.ismp.org/selfassessments/default.asp), may be used to identify opportunities for improvement through a gap analysis.[21] ISMP also offers other risk assessment and best-practice tools that focus on specific areas, such as automated dispensing cabinets (ADCs) and anticoagulation.[22] ASHP also publishes policy positions and guidelines that are national best practices (www.ashp.org/Pharmacy-Practice/Policy-Positions-and-Guidelines). A failure modes and effects analysis (FMEA) and a gap analysis are other methods that can be used to complete a risk assessment. These proactive tools are used to identify the risk of failure before it occurs so that systems can be designed to minimize risk. Examples of where these tools can be applied include when evaluating high-alert medication processes as well as medication-related equipment (**Appendix B**).[8,23]

Reducing the Risk of Errors. Organizations should prospectively design and implement strategies to reduce certain types of errors in order to prevent patient harm. Areas that must be addressed are high-risk populations, high-risk processes, high-alert medications, and easily confused drug names, also known as "look-alike/sound-alike" (LASA) medications.

Two areas of focus are addressed below. High-alert medications are medications that have an increased risk of causing serious patient harm when used in error. A hospital-specific list of high-alert medications may be developed using the ISMP list of high-alert drugs in conjunction with the hospital's patterns of medication use and harm events.[24] Risk-reduction strategies should be implemented that will (1) prevent errors, (2) make errors visible, and (3) mitigate the harm if an error occurs.[25] Strategies will be successful if they effectively address the underlying cause of error and impact as many steps of the medication-use process as possible; a single risk-reduction strategy should not be depended on in most cases. When developing strategies, the literature should be used to identify risk-reduction strategies that have been proven effective, recommended by experts, or implemented successfully elsewhere (**Appendix A**).[26]

Examples of safety strategies include but are not limited to

- Using oral syringes that cannot be connected to i.v. tubing ports along with education on the existence of oral syringes and safe use.
- Using epidural tubing without ports.
- Using smart infusion pumps.
- Using electronic prescribing systems with clinical decision support.
- Implementing barcode technology for the preparation, dispensing, and administration of medications.
- Employing evidence-based standard order sets and protocols.
- Standardizing concentrations, diluents, and container sizes.
- Using scales that only weigh patients in kilograms and documenting weight only in kilograms.
- Using commercially available products instead of compounding.
- Dispensing oral and parenteral medications in the most ready-to-administer form.
- Using oral measuring devices only in metric scale.
- Performing independent double checks on dosing, infusion pump programming, and concentrations when appropriate.
- Utilizing auxiliary labels when appropriate.
- Improving readability of labels.

Medications that are commonly confused due to similarities in name, dosage form, or packaging should also be proactively addressed. Medications that are at risk of error can be identified by reviewing local data on errors and the list of confused drug names published by ISMP.[27] Strategies should be implemented that address LASA medication risks. LASA error prevention strategies include differentiation, improved access to information, reminders, limiting access or use, and redundancies.[28]

Strategies for handling LASA medications include

- Using both brand and generic names when appropriate.
- Using tall-man lettering, color, or font to differentiate.[29]
- Including the indication for use on orders.
- Limiting the use of verbal orders.
- Using read-back processes to minimize errors by spelling the medication name and stating the intended purpose.
- Implementing barcode technology and/or radio frequency identification (RFID) for the preparation, dispensing, and administration of medications.
- Avoiding abbreviating drug names if possible.

Product packaging is another source of look-alike drug errors. Strategies to minimize the risk of error include making items look different by purchasing products from different manufacturers, purchasing different-size containers, storing drugs in separate areas, and using alerts on the product and in the storage area.[28]

The practice of performing independent double checks has been widely promoted in healthcare to identify potential errors before they reach patients.[30] However, misuse and improper execution of this practice could jeopardize medication safety. Independent double checks should be selectively applied to certain medications after careful consideration to avoid excessive use and maximize its intent as an independently performed task. An independent double check requires 2 people and must be conducted independently by the second person to reduce bias and increase effectiveness. Avoid using independent double checks as a sole-reliance strategy. Independent double checks should be implemented in combination with other risk-reduction strategies to reduce the frequency of errors.

Pharmacists should be familiar with which medications are managed via a risk evaluation and mitigation strategy (REMS). REMS is a Food and Drug Administration (FDA)-mandated program that seeks to manage the safe use of a medication with known or potential serious risks. The REMS may include a medication guide, patient package insert, communication plan, elements to ensure safe use, and an implementation system. Requirements of REMS programs are not identical among different medications; thus, it is important for pharmacists to understand the unique aspects that may exist.[31]

Selection and Procurement

Selection and procurement of medications involve appropriately selecting which medications will be stocked in the institution (the formulary) and then safely and effectively obtaining the medications from manufacturers and wholesalers. Best practices for decreasing the risk of errors during selection and procurement can generally be divided into 5 categories: (1) formulary assessment and management, (2) standard concentrations, (3) safety-alert monitoring, (4) safe procurement, and (5) medication shortage management.

Formulary Assessment and Management. A well-designed formulary system will guide clinicians to prescribe the safest and most cost-effective agent for treating a particular disease state or medical issue.[32] Formularies limit the selection of medications available so that clinicians become proficient with the dosing, preparation, and administration practices of a selected number of medications. A streamlined formulary can also help to standardize the content of EHRs, pharmacy information systems, and infusion pump settings/medication libraries. Formularies should be designed to enhance the safe use of medications and not simply as a cost-saving measure.

The "ASHP Guidelines on the Pharmacy and Therapeutics Committee and the Formulary System" provide detailed guidance on formularies and medication evaluation documents (i.e., monographs) and should be consulted for more information.[32] In particular, when preparing an evidence-based formulary review document for a medication, a section should be devoted to medication safety assessment and recommendations. In short, the pharmacist should consider whether the medication being reviewed for addition to the formulary has potential safety issues, such as a complicated admixture or administration process, a similarity in sound or appearance to another medication (i.e., LASA medication), dosing or duration limitations, a REMS program, admixture or administration handling precautions, specific requirements on storage or waste, extravasation management, and significant serious adverse effects that should be monitored. This assessment should include a relevant literature search, including published studies and case reports, manufacturer information, and professional organization and agency websites such as those of ISMP, FDA (e.g., MedWatch reports), accreditation agencies (e.g., Joint Commission), Centers for Disease Control and Prevention (i.e., occupational safe handling—National Institute of Occupational Safety's List of Antineoplastic and Other Hazardous Drugs in Healthcare Settings), and the Environmental Protection Agency (e.g., waste precautions). Health-system pharmacists may choose to develop and use a standard checklist for medication safety review of formulary additions; there are examples on the ASHP Medication-Use Safety Resource Center.[33] If the medication is new and limited information is available, pharmacists need to consider what potential medication safety issues could arise.

When medications with heightened error potential are added to the formulary, strategies to prevent medication errors should be considered. Preferably, these safety enhancements are established and implemented before the initial use of the medication and should be reevaluated as needed.

When planning for formulary additions and changes, the medication's integration into technology should be carefully coordinated. Dosage forms, concentrations, and ordering options should be limited and standardized.

Questions to ask when integrating new formulary medications into technology include the following:

- Should the routes of administration available for selection be limited?
- Are tall-man letters needed to distinguish from other medications?
- Are there significant medication interaction alerts that should be tested for appropriate firing?
- Are additional alerts or warnings needed for laboratory monitoring requirements, pregnancy contraindications, formulary restrictions, or other issues?
- Can appropriate and important lab results be displayed during order entry or verification?
- Are dose range-checking and smart pump-dosing recommendations integrated into the computer system and pumps? Are they correct?
- Should an order set be created to ease prescribing and monitoring requirements?
- Should the item be stored in ADCs?
- Should the medication be able to be overridden in ADCs?
- Are there additional alerts or warnings needed when withdrawing the medication from the ADC?

Standard Concentrations. Hospitals should standardize and limit the number of medication concentrations available; indeed, many regulatory agencies require the use of standardized concentrations. Standardization may help avoid error-prone calculations, reduce waste, streamline inventory, and facilitate the use of premixed i.v. solutions. The "rule of 6" should not be used, as this method for calculating concentrations of continuous infusions led to calculation errors and waste.[34] When more than 1 concentration is needed for medications, the institution should use consistent terminology (e.g., *double strength, maximum concentration*) and consider additional labeling to distinguish between concentrations (e.g., label comments, auxiliary labels). Furthermore, all needed concentrations should be available in the pharmacy verification system; conversely, rarely used or nonformulary concentrations should be removed.

National standardized concentrations should be used when they are available and are therapeutically appropriate. Standardize 4 Safety is a national initiative between ASHP and FDA to develop and implement national standardized concentrations for i.v. and oral liquid medications, both adult and pediatric. These standardized concentrations, as developed, will be available on the Standardize 4 Safety website.[35,36]

Safety-Alert Monitoring. Medication safety evaluation does not end when a medication is added to the formulary. The pharmacy department should continue to monitor the literature for new medication safety warnings, in addition to the review and analysis of the institution's medication error reporting data. Analyses and recommendations for handling safety alerts that impact the institution should be managed via the medication safety committee or the pharmacy and therapeutics committee.

Every institution or hospital system should have an ongoing mechanism to react to medication safety updates. ISMP's website and newsletters are unique resources and provide communication about medication errors and strategies to prevent their reoccurrence.[37] The ISMP website offers much of its content free of charge.

FDA also provides numerous methods to keep up-to-date with medication information. By signing up for the MedWatch E-list (email), clinicians will be notified when MedWatch alerts are released.

The National Alert Network (NAN) should be monitored for urgent advisories about serious errors or information requiring immediate attention. These alerts are distributed via ASHP and ISMP.[38] NAN alerts are incident driven and reach healthcare providers through several national distribution channels.

Safe Procurement. The pharmacy department must be responsible for all procurement of medications within the organization, including less-obvious patient care areas (e.g., diagnostic imaging, procedural areas).[39] Medications should not be brought in from outside sources without collaboration with the pharmacy department (e.g., samples, transfers from other institutions). The "ASHP Guidelines: Minimum Standard for Pharmacies in Hospitals" has a section on medication procurement that includes several safety recommendations, including how to handle medication samples and patients' home medication use in the hospital.[39] In short, samples should not be used for inpatient treatment and only used for outpatient treatment with appropriate policies and procedures in place (e.g., maintenance of records, proper storage). Likewise, a patient's own medications should only be used after prescriber order and pharmacist identification.

Pharmacists should be actively involved in the evaluation of all medication device purchasing and replacement decisions (e.g., pumps) and included in discussions related to devices that utilize medications for operational requirements (e.g., dialysis machines). In addition, patients may be admitted to hospitals with indwelling pumps, such as pain management or insulin pumps, and policy and procedures must be established to ensure safety and continuity of care with these unique medication delivery systems.

The pharmacy department should take a lead role in coordination of outsourcing services and should consult the "ASHP Guidelines on Outsourcing Pharmaceutical Services"[40] and the "ASHP Guidelines on Outsourcing Sterile Compounding Services."[41]

Medication Shortages Management. Hospitals, via the pharmacy department, should have a process to communicate medication shortages, including alternatives and substitution protocols, to prescribers and other clinical staff. The "ASHP Guidelines on Managing Drug Product Shortages in Hospitals and Health Systems" provides detailed guidance.[42] The pharmacy department should take a lead role in developing and managing a contingency plan in close collaboration with affected physicians and health-system committees when faced with severe shortages. Just as when considering the use of a new medication, alternative products should be examined for possible medication safety issues. Oftentimes with shortages, the medication may continue to be available but in a different size, dosage form, or concentration, so medication shortage action plans must examine the implications of these product changes for frontline staff, dispensing system automation, and EHRs. Furthermore, once a shortage is resolved, all system changes that have been made to address the shortage need to be reversed and corrected.

Storage

Careful arrangement of medication storage in the pharmacy and throughout the hospital can help reduce the risk of medication errors. In the pharmacy, product arrangement should minimize unintended selection of the wrong product or dosage form.[43,44] Steps to minimize selection of the wrong product or dosage form in the pharmacy include the following:

- Use barcode or RFID scanning in the pharmacy to ensure correct products are dispensed.
- Provide adequate space for each medication and strength.
- Ensure labels on bottles face forward.
- Designate separate areas for each dosage form or route of administration.
- Separate frequently confused pairs.
- Segregate high-alert medications and LASA medications.
- Use labeling and alerts when appropriate.

Ambiguous nomenclature should be avoided. The same drug nomenclature should be used in all databases used throughout the entire medication-use process (e.g., EHRs, pharmacy information system, infusion pumps, ADCs), using differentiation and screen alerts for medications that may pose a risk for potential errors, such as LASA medications, medications that should not be crushed, and high-alert medications. Wherever possible, generic names of medications should be used, unless the product is a combination product.

Pharmacy inventory should be managed to reduce the risk of errors associated with drug shortages and expired medications. A system for rotating stock should be established, and all areas should be monitored for expired medications and storage at appropriate temperatures. Because managing expired medications can be challenging, a schedule assigning staff to regularly inspect and remove expired medications should be implemented. A process should also be implemented to ensure medications are not used passed the beyond-use date (i.e., reconstituted bulk bottles).

All medications should be stored securely; access to secured medication areas should be limited to authorized personnel.[44]

Medications that should not be stored outside of the pharmacy include

- Concentrated electrolytes (i.e., potassium chloride, 3% sodium chloride)
- Concentrated oral opioid solutions
- Concentrated insulin U-500
- Sterile water in bags
- Concentrated epinephrine multidose vials
- Neuromuscular blocking agents[28]

The use of ADCs on nursing units can reduce the frequency of certain medication errors.[25,43,45,46] The ISMP guidance document can be consulted for ensuring safe use of an ADC.[25,43,45–47] Medications and the quantity that will be stocked in the ADC should be carefully selected. Medications should be in ready-to-use, unit dose, or unit-of-use containers. Avoid medications that are in bulk supply or those that are multidose vials. Do not stock medications that require extensive dilutions or calculations. Barcoding should be used to assist in stocking and restocking the correct medication. Medications should not be removed from storage until immediately before administration, and any doses that are not administered should be returned to controlled storage promptly. Nurses should not return medications to the ADC, returning them only to the ADC return bin. When configuring storage within the ADC, the use of individual, locked, locked-lidded compartments that open when the product is selected is preferred for all medications, if possible, but at a minimum for high-alert medications, reversal agents, and drugs prone to diversion. If matrix bins are used, each medication and strength must have a separate bin. Steps should be taken to differentiate LASA medications within the ADC. This may include a more-secured configuration of lidded drawers or locked-lidded drawers to separate these medications or make the bins more distinctive. Systematic inventory audits should be performed to identify and remove expired and low-usage products. The ADC functionality allows for medications to be vended from the machine after medication order review and verification by the pharmacist, which is the safest scenario. Functionality of override exists for emergency situations, which bypasses the pharmacist's review before nurse vending of the medication. The institution must define and approve the specific criteria to allow for medication overrides in emergency situations and specify which specific medication overrides should be allowed.

Patient Admission

Prescribing errors commonly occur during hospital admission for many reasons, and patients taking numerous medications are at a higher risk for adverse drug events (ADEs), which can include medication errors.[48] The "ASHP Statement on the Pharmacist's Role in Medication Reconciliation" outlines the importance of pharmacists sharing accountability with other hospital and health-system leaders for the ongoing success of the medication reconciliation processes across the continuum of care.[49]

Obtaining a medication history and performing medication reconciliation on admission are crucial, and it is recommended that pharmacy be involved in obtaining an accurate medication history. It is important to standardize this process across the institution in different settings (e.g., outpatient procedures, radiology), have 1 system used for both medication histories and reconciliation, and conduct ongoing education to ensure a safe system for patients.

It is important to have an institutional requirement for the timeframe for completion of medication histories and medication reconciliations. Many institutions require review and reconciliation of the medication list within 24 hours of an inpatient admission. However, high-alert and time-sensitive medications such as anticonvulsants, anticoagulants, antibiotics, and antiparkinsonian agents may need to be reconciled sooner.[50]

Ordering, Transcribing, and Reviewing

Ordering. Ordering errors are failures in the prescribing process that lead to or have the potential to lead to harm to the patient and are committed by credentialed providers, including physicians, nurse practitioners, physician assistants, privileged pharmacists, and others. Common ordering errors include omission, incomplete and unclear orders, wrong drug, wrong time, wrong dose, wrong dosage form, patient allergy, and wrong patient. There are a number of steps that providers must consider when ordering medications: patient assessment, ordering of diagnostic or monitoring tests, diagnoses, patient history, appropriate selection and dose of medication, concomitant therapies, and therapy duration. A single error in any of these steps could result in an ADE. To determine appropriate drug therapy, prescribers should stay abreast of the current state of pharmacotherapy practices and clinical practice guidelines. Prescribers should evaluate the patient's health status and review all existing drug therapy before prescribing new or additional medications. Differentiation between nonpreventable ADEs and medication errors is also a dynamic concept. Growing knowledge about how individual genetic differences result in altered drug metabolism, efficacy, and adverse effects provides a new opportunity to optimize medication use and reduce this category of prescribing errors.

Prescribers should be familiar with the medication-ordering system (e.g., EHR and downtime procedures, written order process, general medication order policy) and available safety-alert capabilities.[51] The following are recommendations for preventing medication ordering errors:

1. Medication orders must be complete and in compliance with the hospital's medication order policy. They should include patient identifiers (name, date of birth, patient number), patient allergies and weight in metric units, generic drug name, trademarked name (if a specific product is required), route and site of administration, dosage form, dose, strength, quantity, frequency of administration, intended duration of therapy, indication for use for as-needed orders, and prescriber's name. For i.v. medications, a concentration, rate, and time of administration should be specified. Prescribers should review all drug orders for accuracy and clarity immediately after they have prescribed them.
2. Care should be taken to ensure that the intent and indication of medication orders is clear. Prescribers should adhere to the following guidelines:
    a. Type or write out instructions and avoid using unapproved abbreviations. For example, use "daily" rather than "q.d." (which could be misinterpreted as q.i.d.) or "units" rather than "u" (which could be misinterpreted as a 0).
    b. Do not use vague or blanket instructions, such as "take as directed" or "resume preop meds," because specific directions can help differentiate among intended medications and clarify instructions for other clinicians.
    c. Limit the number of as-needed orders for the same therapeutic indication, and provide clear directions regarding the order and symptom hierarchy in which as-needed medications are to be used.
    d. Avoid range-of-frequency orders. If allowed by the organization, range-of-dose orders should use objective measures to determine the correct dose.
    e. Specify exact dosage strengths (such as milligrams or milliliters) rather than dosage form units (such as 1 tablet or 1 vial). An exception is for combination drug products, for which the number of dosage form units should be specified, and the combination product name should be identified in the comments field of the medication order.
    f. When applicable, pediatric prescriptions should be prescribed both in units/weight and total individual dose.[52] For example, if the patient weighs 10 kg, order as acetaminophen 100 mg (10 mg/kg).
    g. Prescribe by standard nomenclature, using the drug's generic name or trademarked name (if deemed medically necessary). Avoid the following: coined names (e.g., Dr. Doe's syrup or ketofol), chemical names (e.g., 6-mercaptopurine [instead of mercaptopurine] could result in a 6-fold overdose if misinterpreted), abbreviated drug names (e.g., "AZT" could stand for zidovudine, azathioprine, or aztreonam), drug names where numbers are part of the drug name (e.g., Tylenol #3), acronyms, and apothecary or chemical symbols (unless used as part of specifying a radioactive isotope).
    h. Always use a leading 0 before a decimal expression of <1 (e.g., 0.5 mL). Conversely, a trailing 0 should never be used (e.g., 5.0 mL), since failure to see the decimal could result in a 10-fold overdose. When possible, avoid the use of decimals (e.g., prescribe 500 mg rather than 0.5 g, 25 μg rather than 0.025 mg).
    i. Use the metric system.
3. Maximize the use of computerized prescriber order entry (CPOE). If CPOE is unavailable, written drug or

prescription orders (including signatures) should be legible. Prescribers with poor handwriting should print or type medication or prescription orders. A handwritten order should be completely readable, not merely recognizable through familiarity.

4. All unclear orders should be regarded as potential errors, as staff should not have to interpret what the physician is ordering. The hospital's patient safety culture should require nursing and pharmacy staff to stop processing the order until clarification is provided by the prescriber.
5. Verbal or telephonic medication orders should be reserved only for situations in which it is impossible or impractical for the prescriber to write the order or enter it into the computer (e.g., during an emergency situation, if prescriber is involved in a sterile procedure). The prescriber should dictate verbal orders slowly, clearly, and articulately to avoid confusion. The recipient must read back the order to the prescriber slowly, clearly, and articulately to avoid confusion. When read back, the medication name should be spelled out, and the drug dosage (e.g., 15 mg should be repeated as "one-five") and directions must be confirmed. Avoid using abbreviations during the read-back process.
6. The use of hold orders should be avoided. Instructions with respect to hold orders for medications must be clear. Most often, a hold order is interpreted as an order to discontinue the medication. The hold order must include duration or clearly identified point in time for continuation (e.g., hold until able to tolerate oral diet); otherwise, the medication must be reordered or renewed.
7. If automatic stop orders are used for therapy discontinuations due to safety reasons, active systems or reminders should be established for the prescriber to be notified that therapy will discontinue, with the opportunity to renew the order, if appropriate.
8. Automatic dosing protocols, such as therapeutic class substitutions/interchange, i.v.-to-oral switch, renal dosing, dose rounding, and automatic stop orders, should be clearly written or placed into the patient chart or EHR so interdisciplinary care providers know the originally ordered medication and the equivalent approved dose and frequency of the interchanged medication and can reference the approved conversion chart or protocol if needed.
9. Maximize the use of standard order sets regardless of whether using a paper-based or an EHR. Well-designed order sets integrate and coordinate care by communicating best practices through multiple disciplines, levels of care, and services; promoting evidence-based care; reducing variation and unintentional oversight; enhancing workflow with pertinent instructions that are easily understood and intuitively organized; and reducing unnecessary calls to physicians for clarifications and questions about orders.[53]
10. All new prescribers must have sufficient training and mentoring on medication order entry.

Transcribing. Transcribing errors are defined as any deviation during the transfer of information from an order sheet to documentation forms or medication administration records (MARs). Transcribing involves orders that are manually transcribed into written records (e.g., MAR) and those that are electronically transcribed into the EHR. Some of the contributing factors include incomplete or illegible prescriber orders, incomplete or illegible nurse handwriting, use of error-prone abbreviations, inappropriate defaults in the EHR, and lack of familiarity with drug names, doses, or frequencies. Common transcribing errors include wrong drug name, dose, route, frequency, or patient. An environment that is noisy or poorly lit can also contribute to errors. EHRs with CPOE capability increase the speed and accuracy of transcription, which results in fewer medication errors. Reduction of handwritten orders, verbal orders, and standardized order sets also expedite the transcription of orders without CPOE. The following are recommendations for preventing transcribing medication errors[54]:

1. Clarify the order before the prescriber leaves the patient care unit. If the prescriber has left the unit, contact the prescriber before transcribing the order.
2. Do not process incomplete orders. Orders must contain the information required in the hospital's medication order policy.
3. Minimize the use of error-prone abbreviations and avoid the use of unapproved abbreviations on the MAR.
4. Always use a leading zero before a decimal, and never use a trailing zero after the decimal.
5. Complete the transcription process in a quiet, well-lit area, away from distractions.
6. Implement a system to check the MAR document against active orders whether the MAR is manually or computer generated.
7. Implement a second check system for the transcription.

Reviewing. Order review errors are normally those that are committed during the process where the pharmacist reviews the prescriber's medication order. However, order review errors may also occur when a proper order review is omitted or when the order review does not occur in a timely manner (e.g., hospital pharmacy is not open 24 hours and does not have telepharmacy services or medication order has been overridden). A fundamental responsibility of a pharmacist is to review the medication order to ensure its appropriateness. Pharmacists must prospectively review all medication orders before the preparation and dispensing of medications, with only a few exceptions (e.g., licensed independent practitioner [LIP] present, urgent situation, LIP in emergency room, screening tool for contrast media in radiology). When medications are dispensed without pharmacist review or on override, the LIP assumes the role of the pharmacist in checking the order for appropriateness. Common order review errors include but are not limited to wrong drug, wrong dose, wrong patient, wrong route, wrong rate, wrong diluent, wrong dosage form, wrong time, and missed allergy.

Preparation

Preparation, or admixture, errors are generally considered to occur within the pharmacy department, but they can occur anywhere in the continuum of care when a medication is changed or manipulated from the manufacturer's packaged preparation in any way before being administered to the patient. Common preparation errors include wrong concentration, wrong drug, wrong dose, wrong base solution/diluent, wrong volume, preparations made for the wrong patient, and preparations prepared for administration by the wrong route.

Preparation should occur under proper conditions of sanitation, temperature, light, moisture, ventilation, segregation, and security to ensure medication integrity and personnel safety throughout the hospital.[39]

In most cases, if an item is prepared within the pharmacy and is prepared by a pharmacy technician, an independent double check of the preparation is made by a licensed pharmacist. The same policy may not apply if a pharmacist is preparing the medication or if the item is prepared outside of the pharmacy. Every effort should be made to minimize the compounding of sterile preparations outside of the pharmacy. When compounding does occur outside of the pharmacy, the department of pharmacy should be involved in policies and procedures for items compounded outside the pharmacy and the checking process that is utilized. Ideally, regardless of licensure or job description of the individual who prepares the medication, an independent double check of the preparation should occur. The double check should include verification of the ingredients used, the quantities of the ingredients, and the expiration dates of all components. ISMP recommends performing an independent verification of medications and diluents to ensure the proper ingredients and proper amounts are confirmed before adding them to the final preparation.[55] Doing so eliminates the proxy method of verifying compounded sterile preparations (e.g., utilization of the syringe pullback method as a means to double check the accuracy of prepared medications). Another way to eliminate proxy methods is to use technologies that build barcoding not only into the administration and dispensing phases but also the preparation phase of the medication-use system. In addition to barcoding, pharmacy automation used to improve the safety of the preparation phase includes repackaging equipment, gravimetric verification, compounding technologies, and technology utilized in telepharmacy operations.

Whenever possible, medications should be available for inpatient use in unit-of-use and ready-to-administer packaging without further manipulation by the person administering the medication. Every effort should be made to reduce situations where the person administering the medication has to withdraw doses from containers, reconstitute powdered drug products, split tablets, or perform other similar manipulations. When oral products are not available in unit-of-use packaging, pharmacy staff should repackage these preparations. ASHP's "Technical Assistance Bulletin on Repackaging Oral Solids and Liquids in Single Unit and Unit Dosed Packages" provides detailed guidance on best practices for repackaging.[56] Care should be taken to protect patients and staff if hazardous drugs are being repackaged.[57,58] If barcode technology is integrated into any step of the medication-use process at a hospital, a barcode must be affixed to any repackaged item. The organization should have specific policies and procedures for determining the type of barcode for each repackaged item and how that barcode will be used throughout the medication-use process.

Preparation of medications via feeding tubes is another aspect of preparation, and there are many different types of feeding tubes. Some medications cannot be crushed or chewed, as absorption is disrupted, and some medications cannot be opened for feeding tube use due to biohazard reasons.

Aside from repackaging, compounding is the main mechanism used to prepare medications. Whether nonsterile or sterile compounding is occurring, staff must be adequately trained and facilities must be in compliance with current state and federal standards and regulations to minimize potential for medication errors. Personnel should not only be adequately trained, but must also maintain and document competency on a regular basis for all processes and procedures for which they are responsible. For instance, attention must be paid to calculations, compatibility of preparations, proper storage, and quality-assurance principles. Many compounding errors are due to miscalculations that can result in extreme overdosing or underdosing of a patient, especially in pediatric patients or when high-risk medications like chemotherapy are involved, or can create an incompatibility situation. Incompatibility errors can range from delays in products going into the solution in a timely manner to the combining of 2 drugs creating a dangerous situation for a patient (i.e., calcium and phosphorus binding in parenteral nutrient solutions, creating precipitates). Knowledge of storage requirements, expiration dates of products, and beyond-use dates of preparations is needed to ensure that a properly prepared compound maintains its integrity during the transport and storage phases.

Extemporaneous nonsterile dosage forms include items such as solutions, suspensions, creams, ointments, capsules, suppositories, troches, emulsions, and powders. The medical literature adequately explains the proper processes and procedures that should be followed when preparing these types of products. *United States Pharmacopeia* (*USP*) chapter 795, among other chapters, outlines many important details about the stability and beyond-use dating of nonsterile compounds.[59] This minimum standard should be followed by individuals preparing nonsterile compounds, but the use of additional quality measures is encouraged. In addition, ASHP's "Technical Assistance Bulletin on Compounding Nonsterile Products in Pharmacies" speaks to best practices in this area.[60] Sterile compounding involves products that need to be sterile when they are administered, such as injections of any type including epidural and intrathecal preparations, irrigations for wounds or body cavities, ophthalmic preparations, and aqueous bronchial and nasal inhalations. *USP* chapter 797 outlines the minimum standards for sterile compounding, regardless of the setting or compounding personnel involved. Additional *USP* chapters apply to sterile compounding and should be evaluated as well. For example, *USP* chapter 85 addresses endotoxin testing, *USP* chapter 71 addresses sterility testing, and *USP* chapter 800 addresses compounding of hazardous preparations.[61] Many state boards of pharmacy have adopted *USP* chapter 797 into the state regulations, at least in part, and inspectors survey against this standard. Very specific guidance is provided for environmental quality, responsibilities of compounding personnel, cleaning and disinfecting the compounding area, and facility design in this chapter. ISMP and ASHP have also promulgated sterile compounding guidelines.[62,63]

All of the published guidelines stress that compounding personnel be competent in preparing compounded sterile preparations and understand the levels of environmental and end-process testing and validation required to ensure the quality and safety of the products. Aseptic technique is required in all sterile compounding situations, and personnel must be adequately trained and regularly audited for competency. Risk levels and subsequent beyond-use dates are to be assigned by compounding personnel and are determined by the complexity of the compounding process and the conditions in which the preparation is made.[59]

Automation is often incorporated into sterile compounding, and the equipment is regularly being updated and new technologies continue to enter the market. Compounders (i.e., those used for parenteral nutrition), repeater pumps, cameras or recording devices for quality documentation, robotic systems, and others are used in sterile compounding. I.V. workflow software and technology must be used for the preparation of sterile admixtures as per the i.v. workflow software and technology instructions for use. Compounding personnel must be competent in using, calibrating, cleaning, and updating existing systems. A solid understanding of all checks and balances built into the organization's sterile compounding processes and the reasons for them must be understood by all compounding personnel to minimize the likelihood of bypassing these systems. Similarly, frontline compounding personnel should be involved in FMEA of new technologies used in compounding or other preparation areas.

USP chapter 800 addresses the additional element of protecting the individual preparing the items.[64] In most cases, the preparation of hazardous drugs involves a sterile compounding process, with care taken to avoid exposure of compounding personnel to the hazardous substance. A closed-system transfer device shall be used, as feasible, in the preparation of hazardous drugs. Avoidance of errors in hazardous drug compounding requires similar processes and procedures to those used in nonhazardous drug compounding.

The outsourcing of compounded products is a common practice. Organizations that utilize products made by an outsourced compounding facility should refer to the "ASHP Guidelines on Outsourcing Sterile Compounding Services" and the ASHP Research and Education Foundation's outsourcing sterile products preparation tool.[41,65] These guidance statements provide a mechanism for hospitals to evaluate compounding facilities and determine if practices are aligned with hospital pharmacy leadership decisions to outsource. Similarly, health systems outsourcing radiopharmaceuticals should be familiar with the American Pharmacists Association radiopharmaceutical vendor qualification checklist.[66]

Since neonates, infants, and many young children are unable to swallow solid oral dosages, most medications are needed in a liquid formulation. This requires nonsterile or sterile compounding with often-complex calculations to provide the proper dilution for the patient.

Since many oral pediatric medications are prepared in oral liquid formulations (dilutions, solutions, and suspensions), the potential for confusing an oral syringe and an i.v. syringe exists. Best practices recommend only using oral syringes for oral preparations and never using i.v. syringes for oral medication administration.[52] Similarly, products intended for other routes (e.g., potentially containing particulates or pyrogens or not sterile) should not be dispensed in an i.v. bag to avoid mistaken administration by the parenteral route.

Dispensing

All medications in nonemergency situations should be reviewed by a pharmacist (or advanced pharmacy technician qualified and trained to perform "tech-check-tech") before dispensing. The pharmacist should review the original medication order (either the written order or the electronic order). The pharmacist should ensure that all work performed by supportive personnel or through the use of automated devices is checked by manual or technological means. At a minimum, pharmacists should participate in a self-checking process in reading prescriptions, labeling (drug or ingredients and pharmacist-generated labeling), and dosage calculations. For high-alert drug products (e.g., chemotherapy, pediatric medication, total parenteral nutrition), work should be independently checked by a second individual, preferably another pharmacist.[30] Selective use of this strategy can play an important role in medication safety. Pharmacists must make certain that the following are accurate: drug, labeling, packaging, quantity, dose, and instructions. The double check should be done by a second independent practitioner at a different time, not simultaneously with the first pharmacist.

Hospitals with ADCs often experience medication order overrides when a member of the patient care staff withdraws medications from the ADC before pharmacist review of the medication order if a delay would harm the patient or if the patient experiences a sudden change in clinical status.[67] The practice of overrides bypasses the safety net of pharmacy review and should be minimized.[46] The hospital's pharmacy and therapeutics committee and medication safety committee should develop and implement a list of medications with corresponding indications that are authorized for override and include criteria for appropriate override of medications along with the clinical indication for overriding the medication (e.g., aspirin and chest pain), for specific circumstances, and for monitoring compliance to minimize risk. The ADC security functions should be utilized and programmed to maximize medication security and decrease the frequency of overrides. An override monitoring process should be developed, and audits should be performed to ensure appropriate use by nurses and other authorized staff. Available technology, such as barcoding, that complements the ordering, transcribing, and reviewing section of the medication-use process should be used.[46]

Hospitals that do not offer 24-hour pharmacy service should investigate the possibility of telepharmacy or remote review. If these are not possibilities, a qualified healthcare professional (e.g., head nurse, night nurse supervisor) who can conduct the medication order review in the absence of the pharmacist should be identified. The qualified healthcare professional must be trained on the components of an appropriate medication order.

A pharmacist should conduct a retrospective review of all medication orders generated while the pharmacy was closed (if not conducted by telepharmacy) as soon as a pharmacist is available or the pharmacy opens. A pharmacist verifying orders from another site should have access to drug information and local policies of the non-24-7 site and should have a mechanism to document and communicate problem orders as well as contact the non-24-7 site leadership for orders needing clarification. "ASHP Guidelines on Remote Medication Order Processing" provide clear direction on safe practices.[68]

Administration

Administration Errors. The "5 rights of medication administration"—the right patient, the right drug, the right dose, the right route, and the right time—are often discussed in relation to administration errors.[69,70] The list of "rights" that should be confirmed before administration continues to evolve and is not without controversy since this process still has potential for human error. Common administration errors include wrong patient, wrong route, wrong dosage form, wrong time, wrong dose or rate, and wrong drug.[70] Additional errors in this category may include errors of omission or missed doses. Administration errors that are more specific to i.v. administration include wrong rate or incompatibility at the Y-site of the infusion.

Accidental connections between enteral feeding tubing and epidural and/or i.v. tubing connections can have catastrophic patient effects. Efforts are underway by the Global Enteral Device Supplier Association to design new standards for medical device tubing.[71] The goal of this international working group is to reduce the incidence of tubing misconnections by designing new devices that do not allow connection between unrelated delivery systems. The group is starting with enteral devices.

Practitioners at the bedside are able to prevent a significant number of prescribing and dispensing errors from reaching the patient. When appropriate, independent double checks for high-alert medications should be completed before administration by completing independent calculations and checking the patient's allergies. Before administering the medication to the patient, 2 patient identifiers should be verified along with communicating the indication for the medication to ensure the patient is knowledgeable about his or her medication's indications, duration, and potential adverse effects. This communication can identify potential errors. While nurses are most often the practitioners administering medication, other health professionals—including physicians, pharmacists, respiratory therapists, radiology technologists, and rehabilitation staff—also administer medications in the scope of their practice, and the same safe practices apply.

Barcode-assisted medication administration (BCMA) can improve medication safety by verifying that the right drug is being administered to the right patient.[72] Studies have shown that BCMA technology can help reduce medication administration errors.[73,74]

However, if BCMA is not executed appropriately, medication errors can still occur. If a pharmacy-generated label is placed on the wrong medication or covers the information on a manufacturer's label, the BCMA system will not detect this error. When possible, the original manufacturer barcode that appears directly on the product should be scanned instead of the pharmacy label. FDA currently requires barcodes on containers but does not require that unit dose containers be available for all medications. Since not all manufacturers provide barcoded unit-of-use dosage forms and pharmacies routinely prepare half-tablets, automated repackaging equipment is often used. It is essential that a robust verification process is implemented within the pharmacy to ensure proper labeling and dispensing of these medications.

The effectiveness of BCMA is limited by the degree it is used at the bedside. If workarounds are used, errors will still occur. Common examples of workarounds include silencing alerts, using a second preprinted patient label or medication barcode, manually entering the information when the barcode does not scan correctly, and scanning the medications outside of the patient's room. Evaluating workflow concerns and monitoring BCMA user data on compliance with scanning can assist in combating workarounds.

To ensure BCMA is being used effectively, BCMA reports should be evaluated regularly to assess compliance and identify potential barriers. Direct observation should also be employed to ensure workarounds are not being used. There should also be a process to notify the pharmacy when products are not scanning properly. The pharmacy should dispense patient-specific doses with barcodes whenever possible.

Administration of I.V. Medications via Smart Infusion Pumps. Intravenous medication administration errors account for a large number of medication errors.[74] Technology has been focused on decreasing medication errors related to i.v. administration. Infusion devices include gravity administration pumps, pumps that prevent free flow, and smart or intelligent pumps that include built-in medication libraries or guidelines that provide a range for safe administration doses, concentrations, and rates of administration. As with any technology, the devices are only as smart as the information entered into them and are limited by the degree of adoption by the bedside clinician.

Best practices in the area of smart infusion pumps should include a multidisciplinary approach to standardizing concentrations of i.v. medications, evaluation of interoperability options between the pumps and other technology in the organization, setting the lower and upper dosing limits, and careful use of soft and hard limits. Hard limits cannot be bypassed, so they can be a strategic safety step to reduce dangerous use of i.v. medications. If excessive alerts are created, alert fatigue will occur and key safety information alerts will be bypassed. Determination of the medications to be included in the pump, how the medications are listed (i.e., alphabetically by generic name), which areas of the hospital should use them, and how they are operated should not be made without inclusion of pharmacy, nursing, medical staff, and information technology assistance. Many facilities are challenged due to low compliance with the use of smart pumps and the associated drug libraries. If the end user does not select a drug from the drug library and enter the correct information into the pump, the pump safety features are bypassed. Pumps that utilize barcode scanning linked to autoprogramming of the pump assist with adherence to these features. Similarly, the pumps cannot prevent line switch errors on their own. The basic review of tracing the line back from the infusion site to the channel on the pump should occur.

Data that are available from the pumps vary depending on the pump manufacturer and may require wireless or wired downloads of the data to allow for pump optimization. Policies and procedures for how data downloads and pump queries will be completed should be included in the standard operating procedures for infusion pump use. Similarly, policies and procedures should be determined for how and when medication libraries are updated, who is authorized to approve the changes, and how unique situations such as drug shortages should be handled. The pumps also have continuous quality-improvement data programs that can generate reports and trends of medication alerts overridden, bypassed soft alerts, and the use of the free-text or wildcard function for medications not having standardized entries in the pump. The pharmacy should take a leadership role in analyzing these data to keep the drug library settings for alerts, alarms, and advisories as robust as possible while continually improving the settings to reflect current best practices.

Practitioner Education. Although nurses are the most common healthcare providers to administer medications, they are not the only practitioners to do so. All practitioners responsible for administering medications should be properly trained on administration procedures. Healthcare systems must establish effective medication administration education programs for practitioners. These programs must include proper patient identification; familiarization with the medication ordering, reviewing, preparing, dispensing, and monitoring system; proper utilization of the 5 rights as a team approach and not just the responsibility of 1 member; medication administration devices; metric equivalents; basic dosage and flow rate calculations; administration of high-alert medications; and effective implementation of independent double checks.[69] Education and training should be documented in the staff competency files and conducted periodically or as needed.

Patient Education. Patients and their direct caregivers have the right to know about all aspects of their care, including drug therapy. When patient status allows, healthcare providers should encourage patients to take an active role in their drug therapy by questioning and learning about their treatment regimens in order to act as their advocate and help prevent medication errors. Nurses, pharmacists, or healthcare providers can instruct the patient or direct caregiver on the name and purpose of the prescribed medications, guidelines for safe administration, possible adverse effects, and actions to take if problems occur. Effective communication is imperative and helps ensure better adherence to treatment plans. Basic communication techniques include asking open-ended questions, reflecting patient comments back to them, using the teach-back method, and employing active listening. Patients should be able to explain in their own words how to take their medications and what to expect from the treatment. Clinical staff must be able to recognize a patient's level of health literacy and English language proficiency and take appropriate actions to ensure effective communication.[76] Patients should be instructed to maintain a personal list of all medication therapy including prescribed drugs, nonprescription drugs, home remedies, and medical foods. Patients should also feel free to ask questions about any procedures and treatments received.[77] Educating patients about the safe and effective use of medication promotes patient involvement in healthcare and can help prevent medication errors. It is very important to involve patients in the administration step as they may be helpful in catching errors as well.

Monitoring

Monitoring errors may be categorized as follows:

- Failure to monitor medication effects
- Incorrect interpretation of laboratory data used to monitor medication effects
- Incorrect transcription of laboratory test values
- Incorrect timing of monitoring
- Incorrect timing of serum concentration monitoring

Examples of failing to monitor medication effects include not checking a scheduled blood glucose level and checking the level but not reacting to the level. Incorrect interpretation errors might include checking the blood glucose level but giving the wrong amount of corrective or sliding-scale insulin for the value. Incorrect transcription of laboratory test values may include transposed numbers or numbers being transcribed in the wrong place. Incorrect timing errors may occur when a blood glucose level is taken at the wrong time relative to meals or an aminoglycoside level is not taken as a true trough level. Where possible, guidelines for the correct time to obtain blood for serum concentrations and laboratory values should be created collaboratively by pharmacists, nurses, physicians, and laboratory staff. Critical values should be determined with action alerts generated electronically for clinicians, if possible.

Failure to Monitor. Failure to monitor medication therapy for efficacy and toxicity may result in treatment failure or unrecognized adverse drug reactions. Hospitals and health systems should train staff to identify common adverse effects encountered by patients and have a pathway in place to react to adverse reactions. If an adverse drug reaction occurs, the patient should be stabilized first and then the reaction (e.g., allergy, contraindication, side effect or intolerance) should be documented in the patient's medical record to allow all practitioners caring for the patient access to the event. If warranted, an allergy to the medication should be placed in the medical record. If criteria are met, the adverse reaction should be reported to MedWatch. Further guidance on how to respond to adverse drug reactions can be found in the "ASHP Guidelines on Adverse Drug Reaction Monitoring and Reporting."[78]

Similarly, practitioners should be adequately trained to monitor for efficacy of medications. Monitoring may come in the form of checking vital signs, monitoring blood glucose, monitoring electrocardiograms, or evaluating other laboratory or test results. When an inadequate response to medication is observed, practitioners need to know how to optimize the patient's therapy and the protocol to do so. For instance, in the case of a high blood glucose result, there should be a protocol in place to automatically increase the rate of an insulin infusion to account for the higher blood glucose. If a protocol does not formally exist, all practitioners need to be aware of how and when to alert prescribers to critical levels. Required monitoring for efficacy and toxicity should be built into order panels or order sets whenever possible. Pharmacists can take a leadership role in developing such nursing-driven or pharmacist-driven dosing algorithms or order sets. In the hospital, institutional protocols approved by the pharmacy and therapeutics committee can allow pharmacists or nurses to automatically modify dosing, obtain and administer necessary rescue medications (e.g., naloxone, dextrose 50%), and order laboratory tests for patient safety (i.e., point-of-care blood glucose test).

Incorrect Interpretation. Root causes of incorrect interpretation errors may include distractions, interruptions, workload, lack of training, confusing protocols, and incorrect documentation. Distractions should be minimized when practitioners are evaluating patient data. Interpreting patient data requires focus, an understanding of the process at hand, and easy access to normal ranges. Clear documentation of the values being monitored must exist to facilitate correct interpretation of data. If a protocol exists, the protocol should be clearly written and readily available such that all practitioners can interpret the protocol in the same way. Practitioners should be adequately trained on interpreting patient data.

Incorrect Transcription. Transcribing errors can impact safety when laboratory or point-of-care testing values are recorded incorrectly. These values are critical to patient care decisions and must be documented correctly. Transcription errors include not only transcribing or reporting the wrong laboratory value for a patient but also documenting values for the wrong patient. Contributing factors include lack of technology adoption or utilization, lack of efficient workflow, workload, lack of 2 patient identifiers, and lack of a common place to record data. Many organizations have multiple places where vital signs, pain scores, and bedside blood glucose monitoring are documented. Without a standard place for practitioners to look for this information, the potential for error is present.

Incorrect Timing. Timing of laboratory blood draws and other bedside monitoring is critical for accuracy of patient data. Alerts and orders for specific timing of monitoring can be built into decision support software, but care must be taken not to contribute to alert fatigue. Standardization of medication administration times and pertinent monitoring times should be built into the workflow as much as possible. For instance, many organizations have standard times for monitoring International Normalized Ratios (INRs) in relation to warfarin dosing, along with a standard daily administration time for warfarin. For titratable medications (e.g., heparin, vasopressors, insulin), timing of monitoring should be built into order sets. All values should be documented with time and date so that the practitioner reviewing the data has the proper frame of reference for the values.

Patient Discharge

Pharmacists' involvement in activities before patient discharge provides a valuable opportunity to prevent potential medication errors. Data show that adverse events are a major cause of avoidable hospital readmissions; more postdischarge adverse events are related to medications than other causes.[79] Lack of adherence to medications prescribed at discharge has also contributed to postdischarge ADEs.[80] Common errors include patients unable to obtain their medications at discharge due to availability, transportation, or insurance coverage; patients not scheduling follow-up appointments and laboratory tests; patients being discharged without all prescribed medications or equipment (e.g., blood glucose monitors); lack of monitoring; and confusion regarding how to take the medications and which prehospitalization medications to discontinue. Pharmacists can contribute to positive outcomes by educating and counseling patients to prepare and motivate them to follow their pharmacotherapeutic regimens and monitoring plans after discharge.[77]

Effective, open-ended questioning and active listening are essential skills for obtaining information from and sharing information with patients. Pharmacists have to adapt messages to fit patients' communication skills and primary languages through the use of teaching aids, interpreters, or cultural guides if necessary. Pharmacists also need to observe and interpret the nonverbal messages (e.g., eye contact, facial expressions, body movements, vocal characteristics) patients give during education and counseling sessions. Education and counseling are most effective when conducted in a room or space that ensures privacy and opportunity to engage in confidential communication. Patient education focused on medications (e.g., drug–food interaction, INR monitoring, and adherence for anticoagulation) and complex pharmacotherapeutic regimens (e.g., glucometer, insulin administration, and multiple medications for diabetes) could prevent medication errors and potential readmission. Proper education empowers patients to participate in their healthcare and provides a safeguard against errors.[81] Caregivers and family members should be involved whenever appropriate.

Pharmacists should participate in multidisciplinary discharge committees and be involved in the medication reconciliation process before discharge. Medication reconciliation requires explaining differences between the medications a patient was taking before admission to the hospital and medications prescribed for the patient during hospitalization. At hospital discharge, an accurate list of medications that a patient is to take after discharge should be provided to the patient.[82] Pharmacists can recognize patients who are at high risk or on complex medication regimens for follow-up by an ambulatory care pharmacist. Pharmacists also can take an active role in discharge medication procurement and explanation of insurance plans and coverage to ensure patients have their medications in-hand before leaving the hospital. If this is not possible, the pharmacist can educate the patient on the newly added medications and prescription plan coverage or prior-authorization processes.

The responsibility for the prevention of medical errors rests not only with healthcare professionals and healthcare systems but also with the patients themselves. By being informed of the names of their medications, the reasons for their use, the times they should be administered, and the correct dose, patients can act as the final check in the system. The practice of carrying an updated list of medications can be invaluable in the event of an emergency or if patients cannot speak for themselves. This reduces the chance of miscommunication or misinformation. When patients take an active and informed role in their healthcare, many errors can be prevented.

Evaluation

Healthcare organizations should continuously evaluate their systems and processes in order to prevent medication errors. The "ASHP Guidelines: Minimum Standard for Pharmacies in Hospitals" states, "There shall be an ongoing systematic program for quality assessment and improvement of pharmacy services and the medication-use system."[39] Quality-improvement activities should be routinely performed.

In the planning section, best practices for proactive evaluation of safety by using self-assessments and FMEA are outlined. This section focuses on retrospective evaluation of safety processes:

- RCA
- Medication-use evaluation
- Quality improvement
- Event detection

RCA. RCA is a method used to identify system vulnerabilities after an event or close call and to develop an action plan that will prevent the same event from occurring again or at least minimize the possibility of reoccurrence. This method is used after an event occurs, in contrast to FMEA described previously, which is a proactive method for preempting problems. The implementation and effectiveness of the RCA action items should be monitored.[83] Typically, RCAs are used for serious or significant events that the institution wishes to evaluate in closer detail, but the process may be utilized for any event. Each institution must decide who or what determines when an RCA is conducted. In some states, an RCA may be required for sentinel or other serious events.[84] The RCA should be conducted and recommendations implemented within a timely manner. For sentinel events, the Joint Commission requires that hospitals "prepare a thorough and credible comprehensive systematic analysis and action plan within 45 business days of the event or of becoming aware of the event."[85] An RCA is 1 such comprehensive systemic analysis, but other tools and methodologies may be used.

The health system should identify a standard method and template for performing the RCA and for reporting the results and recommendations. Various RCA resources, experts, and consultants are available. Various templates may be used including the VA National Center for Patient Safety tool and the Joint Commission tool.[86,87] In 2016, the National Patient Safety Foundation released recommendations on conducting an RCA entitled *RCA²: Improving Root Cause Analyses and Actions to Prevent Harm.*[88] The institution should consider implementation of these recommendations, which include leadership involvement, timely review, team membership recommendations, and a risk-based prioritization system to identify events requiring RCA review and actions to be taken.

Pharmacy department leadership should provide adequate time for pharmacy staff to attend the RCA meetings, including any needed training.[89] Medication safety officers and pharmacists should be involved in any RCA that is evaluating a medication-related event. Individuals leading RCAs should undergo training.

Medication-Use Evaluation. Medication-use evaluation is a performance improvement tool that evaluates specific medication issues or medication-use processes with the ultimate goal of improving patient care. For further information, consult the "ASHP Guidelines on the Medication-Use Evaluation."[90] Medication-use evaluation may be used to evaluate and audit a specific high-alert medication, a frequently occurring event, or any other high-alert or error-prone system or medication. Once data collection is completed, data can be evaluated and used to make process improvements, formulary guidelines or restrictions, or decision-support rules to promote best practices.

Quality Improvement. The Health Resources and Services Administration defines quality improvement as "systematic and continuous actions that lead to measurable improvement in healthcare services and the health status of targeted patient groups."[91] Describing the various methods and techniques used in improving healthcare quality is beyond the scope of this guideline. However, pharmacists who participate in medication safety practices should have a working knowledge of the methodologies and tools used in their healthcare system, such as Plan-Do-Study-Act, Lean Production System, Six-Sigma, TeamSTEPPS, and FOCUS-PDCA.[92,93] Changes to processes and systems should follow 1 of these methodologies for optimal planning and success.

Event Detection. To reduce preventable medication errors, clinicians must understand what risks are already present in their institutions. Clinicians may learn of events and close calls from various methods including

- Voluntary reporting
- Direct observation method
- Chart review (e.g., trigger medications, such as antidotes and reversal agents)
- Information technology (e.g., computer alerts, data mining, BCMA compliance, data from i.v. infusion pump)
- Pharmacist therapeutic interventions

Voluntary reporting via paper or electronic means is the most basic and common process for event detection, and every institution should have a method to report all events that either reached the patient or did not reach the patient (close calls). The reporting process should be relatively easy and not cumbersome, and reporting should be encouraged and supported by supervisors. For example, some institutions have implemented a "Good Catch" program where clinicians are rewarded with a small prize and acknowledgment. Staff should be educated as to how medication error reports will be used (for safety improvements, not as a success metric).[94] The culture of the organization is key to ensuring staff are comfortable in reporting. Furthermore, when appropriate, individuals who report events should be notified of safety improvements that have occurred as a result; this information may also be shared more collectively at staff meetings (again, as appropriate). However, because voluntary reporting is dependent on many factors, including patient safety culture, type of reporting system, and staff recognition and knowledge, pharmacists should use a combination of the above methods to detect medication errors.[94] Voluntary reporting often collects the most significant events but does not provide a comprehensive look at adverse events or medication errors.

Pharmacists should also share events with external reporting systems for large-scale tracking and trend analysis. For example, events might be shared with the product manufacturer, equipment and technology vendor, FDA, and ISMP.[8] Institutions may also choose to report events through federal patient safety organizations (PSOs). PSOs were developed under the Patient Safety and Quality Improvement Act of 2005 and encourage clinicians and healthcare organizations to voluntarily report and share quality and patient safety information to enhance quality and safety nationally.[95]

Regardless of how medication errors are discovered, the information should be used to prevent future errors. A multidisciplinary group should evaluate error information where feasible to develop risk-reduction strategies. While it is important to focus on errors that have caused harm to the patient, close calls should also be reviewed.

Conclusion

While medication errors cannot always be prevented, organizations can mitigate and reduce harm through robust system redesign, help employees make safe behavioral choices, and understand why people make the choices they make. If system faults and behavioral choices are understood, risk-reduction strategies can be created. Medication errors can occur at any point of the medication-use system. Health-system pharmacists have the responsibility and expertise to lead and participate in multidisciplinary committees to examine and improve systems currently in place.

References

1. Hepler CD, Strand LM. Opportunities and responsibilities in pharmaceutical care. *Am J Hosp Pharm.* 1990; 47:533–43.
2. National Coordinating Council for Medication Error Reporting and Prevention. About medication errors. www.nccmerp.org/about-medication-errors (accessed 2017 Jun 13).
3. Kohn LT, Corrigan JM, Donaldson MS, eds. To err is human: building a safer health system. Washington, DC: National Academy Press; 1999:ix.
4. Wachter RM. The end of the beginning: patient safety five years after "to err is human." *Health Aff.* 2004; 24:534–45.
5. Wachter RM. Patient safety at ten: unmistakable progress, troubling gaps. *Health Aff.* 2010; 29:1165–73.
6. National Patient Safety Foundation. Free from harm: accelerating patient safety improvement fifteen years after to err is human. www.npsf.org/?page=freefromharm (accessed 2017 Jun 13).
7. Aspden P, Wolcott J, Bootman JL et al. Preventing medication errors: quality chasm series. www.nap.edu/read/11623/chapter/1 (accessed 2017 Jun 13).
8. Smetzer JL, Cohen MR. Medication error reporting systems. In: Cohen MR, ed. Medication errors, 2nd ed. Washington, DC: American Pharmacists Association; 2007:513–50.
9. Reason J. Human error: models and management. *BMJ.* 2000; 320:768–70.
10. American Society of Health-System Pharmacists. ASHP long-range vision for the pharmacy work force in hospitals and health systems. *Am J Health-Syst Pharm.* 2007; 64:1320–30.
11. American Society of Health-System Pharmacists. ASHP statement: role of the medication safety leader. *Am J Health-Syst Pharm.* 2013; 70:448–552.
12. University of Missouri Health System. Caring for the caregiver. www.muhealth.org/about/qualityofcare/office-of-clinical-effectiveness/foryou-team/caring-for-caregivers (accessed 2017 Jun 13).
13. Krzan KD, Merandi J, Morvay S et al. Implementation of "second-victim" program in pediatric hospital. *Am J Health-Syst Pharm.* 2015; 72:563–7.
14. ASHP policy 1524: support for second victims. In: Hawkins B, ed. Best practices: positions and guidance documents of ASHP. 2015–2016 ed. Bethesda, MD: American Society of Health-System Pharmacists; 2015:212.
15. Gragg DN. Designing an internal reporting and learning system. In: Manasse HR, Thompson KK, eds. Medication safety: a guide for health care facilities. Bethesda, MD: American Society of Health-System Pharmacists. 2005:171–83.
16. American Society of Health-System Pharmacists. ASHP statement on reporting medical errors. *Am J Health-Syst Pharm.* 2000; 57:1531–2.
17. May S. Building an effective medication safety team. In: Manasse HR, Thompson KK, eds. Medication safety: a guide for health care facilities. Bethesda, MD: American Society of Health-System Pharmacists; 2005:89–105.
18. Marvin K. The safe use of technology in hospitals and health systems. In: Manasse HR, Thompson KK, eds. Medication safety: a guide for health care facilities. Bethesda, MD: American Society of Health-System Pharmacists; 2005:185–200.
19. Grissinger M, Cohen J, Vaida AJ. Using technology to prevent medication errors. In: Cohen MR, ed. Medication errors, 2nd ed. Washington, DC: American Pharmacists Association; 2007:413–39.
20. ASHP policy positions: automation and information technology. In: Hawkins B, ed. Best practices: positions and guidance documents of ASHP. 2015–2016 ed. Bethesda, MD: American Society of Health-System Pharmacists; 2015:4.
21. Institute for Safe Medication Practices. 2011 ISMP medication safety self-assessment for hospitals. www.ismp.org/selfassessments/Hospital/2011/Abbreviated.pdf (accessed 2017 Jun 13).
22. Institute for Safe Medication Practices. ISMP self-assessments. www.ismp.org/selfassessments/default.asp (accessed 2017 Jun 13).
23. Senders SJ, Smetzer JL, Burkhardt M et al. Health care failure mode and effects analysis. In: Cohen MR, ed. Medication errors, 2nd ed. Washington, DC: American Pharmacists Association; 2007:561–86.
24. Institute for Safe Medication Practices. ISMP's list of high-alert medications. www.ismp.org/Tools/highalertmedications.pdf (accessed 2017 Jun 13).
25. Cohen MR, Smetzer JL, Tuohy NR et al. High-alert medications: safeguarding against errors. In: Cohen MR, ed. Medication errors, 2nd ed. Washington, DC: American Pharmacists Association; 2007:317–412.
26. Institute for Safe Medication Practices. Your high-alert medication list—relatively useless without associated risk-reduction strategies (April 4, 2013). www.ismp.org/resources/your-high-alert-medication-list-relatively-useless-without-associated-risk-reduction (accessed 2018 Jun 25).
27. Institute for Safe Medication Practices. ISMP's list of confused drug names. www.ismp.org/Tools/confuseddrugnames.pdf (accessed 2017 Jun 13).
28. Smetzer JL, Cohen MR. Preventing drug administration errors. In: Cohen MR, ed. Medication errors, 2nd ed. Washington, DC: American Pharmacists Association; 2007:252–64.
29. Institute for Safe Medication Practices. FDA and ISMP lists of look-alike drug names with recommended tall man letters. www.ismp.org/Tools/tallmanletters.pdf (accessed 2017 Jun 13).
30. Institute for Safe Medication Practices. Independent double checks: undervalued and misused: selective use of this strategy can play an important role in medication safety (June 13, 2013). www.ismp.org/newsletters/acutecare/showarticle.aspx?id=51 (accessed 2017 May 31).
31. Food and Drug Administration. Risk Evaluation and Mitigation Strategies (REMS). https://www.fda.gov/drugs/drug-safety-and-availability/risk-evaluation-and-mitigation-strategies-rems (accessed 1 July 2019).
32. American Society of Health-System Pharmacists. ASHP guidelines on the pharmacy and therapeutics committee and the formulary system. *Am J Health-Syst Pharm.* 2008; 65:1272–83.

33. American Society of Health-System Pharmacists. Medication-use safety online tools and resources. www.ashp.org/Pharmacy-Practice/Pharmacy-Topics/Patient-Safety/Medication-Use-Safety (accessed 2017 May 31).
34. Levine S, Cohen MR. Preventing medication errors in pediatric and neonatal patients. In: Cohen MR, ed. Medication errors, 2nd ed. Washington, DC: American Pharmacists Association; 2007:478–81.
35. Food and Drug Administration. Safe Use Initiative. www.fda.gov/Drugs/DrugSafety/SafeUseInitiative (accessed 2017 Jun 13).
36. American Society of Health-System Pharmacists. Standardize 4 Safety Initiative. www.ashp.org/Pharmacy-Practice/Standardize-4-Safety-Initiative (accessed 2017 May 31).
37. Institute for Safe Medication Practices. ISMP Medication Safety Alert! newsletters. www.ismp.org/newsletters/default.asp (accessed 2017 Jun 8).
38. Institute for Safe Medication Practices. Special Error Alerts. www.ismp.org/nan/ (accessed 2017 Jun 8).
39. American Society of Health-System Pharmacists. ASHP guidelines: minimum standard for pharmacies in hospitals. *Am J Health-Syst Pharm.* 2013; 70:1619–30.
40. American Society of Health-System Pharmacists. ASHP guidelines on outsourcing pharmaceutical services. *Am J Health-Syst Pharm.* 1998; 55:1611–7.
41. American Society of Health-System Pharmacists. ASHP guidelines on outsourcing sterile compounding services. *Am J Health-Syst Pharm.* 2015; 72:1664–75.
42. American Society of Health-System Pharmacists. ASHP guidelines on managing drug product shortages in hospitals and health systems. *Am J Health-Syst Pharm.* 2009; 66:1399–406.
43. Cohen MR, Smetzer JL. Preventing dispensing errors. In: Cohen MR, ed. Medication errors, 2nd ed. Washington, DC: American Pharmacists Association; 2007:209–10.
44. Sanborn MD. What to focus on first—prioritizing safety-improvement initiatives. In: Manasse HR, Thompson KK, eds. Medication safety: a guide for health care facilities. Bethesda, MD: American Society of Health-System Pharmacists; 2005:62–5.
45. Institute for Safe Medication Practices. Guidance on the interdisciplinary safe use of automated dispensing cabinets (2008). www.ismp.org/Tools/guidelines/ADC_Guidelines_Final.pdf (accessed 2017 Jun 13).
46. American Society of Health-System Pharmacists. ASHP guidelines on the safe use of automated dispensing devices. *Am J Health-Syst Pharm.* 2010; 67:483–90.
47. Institute for Safe Medication Practices. Guidance on the interdisciplinary safe use of automated dispensing cabinets. www.ismp.org/tools/guidelines/ADC_Guidelines_final.pdf (accessed 2017 May 31).
48. Agency for Healthcare Research and Quality. Patient safety primers: medication errors. http://psnet.ahrq.gov/primer.aspx?primerID=23 (accessed 2017 Jun 8).
49. American Society of Health-System Pharmacists. ASHP statement on the pharmacist's role in medication reconciliation. *Am J Health-Syst Pharm.* 2013; 70:453–6.
50. Cohen MR, Smetzer JL. Delayed administration and contraindicated drugs place hospitalized Parkinson's disease patients at risk; doxorubicin liposomal mix-up; avoid mix-ups between hydroxyprogesterone and medroxyprogesterone. *Hosp Pharm.* 2015; 50:559–63.
51. National Coordinating Council for Medication Error Reporting and Prevention. Recommendations to enhance accuracy of prescription/medication order writing. www.nccmerp.org/recommendations-enhance-accuracy-prescription-writing (accessed 2017 Jun 8).
52. Levine S, Cohen MR, Blanchard NR et al. Guidelines for preventing medication errors in pediatrics. *J Pediatr Pharmacol Ther.* 2001; 6:426–42.
53. Institute for Safe Medication Practices. ISMP's guidelines for standard order sets (2010). www.ismp.org/tools/guidelines/standardordersets.pdf (accessed 2017 Jun 8).
54. Massachusetts Coalition for the Prevention of Medical Errors. Errors in transcribing and administering medications (2001). www.macoalition.org/documents/SafetyFirst3.pdf (accessed 2017 Jun 8).
55. Institute for Safe Medication Practices. Targeted medication safety best practices for hospitals. www.ismp.org/tools/bestpractices/TMSBP-for-Hospitals.pdf (accessed 2017 May 31).
56. American Society of Health-System Pharmacists. ASHP technical assistance bulletin on repackaging oral solids and liquids in single unit and unit dosed packages. *Am J Hosp Pharm.* 1983; 40:451–2.
57. Hazardous drugs—handling in healthcare settings (general chapter 800). In: The United States pharmacopeia, 39th rev., and The national formulary, 34th ed. Rockville, MD: United States Pharmacopeial Convention; 2016.
58. National Institute for Occupational Safety and Health. NIOSH list of antineoplastic and other hazardous drugs in healthcare settings, 2014. www.cdc.gov/niosh/docs/2014-138/pdfs/2014-138.pdf (accessed 2017 Jun 13).
59. Pharmaceutical compounding—nonsterile preparations (general information chapter 795). In: The United States pharmacopeia, 34th rev., and The national formulary, 29th ed. Rockville, MD: United States Pharmacopeial Convention; 2011:330–6.
60. American Society of Hospital Pharmacists. ASHP technical assistance bulletin on compounding nonsterile products in pharmacies. *Am J Hosp Pharm.* 1994; 51:1441–8.
61. United States Pharmacopeial Convention. USP compounding compendium (2014). www.usp.org/sites/default/files/usp_pdf/EN/products/toc-usp-compounding-compendium.pdf (accessed 2017 Jun 13).
62. Institute for Safe Medication Practices. Proceedings of the ISMP Sterile Preparation Compounding Safety Summit: guidelines for safe preparation of sterile compounds (September 19, 2016). www.ismp.org/Tools/guidelines/IVSummit/IVCGuidelines.pdf (accessed 2017 Jun 13).
63. American Society of Health-System Pharmacists. ASHP guidelines on compounding sterile preparations. *Am J Health-Syst Pharm.* 2014; 71:145–66.
64. Hazardous drugs—handling in healthcare settings (general chapter 800). United States Pharmacopeia,

39th rev., and The national formulary, 34th ed. First supplement. Rockville, MD: United States Pharmacopeial Convention; 2016.

65. ASHP Research and Education Foundation. Outsourcing sterile products preparation: contractor assessment tool. www.ashpfoundation.org/MainMenuCategories/AdvancingPractice/SterileProductsTool (accessed 2017 May 31).
66. Radiopharmaceuticals vendor qualification checklist (2014). American Pharmacists Association–Academy of Pharmacy Practice and Management Special Interest Group. www.pharmacist.com/sites/default/files/files/Nuclear%20Pharm%20Qualifaction_Checklist.pdf (accessed 2017 Jun 13).
67. Kowiatek JG, Weber RJ, Skledar S et al. Assessing and monitoring override medications in automated dispensing devices. *Jt Comm J Qual Patient Saf.* 2006; 32:309–17.
68. American Society of Health-System Pharmacists. ASHP guidelines on remote medication order processing. *Am J Health-Syst Pharm.* 2010; 67:672–7.
69. 10 Golden rules for administering drugs safely. In: McGovern K. Preventing medication errors. Springhouse, PA: Springhouse; 1994:2–3.
70. Institute for Safe Medication Practices. The 5 rights, a destination without a map (January 25, 2007) www.ismp.org/newsletters/acutecare/articles/20070125.asp (accessed 2017 May 31).
71. Global Enteral Device Supplier Association. Stay connected homepage. http://stayconnected.org (accessed 2017 Jun 12).
72. American Society of Health-System Pharmacists. ASHP statement on bar-code verification during inventory, preparation, and dispensing of medications. *Am J Health-Syst Pharm.* 2011; 68:442–5.
73. Poon EG, Keohane CA, Yoon CS et al. Effect of bar-code technology on the safety of medication administration. *N Engl J Med.* 2010; 362:1698–707.
74. Seibert HH, Maddox RR, Flynn EA et al. Effect of bar-code technology with electronic medication administration record on medication accuracy rates. *Am J Health-Syst Pharm.* 2014; 71:209–18.
75. Institute for Safe Medication Practices. Proceedings from the ISMP summit on the use of smart infusion pumps: guidelines for safe implementation and use. www.ismp.org/tools/guidelines/smartpumps/comments (accessed 2017 May 22).
76. National Quality Forum. Safe practices for better healthcare—2010 update (April 2010). www.qualityforum.org/Publications/2010/04/Safe_Practices_for_Better_Healthcare_%E2%80%93_2010_Update.aspx (accessed 2017 Jun 13).
77. American Society of Health-System Pharmacists. ASHP guidelines on pharmacist-conducted patient education and counseling. *Am J Health-Syst Pharm.* 1997; 54:431–4.
78. American Society of Health-System Pharmacists. ASHP guidelines on adverse drug reaction monitoring and reporting. *Am J Health-Syst Pharm.* 1995; 52:417–9.
79. Centers for Medicare and Medicaid Services. Partnership for Patients Initiative. https://partnershipforpatients.cms.gov (accessed 2017 Jun 13).
80. Foster AJ, Murff HJ, Peterson JF et al. The incidence and severity of adverse events affecting patients after discharge from the hospital. *Ann Intern Med.* 2003; 138:161–7.
81. Foster SL, Smith EB, Seybold MR. Advanced counseling techniques: integrating assessment and intervention. *Am Pharm.* 1995; NS35:40–8.
82. Gleason KM, Brake H, Agramonte V, Perfetti C. Medications at Transitions and Clinical Handoffs (MATCH) toolkit for medication reconciliation. www.ahrq.gov/sites/default/files/publications/files/match.pdf (accessed 2018 Jun 25).
83. Burkhardt M, Lee C, Taylor L et al. Root cause analysis of medication errors. In: Cohen MR, ed. Medication errors, 2nd ed. Washington, DC: American Pharmacists Association; 2007:67–86.
84. Agency for Healthcare Research and Quality. Root cause analysis (August 2014). http://psnet.ahrq.gov/primer.aspx?primerID=10 (accessed 2017 Jun 13).
85. Joint Commission. Sentinel events. In: Comprehensive accreditation manual for hospitals (January 2016). www.jointcommission.org/assets/1/6/CAMH_24_SE_all_CURRENT.pdf (accessed 2017 Jun 13).
86. VA National Center for Patient Safety. Root cause analysis. www.patientsafety.va.gov/professionals/onthejob/rca.asp (accessed 2017 Jun 13).
87. Joint Commission. Framework for conducting a root cause analysis and action plan (March 21, 2013). www.jointcommission.org/Framework_for_Conducting_a_Root_Cause_Analysis_and_Action_Plan (accessed 2017 Jun 13).
88. National Patient Safety Foundation. RCA^2: improving root cause analyses and actions to prevent harm (January 2016). http://c.ymcdn.com/sites/www.npsf.org/resource/resmgr/PDF/RCA2_v2-online-pub_010816.pdf (accessed 2017 Jun 13).
89. Crea KA. Medication misadventures II: medication and patient safety. In: Malone PM, Kier KL, Stanovich JE, eds. Drug information: a guide for pharmacists. 4th ed. New York: McGraw Hill; 2012.
90. American Society of Health-System Pharmacists. ASHP guidelines on medication-use evaluation. *Am J Health-Syst Pharm.* 1996; 53:1953–5.
91. Health Resources and Services Administration. Quality improvement. www.hrsa.gov/quality/toolbox/methodology/quality_improvement/ (accessed 2017 Jun 13).
92. Agency for Healthcare Research and Quality. WebM&M cases and commentaries. https://psnet.ahrq.gov/webmm (accessed 2017 May 31).
93. Skledar SJ. Continuous quality improvement principles. In: Larson CM, Saine D, eds. Medication safety officer's handbook. Bethesda, MD: American Society of Health-System Pharmacists; 2013:146.
94. Phillips MS. Medication error reporting and analysis. In: Larson CM, Saine D, eds. Medication safety officer's handbook. Bethesda, MD: American Society of Health-System Pharmacists; 2013:243–54.
95. Agency for Healthcare Research and Quality. Patient safety organization program. www.pso.ahrq.gov (accessed 2017 May 31).

Appendix A—High-Alert Medication Checklist

Scoring: Each secondary question receives 1 point if you answer "yes" to 50% or greater of any of the questions.

Questions	Question Scoring		Secondary Questions	Secondary Question Scoring		Frequently Asked Questions
	Yes	No		Yes	No	
1. Does this medication exist on the ISMP High Alert Medication list, or does it need to remain on your current list (if already there)?						Definition of ISMP high-alert medications (or drugs): Medications that bear a heightened risk of causing significant patient harm when they are used in error. Although mistakes may or may not be more common with these drugs, the consequences of an error are more devastating to patients. The current medications on your high alert list should also be reviewed to determine if they need to remain.
2. Have serious errors been reported with this medication internally at your facility? (If it is a medication new to the market, look at other similar medications in the same therapeutic drug class or category), or could the outcome of an error with this medication cause serious patient harm?						Q. How do I evaluate error reports if the medication is new to formulary? A. Evaluate error reports of medications in the same class/category. Serious harm is defined as NCC MERP severity categories F-I.
3. Have errors, reports, alerts, or recommended special restrictions or requirements been reported with this drug by external bodies (e.g., ISMP, FDA)?						Q. Where do I find external sources of error reports for new medications? A. Review reports from ISMP, FDA, Joint Commission, other facilities in your area, listservs and current literature.
4. Does this medication treat a vulnerable patient population? a. Neonates b. Critical Care c. Hematology/Oncology d. Transplant						Q. How should I score this question if my hospital treats patients who are only within these populations (e.g., a children's hospital or a cancer center)? A. Scoring for this question can be deferred if your patients fall into one of these categories.

Appendix A—High-Alert Medication Checklist *(continued)*

Questions	Question Scoring		Secondary Questions	Secondary Question Scoring		Frequently Asked Questions
	Yes	No		Yes	No	
5. Does this medication require special knowledge or precautions in any of the following medication use phases: prescribing, transcribing, storage, dispensing/preparation, administration, monitoring?			Within the **PRESCRIBING** phase: 1. Is this a look-alike, sound-alike drug? 2. Should there be limited concentrations available? 3. Are there multiple formulations available (e.g., extended-release products, liposomal formulations, multiple dosage forms)? 4. Are there standard order sets developed to guide prescribers? 5. Should there be maximum dose limits (forcing function)? 6. Are weight-based dose limits needed? 7. Are there drug information resources? 8. Should the medication be considered restricted access to specialized prescribers (e.g., tPA to neurology)?			
			Within the **TRANSCRIBING** phase: 1. Are verbal orders prohibited?			
			Within the **STORAGE** phase: 1. Are there specific medication security requirements? 2. Should the medication be placed in a locked location or separated from other medications (concentrated electrolytes, controlled substances, neuromuscular blockers)? 3. Should there be limited access (e.g., stored only in the pharmacy, not on a patient care unit)? 4. Are auxiliary warning labels required?			
			Within the **DISPENSING/PREPARATION** phase: 1. Should personnel be trained and credentialed? 2. Are there special handling/transportation precautions? 3. Is the medication available as a unit dose or premade product or does it require compounding? 4. Does this medication require limited distribution or access such as storage in a specialized pharmacy location (e.g., satellite pharmacy [pediatrics, oncology, critical care])? 5. Is an independent double check recommended? 6. Are auxiliary warning labels required?			

Appendix A—High-Alert Medication Checklist *(continued)*

Questions	Question Scoring		Secondary Questions	Secondary Question Scoring		Frequently Asked Questions
	Yes	No		Yes	No	
			Within the **ADMINISTRATION** phase: 1. Should there be a limit or maximum infusion rates (forcing functions)? 2. Should the medication be independently double checked prior to administration? 3. Does this medication require special handling? 4. Does the medication require credentialed personnel for administration? 5. Does the medication require special reconstitution or manipulation immediately prior to administration? 6. Is the route of administration considered high risk (e.g., intrathecal, intravenous). 7. Is the medication a vesicant or is there a heightened risk for extravasation? 8. Does the medication match the indication?			
			Within the **MONITORING** phase: 1. Does the medication have an associated REMS requirement? 2. Is special monitoring required (e.g., labs, vital signs, monitoring equipment)? 3. Is an independent double check required for changes to the infusion rate? 4. Is the medication a vesicant or is there a heightened risk for extravasation? 5. Do the lab results match the patient (correct patient) and were they drawn appropriately (e.g., trough drawn before infusion, not during or after)?			
Total Score for Question Scoring + Secondary Question Scoring						
Final Score						

Appendix B—Self-Assessment Checklist*

- ☐ A medication safety leader has been designated by the institution.
- ☐ A medication safety strategic plan has been developed for the institution.
- ☐ A culture of safety has been supported at the highest level of the organization.
- ☐ An event reporting system is available for voluntary reporting of patient events.
- ☐ A medication safety team/committee has been developed and is multidisciplinary; alternatively, for smaller hospitals, the medication safety "business" can be taken care of at another meeting.
- ☐ The institution has a program or support system available for second victims.
- ☐ Errors and close calls are analyzed and investigated to develop measures to prevent reoccurrence.
- ☐ A clear and transparent process to evaluate errors is used.
- ☐ Programs to support second victims and educate healthcare professionals are in place.
- ☐ Other methods for event detection are considered, such as direct observation method, trigger medications, and using information technology.
- ☐ The institution has a pharmacist position dedicated to medication safety.
- ☐ Pharmacists are involved in technology decisions.
- ☐ Proactive risk assessment tools are used to identify opportunities for improvement.
- ☐ The institution has developed a high-alert medications list. The list is based on the hospital's patterns of medication use and harm events.
- ☐ Risk reduction strategies for high alert medications that do not rely upon a single risk-reduction step have been developed based on literature and best practices.
- ☐ The institution has developed a look-alike/sound-alike list. The list is based on the hospital's patterns of medication use and harm events.
- ☐ Risk reduction strategies for look-alike/sound-alike medications have been developed based on literature and best practices.
- ☐ The pharmacy department has a process for handling medications that are managed by REMS.
- ☐ The pharmacy department has a well-designed formulary system (see ASHP Guidelines).
- ☐ When reviewing a medication for addition to formulary, the formulary review contains a section on medication safety assessment and recommendations; potential safety issues are considered after a relevant literature search.
- ☐ A standard checklist is used to review the safety of a new formulary medication.
- ☐ Strategies are established to prevent errors with high risk medications prior to addition to formulary.
- ☐ When new formulary medications are added to the electronic health record or to pharmacy systems, dosage forms, concentrations and ordering options are limited and standardized.
- ☐ Medication concentrations are standardized.
- ☐ If multiple concentrations are needed, consistent terminology, auxiliary labels, or label comments are used to distinguish between concentrations.
- ☐ The Rule of 6 is not used.
- ☐ National standardized concentrations are used when available and therapeutically appropriate (Standardize 4 Safety initiative).
- ☐ The medication safety committee monitors and reacts to medication safety alerts and updates from the FDA, ISMP, and other organizations and agencies.
- ☐ The pharmacy department is responsible for procurement of all medications within the organization.
- ☐ Sample medications are not used for inpatient treatment.
- ☐ When hospitalized, patients' own medications should only be used after prescriber order and pharmacist identification.
- ☐ Pharmacists are actively involved in the evaluation of all medication device purchasing and replacement decisions (e.g., pumps).
- ☐ Policies and procedures are established to ensure safety and continuity of care with patients who come in with indwelling pumps, such as pain management or insulin pumps.
- ☐ The pharmacy department takes a lead role in coordination of outsourcing pharmaceutical services.
- ☐ The pharmacy has processes in place to communicate medication shortages, including alternatives and substitution protocols, to prescribers and other clinical staff.
- ☐ When alternative products are utilized due to a shortage, they should be examined for possible medication safety issues.
- ☐ Product arrangement minimizes unintended selection of the wrong product or dosage form.
- ☐ The same drug nomenclature used in storage databases is used throughout the entire medication-use process (electronic health records, pharmacy information system, infusion pumps).
- ☐ Differentiation and screen alerts are used for medications with risk for potential errors, such as look-alike medications, medications that should not be crushed, and high-alert medications.
- ☐ A system for rotating stock has been established. All storage areas are monitored for expired medications and appropriate temperatures.
- ☐ A schedule assigning staff to regularly inspect and remove expired medications has been implemented.
- ☐ Medications in automated dispensing cabinets (ADCs) are in ready-to-use, unit dose or unit-of-use containers.
- ☐ Barcoding is used to assist in stocking and restocking medications. If barcode capability is not available, double checks are used by two staff members to help minimize stocking errors.
- ☐ Medications are not removed from storage until immediately prior to administration, and un-administered doses are returned to controlled storage promptly. Nurses do not return medications to ADC stock; only to the ADC return bin.
- ☐ If matrix bins are used, each medication and strength has a separate bin.
- ☐ Medications with look-alike names or similar packaging are not stored near one another.
- ☐ Systematic inventory audits are performed to identify and remove expired and low usage products from ADCs.
- ☐ The institution has defined, and the pharmacy and therapeutics and medication safety committees have approved, the specific criteria to allow for medication override emergency situations for ADCs.

Appendix B—Self-Assessment Checklist* *(continued)*

- ☐ Processes for taking a medication history and performing medication reconciliation on admission is standardized across the institution in different settings, (e.g., outpatient procedures, radiology) and ongoing education is conducted to ensure a safer system for patients.
- ☐ Institutional requirements for the review and reconciliation of the medication list within a set amount of time of an inpatient admission are outlined. High-risk medications, such as anticonvulsants, anticoagulants, and antibiotics should be reconciled sooner.
- ☐ Medication orders include patient identifiers (name, date of birth, patient number), patient allergies, generic drug name, trademarked name (if a specific product is required), route and site of administration, dosage form, dose, strength, quantity, frequency of administration, intended duration of therapy, indication for use, and prescriber's name. For intravenous medications, dilution, rate, and time of administration are specified.
- ☐ Vague or blanket instructions, such as "take as directed" or "resume pre-op meds" are not used for medication orders.
- ☐ Pediatric prescriptions should be prescribed both in units/weight and total individual dose.
- ☐ An independent double check of a preparation occurs regardless of who the preparer is.
- ☐ The pull-back method is avoided as a means to check preparations.
- ☐ For oral products not available in unit-of-use packaging, the preparations are repackaged by pharmacy staff.
- ☐ Frontline compounding personnel are involved in FMEA of new technologies used in compounding or other preparation areas.
- ☐ Oral syringes are only used for oral preparations and IV syringes are never used for oral medication administration.
- ☐ Products intended for other routes (e.g., potentially containing particulates, pyrogens or not sterile) are not dispensed in an IV bag to avoid mistaken administration by the parenteral route.
- ☐ All medications in nonemergency situations are reviewed by a pharmacist before dispensing.
- ☐ For high-risk drug products, (e.g., chemotherapy, pediatric medication, PPN), work is independently checked by a second individual, preferably another pharmacist.
- ☐ The hospital's pharmacy and therapeutics committee and medication safety committee has developed and implemented a list of medications with corresponding indications that are authorized for override. Criteria for appropriate override of medications are included, along with the clinical indication for overriding the medication (i.e., aspirin and chest pain), for specific circumstances. Compliance is monitored to minimize risk.
- ☐ An override monitoring process has been developed and audits are performed to ensure appropriate use by nurses and other authorized staff.
- ☐ BCMA reports are evaluated regularly to assess compliance and to identify potential barriers to ensure BCMA is being used effectively.
- ☐ A process is in place to notify the pharmacy when products are not scanning properly.
- ☐ The pharmacy dispenses patient-specific doses with barcodes whenever possible.
- ☐ Policies and procedures have been determined for how and when medication libraries are updated, who needs to approve the changes, and how unique situations such as drug shortages should be handled.
- ☐ The continuous quality improvement data analytics programs that are generated as reports and trends of medication alerts (overrides, bypass of soft alerts, and use of the free-text or "wildcard" function for medications not having standardized entries in the pump) are analyzed to keep the drug library settings for alerts, alarms, and advisories as robust as possible. Settings are continually updated and improved to encourage and reflect current best practices.
- ☐ All practitioners responsible for administering medications are properly trained on administration procedures.
- ☐ Effective medication administration education programs for practitioners have been established, and training is documented in the staff competency files and conducted periodically or as needed.
- ☐ Guidelines for the correct time to obtain blood for serum concentrations and laboratory values were created collaboratively by pharmacists, nurses, physicians, and laboratory staff.
- ☐ Critical values are determined with action alerts for clinicians and generated electronically.
- ☐ Staff is trained to identify common adverse effects encountered by patients. A pathway is in place to react to adverse reactions.
- ☐ Required monitoring for efficacy and toxicity is built into order panels or order sets whenever possible.
- ☐ Distractions are minimized when practitioners are evaluating patient data.
- ☐ Protocols are clearly written and readily available such that all practitioners can interpret each protocol in the same way.
- ☐ Institutional protocols approved by the pharmacy and therapeutics committee have been implemented to allow pharmacists or nurses to automatically modify dosing, obtain necessary rescue medications (i.e., naloxone, dextrose 50%, insulin), and order laboratory tests for patient safety.
- ☐ A standard place for practitioners to look for vital signs, pain scores, laboratory values, and point-of-care testing values is available.
- ☐ Standardization of medication administration times and pertinent monitoring times is built into the workflow and order sets.
- ☐ Pharmacists participate in multi-disciplinary discharge committees and are involved in the medication reconciliation process prior to discharge.
- ☐ There is an ongoing systematic program for improvement of pharmacy services and the medication-use system utilizing medication use evaluations and quality improvement tools such as Plan-Do-Study-Act (PDSA), Lean Production System, Six-Sigma, TeamSTEPPS® and FOCUS-PDCA.
- ☐ Root cause analyses (RCAs) (or other comprehensive systemic analyses) are performed for serious or significant medication events but may be used for any event that the institution wishes to evaluate in closer detail.
- ☐ Each institution (or pharmaceutical department) has a process for when an RCA is conducted.
- ☐ The institution or pharmaceutical department should consider utilizing the RCA2: Improving Root Cause Analyses and Actions to Prevent Harm recommendations.
- ☐ Regardless, there is a standard method and template for performing the RCA, as well as for reporting of the results and recommendations.
- ☐ Medication safety officers and pharmacists are involved in all RCAs evaluating a medication-related event.

Appendix B—Self-Assessment Checklist* *(continued)*

- ☐ Adequate time is set aside for pharmacy staff (and other hospital personnel) to attend the RCA meetings, including any needed training.
- ☐ Recommendations from a RCA or systemic analysis are monitored to ensure implementation.
- ☐ The institution has a method for voluntary reporting of events.
- ☐ Individuals who report events are notified of safety improvements that have occurred as a result; this information is also shared more collectively at staff meetings.
- ☐ The pharmaceutical department uses other methods to detect medication events, such as trigger tools or analysis of pharmacist therapeutic interventions.
- ☐ Events are shared with external organizations and agencies like the FDA and ISMP.

*This checklist is included for information purposes only and may not be comprehensive.

Developed through the ASHP Section of Inpatient Practitioners and approved by the ASHP Board of Directors on November 8, 2017.

COL Jorge D. Carrillo, Pharm.D., M.S., M.P.H., BCPS, Department of Pharmacy, Womack Army Medical Center, Fort Bragg, NC.

Angela T. Cassano, Pharm.D., BCPS, FASHP, Pharmfusion Consulting, LLC, Midlothian, VA.

Molly Billstein-Leber, Pharm.D., BCPS, Drug Use Policy and Formulary Management, Yale New Haven Health System, New Haven, CT.

Kym Moline, Pharm.D., M.S.A., Medication Safety and Process Excellence, Mercy Health Saint Mary's, Grand Rapids, MI.

Jennifer J. Robertson, Pharm.D., BCPS, Pharmaceutical Department, St. Jude Children's Research Hospital, Memphis, TN.

ASHP gratefully acknowledges the following organizations and individuals for reviewing these guidelines (review does not imply endorsement): American Association of Critical Care Nurses; American Pharmacists Association; South Carolina Society of Health-System Pharmacists; UC Health; Kelly Besco, Pharm.D., FISMP, CPPS; Gregory P. Burger, Pharm.D., CPPS; Michael Dickens; Paul Driver, Pharm.D., BCPS, FASHP; Rosemary Call Duncan, Pharm.D., BCPS; Ashley Duty, Pharm.D., M.S.; Lara K. Ellinger, Pharm.D., BCPS; Jeanne Ezell, M.S., FASHP; Lonnye Finneman, Pharm.D.; Katayoon Kathy Ghomeshi, Pharm.D., BCPS; Paul W. Goebel, Pharm.D., BCPS, BCCCP; Kyle Grose, Pharm.D.; Kathleen Gura, Pharm.D., BCNSP, FASHP, FPPAG, FASPEN; Jim Hayman, M.S., M.B.A., FASHP; Charlene Hope Henry, Pharm.D., M.S., BCPS, CPPS; James M. Hoffman, Pharm.D., M.S., BCPS, FASHP; Herb Hunter, Pharm.D., BCPS; Patricia Kienle, M.P.A., FASHP; Joanne G. Kowiatek, M.P.M., FASHP; Eric C. Kutscher, Pharm.D., M.B.A., BCPP, FASHP; Timothy W. Lynch, Pharm.D., M.S., FASHP, FABC; Charles E. Mahan, Pharm.D., Ph.C.; Natasha Nicol, Pharm.D., FASHP; Marjorie Shaw Phillips, M.S., FASHP; Allison Pollock, Pharm.D., BCPS; James Ponto, M.S., FASHP; Robert Poole, Pharm.D., FPPAG, FCSHP, FASHP; Julia Baker Rawlings, Pharm.D., BCPS, CPPS; James R. Rinehart, M.S., FASHP; Deb Saine, M.S., FASHP, FSMSO; Susan J. Skledar, M.P.H., FASHP; Linda Tyler, Pharm.D.; Dagny Ulrich, Pharm.D., Ph.D.; Elizabeth Wade, Pharm.D., BCPS; Jody Jacobson Wedret, FASHP, FCSHP; Ann E. Wehmeyer, Pharm.D., BCPS; Stacey Wessel; and Maria Zarambo, Pharm.D.

The contributions of Kristen Hughes, Pharm.D., are acknowledged.

The authors have declared no potential conflicts of interest.

These guidelines supersede the ASHP guidelines on preventing medication errors dated June 23, 1993.

Copyright © 2018, American Society of Health-System Pharmacists, Inc. All rights reserved. Contact ASHP for reprint and permissions requests. This content may not be used for commercial purposes without the express written consent of ASHP.

The bibliographic citation for this document is as follows: American Society of Health-System Pharmacists. ASHP guidelines on preventing medication errors in hospitals. *Am J Health-Syst Pharm.* 2018; 75:1493–1517.

ASHP Guidelines on Preventing Medication Errors with Chemotherapy and Biotherapy

Purpose and Definitions

The purposes of these guidelines are to define best practices for the safe use of chemotherapy and biotherapy agents and to assist practitioners in improving their medication-use systems to prevent medication errors and patient harm from these agents. Although the guidelines are intended primarily to address use of chemotherapy and biotherapy agents in cancer treatment, some recommendations may be more broadly applicable across the medication-use system. These guidelines supplement ASHP's Guidelines on Preventing Medication Errors in Hospitals and address error prevention within diverse healthcare settings.[1] Further, these guidelines provide updated general guidance to include a standard definition of a "medication error" and applicable aspects of recommendations from the National Coordinating Council on Medication Error Reporting and Prevention (NCC MERP). NCC MERP's definition of a medication error is:

> any preventable event that may cause or lead to inappropriate medication use or patient harm while the medication is in the control of the healthcare provider, patient, or consumer. Such events may be related to professional practice, healthcare products, procedures, and systems, including prescribing; order communication; product labeling, packaging, and nomenclature; compounding; dispensing; distribution; administration; education; monitoring; and use.[2]

For the purposes of these guidelines, chemotherapy and biotherapy agents are defined as any medication that (1) is listed in section 10:00 of the American Hospital Formulary Service[3] (AHFS) pharmacologic–therapeutic classification system; (2) has at least one FDA-labeled indication to prevent or treat cancer, even if not listed in AHFS 10:00; or (3) is an investigational medication being used to prevent or treat cancer. This definition includes medications administered by any route. For simplicity, the term "chemotherapy" is used throughout these guidelines to refer to any chemotherapy or biotherapy medication that is used for cancer treatment.

The variety of therapies used in the treatment of cancer will only increase as advances are made, and healthcare organizations will confront the challenge of defining the products that require special procedures for safe use. Given the complexity of cancer care, it is recommended that such a list be as inclusive as possible. While these guidelines focus on the safe use of chemotherapy in treating cancer patients, in some situations chemotherapy agents may be used for non-malignant diseases. In general, these additional safety procedures should apply for all uses of a chemotherapy agent, regardless of indication. Although they are specific to use of chemotherapy for cancer treatment, many of the principles of these guidelines also apply to cancer supportive care (e.g., treatment for pain and nausea). Finally, for organizations that conduct clinical research, investigational chemotherapy agents should be included in all safety systems established for FDA-approved chemotherapy agents.

These guidelines provide wide-ranging recommendations for preventing errors with chemotherapy agents in healthcare organizations, with an emphasis on hospitals, infusion centers, and ambulatory care clinics that offer direct pharmacy services. Nevertheless, it is strongly recommended that the guidance also be adopted by other settings, including physician office practices, home care, and patients self-administering oral and injectable therapies at home. Other guidance on the safe use of chemotherapy in the ambulatory setting has been published by the American Society of Clinical Oncology (ASCO) and the Oncology Nursing Society (ONS).[4] These recommendations cover known procedural, technical, and behavioral elements that could systematically reduce a healthcare organization's vulnerabilities to errors. Given use of an electronic medical record (EMR) increased from 3.8% of hospitals in 2007 to 8% in 2011, and computerized provider order entry (CPOE) use increased from 4% of hospitals in 2005 to 34% of hospitals in 2011,[5] additional information on the unique considerations of using CPOE for chemotherapy ordering has been included in these guidelines.

Strict adherence to good practice recommendations is not sufficient. Because the complexities of chemotherapy use afford unlimited opportunities for system failures, continuous diligence to verify accuracy is critical by all persons responsible for medication-use functions for chemotherapy. These guidelines focus on the medication-use responsibilities shared by and unique to specific professional healthcare disciplines, progressing from general to specific applications. The structure of the guidelines, by necessity, includes the repetition of some material, repeated and enhanced in specific sections and recommendations for different healthcare professionals. With the growth in use and number of oral chemotherapy agents on the market, a greater responsibility for care management is now placed on the patient. It is essential that applicable sections of these guidelines extend to patients so they can participate in protecting their own safety.

The guidelines contain the following major sections:

1. Recommendations for healthcare organizations
2. Recommendations for multidisciplinary monitoring of medication use and verification
3. Recommendations for prescribing systems and prescribers
4. Recommendations for medication preparation and dispensing systems and roles for pharmacists
5. Recommendations for medication administration systems and roles for nurses
6. Recommendations for patient education
7. Recommendations for manufacturers and regulatory agencies
8. Recommendations for identifying and managing medication errors

Because of the complexity of and differences in practice settings and organizational arrangements, aspects of these

DOI 10.37573/9781585287048.050

guidelines may be more applicable to some practice settings than others. Pharmacists, physicians, nurses, and other healthcare providers should use their professional judgment in assessing and adapting the guidance to their own settings. These guidelines focus on safe use of a specific type of high-risk medications at various stages of the medication-use process and should be augmented as appropriate by other clinical and practice guidance, including ASHP statements and guidelines.

Background

Although the rate of medication errors for chemotherapy administered in the inpatient setting is not well documented, estimates of the frequency of errors with adult and pediatric chemotherapy in the ambulatory setting have been published. In one study, the overall chemotherapy error rate was 8.1 errors per 100 clinic visits.[6] For adults, errors were associated with 7.1% of clinic visits, and errors were associated with 18.8% of pediatric clinic visits. Errors occurred across all phases of the medication-use system, but administration (56%) and ordering (36%) errors were most common. Another study found a substantially lower rate (3%) of errors in chemotherapy orders in the outpatient infusion center at a major cancer center.[7] The error rate with oral chemotherapy agents is less well studied, but serious medication errors can occur with these therapies across all phases of the medication-use system.[8,9] Taylor and colleagues[10] documented a 9.9% error rate with oral chemotherapy given to pediatric patients with acute lymphoblastic leukemia. In this study, the errors occurred at the prescribing and administration steps.

Regardless of the exact rate of medication errors for chemotherapy agents, the safe use of these therapies presents unique challenges that demand additional safety systems. Chemotherapy agents often have a narrow therapeutic index, and they are used in complex, multidrug regimens. Complex dose calculations and adjustments are required, such as dosing per body surface area (BSA) and frequent adjustment according to renal function, toxicity, and other clinical parameters. Chemotherapy agents can cause serious toxicities at FDA-approved dosages and with FDA-approved administration schedules. Advocates for safe medication use, including oncology pharmacy specialists, have recommended that healthcare organizations improve their medication-use systems specifically to prevent medication errors with chemotherapy.[11–14]

Chemotherapy-related medication-error prevention remains a priority. Increasingly, many chemotherapy agents are administered outside the inpatient or ambulatory care setting. A growing number of patients are self-administering oral chemotherapy agents at home.[15] Thus, error-prevention strategies should be applicable to the diverse settings in which chemotherapy agents are used.

Surveys have indicated a need for improvement in medication-use systems for chemotherapy agents. One survey of major United States cancer centers indicated that the safety systems routinely used for infused chemotherapy agents are rarely applied to oral chemotherapy agents.[16] Another survey replicated this finding and indicated that many other recommended safety practices for chemotherapy agents are not followed.[17]

Recommendations for Healthcare Organizations

Optimal and comprehensive patient care, especially for patients receiving chemotherapy, requires the participation of multiple healthcare disciplines. Systems are necessary to coordinate the functions throughout the medication-use process of prescribing, preparing, dispensing, and administering of chemotherapy, and for educating and counseling patients.

Healthcare organizations where multiple disciplines are represented should establish committees with representatives from each discipline to develop policies and procedures for the medication-use process and to oversee its operation. These policies and procedures should include educational and competency requirements for persons with medication-use responsibilities; general system requirements that minimize vulnerabilities to errors; and periodic auditing of physicians', pharmacists', and nurses' proficiency with the system. Further, near misses and errors involving both commercial and investigational chemotherapy agents should be analyzed in all settings, and problems in the procedures that place patients at risk should be resolved.

Education, Competency, and Credentialing. All practice settings should establish policies and procedures ensuring that healthcare providers who prescribe, prepare, dispense, and administer chemotherapy and monitor patients receiving those medications are competent to perform those functions. For pharmacists and nurses, specific education and experience or board certification in a practice specialty may be included in the institution's credentialing process.

Employers should evaluate prospective employees' training and previous practice experiences for knowledge and mastery of the skills that are essential prerequisites for working with chemotherapy. Prerequisites for preparing and administering chemotherapy should include discipline-appropriate training in how to safely handle chemotherapy agents to protect themselves, co-workers, and patients. Competency to appropriately educate patients and monitor adherence with prescribed therapy should be assessed. Deficiencies in applicants' training and experience must be identified and remedied before new employees assume patient-care responsibilities. Ongoing training for new and current employees should emphasize collaboration among healthcare providers to ensure optimal patient care, outcomes, and worker safety.

All healthcare providers who prescribe, prepare, dispense, and administer chemotherapy and monitor patients receiving those medications should be oriented in their practice setting before commencing patient-care responsibilities. Orientation should include an introduction of new employees to all the departments, service providers, and functions that affect patient care. Each provider's roles and responsibilities should be identified, and expectations should be clarified about how healthcare providers from different disciplines will communicate and work collaboratively with respect to the chemotherapy medication-use process.

Further, healthcare organizations should require that all personnel who prescribe, prepare, dispense, administer, and handle hazardous drugs or contaminated materials, and all persons who may be exposed to hazardous drugs or contaminated materials in the course of their duties, complete job-appropriate training and evaluation. Employees should demonstrate competence, knowledge, and proficiency in techniques and procedures for safely handling (preventing exposure to oneself, other persons, and the environment, and managing accidental exposure) and disposing of hazardous drugs. Those competencies should be reassessed annually or more frequently if performance problems occur. It is the responsibility of medication-use system administrators and supervisory personnel to know the current government restrictions that limit or prohibit some healthcare providers from preparing and administering chemotherapy medications.

Healthcare providers who participate in the chemotherapy medication-use process and those who monitor patients receiving chemotherapy should be knowledgeable and have current information available about each of the following factors, relative to their scope of practice and job duties, on the chemotherapy used in their practice settings:

1. Names of chemotherapy drug formulations.
2. Indications and uses, and whether they comply with the FDA-approved labeling or approved compendia or are part of an investigational protocol.
3. Routes of administration.
4. Administration schedules.
5. Appropriate dosages, including dose adjustments for toxicity and, when applicable, constraints for the maximum dose of medication that can be safely given during a single administration, over a course of treatment, or cumulatively over a lifetime.
6. Appropriate storage conditions.
7. Potential adverse effects.
8. Potential drug interactions.
9. Procedures to use for handling hazardous substances.
10. Strategies for identifying and mitigating the risks of extravasation.

Every practice setting where cancer patients receive chemotherapy should provide opportunities for continuing professional and technical education related to chemotherapy management. A portion of the annual continuing education programs for healthcare providers specializing in oncology should be related to chemotherapy agents and their uses.

Providers who use drug-delivery devices (e.g., intravenous pumps and infusion controllers) to administer chemotherapy agents should be required to demonstrate competencies related to the clinical application, function (general use, operational limits, alarms), and care of these devices; problems that may occur with the devices; and troubleshooting.

Communication and Access to Information. Many errors occurring in the medication-use process are caused or aggravated by inadequate patient-specific information. Patients' medical records should be organized and made readily accessible for use by all providers who prescribe, dispense, and administer chemotherapy to enable independent confirmation that all prerequisite criteria have been met before commencing treatment. In some cases, individual disciplines may keep additional patient records that supplement the patient's primary medical record. For example, it has historically been the responsibility of pharmacists and pharmacies to maintain patient-specific medication profiles and records of medications that were prescribed and dispensed for each patient. Medication profiles for cancer patients should, at a minimum, include the following information:

1. Patient's name and a unique identifying code or number.
2. A brief medical history that identifies a patient's cancer diagnosis.
3. Known drug-related adverse events, allergies, and medication-, nutrient-, and food-related sensitivities.
4. Vital statistics that may affect treatment intensity, particularly those needed to calculate medication doses, including height, weight, BSA, age, sex, and pertinent laboratory values (e.g., serum creatinine, creatinine clearance, liver transaminases).
5. Data about all prescription, over-the-counter, and complementary and alternative medications used by a patient, including:
   - All relevant dates, including when the medication(s) were:
     - Prescribed (if it differs from the date they were prepared and administered).
     - Prepared and dispensed (if it differs from the date the medications were administered).
     - Administered (use planned date for patient self-administered agents).
   - Drug identity
   - Drug dosage and reason(s) for any dose adjustments, as appropriate
   - Total drug dosage administered per unit interval (e.g., day, week, treatment cycle)
   - Administration route
   - Administration schedule as a function of the treatment plan (e.g., every 3 hours, days 1, 8, and 15, with the specific treatment dates)
   - Rate of administration (when relevant)
   - Prescribed duration of use (e.g., number of doses to administer; number of treatment hours, days, or weeks)
   - The product manufacturer's identity, product lot numbers, and (when practicable) expiration dates for drugs dispensed from that facility
6. Additional ingredients and diluting agents and the amounts used in extemporaneously compounded medications.
7. Primary references that describe the treatment regimen.
8. An up-to-date treatment history, including:
   - The treatment cycle or course number for each treatment repetition
   - The dates on which a patient last received treatment
   - How previous treatment was tolerated
   - The cumulative amount of drug previously administered for medications with established absolute cumulative dosage limits (e.g., anthracyclines, bleomycin) or constraints against repeated administration as a function of time

Other settings, such as ambulatory, home, specialty, and managed care organizations are vulnerable to the same communication and interpretation errors that occur in hospitals. These settings and organizational arrangements, however, could introduce additional opportunities for errors of omission and duplication when treatments and other services are provided at multiple locations and by more than one participating provider or group of providers. In hospitals and integrated health systems, patient-specific medical information has traditionally been communicated through a single comprehensive medical record. In contrast, providers in private practice, home care, and managed care organizations generally cannot rely on the availability of a comprehensive medical record, because medication prescribing, preparing, and administering may occur at geographically separate facilities.

Local policies should be developed to ensure that orders for a patient's chemotherapy medications are transmitted accurately and completely, that medication reconciliation takes place at all transitions in care, and that patient confidentiality is protected.[18] Electronic means of communication are recommended to transmit up-to-date, accurate, and comprehensive patient-specific medical information among providers. Thus, data entered into this electronic system by any one provider are immediately available to all. Until a single unifying network becomes available for all healthcare providers, portable printed and electronic records (including an accurate, updated patient medication list) that ensure patient safety and confidentiality must be devised.

Schedule Coordination. Because oncology patients often receive care from more than one healthcare provider, their primary provider, care coordinator, or patient navigator should coordinate patient care with other providers and facilities. Efficient organizational systems should have someone to coordinate a patient's healthcare needs with their various healthcare providers' schedules.

Standardize Medication Ordering. To the extent possible, medication prescribing, preparation, dispensing, and administration should be standardized. Healthcare organizations should adopt and incorporate national standards into their practice. Patient-care facilities should develop and use standardized preprinted medication-order forms or forms that are retrievable from a computerized database for requesting frequently used chemotherapy treatments and treatment-related services. Well-designed standardized, regimen-specific, medication-order forms decrease potential errors by organizing treatment information in a clear, consistent, and uniform format. As discussed further below, CPOE provides standardization opportunities and other potential benefits.

Standardized forms should be developed collaboratively with input from the healthcare providers who prescribe, prepare, and administer chemotherapy medications. Forms should be preprinted with the entire treatment plan and include items such as generic drug names, specifications for drug dosage and dosage modifications as a function of patient-specific variables, and administration routes and schedules. Forms should include the entire treatment plan, including oral medications that may be filled by an outside provider and patient self-administered. Prescription forms should also include space for prescribers to note laboratory test results that affect dosages, administration rates, and treatment duration. These forms may also permit prescribers to schedule laboratory tests and request other services for comprehensive patient care. A multidisciplinary process should be in place for the development, implementation and maintenance of these standard order forms, including independent double checks of the content. (An "independent double check" is a process in which two qualified individuals separately check, alone and apart from each other, an item or action, and then compare results to ensure the desired outcomes.[19]) These forms should include the revision date, as appropriate, to allow everyone involved to identify and validate that they are using the most current version.

Standardized medication-order forms, including prescriptions for oral therapies administered by patients, simplify and expedite medication ordering by requiring prescribers to supply only patient-specific information, such as

1. Patient's name and unique identifying number (e.g., medical record number) or date of birth according to institutional policies regarding patient identification.
2. Date and time the order was generated.
3. Time and date treatments are to be administered.
4. Cycle and day number.
5. Current patient-specific laboratory values (as defined by institutional policy regarding the timeframe for which laboratory test results are considered acceptable to use to determine whether chemotherapy can be initiated).
6. Patient-specific dosing parameters (i.e., height, weight, dosing weight, BSA).
7. Medication generic name.
8. Planned medication dosages and administration rates as a function of patient-specific factors and the calculated doses and rates to be administered.
9. Route of administration (including the venous access device type, if applicable).
10. Patient's allergies and medication and nutrient sensitivities.
11. Prescriber's name and signature.
12. Prescriber's telephone, pager, or fax number (or another means to communicate with the prescriber).

Preprinted forms should specify, by protocol number or publication reference, the treatment that is to be administered.[11,20,21]

For investigational chemotherapy treatments, standardized forms should also include the study name, protocol number, and patient-specific study number, as applicable. Color-coded forms, for example, may be used to designate different types of treatment, such as commercially marketed chemotherapy and investigational medications.

Standardized order forms eliminate many of the issues related to misinterpreting medication orders that are commonly associated with nonstandardized orders; however, healthcare providers must be aware that interpretation errors may still result from illegible handwriting. Multipurpose preprinted forms that list chemotherapy medications alphabetically may also contribute to prescribing errors when two similar drug names appear in close proximity. Since lined paper can obscure the details of a prescriber's orders, preprinted forms should be printed on unlined paper.

Self-replicating forms (e.g., carbon copies, no-carbon required paper) can produce copies that are difficult to read, and these forms should be avoided. Further, poor quality fax transmissions of these order sets should also be avoided. Providers who prepare and administer medications on the basis of a copy of a prescriber's order should be wary of ambiguous notations, artifact markings, and omissions on the copy. Each facility should restrict chemotherapy ordering (e.g., access to medication-order forms) to providers with the appropriate clinical privileges. Healthcare organizations that depend on standardized forms should review all forms on a regularly defined schedule and must ensure that only the most current versions of standardized forms are available and that obsolete forms are recalled and destroyed.

CPOE. CPOE should be implemented to further enhance the safety of the chemotherapy-use process. CPOE offers an opportunity to introduce new safety features into the chemotherapy prescribing process, but implementation of CPOE for chemotherapy providers appears to lag other areas.[5,22,23]

CPOE provides many of the same safety and convenience features as preprinted orders, such as order legibility, standardization across practitioners, chemotherapy scheduling and sequencing, and inclusion of support care medications and some patient demographics. CPOE also provides additional benefits that are not available with a paper system. For example, the ability to control user access to various sections of the system can be very useful in managing prescriber privileges, especially to limit which staff may order chemotherapy or prescribe specific investigational drugs. CPOE improves efficiency by allowing data to be accessed by different providers in different locations at the same time, and it serves as a guide for the ordering provider via clinical decision support features and serves to structure workflow (i.e., specific steps in subsequent preparation, dispensing, and administration). CPOE provides benefits over a paper system, including additional safety checks not possible with paper, but diligence by the prescriber and careful independent checks of the resulting orders are still essential when using CPOE for chemotherapy.

CPOE for chemotherapy must be implemented with great care. CPOE represents a major change in an organization's chemotherapy use process and workflow, and it may introduce new errors that may not have existed in the traditional handwritten process.[24] In a well-established and mature chemotherapy-use system, one must be certain that the dramatic changes produced by CPOE do not threaten the safety of the chemotherapy-use process during the implementation period.

To gain the benefits of CPOE, there are several key principles of implementation and continued development that must be considered, such as standardization, reduction in ambiguity, safety over convenience, and an evaluation of workflow effects.[25,26] When feasible, formal process redesign methods should be applied before implementing CPOE for chemotherapy. Given the patient safety risks involved, a formal failure modes and effects analysis (FMEA) should be considered, as such an approach has been successfully used.[23,27] When reviewing the capabilities of a CPOE system, pertinent patient data must be available to all providers. These data include provider notes, laboratory values, flow sheets that show prior chemotherapy and medications administered, and consent forms, among others. Workflow should be considered when determining how data are displayed and in what order the data are presented. This workflow begins at the point the order is entered by the prescriber, followed by pharmacist review, nurse review, drug administration, and the documentation of the effect on the patient. The number and type of checks required to verify the order should be reviewed with consideration of the CPOE capabilities and workflow. Some institutional chemotherapy policies dictate a final review and approval (informally known as "OK to Give" or final sign-off) of the chemotherapy order by an attending physician or other senior clinician.

Clinical decision support is another important consideration for CPOE.[26] Clinical decision support can guide the prescriber through various phases of the ordering process and include specific chemotherapy considerations based on individual patient parameters, such as laboratory values, comorbid conditions, hydration requirements, and the need for supportive care medications (e.g., antiemetics). Appropriate alerts, such as allergies, drug interactions, duplicate therapies, and maximum doses, should be incorporated as appropriate and be consistent with the institution's overall plan for implementing clinical decision support alerts. The duration of the order set, a cycle or specific weeks of therapy, should be standardized, and clear criteria to treat or continue treatment must be documented for the patient to continue treatment.

Users should plan for improvements and alterations to the CPOE system after implementation. Changes should be considered by a multidisciplinary team and include provider feedback as well as data from continuous monitoring of the order entry process, including safety reporting and near-miss data. Continuous review and improvement are multidisciplinary processes and need to include both clinicians and information systems staff.[28]

Implementing CPOE for chemotherapy is an important step, and CPOE should be leveraged to provide guidance for prescribers ordering chemotherapy. By definition, the prescriber is entering orders directly into the system, and safety can be improved because there is usually no intermediary who must interpret the orders and enter them into another information system. Since CPOE clearly reflects and communicates the intent of the prescriber, properly planned CPOE should give prescribers the ability to select a specific regimen or protocol that delineates the necessary information to produce a clear and accurate drug regimen.[28] These custom ordering screens are typically called "order sets" or "templates," and they are essential to safely using CPOE for chemotherapy.[23]

Depending on the system and resources devoted to order sets, additional information (e.g., requirements for laboratory values, supportive care, dose reductions, or dose-limiting parameters) may be part of the order sets. Information such as dosing (e.g., mg/kg or mg/m^2, diluents, or concentration, if appropriate) should be part of the order set to facilitate dose verification by the pharmacist. The system may also be able to prevent ordering the wrong route of administration or append a warning message to specific orders, averting such potentially deadly mistakes as inadvertently prescribing vincristine intrathecally.

Transitioning complex order sets from paper to a CPOE system poses various challenges. Care must be taken in designing ordering templates, because an undetected design error may result in multiple mistakes. Prescribers and investigators (in the case of an investigational protocol ordering set) should be involved in the checking of the template, and ideally they should be asked to sign off on the particular ordering screens before they are put into wide use. The building of these orders sets is not a simple process, especially pediatric order sets and investigational drug regimens.[29]

Cancer chemotherapy often includes a complicated sequencing of drugs and scheduling of the regimen. Growth factors need to be scheduled at the proper time to be effective and not interfere with the mechanism of action of the chemotherapy or biotherapy regimen. Unfortunately, if there is a delay in the scheduled administration times, some systems may not allow a simple click or two to reschedule multiple days and doses, in contrast to older methods in which a prescriber could just write "delay chemotherapy by 6 hours."

If possible, the CPOE system and electronic health record should allow for an electronic check and documentation of the independent checks by the pharmacist, nurse, and any others involved in the chemotherapy use process. A notation in the system alerting the nurse or prescriber that the order is under review by the pharmacist is very helpful. Systems should allow senior physician final approval (i.e., "OK to give" or final sign-off) before action is taken by the pharmacy.

Careful thought is necessary and critical when using a CPOE system, and the potential for error still exists. Prior to order entry, the prescriber must consider whether a dose reduction is needed based on a change in laboratory values or organ function. If an investigational protocol is involved, the prescriber must select the correct cycle or dose level, if dose escalation is necessary. CPOE systems may be able to guide the prescriber, but they cannot make the correct choice for him or her. Another potential source of error is the auto-calculation feature of some systems. The system can utilize the latest height and weight to calculate BSA or use the patient's weight to calculate the proper dose. However, an incorrect height or weight entry can result in a dosing error. It is easy for prescribers to miss small but significant changes that could result from data entry errors. Systems may be able to prevent data entry error by displaying an alert when data differ from a previous entry by a certain percentage or final dose amount.

Emergency contingency plans for how to communicate chemotherapy orders in the event the CPOE is not available (e.g., power outage, system failure) should be developed and tested. Whenever possible, the contingency plan should replicate the CPOE process (e.g., paper orders replicating CPOE screens) as much as possible to minimize introduction of new risks. Training and awareness of the emergency contingency plan should be part of the orientation and annual competency plan for all providers.

Implementation of a CPOE system presents many new challenges for the health (or patient) care team. Although remotely entering orders in a CPOE system may be convenient for some, it may also reduce the face-to-face contact of writing in the chart during rounds or while on the patient-care unit, reducing the opportunity for personal interactions between healthcare professionals. While CPOE has been shown to prevent prescribing errors, it is not a panacea, and diligence and independent checks are still essential to a safe chemotherapy process using CPOE. Knowing some of its pitfalls in advance will aid in the design and use of all the features available in a CPOE system, especially for high-risk therapies such as chemotherapy. The success of CPOE depends on having high-level administrative, clinical, financial, and information technology support. It is critical front-line staff have a significant role in the development, implementation, and monitoring of CPOE.[28]

Verbal Orders for Chemotherapy Medications. Except for discontinuing treatment, medication-use systems should not permit healthcare providers to use or accept verbal orders to commence or modify a chemotherapy medication.[11,12,30] Verbal communication for chemotherapy orders, whether face-to-face or over the telephone, circumvent an essential checkpoint in the order-verification process, whether they are communicated directly to persons who prepare medications or received and reported by one or more intermediaries.[31]

Stat Orders for Chemotherapy Medications. It is rarely necessary to begin chemotherapy treatment as quickly as possible (i.e., "stat"). In general, stat orders for chemotherapy may compromise essential order-verification safeguards and are almost never appropriate. Except for urgently required treatments, chemotherapy medication preparation and administration should be scheduled when staffing is adequate to ensure that appropriate safety checks are performed during compounding, verification, and administration. It is essential that patient care is not compromised under any circumstances.

Standardize Dosage Calculation. Medication-use systems should establish whether drug dosages should be routinely calculated as a function of actual, ideal (lean), or adjusted body weight and develop standardized criteria that direct dosage calculation as a function of this weight. ASCO has produced guidelines for dosing chemotherapy in obese patients that suggest using actual body weight if the intent is cure.[32] Institutions should consider this information when deciding on dose calculation standards. Institutions should also define policies for other situations, such as in pediatric or hematopoietic stem cell transplant patients, where adjusted-weight dosing is used, or when cure is not the goal. Investigational protocols may specify treatment parameters different from institutional parameters. In all cases, the treatment plans and medication orders should indicate whether patients' actual or ideal body weight was used in calculating drug dosages and identify the equation from which dosages were calculated.

Methods should be standardized for calculating BSA and ideal body weight, rounding calculated results (e.g., drug dosages and administration rates), and changing dosages and administration rates in response to changes in patients' weight and stature. For dosage and administration rates calculated from pharmacokinetic data, the mathematical equations that describe how calculated values were derived should appear in the treatment plans and medication orders.

Standardize the Content of Medication Orders. Standards should be established for the content of an acceptable medication order, requirements for patient-specific measurements, and data that must be included on medication-order forms.[33,34] The following standards are recommended:

1. All orders for patient-care services should be clearly dated and timed.
2. When ordering chemotherapy medications, the generic drug name (as approved by the United States Adopted Names [USAN] program) should be used. Brand names are not acceptable unless they aid in identifying

combination drug products or a particular drug formulation (e.g., to distinguish between liposomal and non-liposomal product formulations).

3. The dosage form should be specified.
4. Orders for medications should include the patient-specific data from which drug doses are calculated (height, weight, BSA, laboratory test results). When drug dosages and schedules are modified for current or anticipated pathologies, treatment plans and medication orders should explicitly identify the factors on which treatment modifications are based. If the order is for chemotherapy as part of the clinical trial, identifying information for the protocol should be included in the order.
5. Drug dosages and calculated doses should be expressed in metric notation. The word units should never be abbreviated in medication orders where drug dosages and administration rates are expressed in biological activity units (e.g., aldesleukin, asparaginase, bleomycin). Leading zeros (e.g., 0.3 mg) should be used for numbers less than one. Trailing zeros should never be used.
6. Medication orders should specify the drug dosage and calculated dose according to the "container rule" (i.e., the specified and calculated dose is the amount prepared in and administered from a single container).[20]
7. Administration vehicle solutions and volumes should be specified, unless standard solutions and volumes have been established.
8. The administration route should be specified.
9. The administration rate should be specified, when relevant.
10. The administration schedule and the duration of treatment should be specified. Treatment plans and medication orders should specify the interval between repeated doses, the days on which each dose is to be given within a treatment cycle or course, and the total length of a treatment cycle or course.
11. The dates and times when drug administration is to commence, or the temporal sequence in which each medication is to be administered, should be specified. When 1200 is written as 12 a.m. or 12 p.m., it may be incorrectly interpreted. Directions indicating events for 1200 should be written as 12:00 noon or 12:00 midnight, or expressed in the 24-hour system.
12. The medical record should contain a justification for the chemotherapy treatment plan (e.g., a reference to FDA product labeling, the primary literature, institutionally approved guidelines, national consensus guidelines, or an investigational protocol); similar information may be included in the medication order to provide additional clarification.
13. Although healthcare providers have traditionally used abbreviations, acronyms, and nicknames to describe chemotherapy medications and treatment regimens, the practice is potentially dangerous and should be avoided. Abbreviations for drug names, scheduling information, and directions for medication use should be prohibited in medication orders. Nonstandard abbreviations, Latin abbreviations, and apothecaries' weights and measures should not be used in orders for chemotherapy medications. Whenever possible, measurement units should be expressed in metric notation.

Therefore, a medication order that complies with these recommendations would appear as follows for a patient with a BSA of 2 m^2: Methotrexate injection 100 mg/m^2/dose = 200 mg in 100 mL 5% dextrose injection/dose, administer by continuous intravenous infusion over 24 hours, every 48 hours for three doses days 1, 3, and 5. Start at 0800 on April 1, 2014.

Establish Dosage Limits and Acceptable Routes of Administration. Medication-use systems should include utilization limits for chemotherapy medications. Constraints should be developed to limit maximum chemotherapy drug dosages and administration routes and schedules. Multidisciplinary peer review should be completed before established drug administration limits are exceeded.[11,12] These constraints should include the maximum amount of a chemotherapy drug that may be administered as a single dose, the maximum amount that may be administered during a defined time interval (including maximum administration rates for parenterally administered medications and maximum dose per day for oral therapy), and the routes by which each drug should be administered.[35] For example, some institutions cap the dose of vincristine at 2 mg or limit the lifetime dose of doxorubicin to 550 mg/m^2 in patients with normal cardiac function.

Constraints for dosage and administration rate may be defined by treatment regimens and protocols and may vary among protocols. In contrast, the types of treatments administered in some practice settings may be consistently similar, permitting the establishment of absolute maximum dose limits within that practice setting.

Limits should also be established for the maximum amount of a chemotherapy drug that may be administered during one treatment course or cycle and, when appropriate, the maximum amount of drug that may be administered to a single patient within his or her lifetime.[11] In addition, dosage limits should be established for chemotherapy medications used in specific combination regimens (defined for each drug) in which clinical toxicities may be exacerbated by combining agents with overlapping adverse-effect profiles.

Chemotherapy drug-use limits should appear prominently in printed treatment descriptions (e.g., protocol summaries, care maps, schematic treatment diagrams) and on printed medication-order forms and computer-based medication-order templates. Active clinical decision support that alerts healthcare providers whenever an order for chemotherapy medications exceeds defined limits would be ideal.[36] For patients who receive chemotherapy medications for which cumulative dosage limits have been established, cumulative dosage data should be constantly updated in their permanent medical records and in any supplementary records. Patients' cumulative dosage data should be audited and independently confirmed by healthcare providers when verifying orders for chemotherapy medications.[11,37]

In each healthcare organization, the medication-use system should include a multidisciplinary committee that oversees matters related to medication-use limits. The committee should proactively develop and establish policies and procedures for resolving disagreements related to patient treatment among providers; whether medications should be prepared, dispensed, and administered if a discrepancy cannot be resolved; and how medication-use-related disputes are to be resolved. Committee membership should comprise all providers who have responsibilities in the medication-use process in the organization.[11]

Investigational Chemotherapy Medications. Cancer patients often receive investigational (i.e., experimental) anticancer treatments at facilities participating in clinical trials. Consideration must be given to ensure that the same safety precautions and checks that are used for FDA-approved chemotherapy therapies apply similarly to prescribing, preparing, dispensing, and administering oral and parenteral investigational medications and monitoring patients who receive those therapies.

Facility administrators should ensure that adequate staff is maintained to support an investigational drug program.[31] Ideally, nurses and pharmacists should be involved early in the process of developing clinical protocols involving the use of commercially marketed and investigational chemotherapy medications.[38] Early involvement helps ensure that chemotherapy regimens are expressed in a fashion to mitigate errors, and investigational medications are prepared and administered in accordance with local policies and procedures. Nurses and pharmacists should be voting members on regulatory and review committees that evaluate the scientific and ethical treatment of patients receiving chemotherapy medications and monitor investigational therapies (e.g., institutional review boards).[11]

Because a protocol governs and supplies the rules for drug use in clinical trials, an up-to-date copy of the study protocol should be available for review at all sites where medications are prepared and administered. All staff should be informed through inservice education programs before new protocols are implemented. Inservice programs and study-related information should be provided by persons associated with the investigational study (e.g., principal investigator, associate investigators, protocol chairperson, study-coordinating personnel). If an investigational protocol is to be conducted at more than one site within a health system, procedures should be developed to ensure that up-to-date information is available at all study sites where patients receive protocol-directed care.

Procedures for supplying healthcare providers with information about patients' dose assignments, drug dosage, and schedule modifications should also be devised. A separate procedure should be established allowing independent dose-checking activity among all disciplines involved in the medication-use process for investigational drugs.

Intrathecal Administration. Administration of chemotherapy via the intrathecal route is necessary for certain treatment regimens. Given the high risk associated with intrathecal administration (e.g., vincristine intrathecal administration is fatal), specific considerations apply to intrathecal administration of chemotherapy:

1. Prescribing should be limited to providers with institutional privileges to prescribe chemotherapy.
2. Drug labels should clearly indicate that the chemotherapy is only intended for intrathecal administration, including ancillary labels. Vinca alkaloid drugs must contain label warnings to avoid intrathecal administration.
3. Medications that will be administered intrathecally should be placed in separate bags from medications administered by other routes (e.g., intravenous, subcutaneous, intramuscular) in the pharmacy. Upon delivery to the unit, intrathecal medications should be stored separately from medications with other routes of administration.
4. Providers administering intrathecal chemotherapy should do so in a setting that has been designated for that procedure. An independent double check by two qualified individuals should be completed prior to administration.

Recommendations for Multidisciplinary Monitoring of Medication Use and Verification

Independent medication-order verification is an essential safeguard that ensures the accuracy and appropriateness of medical treatment. It is imperative that healthcare providers resolve any questions related to medication orders before treatment commences. Providers should recognize that medication-order verification and other system safeguards ensure patients' safety.[11,20,37] Lack of information about patients and their medications has been described as the most frequent cause of medication errors.[24,39] In order to independently verify prescribers' orders for medications, all persons who prepare and administer chemotherapy medications and those who monitor patients who have received chemotherapies should also have access to complete, up-to-date copies of treatment protocols and patient-specific data, including home medication lists.[11,30,37] Drug information and reference materials should be readily available to all persons who provide patient care.

Each healthcare provider has a responsibility to share information with other providers and consultants to ensure patient safety and an optimal treatment outcome. Policies that regulate treatment verification standards should describe how prescribers, medically responsible and senior authorizing physicians, pharmacists and pharmacy technicians, nurses, and other persons who are responsible for transcribing and transmitting medication orders should interact and communicate information.

Providers who prescribe, prepare, dispense, and administer chemotherapy medications should perform independent double checks at defined points in the chemotherapy use process. Treatment-verification systems may incorporate computerized medication-order safety checks but should also include independent manual double checks.[11,31] Ideally, computerized systems (e.g., CPOE) are used to calculate and verify dosages and the rate and route of administration for chemotherapy drug orders and to screen medication orders for compliance with dosage limits. In addition to facilitating chemotherapy-order processing, computer software can also serve as a double check on prescribers' orders. Systems requiring pharmacists to transcribe prescribers' medication orders into a computerized or manual drug-ordering system should have a second person, preferably a pharmacist, recheck all order-processing documents and product labeling before a drug product is dispensed. In situations in which a pharmacist is not available, a prescriber or nurse may serve as the second check.

Providing medications to patients includes five discrete steps: prescribing, preparation, dispensing, administration, and monitoring. The ideal verification system has ten established checkpoints to ensure that an chemotherapy drug is accurately prescribed, prepared, dispensed, and administered to the patient for whom it was intended (**Figure 1**). Different individuals should complete each check so that no single person bears responsibility for checking his or her own work.

Prescribing Chemotherapy Medications (Checkpoint 1). Healthcare providers who prescribe, prepare, and administer chemotherapy drugs should be familiar with the entire treatment regimen. A prescriber should order all the medications necessary for the entire treatment regimen, including hydration and supportive care orders, at the same time and prior to administration of any of the medications. When prescribing chemotherapy regimens based on a patient's weight (or BSA, which relies on weight), weight data and trends in patient weight should be evaluated to be sure the correct information is used. In CPOE, order sets may assist in completing all relevant orders of a treatment regimen at the same time. Requiring all treatment details in advance ensures that orders can be checked for completeness and accuracy and compliance with planned treatment.

Institutions should establish policies regarding whether chemotherapy may be prescribed by physicians-in-training (e.g., medical fellows) and nonphysician healthcare providers with prescribing privileges (e.g., nurse practitioners, physician assistants). If the institution allows prescriptions by these individuals, these orders should be verified by at least one medically responsible person, other than the prescriber, who is knowledgeable about medical oncology.

When orders for chemotherapy drugs must be countersigned by a second medically responsible individual, the person who countersigns the medication orders should critically evaluate each order for a chemotherapy treatment. This is checkpoint 1. The orders should be compared with

FIGURE 1. Medication-order verification system. These established checkpoints ensure a chemotherapy medication is accurately prescribed, prepared, dispensed, administered, and monitored.

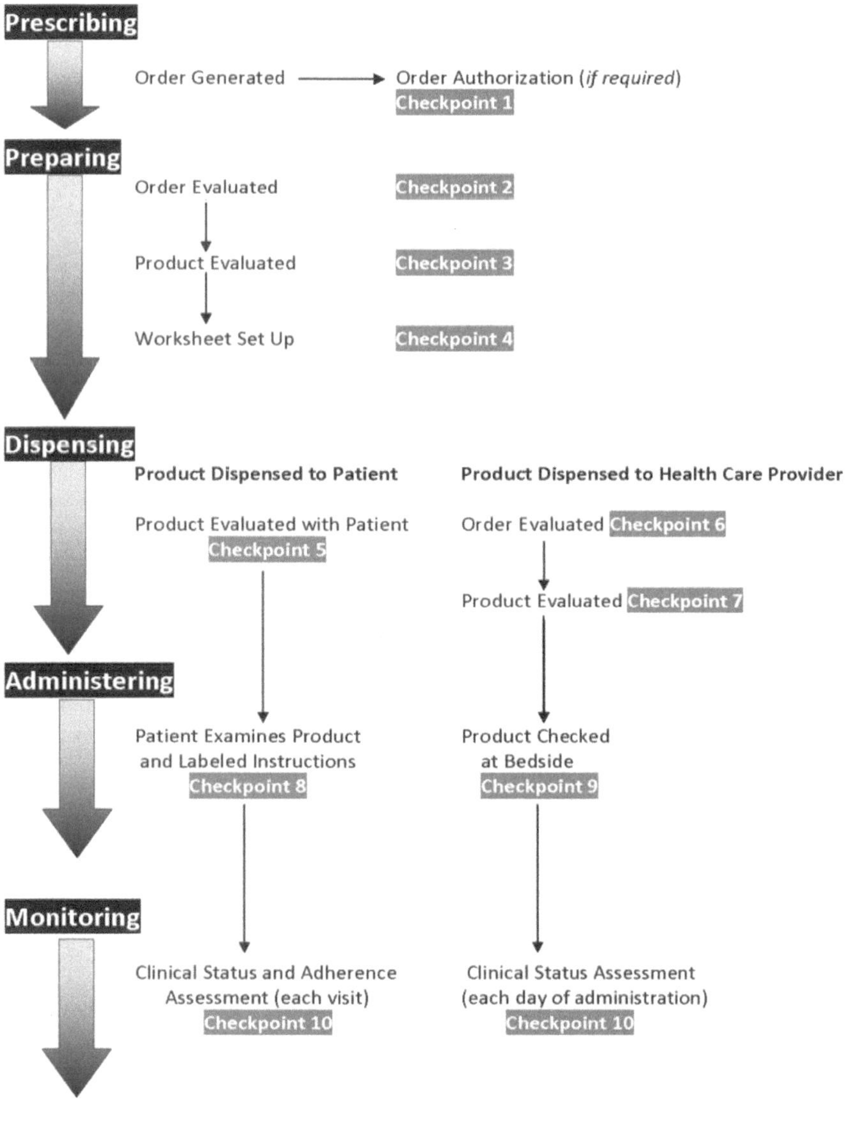

patient-specific data and verified against original reference sources that describe the treatment regimen (e.g., a published article, validated standard reference text, investigational protocol). If the patient is taking part in an investigational study, verification of enrollment onto the trial and of informed consent should be reviewed.

Preparing Chemotherapy Medications (Checkpoints 2–4). Checkpoint 2 requires persons receiving a prescriber's order for chemotherapy medications to review the original medication orders and independently verify them against published standards (e.g., product package labeling, reports published in professional journals, treatment protocols, standard reference textbooks) and determine appropriateness based on patient-specific information. The dose per container and the total course dose should be verified at this checkpoint.

Because erroneous information sometimes appears in published information, orders for noninvestigational chemotherapy medications should be verified against the primary reference in which the specific treatment was described (e.g., published reports, study protocols, meeting proceedings). If a primary reference is not available, the treatment regimen should be confirmed with a resource that previously had been validated as accurately describing the planned treatment (locally compiled handbooks, guides, and compendia) or at least two alternative publications, including reviews and reference textbooks.[11,34] Investigational drug doses and administration schedules must be verified against a study protocol that was approved by all relevant regulatory agencies and study sponsors (e.g., institutional review board, National Cancer Institute, FDA). Protocol amendments should be distributed immediately and be readily available for reference. In addition, order templates should be updated as soon as possible, especially for drug dose or preparation changes.

Although preprinted order forms and CPOE preclude the necessity of repeatedly verifying drug names, dosages, routes, and schedules, all medication orders should be evaluated for completeness, compliance with the planned regimen, and, during repeated courses, deviations from previous treatments by following these recommendations:

1. The date a patient was last treated and the next planned treatment date should be compared to ensure that an appropriate interval has elapsed since treatment was last administered.
2. Measurements from which a patient's medication dosage and administration rate are calculated should be confirmed (e.g., height, weight, BSA). Institutions should develop policies and procedures regarding when patient-specific data (e.g., height, weight, BSA) should be re-measured. It is important to review trends in height and weight as a double check to ensure there were no errors in documentation.
3. Appropriate laboratory test and physical assessment values should be evaluated and primary treatment references should be consulted to determine whether they are within acceptable ranges or if treatment modifications are indicated.
4. A patient's allergy, drug sensitivity, and adverse drug effect histories and his or her current medication profile should be evaluated for potential drug interactions with planned chemotherapy treatment.

For patients who receive treatment in clinical trials in which more than one primary or ancillary treatments are prescribed (e.g., dose- and duration-escalating studies), treatment assignment and dosage and administration schedule modifications should be confirmed with at least one person directly associated with the clinical trial, other than the prescriber (e.g., the principal investigator, an associate investigator, research nurses or pharmacists, a study coordinator or chairperson). The prescriber should be consulted when expected treatment modifications were not ordered or when nonstandard modifications were prescribed.

Instructions for diluents, drug administration sequence and duration, number of doses, and starting date and time should be checked. To ensure that appropriate ancillary and supportive medications that facilitate chemotherapy drug delivery and those required by protocol have been prescribed and are complete and accurate (e.g., premedications, hydration, cytoprotectant and "rescue" medications, antiemetics, hematopoietic growth factors), their orders should be reviewed and confirmed. Discrepancies between prescribed medications and planned treatment should be brought to the prescriber's attention and resolved before medication preparation proceeds.

At checkpoint 3, after treatment orders have been verified, all work related to medication-order processing and preparation accuracy should be routinely documented in a standardized format, either on paper or electronically. Drug preparation work sheets (sometimes referred to as work cards or admixture or compounding logs, sheets, and cards) identify the drug products prepared for each patient and the persons who prepared and checked the medications. Although layout and design may vary among work sheets, and data may be organized as a continuous log in which each drug product appears on separate, consecutive lines or as a separate record for each patient, all work sheets should detail the techniques used in preparing the drug products. They should also identify special preparation and dispensing information, such as the indication of special product containers, requirements for filtration, the need for special diluents, intermediate dilution steps, and how and when administration sets should be attached to the drug product container. Order processing, drug preparation, and processing records should be confirmed by a second individual (preferably a pharmacist).[11,12] The calculations written on preparation work sheets should be independently verified by a second healthcare provider who did not prepare the work sheet. Independent verification should include checking the work sheet for completeness and accuracy of content, with particular attention given to special preparation instructions. A checklist, whether paper or electronic, that identifies the necessary elements in chemotherapy drug preparation may be a helpful reference (**Figure 2**).[11] Technology can serve as a surrogate checklist, if practitioners follow procedures in using appropriately developed and applied software.

At checkpoint 4, drug products should be checked, after preparation, against both the preparation work sheet and the original order by an individual who was not involved in preparing the work sheet. Checklists may also be helpful for this step.[11]

Dispensing Chemotherapy Medications (Checkpoint 5). Checkpoint 5 requires persons dispensing medications to patients or caregivers for outpatient use to verify a patient's identity when a medication is dispensed. Patients who self-administer their medications or personal caregivers should visually examine the medication, confirm whether its appearance meets their expectations, and compare its instructions with information they received from their healthcare providers (e.g., a chemotherapy calendar).

Dispensing and Administering Chemotherapy Medications (Checkpoints 6–9). At checkpoint 6, before starting treatment, each chemotherapy medication should be checked independently against the prescriber's orders by at least two individuals who are trained and competent to administer chemotherapy medications. All dosage- and administration-rate-related calculations should be independently verified. This includes any infusion pump rate settings, which should be checked at the initiation of each container of the infusion, periodically throughout the infusion, and whenever a new nurse assumes care for the patient. Healthcare providers should routinely confirm that the medication will be administered to the intended patient by comparing a patient's name and unique identifying code or number with medication labels (e.g., alpha–numeric characters or bar codes) and that a drug product's identity, ancillary components (e.g., additional medications, diluent, and vehicle solutions), route of administration, and schedule are correct.

At checkpoint 7, healthcare providers should examine the medication container and note whether the content's general appearance is what was expected. Many parenteral chemotherapy products have distinctive colors, and product coloration should be confirmed before administration.

At checkpoint 8, patients who self-administer their medications (or receive it from personal caregivers) should carefully read the container's label to confirm the product's identity and review its instructions for use (schedule of dosing, whether to take with or without food) each time they take a medication.

At checkpoint 9, patients should be encouraged to ask questions about their treatment before its administration and

FIGURE 2. Chemotherapy drug preparation checklists.

Checklist for Initial Setup of Chemotherapy Drug Work Card

This form should be completed on paper or electronically by the pharmacist checking the work card. Place check mark (or N/A) in each space after each check is completed. Your check marks and initials at the bottom of this work sheet are your personal assurance that you checked all these items for accuracy in the setup and transcription of information onto the work card. Each drug requires a separate checklist.

Patient ________________ Drug ______________

Start date ____________

Administration time ____________

Stop date ____________

Duration ____________

Correct drug name ____________

Number of doses _____

Dose ____________

Drug concentration ____________

Drug volume ____________

Diluent ____________

Volume of diluent _____Overfill _____Drug in overfill ____

Expiration time ____________

Special delivery devices (tubing, cassette, container, etc.)

Correct route of administration ______________________

Correct line type, as appropriate ____________________

Correct mixing instructions (special directions, e.g., "Do Not Filter") ____________

Auxiliary label information (e.g., "Do Not Refrigerate," "Use In-line Filter," "For Intrathecal Use Only") _________

Correct total volume ____________

Pharmacist's initials _____________ Date _____________

This record should remain with the work card for the duration of the order and be saved for the supervisor for review after discontinuation of the order.

Supervisor's initials _____________ Date _____________

Continued on next page

FIGURE 2 *(continued)*

Checklist for Preparing and Labeling Chemotherapy Drugs

For each order you check, verify that each element is correct with a check mark.

Patient ____________________ Drug __________

Date ___________

Label check

Patient name is same as on front of work card ________

Drug name on label matches drug name written on back of work card __________

Dose on label matches dose written on back of work card__________

Diluent on label matches diluent written on back of work card __________

Volume of diluent on label matches volume of diluent on back of work card _____

Correct date to prepare __________

Expiration date and time __________

Correct time (expiration date not greater than administration time) __________

For each drug/additive

Correct drug used ______Proper protocol supply ___

Drug concentration in each vial __________

Additives, such as sodium bicarbonate solution, for which large stock bottles are used (which remain in hood) are visually checked, lot number is verified, and technician is asked to verify volume used __________

Drug volume for dose verified __________

Drug lot number on each vial matches lot number written on work card __________

Calculations are checked __________

Drug has not expired __________

For each diluent

Correct diluent _____Volume of diluent ____

Diluent has not expired __________

Special instructions followed

Air purged from bag ___

Tubing affixed/primed to end of line ______

Diluent for reconstitution _____

Correct container ____Proper overfill ___Drug in overfill ___

Final miscellaneous steps

Chemotherapy work card checklist is in card pocket ____

Solution is inspected for impurities/floaters__________

Label is initialed (on left-hand side of label just below last additive or drug) **after** being affixed to correct admixture __________

Total volume to be infused ____ Red chemo i.v. seal ____

"Caution chemo" label ___ Other auxiliary labeling ___

Zip-lock bag ________

Work card is initialed __________

Pharmacist's initials _________ Date __________
Supervisor's initials _________ Date __________

compare its appearance and medication label with information they received about the treatment. Patient identification using two identifiers should occur prior to chemotherapy administration. Whenever possible, barcode-driven administration should be used.[40]

In ambulatory care practice, it is common for patients to receive parenteral chemotherapy medications in a setting where a physician and a nurse (or other healthcare professional) complete all tasks related to prescribing, preparing, administering, and monitoring treatment without a pharmacist's participation. Under these circumstances, the healthcare providers involved should perform independent double checks and be involved in the entire process. The person preparing chemotherapy medications should work from written orders.

Monitoring (Checkpoint 10). Chemotherapy agents are usually expected to produce adverse events, so it is sometimes difficult to detect possible medication errors resulting from failure at one of the prior checkpoints. However, a vigilant healthcare team might discover a potential error sooner if they are knowledgeable about the expected adverse effects and are vigilant for either exaggerated or unexpected adverse effects.

For all chemotherapy agents administered at a healthcare institution, the patient's clinical status should be assessed on each day of chemotherapy administration. Vital signs should be taken and a standardized assessment for possible toxicities should be performed.

For oral chemotherapy agents, assurance that patients understand how to take their chemotherapy medicine should be assessed initially and then at each patient encounter. An assessment for adherence should be performed at each clinic visit. Patients should be taught how to recognize and report expected and unexpected toxicities.

Recommendations for Prescribing Systems and Prescribers

Chemotherapy prescribing is complicated by numerous medical publications that report indications, dosages, and administration schedules inconsistent with FDA-approved product labeling. Chemotherapy treatments frequently involve off-label uses based on preliminary reports, promising information from abstracts, and compendia information. Prescribers must exercise great care in correctly interpreting this information and clearly communicating orders for chemotherapy medications with other healthcare providers.

Health-system administrators should require orders for all chemotherapy medications and other high risk drugs prescribed by physicians-in-training or nonphysician prescribers to be countersigned by a senior physician with expertise in the specialty to safeguard against errors in interpretation and prescribing. Healthcare providers seeking privileges for prescribing chemotherapy drugs should complete an orientation to local policies and procedures related to prescribing chemotherapy before they are permitted to order them for patient care.

Healthcare providers should locally develop standardized dosage and administration schedule modifications for each chemotherapy medication. Treatment modifications may be appropriate for patients with the following characteristics: (1) preexisting pathologies that predispose a patient to adverse effects from treatment with particular chemotherapies (e.g., withholding or decreasing bleomycin dosages in patients with preexisting pulmonary dysfunction or cardiotoxic agents in patients with congestive heart failure); (2) a history of severe, prolonged, or cumulative adverse effects after previous chemotherapy treatments; (3) impaired physiological function that predisposes patients to altered pharmacodynamic responses (e.g., renal or hepatic impairment); (4) low or decreased performance status; and (5) patients on multiple medications with a potential for a drug interaction with a particular chemotherapy.

Healthcare providers should also establish for their institutions standardized guidelines for prescribing drugs that are routinely administered concomitantly with chemotherapy medications. Medication-use guidelines for supportive care and ancillary agents (e.g., antiemetics, hydration, chemoprotectants) should be made accessible to all healthcare providers who prescribe, prepare, and administer chemotherapy drugs and for persons who perform clinical monitoring.

When generating medication orders in a setting where preprinted ordering forms, CPOE, and other electronic and mechanical means (e.g., e-prescribing) are not available, prescribers should legibly print the names of medications, dosages, routes of administration, and administration schedules in plain block letters and Arabic numerals. Medication orders should include the indications for which they are prescribed (e.g., for sore mouth, for nausea, for chronic lymphocytic leukemia).

When chemotherapy treatment (ordering, preparing, and administering) is coordinated at a single location, it is the prescriber's responsibility (or in the conduct of clinical trials, it is the principal investigator's responsibility) to provide information about the treatment (e.g., protocols, publication reprints) to those who prepare and administer medications and monitor patient outcomes. It remains the prescriber's responsibility to answer questions and provide information to other healthcare providers when treatment is implemented in a place that is geographically separate from the prescriber's location. Prescribers, clinical investigators, and medically responsible staff should provide to healthcare providers who prepare and administer chemotherapy medications a complete printed (or electronically reproduced) copy of the treatment regimen.

General Guidelines for Prescribing Chemotherapy Medications.[11,13,20,41] The following are general guidelines for prescribing chemotherapy drugs:

1. Instructions for medication regimens should be explicit, complete, clear, and easy to follow. Treatment regimens should be described accurately and consistently in all written, published, or circulated materials in which chemotherapy medication use is described.
2. The patient's medical record should contain a justification for the chemotherapy treatment plan (e.g., FDA product labeling, a primary literature reference, institutionally approved guidelines, national consensus guidelines, or an investigational protocol).
3. Medication-use systems should require healthcare providers to use standardized vocabulary and nomenclature for describing treatment with chemotherapy medications. "Tall Man" lettering should be used for written and electronic orders.
4. Prescribers should use uniform and consistent notations to express quantifiable amounts (dosage, concentration, volume, and time).
5. Prescribers should never trail a whole number with a decimal point followed by a zero (e.g., write "5 mg," not "5.0 mg").
6. When writing amounts less than one, the expression should be written with a leading zero preceding the decimal point (e.g., "0.125 mg").

7. All treatment plans and medication orders should identify the dosage (as a function of body weight, BSA, or other dosing factors) and the calculated dose. Total course dose should be included in circumstances in which a single infusion container is designed to provide multiple days of treatment (e.g. 7-day cladridine infusion).
8. When treatment day enumeration is arbitrary, day 1 typically describes the day treatment commences. In contrast, hematopoietic progenitor-cell transplantation regimens often include day 0, and significant treatment-related events before and after a progenitor-cell graft is administered are distinguished by negative (minus) and positive (plus) prefixes, respectively.
9. All medications that are a part of the treatment regimen (e.g., oral chemotherapies) should be included, indicating where the product will be filled or dispensed.
10. Recommendations for proper medication storage should also be included. Cancer patients must often travel long distances to receive care, so guidance and support (provision of coolers and ice packets for refrigerated medications) to properly store medications when in transit as well as at home.

In some cases, CPOE can be used to promote best practices (e.g., eliminating the use of trailing and leading zeros [items 4 and 5 above]).

Specific Recommendations for Parenterally Administered Medications.[20] Healthcare providers should adhere to the following guidelines for parenteral chemotherapy drugs:

1. In treatment plans and orders, doses should be expressed as the total amount of medication to be administered from a single container (i.e., the total amount of medication per syringe, bag, or other container).
2. For medication admixtures that can be prepared in more than one way, practitioners should institute *a priori*, standard, and consistent methods directing how each medication will be prepared and administered.
3. When a medication with extended stability is administered from a single container for more than 24 hours, a prescriber's order for treatment should specify the amount of medication to be administered during each 24-hour interval.[20] For example, a medication order for a patient with a BSA of 2 m^2 should read: Drug XYZ (8 mg/m^2/day × 3 days) 48 mg in 150 mL 0.9% sodium chloride injection by continuous intravenous infusion over 72 hours. Start on 04/01/2001 at 0800 (total dose/cycle = 48 mg).

Specific Recommendations for Orally Administered Chemotherapy Medications.[20,42] Prescribing orally administered chemotherapy agents presents unique challenges for healthcare providers due to the greater responsibility placed upon patients to manage their own care and patients' perception that these agents may be less dangerous than parentally administered agents. Healthcare providers should adhere to the following recommendations when oral medications are the prescribed chemotherapy treatment or when oral chemotherapy is included as part of the treatment regimen:

1. In treatment plans and medication orders, drug doses and schedules should be described as the amount of medication to be taken per dose, not as a total daily dose that is to be taken in divided doses.
2. In treatment plans, medication orders, and instructions to a patient, the number of doses to be administered or taken should be clearly identified.
3. Doses for solid orally administered dosage forms should specify whether and how doses are to be rounded to the nearest capsule or tablet strength. If the calculated dose can't be provided based on the available dosage forms, the following alternatives can be considered:
    a Whether tablet formulations should be broken (if not a hazardous drug).
    b. Whether an alternative dosage method or formulation is appropriate.
    c. Whether alternate day dosing is appropriate based on the pharmacokinetic and pharmacodynamic properties of the medication. The goal of alternate day dosing is to fulfill the total weekly dose rather than giving the exact daily dose (e.g., if an agent is to be given 175 mg daily for 2 weeks, but the drug is only available in 50 mg capsules, consider alternate day dosing by giving 200 mg on one day and 150 mg on the next day). If alternate day dosing is used, then instructions that say "take X tablets on odd days and X tablets on even days" should be avoided, as two consecutive odd days may occur when transitioning from one month to another. For example: January 31 and February 1.
4. Only the quantity needed to cover the administration period until the next clinical evaluation should be ordered.
5. If appropriate, instructions should address how medications are to be taken with respect to food ingestion and indicate whether particular types of food may affect medication activity.
6. Oral chemotherapy medication orders should be included with parenteral chemotherapy orders to allow for appropriate screening and safety checks.
7. Oral chemotherapy medication orders should be included on the patient's home medication list to allow for appropriate screening and safety checks.
8. Oral chemotherapy medication orders should be communicated to the pharmacist for appropriate screening and safety checks.
9. Patient instructions should address what to do if a dose is missed.
10. Patients should be provided with explicit instructions regarding what adverse effects to expect, which ones require a telephone call to a provider, and who and where to call.
11. Instructions should describe safe handling, storage, and disposal of oral chemotherapy.
12. Essential ancillary medications and supportive care that accompany a chemotherapy treatment regimen should be explicitly identified.
13. Refills on oral chemotherapy medications should be discouraged, when feasible.
14. Patients should be appropriately educated regarding access and cost issues (e.g., regarding specialty pharmacies, prior authorization, out-of-pocket costs, and options for pharmaceutical manufacturer or copay assistance).

Recommendations for Medication Preparation and Dispensing Systems and Roles for Pharmacists

For each practice setting, persons representing the various healthcare disciplines that prescribe, prepare, and administer chemotherapy medications should participate in planning and managing local medication-use systems.

Standardized Medication Preparation Guidelines. Healthcare providers should establish standardized guidelines for reconstituting, diluting, admixing, packaging, and labeling commonly used chemotherapy and other medications that are routinely administered with chemotherapy. Each practice facility should also establish a standardized method for labeling multidose vials and reconstituted drug products. Standardized medication preparation guidelines should be prominently displayed (e.g., as a chart) for easy accessibility in areas where orders are processed and medications prepared. Policies should be developed for prescribing of oral chemotherapy that are not being dispensed by the health system. Instructions for patient counseling, safe handling, and disposal should be included in these policies.

Policies and procedures should be developed for situations in which medications are prepared at facilities that are geographically removed from where treatment is administered. Procedural protocols should describe requirements for medication packaging, storage conditions during transportation, duration of transport, and handling after delivery. Medication couriers should receive training in organizational policies for handling medications and should immediately report when conditions and handling practices deviate from procedural standards. In addition, handling procedures should ensure patient confidentiality and provide guidelines for emergency situations, such as hazardous-drug spills.

Persons who prepare and dispense chemotherapy medications should ensure timely drug delivery to patients and patient-care areas after receiving written orders. If dispensing is delayed for any reason, healthcare providers awaiting the medications should be notified.[11]

Quality Assurance and Improvement. In collaboration with healthcare providers who prescribe and administer medications, pharmacists and persons who prepare and dispense chemotherapy should take the initiative in developing and managing quality-assurance and quality improvement programs for their medication-use systems. These programs should include surveillance and reporting systems, FMEAs, and root-cause analysis, when appropriate, that track potential and actual medication errors, evaluate the proximal causes of errors among processes and systems, and identify preventive measures.[11,43] The major advantage of multidisciplinary participation is that each discipline's perspectives and methods for conceptualizing system flaws and solutions can be incorporated in designing strategies for preventing medication errors. Confidential reporting is essential to the success of a medication-error surveillance and reporting system. Only by understanding what causes and contributes to errors can the number of errors be reduced. In designing a medication-error surveillance and reporting system, strategic emphasis should be placed on understanding why errors occur and not on blaming or censuring personnel.[44] Further, proactive assessment of the chemotherapy-use process should be conducted.

Orientation on Medication-Error Reduction. Pharmacy supervisors and managers should develop an orientation program about medication errors commonly associated with chemotherapy medications for training of pharmacy personnel who prepare and dispense chemotherapy. Pharmacists should develop ongoing interprofessional educational programs that focus awareness on potential medication errors with chemotherapy medications, strategies for preventing errors, and local and national medication-error reporting and evaluation systems for all practitioners who have direct patient contact.

Pharmacists should engage the support of medical and nursing administrators and supervisors to encourage their staff (particularly those in professional training programs) to complete chemotherapy medication-error awareness programs.[30] Educational programs should be discipline specific. Program content should include medication-error case scenarios, problem-solving to prevent and mitigate medication errors, and discussion about the effects that medication errors have on patients' quality of life and the health system.[11,31]

Standardized Drug Procurement and Storage. Pharmacists who select and procure drugs should strive to minimize or eliminate look-alike drug product containers and limit the availability of different vial sizes for parenteral medications whenever possible.[12] Frequent additions to the variety of available drug products and changes among alternative manufacturers' drug products can contribute to medication-use errors and should be avoided. If it is necessary to change manufacturers, healthcare organizations should develop a process to ensure staff are educated about the new product and that computer systems have the appropriate manufacturer's information. When practical, drug products with similar names and packaging should not be stored next to each other. Medication-use systems that involve a formulary should separate nonformulary products from those that are on the formulary. Healthcare providers should familiarize themselves with chemotherapy drugs that are not on formulary before prescribing, preparing, and administering them.

Standardized Medication Preparation and Dispensing. Chemotherapy medications should be dispensed in ready-to-administer dosage forms whenever possible. Generally, chemotherapy for intermittent parenteral administration should be prepared so that each medication container has only one dose. The risk of incorrect medication use is increased when the amount of drug dispensed in a single container exceeds the amount to be administered during a 24-hour period. It is essential that individuals and committees responsible for developing and overseeing medication-use systems establish guidelines on whether prescribers may order chemotherapy preparations to be administered from a single container for more than 24 hours. In all practices where parenteral drugs with extended stability (more than 24 hours) are sanctioned, it is imperative that the duration of their use is clearly labeled and that healthcare providers are trained to correctly prescribe, prepare, and administer them.[20]

When preparing a chemotherapy admixture, a quantity of medication that most closely approximates the prescribed dose should be segregated from other drug supplies. For treatment regimens that include two or more drugs, especially when medications are to be administered by different routes, the medications should be physically segregated during preparation and when administered. Compounded medications should be prepared one at a time, using standardized techniques whenever possible.

The chemotherapy preparation process should include an independent double check by two separate individuals of the correct drug, diluents, administration containers, and volume measurements before the solutions are transferred to the final administration container. A person other than the individual who selected the components of the preparation (drug and diluent) and measured the volume of diluent solutions used to reconstitute the medications should visually confirm the correct product(s) and measurement(s) before the solutions are transferred from the measuring device to the drug vial for reconstituted drugs and to the final administration container. Post hoc or proxy methods for checking medication preparation, including pulling back syringe plungers to demonstrate the volume of fluid that was injected into the secondary container, should not be used as the sole method for verifying chemotherapy product preparation. Verification may be accomplished by direct visual inspection; remote monitoring through telepharmacy applications (with pictures); or by weighing syringes, other transfer devices, and intermediate product containers before fluid transfer is completed. Whenever possible, methods that allow direct observation of product preparation should be used. The actual original medication vials and diluents that were used during preparation must be present for inspection during the verification process.

Technologies to automate the preparation of sterile products, including chemotherapy, are emerging. Some robotic technologies enclose and automate the entire production process, and these products may provide a variety of benefits to institutions with a sufficient volume of chemotherapy to justify their substantial cost. A more common technology organizes information, manages workflow, adds new checks, and documents parenteral drug therapy preparation through a combination of computer software, barcodes, and cameras. In these systems, the components of a chemotherapy preparation are verified with bar code technology and pictures before preparation, and pictures of the preparation are stored. These systems add additional double checks with the barcode technology and improve documentation of the preparation and other relevant information such as product lot number. In some settings, the photos taken through this technology enable the pharmacist to check chemotherapy preparation outside the sterile area. Like other technologies, automation for parenteral therapies must be carefully implemented to be certain the new technology is not eliminating checks in the process. For example, bar coding the components of a chemotherapy dose does not eliminate the need to check the components of the chemotherapy before they are admixed.

Standardized Medication Labeling. Strict procedures should be established for standardizing medication labeling. A uniform, systematic labeling method should be used, especially when multiple drugs are prepared for a single patient. Medication labels should be mechanically printed (not handwritten). Chemotherapy medications should be labeled immediately after preparation. Oral medications should also be sealed with child-resistant or poisoning-prevention closures.

Chemotherapy agents are administered parenterally by many routes other than the intravenous route (e.g., intrathecally, intrahepatically, intrapleurally, intraarterially). Inadvertent administration by the wrong route can result in serious or fatal consequences (e.g., administering vincristine intrathecally is fatal). Medication-use systems should include policies and procedures that clearly distinguish medications administered by the intravenous route from those intended for administration by other routes. Auxiliary labels may facilitate distinguishing among medications that are administered by particular delivery methods.

Labels for oral dosage forms, rectal suppositories, and topically applied unit-dose products should include *all* of the following information:

1. Patient's name, unique identifying code or number, and location within a treatment facility (when applicable).
2. Date (with or without specifying time) the medication was dispensed.
3. Generic drug name.
4. Dosage form and strength.
5. Amount of medication per dose (when the container dispensed holds more than one dose).
6. Administration route.
7. Detailed instructions to the patient for self-administering the medication (including a dosing calendar when appropriate).
8. Supplemental administration instructions (e.g., starting and completion dates and times; number of doses to administer; cautionary information about when medications are to be taken in relation to food ingestion and other medications; and instructions and warnings regarding administration route, handling precautions, storage conditions, and container closures).
9. The quantity dispensed within each container (the number of tablets, capsules, or suppositories, packaged in a single container).

Labels for injectable dosage form containers should include *all* of the following information:

1. Patient's name, unique identifying code or number, and location within a treatment facility (when applicable).
2. Generic drug name.
3. The amount of medication per container and, when a product container holds more than one dose (e.g., multiple doses for intermittent administration), the amount of medication per dose).[20]
4. How much overfill is added to a container when excess medication and fluid volumes are added to displace air from the tubing lumen ("dead space") in administration sets.
5. Route of administration (for example, medications prescribed for administration other than by the intravenous route—especially those for intrathecal administration—should bear ancillary labels that distinctively identify the intended administration route).
6. The name and amount of all drug additives in a chemotherapy admixture.
7. Diluent (vehicle fluid) name.

8. The volume of fluid to be administered. Adding overfill to the container should be discouraged, but when unavoidable, both the volume to administer and the overfill volume should be specified. Proper education for nurses administering these products is essential to ensure that patients do not receive additional drug.
9. Administration rate and duration. Ideally, both administration rate and duration should be specified. Because administration rates can be calculated from the volume to be administered and duration of administration, duration is the essential component.
10. Supplemental administration instructions, such as starting and completion dates and times; prohibitions about when medications are not to be administered in relation to other medications; and instructions and warnings regarding administration (e.g., information about special requirements for administration sets, including inline filtration, warnings to avoid intrathecal administration with vinca alkaloid drugs, and hazardous- drug warning labels).
11. When it is necessary to prepare more than one medication intended for sequential administration, the container labels should be numbered. The sequence in which each container is to be used and the total number of containers (e.g., bag 1 of 3, bottle 3 of 7) should be indicated.
12. Date (with or without specifying time) the medication was ordered or prepared. Investigational compounds, in particular, should be labeled with the date and time they were prepared.
13. Expiration date and time after which a medication should no longer be used (i.e., beyond-use date and time).
14. Cautionary warnings as required for hazardous drug products.[45]
15. Storage specifications.
16. The name (with or without specifying location or telephone number) of the institution, pharmacy, or practice from which a medication was dispensed and the prescriber's identity.

Credentialing Pharmacists for Chemotherapy Medication-Use Programs. Pharmacy managers and supervisors should require pharmacist employees to complete training and demonstrate competencies related to chemotherapy medication use, evaluating medication orders, preparing chemotherapy medications, safe handling procedures, error surveillance and reporting programs, and local policies as a prerequisite to pharmacist credentialing. Healthcare organizations should periodically reassess pharmacist employees' competencies related to their responsibilities, increasing the frequency of reassessment if performance problems occur.[14]

Roles for Pharmacists. Among primary healthcare providers, pharmacists generally are best positioned to ensure that medications are used rationally and safely and increase others' awareness about medication errors and how to prevent them. Pharmacists should participate in all aspects of patient care related to chemotherapy treatment, including developing policies for safe and appropriate medication use and other services consistent with pharmacist patient care.[11,30] Pharmacists should participate with other primary healthcare providers in multidisciplinary groups that develop, implement, and periodically reevaluate practice-specific procedures and processes for verifying chemotherapy medication orders, resolving procedural questions related to confirming and processing medication orders, and evaluating and resolving disputes among healthcare providers.

Each organization should establish a minimum acceptable level of pharmacist participation in the error-prevention elements of patient care, such as proactively reviewing medication orders, screening laboratory results, providing drug information and patient counseling, and reviewing drug storage conditions.[11,46]

The following roles are recommended for pharmacist participation:

1. Educating healthcare providers about medication errors.
2. Independently verifying medication dosages, routes of administration, and schedules.
3. Participating in multidisciplinary efforts to establish drug-specific utilization constraints that limit maximum doses, administration rates, and administration schedules for chemotherapy medications.
4. Participating in multidisciplinary efforts to standardize the prescribing vocabulary and the development, implementation, and maintenance of standardized order sets.
5. Participating in multidisciplinary efforts to educate patients, their families, and personal caregivers.
6. Participating in multidisciplinary efforts to develop adherence programs and monitor patient adherence to prescribed regimens, including recommendations for supportive care to treat and or mitigate adverse events associated with chemotherapy agents.
7. Participating in multidisciplinary efforts to assist patients with accessing medications (e.g., prior authorization, manufacturer assistance programs, copay assistance programs, coping with drug shortages).
8. Improving communication among healthcare providers and among healthcare providers, patients, and caregivers.
9. Working with pharmaceutical or equipment manufacturers on medication-specific safety strategies.

Drug Information Resources and Education for Providers. Pharmacists should help ensure the availability of up-to-date references on the appropriate use of chemotherapy drugs for all healthcare providers involved in medication use.[11,31] Drug information resources should provide information about:

- Drug products' FDA-approved labeling, compendia-supported indications, and investigational uses.
- Drug-specific precautionary warnings and information about adverse effects, particularly dosage- and schedule- limiting effects.
- Potential interactions with other drugs, disease states, and foods.
- Administration methods, including drug admixture stability and compatibility data.
- Usual adult and pediatric dosages.
- Dosage recommendations for single- and multiple-treatment courses.
- Treatment modifications for persons with concurrent pathologies or end-organ impairment.
- Safety Data Sheets.
- Pharmacokinetically based dosing and monitoring guidelines.

Information and guidelines for handling chemotherapy extravasations and hypersensitivity reactions, including the use of antidotes, should be developed by a multidisciplinary team and be readily available.

Pharmacists should develop and provide discipline-specific educational materials about chemotherapy medication use to healthcare providers who prescribe, prepare, and administer chemotherapy medications. The instructional tools developed for each professional healthcare discipline should complement the materials developed for the other disciplines.[11]

When new chemotherapies, treatment regimens, or treatment protocols are introduced, pharmacists should assume a continuous, proactive leadership role in developing educational programs and materials for healthcare providers, patients, and caregivers.[11,31] Pharmacists should assess the competency of individuals assigned primary responsibility for chemotherapy education to confirm their ability to effectively communicate medication-related information.

For patients whose care is transferred from oncologists to nonspecialist practitioners, oncology pharmacy specialists should develop and provide drug monographs, medication-use summaries, and other treatment-related materials describing how oral and parenteral chemotherapy medications and treatment regimens are to be accomplished.[12,30] The need is especially acute among organizations and practitioners who provide local care for patients enrolled in clinical trials or receiving investigational chemotherapy treatments.

Treatment Protocols. Oncology pharmacy specialists should participate in developing treatment protocols for standard treatments and clinical investigations. In practice settings where chemotherapy medications and treatment regimens are used routinely, pharmacists should initiate the development of tools that standardize the way medications are ordered, thereby facilitating accurate and appropriate prescribing, order interpretation and verification, and medication processing and dispensing.[31,47] Pharmacists should lead initiatives to standardize drug preparation procedures, including reconstitution, dilution, and drug admixture methods for commonly used parenteral chemotherapy medications.[12]

CPOE. Pharmacists should work with information systems personnel, computer programmers, and software vendors to develop CPOE systems. System requirements should include mechanisms for standardizing medication orders, decreasing opportunities for error by minimizing data entry, and screening orders for medication doses and administration schedules that exceed established limits. Pharmacists should advocate for and participate in establishing maximum safe chemotherapy dosage and scheduling limits with physicians, nurses, and other primary healthcare providers. Pharmacists should guide the appropriate use of clinical decision support in CPOE systems for chemotherapy and the medication management process.

Vocabulary and Nomenclature. Pharmacists are uniquely qualified to lead multidisciplinary efforts to develop and implement clear, detailed, standardized vocabulary and nomenclature for chemotherapy treatment regimens, medication orders, and administration instructions. Pharmacists should participate in the early stages of protocol development for standard treatments and clinical investigations to ensure that pharmacotherapeutic regimens are clearly described, easily understood, and incorporate standardized language, content, abbreviations, and units of measure.[11,20,30]

Patient Education and Counseling. Pharmacists should ensure that educational materials used for patient education are comprehensive and routinely updated. When meeting or interviewing patients, their family members, or other home-based caregivers (e.g., completing medication-use and allergy histories, screening blood pressure, performing ongoing treatment response assessment, dispensing medications), pharmacists should provide medication education and counseling. They should verify that patients and their caregivers understand the following:

1. The purpose of the medication and its intended use.
2. The appropriate use and safe handling of medications (e.g., don't place oral chemotherapy agents in a pill box, keep away from children) and administration devices.
3. Appropriate temperature and safe storage conditions.
4. Special precautions to prevent exposure to hazardous materials that may be present in patients' clothing, linens, body fluids, and excreta during and after treatment.
5. The potential interactions with other medications and foods.
6. The critical need for good medication adherence practices.
7. What to do if a dose is missed.
8. Dosing calendars or other supplemental information to improve adherence.
9. Common and possible adverse effects associated with the medication.
10. Methods for preventing, managing, and reporting adverse effects.
11. What to do if potentially serious adverse effects occur, including when to contact a provider, who to contact, and how to reach them.[11,36]
12. How to properly dispose of the medication, container, and supplies.
13. Access and cost issues (specialty pharmacies, prior authorization, out-of-pocket costs, options for pharmaceutical manufacturer or copay assistance, drug shortages).

Pharmacists should provide educational materials to patients and suggest supplemental and alternative information resources, such as the National Cancer Institute information services department (1-800-4-CANCER and www.cancer.gov), the American Cancer Society, libraries, and bookstores.[11] If pharmacists are not available to provide chemotherapy patient education, they should assist in competency assessment of those assigned primary responsibility for that education.

Advocates for Patients' Rights. Pharmacists should encourage patients and their caregivers to participate in their own care and advise patients how to protect themselves from medication errors. Pharmacists should advise patients that they are entitled to satisfactory answers from their healthcare providers. Pharmacists should encourage patients to double-check the details of their treatment, including drug names and dosages, and to request dosage recalculation if their biological measurements change. Pharmacists who participate in developing treatment plans and protocols should ensure that consent-for-treatment forms contain accurate, complete information to secure patients' informed consent. Pharmacists should help to prepare treatment consent forms; provide patients with an accurate and detailed description of their treatment plan in clear, unambiguous, and easily understood language and answers to their questions about the treatment and alternative treatment options; and assess patients' understanding of expected and possible outcomes. Pharmacists should also describe their role as primary care providers and the care they provide.[11,12]

Clinical Intervention, Analysis, and Performance Improvement. In addition to dispensing medications, pharmacists can help improve the quality of patient care by implementing a proactive clinical intervention program and documenting healthcare providers' deviations from planned chemotherapy treatments. Longitudinal data collection, analysis, and reporting can reveal system flaws that contributed to (or failed to prevent) prescribing errors, suggest targets for quality improvement, and validate pharmacists' interventions.

Pharmacists should proactively work with other primary care providers to establish medication-use reporting and surveillance programs. Committees established for this purpose should include representatives from medical, nursing, pharmacy, and risk-management disciplines. Programs should continually evaluate local medication-use systems to identify potential problems and solutions related to medication use and prevent medication errors.[11,43] Such programs in institutions should seek endorsement from appropriate local multidisciplinary committees (e.g., pharmacy and therapeutics, medical executive, and clinical practice committees).

Feedback for Pharmaceutical Manufacturers and Regulators. Pharmacists should work with pharmaceutical manufacturers and the FDA to eliminate ambiguous, confusing, and potentially misleading drug product and treatment information from published resources (e.g., product packaging, package inserts, official compendia, and promotional information). Pharmacists working in the pharmaceutical manufacturing industry should proactively identify preventable causes of product-user errors and adverse effects associated with product labeling, packaging, and promotion.[48] Pharmacists' voluntary participation in national reporting programs can increase the awareness of medication errors and promote error prevention throughout the healthcare system. These aggregate data promote changes in product identity, packaging, labeling, commercial information, and marketing practices that are subject to manufacturers' control and governmental regulation.[11,41]

Recommendations for Medication Administration Systems and Roles for Nurses

Nurses are often the last link in the chain of healthcare providers who provide treatment with chemotherapy medications. To safeguard patients from mistakes that have potentially lethal consequences, evidence-based systems have evolved that promote safety and include[4]:

- Requirements for credentialing persons who administer chemotherapy medications.
- Tools and methods to facilitate documentation and identification of correct medication use.
- Independent verification of medication orders.
- Independent double check of the final product and infusion pump settings.
- Accurate documentation of medication use and effects on patient care.
- Strict compliance with regulations and practice standards.
- Patient education regarding medication safety.

Credentialing Nurses for Chemotherapy Medication-Use Programs. Organizational policies and procedures should require nurse employees to complete training and demonstrate nursing care-related competencies, such as administering chemotherapy medications, caring for patients who have received chemotherapy medications, and knowledge of local policies. Specialty certification (e.g., ONS Oncology Certified Nurse credential, ONS Chemotherapy and Biotherapy Provider Card) is highly encouraged. Nurses may be required to complete additional training and competency assessments before they are permitted to administer experimental medications. Training usually combines didactic and supervised practical instruction. Didactic instruction generally includes training about specific chemotherapy agents, appropriate dosages and dosage ranges, adverse effects and clinical toxicities, administration techniques, and safe handling. Technical experience in administering chemotherapy medications requires demonstrating competence with administering intravenous medications. Healthcare organizations should periodically (at least annually, but more frequently if performance problems occur) reassess nurses' competencies related to their responsibilities.

Standardized Medication Administration Practices. In collaboration with the multidisciplinary team, nurses within an organization should standardize chemotherapy administration practices. It should be determined whether intravenous chemotherapy agents should be infused as a primary or secondary infusion across the organization. Institutions should establish cut-off times to initiate nonurgent chemotherapy administration in relation to the need for adequate staffing.

Medication safety technologies should be implemented to enhance the chemotherapy administration process. ASHP encourages health systems to adopt bar-code-enabled medication administration (BCMA) technology to improve patient safety and the accuracy of medication administration and documentation.[39] Infusion pumps that provide dose and infusion-rate warnings (often called "smart pumps") should also be implemented. Because of unique challenges from chemotherapy (e.g., BSA-based dosing), some organizations' pumps may not immediately provide warnings for chemotherapy, and care must be taken to make enhancements to the technology to accommodate chemotherapy. Appropriate use of both of these technologies provides new checks in the chemotherapy administration process.

Standardized Tools for Recording Medication Administration. Nurses with a variety of experiences have devised and contributed to designing tools to facilitate the prevention of drug administration errors, such as standardized work sheets used to calculate medication dosages and administration rates and checklists of pertinent laboratory results and physiological measurements. Treatment flow sheets provide easily interpretable information about when a patient's previous treatments were administered, whether dosages and medication delivery deviated from planned treatment, and the cumulative amount of medication administered. Thoughtfully designed treatment flow sheets may become part of a patient's permanent medical record and can be an invaluable resource for patient care.

Checking Orders and Equipment for Administering Chemotherapy Medications. Medication orders for chemotherapy require documentation of independent double-checks by two individuals prior to administration.[4] These individuals should be different than the individual who prepared the product. In addition, nurses should evaluate and confirm the functional integrity of vascular access devices (and devices for other administration routes), medication pumps, and other devices that control medication delivery. For adjustable and programmable mechanical and electronic devices, mechanical adjustments or electronic programming for delivering the correct dose at the appropriate rate should be independently verified with another healthcare provider who is knowledgeable about the delivery device before it is used to administer medications.

Recording and Tracking Chemotherapy Use. After medications have been administered, it is a nurse's responsibility to manually or electronically record the activity. The documentation should be in a standardized format and include the patient's name, the names of all medications administered, dosages, administration routes, rates of administration, the date and time administration began, the duration of administration or time that treatment was completed, and whether adverse effects were observed or reported by the patient during or after administration. Communications with patients, other healthcare providers, and personal caregivers should be documented in an objective, chronological narrative style, reporting the dates and times the events occurred, the names of involved persons, and how questions and problems were resolved.

Clinical Intervention, Analysis, and Performance Improvement. Nurses and other personnel should immediately report to medically responsible personnel and their supervisors any instance in which medications were used incorrectly and the events attributable to the error. In response to discovering a medication-use error, a provider's primary responsibility is to ensure the patient's safety. Subsequently, the error and related circumstances should be recorded in accordance with specific policies and procedures. Medication-use error reports (also called occurrence, safety, or incident reports) should be written in an objective, chronological, narrative style without editorial remarks and speculative comments. Comprehensive occurrence reports are useful in discovering and evaluating system flaws and may provide the impetus for improving medication-use systems.

To prevent medication errors, nurses and other personnel who administer chemotherapy medications must comply with policies and procedures that define standards of practice. It is important, however, to periodically reevaluate practice standards in order to assess how well a medication-use system functions, make appropriate changes, and, ultimately, improve patient safety and the quality of care.

Healthcare providers administering chemotherapy medications should not deviate from guidelines for ordering, preparing, and administering chemotherapy agents. Examples of inappropriate practice include borrowing medications from a patient's drug supply to give to another patient and preparing agents without the proper facilities or staff. Medication administration schedules should be followed as closely as possible; providers and caregivers should strive to comply with treatment plans. Drug administration should be documented promptly after it is completed, and providers administering chemotherapy medications should rigorously comply with local requirements for documenting treatment. To prevent the inadvertent duplication of treatment, it is recommended that one individual assume the primary responsibility for each patient during a work period (shift or tour of duty). When one individual cannot assume primary responsibility for each patient during a work period, appropriate hand-off communication is essential.

Nurses and Patient Education. Nurses who administer chemotherapy medications have a prominent role in educating patients about their chemotherapy. Nurses should encourage patients and their personal caregivers to ask questions about their treatment. Patient education guidelines may be included in treatment maps and clinical care plans.

Recommendations for Patient Education

Well-informed patients (and their authorized caregivers) are the vital last link in the safety chain to prevent errors related to chemotherapy medications. Patients are entitled to know all pertinent facts about the medications they receive during their treatment. Healthcare providers charged with educating patients should have demonstrated competency to accurately perform this function. Healthcare providers have an obligation to encourage patients to ask questions and to provide answers.

The following suggestions are offered to help patients and their caregivers ensure optimal outcomes from the cancer therapy medications.

Multifocal Medication Education. Patients need multifocal education about the purpose, adverse effects, schedules, routes of administration, and descriptions (e.g., colors, shapes) for all the medications they will receive during their treatment. This includes the chemotherapy regimen, including both oral and intravenous therapy, and all ancillary and supportive medications, such as antiemetics and medications that hasten bone marrow recovery. In order to ensure patients receive the appropriate education to manage their therapy or its side effects, it is imperative that roles of the various healthcare professionals are defined and that responsibility for primary patient education versus reinforcement of key information is clearly delineated. When patients are well informed and the information they receive is reinforced by nurses, pharmacists, and other caregivers, they are better prepared to detect a misinterpreted medication order and assertively question conflicting information.[49] Healthcare professionals should be sensitive to the emotional aspects of patients with cancer when planning medication education. Education should take place at a time when a patient is able to listen and understand. Medication education should not be attempted when patients are sedated or confused as a result of medications or immediately after receiving their cancer diagnosis.

Patients should participate in their care by asking questions about their cancer treatment and related medications and by confirming the regimen with their nurse before receiving treatment. Healthcare providers should make educational materials available in counseling and treatment areas to encourage patients to learn more about their cancer therapies.

Health-System Procedures Education. Patients should understand the health system's plan for chemotherapy medication-error prevention. They should become familiar with their providers' routine procedures for checking medication orders so that they can understand the safeguards that have been established and why delays may occur before their treatment can be started. For example, patients can remind the person administering chemotherapy to compare medication labels with a patient's identity and can verify their height and weight each time they are measured.

Patient Participation in a Medication-Use System. Patients (or their caregivers) should be knowledgeable about their medications and the ways in which the medications are to be administered according to their treatment plan. In some circumstances, patients should be encouraged to take responsibility for some of their care to help improve their quality of life. Examples include self-administering medications, maintaining the patency of vascular access devices, giving themselves a subcutaneous injection, and troubleshooting a problem with the portable infusion pump. Patients should demonstrate their ability to perform these functions if they are included in the therapy plan. Competency and readiness for self-administration should be assessed for patients prescribed oral chemotherapy.

Each patient should be given a detailed treatment calendar that clearly identifies his or her treatment plan. They should be encouraged to keep their calendar with them to compare the expected treatment with what is being dispensed and administered.

Patients' Responsibilities. Patients should be taught and empowered to detect and to seek help in managing adverse effects that may occur during their cancer treatment. Healthcare providers should be promptly informed about adverse effects experienced during a chemotherapy cycle before the next cycle commences. Patients should keep a list of the medications that they may self-administer to treat these adverse effects. Patients should be encouraged and taught how to report medication errors and near misses that occur as a result of self-administration. Safe handling, storage, and disposal of oral chemotherapy should be taught to the patient or their caregiver.

It is important for healthcare providers to be able to determine potential interactions between a patient's nonchemotherapy medications and the chemotherapy they are to receive. Therefore, patients should be requested to provide to their healthcare team members a list of all medications they are using, including over-the-counter preparations, dietary supplements, and other complementary and alternative medicines. In general, use of any medication should be discussed with their healthcare providers before initiating therapy.

Recommendations for Manufacturers and Regulatory Agencies

Pharmaceutical manufacturers have a responsibility to exercise care in designing product packaging and labeling, determining dosage strengths and dosage forms, and in promoting their products, as these features may contribute to errors in prescribing, product selection, preparation, and administration. Companies that market chemotherapy agents should develop and support educational programs that encourage safe and accurate prescribing, preparation, administration, handling, storage, and disposal of their products. The following guidelines address some of the major areas.

Product Naming, Packaging, Labeling, and Drug Dosage Strengths/Forms. Companies should avoid trademarking drug names that look or sound similar to those of other drug products. Proprietary drug names for new products and product formulations should not be similar to existing generic and proprietary names. Manufacturers should avoid appending letters and numbers to drug names, as this practice can result in potential confusion with dosage strengths, medication quantities, and the amount of medication to be administered.

Product packaging and labeling should provide clear, easily distinguished features to identify a drug and the amount of drug per dosage unit (e.g., tablet, capsule, wafer) and within a product container (e.g., vials, bags, bottles, prefilled syringes). It is particularly important that a drug product's USAN-approved generic name appear more prominently than other information on the product label. Drug names should be printed on both the front and back of the containers and packaging of parenteral drugs; "Tall Man" characters should be used to distinguish between similar drug names. Container labels for drugs that are in solution and for those that require reconstitution or dilution before they are used should identify the total drug content in mass units (or biological activity units) rather than concentration.[19] Product packaging and labeling that include both mass and concentration values should be designed to display mass units more prominently. Product packaging should include a bar code on inner and outer packaging.

Labels should be unique and well designed. Distinguishing colors and contrasting hues facilitate identifying and distinguishing drug products and products in different strengths and concentrations. Warnings and special or unique instructions should be prominently displayed on product packaging and labeling. Unique labeling and packaging techniques should be used to prevent product misidentification and to warn about dosing errors and unique characteristics that predispose medication users to potentially serious or life-threatening toxicities. Examples include the unique way that the Platinol-AQ brand of cisplatin injection (Bristol-Myers Squibb, Princeton, NJ) is packaged to prevent misidentification with carboplatin and the cautionary statements on vials containing vincristine sulfate injection that warn against using the entire contents of a vial for a single patient (on bulk packages) and that intrathecal administration may be fatal.

A statement that declares a drug's approved routes of administration is optional and may or may not appear on product packaging. If the agent is approved for administration by only one route, it must be clearly indicated.

Appropriate storage temperatures or conditions should be clearly visible on drug labeling and packaging.

Drug labeling and packaging must identify the manufacturer's product lot or control number.

Drugs that must be reconstituted and diluted before clinical use should include reconstitution instructions that identify appropriate diluents and volumes.

A manufacturer's drug product preparation date (for experimental drugs) or an expiration date should be clearly visible on the product label.

Special instructions (e.g., "Shake Well," "Do Not Shake," "Albumin Required") and instructions for dilution should appear on product labeling. In cases where important information will not fit on a product label, a package insert, or "pull-away" label may be required as part of the labeling and packaging.

In the case of oral chemotherapy agents, careful consideration should be given to dosage forms and strengths provided. Often patients must combine multiple strengths of a medication to receive their prescribed dosage, thereby increasing the opportunity for a medication error. Many oncology patients have difficulty swallowing and cannot take solid dosage forms. Manufacturers should be responsive to dosing practice patterns and other patient-specific needs of oncology patients that become apparent after medications are released into the market.

Product changes should be widely communicated to prescribers, pharmacists, nurses, and other healthcare providers involved in drug prescribing, preparation, and administration.

Package inserts and product information that describe medical indications, medication doses, administration schedules, safe handling, disposal, and product use should not include abbreviations. This is especially important for drugs used in complex treatment regimens.

Educational Materials and Programs. Pharmaceutical manufacturers and drug product sponsors should be encouraged to provide educational materials and programs that promote and encourage safe use of their drug products. Programs should clearly explain the indications appearing on FDA-approved labeling, dosages, methods for preparation, administration routes and schedules, and safe handling and disposal. Treatment descriptions should be standardized and consistent with guidelines designed to prevent medication-use errors.[20] Medication names and administration information should not be abbreviated in educational and promotional materials.

Restricted Drug Distribution. Chemotherapy agents, particularly newer oral chemotherapy agents, may be subject to restricted distribution. Restricted drug distribution products are available only through a select distribution program in which only prescribers and patients registered with the program are able to prescribe, administer, and receive the product.[50] Restricted distribution can occur due to decisions made by pharmaceutical manufacturers or as a result of Risk Evaluation and Mitigation Strategies (REMS).[51] There are circumstances in which properly implemented constraints on the traditional drug distribution system are appropriate.[52] The primary safety concern is that restricted distribution may adversely affect continuity of care. For example, when patients receive medications from various sources (clinic, local pharmacy, specialty pharmacy), it is difficult to establish a comprehensive medication list for screening of drug interactions, therapeutic duplications, and other important aspects of medication management. Delays in therapy could result when patients must wait for medications to be shipped to their home from a specialty pharmacy. Receiving prescriptions by mail does not allow for a face-to-face interaction between the patient and the pharmacist, where patient concerns and educational deficits may be identified. In addition, specialty pharmacies may not have access to the patient's complete health record and this may compromise the specialty pharmacist's ability to properly verify the order. Given these challenges, when patients can only obtain chemotherapy through a restricted drug distribution system, pharmacists and other providers should proactively provide relevant information to patients and specialty pharmacies to coordinate care. Follow up, such as phone calls, should be conducted to verify that the patient receives the chemotherapy and understands proper use. The ASHP Task Force on Caring for Patients Served by Specialty Suppliers provided recommendations for effectively managing restricted-distribution drugs and other aspects of working with specialty suppliers.[50] The National Comprehensive Cancer Network (NCCN) has also commented on specialty pharmacies and their effects on patient care and medication safety regarding chemotherapy.[53]

Regulatory Oversight. Regulatory agencies have a responsibility to review product packaging, labeling, and advertising to ensure that their content accurately reflects safety and efficacy data and conforms with language that has been approved by the FDA. A key component in those reviews should be that the product packaging and labeling facilitate safe and appropriate use and prevent users from making errors in selecting, preparing, and administering a drug product. Pharmacists should be consulted in screening proprietary drug names, product packaging, and labeling before drug products are approved for commercial use.

Recommendations for Identifying and Managing Medication Errors

Medication-use errors with chemotherapy are distinguished from errors with other types of drugs in two important ways, both of which relate to the inherent toxicity of chemotherapy agents. Individually and categorically, the therapeutic index for chemotherapy drugs is less than that for any other class of drugs. Adverse effects are an expected pharmacodynamic consequence attendant with chemotherapy use, and clinical toxicities may occur and persist at substantially lower dosages and schedules than are therapeutically used. The second characteristic that distinguishes chemotherapy from many other types of drugs is that subtherapeutic doses ("underdoses") of chemotherapy can severely complicate further treatment. Subtherapeutic doses of chemotherapy medications may not only fail to provide a therapeutic benefit but may also compromise patients' ultimate response to therapy by delaying effective treatment until adverse effects are resolved or contributing to cumulative, long-term patient harm from adverse effects. It should be noted that chemotherapy treatments are almost always repeated, and the effect of a medication-use error may not be apparent until long after the error occurs. Consequently, if treatment plans and medication orders are not verified during each treatment cycle, errors may be compounded during repeated cycles and go undetected throughout an entire treatment course. With the increased responsibility placed upon patients to manage oral therapies, it is likely that medication errors will occur with self-administration. Patients should be educated and encouraged to report medication errors to their healthcare providers, who in turn should report the error through the institutional reporting system. Patient reported errors should be handled with the same concern and diligence as an error that occurred in the hospital, clinic, or physician's office.

In addition to the actions already set forth in the ASHP Guidelines on Preventing Medication Errors in Hospitals,[1] the following actions are recommended after detecting a medication error[6]:

1. Implement monitoring and interventions for controlling injurious effects and ensuring patient safety.
2. Determine whether an error could have previously occurred during prior treatment in the same patient and in other patients. Medication preparation work sheets or logs and drug administration records should be evaluated. Unexpected toxicities and an apparent or unaccountable lack of therapeutic and adverse effects should be investigated when it is suspected that a medication error has occurred.
3. Seek the advice of healthcare professionals from various disciplines. The diverse perspective of providers in other disciplines may facilitate discovering and understanding the circumstances that allowed a medication error to occur.
4. Determine whether an immediate temporary or stopgap change in policy or procedure is necessary to prevent recurrence of an error while the proximal cause is being analyzed.
5. Provide immediate professional counseling and support for employees implicated in causing or contributing to an error that results in serious patient harm. Counseling and support should be offered to all personnel who learn that they have been involved in a medication error without regard for how recently the error occurred.
6. Establish procedures to inform and follow up with patients and their families about a medication error.
7. Understand that reporting medication errors and adverse drug reactions is a responsibility that should be shared by all healthcare providers. However, health systems may designate a person or committee to be specifically responsible for reporting and investigating medication errors and adverse drug reactions. In investigational drug studies, a study's principal investigator must report serious adverse events to the trial's sponsors (the drug manufacturer and the investigational new drug application holder) and to the institutional review board that oversees study conduct. Investigational drug sponsors are required to report to the FDA serious adverse effects associated with investigational agents, even if they are caused by a medication-use error. While reporting of medication errors in investigational studies to the institutional review board and the FDA occur, it is imperative they also be reported through the institutional reporting system or committee so that system and process improvement can occur in the setting of investigational studies.
8. Encourage practitioners to report medication errors to a national medication-error tracking program. This allows other providers to learn how medication errors occur and how they can be prevented. Reporting mechanisms for medication-use systems should be standardized by policy. Mechanisms must be developed for ongoing, interprofessional analysis and use of information that is reported to medication-error databases.[54]

Categorizing Medication Errors. In practice settings where a variety of disciplines provide patient care, serious potential and actual errors should be reported to an oversight committee composed of representatives of all the disciplines that provide care. By standardizing the way medication errors are reported, comparisons between reports and databases are facilitated, error trends are more easily identified, and system-based solutions can be developed.[55] Continuous oversight by a multidisciplinary quality-assurance committee promotes continuity and permits all primary patient-care providers to evaluate system flaws and develop and improve the quality of processes and systems that safeguard patient care.[43] Medication-use oversight committees are advised to review medication-error reports from systems other than their own and evaluate their local medication-use system for design characteristics that may permit similar errors.[30,38]

The ASHP Guidelines on Preventing Medication Errors in Hospitals[1] recommend adopting a system for categorizing medication-error severity, such as the one developed by Myers and Hartwig, et al.[54,55] Although this system is generally applicable to errors of occurrence with chemotherapy drugs, it categorizes errors by severity and prioritizes them without consideration for the frequency at which repeated errors occur. Accordingly, errors with the highest severity ranking receive the greatest efforts toward remediation. In contrast, potential errors are assigned a "zero" ranking, the lowest severity level, as they do not reach patients. By relegating potential errors to the lowest priority category, this outcome severity-based system risks trivializing system-design flaws. Errors discovered before they reach patients could cause devastating consequences, yet serious nascent errors are often transformed into potential errors only by serendipitous discovery. Therefore, potential errors should be distinguished from errors of occurrence and subcategorized based on their potential to cause harm.[54,55] However, potential errors should not be taken less seriously than errors of occurrence. When serious potential errors are discovered, the systems and processes that contributed to the errors should be evaluated and their proximal causes identified. The greatest efforts toward remediation of potential errors and errors of occurrence should be concentrated on eliminating the causes of errors that could have and had, respectively, the greatest adverse effects on patients' health.

NCC MERP's definition for medication errors includes any event that may cause or lead to inappropriate medication use.[2] The definition is complemented by the NCC MERP Taxonomy of Medication Errors, a comprehensive expandable tool intended for use in developing databases and analyzing medication-error reports.[56] The Taxonomy provides standardized language and structure for recording and tracking medication-error-related data for errors of occurrence and potential errors. NCC MERP permits interested persons to adopt it as it is presented or adapt it for use in a particular practice setting.

Conclusion

The use of chemotherapy and biotherapy agents presents healthcare organizations with distinct safety challenges that require additional precautions to prevent medication errors. These guidelines provide best practices for the safe use of chemotherapy and biotherapy agents to help practitioners improve their medication-use systems to prevent medication errors and patient harm from these agents. The guidelines describe the medication-use responsibilities shared by and unique to specific professional healthcare disciplines, progressing from general to specific applications. Although the guidelines focus on the safe use of chemotherapy in treatment of cancer patients, in general the recommendations apply for all uses of a chemotherapy agent, regardless of indication. These wide-ranging recommendations focus on preventing errors with chemotherapy agents in hospitals and ambulatory care clinics that offer direct pharmacy services, but the guidance may also be useful in other settings. Because of the complexity of and differences between practice settings and organizational arrangements, aspects of these guidelines may be more applicable to some practice settings than others. Healthcare providers should use their professional judgment in assessing and adapting the recommendations to their own circumstances, keeping in mind that these guidelines address a specific aspect of the medication-use process and should be augmented as appropriate by other clinical and practice guidance.

References

1. American Society of Hospital Pharmacists. ASHP guidelines on preventing medication errors in hospitals. *Am J Hosp Pharm.* 1993; 50:305–14.
2. National Coordinating Council on Medication Error Reporting and Prevention. About medication errors. www.nccmerp.org (accessed 2001 Jun 4).
3. McEvoy GK, ed. AHFS drug information. Section 10:00. Bethesda, MD: American Society of Health-System Pharmacy; 2013.
4. Neuss MN, Polovich M, McNiff K, et al. 2013 updated American Society of Clinical Oncology/Oncology Nursing Society chemotherapy administration safety standards including standards for the safe administration and management of oral chemotherapy. *J Oncol Pract.* 2013 (Mar 1); 9:5s–13s.
5. Pedersen CA, Schneider PJ, Scheckelhoff DJ. ASHP national survey of pharmacy practice in hospital settings: Dispensing and administration—2011. *Am J Health-Syst Pharm.* 2012; 69:768–85.
6. Walsh KE, Dodd KS, Seetharaman K, et al. Medication errors among adults and children with cancer in the outpatient setting. *J Clin Oncol.* 2009; 27:891–6.
7. Gandhi TK, Bartel SB, Shulman LN, et al. Medication safety in the ambulatory chemotherapy setting. *Cancer.* 2005; 104:2477–83.
8. Weingart SN, Toro J, Spencer J, et al. Medication errors involving oral chemotherapy. *Cancer.* 2010; 116:2455–64.
9. Weingart SN, Spencer J, Buia S, et al. Medication safety of five oral chemotherapies: a proactive risk assessment. *J Oncol Pract.* 2011; 7:2–6.
10. Taylor JA, Winter L, Geyer LJ, et al. Oral outpatient chemotherapy medication errors in children with acute lymphoblastic leukemia. *Cancer.* 2006; 107:1400–06.
11. Cohen MR, Anderson RW, Attilio RM, et al. Preventing medication errors in cancer chemotherapy. *Am J Health-Syst Pharm.* 1996; 53:737–46.
12. Attilio RM. Caring enough to understand: the road to oncology medication error prevention. *Hosp Pharm.* 1996; 31:17–26.
13. Beckwith MC, Tyler LS. Preventing medication errors with antineoplastic agents, part 1. *Hosp Pharm.* 2000; 35:511–23.
14. Beckwith MC, Tyler LS. Preventing medication errors with antineoplastic agents, part 2. *Hosp Pharm.* 2000; 35:732–47.
15. Weingart SN, Brown E, Bach PB, et al. NCCN Task Force Report: Oral chemotherapy. *J Natl Compr Canc Netw.* 2008; 6(Suppl 3):S1–S14.
16. Weingart SN, Flug J, Brouillard D, et al. Oral chemotherapy safety practices at US cancer centers: questionnaire survey. *BMJ.* 2007; 334:407.
17. Johnson PE, Chambers CR, Vaida AJ. Oncology medication safety: a 3D status report. *J Oncol Pharm Pract.* 2008; 14:169–80.
18. American Society of Health-System Pharmacists. ASHP statement on medication reconciliation. *Am J Health-Syst Pharm.* 2013; 70:453–6.
19. Institute for Safe Medication Practices [ISMP]. Independent double checks: undervalued and misused. ISMP Medication Safety Alert - Acute Care. June 13, 2013. www.ismp.org/newsletters/acutecare/showarticle.asp?id=51 (accessed 2013 Oct 23).
20. Kohler DR, Montello MJ, Green L, et al. Standardizing the expression and nomenclature of cancer treatment regimens. *Am J Health-Syst Pharm.* 1998; 55:137–44.
21. ISMP Guidelines for Standard Order Sets. www.ismp.org/tools/guidelines/StandardOrderSets.asp (accessed 2012 Aug 12).
22. Pedersen CA, Gumpper KF. ASHP national survey on informatics: assessment of the adoption and use of pharmacy informatics in U.S. hospitals—2007. *Am J Health-Syst Pharm.* 2008; 65:2244–64.
23. Hoffman JM, Baker DK, Howard SC, et al. Safe and successful implementation of CPOE for chemotherapy at a children's cancer center. *J Natl Compr Canc Netw.* 2011; 9:S36–S50.
24. Koppel R, Metlay JP, Cohen A, et al. Role of computerized physician order entry systems in facilitating medication errors. *JAMA.* 2005; 293:1197–203.
25. Shulman LN, Miller RS, et al. Principles of Safe Practice Using an Oncology HER System for Chemotherapy Ordering, Preparation, and Administration, Part 1 of 2. *J Oncol Pract.* 2008; 4:203–6.
26. Shulman LN, Miller RS, et al. Principles of Safe Practice Using an Oncology HER System for Chemotherapy Ordering, Preparation, and Administration, Part 2 of 2. *J Oncol Pract.* 2008; 4:254–7.
27. Kim GR, Chen AR, Arceci RJ, et al. Error reduction in pediatric chemotherapy: computerized order entry and failure modes and effects analysis. *Arch Pediatr Adolesc Med.* 2006; 160:495–8.
28. American Society of Health-System Pharmacists. ASHP guidelines on pharmacy planning for implementation of computerized provider-order-entry systems in hospitals and health systems. *Am J Health-Syst Pharm.* 2011; 68:e9–31.
29. Baker DK, Hoffman JM, Hale G, et al. Analysis of Patient Safety: Converting Complex Pediatric Chemotherapy Ordering Processes from Paper to Electronic System. *Advances in Patient Safety: New Directions and Alternative Approaches.* Volumes 1-4, AHRQ

Publication Nos. 08-0034 (1-4). July 2008. Agency for Healthcare Research and Quality, Rockville, MD. www.ahrq.gov/downloads/pub/advances2/vol2/Advances-Baker_107.pdf (accessed 2012 Sep 26).

30. Kloth DD. Assuring safe care for cancer patients through an organized multidisciplinary team effort. *Hosp Pharm.* 1997; 32(suppl 1):S21–5.
31. Fischer DS, Alfano S, Knobf MT, et al. Improving the cancer chemotherapy use process. *J Clin Oncol.* 1996; 14:3148–55.
32. Griggs JL, Mangu PB, Anderson H, et al. Appropriate chemotherapy dosing for obese adult patients with cancer: American Society of Clinical Oncology Practice Guidelines. *J Clin Oncol.* 2012; 30:1553–61.
33. Lajeunesse JD. Quality assurance methods in chemotherapy production. *Hosp Pharm.* 1997; 32(suppl 1): S8–13.
34. Attilio RM. Strategies for reducing chemotherapy-related medication errors: improving the chemotherapy prescribing, dispensing, and administration process, and the patient's role in ensuring safety. *Hosp Pharm.* 1997; 32(suppl 1):S14–20.
35. Institute for Safe Medication Practices. Guideline for Maximum Adult Dose Limits of Parenteral Chemotherapy. www.medpathways.info/medpathways/tools/content/1_F.pdf (accessed 28 Mar 2013).
36. Hutcherson DA, Gammon DC. Preventing errors with antineoplastic agents: a pharmacist's approach. *Hosp Pharm.* 1997; 32:194–202, 209.
37. United Kingdom Joint Council for Clinical Oncology. Quality control in cancer chemotherapy. Managerial and procedural aspects. Oxford, England: Royal College of Physicians of London, 1994.
38. Cohen MR. Enhancing chemotherapy safety through medication system improvements. *Hosp Pharm.* 1997; 32(suppl 1):S1–7.
39. Leape LL, Bates DW, Cullen DJ, et al. Systems analysis of adverse drug events. *JAMA.* 1995; 274:35–43.
40. American Society of Health-System Pharmacists. ASHP statement on barcode-enabled medication administration technology. *Am J Health-Syst Pharm.* 2009; 66:588–90.
41. USP Quality Review. National council focuses on coordinating error reduction efforts. Rockville, MD: United States Pharmacopeial Convention, 1997 Jan.
42. Goodin S, Griffith N, Chen B, et al. Safe handling of oral chemotherapeutic agents in clinical practice: recommendations from an international pharmacy panel. *J Oncol Prac.* 2011; 7:7–12.
43. Top-priority actions for preventing adverse drug events in hospitals. Recommendations of an expert panel. *Am J Health-Syst Pharm.* 1996; 53:747–51.
44. Pepper GA. Errors in drug administration by nurses. *Am J Health-Syst Pharm.* 1995; 52:390–5.
45. OSHA Training and Education Directive 1.15—Controlling exposure to hazardous drugs. Section V. Chap. 3. Washington, D.C.: U.S. Department of Labor, 1995 Sep 22.
46. Waddell JA, Solimando DA Jr, Strickland WR, et al. Pharmacy staff interventions in a medical center hematology–oncology service. *J Am Pharm Assoc.* 1998; 38:451–6.
47. Thorn DB, Sexton MG, Lemay AP, et al. Effect of a cancer chemotherapy prescription form on prescription completeness. *Am J Hosp Pharm.* 1989; 46:1802–6.
48. Lesar TS, Lomaestro BM, Pohl H. Medication-prescribing errors in a teaching hospital. A 9-year experience. *Arch Intern Med.* 1997; 157:1569–76.
49. Cohen MR. Drug product characteristics that foster drug-use-system errors. *Am J Health-Syst Pharm.* 1995; 52:395–9.
50. American Society of Health-System Pharmacists. Report of the ASHP Task Force on Caring for Patients Served by Specialty Suppliers. *Am J Health-Syst Pharm.* 2010; 67:1650–8.
51. Stubbings JA, Joshi R, Hoffman JM. Risk evaluation and mitigation strategies (REMS): Challenges and opportunities for pharmacists. *Am J Health-Syst Pharm.* 67:1447–54, 2010.
52. ASHP policy position 0714: restricted drug distribution systems. In: Hawkins B, ed. Best practices for hospital and health-system pharmacy: positions and guidance documents of ASHP. 2011–2012 ed. Bethesda, MD: American Society of Health-System Pharmacists; 2011:338. www.ashp.org/DocLibrary/BestPractices/MarketingPositions.aspx (accessed 2012 Jun 07).
53. Schwartz RN, Eng KJ, Frieze DA, et al. National Comprehensive Cancer Network Task Force Report: Specialty Pharmacy. *J Natl Compr Canc Network.* 2010; 8 (Suppl 4):S1–12.
54. Myers CE. Needed: an interdisciplinary approach to drug misadventures. *Am J Health-Syst Pharm.* 1995; 52:367. [editorial]
55. Hartwig SC, Denger SD, Schneider PJ. Severity-indexed, incident report-based medication error-reporting program. *Am J Hosp Pharm.* 1991; 48:2611–6.
56. National Coordinating Council for Medication Error and Reporting (NCC MERP). NCC MERP taxonomy of medication errors (1998). www.nccmerp.org/pdf/taxo2001-07-31.pdf (accessed 2012 Sep 10).

Developed through the ASHP Council on Pharmacy Practice and approved by the ASHP Board of Directors on April 10, 2014. These guidelines supersede ASHP Guidelines on Preventing Medication Errors with Antineoplastic Agents dated April 19, 2002.

Barry Goldspiel, Pharm.D., BCPS, BCOP, FASHP, FISOPP, is Chief, Clinical Pharmacy Specialist Section, Clinical Center Pharmacy Department, National Institutes of Health, Bethesda, MD. James M. Hoffman, Pharm.D., M.S., BCPS, is Medication Outcomes and Safety Officer, Pharmaceutical Sciences, St. Jude Children's Research Hospital, Memphis, TN. Niesha L. Griffith, M.S., FASHP, is Director of Pharmacy and Infusion Services, Arthur G. James Cancer Hospital and Richard J. Solove Research Institute, The Ohio State University, Columbus. Susan Goodin, Pharm.D., BCOP, FASHP, FCCP, is Executive Director, Statewide Affairs, Rutgers Cancer Institute of New Jersey, New Brunswick, and Professor of Medicine, Division of Medical Oncology, Robert Wood Johnson Medical School, New Brunswick. Robert DeChristoforo, M.S., FASHP, is Chief, Clinical Center Pharmacy Department, National Institutes of Health. CAPT Michael Montello, Pharm.D., M.B.A., is Associate Branch Chief for Clinical Trials Technology and Pharmacist Consultant, Clinical Investigations Branch, National Cancer Institute (NCI) Cancer Therapy Evaluation Program, Bethesda, and Project Officer, NCI Cancer Trials Support Unit, Bethesda. Judy L. Chase, Pharm.D.,

FASHP, is Director, Clinical Pharmacy Services, University of Texas M. D. Anderson Cancer Center, Houston. Sylvia Bartel, M.P.H., is Director of Pharmacy and Clinical Support Services, Dana-Farber Cancer Institute, Boston, MA. Jharana Tina Patel, Pharm.D., is Quality Assurance Officer, Clinical Center, National Institutes of Health.

The Hematology/Oncology Pharmacy Association (HOPA) is gratefully acknowledged for reviewing and endorsing these guidelines.

ASHP also gratefully acknowledges the following organizations and individuals for reviewing these guidelines (review does not imply endorsement): Academy of Medical-Surgical Nurses (AMSN); American Nurses Association (ANA); Society of Hospital Pharmacists of Australia (SHPA); Carol Bickford, Ph.D., RN-BC, CPHIMS (ANA); Jeff Brittain, Pharm.D., BCPS; Melissa Dinolfo, Pharm.D., BCOP; Paul S. Driver, Pharm.D., BCPS, FASHP; Glenn T. Etow, Pharm.D.; Jennifer Hagen, Pharm.D.; John Hamiel, Pharm.D.; Mark Holdsworth, Pharm.D., BCOP; Lisa M. Holle, Pharm.D., BCOP (HOPA); Sean Keefe, Pharm.D., BCOP; Jim Lile, Pharm.D.; Neil J. MacKinnon, M.S.Pharm., Ph.D.; Shannon Manzi, Pharm.D.; Patrick McDonnell, Pharm.D.; Cham Nguyen, Pharm.D.; Robert S. Oakley, M.S., FASHP; Karen M. O'Leary, B.S.Pharm. (SHPA); N. Pauline Thomas Parks, M.S.; Nisha Pherwani, Pharm.D., BCOP; Judy Pi, Pharm.D., BCOP; Carol Rollins, M.S., Pharm.D., BCNSP; Andrea N. Sikora, Pharm.D.; Sue Stott, B.S. (AMSN); Thomas V. Thomas, Pharm.D.; Dennis Tribble, Pharm.D.; Siu-Fun Wong, Pharm.D., FASHP, FCSHP; Arlene Wright; Daisy Yang, Pharm.D.; and Maria L. Zarambo, Pharm.D.

The authors have declared no potential conflicts of interest.

Copyright © 2015, American Society of Health-System Pharmacists, Inc. All rights reserved. Contact ASHP for reprint and permissions requests. This content may not be used for commercial purposes without the express written consent of ASHP.

The bibliographic citation for this document is as follows: Goldspiel B, Hoffman JM, Griffith NL, et al. ASHP guidelines on preventing medication errors with chemotherapy and biotherapy. *Am J Health-Syst Pharm.* 2015; 72:e6–35.

Medication Therapy and Patient Care

DOI 10.37573/9781585287048

Organization and Delivery of Services

2302

DIGITAL THERAPEUTICS PRODUCTS

Source: Council on Pharmacy Management

To affirm the essential role of the pharmacist in the team-based evaluation, implementation, use, and ongoing assessment of digital therapeutic products to ensure the safety, effectiveness, and efficiency of medication use; further,

To encourage the pharmacy workforce to promote broader and more equitable use of digital therapeutic products by identifying and addressing barriers to patient and healthcare worker access to those products; further,

To encourage clinicians and researchers to establish evidence-based frameworks to guide use of digital therapeutic products; further,

To advocate that insurance coverage and reimbursement decisions regarding digital therapeutic products be made on the basis of those evidence-based frameworks.

Rationale

Digital health is a broad, multi-faceted term used to describe a broad category of practices, products, and processes. The Food and Drug Administration (FDA) describes digital health as "the broad scope of digital health includes categories such as mobile health (mHealth), health information technology (IT), wearable devices, telehealth and telemedicine, and personalized medicine." The Digital Therapeutics Alliance describes digital therapeutics products, a component of digital health, as products that "deliver evidence-based therapeutic interventions that are driven by high-quality software programs to prevent, manage, or treat a medical disorder or disease. They are used independently or in concert with medications, devices, or other therapies to optimize patient care and health outcomes." Generally, digital therapeutic products are used to monitor indicators of a patient's condition (e.g., blood pressure, hemoglobin A1c) or encourage behaviors (e.g., adherence to medication or behavioral therapies) and share several similar features: a digital interface used by patients, clinicians, and sometimes medical devices; wearable devices that provide information about a patient's conditions to patients, clinicians, or medical devices; integration of disparate sources of data; enhanced patient engagement with their data and treatment; and automated or live digital coaching features to improve patient adherence with medication and/or behavioral therapies. The Access to Prescription Digital Therapeutics Act of 2022 would expand Medicare coverage to prescription digital therapeutics products and would help ensure that these products are tested for safety and efficacy and have a defined FDA approval process.

The proliferation of digital therapeutics products has the potential to create fundamental shifts in patient care. When digital therapeutics products impact medication use, pharmacists can and should participate in the evidence- and team-based decision-making about how those products are selected and used. Pharmacist expertise is essential in the team-based evaluation, implementation, use, and ongoing assessment of those products to ensure the safety, effectiveness, and efficiency of medication use. Pharmacists' medication-use expertise can assist in appropriate patient selection, product prescribing and ordering, and patient education regarding product use.

DOI 10.37573/9781585287048.051

Appropriate use of digital therapeutics products will require healthcare decision-makers (e.g., clinicians, researchers, pharmacy and therapeutics committees, and payers) to establish evidence-based frameworks to guide use of and coverage and reimbursement decisions regarding use. Although evidence used in the approval process for these products should inform these decisions, ongoing research will be required to assess the absolute and comparative safety and effectiveness of digital therapeutics products. In addition, to promote optimal use, members of the pharmacy workforce will require education and training in the evaluation and use of digital therapeutics products.

Finally, one of the major drivers of societal inequities is the digital divide that separates those with access to technology from those without. ASHP encourages the pharmacy workforce to promote broader and more equitable use of digital therapeutic products by identifying and addressing barriers to patient and healthcare worker access to those products.

2309

PAYER-DIRECTED DRUG DISTRIBUTION MODELS

Source: Council on Pharmacy Management

To advocate that insurers and pharmacy benefit managers be prohibited from mandating drug distribution models that introduce patient safety and supply chain risks or limit patient choice.

This policy supersedes ASHP policy 2248.

Rationale

Hospitals and health systems have a responsibility to confirm drug product integrity and pedigree to ensure safe and appropriate administration of drug products. Drug products supplied to a hospital or health system without an institution's direct oversight raise questions about the product's proper storage and pedigree. These drug products include patients' home drug products, including clinician-administered pharmaceuticals (i.e., brown bagging) brought in by the patient or caregiver, and clinician-administered pharmaceuticals shipped from an external pharmacy directly to the location where they are being administered (i.e., white bagging).

Due to patient safety and supply chain risks, hospitals and health systems should advocate for action from boards of pharmacy to directly address payer-mandated drug distribution models and encourage state policymakers to prohibit insurers and PBMs from mandating white and brown bagging, including prohibiting insurers and PBMs from steering patients away from hospitals and health systems that refuse to accept potentially dangerous white-bagged or brown-bagged drug products.

2310

USE OF SOCIAL DETERMINANTS OF HEALTH DATA IN PHARMACY PRACTICE

Source: Council on Pharmacy Management

To encourage the use of patient and community social determinants of health (SDoH) data in pharmacy practice to optimize patient care services, reduce healthcare disparities, and improve healthcare access and equity; further,

To educate the pharmacy workforce and learners about SDoH domains, including their impact on patient care delivery and health outcomes; further,

To encourage research to identify methods, use, and evaluation of SDoH data to positively influence key quality measures and patient outcomes.

This policy supersedes ASHP policy 2249.

Rationale

Social determinants of health (SDoH) are defined by the Centers for Disease Control and Prevention (CDC) as the "conditions in the environments where people are born, live, learn, work, play, worship and age." These conditions can have a significant impact on healthcare outcomes, health equity, and the quality of life for individuals and communities. SDoH have been found to account for 80–90% of modifiable contributors to health outcomes. From a third-party payer perspective, the recent shift of many organizations from fee-for-service to value-based reimbursement models places more emphasis on SDoH, screening, and evidence-based decision-making to prioritize long-term health outcomes. Healthy People 2030, a national program developed by the Office of Disease Prevention and Health Promotion within the U.S. Department of Health and Human Services, includes 355 measurable, data-driven, national objectives to improve the health and well-being of the American public by the year 2030. Healthy People 2030 recognizes five distinct SDoH domains: Economic Stability, Education Access and Quality, Healthcare Access and Quality, Neighborhood and Built Environment, and Social and Community Context. Patient screenings and data collection from multiple data sources to ascertain SDoH would be optimized through the use of standardized codes (e.g., ICD-10-CM Z codes, SNOMED-CT value sets) that are consistent, discrete data elements that are reportable and can be shared with other technologies, leading to actionable intelligence to enhance quality improvement initiatives. To support this goal, there is a need for broader implementation of SDoH health information technology (IT) tools into general practice and development of policies for how to appropriately use SDoH in clinical decision-making. The Office of the National Coordinator for Health Information Technology has identified four priority areas for advancing interoperability and use of SDoH data: standards and data, infrastructure, policy, and implementation. Many health IT and electronic health record (EHR) vendors have invested significant resources in development of SDoH tools and products. Among these products are screening tools, population health metrics, referral and care transition tools, and analytic and reporting tools. Health systems must have access to appropriate technology-based platforms to exchange SDoH data and make referrals for patients at discharge or transfer to another institution. Lack of standardization of data and reporting across health systems makes sharing of best practices and metric goal-setting difficult.

Efforts to address SDoH through pharmacy practice have varied. A 2018 survey of postgraduate pharmacy residents and their program directors found that only 1% of residents and 4% of residency program directors stated they had received education and training on Healthy People 2020. (Chandra RN. Pharmacists' knowledge of social determinants of health in post-graduate pharmacy residency programs. Wright State University; Dayton, OH; 2018.) The pharmacy workforce has opportunities to advance the use of SDoH in pharmacy practice (e.g., consults, medication reconciliation, patient assistance programs) to improve health outcomes.

Tools available within some EHR platforms include those measuring quality of life, suicidal ideation rating, community service referral capabilities, and use of secondary survey data in conjunction with the CDC/ATSDR social vulnerability index to further evaluate population health at a community level. SDoH tools can be categorized as either single domain, such as the Hunger Vital Sign tool to evaluate food insecurity, or multiple domain, such as the WE CARE survey to evaluate education, employment/income, food insecurity, and housing/utility domains. The validity of each tool should be considered before implementing into practice, and more research is needed to determine the utility of specific tools in pharmacy practice. The Pharmacy Quality Alliance (PQA) has developed a Medication Access Framework for Quality Measurement and is evaluating a pharmacy measure concept to address the social determinants of health that hinder patient medication access and contribute to poor health outcomes.

2313

REDUCING HEALTHCARE SECTOR CARBON EMISSIONS TO PROMOTE PUBLIC HEALTH

Source: Council on Pharmacy Practice

To promote reducing carbon emissions from the health care sector through collaboration with other stakeholders; further,

To encourage members of the pharmacy workforce to seek out opportunities to engage in efforts to reduce carbon emissions in their workplaces and communities.

Rationale

ASHP acknowledges the scientific consensus on the adverse impact of carbon emissions on human health and the environment and recognizes the need to reduce carbon emissions, including from the healthcare sector. Climate change negatively impacts human health and increases strain on the healthcare system. Health-related consequences of climate change that lead to increased morbidity and mortality include but are not limited to heat-related illnesses, respiratory illnesses, and vector-borne diseases. The 2015 Lancet Commission on Health and Climate Change concluded that addressing climate change is the greatest public health opportunity of the 21st century and that failure to adequately address climate change could undo most of the past century's progress in global health.

Carbon emissions are a target for addressing climate change. It has been estimated that the healthcare sector is responsible for 8.5% of carbon emissions in the U.S. Sources of healthcare carbon emissions rank as follows: healthcare facility operations (estimated to account for 7% of healthcare sector emissions); purchased sources of energy, heating, and cooling (11%); and healthcare sector procurements or supply chain for services and goods (>80%).

Healthcare organizations have been called upon to reduce their carbon footprint ("decarbonize") as a measure to promote patient and public health. The federal government has goals to decrease carbon emissions by 50% by 2030 and to achieve net-zero levels by 2050. Many healthcare-related organizations have made climate change and decarbonization pledges, including the members of the Medical Society Consortium on Climate & Health and organizations engaged in the National Academy of Medicine (NAM) Action Collaborative on Climate Change. In the fall of 2021, NAM launched the Action Collaborative on Decarbonizing the U.S. Health Sector (the "Climate Collaborative"), mobilizing four work groups: healthcare supply chain and infrastructure; healthcare delivery; health professional education and communication; and policy, financing, and metrics.

The pharmacy workforce has an important role in reducing carbon emissions from healthcare-related sources (Beechinor RJ et al. Climate change is here: what will the profession of pharmacy do about it? *Am J Health-Syst Pharm.* 2022; 79:1393–6). ASHP encourages collaboration with stakeholders that share a commitment to reducing carbon emissions from the healthcare sector and encourages members of the pharmacy workforce to seek out opportunities to engage in efforts to reduce carbon emissions in their workplaces and communities. To fill their roles in reducing carbon emissions, the pharmacy workforce will require education, training, and resources on emissions-reduction strategies. The development of evidence-based strategies will require research and dissemination of information on ways to reduce carbon emissions.

2314

MANIPULATION OF DRUG PRODUCTS FOR ALTERNATE ROUTES OF ADMINISTRATION

Source: Council on Therapeutics

To advocate that the Food and Drug Administration encourage drug product manufacturers to identify changes in pharmacokinetic and pharmacodynamic properties of drug products when manipulated for administration through an alternate delivery system or different route than originally studied, and to make this information available to healthcare providers; further,

To collaborate with stakeholders to increase research on clinically relevant changes to pharmacokinetic and pharmacodynamic properties of drug products when manipulated or administered through a different route and to enhance the aggregation and publication of and access to this data; further,

To research and promote best practices for manipulation and administration of drug products through alternate routes when necessary; further,

To foster pharmacist-led development of policies, procedures, and educational resources on the safety and efficacy of manipulating drug products for administration through alternate routes.

Rationale

Manipulation of a drug product can include crushing, splitting, or suspending it in a solvent, which can alter the pharmaceutical properties of the original dosage form. These manipulations are often performed because a patient requires the medication administered enterally but is unable to take the medication by mouth, requires a dose that is not readily available and so can only be delivered through manipulation, or is unable to swallow or has a feeding tube placed necessitating manipulation. For patients who lose the ability to swallow easily (e.g., due to stroke or cancer), it is sometimes quite difficult to provide all their drug products via liquid formulations or those that can be crushed, due to lack of such products.

Complicating the clinical picture is that in many studies of oral drug products the dose passes through the stomach, exposing it to a specific set of pH conditions. The stomach may be bypassed when drug products are administered via feeding tube to organ systems in the body that may have a different pH, affecting the adsorption, metabolism, or distribution of the drug. Some drug products cannot be administered because they are insoluble in aqueous solutions. In addition, the physical properties of the manipulated formulation may also cause obstruction and clogging of enteral tubes used for feeding and medication administration, leading to undesirable outcomes, including supra- or subtherapeutic concentrations in the body, which could lead for example to organ rejection in transplant patients, loss of viral suppression in HIV-positive patients, or toxicities when manipulating an extended-release tablet. There are also exposure risks to caregivers preparing or administering manipulated drug products that are carcinogenic or teratogenic.

Additionally, there are too few resources that provide guidance on how manipulation may affect the bioavailability of the drug product or whether the manipulated drug product remains bioequivalent with the original dosage form. There is even less research or publicly available information on the clinical effects of manipulated drug products. ASHP encourages manufacturers and independent clinical and practice-based researchers to conduct studies on these subjects and to disseminate this information via journal articles and other easily accessible resources. ASHP also encourages education of the pharmacy workforce and other healthcare providers regarding the basic principles of and drug dosing for manipulated drug products.

2315

RESPONSIBLE MEDICATION-RELATED CLINICAL TESTING AND MONITORING

Source: Council on Therapeutics

To recognize that overuse of clinical testing leads to unnecessary costs, waste, and patient harm; further,

To encourage the development of standardized measures of appropriate clinical testing to better allow for appropriate comparisons for benchmarking purposes and use in research; further,

To promote pharmacist accountability and engagement in interprofessional efforts to promote judicious use of clinical testing and monitoring, including multi-faceted, organization-level approaches and educational efforts; further,

To promote research that evaluates pharmacists' contributions and identifies opportunities for the appropriate ordering of medication-related procedures and tests; further,

To promote the use of interoperable health information technology services and health information exchanges to decrease unnecessary testing.

This policy supersedes ASHP policy 1823.

Rationale

As the prevalence of collaborative practice grows and as pharmacist care expands into direct patient care services, so too do the responsibilities held by these practitioners. In many institutions, pharmacists' responsibilities now include ordering blood draws as a part of initiating a medication regimen, assessing drug levels, monitoring for adverse effects, or ordering imaging such as ultrasound for evaluating a deep vein thrombosis or an electrocardiogram to evaluate a QTc interval.

Overuse of medical care is a long-recognized problem in clinical medicine, and more spending and treatment do not translate into better patient outcomes and health. The number of articles on overuse nearly doubled from 2014 to 2015, indicating that awareness of overuse is increasing, despite little evidence of improved practice, which may mean that the overuse of diagnostic tests and lab monitoring is leading to patient harm and could outweigh benefits. Healthcare continues to be enthralled by high-technology innovation, including both therapies and tests. Once practice norms are established, clinicians are slow to de-implement services, even those that are found to be potentially dangerous. Reasons for excessive ordering of tests by healthcare providers include defensive behavior, fear, uncertainty, lack of experience, the use of protocols and guidelines, routine clinical practice, inadequate educational feedback, and clinician's lack of awareness about the cost of examinations. Inappropriate testing causes unnecessary patient discomfort, may lead to iatrogenic anemia from over-testing, entails the risk of generating false-positive results and unnecessary treatment, leads to overloading of diagnostic services, wastes valuable healthcare resources, and is associated with other inefficiencies in healthcare delivery, thus undermining the quality of health services. Furthermore, ordering unnecessary tests may also disproportionately affect vulnerable populations, including pediatric patients; trigger unnecessary therapies, such as for asymptomatic bacteriuria; and introduce bias, such as when screening for illicit drugs is performed but not as part of a differential diagnosis. A multi-faceted approach is recommended to reduce waste and support the judicious use of clinical testing. Key strategies include use of interoperable health information technology services and health information exchanges; optimization of test ordering through use of clinical decision support systems; provider and pharmacist education; benchmarking; and organization-level guidance, such as through establishment of a laboratory formulary committee that includes formulary control. Additionally, a key limitation of current literature surrounding appropriateness of clinical testing is a lack of standardized definitions of "appropriateness." Guideline and professional organization-endorsed standards may be used to benchmark clinical testing, although variations by country or institutional practices may confound these definitions.

Choosing Wisely is a national program designed to help raise provider and public awareness and garner support for appropriate test utilization, with the goal of promoting conversations between providers and patients about choosing appropriate care in order to reduce both harm and waste. In 2016, ASHP announced its partnership with the ABIM Foundation on the Choosing Wisely campaign, and in 2017 became the first pharmacy organization to contribute recommendations to the campaign. ASHP has continued to support this partnership through regular review and updates of its recommendations.

2319

STANDARDIZATION OF MEDICATION CONCENTRATIONS, DOSING UNITS, LABELED UNITS, AND PACKAGE SIZES

Source: Council on Pharmacy Practice

To support adoption of nationally standardized medication concentrations, dosing units, labeled units, and package sizes for medications administered to adult and pediatric patients, and to advocate that the number of standard concentrations, dosing units, labeled units, and package sizes be limited as much as possible; further,

To encourage interprofessional collaboration on the adoption and implementation of these standards across the continuum of care; further,

To encourage manufacturers and registered outsourcing facilities to provide medications in those standardized concentrations, labeled units, and package sizes.

This policy supersedes ASHP policy 1306.

Rationale

Standardization and simplification are widely accepted methods for reducing variability in processes and risk for error. With increased adoption of intelligent infusion devices, use of standard concentrations has enhanced infusion safety by eliminating most dosing and rate calculations. Standardizing concentrations reduces the potential for errors, particularly during transitions of care; simplifies ordering by providing fewer choices, which decreases provider uncertainty; reduces operational variations, which enhances provider efficiency; and streamlines manufacturing, which accelerates production and allows for the formulation of premixed medications. In addition, broader use of standard concentrations might stimulate industry to offer a broader array of ready-to-administer infusions and facilitate the development of drug libraries.

To improve patient safety and availability of products, units of measure used for ordering, labeling, and administration of medications need to be standardized as well, as do package sizes for liquid formulations. All liquid formulations, including intravenous, oral, and topical formulations, need to be included in the standardization process, and standards specific to pediatric and adult populations are needed and should be limited in number to the extent possible. Development of these standards requires a holistic view of the medication-use process that considers all these aspects, as they all intersect and impact patient safety and the interoperability of automated systems.

In 2015, ASHP launched the Standardize 4 Safety (S4S) initiative. Funded by the U.S. Food and Drug Administration (FDA) and helmed by ASHP, S4S is the first national, interprofessional effort to standardize medication concentrations to reduce errors resulting from confusion over nonstandardized drug concentrations and errors that result from concentration differences when patients transition their care from one setting to another. To date, the expert committees have developed four lists—standardized concentrations for adult continuous infusions, pediatric continuous infusions, compounded oral liquids, and PCA/epidural infusion—and the S4S Initiative offers the pharmacy workforce other resources to help implement standardized concentrations.

2321

MEDICATION ADMINISTRATION BY THE PHARMACY WORKFORCE

Source: Council on Pharmacy Practice

To support the position that the administration of medications is within the scope of pharmacy practice; further,

To advocate that states grant pharmacists and appropriately supervised student pharmacists and pharmacy technicians the authority to administer medications; further,

To support the position that pharmacists should be participants in establishing procedures in their own work settings with respect to the administration of medications (by anyone) and monitoring the safety and outcomes of medication administration.

Note: This policy supersedes ASHP policy 9820.

Rationale

Laws, regulations, and local policies on medication administration vary greatly. Medications are routinely administered by many different practitioners, including nurses, physicians, radiology and nuclear medicine technologists, nurses aides, laboratory technologists, dental hygienists, respiratory therapists, and physical therapists. ASHP believes that administration of medications is within the scope of pharmacy practice and supports laws, regulations, and local policies that allow for it and for medication administration by appropriately trained and supervised student pharmacists and pharmacy technicians. Decisions about pharmacists' involvement in medication administration should be made by individual healthcare organizations, which have an awareness of their resources and the adequacy of their medication administration processes. Patient need should be the primary factor in deciding who administers medications in any institution, and pharmacists should be involved in the institution's decision-making process regarding procedures used to administer medications.

2205

TRANSITIONS OF CARE

Source: Council on Pharmacy Management

To encourage the pharmacy workforce to assume responsibility for medication-related aspects of ensuring the continuity of care as patients move from one care setting to another; further,

To encourage the development, optimization, and implementation of technologies that facilitate sharing of patient-care data across care settings and interprofessional care teams; further,

To advocate that health systems provide sufficient resources to support the important roles of the pharmacy workforce in supporting transitions of care; further,

To encourage payers to provide reimbursement for transitions of care services; further,

To encourage the development of strategies to address the gaps in continuity of pharmacist patient care services, including effective patient engagement.

This policy supersedes ASHP policy 1208.

Rationale

Continuity of patient care is a vital requirement in the appropriate use of medications. Changes in healthcare reimbursement have resulted in an increasing focus on transitions of care from the acute care environment to other settings (e.g., ambulatory care to inpatient care to home care or specialty settings). Pharmacy workforce engagement, as integral members of interprofessional care teams, is pivotal to support health systems focus on reducing readmissions, improving patient satisfaction, and effectively educating patients about their medications. It is important that ASHP advocate for improvements in technologies that facilitate sharing of patient information across various care settings. Further alignment of financial incentives and sufficient resource allocation that encourage and support patient care roles of the pharmacy workforce in the transition of care are also required.

2206

CONTINUOUS PERFORMANCE IMPROVEMENT

Source: Council on Pharmacy Management

To encourage the pharmacy workforce to establish multidisciplinary continuous performance improvement (CPI) processes within their practice settings to assess the effectiveness and safety of patient care services, adherence to standards, and quality and integrity of practice; further,

To encourage the pharmacy workforce to use contemporary CPI techniques and methods for ongoing improvement in their services; further,

To support the pharmacy workforce in their development and implementation of CPI processes.

This policy supersedes ASHP policy 0202.

Rationale

Pharmacy departments should continually strive for medication safety and quality by identifying and prioritizing quality improvement efforts that align with national and health-system goals. The pharmacy workforce can make use of a variety of methods to ascertain goals, aims, and interventions for the system and to influence medication-related goals, aims, and interventions in the pursuit of high-value care and improved patient outcomes. Some of these process improvement methodologies include Six Sigma, Lean Management, Lean Six Sigma, Agile Management, Total Quality Management, and Kaizen. All the process improvement tools share many common features and the philosophy that processes can always be improved. They share the assumption of measurement and statistics being a key to improvement and the faith in the power of the workers closest to a process to be able to improve it. The continuous performance or quality improvement program is structured to assess the effectiveness and safety of patient care services, adherence to standards, and quality and integrity of the practice. It is aligned with the health system's overall plan and system for performance and quality improvement, accrediting organizations, and with payer contractual obligations for quality reporting. Pharmacy departments must have internal procedures for ongoing surveillance and reporting to assess overall appropriateness of services and implement quality improvements as needed to integrate quality metrics that drive quality improvement and refocus efforts on areas of need. The pharmacy department should have process and feedback loop in place that translates analysis to initiatives and initiatives to measured and improved outcomes using appropriate tools derived from implementation science.

2208

PHARMACIST'S ROLE IN TEAM-BASED CARE

Source: Council on Pharmacy Practice

To recognize that pharmacists, as core members and medication-use experts on interprofessional healthcare teams, increase the capacity and efficiency of teams for delivering evidence-based, safe, high-quality, and cost-effective patient-centered care; further,

To advocate to policymakers, payers, and other stakeholders for the inclusion of pharmacists as care providers within team-based care and as the provider of comprehensive medication management services; further,

To assert that all members of the interprofessional care team have a shared responsibility in coordinating the care they provide and are accountable to the patient and each other for the outcomes of that care; further,

To urge pharmacists on healthcare teams to collaborate with other team members in establishing and implementing quality and outcome measures for care provided by those teams.

This policy supersedes ASHP policy 1215.

Rationale

There is a growing consensus among healthcare providers and payers that patient-centered care by a collaborative team is the optimal model of care. A collaborative care model provides pharmacists with an opportunity to contribute their expertise in medication use to improving patient outcomes.

The pharmacy profession appears to be struggling, however, with implementation of this care model. Not unexpectedly, there is a wide variation in the way "team-based care" is interpreted and applied. Therefore, states currently in the process of rewriting practice acts have been challenged to find guidance on the fundamental roles and responsibilities of pharmacists in various care settings. This policy recommendation builds on concepts in ASHP policy 1114, Pharmacist Accountability for Patient Outcomes; sets the expectation for other providers that teams with pharmacists will improve the quality, safety, and efficiency of care; and supports advocacy to the broader healthcare community on the value of care delivery by teams that include pharmacists.

2214

MEDICATION ADHERENCE

Source: Council on Therapeutics

To recognize that medication adherence improves the quality and safety of patient care when the following elements are included: (1) assessment of the appropriateness of therapy, (2) provision of patient education, and (3) confirmation of patient comprehension of information necessary to support safe and appropriate use of prescribed therapies; further,

To advocate that the pharmacy workforce take a leadership role in interdisciplinary efforts to improve medication adherence; further,

To recognize that clinicians, patients, and caregivers share accountability for the outcomes of medication therapies, and that the central role patients and their caregivers have in disease management includes responsibility for following instructions for safe and effective medication use; further,

To encourage development, evaluation, and dissemination of models and tools that improve adherence, including those that combine existing strategies that have demonstrated effectiveness; further,

To oppose misinformation or disinformation that leads patients to decline education and clinical information regarding their medication therapy; further,

To support the development of mechanisms to document medication adherence interventions, including information technology solutions; further,

To advocate for payment models that facilitate an expanded role for the pharmacy workforce in and provide reimbursement for medication adherence efforts.

This policy supersedes ASHP policy 1222.

Rationale

The need to improve medication adherence as a cornerstone of efforts to improve patient care outcomes is widely recognized. A 2010 *New England Journal of Medicine* editorial issued a call to action to improve adherence based on estimates that 50% of all patients are non-adherent, resulting in an estimated $100 billion spent annually on avoidable hospitalizations. ASHP supports programs to improve adherence, but such efforts are not useful, and are perhaps harmful, if they fail to (1) assess the appropriateness of therapy, (2) provide patient education, and (3) ensure patient comprehension of information necessary to support safe and appropriate use of prescribed therapies. Because of their distinct knowledge, skills, and abilities, pharmacists are the ideal clinician to lead interdisciplinary efforts to develop, implement, monitor, and maintain effective strategies for improving medication adherence, and other members of the pharmacy workforce can have important roles in those efforts. Other members of the interdisciplinary team could include physicians, nurses, health psychologists, and social workers. Patients and their caregivers must share accountability with clinicians for medication therapy outcomes, including the responsibility for following instructions for safe and effective medication use. Otherwise, the results from efforts of pharmacists and other clinicians would be negligible. Some interventions to improve medication adherence have shown favorable results, but the greatest success is achieved by models that incorporate multiple strategies reinforced over time. Therefore, the development, evaluation, and dissemination of models that use multimodal approaches are encouraged. The development of information technology solutions and other mechanisms (e.g., digiceuticals) to document interventions intended to improve medication adherence is also recommended. Further, payment models that support an expanded role for the pharmacy workforce in medication adherence efforts should be pursued.

2235

USE OF INCLUSIVE VERBAL AND WRITTEN LANGUAGE

Source: Council on Pharmacy Practice

To recognize that stigmatizing and derogatory language can be a barrier to safe and optimal patient care as well as compromise effective communication among healthcare team members; further,

To promote the use of inclusive verbal and written language in patient care delivery and healthcare communication; further,

To urge healthcare leadership to promote use of inclusive language; further,

To provide education, resources, and competencies for the pharmacy workforce to champion the use of inclusive verbal and written language.

Rationale

Inclusive verbal and written language (i.e., language that is free of stigma, bias, and oppression) is essential for the provision of equitable patient care. The use of derogatory and stigmatizing language in the healthcare environment is a risk to patient safety and a threat to optimal health. In addition, when used among care team members, it introduces a culturally insensitive and noninclusive work environment. Stigmatizing language may fuel and trigger implicit or explicit bias in a healthcare clinician or team member and harm patients, worsen health outcomes, and compromise team dynamics. Derogatory and stigmatizing language may occur between patients and the care team, among care team members, and in medical documentation. Commitment to the use of conscious language—the intentional use of words and terms to create empathetic, inclusive, and non-stigmatizing content—is suggested as an alternative to ensure language and communication does not lead to poorer health outcomes, health inequities, and stigma.

The use of stigmatizing and derogatory language in medical chart documentation becomes even more damaging as patients have increased access to their own health records (Davis B. Derogatory language in charting: the domino effect. *Patient Safety*. 2021; 3:74–8.). Patients may not be empowered to take ownership of their care if stigmatizing and derogatory language is used. The same can apply for verbal communications. The use of argot or slang to disguise the meaning to bystanders may be useful to build bonds between colleagues but is unprofessional and creates judgments about patients not based in facts (Goldman B. Derogatory slang in the hospital setting. *AMA J Ethics*. 2015; 17:167–71).

There are multiple strategies for eliminating the use of stigmatizing language in the course of caring for a patient, such as using person-first and technical language and avoiding the use of sensational or fear-based language. Eliminating derogatory and stigmatizing language from healthcare settings requires leadership commitment across the spectrum of care delivery and an educated and empowered healthcare workforce. Pharmacists, student pharmacists, and pharmacy technicians have a professional duty to provide culturally competent and compassionate patient care and can serve as champions in eliminating the use of stigmatizing language in healthcare.

2236

PHARMACIST PRESCRIBING IN INTERPROFESSIONAL PATIENT CARE

Source: Council on Pharmacy Practice

To advocate that healthcare delivery organizations establish credentialing and privileging processes for pharmacists that delineate scope of practice, support pharmacist prescribing, and ensure that pharmacists who prescribe are accountable, competent, and qualified to do so; further,

To advocate for comprehensive medication management that includes autonomous prescribing authority for pharmacists as part of optimal interprofessional care; further,

To advocate that all pharmacists on the interprofessional team have a National Provider Identifier (NPI); further,

To advocate that payers recognize pharmacist NPIs.

This policy supersedes ASHP policy 1213.

Rationale

Pharmacists are highly trained medication experts skilled in providing comprehensive medication management (CMM) services across the continuum of care. Nearly all states include pharmacist prescribing authority within their state practice acts, although those acts differ in how pharmacist prescribing authority is described, terminology used, and the degree of prescribing autonomy (i.e., autonomous or collaborative). Regulations at the state level are critical to ensuring that pharmacists can seamlessly provide CMM services within the interprofessional team and to the top of their skills and abilities. Pharmacists are a core healthcare team member, well-positioned to provide high-quality, cost-effective care that increases patient access and reduces the burden on other healthcare providers. Hundreds of studies published in peer-reviewed literature, conducted throughout a variety of organizations and health systems, have consistently demonstrated the benefits of pharmacist-directed patient care across a variety of clinical practice settings. A 2010 comprehensive systematic review of 298 studies of U.S. pharmacists' effect as a member of the patient care team found positive results on therapeutic and safety metrics (Chisholm-Burns MA, Kim Lee J, Spivey CA, et al. US pharmacists' effect as team members on patient care: systematic review and meta-analyses. *Med Care*. 2010; 48:923–33).

Autonomous prescribing allows pharmacists to be fully optimized as a part of the interprofessional healthcare team and ensures that their skills are used to the fullest potential to allow them to be responsible and accountable and fully execute CMM treatment plans. Pharmacist prescribing is implicit to interprofessional care delivery, but the form and manner of pharmacist prescribing varies among health systems and organizations. Independent and autonomous drug therapy decision-making by pharmacists is already common and accepted by other licensed practitioners (e.g., physicians, physician assistants, and nurse practitioners). Practitioners participating in interprofessional teams that include pharmacists rely on the knowledge, demonstrated competency, and expertise of those pharmacists for CMM. Pharmacists in specialty practice areas such as anticoagulation management, solid organ transplant, and nutrition support have long functioned in roles in which autonomous prescribing authority has improved clinical outcomes in the management and monitoring of medication therapy. In settings such as the Indian Health Service and Veterans Health Administration systems, prescribing authority for pharmacists providing CMM services has been in place for over 40 years and has demonstrated positive clinical impact and increased patient access across the continuum of care.

Many health systems authorize pharmacists to manage drug therapy by enacting pharmacy and therapeutics committee policies that require use of medical staff protocols and physician oversight for pharmacist-initiated orders. While this model works effectively for specific scenarios (e.g., management of population-specific patients), it does not allow the pharmacist to fully function and fulfill the CMM needs of their patients. Depending on the patient, medication, and degree of trust with the pharmacist, physicians often delegate therapeutic decision-making and medication treatment planning to pharmacists, based on the trust relationship developed through the interprofessional team and shared experiences in successfully dealing with challenging clinical situations, rather than through formal collaborative practice agreements. Common examples of pharmacist prescribing include independently managing symptoms and adverse events in oncology patients, identifying and resolving drug-induced disease or problems, managing anticoagulant therapy for patients whose clinical status falls outside specified parameters, and responding to general directives to simply "fix the problem" when medication therapy is indicated. Further, there are settings of care and pharmacy practice models that allow for autonomous and accountable prescribing authority by pharmacist practitioners as core component of CMM, without the need for collaborative practice authority for specific patients or populations. Pharmacist autonomous prescribing authority should be the gold standard for practice, especially when appropriate credentialing and privileging is in place and there is a separation of duties to ensure that a prescribing pharmacist is not responsible for the processing and dispensing of that medication order.

Pharmacists who prescribe must be recognized by payers and reimbursed for performing these advanced practice services. All pharmacist prescribers on the interprofessional team must possess a National Provider Identifier (NPI) number to monitor the care provided as well as reimburse for services rendered. Credentialing and privileging of individual healthcare providers is essential for determining who is authorized to prescribe and should ensure the appropriate evaluation of the quality of care provided. The credentialing procedures used to establish pharmacists' competency to prescribe must ensure that patients receive treatment from highly qualified caregivers. In addition to verifying appropriate education, licensure, and certification, the process should include:

- The same transparency and rigor applied to other prescribers
- Criteria used to measure patient care quality
- Peer review by similar or higher-level peers (i.e., pharmacist prescribers or other licensed practitioners who are authorized to prescribe)

Healthcare organizations should use privileging methods that establish the scope of practice and clinical services that pharmacists are authorized to provide commensurate with their demonstrated competency within an area or areas of clinical expertise. The practice of credentialing and privileging should be consistent between hospitals health systems, accountable care organizations, and other organizations where the pharmacists function as a part of the interprofessional team. Finally, interdisciplinary health professional training programs should incorporate the concept of pharmacist prescribing in a standard way to ensure consistency amongst pharmacists practicing in similar practice settings and with similar levels of responsibilities.

2238

PATIENT DISABILITY ACCOMMODATIONS

Source: Council on Public Policy

To promote safe, inclusive, and accessible care for patients with disabilities; further,

To advocate for research to enhance capabilities in meeting the needs of patients with disabilities; further,

To advocate for inclusion of caring for patients with disabilities in college of pharmacy and pharmacy technician program curricula and in postgraduate residencies; further,

To support pharmacy workforce training to improve awareness of the barriers patients with disabilities face and ensure equitable care.

Rationale

Current statistics indicate that 20–30% of Americans have some type of disability Many of these patients, regardless of whether their disability is physical or mental, would benefit from the creation and adoption of technology and communication tools that improve how pharmacists and other providers interact with them. Because there is such a broad spectrum of potential patient needs, additional research on appropriate and safe implementation of technology and the creation of new solutions, including solutions to improve health equity, is needed and should be supported by federal, state, and private funding. Further, pharmacy schools and other pharmacy workforce training programs should integrate education on serving patients with disability into their established curricula.

2242

USE OF INTRAVENOUS DRUG PRODUCTS FOR INHALATION

Source: Council on Therapeutics

To encourage healthcare organizations to develop an interdisciplinary team that includes pharmacists and respiratory therapists to provide institutional guidance; safety recommendations regarding preparation, dispensing, delivery, and exposure; and electronic health record support for prescribing and administration of intravenous drug products for inhalational use; further,

To advocate for further research on the pharmacokinetic and pharmacodynamic characteristics of drugs not approved for inhalational administration, devices for administration, and the effects of excipients; further,

To foster the development of educational resources on the safety and efficacy of inhalational administration of drug products not approved for that route and devices for administration; further,

To encourage manufacturers to develop ready-to-use inhalational formulations when evidence supports such use.

Rationale

Practitioners have been increasingly seeking out novel delivery mechanisms for drugs to patients who require a more localized application. This approach has more frequently seen through the nebulization of antibiotics and antifungals that are formulated for intravenous (IV) use as a part of an effort to treat an invasive pulmonary infection in critically ill patients. Nebulization of IV morphine has also been used to provide relief in chronic obstructive pulmonary disease exacerbations, dyspnea in cancer patients, and pain management in trauma patients. Data for these treatment efforts is limited to small patient populations, and the information on the pharmacokinetics, safety, and efficacy of drugs administered by this method remain insufficient. Furthermore, the number of drug products that are formulated exclusively for the purpose of aerosolization is limited, and the degree of pulmonary penetration depends on the properties of antimicrobial formulations, including size, viscosity, surface tension, osmolality, tonicity, and pH. Drug stability, safety for both the patient receiving and the person administering the drug, and the methods of preparation and delivery also bear consideration. The mechanism of nebulization also introduces uncertainty. Because pneumatic nebulizers and ultrasonic nebulizers have different particle size tolerance and deliverability capabilities, susceptibility for contamination may vary, depending on the device used.

Nebulized drugs also present a potential risk to healthcare providers, who may be exposed to drug particles that are expelled through the device when administering the drug. Therefore, an interdisciplinary team that includes representatives from pharmacy and respiratory therapy (as it is often a respiratory therapist who administers the drug in an inpatient setting) is needed to ensure that occupational exposure is minimized, that patients are placed in rooms with proper ventilation, and that, if necessary, caregivers are provided with appropriate masks during administration.

There is evidence that certain drugs delivered by nebulization have a beneficial role in management of patient disease. It important to recognize that nebulized drugs that are not commercially available may be compounded with both sterile and nonsterile ingredients and that, when possible, should be compounded with preservative- and additive-free formulations in order to improve patient tolerability. Due to this variability and potential source for sterile compounding and potential administration errors, where there is evidence that supports the use of compounded nebulized drugs, manufacturers should be encouraged to create a commercially available formulation for delivery via nebulizer.

2251

QUALIFICATIONS AND COMPETENCIES REQUIRED TO PRESCRIBE MEDICATIONS

Source: Council on Education and Workforce Development

To affirm that prescribing is a collaborative process that includes patient assessment, understanding of the patient's diagnoses, evaluation and selection of available treatment options, monitoring to achieve therapeutic outcomes, patient education, and adherence to safe and cost-effective prescribing practices; further,

To affirm that safe prescribing of medications, performed independently or collaboratively, requires competent professionals who complement each others' strengths at each step.

This policy supersedes ASHP policy 1202.

Rationale

Debate about health care providers' evolving scopes of practice, focused primarily on prescribing privileges, has raised the question of what training and competencies should be required of current or potential prescribers. The increasing complexity of medication use, growing diversity of professionals authorized to prescribe, and continuing high incidence of adverse drug events call for the development of standards for prescribing and further development of associated competencies and training requirements.

2252

STANDARD DRUG ADMINISTRATION SCHEDULES

Source: Council on Pharmacy Management

To support the principle that standard medication administration times should be based primarily on optimal pharmacotherapeutics and safe medication administration practices, with secondary consideration of workload, caregiver preference, patient preference, and logistical issues; further,

To encourage the development of hospital-specific or health-system-specific standard administration times through an interdisciplinary process coordinated by the pharmacy; further,

To encourage information technology vendors to adopt these principles in system design while allowing flexibility to meet site-specific patient needs.

This policy supersedes ASHP policy 0707.

Rationale

Administering medications at the right time is one of the original "five rights" of medication administration. To achieve the best patient outcomes, standard medication administration times should be based primarily on optimal pharmacotherapeutics and safe medication administration practices. Standard drug administration times help prevent over- or under-dosing of patient medications, improve communication between disciplines, and reduce workload and potential for errors. For example, appropriate timing of laboratory blood draws and other bedside monitoring is critical for obtaining accurate patient data, and standard administration times decrease the chance for miscommunication.

Although considerations such as workload, caregiver and patient preference, and logistical issues cannot be ignored, they should be only secondary considerations in the interprofessional development of hospital- or health-system-specific standard administration times, a process best coordinated by the pharmacy, as medication-use experts. Healthcare systems should establish interdisciplinary policies and procedures related to standard drug administration times for all practitioners responsible for administering medications. Such policies can help concentrate staffing, optimize workflows, and mitigate potential medication safety gaps.

To promote adoption and avoid dangerous workarounds, standardization of drug administration times and pertinent monitoring times should be built into workflows to the extent possible. Healthcare information technology vendors should design these systems to optimize the safety and operational aspects of the medication-use process while allowing for necessary site-specific individualization.

2108

PATIENT EXPERIENCE

Source: Council on Pharmacy Management

To encourage the pharmacy workforce to evaluate their practice settings for opportunities to improve the experience patients have with healthcare services and with the outcomes of their drug therapy; further,

To educate the pharmacy workforce about the relationship between patient experience and outcomes; further,

To develop or adopt tools that will (1) provide a system for monitoring trends in the quality of pharmacy services to patients, (2) increase recognition of the value of pharmacy services, and (3) provide a basis for making improvements in the process and outcomes of pharmacy services in efforts to engage patients and improve their experience; further,

To promote use of interactive patient technology (e.g., self-learning teaching resources) to augment patient experience and help prioritize and improve the effectiveness of pharmacy services; further,

To facilitate a dialogue with and encourage education of patient experience database vendors to include the value of pharmacy services in the patient experience.

This policy supersedes ASHP policy 1616.

Rationale

A major component of quality of healthcare is patient satisfaction (often referred to as "the patient experience"), which is critical to how well patients respond and adhere to healthcare. Research has identified a clear link between patient outcomes and a positive patient experience. Additionally, the patient experience is a key determinant of quality of care and an important component of pay-for-performance metrics. Pharmacy leaders need to continually assess how pharmacists and pharmacy services support an improved patient experience with their care across the continuum of practice sites, including how pharmacists contribute to team-based care.

A study detailed in a white paper by The Beryl Institute found that hospitals using interactive technology to communicate with patients saw improvement in patient satisfaction scores. Interactive patient technology gives patients faster access to hospital staff and services, including access to health education information about the care they receive and the steps they need to take after discharge. Hospitals using interactive technology realize tangible benefits, which translate into significant, measureable improvements in patient outcomes, the hospital's financial performance, and greater patient engagement, making for an exceptional patient experience.

2109

PHARMACY SERVICES FOR UNINSURED AND UNDERINSURED PATIENTS

Source: Council on Pharmacy Management

To support the principle that all patients have the right to receive care from pharmacists; further,

To declare that pharmacists should play a leadership role in ensuring access to pharmacists' services for indigent or low-income patients who lack insurance coverage or are underinsured; further,

To encourage the pharmacy workforce to work with organizational patient assistance, case management, and care coordination teams to ensure seamless patient care transitions for all patients, including uninsured and underinsured patients; further,

To advocate better collaboration among health systems, community health centers, state and county health departments, and the federal Health Resources and Services Administration in identifying and addressing the needs of indigent and low-income patients who lack insurance coverage or are underinsured.

This policy supersedes ASHP policy 0101.

Rationale

Consistent with ASHP Practice Advancement Initiative 2030 themes for change, patients must have access to: 1) a pharmacist in all settings of care; 2) a collaborative, interprofessional care team that coordinates seamless, convenient, and cost-effective care transitions; and 3) a collaborative, interprofessional care team that identifies, assesses, and resolves barriers to medication access, adherence, and health literacy. These principles apply even for patients who lack insurance coverage or are underinsured. Pharmacists and pharmacy technicians should take leadership roles in ensuring access to pharmacists' services for these patients, working with organizational patient assistance, case management, and care coordination teams to ensure seamless patient care transitions for this vulnerable population. Further, community health centers, state and county health departments, and the federal Health Resources and Services Administration should collaborate in identifying and addressing the needs of these patients.

2110

PATIENT ACCESS TO PHARMACY SERVICES IN SMALL AND RURAL HOSPITALS

Source: Council on Pharmacy Practice

To advocate that critical-access hospitals (CAHs) and small and rural hospitals meet national medication management and patient safety standards, regardless of size or location; further,

To provide resources and tools to assist pharmacists who provide services to CAHs and small and rural hospitals in meeting standards related to safe medication use; further,

To promote allocation policies that address the unique challenges faced by CAHs and small and rural hospital pharmacies in procuring medications and supplies.

This policy supersedes ASHP policy 1022.

Rationale

State legislation has sometimes exempted small or rural hospitals from requirements applied to others. For example, Texas has exempted hospitals with fifty or fewer beds in remote locations from requiring prospective medication order review by a pharmacist. Pharmacist prospective order review is a well-supported safety practice that is required by the Centers for Medicare & Medicaid Services Conditions of Participation, Joint Commission accreditation standards for hospitals, and in state practice acts. ASHP policy supports pharmacist prospective order review as a minimum standard for pharmacies in hospitals and a consistent standard of care for all patients regardless of where that care is provided. Furthermore, ASHP encourages under-resourced facilities, including rural settings, to employ alternative strategies, such as expanded use of telehealth and pharmacy technicians, to meet the challenges they face. In addition, ASHP recognizes that one of the challenges faced by these hospitals is industry allocation practices (e.g, allocations based on previous purchases) and restrictive distribution criteria (e.g., requiring specific facilities, equipment, or staff) that reduce access to medications and other resources in times of critical need. ASHP advocates that those allocation practices be made more flexible to meet patient needs, especially in times of crisis.

2121

UNIVERSAL INFLUENZA VACCINATION

Source: Council on Therapeutics

To advocate for universal annual administration of influenza vaccinations to the United States population; further,

To advocate that annual influenza vaccination be a national public health priority; further,

To support the development of safe, effective, and affordable universal influenza vaccination, with the goal of long-term immunity.

This policy supersedes ASHP policy 0601.

Rationale

Influenza places a significant health burden on the United States, with estimates of 9–35 million illnesses, 4–16 million outpatient medical visits, and 139,000–708,000 hospitalizations each season. The influenza virus evolves and changes each year, with changes in its genome that require adjustments to vaccine viruses each season. Furthermore, the timing of the onset, peak, and end of each flu season varies annually, typically falling in the fall and winter. Evidence from several observational studies demonstrate that higher influenza vaccination is associated with a lower risk of influenza outbreaks, but Healthy People 2030 estimates that only 49.2% of persons 6 months or older were vaccinated for the 2017–18 season. Influenza vaccination in low-risk individuals has also shown to be effective and can prevent many illnesses, deaths, and losses in productivity.

The Clinical Practice Guidelines by the Infectious Diseases Society of America: 2018 Update on Diagnosis, Treatment, Chemoprophylaxis, and Institutional Outbreak Management of Seasonal Influenza emphasize that annual vaccination is the best method for preventing or mitigating the impact of influenza, and the 2030 Infectious Disease Goals for Healthy People 2030 have a goal of minimum vaccination rates of 70%. In 2019, an Executive Order created the National Influenza Vaccine Task Force, which identified that collaborative efforts across the federal government, academia, the private sector, and international stakeholders over the past decade have advanced influenza vaccine technologies. The Task Force also noted that influenza is a public health and national security challenge, with significant gaps remaining in vaccine effectiveness, pace of vaccine production, sustainable manufacturing, and vaccine access and coverage across all populations.

2124

PREVENTING EXPOSURE TO ALLERGENS

Source: Council on Therapeutics

To advocate for pharmacy workforce participation in the collection, assessment, documentation, and reconciliation of a complete list of allergens and intolerances pertinent to medication therapy, including food, excipients, medications, devices, and supplies; further,

To promote the education of the healthcare team and patients on the differences between medication-related allergic reactions and medication intolerances; further,

To encourage vendors of electronic health records to create readily available and distinct data fields with consistent designations for medication allergies and intolerances; further,

To advocate that vendors of medication-related databases incorporate and maintain information about medication-related allergens and cross-reactivity; further,

To encourage the accurate and complete documentation of allergens and intolerances within the electronic medical record, including detailed descriptions of the reactions occurring upon exposure, for the purpose of clinical decision-making; further,

To advocate that pharmacists actively review allergens and intolerances pertinent to medication therapy and minimize patient and healthcare worker exposure to known allergens, as feasible.

This policy supersedes ASHP policy 1619.

Rationale

The common theme of several ASHP policies is that patients may be exposed to potentially life-threatening allergens in items encountered in the medication-use process (e.g., natural rubber latex, drugs, drug product excipients, devices, and supplies). Pharmacy workforce involvement in collection, assessment, and documentation of a complete list of allergens pertinent to the medication-use process, including food, excipients, medications, devices, and supplies, would assist in clinical decision-making. Members of the pharmacy workforce should also minimize patient and healthcare worker exposure to known allergens, for example by limiting or banning the use of latex gloves in pharmacies and striving for latex-safe medication formularies. Although allergy information is becoming more readily accessible though the electronic health record (EHR) and clinical decision support systems, some well-known cross-sensitivities are good candidates to be included in medication-related databases.

Only about 5–10% of all medication-related adverse events are allergic in nature. Patients are often labeled with an allergy to many drugs on the basis of a side effect or intolerances such as headache or GI disturbance. Allergen misidentification and documentation can be detrimental to patient care by preventing the use of optimal drug agents or by causing reexposure to a true allergen. Pharmacists and pharmacy technicians can help clarify and provide detailed documentation in the EHR regarding patient allergens. Furthermore, there is inconsistent standards on how and where allergies are located in the EHR and as such, there should be a consistent and standardized approach to documentation.

2126

USE OF RACE CORRECTION IN CLINICAL ALGORITHMS

Source: Council on Therapeutics

To recognize that clinical algorithms that only use race or ethnicity as a variable can contribute to inequities and adverse outcomes; further,

To oppose the use of race or ethnicity correction in clinical algorithms unless there is strong evidence to support its use; further,

To advocate that health systems remove algorithms based on race or ethnicity from all sources of therapy decisions, medication information, and the electronic health record, where strong evidence does not support its use; further,

To support further research on the impact of race or ethnicity on drug therapy and outcomes; further,

To advocate that if research includes considerations based on race or ethnicity, the reason for its use as a variable be specified; further,

To provide education on the limitations and appropriate use of race- or ethnicity-corrected clinical algorithms; further,

To support uniform documentation in the electronic health record of a patient-identified designation of race or ethnicity.

Rationale

As outlined in the ASHP Statement on Racial and Ethnic Disparities in Health Care, race and ethnicity are social constructs with a cultural rather than a scientific basis. Although patient care can and should be informed by a patient's racial or ethnic identity, healthcare providers need to recognize the limited utility of that information

There are currently numerous clinical algorithms and practice guidelines that use a patient's race or ethnicity to determine outcomes. The clinical algorithms are then used by providers to help guide individualized risk assessments and clinical decisions. In return, these algorithms may direct attention and resources away from racial and ethnic minorities. However, the majority of these clinical algorithms do not have data to support a patient's race or ethnicity as a clinical factor. When a rationale is given and traced to its origins, the answer leads to outdated, suspect racial science, or biased data. Additionally, these algorithms do not take into account socioeconomic factors and other social determinants of health that may have a large influence on health outcomes.

Currently, a patient's race or ethnicity plays a role in a clinical algorithms or practice guidelines in almost every therapeutic class, including cardiology, surgery, nephrology, obstetrics, urology, and oncology. For example, the American Heart Association Get with the Guidelines - Heart Failure adds 3 points to the risk score of a patient that is non-Black. The higher scores in this tool predict higher in-hospital mortality. Ultimately, this tool is used to help guide clinical decisions for allocations of healthcare resources and referral to cardiology. The consequences of adding race to this algorithm would mean less direct patient care due to the patient being deemed as lower risk. There are many other clinical algorithms that adds points to their risk score for a patient that is non-Black, such as the STONE Score, Urinary Tract Infection Calculator, and Osteoporosis Risk SCORE. Another example is the estimated glomerular filtration rate (eGRF) MDRD and CKDEPI equations. Both of these equations report higher eGRF for Black patients than for other patients with the same serum creatinine levels. Originally, this disparity was thought to be due to patients that identify as Black having a higher average serum creatinine. However, there have been some concerns that this is not always true, especially when looking at the complexity of patients' racial backgrounds. Overestimating a patient's renal function can delay the time to referral to a kidney specialist or transplantation. In short, the addition of race to the clinical algorithms leads to less patient-specific interventions and ultimately worse patient outcomes.

Healthcare providers using the clinical algorithms and practice guidelines should be educated on how to critically evaluate the addition of race and ethnicity, along with the consequences of adding race when not clinically appropriate. Many providers do not assess the algorithm prior to implementing the results, which can lead to improper treatment of a patient.

Education on the limitations of the clinical algorithms can help providers and patients overcome the barriers that the addition of race and ethnicity has created. Additionally, the medical community needs to advocate to re-evaluate our current clinical algorithms and evaluate future algorithms to determine if there is an evidence-based reason that race should be included. It is imperative that the medical community, primarily researchers, understand how race and ethnicity affects the outcome before adding it into a clinical algorithm.

Researchers have developed guidelines to follow when trying to rationalize when race and ethnicity should be included or excluded in a study, such as explaining how the category was determined, considering all confounders, and determining whether there is uncertainty in the algorithm. Researchers should then favor the practices that will help close health inequities over practices that might amplify them. Appropriately determining if race should be included in the algorithm will then help decrease the inappropriate clinical implementation of these tools.

Future research is needed to determine the relationship between pharmacogenomics, race, and ethnicity. Most providers and researchers use the standard five races and two ethnicities categories determined by the Office of Management and Budget to categorize people according to race and ethnicity. However, many individuals do not fit into these categories due to their complex racial and ethnic backgrounds, which may ultimately fail to account for genetic differences.

Drug therapy stems from these clinical algorithms and practice guidelines, and pharmacists need to work with other providers to critically evaluate the current tools. Additionally, pharmacists could collaborate with other providers to perform research to help better understand the differences between genomics and race. Therefore, providers could assess when race and ethnicity should be added to future clinical algorithms and practice guidelines.

2128

USE OF UNAPPROVED GENE THERAPY PRODUCTS, DRUGS, BIOLOGICS, AND MEDICAL DEVICES (BIOHACKING)

Source: Council on Therapeutics

To advocate for enhanced government oversight and regulation of use of gene therapy, drugs, biologic products, and medical devices created outside of the Food and Drug Administration approval process (i.e., "biohacking"), and aggressive enforcement of those regulations; further,

To oppose the use of biohacking on vulnerable and at-risk populations and those unable to provide consent; further,

To promote education of healthcare professionals regarding use of biohacking and its implications in the medical setting; further,

To encourage the pharmacy workforce to include questions about the use of biohacking when obtaining medication histories; further,

To encourage the pharmacy workforce to ensure that patients using biohacking are educated about the risks and benefits of these treatments, including lack of regulatory oversight; further,

To recommend that health systems use a consistent method for documenting the use of biohacking in the electronic health record.

Rationale

Biohacking has been defined as "do-it-yourself biology" or "do-it-yourself citizen science merging body modification with technology" (Yetisen AK. *Trends Biotechnol.* 2018; 36:744–7). Biohacking is performed by biology enthusiasts, citizen scientists, and other like-minded individuals and includes neurohacking (focuses on brain stimulation for change); manufacturing of pharmaceutical products; implantation of modified technology; and the genetic modification of bacteria, yeast, plants, and humans (as a form of self-experimentation) to improve oneself or treat a disease.

Genetic biohacking in particular has proven to be easy and affordable, with individuals using inexpensive, semi-professional and portable labs to carry out their experiments, including Clustered Regularly Interspaced Short Palindromic Repeats (CRISPR) technology, which permits the user to edit the genome by removing, adding, or altering sections of DNA. It is estimated that more than 30,000 people are involved in do-it-yourself biology in the United States alone. Furthermore, many see themselves as serving the greater health interests of the patient community at large with the right to experiment and create treatments such as gene therapy as a form of social justice. However, many of these biohackers have little to no formal training in safety and do not obtain ethical reviews of their work as one would in an institution with an internal review board. Although most biohackers currently experiment only on themselves, concern about the practice may grow as the cost of traditional therapies, particularly biologics, increases, luring sick and desperate patients to biohackers in hopes of cheaper or more accessible treatments.

The other concern about the biohacking movement is bioterrorism. The Federal Bureau of Investigation continues to form relationships with labs where genetic experimentation occurs to police this threat, but the concern remains.

Currently in the United States, there is no ban on genome editing outside of licensed laboratories. Although the Food and Drug Administration (FDA) does have jurisdiction over regular raw biological products, traditional drug products, and do-it-yourself CRISPR kits, they have not taken public enforcement action against those conducting genome editing. This may be due to practicality, however, as many biohackers are individuals or work within a small community and are hard to track. Additionally, many current laws are outdated and apply only to agricultural genetic modification. The FDA has issued draft guidance for the regulation of intentionally altered genomic DNA in animals and stated that "any use of CRISPR/Cas9 gene editing in humans [is] gene therapy" and therefore subject to regulation.

Another facet of biohacking that must be addressed is its potential impact on manufacturing. For example, due to the high cost of biosimilar insulins, a community of biohackers has created the Open Insulin Project to develop an insulin production method for personal use. This and similar projects may lead to intellectual property, regulatory, patent, and legal issues that could impact manufacturing.

Another aspect of do-it-yourself biology is implantation of devices into one's body for medical purposes. Many of these devices are used to monitor a medical condition or to optimize drug delivery to manage disease, such as implantation of veterinary chips for monitoring vital signs, use of a wearable artificial kidney that performs dialysis via a coated skin port, and homemade insulin pumps. Pharmacists need to be aware of these devices, as they impact how patients receive medications and how they are treated. At some point in their health journey, patients using these devices are likely to be admitted to a hospital; a mechanism for documentation of this information in the electronic health record is necessary. Furthermore, pharmacists will need to understand the impact these devices have on the pharmacokinetics, pharmacodynamics, and other aspects of drug therapy.

An overall approach that should be considered is that of education of those engaged in the biohacking movement regarding the role of the federal agencies in consumer protection, risks and benefits and establish practice standards and norms that minimize harm.

2134

PATIENT ACCESS TO PHARMACIST CARE WITHIN PROVIDER NETWORKS

Source: Council on Pharmacy Management

To advocate for laws and regulations that require healthcare payer provider networks to include pharmacists providing patient care services within their scope of practice when such services are covered benefits; further,

To advocate for laws and regulations that require healthcare payer provider networks to consider all qualified pharmacists who apply to participate as a provider in the network and to reimburse all participating providers fairly and equitably for services that are a covered benefit; further,

To acknowledge that healthcare payers may develop and use criteria to determine provider access to its networks to ensure the quality and viability of healthcare services provided; further,

To advocate for laws and regulations that would help ensure the same level of patient care within a payer network by requiring healthcare payers to (1) disclose to participating providers and those applying to participate the criteria used to include, retain, or exclude providers; (2) ensure that those criteria are standardized across all network providers; and (3) collect data on how well providers meet those criteria and report that data to providers; further,

To advocate for comparative, transparent sharing of performance and quality measure data based on those criteria.

This policy supersedes ASHP policy 1808.

Rationale

As hospitals and healthcare organizations have become more engaged in developing ambulatory care services, pharmacists providing patient care services within those settings increasingly find themselves excluded from healthcare payer networks. Vertical integration of the healthcare value chain has given payers more control over healthcare costs and has better positioned them to link directly with providers and negotiate value-based contracts. ASHP acknowledges that healthcare payers may develop and use criteria to determine provider access to its networks to ensure the quality of services and the financial viability of providers (i.e., ensuring sufficient patient volume to profitably operate), but when creating provider networks, payers should consider including pharmacists providing patient care services, within their scope of practice, when such services are covered benefits. To ensure equal treatment for healthcare providers, payers should be required to disclose to participating providers and those applying to participate in a provider network the criteria used to include, retain, or exclude providers. When pharmacists obtain provider status, the infrastructure required to implement direct, independent patient care and billing for provider-based services needs to be in place and accessible. Although a possible risk of payer transparency is a reduction in market competition, comparative, transparent sharing of performance and quality measure data, based on standardized criteria, reveals the level of patient care provided and demonstrates to payers and providers where their performance and quality fall in comparison to others. Ensuring that pharmacists have the opportunity to engage and have access to payers and payer networks improves coordination of care and patient access to pharmacists' care.

2137

DOCUMENTATION OF PHARMACIST PATIENT CARE

Source: Council on Pharmacy Practice

To promote the use of standardized, integrated documentation of pharmacist care provision in a patient's health record; further,

To advocate that documentation by pharmacists in the medical record be used for billing and attribution of value without requiring additional documentation from other clinicians; further,

To advocate for standardized measurement of pharmacist care provision and the attribution of those activities to patient-centered outcomes.

Rationale

ASHP has advocated for the importance of documentation of pharmacist care in patient medical records to ensure accurate and complete documentation of the care and services provided to the patient. However, differences in pharmacy practice within and across health systems make it hard to standardize such documentation in the electronic health record (EHR). The differences are caused by diverse clinical practices, EHR permissions, and documentation elements of the care provided by pharmacists. Documentation by the pharmacist may change depending on care settings, the level of care provided, or in respect to reimbursement. As a result, it is hard to validate and evaluate pharmacists' impact on patient outcomes due to the incomplete measurement and attribution of such care and lack of standardized documentation.

Other healthcare providers have released similar statements on documentation within their fields. The American College of Physicians states that physicians should define professional standards regarding clinical documentation and use macros and templates appropriately (Kuhn T, Basch P, Barr M et al. Clinical documentation in the 21st century: executive summary of a policy position paper from the American College of Physicians. *Ann Intern Med.* 2015; 162:301–3). The American Nurses Association (ANA) Principles for Nursing Documentation states that if patient documentation is not timely, accurate, accessible, complete, legible, readable, and standardized, it will interfere with the ability of those who were not involved in and are not familiar with the patient's care to use the documentation (ANA's Principles for Nursing Documentation: Guidance for Registered Nurses. 2010. www.nursingworld.org/~4af4f2/globalassets/docs/ana/ethics/principles-of-nursing-documentation.pdf). The American Speech-Language-Hearing Association (ASHA) states that speech-language pathologists should participate in the development of the templates that they will use for billing and clinical documents so that the information that is necessary is provided (ASHA. Documentation in health care. www.asha.org/PRPSpecificTopic.aspx?folderid=8589935365&section=References).

Other healthcare providers have recognized the benefits of requiring their documentation to be recorded in a standardized form that allows other healthcare stakeholders to quickly access the information. Employing accessible, standardized documentation improves communication and knowledge sharing between providers. Pharmacists are valuable members of the healthcare team that contribute significantly to patient care. More consistency and standardization of a pharmacist's documentation can provide essential information on a patient's care, such as therapeutic drug monitoring, appropriateness and effectiveness of patient's medications, or pain and antibiotic management, for example. Standardized notes enable healthcare team members to review the pharmacist note and become aware of the medication plan. Implementing standardized and integrated documentation across all healthcare providers, especially pharmacists, will allow for increased interactions and information to be shared between healthcare providers to improve overall patient care. In addition, such standardized and integrated documentation by pharmacists should be used for billing and attribution of value without additional documentation requirements from other clinicians.

Implementing a standardized clinical pharmacy documentation system will also inform and enable a measurement approach for evaluation of the impact of pharmacist services. Many institutions use different tools for operational internal and external benchmarking to meet these measures; however, the tools are limited in their use for clinical benchmarking (Rough SS, McDaniel M, Rinehart JR. Effective use of workload and productivity monitoring tools in health-system pharmacy, pt 1. *Am J Health Syst Pharm.* 2010; 67:300–11). Institutions have tried to implement their own clinical pharmacy productivity measures tools to help demonstrate the value of de-centralized pharmacists on patient care teams. However, no current measure or measure set accurately identifies the impact pharmacists have on patient care outcomes or allows comparison and benchmarking across institutions. In response to this need, the ASHP Pharmacy Accountability Measures (PAM) Work Group seeks to identify pharmacy-related clinical quality measures that institutions could use for benchmarking (Andrawis MA, Carmichael J. A suite of inpatient and outpatient clinical measures for pharmacy accountability: recommendations from the Pharmacy Accountability Measures Work Group. *Am J Health Syst Pharm.* 2014; 71:669–78).

The PAM Workgroup evaluated quality measures endorsed by the National Quality Forum (NQF) and curated those selected into six therapeutic areas, which include antithrombotic safety, cardiovascular control, glycemic control, pain management, behavioral health, and antimicrobial stewardship (Andrawis M, Ellison C, Riddle

S et al. Recommended quality measures for health-system pharmacy: 2019 update from the Pharmacy Accountability Measures Work Group. *Am J Health Syst Pharm.* 2019; 76:874–87). Using the NQF-endorsed measures along with appropriate documentation of the care may allow institutions to more readily benchmark performance.

After determining the most appropriate pharmacy quality measures, the documentation of the care provided should be standardized and efficient. Implementing standardized templates and more retrievable data fields in the documentation process has been shown to improve workflow for pharmacists. One study demonstrated that by implementing EHR note templates that allowed retrievable data to be incorporated, pharmacists increased the amount of time providing value-added services from 47% to 72% and in providing direct patient care from 27% to 53% (Ekstrand MJ, Kobany JM, Pestka DL. Leveraging quality improvement principles in comprehensive medication management pharmacy practice: a case example. *J Am Pharm Assoc.* 2020; 60:509–15.e1.).

Finally, pharmacists must also be properly educated on how to use a standardized pharmacy documentation system. In one study, a health system that implemented an improved pharmacist documentation process found that a focused education initiative increased the number of pharmacist- delivered services by 120% while also improving cost avoidance (Rector KB, Veverka A, Evans SK. *Am J Health-Syst Pharm.* 2014; 71:1303–10). Overall, research has shown that focused education has helped improve the standardized documentation of pharmacist care, leading ultimately to better care for patients and demonstrating the value of pharmacy services.

2006

PHARMACIST'S LEADERSHIP ROLE IN ANTICOAGULATION THERAPY MANAGEMENT

Source: Council on Therapeutics

To advocate that pharmacists provide leadership in caring for patients receiving drug products for anticoagulant therapy management; further,

To advocate that pharmacists be responsible for coordinating the individualized care of patients receiving drug products for anticoagulation therapy management; further,

To encourage pharmacists who participate in anticoagulation therapy management to educate patients, caregivers, prescribers, and other members of the interprofessional healthcare team about anticoagulant drug product uses, drug interactions, reversal therapies and strategies, adverse effects, the importance of adhering to therapy, access to care, and recommended laboratory testing and other monitoring.

This policy supersedes ASHP policy 1703.

Rationale

As medication experts, pharmacists are well positioned to play a key role in implementation, maintenance, monitoring, management of complications, risk assessment, and assurance of continuity of care for patients receiving medications for management of anticoagulation therapy. Inappropriate medication-related management of anticoagulants creates unnecessary preventable harm.

Since 2008, The Joint Commission National Patient Safety Goals for hospitals have included a requirement for reducing the likelihood of harm associated with anticoagulant therapy. Healthcare facilities were instructed to assign leadership for ensuring compliance with this requirement, standardize therapeutic practices and protocols, establish monitoring procedures and a drug–food interaction program, individualize care for each patient receiving these treatments, and provide education on the appropriate management of these patients. In 2019, the related elements of performance were revised to address a rise in adverse drug events associated with direct oral anticoagulants (DOACs).

2008

HEALTH-SYSTEM FACILITY DESIGN

Source: Council on Pharmacy Management

To advocate the development and the inclusion of contemporary pharmacy and medication-use specifications in national and state healthcare design standards to ensure adequate space for safe provision of pharmacy products and patient care services; further,

To promote pharmacist involvement in the design-planning and space-allocation decisions of healthcare facilities.

This policy supersedes ASHP policy 0505.

Rationale

Often the design and location of health-system pharmacy departments are less than ideal. Many pharmacy departments do not have adequate square footage, and too often the pharmacy is located in the basement of the hospital, far removed from the patients. The impact of physical space on staff satisfaction may also contribute to staff turnover. Pharmacy design often occurs before pharmacy leadership has an opportunity for input on the design, location, or size.

Healthcare architects and facility engineers need to be knowledgeable in the contemporary and future needs of pharmacy design and the facility requirements for medication use (e.g., medication preparation rooms, temperature monitoring, automated dispensing cabinets). This includes, for instance, the inclusion of technical specifications (including those in applicable compendial standards of the United States Pharmacopeia) for pharmacies in national healthcare design standards.

Regarding facility design, pharmacist collaboration with the Association of Healthcare Engineers and the American Institute of Architects is paramount to design success. The Guidelines for Design and Construction of Hospital and Health Care Facilities is the primary document driving design decisions by architects and healthcare engineers. Research results on optimal, evidenced-based facility design to support safe medication use should be incorporated in new or renovation construction plans.

2033

HEALTH-SYSTEM USE OF ADMINISTRATION DEVICES SUPPLIED DIRECTLY TO PATIENTS

Source: Council on Pharmacy Management

To recommend that hospitals and health systems have a system in place for determining the risk versus benefit of permitting a patient to use his or her own medication administration devices; further,

To advocate that hospitals and health systems have policies and procedures, including the training of staff, on the use and management of medication administration devices and devices that augment medication administration (e.g., continuous glucose monitors); further,

To advocate that hospitals and health systems ensure that pharmacists participate in the identification of medication administration devices brought in by patients and communicate those findings to the interprofessional care team; further,

To advocate for adequate reimbursement for preparation, order review, and other costs associated with the safe provision and administration of medications and use of related devices.

This policy supersedes ASHP policy 0806.

Rationale

The potential exists for serious patient safety and liability issues for healthcare staff when the use of patients' own infusion devices is allowed. Devices unfamiliar to staff are particularly risky and may result in patient harm. There are, however, occasions when the benefits of using patients' own devices may outweigh the risks. Organizational policies and procedures should exist for handling such situations, complemented by expedient methods to gain familiarity and competency demonstration with a device. A pharmacist should be available to verify the medication and the associated device and use a technique (e.g., Situation, Background, Assessment and Recommendation [SBAR], team huddle) for communicating critical information to the interprofessional care team.

2039

COMPLEMENTARY, ALTERNATIVE, AND INTEGRATIVE MEDICINE PRODUCTS

Source: Council on Therapeutics

To promote awareness of the impact of complementary, alternative, and integrative medicine (CAM) products on patient care, particularly drug interactions, medication safety concerns, and the risk of contamination and variability in active ingredient content; further,

To advocate for the documentation of CAM products in the health record to improve transparency and optimize patient safety; further,

To advocate for the inclusion of up-to-date and readily available information about CAM products and their characteristics in medication-related databases; further,

To provide education on the impact of CAM product administration on patient care within healthcare organizations.

This policy supersedes ASHP policy 1511.

Rationale

The terms complementary, alternative, and integrative are sometimes used interchangeably to describe healthcare approaches that are not part of conventional medical care. When a non-mainstream practice is used together with conventional medicine, it is considered complementary. When a non-mainstream practice is used in place of conventional medicine, it is considered alternative. Integrative healthcare often brings conventional and complementary approaches together in a coordinated way and emphasizes a holistic, patient-focused approach to healthcare and wellness. CAM includes the use of natural products such as herbs, vitamins, and minerals sold as dietary supplements. According to the National Center for Complementary and Alternative Medicine (NCCAM), an estimated 38% of adults and 12% of children use some form of CAM.

In the ASHP Statement on the Use of Dietary Supplements, ASHP expresses concern that the widespread, indiscriminate use of dietary supplements presents substantial risks to public health and details the basis of those concerns. Some dietary supplements are inherently unsafe. Product content (both active ingredient and excipients) is not standardized, therapeutic goals are vague, and evidence of efficacy and safety is absent or ambiguous. Lax regulation of dietary supplement manufacturing presents the risk of contamination or adulteration with harmful substances. Numerous dietary supplements interact with medications and may therefore compromise, complicate, or delay effective treatment. Some patients, particularly those who cannot afford expensive medication regimens, may substitute ineffective alternatives for proven medical therapies.

Healthcare organizations take varying approaches to addressing CAM use. Some actively counsel patients against CAM use, others take a more integrative approach and accept the practice, and some even have clinics for referrals. ASHP has long encouraged healthcare organizations to develop an institutional policy regarding the use of dietary supplements that allows pharmacists and other healthcare practitioners to exercise their professional judgment while balancing patient autonomy and institutional concerns. Such policies should include promoting healthcare practitioner awareness of the potential impacts of CAM use and should encourage documentation of CAM use in the patient's health record so pharmacists and other healthcare practitioners have the knowledge and information they need to safely treat and advise patients.

1902

SAFE ADMINISTRATION OF HAZARDOUS DRUGS

Source: Council on Pharmacy Practice

To advocate that all healthcare settings proactively conduct an interprofessional assessment of risk for exposure to hazardous drugs (HDs) during administration, including when closed-system transfer devices (CSTDs) cannot be used; further,

To advocate for pharmacist involvement in the development of policies, procedures, and operational assessments regarding administration of HDs, including when CSTDs cannot be used; further,

To encourage device and pharmaceutical manufacturers and the Food and Drug Administration to foster development of CSTD-compatible, ready-to-administer HD products.

Rationale

Hazardous drugs (HDs) present well-known risks to healthcare workers who handle them. Most HDs are administered orally or intravenously; however, other routes of administration are sometimes used, such as intrathecal, intraventricular, or intravesicular administration, or perfusion into a vessel or organ cavity. These procedures are becoming more common. Healthcare providers are required to use personal protective equipment and other protective devices, such as closed-system transfer devices (CSTDs), when the dosage form allows. The protective precautions required for administration through these routes is well described in United States Pharmacopeia (USP) General Chapter 800, the ASHP

Guidelines on Handling Hazardous Drugs, the Oncology Nursing Society's Safe Handling of Hazardous Drugs, and other sources.

HDs are sometimes administered through other routes (e.g., Ommaya reservoirs, intraperitoneal infusion) for which protective precautions are not as well described or CSTD use is not possible. ASHP encourages all healthcare settings to conduct an interprofessional, proactive assessment of the risk of such procedures to assess the potential exposure risks for healthcare providers and identify mitigating measures. Given their depth of knowledge regarding the handling of HDs, pharmacists should be involved in the development of policies, procedures, and operational assessments regarding administration of HDs in such circumstances. To reduce the risks to healthcare providers, ASHP encourages device and pharmaceutical manufacturers and the Food and Drug Administration to foster the development of CSTD-compatible, ready-to-administer HD drug products. The goal would be that CSTDs be utilized for all routes of administration of HD products as a best practice. However, when such use is not possible, an assessment of risk could identify gaps and ensure there are pharmacy-guided policies to address the handling, compounding, and administration for all healthcare staff coming into contact with HDs during administration via nontraditional routes. Such policies could also address any specialized training for staff in procedural areas, or the availability of a HD-specialized trained staff member to assist in the administration of the drug (e.g., a "chemo nurse").

1809

HEALTH INSURANCE POLICY DESIGN

Source: Council on Pharmacy Management

To advocate that all health insurance policies be designed and coverage decisions made in a way that preserves the patient–practitioner relationship; further,

To advocate that health insurance payers and pharmacy benefit managers provide public transparency regarding and accept accountability for coverage decisions and policies; further,

To oppose provisions in health insurance policies that interfere with established drug distribution and clinical services designed to ensure patient safety, quality, and continuity of care; further,

To advocate for the inclusion of hospital and health-system outpatient and ambulatory care services in health insurance coverage determinations for their patients.

This policy supersedes ASHP policy 1520.

This policy was reviewed in 2023 by the Council on Pharmacy Management and by the Board of Directors and was found to still be appropriate.

Rationale

Evolving practices by health insurers are negatively affecting patient care decisions and impacting the relationships between patients and their care providers. One common health insurance practice restricts management of and access to certain drugs to specialty suppliers. Another problematic practice is that certain drugs are not reimbursed by the insurer when used as part of the patient's hospital or health-system care. Medicare, for example, deems certain drugs as self-administered drugs, which are not reimbursed when provided to a patient because they are not considered integral to the reason for admission. These practices increase the number of patients that "brown bag" medications when they are admitted to a hospital to avoid being charged personally for the uncovered medications. ASHP has identified a number of concerns about these practices, including impact on continuity of care, integrity of the drug supply, patient satisfaction, and public perception of healthcare organizations.

It is the responsibility of the pharmacist to ensure the integrity of drugs used in the care of patients in the healthcare facility in which he or she practices. Having to verify products that patients bring with them from multiple suppliers disrupts the care process. Having patients go unreimbursed for a medication because it was administered in and supplied by the healthcare organization is confusing to the patient and damaging to the patient–provider relationship. More broadly, lack of understanding of the differing payment systems in different care settings leads to public relations challenges. In addition, the lack of transparency regarding how payers make certain coverage determinations and apply performance penalties (e.g., direct and indirect remuneration fees) creates a significant challenge for healthcare providers as they care for patients.

ASHP advocates reforming these insurance practices. Coverage of medications should not interfere with the safe and effective provision of care and should recognize the responsibility of pharmacists to ensure product integrity for care provided where they practice. In addition, ASHP advocates that the Centers for Medicare & Medicaid Services, commercial payers, and others include hospital and health-system outpatient and ambulatory care services in health insurance coverage determinations for their patients.

1811

USE OF INTERNATIONAL SYSTEM OF UNITS FOR PATIENT- AND MEDICATION-RELATED MEASUREMENTS

Source: Council on Pharmacy Practice

To advocate that the U.S. healthcare system adopt and only use the International System of Units (SI units) for all patient- and medication-related measurements and calculations; further,

To advocate that healthcare organizations use clinical decision support systems, equipment, and devices that allow input and display of patient- and medication-related measurements and calculations in SI format only; further,

To advocate that health information technology manufacturers utilize only SI units in their product designs for patient- and medication-related measurements; further,

To promote education in the use of SI units and the importance of using SI units to prevent medical errors.

This policy was reviewed in 2023 by the Council on Pharmacy Practice and by the Board of Directors and was found to still be appropriate.

Rationale

National healthcare, quality, and safety organizations have for years promoted the sole use of SI units for dosing and weight measurements. Errors in conversion from pounds to kilograms have caused two-fold overdosing and significant underdosing, particularly among pediatric patients, where even small dosing changes can have profound effects. Conversion to and from English units of volume (e.g., from milliliters to teaspoons) has long been identified as a source of dosing errors. These types of errors have been reported in all phases of the medication-use process (e.g., prescribing, preparation, dispensing, and administration) in all patient care settings.

Official labeling for U.S. drug products provides weight-based dosing only in SI units (e.g., mg/kg), so use of any other units introduces a risk of error. ASHP endorses national and institutional efforts to standardize the measurement and communication of patient weight using only SI units (i.e., grams and kilograms) but recognizes that other patient measures are sometimes used in dosing and other health-related calculations (e.g., body surface area, creatinine clearance, glomerular filtration rate, body mass index, or adjusted body weight). ASHP therefore advocates sole use of SI units by healthcare providers during prescribing, preparation, dispensing, and administration of medications in all patient care settings. To promote that practice, clinical decision support systems (e.g., electronic health record) and equipment (e.g., scales, stadiometers, infusion pumps) should be structured to allow input and display of patient-related measurements and calculations in SI format only. Finally, education in how to use SI units, and about the importance of using SI units to prevent medical errors, will be required to overcome cultural resistance by healthcare providers, caregivers, and patients regarding SI unit use.

1822

RATIONAL USE OF MEDICATIONS

Source: Council on Therapeutics

To promote evidence-based prescribing and deprescribing for indication, efficacy, safety, duration, cost, and suitability for the patient; further,

To advocate that pharmacists lead interprofessional efforts to promote the rational use of medications, including engaging in strategies to monitor, detect, and address patterns of irrational medication use in patient populations.

This policy supersedes ASHP policy 1312.

This policy was reviewed in 2023 by the Council on Therapeutics and by the Board of Directors and was found to still be appropriate.

Rationale

The World Health Organization (WHO) identifies that rational use of medications requires that "patients receive medications appropriate to their clinical needs, in doses that meet their own individual requirements, for an adequate period of time, and at the lowest cost to them and their community." The overuse, underuse, or misuse of medicines results in wastage of scarce resources and widespread health hazards. Examples of irrational use of medicines include use of too many medicines per patient, inappropriate use of antimicrobials, inadequate dosage, overuse of injections when oral formulations would be more appropriate, failure to prescribe in accordance with clinical guidelines, inappropriate self-medication, decreased access to medicines, and nonadherence to dosing regimens. These actions can negatively affect the quality of patient care, raise healthcare costs, and increase the number of adverse reactions and events, and may cause adverse reactions or negative psychosocial effects.

Strategies to address irrational medication use can be characterized as educational, managerial, economic, or regulatory in nature. Furthermore, the WHO advocates 12 key interventions to promote more rational use of medications:

- establishment of a multidisciplinary national body to coordinate policies on medication use;
- use of clinical guidelines;
- development and use of national essential medications list;
- establishment of drug and therapeutics committees in districts and hospitals;
- inclusion of problem-based pharmacotherapy training in undergraduate curricula;
- continuing in-service medical education as a licensure requirement;
- supervision, audit, and feedback;
- use of independent information on medications;
- public education about medications;
- avoidance of perverse financial incentives;
- use of appropriate and enforced regulation; and
- sufficient government expenditure to ensure availability of medications and staff.

These recommendations are echoed by the Joint Commission of Pharmacy Practitioners, whose tenets of the pharmacists' patient care process include the collection of necessary subjective and objective information about the patient in order to understand the relevant medical/medication history and clinical status of the patient; assessment of information collected and analysis of the clinical effects of the patient's therapy in the context of the patient's overall health goals in order to identify and prioritize problems and achieve optimal care; development of an individualized patient-centered care plan, in collaboration with other healthcare professionals and the patient or caregiver that is evidence-based and cost-effective; implementation of the care plan in collaboration with other healthcare professionals and the patient or caregiver; and monitoring and evaluation of the effectiveness of the care plan and modification of the plan in collaboration with other healthcare professionals and the patient or caregiver as needed. ASHP also supports the use of stewardship programs with pharmacists in a lead role, as these have been shown to demonstrate the rational use of medications.

1824

USE OF BIOMARKERS IN CLINICAL PRACTICE

Source: Council on Therapeutics

To promote appropriate, evidence-based use of biomarkers in clinical practice; further,

To encourage research that evaluates the clinical and safety implications of biomarkers in the care of patients and to guide clinical practice; further,

To promote Food and Drug Administration qualified biomarkers in drug development, regulation, and use in clinical practice; further,

To foster the development of timely and readily available resources about biomarkers and their evidence-based application in clinical practice.

This policy was reviewed in 2023 by the Council on Therapeutics and by the Board of Directors and was found to still be appropriate.

Rationale

Developed jointly by the Food and Drug Administration (FDA) and National Institutes of Health (NIH) through the FDA-NIH Biomarker Working Group, The Biomarkers, EndpointS, and other Tools (BEST) resource serves as a living document to clarify and promote consistent terminology surrounding the use of biomarkers. As defined by the FDA-NIH Biomarker Working Group, a biomarker is "a defined characteristic that is measured as an indicator of normal biological processes, or responses to an exposure or intervention, including therapeutic interventions. Molecular, histologic, radiographic, or physiologic characteristics are types of biomarkers. A biomarker is not an assessment of how a patient feels, functions, or survives." In comparison to a clinical endpoint, a biomarker is strictly objective and quantifiable, whereas a clinical endpoint reflects the subject's well-being and health status from the subject's perspective. Biomarkers are classified by BEST in the following seven categories: susceptibility/risk biomarker, diagnostic biomarker, monitoring biomarker, prognostic biomarker, predictive biomarker, pharmacodynamic/response biomarker, and safety biomarker.

Further, the FDA and its Center for Drug Evaluation and Research are involved in regulating biomarkers in drug development, regulation, and use in clinical practice. Under the FDA **Biomarker Qualification Program**, researchers can request qualification of a biomarker in the use of drug development. The FDA's involvement in biomarker qualifications allows for the development of a regulatory process to investigate the safety and efficacy of biomarkers. Innovative and newly discovered biomarkers are investigated or found unexpectedly in clinical research. Recently published articles demonstrate newly discovered biomarkers that potentially show clinical efficacy; however, there is debate about how to conduct further research to establish a biomarker's clinical efficacy.

This growth in discovery and application of established biomarkers in practice presents several practice issues, including use of recognized biomarkers, collaborating with practitioners concerning newly discovered or rising biomarkers, conducting research on the outcomes of the use of various biomarkers, and integrating use of biomarkers into practice.

1721

CLINICAL SIGNIFICANCE OF ACCURATE AND TIMELY HEIGHT AND WEIGHT MEASUREMENTS

Source: Council on Therapeutics

To encourage pharmacists to participate in interprofessional efforts to ensure accurate and timely patient height and weight measurements are recorded in the patient medical record to provide safe and effective drug therapy; further,

To encourage drug product manufacturers to conduct and publicly report pharmacokinetic and pharmacodynamics research in pediatric, adult, and geriatric patients at the extremes of weight and weight changes to facilitate safe and effective dosing of drugs in these patient populations, especially for drugs most likely to be affected by weight; further,

To encourage independent research on the clinical significance of extremes of weight and weight changes on drug use, as well as the reporting and dissemination of this information via published literature, patient registries, and other mechanisms; further,

To advocate that clinical decision support systems and other information technologies be structured to facilitate prescribing and dispensing of drugs most likely to be affected by extremes of weight and weight changes.

This policy was reviewed in 2022 by the Council on Therapeutics and by the Board of Directors and was found to still be appropriate.

Rationale

Patients who have clinically significant changes in weight during an admission or between physician visits, or who are at an extreme high or low weight, have a higher risk of medication dosing errors that depend on weight body surface area. Accurate heights and weights in SI units (i.e., kilograms, grams, meters, and centimeters) are an integral part of a physical examination for pharmacists to ensure proper dosing of medications. Certain medications require dosing based on body surface area, and there is a need for healthcare organizations to consistently record patients' height, as estimation of height or weight can contribute to potential over or underdosing.

Factors such as clinically significant changes in weight due to fluid overload and subsequent diuresis, patient growth, and weight changes due to changes in caloric consumption complicate the picture of an appropriate weight to record for dosing certain medications. Some healthcare organizations default to a dosing weight that is used for dosing medications alone, while other weight fluctuations recorded on a daily basis are not used to dose medications, whereas other organizations alert pharmacists to a clinically significant change in weight. Leveraging technology to ensure such safeguards are in place is essential, and providing interoperability between the patient's recorded dosing weight and smart pumps is ideal.

Pharmacists are also seeing an increase in the number of patients at both extremes of weight, and there is a lack of information regarding dosing medications for these populations. ASHP advocates that the Food and Drug Administration (FDA) develop guidance for voluntary drug dosing studies in these populations, as the need for this guidance is supported by the complexity of drug dosing that can vary based on drug and patient characteristics. Drug product manufacturers should be encouraged to complete pharmacokinetic and pharmacodynamic dosing studies, and to publicly report the results, especially for drugs for which significant weight extremes may have clinical impact.

1504

PATIENT ADHERENCE PROGRAMS AS PART OF HEALTH INSURANCE COVERAGE

Source: Council on Public Policy

To advocate for the pharmacist's role in patient medication adherence programs that are part of health insurance plans; further,

To advocate those programs that (1) maintain the direct patient pharmacist relationship; (2) are based on the pharmacist's knowledge of the patient's medical history, indication for the prescribed medication, and expected therapeutic outcome; (3) use a communication method desired by the patient; (4) are consistent with federal and state regulations for patient confidentiality; and (5) permit dispensing of partial fills or overfills of prescription medications in order to synchronize medication refills and aid in medication adherence.

This policy was reviewed in 2020 by the Council on Public Policy and by the Board of Directors and was found to still be appropriate.

Rationale

Current payment rules for Medicare Part D plans require a prorated cost-sharing rate for prescriptions dispensed with less than a 30-day supply. This is allowed to avoid waste in the event that a prescription is modified in response to an adverse reaction. Aligning or synchronizing a medication to all of a patient's chronic medications has been proven to improve adherence. Although Medicare has adopted a policy allowing for a daily cost-sharing rate, other payers have not followed suit. ASHP advocates for similar changes in state law and regulation, since such a change would allow for broader synchronization and improved adherence for patients covered by Medicaid and private third-party payers.

1523

PHARMACIST'S ROLE IN POPULATION HEALTH MANAGEMENT

Source: Council on Pharmacy Management

To recognize the importance of medication management in patient-care outcomes and the vital role of pharmacists in population health management; further,

To encourage healthcare organizations to engage pharmacists and pharmacy leaders in identifying appropriate patient cohorts, anticipating their healthcare needs, and implementing the models of care that optimize outcomes for patients and the healthcare organization; further,

To encourage the development of complexity index tools and resources to support the identification of high-risk, high-cost, and other patient cohorts to facilitate patient-care provider panel determinations and workload balancing; further,

To promote collaboration among members of the interprofessional healthcare team to develop meaningful measures of individual patient and population care outcomes; further,

To advocate for education to prepare pharmacists for their role in population health management.

This policy was reviewed in 2020 by the Council on Pharmacy Management and by the Board of Directors and was found to still be appropriate.

Rationale

As hospital and health systems become larger and adjust to new payment models (e.g., readmissions penalties and reduced Medicare payments), the need for health-system and pharmacy leaders to determine the safest, most efficient, and most economical way to care for identified patient populations has become a significant challenge. Pharmacists have an important role in managing medication therapies for individual patients as well as participating in the development of care models for patient populations with the interprofessional teams they work within. The utilization of "big data" by health systems is a growing domain of research, and it will be important for pharmacists and pharmacy leaders to make use of this information when developing strategic plans and resource allocations. Similar to the workload and productivity issues traditionally facing hospital leaders, the need to stratify total patient populations, anticipate their healthcare resource needs, and then assign the best site and model of care to obtain the ideal return on investment for both the patient and organization has become of paramount importance. The need for identifying the ideal patient panel sizes and the demographics of these panels will be important for patients and pharmacists as pharmacists practice more in the ambulatory care environment. To accomplish these goals, pharmacists will require education to prepare for their role in population health management.

1525

STANDARDIZATION OF DOSES

Source: Council on Pharmacy Practice

To recognize that standardization of medication doses reduces medication errors and improves information technology interoperability, operational efficiency, and transitions of care; further,

To encourage development of universal standardized doses for specific patient populations; further,

To encourage healthcare organizations to adopt standardized doses and to promote publication and education about best practices.

Rationale

Standardization and simplification are widely accepted methods for reducing variability in processes with risk for error. Standardization of medication doses reduces waste and improves efficiency. Computer databases could be constructed with standard dosage forms, facilitating information technology interoperability. Simplified instruction for patients and caregivers improves administration in the home as well as patient adherence.

The standardization of liquid doses has been successfully accomplished in hospitals, but standardization of doses is also applicable to parenteral nutrition solutions and other injectable dosage forms. Standardization of doses within a hospital or health system would reduce waste and the potential for errors in those settings. The strict application of pediatric weight-based dosing, for example, leads to a large number of different doses being used, and many of those doses must then be prepackaged dose-by-dose due to limited stability of liquid and injectable dosage forms.

Standardization of doses within organizations would be made easier by the development of universal standardized doses for specific patient populations, which will require substantial research. Additional studies to determine best practices for standardization of medication doses and education of healthcare practitioners are also needed to facilitate broad adoption of this practice.

1401

STANDARDIZATION OF ORAL LIQUID MEDICATION CONCENTRATIONS

Source: Council on Pharmacy Practice

To advocate for the development of nationally standardized drug concentrations for oral liquid medications; further,

To encourage all health care providers and organizations to standardize concentrations of oral liquid medications; further,

To promote effective instruction of patients and caregivers on how to properly measure and administer oral liquid medications.

This policy was reviewed in 2019 by the Council on Pharmacy Practice and by the Board of Directors and was found to still be appropriate.

Rationale

Standardization and simplification are widely accepted methods for reducing variability in processes with risk for error. Many oral liquid medications are available in more than one concentration from manufacturers, and unique pharmacy-compounded formulations also result in a wide variety of concentrations. Standardization at a national level would reduce variability when patients are discharged and have prescriptions filled at pharmacies in the community. Standardization of concentrations within a hospital or health system would reduce the potential for errors in those settings. Standard doses would reduce the potential for error, reduce waste, and improve efficiency. Improved instruction of patients and caregivers would improve proper administration in the home, safely delivering the prescribed dosage of medication.

1419

DOCUMENTATION OF PATIENT-CARE SERVICES IN THE PERMANENT HEALTH RECORD

Source: Council on Pharmacy Management

To advocate for public and organizational policies that support pharmacist documentation of patient-care services in the permanent patient health record to ensure accurate and complete documentation of the care provided to patients and to validate the impact of pharmacist patient care on patient outcomes and total cost of care; further,

To advocate that electronic health records be designed with a common documentation space to accommodate all health care team members and support the communication needs of pharmacy.

This policy was reviewed in 2019 by the Council on Pharmacy Management and by the Board of Directors and was found to still be appropriate.

Rationale

Documentation in the patient record is critical for a complete record for patient care and communication among members of the health care team. Documentation should be done within an electronic health record (EHR) or on paper. When documenting electronically, use of standardized and coded formats will allow for improved patient outcome measurements.

1313

DRUG-CONTAINING DEVICES

Source: Council on Therapeutics

To recognize that use of drug-containing devices (also known as combination devices) has important clinical and safety implications for patient care; further,

To advocate that use of such devices be documented in the patient's medical record to support clinical decisionmaking; further,

To encourage pharmacists to participate in interprofessional efforts to evaluate and create guidance on the use of these products through the pharmacy and therapeutics committee process to ensure patient safety and promote costeffectiveness; further,

To advocate that the Food and Drug Administration (FDA) and device manufacturers increase the transparency of the FDA approval process for drug-containing devices, including access to data used to support approval; further,

To encourage research that evaluates the clinical and safety implications of drug-containing devices to inform product development and guide clinical practice.

This policy was reviewed in 2023 by the Council on Therapeutics and by the Board of Directors and was found to still be appropriate.

Rationale

As defined by the FDA, a combination product is "a product comprised of two or more regulated components, i.e., drug/device, biologic/device, drug/biologic, or drug/device/biologic, that are physically, chemically, or otherwise combined or mixed and produced as a single entity" or "two or more separate products packaged together in a single package or as a unit and comprised of drug and device products, device and biological products, or biological and drug products." Examples include, but are not limited to, antibiotic-loaded bone cement (ALBC), drug-eluting catheters and stents, and hemostatic sponges and other products used for wound care. Drugs in these products have a therapeutic effect, impact overall patient care, and in some instances may result in drug interactions and adverse drug events. For these reasons, ASHP advocates for documentation of the use of these products in patients' medical records.

Pharmacists usually are not involved in decisions about how these products will be used within the health system but often end up playing a role in the set-up, programming, maintenance, and education of patients and providers in the use of devices. In addition to patient safety concerns, other shortcomings of this approach include lost revenue because these products are frequently not accurately billed or tracked as inventory. ASHP encourages pharmacists to participate in interprofessional discussions concerning use of these products and suggested that the pharmacy and therapeutics committee may provide the ideal mechanism to conduct these evaluations.

The FDA provides recommendations for drug-device development in *Guidance for Industry and Staff: Early Development Considerations for Innovative Combination Products*, including a suggestion that additional preclinical or clinical studies may be needed to evaluate "the potential for change in the established or understood safety, effectiveness, and/or dosing requirements" when a previously approved drug product is incorporated into a combination device. However, these studies are recommended, not required, by the FDA, and even when these studies are completed, information from these studies is not widely available or easily accessible. Finally, it is not always apparent why a specific combination product receives a primary product assignment as a device or drug, which is important because this assignment can impact the approval pathway. ASHP advocates that the FDA and manufacturers of drug-containing devices improve the transparency of the approval process and access to information.

There is often little research concerning the interplay of drugs and devices (e.g., the rate and extent of drug release from the device) or pharmacodynamics once these devices are administered, applied, or implanted in the patient. Further, little is known about the contribution of ALBC or antibiotic beads and spacers to antimicrobial resistance. Therefore, ASHP encourages research that could inform product manufacturers during the development process and provide information to clinicians about use of these products in patient care.

1107

PATIENT-REPORTED OUTCOMES TOOLS

Source: Council on Therapeutics

To advocate for expanded use of validated patient-reported outcomes (PRO) tools in clinical research and direct patient care; further,

To support development of validated PRO tools that are sensitive to differences in cultural and health literacy; further,

To encourage additional research on PRO tools, including studies to assess their correlation to overall patient outcomes; further,

To educate clinicians and patients about the appropriate use of PRO tools.

This policy was reviewed in 2021 by the Council on Therapeutics and by the Board of Directors and was found to still be appropriate.

Rationale

The Council supported expanded use of validated patient-reported outcomes (PRO) tools—assessments of patient satisfaction, health-related quality of life, or health status—in clinical research and direct patient care, and the Board and House agreed. Although PRO tools are most often applied in the research setting, the Council, Board, and House believed that their increased application in direct patient care was warranted as a mechanism to integrate the patient perspective into the assessment and management of disease. Use of PRO tools was noted as consistent with the emphasis on patient-centered care advocated by the Institute of Medicine and other quality improvement initiatives. The Council, Board, and House supported the development of validated PRO tools that account for variability in patient cultural and health literacy and encouraged research to better define the relationship between PRO measures and overall patient outcomes. The need for clinician and patient education on the appropriate use of PRO tools was noted, including the importance of instructing clinicians to select PRO tools that are validated in patient populations that are similar to the populations in which they will be used.

1114

PHARMACIST ACCOUNTABILITY FOR PATIENT OUTCOMES

Source: Council on Pharmacy Practice

To affirm that pharmacists are obligated by their covenantal relationship with patients to ensure that medication use is safe and effective; further,

To declare that pharmacists, pursuant to their authority over a specialized body of knowledge, are autonomous in exercising their professional judgment and accountable as professionals and health care team members for safe and effective medication therapy outcomes; further,

To encourage pharmacists to define practices and associated measures of effectiveness that support their accountability for patient outcomes; further,

To promote pharmacist accountability as a fundamental component of pharmacy practice to other health care professionals, standards-setting and regulatory organizations, and patients.

This policy was reviewed in 2021 by the Council on Pharmacy Practice and by the Board of Directors and was found to still be appropriate.

Rationale

The Council, Board, and House agreed that a clear, succinct policy communicating the interrelationship of authority and autonomy with accountability for outcomes, good or bad, is needed. The policy should distill and define ASHP's stance on accountability and draw on concepts implicit in current ASHP policy documents. The Council, Board, and House recognized that authority, autonomy, and accountability are inseparable components of professional practice. Without accountability, the pharmacy profession cedes the ultimate authority for decision-making in matters of medication therapy to prescribers, calling into question whether pharmacy is, in fact, a profession.

The pharmacist's covenantal relationship with patients is described in the Pharmacist's Oath, to which all pharmacy students profess, and which states in part:

- I will consider the welfare of humanity and relief of suffering my primary concerns.
- I will apply my knowledge, experience, and skills to the best of my ability to assure optimal outcomes for my patients.
- I will embrace and advocate changes that improve patient care.

The attributes of professional status are defined by sociological, ethical, and legal expectations in literature on this subject. Those commonly cited include:

- Work is based upon the mastery of a complex body of knowledge and skills; a practice founded upon this knowledge is used in the service of others.
- Members are governed by codes of ethics and profess a commitment to competence, integrity, and . . . promotion of the public good within their domain.
- A social contract exists in which, in exchange for these commitments, society recognizes the profession's authority over the knowledge base, autonomy in practice, and the privilege of self-regulation.
- The profession's members are accountable to those served and society.

Despite strong advocacy by pharmacy thought leaders and a wealth of evidence in its support, the precept that pharmacists are accountable for medication therapy outcomes is not widely accepted by other health care disciplines, nor is it broadly integrated into pharmacy practice. Moreover, many pharmacists may be ambivalent about assuming a role that holds them to high standards of practice and makes them answerable for the welfare of patients.

Accountability is implicit in many ASHP policy documents, most notably in the *ASHP Statement on Pharmaceutical Care*:

> Pharmaceutical care is not a matter of formal credentials or place of work. Rather, it is a matter of a direct personal, professional, responsible relationship with a patient to ensure that the patient's use of medication is optimal and leads to improvements in the patient's quality of life.

The pharmacist's authority over and expertise in use of medications are supported by the Centers for Medicare & Medicaid Services (CMS) Conditions of Participation Interpretive Guidelines, which establish a definition and expectation for pharmaceutical care:

> Pharmaceutical care is defined as the direct, responsible provision of medication-related care for the purpose of achieving definite outcomes that improve a patient's quality of life while minimizing patient risk.

The Statement on the Future Vision of Pharmacy Practice from the Joint Commission of Pharmacy Practitioners (JCPP) is explicit in its expectation for pharmacist autonomy and accountability and states in part:

> **How Pharmacists Will Practice.** Pharmacists will have the authority and autonomy to manage medication therapy and will be accountable for patients' therapeutic outcomes. In doing so, they will communicate and collaborate with patients, care givers, health care professionals, and qualified support personnel. As experts regarding medication use, pharmacists will be responsible for rational use of medications, including the measurement and assurance of medication therapy outcomes.... Working cooperatively with practitioners of other disciplines to care for patients, pharmacists will be . . . valued patient care providers whom health care systems and payers recognize as having responsibility for assuring the desired outcomes of medication use.

The JCPP vision statement encompasses these attributes and clearly illustrates the direction that the pharmacy profession must take. In particular, the Council, Board, and House confirmed that pharmacist accountability is a profession-defining issue that must be urgently addressed, recognizing that the policy is at most a starting point for the transformation that needs to take place in order to realize the JCPP vision.

The Council stated that unless the pharmacy profession commits to actions that translate the policy into practice, pharmacists are at risk of becoming irrelevant. As changes brought about by health care reform are implemented to add value to health care and reduce costs, the extensive training and high salaries of pharmacists cannot be justified if, as noted by the 2007 Council, "pharmacists are responsible and held accountable only for the acquisition, storage, and dispensing of medications."

The Council called on ASHP to be fearless and persistent in promoting and establishing the JCPP vision within the profession. The Council also recommended that ASHP use its influence to create the "pull" for accountability in pharmacy practice by establishing an expectation of pharmacist accountability by other health care providers, standards-setting and regulatory organizations, and payers.

1005

MEDICATION THERAPY MANAGEMENT

Source: Council on Public Policy

To support medication therapy management (MTM) services as defined in Section 3503 of the Patient Protection and Affordable Care Act (PL 111-148); further,

To affirm that MTM is a partnership between the patient (or a caregiver) and a pharmacist, in collaboration with other health care professionals, that promotes the safe and effective use of medications.

This policy was reviewed in 2020 by the Council on Public Policy and by the Board of Directors and was found to still be appropriate.

Rationale

The term "medication therapy management" (MTM) has received widespread use within the pharmacy profession and among health policymakers. The definition of MTM under Part D of the Medicare program is significantly different from the consensus definition developed by national pharmacy organizations, including ASHP, in 2004. Provisions dealing with MTM grant programs contained in Section 3503 of the Patient Protection and Affordable Care Act (PL 111-148) (PPACA) broaden and enhance MTM beyond the Part D definition. Those provisions also refer to collaborative practice agreements as allowed by state practice acts, referred to in ASHP policy and elsewhere as "collaborative drug therapy management" (CDTM). As health care reform evolves and is implemented, it is important to recognize the distinction that state and federal laws and regulations and ASHP policy make between those two terms and to affirm ASHP's support for the broader definition of MTM in PPACA and the central role of pharmacists in MTM.

1023

SCOPE AND HOURS OF PHARMACY SERVICES

Source: Council on Pharmacy Practice

To support the principle that all patients should have 24-hour access to a pharmacist responsible for their care, regardless of hospital size or location; further,

To advocate alternative methods of pharmacist review of medication orders (such as remote review) before drug administration when onsite pharmacist review is not available; further,

To support the use of remote medication order review systems that communicate pharmacist approval of orders electronically to the hospital's automated medication distribution system; further,

To promote the importance of pharmacist access to pertinent patient information, regardless of proximity to patient.

This policy was reviewed in 2020 by the Council on Pharmacy Practice and by the Board of Directors and was found to still be appropriate.

Rationale

Recent legislation in Texas exempts hospitals with fifty or fewer beds in remote locations from requiring prospective medication order review by a pharmacist. Pharmacist prospective order review is a well-supported safety practice that is required by the Centers for Medicare & Medicaid Services

Conditions of Participation, Joint Commission accreditation standards for hospitals, and in state practice acts. Current ASHP policy supports pharmacist prospective order review and a consistent standard of care for all patients regardless of where that care is provided.

0502

HEALTH CARE QUALITY STANDARDS AND PHARMACY SERVICES

Source: Council on Administrative Affairs

To advocate that health care quality improvement programs adopt standard quality measures that are developed with the involvement of pharmacists, are evidence-based, and promote the demonstrated role of pharmacists in improving patient outcomes.

This policy was reviewed in 2020 by the Council on Pharmacy Practice and by the Board of Directors and was found to still be appropriate.

0525

MANDATORY TABLET SPLITTING FOR COST CONTAINMENT

Source: Council on Professional Affairs

To oppose mandatory tablet splitting for cost containment in ambulatory care; further,

To encourage pharmacists, when voluntary tablet splitting is considered, to collaborate with patients, caregivers, and other health care professionals to determine whether tablet splitting is appropriate on the basis of the patient's ability to split tablets and the suitability of the medication (e.g., whether it is scored or is an extended-release product); further,

To urge pharmacists to promote dosing accuracy and patient safety by ensuring that patients are educated on how to properly split tablets; further,

To encourage further research by the United States Pharmacopeia and the Food and Drug Administration on the impact of tablet splitting on product quality.

This policy was reviewed in 2023 by the Council on Pharmacy Practice and by the Board of Directors and was found to still be appropriate.

ASHP Statement on Confidentiality of Patient Health Care Information

The American Society of Health-System Pharmacists (ASHP) believes that all medical information is sensitive and should be given the utmost protection. ASHP supports the adoption into federal law of a minimum standard for protection of individually identifiable patient health information and believes that states should retain the ability to adopt standards that are more stringent than federal law.

ASHP believes that patients should have the right to access and review their medical records and the ability to correct factual errors in those records. Patients should also have the right to know who has access to their medical records and to authorize how their medical information will be used.

The Health Insurance Portability and Accountability Act of 1996 (HIPAA) requires health systems to have written policies and procedures in place to guard against the unauthorized collection, use, or disclosure of individually identifiable patient health information and provide notice of such policies to their patients. All health-system personnel should be trained to understand and comply with those privacy standards.

ASHP strongly believes that pharmacists must have access to patient health records in order to provide quality care and ensure the safe use of medications. Within health systems, all authorized practitioners should be encouraged to communicate freely with each other while maintaining patient confidentiality and privacy. This includes pharmacists practicing across the continuum of practice settings in order to maintain continuity of care. Pharmacists recognize that with access to the patient's health record comes the pharmacist's professional responsibility to safeguard the patient's rights to privacy and confidentiality. Uniquely identifiable patient information should not be exchanged without the patient's authorization for any reason not directly related to treatment, payment, health care operations, or research conducted under an appropriately constituted institutional review board (IRB). ASHP advocates strict governmental protections, with appropriate civil or criminal penalties for violations, to prevent disclosure of individually identifiable patient information outside the health system (i.e., to an unauthorized third party) for any purposes not directly related to treatment, payment, health care operations, or research conducted under an appropriately constituted IRB.

Pharmacists participate extensively in research on drugs. ASHP believes that all research data must be recorded and stored in such a way that the subjects' rights of privacy and confidentiality are protected. IRBs have a responsibility to determine when informed consent is necessary and to establish procedures for obtaining informed consent. Patients should receive a statement describing the parties who may have access to patient-identifiable information (e.g., institutional personnel, business associates, researchers, personnel from study sponsors, employees of government agencies that monitor compliance with regulations). Patient authorization requirements under the privacy regulations of HIPAA must be followed, and patients always have the right to withdraw their consent at any time.

DOI 10.37573/9781585287048.052

ASHP believes that there is no potential for a breach of patient confidentiality when patient information is aggregated for use in legitimate research or statistical measurement and is not uniquely identifiable. Therefore, specific authorization by individual patients for access to this information is not needed.

ASHP believes that pharmacy residency programs and other training programs must implement policies and procedures to ensure the confidentiality of patient medical records while allowing pharmacy students and residents access to these records in the course of their training and presentation of their research.

This statement was reviewed in 2023 by the Council on Public Policy and by the Board of Directors and was found to still be appropriate.

Developed through the ASHP Council on Public Policy and approved by the ASHP Board of Directors on February 22, 2008, and by the ASHP House of Delegates on June 10, 2008.

This statement supersedes the ASHP Statement on the Confidentiality of Patient Health Care Information dated April 21, 1999.

Copyright © 2009, American Society of Health-System Pharmacists, Inc. All rights reserved. Contact ASHP for reprint and permissions requests. This content may not be used for commercial purposes without the express written consent of ASHP.

The bibliographic citation for this document is as follows: American Society of Health-System Pharmacists. ASHP statement on confidentiality of patient health care information. *Am J Health-Syst Pharm.* 2009; 66:411–2.

ASHP Statement on the Health-System Pharmacist's Role in National Health Care Quality Initiatives

Position

The American Society of Health-System Pharmacists (ASHP) believes that pharmacists who practice in hospitals and health systems ("health-system pharmacists") have a critical leadership role in national health care quality-improvement initiatives. Health-system pharmacists possess the knowledge of drug therapy and medication-use systems required to successfully implement quality-assurance and improvement programs. These pharmacists should use their authority over and accountability for medication management systems to align medication use in hospitals and health systems with the national health care quality agenda.

Background

Major reports from the Institute of Medicine (IOM) have demonstrated that the quality and safety environment across the health care industry needs significant transformation. *The Urgent Need to Improve Health Care Quality*[1] suggested that the quality of the health care system in the United States could be accurately measured and that the quality of care was being compromised by the underuse, overuse, and misuse of health care entities. *Crossing the Quality Chasm*[2] built a compelling case that the American health care delivery system requires major restructuring and proposed goals for improving six key dimensions of health care quality: safety, timeliness, effectiveness, efficiency, equity, and patient centeredness (the "STEEP" framework). To achieve these aims, IOM called for fundamental reforms, including new payment methodologies, public reporting, and transparency of quality-improvement data.

Since the release of these reports, health care policymakers, providers, purchasers, payers, consumers, and others have responded in ways that are beginning to change the U.S. health care delivery system. These changes are influenced by a growing number of private and public organizations, including the Joint Commission, Centers for Medicare and Medicaid Services (CMS), National Quality Forum, National Priorities Partnership, Agency for Healthcare Research and Quality, Institute for Healthcare Improvement, and American Health Quality Association, among others. These organizations, alone or in collaboration, identify health care quality measures to set the national health care quality agenda. These quality measures are collected and reported through both mandatory and voluntary reporting systems, and the outcome measurements of a health system may be linked to reimbursement (e.g., through CMS pay-for-performance programs).

Responsibilities of Health-System Pharmacists

Many national health care quality measures are related to medication use.[3] Health-system pharmacists are strategically positioned to integrate practices and procedures that support these quality measures into the medication-use system. To help align medication use in hospitals and health systems with the national health care quality agenda, health-system pharmacists should

- Become familiar with the organizations that influence the national health care quality agenda and monitor those organizations for changes in medication-use-related quality measures.
- Participate in the development, implementation, and evaluation of national and state health care quality-improvement initiatives related to medication use.
- Collaborate with other health care professionals to evaluate medication-use practices in their organizations and develop and implement programs that optimize patient outcomes, improve medication use, and align with the national health care quality agenda, including expanding the scope and reach of pharmacists' services when appropriate.
- Collect, analyze, and report data that measure health care quality related to medication use, and support the public availability of those data.
- Integrate and align information systems in their organizations with the national health care quality agenda.
- Educate other health care practitioners, health care executives, and the public about medication-related health care quality-improvement initiatives and the critical role pharmacists have in those initiatives (e.g., by publishing articles about innovative pharmacy services that improve patient outcomes or medication use).
- Encourage national pharmacy organizations to support, guide, and provide education related to the national health care quality agenda.

Conclusion

The number of mandatory and voluntary health care quality measures related to the use of medications is large and growing. As medication-use experts, health-system pharmacists have a responsibility to become knowledgeable about national health care quality-improvement initiatives and to align their practices accordingly. Because health-system pharmacists possess knowledge of drug therapy and medication-use systems and have authority over and accountability for medication management systems, they have a fundamental leadership role in the development, implementation, and evaluation of health care quality-improvement initiatives.

References

1. Chassin MR, Galvin RW. The urgent need to improve health care quality. Institute of Medicine National Roundtable on Health Care Quality. *JAMA*. 1998; 280:1000–5.
2. Institute of Medicine Committee on Quality of Health Care in America. Crossing the quality chasm: a new health system for the 21st century. Washington, DC: National Academy Press; 2001:43–56.

DOI 10.37573/9781585287048.053

3. Bohenek WS, Grossbart SR. Pharmacists' role in improving quality of care. *Am J Health-Syst Pharm.* 2008; 65:1566–70.

This policy was reviewed in 2013 by the Council on Pharmacy Practice and by the Board of Directors and was found to still be appropriate.

Approved by the ASHP Board of Directors on April 17, 2009, and by the ASHP House of Delegates on June 16, 2009. Developed through the ASHP Council on Pharmacy Practice.

The contributions of Wayne S. Bohenek, Pharm.D., M.S., FASHP, and Jamie S. Sinclair, M.S., to this statement are gratefully acknowledged. The following organizations and individuals are acknowledged for reviewing draft versions of this statement (review does not imply endorsement): Academy of Managed Care Pharmacy (AMCP); Accreditation Council for Pharmacy Education (ACPE); American Pharmacists Association (APhA); South Carolina Society of Health-Systems Pharmacists (SCSHSP); John A. Armitstead, M.S., FASHP; Cathy Baker, Pharm.D.; Frank Briggs, Pharm.D., M.P.H.; Kimberly K. Daugherty, Pharm.D., BCPS; Jeanne Ezell, M.S., FASHP; Linda Gore Martin, Pharm.D., M.B.A., BCPS; Jody Jacobson Wedret, FASHP, FCSHP; Patricia Kienle, M.P.A., FASHP; Julie Kuhle, B.S.Pharm.; Greg Polk, M.B.A.; James A. Ponto, M.S., BCNP, FASHP; Mike Rouse, B.Pharm.(Hons), M.P.S. (ACPE); Marissa Schlaifer, M.S. (AMCP); Sue Skledar, M.P.H., FASHP; Darren M. Triller, Pharm.D.; and Bradley White, Pharm.D., R.N. (SCSHSP).

Copyright © 2010, American Society of Health-System Pharmacists, Inc. All rights reserved. Contact ASHP for reprint and permissions requests. This content may not be used for commercial purposes without the express written consent of ASHP.

The bibliographic citation for this document is as follows: American Society of Health-System Pharmacists. ASHP statement on the health-system pharmacist's role in national health care quality initiatives. *Am J Health-Syst Pharm.* 2010; 67:578–9.

ASHP–SHM Joint Statement on Hospitalist–Pharmacist Collaboration

Position

The American Society of Health-System Pharmacists (ASHP) and the Society for Hospital Medicine (SHM) believe that the rapidly emerging hospitalist model of inpatient care offers new and significant opportunities to optimize patient care through collaboration among hospitalists, hospital pharmacists (hereinafter, "pharmacists"), and other health care providers. The emerging model of care allows for deeper professional relationships among health care providers and promotes a shared interest in and responsibility for direct patient care, indirect patient care, and service activities. ASHP and SHM encourage hospitalists, pharmacists, and health care executives to seek out ways to foster collaboration between hospitalists and pharmacists.

The purpose of this consensus statement is to promote an understanding of the ways hospitalists and pharmacists can jointly optimize the care provided to patients in hospitals, examine opportunities for improving hospitalist–pharmacist alliances that enhance patient care, suggest future directions for collaboration, and identify aspects of such collaboration that warrant further research.

Background

Increases in health care spending and the expanding influence of managed care in the late 1980s and early 1990s resulted in calls for more efficient health care. The movement toward greater efficiency resulted in more emphasis on ambulatory care, fewer hospital admissions, shortened hospital stays, and an overall increase in the acuity of illness of hospitalized patients. The emphasis on ambulatory care increased the number and complexity of physician office visits, and the changing characteristics of office- and hospital-based care placed significant demands on primary care physicians and contributed to the rise of hospital medicine.

In 1996, the term "hospitalist" was introduced to the health care lexicon.[1] A hospitalist was defined as an inpatient physician who manages the care of hospitalized patients and facilitates the transfer of their care back to the primary care physician. The Society of Hospital Medicine has since defined a hospitalist as a physician whose primary professional focus is the general medical care of hospitalized patients and whose activities may include patient care, teaching, research, and leadership related to hospital medicine.[2]

The past decade has seen rapid growth in the number of hospitalists and the use of hospitalists by U.S. hospitals.[3] In 2005, 70% of hospitals with more than 200 beds used hospitalist services, and there were over 16,000 hospitalists in practice.[4] An estimated 20,000 hospitalists were practicing at over 2,600 U.S. hospitals in 2007.[5]

Initially, many physicians expressed concern about the potential for hospitalists to interfere in the relationship between the patient and the primary care physician, as well as about the potential negative impact on continuity of care.[6] However, subsequent studies demonstrated increasing acceptance of hospitalists by primary care physicians, with as many as 89% considering the hospitalist model to be superior to the historical model of hospital care being provided by primary care physicians or by specialists working on rotations.[7,8] Numerous studies demonstrate the value of hospitalists in improving quality of care, decreasing hospital costs and length of stay, and reducing hospital readmissions.[9–21]

As early as 1921, hospital pharmacists in the American Pharmaceutical Association (now the American Pharmacists Association) had formed a committee to address their distinct concerns. During the 1930s, hospital pharmacists began to organize state organizations and to adhere to a set of minimum standards of practice. In 1942, the American Society of Hospital Pharmacists (now the American Society of Health-System Pharmacists [ASHP]) was formed to establish minimum standards of pharmaceutical services in hospitals, provide interchange among pharmacists, promote new pharmaceutical techniques, and aid the medical profession in extending the economic and rational use of medications.[22] As of 2005, there were approximately 50,000 pharmacists practicing in U.S. hospitals.[23]

The modern mission of hospital pharmacy departments is to ensure optimal outcomes from the use of medicines.[24] Although the focus of hospital pharmacy has traditionally been on the safe dispensing of medications, direct patient care by pharmacists (clinical pharmacy) has always been a component of hospital pharmacy practice. Following the rise of pharmaceutical care in the 1980s,[25] these pharmacist services have expanded greatly. It has been estimated that 35–40% of hospital pharmacists are devoted to providing clinical services.[23] A systematic review in 2006 documented improved outcomes when clinical pharmacists interacted with the health care team on patient rounds, interviewed patients, reconciled medications, and provided discharge counseling and follow-up.[26] These findings support those of other studies in which specific clinical pharmacy services were associated with improved therapeutic and economic outcomes.[27–31]

Opportunities for Collaboration Between Pharmacists and Hospitalists

Pharmacists and hospitalists have shared interests that provide strong incentives for collaboration. All health care professionals share, first, a commitment to and responsibility for providing safe and effective patient care. Physicians, pharmacists, and other health care providers have long collaborated in providing direct patient care. The emerging hospitalist model of care offers more opportunities for collaboration because pharmacists and hospitalists also share interest in and responsibility for indirect patient care and service activities—developing the institutional policies, processes, and infrastructure that support patient care.

Direct patient care activities typically performed by hospitalists include obtaining patient histories, conducting physical examinations, making diagnoses, developing treatment plans, monitoring patients' responses to therapy, performing follow-up hospital visits, participating in family

DOI 10.37573/9781585287048.054

meetings, and providing discharge instructions.[32] Specific clinical pharmacy services that have been associated with improved health care outcomes include providing drug information, managing medication protocols and adverse drug reactions, participating in medical rounds, gathering admission medication histories, interviewing patients, reconciling patient medications, and providing discharge counseling and follow-up.[26–31]

Pharmacists should be involved in the care of hospitalized patients and can collaborate with hospitalists in numerous ways, including

- Providing consultative services that foster appropriate, evidence-based medication selection (e.g., during rounds).
- Providing drug information consultation to physicians, nurses, and other clinicians.
- Managing medication protocols under collaborative practice agreements.
- Assisting in the development of treatment protocols.
- Monitoring therapeutic responses (including laboratory test results).
- Continuously assessing for and managing adverse drug reactions.
- Gathering medication histories.
- Reconciling medications as patients move across the continuum of hospital care.
- Providing patient and caretaker education, including discharge counseling and follow-up.

Both hospitalists and pharmacists have a responsibility for ensuring continuity as patients move across settings of care.

In addition to their direct patient care activities, hospitalists add value through their efforts in hospital service activities, student and resident education, and research. Typical service activities include participating in quality-improvement and safety initiatives, developing institutional guidelines and protocols for the treatment of specific diseases, serving on hospital committees (e.g., the pharmacy and therapeutics [P&T] committee), and working with others to introduce new technologies to the hospital setting.[33,34]

Pharmacists also participate in hospital service activities, student and resident education, and research. For example, pharmacists serve on the P&T committee and are directly involved in managing the formulary system that guides an institution's medication use. As medication experts, pharmacists contribute to the development and implementation of patient care guidelines and other medication-use policies. Pharmacist expertise is also integral to many quality-improvement efforts (e.g., surgical infection prophylaxis) and to technology initiatives (e.g., bedside medication scanning and computerized prescriber-order-entry systems). Pharmacist provision of inservice education on medications and medication use is invaluable for all health care providers.

These overlapping responsibilities provide hospitalists and pharmacists with opportunities to collaborate on activities that can have a profound effect on care in the hospital. Hospitalists and pharmacists can work together to ensure that care is evidence-based, cost-effective, and adherent to national guidelines; establish an institutional culture of safety; develop and implement quality-improvement initiatives; meet accreditation standards; and, in many cases, foster the institution's education and research initiatives. Health professional education and research offer the opportunities to improve patient care provided not just by a single hospital but by other facilities as well.

Opportunities to Improve Collaboration

ASHP and SHM believe that there are opportunities for improving collaboration between hospitalists and pharmacists. Barriers to collaboration include real and perceived professional boundaries, poor integration of technology systems, inadequate pharmacist and hospitalist staffing, time constraints, inadequate funding and resources, lack of third-party compensation for clinical pharmacy services, and the competing obligations weighing on both professions.

Real and perceived professional boundaries can be addressed by clear communication and by enhanced interdisciplinary educational opportunities for all members of the health care team.[35–38] ASHP and SHM believe that, while hospitalists should serve as the primary leaders of hospital care teams, all health care professionals should be willing to assume a leadership role in treating patients and, when appropriate, accept leadership by other team members. Like all members of the care team, pharmacists require timely access to hospitalists for consultation, as well as access to patient information. The vital flow of information and communication among health care providers should be conducive to collaborating and improving patient outcomes. ASHP and SHM believe that properly applied, well-integrated technologies (e.g., electronic medical records and personal digital assistants with clinical decision support systems, including drug information) can enhance communication among all members of the health care team.

Hospitalists and pharmacists can work together to overcome limitations created by inadequate funding and staffing by providing evidence to health care executives of the value of clinical pharmacist positions and pharmacist–hospitalist collaboration. This evidence should examine the impact of these positions and such collaboration on therapeutic, safety, humanistic, and economic outcomes. Collaboration among all members of the health care team would also be encouraged by reforming the current fee-for-service reimbursement practices to base payment for care delivery on overall treatment goals (e.g., a payment rate based on diagnosis).

Conclusion

An interdisciplinary approach to health care that includes physicians, pharmacists, nurses, and other health care professionals will improve the quality of patient care. Hospitalists and pharmacists need to collaborate with each other and with other health care professionals to optimize outcomes in hospitalized patients. ASHP and SHM believe that hospitalist–pharmacist alliances should be encouraged and that the systems and technologies that enable collaboration, and the incentives for such collaboration, should be enhanced.

References

1. Wachter RM, Goldman L. The emerging role of "hospitalists" in the American health care system. *N Engl J Med.* 1996; 335:514–7.

2. Society of Hospital Medicine. Definition of a hospitalist. www.hospitalmedicine.org/Content/NavigationMenu/AboutSHM/DefinitionofaHospitalist/Definition_of_a_Hosp.htm (accessed 2007 May 29).
3. Kralovec PD, Miller JA, Wellikson L, et al. The status of hospital medicine groups in the United States. *J Hosp Med.* 2006; 1:75–80.
4. AHA hospital statistics. Chicago: American Hospital Association; 2005.
5. Hospital medicine specialty shows 20 percent growth. SHM analysis of 2005 American Hospital Association survey data. www.hospitalmedicine.org/AM/Template.cfm?Section=Press_Releases&Template=/CM/ContentDisplay.cfm&ContentID=12507 (accessed 2007 May 29).
6. Sox HC. The hospitalist model: perspectives of the patient, the internist, and internal medicine. *Ann Intern Med.* 1999; 130:368–72.
7. Auerbach AD, Nelson EA, Lindenauer PK, et al. Physician attitudes toward and prevalence of the hospitalist model of care: results of a national survey. *Am J Med.* 2000; 109:648–53.
8. Fernandez A, Grumbach K, Goitein L, et al. Friend or foe? How primary care physicians perceive hospitalists. *Arch Intern Med.* 2000; 160:2902–8.
9. Wachter RM, Katz P, Showstack J, et al. Reorganizing an academic medical service: impact on cost, quality, patient satisfaction, and education. *JAMA.* 1998; 279:1560–5.
10. Diamond HS, Goldberg E, Janosky JE. The effect of full-time faculty hospitalists on the efficiency of care at a community teaching hospital. *Ann Intern Med.* 1998; 129:197–203.
11. Stein MD, Hanson S, Tammaro D, et al. Economic effects of community versus hospital-based faculty pneumonia care. *J Gen Intern Med.* 1998; 13:774–7.
12. Craig DE, Hartka L, Likosky WH, et al. Implementation of a hospitalist system in a large health maintenance organization: the Kaiser Permanente experience. *Ann Intern Med.* 1999; 130:355–9.
13. Freese RB. The Park Nicollet experience in establishing a hospitalist system. *Ann Intern Med.* 1999; 130:350–4.
14. Rifkin WD, Connor DS, Silver A, et al. Comparison of hospitalists and primary care internists in the care of patients with pneumonia. *J Gen Intern Med.* 1999; 14(suppl):S118.
15. Rifkin WD, Connor DS, Silver A, et al. Comparing hospitalists' and community-based primary care physicians' care of patients with pneumonia. *J Gen Intern Med.* 2001; 16(suppl):S215.
16. Davis KM, Koch KE, Harvey JK, et al. Effects of hospitalists on cost, outcomes, and patient satisfaction in a rural health system. *Am J Med.* 2000; 108:621–6.
17. Halpert AP, Pearson SD, LeWine HE, et al. The impact of an inpatient physician program on quality, utilization, and satisfaction. *Am J Manag Care.* 2000; 6:549– 55.
18. Bellet PS, Whitaker RC. Evaluation of a pediatric hospitalist service: impact on length of stay and hospital charges. *Pediatrics.* 2000; 105:478–84.
19. Landrigan C, Srivastava R, Muret-Wagstaff S, et al. Outcomes of hospitalization in pediatric patients insured by HMOs: comparison of care by hospitalists and traditional academic providers. *Pediatr Res.* 2000; 47:204A. Abstract.
20. Srivastava R, Landrigan C, Muret-Wagstaff S, et al. Impact of a managed care hospitalist system in academic pediatrics. *Pediatr Res.* 2000; 47:228A. Abstract.
21. Srivastava R, Landrigan C, Muret-Wagstaff S, et al. Cost savings for patients with acute conditions cared for by pediatric hospitalists in a tertiary care center. *Pediatr Res.* 2001; 49:125A. Abstract.
22. Zellmer WA. Overview of the history of pharmacy in the United States. In: Brown TR, ed. Handbook of institutional pharmacy practice. Bethesda, MD: American Society of Health-System Pharmacists; 2006:19–32.
23. Pedersen CA, Schneider PJ, Scheckelhoff DJ. ASHP national survey of pharmacy practice in hospital settings: dispensing and administration—2005. *Am J Health-Syst Pharm.* 2006; 63:327–45.
24. Zellmer WA. Perspectives on Hilton Head. *Am J Hosp Pharm.* 1986; 43:1439–43.
25. American Society of Hospital Pharmacists. ASHP statement on pharmaceutical care. *Am J Hosp Pharm.* 1993; 50:1720–3.
26. Kaboli PJ, Hoth AB, McClimon BJ, et al. Clinical pharmacists and inpatient medical care: a systematic review. *Arch Intern Med.* 2006; 166:955–64.
27. Bond CA, Raehl CL, Franke T. Interrelationships among mortality rates, drug costs, total cost of care, and length of stay in United States hospitals: summary and recommendations for clinical pharmacy services and staffing. *Pharmacotherapy.* 2001; 21:129–41.
28. Bond CA, Raehl CL, Franke T. Clinical pharmacy services, hospital pharmacy staffing, and medication errors in United States hospitals. *Pharmacotherapy.* 2002; 22:134–47.
29. Bond CA, Raehl CL. Clinical pharmacy services, pharmacy staffing, and adverse drug reactions in United States hospitals. *Pharmacotherapy.* 2006; 26:735–47.
30. Schumock GT, Butler MG, Meek PD, et al. Evidence of the economic benefit of clinical pharmacy services: 1996–2000. *Pharmacotherapy.* 2003; 23:113–32.
31. Kucukarslan SN, Peters M, Mlynarek M, et al. Pharmacists on rounding teams reduce preventable adverse drug events in hospital general medicine units. *Arch Intern Med.* 2003; 163:2014–8.
32. O'Leary KJ, Liebovitz DM, Baker DW. How hospitalists spend their time: insights on efficiency and safety. *J Hosp Med.* 2006; 1:88–93.
33. Hauer KE, Wachter RM. Implications of the hospitalist model for medical students' education. *Acad Med.* 2001; 76:324–30.
34. Plauth WH III, Pantilat SZ, Wachter RM, et al. Hospitalists' perceptions of their residency training needs: results of a national survey. *Am J Med.* 2001; 111:247–54.

35. Committee on the Health Professions Education Summit. Health professions education: a bridge to quality. Washington, DC: National Academy Press; 2003.
36. Cooper H, Carlisle C, Gibbs T, et al. Developing an evidence base for interdisciplinary learning: a systematic review. *J Adv Nurs.* 2001; 31:228–37.
37. Horsburgh M, Lamdin R, Williamson E. Multiprofessional learning: the attitudes of medical, nursing, and pharmacy students to shared learning. *Med Educ.* 2001; 35:876–83.
38. Crawford GB, Price SD. Team working: palliative care as a model of interdisciplinary practice. *Med J Aust.* 2003; 179:S32–4.

This statement was reviewed in 2012 by the Council on Pharmacy Practice and by the Board of Directors and was found to still be appropriate.

Approved by the ASHP Council on Pharmacy Practice on September 24, 2007, by the ASHP Board of Directors on September 27, 2007, by the SHM Board of Directors on September 26, 2007. Developed through the American Society of Health-System Pharmacists Research and Education Foundation through a sponsorship from sanofi-aventis, Inc.

Daniel J. Cobaugh, Pharm.D., FAACT, DABAT (Corresponding Author, ASHP); Alpesh Amin, M.D., MBA, FACP (Corresponding Author, SHM); Thomas Bookwalter, Pharm.D. (ASHP, SHM); Mark Williams, M.D., FACP (SHM), Patricia Grunwald, Pharm.D. (ASHP); Cynthia LaCivita, Pharm.D. (ASHP); and Bruce Hawkins, B.A., B.S. (ASHP) are gratefully acknowledged for drafting this statement.

Copyright © 2008, American Society of Health-System Pharmacists, Inc. All rights reserved. This content may not be used for commercial purposes without the express written consent of ASHP.

The bibliographic citation for this document is as follows: American Society of Health-System Pharmacists. ASHP–SHM joint statement on hospitalist–pharmacist collaboration. *Am J Health-Syst Pharm.* 2008; 65:260–3.

ASHP Statement on Pharmaceutical Care

The purpose of this statement is to assist pharmacists in understanding pharmaceutical care. Such understanding must precede efforts to implement pharmaceutical care, which ASHP believes merit the highest priority in all practice settings.

Possibly the earliest published use of the term pharmaceutical care was by Brodie in the context of thoughts about drug use control and medication-related services.[1,2] It is a term that has been widely used and a concept about which much has been written and discussed in the pharmacy profession, especially since the publication of a paper by Hepler and Strand in 1990.[3–5] ASHP has formally endorsed the concept.[6] With varying terminology and nuances, the concept has also been acknowledged by other national pharmacy organizations.[7,8] Implementation of pharmaceutical care was the focus of a major ASHP conference in March 1993.

Many pharmacists have expressed enthusiasm for the concept of pharmaceutical care, but there has been substantial inconsistency in its description. Some have characterized it as merely a new name for clinical pharmacy; others have described it as anything that pharmacists do that may lead to beneficial results for patients.

ASHP believes that pharmaceutical care is an important new concept that represents growth in the profession beyond clinical pharmacy as often practiced and beyond other activities of pharmacists, including medication preparation and dispensing. All of these professional activities are important, however, and ASHP continues to be a strong proponent of the necessity for pharmacists' involvement in them. In practice, these activities should be integrated with and culminate in pharmaceutical care provided by individual pharmacists to individual patients.

In 1992, ASHP's members urged the development of an officially recognized ASHP definition of pharmaceutical care.[9] This statement provides a definition and elucidates some of the elements and implications of that definition. The definition that follows is an adaptation of a definition developed by Hepler and Strand.[3]

Definition

The mission of the pharmacist is to provide pharmaceutical care. Pharmaceutical care is the direct, responsible provision of medication-related care for the purpose of achieving definite outcomes that improve a patient's quality of life.

Principal Elements

The principal elements of pharmaceutical care are that it is *medication related*; it is *care* that is *directly provided* to the patient; it is provided to produce *definite outcomes*; these outcomes are intended to improve the patient's *quality of life*; and the provider accepts personal *responsibility* for the outcomes.

Medication Related. Pharmaceutical care involves not only medication therapy (the actual provision of medication) but also decisions about medication use for individual patients. As appropriate, this includes decisions *not* to use medication therapy as well as judgments about medication selection, dosages, routes and methods of administration, medication therapy monitoring, and the provision of medication-related information and counseling to individual patients.

Care. Central to the concept of care is caring, a personal concern for the well-being of another person. Overall patient care consists of integrated domains of care including (among others) medical care, nursing care, and pharmaceutical care. Health professionals in each of these disciplines possess unique expertise and must cooperate in the patient's overall care. At times, they share in the execution of the various types of care (including pharmaceutical care). To pharmaceutical care, however, the pharmacist contributes unique knowledge and skills to ensure optimal outcomes from the use of medications.

At the heart of any type of patient care, there exists a one-to-one relationship between a caregiver and a patient. In pharmaceutical care, the irreducible "unit" of care is one pharmacist in a direct professional relationship with one patient. In this relationship, the pharmacist provides care directly to the patient and for the benefit of the patient.

The health and well-being of the patient are paramount. The pharmacist makes a direct, personal, caring commitment to the individual patient and acts in the patient's best interest. The pharmacist cooperates directly with other professionals and the patient in designing, implementing, and monitoring a therapeutic plan intended to produce definite therapeutic outcomes that improve the patient's quality of life.

Outcomes. It is the goal of pharmaceutical care to improve an individual patient's quality of life through achievement of definite (predefined), medication-related therapeutic outcomes. The outcomes sought are

1. Cure of a patient's disease.
2. Elimination or reduction of a patient's symptomatology.
3. Arresting or slowing of a disease process.
4. Prevention of a disease or symptomatology.

This, in turn, involves three major functions: (1) identifying potential and actual medication-related problems, (2) resolving actual medication-related problems, and (3) preventing potential medication-related problems. A medication-related problem is an event or circumstance involving medication therapy that actually or potentially interferes with an optimum outcome for a specific patient. There are at least the following categories of medication-related problems[3]:

- *Untreated indications.* The patient has a medical problem that requires medication therapy (an indication for medication use) but is not receiving a medication for that indication.
- *Improper drug selection.* The patient has a medication indication but is taking the wrong medication.
- *Subtherapeutic dosage.* The patient has a medical problem that is being treated with too little of the correct medication.

DOI 10.37573/9781585287048.055

- *Failure to receive medication.* The patient has a medical problem that is the result of not receiving a medication (e.g., for pharmaceutical, psychological, sociological, or economic reasons).
- *Overdosage.* The patient has a medical problem that is being treated with too much of the correct medication (toxicity).
- *Adverse drug reactions.* The patient has a medical problem that is the result of an adverse drug reaction or adverse effect.
- *Drug interactions.* The patient has a medical problem that is the result of a drug–drug, drug–food, or drug–laboratory test interaction.
- *Medication use without indication.* The patient is taking a medication for no medically valid indication.

Patients may possess characteristics that interfere with the achievement of desired therapeutic outcomes. Patients may be noncompliant with prescribed medication use regimens, or there may be unpredictable variations in patients' biological responses. Thus, in an imperfect world, intended outcomes from medication-related therapy are not always achievable.

Patients bear a responsibility to help achieve the desired outcomes by engaging in behaviors that will contribute to—and not interfere with—the achievement of desired outcomes. Pharmacists and other health professionals have an obligation to educate patients about behaviors that will contribute to achieving desired outcomes.

Quality of Life. Some tools exist now for assessing a patient's quality of life. These tools are still evolving, and pharmacists should maintain familiarity with the literature on this subject.[10,11] A complete assessment of a patient's quality of life should include both objective and subjective (e.g., the patient's own) assessments. Patients should be involved, in an informed way, in establishing quality-of-life goals for their therapies.

Responsibility. The fundamental relationship in any type of patient care is a mutually beneficial exchange in which the patient grants authority to the provider and the provider gives competence and commitment to the patient (accepts responsibility).[3] Responsibility involves both moral trustworthiness and accountability.

In pharmaceutical care, the direct relationship between an individual pharmacist and an individual patient is that of a professional covenant in which the patient's safety and well-being are entrusted to the pharmacist, who commits to honoring that trust through competent professional actions that are in the patient's best interest. As an accountable member of the health-care team, the pharmacist must document the care provided.[4,7,12,13] The pharmacist is personally accountable for patient outcomes (the quality of care) that ensue from the pharmacist's actions and decisions.[1]

Implications

The idea that pharmacists should commit themselves to the achievement of definite outcomes for individual patients is an especially important element in the concept of pharmaceutical care. The expectation that pharmacists personally accept responsibility for individual patients' outcomes that result from the pharmacists' actions represents a significant advance in pharmacy's continuing professionalization. The provision of pharmaceutical care represents a maturation of pharmacy as a clinical profession and is a natural evolution of more mature clinical pharmacy activities of pharmacists.[14]

ASHP believes that pharmaceutical care is fundamental to the profession's purpose of helping people make the best use of medications.[15] It is a unifying concept that transcends all types of patients and all categories of pharmacists and pharmacy organizations. Pharmaceutical care is applicable and achievable by pharmacists in all practice settings. The provision of pharmaceutical care is not limited to pharmacists in inpatient, outpatient, or community settings, nor to pharmacists with certain degrees, specialty certifications, residencies, or other credentials. It is not limited to those in academic or teaching settings. Pharmaceutical care is not a matter of formal credentials or place of work. Rather, it is a matter of a direct personal, professional, responsible relationship with a patient to ensure that the patient's use of medication is optimal and leads to improvements in the patient's quality of life.

Pharmacists should commit themselves to continuous care on behalf of individual patients. They bear responsibility for ensuring that the patient's care is ongoing despite work-shift changes, weekends, and holidays. An important implication is that a pharmacist providing pharmaceutical care may need to work as a member of a team of pharmacists who provide backup care when the primary responsible pharmacist is not available. Another is that the responsible pharmacist should work to ensure that continuity of care is maintained when a patient moves from one component of a health-care system to another (e.g., when a patient is hospitalized or discharged from a hospital to return to an ambulatory, community status). In the provision of pharmaceutical care, professional communication about the patient's needs between responsible pharmacists in each area of practice is, therefore, essential. ASHP believes that the development of recognized methods of practicing pharmaceutical care that will enhance such communication is an important priority for the profession.

Pharmaceutical care can be conceived as both a purpose for pharmacy practice and a purpose of medication use processes. That is, a fundamental professional reason that pharmacists engage in pharmacy practice should be to deliver pharmaceutical care. Furthermore, the medication use systems that pharmacists (and others) operate should be designed to support and enable the delivery of pharmaceutical care by individual pharmacists. ASHP believes that, in organized health-care settings, pharmaceutical care can be most successfully provided when it is part of the pharmacy department's central mission and when management activity is focused on facilitating the provision of pharmaceutical care by individual pharmacists. This approach, in which empowered frontline staff provide direct care to individual patients and are supported by managers, other pharmacists, and support systems, is new for many pharmacists and managers.

An important corollary to this approach is that pharmacists providing pharmaceutical care in organized health-care settings cannot provide such care alone. They must work in an interdependent fashion with colleagues in pharmacy and other disciplines, support systems and staff, and managers.[7]

It is incumbent on pharmacists to design work systems and practices that appropriately focus the efforts of all activities and support systems on meeting the needs of patients. Some patients will require different levels of care, and it may be useful to structure work systems in light of those differences.[16,17] ASHP believes that the provision of pharmaceutical care and the development of effective work systems to document and support it are major priorities for the profession.

In the provision of pharmaceutical care, pharmacists use their unique perspective and knowledge of medication therapy to evaluate patients' actual and potential medication-related problems. To do this, they require direct access to clinical information about individual patients. They make judgments regarding medication use and then advocate optimal medication use for individual patients in cooperation with other professionals and in consideration of their unique professional knowledge and evaluations. Pharmaceutical care includes the active participation of the patient (and designated caregivers such as family members) in matters pertinent to medication use.

The acknowledgment of pharmacists' responsibility for therapeutic outcomes resulting from their actions does not contend that pharmacists have exclusive authority for matters related to medication use. Other health-care professionals, including physicians and nurses, have valuable and well-established, well-recognized roles in the medication use process. The pharmaceutical care concept does not diminish the roles or responsibilities of other health professionals, nor does it imply any usurping of authority by pharmacists. Pharmacists' actions in pharmaceutical care should be conducted and viewed as collaborative. The knowledge, skills, and traditions of pharmacists, however, make them legitimate leaders of efforts by health-care teams to improve patients' medication use.

Pharmaceutical care requires a direct relationship between a pharmacist and an individual patient. Some pharmacists and other pharmacy personnel engage in clinical and product-related pharmacy activities that do not involve a direct relationship with the patient. Properly designed, these activities can be supportive of pharmaceutical care, but ASHP believes it would be confusing and counterproductive to characterize such activities as pharmaceutical care. ASHP believes that clinical and product-related pharmacy activities are essential, however, and are as important as the actions of pharmacists interacting directly with patients.

Pharmaceutical educators must teach pharmaceutical care to students.[18] Providers of continuing education should help practicing pharmacists and other pharmacy personnel to understand pharmaceutical care. Students and pharmacists should be taught to conceptualize and execute responsible medication-related problem-solving on behalf of individual patients. Curricula should be designed to produce graduates with sufficient knowledge and skills to provide pharmaceutical care competently.[8,18] Initiatives are under way to bring about these changes.[8] Practicing pharmacists must commit their time as preceptors and their workplaces as teaching laboratories for the undergraduate and postgraduate education and training necessary to produce pharmacists who can provide pharmaceutical care.[8]

Research is needed to evaluate various methods and systems for the delivery of pharmaceutical care.

Pharmaceutical care represents an exciting new vision for pharmacy. ASHP hopes that all pharmacists in all practice settings share in this vision and that the pharmaceutical care concept will serve as a stimulus for them to work toward transforming the profession to actualize that vision.

References

1. Brodie DC. Is pharmaceutical education prepared to lead its profession? The Ninth Annual Rho Chi Lecture. *Rep Rho Chi.* 1973; 39:6–12.
2. Brodie DC, Parish PA, Poston JW. Societal needs for drugs and drug-related services. *Am J Pharm Educ.* 1980; 44:276–8.
3. Hepler CD, Strand LM. Opportunities and responsibilities in pharmaceutical care. *Am J Hosp Pharm.* 1990; 47:533–43.
4. Penna RP. Pharmaceutical care: pharmacy's mission for the 1990s. *Am J Hosp Pharm.* 1990; 47:543–9.
5. Pierpaoli PG, Hethcox JM. Pharmaceutical care: new management and leadership imperatives. *Top Hosp Pharm Manage.* 1992; 12:1–18.
6. Oddis JA. Report of the House of Delegates: June 3 and 5, 1991. *Am J Hosp Pharm.* 1991; 48:1739–48.
7. American Pharmaceutical Association. An APhA white paper on the role of the pharmacist in comprehensive medication use management; the delivery of pharmaceutical care. Washington, DC: American Pharmaceutical Association; 1992 Mar.
8. Commission to Implement Change in Pharmaceutical Education. A position paper. Entry-level education in pharmacy: a commitment to change. *AACP News.* 1991; Nov (Suppl):14
9. Oddis JA. Report of the House of Delegates: June 1 and 3, 1992. *Am J Hosp Pharm.* 1992; 49:1962–73.
10. Gouveia WA. Measuring and managing patient outcomes. *Am J Hosp Pharm.* 1992; 49:2157–8.
11. MacKeigan LD, Pathak DS. Overview of health-related quality-of-life measures. *Am J Hosp Pharm.* 1992; 49:2236–45.
12. Galinsky RE, Nickman NA. Pharmacists and the mandate of pharmaceutical care. *DICP Ann Pharmacother.* 1991; 21:431–4.
13. Angaran DM. Quality assurance to quality improvement: measuring and monitoring pharmaceutical care. *Am J Hosp Pharm.* 1991; 48:1901–7.
14. Hepler CD. Pharmaceutical care and specialty practice. *Pharmacotherapy.* 1993; 13:64S–9S.
15. Zellmer WA. Expressing the mission of pharmacy practice. *Am J Hosp Pharm.* 1991; 48:1195. Editorial.
16. Smith WE, Benderev K. Levels of pharmaceutical care: a theoretical model. *Am J Hosp Pharm.* 1991; 48:540–6.
17. Strand LM, Cipole RJ, Morley PC,, et al. Levels of pharmaceutical care: a needs-based approach. *Am J Hosp Pharm.* 1991; 48:547–50.
18. O'Neil EH. Health professions education for the future: schools in service to the nation. San Francisco, CA: Pew Health Profession Commission; 1993.

This statement was reviewed in 1998 by the Council on Professional Affairs and the ASHP Board of Directors and was found to still be appropriate.

Approved by the ASHP Board of Directors, April 21, 1993, and by the ASHP House of Delegates, June 9, 1993. Developed by the ASHP Council on Professional Affairs.

Copyright © 1993, American Society of Hospital Pharmacists, Inc. All rights reserved. Contact ASHP for reprint and permissions requests. This content may not be used for commercial purposes without the express written consent of ASHP.

The bibliographic citation for this document is as follows: American Society of Hospital Pharmacists. ASHP statement on pharmaceutical care. *Am J Hosp Pharm.* 1993; 50:1720–3.

ASHP Statement on the Roles of Pharmacy Technicians

Position

ASHP recognizes that well-educated and highly skilled pharmacy technicians have important roles and responsibilities in the pharmacy profession and that a safe and effective medication-use process depends significantly on the skills, knowledge, and competence of those pharmacy technicians. To properly fill these roles, pharmacy technicians require standardized education, training, and competence assessment. ASHP advocates that states encourage this education, training, and assessment through the development and adoption of uniform state laws and regulations requiring licensure of pharmacy technicians.

Background

Pharmacy technicians practice in a variety of settings and have diverse roles and responsibilities, ranging from those suitable for technicians meeting minimum requirements for education, training, and experience to complex, advanced, or specialized roles that require additional education, training, and demonstration of competence. Because pharmacy technicians are the foundation of pharmacy's distributive functions and are utilized in clinical functions where appropriate, pharmacy must strongly support the development of uniform education, training, registration, certification, and recertification of pharmacy technicians. Standardization will be required at all levels of pharmacy technician practice.

The role of pharmacy technicians is a significant focus of the ASHP Pharmacy Practice Model Initiative (PPMI). The goal of the PPMI is "to significantly advance the health and well-being of patients by developing and disseminating a futuristic practice model that supports the most effective use of pharmacists as direct patient care providers."[1] ASHP strongly believes that advancing the roles of pharmacists will require changes in the way that pharmacy technicians are educated, trained, regulated, and incorporated into pharmacy practice, dependent on their capabilities. The consensus of the Pharmacy Practice Model Summit called for standardization in scope of practice, competencies, education and training, licensure, and certification of pharmacy technicians.[2] One of the recommendations from the ASHP Ambulatory Care Conference and Summit recognized that to "promote efficiency and improve access to patient care, pharmacists who provide ambulatory care services should optimize the role of certified pharmacy technicians and other members of the healthcare team."[3]

Purpose

The purpose of this statement is to outline the evolving roles and responsibilities of pharmacy technicians, describe a model for educating and certifying pharmacy technicians, and propose a legal and regulatory structure that reflects the evolving nature of pharmacy technicians' responsibilities.

Roles and Responsibilities of Pharmacy Technicians

ASHP recognizes that pharmacy technicians have many different roles in a variety of healthcare settings, with varying levels of responsibility and complexity, from those suitable for technicians just entering the work force to advanced or specialized roles that require additional education, training, experience, and competence.

Entry-Level Pharmacy Technicians. The following are categories of competencies that pharmacy technicians must possess for entry to practice:

1. Pharmacology for technicians
2. Pharmacy law and regulations
3. Compounding
   a. Low- or medium-risk level sterile compounding
   b. Nonsterile compounding
4. Basic safe medication practices
5. Pharmacy quality assurance
6. Medication order entry and distribution
7. Pharmacy inventory management
8. Pharmacy billing and reimbursement
9. Medication-use system technology

Advanced Pharmacy Technicians. Advanced pharmacy technicians who have additional education, training, and competencies may perform tasks that require more responsibility. Under the supervision of pharmacists and/or with the approval of state boards of pharmacy, advanced pharmacy technicians may be involved in, but not limited to, the following roles:

1. Advanced medication systems, including "tech-check-tech" programs
2. Purchasing or fiscal management
3. Management or supervision of other pharmacy technicians
4. Medication history assistance
5. Medication therapy management assistance
6. Quality improvement
7. Immunization assistance
8. Hazardous drug handling
9. Patient assistance programs
10. Pharmacy technician education and training
11. Community outreach
12. Drug utilization evaluation and/or adverse-drug-event monitoring
13. Industry
14. Informatics[4]

In today's era of rapid evolution of healthcare, declining reimbursements, and increasing complexity of the healthcare market, pharmacy technicians will need to advance to a level of operations management that has not been previously required. Pharmacists and pharmacy technicians

DOI 10.37573/9781585287048.056

must work synergistically in targeted initiatives to provide patient care services, understanding their potential roles to maximize the utilization of resources.[5] The integration of pharmacy technicians into pharmacy care teams has been demonstrated in database and interface management and in an analyst role, with the goal of achieving the highest level of care for patients.[6] These roles include preparing and analyzing reports as well as benchmarking by educated and trained pharmacy technicians, who provide information to pharmacists ready for decision-making. These pharmacy technicians require standardized education to develop a sufficient knowledge of medications and the medication-use process, documentation systems, and databases.

In management, pharmacy technicians are an untapped resource, though some are already performing leadership roles, such as operations manager, independently.[7] These individuals are essential to pharmacy services, as they can provide leadership in supervisory roles and tasks,[7,8] freeing pharmacists to devote their attention to other areas of patient care.[9] ASHP believes there must be an emphasis within leadership teams to ensure the success of these technician leaders through the elimination of perceived technician practice barriers, enhancement of educational opportunities, and provision of increased mentoring sessions.

Specialized Pharmacy Technicians. ASHP recognizes the need for specialized certification of pharmacy technicians who perform activities involving greater degrees of complexity and risk. Any pharmacy technician in an area of pharmacy practice designated for specialty certification by the Pharmacy Technician Certification Board (PTCB) must have successfully completed the appropriate certifications before practicing in that specialty area. ASHP further recommends that any pharmacy technician in an area of pharmacy practice designated for other specialty or advanced certification have successfully completed the appropriate certifications before practicing in that specialty area. PTCB plans careful evaluation and recognition of emerging specialties as practice and patient needs evolve.

Education and Training of Pharmacy Technicians

Current Educational Models. National standards for the education and training of pharmacy technicians exist[10]; however, they have not been widely adopted. Technicians attain the necessary knowledge base in a variety of ways, ranging from on-the-job training to online or publication-based training, employer-based structured didactic learning, and formalized study with programs that may or may not have proper professional accreditation status.

Future Models. To obtain the pharmacy technician work force of the future, pharmacy must attract the highest-quality candidates. To attract the best possible candidates, ASHP advocates that pharmacy technician education ultimately require a minimum of an associate's degree from an accredited source. ASHP also supports testing candidates in reading, oral and written English communication, and math upon entry into a technician program to establish a minimum baseline of performance.

ASHP recognizes that differing roles for pharmacy technicians will require advanced education and training beyond that of an entry-level technician. Education and training requirements must reflect the responsibilities that technicians will have in their daily activities. Ongoing competence assessment must be a component of advanced or specialized technician roles. In addition to meeting the requirements to become PTCB certified, pharmacy technicians also must undergo site-specific training to the specific roles and responsibilities that they will perform. When a new role is introduced, additional training specific to that new position must be completed. Quality measures must be employed to assess the accuracy of the pharmacy technician's performance.

ASHP advocates that all pharmacy technicians, from entry-level to specialty-trained technicians, complete a pharmacy technician training program accredited by ASHP and the Accreditation Council for Pharmacy Education (ACPE) through the Pharmacy Technician Accreditation Commission as a requirement for earning PTCB certification. Further, ASHP advocates that pharmacy technicians be PTCB certified and maintain their certification through mandated continuing education and recertification. In addition, changes to the PTCB certification process over the coming years will elevate PTCB's standards for national certification and recertification, including a requirement for completion of an ASHP-/ACPE-accredited education program by 2020 and modifications to the continuing-education requirements for recertification.[11]

Laws and Regulations Regarding Pharmacy Technician Licensure

Currently, only a handful of states require pharmacy technician licensure, several states do not require either licensure or registration, and the majority require registration of pharmacy technicians. ASHP advocates the development and adoption of uniform state laws and regulations regarding pharmacy technicians. ASHP strongly advocates that those laws and regulations eventually require that pharmacy technicians be licensed by state boards of pharmacy to grant technicians permission to engage in the full scope of responsibilities authorized by the state.

ASHP advocates that pharmacy technicians must be certified by PTCB as a prerequisite to licensure by their state board of pharmacy. The National Association of Boards of Pharmacy and ASHP advocate that pharmacy technicians become certified by PTCB before being licensed or registered by state boards of pharmacy.[12]

ASHP advocates that (1) licensure of technicians must not permit the independent, unsupervised practice of pharmacy technicians, (2) all pharmacy functions must be performed under the supervision of a licensed pharmacist, and (3) licensed pharmacists and technicians must be held mutually accountable for the quality of pharmacy services provided.

Conclusion

ASHP supports the advancement of pharmacy technician roles and responsibilities to aid pharmacists in providing optimal patient care. In order to be effective in these roles and responsibilities, it is imperative that pharmacy technicians have standardized education, training, certification, and licensing requirements.

References

1. American Society of Health-System Pharmacists. Pharmacy Practice Model Initiative overview. www.ashpmedia.org/ppmi/overview.html (accessed 2015 Sep 4).
2. American Society of Health-System Pharmacists. The consensus of the Pharmacy Practice Model Summit. *Am J Health-Syst Pharm.* 2011; 68:1148–52.
3. American Society of Health-System Pharmacists. Recommendations of the summit. *Am J Health-Syst Pharm.* 2014; 71:1390–1.
4. American Society of Health-System Pharmacists. ASHP statement on the pharmacy technican's role in pharmacy informatics. *Am J Health-Syst Pharm.* 2014; 71:247–50.
5. Weber E, Hepfinger C, Koontz R, et al. Pharmacy technicians supporting clinical functions. *Am J Health-Syst Pharm.* 2005; 62:2466–72.
6. Ervin KC, Skledar S, Hess M et al. Data analyst technician: an innovative role for the pharmacy technician. *Am J Health-Syst Pharm.* 2001; 58:1815–8.
7. Thompson J, Swarthout MD. Developing pharmacy technicians across the leadership spectrum. *Am J Health-Syst Pharm.* 2012; 69:2040–2.
8. Shane R. Advancing technician roles: an essential step in pharmacy practice model reform. *Am J Health-Syst Pharm.* 2011; 68:1834–5.
9. American Society of Health-System Pharmacists. ASHP long-range vision for the pharmacy work force in hospitals and health systems. *Am J Health-Syst Pharm.* 2007; 64:1320–30.
10. American Society of Health-System Pharmacists. Accreditation standards for pharmacy technician education and training programs (April 2013). www.ashp.org/DocLibrary/Accreditation/Regulations-Standards/Pharmacy-Technician-Education-and-Training-Programs.pdf (accessed 2015 Sep 4).
11. Pharmacy Technician Certification Board. Certification program changes. www.ptcb.org/about-ptcb/crest-initiative (accessed 2015 Sep 4).
12. National Association of Boards of Pharmacy. Report of the Task Force on Standardized Pharmacy Technician Education and Training (September 2009). www.nabp.net/news/assets/08TF_Standard_Pharm_Tech_Educ_Training.pdf (accessed 2015 Sep 4).

Approved by the ASHP Board of Directors on September 18, 2015, and by the ASHP House of Delegates on November 20, 2015. Developed through the ASHP Section of Inpatient Care Practitioners Advisory Group on Advancing Pharmacy Practice with Technicians.

The authors have declared no potential conflicts of interest.

Jennifer M. Schultz, Pharm.D., FASHP, Pharmacy Department, Bozeman Health Deaconess Hospital, Bozeman, MT.

Cynthia Kay Jeter, B.S., CPP, CPhT, BGS, McKesson Pharmacy Optimization, Springdale, AR.

Jan M. Keresztes, B.S.Pharm., Pharm.D., South Suburban College, South Holland, IL.

Naomi M. Martin, M.S. Health-System Management, B.S.Pharm., Comprehensive Pharmacy Services, Indianapolis, IN.

Terri K. Mundy, B.S.Pharm., Bossier Parish Community College, Bossier City, LA.

Jeffrey S. Reichard, Pharm.D., M.S., BCPS, Novant Health, Chapel Hill, NC.

Jennifer D. Van Cura, Pharm.D., Cardinal Health, Innovative Delivery Solutions, Houston, TX.

ASHP gratefully acknowledges the following organizations and individuals for reviewing these guidelines (review does not imply endorsement): American Association of Colleges of Pharmacy; American Pharmacists Association; Canadian Society of Hospital Pharmacists; Idaho Society of Health-System Pharmacists; New Hampshire Society of Health-System Pharmacists; Pharmacy Technician Certification Board; Pharmacy Technician Educators Council; Thomas S. Achey, Pharm.D.; Tolulope Akinbo, Pharm.D., M.P.H.; Sandra Andrews, CPhT, BLS; John Armitstead, M.S., FASHP; Nicole Avant, Pharm.D.; Ann Barnes, Pharm.D.; Megan Brafford, Pharm.D., BCOP; Dominick A. Caselnova III, M.H.A.; Angela T. Cassano, Pharm.D., BCPS, FASHP; John S. Clark, Pharm.D., M.S., BCPS, FASHP; Gwyn Collier, CPhT, MCPhT, M.B.A.; Debra Cowan, Pharm.D., FASHP; Travis B. Dick, Pharm.D., M.B.A., BCPS; Lonnye Finneman; Rena Gosser, Pharm.D.; Jacquelyn Grahm, B.S., CPhT; Kathleen M. Gura, Pharm.D., BCNSP, FASHP, FPPAG, FASPEN; Tracy Hagemann, Pharm.D., FCCP, FPPAG; John B. Hertig, Pharm.D., M.S., CPPS; Stephen K. Hetey, M.S., FASHP; Stan Kent, M.S.; Susan Kleppin; James Lee, Pharm.D., BCACP; Janet Liles, CPHT, MSHS; Brandon Nemecek; Judy Neville; Stephanie C. Peshek, Pharm.D., M.B.A., M.S., FASHP; Barbara Petroff, M.S., FASHP; James Ponto, M.S., FASHP; Timothy Reilly, Pharm.D., BCPS, CGP, FASCP; Kelly Sennett, Pharm.D.; Jamie S. Sinclair, M.S., FASHP; Paul Wittmer, M.B.A.; and Roger Woolf, Pharm.D.

Copyright © 2016, American Society of Health-System Pharmacists, Inc. All rights reserved. Contact ASHP for reprint and permissions requests. This content may not be used for commercial purposes without the express written consent of ASHP.

The bibliographic citation for this document is as follows: American Society of Health-System Pharmacists. ASHP statement on the roles of pharmacy technicians. *Am J Health-Syst Pharm.* 2016; 73:928–30.

ASHP Guidelines on Documenting Pharmaceutical Care in Patient Medical Records

Purpose

The professional actions of pharmacists that are intended to ensure safe and effective use of drugs and that may affect patient outcomes should be documented in the patient medical record (PMR). These guidelines describe the kinds of information pharmacists should document in the PMR, how that information should be documented, methods for obtaining authorization for pharmacist documentation, and the important role of training and continuous quality improvement (CQI) in documentation.

Background

Pharmaceutical care is the direct, responsible provision of medication-related care for the purpose of achieving definite outcomes that improve a patient's quality of life.[1] A core principle of pharmaceutical care is that the pharmacist accepts professional responsibility for patient outcomes.[2] Integrating pharmaceutical care into a patient's overall health care plan requires effective and efficient communication among health care professionals. As an integral member of the health care team, the pharmacist must document the care provided. Such documentation is vital to a patient's continuity of care and demonstrates both the accountability of the pharmacist and the value of the pharmacist's services. Moreover, because clinical services (e.g., those incident to a physician's services) are generally considered reimbursable only when they are necessary for the medical management of a patient and when the service provided and the patient's response are carefully documented, thorough documentation may increase the likelihood of reimbursement. Early implementation of such documentation practices may help health-system pharmacies cope with documentation requirements in the event pharmacists' clinical services become reimbursable.

The PMR's primary purpose is to convey information for use in patient care; it serves as a tool for communication among health care professionals. Information in the PMR may also be used in legal proceedings (e.g., as evidence), education (e.g., for training students), research (e.g., for evaluating clinical drug use), and quality assurance evaluations (e.g., to ascertain adherence to practice standards).[3]

Clinical recommendations made by a pharmacist on behalf of the patient, as well as actions taken in accordance with these recommendations, should be documented in a permanent manner that makes the information available to all the health care professionals caring for the patient. ASHP believes that, to ensure proper coordination of patients' medication therapies, health care systems must be designed to enable, foster, and facilitate communication and collaboration among health care providers.[2] Health care systems must not erect barriers to that communication or to the exercise of the professional judgment of health care providers.

Although telephone calls and other oral communication may be necessary for immediate interventions, they do not allow for the dissemination of information to care providers who are not a part of the conversation. Such interventions should be documented in the PMR as soon as possible after the acute situation has settled. For less urgent and routine recommendations, timely documentation is also preferred, because delays in response to telephone calls or pager messages may lead to miscommunicated or undocumented recommendations. Unofficial, temporary, or removable notes placed in the PMR do not provide a standard of acceptable communication or documentation and therefore are discouraged. Documentation that is not a part of the PMR (e.g., documentation in pharmacy records) may provide a degree of risk reduction; however, such documentation does not provide important information to other care providers and can interrupt continuity of care when the patient is discharged or transferred.

Documenting Pharmaceutical Care

Pharmacists should be authorized and encouraged to make notations in the PMR for the purpose of documenting their findings, assessments, conclusions, and recommendations.[2] ASHP believes that all significant clinical recommendations and resulting actions should be documented in the appropriate section of the PMR. The pharmacy department should establish policies and procedures for documenting information in the PMR. Such policies and procedures will help pharmacists exercise good judgment in determining what information to document in the PMR and how to present it.

Examples of information a pharmacist may need to document in the PMR include, but are not limited to, the following:

1. A summary of the patient's medication history on admission, including medication allergies and their manifestations.
2. Oral and written consultations provided to other health care professionals regarding the patient's drug therapy selection and management.
3. Physicians' oral orders received directly by the pharmacist.
4. Clarification of drug orders.
5. Adjustments made to drug dosage, dosage frequency, dosage form, or route of administration.
6. Drugs, including investigational drugs, administered.
7. Actual and potential drug-related problems that warrant surveillance.
8. Drug therapy-monitoring findings, including
    a. The therapeutic appropriateness of the patient's drug regimen, including the route and method of administration.
    b. Therapeutic duplication in the patient's drug regimen.
    c. The degree of patient compliance with the prescribed drug regimen.
    d. Actual and potential drug–drug, drug–food, drug–laboratory test, and drug–disease interactions.

DOI 10.37573/9781585287048.057

e. Clinical and pharmacokinetic laboratory data pertinent to the drug regimen.
f. Actual and potential drug toxicity and adverse effects.
g. Physical signs and clinical symptoms relevant to the patient's drug therapy.

9. Drug-related patient education and counseling provided.

Documentation by pharmacists should meet established criteria for legibility, clarity, lack of judgmental language, completeness, need for inclusion in the PMR (versus an alternative form of communication), appropriate use of a standard format (e.g., SOAP [subjective, objective, assessment, and plan] or TITRS [title, introduction, text, recommendation, and signature]), and how to contact the pharmacist (e.g., a telephone or pager number).[4]

The authority to document pharmaceutical care in the PMR comes with a responsibility to ensure that patient privacy and confidentiality are safeguarded and the communication is concise and accurate. Local, state, and federal guidelines and laws (including the Health Insurance Portability and Accountability Act of 1996 [HIPAA]) and risk management sensitivities should be considered. Nonjudgmental language should be used, with care taken to avoid words that imply blame (e.g., *error, mistake, misadventure,* and *inadvertent*) or substandard care (e.g., *bad, defective, inadequate, inappropriate, incorrect, insufficient, poor, problem,* and *unsatisfactory*).[3] Facts should be documented accurately, concisely, and objectively; such documentation should reflect the goals established by the medical team.

Documentation of a formal consultation solicited by a physician or other health care provider may include direct recommendations or suggestions as appropriate. However, unsolicited informal consultations, clinical impressions, findings, suggestions, and recommendations should generally be documented more subtly, with indirect recommendations presented in a way that allows the provider to decline the suggestion without incurring a liability. For example, the phrase "may want to consider" creates an opportunity for the suggestion to be acted upon or not, depending on presenting clinical factors.

Obtaining Authorization to Document Pharmaceutical Care

The authority to document pharmaceutical care in the PMR is granted by the health care organization in accordance with organizational and medical staff policies. Although documenting pharmaceutical care in the PMR is a pharmacist's professional responsibility, physicians and other health care professionals may not be accustomed to or open to this practice.

The following steps are recommended for obtaining authorization to document pharmaceutical care in the PMR:

1. Determine the existing organizational and medical staff policies regarding authority for documentation in the PMR. These policies may provide specific guidance on how to proceed.
2. Ascertain whether other nonphysician and nonnurse providers in the organization or affiliated organizations have been granted authority to document patient care activities in the PMR. If so, consult them regarding the process used to establish the authority.
3. Identify physicians in the organization who are willing to support documentation of pharmaceutical care in the PMR.
4. Identify the committees in the organization whose recommendations or decisions will be required to establish authority for pharmacists to document pharmaceutical care in the PMR. Determine the necessary sequence of these approvals. Committees typically involved include the pharmacy and therapeutics (P&T) committee, the executive committee of the medical staff, a quality-assurance committee (e.g., the CQI committee), and the medical records committee.
5. Determine the accepted method and format for submitting a proposal requesting authority to document pharmaceutical care in the PMR. In some organizations, a written proposal may be required. If so, determine the desired format (length, style, and necessary justification) and deadlines for proposal submission. An oral presentation to the deciding bodies may be required. If so, determine in advance the desired presentation format and supporting materials desired by these bodies.
6. Draft a written plan describing
   a. Examples of information to be documented in the PMR. It may be helpful to describe how this important information may be lost or miscommunicated if it is not documented in the PMR.
   b. The locations within the PMR where documentation will be made and any special format or forms proposed. New forms will have to comply with HIPAA regulations and will require review and approval by specific organizational or medical staff committees. To achieve the goal of effective communication among all the members of the health care team, compartmentalization of the PMR should be avoided.
   c. The persons who will be documenting pharmaceutical care in the PMR (i.e., pharmacists, residents, or students). If pharmacy residents or students will be making notations in the PMR, procedures regarding authority and cosignatures will also have to be described.
7. Review the draft plan with the chair of the P&T committee, the director of nursing, the director of medical records, and other appropriate administrative personnel, such as the organization's risk management officer and legal counsel.
8. Seek the endorsement and recommendation of the P&T committee.
9. In appropriate sequence, seek the endorsement or decision of any other committees necessary for ultimate approval. Monitor the proposal's course through the various committees and provide assistance, clarification, or additional data as necessary.
10. When the final approving body grants PMR documentation authority, participate in the required policy development and the communication of the new policy to the individuals or departments in the organization that will be affected by the change (e.g., nurses, the medical staff, the quality-assurance staff, and the medical records department).

Training and CQI

Pharmacist documentation in the PMR is a skill that requires ongoing training and evaluation.[4] A temporary committee may be formed to manage the initial training required to implement pharmacist documentation in the PMR. That committee may consider offering presentations by physicians or other members of the health care team to provide their perspective on how to effectively communicate using the PMR. The information in those presentations may be reinforced by workshops on documentation skills. Presentation and workshop topics may include the choice of communication method (i.e., when documentation in the PMR is preferred to other means of communication), the documentation format (e.g., SOAP or TITRS), documentation etiquette, and legal requirements.[4] Documentation skills should be demonstrated before a pharmacist is allowed to make notations in the PMR.[4] The ASHP Clinical Skills Program is another tool for training pharmacists to use the PMR.[3]

Documentation of pharmaceutical care should also be one of the many functions addressed in CQI efforts. Pharmacy department CQI efforts should include the development of quality indicators that can be used to evaluate pharmacist documentation in the PMR.[4] Other CQI efforts might analyze and improve systemwide policies and procedures for documenting medication use.[5] Periodic review of organizational policies and procedures will allow for their revision in response to changes in health care and advances in technology, including the availability of an electronic PMR.[6,7]

References

1. Hepler CD, Strand LM. Opportunities and responsibilities in pharmaceutical care. *Am J Hosp Pharm.* 1990; 47:533–43.
2. American Society of Hospital Pharmacists. ASHP statement on pharmaceutical care. *Am J Hosp Pharm.* 1993; 50:1720–3.
3. Shepherd MF. Professional conduct and use of patient medical records. In: ASHP Clinical Skills Program, module 1: reviewing patient medical charts. Bethesda, MD: American Society of Hospital Pharmacists; 1992:38–41.
4. Lacy CF, Saya FG, Shane RR. Quality of pharmacists' documentations in patients' medical records. *Am J Health-Syst Pharm.* 1996; 53:2171–5.
5. Matuschka P. Improving documentation of preoperative antimicrobial prophylaxis. *Am J Health-Syst Pharm.* 1998; 55:993–4.
6. Lau A, Balen RM, Lam R,, et al. Using a personal digital assistant to document clinical pharmacy services in an intensive care unit. *Am J Health-Syst Pharm.* 2001; 58:1229–32.
7. Gordon W, Malyuk D, Taki J. Use of health-record abstracting to document pharmaceutical care activities. *Can J Hosp Pharm.* 2000; 53:199–205.

These guidelines were reviewed in 2008 by the Council on Pharmacy Practice and by the Board of Directors and were found to still be appropriate.

Approved by the ASHP Board of Directors, February 20, 2003. Revised by the ASHP Council on Professional Affairs. Supercedes the ASHP Guidelines for Obtaining Authorization for Documenting Pharmaceutical Care in Patient Medical Records dated November 16, 1988.

Copyright © 2003, American Society of Health-System Pharmacists, Inc. All rights reserved. Contact ASHP for reprint and permissions requests. This content may not be used for commercial purposes without the express written consent of ASHP.

The bibliographic citation for this document is as follows: American Society of Health-System Pharmacists. ASHP guidelines on documenting pharmaceutical care in patient medical records. *Am J Health-Syst Pharm.* 2003; 60:705–7.

ASHP Guidelines on Pharmacist-Conducted Patient Education and Counseling

Purpose

Providing pharmaceutical care entails accepting responsibility for patients' pharmacotherapeutic outcomes. Pharmacists can contribute to positive outcomes by educating and counseling patients to prepare and motivate them to follow their pharmacotherapeutic regimens and monitoring plans. The purpose of this document is to help pharmacists provide effective patient education and counseling.

In working with individual patients, patient groups, families, and caregivers, pharmacists should approach education and counseling as interrelated activities. ASHP believes pharmacists should educate and counsel all patients to the extent possible, going beyond the minimum requirements of laws and regulations; simply offering to counsel is inconsistent with pharmacists' responsibilities. In pharmaceutical care, pharmacists should encourage patients to seek education and counseling and should eliminate barriers to providing it.

Pharmacists should also seek opportunities to participate in health-system patient-education programs and to support the educational efforts of other health care team members. Pharmacists should collaborate with other health care team members, as appropriate, to determine what specific information and counseling are required in each patient care situation. A coordinated effort among health care team members will enhance patients' adherence to pharmacotherapeutic regimens, monitoring of drug effects, and feedback to the health system.

ASHP believes these patient education and counseling guidelines are applicable in all practice settings—including acute inpatient care, ambulatory care, home care, and long-term care—whether these settings are associated with integrated health systems or managed care organizations or are freestanding. The guidelines may need to be adapted; for example, for use in telephone counseling or for counseling family members or caregivers instead of patients. Patient education and counseling usually occur at the time prescriptions are dispensed but may also be provided as a separate service. The techniques and the content should be adjusted to meet the specific needs of the patient and to comply with the policies and procedures of the practice setting. In health systems, other health care team members share in the responsibility to educate and counsel patients as specified in the patients' care plans.

Background

The human and economic consequences of inappropriate medication use have been the subject of professional, public, and congressional discourse for more than two decades.[1–5] Lack of sufficient knowledge about their health problems and medications is one cause of patients' nonadherence to their pharmacotherapeutic regimens and monitoring plans; without adequate knowledge, patients cannot be effective partners in managing their own care. The pharmacy profession has accepted responsibility for providing patient education and counseling in the context of pharmaceutical care to improve patient adherence and reduce medication-related problems.[6–9]

Concerns about improper medication use contributed to the provision in the Omnibus Budget Reconciliation Act of 1990 (OBRA '90) that mandated an offer to counsel Medicaid outpatients about prescription medications. Subsequently, states enacted legislation that generally extends the offer-to-counsel requirement to outpatients not covered by Medicaid. Future court cases may establish that pharmacists, in part because of changing laws, have a public duty to warn patients of adverse effects and potential interactions of medications. The result could be increased liability for pharmacists who fail to educate and counsel their patients or who do so incorrectly or incompletely.[10]

Pharmacists' Knowledge and Skills

In addition to a current knowledge of pharmacotherapy, pharmacists need to have the knowledge and skills to provide effective and accurate patient education and counseling. They should know about their patients' cultures, especially health and illness beliefs, attitudes, and practices. They should be aware of patients' feelings toward the health system and views of their own roles and responsibilities for decision-making and for managing their care.[11]

Effective, open-ended questioning and active listening are essential skills for obtaining information from and sharing information with patients. Pharmacists have to adapt messages to fit patients' language skills and primary languages, through the use of teaching aids, interpreters, or cultural guides if necessary. Pharmacists also need to observe and interpret the nonverbal messages (e.g., eye contact, facial expressions, body movements, vocal characteristics) patients give during education and counseling sessions.[12]

Assessing a patient's cognitive abilities, learning style, and sensory and physical status enables the pharmacist to adapt information and educational methods to meet the patient's needs. A patient may learn best by hearing spoken instructions; by seeing a diagram, picture, or model; or by directly handling medications and administration devices. A patient may lack the visual acuity to read labels on prescription containers, markings on syringes, or written handout material. A patient may be unable to hear oral instructions or may lack sufficient motor skills to open a child-resistant container.

In addition to assessing whether patients know *how* to use their medications, pharmacists should attempt to understand patients' attitudes and potential behaviors concerning medication use. The pharmacist needs to determine whether a patient is willing to use a medication and whether he or she intends to do so.[13,14]

Environment

Education and counseling should take place in an environment conducive to patient involvement, learning, and acceptance—one that supports pharmacists' efforts to establish caring

DOI 10.37573/9781585287048.058

relationships with patients. Individual patients, groups, families, or caregivers should perceive the counseling environment as comfortable, confidential, and safe.

Education and counseling are most effective when conducted in a room or space that ensures privacy and opportunity to engage in confidential communication. If such an isolated space is not available, a common area can be restructured to maximize visual and auditory privacy from other patients or staff. Patients, including those who are disabled, should have easy access and seating. Space and seating should be adequate for family members or caregivers. The design and placement of desks and counters should minimize barriers to communication. Distractions and interruptions should be few, so that patients and pharmacists can have each other's undivided attention.

The environment should be equipped with appropriate learning aids, e.g., graphics, anatomical models, medication administration devices, memory aids, written material, and audiovisual resources.

Pharmacist and Patient Roles

Pharmacists and patients bring to education and counseling sessions their own perceptions of their roles and responsibilities. For the experience to be effective, the pharmacist and patient need to come to a common understanding about their respective roles and responsibilities. It may be necessary to clarify for patients that pharmacists have an appropriate and important role in providing education and counseling. Patients should be encouraged to be active participants.

The pharmacist's role is to verify that patients have sufficient understanding, knowledge, and skill to follow their pharmacotherapeutic regimens and monitoring plans. Pharmacists should also seek ways to motivate patients to learn about their treatment and to be active partners in their care. Patients' role is to adhere to their pharmacotherapeutic regimens, monitor for drug effects, and report their experiences to pharmacists or other members of their health care teams.[12,15] Optimally, the patient's role should include seeking information and presenting concerns that may make adherence difficult.

Depending on the health system's policies and procedures, its use of protocols or clinical care plans, and its credentialing of providers, pharmacists may also have disease management roles and responsibilities for specified categories of patients. This expands pharmacists' relationships with patients and the content of education and counseling sessions.

Process Steps

Steps in the patient education and counseling process will vary according to the health system's policies and procedures, environment, and practice setting. Generally, the following steps are appropriate for patients receiving new medications or returning for refills[12–21]:

1. Establish caring relationships with patients as appropriate to the practice setting and stage in the patient's health care management. Introduce yourself as a pharmacist, explain the purpose and expected length of the sessions, and obtain the patient's agreement to participate. Determine the patient's primary spoken language.
2. Assess the patient's knowledge about his or her health problems and medications, physical and mental capability to use the medications appropriately, and attitude toward the health problems and medications. Ask open-ended questions about each medication's purpose and what the patient expects, and ask the patient to describe or show how he or she will use the medication.

   Patients returning for refill medications should be asked to describe or show how they have been using their medications. They should also be asked to describe any problems, concerns, or uncertainties they are experiencing with their medications.
3. Provide information orally and use visual aids or demonstrations to fill patients' gaps in knowledge and understanding. Open the medication containers to show patients the colors, sizes, shapes, and markings on oral solids. For oral liquids and injectables, show patients the dosage marks on measuring devices. Demonstrate the assembly and use of administration devices such as nasal and oral inhalers. As a supplement to face-to-face oral communication, provide written handouts to help the patient recall the information.

   If a patient is experiencing problems with his or her medications, gather appropriate data and assess the problems. Then adjust the pharmacotherapeutic regimens according to protocols or notify the prescribers.
4. Verify patients' knowledge and understanding of medication use. Ask patients to describe or show how they will use their medications and identify their effects. Observe patients' medication-use capability and accuracy and attitudes toward following their pharmacotherapeutic regimens and monitoring plans.

Content

The content of an education and counseling session may include the information listed below, as appropriate for each patient's pharmacotherapeutic regimen and monitoring plan.[8,9,20] The decision to discuss specific pharmacotherapeutic information with an individual patient must be based on the pharmacist's professional judgment.

1. The medication's trade name, generic name, common synonym, or other descriptive name(s) and, when appropriate, its therapeutic class and efficacy.
2. The medication's use and expected benefits and action. This may include whether the medication is intended to cure a disease, eliminate or reduce symptoms, arrest or slow the disease process, or prevent the disease or a symptom.
3. The medication's expected onset of action and what to do if the action does not occur.
4. The medication's route, dosage form, dosage, and administration schedule (including duration of therapy).
5. Directions for preparing and using or administering the medication. This may include adaptation to fit patients' lifestyles or work environments.

6. Action to be taken in case of a missed dose.
7. Precautions to be observed during the medication's use or administration and the medication's potential risks in relation to benefits. For injectable medications and administration devices, concern about latex allergy may be discussed.
8. Potential common and severe adverse effects that may occur, actions to prevent or minimize their occurrence, and actions to take if they occur, including notifying the prescriber, pharmacist, or other health care provider.
9. Techniques for self-monitoring of the pharmacotherapy.
10. Potential drug–drug (including nonprescription), drug–food, and drug–disease interactions or contraindications.
11. The medication's relationships to radiologic and laboratory procedures (e.g., timing of doses and potential interferences with interpretation of results).
12. Prescription refill authorizations and the process for obtaining refills.
13. Instructions for 24-hour access to a pharmacist.
14. Proper storage of the medication.
15. Proper disposal of contaminated or discontinued medications and used administration devices.
16. Any other information unique to an individual patient or medication.

These points are applicable to both prescription and nonprescription medications. Pharmacists should counsel patients in the proper selection of nonprescription medications.

Additional content may be appropriate when pharmacists have authorized responsibilities in collaborative disease management for specified categories of patients. Depending on the patient's disease management or clinical care plan, the following may be covered:

1. The disease state: whether it is acute or chronic and its prevention, transmission, progression, and recurrence.
2. Expected effects of the disease on the patient's normal daily living.
3. Recognition and monitoring of disease complications.

Documentation

Pharmacists should document education and counseling in patients' permanent medical records as consistent with the patients' care plans, the health system's policies and procedures, and applicable state and federal laws. When pharmacists do not have access to patients' medical records, education and counseling may be documented in the pharmacy's patient profiles, on the medication order or prescription form, or on a specially designed counseling record.

The pharmacist should record (1) that counseling was offered and was accepted and provided or refused and (2) the pharmacist's perceived level of the patient's understanding.[9] As appropriate, the content should be documented (for example, counseling about food–drug interactions). All documentation should be safeguarded to respect patient confidentiality and privacy and to comply with applicable state and federal laws.[10]

References

1. Smith MC. Social barriers to rational drug therapy. *Am J Hosp Pharm.* 1972; 29:121–7.
2. Priorities and approaches for improving prescription medicine use by older Americans. Washington, DC: National Council on Patient Information and Education; 1987.
3. Manasse HR Jr. Medication use in an imperfect world: drug misadventuring as an issue of public policy, part 1. *Am J Hosp Pharm.* 1989; 46:929–44.
4. Manasse HR Jr. Medication use in an imperfect world: drug misadventuring as an issue of public policy, part 2. *Am J Hosp Pharm.* 1989; 46:1141–52.
5. Johnson JA, Bootman JL. Drug-related morbidity and mortality: a cost-of-illness model. *Arch Intern Med.* 1995; 155:1949–56.
6. Summary of the final report of the Scope of Pharmacy Practice Project. *Am J Hosp Pharm.* 1994; 51:2179–82.
7. Hepler CD, Strand LM. Opportunities and responsibilities in pharmaceutical care. *Am J Hosp Pharm.* 1990; 47:533–42.
8. Hatoum HT, Hutchinson RA, Lambert BL. OBRA 90: patient counseling—enhancing patient outcomes. *US Pharm.* 1993; 18(Jan):76–86.
9. OBRA '90: a practical guide to effecting pharmaceutical care. Washington, DC: American Pharmaceutical Association; 1994.
10. Lynn NJ, Kamm RE. Avoiding liability problems. *Am Pharm.* 1995; NS35(Dec):14–22.
11. Herrier RN, Boyce RW. Does counseling improve compliance? *Am Pharm.* 1995; NS35(Sep):11–2.
12. Foster SL, Smith EB, Seybold MR. Advanced counseling techniques: integrating assessment and intervention. *Am Pharm.* 1995; NS35(Oct):40–8.
13. Bond WS, Hussar DA. Detection methods and strategies for improving medication compliance. *Am J Hosp Pharm.* 1991; 48:1978–88.
14. Felkey BG. Adherence screening and monitoring. *Am Pharm.* 1995; NS35(Jul):42–51.
15. Herrier RN, Boyce RW. Establishing an active patient partnership. *Am Pharm.* 1995; NS35(Apr):48–57.
16. Boyce RW, Herrier RN, Gardner M. Pharmacist-patient consultation program, unit I: an interactive approach to verify patient understanding. New York: Pfizer Inc.; 1991.
17. Pharmacist-patient consultation program, unit II: counseling patients in challenging situations. New York: Pfizer Inc.; 1993.
18. Pharmacist-patient consultation program, unit III: counseling to enhance compliance. New York: Pfizer Inc.; 1995.
19. Boyce RW, Herrier RN. Obtaining and using patient data. *Am Pharm.* 1991; NS31(Jul):65–70.
20. Herrier RN, Boyce RW. Communicating risk to patients. *Am Pharm.* 1995; NS35(Jun):12–4.
21. APhA special report: medication administration problem solving in ambulatory care. Washington, DC: Ameri-can Pharmaceutical Association; 1994.

This guideline was reviewed in 2011 by the Council on Pharmacy Practice and by the ASHP Board of Directors and was found to still be appropriate.

Approved by the ASHP Board of Directors, November 11, 1996. Revised by the ASHP Council on Professional Affairs. Supersedes the ASHP Statement on the Pharmacist's Role in Patient-Education Programs dated June 3, 1991, and ASHP Guidelines on Pharmacist-Conducted Patient Counseling dated November 18, 1992.

Copyright © 1997, American Society of Health-System Pharmacists, Inc. All rights reserved. Contact ASHP for reprint and permissions requests. This content may not be used for commercial purposes without the express written consent of ASHP.

The bibliographic citation for this document is as follows: American Society of Health-System Pharmacists. ASHP guidelines on pharmacist-conducted patient education and counseling. *Am J Health-Syst Pharm.* 1997; 54:431–4.

ASHP Guidelines on the Pharmacist's Role in the Development, Implementation, and Assessment of Critical Pathways

Purpose

The purpose of these guidelines is (1) to describe the pharmacist's role in the development, implementation, and assessment of critical pathways (CPs) and (2) to help pharmacists prepare for that responsibility. Because pharmacotherapy is a central component of many CPs, pharmacists should take leadership roles in the development, implementation, and assessment of CPs. By assuming leadership roles, pharmacists can help improve patient outcomes, contribute to cost-effective patient care, and promote multidisciplinary approaches to patient care and performance improvement. Although pharmacist involvement in the early stages of CP development is crucial to success, CP development is generally cyclical, and pharmacists should seek opportunities to become involved at any stage in the cycle of CP development, implementation, and assessment.

Summary of Guidelines. Because pharmacotherapy is a central component of many critical pathways, pharmacists should take leadership roles in their development, implementation, and assessment.

Pharmacists can improve the development of critical pathways by ensuring the evidence-based selection of medications, establishing measures for monitoring patients for drug efficacy and adverse effects, and evaluating the proposed critical pathway for patient safety.

Pharmacists can improve the implementation of critical pathways by documenting processes and outcomes, ensuring proper patient selection and medication use, monitoring patients for drug efficacy and adverse effects, and providing for continuity of care. Pharmacists can improve the assessment of critical pathways by measuring and analyzing processes and outcomes, disseminating the results of those analyses, and reviewing the critical pathways' pharmacotherapy to keep pace with changes in best practices.

Background

The development of CPs has been stimulated by the desire to improve patient outcomes by applying evidence-based clinical practice guidelines; increased interest in measuring and improving the quality of health care, including continuous-quality-improvement (CQI) initiatives; and managed care and other market-driven health care reforms. CPs can be defined as patient care management plans that delineate key steps along an optimal treatment timeline to achieve a set of predetermined intermediate and ultimate goals for patients who have clearly defined diagnoses or require certain procedures.[1] CPs have also been called care guides, clinical pathways, clinical care plans, and care maps.[2] CPs derive from the industrial engineering concept of critical paths[3] and were originally associated with inpatient acute care and used primarily by nurses. CPs have evolved to incorporate the spectrum of patient care providers and settings and to include CQI concepts.[4] CPs and similar tools are developed in many facilities for many purposes.[5–20] Although dismissed by some critics as "cookbook medicine," CPs have in some cases been shown to improve patient outcomes[21–26] and to reduce health care expenses.[27–36] ASHP believes that carefully developed and skillfully managed CPs can improve the care of patients across the spectrum of health-system settings, as well as improve the allocation of scarce health care resources.

Typical CP Process

Each health system will use a process of CP development, implementation, and assessment that meets its own needs within its own structure, culture, practice settings, and policies and procedures, but these processes do share common elements. Typically, once a disease or procedure is selected for CP development, a multidisciplinary team analyzes its current management (including process variances, costs, and outcomes), evaluates the scientific literature, and develops a plan of care. The planned actions for each discipline on the health care team are mapped on a timeline for the specific disease or procedure.[37] Pharmacists perform the following functions in a typical CP: oversee the selection of medications by using an evidence-based approach, develop the criteria for medication selection or dosages, monitor patients for drug efficacy and adverse effects (or establish parameters for monitoring), and ensure continuity of care across the health system. The following describes common steps in the development, implementation, and assessment of CPs.[3]

1. *Select diagnoses and procedures.* Diagnoses and procedures selected for CP development usually include those with high process variability, high cost, high patient volume, and high risk. CPs can be developed for common or specialized diagnoses (e.g., myocardial infarction, diabetes mellitus) or procedures (e.g., transurethral prostatectomy, coronary artery bypass grafting), for diagnoses that are likely to cause changes in health status (e.g., uncontrolled asthma), and for diseases requiring complicated pharmacotherapeutic regimens (e.g., AIDS). The criteria for selection should be developed with input from administrative and clinical leaders to ensure institutionwide acceptance and should be based on scientific evidence.
2. *Appoint a development team.* The development team should include key health care providers from all organizational components involved in the CP. The importance of a multidisciplinary approach to CP development cannot be overemphasized. If possible, consideration should be given to including a patient representative on the CP development team. Although insurance carriers and managed care providers may not have representatives on the development team, their protocols or guidelines should be evaluated by the team for inclusion in the CP as appropriate.

DOI 10.37573/9781585287048.059

3. *Conduct a search of the scientific literature.* A literature and database search conducted early in the process will help identify measures for assessing current processes and outcomes and will help ensure an evidence-based approach to the CP.
4. *Document current processes and outcomes.* The current processes, costs, variances, and outcomes need to be documented, usually through flow charting of the current process, retrospective chart review, and benchmarking. Benchmarking may be internal or external to the health system. Depending on the health system's resources, benchmarking may rely on chart review or may use computerized databases that compare physicians' use of resources, health-system costs, and outcomes for specific diagnosis-related groups. This step identifies the health system's practice and compares it with published clinical guidelines that are preferably consensus based (e.g., guidelines from the Agency for Healthcare Research and Quality or the American Heart Association). The team developing the CP should use an evidence-based approach to identify, discuss, and resolve the gaps between clinical guidelines and current local practice. Input from the practitioners who will be involved in the CP is crucial to the success of this process evaluation and CP development in general.
5. *Develop the CP.* Multidisciplinary, standardized development of the CP ensures integration of care and elimination of duplication and oversights. The CP should state its goals, define actions essential to achieving those goals, provide for patient education, outline assessment of patient safety, identify measures of conformance and outcomes, and describe required documentation. The actions and resources required for implementation should be discussed and agreed upon by all disciplines involved.
   a. Goals and outcomes
      - Define the specific goals or measurable outcomes of the CP (e.g., decreased length of stay, decreased ventilator time, reduced overall patient cost, decreased pain scores, early ambulation).
      - Select the areas of focus or categories of actions essential to achieving the goals and outcomes. To ensure consistency and continuity, these areas of focus should be standardized for all CPs developed within a health system; examples of focus areas are treatments, medications, and patient education and counseling.
      - Determine the appropriate time frame. This will vary according to the disease or procedure being addressed and the practice setting (e.g., emergency room, ambulatory care clinic, acute care hospital). The time frame may be specified in minutes, hours, days, or phases. A workload assessment may be required to develop appropriate time frames.
      - Define the activity for the focus area under the appropriate time frame (e.g., "pharmacist provides medication-use education and counseling on discharge day").

   b. Patient education
      - Modify the CP, using lay terms in the patient's primary language, to educate the patient about activities to be performed, time frames, and expected outcomes. In some practice settings, the patient may be an active partner in CP decision-making and implementation.

   c. Patient safety
      - Identify potential risks to the patient that may arise from use of the CP. For example, the CP could be subjected to the institution's failure-mode and effects analysis, or the medication safety self-assessment tool of the Institute for Safe Medication Practices could be used to assess the safety of the practices outlined in the CP.[38]

   d. Monitoring
      - Identify measures of conformance and variance so that the CP and the resulting outcomes can be continuously improved. Variances are deviations from the CP that may be positive or negative, avoidable or unavoidable, consequential or inconsequential. Sources of variances include patient responses to medications, physician decisions, and system breakdowns.

   e. Documentation
      - Develop a single, multidisciplinary work sheet or other tool that describes the CP's actions and time frames and provides spaces for documenting that actions were performed.[12] Describe how this tool will be used and how data will be collected.
6. *Obtain approval for the CP and educate participants.* To ensure global acceptance among all health care provider groups, the CP should be approved by appropriate committees, especially those of the medical staff. The impact of CP implementation on practitioner workloads will require careful consideration, and departmental policies or procedures may need to be modified. The pharmacy and therapeutics (P&T) committee should review pharmacotherapeutic issues associated with the CP early enough during development that therapeutic concerns can be addressed as they arise rather than after the CP is implemented. After the CP is approved, all health care team members involved in the care of the patients affected by the CP should be educated about the anticipated outcomes, specific actions and time frames, and professional responsibilities associated with the CP.
7. *Implement the CP.* After the necessary education and training of providers, the CP is available for use. Starting the CP as a pilot project for a small number of patients may provide valuable initial assessments that will facilitate wider implementation. Staff members should be designated to identify patients suitable for the CP and to guide their enrollment and the CP's use. Patients enrolled in a CP are assigned to a health care team whose members have specific responsibilities for actions and time frames.
8. *Assess the CP.* Because not all consequences of a CP are foreseeable, CPs require periodic assessment. Assessments after a few days or weeks of use may gauge only

the feasibility of the CP and not its success in achieving desired goals, but they should identify unexpected problems that may require modifications to the CP. Surveys of health care practitioners may be useful in such initial assessments. Assessments after a few months of use may provide an initial perspective on the CP's success but may not be sufficient to fully evaluate outcomes. Assessments after longer periods should produce evidence supporting the CP's original goals. Regular analysis of the results and variances, as well as new information (e.g., new indications for medications) and technologies (e.g., new pharmacotherapy), provides data for a root-cause analysis and continuous improvement of the CP.

9. *Disseminate the results of the assessment.* The results of the assessment should be shared not just with health-system managers or members of the CP development or oversight committees but with all staff involved in the CP. Widespread dissemination allows for more suggestions for improvement from all members of the health care team and encourages acceptance of any alterations in the CP required by the assessment. Publishing the results in a journal, sharing the experience with a practice network, or presenting the results at a meeting expands the general pool of knowledge concerning CPs.

Pharmacist Involvement

These guidelines suggest actions to help prepare pharmacists and pharmacy departments for involvement in the development, implementation, and assessment of CPs at various levels of care and in different practice settings. The applicability of these guidelines depends on a pharmacist's or pharmacy department's current level of involvement in patient care and CPs. Pharmacists should focus on incorporating contemporary pharmaceutical care principles (e.g., assessing medication orders, developing pharmacotherapeutic regimens and monitoring plans, educating and counseling patients, calculating doses according to pharmacokinetic principles, conducting medication-use evaluations [MUEs], and managing anticoagulation therapy) in the development, implementation, and assessment of CPs.[39–42]

Preparing for Involvement in CP Development. Pharmacists should learn about their health system's approach to CP development and assess their readiness for involvement. They should

1. Review the health system's current strategic plan with respect to CPs. Because CPs are inherently collaborative, pharmacists should try to understand this strategic plan from the perspective of other health care providers, seeking advice from them when necessary. When reviewing the strategic plan, pharmacists should also consider the needs of specific patient populations served by their institutions.
2. Educate the pharmacy staff on the purposes and processes of CP development and the contents of CPs. The patient care decisions required in CPs demand clinical knowledge, and the pharmacotherapy involved should be based on evidence in the scientific literature. This clinical knowledge is fundamental to the CP. An effective contributor to the CP process needs to first acquire the clinical knowledge on which the CP is based and then use CQI, teamwork, negotiation, and administrative skills to develop, implement, and assess the CP.
3. Discuss CP experiences with pharmacy colleagues within and outside the health system. Pharmacists should create a forum within the health system for ongoing dialogue about CPs; for example, CPs could be made a regular agenda item for the P&T committee meeting and for other multidisciplinary clinical and departmental meetings.
4. Monitor pharmacy, nursing, quality management, health-system, health care, and management literature for ideas on CP development, implementation, and assessment. CPs from other institutions may be used as examples of and frameworks for mapping care, but they should not be adopted directly, because acceptance and use are greater when CPs are developed or adapted by their users.
5. Identify opportunities for contributing, through the provision of pharmaceutical care, to the health system's patient care delivery and improvement efforts.

Initiating Involvement. Pharmacists should begin their involvement in the CP process in ways most appropriate to their health system's structure, culture, practice settings, and policies and procedures. Involvement may vary substantially from one health system to another, but in general pharmacists should

1. Develop relationships with nursing, medical, dietary, laboratory, quality management, risk management, respiratory care, and other personnel through routine meetings, nursing and medical forums, and other multidisciplinary opportunities. These relationships should be used to promote pharmacists' contributions to collaborative patient care. The pharmacy department should support the use of CPs as an effective way to integrate and align services, processes, and costs.
2. Support or initiate the implementation of a multidisciplinary team for CP development and oversight and ensure that the pharmacy department and the P&T committee are represented on the oversight committee.
3. Seek leadership roles on the health system's CP oversight committee and development teams but be willing to accept subordinate roles. For example, pharmacists should be willing to lead or assist with literature evaluation for the health system's CP development teams.
4. Identify qualities required for the pharmacist's role and develop a consistent process for selecting the most appropriate pharmacists to participate on the various CP development teams.
5. Ensure the ongoing involvement of the P&T committee in the CP process. The P&T committee can facilitate the process by
   - Reviewing and endorsing the pharmacotherapy proposed for inclusion in each CP.
   - Establishing a standing P&T subcommittee or liaison position to assist CP development teams. The subcommittee or liaison would have the opportunity to educate the CP team about the formulary process, the process for MUE, the appropriate use of restricted medications, and other critical medication-use issues.

- Publishing CPs and information about the health system's experiences with CPs in the P&T committee newsletter.
- Developing the drug therapy portion of the CP assessment into an MUE.

6. Emphasize to pharmacists, other health care providers, and health-system administrators pharmacists' responsibility for implementing CP steps that involve pharmacotherapeutic regimens and monitoring, medication distribution, and patient education and counseling.
7. Initiate, after appropriate approvals, the development of the pharmacotherapeutic components of CPs.
8. Offer to evaluate and adapt the pharmacotherapeutic components of existing protocols and guidelines for CPs under development. Maintain a pharmacotherapy database to facilitate CP updates when new medications and pharmacotherapeutic alternatives become available.
9. Develop patient education and counseling materials for the pharmacotherapeutic components of CPs and develop plans for pharmacists or other members of the health care team to provide education and counseling to patients.
10. Advocate the development and use of preprinted medication orders (hard copy or electronic) and consistent use of terminology (e.g., generic drug names, decimals and units of measurement, and standardized terms and abbreviations) within the CP.
11. Be proactive in anticipating alternative processes or drug regimens that may be required in unusual circumstances, such as drug shortages.

Maintaining Involvement. Pharmacists' continued involvement in CPs will depend on their ability to demonstrate their contributions to patient care delivery and improvement to the CP oversight committee and development teams and to the health system's administration. To accomplish this, pharmacists can

1. Monitor the literature of pharmacy, nursing, quality management, health systems, health care, and management for ideas on CP development, implementation, and assessment.
2. Identify new areas for CP development on the basis of medication-use data (e.g., medication error data and MUE findings).
3. Incorporate CPs into the pharmacy department's culture by building responsibilities and performance expectations for CP development, implementation, and assessment into pharmacists' job descriptions.
4. Identify and train pharmacy staff on their roles and responsibilities for implementing the pharmaceutical care components of CPs.
5. Provide objective clinical input that is based on scientific evidence.
6. Ensure consistent use of terminology (e.g., generic drug names, decimals and units of measurement, and standardized terms and abbreviations), rational medication use, and appropriate monitoring. This could be done by the P&T committee or by a pharmacist who coordinates and reviews the pharmacotherapeutic efforts of all CPs.
7. Maintain good working relationships with CP development teams. The pharmacist member should be confident, assertive, cooperative, and effective in communicating with other health care providers.
8. Develop and maintain clinical and management skills through ongoing self-education.

Contributing to the CQI Aspects of CPs. The pharmacist should ensure that the pharmaceutical care actions of the CP contribute to patient satisfaction, desired clinical outcomes, and financial goals by

1. Monitoring the literature for best-practice results relating to specific disease states (as defined by federal diagnosis-related-group classification) and comparing these results with the health system's experience.
2. Ensuring that an internal system of CP tracking and therapeutic review is in place for the rapid insertion of new, more effective therapies into the CP and that CPs are integrated into the institution's CQI processes.
3. Assisting the development of patient satisfaction surveys.
4. Monitoring the results of the CPs and using them to perform MUEs.[42] Since patients enrolled in CPs are receiving predetermined pharmacotherapeutic regimens and monitoring, this is an excellent opportunity to perform disease- and outcome-oriented MUEs. The pharmacist should review the variances and outcomes associated with the CP, determine the effects of pharmacotherapy, and use this analysis to modify the CP. The pharmacotherapeutic component must be specific enough (e.g., specifying the medication and dosage) that its influence on the outcomes can be determined with confidence.
5. Ensuring that CPs are updated when there are changes in institutional practices (e.g., formulary changes) or when external practices change (e.g., guidelines are revised, dosage or monitoring recommendations are revised).

Ensuring the Continuity of a CP. Many CPs require continuity of care across various levels of care and practice settings. Such CPs should specify referral patterns among the levels of care and practice settings. To help accomplish this, pharmacists can

1. Ensure that members of all organizational components are included in the development and assessment of the CP as appropriate for the particular disease or procedure. Included might be personnel in the emergency department, the operating room, the intensive care unit, the step-down unit, the general nursing unit, the rehabilitation unit, the long-term-care facility, the ambulatory care clinic, the laboratory, and the home care service.
2. Develop relationships with ambulatory care, home care, and long-term-care pharmacists and other health care providers to foster the seamless provision of pharmaceutical care by inviting pharmacist members of managed care organizations to participate in CP development, exchanging CPs with the managed care organizations, and creating work teams to ensure the continuity of care.
3. Organize interdisciplinary sharing of information (e.g., recent laboratory test results) and documentation that are useful to all health care providers.

4. Develop a plan to communicate and monitor both internal and external CPs so that pharmacists have a full understanding of the CP process and can evaluate and adjust the CP as necessary when new therapeutic modalities emerge. Optimize this by using electronic and Internet technology to rapidly insert new pharmacotherapies into CPs when appropriate and evaluate which pharmacotherapies are included in which CPs to ensure consistency in medication management.
5. Initiate dialogue among pharmacists to ensure the continuity of the individual patient's CP. For example, when a patient is admitted, the hospital pharmacist should, if necessary and with the patient's permission, contact the patient's community pharmacist or managed care company to obtain information as allowed under local, state, and federal laws (e.g., the Health Insurance Portability and Accessibility Act). The pharmacist should document an accurate medication history (prescription and nonprescription products, dietary supplements, and home remedies), the patient's history of adverse drug reactions and allergies, the patient's medication-taking behaviors (adherence, health beliefs, and social and cultural issues), and any self-monitoring. This does not obviate the requirement for the pharmacist to establish a professional relationship with the patient and to obtain information directly. When the patient is discharged, the hospital pharmacist could (in accordance with the institution's policies and procedures and with the patient's permission) prepare an original discharge summary or append to the physician's discharge summary any necessary notes regarding medications. An appropriate member of the discharge team should forward the discharge summary to relevant health care providers (e.g., physicians, home care nurses, and community or home care pharmacists). The summary should include the patient's chief complaint, the patient's height and weight, a history of the present illness (including the hospital course), pregnancy and lactation status, prescription and nonprescription medications on admission and at discharge, patient education and counseling, the monitoring plan (including patient self-monitoring and a plan for long-term monitoring of the patient's pharmacotherapeutic regimen), and a person to contact if the patient has questions. The pharmacist should check any discharge prescriptions against the indications listed in the discharge summary.

The Pharmacist's Responsibility

Carefully developed and skillfully managed CPs can improve the quality of care and the allocation of health care resources. Because pharmacotherapy is a central component of many CPs, pharmacists can help improve patient outcomes, contribute to cost-effective patient care, and promote team approaches to patient care and performance improvement by incorporating contemporary pharmaceutical care principles, activities, and services into the development, implementation, and assessment of CPs. Health systems will develop CPs in ways that are most appropriate to their patient populations, organizational structure, culture, and environment, so it is the responsibility of health-system pharmacists to identify opportunities to become involved in and improve the CPs in their institutions.

References

1. Darer J, Pronovost P, Bass E. Use and evaluation of critical pathways in hospitals. *Eff Clin Pract.* 2002; 5:114–9.
2. Lumsdon K, Hagland M. Mapping care. *Hosp Health Netw.* 1993; 67:34–40.
3. Coffey RJ, Richards JS, Remmert CS,, et al. An introduction to critical paths. *Qual Manag Health Care.* 1992; 1:45–54.
4. Jaggers LD. Differentiation of critical pathways from other health care management tools. *Am J Health-Syst Pharm.* 1996; 53:311–3.
5. Koch KE. Opportunities for pharmaceutical care with critical pathways. *Top Hosp Pharm Manag.* 1995; 14:1–7.
6. Stevenson LL. Critical pathway experience at Sarasota Memorial Hospital. *Am J Health-Syst Pharm.* 1995; 52:1071–3.
7. Gousse GC, Rousseau MR. Critical pathways at Hartford Hospital. *Am J Health-Syst Pharm.* 1995; 52:1060–3.
8. Shane R, Vinson B. Use of critical pathways and indicators in pharmacy practice. *Top Hosp Pharm Manag.* 1995; 14:55–67.
9. Gouveia WA, Massaro FJ. Critical pathway experience at New England Medical Center. *Am J Health-Syst Pharm.* 1995; 52:1068–70.
10. Saltiel E. Critical pathway experience at Cedars-Sinai Medical Center. *Am J Health-Syst Pharm.* 1995; 52:1063–8.
11. Nelson SP. Critical pathways at University of Iowa Hospitals and Clinics. *Am J Health-Syst Pharm.* 1995; 52:1058–60.
12. Marrie TJ, Lau CY, Wheeler SL,, et al. A controlled trial of a critical pathway for treatment of community-acquired pneumonia. CAPITAL Study Investigators. Community-Acquired Pneumonia Intervention Trial Assessing Levofloxacin. *JAMA.* 2000; 283:749–55.
13. Cannon CP, Hand MH, Bahr R,, et al. Critical pathways for management of patients with acute coronary syndromes: an assessment by the National Heart Attack Alert Program. *Am Heart J.* 2002; 143:777–89.
14. Jones S. A clinical pathway for pediatric gastroenteritis. *Gastroenterol Nurs.* 2003; 26:7–18.
15. Nierman DM. A structure of care for the chronically critically ill. *Crit Care Clin.* 2002; 18:477–91.
16. Kercsmar CM, Myers TR. Clinical pathways in treatment of asthma. *Curr Opin Allergy Clin Immunol.* 2002; 2:183–7.
17. Mavroukakis SA, Muehlbauer PM, White RL Jr,, et al. Clinical pathways for managing patients receiving interleukin 2. *Clin J Oncol Nurs.* 2001; 5:207–17.
18. Zevola DR, Raffa M, Brown K. Using clinical pathways in patients undergoing cardiac valve surgery. *Crit Care Nurse.* 2002; 22:31–9, 44–50.
19. Rymer MM, Summers D, Soper P. Development of clinical pathways for stroke management: an example from Saint Luke's Hospital, Kansas City. *Clin Geriatr Med.* 1999; 15:741–64.

20. Bisanz A, DeJesus Y, Saddler DA. Development, implementation, and ongoing monitoring of pathways for the treatment of gastrointestinal cancer at a comprehensive cancer center. *Gastroenterol Nurs.* 1999; 22:107–14.
21. Sesperez J, Wilson S, Jalaludin B,, et al. Trauma case management and clinical pathways: prospective evaluation of their effect on selected patient outcomes in five key trauma conditions. *J Trauma.* 2001; 50:643–9.
22. Mamolen NL, Brenner PS. The impact of a burn wound education program and implementation of a clinical pathway on patient outcomes. *J Burn Care Rehabil.* 2000; 21:440–5.
23. Crane M, Werber B. Critical pathway approach to diabetic pedal infections in a multidisciplinary setting. *J Foot Ankle Surg.* 1999; 38:30–3.
24. Baker CM, Miller I, Sitterding M,, et al. Acute stroke patients comparing outcomes with and without case management. *Nurs Case Manag.* 1998; 3:196–203.
25. Holtzman J, Bjerke T, Kane R. The effects of clinical pathways for renal transplant on patient outcomes and length of stay. *Med Care.* 1998; 36:826–34.
26. Petitta A, Kaatz S, Estrada C,, et al. The transition to medication system performance indicators. *Top Hosp Pharm Manag.* 1995; 14:20–6.
27. Johnson KB, Blaisdell CJ, Walker A,, et al. Effectiveness of a clinical pathway for inpatient asthma management. *Pediatrics.* 2000; 106:1006–12.
28. Philbin EF, Rocco TA, Lindenmuth NW,, et al. The results of a randomized trial of a quality improvement intervention in the care of patients with heart failure. The MISCHF Study Investigators. *Am J Med.* 2000; 109:443–9.
29. Murphy M, Noetscher C, Lagoe R. A multihospital effort to reduce inpatient lengths of stay for pneumonia. *J Nurs Care Qual.* 1999; 13:11–23.
30. Dzwierzynski WW, Spitz K, Hartz A,, et al. Improvement in resource utilization after development of a clinical pathway for patients with pressure ulcers. *Plast Reconstr Surg.* 1998; 102:2006–11.
31. Boykin JV Jr, Crossland MC, Cole LM. Wound healing management: enhancing patient outcomes and reducing costs. *J Healthc Resour Manag.* 1997; 15:22,24–6.
32. Leibman BD, Dillioglugil O, Abbas F,, et al. Impact of a clinical pathway for radical retropubic prostatectomy. *Urology.* 1998; 52:94–9.
33. Bailey R, Weingarten S, Lewis M,, et al. Impact of clinical pathways and practice guidelines on the management of acute exacerbations of bronchial asthma. *Chest,* 1998; 113:28–33.
34. Uchiyama K, Takifuji K, Tani M,, et al. Effectiveness of the clinical pathway to decrease length of stay and cost for laparoscopic surgery. *Surg Endosc.* 2002; 16:1594–7.
35. Wilson SD, Dahl BB, Wells RD. An evidence-based clinical pathway for bronchiolitis safely reduces antibiotic overuse. *Am J Med Qual.* 2002; 17:195–9.
36. Smith DM, Gow P. Towards excellence in quality patient care: a clinical pathway for myocardial infarction. *J Qual Clin Pract.* 1999; 19:103–5.
37. Kirk JK, Michael KA, Markowsky SJ,, et al. Critical pathways: the time is here for pharmacist involvement. *Pharmacotherapy.* 1996; 16:723–33.
38. Institute for Safe Medication Practices. Medication safety self-assessment. www.ismp.org/pages/mssacaprdf.html (accessed 2003 May 16).
39. American Society of Hospital Pharmacists. ASHP statement on pharmaceutical care. *Am J Hosp Pharm.* 1993; 50:1720–3.
40. American Society of Hospital Pharmacists. ASHP statement on principles for including medications and pharmaceutical care in health care systems. *Am J Hosp Pharm.* 1993; 50:756–7.
41. American Society of Health-System Pharmacists. ASHP guidelines on a standardized method for pharmaceutical care. *Am J Health-Syst Pharm.* 1996; 53:1713–6.
42. American Society of Health-System Pharmacists. ASHP guidelines on medication-use evaluation. *Am J Health-Syst Pharm.* 1996; 53:1953–5.

These guidelines were reviewed in 2009 by the Council on Pharmacy Practice and by the Board of Directors and were found to still be appropriate.

Approved by the ASHP Board of Directors on April 15, 2004. Developed by the ASHP Council on Professional Affairs. Supersedes the "ASHP guidelines on the pharmacists' role in the development of clinical care plans" dated November 16, 1996.

Copyright © 2004, American Society of Health-System Pharmacists, Inc. All rights reserved. Contact ASHP for reprint and permissions requests. This content may not be used for commercial purposes without the express written consent of ASHP.

The bibliographic citation for this document is as follows: American Society of Health-System Pharmacists. ASHP guidelines on the pharmacist's role in the development, implementation, and assessment of critical pathways. *Am J Health-Syst Pharm.* 2004; 61:939–45.

ASHP Guidelines on a Standardized Method for Pharmaceutical Care

Need for a Standardized Method

The purpose of this document is to provide pharmacists with a standardized method for the provision of pharmaceutical care in component settings of organized health systems. Since the introduction of the pharmaceutical care concept[1] and the development of the ASHP Statement on Pharmaceutical Care,[2] considerable variation in pharmacists' provision of pharmaceutical care has been noted. ASHP believes pharmacists need a standardized method for providing pharmaceutical care.

This document describes a standardized method based on functions that all pharmacists should perform for individual patients in organized health systems. The use of this method would foster consistency in the provision of pharmaceutical care in all practice settings. It would support continuity of care both within a practice setting (e.g., among pharmacists on different work shifts caring for an acutely ill inpatient) and when a patient moves among practice settings (e.g., when an inpatient is discharged to home or ambulatory care). Further, a standardized method would establish consistent documentation so that patient-specific and medication-related information could be shared from pharmacist to pharmacist and among health professionals.

The need to identify the functions involved in pharmaceutical care and the critical skills necessary to provide it was discussed at the San Antonio consensus conference in 1993.[3] Functions for the provision of pharmaceutical care were identified by the practitioner task force of the Scope of Pharmacy Practice Project.[4] Those functions have been defined in more detail in the pharmacotherapy series of the ASHP Clinical Skills Program.[5–9]

These Guidelines are not specific to any practice setting. ASHP believes this standardized method can be used in acute care (hospitals), ambulatory care, home care, long-term care, and other practice settings. Functions can be tailored as appropriate for a given practice setting. It is recognized that the degree of standardization and tailoring appropriate for a given work site will depend on the practice environment, the organization of services (e.g., patient-focused or department-focused), working relationships with other health professionals, the health system's and patient's financial arrangements, and the health system's policies and procedures. ASHP believes the use of the systematic approaches encouraged by these guidelines will assist pharmacists in implementing and providing pharmaceutical care in their work sites.

Functions of Pharmaceutical Care

ASHP believes that a standardized method for the provision of pharmaceutical care should include the following:

- Collecting and organizing patient-specific information.
- Determining the presence of medication-therapy problems.
- Summarizing patients' health care needs.
- Specifying pharmacotherapeutic goals.
- Designing a pharmacotherapeutic regimen.
- Designing a monitoring plan.
- Developing a pharmacotherapeutic regimen and corresponding monitoring plan in collaboration with the patient and other health professionals.
- Initiating the pharmacotherapeutic regimen.
- Monitoring the effects of the pharmacotherapeutic regimen.
- Redesigning the pharmacotherapeutic regimen and monitoring plan.

These major functions have been adapted, in part, from the pharmacotherapy series of the ASHP Clinical Skills Program and the final report of the ASHP Model for Pharmacy Practice Residency Learning Demonstration Project.

Collecting and Organizing Pertinent Patient-Specific Information. Information should be collected and used as a patient-specific database to prevent, detect, and resolve the patient's medication-related problems and to make appropriate medication-therapy recommendations. The database should include the following sections, each containing specific types of information to the extent that it is relevant to medication therapy:

Demographic
- Name
- Address
- Date of birth
- Sex
- Religion and religious affiliation
- Occupation

Administrative
- Physicians and prescribers
- Pharmacy
- Room/bed numbers
- Consent forms
- Patient identification number

Medical
- Weight and height
- Acute and chronic medical problems
- Current symptoms
- Vital signs and other monitoring information
- Allergies and intolerances
- Past medical history
- Laboratory information
- Diagnostic and surgical procedures

Medication therapy
- Prescribed medications
- Nonprescription medications
- Medications used prior to admission
- Home remedies and other types of health products used
- Medication regimen
- Compliance with therapy
- Medication allergies and intolerances

DOI 10.37573/9781585287048.060

Concerns or questions about therapy
Assessment of understanding of therapy
Pertinent health beliefs

Behavioral/lifestyle
Diet
Exercise/recreation
Tobacco/alcohol/caffeine/other substance use or abuse
Sexual history
Personality type
Daily activities

Social/economic
Living arrangement
Ethnic background
Financial/insurance/health plan

Objective and subjective information should be obtained directly from patients (and family members, other caregivers, and other health professionals as needed). A physical assessment should be performed as needed. In addition, information can be obtained by reviewing the patient's health record and other information sources.

Information in the patient's health record should be understood, interpreted, and verified for accuracy before decisions are made about the patient's medication therapy. With access to the patient's health record comes the professional responsibility to safeguard the patient's rights to privacy and confidentiality. The Privacy Act of 1974,[10] professional practice policies,[11,12] and policies and procedures of organized health systems provide guidance for the pharmacist in judging the appropriate use of patient-specific information.

The patient (as well as family members, caregivers, and other members of the health care team as needed) should be interviewed. This is necessary for the pharmacist to establish a direct relationship with the patient, to understand the patient's needs and desired outcome, to obtain medication-related information, and to clarify and augment other available information. Pharmacists in many practice settings, including ambulatory care, may need to perform physical assessments to collect data for assessing and monitoring medication therapy.

Information, including clinical laboratory test results, gathered or developed by other members of the health care team may not be in the patient's health record. Therefore, to ensure that the patient information is current and complete, other sources should be checked. Other sources may include medication profiles from other pharmacies used by the patient.

Although it is ideal to have a comprehensive database for all patients, time and staffing limitations may necessitate choices regarding the quantity of information and the number of patients to follow. Choices could be determined by the health system's policies and procedures, by clinical care plans, or by disease management criteria in the patient's third-party health plan.

Systems for recording patient-specific data will vary, depending on pharmacists' preferences and practice settings. Electronic documentation is recommended. Some information may already be in the patient's health record. Therefore, when authorized, the additional information gathered by the pharmacist should be recorded in the patient's health record so that it can be shared with other health professionals. Abstracted summaries and work sheets may also be useful.

Determining the Presence of Medication-Therapy Problems. Conclusions should be drawn from the integration of medication-, disease-, laboratory test-, and patient-specific information. The patient's database should be assessed for any of the following medication-therapy problems:

- Medications with no medical indication
- Medical conditions for which there is no medication prescribed
- Medications prescribed inappropriately for a particular medical condition
- Inappropriate medication dose, dosage form, schedule, route of administration, or method of administration
- Therapeutic duplication
- Prescribing of medications to which the patient is allergic
- Actual and potential adverse drug events
- Actual and potential clinically significant drug–drug, drug–disease, drug–nutrient, and drug–laboratory test interactions
- Interference with medical therapy by social or recreational drug use
- Failure to receive the full benefit of prescribed medication therapy
- Problems arising from the financial impact of medication therapy on the patient
- Lack of understanding of the medication therapy by the patient
- Failure of the patient to adhere to the medication regimen

The relative importance of problems must be assessed on the basis of specific characteristics of the patient or the medication. Checklists, work sheets, and other methods may be used to determine and document the presence of medication-therapy problems. The method should be proactive and should be used consistently from patient to patient.

Summarizing Patients' Health Care Needs. The patient's overall needs and desired outcomes and other health professionals' assessments, goals, and therapy plans should be considered in determining and documenting the medication-related elements of care that are needed to improve or prevent deterioration of the patient's health or well-being.

Specifying Pharmacotherapeutic Goals. Pharmacotherapeutic goals should reflect the integration of medication-, disease-, laboratory test-, and patient-specific information, as well as ethical and quality-of-life considerations. The goals should be realistic and consistent with goals specified by the patient and other members of the patient's health care team. The therapy should be designed to achieve definite medication-related outcomes and improve the patient's quality of life.

Designing a Pharmacotherapeutic Regimen. The regimen should meet the pharmacotherapeutic goals established with the patient and reflect the integration of medication-, disease-, laboratory test-, and patient-specific information; ethical and quality-of-life considerations; and pharmacoeconomic principles. It should comply with the health system's medication-use policies, such as clinical care plans and disease management plans. The regimen should be designed for optimal medication use within both the health system's and the patient's capabilities and financial resources.

Designing a Monitoring Plan for the Pharmacotherapeutic Regimen. The monitoring plan should effectively evaluate achievement of the patient-specific pharmacotherapeutic goals and detect real and potential adverse effects. Measurable, observable parameters should be determined for each goal. Endpoints should be established for assessing whether the goal has been achieved. The needs of the patient, characteristics of the medication, needs of other health care team members, and policies and procedures of the health care setting will influence the monitoring plan.

Developing a Pharmacotherapeutic Regimen and Corresponding Monitoring Plan. The regimen and plan developed in collaboration with the patient and other health professionals should be systematic and logical and should represent a consensus among the patient, prescriber, and pharmacist. The approach selected should be based on consideration of the type of practice setting, its policies and procedures, practice standards, and good professional relations with the prescriber and patient. The regimen and monitoring plan should be documented in the patient's health record to ensure that all members of the health care team have this information.

Initiating the Pharmacotherapeutic Regimen. Depending on the regimen and plan, the pharmacist could, as appropriate, implement all or portions of the pharmacotherapeutic regimen. Actions should comply with the health system's policies and procedures (e.g., prescribing protocols) and correspond to the regimen and plan. Orders for medications, laboratory tests, and other interventions should be clear and concise. All actions should be documented in the patient's health record.

Monitoring the Effects of the Pharmacotherapeutic Regimen. Data collected according to the monitoring plan should be sufficient, reliable, and valid so that judgments can be made about the effects of the pharmacotherapeutic regimen. Changes in patient status, condition, medication therapy, or nonmedication therapy since the monitoring plan was developed should be considered. Missing or additional data should be identified. Achievement of the desired endpoints should be assessed for each parameter in the monitoring plan. A judgment should be made about whether the pharmacotherapeutic goals were met. Before the pharmacotherapeutic regimen is adjusted, the cause for failure to achieve any of the pharmacotherapeutic goals should be determined.

Redesigning the Pharmacotherapeutic Regimen and Monitoring Plan. Decisions to change the regimen and plan should be based on the patient's outcome. When clinical circumstances permit, one aspect of the regimen at a time should be changed and reassessed. Recommendations for pharmacotherapeutic changes should be documented in the same manner used to document the original recommendations.

Pharmacist's Responsibility

An essential element of pharmaceutical care is that the pharmacist accepts responsibility for the patient's pharmacotherapeutic outcomes. The same commitment that is applied to designing the pharmacotherapeutic regimen and monitoring plan for the patient should be applied to its implementation. The provision of pharmaceutical care requires monitoring the regimen's effects, revising the regimen as the patient's condition changes, documenting the results, and assuming responsibility for the pharmacotherapeutic effects.

References

1. Hepler CD, Strand LM. Opportunities and responsibilities in pharmaceutical care. *Am J Hosp Pharm.* 1990; 47:533–43.
2. American Society of Hospital Pharmacists. ASHP statement on pharmaceutical care. *Am J Hosp Pharm.* 1993; 50:1720–3.
3. Implementing pharmaceutical care. Proceedings of an invitational conference conducted by the American Society of Hospital Pharmacists and the ASHP Research Foundation. *Am J Hosp Pharm.* 1993; 50: 1585–656.
4. Summary of the final report of the Scope of Pharmacy Practice Project. *Am J Hosp Pharm.* 1994; 51:2179–82.
5. Shepherd MF. Clinical skills program pharmacotherapy series module 1. Reviewing patient medical charts. Bethesda, MD: American Society of Hospital Pharmacists; 1992.
6. Mason N, Shimp LA. Clinical skills program pharmacotherapy series module 2. Building a pharmacist's patient data base. Bethesda, MD: American Society of Hospital Pharmacists; 1993.
7. Mason N, Shimp LA. Clinical skills program–module 3. Constructing a patient's drug therapy problem list. Bethesda, MD: American Society of Hospital Pharmacists; 1993.
8. Jones WN, Campbell S. Clinical skills program pharmacotherapy series module 4. Designing and recommending a pharmacist's care plan. Bethesda, MD: American Society of Hospital Pharmacists; 1994.
9. Frye CB. Clinical skills program pharmacotherapy series module 5. Monitoring the pharmacist's care plan. Bethesda, MD: American Society of Hospital Pharmacists; 1994.
10. PL 93-579. 5 U.S.C.A. 552a (88 Stat. 1896).
11. ASHP guidelines for obtaining authorization for documenting pharmaceutical care in patient medical records. *Am J Hosp Pharm.* 1989; 46:338–9.
12. Principles of practice for pharmaceutical care. Washington, DC: American Pharmaceutical Association; 1995.

Approved by the ASHP Board of Directors, April 24, 1996. Developed by the ASHP Council on Professional Affairs.

Copyright © 1996, American Society of Health-System Pharmacists, Inc. All rights reserved. Contact ASHP for reprint and permissions requests. This content may not be used for commercial purposes without the express written consent of ASHP.

The bibliographic citation for this document is as follows: American Society of Health-System Pharmacists. ASHP guidelines on a standardized method for pharmaceutical care. *Am J Health-Syst Pharm.* 1996; 53:1713–6.

ASHP Principles for COVID-19 Vaccine Distribution, Allocation, and Mass Immunization

Vaccinating against the severe acute respiratory syndrome coronavirus 2 (SARS-CoV-2) is a highly anticipated countermeasure to the coronavirus disease 2019 (COVID-19) global pandemic. High COVID-19 vaccination rates are essential to protect our communities from worsening and future outbreaks. Mass distribution, allocation, and administration of hundreds of millions of doses of vaccine will require extraordinary planning and execution. Although this may be the largest single vaccination effort the global community has ever undertaken, there are best practices and lessons learned in pandemic preparedness, supply chain management, distribution, and clinical practice to guide us as we immunize against SARS-CoV-2.

Deliberate planning and collaboration with domestic and international partners is paramount to efficiently coordinate vaccine distribution and administration to hundreds of millions of people. ASHP offers the following 10 principles for COVID-19 vaccine development, distribution, allocation, mass vaccination, monitoring, and surveillance.

1. **Enforce a transparent and rigorous process for vaccine development, approval, and post-marketing surveillance.**

   The need for vaccine development to advance at an unprecedented rate requires special safeguards to ensure patient safety and instill public trust. Ethical, rigorous, and transparent procedures for informed consent, inclusion of key populations, evidence evaluation for safety and efficacy, and sustained surveillance are critical. Although vaccine candidates will have undergone multiple phases of testing before approval, it is not possible to detect all potential adverse effects and/or additional factors that may affect vaccine effectiveness during pre-marketing clinical trials. Therefore, rigorous post-marketing surveillance is required to monitor the safety and effectiveness of COVID-19 vaccines.

2. **Collaborate and coordinate with domestic and international public health partners to establish and implement a framework for the ethical and equitable global distribution of COVID-19 vaccines.**

   Despite differences in international, federal, state, and local health policy, regulatory frameworks, and practice models, a concerted effort to ensure widespread global vaccination is necessary to contain COVID-19 and limit continued devastation of public health, economies, and geopolitical relations. Effective communication, collaboration, and coordination with government agencies, public health organizations, regulatory agencies, and health departments are critical to synchronize lines of effort and ensure a successful mass immunization campaign.

3. **Engage, prepare, and protect the immunizer workforce.**

   A robust, trained workforce of immunizers ready and available to administer COVID-19 vaccines is vital to mass immunization efforts. Assembling such a workforce will require mobilization of traditional and nontraditional immunizers, including appropriately trained and supervised clinical learners such as pharmacy, nursing, physician assistant, and medical students to assist with patient screening and referral as well as vaccine preparation and/or administration. To safely accomplish mass immunization, shortages of personal protective equipment must be mitigated to protect the immunizing workforce and maximize infection control efforts.

4. **Expand patient access to COVID-19 vaccines by leveraging a highly qualified and empowered clinical pharmacy workforce in all settings of care.**

   Pharmacists and pharmacy technicians contribute significantly to vaccine awareness and immunization rates through clinical efforts such as patient screening and education, vaccine administration, and accurate reporting of adverse events. The pharmacy workforce should be mobilized nationwide to administer COVID-19 vaccines and as clinical team members in the community. State and federal legal, scope of practice, and reimbursement barriers that prevent or limit pharmacist COVID-19 vaccine administration must be removed.

5. **Adhere to established best practices for proper storage and handling of COVID-19 vaccines throughout the supply chain, from distribution to patient administration.**

   Vaccine supply chain capacity and integrity are dependent not only on manufacturing but also on availability of vaccine components and ancillary resources (e.g., vials, syringes, alcohol swabs), cold-chain management, distribution strategies, and storage. To distribute COVID-19 vaccines effectively, storage procedures must be employed to ensure maximum shelf-life capacity and minimize deterioration and waste of what will likely be a constrained supply of vaccine. Another important aspect of judicious vaccine allotment includes the ability to track and monitor vaccine distribution at the organizational, state, federal, and international level. Efforts to track and trace COVID-19 vaccines in a manner that promotes real-time, reliable tracking while minimizing reporting inefficiencies is required.

6. **Ensure equitable allocation of COVID-19 vaccines across populations and communities, prioritized for greatest public health impact.**

   In anticipation of a constrained supply of vaccine immediately after approval, efforts to prioritize and target vaccination of the most vulnerable populations and critical occupational groups, including healthcare and other essential workers, are required. Enabling and operationalizing multiple, broad access points of administration (e.g., physician offices, pharmacies, churches, community centers) will ensure vaccination efforts reach vulnerable and at-risk populations. Systematic approaches to evaluating whether distribution strategies align with allocation decisions must be considered. This information will inform ongoing

DOI 10.37573/9781585287048.061

prioritization adjustments as more vaccine becomes available for the general population.

7. **Achieve high acceptance and uptake of COVID-19 vaccines by minimizing vaccine hesitancy and misinformation.**

   Hesitancy and misinformation surrounding administration of a COVID-19 vaccine are significant barriers to vaccination rates. Ensuring a coordinated, transparent nationwide education campaign that is culturally and health-literacy sensitive from public health experts, community organizers, and the healthcare community will be vital in gaining and maintaining trust within the community. Pharmacists, as one of the most trusted and accessible healthcare providers, serve as vaccine champions ready to educate the public. ASHP is committed to providing evidence-based information to pharmacists, other health professionals, and the public related to the safe and effective use of COVID-19 vaccines. Furthermore, ASHP is committed to countering misinformation about COVID-19 vaccines while expanding public outreach and building trust.

8. **Seek innovative solutions for adverse drug event monitoring and documentation to improve the thoroughness, accuracy, and usefulness of data collection for improved vaccine safety.**

   To meet the challenge of COVID-19 in the United States and worldwide, multiple types of vaccines with different risk profiles are anticipated. Although adverse events to vaccines are rare compared to the millions of doses administered yearly, it will be critical to identify any adverse event signals with accuracy and expediency. The national Vaccine Adverse Event Reporting System and state immunization information systems are important tools to detect concerning safety signals and track administered doses from multiple suppliers. These programs must receive the necessary resources to enable real-time, efficient, and interoperable reporting processes. Prioritization of accurate and timely reporting of any adverse events due to COVID-19 vaccine administration will assist healthcare personnel in providing the best care and prevention services to their patients and ensure individuals feel empowered regarding their self-care decisions.

9. **Ensure patient access to COVID-19 vaccines by preventing and removing financial barriers.**

   Cost and reimbursement barriers for COVID-19 vaccine administration will reduce the impact of sustained immunization efforts within communities. High costs for patients and reimbursement barriers for immunizers will negatively affect patient access and result in lower vaccination rates. To mitigate these impacts, it is important to identify potential financial barriers and work collectively to ensure reasonable costs and fair reimbursement.

10. **Remain vigilant with continued research and comprehensive surveillance procedures for COVID-19 vaccine use, safety, and effectiveness.**

    Ongoing research and surveillance will expand the body of evidence related to COVID-19 vaccine use, safety, and effectiveness as well as inform current and future mass immunization efforts. ASHP calls for the support of research and the development of measures to evaluate the impact of vaccination on population protection from SARS-CoV-2, allocation to vulnerable populations, mobilization of the immunizer workforce, and other population and global health indicators.

Summary

It is imperative that COVID-19 vaccines are distributed in an ethical, equitable, and efficient manner to maximize population protection from SARS-CoV-2. To achieve this goal, extraordinary efforts will be required to coordinate, prepare, and mobilize an immunization workforce while operationalizing the critical infrastructure for the vaccine supply chain. ASHP acknowledges the multifaceted approaches required for the continuum of mass immunization efforts and is committed to advancing resources and support.

Approved by the ASHP Board of Directors on August 31, 2020.

Copyright © 2020, American Society of Health-System Pharmacists, Inc. All rights reserved. Contact ASHP for reprint and permissions requests. This content may not be used for commercial purposes without the express written consent of ASHP.

The bibliographic citation for this document is as follows: American Society of Health-System Pharmacists. ASHP principles for COVID-19 vaccine distribution, allocation, and mass immunization. *Am J Health-Syst Pharm.* 2020; 77:2112–3.

Specific Practice Areas

2305

EDUCATION ABOUT PERFORMANCE-ENHANCING SUBSTANCES

Source: Council on Pharmacy Practice

To encourage pharmacists to engage in and advise community outreach efforts informing the public on the risks associated with the use of performance-enhancing substances, including but not limited to medications; further,

To educate patients on the importance of disclosing the use of performance-enhancing substances that may or may not be prescribed for legitimate medical indications; further,

To encourage pharmacists to advise athletic authorities, athletes, the community, and healthcare providers on the dangers of performance-enhancing substances and other products that are prohibited in competition; further,

To advocate for the role of the pharmacist in all aspects of performance-enhancing substances control.

This policy supersedes ASHP policy 1305.

Rationale

The risks of using performance-enhancing substances (PES) are well documented in sports medicine journals and other biomedical literature. The U.S. Anti-Doping Agency (USADA) maintains a comprehensive list of performance-enhancing substances that are banned for U.S. athletes competing in the Olympics. In addition to anabolic steroids, the list includes hormones and hormone-like substances (e.g., insulin, tamoxifen); beta-2 agonists; diuretics; red blood cells (RBC) in any form and RBC enhancers; agents that alter genes or genetic expression; stimulants (including caffeine and nicotine); narcotics; cannabinoids; and glucocorticoids. Certain dietary supplements that are known to contain prohibited substances are also banned. The U.S. Food and Drug Administration has also identified dietary supplements that contain pathogens (e.g., Salmonella), contaminants (e.g., lead or mercury), or undeclared prescription drug ingredients (e.g., ephedrine, sildenafil, or dexamethasone).

Although such authorities as the National Collegiate Athletic Association and the USADA have implemented bans on use of these agents and drug testing policies to enforce them, these strategies have been only partially effective in curbing the use of PES. In addition, use of PES has spread beyond professional athletes to military personnel, recreational body builders, professional entertainers, and others wishing to lose weight, increase muscle mass, improve alertness, and increase stamina.

Pharmacists, as medication-use experts and the most-accessible healthcare provider in many communities, can play an important role in community outreach efforts to provide education regarding the use of performance-enhancing substances, including medications, and the importance of disclosing any such use to their healthcare providers.

2324

POINT-OF-CARE TESTING AND TREATMENT BY PHARMACISTS

Source: Council on Therapeutics

To advocate for laws, regulations, and development of specific, structured criteria that include performing diagnostic point-of-care testing (POCT), interpreting test results, prescribing, dosing, and dispensing as clinically indicated by POCT within pharmacists' scope of practice, or referral; further,

To support the tracking of reportable diseases through pharmacist-managed POCT and reporting to public health agencies when appropriate; further,

To promote training and education of the pharmacy workforce to competently engage in POCT and related patient care services; further,

To foster research on patient access and public health improvements, cost savings, and revenue streams associated with pharmacist-managed POCT and related patient care services.

This policy supersedes ASHP policy 2229.

Rationale

Point-of-care testing (POCT) is laboratory testing that takes place at or near the site where the patient is located. These tests are quality-assured pathology services using analytical tools such as blood gas; critical care analyzers; and meters for glucose, urinalysis, and other metabolites. They can be used for both communicable and noncommunicable disease states, including influenza A and B, strep throat, diabetes mellitus, hypertension, anticoagulation, congestive heart failure, and stroke. POCT can be performed by patients in their home, using for example a device that monitors international normalized ratio (INR) for warfarin management, or in the field by healthcare providers, such as rapid strep testing in community pharmacies. POCT devices fall under the Federal Food, Drug, and Cosmetic Act and therefore are also subject to pre- and post-marketing surveillance and review.

As the shortage of primary care providers continues and POTC technology improves, there is ample opportunity to expand the pharmacy workforce's roles in disease screening, identification, and management. POCT provides fast results, which can reduce the time to therapeutic intervention through test-to-treat services, often at a lower cost to patients than an office visit. Pharmacists are well positioned to conduct risk assessments, provide appropriate treatment and referrals when necessary, provide disease state monitoring services, and in turn, improve adherence and identify unnecessary or inappropriate medications. For example, the availability of rapid influenza tests allows pharmacists to quickly diagnose and recommend treatment for influenza A and B, which has been found to reduce the time to first dose of antiviral drugs among individuals with influenza-like illness, compared to those referred to other providers. The combined benefits of telehealth and test-to-treat services should not be discounted. Newer technology that patients can use in the home, including smart scales that monitor changes in weight for congestive heart failure patients, home blood glucose monitoring systems for diabetic patients, and INR monitoring have already demonstrated improved patient outcomes in conjunction with pharmacist care. Numerous studies demonstrate that home POCT can be implemented to streamline healthcare services to patients with chronic and acute disease states and also limit hospital

DOI 10.37573/9781585287048.062

admissions, readmissions, and delays in care and can ultimately lead to better outcomes as well as cost savings for patients and providers.

State legislation concerning pharmacist-managed POCT varies widely. For example, in California, pharmacists are able to perform routine patient assessment procedures through POCT that includes testing for human immunodeficiency virus (HIV) antibodies, total cholesterol, glucose and hemoglobin A1c levels, opiates, blood ketones, thyroid-stimulating hormone, hematocrit, and prothrombin time. Most common is legislation that permits pharmacists in collaborative practice agreements to perform rapid testing to diagnose group A streptococcal pharyngitis and prescribe antimicrobial therapy when a test is positive. This practice model has been shown to decrease the cost of diagnosis and treatment for children and adults and has demonstrated increased patient satisfaction.

ASHP advocates development of specific and structured criteria for pharmacist prescribing, dosing, and dispensing of antimicrobials for this purpose, under a variety of models (e.g., autonomous prescribing authority for pharmacists, delegation protocols, or collaborative practice agreements). A 2018 study found that 69% of pharmacists are willing to perform POCT in a community pharmacy setting, and 86% either strongly agreed or agreed to be willing to recommend appropriate treatment for influenza and group A streptococcal pharyngitis. With collaborative practice agreements in place, patients can bypass visiting a primary care provider, empowering pharmacists to assume an active role not only in treating patients but also in promoting public health by reporting positive cases to local health departments, should rapid testing and reporting be a requirement of dispensing. A Washington State University study demonstrated that after a POCT training module, student pharmacists were not only able to proficiently perform POCT for group A streptococcal pharyngitis, influenza, and HIV, but also showed an increased willingness to perform and recommend the tests, which could expand access.

2327

THERAPEUTIC AND PSYCHOSOCIAL CONSIDERATIONS OF PATIENTS ACROSS THE GENDER IDENTITY SPECTRUM

Source: Council on Therapeutics

To recognize the role of gender-affirming care in achieving health equity and reducing health disparities; further,

To advocate that gender identity is a critical component of medication and disease management of patients across the gender identity spectrum; further,

To advocate for equitable access to gender-affirming care, including access to a pharmacist who ensures safe and effective medication use; further,

To promote research, development, and implementation of therapeutic and biopsychosocial best practices in the care of patients across the gender identity spectrum; further,

To encourage the incorporation of specific education and training regarding patient gender identity into educational standards and competencies for the pharmacy workforce; further,

To encourage easily accessed, structured documentation of a patient's sex assigned at birth, self-identified gender, chosen name, personal pronouns, and relevant medical history in electronic health records; further,

To affirm that healthcare workers should be able to provide gender-affirming care per their clinical judgment and their conscience without fear of legal consequence, workplace sanctions, social stigmatization, harassment, or harm.

This policy supersedes ASHP policy 1718.

Rationale

Transgender people are at risk for health and access inequities as a direct result of biases and stigma. Insurance coverage for medication therapies, corrective surgeries, and associated medical needs such as mental health and endocrine services may be limited or nonexistent due to these discriminatory barriers.

In its National Survey on LGBTQ Youth Mental Health 2020, which surveyed over 40,000 lesbian, gay, bisexual, transgender, queer, and questioning (LGBTQ) young people, the Trevor Project found that 29% of those who responded experienced housing instability; 40% seriously considered attempting suicide in the past 12 months, with more than half of transgender and nonbinary youth having seriously considered suicide; 68% reported symptoms of generalized anxiety disorder in the past 2 weeks, including more than 75% of transgender and nonbinary youth; and 48% reported engaging in self-harm in the past 12 months, including over 60% of transgender and nonbinary youth. The authors also reported that 60% of respondents identified that the ability to afford care was the strongest barrier to receiving mental health care, and that nearly half of transgender and nonbinary youth did not receive wanted mental healthcare due to concerns related to the LGBTQ competence of providers. Further, they found that when transgender and nonbinary youth had access to binders, shapewear, and gender-affirming clothing, they reported lower rates of suicide attempts compared to transgender and nonbinary youth without access. These findings are echoed by Safer and colleagues, who also identify a lack of providers who are sufficiently knowledgeable on the topic, financial barriers, discrimination, lack of cultural competence by providers, health-system barriers, and socioeconomic barriers to this patient population.

There are guidelines to help practitioners identify the health and biopsychosocial needs of transgender and gender-nonbinary people as well as inclusive language guidelines for all practitioners to incorporate into their lexicon.

Patients electing to transition from their sex assigned at birth to their self-identified gender may have surgeries and take higher doses of hormones to change their physical appearance to reflect their self-identified sex. These patients have significant requirements for therapeutic drug monitoring, as certain lab values may appear out of normal limits but are clinically appropriate for the transgender patient, and the risk of drug-drug interactions may be higher because medications may be taken at higher than normal doses. These patients may be more at risk for adverse effects, including thyroid disorders, and may more frequently require anticoagulation and management of diabetes as a result of medication therapy. Other unique needs of these patients include cardiovascular and thrombotic risk assessment, screening for certain types of cancers should they elect to keep their gonadal organs, and other associated primary care screenings associated with their birth sex. Considerations for transgender patients who wish to have children will add the complexity of fertility as well as attention to use of teratogenic medications to their needs. Because of the unique and complex healthcare needs of transgender patients, it is essential that they have adequate access to appropriate care, including pharmacist care. To help ensure appropriate patient identification, assessment, and treatment, a patient's sex assigned at birth, self-identified gender, chosen name, personal pronouns, and (if applicable) gender-confirming therapies or procedures should be documented in a structured way in electronic health records. This documentation also helps healthcare providers address another of the unique biopsychosocial needs of transgender patients; like other healthcare providers, pharmacists should address transgender patients by their self-identified gender and chosen name and personal pronouns.

Those caring for these patients should be knowledgeable regarding the clinical, social, and access needs of this patient population. Student pharmacists, pharmacy residents, pharmacists, and pharmacy technicians therefore should all be trained to appropriately care for this patient population. The Affordable Care Act prohibits pharmacists from making their own decisions about the suitability of a prescribed medication in situations that would constitute discrimination against patients. Although ASHP policy 0610, Pharmacist's Right of Conscience and Patient's Right of Access to Therapy, recognizes the pharmacist's right of conscience, the policy also recognizes "the patient's right to obtain legally prescribed and medically indicated treatments" and states that "a pharmacist exercising the right of conscience must be respectful of, and serve the legitimate healthcare needs and desires of, the patient, and shall provide a referral without any actions to persuade, coerce, or otherwise impose on the patient the pharmacist's values, beliefs, or objections." In addition, ASHP believes that healthcare workers should be able to provide care per their clinical judgment and their conscience without fear of legal consequence, workplace sanctions, social stigmatization, harassment, or harm.

2328

REMOVAL OF INJECTABLE PROMETHAZINE FROM HOSPITAL FORMULARIES

Source: Council on Therapeutics

To advocate that injectable promethazine be removed from hospital formularies; further,

To encourage regulatory and safety bodies to review patient safety data and conduct research on adverse events related to administration of injectable promethazine; further,

To encourage manufacturers to produce injectable promethazine in package sizes and concentrations that reduce risk.

This policy supersedes ASHP policy 1831.

Rationale

In its 2020–2021 Targeted Medication Best Practices for Hospitals, the Institute for Safe Medication Practices (ISMP) included a recommendation to eliminate injectable promethazine from hospitals. This recommendation includes removal of injectable promethazine from all areas of the hospital, including the pharmacy; classification of injectable promethazine as a nonstocked, nonformulary medication; implementation of a medical staff-approved automatic therapeutic substitution policy; conversion of all injectable promethazine orders to another antiemetic; and removal of injectable promethazine from all computerized medication order screens and from all order sets and protocols. In 2018, only 56% of ISMP Survey respondents believed promethazine to be a high-alert medication, which was a *decrease* from 59% in 2014. The 2018 survey also found that 54% of respondents also thought that "IV promethazine" should be changed to "injectable promethazine," also underscoring the need for broader protections from intravenous administration use. This recommendation reiterated the identical 2018–2019 ISMP Best Practice recommendation, which was a change from previous ones in which ISMP promoted safe use by raising awareness about risks associated with intravenous (IV) promethazine administration. Despite the efforts to improve the safety of injectable promethazine use, sporadic and significant patient harm continues to occur.

Promethazine is a known vesicant that can cause tissue damage and necrosis when extravasation occurs during IV administration, and it has negative effects on cardiac conduction. Although therapeutic alternatives are available for most indications, the alternative therapies are also not without risk and may not be as effective in some clinical situations. Processes to limit the potential for patient harm when IV administration of promethazine is indicated include but are not limited to use of therapeutic alternatives (e.g., 5-HT_3 receptor antagonists, antipsychotic agents, antihistamines); use of alternate routes and modalities of administration (e.g., oral, rectal); and restrictions on use (e.g., nonformulary, nonstocked status and removal from order sets and protocols). While prior guidance provided practice recommendations to mitigate the risk of injectable promethazine use (e.g., minimum drug dilution, continuous nurse monitoring of infusion, administration through a running IV line), a 2006 ISMP survey of hospitals revealed poor adherence to these recommendations, despite the well-documented risks of circumventing them. Although medication regimens for some specific patient populations may include injectable promethazine, many guidelines for management of disease states in which promethazine may have a role do not recommend injectable promethazine as an agent of initial choice, indicating it should be used as last line/salvage therapy. Often, these guidelines do not include injectable promethazine as a therapeutic option at all; given the number and variety of suitable alternatives, the risks of using this medication outweigh the benefits.

In addition, because ISMP has recommended injectable promethazine's removal from formularies, there is not much data on its safety and efficacy, as implementation of the recommendation has varied across the U.S., and what data is available has been mostly anecdotal or case-based reports. ASHP encourages regulatory and safety bodies to review patient safety data and conduct research on adverse events related to administration of injectable promethazine. Finally, ASHP encourages manufacturers to produce injectable promethazine in package sizes and concentrations that reduce risk in a similar manner to those recommended by ISMP for administration of electrolytes (e.g., use of prediluted standardized solutions).

2211

NALOXONE AVAILABILITY

Source: Council on Therapeutics

To recognize the public health benefits of naloxone for opioid reversal; further,

To support efforts to safely expand patient and public access to naloxone through independent pharmacist prescribing authority, encouraging pharmacies to stock naloxone, supporting availability of affordable formulations of naloxone (including zero-cost options), and other appropriate means; further,

To advocate for statewide naloxone standing orders to serve as a prescription for individuals who may require opioid reversal or those in a position to aid a person requiring opioid reversal; further,

To support and foster standardized education and training on the role of naloxone in opioid reversal and its proper administration, safe use, and appropriate follow-up care, and dispelling common misconceptions to the pharmacy workforce and other healthcare professionals; further,

To support the use of objective clinical data, including leveraging state prescription drug monitoring programs and clinical decision-making tools, to facilitate pharmacist-initiated screenings to identify patients who may most benefit from naloxone prescribing; further,

To encourage the co-prescribing of naloxone with all opioid prescriptions; further,

To support legislation that provides protections for those seeking or providing medical help for overdose victims.

This policy supersedes ASHP policy 2014.

Rationale

According to the Centers for Disease Control and Prevention (CDC), prescription drug abuse is a national epidemic. Deaths from prescription opioid overdose number 10,000 per year; in contrast, deaths from heroin overdose number 2000. People at risk for opioid overdose include not only substance abusers, but also opioid-naive patients, such as those being admitted for or discharged from ambulatory surgery.

Naloxone is a competitive opioid antagonist that rapidly rescues patients from opioid overdose by displacing mu2 opioid receptors in the central nervous system. Naloxone has an excellent safety profile. The World Health Organization includes naloxone on its model list of essential medicines.

Evidence has demonstrated a clear public health benefit from expanding access to naloxone. Naloxone is currently distributed without a prescription via standing orders, collaborative practice agreements, or pharmacist prescribing authority in all 50 states to ensure liberal access to this lifesaving drug. Several states have also started to permit pharmacy technicians to dispense naloxone under these provisions as well.

Currently there are several formulations of naloxone on the market, which vary in strength and route of administration, including subcutaneous injection (which caregivers or peers may have difficulty administering properly) and intranasal formulations. Studies have shown that intranasal naloxone is as effective as injectable routes in rapid opioid reversal. However, its cost ($130–300 per kit) presents a barrier to widespread use. ASHP encourages the Food and Drug Administration to explore ways to get more user-friendly and less-costly formulations to the market for patients and caregivers. Recognizing that naloxone should not be cost-prohibitive, efforts should be made to fully subsidize the cost of this lifesaving medication.

Despite expanded access to naloxone, there are still significant barriers to its widespread use, including hesitancy among pharmacists to dispense naloxone. Uniform education for those administering the drug, training on safe administration, and recommendations on follow-up care with abuse treatment programs for treated individuals is needed.

Furthermore, although great strides have been made in many areas to improve naloxone access, it is necessary to recognize areas of practice where such efforts are inadequate as a one-size-fits-all model. While pharmacists in all 50 U.S. states now have the ability to participate in naloxone prescribing in some form, barriers to access may still exist, such as in rural communities with no physician willing to participate in a collaborative practice agreement, or indeed, perhaps no physician whatsoever. To that end, pharmacists' naloxone prescribing authority should be independent (i.e., not requiring a protocol or collaborative practice agreement to be in place). Where there are barriers to such independent authority, ASHP should advocate for legislation that promotes standing orders for naloxone as a part of patient care, much as ASHP advocates for pharmacists' independent prescribing authority for medication-assisted treatment (ASHP policy 1909).

Pharmacists should make every effort to intervene on behalf of their patients' safety; therefore, pharmacist education regarding use of naloxone should begin in the didactic curriculum in schools of pharmacy and be part of an ongoing effort for pharmacists as lifelong learners. Current literature suggests that one key barrier to expanded pharmacist involvement in naloxone prescribing is a lack of confidence—which may be addressed by increased education—and also by persistent misconceptions, such as the notion that increased naloxone availability will promote opioid misuse. Because the pernicious nature of this idea is so harmful, it should be highlighted for targeted educational efforts.

Significant access and racial prescribing disparities have been noted in clinical literature regarding naloxone (Dayton L et al. Racial Disparities in Overdose Prevention among People Who Inject Drugs. *J Urban Health* 2020; 97:823–30). Encouraging pharmacists to be proactive in making clinical interventions is important, but safeguarding patients to protect them from the harms of bias is essential in ensuring equitable access to this medication. Whenever possible, pharmacists should use objective measures (e.g., history of overdose, polypharmacy including multiple CNS-depressing agents, high morphine milligram equivalents per day) to identify high-risk patients and make proactive interventions to provide naloxone to them.

Finally, encouraging co-prescribing of naloxone with every opioid prescription aligns ASHP with the American Medical Association, CDC guidelines, and other organizations that recommend prescribing or co-prescribing naloxone to reduce the risk of overdose deaths. Laws, including medical amnesty and those that provide protection against legal liability for persons administering naloxone (i.e., Good Samaritan laws), are needed as well as laws protecting individuals who call for help for someone who has overdosed from prosecution from minor drug possession or drug paraphernalia.

2212

SAFE AND EFFECTIVE THERAPEUTIC USE OF INVERTEBRATES

Source: Council on Therapeutics

To recognize use of medical invertebrates (e.g., maggots and leeches) as an alternative treatment in limited clinical circumstances; further,

To educate pharmacists, other providers, patients, and the public about the risks and benefits of medical invertebrates use and about best practices for use; further,

To advocate that pharmacy departments, in cooperation with other departments, provide oversight of medical invertebrates to assure appropriate formulary consideration and safe procurement, storage, use, and disposal; further,

To encourage independent research and reporting on the therapeutic use of medical invertebrates.

This policy supersedes ASHP policy 1724.

Rationale

Medical invertebrates, including leeches and maggots, are used as a therapeutic intervention for various indications, including in treatment of extravasation injury, post-plastic-surgery salvage, relief of vascular congestion, macroglossia, compartment syndrome, pain management, and debridement therapy. The use of medical invertebrates is not without risk. There have been reports of local and systemic infections with use of leeches and transmission of communicable disease if not handled properly, and use may mask coagulopathies. Antimicrobial prophylaxis may be required, and there are also drug-invertebrate interactions that may impact the effectiveness of invertebrate therapy. There is also limited research on the efficacy of these therapies that lead to varied practice and unsubstantiated claims. In addition, leeches may present a biohazard. Application or manipulation may require expulsion of blood to encourage reattachment, and there have been cases in which engorged leeches have fallen off patients, potentially exposing caregivers and other patients to blood.

To promote safe use of medical invertebrates, pharmacy departments, in cooperation with other health-system departments, should assure appropriate formulary consideration and safe procurement, storage, use (e.g., control, prescribing, preparation, dispensing, administration, application, manipulation, documentation, consideration for antimicrobial prophylaxis, clinical and regulatory monitoring), and disposal.

2213

CRITERIA FOR MEDICATION USE IN GERIATRIC PATIENTS

Source: Council on Therapeutics

To support comprehensive medication management, including assessment of physiologic and pharmacokinetic factors, as a central component of providing safe and effective medication therapy to geriatric patients; further,

To oppose use of the Beers criteria or similar criteria by the Centers for Medicare & Medicaid Services, other accreditation and quality improvement entities, and payers as the sole indicator to assess the appropriateness of prescribing for geriatric patients based on known limitations in the evidence evaluating the association between use of medications listed in such criteria and subsequent adverse drug events; further,

To advocate for the development, refinement, and validation of new criteria that consider drug-, disease-, and patient-specific factors, and criteria and quality measures that demonstrate the ability to decrease the occurrence of adverse drug events in geriatric patients; further,

To support research to assess the clinical application of existing and proposed criteria, including assessment of their correlation to patient outcomes and strategies for implementation; further,

To encourage inclusion of validated criteria in clinical decision support systems and other information technologies to facilitate prescribing and deprescribing for geriatric patients; further,

To acknowledge that such criteria are intended as a guide and should not replace the clinical judgment of pharmacists and other clinicians.

This policy supersedes ASHP policy 1221.

Rationale

Criteria have been developed to identify high-risk drugs that should be avoided in geriatric patients (i.e., those 65 years of age or older) based on the potential for these therapies to cause adverse drug events that can result in falls, hospitalizations, and other incidents that lead to significant morbidity and mortality in this patient population. Those criteria include the 2019 iteration of the Beers criteria and the Screening Tool of Older Persons' Potentially Inappropriate Prescriptions, or STOPP (version 2 of the STOPP/START criteria was published in 2015). Although ASHP supports the intent of these criteria to prevent patient harm, safe and effective use of medications in geriatric patients requires the more thorough assessment associated with pharmacist-provided comprehensive medication management. ASHP opposes adoption of the Beers criteria by the Centers for Medicare & Medicaid Services (CMS) and other accreditation and quality improvement organizations as a tool to assess prescribing in long-term care and other settings, noting concerns about the development and validation of that tool. More importantly, studies evaluating the clinical application of the 2003 iteration of the Beers criteria have not demonstrated a reduction in adverse events when that tool is used. The American Geriatric Society publishes an update every three years, with the most recent update occurring in 2019. Although the update addressed some concerns (e.g., removal of drugs no longer available, drug-drug interactions), some of the criteria's shortcomings (e.g., lack of validation) remain unresolved. In that regard, STOPP, which is based on organ systems and accounts for patients' concomitant disease, is considered more useful. Studies evaluating STOPP, though small in number and consisting of heterogeneous study populations and implementation plans, project a favorable impact on patient outcomes. ASHP encourages additional work to develop, refine, and validate this and similar evidence-based criteria.

Quality indicators for appropriate medication use in older adults were identified as part of the Assessing Care of Vulnerable Elders (ACOVE) project. The indicators provide suggestions for improving prescribing practices and identify medications that require monitoring or should be avoided in vulnerable elders. Practical indicators that can be reviewed from patient encounters and transitions of care include maintenance of a medication list, periodic drug therapy review, assessing response to therapy, drug monitoring, and patient education. Review of these indicators may facilitate benchmarking and consideration of discontinuing unnecessary medications, dose reduction, and consideration of nonpharmacologic alternative strategies.

Further, there is a need for practice-based research to evaluate the application of such criteria and inclusion of validated criteria in clinical decision support systems and other information technologies is necessary to facilitate the use of these criteria in clinical practice. Finally, these tools are intended to serve as a guide or screening tool and should not replace the clinical judgment of pharmacists and other clinicians.

2220

PROMOTING TELEHEALTH PHARMACY SERVICES

Source: Council on Pharmacy Practice

To advocate for innovative telehealth pharmacy practice models that (1) enable the pharmacy workforce to promote clinical patient care delivery, patient counseling and education, and efficient pharmacy operations; (2) improve access to pharmacist comprehensive medication management services; (3) advance patient-centric care and the patient care experience; and (4) facilitate pharmacist-led population and public health services and outreach; further,

To advocate for removal of barriers to access to telehealth services; further,

To advocate for laws, regulations, and payment models for telehealth services that are equitable to similar services provided in person by health systems, with appropriate accountability and oversight; further,

To encourage comparative effectiveness and outcomes research on telehealth pharmacy services.

Rationale

The definitions and terminology used to describe telehealth vary. Many refer to virtual health, telehealth, telemedicine, and/or telepharmacy interchangeably. The Centers for Medicare & Medicaid Services (CMS) describes telemedicine as a means for improving a patient's health by permitting two-way, real-time, interactive communication between a patient and a healthcare provider who are geographically separated. ASHP defines telepharmacy as a method used in pharmacy practice in which a pharmacist utilizes telecommunications technology to oversee aspects of pharmacy operations or provide patient care services.

Telehealth is part of a larger digital transformation in healthcare. Patients are increasingly making decisions about who delivers their care and engaging in the delivery of that care digitally. As a result, hospitals and health systems need a strategy for their own digital transformation and to meet patient demands. In general, telehealth includes a broader scope of remote healthcare services than telemedicine and telepharmacy; therefore, ASHP considers telehealth to be the overarching term for the remote delivery of patient care services.

The availability of telehealth services in rural areas facilitates greater access to care by eliminating the need to travel long distances to see a qualified healthcare provider. It promises to save patients time and money, reduces patient transfers, emergency department and urgent care center visits, and delivers savings to payers (American Hospital Association [AHA]. Fact Sheet: Telehealth; AHA. Optimizing Pharmacy Services: Managing your hospital pharmacy during the COVID-19 pandemic and beyond). Pharmacists' role in telehealth is instrumental, as telehealth serves are a valuable tool for the profession of pharmacy to extend its reach to patients for the provision of medication management and complex patient care (AHA. Optimizing Pharmacy Services: Managing your hospital pharmacy during the COVID-19 pandemic and beyond; ASHP Statement on Telepharmacy). Telehealth services have grown significantly over recent years, especially during the COVID-19 pandemic. Telehealth services have the potential to improve patient access to care, cost efficiencies, and quality while meeting consumer demand. They also offer patients the convenience of remote drug therapy monitoring, authorization for prescriptions, patient counseling, and monitoring patients' compliance with prescriptions, and they can be offered remotely to patients with diabetes, congestive heart failure, and other chronic diseases. Pharmacists may also use telehealth when suitable to remotely verify sterile compounding, offer pre- and postoperative medication order review, provide interactive postoperative patient medication counseling, or deliver drug information to a facility that is geographically isolated (ASHP Statement on Telepharmacy). To ensure the best patient care outcomes and most efficient use of healthcare resources, additional research will be needed to compare telehealth pharmacy services with those offered in person.

2224

DRUG DESENSITIZATION

Source: Council on Therapeutics

To encourage an allergy reconciliation process to ensure allergy documentation is accurate and complete for drug desensitization; further,

To advocate for pharmacist involvement in the interdisciplinary development of institutional drug desensitization policies and procedures; further,

To support the creation and implementation of drug desensitization order sets and safeguards in the electronic health record to minimize potential error risk; further,

To recommend appropriate allocation of resources needed for the drug desensitization process, including adequate availability of allergic reaction management resources near the desensitization location; further,

To support the education and training of pharmacists regarding allergy reconciliation, drug desensitization processes, and allergic reaction prevention and management; further,

To recommend patient education and appropriate documentation in the electronic health record of the outcomes of the drug desensitization process.

Rationale

Only about 5–10% of all drug-related adverse events are allergic in nature. Patients are often labeled with an allergy on the basis of a side effect or intolerances such as headache or gastrointestinal disturbance. Allergen misidentification and documentation can be detrimental to patient care by preventing the use of optimal drugs or by causing re-exposure to a true allergen. However, when a patient has a true allergy, and the drug is required for treatment, drug desensitization is often the next step in patient care.

Drug desensitization is a procedure that transiently alters a patient's immune response to a drug to permit an allergic patient to receive the sensitizing drug safely. Approaches to desensitization are often drug- and protocol-specific and vary widely (e.g., in the length of sensitization based on patient-specific factors such as immune response, body composition, height, and weight). This approach to patient care is not without risk or controversy, as the mechanism of drug desensitization is not completely understood but the procedure is often deemed essential to patient care when a specific drug is the only appropriate therapy for a patient. Drug concentrations and dilutions are often not standardized, and depending on the drug, can be a source of significant error, particularly with high-risk medications such as chemotherapeutic agents. Sources of error that have been cited in the literature include compounding errors, order entry into the electronic health record, lack of standardized order sets, variability in concentrations of sensitizing doses, allergic reaction prevention, and documentation of desensitization outcomes.

2240

POST-INTENSIVE CARE SYNDROME

Source: Council on Therapeutics

To recognize that multidimensional rehabilitation is essential for recovery after intensive care; further,

To support research on and dissemination of best practices in the prevention, identification, and treatment of post-intensive care syndrome (PICS) in patients of all ages; further,

To advocate that health systems support the development and implementation of interdisciplinary clinics, inclusive of pharmacists, to treat patients with PICS, including provisions for telehealth and innovative practice models to meet the needs of patients with PICS; further,

To advocate for the integration of post-ICU patient and ICU caregiver support groups; further,

To provide education on the role of the pharmacist in caring for patients with PICS.

Rationale

Post-intensive care unit (post-ICU) rehabilitation is essential for recovery after critical illness. Post-intensive care syndrome (PICS) is a conglomerate of new or worsening multidimensional impairments in physical, psychological, cognitive, and social status arising from critical illness that continue after hospital discharge. PICS is associated with high morbidity among patients discharged from ICUs, with 30–80% of patients having issues with remembering, paying attention, solving problems, or organizing and working on complex tasks.

The burden of PICS continues to grow. With only up to 50% of patients with PICS able to return to work within the first year, some are unable to return to the jobs they had before their illness and need help with activities after leaving the hospital. While PICS is widely discussed across medical disciplines, it not well defined, nor are ways to prevent and treat this disorder well researched. It is recognized that patients with PICS require a multidimentional, interdisciplinary treatment effort, including cognitive rehabilitation, mental health treatment, and intensive transitions of care interventions, as patients may be discharged on medications that should not be continued and they may need support to resume daily activities. The rapid COVID-19-related increase in patients requiring the use of ICUs has exacerbated the demand for high-quality PICS care, but the simultaneous expansion of telemedicine and other innovative patient care models has shown that rapid changes in team-based care can be achieved with the proper incentives and flexibilities.

2245

SUBSTANCE USE DISORDER

Source: Council on Therapeutics

To affirm that a patient with a substance use disorder (SUD) has a chronic condition with associated neurodevelopmental, physiologic, and psychosocial changes; further,

To recognize that dehumanizing language and stigmatization regarding SUD and persons who use drugs (PWUD) create barriers to healthcare access and result in poor clinical outcomes; further,

To recognize the disproportionately harmful health impact that criminalization and policing practices related to SUD and PWUD have had on communities, particularly those of color; further,

To advocate for destigmatization efforts and elimination of barriers to care for SUD and PWUD; further,

To support risk mitigation and harm reduction strategies, including syringe services programs, recognizing the roles they have in public health efforts to reduce infectious disease burden, improve access to healthcare, improve patient trust, and reduce expenditures; further,

To advocate for expansion of comprehensive medication management services provided by pharmacists for prevention, treatment, and recovery services within the interprofessional care team and throughout the continuum of care; further,

To support pharmacists leading community-based comprehensive preventive health and treatment programs; further,

To encourage the inclusion of longitudinal SUD training in didactic pharmacy curricula, starting with an early initiation of education; use of evidence-based practices, including risk mitigation, harm reduction, and destigmatizing communication strategies; and increasing experiential education pertaining to SUD; further,

To support and foster standardized education and training on SUD, including dispelling common misconceptions to the pharmacy workforce and other healthcare professionals.

This policy supersedes ASHP policy 9711.

Rationale

Substance use disorder (SUD) is a public health crisis that has grown to epidemic levels in the United States over the past 30 years. The Department of Health and Human Services recognized it as a public health emergency in 2017. In 2019, over 70,000 people died from drug overdoses, and between June 2019 and June 2020, overdoses of synthetic opioids caused over 48,000 deaths. Additionally, the Centers for Disease Control and Prevention (CDC) estimates that the economic burden of prescription opioid misuse alone in the United States is $78.5 billion a year, including the costs of healthcare, lost productivity, addiction treatment, and criminal justice involvement. The National Academy of Medicine and the Department of Health and Human Services identify several populations that are at risk for SUD, including justice-involved populations; those living in rural areas; people who inject drugs; pregnant patients; children born to SUD; and those with lower incomes, insecure housing, and lacking access to health insurance. Additionally, researchers have demonstrated links between the increase in opioid overdoses and the rate of opioid prescriptions, particularly in populations in which overdoses had not been seen before. Age-adjusted rates of opioid overdose deaths from 1990 to

2017 have increased sixfold among Whites, climbed from 3.5 to 6.8 overdoses per 100,000 people among Hispanics, and among Blacks has increased from 3.5 to 12.9 per 100,000 people in the U.S. The age-adjusted rate of overdose deaths increased by 31% from 2019 (21.6 per 100,000) to 2020 (28.3 per 100,000). When considering infectious diseases, SUD had also been cited as a cause for a tripling of hepatitis C cases from 2010 to 2017 as well as increases in hepatitis B, human immunodeficiency virus, bacterial, and fungal bloodstream infections, as well as sexually transmitted infections and endocarditis.

SUD is a chronic condition with associated neurological and physiological changes, not a personal choice. Dehumanizing language and stigmatization regarding SUD and people who use drugs (PWUD) create barriers to healthcare access and result in poor clinical outcomes. In addition, criminalization and policing practices related to SUD and PWUD have disproportionately harmful health impact on communities of color.

The best approach to managing SUD is a multifaceted one that requires involvement at the community, hospital and health system, legislative, government, and provider levels. Programs must also include stakeholders from these levels at the planning, implementation, and enduring service stages to optimize uptake, adoption, and sustainability. Pharmacists are an essential team member as part of interprofessional teams and providing comprehensive medication management (CMM) for patients with SUD. Pharmacists are integrated as key team members across the continuum of care from community pharmacies, health systems, and ambulatory care settings. Clear communication and coordination are also crucial so that successes and failures can be assessed, modified, or discontinued to suit the goals of prevention, treatment, harm reduction, and recovery.

Harm reduction strategies including syringe service programs have proven effective, not only in preventing deaths from injectable drug overdoses and infections but also as a site of care for providing such additional services as vaccinations, testing, referral to infectious disease care and substance use treatment, and access to and disposal of needles, syringes, and other injection equipment. Elimination of barriers to sterile syringe access, including discouraging prescription or logbook requirements and providing methods of syringe disposal, promotes access to healthcare.

Education and tools for the pharmacy workforce that assist in supporting the needs of PWUD and patients with SUD should also incorporate specifics about destigmatization, person-first language, harm reduction strategies, evidence-based practices, social determinants of health, and ways to provide trauma-informed and culturally sensitive care to patients. Education should include efforts to recognize bias and misinformation, as these contribute to the stigma that serves as a major barrier in treating SUD.

2247

PHARMACY WORKFORCE'S ROLE IN VACCINATION

Source: Council on Pharmacy Practice

To affirm that the pharmacy workforce has a role in improving public health and increasing patient access to vaccinations by promoting and administering appropriate vaccinations to patients and employees in all settings; further,

To collaborate with key stakeholders to support the public health role of the pharmacy workforce in the administration of adult and pediatric vaccinations; further,

To advocate that states grant pharmacists and appropriately supervised student pharmacists the authority to initiate and administer all adult and pediatric vaccinations; further,

To advocate that states grant appropriately supervised pharmacy technicians the authority to prepare and administer all adult and pediatric vaccinations; further,

To advocate for the inclusion of pharmacist-provided vaccination training in college of pharmacy curricula and pharmacy technician-provided vaccination training in technician training programs; further,

To advocate that members of the pharmacy workforce who have completed a training and certification program acceptable to state boards of pharmacy and meeting the standards established by the Centers for Disease Control and Prevention may provide such vaccinations; further,

To advocate that state and federal health authorities establish centralized databases for timely documentation of vaccine administrations that are interoperable and accessible to all healthcare providers; further,

To advocate that state and federal health authorities require all vaccination providers to report their documentation to these centralized databases, if available; further,

To encourage the pharmacy workforce to educate all patients, their caregivers, parents, guardians, and healthcare providers to promote vaccine confidence and convey the importance of vaccinations for disease prevention; further,

To encourage the pharmacy workforce to seek opportunities for involvement in disease prevention through community vaccination programs; further,

To foster education, training, and the development of resources to assist the pharmacy workforce and other healthcare professionals in building vaccine confidence; further,

To advocate for adequate staffing, resources, and equipment for the pharmacy workforce to support vaccination efforts to ensure patient safety; further,

To advocate for appropriate reimbursement for vaccination services rendered; further,

To work with federal, state, and local governments and others to improve the vaccine development and supply system in order to ensure an adequate and equitably distributed supply of vaccines.

This policy supersedes ASHP policies 1309 and 2122.

Rationale

Increasing adult and pediatric patients' access to vaccinations is an important public health challenge. The unique training and expertise of members of the pharmacy workforce in all aspects of the medication-use system can help expand patients' access to vaccinations and promote disease prevention in all practice settings. Hospital and health-system pharmacists, student pharmacists, and pharmacy technicians provide care to a patient population that is vulnerable and often critically ill, and such patients are especially dependent on herd immunity. Patients in rural areas, where a pharmacy may provide the only convenient access to a healthcare professional, will benefit from increased pharmacist vaccination authority.

Although all states permit pharmacist administration of some vaccines, state laws differ in the range of vaccines pharmacists may administer and the patient populations they are permitted to vaccinate. During the COVID-19 public health emergency, new regulatory flexibility under the Public Readiness and Emergency Preparedness (PREP) Act allowed pharmacy technicians and pharmacy students, under the supervision of a licensed pharmacist, to administer COVID-19 and pediatric vaccinations. Permanently allowing trained and certified pharmacists, including student pharmacists, to order and administer all adult and pediatric vaccines (e.g., by eliminating the requirement that some pharmacist-provided vaccinations be conducted within a collaborative drug therapy management agreement) would encourage standardization of pharmacy vaccination practice within and among states, as would permitting appropriately supervised pharmacy technicians to prepare and administer vaccinations. ASHP also advocates for appropriate reimbursement for all vaccination services.

Only pharmacists, student pharmacists, and pharmacy technicians who undergo appropriate training and certification should be authorized by state boards to provide vaccinations. To ensure their consistency and quality, those training and certification programs should meet Centers for Disease Control and Prevention standards.

To aid in sharing important patient vaccination information, centralized and interoperable databases of patient vaccinations should be established, and all authorized vaccination providers, including pharmacists, student pharmacists, and pharmacy technicians, should be required by law or regulation to document their vaccinations in those databases in a timely manner when they become available.

Pharmacists, student pharmacists, pharmacy technicians, and pharmacy educators should embrace their role in this important public health effort by providing education about the importance of vaccination in disease prevention, participating in community vaccination programs, and training vaccination providers.

The pharmacy workforce has an integral role in promoting disease prevention and health equity by promoting vaccine confidence. The CDC defines vaccine confidence as "the trust that patients, their families, and providers have in recommended vaccines, the providers who administer vaccines, and the processes and policies that lead to vaccine development, licensure or authorization, manufacturing, and recommendations for use." Building vaccine confidence can involve helping patients, caregivers, healthcare providers, and members of the public overcome vaccine hesitancy, which is a delay in acceptance or refusal of vaccination despite availability of vaccination services. Vaccine hesitancy is complex and context specific, varying across time, place, and vaccines, and is influenced by factors such as complacency, convenience, and confidence. Vaccine-hesitant patients, healthcare providers, and caregivers have been found to be responsive to vaccine information, consider vaccination, and are not opposed to all vaccines, and therefore would benefit from counseling.

The pharmacy workforce, and in particular its leaders, also has an important role in working with federal, state, and local government, the pharmaceutical industry, and other stakeholders to improve the vaccine development and supply system to ensure a consistent and adequate supply of vaccines, and to ensure that vaccines supplies are equitably distributed to promote public health by reducing disparities in vaccine access.

2250

ACCESS TO REPRODUCTIVE HEALTH SERVICES

Source: House of Delegates

To recognize that reproductive healthcare includes access to and safe use of medications; further,

To recognize that reproductive health services include pre-conception, conception, post-conception, and termination of pregnancies; further,

To advocate for access to safe, comprehensive reproductive healthcare for all patients, including historically underserved patient groups such as patients of color, those with limited means, and those living in rural areas; further,

To affirm that healthcare workers should be able to provide reproductive healthcare per their clinical judgment and their conscience without fear of legal consequence, workplace sanctions, social stigmatization, harassment, or harm.

Rationale

Reproductive health has been defined as "a state of complete physical, mental and social well-being and not merely the absence of disease or infirmity, in all matters relating to the reproductive system and to its functions and processes," and reproductive healthcare has been defined as "the constellation of methods, techniques and services that contribute to reproductive health and well-being by preventing and solving reproductive health problems." (International Conference on Population and Development Programme of Action, Twentieth Anniversary Edition, United Nations Population Fund, Sep 2014). In the U.S., the term "reproductive health services" is defined in 18 USC § 248(e)(5) as "medical, surgical, counselling or referral services relating to the human reproductive system, including services relating to pregnancy or the termination of a pregnancy." Reproductive health services include pre-conception, conception, post-conception care, including termination of pregnancies, and reproductive healthcare includes access to and safe use of medications.

ASHP advocates for access to safe, comprehensive reproductive healthcare for all patients, including historically underserved patient groups. Studies show that there have been longstanding disparities in access to and outcomes from reproductive health services in the U.S., especially for racial and ethnic minorities. For example, black women have the highest maternal morbidity and mortality rates in the country. These disparities include contraceptive use, reproductive cancers, preterm deliveries, and maternal morbidity and mortality. (Sutton MY, Anachebe NF, Lee R et al. Racial and ethnic disparities in reproductive health services and outcomes, 2020. *Obstet Gynecol.* 2021; 137:225–33.)

On June 24, 2022, the Supreme Court of the United States overturned Roe v. Wade, freeing states to restrict or outlaw abortion. Thirteen states had implemented trigger laws that would outlaw abortion almost immediately, and 26 states were expected to ban or severely restrict access to abortion. These state laws are likely to impact patient access to necessary treatments, including medications, and the practice of pharmacy, in the following ways:

- *Access to necessary treatments:* Pharmacists are involved in treating patients with ectopic pregnancy or pregnant patients with cancer diagnoses. These laws could limit patient access to lifesaving treatments because of the risk of legal liability for providers. Pharmacists have a role in providing medications for these treatments as well as supporting patients' mental health and well-being related to reproductive health.

- *Access to medications:* A number of companies have formed that provide telehealth access to medications used to induce abortion. There are likely to be challenges to interstate mail order of these medications. In addition, some overseas companies also provide these medications, which raises questions about foreign importation of medications. ASHP opposes wholesale importation of medications from other countries due to supply chain security concerns but does not object to patients ordering from legitimate foreign pharmacies for their personal needs. Further, medications (e.g., misoprostol) that are used off-label as abortifacients but have other clinical uses may become harder for patients to access because providers fear the legal liability for prescribing or dispensing these medications. Finally, access to medications is a national security issue. For examples, the Department of Defense is required by law to make contraceptive services available to all female active-duty service members.
- *Clinician judgment:* Restrictions on medication abortion function as limitations on clinicians' professional judgment. As noted above, because some medications can be used off-label as abortifacients, it is possible that there will be increased scrutiny of the prescribing and dispensing of certain medications. Further, some states are pursuing laws that would allow citizens a private right of action against a clinician who assists in an abortion (i.e., "bounty laws"). These laws could create civil and/or criminal liability against clinicians who prescribe or dispense abortion medications.

In addition to these concerns, other procedures that are not abortion but might result in destruction of an embryo (e.g., in vitro fertilization therapy) could fall into an uncertain legal zone. Medications used to induce labor to protect a pregnant patient could be restricted. Because the decision in *Roe v. Wade* was based on a constitutional right to privacy, other privacy-related rulings are now in question, including Griswold v. Connecticut, which allowed access to contraception.

The decision to terminate a pregnancy is a complicated, difficult, and often extremely emotional choice for patients and healthcare providers, and it often involves weighing the risks to the pregnant patient. Under some state laws, pregnant patients could be prosecuted for seeking lifesaving treatment, and healthcare providers involved in these difficult decisions and providing necessary treatments could be subject to unjust criminal prosecution. ASHP believes that healthcare workers should be able to provide reproductive healthcare per their clinical judgment and their conscience without fear of legal consequence, workplace sanctions, social stigmatization, harassment, or harm.

2254

PAIN MANAGEMENT

Source: Council on Therapeutics

To advocate for improved access to equitable and patient-centered pain care for all patient populations; further,

To advocate that pharmacists actively participate in the development and implementation of multimodal pain management stewardship programs, policies, protocols, and research; further,

To support pharmacist participation and collaboration in interprofessional healthcare teams for selecting appropriate drug therapy regimens, educating patients and caregivers, monitoring patients, and continually assessing outcomes of pain management therapy; further,

To advocate that pharmacists lead efforts to prevent inappropriate use of pain therapies, including engaging in strategies to detect and address patterns of medication use that can increase the risk of serious adverse events; further,

To foster the development of educational resources on multimodal pain therapy, substance use disorder, and prevention of adverse effects; further,

To encourage and support the education of the pharmacy workforce and other healthcare providers regarding the principles of multimodal pain management and substance use disorder, including approaches to reduce stigma, improve access to care, and improve general health and well-being.

This policy supersedes ASHP policy 1722.

Rationale

Currently there are over 100 million adults in the United States affected by acute and chronic pain. ASHP emphasizes the importance of individualized patient-centered care in the diagnosis and treatment of acute and chronic pain. A multimodal and interprofessional team approach should be implemented to target outcomes that focus on improvement in function and quality of life. Pain management requires ongoing assessment of the care plan, and pharmacists are well poised to fill a key role in appropriate treatment and optimization of pain with multimodal treatment strategies. Pain therapies, in particular, have the potential for serious adverse events. ASHP is cognizant of the delicate balance between undertreatment of pain and barriers that can occur with the implementation of strategies that restrict or limit access to treatment.

ASHP advocates increased awareness of the risks of pain therapies, and encourages pharmacists to take a lead role in implementing harm reduction strategies through individual clinician efforts (e.g., prescriber and patient education on medication risk, ensuring access to naloxone when applicable) and system-based approaches (e.g., use of information technology systems to monitor for trends that suggest unsafe prescribing or patient use). ASHP also supports the inclusion of pharmacists as key members of interprofessional care teams that specialize in pain management and stewardship. Finally, ASHP advocates for the inclusion of pharmacists in pain research as pharmacists are well poised to fill a key role in research initiatives across the spectrum of pain management.

2102

USE OF ANTIMICROBIALS IN SURGICAL WOUNDS AND PROCEDURES

Source: Council on Therapeutics

To oppose the use of antimicrobial agents in surgical wounds and procedures not based on evidence; further,

To encourage further research to assess the efficacy, safety, and risks of resistance development of antimicrobials used in surgical wounds and procedures; further,

To foster evidence-based recommendations on the use of antimicrobial agents in surgical wounds and procedures and on how to prepare those agents according to appropriate sterile practices; further,

To advocate that antimicrobial stewardship programs review and monitor the use of antimicrobial agents in surgical wounds and procedures; further,

To encourage pharmacists to educate prescribers on adverse outcomes and reactions associated with the use of antimicrobials in surgical wounds and procedures; further,

To support clear and consistent documentation of antimicrobial agents used for surgical wounds and procedures in the electronic health record.

Rationale

The addition of antimicrobials to irrigation solutions during surgical procedures in an effort to prevent surgical site infections has been a long-standing surgical practice. Antibiotics are the most common additives to surgical irrigation fluids, but recent data has shown no clinical benefit compared with saline irrigation, likely due to the mechanism of antibiotics needing a longer exposure time than is allowed during irrigation. Further, the use of topical antibiotics in the open surgical wound is often not monitored and has not been subject to any evidence-based standardization of care. When mixing practices were surveyed across hospitals and health systems, most respondents from facilities in which the solutions were mixed in the operating room (OR) were unaware of who was doing the mixing; of those who were aware, surgical scrub technicians or OR nurses were the individuals most often reported to be doing the mixing.

The results of numerous surveys of surgeons has indicated that the practice of using topical antibiotics intraoperatively, in both irrigation fluids and powders, is widespread. This practice stemmed from the belief that applying antibiotics locally would minimize toxicity and resistance. However, newer data suggest that there is a potential for toxicities and systemic exposure leading to resistance associated with these practices. Because of this, the Infectious Diseases Society of America, Society for Healthcare Epidemiology of America, Surgical Infection Society, American Society of Health-System Pharmacists, World Health Organization, American College of Surgeons, and the International Consensus on Orthopedic Infections all recommend against the use of topical antimicrobial irrigation. Despite these recommendations, this practice is still prevalent throughout hospitals and health systems. Complicating the picture is that neither the Joint Commission nor the Centers for Medicare and Medicaid Services have addressed the use of topical antibiotics.

Due to the risks of topical use and the lack of evidence supporting it, this practice should be an essential part of antimicrobial stewardship programs. All antibiotics sent from pharmacy to the OR, including those intended for topical use, should be documented clearly in the electronic health record, including type and amount used, and should be part of comprehensive surveillance for patient outcomes for surgical site infections, allergic reactions, resistance trends, management of shortages, and toxicity adverse events related to topical surgical administration of antibiotics.

2125

TOBACCO, TOBACCO PRODUCTS, AND ELECTRONIC NICOTINE DELIVERY SYSTEMS

Source: Council on Therapeutics

To discourage the use of tobacco, tobacco products, and electronic nicotine delivery systems due to their long-term adverse health effects; further,

To oppose the distribution and sale of tobacco, tobacco products, and electronic nicotine delivery systems by pharmacies or facilities that contain a pharmacy; further,

To advocate for tobacco-free environments in hospitals and health systems; further,

To promote legislation that supports pharmacist prescriptive authority for tobacco-cessation medications; further,

To promote the pharmacist's interprofessional role in tobacco-cessation counseling and comprehensive medication management; further,

To join with other interested organizations in statements and expressions of opposition to the use of tobacco, tobacco products, and electronic nicotine delivery systems; further,

To educate the public and patients on the risks of nicotine consumption through traditional and electronic delivery systems.

This policy supersedes ASHP policy 1625.

Rationale

Pharmacists, as healthcare providers, have long discouraged the use of tobacco and tobacco products as a threat to public health. Electronic nicotine delivery systems (e.g., vaporizers, vape pens, hookah pens, and electronic cigarettes and pipes) are relatively new and unregulated delivery systems for nicotine. The contents of these systems include flavorings, propylene glycol, glycerin, and other unknown ingredients, and the long-term effects of their use have not been studied. Given these uncertainties, pharmacists should discourage their use as well. In addition, ASHP opposes the distribution or sale of tobacco, tobacco products, and electronic nicotine delivery systems by pharmacies or facilities that contain a pharmacy (e.g., grocery or retail stores) and advocates that hospitals and health systems be tobacco-free environments.

Furthermore, pharmacists have a role in recommending and managing drug therapy to support cessation of nicotine-containing products, including tobacco and electronic nicotine delivery systems, as described in the ASHP Therapeutic Position Statement on Cessation of Tobacco Use. Newer therapies, including varenicline, are associated with more and evolving safety risks when compared to nicotine replacement therapies. Given the complexity of drug therapy, pharmacists should play a central role in ensuring the safe and appropriate use of these therapies.

2127

TESTING AND DOCUMENTATION OF PENICILLIN ALLERGY AS A COMPONENT OF ANTIMICROBIAL STEWARDSHIP

Source: Council on Therapeutics

To advocate that state board of pharmacy regulations include penicillin allergy skin testing under pharmacists' scope of practice; further,

To advocate involvement of pharmacists in the clarification and assessment of penicillin allergy, intolerance, and adverse drug events; further,

To advocate for documentation and de-labeling of penicillin allergies, intolerances, reactions, and severities in the medical record when appropriate to facilitate optimal antimicrobial selection; further,

To recommend the use of penicillin skin testing, graded antibiotic challenges, and oral direct challenges in appropriate candidates when clinically indicated to optimize antimicrobial selection; further,

To support the education and training of pharmacists in the assessment, management, and documentation of penicillin allergies, intolerances, and adverse events; further,

To advocate for reimbursement for pharmacists' patient care services involved in penicillin allergy skin testing; further,

To educate patients, healthcare providers, and the public about the risks of inaccurate penicillin allergy labeling and the role of pharmacists in health-record reconciliation and the value of pharmacist-driven health-record reconciliation, including penicillin skin testing.

This policy supersedes ASHP policy 1921.

Rationale

Approximately 10% of all patients in the United States report having a penicillin allergy; however, only 1 in 10 patients with a labeled penicillin allergy are truly allergic. Furthermore, approximately 80% of patients with an IgE-mediated penicillin allergy lose their sensitivity after 10 years. Specific rates of cross-reactivity between penicillins and cephalosporins vary depending on specific resources, although the likelihood of cross-reactivity is lower than previously described. Historically, it has been estimated that 10% of patients with a true penicillin allergy will experience an allergic reaction if administered a cephalosporin, but this data is from early cross-reactivity studies with potential contamination of early cephalosporin products with penicillin G. More recent data suggest cross-reactivity rates of less than 1%. Cross-reactivity is more closely associated with structurally similar R-1 side chains than with the beta-lactam ring itself.

Penicillin allergies have led to considerable public health risks and unintended consequences, including receipt of more broad-spectrum antibiotics, suboptimal therapy for infectious disease management, more antibiotic-related costs, increased risk of adverse effects, and increased risk of methicillin-resistant *Staphylococcus aureus* and *Clostridioides difficile*. As such, structured and thorough interview assessments with appropriate documentation and de-labeling of penicillin allergies are necessary to combat these potential negative consequences of labeled penicillin allergies. Penicillin skin testing and graded or oral challenges are excellent opportunities to assist in the assessment and delabeling of penicillin allergies. Although pharmacists are well positioned to be involved in these processes, state boards of pharmacy have different regulations regarding whether penicillin skin testing is within pharmacists' scope of practice. Penicillin allergy assessment, management, and documentation are excellent opportunities to improve pharmacist involvement in patient care and to improve antimicrobial stewardship initiatives for health systems, and offer a potential opportunity for pharmacists to bill for their services.

The American Academy of Allergy, Asthma, and Immunology, as part of the Choosing Wisely campaign, recommends against the overuse of non-beta-lactam antibiotics in patients with a history of penicillin allergy, without appropriate evaluation. In a research abstract from the Canadian Society of Allergy and Clinical Immunology meeting in 2014, researchers found that only 15% of hospital-discharged patients notified a family physician of a negative penicillin allergy evaluation; at the same time, 30% were still listed as penicillin allergic upon readmission to the hospital. Additionally, the existence of a pharmacist-provided allergy skin test has proven to positively impact patient care by optimizing antibiotic regimens and accelerate discharges for patients while reducing healthcare costs.

2135

ROLE OF THE PHARMACY WORKFORCE IN PANDEMIC PREPAREDNESS AND RESPONSE

Source: Council on Pharmacy Practice

To advocate that all healthcare organizations include pandemic preparedness in emergency preparedness planning; further,

To encourage all healthcare organizations to be actively engaged with their regional healthcare coalitions and to promote collaboration and communication among healthcare workers, healthcare organizations, government agencies, industry, and other stakeholders in pandemic preparedness and response; further,

To promote pharmacy workforce involvement in networks at the federal, state, local, and institutional levels for emergency response; further,

To advocate that pharmacy personnel be included as leaders on teams responsible for pandemic preparedness planning and response at the federal, state, local, and institutional levels, and that they integrate such planning into emergency preparedness planning for their workplaces; further,

To encourage all healthcare organizations to establish criteria for evidence-based medication-use decisions, even when such evidence is scarce, incomplete, or conflicting, and recognize the unique role that pharmacy personnel have in ensuring the safe and effective use of medications based on best available evidence and resources; further,

To advocate that healthcare organizations recognize the unique and collective stress a pandemic places on healthcare workers and provide suitable resources to maintain workers' well-being and resilience; further,

To support research on and provide resources and education to aid the pharmacy workforce in preparing for and responding to pandemics.

Rationale

ASHP has long advocated "that hospital and health-system pharmacists must assertively exercise their responsibilities in preparing for and responding to disasters, and the leaders of emergency planning at the federal, regional, state, and local levels must call on pharmacists to participate in the full range of issues related to pharmaceuticals." (ASHP Statement on Emergency Preparedness)

The Coronavirus Disease 2019 (COVID-19) global pandemic differs from other types of disasters in significant respects, testing the resiliency of the healthcare system and workforce. Treating patients with a novel viral pathogen has driven rapid evolution in therapies, forcing healthcare providers to make patient care decisions based on scarce, incomplete, or conflicting information. These decisions have sometimes been complicated by shortages of crucial drugs, equipment, or staff, creating a crisis standard of care in which difficult patient care decisions must be made. The patient surges that healthcare organizations have had to manage have lasted significantly longer than those of other disasters. Healthcare workers have faced stressful patient care situations and extended shifts for a longer period of time than in other disasters. In addition, the fear of infection and of spreading that infection to family members and others has added additional stress. Infection control procedures have shut down some areas of healthcare operations, forcing healthcare workers into unfamiliar roles and care settings.

ASHP advocates that the lessons learned from the COVID-19 pandemic be shared broadly and incorporated into emergency planning at the federal, state, local, institutional, and pharmacy department levels. All healthcare organizations should be actively engaged with their regional healthcare coalitions, and pharmacy leaders, with their unique understanding of medication-use processes, should be relied upon to provide strategic direction on the full range of issues related to medication use, especially when evidence is scarce, incomplete, or conflicting, and drugs or other critical resources are in shortage. The pharmacy workforce should incorporate the lessons learned in its emergency planning efforts, integrating those efforts into the efforts of emergency response networks at the federal, state, local, and institutional levels. ASHP pledges to promote collaboration and communication among the various stakeholders in pandemic preparedness and response, and to provide resources and education to aid the pharmacy workforce and others in preparing for and responding to pandemics, including resources regarding novel therapies, shortages of drugs and other critical supplies, and healthcare worker well-being and resilience.

2136

ROLE OF THE PHARMACY WORKFORCE IN SUPPORTING PATIENT ACCESS TO MEDICAL SUPPLIES

Source: Council on Pharmacy Practice

To support patient access to medical supplies as part of a comprehensive treatment plan; further,

To advocate for policies that empower pharmacy personnel to facilitate patient access to and effective use of medical supplies, including reimbursement policies; further,

To educate pharmacists, other healthcare professionals, payers, and policymakers about the role of pharmacy personnel in helping patients obtain and use medical supplies; further,

To collaborate with other healthcare professional and patient advocacy organizations to advocate for expanded patient access to medical supplies.

For purposes of this policy, "medical supplies" includes durable medical equipment, Food and Drug Administration-approved medical devices, and other nondurable disposable healthcare materials.

Rationale

Pharmacists and pharmacy technicians have the knowledge and skills to support patient access to medical supplies and equipment, durable medical equipment (DME), and medical devices. These tools, like medications, are essential components to a patient's personalized care plan. Although many providers combine medical supplies and equipment, DME, and medical devices under the umbrella term "medical supplies," as is done here for purposes of this policy, there are critical differences between them that determine how these items are accessed and reimbursed. Under Centers for Medicare & Medicaid Services (CMS) rules, "medical supplies and equipment" (e.g., bandages and gauzes) are nondurable disposable healthcare materials used to serve a medical purpose that cannot be used in the absence of illness or injury or repeatedly by different individuals. CMS typically does not consider medical supplies and equipment as a covered benefit. DME (e.g., blood sugar monitors, blood sugar test strips, continuous glucose monitors, and infusion pumps and supplies) are durable healthcare materials used at home that can withstand repeated use, provide a medical purpose, and are not used in the absence of an illness or injury. In contrast to medical supplies and equipment, DME is covered under Medicare Part B. Finally, the Food and Drug Administration (FDA) defines a medical device as an instrument, apparatus, implement, machine, contrivance, implant, in vitro reagent, or other similar or related article, including a component part, or accessory (FDA. Medical Devices. Available at: **https://www.fda.gov/medical-devices**. Accessed August 20, 2020).

Pharmacists are experts in initiating and managing a patient's comprehensive medication management (CMM) plan. A CMM is an individualized care plan that helps patients achieve specific goals of therapy. The patient-centered medical home: integrating comprehensive medication management to optimize patient outcomes resource guide, 2nd ed. (**www.pcpcc.org/sites/default/files/media/medmanagement.pdf**). Any intervention that supplements medication goals and improves a patient's quality of life and patient outcomes should be considered in the CMM process and plan, including use of medical supplies and equipment, DME, and medical devices, and provide an opportunity for a pharmacist or pharmacy technician to improve patient care.

ASHP has long advocated for the role pharmacists have in helping patients obtain and properly use drug delivery systems and devices. The ASHP Statement on the Pharmacist's Role with Respect to Drug Delivery Systems and Administration Devices states:

> Pharmacists bear a substantial responsibility for ensuring optimal clinical outcomes from drug therapy and are suited by education, training, clinical expertise, and practice activities to assume responsibility for the professional supervision of drug delivery systems and administration devices. As a natural extension of efforts to optimize drug use, pharmacists should participate in organizational and clinical decisions with regard to these systems and devices.

Extension of those responsibilities to medication-related medical supplies and equipment, DME, and medical devices is a natural progression in pharmacist patient care. There are many actions that pharmacists can implement to help improve patient outcomes in regards to medical supplies and equipment, DME, and medical devices. To increase patient access, pharmacists can collaborate with patients and physicians to determine which device to use based on patient indication, preferences, and product specifications. Pharmacists could also collaborate with CMS and other insurance plans to ensure that patients have adequate coverage of DME along with advocating to allow pharmacists to submit claims for reimbursement. Furthermore, ASHP could collaborate with patient advocacy organizations and disease specific organizations (e.g., American Diabetes Association) to advocate for increased patient access to specific medical supplies and equipment.

Additionally, pharmacists can advocate for broader pharmacy management of medical supplies and equipment, DME, and medical devices along with medications as a part of the patient's CMM plan. Pharmacists can support patient access through documentation required for coverage, provide education on how to use the device, monitor the device for safety and efficacy, and interpret results if applicable. Collaborative practice agreements and credentialing and privileging are two ways pharmacists can use data provided from the devices to help make necessary changes to the patient's medication plan. Pharmacists' expertise should be leveraged to help patients procure and manage their medical supplies and equipment, DME, and medical devices to provide all-encompassing comprehensive medication management.

2001

SAFETY AND EFFECTIVENESS OF ETHANOL FOR PREVENTION OR TREATMENT OF ALCOHOL WITHDRAWAL SYNDROME

Source: Council on Therapeutics

To oppose the use of oral or intravenous ethanol for the prevention or treatment of alcohol withdrawal syndrome (AWS) because of its poor effectiveness and safety profile; further,

To support hospital and health-system efforts that prohibit the use of oral or intravenous ethanol therapies to prevent or treat AWS; further,

To support the removal of oral or intravenous ethanol from hospital and health systems for the prevention and treatment of AWS; further,

To educate clinicians about evidence-based therapies for AWS.

This policy supersedes ASHP policy 1514.

Rationale

AWS can delay patient recovery and interfere with response to therapy. Based on a review of the available evidence, including treatment guidelines from the American Society of Addiction Medicine (ASAM), ASHP opposes the use of oral or intravenous ethanol to prevent or treat AWS. Limited and conflicting evidence of effectiveness, inability to achieve accurate and consistent dosing and blood levels, and the availability of safer and more effective therapies are among the reasons to oppose use of ethanol to prevent or treat AWS symptoms. Benzodiazepines are the preferred drugs for the treatment of AWS, along with other supportive and adjunctive therapies as clinically appropriate. Guidelines from the American Association of Family Physicians recommend benzodiazepines on a fixed schedule for AWS, outpatient detoxification, and enrollment in an alcohol treatment program. ASHP supports efforts to prohibit use of ethanol for AWS and advocates education to a variety of healthcare practitioner audiences to increase awareness of appropriate evidence-based therapies.

2003

ANTICANCER TREATMENT PARITY

Source: Council on Therapeutics

To support anticancer treatment parity legislation at both the state and federal level that ensures equality of access and insurance coverage for all anticancer drug products approved by the Food and Drug Administration (FDA); further,

To advocate all insurers and manufacturers design plans containing limits on out-of-pocket expenditure so that patient cost sharing for anticancer treatment is equivalent, regardless of treatment modality or route of administration; further,

To encourage the development of policies and endorse practices that contribute to a decrease in anticancer treatment costs to the consumer; further,

To continue to foster the development of best practices, including adherence monitoring strategies, and education on the safe use and management of anticancer agents, regardless of route of administration.

This policy supersedes ASHP policy 1516.

Rationale

An estimated $200 billion will be spent on cancer care by 2020, and a recent survey showed if faced with a cancer diagnosis, 57% of Americans say they would be most concerned about either the financial impact on their families or about paying for treatment. Additionally, there is an increase in insurance premiums, co-pays, co-insurance, and deductibles. Most insured cancer patients in the U.S. are responsible for a portion of the cost of their anticancer agents, which can be significant. The average out-of-pocket expense for Medicare patients with cancer is 23.7% of household income. Cancer survivors are 2.7 times more likely to file for bankruptcy.

Traditionally, intravenous (IV) and injected treatments were the primary methods of chemotherapy delivery. Patient-administered anticancer agents have become more prevalent and are now the standard of care for many types of cancer. Oral anticancer agents account for approximately 35% of the oncology development pipeline. Many oral anticancer agents do not have infusible or injectable alternatives, and are the only treatment option for some cancer diagnoses. Oral agents have been embraced because of convenience, efficacy, and safety, but because insurers cover them differently than intravenous drugs, prescribing oral anticancer agents can impose burdensome levels of cost-sharing on patients.

While IV anticancer treatments are covered under a health plan's medical benefit, often requiring patients to pay a minimal co-pay or no cost at all for the medication, oral anticancer agents are usually covered under the pharmacy benefits. This results in increased out-of-pocket costs. Cost sharing of oral specialty drugs has increased from 3% in 2004 to 25% in 2013, and continues to rise.

The impact of rising out-of-pocket prescription costs for cancer patients can negatively affect adherence and subsequently treatment outcomes. Co-pays can be hundreds or thousands of dollars per month and, as a result, almost 10% of patients choose not to fill their initial prescriptions for oral anticancer agents. A study of claims data from more than 38,000 people who received a new prescription for one of 38 oral anticancer agents from 2014 to 2015 found that, as out of-pocket costs rose, fewer patients filled their prescriptions. When the required co-pay was less than $10, only 10% of patients failed to pick up their prescriptions. This increased to 32% for patients whose out-of-pocket costs were between $100 and $500, and to 41% when costs were between $500 and $2000. When the out-of-pocket costs exceeded $2000, nearly half of patients (49%) never filled their prescriptions. Delayed initiation of treatment was also significantly higher for those with higher cost-sharing burdens.

Oral parity is a proposed legislative solution to alleviate coverage discrepancies between oral and intravenous anticancer agents. Parity laws are currently state laws designed to ensure that orally administered agents for treating cancer are not more costly for patients than anticancer agents given via infusion at a clinic or hospital. At this point, 43 states and Washington, DC, have enacted parity laws that require patients to pay no more for an oral cancer treatment than they would for an infusion.

However, state parity laws only apply to certain commercial health insurance plans, including those purchased by small groups and individuals. Self-funded patients, patients covered by health plans that fall under federal law (large, multi-state health plans), or those covered by Medicare and other federally funded insurance plans are not eligible. An estimated fifty percent of cancer patients are currently not protected under state parity laws.

The Cancer Drug Parity Act of 2019 (H.R. 1730, introduced on March 13th, 2019; formerly introduced in 2017 as H.R. 1409) would require any health plan that currently provides coverage for cancer treatment to provide coverage for self-administered anticancer agents at a cost no less favorable than the cost of IV, port-administered, or injected anticancer agents.

There may be false patient perception that oral anticancer agents are less dangerous than IV chemotherapy, furthering supporting the important role of the pharmacist in educating the patients about the agent, its adverse effects, how to manage toxicities, and when to contact their healthcare team. Pharmacists monitor oral chemotherapy treatments to prevent medication and food interactions, adverse drug reactions, and medication errors. Pharmacists are also positioned to play an integral role in shared decision-making and assisting with procurement.

Treatment of cancer also continues to evolve, and many agents may not fall under the category of traditional chemotherapy (e.g., biologic agents, antimicrobials, and others). As a result, practitioners and legislatures have moved away from the singular term chemotherapy and use chemotherapy, anticancer and cancer drug interchangeably, with anticancer being the preferred term.

2009

ROLE OF THE PHARMACY WORKFORCE IN IDENTIFYING AND CARING FOR VICTIMS OF HUMAN TRAFFICKING

Source: Council on Pharmacy Practice

To recognize that human trafficking is a significant public health problem in the U.S.; further,

To affirm that the pharmacy workforce has important roles in identifying and caring for victims of human trafficking; further,

To foster education, training, and the development of resources to prepare the pharmacy workforce for their roles in identifying and caring for victims of human trafficking.

Rationale

The U.S. Department of Health and Human Services Office on Trafficking in Persons (OTIP) describes human trafficking as a form of modern slavery that "occurs when a trafficker exploits an individual with force, fraud, or coercion to make them perform commercial sex or work." OTIP outlines two types of trafficking: labor trafficking, in which individuals are compelled to work or provide services; and sex trafficking, in which "adults are compelled to engage in commercial sex by force, fraud, or coercion or minors are compelled to perform a commercial sex act regardless of the presence of force, fraud, or coercion."

Combating human trafficking is one of the central goals of the American Hospital Association Hospitals Against Violence Initiative. All healthcare providers have a role in identifying and caring for victims of human trafficking. These roles include recognizing indicators of human trafficking; being aware of common healthcare issues faced by human trafficking victims; providing for a patient's medical and nonmedical needs while providing a safe and comfortable environment; complying with applicable laws regarding reporting of suspected human trafficking, including child abuse; and providing care and resources for survivors of human trafficking.

2017

ROLE OF THE PHARMACY WORKFORCE IN PREVENTING ACCIDENTAL AND INTENTIONAL FIREARM INJURY AND DEATH

Source: Council on Pharmacy Practice

To recognize that accidental and intentional firearm injury and death in the U.S. is a public health crisis; further,

To affirm that the pharmacy workforce has important roles in the comprehensive public health and medical approach to reducing death and disability from firearm injury.

Rationale

A formulary is a continually updated list of medications and related information, representing the clinical judgment of pharmacists, physicians, and other experts in the diagnosis and treatment of disease and promotion of health. A formulary includes, but is not limited to, a list of medications, standardized medication concentrations, and medication-associated products or devices, medication-use policies, important ancillary drug information, decision-support tools, and organizational guidelines. The multiplicity of medications available, the complexities surrounding their safe and effective use, and differences in their relative value make it necessary for healthcare organizations to have medication-use policies that promote rational, evidence-based, clinically appropriate, safe, and cost-effective medication therapy. The formulary system is the ongoing process through which a healthcare organization establishes policies on the use of drugs, therapies, and drug-related products and identifies those that are most medically appropriate and cost-effective to best serve the health interests of a given patient population.

As described in more detail in the ASHP Statement on the Pharmacy and Therapeutics Committee and the Formulary System, a fundamental characteristic of the formulary system is that all decisions are made based on factors that result in optimal patient care, include the involvement of appropriate healthcare professionals, and are not based solely on economic factors.

Formulary management techniques may differ under an integrated or network system versus an individual healthcare entity. Standardized drug formularies within integrated health systems increase coordination complexity, but help drive standardized medication use processes across sites of care.

Additionally, insurance coverage of medications should not interfere with the safe and effective provision of care. For example, some hospitals are currently being forced to administer a specific payer-preferred biosimilar drug to a covered patient, which requires hospitals to stock a different product for each payer and then ensure the correct one is dispensed. This costly and resource-intensive practice also has medication safety implications and negatively affects supply chain efficiency. Biosimilar drugs are considered to be therapeutically equivalent, but the current Food and Drug Administration (FDA) approval process does not include a determination of interchangeability between reference and biosimilar products. Because the substitution of a biosimilar for a reference product is a decision outside the FDA regulatory process, it is therefore a matter of state pharmacy law. The obligation to have a specific payer-preferred biosimilar results in hospitals and health systems devoting significant resources to procure, store, label, and dispense payer-preferred biosimilars. This duplication adds complexity to the medication-use process, and as more biosimilars become available, the potential for harmful medication errors will increase. The use of biosimilars was a key cost-reduction concept in the Affordable Care Act. However, in May 2018, the price linkage cost-reduction concept within Medicare Part B was rescinded. Going forward, reimbursement will be based on the specific biosimilar product pricing. The full impact of this change for individual healthcare organizations will depend on patient and payer mix. Biosimilars that are priced at a lower acquisition cost compared to the innovator product are likely to stagnate or lose market share due to a low reimbursement margin. As a result, pricing of biosimilars may increase to make the reimbursement margin competitive with the innovator product, leaving healthcare organizations in search of other cost reduction opportunities.

2018

SAFE USE OF TRANSDERMAL SYSTEM PATCHES

Source: Council on Pharmacy Practice

To encourage hospitals and health systems to implement policies and procedures to ensure safe use of transdermal system patches; further,

To advocate for enhanced patient and consumer education and product safety requirements for transdermal system patches; further,

To encourage manufacturers of transdermal system patches to collaborate with pharmacists and other stakeholders to identify and implement packaging, labeling, and formulation changes that prevent accidental exposure and facilitate safe disposal.

This policy supersedes ASHP policy 1404.

Rationale

There have been many reports of errors associated with and abuse or misuse of transdermal system patches. Pharmacists are in a unique position to improve the safe use of these products by encouraging implementation of best practices such as electronic health record builds; regular nursing checks for transdermal patches; and policies for ordering, handling, and disposal of these products. Better patient and consumer education specific to this unique dosage form, especially for outpatient use, is also an important component of safe use. Manufacturers could also take additional steps to prevent misuse of these products by collaborating with pharmacists and other stakeholders to identify and implement packaging, labeling, and formulation changes that would facilitate safe disposal and prevent accidental exposure.

2029

PRESERVING PATIENT ACCESS TO PHARMACY SERVICES BY MEDICALLY UNDERSERVED POPULATIONS

Source: Council on Pharmacy Management

To advocate for funding and innovative payment models to preserve patient access to acute and ambulatory care pharmacy services by rural or medically underserved populations; further,

To support the use of telehealth to maintain pharmacy operations and pharmacist-led comprehensive medication management that extend patient care services to and enhance continuity of care for rural or medically underserved populations; further,

To advocate that the advanced communication technologies required for telehealth be available to rural or medically underserved populations; further,

To advocate for funding of loan forgiveness or incentive programs that recruit pharmacists and pharmacy technicians to practice in rural or medically underserved populations.

Rationale

Medically Underserved Areas (MUAs) and Medically Underserved Populations (MUPs) are areas or populations designated by the Health Resources and Services Administration as having too few primary care providers, high infant mortality, high poverty, or a high elderly population. Whereas MUAs are a geographic designation, MUPs have a shortage of primary care health services for a specific population subset within an established geographic area. MUPs may face economic, cultural, or linguistic barriers to healthcare; examples include low-income, Medicaid-eligible, homeless, migrant or seasonal worker, or Native American populations. Many federal programs use different types of shortage designations to determine eligibility. The Health Center Program and Physician J-1 Visa Waiver Program, for example, use both MUA and MUP, whereas the CMS Rural Health Clinic Program only uses MUA. Trends within the healthcare industry are also increasing the number of MUPs. Waning interest in primary care practice among medical graduates and the fiscal challenges of providing care in areas with declining populations or fewer insured patients contribute to this problem.

Increasing hospital closures are not a recent phenomenon-rural areas have been closing hospitals for decades. For instance, 140 rural hospitals closed between 1985 and 1988 after the implementation of Medicare's Inpatient Prospective Payment System. This payment model led to large Medicare losses and increased financial distress for many rural hospitals, ultimately resulting in numerous hospital closings.

Today, many rural hospitals are facing a similar fate. Nationally, 430 rural hospitals are at high financial risk due to low reimbursement rates and decreasing local populations. These factors make it difficult for hospitals to cover fixed costs, let alone remain up to date with technological advances and emerging healthcare practices.

Since 2010, 99 hospitals in rural areas and MUAs in the U.S. have closed. Between 2013 and 2017 alone, 64 rural hospitals closed, which is more than twice as many as the previous 5-year period. Hospital closures disproportionality affected rural hospitals in the South (64% of rural hospital closures) and are more prevalent in states that did not expand Medicaid coverage. It is estimated that hundreds more hospitals are at risk of closing; therefore, the impact of these closures on access to and continuity of care should be assessed.

Although hospital closures in rural areas have numerous consequences, reduced access to care for the populations served is the most obvious one. An analysis by the Medicare Payment Advisory Commission determined that one third of hospitals that have closed since 2013 are more than 20 miles from the next closest hospital. An issue brief published by The Kaiser Commission on Medicaid and the Uninsured found a major impact of hospital closure to be loss of access to emergency care in the community; more specifically, a lack of access for people with acute mental health or addiction treatment needs was found.

Other consequences of rural hospital closures are focused around accessibility of physicians and other healthcare providers. Regardless of hospital closures, rural communities commonly struggle to recruit and retain healthcare providers. Retention of these providers becomes increasingly difficult when a hospital closes due to providers relocating to an alternative hospital or clinic location. As a result, communities are often left without vital healthcare providers and exacerbated gaps in access to specialty care. For instance, specialists who visited the local hospital on a regular basis become unavailable to residents in the area after the hospital closes, or residents lose their access point for referrals to subspecialists. In addition, once hospitals close other resources dwindle, such as home health, pharmacy, hospice, and emergency medical services care, thus leading to hospital deserts and a dramatic decrease in access to and continuity of care for residents.

With the number of hospital deserts increasing, residents are forced to seek care elsewhere, if at all. In a 2018 Government Accountability Office report, elderly and low-income populations were more likely to be negatively impacted by rural hospital closures, and these populations were also found to be more likely to delay or forgo care after a hospital closure if the patient had to travel longer distances.

It is important to note that not all rural hospital closures lead to a complete depletion in access to care for residents. There has been some success with transitions to community-based primary care following a hospital closure. In this scenario local residents still have access to primary care services, but not necessarily critical services, such as those necessary for cardiac arrest or stroke. Currently there is no systematic approach to determine which services are critical to provide locally or virtually, and not every hospital closing can be smoothly transitioned into a primary care facility to address residents' healthcare needs.

2035

ROLE OF THE PHARMACY WORKFORCE IN VIOLENCE PREVENTION

Source: Council on Pharmacy Practice

To recognize that violence in the U.S. is a public health crisis; further,

To affirm that the pharmacy workforce has important roles in a comprehensive public health and medical approach to violence prevention, including leadership roles in their communities and workplaces; further,

To encourage members of the pharmacy workforce to seek out opportunities to engage in violence prevention efforts in their communities and workplaces; further,

To promote collaboration between the pharmacy workforce and community and healthcare organizations in violence prevention efforts; further,

To foster education, training, and the development of resources to prepare the pharmacy workforce for their roles in violence prevention; further,

To support research and dissemination of information on the effectiveness of pharmacy-focused violence-prevention strategies.

Rationale

The World Health Organization defines violence as "the intentional use of physical force or power, threatened or actual, against oneself, another person, or against a group or community, that either results in or has a high likelihood of resulting in injury, death, psychological harm, maldevelopment or deprivation." The Centers for Disease Control and Prevention (CDC) reports that in the U.S. 7 people die a violent death each hour—47,000 from suicide and 19,500 from homicide annually—and a 2015 report found more than 2.5 million violence-related injuries annually. The CDC estimates that violence costs the U.S. $9 billion annually in medical costs and lost work, and a separate estimate places the cost of violence as a whole to U.S. hospitals and health systems at $2.7 billion dollars in 2016. The staggering human loss and soaring costs have led numerous organizations of healthcare and public health professionals to label violence a public health crisis and take action to address violence as a public health problem. One prominent example is the American Hospital Association Hospitals Against Violence Initiative, which provides examples and best practices to address its three central topics: workforce and workplace violence, combating human trafficking, and preventing youth violence.

ASHP believes that members of the pharmacy workforce have "a responsibility to participate in global, national, state, regional, and institutional efforts to promote public health" and that the pharmacy workforce has important roles in primary, secondary, and tertiary interventions to prevent violence. The CDC National Center for Injury Prevention and Control, Division of Violence Prevention states that the different forms of violence they identify—child abuse and neglect, youth violence, intimate partner violence, sexual violence, elder abuse, and suicidal behavior—are strongly connected and share common risk and protective factors. Interventions the pharmacy workforce could be involved in include but are not limited to:

- Improving access to mental health services, including treatment for substance use disorder

- Screening to identify victims of or individuals at risk of violence
- Providing trauma informed care
- Providing lethal means counseling
- Supporting hotlines and community support systems for people in crisis
- Providing or promoting Stop-the-Bleed bystander training
- Participating in or promoting community- or hospital-based violence prevention organizations

To fill these important roles, members of the pharmacy workforce will need appropriate education, training, and resources. Although some education, training, and resources are appropriate for different healthcare providers, ASHP is committed to the development of resources to prepare the pharmacy workforce for pharmacy-specific roles in violence prevention and to supporting research and dissemination of information on the effectiveness of pharmacy-focused violence-prevention strategies. In addition, institutional and community leaders need to be aware of the pharmacy workforce's commitment to preventing violence. ASHP is committed to raising awareness with other stakeholders of the profession's commitment to collaborate to end the cycle of violence in their institutions and communities.

2041

SAFETY OF INTRANASAL ROUTE AS AN ALTERNATIVE ROUTE OF ADMINISTRATION

Source: Council on Therapeutics

To encourage the development of institutional guidance and advocate for further research on the pharmacokinetic and pharmacodynamic characteristics of drugs not approved for intranasal administration; further,

To foster the development of educational resources on the safety of intranasal administration of drugs not approved for that route; further,

To encourage manufacturers to develop intranasal formulations in ready-to-use devices.

This policy supersedes ASHP policy 1601.

Rationale

Intranasal administration can be used for systemic drug delivery and is the delivery route of choice in specific circumstances. Intranasal administration is often the route of choice in the emergency department due to access issues, safety concerns, and the characteristics of specific patient populations (e.g., children). Soluble drugs such as naloxone can be converted for intranasal administration without altering the substance simply by use of an aerosolizer. The intranasal route is frequently used to treat pain when oral and intravenous routes are not optimal, and intranasal midazolam is often used for sedation in the pediatric population, although that route of administration has not been approved by the Food and Drug Administration. Certain rescue medications such as naloxone can also be administered intranasally and may be preferred for intravenous drug users. Vaccines are also commonly administered via the intranasal route.

Because many of these drugs are not approved for intranasal administration, there are varying degrees of evidence for use in specific cases. There is also varying evidence regarding the degree of systemic absorption of intranasally administered drugs that are not formulated for that route. A large number of characteristics may affect systemic distribution from the intranasal route, such as the presence of preservatives and viscosity of the agents. Given the interest in and potential benefits of intranasal administration, further research on the pharmacokinetics and pharmacodynamics of that route is needed.

In recent years, intranasal administration has become a part of routine practice, but a pre-made, ready-to-administer device has not been developed. Medication is often administered through an ancillary device such as an atomizer to optimize delivery, but these devices are not always available and have been on backorder in the past. By encouraging manufactures to develop intranasal formulations in ready-to-use devices, patient-specific doses could be administered, allowing patients or caregivers to administer medications in a less-invasive or labor-intensive method.

1901

SUICIDE AWARENESS AND PREVENTION

Source: Council on Education and Workforce Development, Council on Pharmacy Management, Council on Pharmacy Practice, Council on Public Policy, and Council on Therapeutics

To support the goal of zero suicides; further,

To collaborate with key stakeholders in support of suicide awareness and prevention; further,

To acknowledge that optimal suicide awareness and prevention efforts focus both on patients and on the healthcare workforce; further,

To recognize that pharmacists, as key providers on the patient care team, are integral to suicide awareness and prevention efforts, and to acknowledge the vital role of other members of the pharmacy workforce in those efforts; further,

To foster the use and development of clinically validated tools to aid the pharmacy workforce in assessing the influence of medications and other factors on suicidality; further,

To provide education that assists the pharmacy workforce in their continuing professional development efforts related to suicide awareness and prevention; further,

To support the inclusion of suicide awareness and prevention principles throughout pharmacy curricula and postgraduate educational and training programs; further,

To encourage efforts that support universal education and training of healthcare providers in suicide awareness and prevention; further,

To advocate for adequate government and healthcare organization funding for suicide awareness and prevention; further,

To enhance awareness of local, state, and national suicide awareness and prevention resources, including the National Suicide Prevention Lifeline funded by the Substance Abuse and Mental Health Services Administration; further,

To foster education and research on suicide awareness and prevention.

Rationale

The high and increasing number of suicides in the U.S. has created a call for national action. The U.S. Surgeon General and the National Action Alliance for Suicide Prevention, in the 2012 National Strategy for Suicide Prevention, provided general guidance for various societal approaches, including public awareness and development of effective clinical practices targeting suicide prevention. The National Strategy set an aspirational zero suicides goal for healthcare services, which will require a system-wide effort to improve healthcare's approach to suicide prevention, including clinician training and implementation of better referral systems.

The responsibility for healthcare professionals to become involved in suicide prevention extends beyond those specializing in mental health services, as suicide may be viewed as a response to multiple biological, psychological, interpersonal, environmental, and societal influences that interact with one another and may change over time. Suicide prevention, when viewed as the collective efforts of government, public and private organizations, and care providers to reduce the incidence of suicide, requires a correspondingly broad response by healthcare professionals. In 2016, the Joint Commission published a Sentinel Event Alert urging healthcare organizations to develop policies, staff education, and comprehensive care plans to utilize suicide risk assessment tools and support patients with suicide risk factors. The Joint Commission urged all healthcare organizations to develop clinical environment readiness by identifying, developing, and integrating comprehensive behavioral health, primary care, and community resources to assure continuity of care for individuals at risk for suicide.

In addition, concern over drug-associated suicidal ideation and behavior has been increasing over the last decade. In 2012, the Food and Drug Administration (FDA) issued draft guidance on assessing the occurrence of suicidal ideation and behavior in clinical drug trials. Over 800 drugs have been linked to an increased risk of suicidal thoughts and depression, from central nervous system agents to antimicrobials. The ASHP Medications and Suicidality Web Resource Center contains guidelines and publications concerning drug-associated suicidality and maintains links to information on individual drugs associated with depression and suicidality.

ASHP encourages continued research on suicidal ideation and behavior in clinical trials and supports safety measures by manufacturers and FDA (e.g., risk evaluation and mitigation strategies, boxed warnings) when appropriate.

Given the leading role of pharmacists in overseeing safe medication use, the dangers of medications relating to suicide risk, and the high degree of pharmacist interaction with patients, pharmacists are well positioned to play a key role in suicide awareness and prevention efforts. The pharmacist's role could include, for example, ensuring appropriate use of medications in management of mental health and other medical conditions; identifying patients at risk for suicide, and evaluating that suicide risk; and recommending care, making referrals, and following up on referrals with patients and providers. Strategies could range from evaluating patients' prescribed medications and identifying those that increase risk for suicidality; to counseling patients, caregivers, and other healthcare providers about those risks; to educating the public about the dangers of unused medications and the need for proper disposal. Clinical pharmacy specialists trained in behavioral health could also be incorporated into behavioral health programs to serve as a resource to the healthcare team. Other pharmacy practitioners (student pharmacists and pharmacy technicians) could perform vital services in suicide awareness and prevention efforts as well, such as medication reviews. The goal of zero suicides will also require a combined effort from individual healthcare workers and the healthcare system as a whole to sustain clinician well-being and resilience, as further described in ASHP policy 1825, Clinician Well-Being and Resilience.

To ensure that pharmacy practitioners have the competence and confidence to properly fill these key roles, ASHP is committed to providing education and tools to assist pharmacy practitioners in suicide awareness and prevention efforts. Further, ASHP advocates inclusion of suicide awareness and prevention in college of pharmacy curricula and postgraduate educational and training programs, through a multimodal approach. ASHP also advocates universal suicide awareness and prevention training for healthcare providers, including pharmacists, via mandatory state education requirements and other means. Adequate government and private-sector funding of suicide awareness and prevention efforts will be required to promote the success of suicide awareness and prevention efforts. ASHP joins other organizations in supporting efforts to promote awareness of local, state, and national suicide awareness and prevention resources, including the National Suicide Prevention Lifeline (1-800-273-TALK [8255]), with the ultimate goal of making the Lifeline number as memorable as the 911 emergency hotline. The Lifeline, accessible via phone and chat (https://suicidepreventionlifeline.org/), is a national network of 150 local crisis centers that provides free and confidential emotional support to people in suicidal crisis or emotional distress 24 hours a day, 7 days a week. Finally, ASHP urges research on suicide awareness and prevention, including research on patient assessment tools, the role of genomic testing in drug approval and patient care, and practice models and strategies to identify and manage patients at risk for suicide.

1910

THERAPEUTIC USE OF CANNABIDIOL

Source: Council on Therapeutics

To support continued research and to provide education on the therapeutic uses, adverse effects, and drug interactions of cannabidiol (CBD); further,

To oppose use of CBD-containing products not regulated by the Food and Drug Administration; further,

To advocate for enhanced public education regarding safe use of CBD-containing products.

Rationale

In June 2018, the Food and Drug Administration (FDA) approved Epidiolex, an oral solution containing cannabidiol (CBD), for the treatment of seizures associated with Lennox-Gastaut syndrome and Dravet syndrome, in patients two years of age and older. Epidiolex is the first prescription formulation of a highly purified component of the Cannabis sativa plant. Because it does not contain a significant amount of tetrahydrocannabinol, the intoxicating substance in Cannabis sativa, in September 2018 the Drug Enforcement Administration placed Epidiolex in schedule V of the Controlled Substances Act (CSA), the least restrictive schedule of the Act.

Given the patchwork of state legislation regarding recreational and medical cannabis, there is a robust but largely unregulated industry in cannabis derivatives, including products promoted as containing CBD. These formulations range from lotions for topical application to oils for enteral consumption, and their components and CBD concentrations vary, leading to questions about their safety. FDA has issued over 40 warning letters to firms marketing products that allegedly contain CBD. As part of these actions, FDA has tested the chemical content of cannabinoid compounds in some of the products, finding that many do not contain the levels of CBD claimed.

With CBD's easy availability came spurious claims regarding its efficacy in treating a number of maladies. Faced with the unique challenge of regulating an approved drug and widely available formulations of a similar product, FDA is currently considering a two-pronged approach that would:

1. Regulate products that make therapeutic claims as new drugs, evaluating them for both safety and efficacy (e.g., Epidiolex)
2. Allow the continued marketing of CBD-containing products that do not make therapeutic claims, with limited regulation for safety (e.g., as dietary supplements)

ASHP opposes use of CBD-containing products not regulated by FDA in research and patient care. Further, due to concerns that patients may substitute unapproved cannabis-derivative products for the FDA-approved drug or confuse the two, ASHP advocates for enhanced patient and public education regarding safe use of CBD-containing products, and encourages pharmacists take a leadership role in those efforts. ASHP encourages research on the potential therapeutic uses, adverse effects, and drug interactions of CBD, and is committed to providing education to pharmacists and other healthcare providers on those topics.

1725

DRUG DOSING IN EXTRACORPOREAL THERAPIES

Source: Council on Therapeutics

To encourage research on the pharmacokinetics and pharmacodynamics of drug dosing in extracorporeal therapies; further,

To support development and use of standardized models of assessment of the pharmacokinetics and pharmacodynamics of drug dosing in extracorporeal therapies; further,

To collaborate with stakeholders in enhancing aggregation of data on the pharmacokinetics and pharmacodynamics of drug dosing in extracorporeal therapies; further,

To encourage the education of the pharmacy workforce and other healthcare providers regarding the basic principles of and drug dosing in extracorporeal therapies.

This policy supersedes ASHP policy 1606.

Rationale

There are few resources and recommendations for drug dosing in patients receiving the varied forms of extracorporeal therapies, including renal replacement therapy, extracorporeal membrane oxygenation (ECMO) support, apheresis, plasmapheresis, molecular adsorbent recirculating system (MARS) support, single pass albumin dialysis (SPAD), fractionated plasma separation and adsorption (PROMETHEUS), therapeutic plasma exchange (TPE), extracorporeal liver assist device (ELAD) support, modular extracorporeal liver (MELS) support, peritoneal dialysis, and use of ventricular assist devices.

Appropriate dosing is very important in optimizing patient outcomes and achieving goals of therapy. Often drug properties are used to make educated guesses on appropriate dosing and are based on estimations of clearance. In the critically ill population, serious infections and renal issues often occur simultaneously. Solute removal has a significant impact on dosing and appropriate dosing. Many patient characteristics and device variables need to be considered when dosing patients receiving these therapies. These factors include flow rate, membrane pore size, volume of distribution, and patient status. Protein binding helps sustain the drug in tissue, and drugs with a large molecular weight may clog the porous membranes.

Research on drug removal by these extracorporeal means is scarce, and ASHP encourages independent clinical and practice-based research to further define clinical use of drugs for patients receiving these modes of treatment as well as clinician reporting of patient experience via published articles and clinical registries. ASHP also encourages education of the pharmacy workforce and other healthcare providers regarding the basic principles of and drug dosing in extracorporeal therapies.

1603

STEWARDSHIP OF DRUGS WITH POTENTIAL FOR ABUSE

Source: Council on Therapeutics

To advocate for the inclusion of a clinically appropriate indication of use, the intended duration, and the goals of therapy when prescribing drugs with potential for abuse; further,

To encourage pharmacists to engage in interprofessional efforts to promote the appropriate, but judicious, use of drugs with the potential for abuse, including education, monitoring, assessment of clinical progress, and discontinuation of therapy or dose reduction, where appropriate; further,

To advocate that pharmacists lead efforts to prevent inappropriate use of drugs with potential for abuse, including engaging in strategies to detect and address patterns of use in patient populations at increased risk for adverse outcomes; further,

To facilitate the development of best practices for prescription drug monitoring programs and drug take-back disposal programs for drugs with potential for abuse.

Rationale

Drug abuse in the U.S. has reached epidemic proportions. In 2011, 110 people died every day from drug poisonings, and prescription drugs were involved in 41,300 deaths. According to the CDC, almost 5% of the U.S. population over 12 years used opioid pain relievers for non-medical reasons in 2010. The CDC estimates the cost to insurance companies to be 70 billion annually. The Centers for Disease Control and Prevention (CDC) and White House continue to prioritize drug abuse issue as a national concern. SAMHSA has released a toolkit on opioid overdose, and state prescription drug monitoring programs are increasingly sharing information among states. In 2013, ASHP and others successfully advocated for the rescheduling of hydrocodone combination products due to safety concerns. ASHP has also advocated broader access to naloxone for opioid reversal as part of the nation's collective efforts to reduce harm from drugs of abuse.

Drugs of abuse consist of a variety of classes of medications and are not limited to opioids, however. The Substance Abuse and Mental Health Services Administration (SAMHSA) acknowledges that drugs of abuse include sedatives, stimulants, and antidepressants, in addition to opioids. Despite their risk for abuse, prescription medications for short-term symptomatic reliefs are often refilled well beyond recommended treatment time periods. Counseling on chronic long-term therapy is important for those prescribed these drugs, which may require well-planned titration schedules for safe and effective discontinuation. Patients may not have sufficient information on discontinuation of therapy and disposal of agents.

Including a clinically appropriate indication of use, the intended duration, and the goals of therapy in the health record when drugs with potential for abuse are prescribed will foster the appropriate but judicious use of those drugs. Pharmacists, as medication-use experts, should engage in efforts to prevent inappropriate use of drugs with potential for abuse by promoting education, monitoring, assessment of clinical progress, and discontinuation of therapy or dose reduction, where appropriate, and should provide leadership in developing strategies to prevent adverse outcomes from drugs with potential for abuse and optimize prescription drug monitoring programs and drug take-back disposal programs for those drugs as well.

1604

APPROPRIATE USE OF ANTIPSYCHOTIC DRUG THERAPIES

Source: Council on Therapeutics

To advocate for the documentation of appropriate indication and goals of therapy to promote the judicious use of antipsychotic drugs and reduce the potential for harm; further,

To support the participation of pharmacists in the management of antipsychotic drug use, which is an interprofessional, collaborative process for selecting appropriate drug therapies, educating patients or their caregivers, monitoring patients, continually assessing outcomes of therapy, and identifying opportunities for discontinuation or dose adjustment; further,

To advocate that pharmacists lead efforts to prevent inappropriate use of antipsychotic drugs, including engaging in strategies to detect and address patterns of use in patient populations at increased risk for adverse outcomes.

Rationale

Antipsychotic drugs are often prescribed and continued in nursing homes after transition from other care settings without appropriate justification. Although there is currently no FDA-approved drug for behavioral and psychological symptoms of dementia (BPSD), antipsychotic drugs are consistently used off-label for BPSD. According to the Agency for Healthcare Research and Quality, there is medium-level evidence to suggest effectiveness of olanzapine, risperidone, and quetiapine to reduce agitation and behavioral disturbances for people with dementia. Some nursing homes are turning away patients with these conditions because of changes to the CMS Five-Star Quality Rating System for nursing homes, which includes two quality measures on antipsychotic drug use. These quality measures exclude patients with schizophrenia, Huntington's disease, and Tourette syndrome.

Antipsychotic drugs have a black-box warning for increased mortality in the elderly population. In certain patients there is a benefit for use, and these patients may require more intense monitoring and assessment. Some studies suggest a significant increase in cognitive function for Alzheimer's patients with aggressive behavior (Vigen 2011). Another study (Bonner 2015) looked at rationales for prescribing and found vague, generalized indications such as anger and agitation, which is not appropriate, according to guidelines. Nonpharmacological interventions are also supported in managing BPSD. These interventions may be more appropriate in the elderly population, despite being time consuming and labor-intensive.

1605

SAFETY OF EPIDURAL STEROID INJECTIONS

Source: Council on Therapeutics

To encourage healthcare providers to 1) inform patients about the significant risks and potential lack of efficacy of epidural steroid injections, 2) request their informed consent, and 3) inform patients of alternative therapies and their risks and benefits; further,

To recommend pharmacist involvement in the medication-use process associated with epidural steroid injections when such injections are medically necessary.

Rationale

Use of epidural steroid injections to treat low back pain is increasing, despite not being a labeled indication and sparse literature confirming the safety and efficacy of the treatment. These drugs, in this route of administration, have narrow therapeutic indices, and there are quality assurance issues related to the compounding of the preparations used in epidural injections. The safety of epidural steroid injections has been referred to in the FDA Safe Use Initiative (SUI), in which 13 stakeholders were involved in assessing evidence of neurological complications of injections. Several recommended practices resulted, including a controversial preference for nonparticulate steroid injections for use in cervical transforaminal injections. In addition to the concerns about particulates in the injections, there are very significant safety concerns due to the proximity of intrathecal, epidural, and subdural spaces and how the injections are administered. Skillful technique is required to appropriately administer these drugs. Radiographic contrast is often used to guide the needle to injection sites. Improper technique can cause vasospasm and stroke, which is not related to particulates in the injection.

In April 2014 the FDA released a drug safety communication stating that rare and serious neurological effects can result from epidural steroid injections. The safety communication noted that "the effectiveness and safety of epidural administration of corticosteroids have not been established, and FDA has not approved corticosteroids for this use" and recommended that healthcare providers "discuss with patients the benefits and risks of epidural corticosteroid injections and other possible treatments." ASHP concurs with those recommendations and encourages use of an informed consent process in addition to other institutional protocols, including pharmacist involvement in the medication-use process when such injections are medically necessary, to promote the safe use of epidural steroid injections.

1607

USE OF METHADONE TO TREAT PAIN

Source: Council on Therapeutics

To acknowledge that methadone has a role in pain management and that its pharmacologic properties present unique risks to patients; further,

To oppose the payer-driven use of methadone as a preferred treatment option for pain; further,

To advocate that pain management experts, payers, and manufacturers collaborate to provide educational programs for healthcare professionals on treating pain with opioids, including the proper place in therapy for methadone; further,

To advocate that all facilities that dispense methadone, including addiction treatment programs, participate in state prescription drug monitoring programs.

Rationale

Over 16,000 people die each year in the U.S. from opioid overdose. Although methadone accounts for only two percent of opioid prescriptions each year, it is estimated to be responsible for over one third of overdose deaths, according to a 2012 Mortality and Morbidity Weekly Report (MMRW) Vital Signs report. The use of methadone to treat pain and its contribution to overdose deaths is an urgent public health concern.

Methadone was approved in 1947 as an analgesic and antitussive, and in 1972 it received approval for use in treating opioid addiction. In 1995, over 100,000 people in the U.S. received addiction treatment with methadone.

There are significant risks associated with the use of methadone for pain management because of its pharmacokinetic and pharmacodynamic properties. Methadone has a long half-life and short duration of analgesic effect. The respiratory effects last longer, and there is also a risk of QT interval prolongation. In 2006, the FDA released a medication safety alert on the dangers of methadone use for the treatment of pain that included a black-box warning and increased the recommended dosing interval from 3 to 8 hours. In 2008, the Drug Enforcement Agency requested manufacturers to restrict distribution of high-dose formulations to addiction treatment programs and hospitals. Federal regulations restrict the dispensing of methadone; for example, dispensing for opioid addiction treatment is limited to programs certified by the Substance Abuse and Mental Health Services Administration (SAMHSA) and for emergency situations to bridge patients to a treatment program.

Despite these dangers, 30 state Medicaid programs include methadone on the preferred drug list for treatment of pain, primarily due to its low cost. The Centers for Disease Control and Prevention (CDC) has recommended that insurance companies and other payers remove methadone from the preferred lists for treating noncancer pain. Several organizations and federal agencies have recommended against the use of methadone as a first-line agent to treat pain, including the FDA, CDC, the American Academy of Pain Medicine (AAPM), and the American Society of Interventional Pain Physicians. In May 2015, the Energy and Commerce Committee of the U.S. Senate held a hearing to assess what the federal government is doing to combat the opioid abuse epidemic and identified use of methadone for treatment of pain as a concern. ASHP joins AAPM in advocating that pain management experts, payers, and manufacturers collaborate to provide educational programs on best practices for prescribing opioids, including methadone.

1527

PHARMACIST'S ROLE IN URGENT AND EMERGENCY SITUATIONS

Source: Council on Pharmacy Practice

To affirm that pharmacists should participate in planning and providing emergency treatment team services; further,

To advocate that pharmacists participate in decision-making about the medications and supplies used in medical emergencies; further,

To advocate that pharmacists serve in all emergency responses, and that those pharmacists receive appropriate training and maintain appropriate certifications.

Rationale

Pharmacists have a leadership role in many hospitals in planning for emergency treatment team services. ASHP National Survey data show that approximately 40% of hospitals have pharmacist participation in cardiopulmonary resuscitation (CPR) teams. This role includes developing policy on the contents of code carts and other supplies as well as establishing the role of the pharmacist in supporting these services. The literature demonstrates that pharmacists can make significant contributions to CPR and other emergency response teams as medication-use leaders and as participants, and there is evidence that better patient outcomes result when pharmacists participate. Pharmacists participating in this role should receive appropriate training and certification (e.g., Basic Life Support, Advanced Cardiopulmonary Life support, and Pediatric Acute Life Support).

This policy was reviewed in 2020 by the Council on Pharmacy Management and by the Board of Directors and was found to still be appropriate.

1402

SAFE USE OF RADIOPHARMACEUTICALS

Source: Council on Pharmacy Practice

To affirm that radiopharmaceuticals require the same standards for safe medication use as other medications, including but not limited to standards for procurement, storage and control, prescribing, preparation, dispensing, administration, documentation, clinical and regulatory monitoring, disposal, and formulary consideration; further,

To advocate that pharmacy departments, in cooperation with departments of nuclear medicine, radiology, and radiation safety, provide oversight of radiopharmaceuticals to assure safe use; further,

To advocate for incorporation of information on radiopharmaceuticals into college of pharmacy curricula and increased pharmacy continuing education on radiopharmaceuticals.

This policy was reviewed in 2019 by the Council on Pharmacy Practice and by the Board of Directors and was found to still be appropriate.

Rationale

Many hospitals utilize radiopharmaceuticals for diagnostic imaging tests or for treatment. Most hospitals outsource the preparation of injectable and oral radiopharmaceuticals to external suppliers. Because of the unique nature of these drugs and their narrow scope of use, the pharmacy department is often not involved with their acquisition, handling, or disposal. Reports of improper handling, storage, and disposal suggest that these products should have similar oversight as other drug products used in hospitals, and that pharmacists, pharmacy students, and pharmacy technicians require education regarding their safe use.

1214

PHARMACIST'S ROLE IN ACCOUNTABLE CARE ORGANIZATIONS

Source: Council on Pharmacy Practice

To recognize that pharmacist participation in collaborative health care teams improves outcomes from medication use and lowers costs; further,

To advocate to health policymakers, payers, and other stakeholders for the inclusion of pharmacists as health care providers within accountable care organizations (ACOs) and other models of integrated health care delivery; further,

To advocate that pharmacist-provided care (including care coordination services) be appropriately recognized in reimbursement models for ACOs; further,

To advocate that pharmacists be included as health care providers in demonstration projects for ACOs; further,

To encourage comparative effectiveness research and measurement of key outcomes (e.g., clinical, economic, quality, access) for pharmacist services in ACOs; further,

To encourage pharmacy leaders to develop strategic plans for positioning pharmacists in key roles within ACOs.

Rationale

The Affordable Care Act of 2009 encourages the formation of accountable care organizations (ACOs). Similar in concept to health maintenance organizations, these entities consist of alliances between physicians, other health care providers, and hospitals that provide comprehensive and coordinated health care to a population of patients. ACOs emphasize primary and preventive care, are provider-led, and receive reimbursement linked to increasing health care quality and lowering per capita costs. The ACO model is based on the premise that care coordinated in this manner and incentivized by a shared-risk reimbursement model will improve health care quality and slow the growth of health care spending. One significant deterrent to pharmacist participation in the fee-for-service care model, lack of provider status, is less of a barrier in the ACO model because reimbursement is tied to quality and reduced costs rather than specific services.

Integrated systems present an important opportunity for pharmacists to demonstrate their value to the quality of care. Pharmacists could contribute to the success of ACOs by providing the following patient care services:

- Developing, implementing, and monitoring patient-specific, evidence-based drug therapy as an active participant in team-based care.
- Improving transitions in care with coordinated MTM services for patients in the hospital as well as postdischarge in ambulatory clinics and physician practices.
- Monitoring the therapy of patients with multiple chronic conditions or complex medication regimens.
- Preventing and managing adverse drug events.

Although a number of ACOs have already evolved from existing disease management and medical home programs, not much is known about the elements of success for ACOs, and implementation is likely to be challenging. To establish these elements of success, pharmacists will need to be included in ACO demonstration projects and pharmacist services will need to be the subject of research on ACO effectiveness.

As pharmacists assume the expanded roles outlined in the PPMI recommendations, pharmacy leaders should use their expertise to explore innovative strategies to meet the broader goals of ACOs. This payment model is an opportunity to demonstrate how pharmacists can help these organizations reach clinical and financial performance targets set by the Centers for Medicare & Medicaid Services (CMS), i.e., improved patient results and lower health care costs. Pharmacy managers and other pharmacy leaders should prepare now to participate in emerging ACOs by developing strategic plans for positioning pharmacists in roles where their expertise can be best applied to these goals.

This policy was reviewed in 2017 by the Council on Pharmacy Practice and by the Board of Directors and was found to still be appropriate.

0902

PHARMACIST'S ROLE IN PROVIDING CARE FOR AN AGING POPULATION

Source: Council on Pharmacy Practice

To encourage expansion of geriatric health care services; further,

To foster expanded roles for pharmacists in caring for geriatric patients; further,

To support successful innovative models of team-based, interdisciplinary geriatric care; further,

To increase training of pharmacists in caring for geriatric patients within college of pharmacy curricula, in ASHP-accredited postgraduate-year-one residencies, and through the expansion of the number of ASHP-accredited postgraduate-year-two geriatric pharmacy residency programs.

This policy was reviewed in 2019 by the Council on Pharmacy Practice and by the Board of Directors and was found to still be appropriate.

Rationale

The 2008 report from the Institute of Medicine, Retooling for an Aging America: Building the Health Care Workforce, predicts a pending crisis caused by an inadequate workforce for a rapidly increasing elderly patient population and highlights issues significant for pharmacy. Although older adults currently make up only about 12% of the U.S. population, they account for approximately 26% of all physician office visits, 35% of all hospital stays, 34% of all prescriptions, 38% of all emergency medical service responses, and 90% of all nursing-home use. By 2030, the number of adults age 65 and older will have doubled to 70 million, or 20% of total population, which will place even more demands on an already undermanned workforce.

The report recommends three major immediate actions to retool the workforce: enhancing the competence of all health care practitioners in geriatric care, increasing the recruitment and retention of geriatric specialists and caregivers, and redesigning models of care to broaden provider and patient roles to achieve greater flexibility. The report discusses the significant role of pharmacists in counseling, monitoring of medication-related problems, and support of medication adherence. Many elderly people have a number of drug-related issues as well as cognitive impairment and complex needs. These factors increase the amount of expertise, time, and attention required to deliver appropriate care. The pharmacist's role on patient care teams and in medication therapy management will become more important with increasing numbers of frail or chronically ill patients being treated with medication. Many pharmacists may not have received sufficient training to assume this role. While professional education for pharmacists provides basic competence for medication management in the elderly, education in geriatrics may vary widely, and there are comparatively few geriatric pharmacy specialists, as only 10 programs currently offer ASHP-accredited geriatric pharmacy residency training.

0908

PHARMACIST ROLE IN THE HEALTH CARE (MEDICAL) HOME

Source: Council on Public Policy

To advocate to health policymakers, payers, and other stakeholders for the inclusion of pharmacists as a care provider within the health care (medical) home model; further,

To ensure that there are appropriate reimbursement mechanisms for the care that pharmacists provide (including care coordination services) within the health care home model; further,

To advocate to the Centers for Medicare & Medicaid Services that pharmacists be included in demonstration projects for the health care home model; further,

To encourage comparative effectiveness research and measurement of key outcomes (e.g., clinical, economic, quality, access) for pharmacist services in the health care home model.

This policy was reviewed in 2019 by the Council on Public Policy and by the Board of Directors and was found to still be appropriate.

Rationale

The concept of a "health care home," also referred to as a "medical home," was first described by the American Academy of Pediatrics in 1992. The health care (medical) home model emphasizes care coordination from a medical practice and uses an interdisciplinary health care team approach to managing a patient's overall health. A recent Medicare Payment Advisory Commission (MedPAC) report discussed a health care home program in Medicare and stated that medication reviews conducted by a health care home would ideally be coordinated by a pharmacist. As the Centers for Medicare & Medicaid Services (CMS) begins health care home demonstration projects, it is important that a pharmacist be included in the health care home model and that pharmacists be factored into the compensation for services provided. To determine the effectiveness of the care that is delivered, research and measurement of key outcomes are important elements of any demonstration or permanent delivery model.

0912

SAFE AND EFFECTIVE USE OF HEPARIN IN NEONATAL PATIENTS

Source: Council on Therapeutics

To support the development and use of nationally standardized concentrations of heparin when used for maintenance and flush of peripheral and central venous lines in neonatal patients; further,

To advocate that hospitals and health systems use manufacturer-prepackaged heparin flush products to improve the safe use of heparin in neonatal patients.

This policy was reviewed in 2019 by the Council on Therapeutics and by the Board of Directors and was found to still be appropriate.

Rationale

The preferential use of saline to maintain peripheral lines and devices in adult patients has largely become the standard of care, but use of heparin in neonates continues because of a lack of consensus and perceived and actual limitations in the evidence in published literature. However, fatal medication errors caused by the use of heparin in this patient population have brought to the forefront concern that the risks of using heparin for this purpose may outweigh the potential benefits. The ASHP Therapeutic Position Statement on the Institutional Use of 0.9% Sodium Chloride Injection to Maintain Patency of Peripheral Indwelling Intermittent Infusion Devices provides evidence for the use of sodium chloride as the preferred solution for maintaining peripheral lines in adult patients but does not address the use of sodium chloride versus heparin in patients younger than 12 years of age, because at the time of publication there was a lack of sufficient evidence regarding the effectiveness of sodium chloride solution for flushing peripheral lines or maintaining their patency in neonatal and pediatric patient populations.

ASHP's Council on Therapeutics has reviewed evidence from evaluations of the use of 0.9% sodium chloride and heparin to maintain and flush arterial and central lines in neonatal patients and reports of medication errors that involved heparin. The advantages of saline include greater compatibility than heparin with concurrently administered drug therapies, lower product costs, fewer potential adverse drug events (e.g., heparin-induced thrombocytopenia, a rare but potentially fatal event for neonatal patients), and prevention of potential medication errors related to improper selection or dilution of heparin products. Advantages of heparin use include extended line patency and a beneficial antithrombotic effect at the insertion site. The data are conflicting and insufficient to support the recommendation of a preferred solution for line maintenance in neonatal patients at this time. The development of standardized concentrations of heparin to decrease practice variation and the use of manufacturer-prepackaged products are the best ways to improve the safe use of heparin in neonatal patients.

0307

PHARMACIST SUPPORT FOR DYING PATIENTS

Source: Council on Professional Affairs

To support the position that care for dying patients is part of the continuum of care that pharmacists should provide to patients; further,

To support the position that pharmacists have a professional obligation to work in a collaborative and compassionate manner with patients, family members, caregivers, and other professionals to help fulfill the patient care needs, especially the quality-of-life needs, of dying patients of all ages; further,

To support research on the needs of dying patients; further,

To provide education to pharmacists on caring for dying patients, including education on clinical, managerial, professional, and legal issues; further,

To urge the inclusion of such topics in the curricula of colleges of pharmacy.

This policy was reviewed in 2018 by the Council on Pharmacy Practice and by the Board of Directors and was found to still be appropriate.

ASHP Statement on Pharmacist Prescribing of Statins

Position

The American Society of Health-System Pharmacists (ASHP) believes that existing models for over-the-counter (OTC) dispensing do not provide the safeguards required to ensure the safe and effective use of 3-hydroxy-3-methylglutaryl coenzyme A (HMG-CoA) reductase inhibitors ("statins") as part of a multimodal approach to preventing atherosclerotic cardiovascular disease (ASCVD). ASHP supports the goal of more widespread use of ASCVD-preventive therapies, including statin therapy, and encourages consideration of pharmacist prescribing models for statins that would advance ASCVD prevention.

ASHP launched the Practice Advancement Initiative (PAI) in 2015 with the objective of significantly advancing the health and well-being of patients in hospitals and health systems by developing and disseminating optimal pharmacy practice models that are based on the effective use of pharmacists as direct patient care providers.[1] In 2020, ASHP updated the initial PAI recommendations with the ASHP PAI 2030 recommendations.[2] These recommendations included 59 recommendations focused on patient-centered care; pharmacists' and pharmacy technicians' roles, education, and training; technology and data science; and leadership in medication use and safety. Recommendation B2 states that pharmacists should leverage and expand their scopes of practice, including prescribing, to optimize patient care. ASHP believes statins are an ideal candidate for dispensing under pharmacist prescribing models.

Background

ASHP supports the use of statins to lower cholesterol and reduce morbidity and mortality in patients at risk for cardiovascular events. Elevated cholesterol, specifically low-density lipoprotein cholesterol (LDL-C), is an important risk factor for the development of ASCVD. ASHP has recommended that evaluation and management of lipid disorders be guided by the recommendations of the American Heart Association/American College of Cardiology (AHA/ACC) guidelines on the management of blood cholesterol.[3] Statins are considered the drug of choice for most patients with dyslipidemia who require lipid-lowering therapy for both primary and secondary prevention of ASCVD. Statins are effective in lowering elevated LDL-C, and studies have demonstrated that statins reduce the risk of ASCVD events in patients without known ASCVD (primary prevention). In addition, statins have been shown to reduce ASCVD events and mortality in patients with ASCVD (secondary prevention). Cardiovascular disease is the leading cause of death for both men and women in the United States, and ASCVD is responsible for nearly 80% of all deaths from cardiovascular disease.[4] Individuals with multiple cardiovascular risk factors and a low LDL-C derive an absolute benefit in reducing risk of ASCVD for a given milligram-per-deciliter lowering of LDL-C. In patients being treated for primary prevention with intermediate risk (7.7–19.9% 10 year predicted risk) of an ASCVD event, the percent LDL-C lowering is targeted at 30–49% and ≥50% for high-risk patients (≥20% 10-year predicted risk).[5] Further, for secondary prevention in patients with established ASCVD, the percent LDL-C lowering is targeted at ≥50% along with an LDL-C threshold of <70 mg/dL to consider adding non-statin therapy to maximally tolerated statin therapy.

The effectiveness of statins in reducing LDL-C has prompted calls for more widespread use, including suggestions for a reclassification of statins as an OTC medication. Although ASHP does not support reclassification to OTC status as that status is currently constructed, ASHP does support alternative approaches that expand pharmacists' scopes of practice, including prescribing of statins, to optimize patient care to reduce risk of ASCVD.

Current OTC Model

To approve a reclassification to OTC status, Food and Drug Administration reviewers must find that (1) a drug is safe and effective in its proposed use(s), (2) the benefits of the drug outweigh its risks, and (3) consumers will be able to use the drug's labeling (e.g., its package insert) to safely use the medication in an OTC setting.[6] Because statins do not meet the third criterion of this test, they are not suitable for OTC status as that class is currently regulated.

ASHP believes that any statin dispensing model should be based on AHA/ACC guidelines for primary and secondary prevention of ASCVD.[3] These guidelines provide both disease-specific and risk-factor-based prescribing criteria to achieve safe and effective use. ASHP believes that *before* a patient begins statin therapy, a cardiac risk assessment should be performed by a competent healthcare professional in order to

- Determine the patient's LDL-C value, which can be used as a baseline value if the patient is a candidate for treatment.
- Assess the individual for other cardiovascular risk factors such as smoking, diabetes, hypertension, diet, weight, amount of exercise, and family history of cardiovascular disease.
- Assess patient with the 10-year ASCVD risk score if a primary prevention patient.

ASHP believes that *after* a patient begins statin therapy, there should be an assessment with the patient to evaluate for both safety and effectiveness of the statin therapy in order to

- Determine the patient's LDL-C lowering seen with the statin therapy at 4–12 weeks post-initiation to evaluate if the patient achieved the desired response.
- Assess the individual for any potential adverse effects from the statin therapy (e.g., statin-associated muscle symptoms, hyperglycemia) and develop a plan for further monitoring and management if an ADE occurs.
- Counsel the patient on the importance of medication adherence with statin therapy to achieve the goal of lower ASCVD risk.

One of the studies that has examined the use of statins in a simulated OTC setting, the CUSTOM study,[7] was an open-label study designed to observe consumers' initial and continued use of a statin to lower LDL-C. Although

DOI 10.37573/9781585287048.063

the results may indicate that some individuals in the study sample were able to use an OTC statin as directed, the study was, by the investigators' own admission, not designed to evaluate clinical outcomes and therefore not able to demonstrate efficacy. The study certainly did not prove that the existing OTC model would provide the level of counseling required to reduce cardiovascular risk factors other than LDL-C levels.

A more recent study by Nissen et al.[8] evaluated whether a technology-assisted, self-selection process for nonprescription statin therapy had concordance with a clinician assessment for statin eligibility. In this study of 500 patients, 96.2% concordance was seen between the patient and clinician selection as either "OK to use," "not right for you," or "ask a doctor." Further, 91.6% of the 96.2% concordance was for the "not right for you" or "ask a doctor" category, indicating that this tool may help determine when a patient is statin ineligible. However encouraging those results might seem, caution should be exercised in extrapolating such information to a larger population, especially information regarding safety. An accompanying article pointed out several shortcomings of the study:

- the study population was self-selected and may differ from the general population;
- the study cohort was relatively young, and few participants had actual indications for primary prevention statin therapy;
- the study tool did not consider the complex algorithms required for evaluation of different statin doses or nonstatin lipid therapies;
- the study could not assess the impact of the tool on actual patient initiation of or adherence to statin therapy, the latter of which has proven especially problematic.[9]

The adverse effects of drugs should always be assessed, especially if the drugs that cause them are easily available to the public. A system that relies on the voluntary reporting of such adverse effects by patients may be inadequate to protect the public or detect subtle signals. It is imperative that the decision to reclassify a statin to nonprescription status include a wide margin of safety. After statin therapy starts, ongoing evaluations should assess the patient's response, reassess risk factors, and monitor for and report adverse drug events. The existing model for OTC medications would place the entire burden for performing this evaluation and reassessment on the patient. Most patients are likely to be unfamiliar with the system used to report an adverse drug event (ADE), if the ADE is even recognized. Although ADEs from prescription statins are rare, particularly at lower doses, they can occur months or years after therapy is initiated. Since OTC status would encourage wider use of statins, these drugs might be used by individuals with multiple disease states or those taking potentially interacting medications (e.g., cyclosporine, diltiazem, verapamil, macrolide antibiotics, azole antifungals, or protease inhibitors). Because statins are a chronic therapy, new risks may be introduced as the patient's health varies, requiring vigilance on the part of the patient as well as healthcare providers.

ASHP concludes, for these reasons, that reclassification of statins to OTC status as currently constructed is not advisable but advocates that alternative models for dispensing these valuable drugs be explored.

Pharmacist Prescribing Models

ASHP supports the role of pharmacists in developing collaborative practice agreements (CPAs) with licensed providers to optimize care for care for patients. A CPA has been defined as ". . . a formal agreement in which a licensed provider makes a diagnosis, supervises patient care, and refers patients to a pharmacist under a protocol that allows the pharmacist to perform specific patient care functions."[10] Collaborative drug therapy management (CDTM) with physicians and other healthcare providers via CPAs allows qualified pharmacists with an advanced scope of practice to initiate, adjust, and discontinue medications; order and monitor laboratory studies; and perform limited physical assessments for various conditions (e.g. diabetes, hypertension, hyperlipidemia).[11] The privileges of pharmacists vary by state, practice site, and payer. For example, in some states they are recognized as an Advanced Practice Pharmacist (APP), a Clinical Pharmacist Practitioner (CPP), or a Pharmacist Clinician (PhC).

A number of pharmacist-led programs to increase statin prescribing both for the primary and secondary prevention of ASCVD have demonstrated significant improvements in statin use across different clinical settings through use of CPAs, CDTM, or statewide protocols.[12–13] One study that evaluated the impact of a pharmacist population health initiative across 10 primary care clinics in Washington demonstrated that a protocolized prescribing authority initiative resulted in a 50% increase in initiation of statin therapy for secondary prevention of ASCVD.[14] This literature not only shows the impact that pharmacists with statin prescribing authority through CPAs, CDTM, and statewide protocols can have, but also highlights the need to expand these prescribing models to reduce patients' CV risk through primary and secondary prevention of ASCVD.

Pharmacogenomics of Statin Therapy

Muscle toxicities are among the most common side effects of statins. Statins' effects on muscles range from mild myalgias to life-threatening rhabdomyolysis. Statins exert their effect in the liver by active transport of the drug into hepatocytes by *SLCO1B1* (also known as *OATP*). People who have poor *SLCO1B1* function are at increased risk for the development of myopathies to life-threatening rhabdomyolysis. Atorvastatin, fluvastatin, lovastatin, pitavastatin, pravastatin, rosuvastatin, and simvastatin have the most evidence for alterations in pharmacotherapy based on *SLCO1B1* genotype. The Clinical Pharmacogenomics Implementation Consortium guideline for statins discusses the risk of statin-associated musculoskeletal symptoms in patients who have been genotyped for *SLCO1B1*, *CYP2C9*, or *ABCG2*.[15] Knowledge of a person's *SLCO1B1* genotype test result prior to initiation of statin therapy can help in initial agent and dosage selection. Identification of a clinical laboratory performing *SLCO1B1* genotyping can be done by reviewing the National Center for Biotechnology Information genetic testing registry resource.[16]

Conclusion

ASHP supports pharmacist prescribing models for statins that ensure their safe and effective use as part of a multimodal approach to ASCVD prevention. Given the complexities of therapies to prevent ASCVD, ASHP encourages consideration of pharmacist statin prescribing models rather than any OTC distribution for statins.

References

1. Engels MJ, Chaffee BW, Clark JS. Comparison and alignment of an academic medical center's strategic goals with ASHP initiatives. *Am J Health-Syst Pharm.* 2015; 72:2065–2078.
2. ASHP Practice Advancement Initiative 2030: New recommendations for advancing pharmacy practice in health systems. *Am J Health-Syst Pharm.* 2020; 77:113–121. https://doi.org/10.1093/ajhp/zxz271
3. Grundy SM, Stone NJ, Bailey AL et al. 2018 AHA/ACC/AACVPR/AAPA/ABC/ACPM/ ADA/AGS/APhA/ASPC/NLA/PCNA Guideline on the Management of Blood Cholesterol: A Report of the American College of Cardiology/American Heart Association Task Force on Clinical Practice Guidelines. *J Am Coll Cardiol.* 2019; 73(24):e285-e350. doi: 10.1016/j.jacc.2018.11.003. Epub 2018 Nov 10. Erratum in: *J Am Coll Cardiol.* 2019; 73(24):3237–3241. PMID: 30423393.
4. Tsao CW, Aday AW, Almarzooq ZI, et al. Heart disease and stroke statistics—2022 update: a report from the American Heart Association. *Circulation.* 2022;145:e00–e00. DOI: 10.1161/CIR.0000000000001052.
5. American College of Cardiology. ASCVD Risk Estimator Plus. Accessed January 19, 2022. https://tools.acc.org/ascvd-risk-estimator-plus/#!/calculate/estimate/
6. Reinberg S. FDA panel nixes over-the-counter sale of cholesterol drug. HealthDay. Published January 14, 2005. Accessed September 5, 2022. http://consumer.healthday.com/public-health-information-30/foodand-drug-administration-news-315/fda-panel-nixes-over-the-counter-saleof-cholesterol-drug-523436.html
7. Melin JM, Struble WE, Tipping RW, et al. A consumer use study of over-the-counter lovastatin (CUSTOM). *Am J Cardiol.* 2004; 94:1243–1248.
8. Nissen SE, Hutchinson HG, Wang TY, et al. Technology-assisted self-selection of candidates for nonprescription statin therapy. *J Am Coll Cardiol.* 2021; 78:1114–1123.
9. Pagidipati NJ, Peterson ED. Should cardiovascular preventive therapy be over-the-counter? *J Am Coll Cardiol.* 2021; 78:1124–1126. doi:10.1016/j.jacc.2021.07.020
10. Centers for Disease Control and Prevention. *Advancing Team-Based Care Through Collaborative Practice Agreements.* Accessed February 10, 2022. https://www.cdc.gov/dhdsp/pubs/docs/cpa-team-based-care.pdf
11. Turingan EM, Bates JS, Amerine LB. Integration of physical assessment into pharmacy practice. *Am J Health-Syst Pharm.* 2018;75:169–170.
12. Elkomos M, Jahromi R, Kelly MS. Pharmacist-led programs to increase statin prescribing: a narrative review of the literature. *Pharmacy (Basel).* 2022;10(1):13. doi:10.3390/pharmacy10010013
13. Dixon DL, Khaddage S, Bhagat S, et al. Effect of pharmacist interventions on reducing low-density lipoprotein cholesterol (LDL-C) levels: a systematic review and meta-analysis. *J Clin Lipidol.* 2020;14:282–292.
14. Haby HE, Alm RA, Corona AR, Hall AC. Population health model for pharmacist assessment and independent prescribing of statins in an ambulatory care setting. *J Am Pharm Assoc.* 2020;60:130–137.
15. Cooper-DeHoff RM, Niemi M, Ramsey LB, et al. The Clinical Pharmacogenetics Implementation Consortium (CPIC) guideline for *SLCO1B1*, *ABCG2*, and *CYP2C9* and statin-associated musculoskeletal symptoms. *Clin Pharmacol Ther.* Published online February 12, 2022. doi:10.1002/cpt.2557.
16. National Center for Biotechnology Information. Genetic Testing Registry. Accessed February 10, 2022. https://www.ncbi.nlm.nih.gov/gtr/

Approved by the ASHP Board of Directors on March 23, 2022, and by the ASHP House of Delegates on May 19, 2022. Developed through the ASHP Council on Therapeutics. Supersedes the ASHP statement on the over-the-counter availability of statins dated June 14, 2005.

The authors have declared no potential conflicts of interest.

Joel C. Marrs, PharmD, FASHP, FCCP, FNLA, BCPS-AQ Cardiology, BCACP, CLS, ASH-CHC, Billings Clinic, Billings, MT, University of Colorado School of Medicine, Aurora, CO.

Cyrine-Eliana Haidar, PharmD, BCPS, BCOP, St. Jude Children's Research Hospital, Memphis, TN.

Copyright © 2022, American Society of Health-System Pharmacists, Inc. All rights reserved. Contact ASHP for reprint and permissions requests. This content may not be used for commercial purposes without the express written consent of ASHP.

The bibliographic citation for this document is as follows: American Society of Health-System Pharmacists. ASHP statement on pharmacist prescribing of statins. *Am J Health-Syst Pharm.* 2022; 79:2182–4.

ASHP-SIDP Joint Statement on the Pharmacist's Role in Antimicrobial Stewardship

Position

The American Society of Health-System Pharmacists (ASHP) and the Society of Infectious Diseases Pharmacists (SIDP) jointly believe that all pharmacists have a responsibility to promote antimicrobial stewardship (AMS) and optimize antimicrobial use. Pharmacists qualified through education, training, or experience in infectious diseases (ID) and/or AMS should be recognized as appropriate leaders, or ideally co-leaders, of AMS programs (ASPs). Training in ID and AMS through ID specialty training, a certificate program, or other AMS training is essential to equip ASP leaders with the necessary tools to successfully advocate for and direct appropriate antimicrobial use, educate the public, and empower other healthcare professionals to engage in AMS efforts.

Background

Pharmacists have long been at the forefront of the creation, development, and advancement of AMS by influencing antimicrobial prescribing to improve patient outcomes, reducing antimicrobial-related adverse events, encouraging cost-effective care, and minimizing the development of antimicrobial resistance.[1,2] Over the past several years, U.S. accrediting bodies, regulatory agencies, and quality-assurance organizations recognized the importance of AMS by adopting ASP minimum standards into quality criteria.[3–11] Pharmacists' knowledge and importance in leading ASP implementation efforts were specifically recognized in 2019, when "drug expertise" was changed to "pharmacist expertise" as a Centers for Disease Control and Prevention (CDC) Core Element for Hospital Antimicrobial Stewardship Programs.[12] The CDC also emphasizes the importance of pharmacist expertise as a priority for hospital core element implementation and in expanded guidance for settings beyond acute care.[13–17] Still, AMS is an interprofessional effort in every setting, and healthcare professionals should be guided by the knowledge and expertise of pharmacy leaders, ideally in co-leadership roles with ID physicians.[18]

ASHP and SIDP previously published separate statements on the pharmacist's role in AMS.[19–21] In general, ASHP statements express basic philosophy and are concise responses to specific therapeutic issues. Both organizations endorse evidence-based guidelines published by the Infectious Diseases Society of America (IDSA), the Pediatric Infectious Diseases Society (PIDS), and the Society for Healthcare Epidemiology of America (SHEA) for implementation and measurement of AMS interventions in inpatient populations.[3]

This current statement is a combined effort to incorporate and expand upon earlier ASHP and SIDP statements to address recent regulatory, scientific, policy, and practice-based advances. The following adaptable framework aligns with national AMS guidance and standards and provides an overview of the evolving roles and responsibilities of AMS/ID pharmacists as ASP leaders or co-leaders. The recommendations in this joint statement represent a consensus of professional judgment, expert opinion, and documented evidence. They are written to establish reasonable goals, to be progressive and challenging, yet attainable as best practices in applicable settings. Healthcare professionals are encouraged to exercise their professional judgment in assessing and adapting these recommendations to meet the specific needs of their healthcare organizations. Many recommendations in this document are based on U.S. published guidance; nevertheless, AMS advancement requires worldwide effort.

Leadership Responsibilities

Leadership support is critical to the success of ASPs.[4–9,12–17] Pharmacy, executive, and operational leadership can facilitate the success of ASPs in a variety of ways, including but not limited to the following:

1. Establishing AMS as a site and organizational priority, as demonstrated through ASP implementation and sustained, quantifiable support, including identification of an ASP point-of-contact within the executive and operational leadership group(s) and public communication with employees.
2. Allocating dedicated resources required for a sustainable infrastructure that supports local and national ASP activities, including required participation in the National Healthcare Safety Network's Antimicrobial Use and Resistance (AUR) Module.[22] If local resources are limited, funding of remote consultation or telemedicine with AMS experts should be considered.[15]
    a. Resources can include but are not limited to adequate pharmacist and key support personnel full-time equivalents, salary support, protected time, support for initial training and education as well as continued professional development, information technology (IT) solutions, clinical decision support (CDS), and data analytics.[7,23–25]
3. Appointing a pharmacist qualified through substantial education, training, or experience in ID and/or AMS, combined with strong communication and leadership skills, as the leader or co-leader of the ASP. If such an individual is unavailable, executive and pharmacy leaders should provide resources to train current practitioners, including formal or informal mentorship programs.[17]
4. Including AMS responsibilities in employment contracts, job descriptions, and/or job titles.
5. Prioritizing and ensuring accountability by including AMS activities and outcomes in quality and patient safety metrics and incorporating or incentivizing AMS-related actions in performance reviews.[26]
6. Facilitating integration and collaboration among all stakeholders responsible for AMS, as applicable, at

DOI 10.37573/9781585287048.064

each practice setting. This includes but is not limited to the infection prevention and control program, microbiology laboratory, IT, pharmacy services, quality improvement, medical staff, nursing services, and interprofessional committees.

7. Optimizing daily practice models to ensure a consistent, interprofessional team approach to AMS endeavors, including optimization of pharmacy practice models to facilitate and support AMS efforts with all pharmacists.
8. Acting on improvement opportunities identified by ASPs and facilitating appropriate follow-up to ensure continuous quality improvement and patient safety.
9. Endorsing and supporting policies or formal procedures that sustain local, sub-national, or national AMS action plans.
10. Promoting collaboration within the pharmacy and therapeutics committee (or equivalent structure) and/or quality department, which may include leading or co-leading an ID- or AMS-related subcommittee.[12]

Responsibilities of Pharmacists

AMS/ID pharmacists' responsibilities include promoting the optimal use of antimicrobials; tracking, analyzing, and reporting antimicrobial data; and educating healthcare professionals, patients, and the public. Pharmacist leaders of ASPs should not only lead by example, but also empower other pharmacy colleagues to address AMS interventions within their daily workflows. A team approach to daily AMS activities can improve program efficiency and expand the reach of the ASP.

Promoting Optimal Use of Antimicrobial Agents

Actions. The implementation of specific actions promotes optimal antimicrobial use. Actions may vary based on the setting, patient population, and available resources. Several interventions have been associated with improved antimicrobial use and are considered priority interventions, particularly in the hospital setting.[12,13] Examples of pharmacist-driven actions include, but are not limited to, the following:

1. Guidelines, protocols, policies, and collaborative practice agreements specific to the treatment facility and setting.
2. Prospective audit and feedback.
3. Preauthorization.
4. Implementation and optimization of IT solutions and CDS.
5. Microbiology laboratory integration and collaboration, including implementation of diagnostic stewardship.
6. Antimicrobial formulary management (e.g., mitigating shortages, agent selection).
7. Facilitating selection of antimicrobial regimens and monitoring plans for transitions of care and outpatient antimicrobial management.[27]
8. Participation in antimicrobial awareness campaigns.

Tracking and Reporting. Tracking and reporting antimicrobial use and resistance, the impact of interventions, and process and outcome measures are cornerstones of identifying opportunities for improvement and disseminating the impact of ASPs.[5,12–16] ASHP and SIDP recommend pharmacist leaders of ASPs do the following:

1. Determine meaningful and required measures to track and work with leadership and dedicated data analysts to identify the necessary resources to obtain, analyze, and report data.[28]
2. Guide the routine and accurate tracking and reporting of selected measures, programmatic strategies, achievements, and opportunities, which is crucial to evaluating and advancing an ASP. Routine feedback compiled and presented by the ASP leaders and/or provider self-assessment of antimicrobial prescribing practices is recommended.[14]
3. Collaborate with microbiology personnel for antibiogram development, reporting, and tracking. Antibiograms should follow current best practice recommendations and guide antimicrobial selection and protocol/guideline development and maintenance.[29,30]

Education and Training for Pharmacists Involved in AMS

Pharmacists qualified through education, training, or experience in ID or AMS have the knowledge, skills, and confidence to promote AMS in a variety of settings. In addition to having ID knowledge, training specific to AMS is crucial to the development of a robust and sustainable ASP. ASHP and SIDP recommend the following regarding education and training for pharmacists involved in AMS:

1. Pharmacy leaders of ASPs should have AMS-specific education or substantial experience in the field.
   a. Examples include a postgraduate year 2 (PGY2) ID residency, an ID fellowship with clinical AMS experience, or successful completion of an AMS certificate program appropriate to the practice setting. ASHP and SIDP recognize that factors in some settings may require pharmacists without such training to assume AMS responsibilities. Support for AMS-specific training, education, or mentoring should be provided.
   b. Accrediting, regulatory, and quality assurance organizations should incorporate qualification standards and pharmacy expertise into their regulatory framework.
   c. Federal support of PGY2 ID pharmacy residency training programs is needed to ensure a highly trained workforce and support the expansion of AMS across healthcare settings.
2. All pharmacists involved in AMS should seek continuing education related to AMS as part of regular credentialing maintenance, state licensure, or professional development.
3. Pharmacist leaders of ASPs are encouraged to obtain Board of Pharmacy Specialties certification in ID (BCIDP) and maintain up-to-date knowledge with emerging AMS initiatives.
4. General AMS education should be embedded within the curricula of colleges of pharmacy, including interprofessional AMS-related activities.

Pharmacists as AMS Educators

Pharmacists involved in AMS have an obligation to provide accurate, up-to-date information about AMS to interprofessional healthcare teams, patients, caregivers, and the public, and can help meet standards related to education.[5,6] Specific activities may include, but are not limited to, the following:

1. Tailoring AMS education to the target audience to optimize antimicrobial use through appropriate communication methods (e.g., case-based teaching, newsletters). Engaging other healthcare providers in providing AMS education to patients and caregivers can provide another avenue for dissemination of AMS principles.
2. Leading and collaborating on the development of local, regional, or national guidelines or guidance documents for antimicrobial monitoring and the management of infections to promote AMS principles.
3. Leading and collaborating on research or quality-improvement projects (e.g., analyzing and sharing results to advance the field, demonstrate value, and help determine how to optimize ASP implementation and effectiveness).
4. Participating in public health education, advocacy, and awareness programs aimed at promoting AMS, including topics such as prudent antimicrobial use, when antimicrobials have a role (e.g., viral vs. bacterial infections), and the negative consequences of antimicrobial overuse.

Conclusion

ASHP and SIDP jointly believe that while ID and/or AMS pharmacists have a responsibility to lead, or ideally, co-lead ASPs, all pharmacists have a responsibility to promote AMS efforts. The pharmacist's leadership ability should be recognized in all settings where antimicrobials are prescribed. ASHP and SIDP jointly believe that pharmacists have the expertise and skills to optimize antimicrobial use at the patient level and to advance the field on a broad scale, including AMS education, guideline development, and research endeavors.

References

1. Shlaes DM, Gerding DN, John JF Jr, et al. Society for Healthcare Epidemiology of America and Infectious Diseases Society of America Joint Committee on the Prevention of Antimicrobial Resistance: guidelines for the prevention of antimicrobial resistance in hospitals. *Clin Infect Dis.* 1997; 25:584–599. doi:10.1086/513766.
2. Dellit TH, Owens RC, McGowan JE Jr, et al. Infectious Diseases Society of America and the Society for Healthcare Epidemiology of America guidelines for developing an institutional program to enhance antimicrobial stewardship. *Clin Infect Dis.* 2007; 44:159–177. doi:10.1086/510393.
3. Barlam TF, Cosgrove S, Abbo LM, et al. Implementing an antibiotic stewardship program: guidelines by the Infectious Diseases Society of America and the Society for Healthcare Epidemiology of America. *Clin Infect Dis.* 2016; 62:e51–e77. doi:10.1093/cid/ciw118.
4. The Joint Commission. Approved: new antimicrobial stewardship standard (2016). https://www.jointcommission.org/-/media/enterprise/tjc/imported-resource-assets/documents/new_antimicrobial_stewardship_standardpdf.pdf (accessed 10 Feb 2023).
5. The Joint Commission. New and revised requirements for antibiotic stewardship. R3 report. https://www.jointcommission.org/-/media/tjc/documents/standards/r3-reports/r3_antibioticstewardship_july2022_final.pdf (accessed 14 Oct 2022).
6. The Joint Commission. Antimicrobial stewardship in ambulatory care. R3 report. https://www.jointcommission.org/-/media/tjc/documents/standards/r3-reports/r3_23_antimicrobial_stewardship_amb_6_14_19_final2.pdf (accessed 10 Feb 2023).
7. Medicare and Medicaid Programs; hospital and critical access hospital (CAH) changes to promote innovation, flexibility, and improvement in patient care, Fed. Reg. 39448 (June 16, 2016) (amending 42 CFR 482 and 485). https://www.govinfo.gov/content/pkg/FR-2016-06-16/pdf/2016-13925.pdf (accessed 10 Feb 2023).
8. Safety & Oversight Group, Centers for Medicare & Medicaid Services. QSO-22-20-Hospitals: infection prevention and control and antibiotic stewardship program interpretive guidance update. https://www.cms.gov/files/document/qso-22-20-hospitals.pdf (accessed 10 Feb 2023).
9. National Quality Partners. National Quality Partners playbook: antimicrobial stewardship in acute care: a practical playbook. https://www.qualityforum.org/Publications/2016/05/National_Quality_Partners_Playbook__Antibiotic_Stewardship_in_Acute_Care.aspx (accessed 10 Feb 2023).
10. The Leapfrog Group. Giant leaps for patient safety. https://www.leapfroggroup.org/ (accessed 10 Feb 2023).
11. Medicare and Medicaid programs; reform of requirements for long-term care facilities. Final rule. 81 Fed. Reg. 68688 (October 4, 2016) (amending 42 CFR 405, 431, 447, 482, 483, 485, 488, and 489). https://www.govinfo.gov/content/pkg/FR-2016-10-04/pdf/2016-23503.pdf (accessed 10 Feb 2023).
12. Centers for Disease Control and Prevention. Core Elements of Hospital Antibiotic Stewardship Programs. Published 2019. https://www.cdc.gov/antibiotic-use/healthcare/pdfs/hospital-core-elements-H.pdf (accessed 10 Feb 2023).
13. Centers for Disease Control and Prevention. Priorities for hospital core element implementation. https://www.cdc.gov/antibiotic-use/core-elements/hospital/priorities.html (accessed 10 Feb 2023).
14. Sanchez GV, Fleming-Dutra KE, Roberts RM et al. Core elements of outpatient antibiotic stewardship. *MMWR Recomm Rep.* 2016; 65:1–12. doi:10.15585/mmwr.rr6506a1.
15. Centers for Disease Control and Prevention. Implementation of antibiotic stewardship core elements at small and critical access hospitals. https://www.cdc.gov/antibiotic-use/core-elements/small-critical.html (accessed 10 Feb 2023).

16. Centers for Disease Control and Prevention. Core elements of antibiotic stewardship for nursing homes. https://www.cdc.gov/antibiotic-use/core-elements/nursing-homes.html (accessed 10 Feb 2023).
17. Centers for Disease Control and Prevention. The core elements of human antibiotic stewardship programs in resource-limited settings: national and hospital levels. https://www.cdc.gov/antibiotic-use/core-elements/resource-limited.html (accessed 10 Feb 2023).
18. Dodds-Ashley E, Davis SL, Heil EL, et al. Best care for patients achieved through multidisciplinary stewardship. Letter. *Clin Infect Dis.* 2018; 67:1637. doi:10.1093/cid/ciy392.
19. American Society of Health-System Pharmacists. ASHP statement on the pharmacist's role in antimicrobial stewardship and infection prevention and control. *Am J Health-Syst Pharm.* 2010; 67:575–577. doi:10.2146/sp100001.
20. Heil EL, Kuti JL, Bearden DT, et al. The essential role of pharmacists in antimicrobial stewardship. *Infect Control Hosp Epidemiol.* 2016; 37:753–754. doi:10.1017/ice.2016.82.
21. Blanchette L, Gauthier T, Heil E, et al. The essential role of pharmacists in antibiotic stewardship in outpatient care: an official position statement of the Society of Infectious Diseases Pharmacists. *J Am Pharm Assoc (2003).* 2018; 58:481–484. doi:10.1016/j.japh.2018.05.013.
22. Centers for Disease Control and Prevention. Antimicrobial use and resistance (AUR) options. https://www.cdc.gov/nhsn/psc/aur/index.html (accessed 15 Feb 2023).
23. Greene MH, Nesbitt WJ, Nelson GE. Antimicrobial stewardship staffing: how much is enough? *Infect Control Hosp Epidemiol.* 2020; 41:102–112. doi:10.1017/ice.2019.294.
24. Doernberg SB, Abbo LM, Burdette SD, et al. Essential resources and strategies for antibiotic stewardship programs in the acute-care setting. *Clin Infect Dis.* 2018; 67:1168–1174. doi:10.1093/cid/ciy255.
25. Echevarria K, Groppi J, Kelly AA, et al. Development and application of an objective staffing calculator for antimicrobial stewardship programs in the Veterans Health Administration. *Am J Health-Syst Pharm* 2017; 74:1785–1790. doi:10.2146/ajhp160825.
26. Yoshikawa Y, Feldhaus I, Özçelik E, et al. Financial strategies targeting healthcare providers to promote the prudent use of antibiotics: a systematic review of the evidence. *Int J Antimicrob Agents.* 2021; 58:106446. doi:10.1016/j.ijantimicag.2021.106446.
27. Rivera CG, Mehta M, Ryan KL, et al. Role of infectious diseases pharmacists in outpatient intravenous and complex oral antimicrobial therapy: Society of Infectious Diseases Pharmacists insights. *J Am Coll Clin Pharm.* 2021; 4:1161–1169. doi:10.1002/jac5.1473.
28. Clinical and Laboratory Standards Institute. *Analysis and Presentation of Cumulative Antimicrobial Susceptibility Test Data.* 5th ed. CLSI guideline M39. Clinical and Laboratory Standards Institute; 2022.
29. European Committee on Antimicrobial Susceptibility Testing. Breakpoint tables for interpretation of MICs and zone diameters, version 12.0, 2022.

Developed through the ASHP Council on Pharmacy Practice and the SIDP Guidelines Committee and approved by the SIDP Board of Directors on March 14, 2023, and the ASHP Board of Directors on April 5, 2023. This statement supersedes the ASHP Statement on the Pharmacist's Role in Antimicrobial Stewardship and Infection Prevention and Control dated June 16, 2009, and the joint ASHP-SIDP position paper, "The Essential Role of Pharmacists in Antimicrobial Stewardship," dated April 1, 2016.

ASHP and SIDP gratefully acknowledge the following individuals for reviewing this document (review does not imply endorsement): Nicole M. Acquisto, PharmD, FASHP, FCCM, FCCP, BCCCP; Victoria Adams-Sommers, PharmD, BCPS-AQ-ID; Daniel Anderson, PharmD, BCIDP; Christina Andrzejewski, PharmD, BCPS, BCIDP; Sohail Azam, PharmD; Amanda Barner, PharmD, BCPS, BCIDP; Lauren Biehle, PharmD, BCPS, BCIDP; Amanda Binkley, PharmD, BCIDP, AAHIVP; Laura Bio, PharmD, BCPS, BCIDP; James Bird, PharmD, BCCCP; Daniel B. Chastain, PharmD, BCIDP, AAHIVP; Tom Dilworth, PharmD, BCPS-AQ-ID; Richard Drew, PharmD, MS; Susan B. Egbert, PharmD; Sarah Embrey, PharmD, BCPS; Taryn A. Eubank, PharmD, BCIDP; Josh Eudy, PharmD, BCIDP; Jillian Foster, PharmD, MBA, FASHP, FACHE; Debra A. Goff, PharmD; Alan Gross, PharmD, FCCP, BCIDP, BCPS; Stephanie Harding, PharmD, BCIDP, BCPS; Cynthia R Hennen, BSPharm; Crystal K. Hodge, PharmD, BCIDP, BCPS; Justin Hooper, PharmD, BCPS; Dan Ilges, PharmD, BCIDP; Aleena Issac, PharmD; Jacob Jarboe, PharmD candidate; Asmaa Kamal, MSc, BCPS; Jarrod W. Kile, RPh, BCPS; Nina Kleinschmidt, PharmD, BCPS; Kelli Kronsberg, PharmD, BCPS, BCIDP; Bradley Lauver, PharmD, BCPS, BCIDP; Ann Lloyd, PharmD, BCPS, BCIDP; David L. Lourwood, PharmD, BCPS, FCCP; Aleksandr Lyakhovetskiy, PharmD, BCPS; Justin Ma, PharmD; Monica Mahoney, PharmD, BCPS, BCIDP, FCCP, FIDSA, FIDP; Chris Martens, PharmD, BCIDP; Linda Gore Martin, PharmD, MBA, BCPS, FASHP; James McCracken, PharmD, BCIDP, AAHIVP; Chris McKnight, PharmD, MBA, BCPS; Karen Michaud, PharmD BCPS; Jennifer Miles, PharmD, CPh, BCACP, BCMTMS, LSSGB; LeAnne Moore, PharmD, BCPS, BCIDP; Mandana Naderi, PharmD, BCIDP; Rama Nasef, PharmD, BCIDP; Melinda M. Neuhauser, PharmD, MPH, FCCP, FASHP; Clara Ni, PharmD, BCIDP; Tristan O'Driscoll, PharmD, MPH; Richard Pacitti, PharmD, MBA, FASHP; Andrea Pallotta, PharmD, BCIDP; Fred J. Pane, BSPharm, FASHP, FABC; Sonal Patel, PharmD, BCIDP; Matthew F. Pearsall, BSPharm, PharmD; Marcus C. Ravnan, PharmD; Jennifer L. Richardson, PharmD, BCPS; Ashley Rizzo, PharmD; Hunter O. Rondeau, PharmD; Craig Sastic, PharmD, MBA, BCPS; Daryl Schiller, PharmD, BCPS, FASHP; T. Lance Smith, PharmD, BCIDP; Matthew Song, PharmD, BCIDP; Ryan Stevens, PharmD, BCIDP; Elena Swingler, PharmD, MBA, BCIDP; Tristan Timbrook, PharmD, MPH, MBA, BCIDP; Noreen Chan Tompkins, PharmD, BCPS-AQ ID, APH; Kendall J. Tucker, PharmD, MS, BCPS, BCIDP; William R. Truong, PharmD, BCIDP, BCPS, AAHIVP; Tyler A. Vest, PharmD, MS, BCPS, BCSCP; Erin Weslander, PharmD, BCIDP; Tracy Zembles, PharmD; and Anna Y. Zhou, PharmD, BCIDP.

Curtis D. Collins, PharmD, MS, BCPS, BCIDP, FASHP, Trinity Health Ann Arbor, Ann Arbor, MI

Lisa E. Dumkow, PharmD, BCIDP, Trinity Health Saint Mary's, Grand Rapids, MI

Wesley D. Kufel, PharmD, BCIDP, BCPS, AAHIVP, Binghamton University, Binghamton, NY

Cynthia T. Nguyen, PharmD, BCIDP, University of Chicago Medicine, Chicago, IL

Jamie L. Wagner, PharmD, BCPS, BCIDP, University of Mississippi School of Pharmacy, Jackson, MS

The authors wish to disclose the following potential conflicts of interest within the last 12 months: Dr. Collins reports service with the National Quality Forum and the Board of Pharmacy Specialties and a consulting arrangement with ASHP Consulting. Dr. Kufel received a research grant from Merck & Co and reports service with the Board of Pharmacy Specialties. The organizations wish to disclose the following potential conflicts of interest: ASHP accredits pharmacy residency programs, including PGY2 infectious disease residencies, and develops board certification resources. SIDP offers certificate programs in antimicrobial stewardship, board certification resources, educational programming and funding for postgraduate training in infectious diseases pharmacy.

Copyright © 2023, American Society of Health-System Pharmacists, Inc. All rights reserved. Contact ASHP for reprint and permissions requests. This content may not be used for commercial purposes without the express written consent of ASHP.

The bibliographic citation for this document is as follows: American Society of Health-System Pharmacists. ASHP statement on the pharmacist's role in antimicrobial stewardship. *Am J Health-Syst Pharm*. 2023;80:1577–81.

ASHP Statement on the Pharmacist's Role in Clinical Pharmacogenomics

Position

The American Society of Health-System Pharmacists (ASHP) believes pharmacogenomic testing can improve medication-related outcomes across the continuum of care in all healthsystem practice settings. These improvements include improved clinical outcomes, decreased side effects, lower cost of treatment, increased medication adherence, more appropriate selection of therapeutic agents, decreased length of treatment, and enhanced patient safety.[1–4] Because of their distinct knowledge, skills, and abilities, pharmacists are uniquely positioned to lead interprofessional efforts to develop processes for ordering pharmacogenomics tests and for reporting and interpreting test results. Pharmacists are also singularly qualified to lead efforts to guide optimal drug selection and drug dosing and provide patient as well as provider education based on those results. Pharmacists therefore have a fundamental responsibility to ensure that pharmacogenomic testing is performed when needed and the results are utilized to optimize medication therapy.[1] Pursuant to this leadership role, pharmacists share accountability with other health-system leaders, such as physicians, laboratory professionals, and genetic counselors, for the ongoing implementation and application of pharmacogenomics across the continuum of care. Because test results will have implications throughout a patient's lifetime, all pharmacists should serve as advocates for preemptive and reactive testing and have a basic understanding of pharmacogenomics in order to provide appropriate patientcare recommendations. ASHP therefore encourages pharmacist education on the use of pharmacogenomics and advocates inclusion of pharmacogenomics and its application to the therapeutic decision-making process in student and resident training, continuing education offerings, and Board of Pharmacy Specialties certification processes. Some advanced pharmacist functions in applying clinical pharmacogenomics may require specialized education, training, or experience.

Background

Clinical pharmacogenomics uses genetic information to guide optimal drug selection and drug dosing for patients to maximize therapeutic effects, improve outcomes, and minimize toxicity.[3] Although early applications of pharmacogenomics were in the oncology and cardiology realms, the use of pharmacogenomic data has expanded to other across therapeutic areas, for example psychiatry, neurology, and infectious diseases.[5–8]

Pharmacogenomic testing can be performed reactively or preemptively. Reactive testing generally occurs when a patient is experiencing adverse effects unexplained by dose or drug-drug or drug-disease interactions, or when the use of a drug that is affected by pharmacogenomic variations is anticipated. In contrast, preemptive testing occurs when patients are genotyped prior to developing an indication for specific pharmacotherapy; usually multiple pharmacogenomics genes are assessed at the same time. Preemptive testing yields the highest value and quality of care for the patient by preventing undesirable drug responses such as toxicity or therapeutic failure.[9]

Application of pharmacogenomics information requires an understanding of how genetic variations impact the pharmacokinetic and pharmacodynamics properties of a drug and prevent the occurrence of adverse drug events. The combined influence of factors such as age, sex, race, ethnicity, diet, pathophysiologic conditions, and current medication use, as well as their relationship to genetic variability, must also be understood. The development of patient-individualized therapeutic regimens should therefore include an assessment of the patient's pharmacogenomics profile in addition to their allergy and adverse reaction history, drug interactions, dietary and lifestyle factors, patterns of adherence, and other therapeutic drug-monitoring parameters.[10] There are more than a dozen comprehensive, ASHP-endorsed therapeutic guidelines from the Clinical Pharmacogenetics Implementation Consortium (CPIC) to guide pharmacotherapy decisions when pharmacogenomic information is available.[11–13] From a regulatory perspective, the Food and Drug Administration also provides a list of drugs for which pharmacogenomic markers are included in the drug labeling[14] as well as a table of pharmacogenomics associations.[15] Pharmacogenomic information is emerging in other sources, such as specialty guidelines and widely used drug information resources, so pharmacists should consult a variety of evidence-based resources in therapeutic decision-making.

The pharmacist's patient-care responsibilities include education as well as appropriate and cost-conscious medication selection and monitoring, which now increasingly include pharmacogenomic profile assessment. The purpose of this statement is to describe pharmacists' responsibilities and accountabilities in the field of clinical pharmacogenomics.

Pharmacists' Responsibilities

Pharmacists' responsibilities for pharmacogenomics include promoting the optimal use and timing of pharmacogenomic tests; interpreting pharmacogenomic test results; and educating healthcare professionals, patients, and the public about the field of pharmacogenomics. The following are responsibilities that should be part of any clinical pharmacogenomics program:

- Advocating for the rational and ethical use of pharmacogenomics testing as part of routine patient care.[16]
- Ordering pharmacogenomics tests, when appropriate, and providing test result interpretation and clinical guidance for the return of pharmacogenomic results to providers and patients in collaboration with other healthcare professionals.
- Optimizing medication therapy based on pharmacogenomic test results.
- Providing information and educating healthcare professionals, patients, and members of the public on the evidence-based, clinical application of pharmacogenomics.

DOI 10.37573/9781585287048.065

- Supporting and participating in research, consortia, and networks that guide and accelerate the application of pharmacogenomics in clinical practice.
- Facilitating the seamless integration of pharmacogenomics in the electronic health record (EHR) with clinical decision support.
- Promoting EHR interoperability and portability of patient-specific pharmacogenomic test results across health systems and to pharmacies.[17,18]

Using these responsibilities as a guide, ASHP has developed the following recommendations for pharmacists' roles in pharmacogenomics.

Pharmacists' Roles

All pharmacists should have a basic understanding of pharmacogenomics to provide patient care incorporating pharmacogenomic recommendations regarding medication response. Elements of a basic understanding of pharmacogenomics should enable pharmacists to perform the following responsibilities:

- Recommending or ordering preemptive or reactive pharmacogenomic testing to aid in the process of drug and dosage selection.
- Designing patient-specific drug and dosage regimens based on a person's pharmacogenomic profile and other pertinent factors, such as the pharmacokinetic and pharmacodynamic properties of the drug, drug-drug and drug-gene interactions, comorbidities, patient demographics, and laboratory data to optimize patient outcomes.
- Educating healthcare professionals about pharmacogenomic principles and appropriate indications for cost-effective pharmacogenomic testing.[19]
- Communicating pharmacogenomicsbased drug therapy recommendations to the healthcare team, including documentation of and interpretation of results in the patient's health record.[17,18,20]
- Providing resources and education that empower patients to make informed healthcare decisions about undergoing pharmacogenomic testing and understanding their test results.[21]
- Ensuring pharmacogenomic test results are handled in an ethical manner and that patients are provided access to their genetic data when applicable.
- Pharmacists with specialized education, training, or experience in pharmacogenomics should also assume the following additional roles:
- Developing institutional guidelines and processes for or leading the use and implementation of a clinical pharmacogenomic program.
- Applying collaborative drug therapy management principles to a clinical pharmacogenomics program, including advocating for the reimbursement of testing and pharmacist interpretation by health insurance plans.
- Serving as a subject matter expert for clinical pharmacogenomics. Pharmacists who practice in the oncology setting should also incorporate results of tumor genomics (somatic variations) to personalize and optimize pharmacotherapy. Pharmacists typically have leadership roles on institutional tumor boards in this practice setting.
- Contributing to the evaluation and implementation of clinical pharmacogenomics testing as an integral part of medication therapy.
- Promoting collaborative relationships with healthcare professionals and key departments within the institution to encourage the development and appropriate use of pharmacogenomic principles in patient care.
- Advocating for the use of standardized pharmacogenomic nomenclature, including the use of standardized terms from the Systematized Nomenclature of Medicine—Clinical Terms (SNOMED CT) and Logical Observation Identifiers Names and Codes (LOINC) in EHRs.[22,23]
- Developing pharmacogenomic-specific clinical decision support tools in EHR systems that guide prescribers on the appropriate use and dosing of medicines based on a patient's pharmacogenomics profile.[24–26]
- Encouraging EHR vendors to assist in the seamless integration of pharmacogenomics in the EHR and promote interoperability and portability of pharmacogenomic data.
- Developing and planning pharmacogenomic-specific advanced training opportunities for pharmacists and other healthcare professionals.
- Establishing processes for communicating patient-specific results with healthcare professionals, including documentation of results in the patient's health record and informing healthcare providers outside of the institution whose care would be impacted by the results.
- Developing a process for return of results to patients, including patient-specific educational materials explaining the importance and lifelong significance of their pharmacogenomic test results.
- Developing processes to document patient outcomes and economic benefits as a result of pharmacogenomic testing.
- Establishing a process for reinterpretation and updating of pharmacogenomics test results based on the emergence of new findings.
- Designing and conducting pharmacogenomics research.
- Actively contributing to the body of knowledge in pharmacogenomics by publishing articles on the topic in the biomedical literature.

Future Directions

As pharmacogenomic testing continues to evolve, genotyping will likely be performed using next-generation sequencing (NGS) technologies, and more patients will get tested for a larger number of variants.[27] Pharmacists will need to have a basic understanding of NGS, including its limitations and how to address variants of unknown significance.[28] The roles of pharmacists must therefore expand and evolve as well, including but not limited to the following:

- Routinely utilizing a patient's pharmacogenomic test results as standard practice within comprehensive medication management workflows.

- Working closely with other medical specialties (e.g., close collaboration with medical geneticists or genetic counselors) to provide pharmacogenomics expertise and return of results to patients when broad testing (e.g., whole-genome sequencing) is ordered.
- Assessment of the economic value of clinical pharmacogenomics and pharmacogenomics test reimbursement policies. Payer policies are maturing and are expected to expand as further evidence is generated. The unique expertise of pharmacists will be essential in the development of these best practices policies.[29–31]
- Data interoperability and sharing of pharmacogenomic test results with other healthcare institutions, including community pharmacies, will be a critical factor to enable continuing use of the information over a patient's lifetime.
- For pharmacists who practice in the oncology setting, aiding in the replication of the successful principles of germline pharmacogenomics integration in the EHR to somatic variations will help optimize medication therapy.

Conclusion

ASHP believes all pharmacists have a responsibility to take a prominent role in the rational, ethical use and clinical application of pharmacogenomics. Clinical pharmacogenomics initiatives should be spearheaded by pharmacists to promote safe, effective, and cost-efficient medication use. Pharmacists should also lead the efforts of patient and interprofessional pharmacogenomic education.

References

1. Swen JJ, Nijenhuis M, de Boer A, et al. Pharmacogenetics: from bench to byte—an update of guidelines. *Clin Pharmacol Ther.* 2011;89(5):662–673.
2. KNMP. Pharmacogenetics. Accessed February 15, 2021. https://www.knmp.nl/patientenzorg/medicatiebewaking/farmacogenetica/pharmacogenetics-1/pharmacogenetics
3. Manolio TA, Chisholm RL, Ozenberger B, et al. Implementing genomic medicine in the clinic: the future is now. *Genet Med.* 2013;15(4):258–267.
4. Berm EJ, de Looff M, Wilffert B, et al. Economic evaluations of pharmacogenetic and pharmacogenomic screening tests: a systematic review. Second update of the literature. *PLoS One.* 2016;11:e0146262. Accessed February 15, 2021. doi.org/10.1371/journal.pone.0146262
5. Ramsey LB, Ong HH, Schildcrout JS, et al. Prescribing prevalence of medications with potential genotype-guided dosing in pediatric patients. *JAMA Netw Open.* 2020;3:e2029411. doi:10.1001/jamanetworkopen.2020.29411
6. Samwald M, Xu H, Blagec K, et al. Incidence of exposure of patients in the United States to multiple drugs for which pharmacogenomic guidelines are available. *PLoS One.* 2016;11(10):e0164972. Accessed February 15, 2021. https://doi.org/10.1371/journal.pone.0164972
7. Chanfreau-Coffinier C, Hull LE, Lynch JA, et al. Projected prevalence of actionable pharmacogenetic variants and level a drugs prescribed among US Veterans Health Administration pharmacy users. *JAMA Netw Open.* 2019;2:e195345. doi:10.1001/jamanetworkopen.2019.5345
8. Hicks JK, Rouby NE, Ong HH, et al. Opportunity for genotype-guided prescribing among adult patients in 11 U.S. health systems. *Clin Pharmacol Ther.* Published online January 11, 2021. Accessed February 15, 2021. doi.org/10.1002/cpt.2161
9. Roden DM, Van Driest SL, Mosley JD, et al. Benefit of preemptive pharmacogenetic information on clinical outcome. *Clin Pharmacol Ther.* Published online March 13, 2018. Accessed January 14, 2021. doi.org/10.1002/cpt.1035
10. ASHP policy position 1104: pharmacogenomics. In: Hawkins B, ed. *ASHP Best Practices: Positions and Guidance Documents of ASHP.* 2020–2021 ed. American Society of Health-System Pharmacists; 2020:212. Accessed January 19, 2021. https://www.ashp.org/-/media/assets/policy-guidelines/docs/policy-positions/policy-positionsformulary-management.ashx
11. Relling MV, Klein TE, Gammal RS, et al. The Clinical Pharmacogenetics Implementation Consortium: 10 years later. *Clin Pharmacol Ther.* 2019;107:171–175. doi:10.1002/cpt.1651
12. Clinical Pharmacogenetics Implementation Consortium (CPIC). Drug-gene pairs. Accessed January 19, 2021. https://cpicpgx.org/genes-drugs/
13. American Society of Health-System Pharmacists. Endorsed documents. Accessed January 19, 2021. https://www.ashp.org/Pharmacy-Practice/Policy-Positions-and-Guidelines/Browse-by-Document-Type/Endorsed-Documents
14. Food and Drug Administration. Table of pharmacogenomic biomarkers in drug labeling. Accessed January 14, 2021. www.fda.gov/drugs/science-and-research-drugs/tablepharmacogenomic-biomarkers-druglabeling
15. Food and Drug Administration. Table of pharmacogenetic associations. Accessed January 14, 2021. www.fda.gov/medicaldevices/precision-medicine/table-pharmacogenetic-associations
16. Butnariu A, Samasca G, Lupan I. Ethical implications in pharmacogenetics and pharmacogenomics. *Medical Connections.* 2015;10:41–44. Accessed January 14, 2021. https://www.researchgate.net/publication/299662333_Ethical_implications_in_pharmacogenetics_and_pharmacogenomic
17. Hicks JK, Dunnenberger HM, Gumpper KF, et al. Integrating pharmacogenomics into electronic health records with clinical decision support. *Am J Health-Syst Pharm.* 2016;73:1967–1976. doi:10.2146/ajhp160030
18. Hoffman JM, Flynn AJ, Juskewitch JE, et al. Biomedical data science and informatics challenges to implementing pharmacogenomics with electronic health records. *Ann Rev Biomed Data Sci.* 2020;3:289–314. Published online April 27, 2020. Accessed January 14, 2021. doi.org/10.1146/annurev-biodatasci-020320-093614

19. Feero WG, Kuo GM, Jenkins JR, et al. Pharmacist education in the era of genomic medicine. *J Am Pharm Assoc.* 2012;52:e113-e121.
20. Liu M, Vnencak-Jones CL, Roland BP, et al. A tutorial for pharmacogenomics implementation through end-to-end clinical decision support based on ten years of experience from *PREDICT. Clin Pharmacol Ther.* Published online October 13, 2020. doi:10.1002/cpt.2079
21. Feldman EA. The Genetic Information Nondiscrimination Act (GINA): public policy and medical practice in the age of personalized medicine. *J Gen Intern Med.* 2012;27(6):743–746. doi:10.1007/s11606-012-1988-6
22. Welch BM, Kawamoto K. Clinical decision support for genetically guided personalized medicine: a systematic review. *J Am Med Inform Assoc.* 2013;20(2):388–400.
23. Pulley JM, Denny JC, Pederson JF, et al. Operational implementation of prospective genotyping for personalized medicine: the design of the Vanderbilt PREDICT project. *Clin Pharmacol Ther.* 2012;92:87–95.
24. Bell GC, Crews KR, Wilkinson MR, et al. Development and use of active clinical decision support for preemptive pharmacogenomics. *J Am Med Inform Assoc.* 2014;21(e1):e93-e99. doi:10.1136/amiajnl-2013-001993
25. Caudle KE, Dunnenberger HM, Freimuth RR, et al. Standardizing terms for clinical pharmacogenetic test results: consensus terms from the Clinical Pharmacogenetics Implementation Consortium (CPIC). *Genet Med.* 2017;19:215–223. doi:10.1038/gim.2016.87
26. Caudle KE, Keeling NJ, Klein TE, et al. Standardization can accelerate the adoption of pharmacogenomics: current status and the path forward. *Pharmacogenomics.* 2018;19:847–60. doi:10.2217/pgs-2018-0028
27. Yang W, Wu G, Broeckel U, et al. Comparison of genome sequencing and clinical genotyping for pharmacogenes. *Clin Pharmacol Ther.* 2016;100:380–388. doi:10.1002/cpt.411
28. Hippman C, Nislow C. Pharmacogenomic testing: clinical evidence and implementation challenges. *J Pers Med.* 2019;9:40. doi:10.3390/jpm9030040
29. Empey PE, Pratt VM, Hoffman JM, et al. Expanding evidence leads to new pharmacogenomics payer coverage. *Genet Med.* Published online February 24, 2021. doi:10.1038/s41436-021-01117-w
30. Hart MR, Garrison LP Jr, Doyle DL, et al. Projected cost-effectiveness for 2 genedrug pairs using a multigene panel for patients undergoing percutaneous coronary intervention. *Value Health.* 2019;22:1231–1239. doi:10.1016/j.jval.2019.05.015
31. Dong OM, Wheeler SB, Cruden G, et al. Cost-effectiveness of multigene pharmacogenetic testing in patients with acute coronary syndrome after percutaneous coronary intervention. *Value Health.* 2020;23:61–73. doi:10.1016/j.jval.2019.08.002

Developed through the ASHP Section of Clinical Specialists and Scientists Section Advisory Group on Emerging Sciences, and approved by the ASHP Board of Directors on March 29, 2021, and by the ASHP House of Delegates on May 19, 2021. This statement supersedes a previous version dated June 1, 2014.

ASHP gratefully acknowledges the following individuals for reviewing the current version of the statement (review does not imply endorsement): Jill S. Bates, PharmD, MS, BCOP, FASHP; Philip E. Empey, PharmD, PhD; Barry R. Goldspiel, PharmD, BCOP, BCPS, FASHP, FHOPA; and Jasmine Luzum, PharmD, PhD, BCPS. The contributions of Cyrine-Eliana Haidar, PharmD, BCPS, BCOP; James M. Hoffman, PharmD, MS; and Samuel G. Johnson, PharmD, FCCP, BCPS-AQ Cardiology to the previous version of this statement are also gratefully acknowledged.

The authors have declared no potential conflicts of interest.

Cyrine-Eliana Haidar, PharmD, BCPS, BCOP, St. Jude Children's Research Hospital, Memphis, TN.

Natasha Petry, PharmD, MPH, BCACP, North Dakota State University, Sanford Health, Fargo, ND.

Carolyn Oxencis, PharmD, BCOP, Medical College of Wisconsin, Milwaukee, WI.

Janine S. Douglas, PharmD, BCPS, The University of Texas MD Anderson Cancer Center, Houston, TX.

James M. Hoffman, PharmD, MS, St. Jude Children's Research Hospital, Memphis, TN.

Copyright © 2022, American Society of Health-System Pharmacists, Inc. All rights reserved. Contact ASHP for reprint and permissions requests. This content may not be used for commercial purposes without the express written consent of ASHP.

The bibliographic citation for this document is as follows: American Society of Health-System Pharmacists. ASHP statement on the pharmacist's role in clinical pharmacogenomics. *Am J Health-Syst Pharm.* 2022;79:704–707.

ASHP Statement on the Pharmacist's Role in Clinical Pharmacokinetic Monitoring

The American Society of Health-System Pharmacists (ASHP) believes that clinical pharmacokinetic monitoring is a fundamental responsibility of all pharmacists providing pharmaceutical care. Clinical pharmacokinetic monitoring is an integral component of pharmaceutical care for selected patients based on their specific pharmacotherapy, disease states and related factors, and treatment goals. ASHP believes that clinical pharmacokinetic monitoring is essential to achieving positive outcomes for these patients across the continuum of care and in all practice settings of health systems. Examples of such outcomes include decreased mortality, decreased length of treatment, decreased length of hospital stay, decreased morbidity (either improved symptoms of disease or improved recuperation), and decreased adverse effects from drug therapy.

Background

Clinical pharmacokinetics is the process of applying pharmacokinetic principles to determine the dosage regimens of specific drug products for specific patients to maximize pharmacotherapeutic effects and minimize toxic effects. Application of these principles requires an understanding of the absorption, distribution, metabolism, and excretion characteristics of specific drug products in specific diseases and patient populations. The influence of factors such as age, sex, diet, pathophysiologic conditions, and concomitant use of other drug products must also be understood. The development of patients' individualized dosage regimens should be based on integrated findings from monitoring both the drug concentration-versus-time profiles in biological fluids and the pharmacologic responses to these drug products.

Within the pharmaceutical care process, pharmacists' clinical functions include appropriate and cost-conscious therapeutic drug monitoring and provision of clinical pharmacokinetic assessments. Clinical pharmacokinetic monitoring is necessary when the range between minimal effectiveness and toxicity is narrow and the results of the drug assay provide significant information for clinical decision-making. In the absence of drug concentration measurements, patient-specific characteristics and physiological markers should be used to provide clinical pharmacokinetic assessments and make dosage-regimen recommendations.

Responsibilities

The following responsibilities should be part of clinical pharmacokinetic services or monitoring conducted by pharmacists:

1. Designing patient-specific drug dosage regimens based on the pharmacokinetic and pharmacologic characteristics of the drug products used, the objectives of drug therapy, concurrent diseases and drug therapy, and other pertinent patient factors (e.g., demographics, laboratory data) that improve the safety and effectiveness of drug therapy and promote positive patient outcomes.
2. Recommending or scheduling measurements of drug concentrations in biological fluids (e.g., plasma, serum, blood, cerebrospinal fluid) or tissues in order to facilitate the evaluation of dosage regimens.
3. Monitoring and adjusting dosage regimens on the basis of pharmacologic responses and biological fluid and tissue drug concentrations in conjunction with clinical signs and symptoms or other biochemical variables.
4. Evaluating unusual patient responses to drug therapy for possible pharmacokinetic and pharmacologic explanations.
5. Communicating patient-specific drug therapy information to physicians, nurses, and other clinical practitioners and to patients orally and in writing, and including documentation of this in the patient's health record.
6. Educating pharmacists, physicians, nurses, and other clinical practitioners about pharmacokinetic principles and appropriate indications for clinical pharmacokinetic monitoring, including the cost-effective use of drug concentration measurements.
7. Developing quality assurance programs for documenting improved patient outcomes and economic benefits resulting from clinical pharmacokinetic monitoring.
8. Promoting collaborative relationships with other individuals and departments involved in drug therapy monitoring to encourage the development and appropriate use of pharmacokinetic principles in pharmaceutical care.

Pharmacists with specialized education, training, or experience may have the opportunity to assume the following additional responsibilities:

1. Designing and conducting research to expand clinical pharmacokinetic knowledge and its relationship to pharmacologic responses, exploring concentration–response relationships for specific drugs, and contributing to the evaluation and expansion of clinical pharmacokinetic monitoring as an integral part of pharmaceutical care.
2. Developing and applying computer programs and point-of-care information systems to enhance the accuracy and sophistication of pharmacokinetic modeling and applications to pharmaceutical care.
3. Serving as an expert consultant to pharmacists with a general background in clinical pharmacokinetic monitoring.

Readers are referred to ASHP's more thorough publications on the subject of clinical pharmacokinetic monitoring, including *Clinical Pharmacokinetics Pocket Reference* and *Concepts in Clinical Pharmacokinetics: A Self-Instructional Course.*

DOI 10.37573/9781585287048.066

This statement was reviewed in 2013 by the Council on Pharmacy Practice and by the Board of Directors and was found to still be appropriate.

Approved by the ASHP Board of Directors, November 15, 1997, and by the ASHP House of Delegates, June 3, 1998. Revised by the ASHP Council on Professional Affairs. Supersedes a previous version approved by the House of Delegates on June 5, 1989.

Copyright © 1998, American Society of Health-System Pharmacists, Inc. All rights reserved. Contact ASHP for reprint and permissions requests. This content may not be used for commercial purposes without the express written consent of ASHP.

The bibliographic citation for this document is as follows: American Society of Health-System Pharmacists. ASHP statement on the pharmacist's role in clinical pharmacokinetic monitoring. *Am J Health-Syst Pharm.* 1998; 55:1726–7.

ASHP Statement on the Pharmacist's Role in Medication Reconciliation

Position

The American Society of Health-System Pharmacists (ASHP) believes that an effective process for medication reconciliation reduces medication errors and supports safe medication use by patients. ASHP encourages hospitals and health systems, including community-based providers and managed care systems, to collaborate in organized, multidisciplinary medication reconciliation programs to promote continuity of patient care. ASHP further believes that pharmacists, because of their distinct knowledge, skills, and abilities, are uniquely qualified to lead interdisciplinary efforts to establish and maintain an effective medication reconciliation process in hospitals and across health systems. Pharmacists should lead or assume key roles in the following essential components of medication reconciliation: developing policies and procedures, implementing and continuously improving medication reconciliation processes, training and assuring the continuing competency of those involved in medication reconciliation, providing operational and therapeutic expertise in the development of information systems that support medication reconciliation, and advocating for medication reconciliation programs in the community. Pursuant to their leadership role, pharmacists share accountability with other hospital and health-system leaders for the ongoing success of medication reconciliation processes across the continuum of care.

Background

The term "medication reconciliation" is defined by the Joint Commission as "the process of comparing the medications a patient is taking (and should be taking) with newly ordered medications" in order to resolve discrepancies or potential problems.[1] The goals of medication reconciliation are to obtain and maintain accurate and complete medication information for a patient and use the information within and across the continuum of care to ensure safe and effective medication use. Although it is sometimes associated with survey and accreditation activities, medication reconciliation is an important component of patient safety and has demonstrated effectiveness in preventing adverse drug events. When organizations do not consistently and reliably reconcile patient medications across the continuum of care, medication errors and adverse drug events occur: approximately half of all hospital-related medication errors and 20% of all adverse drug events have been attributed to poor communication at the transitions and interfaces of care.[2,3]

In 1999, the Institute of Medicine report *To Err Is Human: Building a Safer Health System*[4] identified medication errors as the most common type of health-system error, contributing to several thousand deaths each year. The fiscal impact of these errors is also significant. With reported costs of $2595–4685 per adverse drug event, drug-related morbidity and mortality were estimated to cost over $177 billion in 2000 alone.[5]

Reports and studies such as these had a profound impact on the medical community, and the call for action was immediate. Organizations such as the Institute for Healthcare Improvement, the Agency for Healthcare Research and Quality, and the Joint Commission launched initiatives for performance improvement and established higher expectations through new regulatory standards for improved communication between providers and patients and across health care systems.

In 2005, the Joint Commission made medication reconciliation a focus of one of its National Patient Safety Goals. The initial goal included a number of detailed and specific requirements, which made implementation challenging and resulted in numerous findings of noncompliance during survey. In response, the Joint Commission affirmed the importance of the goal but suspended it in 2009 and 2010 for extensive revision. After a comprehensive literature review and analysis of data collected by surveyor teams, a modified goal was released in 2011, and scoring of the goal began in July 2011.[6] The revised goal sets an expectation for maintaining accurate medication information at critical risk points in the medication-use process while allowing organizations latitude to define processes and encouraging performance improvement.

The purpose of this statement is to describe pharmacists' responsibilities and accountabilities in medication reconciliation practices.

Pharmacists' Responsibilities

When performed by pharmacists, medication reconciliation can reduce the frequency and severity of hospital medication errors that could potentially result in patient harm.[7] Pharmacists have demonstrated high rates of patient interventions; interventions per patient; and documentation of medications, medication interactions, drug-related admissions, and previous drug failures.[8]

ASHP and the American Pharmacists Association began a collaborative effort in 2007 and 2008 to create a shared vision for the role of the pharmacist in medication reconciliation processes.[9] That vision recognizes that pharmacists should take a leadership role in improving medication reconciliation, acting as both advocates and medication experts, to provide information to and educate patients and health care providers. Specifically, pharmacists' responsibilities were described as including but not being limited to

- Providing leadership in designing and managing patient-centered medication reconciliation systems.
- Educating patients and health care professionals about the benefits and limitations of the medication reconciliation process.
- Serving as patient advocates throughout transitions of care.

Using this vision as a guide, ASHP has developed the following recommendations for pharmacists' functions in medication reconciliation activities.

DOI 10.37573/9781585287048.067

Pharmacists' Functions

Although medication reconciliation is required at key transitions of care, activities associated with medication reconciliation should be considered part of ongoing care provided to a patient. Beyond active participation in medication reconciliation activities, pharmacists have five fundamental functions in medication reconciliation: developing policies and procedures regarding medication reconciliation processes, implementing and continuously improving those processes, training and assuring the continuing competency of those involved in medication reconciliation, providing operational and therapeutic expertise in the development of information systems that support medication reconciliation, and advocating for medication reconciliation programs in the community. The extent of pharmacist involvement in these functions will depend on the resources available.

Policy and Procedure Development. Pharmacists should provide leadership and participate in establishing policies and procedures that encourage (a) provision of patient care services that include medication reconciliation processes, (b) implementation and operation of an evidence-based medication reconciliation system that optimizes available resources, (c) education of organization staff on the importance of medication reconciliation as a patient safety initiative, and (d) promotion of medication reconciliation as a focus of performance-improvement activities.

Implementation and Performance Improvement. Pharmacists should lead or participate in organizational implementation of and performance-improvement efforts regarding medication reconciliation activities. These activities may include but are not limited to (a) establishing a medication reconciliation implementation task force or redesign team, (b) creating a vision and expectations for medication reconciliation activities, (c) securing executive-level commitment to or sponsorship of medication reconciliation resource needs, (d) identifying barriers that are preventing, or potential barriers that may prevent, safe and effective medication reconciliation procedures within their practice model, as well as possible solutions, (e) guiding workflow development that integrates operational and clinical needs, (f) establishing roles and responsibilities of health care providers in medication reconciliation processes, including pharmacy technicians, pharmacy students, and other medical support personnel, (g) ensuring that competency-based training for all personnel involved in medication reconciliation procedures is established, (h) creating or assisting in the development of standardized documentation templates for medication lists and reconciliation, (i) ensuring that established procedures meet regulatory requirements and organizational policy, and (j) developing a method for ongoing medication reconciliation system evaluation.

Training and Competency Assurance. Pharmacists should lead or participate in (a) identifying all health care providers and support staff involved in medication reconciliation activities, (b) creating competency training and skills assessment that are specific to each staff member's roles and responsibilities in medication reconciliation (e.g., conducting a medication interview, taking a medication history, performing medication reconciliation), (c) providing education and performing assessments to ensure the competency of those who document and perform medication reconciliation activities, and (d) providing didactic or simulated training for medication history and reconciliation procedures.

Information Systems Development. As more organizations adopt computerized provider order entry, electronic medical records, and other information systems, pharmacists should ensure that the systems support medication reconciliation throughout the continuum of care. Consideration should be given to establishing methods for data extraction from the medical record that allow for internal and external reporting of measures related to medication reconciliation.

Advocacy. Pharmacists should provide information about medication reconciliation to health care providers, patients, and the community, and they should evaluate the effectiveness of these advocacy efforts on the medication reconciliation process. Activities may include clinical grand rounds, professional conferences, patient counseling, and mass communications such as newsletters and public service announcements. These efforts should (a) demonstrate the effectiveness of sound medication reconciliation processes in improving patient safety and reducing health care costs, (b) emphasize the importance of timely and accurate communication of medication information between patients and their health care providers, (c) clarify and describe the important role of technology and electronic medical records that support medication reconciliation documentation and reconciliation, (d) provide strategies for preventing medication adverse events related to overuse, misuse, omission, duplication, or other discrepancies found during medication reconciliation processes, (e) highlight the importance of completing a full and accurate medication history, including supplement use, prior to prescribing or administering a new medication, and (f) describe opportunities for pharmacist extenders, such as pharmacy technicians and students, to participate in medication reconciliation activities.

Resource Constraints. Although the literature demonstrates the important role of pharmacists in successful medication reconciliation processes across the continuum of care, significant resources are needed to perform medication reconciliation skillfully and efficiently, which suggests opportunities for expanding the roles of pharmacy residents, students, and technicians. When properly trained, these individuals can participate in the documentation of medication histories, which should then be reviewed by the pharmacist for accuracy prior to medication reconciliation, as described in the ASHP Pharmacy Practice Model Initiative Summit Recommendations.[10] In one study, potential errors due to incomplete or incorrect information, illegible orders, and serious drug interactions were reduced by 82% by having pharmacy technicians obtain medication histories.[11]

When confronted with limited resources, pharmacists should at a minimum participate in and guide interdisciplinary efforts to develop and define policies and procedures for their organizations, standardize workflows for electronic documentation, promote safe practices to the community, and, most importantly, engage health care leadership in efforts to ensure medication reconciliation processes are successful.

Conclusion

An effective process for medication reconciliation reduces medication errors and supports safe medication use. Pharmacists are uniquely qualified to lead interdisciplinary efforts to establish and maintain an effective medication reconciliation process in hospitals and across health systems and should lead or assume key roles in the essential components of medication reconciliation. Because of their crucial role, pharmacists share accountability with other hospital and health-system leaders for the ongoing success of medication reconciliation processes across the continuum of care.

References

1. Joint Commission. National Patient Safety Goals effective January 1, 2012. NPSG.03.06.01. www.jointcommission.org/assets/1/6/NPSG_Chapter_Jan2012_HAP.pdf (accessed 2012 Feb 2).
2. Barnsteiner JH. Medication reconciliation: transfer of medication information across settings: keeping it free from error. *J Infus Nurs.* 2005; 28(suppl 2):31–6.
3. Rozich J, Roger R. Medication safety: one organization's approach to the challenge. *J Clin Outcomes Manag.* 2001; 8:27–34.
4. Kohn LT, Corrigan JM, Donaldson MS, eds. To err is human: building a safer health system. Washington, DC: National Academy Press; 1999.
5. Bates DW, Spell N, Cullen DJ, et al. The cost of adverse drug events in hospitalized patients. *JAMA.* 1997; 277:307–11.
6. Joint Commission. 2011 National Patient Safety Goals. www.jointcommission.org/standards_information/npsgs.aspx. (accessed 2011 Dec 13).
7. Gleason KM, Groszek JM, Sullivan C, et al. Reconciliation of discrepancies in medication histories and admission orders of newly hospitalized patients. *Am J Health-Syst Pharm.* 2004; 61:1689–95.
8. Gurwich EL. Comparison of medication histories acquired by pharmacists and physicians. *Am J Hosp Pharm.* 1983; 40:1541–2.
9. Chen D, Burns A. ASHP–APhA Medication Reconciliation Initiative Workgroup Meeting, February 12, 2007: summary and recommendations. www.ashp.org/s_ashp/docs/files/MedRec_ASHP_APhA_Wkgrp_MtgSummary.pdf (accessed 2012 Feb 1).
10. American Society of Health-System Pharmacists. Pharmacy Practice Model Initiative Summit recommendations. Recommendation D3a. February 1, 2011. www.ashp.org/DocLibrary/PPMI/Summit-Recommendations.aspx (accessed 2012 Feb 1).
11. Michels R, Meisel S. Program using pharmacy technicians to obtain medication histories. *Am J Health-Syst Pharm.* 2003; 60:1982–6.

Approved by the ASHP Board of Directors on April 13, 2012, and by the ASHP House of Delegates on June 10, 2012. Developed through the ASHP Council on Pharmacy Practice.

This statement was drafted by Michelle M. Thoma, Pharm.D., who declared no potential conflicts of interest.

ASHP gratefully acknowledges the following individuals and organizations for reviewing drafts of this statement (review does not imply endorsement): Academy of Managed Care Pharmacy (AMCP); Paul Barrett, Pharm.D., M.P.A., BCPS, FASHP; Julie Cooper, Pharm.D., BCPS; Jean Douglas, Pharm.D.; Michael S. Edwards, Pharm.D., M.B.A., BCOP, FASHP; Kristine M. Gleason, B.S.Pharm.; Kayla Hansen, Pharm.D., M.S.; Becky Harvey, Pharm.D.; John Hertig, Pharm.D., M.S.; Justin Julius, Pharm.D.; Nishaminy Kasbekar, Pharm.D., FASHP; Carlo Lupano, B.S.Pharm., M.B.A., CCP; Ashley M. Overy, Pharm.D.; Fred J. Pane, B.S.Pharm., FASHP; Barbara Petroff, M.S., FASHP; James Ponto, M.S., FASHP; Curt W. Quap, M.S., FASHP; Elizabeth Sampsel, Pharm.D., M.B.A., BCPS (AMCP); Jamie S. Sinclair, M.S., FASHP; Richard L. Stambaugh, Pharm.D., M.S., BCPS; Robert L. Stein, Pharm.D., J.D.; and Jeffrey Stroup, Pharm.D., BCPS, AAHIVE.

Copyright © 2013, American Society of Health-System Pharmacists, Inc. All rights reserved. Contact ASHP for reprint and permissions requests. This content may not be used for commercial purposes without the express written consent of ASHP.

The bibliographic citation for this document is as follows: American Society of Health-System Pharmacists. ASHP statement on the pharmacist's role in medication reconciliation. *Am J Health-Syst Pharm.* 2013; 70:453–6.

ASHP Statement on the Pharmacist's Role in Public Health

Position

Pharmacists play a vital role in maintaining and promoting public health. All pharmacists have a responsibility to participate in global, national, state, regional, and institutional efforts to promote public health and to integrate the goals of those initiatives into their practices. Furthermore, pharmacists have a responsibility to work with public health planners to ensure their involvement in public health policy decision-making and in the planning, development, and implementation of public health efforts.

The primary objectives of this statement are to (1) increase awareness of pharmacists' contributions to public health, (2) educate pharmacists about public health and their role in promoting public health, (3) describe the role of pharmacists in public health planning and promotion, and (4) identify new opportunities for pharmacists' involvement in future public health initiatives. This statement does not provide an exhaustive review of pharmacists' public health activities. Its intent is to stimulate dialogue about the role that pharmacists can play in improving public health in the United States. The statement is also meant to draw attention to and highlight the significance of enhanced and proactive communication between the public health sector and the pharmacy profession's leaders and stakeholders representing national and state affiliates, colleges of pharmacy, and health systems to advocate the pharmacist's role in public health.

Background

Public health is a science-based field designed to "protect and improve the health of people and their communities."[1] In contrast to clinical medicine, public health concentrates on whole populations and communities, working to improve the places where they "live, learn, work and play,"[2] through health-promoting policies, prevention, interventions, and education.

These goals are accomplished through an upstream approach, or what could be considered "upstream healthcare." Public health recognizes four levels of prevention: primordial, primary, secondary, and tertiary.[3] Primordial prevention is prevention of risk factors for disease, illness, injury, or poor health outcomes from ever developing; primary prevention is the prevention of disease, illness, injury, or poor health outcomes from occurring; secondary prevention focuses on reducing the impact of disease, illness, injury, or poor health outcomes; and tertiary prevention focuses on minimizing the long-term impact of disease, illness, injury, and poor health outcomes.[3] While all four levels of prevention are recognized and used in public health, primordial and primary prevention are considered largely upstream, whereas secondary and tertiary prevention are considered more downstream. Public health focuses heavily on upstream efforts while also working closely with the medical community and others to positively impact downstream work. Examples of the different types of prevention can be found in **Table 1**.

There are many factors that contribute to the overall health of a community or population. To understand how best to prevent the risk factors of disease, illness, injury, and poor health outcomes from ever developing, one must first understand the many factors that contribute to overall health, referred to as "determinants of health." While there are many determinants of health, most can be grouped into five primary categories: social factors, referred to as "social determinants of health"; policy; health services; individual behavioral choices; and biology and genetics[4]:

- **Social determinants of health** include but are not limited to socioeconomic status, employment status, educational attainment, cultural and physical environment, family influence, intimate partners, social groups, and religious groups.
- **Policy** includes but is not limited to economic policies, political policies, justice policies, educational policies, health policies, work policies, and neighborhood and zoning policies.
- **Health services** include but are not limited to access to services, quality of services, cost of services, insurance coverage, language access, health programs, and time and means of access.
- **Individual behavioral choices** include but are not limited to diet; physical activity; alcohol, drug, or tobacco use; handwashing; sexual activity; stress management; sleep; and therapy adherence issues.
- **Biology and genetics** include but are not limited to age; gender; sex; biological response to stimuli, stress, or medications; and genetic predispositions.

The combination of these factors heavily influences the overall health of individuals, communities, and populations, making healthy living either easier or more difficult.[2] These factors are closely intertwined, with no single determinant independent of the others. One study ranked the relative contributions of determinants of health to overall health as follows: behavior, 40%; genetics, 30%; social factors 15%; healthcare, 10%; and environmental factors, 5%.[5] As Shermock[6] points out, "[e]ven if we get the part that healthcare practitioners typically focus on *completely right*, that still leaves 90% of what determines health unaccounted for."

Public health seeks to understand the determinants of health and their influence on risk factors, disease, illness, injury, and negative health outcomes through research. That knowledge is then used to improve the determinants of health and remove the barriers to healthy living, making the healthy choice the easier one.

Public Health Activities of Pharmacists

In 2006, the American Public Health Association (APHA) outlined the public health role of the pharmacist in a statement[7] building on two previous APHA publications.[8,9] In 2013, the American Association of Colleges of Pharmacy recognized the important role pharmacists can play in public health by including population-based care and reducing

DOI 10.37573/9781585287048.068

TABLE 1.
Examples of Prevention

Upstream ←		Downstream →	
Primordial Prevention (prevent risk factors)	**Primary Prevention (prevent illness/injury)**	**Secondary Prevention (reduce impact)**	**Tertiary Prevention (chronic impact)**
Banning smoking in public areas, smoking education programs	Anti-smoking campaigns, taxes on cigarettes, smoking cessation programs, patches, gum	Treatment for smoking related illness, medical intervention, patient counseling	Disease management, respiratory treatment, therapies and screenings
Eliminating food deserts, nutrition education, healthy cooking classes, dietary guidelines	Increasing access to farmers' markets, health screenings	Individual nutrition counseling, medical intervention for diet-related illness, vitamins	Disease management, health monitoring
Laws and regulations against human trafficking, education regarding human trafficking, establishment of safe internet practices	Establishment of human trafficking hotline, raising awareness among the public, establishment of sentinel reporting, education programs for healthcare providers as well as police officers and other public servants	Screening for trafficking as part of all healthcare provider interactions, treatment of injuries and illnesses	Establishment of resources and safe havens for victims, mental health counseling
Opioid education programs, safe practices to avoid illness and injury	Improved opioid prescribing policies, opioid disposal locations and policies etc., patient education	Monitoring opioid use (both systemically and individually), early intervention	Medication-assisted therapy, access to treatment centers, monitoring

health disparities and inequalities in its Center for Advancement in Pharmaceutical Education (CAPE) Educational Outcomes.[10] These outcomes also emphasized the pharmacist's role in the public health components of "design[ing] prevention, intervention, and educational strategies for individuals and communities to manage chronic disease and improve health and wellness."[10]

The public health duties that an individual pharmacist performs will vary, based on the individual's experience, abilities, training, and work setting. All pharmacists, working alone or in collaboration with healthcare colleagues and administrators, can contribute to the promotion of public health. ASHP has described roles pharmacists have in specific public health–related activities, including antimicrobial stewardship and infection control[11]; substance abuse prevention, education, and treatment[12]; prevention of controlled substances diversion[13]; managing drug product shortages[14]; immunization[15]; tobacco cessation[16]; and emergency preparedness and response.[17]

The following are examples of other activities that pharmacists can engage in to promote public health:

- Promoting population health.
- Developing disease prevention and control programs (including chronic disease or disease treatment programs).
- Promoting medication safety efforts in their institutions and communities.
- Engaging in opioid stewardship efforts, including prevention, intervention, and treatment.
- Developing health-education policies and programs within their institutions that address the needs of patients, other healthcare professionals, community leaders, and the public, individually and as members of committees with purview over public health–related activities; and participating as members of public health organizations and chapters in pharmacy organizations.
- Advocating for sound legislation, regulations, and public policy regarding disease prevention and management.
- Engaging in public health–related research and education programs, initiating campaigns to disseminate new knowledge, and providing training programs that include basic population health tools such as statistical analysis, epidemiology, disease surveillance techniques, risk reduction strategies, and insights into methodology.[18]

Population Health. Although pharmacists have a role in both, it is important to distinguish population health from community health. Community health "encompasses population groups and the locus (e.g., place, venue, or other unit) of programs, interventions, and other actions,"[19] typically implying a geographic basis. In contrast, population health focuses on groups of individuals defined by specific characteristics other than geography, such as a health determinant or disease state. For example, Kindig and Stoddart[20] defined population health as "the health outcomes of a group of individuals, including the distribution of such outcomes within the group." They proposed that the field of population health includes policies and interventions that link health outcomes and patterns of health determinants. Evans, Barer, and Marmor[21] described factors in the social environment, external to the healthcare system, that exert a major and potentially modifiable influence on the health of populations.

Efforts to improve population health have been defined in different ways. The Institute for Healthcare Improvement Triple Aim Initiative uses the term "population health management" to describe "the work by healthcare organizations to improve outcomes for individual patients to maximize population health," whereas the National Academy of Medicine prefers the term "population health improvement" to describe "work to identify and improve aspects of or contributors to population health, expanding the focus beyond traditional healthcare delivery systems."[22] Homsted et al[23] provide a process-based definition of population health management:

> The active process of strategically utilizing health determinant data for a defined cohort to design, coordinate, and deliver high-quality, cost-effective, patient-centered care across the continuum, through optimizing communication, collaboration, and utilization of available resources with the goal of creating and sustaining health.

Population health management, a subset of population health, focuses on the comprehensive care of a specific population to implement needed services and interventions to improve the population's health.[24] Pharmacists can participate in population health management by being able to identify the needs of a population and implement necessary changes by, for example, performing medication reviews (especially of risky or costly medications) and working with other healthcare providers to develop care paths and chronic disease state management programs.[25] Given the importance of behavior as a determinant of health, pharmacists can improve population health through concerted actions to improve adherence to medication, diet, and exercise regimens, and through efforts to discourage harmful behaviors such as tobacco use, substance abuse, and high-risk sexual activity. Pharmacists practicing in ambulatory care and primary care settings are particularly well positioned to help ensure patients have received appropriate preventive care, such as well care visits, immunizations, and screenings (e.g., mammograms, colonoscopies). Those pharmacists also have a role in population health management by contributing to team-based monitoring and education of patients about healthy lifestyle choices and screening for social determinants of health.[26]

Medication therapy management (MTM) programs provide one example of a role pharmacists can have a role in population health management. MTM broadly encompasses a range of healthcare services provided by pharmacists that optimize patient outcomes. Pharmacists can expand their roles by leveraging provider status to improve public health through MTM.[27] MTM can be used to identify and resolve drug therapy problems. Pharmacists can develop comprehensive individual care plans, identify and meet vaccination needs, and improve health outcomes through adherence and management of chronic diseases. MTM has the potential to go beyond the treatment and management of diseases and provide pharmacists an opportunity to identify social determinants of health during patient care conversations (e.g., identifying social determinants of health such as food insecurities may shed light on why a patient skips meals and insulin, leading to uncontrolled diabetes) and help address them. Identifying social determinants of health that are impacting patient outcomes and advocating for these patients is an important aspect of MTM, and the future of pharmacy must incorporate social determinants of health principles if the profession is to treat the whole patient and meet the needs of an integrated and multiprofessional healthcare system.

Some of the leading health initiatives of Healthy People 2030 include smoking cessation, fall risk assessment, vaccinations, and medical product safety,[28] which can all be addressed during MTM services provided by pharmacists. Motivational interviewing should be utilized for those who are actively smoking, and benefits of quitting discussed during MTM sessions. This activity, along with identifying needed vaccines and potential fall risks, could improve public health and patient outcomes.

The CAPE 2013 outcomes emphasize the importance of this ability for future pharmacists to be trained in identifying and critically analyzing information that may impact patient-centered and population-based care.[10] As the volume of population and patient data grows, along with the ability to analyze that data using tools such as machine learning, human language processing, and harvesting of data from health apps and social media, well-trained pharmacists will be able to harness the power of big data to care for populations more efficiently and effectively.

Disease Prevention and Control. Pharmacists can be involved in disease prevention and control in many ways. For example, they can help develop institutional screening programs to check immunization status and identify undiagnosed medical conditions (e.g., hypertension, diabetes, hyperlipidemia, depression, substance abuse, behavioral health issues). Pharmacists have gained authority in many parts of the United States to administer immunizations, sometimes with a prescription from a physician, but often just at the request of the patient, and are making it a routine part of offered services. The goals for disease prevention in Healthy People 2020 were focused on the diseases and conditions listed above.[29] Healthy People 2020 also introduced Leading Health Indicators,[30] which included social determinants of health.

In Healthy People 2030, more attention is focused on preventing disease through attention to upstream influences on health, such as social determinants.[28] Healthy People 2030 continues to emphasize helping people prevent conditions that have a high impact on costs and quality of life, such as chronic disease, behavioral health, and equity, or the equal opportunity to be the healthiest a person can be. Pharmacists can encourage and model behaviors to mitigate threats that are high risk to public health, such as anthrax, botulism, plague, and smallpox, as well as currently emerging diseases spread by viral and bacterial vectors, such as Zika, HIV, influenza (e.g., H1N1), and coronaviruses. These behaviors include handwashing, social distancing, mask wearing, immunization, and not working when symptomatic.[31] **Table 2** provides a list of ways to prepare for specific pharmacy public health roles in epidemic or pandemic response.

TABLE 2.
Preparing for Specific Pharmacy Public Health Roles in Epidemic/Pandemic Response[a]

Role in Communication and Information		
To prepare for	**Cause**	**Issues**
Counseling visitors and family members	Concerned and anxious due to fear of unknown	• Prepare for increased phone calls and directing of family members that come to the facility to visit
Poor or confusing communication or information, misinformation	Health officials may update information frequently to adjust to evolving situation; different authorities may say conflicting or confusing things	• Communicate and collaborate with institution, local, and/or state Incident Command Centers for coordinated and informed response • Seek reliable information sources • Seek local information for current quarantine or treatment recommendations • Be an advocate for local citizens and be vigilant for emerging issues • Keep staff well informed through frequent communication via various channels and provide a forum to address questions and concerns
Informing the pharmacy workforce	Information sharing to ensure a ready and engaged workforce	• Stay up to date on the latest information about signs and symptoms, diagnostic testing, and case definitions for the epidemic/pandemic disease • Share information with pharmacists at other institutions experiencing the same crisis • Use network groups to keep colleagues at other institutions abreast of new information, guidelines, and issues • Perform literature searches and communicate with drug manufacturers to obtain unpublished information on file for emerging and investigational regimens
Role in Supply Chain Management		
To prepare for	**Cause**	**Issues**
Challenges securing anticipated stocks of medications and supplies	Supply chain disruption	• Report unusual sales volumes for medications or patient complaints • Determine mechanisms for obtaining drugs not available on market (e.g., emerging investigational therapies) during regular and off-hours • Report supply chain issues (e.g., drug shortages, PPE) to key facility staff and contact local/state health departments
Role in Pharmacy Operations		
To prepare for	**Cause**	**Issues**
Supplying rapid response kits	Timely access to treatment	• For supportive care and as investigational therapies emerge, prepare rapid response kits containing information such as management algorithms, drug dosing and administration guidelines, and pharmacist contact numbers • Make kits available in relevant patient care units such as emergency departments and intensive care units
Leadership in medication use and safety	Safe patient care	• Ensure that appropriate education and drug administration and dosing guidelines are available to guide medical, nursing, and pharmacy staff
Role in Infection Prevention and Control		
To prepare for	**Cause**	**Issues**
Requests to dispose of potentially contaminated medications and supplies	Family members of potential disease cases may have unused medications they want to throw away	• Determine local/state health department recommendations for disposing of unused medication products and supplies that have been dispensed to a patient
Updating policies and procedures	Integrity of drug supply	• Develop or revise policies and procedures pertaining to drug delivery to meet infection control precautions
Protecting workforce from exposure	• Healthcare workers are more likely to become infected if they work closely with patients with infectious diseases • Limiting exposure time and closeness can help prevent infection	• Orient and educate workforce regarding infection control precautions • Use standard respiratory precautions • Handle items associated with potentially exposed patients while wearing gloves • Frequent hand washing • Use face masks if counseling symptomatic patients • Ensure that appropriate pharmacy staff have been medically cleared, fit-tested, and trained for respirator use • Use telephone for counseling • Drop off prescriptions at home • Bill via credit card to avoid handling checks or money

Monitoring pharmacy staff	Fever, cough, and shortness of breath are early signs and symptoms of some infectious diseases	• Be prepared to take temperature of workers once a shift • If fever, cough, and shortness of breath are present, send worker to designated treatment site • If a family member is sick, put employee on sick leave • Notify occupational health services
Role in Patient Care		
To prepare for	**Cause**	**Issues**
Patient/visitor surge	Patients may seek other sources of care and information if local hospitals closed or under quarantine	• Adjust staffing to handle increased traffic, phone calls, and other electronic communications (e.g., social media) • Manage staff to accommodate revised or expanded responsibilities with appropriate sleep/rest cycles • Prepare information for patients/visitors for education and awareness programs • Report patient surges to key facility staff and public health officials
Treating sicker patients	Patients may be sicker than usual but barred from hospitals	• Review latest CDC information for education and awareness programs • Help triage patients in accordance with institution emergency preparedness plan • Inform key facility staff and contact local/state health departments for latest guidance and instructions (e.g., home quarantine)
Caring for the worried well	Patients who have respiratory symptoms but no history of exposure	• Provide information and reassurance through education and awareness programs • Remind patients to get other appropriate vaccines
Requests for ineffective prevention and treatment options	Remedies for self-treating a disease may be requested by patients even though they are not effective	• Provide patients with most current treatment and prevention information.
Team-based care	Interprofessional expertise needed	• Collaborate with key players (e.g., microbiologist) and communicate on interprofessional issues needed to optimize patient care • Be proactive and flexible in assuming new responsibilities within a pharmacists scope of practice

Abbreviations: CDC, Centers for Disease Control and Prevention; PPE, personal protective equipment.

[a]Source: Adapted from Tables 3.5 and 3.6 in Carter J, Slack M. *Pharmacy in Public Health: Basics and Beyond.* American Society of Health-System Pharmacists; 2009.

All healthcare professionals, including pharmacists, have become increasingly concerned about the effect of stress on the overall health of people and interested in promoting ways to reduce stress (e.g., regular exercise, yoga, increasing time in nature, comfort animals). As Healthy People stakeholders, pharmacists can use and make their patients aware of available resources and services by providing website links, data, interactive tools, and reports as passive offerings in clinic and community pharmacies. Pharmacists can more actively manage disease prevention through collaborative care agreements, prescribing, therapeutic medication management, and counseling.

Medication Safety. Medication safety is one of pharmacists' primary responsibilities.[32,33] Adverse medication events are estimated to cost the United States more than $30 billion a year and inflict incalculable loss and suffering on victims.[34] By providing focused and comprehensive medication instruction to individual patients and groups of patients, pharmacists can help reduce emergency room visits and hospital admissions by up to 30%.[34] The pharmacist's role in medication safety and preventable adverse events from medications align with the national public health goals outlined in Healthy People 2030,[28] which include reducing emergency department visits for overdoses from medications. Pharmacists are ideally suited to serve in leadership roles as an expert resource for medication safety by virtue of their education and training and their responsibility for ensuring medication safety through use of technologies such as barcoding, computerized provider order entry systems, infusion pumps, and clinical decision support. Pharmacists can improve medication-related processes and develop strong medication-safety practices utilizing Just Culture principles[35] to facilitate high-reliability organizations[36] through engagement in facility-wide committees (e.g., medication safety or pharmacy and therapeutics committees).[37,38] Pharmacists can also promote adherence and effective medication use through initiatives in the community and local organizations. The 2013 CAPE outcomes include an increasing role for pharmacists in improving the safety of medications at each step in the medication-use system and in transitions of care.[10] Pharmacists are responsible for monitoring the medication-use system and reporting of medication-related adverse events because of their unique expertise in this area. Pharmacists are often an inherent part of transitions of care (e.g., through community pharmacies, managed-care facilities, long-term care), so they can play a significant role in ensuring medication safety by counseling patients, identifying potential medication-related adverse drug events, and putting in place strategies to prevent those events (e.g., notifying pharmacy colleagues in a setting that a patient is transferring to, or raising awareness of possible threats to medication safety for specific patients). Pharmacists' ability to problem-solve and decrease future medication-related adverse events is beneficial to public health at large.

Efforts to Address the Opioid Epidemic. ASHP has described roles and responsibilities pharmacists have in substance abuse prevention, education, and assistance[12] and prevention of controlled substances diversion.[13] The scope and nature of the opioid epidemic warrant particular focus. Healthcare professionals have come to embrace what is termed "pain management and opioid stewardship," recognizing that "opioid stewardship is an integral . . . part of an overall pain management and stewardship strategy" and that behavioral and socioeconomic aspects of care should be "recognized as an overarching component that needs to be addressed across the spectrum of patients."[39] Pharmacists are well positioned in the healthcare and local communities to collaborate with other providers in the treatment of acute and chronic pain working to apply opioid-alternative therapies when possible. In addition, pharmacists should be engaged to recommend appropriate opioid dosage regimens that decrease overprescribing and reduce the risks of abuse and addiction when necessary. Pharmacists, as part of the interprofessional team, have roles in prevention, intervention, and treatment of opioid abuse and addiction that include but are not limited to the following.

Prevention

- Collaborating with healthcare colleagues to take an interprofessional approach to pain management and opioid stewardship that incorporates evidence-based non-opioid therapies and reduces the risks of abuse, misuse, and addiction.
- Adopting communication and educational approaches to explain dosing instructions to patients in ways that avoid or reduce common problems that stem from opioid misuse or overuse.
- Leading efforts to prevent diversion of controlled substances.[13]
- Working with other healthcare professionals, governmental agencies, and civic organizations to destigmatize opioid use disorder and foster development of treatment programs.
- Using and advocating for the enhancement of state prescription drug monitoring programs.
- Participating in public substance abuse education and prevention programs.

Intervention

- Assisting in the identification of individuals, coworkers, and others who may be having problems related to opioid abuse.
- Dispensing and administering naloxone, and training caregivers to administer and at-risk patients to self-administer naloxone.
- Working with local school districts to provide programming and encourage peer interventions as well as opportunities for counseling with the pharmacist on options for treatment.

Treatment

- Seeking out education and training in the use of medications used in medication-assisted treatment of opioid use disorder (e.g., methadone, buprenorphine, buprenorphine/naloxone, naltrexone).
- Optimizing therapy outcomes by gathering vital clinical and health screening information about patients.

Laws regarding the prescribing, dispensing, and use of naloxone have changed dramatically in recent years. By 2019, every state in the United States had some form of immediate availability for naloxone in pharmacies.[40] Healthcare organizations have created training modules for pharmacists on how to use and administer the drug.

Health Education. Another way pharmacists advance public health is by developing, promoting, and implementing education programs aimed across life's stages.[41] Pharmacists have acted as health educators on a variety of topics (**Table 3**).[42–53] In their role as health educators, pharmacists can assess and improve the health literacy of individuals and groups to improve adherence to medication, diet, and exercise regimens; reduce medication-related adverse events; enhance the individual's role in their care and health; and build trust with pharmacists and the healthcare system. Pharmacists who serve as faculty in health professions schools and colleges have a stake in promoting Healthy People 2030. There is a responsibility on their part to integrate strategies on prevention into curricula and interprofessional experiences for the learner. Employing interactive techniques and tools such as games, simulations, and personal fitness devices encourages engagement and commitment by individuals to activities such as exercise and maintaining healthy diets.

Public Health Policy. Pharmacists should participate in public health policy development, from local boards of health to national programs.[54] By linking disease prevalence, medication utilization, and the determinants of disease, pharmacists can place prevention within a larger context. Medication use plays a central role in health and health policy, especially policy directed at chronic disease, which must be formulated with a broad understanding of the relationship between medication therapy and the many other factors that affect disease outcomes. Since medication use increases as patients age, pharmacists' unique perspective on healthcare policy will become more important as the average age of the U.S. population rises.[55]

As medication-use experts and experienced health-system administrators, pharmacists can and should contribute to the development of public health-related legislation and regulation and should be involved in public program oversight and administration. Legislators, regulators, and program managers at all levels of government should be educated to utilize this expertise. Pharmacists, as individuals and through their professional associations, state and local boards of health, and state boards of pharmacy, are encouraged to participate in legislative, regulatory, and oversight processes.

Pharmacists will need knowledge of the policy and financial drivers of public health to engage in advocacy efforts to improve population outcomes.[56] To be most effective, pharmacists need to be trained to take leadership roles in public health policy. Postgraduate year 2 pharmacy

TABLE 3.
Examples of Patient Education Programs, Goals, Methods, and Alignment with Healthy People 2030 Goals

Patient Education Programs	Goals	Method	Aligns with Healthy People 2030 Goal
Birth Control[42]	Provide Women's Health services	Individual	Yes
Chronic Disease	Education Prevention Management	Individual Group Special Populations	Yes
Immunization[43,44]	Prevention Reduce epidemics Provide services Improve health of a nation	Individual Group Special Populations Community Awareness	Yes
Medication Safety[45,46]	Improve Patient Outcome Improve Health Literacy	Individual Health Literacy Assess Group Special Populations Community Awareness	Yes
Mental Health[47,48]	Reduce Stigma Direct individual to services Provide services Prevention	Individual Group Special Populations Community Awareness	Yes
Nutrition	Reduce disease Reduce cost to health system Better individual Health	Individual Group Community Awareness	Yes
Oral Chemotherapy[49]	Improve Patient Outcome	Individual	
Substance Abuse[50,51]	Prevention Direct individual to services Provide services Improve health of a nation	Individual Groups Special Populations Community Awareness Flyers or Brochures	Yes
Tobacco Cessation[52]	Reduce disease Reduce cost to health system Better individual Health	Individual Group Resources	Yes
Resources[53]	Improve Literacy and Guide to Resources and Support for: • Human Trafficking • Partner and Child Abuse • Community Wellness Services	Individual Groups Brochures and Flyers	

residencies are now available in Population Health Management and Data Analytics Pharmacy, and dual PharmD/MPH degrees are available, as are executive programs in public health practice.

Research and Training. Pharmacists should be encouraged to pursue more advanced training and gather credentials that will give them added credibility in addressing broad public health initiatives. Pharmacists should strive to be proficient in research methodology, pharmacoepidemiology, and biostatistics, and how these areas apply to public health decision-making. Pharmacists should actively seek experience in the design, implementation, analysis, and interpretation of clinical studies (both observational and experimental), which can be achieved through both pharmacy curricula and professional education.

Pharmacy curricula should be developed in such a way to include public health, biostatistics, and research design.[57] Inclusion of the content can help assure that future pharmacists have a strong working knowledge of public health principles as well as population health. It is essential that both experiential and didactic training for students, residents, and research fellows include exposure to research in public health policy, pharmacoepidemiology, pharmacoeconomics, health-related quality of life, and evidence-based medicine, with potential opportunities for publication and/or presentation of their work.

Professional education of practicing pharmacists may include refreshers on biostatistics, research, and public health trends, with a focus on the application and analysis of research findings in the clinical setting. Mentoring and collaborative research projects across multiple disciplines is encouraged. Pharmacists can play an important role in data monitoring committees. There are certificate and graduate education programs available for pharmacists to advance their knowledge and skills in the above-mentioned areas of practice.

Pharmacists should seek out opportunities to participate in collaborative research.[58] They are also well suited to serve on institutional review boards, medication safety committees, and pharmacy and therapeutics committees. It is recommended that pharmacists work directly with public health policymakers and other key stakeholders (e.g., leaders in professional organizations, medical centers, academic institutions, governmental agencies, and third-party payers) to learn about processes and to advance their knowledge in order to promote optimal pharmacotherapy.

Future Roles

Some of the future roles of pharmacists in public health will look very similar to their current roles. Safe dispensing of drugs will remain a core responsibility of the profession, but changes in laws regarding dispensing will allow pharmacists to proactively dispense knowledge about medications and increase their primary care responsibilities. Pharmacists will continue to provide easy access to vaccinations and partner with other care providers in grassroots public health campaigns, particularly for underserved populations. Pharmacists will remain key healthcare providers in tobacco cessation. As advances in technology make disease screening more accessible, pharmacists will play an increasingly important role in education and screening for conditions such as obesity, hypertension, heart disease, substance abuse, sexually transmitted diseases, and others. With appropriate changes in law and regulation to confer provider status for pharmacists, interpretation of screening test results and referral to other healthcare providers will fall within the pharmacist's responsibilities. Recognition of pharmacists as healthcare providers and reimbursement for their services would also empower pharmacists to screen for food insecurity, physical or sexual abuse, human trafficking, substance use disorders, and mental health issues.

Advances in informatics will permit aggregation and application of population and patient-specific data in ways that will encourage development of population-specific, evidence-based screening and disease management programs. Pharmacists should gain awareness of how artificial intelligence can illuminate the relationships between risk factors, prevention, treatment, and patient outcomes to better predict successful interventions. The burgeoning field of pharmacogenomics has already demonstrated its value in patient-focused pharmacotherapy, as genotyping has enabled prescribers and pharmacists to reduce treatment failures and prevent adverse drug reactions in large groups of people. As pharmacogenomics and the rapidly expanding field of population genetics become even more important, pharmacists, as medication-use experts, will apply these new tools not simply to improve patient-specific pharmacotherapy but to advance public health through population health management.

Conclusion

Pharmacists play a vital role in maintaining and promoting public health. Pharmacists can improve public health by promoting population health; developing and implementing disease prevention and control programs; advancing medication safety practices; engaging in opioid stewardship; developing health-education policies and programs; advocating for relevant and impactful legislation, regulations, and public policy regarding public health; engaging in public health–related research and education programs; initiating campaigns to disseminate new knowledge; and providing training that includes basic population health tools. All pharmacists have a responsibility to participate in global, national, state, regional, and institutional efforts to promote public health. Pharmacists should integrate the public health practices outlined in this statement into their practices and be empowered by their employers and policymakers to contribute to and improve public health efforts. To more fully utilize their unique expertise, pharmacists should be involved in public health policy decision-making and in the planning, development, and implementation of public health efforts.

References

1. CDC Foundation. What is public health? Accessed July 24, 2020. https://www.cdcfoundation.org/what-public-health
2. American Public Health Association. What is public health? Accessed July 24, 2020. https://apha.org/what-is-public-health
3. Pandve HT. Quaternary prevention: need of the hour. *J Family Med Prim Care*. 2014;3:309–310.
4. Office of Disease Prevention and Health Promotion, US Department of Health and Human Services. Determinants of health. Accessed July 24, 2020. https://www.healthypeople.gov/2020/about/foundation-health-measures/Determinants-of-Health
5. McGinnis JM, Williams-Russo P, Knickman TR. The case for more active policy attention to health promotion. *Health Aff (Millwood)*. 2002;21:78–93.
6. Shermock KM. Population health management: challenges and opportunities for pharmacy. Editorial. *Am J Health-Syst Pharm*. 2017;74:1398–1399. doi:10.2146/ajhp170530
7. American Public Health Association. The role of the pharmacist in public health. Accessed July 24, 2020. http://www.apha.org/policies-and-advocacy/public-health-policy-statements/policy-database/2014/07/07/13/05/the-role-of-the-pharmacist-in-publichealth
8. American Public Health Association. APHA policy 8024: the role of the pharmacist in public health. *Am J Public Health*. 1981;71:213–216.
9. Cain RM, Kahn JS. The pharmacist as a member of the health team. *Am J Public Health*. 1971;61:2223–2228.
10. Medina MS, Plaza CM, Stowe CD, et al. Center for the Advancement of Pharmacy Education 2013 Educational Outcomes. *Am J Pharm Educ*. 2013;77(8):1–10. doi:10.5688/ajpe778162.
11. American Society of Health-System Pharmacists. ASHP statement on the pharmacist's role in antimicrobial stewardship and infection prevention and control. *Am J Health-Syst Pharm*. 1998;55:1724–1726. Accessed January 23, 2019. https://www.ashp.org/-/media/assets/policy-guidelines/docs/statements/pharmacists-roleantimicrobial-stewardship.ashx
12. American Society of Health-System Pharmacists. ASHP statement on the pharmacist's role in substance abuse prevention, education, and assistance. *Am J Health-Syst Pharm*. 2010;67:575–577. Accessed January 23, 2019. https://www.ashp.org/-/media/assets/policy-guidelines/docs/statements/pharmacistsrole-substance-abuse-preventioneducation-assistance.ashx

13. American Society of Health-System Pharmacists. ASHP guidelines on preventing diversion of controlled substances. *Am J Health-Syst Pharm.* 2017;74:325–348. Accessed January 23, 2019. https://www.ashp.org/-/media/assets/policy-guidelines/docs/guidelines/preventing-diversion-ofcontrolled-substances.ashx
14. American Society of Health-System Pharmacists. ASHP guidelines on managing drug product shortages. *Am J Health-Syst Pharm.* 2018;75:e593-e601. Accessed January 23, 2019. https://www.ashp.org/-/media/assets/policyguidelines/docs/guidelines/managingdrug-product-shortages.ashx
15. American Society of Health-System Pharmacists. ASHP guidelines on the pharmacist's role in immunization. *Am J Health-Syst Pharm.* 2003;60:1371–1377. Accessed January 23, 2019. https://www.ashp.org/-/media/assets/policy-guidelines/docs/guidelines/pharmacists-role-immunization.ashx
16. American Society of Health-System Pharmacists. ASHP therapeutic position statement on smoking cessation. *Am J Health-Syst Pharm.* 1999;56:460–464. Accessed January 23, 2019. https://www.ashp.org/-/media/assets/policyguidelines/docs/therapeutic-positionstatements/cessation-tobacco-use.ashx
17. American Society of Health-System Pharmacists. ASHP statement on the role of health-system pharmacists in emergency preparedness. *Am J Health-Syst Pharm.* 2003;60:1993–1995. Accessed January 23, 2019. https://www.ashp.org/-/media/assets/policy-guidelines/docs/statements/role-of-health-system-pharmacists-inemergency-preparedness.ashx
18. Benjamin GC. Ensuring population health: an important role for pharmacy. *Am J Pharm Educ.* 2016;80(2):19.
19. Goodman RA, Bunnell R, Posnera SF. What is "community health"? Examining the meaning of an evolving field in public health. *Prev Med.* 2014;67 (suppl 1):S58-S61. doi:10.1016/j.ypmed.2014.07.028
20. Kindig D, Stoddart G. What is population health? *Am J Public Health.* 2003;93:380–383.
21. Evans RG, Barer ML, Marmor TR. *Why Are Some People Healthy and Others Not? The Determinants of Health Populations.* Transaction Publishers; 1994.
22. Swarthout M, Bishop MA. Population health management: review of concepts and definitions. *Am J Health-Syst Pharm.* 2017;74:1405–1411. doi:10.2146/ajhp170025
23. Homsted FA, Magee CE, Nesin N. Population health management in a small health system: impact of controlled substance stewardship in a patient-centered medical home. *Am J Health-Syst Pharm.* 2017;74:1468–1475.
24. Rivo ML. It's time to start practicing population-based health care: you don't have to be part of an integrated delivery system to optimize care for populations of patients with common conditions. *Fam Pract Manag.* 1998;5:37–46.
25. Sanborn MD. Population health management and the pharmacist's role. Editorial. *Am J Health-Syst Pharm.* 2017;74:1400–1401. doi:10.2146/ajhp170157
26. Knoer SJ, Swarthout MD, Sokn E, et al. The Cleveland Clinic Pharmacy Population Health Management Summit. *Am J Health-Syst Pharm.* 2018;75:1421–1429. doi:10.2146/ajhp180081
27. Casserlie LM, Dipietro Mager NA. Pharmacists' perceptions of advancing public health priorities through medication therapy management. *Pharm Pract (Granada).* 2016;14(3):792. doi:10.18549/PharmPract.2016.03.79
28. Office of Disease Prevention and Health Promotion, US Department of Health and Human Services. Healthy People 2030 framework. Accessed November 26, 2019. www.healthypeople.gov/2020/About-Healthy-People/Development-Healthy-People-2030/Framework
29. Office of Disease Prevention and Health Promotion, US Department of Health and Human Services. Healthy People 2020 topics & objectives. Accessed November 26, 2019. www.healthypeople.gov/2020/topics-objectives
30. Office of Disease Prevention and Health Promotion, US Department of Health and Human Services. Healthy People 2020 Leading Health Indicators. Accessed November 26, 2019. https://www.healthypeople.gov/2020/Leading-Health-Indicators
31. Centers for Disease Control and Prevention. Guidance for pharmacies: guidance for pharmacists and pharmacy technicians in community pharmacies during the COVID-19 response. Accessed December 8, 2020. https://www.cdc.gov/coronavirus/2019-ncov/hcp/pharmacies.html
32. Anderson J, Venepalli NK, Fleming PJ, et al. Documentation of pharmacist-provided patient education for oral chemotherapy [abstract]. *J Clin Oncol.* 2016;34:237. doi:10.1200/jco.2016.34.7_suppl.237
33. Schnipper JL, Kirwin JL, Cotugno MC, et al. Role of pharmacist counseling in preventing adverse drug events after hospitalization. *Arch Intern Med.* 2006;166:565–571. doi:10.1001/archinte.166.5.565
34. Sultana J, Cutroneo P, Trifiro G. Clinical and economic burden of adverse drug reactions. *J Pharmacol Pharmacother.* 2013;4(suppl 1): s73-s77.
35. Boysen PG Jr. Just culture: a foundation for balanced accountability and patient safety. *Ochsner J.* 2013;13:400-406.
36. Chassin MR, Loeb JM. High-reliability health care: getting there from here. *Milbank Q.* 2013;91:459–490.
37. Carrillo JD, Cassano AT, Billstein-Leber M, et al. ASHP guidelines on preventing medication errors in hospitals. *Am J Health-Syst Pharm.* 2018;75:1493–1517.
38. Gorbach C, Blanton L, Lukawski B, et al. Benchmarking and medication error rates. *Am J Health-Syst Pharm.* 2016;73:746–747. doi:10.2146/ajhp150961
39. American Society of Health-System Pharmacists. Report of the ASHP Opioid Task Force. *Am J Health-Syst Pharm.* 2020;77:1158–1165. doi:10.1093/ajhp/zxaa117
40. Temple University Center for Public Health Law Research. Naloxone overdose prevention laws. Accessed July 24, 2020. http://pdaps.org/datasets/laws-regulating-administration-ofnaloxone-1501695139

41. Office of Disease Prevention and Health Promotion, US Department of Health and Human Services. Healthy People 2020: access to health services across the life stages. Accessed August 20, 2020. https://www.healthypeople.gov/node/6067/determinants
42. Young S, Griffin B, Vest K. Active-learning instruction on emergency contraception counseling. *Am J Pharm Educ.* 2013;77:104. doi:10.5688/ajpe775104
43. Bach AT, Goad JA. The role of community pharmacy-based vaccination in the USA: current practice and future directions. *Integr Pharm Res Pract.* 2015;4:67–77. doi:10.2147/IPRP.S63822
44. Bluml BM, Brock KA, Hamstra S, et al. Evaluation of the impact of an innovative immunization practice model designed to improve population health: results of the Project IMPACT Immunizations Pilot. *Pop Hlth Manag.* 2018;21:55–62. doi:10.1089/pop.2017.0049
45. Goldstone LW, Saldaña SN, Werremeyer A. Pharmacist provision of patient medication education groups. *Am J Health-Syst Pharm.* 2015;72:487–492. doi:10.2146/ajhp140182
46. Schnipper JL, Kirwin JL, Cotugno MC, et al. Role of pharmacist counseling in preventing adverse drug events after hospitalization. *Arch Intern Med.* 2006; 166:565–71. doi:10.1001/archinte.166.5.565
47. National Council for Mental Wellbeing. Pharmacists on the front lines with mental health first aid. Published December 13, 2018. Accessed January 24, 2020. www.mentalhealthfirstaid.org/2018/12/pharmacists-on-the-front-lines-withmental-health-first-aid/
48. Werremeyer AB. Editorial: patient education by pharmacists. *Mental Hlth Clinician.* 2012;2:74–76. Doi:10.9740/mhc.n117725
49. Anderson J, Venepalli NK, Fleming PJ, et al. Documentation of pharmacist-provided patient education for oral chemotherapy. *J Clin Oncol.* 2016;34 (suppl 7):237. doi:10.1200/jco.2016.34.7_suppl.237.
50. Tadros A, Layman SM, Davis SM, et al. Emergency department visits by pediatric patients for poisoning by prescription opioids. *Am J Drug Alcohol Abuse.* 2016;42:550–555. doi:10.1080/00952990.2016.1194851
51. CVSHealth. Educating teens & parents about opioid abuse. Accessed November 26, 2019. https://cvshealth.com/thought-leadership/educating-teens-about-opioid-abuse
52. Greenhalgh T, Macfarlane F, Steed L, et al. What works for whom in pharmacist-led smoking cessation support: realist review. *BMC Med.* 2016;14:209. doi:10.1186/s12916-016-0749-5
53. Thomas S. Health literacy in the pharmacy. *Pharmacy Times.* Published August 9, 2016. Accessed July 24, 2020. www.pharmacytimes.com/contributor/swana-thomas-pharmdmph-candidate-2018/2016/08/health-literacy-in-the-pharmacy
54. Little J, Ortega M, Powell M, Hamm M. ASHP statement on advocacy as a professional obligation. *Am J Health-Syst Pharm.* 2019;76:251–254.
55. Georgetown University Health Policy Institute. Prescription drugs. Accessed July 24, 2020. https://hpi.georgetown.edu/rxdrugs/#
56. Lavigne JE, Brown J, Matzke GR. Population health and medicine: policy and financial drivers. *Am J Health-Syst Pharm.* 2017;74:1413–1421. doi:10.2146/ajhp161051
57. Truong H-A, Patterson BY. Professional and educational initiatives, supports, and opportunities for advanced training in public health. *Am J Pharm Educ.* 2010;74(7):122. Accessed November 27, 2019. https://www.ajpe.org/doi/pdf/10.5688/aj7407122
58. Fincham JE. Public health teaching and research in the academy. *Am J Pharm Educ.* 2010;74(5):93. Accessed November 27, 2019. https://www.ajpe.org/doi/pdf/10.5688/aj740593

Other Resources

Pharmacists looking for further involvement in public health have many options. First, training and competence in public health disciplines are invaluable for understanding the field of public health and its applications to pharmacy practice. Accredited schools of public health offer traditional didactic classes, and some have courses or continuing education available online that will give the beginner a clearer understanding of the four traditional areas of public health practice: health administration and policy, health education, biostatistics, and epidemiology. Pharmacists who wish to pursue a degree in public health can also do so online at a growing number of schools of public health.

Pharmacists with an interest in federal public health initiatives can start with one of three main points of access. The first is the Centers for Disease Control and Prevention (www.cdc.gov), the largest repository of documents, program descriptions, and contacts in the realm of prevention. Major efforts aimed at disease surveillance, infectious disease control, immunization, health education, chronic disease maintenance, and disease-related data management provide an ample and readily available source of information. The second major source of information is the Office of Disease Prevention and Health Promotion (https://health.gov/), which provides access to Healthy People and MyHealthfinder (a personalized screening tool) as well as information about food and nutrition, physical activity, health literacy, and healthcare quality. Finally, the Agency for Healthcare Research and Quality website (www.ahrq.gov) has a section on prevention (https://www.ahrq.gov/prevention/index.html) that provides information on a variety of topics as well as access to information from the U.S. Preventive Services Task Force and the Guide to Clinical Preventive Services.

State government websites provide public health information for their respective states. State entities serve as the main policymaking entity for public health priorities and strategies, provide a conduit for federal public health dollars, and are the main repository of health information and data for the state. States often organize a range of advisory groups, task forces, and planning committees whose output shapes their public health agenda. These entities also provide input and direction for state legislative bodies to address, legislate, and fund.

On the local level, departments of health serve as the main government entities involved in public health. Aside from their usual routine of immunizations and restaurant inspections, these boards serve as the policymakers for disaster response and provision of primary care to underserved populations. They receive federal and state dollars that are used to fund public health efforts. They are closest to the general population both in their makeup and in their efforts at improving the public's health. Pharmacists interested in learning more about public health and the types of activities that community public health agencies are involved in can register for a free interactive tutorial at www.nynj-phtc.org/orientation.

Below is a list of websites that provide information related to public health.

Public Health Organizations

- World Health Organization (www.who.int)
- Pan American Health Organization (www.paho.org)
- American Public Health Association (www.apha.org)
- Association of State and Territorial Health Officials (www.astho.org)
- National Association of County and City Health Officials (www.naccho.org)
- Public Health Foundation (www.phf.org)
- Association of Schools of Public Health (www.asph.org)
- Association for Prevention Teaching and Research (www.aptrweb.org/)

Federal Health Agencies

- U.S. Department of Health and Human Services (www.dhhs.gov)
- Office of the Surgeon General, Public Health Reports (https://www.hhs.gov/surgeongeneral/reports-and publications/publichealthreports/index.html)
- Centers for Disease Control and Prevention (www.cdc.gov)
- Food and Drug Administration (www.fda.gov)
- Health Resources and Services Administration (www.hrsa.gov)
- National Institutes of Health (www.nih.gov)
- Agency for Healthcare Research and Quality (www.ahrq.gov)
- Environmental Protection Agency (www.epa.gov)

Developed through the ASHP Council on Pharmacy Practice and approved by the ASHP Board of Directors on March 26, 2021, and by the ASHP House of Delegates on May 19, 2021. This statement supersedes the ASHP Statement on the Role of Health-System Pharmacists in Public Health dated June 24, 2007.

ASHP gratefully acknowledges the following individuals for reviewing the current version of the statement (review does not imply endorsement): Michael Dickens, RPh; Linda Gore Martin, PharmD, MBA, BCPS, FASHP; and Paul L Ranelli, PhD, BSPharm, MSc. The contributions of the following individuals to previous versions of this statement are gratefully acknowledged: Vaiyapuri Subramaniam, PharmD, MS, FASHP, FASCP, FCP, FFIP; Karim Anton Calis, PharmD, MPH, FASHP, FCCP; Robert C. Dombrowski, PharmD, BCPS; Timothy J. Ives, PharmD, MPH, BCPS, FCCP, FASHP, CPP; Linda Gore Martin, PharmD, MBA, BCPS; CAPT Carlene McIntyre, PharmD; CAPT (Ret) Steven R. Moore, MPH, FRSH, FASHP, CPHP; Ruth E. Nemire, PharmD; Frank Pucino, PharmD, BCPS, FASHP, FDPGEC; Ashok Ramalingam, BPharm, MTech, DPharm, DCA, PhD; Paul L. Ranelli, PhD, FAFPE, FAPhA; CAPT Sharon K. Gershon, PharmD; and CDR Charlie V. Hoppes, MPH, CPHP.

The authors have declared no potential conflicts of interest.

Ginger Cameron, MPH, PhD, Purdue University, Global, West Lafayette, IN.

Rachel N. Chandra, PharmD, MPH, Dayton Veterans Affairs Medical Center, Dayton, OH.

Marianne F. Ivey, PharmD, MPH, FASHP, FFIP, University of Cincinnati, Cincinnati, OH.

CDR Sadhna Khatri, PharmD, MPH, MS, MEd, U.S. Public Health Service, Washington, DC, and Center for Drug Evaluation and Research, Food and Drug Administration, Silver Spring, MD.

Ruth E. Nemire, PharmD, EdD, FCCP, FNAP, CRQM, Larkin University College of Pharmacy, Miami, FL.

CAPT John Quinn, RPh, MS, U.S. Public Health Service, Washington, DC, and Center for Drug Evaluation and Research, Food and Drug Administration, Silver Spring, MD.

Vaiyapuri Subramaniam, PharmD, MS, FASHP, FASCP, FCP, FFIP, Executive Board of Directors, Washington Metropolitan Society of Health-System Pharmacists, Silver Spring, MD, and Board of Visitors, Howard University College of Pharmacy, Washington, DC.

Copyright © 2022, American Society of Health-System Pharmacists, Inc. All rights reserved. Contact ASHP for reprint and permissions requests. This content may not be used for commercial purposes without the express written consent of ASHP.

The bibliographic citation for this document is as follows: American Society of Health-System Pharmacists. ASHP statement on the pharmacist's role in public health. *Am J Health-Syst Pharm.* 2022;79:388–399.

ASHP Statement on the Pharmacist's Role in Substance Abuse Prevention, Education, and Assistance

Position

The American Society of Health-System Pharmacists (ASHP) believes that pharmacists have the unique knowledge, skills, and responsibilities for assuming an important role in substance abuse prevention, education, and assistance. Pharmacists, as healthcare providers, should be actively involved in reducing the negative effects that substance abuse has on society, health systems, and the pharmacy profession. Further, ASHP supports efforts to rehabilitate pharmacists and other health-system employees whose mental or physical impairments are caused by substance abuse.

Background

The term *substance abuse* is commonly used to describe the hazardous or addictive use of psychoactive substances with either addictive, typically depressing or stimulating, or perception distorting properties. The American Psychiatric Association's *Diagnostic and Statistical Manual of Mental Disorders (DSM), Fifth Edition,* includes substance use disorders, typically considered addictions with severity categories, and substance–induced disorders, typically intoxication or withdrawal, in its Substance-Related and Addictive Disorders chapter.[1] Examples include alcohol; tobacco; "street" drugs, such as marijuana, LSD (lysergic acid diethylamide), PCP (phencyclidine), cocaine, methamphetamine, methylenedioxymethamphetamine (commonly known as MDMA, ecstasy, or molly), inhalants, GHB (gammahydroxybutyrate), heroin, synthetic marijuana (also known as K2 or spice), salvia, and bath salts; and the nonmedical use or overuse of psychoactive and other prescription and nonprescription drugs (e.g., hydrocodone, oxycodone, ketamine, methadone, dextromethorphan).

Substance abuse is a major societal problem. The 2012 National Household Survey on Drug Use and Health (NSDUH), a primary source of statistical information on drug abuse in the U.S. population, estimated that (1) 23.9 million Americans (or 9.2% of the population 12 years of age or older) had used an illicit drug[a] in the past month, (2) 2.8 million Americans were dependent on or abused both illicit drugs and alcohol, (3) 4.5 million Americans were dependent on or abused illicit drugs but not alcohol, and (4) 14.9 million Americans were dependent on alcohol.[2] In earlier studies, investigators used the *DSM, Fourth Edition, (DSM-IV)* criteria to assess the prevalence of substance abuse and dependence disorders in the United States.[3,4] They reported the following lifetime prevalence figures: 30.3% for alcohol-use disorders,[3] 10.3% for drug-use disorders,[4] 12.5% for alcohol dependence (alcoholism) (17.4% for men, 8.0% for women),[3] and 2.6% for dependence on other drugs (drug addiction), excluding tobacco (3.3% for men, 2.0% for women).[4] Studies suggest that the prevalence of drug abuse among health professionals appears to be similar to that in the general population.[5–7] However, given their access to drugs, health professionals abuse prescription drugs more often and street drugs less often compared with the general population.

Substance abuse frequently coexists with and complicates other psychiatric disorders and is a common and often unrecognized cause of physical morbidity. Intravenous drug abuse is a major factor in the spread of human immunodeficiency virus and hepatitis. Alcohol is a major factor in the development of cirrhosis of the liver, and tobacco is a key contributor to emphysema and lung cancer. Collectively, substance abuse contributes significantly to morbidity and mortality in the U.S. population and to the cost of healthcare.

Substance abuse is also a serious workplace problem. The 2012 NSDUH survey found that approximately 14.6 million Americans reporting past-month illicit drug use were currently employed full- or part-time.[2] Substance abuse by employees of healthcare organizations leads to reduced productivity, increased absenteeism, drug diversion, and, almost certainly, increased accidents and medication misadventures. Consequently, it affects the quality of patient care, liability, and operational and healthcare costs.

The abuse, or nonmedical use, of prescription medications has also become a prevalent issue. In 2012, the NSDUH survey found that nonmedical use of prescription drugs among youths age 12–17 years and young adults age 18–25 years was the second most prevalent illicit drug-use category, with marijuana being the first.[2] The survey also found that over half of all prescription drug abusers had obtained the prescription medication "from a friend or relative for free," compared with 3.9% who had obtained the medication from a drug dealer or stranger.

Pharmacists have unique, comprehensive knowledge about the safe and effective use of medications and about the adverse effects of their inappropriate use. When providing pharmaceutical care to individual patients, pharmacists assess the appropriateness of pharmacotherapy, counsel patients, and monitor medication-use outcomes. Health-system pharmacists are responsible for ensuring a safe and effective medication-use system, including legal and organizational responsibilities for medication distribution and control across the continuum of practice settings within healthcare organizations. With this combination of knowledge and organizational responsibilities, pharmacists are prepared to serve in leadership and service roles in substance abuse prevention and education and assist in a variety of patient care, employee health, and community activities.

Responsibilities

The scope of substance abuse–related responsibilities of pharmacists varies with the healthcare organization's mission, policies and procedures, patient population, and community. The responsibilities listed below should be adapted

[a]The NSDUH obtains information on nine categories of illicit drug use: use of marijuana, cocaine, heroin, hallucinogens, and inhalants, as well as the nonmedical use of prescription-type pain relievers, tranquilizers, stimulants, and sedatives.

DOI 10.37573/9781585287048.069

to meet local needs and circumstances. Each responsibility is intended to be applicable to any substance of abuse; therefore, specific substances are generally not mentioned.

Prevention. Pharmacists should be involved in substance abuse prevention by performing the following activities:

1. Participating in or contributing to the development of substance abuse prevention and assistance programs within healthcare organizations. A comprehensive program should consist of (a) a written substance abuse policy, (b) an employee education and awareness program, (c) a supervisor training program, (d) an employee assistance program, (e) peer support systems, such as pharmacist recovery networks, and (f) drug testing.[8]
2. Participating in public substance abuse education and prevention programs (e.g., in primary and secondary schools, colleges, churches, and civic organizations) and stressing the potential adverse health consequences of the misuse of legal drugs and the use of illegal drugs.
3. Opposing the sale of alcohol and tobacco products by pharmacists and in pharmacies.
4. Establishing a multidisciplinary controlled-substance inventory system, in compliance with statutory and regulatory requirements, that discourages diversion and enhances accountability. Where helpful, for example, procedures might require the purchase of controlled substances in tamper-evident containers and maintenance of a perpetual inventory and ongoing surveillance system.
5. Working with local, state, and federal authorities in controlling substance abuse, including participation in state prescription drug monitoring programs, encouraging participation in appropriate prescription disposal programs, complying with controlled-substance reporting regulations, and cooperating in investigations that involve the misuse of controlled substances, especially diversion from a healthcare organization.
6. Working with medical laboratories to (a) identify substances of abuse by using drug and poison control information systems, (b) establish proper specimen collection procedures based on knowledge of the pharmacokinetic properties of abused substances, and (c) select proper laboratory tests to detect the suspected substances of abuse and to detect tampering of samples.
7. Discouraging prescribing practices that enable or foster drug abuse behavior (e.g., prescribing a larger quantity of pain medication than is clinically needed for treatment of short-term pain).
8. Collaborating with outpatient and ambulatory care providers to prevent substance abuse after discharge.

Education. Pharmacists should be involved in substance abuse education by performing the following activities:

1. Providing information and referral to support groups appropriate to the needs of people whose lives are affected by their own or another person's substance abuse or dependency.
2. Providing recommendations about the appropriate use of mood-altering substances to healthcare providers and the public, including those persons recovering from substance dependency and their caregivers.[9]
3. Fostering the development of undergraduate and graduate college of pharmacy curricula and pharmacy technician education on the topic of substance abuse prevention, education, and assistance.[10]
4. Providing substance abuse education to fellow pharmacists, other healthcare professionals, and other employees of their healthcare organization.
5. Instructing drug abuse counselors in drug treatment programs about the pharmacology of abused substances and medications used for detoxification.
6. Promoting and providing alcohol risk-reduction education and activities.
7. Maintaining professional competency in substance abuse prevention, education, and assistance through formal and informal continuing education.
8. Providing postgraduate training in addictions, pain management, and palliative care where feasible.
9. Conducting research on substance abuse and addiction.
10. Educating patients about the correct storage, handling, and disposal of prescription medications.

Assistance. Pharmacists should be involved in substance abuse assistance by performing the following activities:

1. Assisting in the identification of patients, coworkers, and other individuals who may be having problems related to their substance abuse, and referring them to the appropriate people for evaluation and treatment.
2. Participating in multidisciplinary efforts to support and care for the healthcare organization's employees and patients who are recovering from substance dependency.
3. Supporting and encouraging the recovery of health professionals with alcoholism or other drug addictions. Major elements of an employer's support program might include (a) being willing to hire or retain employees, (b) participating in monitoring and reporting requirements associated with recovery or disciplinary contracts, (c) maintaining an environment supportive of recovery, (d) establishing behavioral standards and norms among all employees that discourage the abuse of psychoactive substances, including alcohol, and (e) participating in peer-assistance programs.
4. Collaborating with other healthcare providers in the development of the pharmacotherapeutic elements of drug detoxification protocols.
5. Providing pharmaceutical care to patients being treated for substance abuse and dependency.
6. Maintaining knowledge of professional support groups (e.g., state- and national-level pharmacist recovery networks) and other local, state, and national organizations, programs, and resources available for preventing and treating substance abuse (**appendix**).
7. Refusing to allow any student or employee, including health professionals, to work, practice, or be onsite for rotations within the healthcare organization while his or her ability to safely perform his or her responsibilities is impaired by drugs, including alcohol. The refusal should follow the organization's policies and procedures, the principles of ethical and responsible pharmacy practice, and statutory requirements. Practice should not be precluded after appropriate treatment and monitoring, if approved by the treatment provider or contract monitor (or both, when applicable).

References

1. American Psychiatric Association. Diagnostic and statistical manual of mental disorders. 5th ed. Arlington, VA: American Psychiatric Association; 2013.
2. Substance Abuse and Mental Health Services Administration. Results from the 2012 National Survey on Drug Use and Health: summary of national findings (September 2013). www.samhsa.gov/data/sites/default/files/NSDUHresults2012/-NSDUHresults2012.pdf (accessed 2016 Jan 21).
3. Hasin DS, Stinson FS, Ogburn E, Grant BF. Prevalence, correlates, disability, and comorbidity of DSM-IV alcohol abuse and dependence in the United States: results from the National Epidemiologic Survey on Alcohol and Related Conditions. *Arch Gen Psychiatry.* 2007; 64:830–42.
4. Compton WM, Thomas YF, Stinson FS, Grant BF. Prevalence, correlates, disability, and comorbidity of DSM-IV drug abuse and dependence in the United States: results from the National Epidemiologic Survey on Alcohol and Related Conditions. *Arch Gen Psychiatry.* 2007; 64:566–76.
5. McAuliffe WE, Santangelo SL, Gingras J et al. Use and abuse of controlled substances by pharmacists and pharmacy students. *Am J Hosp Pharm.* 1987; 44:311–7.
6. Sullivan E, Bissell L, Williams E. Chemical dependency in nursing: the deadly diversion. Menlo Park, CA: Addison-Wesley; 1988.
7. Bissell L, Haberman PW, Williams RL. Pharmacists recovering from alcohol and other drug addictions: an interview study. *Am Pharm.* 1989; NS29(6):19–30. [Erratum, *Am Pharm.* 1989; NS29(9):11.]
8. Substance Abuse and Mental Health Services Administration. Making your workplace drug-free: a kit for employers (2007). http://store.samhsa.gov/shin/content//SMA07-4230/SMA07-4230.pdf (accessed 2014 Jun 24).
9. Davis NH. Dispensing and prescribing cautions for medical care during recovery from alcohol and drug addiction. *J Pharm Pract.* 1991; 6:362–8.
10. DeSimone EM, Kissack JC, Scott DM et al. Curricular guidelines for pharmacy: substance abuse and addictive disease. www.aacp.org/resources/education/Documents/CurricularGuidelinesforPharmacy-SubstanceAbuseandAddictiveDisease.pdf (accessed 2014 May 27).

Appendix—Other Resources

Hogue MD, McCormick DD, eds. Points of light: a guide for assisting chemically dependent health professional students. Washington, DC: American Pharmaceutical Association; 1996.

American Association of Colleges of Pharmacy Special Committee on Substance Abuse and Pharmacy Education. American Association of Colleges of Pharmacy guidelines for the development of addiction and related disorders policies for colleges and schools of pharmacy. www.aacp.org/career/grants/Documents/Guidelines%20for%20the%20Development%20of%20Addiction%20and%20Related%20Disorders%20Policies%20for%20Schools%20and%20Colleges%20of%20Pharmacy.pdf (accessed 2014 Jun 24).

Tucker DR, Gurnee MC, Sylvestri MF et al. Psychoactive drug use and impairment markers in pharmacy students. *Am J Pharm Educ.* 1988; 52:42–7.

Miederhoff PA, Voight FB, White CE. Chemically impaired pharmacists: an emerging management issue. *Top Hosp Pharm Manage.* 1987; 7:75–83.

Kriegler KA, Baldwin JN, Scott DM. A study of alcohol and other drug use behaviors and risk factors in health profession students. *J Am Coll Health.* 1994; 42:259–65.

Haberman P. Alcoholism in the professions. Troy, MI: Performance Resource; 1991.

Bissell L, Royce JE. Ethics for addiction professionals. Center City, MN: Hazelden Foundation; 1994.

Colvin R. Prescription drug addiction: the hidden epidemic. Omaha, NE: Addicus; 2002.

Crosby L, Bissell L. To care enough: intervention with chemically-dependent colleagues. Minneapolis: Johnson Institute; 1989.

Johnson VE. Intervention: how to help someone who doesn't want help. A step-by-step guide for families and friends of chemically-dependent persons. Minneapolis: Johnson Institute; 1989.

Rinaldi RC, Steindler EM, Wilford BB et al. Clarification and standardization of substance abuse terminology. *JAMA.* 1988; 259:555–7.

Brown ME, Trinkoff AM, Christen AG, Dole EJ. Impairment issues for health care professionals: review and recommendations. *Subst Abus.* 2002; 23(suppl):155–65.

Dole EJ, Tommasello AC. Recommendations for implementing effective substance abuse education in pharmacy practice. *Subst Abus.* 2002; 23(suppl):263–71.

Lafferty L. Hunter TS, Marsh WA. Knowledge, attitudes and practices of pharmacists concerning prescription drug abuse. *J Psychoactive Drugs.* 2006; 38:229–32.

Baldwin JN, Scott DM, Agrawal S et al. Assessment of alcohol and other drug use behaviors in health professions students. *Subst Abus.* 2006; 27:25–35.

American Pharmacists Association. Pharmacists' role in addressing opioid abuse, addiction, and diversion. *J Am Pharm Assoc.* 2014; 54:e5–15.

Lord S, Downs G, Furtaw P et al. Nonmedical use of prescription opioids and stimulants among student pharmacists. *J Am Pharm Assoc.* 2009; 49:519–28.

American Pharmacists Association. Addiction and substance abuse in the pharmacy professions: from discovery to recovery. *Pharm Today.* 2013; 19:62–72.

Merlo LJ, Cummings SM, Cottler LB. Recovering substance-impaired pharmacists' views regarding occupational risks for addiction. *J Am Pharm Assoc.* 2012; 52:480–91.

Baldwin JN. Substance abuse care. In: Allen LV, ed. Remington: the science and practice of pharmacy. 22nd ed. London, UK: Pharmaceutical; 2013:2613–9.

Kenna GA, Baldwin JN, Trinkoff A et al. Substance use disorders in health care professionals. In: Johnson BA, ed. Addiction medicine: science and practice. New York: Springer; 2011:1375–98.

Baldwin JN, Scott DM, DeSimone EM et al. Substance use attitudes and behaviors at three pharmacy colleges. *Subst Abus.* 2011; 32:27–35.

National Clearinghouse for Alcohol and Drug Information (NCADI). The clearinghouse is a federally funded service that assists in finding information on all aspects of substance abuse. Many publications and educational materials are available free of charge from NCADI. Telephone: 800-729-6686; website: http://store.samhsa.gov/home.

Center for Substance Abuse Prevention (CSAP) Workplace Helpline (for employers). Telephone: 800-967-5752; e-mail: dwp@samhsa.hhs.gov.

National Association of State Alcohol and Drug Abuse Directors (NASADAD). This association coordinates and encourages cooperative efforts between the federal government and state agencies on substance abuse. NASADAD serves as a resource on state drug programs and can provide contacts in each state. Website: www.nasadad.org.

Community organizations are available to help with drug or alcohol problems. Treatment counselors may be valuable in developing assistance policies and in providing professional education about treatment and referral systems. Community drug abuse prevention organizations may be helpful in prevention efforts, including community drug education. Check your local telephone directory under headings such as *Alcoholism Information and Treatment, Drug Abuse Information and Treatment, and Counselors.*

Twelve-step groups (usually available locally unless otherwise noted; listed telephone numbers and websites are for national headquarters):

- Adult Children of Alcoholics is for adults who, as children, lived with alcoholic parents. Telephone: 562-595-7831; website: www.adultchildren.org.
- Al-Anon provides information on alcoholism and alcohol abuse and refers callers to local Al-Anon support groups established to help people affected by others' alcohol misuse. Telephone: 757-563-1500; website: www.al-anon.org.
- Alateen is for adolescents affected by alcoholics. Website: www.al-anon.alateen.org/for-alateen.
- Alcoholics Anonymous provides information and support to recovering alcoholics. Telephone: 212-870-3400; website: www.alcoholicsanonymous.org.
- Cocaine Anonymous is for individuals with cocaine dependencies. Telephone: 310-559-5833; website: www.ca.org.
- International Doctors in Alcoholics Anonymous (IDAA) includes pharmacists in recovery, regardless of degree (a national group that has an annual conference and recovery resources for doctoral degree health professionals). Website: www.idaa.org; IDAA executive director e-mail: executive@idaa.org.
- Nar-Anon helps people affected by another's drug misuse. Telephone: 800-477-6291; e-mail: wso@nar.anon.org.
- Narcotics Anonymous provides information and support to recovering substance abusers. Telephone: 818-773-9999; website: www.na.org.

Advocacy and professional substance abuse education

- Pharmacist Recovery Networks exist in most states in the United States to assist pharmacists (and often also pharmacy technicians and sometimes pharmacy students) with addictions or who are in addiction recovery. The www.usaprn.org website includes information about these programs by state as well as information about other recovery-related resources.
- The Pharmacy Section (cosponsored by the American Pharmacists Association [APhA] and APhA Academy of Students of Pharmacy) of the University of Utah School on Alcoholism and Other Drug Dependencies was a one-week seminar held each summer until 2014. The section was reconstituted as the APhA Institute on Alcoholism and Drug Dependencies in 2015 (www.pharmacist.com/apha-institute-alcoholism-and-drug-dependencies).

Approved by the ASHP Board of Directors on April 10, 2015, and by the ASHP House of Delegates on June 7, 2015. Developed through the ASHP Council on Pharmacy Practice. This statement supersedes a previous version dated June 2, 2013.

Copyright © 2016, American Society of Health-System Pharmacists, Inc. All rights reserved. Contact ASHP for reprint and permissions requests. This content may not be used for commercial purposes without the express written consent of ASHP.

Jeffrey N. Baldwin, Pharm.D., and Chelsea Leeper, Pharm.D., are gratefully acknowledged for revising this statement.

The bibliographic citation for this document is as follows: American Society of Health-System Pharmacists. ASHP statement on the pharmacist's role in substance abuse prevention, education, and assistance. *Am J Health-Syst Pharm.* 2016; 73:e267–70.

ASHP Statement on Racial and Ethnic Disparities in Health Care

Position

Health disparities continue to be a major public health problem confronting the U.S. health care system. These disparities arise from a complex set of factors, including social and economic inequality, cultural and linguistic barriers, and persistent racial and ethnic discrimination. Evidence continues to emerge, however, that some health disparities are attributable to differences in the quality of health care provided to different racial and ethnic groups. The American Society of Health-System Pharmacists (ASHP) believes that all patients, regardless of race, ethnicity, sex, age, sexual orientation, religion, physical or mental disability (or impairment), education, socioeconomic status, diagnosis, or limitations in access, have the right to high-quality health care that reflects knowledge of, sensitivity to, and respect for their differences.

Pharmacists who practice in hospitals and health systems ("health-system pharmacists"), working individually and in coordination with interested organizations and other health care professionals, can play a leading role in building culturally competent systems of care to reduce racial and ethnic disparities in health care by

- Increasing awareness of these disparities among health care providers, health-system administrators, legislators, regulators, third-party payers, and the public.
- Promoting a more diverse and culturally competent health care work force and environment.
- Ensuring effective communication with patients and among providers.
- Fostering consistent use of multidisciplinary teams and evidence-based guidelines for patient care.
- Collecting and reporting data on health care access, utilization, and outcomes by racial and ethnic minorities and measuring progress toward reducing health care disparities.
- Researching, identifying, and disseminating best practices for providing culturally competent care and reducing disparities in health care.

Background

The Institute of Medicine (IOM) defines racial and ethnic disparities in health care as "racial or ethnic differences in the quality of healthcare that are not due to access-related factors or clinical needs, preferences, and appropriateness of intervention."[1] IOM states that "evidence of racial and ethnic disparities in healthcare is . . . remarkably consistent across a range of illnesses and healthcare services." More than 600 articles documenting racial or ethnic variations in health care have been published in the past three decades.[2] With the majority of U.S. population growth between now and 2050 expected to come from racial and ethnic minority Americans and immigrants, our health care system must soon learn how to address the effects that race and ethnicity can have on health care. Eliminating health disparities is so important that it is one of only two overarching goals for the Healthy People 2010 objectives.[3]

Culture has been defined by IOM as "the accumulated store of shared values, ideas (attitudes, beliefs, values, and norms), understandings, symbols, material products, and practices of a group of people."[1] Ethnicity refers to "a shared culture and way of life, especially as reflected in language, folkways, religious and other institutional forms, material culture such as clothing and food, and cultural products such as music, literature, and art."[1] An ethnic group is a collection of people "socially distinguished or set apart, by others or by itself, primarily on the basis of cultural or national-origin characteristics."[1] Like ethnicity, race has been described as a sociocultural concept used to distinguish groups of people (in this case, those who share certain physical characteristics) and treat them differently.

ASHP recognizes the need to address all forms of health disparities and believes that health-system pharmacists can take an important step in addressing these broader disparities by assuming a leadership role in the national campaign to eliminate racial and ethnic disparities in health care. Health-system pharmacists, like other health professionals, have espoused a tradition of nondiscriminatory health care practice.[4,5] Because medication therapy management is central to many of the health disparities cited by IOM (e.g., treatment for pain, HIV infection, diabetes, end-stage renal disease, kidney transplantation),[1] health-system pharmacists have opportunities to directly address these disparities. As health-system administrators and members of multidisciplinary health care teams, health-system pharmacists have an important role to play in implementing the institutional changes necessary to eliminate racial and ethnic disparities in health care. ASHP believes that health-system pharmacists have a professional and moral responsibility to address racial and ethnic disparities in health care.

General Principles

The following three principles should guide the actions of health-system pharmacists in efforts to eliminate racial and ethnic disparities in health care: (1) all patients have the right to high-quality care, (2) medication-use practices should reflect knowledge of, sensitivity to, and respect for the race and culture of the patient, and (3) health-system pharmacists have a vital role to play in eliminating racial and ethnic disparities in health care.

All Patients Have the Right to High-Quality Care. A long-standing policy position of ASHP holds that "all patients have the right to . . . high-quality pharmaceutical care."[4] ASHP believes that all patients have the right to receive care from pharmacists and that health-system pharmacists should play a leadership role in ensuring patient access to pharmacists' services.[6] The Code of Ethics for Pharmacists issued by the American Pharmacists Association states that the pharmacist "places concern for the well-being of the patient at the center of professional practice" and "seeks justice in the distribution

DOI 10.37573/9781585287048.070

of health resources."[5] Racial and ethnic disparities in health care are antithetical to the core principles of pharmacy and must be eliminated.

Medication-Use Practices Should Reflect Knowledge of, Sensitivity to, and Respect for the Race and Culture of the Patient. Culture strongly influences how a person interacts with the world. Failing to account for the patient's race or cultural beliefs and values in health care decisions can lead to negative health consequences. Providers may miss screening opportunities because they are unfamiliar with the prevalence of conditions among racial or ethnic groups. They may fail to consider different responses to medications that exist in different populations. Potential harmful interactions between medications and traditional remedies used by the patient may be overlooked. Finally, miscommunication due to cultural, linguistic, or literacy differences between providers and patients regarding symptoms, medications, supplements, or the use of devices may lead to faulty diagnoses, unnecessary laboratory testing, medication-related errors, decreased adherence to therapy, or missed opportunities for early detection and preventive measures.[7]

The Code of Ethics for Pharmacists states that "in all cases" the pharmacist "respects personal and cultural differences among patients."[5] Clinicians who want to provide the best care for their patients must understand the role of culture and its potential impact on health outcomes and the provider–patient relationship.

Health-System Pharmacists Have a Vital Role to Play in Eliminating Racial and Ethnic Disparities in Health Care. In their roles as medication-use experts, patient care providers, and health-system administrators, health-system pharmacists have the knowledge, skills, and opportunities to contribute to efforts to eliminate racial and ethnic disparities in health care.

Pharmacists' Roles in Eliminating Disparities

IOM has made recommendations to eliminate racial and ethnic disparities in health care.[1] The IOM recommendations most relevant to health-system pharmacists are listed in the **appendix**. ASHP would add to that list that pharmacists can and should engage in research on disparities in health care. ASHP encourages all health care professionals and administrators to embrace these recommendations and urges health-system pharmacists to take the following actions to help eliminate health care disparities.

Increase Awareness of Disparities. One elemental barrier to eliminating racial and ethnic disparities in health care may be a lack of awareness of their existence and their impact on society. Polls show that a significant majority of Americans believe that African Americans receive the same quality of health care as whites,[1,8] despite ample evidence to the contrary.[1] Efforts to eliminate racial and ethnic disparities in health care must begin with the acknowledgment that there is a problem. Health-system pharmacists should lead efforts to increase awareness of health disparities among health care providers, health-system administrators, legislators, regulators, third-party payers, and the public. Pharmacists can increase awareness of health disparities by encouraging their health care organizations to make the elimination of disparities in health care a key component of the organization's mission. They can help their institutions foster an environment that promotes input from and involvement by all members of the organization in addressing this component of the organizational mission. In addition, pharmacists can help develop inhouse and community programs to promote cultural understanding and appreciation of the importance of diversity. They can also partner with community groups, governmental agencies, health care provider organizations, payers, and others to increase awareness of specific diseases among certain populations and encourage innovation and creativity in evaluating and disseminating approaches to eliminating disparities in health care.

Create a More Diverse Health Care Work Force. Increased racial and ethnic diversity among health care professionals may be associated with improved access to care for racial and ethnic minority patients, greater patient choice of and satisfaction with health care professionals, more effective patient–clinician communication, and enhanced educational experiences for students in the health professions.[9] Racial and ethnic diversity in the health care work force has been well correlated with the delivery of quality care to diverse patient populations. For minority patients, racial concordance between patient and physician is associated with greater patient satisfaction and higher self-rated quality of care.[10] Spanish-speaking patients, for example, report more satisfaction with care from Spanish-speaking providers.[11]

In 2002, the American Hospital Association's Commission on Workforce for Hospitals and Health Systems reported that although the national labor force is becoming more diverse, hospital employees remain disproportionately female and Caucasian.[12] The Commission recommended working aggressively to develop a work force that more fully represents changing U.S. demographics. IOM has also cited a continuing shortage of minorities among health care professionals.[9]

ASHP is committed to developing a diverse work force of health-system pharmacists.[13] In June 2003, the ASHP Board of Directors established the Ad Hoc Committee on Ethnic Diversity and Cultural Competence, which has recommended six major goals and developed long-term strategic action plans for each goal.[14] ASHP members are encouraged to participate in these efforts and to monitor their progress at ASHP's Health Disparities Web Resource Center (www.ashp.org/s_ashp/cat1c.asp?CID=4266&DID=7523).

Promote Culturally Competent Care and Services. Many cultures take a different approach to health than is found in allopathic ("western") medicine. Perceptions of illness and disease vary by culture, and culture may influence a person's health-seeking behavior, approach to seeking out health care providers, and treatment preferences. As allopathic medicine increasingly emphasizes evidence-based approaches, health care practitioners will more frequently confront the cultural divide between the demands of their profession and the closely held beliefs of their patients. Cultural competency is rapidly becoming a quality and risk management issue for hospitals and health systems. ASHP is committed to developing a culturally sensitive, competent, and respectful work force.[15]

The Department of Health and Human Services (HHS) states that a culturally competent health care practitioner is

- Knowledgeable about cultural differences and their impact on attitudes and behaviors.
- Sensitive, understanding, nonjudgmental, and respectful in dealings with peoples whose culture is different from one's own.
- Flexible and skillful in responding and adapting to different cultural contexts and circumstances.[16]

HHS's Office of Minority Health has developed a set of standards for culturally and linguistically appropriate services in health care to provide a consistent and comprehensive approach to cultural and linguistic competence in health care.[17] These standards offer a framework for implementing services and organizational structures to help health care organizations and providers, including pharmacists, respond to the cultural and linguistic issues presented by diverse populations. ASHP believes these standards should be used to assess staff competence and to guide organizations' educational programming and strategic planning. Education on cultural competency issues is encouraged in preceptor training sessions, residency standards, and leadership orientation at ASHP and affiliate levels. The Accreditation Council for Pharmaceutical Education now requires that schools and colleges of pharmacy include cultural competency in their curricula.[18] Approaches to the subject could include standalone courses in health disparities and cultural competence, inclusion of traditional healers in the educational process, and infusion of the concept of cultural competence throughout the curriculum (e.g., through case studies that include diverse populations). ASHP believes that experiential learning should also include practice experiences with racial and ethnic minorities, medically underserved populations, and patient populations whose cultures incorporate the use of traditional healers and complementary or alternative medicine (e.g., folk medicine, home remedies).

The Code of Ethics for Pharmacists states that "A pharmacist maintains professional competence."[5] ASHP believes that cultural competence is among the competencies that pharmacists, residents, fellows, students, and technicians have an obligation to develop and maintain.

Ensure Effective Communication with Patients and Among Providers. The Code of Ethics for Pharmacists states that "a pharmacist communicates with patients in terms that are understandable."[5] ASHP guidelines recommend that pharmacists "know about their patients' cultures, especially health and illness beliefs, attitudes, and practices," and "adapt messages to fit patients' language skills and primary languages, through the use of teaching aids, interpreters, or cultural guides if necessary."[19] Persons with the most health problems and the greatest need for self-management skills often have the poorest health literacy. Health-system pharmacists providing direct patient care should be able to assess the health literacy of patients and provide appropriate education.[20]

Lack of interpretation services or culturally and linguistically appropriate health education materials is associated with patient dissatisfaction, poor comprehension and compliance, and ineffective or lower quality of patient care.[21–23] Health care providers rely heavily on the use of the written word to communicate, a circumstance that contributes to health care disparities.[1] When interpretation services are used, practitioners should ensure their quality. Fluency in language is not necessarily sufficient to provide adequate interpretation of the complex concepts involved in medical decision-making. Interpretation by family members also raises issues of patient confidentiality and autonomy.

Communication with patients needs to be culturally and linguistically appropriate. For example, although Spanish is the primary language of many cultures, simply translating educational material into Spanish may not provide the cultural context to make the education effective.

Health-system pharmacists should also utilize their medication-use expertise to help their institutions and communities develop culturally and linguistically appropriate public education campaigns. These campaigns could address health risks prevalent in racial and ethnic minority populations served by the hospital and explain preventive measures and health care services available to those populations.

Health care professionals also need to recognize that racial and cultural differences may affect communication among providers. Health-system pharmacists should take steps to ensure that provider-to-provider communication is effective and reflects the respect for colleagues expressed in the Code of Ethics for Pharmacists.[5]

Utilize Multidisciplinary Teams and Evidence-Based Guidelines. Multidisciplinary team approaches to health care improve health outcomes for majority and minority patients being treated for a range of diseases.[1] ASHP believes pharmacists should be integral participants in the development of multidisciplinary action plans for patient care, disease management plans, and health management plans.[24] Evidence-based guidelines "offer the advantages of consistency, predictability, and objectivity,"[1] but their use must be balanced with the need for clinical flexibility, especially when there is evidence of different outcomes or responses among racial or ethnic groups.

Collect and Monitor Data on Health Disparities. Standardized collection of data regarding access to medications, drug utilization, and medical and cost-effectiveness outcomes from medication therapy management by racial and ethnic minorities would promote research on disparities in health care and help institutions monitor the progress of their efforts to eliminate those disparities.[25] Pharmacists should be active partners with health care administrators and other health professionals in developing measures of progress against health care disparities in institutional performance measures, which should be a key component of the organization's mission.[26]

Research Disparities in Health Care. Health-system pharmacists can research, identify, and disseminate best practices for providing culturally competent care and reducing disparities in health care. Priority areas for research include racial and ethnic groups' access to medications, drug utilization, and medical and cost-effectiveness outcomes from medication therapy management. Pharmacists must keep pace with research regarding disparities in health care, programs to provide culturally competent care to patients, and new educational approaches to improving patient care. It is also important that pharmacy develop researchers to investigate health care disparities and cutting-edge practitioners to translate those research findings into practice.

Conclusion

ASHP believes racial and ethnic disparities in health care are antithetical to the core principles of pharmacy. All patients have the right to high-quality health care that reflects knowledge of, sensitivity to, and respect for their differences. Health-system pharmacists, working individually and in coordination with interested organizations and other health care professionals, can and must play a vital role in efforts to eliminate racial and ethnic disparities in health care.

References

1. Smedley BD, Stith AY, Nelson AR, eds. Unequal treatment: confronting racial and ethnic disparities in health care. Washington, DC: National Academy Press; 2003.
2. Rubenstein LS. Racial disparities and health: Physicians for Human Rights testimony to Congressional Black Caucus. March 18, 2003. www.phrusa.org/research/methics/caucus_0303.html (accessed 2006 Dec 1).
3. U.S. Department of Health and Human Services. Healthy People 2010. www.healthypeople.gov/default.htm (accessed 2005 Nov 4).
4. ASHP policy position 9006: nondiscriminatory pharmaceutical care. In: Hawkins B, ed. Best practices for hospital and health-system pharmacy: positions and guidance documents of ASHP. Bethesda, MD: American Society of Health-System Pharmacists; 2006:82.
5. American Pharmacists Association. Code of Ethics for Pharmacists. www.pharmacist.com/AM/PrinterTemplate.cfm?Section=Search1&template=/CM/HTMLDisplay.cfm&ContentID=2903 (accessed 2008 Jan 7).
6. ASHP policy position 0101: pharmacy benefits for the uninsured. In: Hawkins B, ed. Best practices for hospital and health-system pharmacy: positions and guidance documents of ASHP. Bethesda, MD: American Society of Health-System Pharmacists; 2006:161.
7. Brach C, Fraser I. Can cultural competency reduce racial and ethnic health care disparities? A review and conceptual model. *Med Care Res Rev.* 2000; 57(suppl 1):181–217.
8. Harvard Forums on Health. Americans speak out on disparities in health care. www.phsi.harvard.edu/health_reform/poll_media_report_disparities.pdf (accessed 2004 Dec 10).
9. Committee on Institutional and Policy-Level Strategies for Increasing the Diversity of the U.S. Healthcare Workforce. In the nation's compelling interest: ensuring diversity in the health care workforce. Washington, DC: National Academy Press; 2004.
10. Saha S, Komaromy M, Koepsell TD, et al. Patient-physician racial concordance and the perceived quality and use of health care. *Arch Intern Med.* 1999; 159:997–1004.
11. Morales LS, Cunningham WE, Brown JA, et al. Are Latinos less satisfied with communication by health care providers? *J Gen Intern Med.* 1999; 14:409–17.
12. American Hospital Association Commission on Workforce for Hospitals and Health Systems. In our hands: how hospital leaders can build a thriving workforce. www.aha.org/aha/key_issues/workforce/commission/InOurHands.html (accessed 2004 Dec 10).
13. ASHP policy position 0409: cultural diversity among health care providers. In: Hawkins B, ed. Best practices for hospital and health-system pharmacy: positions and guidance documents of ASHP. Bethesda, MD: American Society of Health-System Pharmacists; 2006:253.
14. Report of the ASHP Ad Hoc Committee on Ethnic Diversity and Cultural Competence. *Am J Health-Syst Pharm.* 2005; 62:1924–30.
15. ASHP policy position 0314: cultural competence. In: Hawkins B, ed. Best practices for hospital and health-system pharmacy: positions and guidance documents of ASHP. Bethesda, MD: American Society of Health-System Pharmacists; 2006:75.
16. Department of Health and Human Services Administration on Aging. Achieving cultural competence: a guidebook for providers of services to older Americans and their families. www.aoa.gov/prof/adddiv/cultural/CC-guidebook.pdf (accessed 2004 Dec 10).
17. U.S. Department of Health and Human Services. Final report: national standards for culturally and linguistically appropriate services in health care (2001). www.omhrc.gov/omh/programs/2pgprograms/finalreport.pdf (accessed 2004 Dec 10).
18. Accreditation standards and guidelines for the professional program in pharmacy leading to the doctor of pharmacy degree. Chicago: Accreditation Council for Pharmaceutical Education; 2006.
19. American Society of Health-System Pharmacists. ASHP guidelines on pharmacist-conducted patient education and counseling. *Am J Health-Syst Pharm.* 1997; 54:431–4.
20. ASHP policy position 0510: communication among health-system pharmacy practitioners, patients, and other health care providers. In: Hawkins B, ed. Best practices for hospital and health-system pharmacy: positions and guidance documents of ASHP. Bethesda, MD: American Society of Health-System Pharmacists; 2006:74.
21. Erizinger S. Communication between Spanish-speaking patients and their doctors in medical encounters. *Cult Med Psychiatry.* 1991; 15:91–101.
22. Carrasquillo O, Orav EJ, Brennan TA, et al. Impact of language barriers on patient satisfaction in an emergency department. *J Gen Intern Med.* 1999; 14:82–7.
23. Perez-Stable EJ, Napoles-Springer A, Miramontes JM. The effects of ethnicity and language on medical outcomes of patients with hypertension or diabetes. *Med Care.* 1997; 35:1212–9.
24. ASHP policy position 9804: multidisciplinary action plans for patient care. In: Hawkins B, ed. Best practices for hospital and health-system pharmacy: positions and guidance documents of ASHP. Bethesda, MD: American Society of Health-System Pharmacists; 2006:161.

25. Ver Ploeg M, Perrin E, eds. Eliminating health disparities: measurement and data needs. Washington, DC: National Academy Press; 2004.
26. The Commonwealth Fund. Enhancing public hospitals' reporting of data on racial and ethnic disparities in care. www.cmwf.org/publications/publications_show.htm?doc_id=452681&#doc452681 (accessed 2007 Jan 31).

Appendix—Institute of Medicine Recommendations Most Pertinent to Hospital and Health-System Pharmacy Practice[1]

General Recommendations
Recommendation 2-1. Increase awareness of racial and ethnic disparities in healthcare among the general public and key stakeholders.
Recommendation 2-2. Increase healthcare providers' awareness of disparities.

Legal, Regulatory, and Policy Interventions
Recommendation 5-3. Increase the proportion of underrepresented U.S. racial and ethnic minorities among healthcare professionals.

Health-System Interventions
Recommendation 5-6. Promote the consistency and equity of care through use of evidence-based guidelines.
Recommendation 5-9. Support the use of interpretation services where community need exists.
Recommendation 5-11. Implement multidisciplinary treatment and preventive care teams.

Patient Education and Empowerment
Recommendation 5-12. Implement patient education programs to increase patients' knowledge of how to best access care and participate in treatment decisions.

Cross-Cultural Education in the Health Professions
Recommendation 6-1. Integrate cross-cultural education into the training of all current and future health professionals.

Data Collection and Monitoring
Recommendation 7-1. Collect and report data on healthcare access and utilization by patients' race, ethnicity, socioeconomic status, and, where possible, primary language.
Recommendation 7-2. Include measures of racial and ethnic disparities in performance measurement.
Recommendation 7-3. Monitor progress toward the elimination of healthcare disparities.
Recommendation 7-4. Report racial and ethnic data by OMB categories, but use subpopulation groups where possible.

This statement was reviewed in 2011 by the Council on Pharmacy Practice and by the Board of Directors and was found to still be appropriate.

Developed through the ASHP Council on Pharmacy Practice and approved by the ASHP Board of Directors on April 16, 2007, and by the ASHP House of Delegates on June 24, 2007.

Copyright © 2008, American Society of Health-System Pharmacists, Inc. All rights reserved. Contact ASHP for reprint and permissions requests. This content may not be used for commercial purposes without the express written consent of ASHP.

The bibliographic citation for this document is as follows: American Society of Health-System Pharmacists. ASHP statement on racial and ethnic disparities in health care. *Am J Health-Syst Pharm.* 2008; 65:728–33.

ASHP Statement on the Role of Pharmacists in Primary Care

Position

ASHP believes that pharmacists have a role in meeting the primary care needs of patients directly and in collaboration with other healthcare providers. Primary care pharmacy practice is the provision of integrated, accessible healthcare services by pharmacists who are accountable for addressing medication needs, developing sustained partnerships with patients, and practicing in the context of family and community.[1] Primary care pharmacy practice is accomplished through the provision of direct patient care and medication management services (MMS) for ambulatory patients, development of long-term relationships, coordination of care, patient advocacy, wellness and health promotion, triage and referral, and patient education and self-management. The primary care pharmacist provides primary care services in a variety of settings, including institutional, private, and community-based clinics. Primary care pharmacists help offset deficits in the primary care workforce caused by a shortage of physicians and other healthcare providers, particularly for underserved populations, by providing MMS in interdisciplinary team-based settings as well as in areas such as telehealth, population health, transitions of care, employer-based services, lifestyle medicine, accountable care organizations, and public health. Primary care pharmacists are often embedded into the primary care practice to provide MMS.

Many states allow pharmacists to partner with physicians via collaborative practice agreements (CPAs) that enable physicians to delegate specific tasks (e.g., initiation, titration, and discontinuation of medications; laboratory monitoring of therapy; medication and disease state monitoring) to a pharmacist. ASHP supports passage of federal and state laws and regulations that authorize pharmacists as providers within collaborative practice and that facilitate reimbursement for services provided by pharmacists.[2] Further, ASHP advocates that pharmacists be recognized as providers in federal, state, and third-party payment programs. Provider recognition would facilitate direct billing for services provided, similar to billing by physicians, nurse practitioners, clinical nurse specialists, and physician assistants.[3] Until that recognition is obtained, ASHP encourages healthcare organizations to use a variety of models to ensure the financial sustainability of services provided by primary care pharmacists, such as through indirect funding, incident-to billing, and increased use of the limited direct insurance billing opportunities available. Several states have passed pharmacist provider status laws or reimbursement parity laws allowing for reimbursement for direct patient care pharmacist services by state Medicaid and/or commercial plans.[4]

As pharmacists become core members of the primary care workforce, credentialing and privileging with payers and healthcare organizations will be essential. As credentialed providers, pharmacists are able to both provide patient care services and contribute to the financial sustainability of those services. Privileging protects their employing organizations from legal risk and ensures patients receive care from qualified and competent providers. ASHP recommends the use of credentialing and privileging in a manner consistent with other healthcare professionals to assess a pharmacist's competence to engage in patient care services.[5] Credentialing and privileging systems already exist for physicians, physician assistants, and nurse practitioners, but are far less common for pharmacists. Integration of pharmacists into existing processes will enable the profession to function collaboratively and in parallel with their colleagues and assist in preparing for pharmacist provider status. There are many opportunities for pharmacists who practice in primary care settings to seek additional credentials beyond a pharmacy degree and licensure, and certain credentials may be required to obtain specific privileges to provide MMS. The variety of state requirements to provide primary care pharmacist services can be a barrier to patient access to those services, thus standardized credentialing is needed.

Primary Healthcare

A 2021 National Academies of Science, Engineering and Medicine report defined high-quality primary care as "the provision of whole-person, integrated, accessible, and equitable health care by interprofessional teams that are accountable for addressing the majority of an individual's health and wellness needs across settings and through sustained relationships with patients, families, and communities."[6] The report stated that high-quality primary care is a critical component to achieving the quadruple aims of healthcare: enhancing the patient experience, improving population health, reducing costs, and improving the health care team experience.[6]

Primary healthcare is a comprehensive and holistic care approach to health and well-being that is centered on and tailored to the needs of individuals, families, and communities. The World Health Organization (WHO) has developed a three-component definition of primary care:

1. Meeting people's health needs through comprehensive promotive, protective, preventive, curative, rehabilitative, and palliative care throughout the life cycle, prioritizing key healthcare services aimed at individuals/families through primary care and the population through public health functions as the central elements of integrated health services.
2. Systematically addressing the determinants of health (social, economic, environmental, as well as people's characteristics and behaviors) through evidence-informed public policies and actions across all sectors.
3. Empowering individuals, families, and communities to optimize their health, as advocates for policies that promote and protect health and well-being, as co-developers of health and social services, and as self-carers and caregivers to others.[7]

Primary care pharmacy practice is the provision of integrated, accessible healthcare services by pharmacists who

DOI 10.37573/9781585287048.071

are accountable for addressing medication needs, developing sustained partnerships with patients, and practicing in the context of family and community.[1] This practice is accomplished through direct patient care and medication management for ambulatory patients, development of long-term relationships, coordination of care, patient advocacy, wellness and health promotion, triage and referral, and patient education and self-management. The primary care pharmacist may practice in institutional, private, and community-based clinics involved in the provision of direct care to diverse patient populations.

Services Provided by Primary Care Pharmacists

Primary care pharmacists may help to offset deficits in the primary care workforce, including the physician shortage, by providing MMS in interdisciplinary team-based settings as well as areas such as telehealth, population health, transitions of care, employer-based services, lifestyle medicine, and public health. Clinical pharmacy services may include:

- Immunizations and travel vaccines.
- Medication therapy management (MTM).
- Collaborative drug therapy management (CDTM).
- Comprehensive medication management (CMM).
- Focused specialty management of chronic diseases (e.g., anticoagulation, diabetes, heart failure).
- Management of complex acute conditions or exacerbation of chronic conditions (e.g., urinary tract infection, chronic obstructive pulmonary disease, asthma).
- Provision of personalized medicine (e.g. pharmacogenomics)
- Patient counseling, education, and training.

Examples of practice settings in which pharmacists provide primary care services include:

- Accountable care organizations (ACOs)
- Community-based or free clinic
- Community pharmacy
- Federally Qualified Health Center (FQHC)
- Hospital-based outpatient clinic
- Indian Health Service clinic
- Managed care integrated system
- Outpatient clinic associated with academic medical center
- Patient-centered medical home (PCMH)
- Private practice physician clinic
- Rural health clinic (RHC)
- Self-insured employee clinic
- Veterans Affairs (VA) medical center

MMS. Primary care pharmacists are often embedded into the primary care practice to provide MMS. MMS has been defined by the Joint Commission of Pharmacy Practitioners (JCPP) as "*a spectrum of patient-centered, pharmacist-provided, collaborative services that focus on medication appropriateness, effectiveness, safety, and adherence with the goal of improving health outcomes.*"[8] For the purposes of this statement, MMS "encompasses a variety of terms, such as medication therapy management (MTM), comprehensive medication management (CMM), and collaborative medication management," as in the JCPP definition.[3] The pharmacist may be an employee of the practice, a department of pharmacy, or a health professions school or college, and may dedicate a part- or full-time effort to providing clinical pharmacy services. Care may be provided face-to-face or via telehealth visits to manage medications for patients with chronic illnesses such as hypertension, diabetes, chronic heart failure, asthma, chronic obstructive pulmonary disease, anticoagulation, osteoporosis, and many others. Primary care pharmacists often provide patient education about lifestyle choices or conduct annual wellness visits (AWVs) for patients with Medicare. Many states allow pharmacists to collaborate with physicians through CPAs that enable physicians to delegate specific tasks such as medication initiation, titration, or discontinuation; laboratory monitoring of drug therapy; and referral for medication and disease state management to the pharmacist.

Transitions of Care Services. The term *transitions of care* refers to the movement of patients between healthcare practitioners, settings, and home as their condition and care needs change.[9] During transitions, medication regimens are frequently changed and may include medication discontinuation, dosage changes, and new prescriptions that can be confusing for patients and caregivers to manage. Poor-quality transitions contribute to medication errors, hospital readmissions, and increased healthcare costs.[9] Pharmacists in the primary care setting can support patients and caregivers as they adjust to new diagnoses, care plans, and medications.

Established Transitional Care Management (TCM) Current Procedural Terminology (CPT) codes allow for billing of transitions of care services, providing a mechanism for reimbursement.[10,11] There are three required elements to bill for TCM services:

1. Interactive communication (e.g., phone, text, email) must occur with the patient or caregiver within 2 days of discharge by a licensed clinical staff member, which can be the primary care pharmacist.
2. Medical decision making of moderate to high complexity occurs during the service period.
3. The patient has a face-to-face or telehealth visit within 7-14 days of discharge.

Services during TCM visits often include reviewing medical records, reconciling medications, coordinating future visits, and providing patient education. Pharmacists may be involved with all components of TCM, but the services can only be billed by a physician or a qualified nonphysician provider such as a nurse practitioner or physician assistant according to current Centers for Medicare & Medicaid Services (CMS) rules. Inclusion of pharmacists in the definition of a nonphysician provider would allow pharmacists to perform these services, among others, and reduce the burden on primary care providers.

ASHP and the American Pharmacists Association (APhA) collaborated to develop the Medication Management in Care Transitions (MMCT) Best Practices that spotlight transitions of care models in pharmacy practice and provide resources for pharmacy leaders.[12] Successful programs improved patient satisfaction scores and decreased readmission rates and medication discrepancies.[12] A descriptive study that evaluated the impact of care transitions intervention on clinical, organizational, and financial outcomes found that adding a pharmacist to the care transitions team decreased hospital readmissions compared to usual care (9 vs. 26%) and prevented 103 admissions per year, translating to an annual savings of over $1 million.[13]

Services Offered through Employer-Based Health Plans. Employers may offer chronic disease management or healthy lifestyle programs to employees as part of their human resources benefits package. Pharmacists are essential team members who can provide chronic disease medication management to employees enrolled in self-insured health plans. The Asheville Project demonstrated that pharmacists who cared for City of Asheville employees with diabetes improved patient satisfaction with their healthcare, decreased healthcare costs, and increased the number of patients who achieved hemoglobin A1c, lipid, and blood pressure goals.[14] An evaluation of a national employer-based program offered by 10 organizations in 70 different communities indicated that pharmacists improved other diabetes-related population health metrics, including monofilament examinations, annual dilated eye examinations, foot self-exams, glucose self-monitoring, weekly exercise, and annual influenza vaccines.[15]

Population Health Services. A shift to population health strategies in primary care has been driven by increasing healthcare costs, emphasis on fee-for-service over value-based care, and lack of widespread prevention initiatives. Primary care pharmacists who dedicate their time to population health management focus on improving the quality of care for specific patient populations. Specific population health metrics that warrant improvement are identified by leaders within the PCMH, the ACO, through community health assessments, or by payers such as Medicare, Medicaid, and private insurers. Demonstration in improved quality metrics may be linked with pay-for-performance payment bonuses, or shared savings incentives. For example, if a metric of importance to the practice is to improve the quality of care for patients with diabetes, primary care pharmacists can provide MMS for high-risk patients to improve attainment of hemoglobin A1c goals.[16]

Public Health Services. Expertise in the domain of public health is increasingly important for the primary care pharmacist due to the impact of public care challenges such as the opioid epidemic, unintended pregnancy with resultant negative maternal fetal outcomes, tobacco abuse, and the COVID-19 pandemic. The Opioid and Naloxone Education (ONE) program has demonstrated the ability of pharmacists to ensure safe opioid use, and prevent opioid misuse and abuse, through implementing naloxone prescribing while utilizing the pharmacist's patient care process.[17] A growing number of states allow pharmacists to prescribe hormonal contraception as a strategy to increase access to care and decrease negative maternal outcomes.[18] Oregon pharmacists prescribing hormonal contraception prevented 51 unintended pregnancies and saved Oregon Medicaid over $1.6 million.[19] As of February 2021, six states (Idaho, Colorado, Indiana, West Virginia, Vermont, North Dakota, and New Mexico) have authorized pharmacists to prescribe all FDA-approved tobacco cessation products, including varenicline, to combat the negative impact of smoking on public health; Oregon and North Dakota are currently developing regulations to implement authorizing legislation.[20]

Pharmacists in primary care settings are also well-positioned to identify immunization needs of patients, provide education to promote vaccine confidence, and administer vaccines. During the COVID-19 pandemic, the U.S. Department of Health and Human Resources authorized immunizing pharmacists to administer childhood vaccines[21] and COVID-19 vaccines[22] as part of the Public Readiness and Emergency Preparedness (PREP) Act.

Telehealth. The Health Resources and Services Administration (HRSA) defines telehealth as "the use of electronic information and telecommunication technologies to support long-distance clinical health care, patient and professional health-related education, health administration and public health."[23] Telehealth has been used for a variety of patient populations, including veterans, rural patients, and patients with psychiatric conditions. The COVID-19 pandemic accelerated the delivery of primary care services by telehealth. The federal government established temporary measures in 2020 to increase access to telehealth during the pandemic through the Coronavirus Preparedness and Response Supplemental Appropriations Act. In addition, CMS relaxed rules for supervision of auxiliary personnel to allow physicians to provide "virtual" supervision in order to promote social distancing and protect frontline healthcare workers.

Telehealth visits may be billed by physicians and non-physician providers and are paid at the same fee-for-service rate as in-person visits for Medicare recipients. Pharmacists may be able to bill using certain approved telephone codes. Reimbursement may vary for Medicaid and private insurance.

Special Practice Settings and Patient Populations

Rural Health. Rural areas make up approximately 97% of the land area in the U.S., yet account for just a little over 19% of the total U.S. population.[24] People living in rural areas are often underserved and experience significant health disparities that can vary between geographical regions and across socioeconomic spectra. Many of the health-related challenges faced by rural America are amplified by the lack of adequate services, particularly primary care providers and medical specialists. Approximately 90% of Americans live within 5 miles of a community pharmacy, creating additional opportunities for pharmacists to partner with primary care providers and provide clinical pharmacy services for rural, underserved patients.[25]

The expansion of pharmacist-delivered services in rural settings is an important strategy to target health disparities that are more common causes of mortality for people who live in rural communities than those living in urban areas. Chronic disease state management, MMS, health screenings, tobacco cessation management and prescribing, medication-assisted treatment of opioid use disorders, and lifestyle coaching through diabetes prevention programs are examples of services that address these common health disparities and can be led by pharmacists or enhanced through interprofessional collaboration with pharmacists as allowed under state-specific pharmacy practice acts. Unique training programs focused on rural pharmacy health exist at several colleges of pharmacy that focus on preparing pharmacists for leadership roles in small and rural communities.[26]

Many health systems that serve rural America receive reimbursement through all-inclusive payment models by Medicare and many state bill Medicaid plans. However, the lack of pharmacist recognition as an independent billable provider by the majority of payers, including Medicare, can challenge the financial feasibility of advanced pharmacist services within these settings.[27] Pharmacists can assist or serve a key role in grant-funded projects and programs and, in the case of government-funded grants, can lead to perpetual funding to rural health providers such as FQHCs, RHCs, and the Indian Health Service as a mechanism to defray pharmacist costs. Examples of sustainable practice models that incorporate pharmacist-delivered care in rural areas include the following:

1. Synchronous or co-visits between a pharmacist and a primary care practitioner who is recognized as an independent billable provider.
2. Visits with a pharmacist independent of other health professionals.
3. Pharmacist involvement in comprehensive care services as part of the PCMH or ambulatory primary care clinic care team.
4. Population health services that focus on quality improvement and can increase reimbursement to the health system or collaborating primary care provider through individual visits with the pharmacist face-to-face or via telehealth, including remote physiologic monitoring (examples of quality improvement measures include blood pressure control, warfarin monitoring, glycemic control, rates of influenza immunizations, and adherence to medication refills [e.g., statin therapy, antiplatelet medications, oral glucose-lowering medications]).
5. Pharmacists involved in accredited Diabetes Self-Management Training (DSMT) programs.

Partnerships between primary care providers and local community pharmacies, critical access pharmacies, or academic institutions can increase access to essential services such as immunization delivery, point-of-care testing, and disease state education and management to people living in rural areas with limited access to primary care providers.[28–30]

FQHCs. FQHCs are considered safety net health providers of outpatient clinical services that receive funding from the HRSA Health Center Program to provide care to individuals in underserved areas.[31] The primary purpose of FQHCs is the provision of primary care services in underserved urban and rural communities. FQHCs are typically located in community health centers but are also found in public housing primary care centers, outpatient health programs operated by a tribe or urban Indian organization, migrant health centers, and healthcare for the homeless centers. Among the requirements of FQHCs are the provision of a sliding fee scale system for uninsured patients with incomes below 200% of the federal poverty guidelines, provision of comprehensive healthcare services (which include medical, pharmacy, dental, and behavioral health), an ongoing quality assurance program, and a governing board of directors.[32]

FQHCs often need to meet the challenges of geographic, social, economic, linguistic, and cultural patient barriers. Primary care pharmacists working in clinical roles within an FQHC can have a tremendous impact on the care of this underserved patient population. Socioeconomic and cultural/language barriers present unique challenges to medication therapy that pharmacists are well suited to help overcome. Chronic diseases are common, noting a high prevalence of hypertension, diabetes and tobacco use. The Uniform Data System requires FQHCs to report on quality of care measures, therefore providing an opportunity for pharmacists to assist in the design and implementation of clinical services aimed at meeting quality benchmarks, as well as participate in the reporting process.

FQHCs differ from traditional primary care practices in the way that payment is issued for primary care encounters. An encounter payment is issued under the FQHC Prospective Payment System (PPS) from CMS that includes medical services, supplies, and overall service coordination provided to patients. The specific payment amount is unique to each FQHC and is determined based on reasonable costs and cost reporting. Because the PPS is provided through CMS, only practitioners who are recognized as healthcare providers by Medicare are eligible to bill directly for services. Because pharmacists are not recognized as healthcare providers federally, any eligible services provided by a pharmacist may not be billed directly but must rather be billed by an eligible healthcare provider. Despite the limited opportunities for pharmacists to promote sustainability through direct revenue, such as Medicare AWVs, there are many primary care services provided by pharmacists in FQHCs that benefit the practice. FQHCs that participate in the 340B program, which provides medication cost savings to uninsured and underinsured patients as well as savings to the pharmacy, commonly leverage the savings to support clinical pharmacy services (e.g., hiring or salary support of a clinical pharmacist). Examples of services provided by pharmacists in FQHCs include:

- MTM
- 340B Program
- Specialty Pharmacy Services
- Spirometry
- Chronic Care Management (CCM) and Principal Care Management (PCM)
- Diabetes Self-Management Training (DSMT)
- Value-Based Care
- Quality Improvement/PCMH
- CDTM/Contract Agreements/Consult Agreements
- Population Health
- Medicare AWVs
- TCM

Additional detailed information can be found in the ASHP Resource Center document, "Opportunities for Sustainable Pharmacy Services in Federally Qualified Health Centers."[33]

Billing and Reimbursement for Primary Care Pharmacy Services

The National Academy of Sciences recommends that payers, including Medicaid, Medicare, commercial insurers, and self-insured employers, should shift payments toward a hybrid model that includes fee-for-service and capitated payments, and that these models should pay prospectively for interprofessional, integrated, team-based care.[6] Financial sustainability for services provided by primary care pharmacists may be achieved using a variety of models. Due to lack of federal provider status for pharmacists and subsequent inability to directly bill Medicare as primary care providers, organizations and practices have become creative in maintaining financial sustainability of primary care pharmacist services. Some settings utilize indirect funding, while others take advantage of some of the limited direct insurance billing opportunities to fund pharmacists in primary care settings. Direct billing opportunities will vary based on the setting, hospital-based versus physician-based practices, as well as state-specific laws and regulations. Medicare, Medicaid, and commercial health plans may reimburse pharmacists for certain services, while some will require direct contracting with the health plan. Several states have passed pharmacist state provider status laws and/or reimbursement parity laws allowing for reimbursement for direct patient care pharmacist services by state Medicaid and/or commercial plans.[4] Some examples of direct and indirect billing methods are listed in **Box 1**.

BOX 1. Examples of Direct and Indirect Funding Methods[34]

Indirect Billing	Direct Billing
Funding by Colleges of Pharmacy/ Academic Health Centers: shared pharmacy practice faculty in primary care settings Affordable Care Organizations/ Managed Care Insurance Plans • Quality improvement/achieving quality metrics • Reducing medication adverse events/ improving disease management 340B Drug Program Covered Entities: Reinvestment of 340B drug cost savings in salary for clinical pharmacists[35]	Medicare Part B/D: • Annual Wellness Visits • Chronic Care Management • Facility Fee Billing (hospital-based clinics)[36] • Incident-to (physician-based clinics)[37] • MTM contract with Medicare Part D plans[38] • Transitional Care Management Medicaid or Commercial Health Plans: • State law dependent[39,40]

Credentialing and Privileging

As pharmacists look to fill gaps in the primary care workforce and create financially sustainable practices, credentialing and privileging with payers and healthcare organizations are essential. Credentialing and privileging are two separate processes. Credentialing is the process by which an individual's credentials (i.e., academic, license, certifications) are verified to reflect that they have the appropriate training to practice as a pharmacist. Privileging evaluates and authorizes providers to deliver care within a requested scope of practice. For example, if a pharmacist is practicing in a specialty clinic such as hematology/oncology, they would have a different scope than when practicing in a primary care setting. The privileging process ensures individuals have the training and competency to provide the requested services in a particular specialty. Often this verification is obtained through a peer evaluation process, whereby colleagues provide feedback on the provider's clinical knowledge, skills, and professional performance.

With the expanding roles of pharmacists, growth in specialization, and the increased complexity of healthcare, the credentialing and privileging process is more important than ever. Credentialing is required by payers in order for providers to bill for services. As credentialed providers, pharmacists are able to both provide patient care services and contribute to the financial sustainability of the service. Privileging protects the organization from legal risk and ensures patients receive care from qualified and competent providers. These systems already exist for pharmacists, physician, physician assistant, and nurse practitioner colleagues; integration of pharmacists into existing processes will enable the profession to function in parallel and collaboratively with our colleagues and assist in preparing for provider status.

Credentials Beyond Pharmacy Degree and State Licensure

There are multiple opportunities for pharmacists who practice in primary care settings to seek additional credentials beyond the pharmacy degree and licensure, and certain credentials may be required to obtain specific privileges to provide MMS. For example, pharmacists who prescribe hormonal contraception or who serve as immunizing pharmacists must complete training and/or certificate programs to be eligible to provide those services in their state. Certain requirements must also be met in order to enter into CPAs and vary by state. Pharmacists who practice under a CPA in New Mexico, California, Montana, and North Carolina are recognized as Pharmacist Clinician (NM), Advanced Practice Pharmacist (CA), and Clinical Pharmacist Practitioner (NC and MT). The wide variety of state requirements to provide primary care pharmacy services serves as a barrier for patient access to services, and advocacy to standardize credentialing is needed.

Employers may require that primary care pharmacists complete a postgraduate year 1 (PGY1) and/or a PGY2 residency training program. They may also require board certification through the Board of Pharmacy Specialties or completion of an interprofessional certificate, such as the Certified Asthma Educator (AE-C), Certified Diabetes Care and Education Specialist (CDCES, formerly Certified Diabetes Educator or CDE), or Certified Anticoagulation Care Provider (CACP), among others. A listing of board certification opportunities along with eligibility criteria for examination are listed in the **appendix**. All board certification programs listed incur an examination fee, and pharmacists must achieve a passing score on the examination and meet ongoing requirements for renewal. Benefits of board certification include greater marketability, enhanced confidence, improved competence, increased responsibility, and a competitive edge in job placement and advancement.[41] The Council on Credentialing in Pharmacy has established guiding principles for post-licensure credentialing of pharmacists.[42]

Conclusion

There are many avenues in which pharmacists can become involved in primary care practice. Identifying the ideal practice model and service offering will involve collaboration with other healthcare providers as well as identifying a patient population and target outcome. Achievement of federal provider status will allow pharmacists the ability to bill Medicare and create sustainable services and financial stability, as has been demonstrated in states with active provider status laws. As pharmacists become more involved in primary care practice, healthcare will move closer towards the goal of optimal, safe, and effective use of medications for all people all of the time.

References

1. Committee on the Future of Primary Care, Division of Health Services, Institute of Medicine; Donaldson MS, Yordy KD, Lohr KN, et al., eds. *Primary Care: America's Health in a New Era.* National Academy Press; 1996.
2. ASHP policy 1715, collaborative practice. In: Hawkins B, ed. *Best Practices: Positions and Guidance Documents of ASHP.* 2020–2021 ed. American Society of Health-System Pharmacists; 2021. www.ashp.org/Pharmacy-Practice/Policy-Positions-and-Guidelines/Browse-by-Document-Type/Policy-Positions
3. ASHP policy 1502, pharmacist recognition as a healthcare provider. In: Hawkins B, ed. *Best Practices: Positions and Guidance Documents of ASHP.* 2020–2021 ed. American Society of Health-System Pharmacists; 2021. www.ashp.org/Pharmacy-Practice/Policy-Positions-and-Guidelines/Browse-by-Document-Type/Policy-Positions
4. National Alliance of State Pharmacy Associations. 2021 state provider status mid-year legislative update. Published June 7, 2021. Accessed December 15, 2021. https://naspa.us/2021/06/2021-state-provider-status-mid-year-legislative-update/
5. ASHP policy 2011, credentialing and privileging by regulators, payers, and providers of collaborative practice. In: Hawkins B, ed. *Best Practices: Positions and Guidance Documents of ASHP.* 2020–2021 ed. American Society of Health-System Pharmacists; 2021. www.ashp.org/Pharmacy-Practice/Policy-Positions-and-Guidelines/Browse-by-Document-Type/Policy-Positions
6. National Academies of Sciences, Engineering, and Medicine 2021. *Implementing High-Quality Primary Care: Rebuilding the Foundation of Health Care.* National Academies Press; 2021. https://doi.org/10.17226/25983.
7. World Health Organization. Primary health care. Accessed August 20, 2021. https://www.who.int/news-room/fact-sheets/detail/primary-health-care
8. Joint Commission of Pharmacy Practitioners. Medication management services definition and key points. Published March 14, 2018. Accessed August 20, 2021 https://jcpp.net/wp-content/uploads/2018/05/Medication-Management-Services-Definition-and-Key-Points-Version-1.pdf
9. The Joint Commission. Transitions of care: the need for a more effective approach to continuing patient care. Published 2012. Accessed August 20, 2021. https://flbog.sip.ufl.edu/risk-rx-article/transitions-of-care-theneed-for-a-more-effective-approachto-continuing-patient-care/
10. Cavanaugh J, Olson J, Parrott AM. Billing for transitional care management visits. Published June 2018. Accessed August 20, 2021. https://www.ashp.org/-/media/assets/pharmacy-practice/resource-centers/ambulatory-care/transitional-care-management-codes.ashx
11. Medicare Learning Network. Transitional care management services. Published July 2021. Accessed January 31, 2022. https://www.cms.gov/Outreach-and-Education/Medicare-Learning-Network-MLN/MLNProducts/Downloads/Transitional-Care-Management-Services-Fact-Sheet-ICN908628.pdf
12. American Society of Health-System Pharmacists and American Pharmacists Association. ASHP-APhA medication management in care transitions best practices. Published 2013. Accessed August 20, 2021. https://www.ashp.org/-/media/assets/pharmacy-practice/resource-centers/quality-improvement/learn-about-quality-improvement-medication-management-care-transitions.ashx
13. Cavanaugh J, Pinelli N, Eckel S, et al. Advancing pharmacy practice through an innovative ambulatory care transitions program at an academic medical center. *Pharmacy (Basel).* 2020; 8:40.
14. Garrett DG, Bluml BM. Patient self-management program for diabetes: first-year clinical, humanistic, and economic outcomes. *J Am Pharm Assoc.* 2005;45:130–137.
15. Bunting BA, Nayyer D, Lee C. Reducing health care costs and clinical outcomes using an improved Asheville Project model. *Innov Pharm.* 2015; 6:article 227.
16. ASHP Section of Ambulatory Care Practitioners Advisory Group on Clinical Practice Advancement. FAQ: getting started with population health management. Published March 2021. Accessed September 14, 2021. https://www.ashp.org/-/media/assets/pharmacy-practice/resource-centers/ambulatory-care/population-health-faq.pdf
17. Skoy E, Eukel H, Werremeyer A, et al. Implementation of a statewide program within community pharmacies to prevent opioid misuse and accidental overdose. *J APhA.* 2020;60(1):117–121.
18. Birth Control Pharmacist. New report released on state efforts to expand access to contraception in pharmacies. Published December 21, 2019. Accessed August 20, 2021. https://birthcontrolpharmacist.com/2019/12/21/report/
19. Rodriguez MI, Hersh A, Anderson LB, et al. Association of pharmacist prescription of hormonal contraception with unintended pregnancies and Medicaid costs. *Obstet Gynecol.* 2019;133:1238-1246.10.

20. National Alliance of State Pharmacy Associations. Pharmacist prescribing: tobacco cessation aids. Published February 10, 2021. Accessed August 19, 2021. https://naspa.us/resource/tobacco-cessation/
21. Department of Health and Human Services. HHS expands access to childhood vaccines during COVID-19 pandemic. Accessed August 19, 2021. https://www.hhs.gov/about/news/2020/08/19/hhs-expands-access-childhood-vaccines-during-covid-19-pandemic.html
22. Department of Health and Human Services. Trump administration takes action to expand access to COVID-19 vaccines. Accessed August 19, 2021. https://www.hhs.gov/about/news/2020/09/09/trump-administration-takes-action-to-expand-access-to-covid-19-vaccines.html
23. Health Resources and Services Administration. Office for the Advancement of Telehealth. Accessed August 20, 2021. https://www.hrsa.gov/rural-health/telehealth
24. Ratcliffe M, Burd C, Holder K, et al. *Defining rural at the U.S. Census Bureau*. Published December 2016. Accessed August 20, 2021. https://www2.census.gov/geo/pdfs/reference/ua/Defining_Rural.pdf
25. Kelling SE. Exploring accessibility of community pharmacy services. *Innov Pharm*. 2015;6: article 210. Accessed August 20, 2021. https://pubs.lib.umn.edu/index.php/innovations/article/view/392
26. Scott MA, Kiser S, Park I, et al. Creating a new rural pharmacy workforce: development and implementa tion of the Rural Pharmacy Health Initiative. *Am J Health Syst Pharm*. 2017;74:2005–2012. doi: 10.2146/ajhp160727.
27. Centers for Medicare & Medicaid Services. Medicare claims processing manual, chapter 9: rural health clinics/ federally qualified health centers. Revised September 18, 2020. Accessed August 20, 2021. https://www.cms.gov/Regulations-and-Guidance/Guidance/Manuals/Downloads/clm104c09.pdf
28. Como M, Carter CW, Larose-Pierre M, et al. Pharmacist-led chronic care management for medically underserved rural populations in Florida during the COVID-19 pandemic. *Prev Chronic Dis*. 2020; 17:200265. doi: http://dx.doi.org/10.5888/pcd17.200265
29. Office of the Secretary, Department of Health and Human Services. Third amendment to declaration under the Public Readiness and Emergency Preparedness Act for medical countermeasures against COVID–19. Fed Reg. 52136. Published August 24, 2020. Accessed August 20, 2021. https://www.govinfo.gov/content/pkg/FR-2020-08-24/pdf/2020-18542.pdf
30. Office of the Assistant Secretary for Health, Department of Health and Human Services. Guidance for licensed pharmacists, COVID-19 testing, and immunity under the PREP Act. Published April 8, 2020. Accessed August 20, 2021. https://www.hhs.gov/sites/default/files/authorizing-licensed-pharmacists-to-order-and-administer-covid-19-tests.pdf
31. Health Resources & Services Administration. Federally Qualified Health Centers: eligibility. Accessed August 20, 2021. https://www.hrsa.gov/opa/eligibility-and-registration/health-centers/fqhc/index.html
32. Centers for Medicare & Medicaid Services. Federally Qualified Health Center. Accessed August 20, 2021. https://www.cms.gov/Outreach-and-Education/Medicare-Learning-Network-MLN/MLNProducts/downloads/fqhcfactsheet.pdf
33. Maack B, Awad M, Rosselli J. Opportunities for sustainable pharmacy services in Federally Qualified Health Centers. Published January 2022. Accessed January 31, 2022. https://www.ashp.org/pharmacy-practice/resource-centers/ambulatory-care/compensation-and-sustainable-business-models
34. American Society of Health-System Pharmacists. Compensation and sustainable business models. Accessed August 20, 2021. https://www.ashp.org/Pharmacy-Practice/Resource-Centers/Ambulatory-Care/Compensation-and-Sustainable-Business-Models
35. Office of Pharmacy Affairs, Health Resources & Services Administration. 340B Drug Pricing Program. Accessed August 20, 2021. https://www.hrsa.gov/opa/index.html
36. Parrott A, Kline E, Renaurer M, et al. FAQ: facility fee billing. Published August 2021. Accessed September 14, 2021. https://www.ashp.org/-/media/assets/pharmacy-practice/resource-centers/ambulatory-care/Facility-Billing.pdf
37. American Society of Health-System Pharmacists. Pharmacist billing/coding quick reference sheet for services provided in physician-based clinics. Accessed August 20, 2021. https://www.ashp.org/-/media/assets/pharmacy-practice/resource-centers/ambulatory-care/billing-quick-reference-sheet.ashx
38. Centers for Medicare & Medicaid Services. Medication therapy management. Accessed August 20, 2021. https://www.cms.gov/Medicare/Prescription-Drug-Coverage/PrescriptionDrugCovContra/MTM
39. Pharmaceutical Reimbursement Parity, HB 42 (New Mexico). New Mexico Legislature. Accessed August 20, 2021. https://www.nmlegis.gov/Legislation/Legislation?Chamber=H&LegType=B&LegNo=42&year=20
40. Engrossed Substitute, SB 5557. Accessed August 20, 2021. http://lawfilesext.leg.wa.gov/biennium/2015-16/Pdf/Bills/Senate%20Passed%20Legislature/5557-S.PL.pdf
41. Board of Pharmacy Specialties. Making a difference. Accessed August 20, 2021. https://www.bpsweb.org/impact-of-bps-certification/making-a-difference/
42. Council on Credentialing in Pharmacy. Credentialing and privileging of pharmacists. *Am J Health-Syst Pharm*. 2014;71:1891–1900.

Appendix—Board Certification Opportunities for Primary Care Pharmacists

Credential	Certification Body	Eligibility Criteria for Examination
Ambulatory care		
Board Certified Ambulatory Care Pharmacist (BCACP)	Board of Pharmacy Specialties https://www.bpsweb.org/bps-specialties/ambulatory-care/	• Graduation from an ACPE-accredited pharmacy program • Current license to practice • Demonstration of ambulatory care practice experience
Anticoagulation		
Certified Anticoagulation Care Provider (CACP)	National Certification Board for Anticoagulation Care Providers www.ncbap.org	• Must hold professional license for 2 years • Registered nurse, nurse practitioner, registered pharmacist, physician, or physician assistant • 750 hours of active antithrombotic management within the 18 months prior to taking the examination
Asthma		
Certified Asthma Educator (AE-C)	National Asthma Educator Certification Board https://naecb.com/	• Licensed healthcare professionals such as pharmacists, physicians, physician assistants, nurses, respiratory therapists, pulmonary function technologists, social workers, health educators, physical therapists, and occupational therapists • Individuals providing direct patient asthma education, counseling or coordinating services with a minimum of 1,000 hours experience in these activities
Diabetes		
Board Certified Advanced Diabetes Management (BC-ADM)	Association of Diabetes Care and Education Specialists https://www.diabeteseducator.org/education/certification/bc_adm	• Registered nurse, nurse practitioner, clinical nurse specialists, registered dietician, pharmacist, physician assistant, physician • 500 clinical practice hours within 48 months of taking the examination
Certified Diabetes Care and Education Specialist (CDCES)[a]	Certification Board for Diabetes Care and Education https://www.cbdce.org/	• Qualifying healthcare professional: registered nurse, nurse practitioner, registered dietician, pharmacist, physician assistant, physician, and others • 2 years of prior professional experience • A minimum of 1,000 hours providing diabetes care and education in the previous 4 years with a minimum of 400 hours in the previous year • A minimum of 15 hours of approved continuing education focused on diabetes in the previous 2 years
Geriatrics		
Board Certified Geriatric Pharmacist (BCGP)	Board of Pharmacy Specialties https://www.bpsweb.org/bps-specialties/geriatric-pharmacy/	• Graduation from an ACPE-accredited pharmacy program • Current license to practice • Demonstration of geriatric practice experience
HIV		
HIV Pharmacist (AAHIVP)	American Academy of HIV Medicine https://aahivm.org/hiv-pharmacist/	• Pharmacist licensure • Documentation of direct HIV care for 25 patients living with HIV within the preceding 36 months • Participate in the Academy's Clinical Consult Form • Complete a minimum of 45 credits or activity hours of HIV and/or HCV-related continuing education within the preceding 36 months
Lipids		
Clinical Lipid Specialist (CLS)	Accreditation Council for Clinical Lipidology https://www.lipidspecialist.org/certchoose/cls/	• Completed a minimum of 10 continuing education credit hours in clinical lipidology in the previous 2 years • Physicians, nurses, nurse practitioners, physician assistants, pharmacists, registered dieticians/nutritionists, clinical exercise physiologists/specialists • 2,000 hours of demonstrated clinical experience in the management of patients with lipid or other related disorders • Additional training requirements

Appendix—Board Certification Opportunities for Primary Care Pharmacists *(continued)*

Credential	Certification Body	Eligibility Criteria for Examination
Medication therapy management		
Board Certified Medication Therapy Management Specialist (BCMTMS)	The National Board of Medication Therapy Management (NBMTM) https://www.nbmtm.org/bcmtms/	• Pharmacy degree • Pharmacy license • 2 years of experience in MTM experience or NBMTM training
Psychiatry		
Board Certified Psychiatric Pharmacist (BCPP)	Board of Pharmacy Specialties https://www.bpsweb.org/bps-specialties/psychiatric-pharmacy/	• Graduation from an ACPE-accredited pharmacy program • Current license to practice • Defined practice experiences or PGY2 psychiatric pharmacy residency

Abbreviations: ACPE, Accreditation Council for Pharmacy Education; HCV, hepatitis C virus; PGY2, postgraduate year 2.

[a]Previously designated Certified Diabetes Educator (CDE).

Developed through the ASHP Section of Ambulatory Care Pharmacists and approved by the ASHP Board of Directors on February 24, 2022, and by the ASHP House of Delegates on May 19, 2022. This statement supersedes the ASHP Statement on the Pharmacist's Role in Primary Care dated June 7, 1999.

ASHP gratefully acknowledges the following individuals for reviewing the current version of the statement (review does not imply endorsement): Jaclyn A. Boyle, Pharm.D., M.B.A., BCACP; Jamie J. Cavanaugh, Pharm.D., CPP; Christina E. DeRemer, Pharm.D., BCACP, BCPS, TTS, FASHP; Ashley M. Parrott, Pharm.D., M.B.A., BCPS, BCACP; Jessica W. Skelley, Pharm.D., BCACP; and Daniel B. Truelove, Pharm.D., BCACP, BCPS. The contributions of Kimberly A. Galt, Pharm.D., FASHP; Richard F. Demers; and Richard N. Herrier, Pharm.D.; to the previous version of this statement are also gratefully acknowledged.

The authors have declared no potential conflicts of interest.

Melanie A. Dodd, Pharm.D., PhC, BCPS, FASHP, The University of New Mexico College of Pharmacy, Albuquerque, NM.

Seena L. Haines, Pharm.D., BCACP, NBC-HWC, CHWC, FNAP, FCCP, FAPhA, FASHP, The University of Mississippi School of Pharmacy, Jackson, MS.

Brody Maack, Pharm.D., BCACP, CTTS, North Dakota State University School of Pharmacy, Fargo, ND.

Jennifer L. Rosselli, Pharm.D., BCPS, BCACP, BC-ADM, CDCES, Southern Illinois University Edwardsville School of Pharmacy, Edwardsville, IL, SIHF Healthcare, Belleville and O'Fallon, IL.

J. Cody Sandusky, Pharm.D., Harrisburg Medical Center, Harrisburg, IL.

Mollie Ashe Scott, Pharm.D., BCACP, CPP, FASHP, UNC Eshelman School of Pharmacy, Asheville, NC.

Betsy Bryant Shilliday, Pharm.D., CDCES, CPP, BCACP, FASHP, UNC Health and UNC Faculty Physicians, Chapel Hill, NC.

Copyright © 2022, American Society of Health-System Pharmacists, Inc. All rights reserved. Contact ASHP for reprint and permissions requests. This content may not be used for commercial purposes without the express written consent of ASHP.

The bibliographic citation for this document is as follows: American Society of Health-System Pharmacists. ASHP statement on the role of pharmacists in primary care. *Am J Health-Syst Pharm.* 2022; 79:2070–8.

ASHP Statement on the Role of the Pharmacy Workforce in Emergency Preparedness

In recent years, there have been many events that caused a large number of casualties and burdened the healthcare system in unique ways. Since the tragic events of September 11, 2001, the United States has endured natural disasters such as hurricanes, wildfires, floods, and earthquakes; cared for the victims of industrial and traffic accidents, mass shootings, and building collapses; and responded to a pandemic that overwhelmed local hospital and health-system capacities. These events have focused attention on the variety of threats that can strain the healthcare system. As we try to mitigate the burden of these threats to providing patient care, local, national, and global resources must be prepared to pivot their emergency preparedness plans to strengthen countermeasures and prepare team members for the inevitability of another disruption to our healthcare system. While continuity of core services will always be the priority, hospitals and health systems should strive to be able to continue to provide the same level of care during and post-disaster as they did pre-disaster.

Healthcare systems must continue to engage their employees, leaders, and communities to prepare for these unforeseen events to alleviate extended disruption of services for their patients in a time of need. Communities look to healthcare systems for support and guidance during times of uncertainty, and providing a safety net during trying times should be a priority to ensure long-term consequences of emergencies are abated. As governments and healthcare systems have developed countermeasures and strategies to respond to these threats, it is clear that the pharmacy workforce has an essential role in emergency preparedness. Their clinical and operational knowledge have been a critical part of the response to many different emergencies. As the threats to providing patient care evolve, the pharmacy workforce must be poised to strengthen emergency-preparedness plans and train team members for the next inevitable disruption to our healthcare system.

Position

The American Society of Health-System Pharmacists (ASHP) believes that members of the pharmacy workforce (ie, pharmacists, pharmacy residents, pharmacy interns, pharmacy technicians, and other nonpharmacist support staff) must assertively exercise their responsibilities in preparing for and responding to emergencies. Leaders of emergency planning at the federal, regional, state, and local levels (both governmental and institutional) must know to call on the pharmacy workforce to help prepare for and respond to emergencies involving pharmaceuticals or pharmacotherapy. For the purposes of this statement, ASHP uses the Federal Emergency Management Agency (FEMA) definition of emergency: any incident, whether natural, technological, or human-caused, that requires responsive action to protect life or property.[1] Emergencies include naturally occurring incidents (eg, floods, hurricanes, tropical storms, tornadoes, earthquakes, tsunamis, wildland and urban fires); human-caused incidents (eg, explosions; hazardous materials spills; chemical or radiation releases; terrorist attacks and threats; civil unrest; mass shootings; and airplane, train, or automobile crashes); and technological disasters (eg, computer ransomware attacks and downtimes, utility failures such as loss of electricity, water, or gas supply). For the purposes of this statement, *emergency scenarios* are expected or supposed emergency situations or sequences of events used in planning. Health-system and hospital pharmacy staff should prepare for both transient emergency scenarios (eg, mass casualty events) and enduring emergency scenarios, such as pandemics. All members of the pharmacy workforce have a role to play in emergency preparedness and response.

General Principles

1. On the basis of their education, training, experience, and legal responsibilities, pharmacists and pharmacy technicians should have a key role in the risk assessment, planning, and execution of pharmaceutical distribution and drug therapy management of patients during all types of emergency scenarios and in all 5 areas of emergency preparedness (prevention, mitigation, preparedness, response, and recovery).
2. Pharmacists should participate in and assume key roles on emergency management and response teams by (a) developing guidelines for the prevention or diagnosis and treatment of casualties and exposed individuals; (b) selecting pharmaceuticals and related supplies (eg, medications and items necessary for administration) for national and regional stockpiles as well as local emergency inventories in emergency-preparedness programs; (c) ensuring appropriate education and counseling of individuals who receive pharmaceuticals from an emergency supply in response to an event, including assisting in the consent and education process for medications approved through the FDA emergency use authorization process; (d) developing guidelines for the allocation of pharmaceuticals when demand is greater than supply; (e) administering medications, if needed and when appropriate; and (f) designing and implementing exercises to assess readiness and vulnerabilities that may identify potential improvements.
3. Pharmacy team members who assume leadership roles on emergency management and response teams should be familiar with the National Incident Management System Preparedness Cycle[2] and have completed FEMA training to assume leadership roles on health-system, regional, or state emergency management committees.
4. The expertise of the pharmacy workforce includes (a) ensuring proper packaging, storage, handling, labeling, and dispensing of emergency supplies of pharmaceuticals; and (b) ensuring appropriate deployment of emergency supplies of pharmaceuticals.

DOI 10.37573/9781585287048.072

5. Pharmacy team members should develop contingency staffing plans to ensure patients have access to medications during all types of events.
6. Pharmacists should collaborate with public health officials and health-system and hospital leaders on appropriate messages to convey to the public regarding the use of essential pharmaceuticals in response to emergencies, including pandemics and mass exposure events. Special consideration should be given to disease prevention, public health outcomes, adverse effects, drug-drug interactions, contraindications, the effectiveness of alternative pharmaceuticals, and the potential development of drug-resistant infectious agents.
7. In the event of an emergency that requires drug therapy (eg, a pandemic or radiation exposure), pharmacists should collaborate with physicians and other prescribers in managing or prescribing the drug therapy of individual affected patients.

Advice to Hospital and Health-System Pharmacy Directors

Every hospital and health-system pharmacy director (or designee) should

1. Participate in an organizational hazard vulnerability analysis.
2. Become well informed about the potential local hazards and risks for emergency scenarios and the related diagnostic and treatment issues.
3. Become thoroughly informed about federal, regional, state, local, and institutional plans for emergency preparedness, especially those related to the distribution, control, and use of pharmaceuticals and related supplies.
4. Ensure that the pharmaceutical components of the institution's emergency plans are coordinated with the overall local preparedness plans involving other institutions, community pharmacies, wholesalers, as well as coordinated with federal, regional, and state plans.
5. Ensure that the appropriate pharmaceuticals and related equipment and supplies[3] are in stock at the institution, consistent with the overall local emergency-preparedness plan, which should account for the interim between the occurrence of an emergency scenario and the receipt of federal or state assistance.
6. Ensure that information about the appropriate use of pharmaceuticals in response to an emergency scenario is available to health professionals and leaders in the institution.
7. Collaborate with institutional ambulatory pharmacies to develop a comprehensive plan to ensure patients have access to discharge and maintenance medication supplies.
8. Ensure that the institution does not engage in stockpiling of pharmaceuticals without regard to local emergency-preparedness plans that are designed to meet the needs of the whole community.
9. Ensure that pharmacy personnel are trained to implement the institution's emergency plans.
10. Clearly define the emergency preparedness and response roles for each member of their pharmacy workforce and ensure that each team member understands their roles.

Advice to Other Members of the Hospital and Health-System Pharmacy Workforce

All members of the hospital and health-system pharmacy workforce should

1. Become well informed about the potential local hazards and risks for emergency scenarios and the related diagnostic and treatment issues.
2. Become thoroughly informed of local and institutional plans for emergency preparedness and response, especially those related to the distribution, control, and use of pharmaceuticals.
3. Consider volunteering in advance of an emergency to assist in (a) distributing emergency supplies of pharmaceuticals, (b) dispensing and administering medications and immunizations, and (c) managing the drug therapy of individual victims.
4. Be familiar, at a minimum, with their institution's command structure and communication plan and, ideally, with the FEMA Incident Command Structure.[4]
5. Engage in system emergency preparedness drills, tabletop discussions, and education opportunities for staff to improve staff familiarity with processes and to increase readiness in the case of an emergency.
6. Strongly discourage individuals from developing personal stockpiles of pharmaceuticals for use in the event of chemical, biological, or radiological/nuclear emergency scenarios.

Health-system and hospital pharmacists should

1. Develop and maintain first-aid skills and basic life support (BLS) certification. Additional certification may be required for administering injectable medications, such as vaccines (eg, advanced cardiovascular life support [ACLS] or vaccine-specific certifications).
2. Consider additional emergency preparedness training, such as basic disaster life support (BDLS), advanced disaster life support (ADLS), or advanced hazmat life support (AHLS) training, as pertinent to their roles in routine and emergency care.
3. Consider engagement in your system's emergency preparedness committee as well as other local and state organizations that distribute resources in the event of an emergency scenario.
4. Share evidence-based information on pharmaceuticals used to respond to emergencies with professional colleagues and patients.

Health-system and hospital pharmacy technicians should

1. Become familiar with the pharmacy technician-specific responsibilities required by the department to respond to emergency scenarios.
2. Engage directly in or with representatives from emergency preparedness committees to better understand health-system and hospital expectations for pharmacy technicians and provide input as needed.

Advice to Hospital and Health-System Administrators

Hospital and health-system administrators should

1. Expect the pharmacy director or designee to participate in the development and implementation of local, state, regional, and federal emergency-preparedness plans.
2. Collaborate with the pharmacy director or designee in their participation in preparing the institution's hazards vulnerability assessment and emergency-preparedness plan.
3. Promote the inclusion of the pharmacy workforce in the organization's emergency management governance committees.
4. Encourage the pharmacy workforce to be active participants within the organization's command/control response framework, and promote cohesive development of service-line-specific plans that support the continuity of critical department functions and resources during a prolonged event.
5. Collaborate with the pharmacy director or designee to coordinate the institution's participation in the building of appropriate emergency pharmaceutical resources for use in the hospital, health system, and community. This includes ensuring that institutional supplies of pharmaceutical resources are coordinated with the local plan.
6. Advocate that local preparedness-planning officials involve the pharmacy workforce in the full range of planning related to pharmaceuticals, related supplies, and patient care.
7. Encourage and enable the pharmacy workforce employed by the institution to participate in local, state, regional, and federal emergency-preparedness planning and to volunteer for community service in the event of emergencies.
8. Consider creating and maintaining emergency preparedness kits (eg, necessary medications and supplies) to dispense to remote locations based on your hospital's assessment of potential surge size and likely emergency scenarios that could arise.
9. Encourage pharmacy workforce participation in the development and enhancement of the enterprise's business continuity program to optimize the efficacy of pharmacy's role in an extended response or downtime.
10. Provide guidance and frameworks for the pharmacy workforce to participate in emergency-preparedness plan development that aligns with broader goals (eg, those of the hospital, health-system, or regional plans).

Advice to Other Healthcare Providers (eg, the Interprofessional Care Team)

Other healthcare providers should

1. Encourage the involvement of the pharmacy department in the development and implementation of emergency response plans.
2. Reinforce the message that pharmacists are an essential part of the team responsible for developing drug treatment guidelines in response to an emergency scenario.
3. Be aware for planning and response purposes that the pharmacy department has a business continuity plan to provide uninterrupted services as part of the emergency management plan.
4. Recognize that pharmacists have expertise that can aid in planning for and responding to a variety of emergency scenarios (eg, modifying drug regimens during emergencies; planning and implementing vaccination programs, including administering vaccines; providing wound care and first aid for minor ailments).
5. Encourage pharmacist participation in post-event reporting (eg, after-action reviews).
6. Involve appropriately trained pharmacists in medical emergencies.

Advice for Emergency-Preparedness Planners

Emergency-preparedness planners at the federal, regional, state, and local levels should

1. Consult with qualified pharmacists in all areas in which the pharmacist's expertise would contribute to the creation and execution of workable plans.
2. Inform pharmacists through state and national pharmacy organizations as well as other applicable channels of plans for deployment of emergency pharmaceutical supplies. This includes both medications and supplies necessary for administration and monitoring therapy so that appropriate mitigation plans can be made.
3. Consult with qualified pharmacists on messages that should be conveyed to the public about the appropriate use of pharmaceuticals in the event of an emergency scenario.
4. Communicate the role and expectations of the pharmacy workforce during an incident. The execution of operational plans relies on the inclusion of pharmacy-specific subject matter expertise in order to maintain continuity of safe patient care.

Advice to Government Agencies

Federal, state, and local government agencies should

1. Recognize the expertise and knowledge of the pharmacy workforce in the use and distribution of medications and should incorporate pharmacists into planning for all emergency scenarios involving disease screening, medication management, and pharmacotherapy.
2. Recognize pharmacists as medication experts, able during emergency scenarios to advise about making modifications to drug regimens during emergency scenarios.
3. Be prepared to allow and provide temporary authorization that facilitates pharmacists and pharmacy technicians practicing in another state and allows states to efficiently grant temporary or emergency licensure during emergency scenarios.
4. In coordination with health systems, build and maintain relationships that foster collaboration in the event of an emergency scenario.

Advice to State Societies of Health-System Pharmacists

State societies of health-system pharmacists should

1. Be a resource to state and local emergency-preparedness planning officials, especially in identifying qualified members of the pharmacy workforce to participate in emergency- preparedness planning and response.
2. Collaborate with other disciplines to identify and plan the pharmacy workforce's response to all types of emergency scenarios.
3. Create a statement for their membership of information unique to the state regarding pharmacists' participation in emergency-preparedness planning and deployment efforts.
4. Provide opportunities for the state's pharmacy workforce to participate in local and/or state training and exercises to improve knowledge and competence for incident management and all types of emergency scenarios.
5. Encourage the pharmacy workforce to join established networks of healthcare professionals to be deployed in emergency scenarios.
6. Collaborate with the pharmacy workforce to communicate information about and resources for public health emergency scenarios.

Advice to Educators

Educators (eg, students, college of pharmacy administrators and faculty, residents, residency program directors, and pharmacy technician educators) should

1. Recognize that emergency preparedness knowledge is a critical component of a well-rounded pharmacist and incorporate emergency preparedness topics in both didactic and experiential learning for both students and residents; pharmacy technician educators and trainers should provide students and trainees with general knowledge on basic safety and emergency-preparedness procedures applicable to pharmacy services.[5,6]
2. Be familiar with the 5 areas of emergency preparedness, how they fit into the local emergency management plan, and how to implement them in an emergency scenario.
3. Define where pharmacy and pharmacy technician educators and students could support public health (eg, participating in education, community outreach, vaccination, and testing) and develop frameworks for deploying support when needed.
4. Establish a relationship with the department of health or the local community (eg, through registration) as a resource to the community or local health system or hospital during an emergency scenario.
5. Consult with professional organizations such as ASHP and American Association of Colleges of Pharmacy for guidance regarding the role pharmacy educators could play and the expertise they could provide in advising about local, state, and national health emergencies whenever a response from colleges of pharmacy is required.
6. Act as liaisons responsible for interacting with emergency response agencies, outside relief agencies, other hospitals and clinics, and potentially law enforcement.

Commitments Made by ASHP

In support of the efforts of the pharmacy workforce in emergency preparedness, ASHP will

1. Maintain an electronic communications network of hospital pharmacy department directors that can be used to transmit urgent information related to emergency preparedness and medical countermeasures.
2. Disseminate promptly to ASHP members and others in the healthcare community important new information related to pharmacy workforce involvement in emergency preparedness.
3. Disseminate to ASHP members and others in the healthcare community timely evidence-based and supply chain-related information about pharmaceuticals used when responding to emergency scenarios.
4. Meet with government officials and others when necessary to clarify promptly important issues that affect the involvement of the pharmacy workforce in emergency preparedness and medical countermeasures.

Future Directions for the Pharmacy Profession

To promote effective emergency preparedness and response in the US, the pharmacy profession should

1. Advocate that emergency-preparedness planners address the impact of emergencies on disadvantaged communities and the need to focus on emergency response as a community or national effort rather than one managed in silos.
2. Encourage domestic production of resources necessary to respond to emergency scenarios, promote increased diversity and redundancy in manufacturing of those resources, and advocate for acquisition and storage policies that facilitate the availability of those resources at the time of need.
3. Encourage elected officials to clarify responsibility for obtaining, monitoring, and allocating resources in the event of an emergency on a community and national level and empower those responsible to respond in a timely manner without excessive bureaucratic barriers or delays.
4. Leverage technology to provide continuation of services with remote staff wherever possible, including safe and effective access and sharing of patient information using personal computers, policies regarding computer usage, and loss of systems both within and outside the hospital and health system.
5. Share information (via publications and presentations) on leadership, training models, practice models, outcome measures, and employee well-being as it relates to emergency preparedness.
6. Increase health literacy and emergency preparedness education efforts in the general population based on hazard vulnerability analyses.
7. Develop robust emergency preparedness guidelines to shape future practice in this area.

Conclusion

The pharmacy workforce has unique expertise that is vital in preparing for and responding to emergencies. Like other healthcare providers, members of the pharmacy workforce have a moral and professional responsibility to participate in federal, state, regional, and institutional emergency preparedness and response efforts. To take full advantage of their unique expertise, members of the pharmacy workforce should be involved in emergency preparedness decision-making and in the implementation of emergency responses. The pharmacy workforce should integrate the practices outlined in this statement into their activities and be empowered by their employers and policymakers to contribute to and enhance emergency preparedness efforts. To carry out these responsibilities, the pharmacy profession needs to bolster educational efforts on the topic and develop robust guidelines and other resources to support the pharmacy workforce's role in emergency preparedness and response.

References

1. Federal Emergency Management Agency. Glossary. Accessed March 3, 2022.
2. Federal Emergency Management Agency. National Incident Management System. Accessed March 3, 2022. https://www.fema.gov/emergency-managers/nims
3. Food and Drug Administration. Drug and biologic essential medicines, medical countermeasures, and critical inputs for the list described in section 3(c) of the Executive Order 13944. Accessed March 3, 2022. https://www.fda.gov/media/143406/download
4. Federal Emergency Management Agency. ICS organizational structure and elements. Accessed March 3, 2022. https://training.fema.gov/emiweb/is/icsresource/assets/ics%20organizational%20structure%20and%20elements.pdf
5. American Society of Health-System Pharmacists. Accreditation standards for pharmacy technician education and training. Accessed March 3, 2022. https://www.ashp.org/professional-development/technician-program-accreditation/accreditation-standards/accreditation-standards-for-pharmacy-technician-education-and-training-programs
6. Griebe K, Jiang C, To L, et al. Pharmacy emergency preparedness training as a PGY2 longitudinal rotation. *Am J Health-Syst Pharm*. 2021;78:669–673. doi:10.1093/ajhp/zxab044

Approved by the ASHP Board of Directors on March 24, 2022, and by the ASHP House of Delegates on May 19, 2022. Developed through the ASHP Council on Pharmacy Practice. Supersedes the ASHP statement on the role of health-system pharmacists in emergency preparedness dated June 2, 2002.

ASHP gratefully acknowledges Batoul Senhaji-Tomza, PharmD, MPH, for his contributions to this statement.

The authors have declared no potential conflicts of interest.

Megan Corrigan, PharmD, MPH, BCPS, Advocate Aurora Health, Elmhurst, IL.

Nancy C. MacDonald, PharmD, BCPS, FASHP, Henry Ford Hospital, Detroit, MI.

Megan Musselman, PharmD, MS, BCPS, BCCCP, DPLA, FCCP, North Kansas City Hospital

Kansas City, MO.

Joseph Pinto, MS, MHA, DPLA, RPh, Mount Sinai Health System, New York, NY.

Mark Skildum, PharmD, MBA, BCPS, DPLA, Allina Health, St Paul, MN

Andrew P. Smith, PharmD, MBA, BCPS, BCCCP, Scripps Mercy Hospital, San Diego, CA.

Copyright © 2022, American Society of Health-System Pharmacists, Inc. All rights reserved. Contact ASHP for reprint and permissions requests. This content may not be used for commercial purposes without the express written consent of ASHP.

The bibliographic citation for this document is as follows: American Society of Health-System Pharmacists. ASHP statement on the role of the pharmacy workforce in emergency preparedness. *Am J Health-Syst Pharm*. 2022;79:2185–2189.

ASHP Statement on the Use of Dietary Supplements

Position

The American Society of Health-System Pharmacists (ASHP) believes that the widespread, indiscriminate use of dietary supplements presents substantial risks to public health and that pharmacists have an opportunity and a professional responsibility to reduce those risks. ASHP recognizes that patients may choose to use legally available dietary supplements, but believes that the decision to use substances that may be pharmacologically active should always be based on reliable information about their safety and efficacy. The current regulatory framework governing dietary supplements does not provide consumers or health care providers with sufficient information on safety and efficacy to make informed decisions. Furthermore, standards for product quality are currently inadequate. ASHP recognizes the concerns raised by the dietary supplement industry regarding regulating dietary supplements as nonprescription drugs because of the industry's inability to patent product ingredients. Still, ASHP urges Congress to amend the Dietary Supplement Health and Education Act of 1994 (DSHEA) to require that the Food and Drug Administration (FDA) develop a regulatory scheme to ensure that dietary supplements are safe and effective. ASHP believes that dietary supplements, at a minimum, should (1) receive FDA approval for evidence of safety and efficacy, (2) meet manufacturing standards for identity, strength, quality, purity, packaging, and labeling, and (3) undergo mandatory postmarketing reporting of adverse events, including drug interactions.

ASHP strongly encourages in vitro and clinical studies of interactions between dietary supplements and medications. Because of the demonstrated risk of these interactions, ASHP discourages the concurrent use of dietary supplements and drug therapy, especially those therapies for which failure may have irreversible consequences (e.g., immunosuppressive therapy, cancer chemotherapy, treatment for human immunodeficiency virus infection, anticoagulation therapy, and hormonal contraceptive therapy).

ASHP believes that the criteria used to evaluate dietary supplements for inclusion in health-system formularies should be as rigorous as those established for nonprescription drugs and that the self-administered use of dietary supplements during a health-system stay may increase risks to patients and liabilities to health care professionals and institutions.

ASHP urges pharmacists and other health care practitioners to integrate awareness of dietary supplement use into everyday practice and encourages pharmacists to increase efforts to prevent interactions between dietary supplements and drugs. ASHP also supports the education of pharmacists and other health care practitioners in the taxonomy, formulation, pharmacology, and pharmacokinetics of dietary supplements and believes that such education should be required in college of pharmacy curricula.

Background

Dietary supplements are defined in DSHEA as products "intended to supplement the diet" that contain vitamins, minerals, herbs or other botanicals, amino acids; "a dietary substance for use by man to supplement the diet by increasing the total daily intake"; or "a concentrate, metabolite, constituent, extract, or combinations of these ingredients."[1]

Evidence of variability in dietary supplement content[2–8] has spurred efforts to standardize products. Current federal regulations regarding the manufacture of dietary supplements are not adequate.[9] Some manufacturers voluntarily follow good manufacturing practices (GMPs) devised by their own trade groups (e.g., the National Nutritional Foods Association GMP Certification Program[10]), and the U.S. Pharmacopeia (USP) has created voluntary standards for a handful of dietary supplements.[11] Manufacturers that wish to carry the "USP approved" seal on their product labels have to subject their products to testing by USP. The creation of these voluntary programs reflects a widespread concern, even on the part of dietary supplement manufacturers, that production processes must be regulated. Although FDA has had the authority to establish dietary supplement GMPs for almost a decade, it issued its first proposed rule on the topic in 2003.[12]

DSHEA does not require FDA to review evidence of the efficacy or safety of dietary supplements, so manufacturers have no burden to prove that their products are effective or safe. Although dietary supplement labeling cannot claim activity in the treatment of a specific disease or condition, claims that suggest an effect on the "structure or function of the body" are allowed.[1] For example, dietary supplements containing echinacea can be labeled as supporting immune health (as a "function") but cannot be labeled as preventing or ameliorating colds (treating a disease). Regardless of this distinction between function and treatment, consumers are bombarded by the lay press (and even some scientific literature) with what can only be described as specific-disease indications for dietary supplements (e.g., glucosamine for osteoarthritis, black cohosh for menopausal symptoms, and St. John's wort for depression).

The health claims allowed in dietary supplement labeling by current interpretation of DSHEA create further confusion for consumers. FDA's attempt to hold these health claims to the same scientific standard required for conventional foods was struck down in *Pearson* v. *Shalala,* so FDA must permit dietary supplement labels to carry "qualified" health claims based on equivocal scientific evidence.[13]

Although DSHEA does require that dietary supplements be safe, it does not require prospective testing to ensure safety. To remove a product from the market, FDA must prove that the product is unsafe. Under DSHEA, some dietary supplements that were banned from the U.S. market because of concerns about their safety have been allowed to return (e.g., sassafras tea, dehydroepiandrosterone). Demonstrably unsafe products have made their way onto the market, and fatal adverse reactions have been reported.[14,15]

Establishing the safety record of dietary supplements has been complicated by the lack of systematically collected data about their adverse reactions. The MedWatch system has been used to a limited extent to report adverse events related to dietary supplement use, but, nine years after the passage of DSHEA, FDA is still developing an

DOI 10.37573/9781585287048.073

adverse-reaction-reporting system for dietary supplements. Despite the limited data, however, the number of case reports of interactions between dietary supplements and medications is growing.[16–21] The safety of dietary supplements for special populations (e.g., children, pregnant women, people with impaired organ or immunologic function) has also not been demonstrated.

Dangers to Public Health

It has been estimated that 40% of the U.S. population uses dietary supplements often and that almost twice as many have used at least 1 of the estimated 29,000 dietary supplements on the market.[22] Out-of-pocket expenditures on dietary supplements total approximately $18 billion annually.[23] Such widespread and indiscriminate use of dietary supplements presents five dangers to the public health:

1. Some dietary supplements are inherently unsafe when ingested orally (e.g., chaparral, ephedra, comfrey, tiractricol, aristolochic acid, pennyroyal).[24–28]
2. Lax regulation of dietary supplement manufacturing presents the risk of contamination or adulteration with harmful substances, including carcinogens,[29–32] and of dangerous variability in active ingredient content among products.[2–8]
3. The use of dietary supplements may compromise, delay, or supplant treatment with therapies of proven efficacy.[16–21,25]
4. Dietary supplements may present dangers to special populations (e.g., children, pregnant women, patients undergoing surgery, patients with impaired organ or immunologic function).
5. Spending on dietary supplements represents an enormous health-related expenditure of unsubstantiated value.[33]

Since the mid-19th century, the federal government has exercised its responsibility to protect Americans from hazardous or adulterated foods and medicines. ASHP believes that, with the passage and implementation of DSHEA, the federal government has abandoned its duty to create a regulatory scheme for dietary supplements that adequately protects the health of consumers. Under DSHEA, consumers and health care practitioners are not provided with the information they need to use dietary supplements safely. To reduce the dangers posed by the current regulatory framework, Congress should amend DSHEA to

1. Require that dietary supplements undergo FDA approval for evidence of safety and efficacy,
2. Mandate FDA-approved dietary supplement labeling that describes safe use in a clear, standardized format, including the potential for interaction with medications and cautions for special populations,
3. Require FDA to promulgate and enforce GMPs for dietary supplements,
4. Require that dietary supplements meet FDA-established standards for identity, strength, purity, and quality, and
5. Empower FDA to establish and maintain an adverse-event-reporting system specifically for dietary supplements, and require dietary supplement manufacturers to report suspected adverse reactions to FDA.

Implications for Practice

Although examples of persons rejecting potentially life-saving medical interventions in favor of alternative therapies can be found in the medical and lay press,[34] the presumption that most users of dietary supplements reject traditional treatments is unfounded. One survey found that most individuals who use alternative therapies for a specific symptom or disease are also receiving care and prescription medications from a physician or surgeon.[35] In a more recent nationwide survey, almost 20% of adults taking prescription drugs reported that they were taking at least one dietary supplement, not including vitamin or mineral supplements.[36]

Pharmacists and other health care practitioners therefore have an opportunity to reduce the risks associated with dietary supplement use. Health care providers face unfamiliar challenges in this effort, however, because much of the information they typically use to establish pharmaceutical treatment regimens is lacking for dietary supplements. Product content is not standardized, therapeutic goals are vague, and evidence of efficacy and safety is absent or ambiguous. ASHP believes that pharmacists, as medication-use experts and accessible members of the health care team, are uniquely qualified and positioned to counsel patients using or considering the use of dietary supplements. Despite their professional responsibility to provide patients with sound advice, pharmacists (like other health care providers) are frustrated by the lack of reliable information about the safety and efficacy of dietary supplements. Pharmacists have shown that they can improve medication safety by identifying and preventing adverse drug events,[37] and they could play a similar role in preventing adverse events due to dietary supplement use if they had sound, evidence-based professional resources.

Incorporate Awareness of Dietary Supplement Use into Practice. ASHP urges pharmacists and other health care practitioners to integrate awareness of dietary supplement use into everyday practice. ASHP believes that all health systems should have an institutional policy regarding the use of dietary supplements. Such policies should allow pharmacists and other health care practitioners to exercise their professional judgment and try to balance patient autonomy and institutional concerns.

Patient Counseling. Although most consumers of alternative therapies also take prescription medications,[35] one survey found that 72% of respondents who used alternative therapies did not report that use to their health care providers.[38] Pharmacists and other health care practitioners must therefore routinely inquire about a patient's current or planned use of dietary supplements, providing examples so that patients understand what is meant (e.g, asking "Do you use dietary supplements, such as St. John's wort or gingko?").[39] This information will allow pharmacists and other health care practitioners to counsel the patient about dietary supplement use and monitor for adverse reactions and drug interactions.

When counseling patients about dietary supplements, the concept of *caveat emptor* (buyer beware) must be emphasized because the content and safety of dietary supplements are not well regulated. ASHP believes that all pharmacists, at a minimum, should be familiar with the pharmacology and pharmacokinetics of common dietary supplements that might contraindicate concurrent use with a therapeutic regimen (i.e., proven and potential pharmacokinetic and pharmacodynamic interactions with prescription and nonprescription medications) to the extent that sound evidence exists. To provide informed counsel to patients using or considering the use of dietary supplements, pharmacists further need to be familiar with the following:

- The typical uses of common dietary supplements and the scientific literature regarding their efficacy and safety.
- The proven and potential interactions between common dietary supplements and prescription and nonprescription medications.
- The methods of therapeutic monitoring for common dietary supplements, including signs and symptoms of potential adverse effects and toxicities.
- The proven and potential effects of certain disease states on supplement absorption, distribution, and elimination.
- The safety of using dietary supplements before or after surgery.

Despite the shortcomings of the data on dietary supplements, the limited references on the topic that are available should be consulted.[40–45]

Patients stabilized on a combination of a supplement and medication should be cautioned not to suddenly discontinue the use of either without first consulting with the prescriber. The potential for adverse effects from an interaction exists both when a dietary supplement is discontinued and when it is initiated.

Dietary supplement sales have a very high potential for profit. Despite the expectation that pharmacies should receive a profit from the sale of products, professional ethics mandate that any recommendations or purchasing suggestions be made with the well-being of the customer or patient as the primary concern. Pharmacists should also review promotional and reference materials promulgated in or by their workplaces to ensure that these materials are evidence based and not misleading or deceptive. The scientific literature about the safety and efficacy of dietary supplements is updated continually. Pharmacists have a responsibility to continually monitor that literature and incorporate the evolving knowledge into their care for and advice to patients.

Inclusion in Formularies. ASHP believes that the criteria used to evaluate dietary supplements for inclusion in health-system formularies should be as rigorous as those established for prescription and nonprescription drugs. The Joint Commission on Accreditation of Healthcare Organizations (JCAHO) has recommended that medical staff weigh the patient care implications of dietary supplements with the same rigor applied to prescription and nonprescription medications,[46] and all JCAHO medication management standards apply to dietary supplements, as well as prescription and nonprescription drugs.[47] ASHP believes that the decision to include any product in a health-system formulary should be based on comparative data regarding efficacy, adverse effects, cost, and potential therapeutic advantages and deficiencies.[48] The lack of definitive evidence of efficacy and safety and the demonstrated variability in product content make most dietary supplements unsuitable for inclusion in health-system formularies.[49] More research is needed to determine the relative effectiveness of dietary supplements and their safety for all patient populations, especially drug–supplement interactions.

The shortcomings that make most dietary supplements unsuitable for inclusion in formularies also argue strongly against their self-administered use by patients during a health-system stay. ASHP believes that the use of self-administered medications should be avoided to the extent possible[50] and that pharmacists should identify all drug products before their use.[15] There is currently no way to definitively determine the content of dietary supplements brought into health systems. In addition, discontinuing supplement use may be advisable as part of the diagnostic workup, and the possibility that supplement use may have contributed to hospitalization should be considered.

If an institution decides, as a matter of patient autonomy, to allow the use of dietary supplements, such use should require a prescribed order for the specific dietary supplement in the patient medical record and pharmacist review and verification of the order. Health systems should be aware that the use of dietary supplements may expose patients to risks, and the health system and staff should take steps to reduce potential liability (e.g., require patients to sign a liability waiver for dietary supplement use) and decrease those risks.

Conclusion

Current regulation of the manufacture and labeling of dietary supplements fails to address substantial risks to the public health. As the activity of some dietary supplements has become apparent, so have their dangers and the shortcomings of the current regulatory framework. These laws and regulations should be revised, with the primary goal of providing consumers and health care practitioners with the information they need to use dietary supplements safely and effectively. In short, dietary supplements should be regulated in a manner that ensures that they are safe and effective. Regardless of the shortcomings of the current regulatory framework, pharmacists have an opportunity and a professional responsibility to reduce the risks presented by dietary supplement use.

References

1. Dietary Supplement Health and Education Act of 1994 (SB 784). http://thomas.loc.gov/ (accessed 2003 Apr 1).
2. Gurley BJ, Wang P, Gardner SF. Ephedrine-type alkaloid content of nutritional supplements containing *Ephedra sinica* (Ma-huang) as determined by high performance liquid chromatography. *J Pharm Sci.* 1998; 87:1547–53.
3. Harkey MR, Henderson GL, Gershwin ME, et al. Variability in commercial ginseng products: an analysis of 25 preparations. *Am J Clin Nutr.* 2001; 73:1101–6.
4. Parasrampuria J, Schwartz K, Petesch R. Quality control of dehydroepiandrosterone dietary supplement products. *JAMA.* 1998; 280:1565. Letter.
5. Feifer AH, Fleshner NE, Klotz L. Analytical accuracy and reliability of commonly used nutritional supplements in prostate disease. *J Urol.* 2002; 168:150–4.

6. De los Reyes GC, Koda RT. Determining hyperforin and hypericin content in eight brands of St. John's wort. *Am J Health-Syst Pharm.* 2002; 59:545–7.

7. Glisson JK, Rogers HE, Abourashed EA, et al. Clinic at the health food store? Employee recommendations and product analysis. *Pharmacotherapy.* 2003; 23:64–72.

8. Gurley BJ, Gardner SF, Hubbard MA. Content versus label claims in ephedra-containing dietary supplements. *Am J Health-Syst Pharm.* 2000; 57:963–9.

9. Fontanarosa PB, Rennie D, DeAngelis CD. The need for regulation of dietary supplements—lessons from ephedra. *JAMA.* 2003; 289:1568–70. Editorial.

10. National Nutritional Foods Association. NNFA GMP certification program overview. www.nnfa.org/services/science/gmp.htm (accessed 2003 Dec 12).

11. U.S. Pharmacopeia. U.S. Pharmacopeia dietary supplement verification program. www.usp-verified.org (accessed 2004 May 13).

12. Food and Drug Administration. Current good manufacturing practice in manufacturing, packing, or holding dietary ingredients and dietary supplements. Proposed rule. *Fed Regist.* 2003; 68:12157–263.

13. *Pearson* v. *Shalala,* 164 F.3d 650 (D.C. Cir. 1999).

14. Food and Drug Administration. Illnesses and injuries associated with the use of selected dietary supplements. www.cfsan.fda.gov/~dms/ds-ill.html (accessed 2003 Feb 14).

15. Palmer ME, Haller C, McKinney PE, et al. Adverse events associated with dietary supplements: an observational study. *Lancet.* 2003; 361:101–6.

16. Williamson EM. Drug interactions between herbal and prescription medicines. *Drug Saf.* 2003; 26:1075–92.

17. Fugh-Berman A. Herb–drug interactions. *Lancet.* 2000; 355: 134–8.

18. Yue QY, Bergquist C, Gerdén B. Safety of St. John's wort *(Hypericum perforatum). Lancet.* 2000; 355:576–7. Letter.

19. Brazier NC, Levine MA. Drug–herb interaction among commonly used conventional medicines: a compendium for health care professionals. *Am J Ther.* 2003; 10:163–9.

20. Izzo AA, Ernst E. Interactions between herbal medicines and prescribed drugs: a systematic review. *Drugs.* 2001; 61:2163–75.

21. Piscitelli SC, Burstein AH, Chaitt D, et al. Indinavir concentrations and St. John's wort. *Lancet.* 2000; 355:547–8. Letter. [Erratum, *Lancet.* 2001;357:1210.]

22. Office of the Inspector General. Dietary supplement labels: key elements. Report OEI-01-01-00120. http://oig.hhs.gov/oei/reports/oei-01-01-00120.pdf (accessed 2004 May 13).

23. Annual overview of the nutrition industry VII. *Nutr Bus J.* 2002; 7(May/Jun):1–11.

24. Food and Drug Administration. Dietary supplements: warnings and safety information. www.cfsan.fda.gov/~dms/ds~warn.html (accessed 2004 May 21).

25. De Smet PA. Herbal remedies. *N Engl J Med.* 2002; 347:2046–56.

26. Blumenthal M, ed. The complete German Commission E monographs—therapeutic guide to herbal medicines. Austin, TX: American Botanical Council; 1998:116,125–6.

27. Nortier JL, Martinez MC, Schmeiser HH, et al. Urothelial carcinoma associated with the use of a Chinese herb (*Aristolochia fangchi*). *N Engl J Med.* 2000; 342:1686–92.

28. Shekelle PG, Hardy ML, Morton SC, et al. Efficacy and safety of ephedra and ephedrine for weight loss and athletic performance: a meta-analysis. *JAMA.* 2003; 289:1537–45.

29. Slifman NR, Obermeyer WR, Musser SM, et al. Contamination of botanical dietary supplements by *Digitalis lanata. N Engl J Med.* 1998; 339:806–11.

30. Food and Drug Administration. Letter to health care professionals: FDA concerned about botanical products, including dietary supplements, containing aristolochic acid. http://vm.cfsan.fda.gov/~dms/ds-botl2.html (accessed 2003 Apr 1).

31. De Smet PA. Toxicological outlook on the quality assurance of herbal remedies. In: De Smet PA, Keller K, Hansel R, et al., eds. Adverse effects of herbal drugs. Vol. 1. Berlin: Springer-Verlag; 1992:1–72.

32. De Smet PA. The safety of herbal products. In: Jonas WB, Levin JS, eds. Essentials of complementary and alternative medicine. Philadelphia: Lippincott Williams & Wilkins; 1999:108–47.

33. De Smet PA. Health risks of herbal remedies. *Drug Saf.* 1995; 13:81–93.

34. Eisenberg DM, Davis RB, Ettner SL, et al. Trends in alternative medicine use in the United States, 1990–1997: results of a follow-up national study. *JAMA.* 1998; 280:1569–75.

35. Astin JA. Why patients use alternative medicine: results of a national study. *JAMA.* 1998; 279:1548–53.

36. Kaufman DW, Kelly JP, Rosenberg L, et al. Recent patterns of medication use in the ambulatory adult population of the United States: the Slone survey. *JAMA.* 2002; 287:337–44.

37. Leape LL, Cullen DJ, Clapp M, et al. Pharmacist participation on physician rounds and adverse drug events in the intensive care unit. *JAMA.* 1999; 282:267–70.

38. Eisenberg DM, Kessler RC, Van Rompay MI, et al. Perceptions about complementary therapies relative to conventional therapies among adults who use both: results from a national survey. *Ann Intern Med.* 2001; 135:344–51.

39. Ang-Lee MK, Moss J, Yuan CS. Herbal medicines and perioperative care. *JAMA.* 2001; 286:208–16.

40. Chambliss WG, Hufford CD, Flagg ML, et al. Assessment of the quality of reference books on botanical dietary supplements. *J Am Pharm Assoc.* 2002; 42:723–34.

41. Haller CA, Anderson IB, Kim SY, et al. An evaluation of selected herbal reference texts and comparison to published reports of adverse herbal events. *Adverse Drug React Toxicol Rev.* 2002; 21:143–50.

42. Kemper KJ, Amata-Kynvi A, Sanghavi D, et al. Randomized trial of an internet curriculum on herbs and other dietary supplements for health care professionals. *Acad Med.* 2002; 77:882–9.

43. Sweet BV, Gay WE, Leady MA, et al. Usefulness of herbal and dietary supplement References. *Ann Pharmacother.* 2003; 37:494–9.
44. Office of Dietary Supplements. International Bibliographic Information on Dietary Supplements (IBIDS) database. http://ods.od.nih.gov/showpage.aspx?pageid=48 (accessed 2003 Dec 11).
45. Memorial Sloan-Kettering Cancer Center. AboutHerbs Web site. www.mskcc.org/mskcc/html/11570.cfm (accessed 2003 Dec 11).
46. Rich DS. Ask the Joint Commission: understanding JCAHO requirements for hospital pharmacies. St. Louis: Facts and Comparisons; 2002:132–3.
47. Medication management standards. In: Comprehensive accreditation manual for hospitals, 2004 update. Oakbrook Terrace, IL: Joint Commission on Accreditation of Healthcare Organizations; 2004:MM1–20.
48. American Society of Hospital Pharmacists. ASHP technical assistance bulletin on the evaluation of drugs for formularies. *Am J Hosp Pharm.* 1988; 45:386–7.
49. Ansani NT, Ciliberto NC, Freedy T. Hospital policies regarding herbal medicines. *Am J Health-Syst Pharm.* 2003; 60:367–70.
50. American Society of Hospital Pharmacists. ASHP technical assistance bulletin on hospital drug distribution and control. *Am J Hosp Pharm.* 1980; 37:1097–1103.
51. American Society of Health-System Pharmacists. ASHP guidelines: minimum standard for pharmacies in hospitals. *Am J Health-Syst Pharm.* 1995; 52:2711–7.

This statement was reviewed in 2014 by the Council on Pharmacy Practice and by the Board of Directors and was found to still be appropriate.

Approved by the ASHP Board of Directors on April 14, 2004, and by the ASHP House of Delegates on June 20, 2004. Developed through the ASHP Council on Professional Affairs. Supersedes ASHP policies 0223, 0304, and 0324.

Copyright © 2004, American Society of Health-System Pharmacists, Inc. All rights reserved. Contact ASHP for reprint and permissions requests. This content may not be used for commercial purposes without the express written consent of ASHP.

The bibliographic citation for this document is as follows: American Society of Health-System Pharmacists. ASHP statement on the use of dietary supplements. *Am J Health-Syst Pharm.* 2004; 61:1707–11.

ASHP Guidelines on Emergency Medicine Pharmacist Services

The American Society of Health-System Pharmacists (ASHP) published its first statement on pharmacy services to the emergency department (ED) in 2008.[1] Best practices continue to evolve since then with numerous publications demonstrating that emergency medicine pharmacist (EMP) participation in patient care improves its safety and efficacy. In 2011, ASHP aimed to establish both a consistent approach and ideal practice model for emergency medicine (EM) pharmacy with its publication of the ASHP Guidelines on Emergency Medicine Pharmacist Services,[2] which was developed by the ASHP Section Advisory Group on Emergency Care.

A group of emergency medicine clinical pharmacy specialist content experts identified by ASHP developed these revised guidelines. The core writers group completed a literature search for updated supporting evidence. A modified Delphi process was then applied to review the recommendations and create a peer consensus in this document. The purpose of these guidelines is to provide a framework reference to guide hospitals, health systems, and, particularly, departments of pharmacy that are planning to initiate, expand, or optimize pharmacy services in the ED. The recommendations in these guidelines represent a consensus of professional judgment, expert opinion, and published evidence. They are written to establish reasonable goals, to be progressive and challenging, yet attainable as best practices in applicable settings. They do not represent minimum levels of practice, and readers are encouraged to exercise their professional judgment in assessing and adapting these recommendations to meet the specific needs of their healthcare organizations.

This revision of the ASHP guidelines has a two-fold aim. The first goal is to combine the ASHP statement and guidelines into a single document.[1,2] Merging these two foundational documents provides one overarching resource for recommendations on how to establish, maintain, and optimize EM pharmacy services in alignment with ASHP's goals. The second goal is to provide an updated roadmap for the functions that are vital to quality EM pharmacy services. One noteworthy difference in this edition is the removal of the concepts "essential" and "desirable."[2] All of the services and responsibilities identified in this document are considered essential, or vital, to EMPs' ability to provide patient-focused pharmacy services in the ED. Recognizing that there will be limitations that may affect an institution's ability to incorporate all of the recommendations stated, these updated guidelines are a framework for reference. Review of this document in collaboration with ED and pharmacy administrators and interdisciplinary EM clinical staff, along with professional judgment of the EMP, should be taken into consideration when determining how to best implement the recommendations in these guidelines at an individual institution.

Increased Demand for Specialized Emergency Medicine Pharmacy Services

EM pharmacy practice continues to expand, demonstrated not only by the number of EMP specialists working in hospitals, but also by the increase availability of specialty residency training programs. The number of accredited training positions dedicated to EM has risen from a mere three in 2007 to 70 in 2020.[3] This represents a more than 2,000% increase in specialty training positions in just over a decade.

In addition, national medical organizations, including the American College of Emergency Physicians (ACEP) and the American College of Medical Toxicology (ACMT), have published position statements endorsing the value of EMPs and formally recognized the impact of EMPs on the evaluation and management of EM and toxicology patients.[4,5]

Factors Affecting Emergency Medicine Pharmacy Practice

Although EM pharmacy services are now considered standard of care in many U.S. institutions, operational and clinical variables make a one-size-fits-all approach to EM pharmacy practice challenging. Ideally, all EDs would have access to EMPs with specialized training in direct patient care roles 24 hours per day, 7 days per week, and there would be sufficient EMP staffing to allow time for both dedicated direct and indirect patient care activities. However, this is often not feasible, based on the staffing capabilities of departments of pharmacy. Furthermore, organizations have different clinical and operational priorities based on practice site-specific variables. Examples of variables that impact the operational aspects of EM pharmacy practice may include, but are not limited to, type and setting of the institution (e.g., academic vs. community setting, urban vs. rural, critical access hospital), size of the ED and number of annual visits, patient population served and specialty services available (e.g., pediatrics, geriatrics, trauma, burn, stroke, and interventional medicine). Other factors that can impact the operations of EMPs also include the number of FTEs dedicated to EM patient care, hours of service provided, whether an ED pharmacy satellite is available for medication preparation and dispensing, EMP role in medication order verification prior to dispensing and pharmacy technician support dedicated to the ED.

In addition to operations, factors that may impact the scope of clinical services provided by EMPs also vary widely and can include, but are not limited to both direct patient care (i.e., bedside presence) and indirect patient care services such quality and safety and other administrative responsibilities. The number of indirect care responsibilities and whether dedicated time away from direct patient care in the ED is provided can have a significant impact on EMP resource allocation and varying roles and responsibilities. It is important to recognize that EDs may function very differently, despite the universal goal of safe, optimized medication therapy-related patient care.

Patient Care

The Institute of Medicine report, Hospital-Based Emergency Care: At the Breaking Point,[6] recommends including clinical pharmacists on the EM care team to ensure patients'

DOI 10.37573/9781585287048.074

medication needs are appropriately met, to lead system changes to reduce or eliminate medication errors, and to evaluate the cost-effectiveness of medication therapy for the patient and hospital.[6] As part of the interdisciplinary EM care team, pharmacists provide care to patients through a variety of direct bedside clinical activities as well as indirect patient care initiatives to ensure safe and effective medication therapy management in the ED setting.

In the past 10 years there has been a culture shift in which pharmacists in this practice setting focus more of their time performing clinical activities as evidenced by a survey published in 2016. Thomas and colleagues reported that of the 187 survey respondents, greater than 90% were engaged in routine clinical activities in the ED, which is in contrast to a similar 2009 study where only 50% of respondents were.[7] Conversely, in 2009 the majority of respondents were spending their time on operational efforts. While clinical activities are a continuously growing primary focus of EMPs, additional job functions are a necessary and vital component of EMP responsibilities. Given this information and the expanded training opportunities for this specialty practice, the activities in these guidelines are listed in order of how much time pharmacists across the nation on average report being involved in them. This approach may help guide new practitioners while still leaving space for individualizing practice to each EMP's unique environment.

Direct Patient Care Activities. The majority of medication errors occur in the prescribing and administration phases of the medication-use process; therefore, it is critical for EMPs to be involved in direct patient care activities, including medication selection and the prescribing process.[8–12] EMPs are most effective in doing this when physically present in the ED. EMPs, in collaboration with other EM providers, should be accountable for ensuring optimized medication therapy regimens and therapeutic outcomes based on emerging literature, treatment guidelines, and quality measures established by accrediting bodies. EMPs should create a triage system to focus their patient care efforts on those with critical illnesses or urgent needs, on high-risk patient populations, or on specific classes of medications most associated with medication errors.

Medication Information. The most common cause of medication errors is a lack of information related to medication therapy.[13] Provision of medication information is therefore a vital role in the practice of all pharmacists, including EMPs. ED-based studies demonstrate that the dissemination of medication information to providers, nurses and other hospital staff is an important service provided by EMPs, though only half of pharmacy departments reported performing this function.[14–17] In addition, EM healthcare clinicians report that they are more likely to utilize the resources of a pharmacist when that pharmacist is located in the ED rather than the central pharmacy department.[16]

The medication information needs of the ED cover a broad spectrum of clinical scenarios and may include questions related to medication selection, dose, and administration; adverse medication reactions; intravenous (IV) compatibility; medication interactions; and identification of unknown medications.[18] EMPs should ensure that access to appropriate primary, secondary, and tertiary references is available to respond to both emergent and non-emergent medication information requests. EMPs must be able to retrieve the answers to medication information questions quickly and accurately using readily available resources, such as computer workstations, mobile applications, textbooks, or other agile resources. A dedicated EMP computer workstation in close proximity to the clinical patient care area and provider care teams, with full internet connectivity can help to ensure the EMP has fast access to both patient information and online resources needed to answer the wide breadth of questions encountered in the ED.

Resuscitation. EMPs should be present during all critical and acute resuscitative efforts in the ED. Initial studies of the role of EMPs in the resuscitation of trauma patients found improved safety from decreased preventable adverse medication events and expedited time to medication administration.[19–22] In addition to trauma resuscitation, EMPs provide value in a number of clinical emergencies, such as stroke, myocardial infarction, cardiac and respiratory arrest, airway compromise requiring rapid sequence intubation and post-intubation care, and other medical emergencies. The role of EMPs in resuscitation may include a variety of responsibilities including, but not limited to:

- Assisting clinicians with differential diagnosis, particularly when related to a potential medication-related cause
- Ensuring appropriate medication selection and dose; answering medication information questions
- Making recommendations for alternative routes of administration when appropriate; preparing medications for immediate administration[23]
- Ensuring appropriate administration of or administering medications pursuant to local scope of practice
- Obtaining medications that are not readily available in the ED
- Completing resuscitation documentation[24,25]

In addition, EMPs should ensure that processes are in place to maintain an appropriate and readily available supply of necessary emergency medications in the ED. Multiple studies support the positive impact of EMPs on specific outcomes in resuscitation. Examples in a variety of acute patient presentations include:

- Increased compliance with advanced cardiac life support (ACLS) guidelines[24]
- Reduced time to administration of antibiotics for patients presenting with sepsis[26,27]
- Reduced time to analgesia for trauma patients[28]
- Reduced time to sedation and analgesia after rapid sequence intubation[29,32]
- Reduced time to thrombolysis for acute ischemic stroke[33,34]
- Improved door-to-balloon time for MI[22]

EMPs have also demonstrated improvement in antibiotic selection and timeliness for patients with open fractures when responding to traumas.[35]

Pharmacist involvement in toxicologic emergencies was first described in the literature more than 30 years ago.[36,37] EMPs should be familiar with the recognition and treatment of patients experiencing a toxicologic emergency. Their role should include recognition of characteristic physical signs and symptoms noted in the physical examination, laboratory parameters, and other diagnostic evaluations (e.g., toxidromes) that can result from a wide range of substances, including prescription and over-the-counter medications, illicit drugs, naturally occurring poisons (e.g., those from plants, mushrooms, or envenomations), and various chemicals.[38,39] When a patient with a suspected toxicologic emergency presents to the ED, EMPs should assist in obtaining a thorough and accurate medication history and a history of present illness, as well as in identifying potential causative agents; assist in the selection and preparation of specific antidotes and other supportive therapies; and provide recommendations for monitoring antidote effectiveness and safety. These services should be provided in collaboration with clinical and medical toxicologists, when available, and local or regional poison control centers. Finally, EMPs should serve as a resource to the pharmacy department in ensuring that an adequate inventory of toxicologic antidotes and supportive therapies are available in the institution.[40,41]

In preparing to become a member of the resuscitation team, EMPs should seek out training and certification in the conditions applicable to their practice settings. Several training opportunities and certification programs are available and include but are not limited to the following:

- American Stroke Association National Institutes of Health Stroke Scale
- American Heart Association (AHA) Basic Life Support (BLS)
- AHA ACLS, AHA Pediatric Advanced Life Support (PALS)
- American College of Surgeons Advanced Trauma Life Support (ATLS)
- American Academy of Clinical Toxicology Advanced HAZMAT Life Support (AHLS)
- Emergency Neurological Life Support (ENLS)
- Board certification as a Diplomate of the American Board of Applied Toxicology (DABAT)

At a minimum, all EMPs should achieve and maintain up-to-date certification in BLS, ACLS, and PALS as appropriate, based on the patient populations they serve. Board certification is strongly encouraged to ensure ongoing expertise in a wide variety of disease states and patient populations.

High-Alert Medications and Procedures. EMPs should be present at the bedside to facilitate the delivery of patient care involving high-alert medications or procedures. Participation should include assisting in the appropriate selection of medications and corresponding doses, preparation of medications, patient monitoring, and medication administration as acceptable per state laws and hospital policies. EMPs should participate in efforts to improve the safety of procedures that utilize high-risk medications. These efforts should include evaluation of current processes and the development of new or improved processes and systems that prevent or reduce potential harm and errors. The EMP's role may include aiding in the development of policies and protocols, with a focus on appropriate medication selection, use, monitoring, and management. Recommendations for reducing errors associated with high-alert medications and procedures are available.[11,42–44] For example, use of medication infusion systems with smart infusion technology software and double checks on high-alert medications may be considered.[42,43] In addition, EMPs should provide education and training related to high-alert medications to ED healthcare providers.

Medication Procurement and Preparation. Medication procurement in the ED presents challenges that differ significantly from those in other areas of the hospital. Because of the urgent treatment needs of patients in the ED, several critical medications must be readily available. EMPs should be an integral part of the medication procurement and preparation process for medications used in the ED, as dispensing medications is one of the five stages of the medication-use process that EMPs can influence to prevent medication errors.[11] EMPs may serve as liaisons between the pharmacy department and ED regarding the development or revision of processes associated with medication procurement, or they may play a more active role in medication procurement and preparation based on operational workflows.

The options available for medication procurement vary widely and should be based on both physical layout (i.e., proximity of the ED to centralized pharmacy areas) and operational workflows. Medications may be available in automated dispensing devices, in emergency kits, from the inpatient centralized pharmacy department, or from a satellite pharmacy within the ED. EMPs should be involved in the decision-making process regarding which medications will be made available immediately within the ED.[45,46] Medications identified as appropriate and necessary for frequent use in the ED should be stored in automated dispensing devices or another location as designated safe by the institution, with appropriate alerts to prevent medication errors.[46] EMPs may assist in the evaluation and management of these medications, including monitoring for appropriate usage, inventory levels, override list optimization, and medication storage per both hospital and regulatory body requirements. Optimization of available medications should occur at regular intervals based on changes in prescribing practices, guideline or protocol recommendations, medication availability, and formulary changes. Inventory and storage replacement should be maintained by pharmacy technician support and should not be the direct responsibility of EMPs.

EMPs should be involved with the institution's formulary review and process-improvement committees to assist with medication reviews of new formulary agents and for revisions to the current formulary regarding medications used in the ED. Furthermore, data from medication-use evaluations (MUEs), safety monitoring, and monitoring for adherence to national quality indicators should be used to assist in evaluating medication procurement and preparation processes.

The burden of extended inpatient boarding in the ED, in addition to ongoing high ED patient volumes, requires EMPs to consider the differing medication distribution needs of both outpatient and inpatient populations co-located in the ED. Similarly, the EMP should be prepared to recognize seasonal fluctuations in medication usage, communicating with purchasers and adjusting stocks accordingly.

Medication shortages are commonplace, and EMPs may spend significant amounts of time monitoring for medication availability and providing up-to-date alerts and recommendations to EM clinicians. EMPs should work closely with pharmacy supply chain staff and their institution's formulary management committee to help plan for alternative therapy recommendations as soon as relevant medication shortages are identified.

Medication Order Review. The Joint Commission standards state that all medication orders should undergo prospective order review by a pharmacist prior to administration of the medication to the patient, with two exceptions:

1. If a delay in administration would harm the patient; and,
2. If a licensed independent practitioner is present to oversee the ordering, preparation, and administration of the medication.[47]

Although many medication orders in the ED fall under the above exceptions, the level of assessment during medication order review should be consistent with that provided for patients elsewhere in the hospital. The ED medication order review process will vary between EDs and should be determined by each institution based on its identified needs, staffing structure, and embedded medication-use systems, as well as site-specific interpretation of requirements by regulatory and accrediting organizations.

The specific role of an EMP may not focus on the ED medication order review process alone but rather should parallel the role of other pharmacy specialists providing direct patient care services within the institution.[48–51] A workflow should be developed to ensure that there is adequate pharmacist support for timely review of medication orders that are not verified by an EMP.[52,53]

Most medication orders in the ED are one-time orders, so an EMP's intervention is most valuable if performed prior to medication administration. Ideally, all orders for high-risk medications would receive prospective review, but optimal medication use in the ED requires a balance between ensuring patient safety and preventing delays in patient care. EMPs should incorporate a triage system into the medication-order review process to help prioritize evaluation of high-risk medications, high-risk patient populations, and emergent or urgent situations, followed by more routine medication orders. When evaluating medication orders, EMPs should focus on key factors such as appropriateness of the medication and doses, potential medication interactions, and patient-specific factors.[47] Prospective order review by an EMP can significantly decrease medication error rates.[8] Approximately one third of the total medication error interceptions by an EMP occur during medication order review, but the majority occur during consultative activities, often during bedside care; therefore, with limited time or resources, medication order review should not be the highest priority for EMPs.[54] Irrespective of the strategy used to identify medication errors, a high proportion intercepted by EMPs are considered significant or serious.[55]

Medication Therapy Monitoring. EMPs should provide recommendations for monitoring parameters for both effectiveness and safety of medications administered in the ED. Given the number of patients in the ED and competing interests for an EMP's time, focusing on high-risk medications should be prioritized (e.g., vasopressors, IV antihypertensives, insulins, analgesic and sedative agents, anti-thrombotics and hemostatic agents). EMPs should work closely with nursing staff and re-assess patients on these medications to ensure proper response, safety, and monitoring is completed. When appropriate, EMPs should follow up with providers to escalate and de-escalate care.

The identification and assessment of monitoring parameters related to medication therapy are essential steps in the medication-use process. They will determine whether the therapy selected was safe and effective, was suboptimal, or failed and changes to the regimen are needed. Pharmacist participation in monitoring medication therapy improves clinical outcomes in a variety of settings, including treatment selection, adjustment, and monitoring of chronic disease state therapies, such as diabetes mellitus, hypertension, and hyperlipidemia, and from therapeutic medication monitoring of antimicrobial and anticoagulant therapy in the hospital setting.[56–59] These clinical outcomes include reduced medication errors, lower adverse event rates, increased medication adherence, and increased medication appropriateness, and these outcomes can be translated to the ED setting with EMP services.[59]

To help address chronic therapy issues, EMPs as appropriate, should assess home medications of ED patients and quickly identify any laboratory tests needed to ensure the ED visit is not related to medication effects. Protocols can be implemented for pharmacists to order drug level tests as appropriate as well as any laboratory tests that may be associated with that medication's assessment; such protocols are instrumental in both the critically ill and general ED population.

Documentation. Pharmacist interventions in the inpatient setting improve patient outcomes through optimized pharmacotherapy regimens, monitoring of medication therapy, and avoidance of adverse medication events.[58] In addition, pharmacist participation in patient care significantly reduces the costs associated with medication therapy.[60,61] In the ED specifically, EMPs improve the medication-use process and patient care by providing recommendations about medication therapy, serving as a medication information resource, and improving patient safety.[8,14,62–67] Cost avoidance has also been documented in several studies.[68–72]

EMPs should be diligent in documenting interventions provided during patient care and other activities (e.g., education). Documentation can include both internal pharmacy documentation for cost justification purposes or patient care notes in the electronic medical record for handoff to other medical professionals. Allergy documentation, therapy plans, and patient education are some examples of activities that can be documented in the medical record. They should regularly review intervention documentation to identify trends, which may indicate a need to educate ED healthcare providers or change medication-use procedures. Finally, cost-avoidance documentation may provide the justification needed for further expansion of EMP services.

Healthcare institutions should support EMPs by providing the means to document interventions. Different media are used to document interventions, including personal digital assistants, software programs on institutional intranets, and manual paper systems.[73–78] Electronic systems offer more complete, readily retrievable documentation and shorter entry times than manual systems, without the risk of loss associated with paper records.[79,80] In addition, electronic documentation systems offer the benefit of associating cost avoidance with the documented intervention and making it readily available for data capture.[70] Although determining true cost avoidance can be difficult, there is some guidance available for quantifying this metric with pharmacist interventions.[15,60,61,81–84] In addition to these benefits, electronic documentation of EMP interventions may improve communication with other healthcare providers caring for the patient after transitioning to admitted status. The EMP can enhance transitions of care by documentation of medication therapy issues or monitoring needs for the next pharmacist or healthcare team member assuming care to follow up and ensure appropriate therapy is continued.

EMPs also increase the rate of medication error reporting, which, in turn, supports an institution's ability to identify issues contributing to errors and implement measures to prevent future errors.[66] Because up to 90% of adverse events in hospitals go undetected and occur in up to one third of all hospital admissions, error prevention is vital.[85]

Patient and Caregiver Education. EMPs are uniquely qualified to provide medication education and information to patients and their caregivers and should play a key role in the delivery of medication information.[68,86] EMPs should develop a system of triage for patient education so that counseling is focused on patients who will be discharged from the ED with a new or high-risk medication or whose visit to the ED was the result of a medication adverse event or error. EMPs may also rely on other EM healthcare providers to identify patients in need of medication education. The medication education provided to patients and caregivers in the ED is diverse and may include information related to the use of a new device or new medication, the importance of medication adherence in disease-state management, or prevention and management of adverse medication events. Education should include oral or written materials and should be documented in the patient's medical record. EMPs should confirm patient and caregiver understanding of the medication education provided.

Care of Boarded Patients. ED overcrowding is common.[87,88] There are many obstacles and processes that factor into the timely transfer of admitted patients from the ED to an inpatient bed.[89] Overcrowding in the ED often results in ED staff providing care to patients for long periods of time while patients await admission or physical transfer to an inpatient bed or to another institution for a different level of care (i.e., boarding). [90] The needs of a boarded patient can vary from simple requests for as-needed medications to complex needs such as critical care management. In addition, EM clinicians may be tasked with the responsibility of initiating and maintaining inpatient levels of care, including routine medications and chronic disease state management. EM clinicians are not specifically trained to provide inpatient care for extended lengths of stay. EMPs are challenged in trying to support prescribers by ensuring thorough medication therapy management on complex boarded patients while continuing to focus efforts on the urgent or emergent needs of newly arrived ED patients.

Processes should be developed, based on institutional resources, to address the needs of boarded patients. Pharmacists and pharmacy departments should evaluate all available resources to support the ongoing level of care needed for inpatients that remain located in the ED (e.g., an EMP or the pharmacist assigned to the area to which the patient will be admitted, or a combination of both, may assume responsibility for the medication-related needs of boarded patients). By supporting this patient influx with additional pharmacist resources, EMPs can maintain their primary role in ensuring the safety and effectiveness of the medication-use process for ED patients. When staffing levels are insufficient (e.g., when only a single EMP is present in the ED) or when the boarding area is physically separated from the ED, the responsibility of caring for boarded patients could be assigned to the inpatient pharmacist. Ideally, to ensure continuity of care, the inpatient pharmacist providing care to the boarded patient would be the same pharmacist responsible for providing care after admission. The services provided to boarded patients by EMPs will depend on the level of services offered by the institution. At a minimum, EMPs should review the medication profile of boarded patients, with a focus on high-risk medications, medication dosing and procurement, and monitoring, as necessary. When it is necessary to initiate a standing medication order for a boarded patient, the responsible pharmacist should review medications administered in the ED and those taken prior to arrival at the ED to prevent duplications in therapy.

Transitions of Care. EMPs can provide a variety of transitions of care (TOC) services. Responsibility for follow-up may be left solely to patients, who often face barriers to receiving ongoing primary care. EMPs should help bridge this gap by ensuring patients understand any changes made to their medication regimen and helping to identify at risk patients for the team to ensure proper follow-up with their primary care physicians or post-discharge clinics. For example, discharge education for anticoagulation provided by an EMP for ED patients resulted in greater patient understanding and decreased return visits.[91] Pharmacist-run TOC programs for patients presenting to the ED with a chief complaint of chronic obstructive pulmonary disease, chronic heart failure, or an asthma exacerbation can provide useful interventions and referral follow-up in an ambulatory care clinic or home-based medication management program.[92]

EMPs have demonstrated to ED staff that EMP review of ED discharge prescriptions can improve patient safety, optimize medication regimens, and improve patient satisfaction.[93] If EMPs are unable to provide this resource, they can serve as liaisons for physicians and triage calls from outpatient pharmacies. EMPs can field the call and identify the options to fix the issue with the discharge prescription, discuss with a physician, and communicate the decision to the outpatient pharmacy. Such a process could more efficiently provide corrective actions to prescription issues and lead to faster patient care by reducing the amount of physician time spent on these issues.

EMPs can also take an active role in discharge culture review. Many EDs are responsible for managing positive culture results from patients discharged without hospital admission. EMP involvement in ED culture follow-up can decrease time to positive culture review and time to patient or primary care provider notification,[94] lead to a reduction in ED revisits,[95,96] and result in improved appropriateness of changes in therapy.[97] Institutional support for pharmacist-led innovative programs targeting reduced return visits and admissions is important. Pharmacist integration into home-hospital services that facilitate continued treatment at home has demonstrated potential.[98,99] One group targeted ED discharge patients at high risk for not filling antimicrobial prescriptions, provided a full course at no charge to the patient, and demonstrated 50% reduction in return visits within the subsequent 7 days compared to standard of care.[100]

Medication Histories and Medication Reconciliation. Medication reconciliation research has identified several barriers to obtaining an accurate medication history in the ED.[101–107] In many cases, ED staff are required to contact multiple sources, including primary care physician offices, pharmacies, and family members to obtain a medication history, and even these burdensome efforts may not result in an accurate home medication list.

Although pharmacy personnel are the health professionals who obtain the most accurate home medication list,[108–111] dedicating a pharmacist solely to medication history collection is not the best allocation of pharmacist resources in the ED. EMPs should assist in the development and implementation of a risk-stratification protocol for identifying and determining which ED patients need a medication history. In general, medication histories should be obtained for patients with known or suspected toxicologic emergencies, with known or suspected adverse events from home medications, or with complicated medication histories that will influence ED clinical decision-making.

Auxiliary pharmacy staff (pharmacy students hired through work/study programs or pharmacy technicians) can also be effective in obtaining accurate home medication histories; when possible, they should be incorporated into medication reconciliation procedures.[112–115] Quality reviews of medication histories completed by auxiliary pharmacy staff should be conducted to assess accuracy and to provide guidance for further training opportunities. EMPs may take an active role in providing oversight of such programs in the ED setting.

Opportunities for Growth in EMP Patient Care. Despite improved integration of pharmacists into the emergency care team, there are still opportunities for growth and utilization. Thomas and colleagues reported that 69% of survey respondents provide an EMP for more than 8 hours/day, but 35% of respondents do not provide an EMP on weekends.[7] One editorial advocated for expansion of clinical pharmacists to EDs and argued the current volume of the EMP workforce is inadequate for high-risk patient populations.[116] These inadequacies continue, as there are many challenges to implementation of a dedicated EMP or expansion of current EMP services. Because EMPs do not generate a direct source of revenue, it may be difficult for administrators to realize the added value and cost savings an EMP may provide. However, the quality and efficiency benefits of EMPs, in addition to their contribution to patient safety, may more than offset the costs.[117]

Administrative Responsibilities

As a practitioner in the ED setting, an EMP should help identify and lead quality improvement initiatives relating to direct patient care, medication safety, compliance with hospital and regulatory policies, and adherence to national practice recommendations and guidelines.[118–120] EMPs, or other pharmacy representatives, should be extensively involved with quality-improvement initiatives in the ED and prehospital setting.[121] Participation in interdisciplinary committees with EM healthcare providers and hospital administrators (e.g., pharmacy and therapeutics, infection control, or disaster preparedness committees) will provide EMPs with an avenue for improving patient care processes in the ED. In addition, EMPs have a unique understanding of formulary management, operational issues and ED workflow that may impact therapeutic decision-making. Treatment pathways and medication-use policy should be congruent with nationally accepted practice guidelines and quality indicators. Finally, EMPs can contribute at the system level to assist in implementing safeguards at the point of prescribing and administration, reducing the risk of medication errors and optimizing medication use practices.[122]

Medication Safety. EMPs play an important role in monitoring and ensuring patient and medication safety in the ED. By its nature, the ED environment is at high risk for patient and medication near misses and adverse events.[123] EMPs should encourage and assist in maintaining a safe environment for medication and patient safety, and establish an ongoing continuous review cycle for potential process improvements. Such a review could include proactive and continuous monitoring of medication practices; identification of errors and high-risk medications for monitoring; addressing hazardous conditions with potential for harm; and documentation and review of medication errors, adverse medication events, and near misses.[19,80,124]

Medication errors and adverse drug reactions that occur in the ED should be reviewed by EMPs, in an interdisciplinary collaboration with other healthcare providers and hospital executives, to identify potential sources of error, contributing factors related to the error, and potential solutions for preventing similar errors. Performance of a root cause analysis (RCA) could identify potential error trends or system failures and contribute to the development of safe medication practices and processes for prevention of future events. RCAs can lead to MUEs of commonly used medications in the ED, as well as those associated with errors.[125,126] Completion of RCAs and MUEs should result in education and future policy or guidelines development. EMPs should be responsible for the development and provision of education to EM healthcare providers on potential sources of errors, the risks associated with errors, and ways to prevent similar errors in the future.

Performance and Quality Improvement. EMPs have the opportunity and responsibility to collaborate with interdisciplinary teams throughout the health system to ensure best practices throughout the entire institution. By participating or taking on a leadership role in institutional committees and performance improvement initiatives, EMPs can have a significant impact in advancing the role of clinical pharmacists in patient care. EMPs demonstrate value in several administrative or indirect care activities, including regulatory compliance, adherence to core measures for maintenance of hospital certifications (such as stroke, MI, trauma, and sepsis), and the creation of medication-use policy and disease state management pathways. In addition, EMPs should focus a significant portion of their time on developing and enhancing medication ordering and order set development in electronic health records.

When the ED is evaluating various technologies as part of the medication-use process, the EMP should assist in selection, development, implementation, and assessment of the technology. EMP involvement may include, but is not limited to, automated dispensing devices location and inventory optimization, infusion pump selection, implementation of smart pump technology and medication library updates, communicating on-going issues with technology updates, crash cart stocking recommendations, or implementation of medication kits for management of emergencies such as anaphylaxis and rapid sequence intubation.

Emergency Preparedness. With expertise in pharmacology and toxicology, EMPs are well suited to prepare for and respond to emergencies, such as natural disasters; disease outbreaks; biological, radiological, or chemical exposures; mass casualty incidents (MCI); and acts of terrorism. It is essential that EMPs, in conjunction with the department of pharmacy and institutional leadership, participate in emergency preparedness planning.[127–130] Planning and involvement should occur at a minimum at the institutional level, with participation ideally expanding to include community emergency preparedness efforts and beyond. Knowledge of local, state, regional, and national emergency preparedness plans, programs, and support systems, such as mass prophylaxis plans, antidote stocking policies, and the Strategic National Stockpile and CHEMPACK, is paramount in the development and successful implementation of institution-specific emergency preparedness plans.[131] EMPs can also participate in evaluating contingency planning needs for mass discharge of inpatients with "take-home pack" style medications (e.g., what medications are included, how many days' supply, dispensation plan). Planning for care of employees and their families with prophylaxis and treatment to allow them to continue caring for patients during disasters may also be part of the institution's emergency preparedness plan.

Furthermore, hospitals should maintain their own supply of antidotes congruent with national consensus guidelines for lesser exposures. ASHP advises that emergency response planners at the federal, regional, state, and local levels call on pharmacists to participate in the full range of planning issues related to pharmaceuticals, including development of a disaster formulary and inventory management; medication procurement, distribution, and use; and stockpile maintenance and acquisition.[41,127,129] EMPs can take a leadership role in ensuring the preparedness level of their institution(s) with respect to medication assessment and needs.

Actively participating in emergency preparedness events, such as disaster or MCI drills, strengthens the ability of EMPs to effectively identify opportunities for improvement within the disaster plan. Another valuable opportunity for EMPs is participation within institutional hospital emergency preparedness response teams. EMPs and leadership in the pharmacy department should work together in the development of pharmacy-specific plans that parallel institution-specific plans. Education of ED and pharmacy staff related to emergency preparedness should be among the responsibilities of EMPs.

EMPs should play a pivotal role not only in the development of emergency operations plans, but also in the provision of clinical services during a disaster or emergency.[132] Ensuring the efficacy and safety of the medication-use process is a natural role for pharmacists because treatment of disaster victims invariably involves the use of pharmacologic agents.[128,133]

As appropriate, EMPs should seek out training and certification in emergency preparedness, such as certification for Advanced Hazmat Life Support (AHLS), Basic Disaster Life Support, Advanced Disaster Life Support, and the Federal Emergency Management Agency (FEMA) National Incident Management System training program. In addition, local training programs funded by FEMA exist and are a great resource for hospitals to initiate hospital emergency response teams trained to respond to mass casualty incidents or disasters that may occur inside or outside the institution. Connecting with the institution's emergency preparedness coordinator as well as the local healthcare incident liaison can also create opportunities for EMP involvement in local training programs and drills. FEMA's Center for Disaster Preparedness in Anniston, Alabama, offers courses year-round, with many, such as Healthcare Leadership for Mass Casualty Incidents, which are directly applicable to EMPs. These training programs help to build and strengthen the EMP's knowledge and ability to not only respond, but also help take a leadership role in coordinating necessary response efforts from pharmacy staff.

Interdisciplinary Education. The role of EMPs in education can be variable and broad, and it has been mentioned in conjunction with other responsibilities throughout these guidelines. As appropriate for the specific institutional setting, EMPs should play an active role in the education of pharmacy staff, including pharmacists, students, and residents, in addition to other healthcare professionals, such as physicians, medical residents, advanced practice providers, nurses, and emergency medical services personnel. The types and levels of education will vary when balancing patient care and administrative workload. Provision of education to EM healthcare staff, at a minimum, should include information on the appropriate use of medications, improvement in quality and effective medication use, and patient and medication safety. Education may include, but is not limited to, formal sessions (e.g., in-service or didactic presentation at a conference) or participation in courses such as BLS, ACLS, or PALS; emergency preparedness; disaster management; poisoning prevention and treatment[5]; and immunizations. Participation in formal education sessions may strengthen the relationship with other EM healthcare providers and serves as a method of continuous learning for EMPs. Given the nature of the ED environment, EMPs have a unique opportunity to provide continuous, on-the-spot education via daily interdisciplinary interaction in the ED, particularly at the bedside, which is an efficient, effective tool for education of staff.

Training the Pharmacist Workforce. Participation in the didactic and experiential education of Doctor of Pharmacy students is a strongly encouraged, routine part of practice that also supports the development of the profession.[134] Precepting pharmacy residents in EM learning experiences supports the overall development of direct patient care practitioners and provides exposure to the practice of EM pharmacy. To support the growth of EM pharmacy services, the continued development and expansion of EM residency programs is necessary. EMPs must be leaders in this endeavor, using their unique skills and expertise in this practice setting to train the next generation. Although the number of postgraduate year two (PGY2) residency programs in EM has increased significantly in recent years, ASHP advocates for continued emphasis on the expansion of the number of

EM-based training opportunities for pharmacists, pharmacy students, and residents. Colleges of pharmacy are encouraged to provide EM-based educational opportunities for students.[135] With the expansion of EM pharmacy services among health systems, expanding coverage hours, and the increasing role of EMPs in administrative activities, the need for additional qualified pharmacists increases. New EMPs should focus on developing current services, with plans to develop advanced residency training programs after the service model is established and the practice experience is significant. Expansion of PGY2 EM pharmacy residency programs will assist in filling the demand gap of highly trained EMPs providing 24-hour clinical pharmacy services. Such residency programs should meet ASHP residency quality standards.[136] These programs should prepare future EMPs for board certification in the specialty most appropriate for their practice.[137] Achievement of the goals, objectives, and expected outcomes of such training can result in a greater ability to provide around-the-clock or on-call EM clinical pharmacist services.[138]

Pharmacy resident and student precepting is a typical part of the job for many EMPs; however, faculty appointments at schools of pharmacy or medicine present unique possibilities to educate students, residents, and faculty in a more formal setting.

In addition, EMPs should identify opportunities to provide education and training for currently practicing pharmacists not specialized in EM. To train pharmacists not specialized in EM, institutions should create a checklist and minimum competency standards to prepare their staff for the ED environment and ensure they are set up for success in this challenging arena. Training should at a minimum consist of knowledge of pharmacist roles in resuscitations and direct patient care activities, appropriate certifications (e.g., ACLS, BLS, PALS), knowledge of common EM medications and antidotes, how to triage and prioritize direct patient care in the ED, and other institution-specific practices in the ED setting. Such training may help fill clinical practice gaps and allow for additional support in ED coverage models.

Research and Professional Development

EMPs should also assume roles in EM-based research and scholarly activity; in professional development, service, and leadership; and in defining future roles for EMPs.

EM-Based Research and Scholarly Activity. The Institute of Medicine provides a framework for EM research that further delineates specific areas of focus.[139] Those areas have been identified as EM research (i.e., research conducted in the prehospital or ED setting by EM specialists); trauma/injury control research (i.e., research of the acute management of trauma injury), and research contributions that are not specific to but nevertheless impact the care of patients in the ED setting. As a specialty, EM has already helped to define a scope of research priorities over the years.[140–144] What is less clearly defined is how EMPs can support research efforts, through interdisciplinary participation in ongoing EM research or identifying opportunities to lead research in medication therapy and pharmacy specialty care outcomes in the ED setting.

The EM-based pharmacy research compendium continues to grow, exploring the impact of various clinical activities, including anticoagulation reversal, toxicology, naloxone distribution programs, emergency response team participation, and pain management.[28, 145–148] Other studies describe progress in the medication-use process and EM-based pharmacy activities.[7,117] Although these studies contribute new knowledge that addresses the varied scope and range of EM pharmacy services, additional information and analysis are still necessary. As a profession and specialty practitioner group, EMPs must continue to provide the necessary evidence that demonstrates the benefit EMPs provide to care in the emergent environment. In addition, EMPs must challenge themselves to incorporate the research priorities described by the Institute of Medicine into their scholarly work, which would require EMPs to think on a broader scope, not only about research topics but also about how to best carry out this work on a larger scale with limited resources. Studies that generate data on therapeutic, safety, humanistic, and economic outcomes of EM pharmacist-mediated process changes are needed. Although not an exhaustive list, specific areas of needed research expansion include the following:

- Alternative strategies for providing 24/7 access to EMP services:
    - Leveraging non-EMP staff to assist with EMP services.
    - Pharmacy resident resources and patient outcomes.
- Clinical and operational outcomes of electronic medical record interventions:
    - Impact of EMP electronic medical record development and maintenance on patient safety.
    - Impact of order set or clinical pathway development on patient outcomes.
- Clinical outcomes of ED-specific, medication-related interventions:
    - Evaluating clinical programs for economic outcomes.
    - Exploration of tangible cost savings or revenue generation.
    - Impact of antimicrobial stewardship.
    - Impact of opioid stewardship and substance use disorder treatments.
    - Impact of medication use on disposition and ED throughput metrics.
    - Medication efficacy and safety outcomes of high-risk medications in the ED with EMP bedside monitoring.
    - Patient outcomes of ED-specific medication therapy management in transitions of care.
- Disaster response:
    - Pharmacist-specific impact in disaster response.
- Public and population health initiatives and outcomes.

Development of a collaborative, interdisciplinary research network among EMPs would facilitate enhanced evaluation of clinical and professional questions of interest.[149] Research networks can help by providing larger and more diverse patient populations in which to conduct research. The ability to collaborate with other EMPs from different practice settings may also help to strengthen the depth and breadth of research being conducted, resulting in studies that have the potential to impact change in EM practice. In addition, EMPs should collaborate with EM clinicians, nursing, clinical staff, and relevant others in research activities.

Professional Development, Service, and Leadership Duties. Hospitals and health systems are encouraged to support EM-based educational programs that produce experts in the field. Postgraduate training of pharmacists will provide a pipeline of clinicians, educators, leaders, and scientists who are experts in and committed to quality emergency care, as well as the expansion of this specialty service. The leadership role of EMPs should include responsibilities to both the pharmacy department and ED. Involvement in administrative processes of both departments allows EMPs to serve as a liaison between the groups to support joint endeavors.

Furthermore, participation in professional organizations at the local, state, and national level is essential for the continued growth of the practice of EM pharmacy. At the local level, EMPs may collaborate to develop a local support network for training and research and can provide new practitioners with avenues for learning. At the state level, legislative and professional advocacy may help educate government officials and other healthcare professionals about EM pharmacy practice. At the national level, collaboration among EMPs increases their strength as a group; serves to challenge existing programs to improve; assists new programs in their development; and allows collaboration as a group to affect the stature, practice, and further development of EM pharmacy practice. In addition to promotion from ASHP, pharmacy professionals are encouraged to create strong interdisciplinary partnerships with medical providers, residents, and students. Such collaboration has recently yielded the recognition and endorsement of EM pharmacy services by the American College of Emergency Physicians (ACEP) and American College of Medical Toxicology (ACMT), as demonstrated by statements of support from both organizations.[1,2] By engaging at a national organization level with other disciplines in emergency care, EMPs continue to build the backbone of support needed to encourage funding and resources for expanded EMP practice at the institutional level.

Future Efforts. EMPs have demonstrated their value in providing well-rounded clinical and operational medication therapy related services in the ED setting. Their unique training and expertise ensures improved patient safety and optimized patient outcomes in direct patient care. As the future of pharmacy evolves, so too must the EMP. Expanding both the scope of practice and the role within the patient care continuum is important to sustaining and maximizing the benefits of this clinical specialty. In the next decade, EMPs should engage in activities that serve both the needs of the healthcare team and public health efforts at large. Although some of these efforts are already underway, it will be incumbent upon EMPs to help advance the goals of provider status and collaborative practice agreements, allowing practice at the highest level of licensure.

In addition, public health is an area in which EMPs can contribute. Examples include the following:

- Providing structure to opioid crisis services, such as naloxone distribution and counseling[147,150] and pharmacist-initiated medication assisted therapy
- Reducing antimicrobial resistance and reducing sepsis mortality with improved ED-specific antimicrobial stewardship interventions and monitoring[151]
- Improving stroke management and meeting core metrics for better patient outcomes
- Establishing ED-based pharmacist medication therapy monitoring consult services as a bridge to the outpatient clinic setting; increasing access to EMP services with alternative strategies, such as offsite resources and telemedicine[152]
- Developing leadership roles in emergency preparedness and crisis response

EMPs must take the lead in setting the expectation for engagement in clinical and operational ED based services in the future.

Conclusion

The specialized role of EMPs within the scope of pharmacy services continues to be a unique and vital component ofboth pharmacy services and EM practice. Through a combination of the integral services described in this document, EMPs are able to help ensure the safety and optimization of medical care to patients in the ED. In addition, EMP involvement in administrative, educational, professional development and research activities, both within and outside their respective ED setting, are vital to EM practice, the pharmacy profession, and, most importantly, patient care. Where possible, we encourage pharmacy and hospital leadership to use these guidelines as a tool to help provide the necessary support for development and expansion of EMP services.

References

1. American Society of Health-System Pharmacists. ASHP statement on pharmacy services to the emergency department. *Am J Health-Syst Pharm.* 2008;65:2380–3.
2. American Society of Health-System Pharmacists. ASHP guidelines on emergency medicine pharmacist services. *Am J Health-Syst Pharm.* 2011;68(23):e81–95.
3. American Society of Health-System Pharmacists. ASHP Residency Directory. https://accreditation.ashp.org/directory/#/program/residency. Accessed June 29.
4. American College of Emergency Physicians. Clinical policy statement: clinical pharmacist services in the emergency department. *Ann Emerg Med.* 2015;66:444–445.
5. Farmer BM, Hayes BD, Rao R, et al. The role of clinical pharmacists in the emergency department. *J Med Toxicol.* 2018;14:114–116.
6. Berger E. Breaking point: report calls for congressional rescue of hospital emergency departments. *Ann Emerg Med.* 2006; 48:140–142.
7. Thomas MC, Acquisto NM, Shirk MB, et al. A national survey of emergency pharmacy practice in the United States. *Am J Health-Syst Pharm.* 2016;73:386–394.
8. Brown JN, Barnes CL, Beasley B et al. Effect of pharmacists on medication errors in an emergency department. *Am J Health-Syst Pharm.* 2008;65:330–333.
9. Patanwala AE, Warholak TL, Sanders AB, et al. A prospective observational study of medication errors in a tertiary care emergency department. *Ann Emerg Med.* 2010;55:522–526.

10. Flynn EA, Barker K, Barker B. Medication-administration errors in an emergency department. *Am J Health-Syst Pharm.* 2010;67:347–348.
11. Peth H. Medication errors in the emergency department: a systems approach to minimizing risk. *Emerg Med Clin North Am.* 2003;21:141–158.
12. DeFrates SR, Weant KA, Seamon JP, et al. Emergency pharmacist impact on health care-associated pneumonia empiric therapy. *J Pharm Pract.* 2013; 26:125–130.
13. Leape LL, Bates DW, Cullen DJ, et al. Systems analysis of adverse drug events. ADE prevention study group. *JAMA.* 1995;274:35–43.
14. Wymore ES, Casanova TJ, Broekemeier RL, et al. Clinical pharmacist's daily role in the emergency department of a community hospital. *Am J Health-Syst Pharm.* 2008; 65:395–6, 398–399.
15. Whalen FJ. Cost justification of decentralized pharmaceutical services for the emergency room. *Am J Hosp Pharm.* 1981;38:684–687.
16. Fairbanks RJ, Hildebrand JM, Kolstee KE, et al. Medical and nursing staff highly value clinical pharmacists in the emergency department. *Emerg Med J.* 2007;24:716–718.
17. Thomasset KB, Faris R. Survey of pharmacy services provision in the emergency department. *Am J Health-Syst Pharm.* 2003;60:1561–1564.
18. Rosenber JM, Koumis T, Nathan JP. Current status of pharmacist-operated drug information centers in the United States. *Am J Health-Syst Pharm.* 2004;61:2023–32.
19. Patanwala AE, Hays DP. Pharmacist's activities on a trauma response team in the emergency department. *Am J Health-Syst Pharm.* 2010;67:1536–8.
20. Kalina M, Tinkoff G, Gleason W, et al. A multidisciplinary approach to adverse drug events in pediatric trauma patients in an adult trauma center. *Pediatr Emerg Care.* 2009;25:444–446.
21. Kelly-Pisciotti S, Hays DP, O'Brien TE. Pharmacists enhancing patient safety during trauma resuscitations [platform presentation]. *American Society of Health System Pharmacists Midyear Clinical Meeting;* 2009.
22. Acquisto NM, Hays DP, Fairbanks RJ, et al. The outcomes of emergency pharmacist participation during acute myocardial infarction. *J Emerg Med.* 2012;42:371–378.
23. Corio JL, Sin JH, Hayes, BD et al. Impact of a pharmacist-driven prothrombin complex concentrate protocol on time to administration in patients with warfarin-associated intracranial hemorrhage. *West J Emerg Med.* 2018. doi:10.5811/westjem.2018.6.37932.
24. Draper HM, Eppert JA. Association of pharmacist presence on compliance with advanced cardiac life support guidelines during in-hospital cardiac arrest. *Ann Pharmacother.* 2008;42:469–474.
25. Shimp LA, Mason NA, Toedter NM. Pharmacist participation in cardiopulmonary resuscitation. *Am J Health-Syst Pharm.* 1995;52:980–984.
26. Flynn JD, McConeghy KW, Flannery AH, et al. Utilization of pharmacist responders as a component of a multidisciplinary sepsis bundle. *Ann Pharmacother.* 2014;48:1145–1151.
27. Moussavi K, Nikitenko V. Pharmacist impact on time to antibiotic administration in patients with sepsis in an ED. *Am J Emerg Med.* 2016;34:2117–2121.
28. Montgomery K, Hall AB, Keriazes G. Pharmacist's impact on acute pain management during trauma resuscitation. *J Trauma Nurs.* 2015;22:87–90.
29. Robey-Gavin E, Abuakar L. Impact of clinical pharmacists on initiation of postintubation analgesia in the emergency department. *J Emerg Med.* 2016;50:308–314.
30. Amini A, Faucett EA, Watt JM, et al. Effect of a pharmacist on timing of postintubation sedative and analgesic use in trauma resuscitations. *Am J Health-Syst Pharm.* 2013;70:1513–1517.
31. Johnson EG, Meier A, Shirakbari A, et al. Impact of rocuronium and succinylcholine on sedation initiation after rapid sequence intubation. *J Emerg Med.* 2015; 49:43–49.
32. Kilber E, Jarrell DH, Sakles JC, et al. Analgosedative interventions after rapid sequence intubation with rocuronium in the emergency department. *Am J Emerg Med.* 2018;36:1129–1133.
33. Rech MA, Bennett S, Donahey E. Pharmacist participation in acute ischemic stroke decreases door-to-needle time to recombinant tissue plasminogen activator. *Ann Pharmacother.* 2017;51:1084–1089.
34. Montgomery K, Hall AB, Keriazes G. Impact of an emergency medicine pharmacist on time to thrombolytics in acute ischemimc stroke. *Am J Emerg Med.* 2016;34:1997–1999.
35. Harvey S, Brad Hall A, Wilson K. Impact of an emergency medicine pharmacist on initial antibiotic prophylaxis for open fractures in trauma patients. *Am J Emerg Med.* 2018;36:290–293.
36. Czajka PA, Skoutakis VA, Wood GC. Clinical toxicology consultation by pharmacists. *Am J Health-Syst Pharm.* 1979;36:1087–1089.
37. Roberts RW, Russell WL. A pharmacist-based toxicology service. *Ann Pharmacother.* 2007;41:1719–1724.
38. Bronstein AC, Spyker DA, Cantilena LR, Jr, et al. 2008 annual report of the American Association of Poison Control Centers' national poison data system (NPDS): 26th annual report. *Clin Toxicol (Phila).* 2009;47:911–1084.
39. Gummin DD, Mowry JB, Spyker DA, et al. 2016 annual report of the American Association of Poison Control Centers' National Poison Data System (NPDS): 34th annual report. *Clin Toxicol (Phila).* 2017;55:1072–1252.
40. Dart RC, Borron SW, Caravati EM, et al. Expert consensus guidelines for stocking of antidotes in hospitals that provide emergency care. *Ann Emerg Med.* 2009;54(3):386–394.e1.
41. Dart RC, Goldfrank LR, Erstad BL, et al. Expert consensus guidelines for stocking of antidotes in hospitals that provide emergency care. *Ann Emerg Med.* 2018;71(3):314–325.e1.
42. Sentinal event alert, issue 11: High-alert medications and patient safety. https://www.jointcommission.org/assets/1/18/SEA_11.pdf. Accessed June 29, 2020
43. Wilson K, Sullivan M. Preventing medication errors with smart infusion technology. *Am J Health-Syst Pharm.* 2004;61:177–183.
44. Federico F. Preventing harm from high-alert medications. *Jt Comm J Qual Patient Saf.* 2007;33:537–542.

45. Lo A, Zhu JN, Richman M, et al. Effect of adding piperacillin-tazobactam to automated dispensing cabinets on promptness of first-dose antibiotics in hospitalized patients. *Am J Health-Syst Pharm.* 2014;71:1663–1667.
46. American Society of Health-System Pharmacists [ASHP]. ASHP guidelines on the safe use of automated dispensing devices. *Am J Health-Syst Pharm.* 2010; 67:483–490.
47. The Joint Commission. Medication management standard MM.5.01: preparing and dispensing (standard No. 5.01.01). https://e-dition.jcrinc.com/Frame.aspx. Accessed June 29, 2020.
48. Pedersen CA, Schneider PJ, Scheckelhoff DJ. ASHP national survey of pharmacy practice in hospital settings: dispensing and administration-2008. *Am J Health-Syst Pharm.* 2009;66:926–946.
49. Bond C, Raehl C, Franke T. Clinical pharmacy services and hospital mortality rates. *Pharmacotherapy.* 1999;19:556–564.
50. Bond C, Raehl C. Clinical pharmacy services, staffing, and adverse drug reactions in United States hospitals. *Pharmacotherapy.* 2006; 26:735–737.
51. Bond C, Raehl C. Clinical pharmacy services, pharmacy staffing and hospital mortality rates. *Pharmacotherapy.* 2007;27:481–493.
52. Gruen RL, Jurkovich GJ, McIntyre LK, et al. Patterns of errors contributing to trauma mortality: lessons learned from 2,594 deaths. *Ann Surg.* 2006; 244:371–380.
53. Barra ME, Culbreth SE, Sylvester KW. Utilization of an integrated electronic health record in the emergency department to increase prospective medication order review by pharmacists. *J Pharm Pract.* 2018;31:636–641.
54. Patanwala AE, Sanders AB, Thomas MC, et al. A prospective, multicenter study of pharmacist activities resulting in medication error interception in the emergency department. *Ann Emerg Med.* 2012;59:369–373.
55. Patanwala AE, Hays DP, Sanders AB, et al. Severity and probability of harm of medication errors intercepted by an emergency department pharmacist. *Int J Pharm Pract.* 2011;19:358–362.
56. Tully MP, Seston EM. Impact of pharmacists providing a prescription review and monitoring service in ambulatory care or community practice. *Ann Pharmacother.* 2000;34:1320–1331.
57. Coast-Senior EA, Kroner BA, Kelley CL, et al. Management of patients with type 2 diabetes by pharmacists in primary care clinics. *Ann Pharmacother.* 1998;32:636–641.
58. Kaboli PJ, Hoth AB, McClimon BJ, et al. Clinical pharmacists and inpatient medical care: a systematic review. *Arch Intern Med.* 2006;166:955–964.
59. Chisholm-Burns MA, Graff Zivin JS, Lee JK, et al. Economic effects of pharmacists on health outcomes in the United States: a systematic review. *Am J Health-Syst Pharm.* 2010;67:1624–1634.
60. McMullin ST, Hennenfent JA, Ritchie DJ. A prospective, randomized trial to assess the cost impact of pharmacist-initiated interventions. *Arch Intern Med.* 1999;159:2306–2309.
61. Kinky DE, Erush SC, Laskin MS, et al. Economic impact of a drug information service. *Ann Pharmacother.* 1999;33:11–16.
62. Elenbaas RM, Waeckerle JF, McNabney WK. The clinical pharmacist in emergency medicine. *Am J Hosp Pharm.* 1977;34:843–846.
63. Elenbaas RM. Role of the pharmacist in providing clinical pharmacy services in the emergency department. *Can J Hosp Pharm.* 1978;31:123–125.
64. Culbertson V, Anderson RJ. Pharmacist involvement in emergency room services. *Contemp Pharm Pract.* 1981;4:167–176.
65. Mialon PJ, Williams P, Wiebe RA. Clinical pharmacy services in a pediatric emergency department. *Hosp Pharm.* 2004;39:121–124.
66. Weant KA, Sterling E, Winstead PS, et al. Establishing a pharmacy presence in the ED. *Am J Emerg Med.* 2006;24:514–515.
67. Rothschild JM, Churchill W, Erickson A, et al. Medication errors recovered by emergency department pharmacists. *Ann Emerg Med.* 2010;55:513–521.
68. Fairbanks RJ, Hays DP, Webster DF, et al. Clinical pharmacy services in an emergency department. *Am J Health-Syst Pharm.* 2004;61:934–937.
69. Levy DB. Documentation of clinical and cost-saving pharmacy interventions in the emergency room. *Hosp Pharm.* 1993;28:624–627, 630–634, 653.
70. Ling JM, Mike LA, Rubin J, et al. Documentation of pharmacist interventions in the emergency department. *Am J Health-Syst Pharm.* 2005;62:1793–1797.
71. Lada P, Delgado G, Jr. Documentation of pharmacists' interventions in an emergency department and associated cost avoidance. *Am J Health-Syst Pharm.* 2007;64:63–68.
72. Aldridge VE, Park HK, Bounthavong M, et al. Implementing a comprehensive, 24-hour emergency department pharmacy program. *Am J Health-Syst Pharm.* 2009;66:1943–1947.
73. Reilly JC, Wallace M, Campbell MM. Tracking pharmacist interventions with a hand-held computer. *Am J Health-Syst Pharm.* 2001;58:158–161.
74. Silva MA, Tataronis GR, Maas B. Using personal digital assistants to document pharmacist cognitive services and estimate potential reimbursement. *Am J Health-Syst Pharm.* 2003;60:911–915.
75. Simonian AI. Documenting pharmacist interventions on an intranet. *Am J Health-Syst Pharm.* 2003;60:151–155.
76. Lau A, Balen RM, Lam R, et al. Using a personal digital assistant to document clinical pharmacy services in an intensive care unit. *Am J Health-Syst Pharm.* 2001;58:1229–1932.
77. Bosinski TJ, Campbell L, Schwartz S. Using a personal digital assistant to document pharmacotherapeutic interventions. *Am J Health-Syst Pharm.* 2004;61:931–934.
78. Mason RN, Pugh CB, Boyer SB. Computerized documentation of pharmacists' interventions. *Am J Health-Syst Pharm.* 1994;51:2131–2138.
79. Schumock GT, Hutchinson RA, Bilek BA. Comparison of two systems for documenting pharmacist

interventions in patient care. *Am J Hosp Pharm.* 1992;49:2211–2214.

80. Zimmerman CR, Smolarek RT, Stevenson JG. A computerized system to improve documentation and reporting of pharmacists' clinical interventions, cost savings, and workload activities. *Pharmacotherapy.* 1995;15:220–227.
81. Spigiel RW, Anderson RJ. Comprehensive pharmaceutical services in the emergency room. *Am J Hosp Pharm.* 1979;36:52–56.
82. Kopp BJ, Mrsan M, Erstad BL, et al. Cost implications of and potential adverse events prevented by interventions of a critical care pharmacist. *Am J Health-Syst Pharm.* 2007;64:2483–2487.
83. Mutnick AH, Sterba KJ, Peroutka JA, et al. Cost savings and avoidance from clinical interventions. *Am J Health-Syst Pharm.* 1997;54:392–396.
84. Schneider PJ, Gift MG, Lee YP, et al. Cost of medication-related problems at a university hospital. *Am J Health-Syst Pharm.* 1995;52:2415–2418.
85. Classen DC, Resar R, Griffin F, et al. 'Global trigger tool' shows that adverse events in hospitals may be ten times greater than previously measured. *Health Aff (Millwood).* 2011;30:581–589.
86. Randolph TC, Parker A, Meyer L, et al. Effect of a pharmacist-managed culture review process on antimicrobial therapy in an emergency department. *Am J Health-Syst Pharm.* 2011;68:916–919.
87. Andrulis DP, Kellermann A, Hintz EA, et al. Emergency departments and crowding in United States teaching hospitals. *Ann Emerg Med.* 1991;20:980–986.
88. Olshaker JS, Rathlev NK. Emergency department overcrowding and ambulance diversion: the impact and potential solutions of extended boarding of admitted patients in the emergency department. *J Emerg Med.* 2006;30:351–356.
89. Kulstad EB, Sikka R, Sweis RT, et al. ED overcrowding is associated with an increased frequency of medication errors. *Am J Emerg Med.* 2010;28:304–309.
90. Farley HL, Kwun R; Emergency Medicine Practice Committee. *Emergency Department Overcrowding: High Impact Solutions.* Irving, TX: American College of Emergency Physicians; May 2016. wwww.acep.org/globalassets/sites/acep/media/crowding/empc_crowding-ip_092016.pdf. Accessed June 29, 2020.
91. Zdyb EG, Courtney DM, Malik S, et al. Impact of discharge anticoagulation education by emergency department pharmacists at a tertiary academic medical center. *J Emerg Med.* 2017;53:896–903.
92. Hohner E, Ortmann M, Murtaza U, et al. Implementation of an emergency department-based clinical pharmacist transitions-of-care program. *Am J Health-Syst Pharm.* 2016;73:1180–1187.
93. Cesarz JL, Steffenhagen AL, Svenson J, et al. Emergency department discharge prescription interventions by emergency medicine pharmacists. *Ann Emerg Med.* 2013;61:209–214.e1.
94. Baker SN, Acquisto NM, Ashley ED, et al. Pharmacist-managed antimicrobial stewardship program for patients discharged from the emergency department. *J Pharm Pract.* 2012;25:190–194.
95. Dumkow LE, Kenney RM, MacDonald NC, et al. Impact of a multidisciplinary culture follow-up program of antimicrobial therapy in the emergency department. *Infect Dis Ther.* 2014;3:45–53.
96. Randolph TC. Expansion of pharmacists' responsibilities in an emergency department. *Am J Health-Syst Pharm.* 2009; 66:1484–1487.
97. Miller K, McGraw MA, Tomsey A, et al. Pharmacist addition to the post-ED visit review of discharge antimicrobial regimens. *Am J Emerg Med.* 2014; 32:1270–1274.
98. Raman-Wilms L. Transition from hospital to home: can pharmacists' interventions improve patients' outcomes? *Can J Hosp Pharm.* 2010; 63:408–409.
99. Trang J, Martinez A, Aslam S, et al. Pharmacist advancement of transitions of care to home (PATCH) service. *Hosp Pharm.* 2015; 50:994–1002.
100. Hayes BD, Zahama L, Winters ME. To-go medications for decreasing ED return visits. *Am J Emerg Med.* 2012; 30:2011–2014.
101. Cornish PL, Knowles SR, Marchesano R, et al. Unintended medication discrepancies at the time of hospital admission. *Arch Intern Med.* 2005; 165:424–429.
102. Eppert HD, Eppert JA. In response to "the unexpected challenges of accurate medication reconciliation." *Ann Emerg Med.* 2009; 53:548–549.
103. Gleason KM, Groszek JM, Sullivan C, et al. Reconciliation of discrepancies in medication histories and admission orders of newly hospitalized patients. *Am J Health-Syst Pharm.* 2004;61:1689–1695.
104. Miller SL, Miller S, Balon J et al. Medication reconciliation in a rural trauma population. *Ann Emerg Med.* 2008;52:483–491.
105. Santell JP. Reconciliation failures lead to medication errors. *Jt Comm J Qual Patient Saf.* 2006;32:225–229.
106. Schenkel S. The unexpected challenges of accurate medication reconciliation. *Ann Emerg Med.* 2008;52:493–495.
107. Tam VC, Knowles SR, Cornish PL, et al. Frequency, type and clinical importance of medication history errors at admission to hospital: a systematic review. *CMAJ.* 2005;173:510–515.
108. Becerra-Camargo J, Martinez-Martinez F, Garcia-Jimenez E. A multicentre, double-blind, randomised, controlled, parallel-group study of the effectiveness of a pharmacist-acquired medication history in an emergency department. *BMC Health Serv Res.* 2013;13:337.
109. Carter MK, Allin DM, Scott LA, et al. Pharmacist-acquired medication histories in a university hospital emergency department. *Am J Health-Syst Pharm.* 2006;63:2500–2503.
110. Nester TM, Hale LS. Effectiveness of a pharmacist-acquired medication history in promoting patient safety. *Am J Health-Syst Pharm.* 2002;59:2221–2225.
111. Reeder TA, Mutnick A. Pharmacist-versus physician-obtained medication histories. *Am J Health-Syst Pharm.* 2008;65:857–60.
112. Lubowski TJ, Cronin LM, Pavelka RW, et al. Effectiveness of a medication reconciliation project conducted by PharmD students. *Am J Pharm Educ.* 2007;71:94.

113. Mersfelder TL, Bickel RJ. Inpatient medication history verification by pharmacy students. *Am J Health-Syst Pharm*. 2008;65:2273–2275.
114. Hayes BD, Donovan JL, Smith BS et al. Pharmacist-conducted medication reconciliation in an emergency department. *Am J Health-Syst Pharm*. 2007;64:1720–1723.
115. Michels RD, Meisel SB. Program using pharmacy technicians to obtain medication histories. *Am J Health-Syst Pharm*. 2003;60:1982–1986.
116. Cobaugh DJ, Schneider SM. Pharmacists in the emergency department: encouraging and discouraging findings. *Am J Health-Syst Pharm*. 2016;73:357.
117. Morgan SR, Acquisto NM, Coralic Z, et al. Clinical pharmacy services in the emergency department. *Am J Emerg Med*. 2018; 36:1727–1732.
118. DeWitt KM, Weiss SJ, Rankin S et al. Impact of an emergency medicine pharmacist on antibiotic dosing adjustment. *Am J Emerg Med*. 2016;34:980–984.
119. Faine BA, Mohr N, Dietrich J et al. Antimicrobial therapy for pneumonia in the emergency department: the impact of clinical pharmacists on appropriateness. *West J Emerg Med*. 2017;18:856–863.
120. Lingenfelter E, Drapkin Z, Fritz K et al. ED pharmacist monitoring of provider antibiotic selection aids appropriate treatment for outpatient UTI. *Am J Emerg Med*. 2016;34:1600–1603.
121. Groth CM, Acquisto NM. Pharmacists as members of the rapid response team. *J Pharm Pract*. 2016;29:116–20.
122. Cohen V. *Safe and effective medication use in the emergency department*. Bethesda, MD: American Society of Health-System Pharmacists; 2009.
123. Farmer BM. Patient safety in the emergency department. *Emerg Med J*. 2016;48:396–404.
124. Ratz Y, Shafir I, Berkovitch S et al. The importance of the pharmacist in reporting adverse drug reactions in the emergency department. *J Clin Pharmacol*. 2010;50:1217–1221.
125. Phillips MS, Gayman JE, Todd MW. ASHP guidelines on medication-use evaluation. *Am J Health-Syst Pharm*. 1996;53:1953–1955.
126. American Society of Health-System Pharmacists. ASHP guidelines on the pharmacist's role in the development, implementation, and assessment of critical pathways. *Am J Health-Syst Pharm*. 2004;61:939–945.
127. American Society of Health-System Pharmacists. ASHP statement on the role of health-system pharmacists in emergency preparedness. *Am J Health-Syst Pharm*. 2003; 60:1993–1995.
128. Setlak P. Bioterrorism preparedness and response: emerging role for health-system pharmacists. *Am J Health-Syst Pharm*. 2004;61:1167–1175.
129. Alkhalili M, Ma J, Grenier S. Defining roles for pharmacy personnel in disaster response and emergency preparedness. *Disaster Med Public Health Prep*. 2017;1:496–504.
130. Awad NI, Cocchio C. Assessment of hospital pharmacy preparedness for mass casualty events. *P T*. 2015;40:264–267.
131. Centers for Disease Control and Prevention. Strategic National Stockpile. https://www.phe.gov/about/sns/Pages/default.aspx. Accessed June 29, 2020.
132. U.S. Federal Emergency Management Administration. Center for Domestic Preparedness. https://cdp.dhs.gov. Accessed June 29, 2020.
133. Bell C, Daniel S. Pharmacy leader's role in hospital emergency preparedness planning. *Hosp Pharm*. 2014; 49:398–404.
134. Vollman KE, Adams CB, Shah MN, et al. Survey of emergency medicine pharmacy education opportunities for students and residents. *Hosp Pharm*. 2015;50:690–699.
135. Gimbar RP, Rynn KO. Designing an emergency medicine pharmacy rotation. *Am J Health-Syst Pharm*. 2018;75:602–605.
136. American Society of Health-System Pharmacists. ASHP accreditation standard for postgraduate year two (PGY2) pharmacy residency programs. https://www.ashp.org/Professional-Development/Residency-Information/Residency-Program-Resources/Residency-Accreditation/Accreditation-Standards-for-PGY2-Pharmacy-Residencies. Accessed June 29, 2020.
137. Board of Pharmaceutical Specialties. BPS announces emergency medicine pharmacy practice analysis task-force appointments. https://www.bpsweb.org/2020/06/10/board-of-pharmacy-specialties-seeks-pharmacists-to-serve-on-its-emergency-medicine-pharmacy-specialty-council/. Accessed June 29, 2020.
138. American Society of Health-System Pharmacists. Educational outcomes, goals, and objectives for post-graduate year two (PGY2) pharmacy residencies in emergency medicine. https://www.ashp.org/-/media/assets/pharmacy-practice/resource-centers/emergency-care/education-outcomes-goals-objectives-postgraduate-year-two-pharmacy-residencies-em.ashx. Accessed June 29, 2020.
139. Institute of Medicine of the National Academies Committee on the Future of Emergency Care in the United States Health System. Enhancing the emergency care research base. In: *Hospital-Based Emergency Care: At the Breaking Point*. Washington DC: National Academy Press; 2006:291–320.
140. Aghababian RV, Barsan WG, Bickell WH. Research directions in emergency medicine. *Am J Emerg Med*. 1996;14:681–683.
141. Hoyt DB, Holcomb J, Abraham E. Working group on trauma research program summary report: National Heart Lung Blood Institute (NHLBI), National Institute of General Medical Sciences (NIGMS), and National Institute of Neurological Disorders and Stroke (NINDS) of the National Institutes of Health (NIH), and the Department of Defense (DOD). *J Trauma*. 2004;57:410–415.
142. Becker LB, Weisfeldt ML, Weil MH. The PULSE initiative: scientific priorities and strategic planning for resuscitation research and life saving therapies. *Circulation*. 2002; 105:2562–70.
143. Maio RF, Garrison HG, Spaite DW. Emergency medical services outcomes project I (EMSOP I): prioritizing conditions for outcomes research. *Ann Emerg Med*. 1999; 33:423–32.
144. Seidel JS, Henderson D, Tittle S. Priorities for research in emergency medical services for children: results of a consensus conference. *Ann Emerg Med*. 1999; 33:206–10.

145. Astrup G, Sarangarm P, Burnett A. Fixed dose 4-factor prothrombin complex concentrate for the emergent reversal of warfarin: a retrospective analysis. *J Thromb Thrombolysis*. 2018; 45:300–5.
146. Weant KA, Bowers RC, Reed J, et al. Safety and cost-effectiveness of a clinical protocol implemented to standardize the use of Crotalidae polyvalent immune fab antivenom at an academic medical center. *Pharmacotherapy*. 2012; 32:433–40.
147. Kaucher KA, Acquisto NM, Broderick KB. Emergency department naloxone rescue kit dispensing and patient follow-up. *Am J Emerg Med*. 2018; 36:1503–1504.
148. Groth ME, McMillian WD, Wolfson DL. Pharmacist input into statewide treatment protocols for emergency medical services. *Am J Health-Syst Pharm*. 2015; 72:61–3.
149. Lipowski EE. Developing great research questions. *Am J Health-Syst Pharm*. 2008; 65:1667–1670.
150. Zschoche JH, Nesbit S, Murtaza U, et al. Development and implementation of procedures for outpatient naloxone prescribing at a large academic medical center. *Am J Health-Syst Pharm*. 2018; 75:1812–1820.
151. Trinh TD, Klinker KP. Antimicrobial stewardship in the emergency department. *Infect Dis Ther*. 2015; 4(Suppl 1):39–50.
152. Gernant SA, Snyder ME, Jaynes H, et al. The effectiveness of pharmacist-provided telephonic medication therapy management on emergency department utilization in home health patients. *J Pharm Technol*. 2016; 32:179–184.

Approved by the ASHP Board of Directors on August 21, 2020. Developed through the ASHP Section of Clinical Specialists and Scientists. These guidelines supersede the ASHP Guidelines on Emergency Medicine Pharmacist Services dated July 8, 2011, and the ASHP Statement on Pharmacist Services to the Emergency Department dated June 10, 2008.

ASHP gratefully acknowledges the following organizations and individuals reviewing these guidelines (review does not imply endorsement): American College of Clinical Pharmacy; American Pharmacists Association; Iowa Pharmacy Association; CaroMont Regional Medical Center Emergency Medicine Clinical Pharmacy Team; Maryland Society of Health-System Pharmacists; Society of Critical Care Medicine; Sandra Bardas, BSP, RPh, FCSHP; Alyson T. Basting, Pharm.D., BCCCP; Carol J. Bickford, Ph.D., RN-BC, CPHIMS, FAMIA, FHIMSS, FAAN; Joel M. Boerth, Pharm.D., BCPP; Timmi Anne Boesken, M.H.A., CPht; Stephanie A. Buckingham, Pharm.D., BCPS; Jaxson Burkins, Pharm.D., BCPS; J Campbell, Pharm.D., BCPS, BCCCP; Michael Dejos, Pharm.D., BCPS, LSSBB, Christopher J. Edwards, Pharm.D., BCPS; Amanda Eger, Pharm.D.; Madeline Foertsch, Pharm.D., BCCCP; Paige Garber, Pharm.D., BCCCP; Renee Petzel Gimbar, Pharm.D.; Roy Guharoy, Pharm.D., MBA, FCCP, FASHP; Nicole Harger, Pharm.D., BCCCP; Molly Howell, Pharm.D., BCPS, BCCCP; Nkem Iroh, Pharm.D, M.B.A., BCPS; Gavin D. Jones, Ph.D., Pharm.D., BCPS; Kevin Kaucher, Pharm.D., BCCCP; Jamie Kerestes, Pharm.D., BCCCP; Eric C. Kutscher, Pharm.D., MBA, FASHP; Ronald E. Lay, M.S. RPh, FASHP, Chung-Shien Lee, Pharm.D., BCPS, BCOP; Abbie Lyden, Pharm.D., BCPS; Nancy MacDonald, Pharm.D., BCPS, FASHP; Julian B. McCreary, Pharm.D., BCPS; Patrick J. McDonnell, Pharm.D., FASHP; Katie Clark McKinney, Pharm.D., MS, BCPS, FACHE, FASHP; Scott Morrison, R.Ph., BCPS, Jessica Nesheim, Pharm.D., BCPS; Jenny Nguyen, Pharm.D. Candidate 2020; Richard Ogden Jr., Pharm.D., M.B.A., BCPS, Amanda Peck, Pharm.D.; Marianne Pop, Pharm.D., BCPS; Megan Rech, Pharm.D., M.S., BCPS, BCCCP; James R. Rinehart, R.Ph., M.S., FASHP; Chris Roberts, Pharm.D., M.B.A., BCPS; Patrick Ryan, Pharm.D., BCCCP; Ashley Schaber, Pharm.D., M.B.A., BCPS, NCPS, Ravipal Singh, Pharm.D., BCCCP; Paul M. Szumita, Pharm.D., FASHP, FCCM, BCCCP, BCPS; Michael C. Thomas, Pharm.D., BCPS, FCCP; Kyle A. Weant, Pharm.D., BCPS, BCCCP, FCCP; Kelsey Williams, Pharm.D., Jessica Winter, Pharm.D., BCPS, BCCCP; Robert M. Woods, Pharm.D., BCPS; Tyler Vest, Pharm.D., M.S., BCPS; Karin Zepf, Pharm.D., BCPS

Melinda J. Ortmann, Pharm.D., BCPS, Department of Pharmacy, The Johns Hopkins Hospital Baltimore, MD.

Elizabeth Giesler Johnson, Pharm.D., BCPS, Department of Pharmacy, John Peter Smith Hospital Fort Worth, TX.

Daniel H. Jarrell, Pharm.D., BCPS, BCCCP, Department of Pharmacy, Banner—University Medical Center Tucson, Department of Pharmacy Practice and Science, The University of Arizona Tucson, AZ.

Matt Bilhimer, Pharm.D., BCPS, Department of Pharmacy, Olathe Medical Center, Olathe, KS.

Bryan D. Hayes, Pharm.D., DABAT, FAACT, FASHP, Department of Emergency Medicine, Harvard Medical School, Department of Pharmacy, Massachusetts General Hospital, Boston, MA.

Aimee Mishler, Pharm.D., BCPS, Department of Pharmacy, Valleywise Health, Phoenix, AZ.

Robert S. Pugliese, Pharm.D., BCPS, Department of Pharmacy, Thomas Jefferson University Hospital, Philadelphia, PA, Department of Pharmacy, Thomas Jefferson University, Philadelphia, PA.

Taylor A. Roberson, Pharm.D., BCPS, Department of Pharmacy, OhioHealth Grant Medical Center, Columbus, OH.

Giles Slocum, Pharm.D., BCCCP, Department of Pharmacy, Rush University Medical Center, Department of Emergency Medicine, Rush University Medical Center, Chicago, IL.

Andrew P. Smith, Pharm.D., MBA, BCPS, BCCCP, Department of Pharmacy, Scripps Mercy Hospital, San Diego, CA.

Katie Yabut, Pharm.D., BCPS, Department of Pharmacy, Legacy Mount Hood Medical Center Portland, OR.

David E. Zimmerman, Pharm.D., BCPS, BCCCP, Department of Pharmacy, Duquesne University School of Pharmacy, Department of Pharmacy, UPMC-Mercy, Pittsburgh, PA.

Copyright © 2021, American Society of Health-System Pharmacists, Inc. All rights reserved. Contact ASHP for reprint and permissions requests. This content may not be used for commercial purposes without the express written consent of ASHP.

The bibliographic citation for this document is as follows: American Society of Health-System Pharmacists. ASHP guidelines on emergency medicine pharmacist services. *Am J Health-Syst Pharm*. 2021; 78:261–265.

ASHP Guidelines on Perioperative Pharmacy Services

Historically, pharmacy involvement in perioperative areas primarily consisted of providing medication stock for access by operating room (OR) staff, confirming appropriate storage conditions, checking expiration dates, submitting billing, and maintaining controlled substance accountability. In the early 1980s, pharmacists recognized the need for increased involvement and OR satellite pharmacies began to appear, particularly in academic institutions.[1] Even so, the focus remained primarily on medication distribution and regulatory compliance. Evolving standards from regulatory and accrediting agencies as well as the need for improved charge capture and greater controlled substance accountability over the last decade drove increased pharmacy involvement in the perioperative medication-use process. Ongoing rapid changes in healthcare now demand that our attention be turned toward incorporating additional activities, such as supporting institutional quality and safety goals, developing perioperative treatment algorithms and order sets, and collaborating with the perioperative team to provide patient-centered, medication-related care in inpatient and outpatient settings. Finally, the challenge of cost-effective perioperative medication use has never been greater, with the movement from fee-for-service payment to value-based payment systems.

Purpose

In 1991, the first ASHP Technical Assistance Bulletin on Surgery and Anesthesiology Pharmaceutical Services was published.[2] It was revised in 1998 and published as the ASHP Guidelines on Surgery and Anesthesiology Pharmaceutical Services, and it was reviewed without revision in 2003. This updated guideline is intended to provide guidance to health systems on perioperative pharmacy services.

Two levels of perioperative pharmacy services are described: essential services, which should be in place in every healthcare setting; and desirable best practices, which must be tailored to the changing demands of healthcare, specific needs of the institution, and available resources.

Services to perioperative areas as well as to procedural areas may be provided from an OR satellite pharmacy but may also be provided from a central or other satellite pharmacy location. While an OR satellite pharmacy with dedicated staff facilitates the development of the specialized expertise and close collaboration with OR personnel, these guidelines are intended for any pharmacy serving the areas noted above. Some or all of the services described may be provided by a dedicated perioperative pharmacist, a management or leadership-level pharmacist, or other pharmacy staff. Pharmacists may also use telepharmacy when suitable to remotely verify sterile compounding verification, pre- and postoperative medication order review, interactive postoperative patient medication counseling, or provide drug information to a facility that is geographically isolated.[3] Consequently, the terms *pharmacy, satellite pharmacy, perioperative environment*, and *perioperative pharmacist* are used in the broadest sense.

The Perioperative Environment

To understand and optimize the unique role of the perioperative pharmacist, significant differences found in the perioperative environment must be recognized, specifically the following:

1. The medication-use process is fundamentally different from that in the patient care unit. Medications are administered by anesthesia care providers (ACPs) (anesthesiologists, certified registered nurse anesthetists [CRNAs], and anesthesiologist assistants), surgeons, others (e.g., perfusionists, physician assistants), and, very rarely, nurses.
2. Medications are almost always administered by licensed independent practitioners such as ACPs or surgeons.
3. A significant proportion of medications are high-alert medications.
4. Medications may be used for off-label indications or administered by routes with which pharmacists may be unfamiliar.
5. Multiple unique documentation systems exist within the perioperative setting.

Medications administered by the surgeon are typically identified by the individual surgeon's case-specific preference card, requested and obtained by the circulating nurse, placed on the sterile field, and administered by the surgeon or physician assistant as needed. There is often no pharmacist review prior to administration, particularly for commonly requested medications such as local anesthetics and topical hemostats. Some medications may be time sensitive, with reliance on verbal communication if the patient requires rapid intraoperative intervention and the surgeon is scrubbed in with his or her full attention on the patient. Pharmacy oversight in the OR may be complicated by medications, glues, and other agents in supply kits, which may be acquired through OR purchasing or a centralized supply department.

Medications administered by ACPs differ from those used by surgeons, with few exceptions (e.g., local anesthetics). ACPs are typically the only practitioner involved in the entire medication-use process—prescribing, formulating and preparing, dispensing, administering, and monitoring the medication. The protection afforded by double checks (pharmacist, nurse, pharmacy technician) and barcode medication scanning that exists in most areas of the hospital is not present. Medications typically administered by ACPs are provided in one of 2 ways: (1) a drug tray stored in a drawer of the anesthesia cart or (2) individual bins or pockets in drawers of an automated anesthesia cart (AAC). Infusions, irrigations, or compounded/diluted high-risk medications are best prepared by pharmacy as needed.

Essential Roles of the Perioperative Pharmacist

Drug therapy management services that are consistently provided to all hospitalized patients should also be provided for patients in the perioperative area if applicable and to

DOI 10.37573/9781585287048.075

the fullest extent possible. These services are available for review elsewhere, including the ASHP Guidelines: Minimum Standard for Pharmacies in Hospitals.[4] Essential roles of the perioperative pharmacist or pharmacy team include the following:

- Medication procurement, preparation, distribution, and flow
- Promotion of safe medication use according to regulations and institutional policies
- Controlled substance management and surveillance
- Preoperative and postanesthesia care unit (PACU) order review
- Provision of drug information and education
- Performance improvement and quality assurance
- Leadership duties and professional service
- Financial management

Medication Procurement, Preparation, Distribution, and Flow

Procurement and Preparation. It is important to know the procurement pathway of all medications used in the perioperative environment. For example, medications may be included in procedural kits procured by OR purchasing or the central supply department (e.g., 1.5% lidocaine with epinephrine in an epidural kit, 0.75% hyperbaric bupivacaine in a spinal kit). Medications may also be supplied by the manufacturer of a particular diagnostic, surgical, or robotic instrument, or as part of a vendor-assembled tray. Regardless of procurement pathway, medications should be appropriately stored and controlled. Collaboration between pharmacy, central supply, anesthesiology, and surgical services is recommended to identify these items and ensure appropriate storage and control.

In the perioperative setting it is not unusual to receive requests for medications that are not commercially available. Such requests place additional pressure on the pharmacy to obtain these unavailable medications by either in-house compounding (many of which may be high risk) or outsourcing. It is critical to proceed carefully with these requests to avoid serious or catastrophic consequences. Guidance on outsourcing sterile products may be found in the ASHP Research and Education Foundation's vendor assessment tool for outsourcing sterile product preparation (http://outsourcingassessment.org/).

Drug Shortages. Federal regulations, product changes, and supply-chain issues leading to shortages have had a significant impact in the perioperative setting.[5] As in other areas, there are medications commonly used perioperatively that are the standard of care. When these medications are unavailable, even for short periods of time, there is potential for significant impact on patient care. In a 2013 survey of approximately 2,500 CRNAs, 90% reported that their institutions were currently experiencing shortages, and approximately 6% of CRNAs reported that a drug shortage was responsible for procedure cancellations.[6] Drug shortages have had such an impact on anesthesiologists' practice that the Anesthesia Quality Institute Anesthesia Incident Reporting System contains a required field to report if the event was impacted by a drug shortage.[7]

An interdisciplinary, collaborative approach to discuss alternatives and strategies with those most impacted by a critical shortage (i.e., ACPs or surgeons) is critical to ensuring patient safety during the time of a drug shortage. Strategies may be pharmacy-based (e.g., centralization of medication supply, preparation of unit doses from bulk medication or compounded) or involve other disciplines (e.g., develop and implement temporary restrictions, use alternative products or medications).[8,9] Use of technology (automated anesthesia information management systems [AIMS]), multiple conservation strategies involving ACPs or surgeons, timely communication, and close monitoring are necessary to ensure that a critical drug in short supply for a prolonged period of time will be available to all patients for whom it is an optimal choice.[8]

Distribution. In the perioperative setting, medications may be distributed to the PACU and preoperative units, or to the operating or procedural rooms. Medications distributed to the PACU and preoperative units should be dispensed manually (i.e., direct delivery from pharmacy of compounded or unit-of-use medications) or through an automated dispensing device. Careful review of state and hospital accrediting body rules or guidelines should be considered when determining whether to profile an automated dispensing cabinet (ADC) in 1 or both units. For safety purposes, it is recommended that ADCs in the nursing units be profiled; however, profiling of medications in the preoperative unit can be challenging when turnover of patients is high. Some ADCs and electronic health record systems have the ability to allow automatic medication-order verification, which verifies a medication order when entered into the electronic health record and allows the medication to be immediately available to the nurse for dispensing. The system would still then allow the pharmacy final review of the medication order. However, such a system does not prevent a nurse or provider from removing and administering the medication prior to the pharmacy review, but instead allows the opportunity for the pharmacy to review an order and potentially catch and correct an error if identified. Such a system may be helpful for a PACU or preoperative unit to maintain medication profiling while allowing flexibility with timeliness of order verification. Without automatic order verification, profiling ADCs may not be feasible and should be carefully reviewed to determine the associated safety risk–benefit ratio.

Distribution to the OR setting may be accomplished by using (1) a manual dispensing system (e.g., drug trays or boxes, pharmacy-prepared infusions, airway emergency kits, and compounded or diluted high-risk drugs); (2) automated dispensing devices (e.g., ADCs, AACs); or (3) a combination of manual and automated dispensing systems. When manual systems are used, the pharmacy should be responsible for stocking, tracking, and delivering drug trays and boxes. To the fullest extent possible, the pharmacy should prepare infusions as well as compounded or diluted high-risk drugs used in the OR.[10,11] Each institution should evaluate all options (i.e., cleanroom-prepared, satellite pharmacy-prepared, provider-prepared, or outsourced product), then determine the best method for providing each infusion, compounded, or diluted high-risk drug in a timely manner with minimal waste.[12]

Automated dispensing devices can improve accountability and storage of medications, as well as improve accuracy and timeliness of medication distribution.[13] In the OR setting, ADCs are generally not pharmacy profiled (as they are in patient-care units, where medication orders are placed and reviewed) and create limitations such as configuration, storage space, and proximity to the end user. Smaller ADCs may be located within each OR suite and contain medications frequently administered by ACPs (e.g., controlled substances) and surgeons (e.g., local anesthetics, topical hemostats). Another option for ACPs would be an AAC in each OR suite and anesthetizing location.

Regardless of the medication distribution system used, the following conditions apply:

- The medication distribution system must ensure medication security by (1) limiting access to authorized persons only, (2) locking all controlled substances while in the OR in an enclosed area not accessible by unauthorized individuals when not under the direct control of the ACP, and (3) including procedures to ensure ACPs have immediate access to emergency drugs while preventing unauthorized access. Anesthesia carts and machines may remain unlocked and medications other than controlled substances left in or on top of an unlocked anesthesia cart or machine immediately prior to, during, and immediately after surgical cases when authorized OR personnel are in the OR suite.[14] Auto-locking anesthesia carts should be set to the narrowest window of time appropriate for the setting. Carts located in offsite anesthetizing areas or procedural rooms should be locked at all times, with medications inaccessible when not in use. The medication-distribution system will have benefits and challenges. For example, medication trays or ADCs can be standardized and exchanged, refilled after each case or on a daily basis, but will often require a manual pharmacy check and manual tracking of medications. ADCs improve medication inventory and tracking but are often insufficient in number, limited in space, not optimally located, dependent on accurate removal by the ACP, and labor intensive to stock.
- The medication distribution system must be developed with the end users to optimize accurate medication selection and stocking and to provide an acceptable level of efficiency and safety.

Promotion of Safe Medication Use According to Regulations and Institutional Policies, and Medication Errors

The OR is a complex, dynamic, time-sensitive, and sometimes chaotic environment. The anesthetic plan for a patient is largely executed by a carefully selected series of medications administered in anticipation of or in response to specific events during the surgical procedure. ACPs have complete responsibility for all steps in the medication-use process from preparation to monitoring and hand-off. Furthermore, many recommended safe medication-use practices are difficult or impossible to implement in the OR.[15] In the OR, AACs and machines do not select and dispense medications for each patient based on a physician order (via computer order entry and clinical decision support) and pharmacist verification. Barcode medication administration to confirm the right drug and dose, as well as documentation of medication administration, is rarely available in the OR. Such critical differences can result in different types of medication errors occurring in the OR than elsewhere in the hospital, where such medication-use practices are in place. The most common types of anesthesia medication errors are:

- Wrong dose as a result of miscalculation of dose, concentration, or infusion rate[10,16,17]
- Wrong drug due to accidental administration of the wrong syringe ("syringe swap") or vial or ampule swap during medication preparation[10,17]
- Extra dose[10]
- Omitted dose/failure to act[10,16]

The Society for Pediatric Anesthesia created Wake Up Safe (http://wakeupsafe.org/), a multicenter collaborative quality improvement initiative. When a medication error that harmed or has the potential to harm occurs in a participating institution, a team of pediatric anesthesiologists analyzes the medication error, arrives at a consensus, and reports the error to Wake Up Safe. Lobaugh and colleagues[17] reviewed 6 years of medication errors reported to Wake Up Safe. The most common medication error was administration of the wrong dose (30%), followed by accidental administration of the wrong syringe ("syringe swap") (18%), wrong dose prepared (15%), and vial or ampule swap during drug preparation (9%). Of the 276 medication errors analyzed,

- >80% reached the patient.
- >50% caused patient harm, with 5% requiring a life-sustaining intervention.
- Approximately 20% involved medications prepared as infusions.
- 97% were perceived by the reporting institution as being preventable.

The literature has demonstrated that fatal or potentially fatal anesthesia medication errors occur, and that such errors include wrong route, miscalculation of a dilution, failure to dilute, infusion pump programming error, administering a medication to a patient with a known allergy, and failure to flush the line after a drug is administered.[10]

Relying on voluntary reporting alone provides a partial view because the vast majority of medication errors are not reported.[18] Webster and colleagues reported that 0.36% to 4% of anesthesia cases have reportable medication errors.[19] A more reliable method of medication error data collection is direct observation. Merry and colleagues[20] found a medication error rate of 11.6% (1 error in every 11.6 medications administered) using direct observation when a paper anesthesia recordkeeping system was used. Also using direct observation, Nanji and colleagues[16] found that approximately 1 in 20 medication administrations and every second operation resulted in a medication error or adverse drug event. Approximately one-third of the errors did not result in any observed patient harm, and the remaining two thirds had the potential for patient harm. The most prevalent medication errors that led to an adverse drug event were inappropriate medication doses (47.1%) and omitted medications or failure to act (31.4%). The most common medication errors associated with a potential adverse drug event were labeling error (22.9%), wrong dose error (22.9%), and omitted medications or failure to act (17.6%). There were no significant differences in the medication error rates between resident physicians, nurse anesthetists, and attending anesthesiologists (5.1%, 5.5%, and 4.5%, respectively; $p = 0.79$), demonstrating that medication errors are not rare, inconsequential events caused by inexperienced ACPs.

Medication Safety Strategies. Select OR medication safety strategies include the following:

- Medications, medication tray, or medication cart:
  - Avoid look-alike medications when possible; if not possible, do not store in proximity, and add alert labels.[10]
  - Use single-use vials; discard multidose vials at end of case; use only preservative-free local anesthetic products.[10]
  - Stock only 1 drug concentration on cart; include alert label on concentrated or high-alert drugs.[10]
  - Standardize medication trays, clearly label divisions, and place drugs to minimize confusion and hidden labels.[10,11,21]
  - Store regional anesthesia drugs in a separate regional cart.[10]
- Medication administration:
  - Label all medications using standardized preprinted labels or labels generated by barcode scan of vial in accordance with standards established by ASTM International, the International Organization for Standardization, and the Institute for Safe Medication Practices.[10,11,22]
  - Minimize provider-prepared syringes when possible; use prefilled syringes and premixed intravenous (i.v.) solutions when possible; use compounded and diluted drugs prepared by pharmacy[10,11]; and perform 2-person or careful single-person double check if ACP prepares dilutions of high-alert drugs.[10]
  - Read and verify every vial, ampule, and syringe label before administration.[10]
  - Administer infusions via smart pumps that have a drug library with guardrails and alerts, and that are standardized across units to eliminate the need to change infusion solutions, rates, or area of the drug library when a patient moves between the OR, PACU, intensive care unit, and the floor[10,11]; upper and lower limits may be customized based on the patient care area (e.g., OR, intensive care unit, floor); infusion concentrations should be standardized.
  - Connect infusions to the most proximal intravenous port.[16]
  - Standardize route-specific, color-coded tubing (yellow epidural, red arterial line), and label all infusion lines.[10,11]
  - Pass only 1 medication at a time in the sterile field; for all medications, check, label, and verify aloud by 2 persons; segregate topical or irrigation fluids (e.g., do not place in parenteral syringe).[10]
  - Ensure adequate venous access and safe administration of magnesium and oxytocin during transfer to the OR for emergency cesarean delivery.[23]
- Pharmacy:
  - Assign a pharmacist or pharmacists to support the OR or perioperative team; ensure that a pharmacist is available 24/7 for questions, that the pharmacist participates in educational activities, and that the OR pharmacist receives specialized education on fundamental OR concepts.[10,11]
  - Stock and manage anesthesia and other medication trays.[10]
  - Alert staff, especially ACPs, to changes in how drugs are supplied (e.g., new labels or concentrations)—one method of doing this is by adding alert labels on new drugs.[10]
  - Provide cognitive aids, rescue protocols, and infusion rate charts to ACPs.
- Governance:
  - Formalize the process of decision-making, implementing decisions, educating staff, and monitoring.[24]
  - Provide anesthesiology department representation on the medication safety committee, keeping in mind that crucial differences between anesthesia medications and those used elsewhere may warrant a separate anesthesia medication safety committee.[24]

Standardization and visual cues are important examples of system-based approaches to anesthesia medication safety. Standardization is a framework that provides recognizable patterns and should not always be interpreted as a single uniform approach for all areas within the OR or between the OR and non-OR areas. Standard medication setups can vary with the type of case (e.g., adult, child, neonate, open heart, or obstetric), and having more than one standard concentration is often necessary to meet patient care needs. ACPs identify the correct medication syringe by a number of factors—text, shape, size, color, and location—often with minimal cognitive processing. This observation may explain why Fasting and Gisvold[25] found that color-coded syringe labels alone did not eliminate syringe swap and that nearly all (27/28; 96%) syringe swaps occurred between syringes of the same size. Grigg and colleagues[26] created an anesthesia medication template (AMT) that defined a formal way of organizing and identifying medication syringes in the anesthesia workspace. In Phase 1 of the study, ACPs participated in simulated scenarios to evaluate the time to locate and complete scripted administrations of different medications in 2 emergency scenarios (anaphylaxis and laryngospasm), using the AMT and a control setup. All medication errors were dosing errors; the correct medication was administered every time. Surprisingly, there were fewer dosing errors when the AMT was used compared with the control setup at 2.4 (95% confidence interval [CI], 1.0–6.1) versus 10.4 (95% CI, 6.6–16.0) errors per 100 medication administrations. The authors proposed that the cognitive load theory may explain why reorganizing medication syringes with the AMT could help with dose calculation. Specifically, searching for the correct medication, calculating the correct dose, and converting the dose to a volume to administer has a lower processing requirement when the AMT is used compared with performing the same functions when the control setup is used. In Phase 2 of this study (implementation of the AMT in clinical practice), the number of medication errors related to the AMT (syringe swap, preparation, miscalculation, timing) decreased from 0.97 (95% CI, 0.64–1.48) pre-AMT implementation to 0.35 (95% CI, 0.17–0.70) errors per 100 anesthetics postimplementation. Other medication safety initiatives were initiated prior to AMT implementation and included reorganization of medication trays, medication practice guidelines with standard syringe sizes and concentrations, and a 2-provider infusion checklist to reduce infusion pump-related errors. The authors concluded that medication safety in the OR is a complex problem that will benefit from a multifaceted approach such as color coding, prefilled syringes, barcoding, and cognitive aids.[26]

Technology solutions that can promote medication safety and should be considered include systems that integrate technologies such as radio frequency identification and cloud-based software; automated barcode medication scanning with audible prompt and real-time medication identification; dose measurement and wireless communication with the electronic anesthesia record to document medication administration; or label generation from point-of-care barcode scan of a medication vial or ampule. Merry and colleagues[20] described the impacts on documentation and administration medication errors when a conventional medication system is replaced with a multimodal medication system. The multimodal medication system included (1) medication trays designed to promote a well-organized workspace and aseptic technique; (2) prefilled syringes for the most commonly used medications; (3) large, legible, color-coded medication labels; and (4) a barcode reader with auditory and visual verification before administration and real-time documentation in the anesthesia record. The conventional system included (1) standard medication tray/cart; (2) standard tray to hold syringes; (3) all medications prepared by ACP; and (4) manual documentation by ACP in anesthesia record. The mean error rate when using the multimodal system was 21% lower than when using the conventional system (mean error rate of 1 in 11.6 medication administrations with the conventional system versus 1 in 9.1 with the multimodal system). Furthermore, when the ACP complied with 2 key elements (scanning the medication barcode before administering and keeping the voice prompt active), the mean error rate was even lower (6.0 medication errors per 100 administrations when the ACP complied versus 9.7 per 100 administrations when the ACP did not comply with these 2 key elements). As with all system implementation initiatives, especially those that involve technology, early and continuous involvement of end users, full evaluation of pros and cons, a complete cost analysis, and a vendor site visit are recommended before proceeding.

Promotion of a nonpunitive culture with open disclosure is essential to encourage robust reporting, analysis, and interventions.[10,27] Medication errors that occur in the perioperative setting should be reported via the standard hospital adverse drug or medication event reporting system, AIMS, or Anesthesia Quality Institute Anesthesia Incident Reporting System.[28] A method should be in place for routine review of all reported events, as well as a process to monitor medication error trends and the impact of interventions. There should also be a process to determine the root cause and failure modes associated with significant or serious errors. Case review of serious errors should be routine practice within the anesthesiology department's quality assurance division, as well as through medication safety committees and formal presentations at departmental morbidity and mortality conferences when appropriate. Errors due to manufacturer labeling or packaging should be reported to the Food and Drug Administration via the MedWatch program (https://www.fda.gov/Safety/MedWatch/default.htm) and to the Institute for Safe Medicine Practices (https://www.ismp.org/report-medication-error). When appropriate, laboratory analysis of causative agents or concentrations of medications in specific products involved in an incident should be performed.

Incorporation of the culture of safe medication handling in the OR, safe worker behavior, and safe work environment should be included in a hospital or health system's patient safety goals. An interdisciplinary team, with significant representation from ACPs, should lead efforts to maintain and improve medication safety in the perioperative environment, focusing on system issues that have an opportunity for modification and improvement that would reduce the likelihood of a medication error by the ACP and OR staff. The team should:

1. Identify and document errors, adverse events, near misses, and high-alert practices.
2. Systematically review such events and conduct root cause analysis when appropriate.
3. Identify and correct hazardous conditions.
4. Define best practices by policy or guideline to prevent similar events in the future.
5. Provide staff education (simulation-based if possible).
6. Conduct ongoing monitoring to assess success of educational efforts and recent system or process changes.

The team should also prepare a report to present to upper management (e.g., quality and safety leadership or perioperative leadership) regarding significant events, as well as trends that have been identified. Follow-up should be in place for rapid-cycle feedback when breaches in practice or medication errors occur. This follow-up could include, but is not limited to, review by the perioperative pharmacist, anesthesiology quality assurance, medication safety committee, alert management, OR steering committee, and patient safety committee.

Contamination Issues. Pharmacists should participate in the institution's infection control department to ensure surgical services personnel and ACPs follow safe medication practices, such as aseptic technique when preparing, transferring (to sterile field), and administering medications; single medication withdrawal; and single patient administration of medications. The Anesthesia Patient Safety Foundation Consensus Recommendations for Improving Medication Safety in the Operating Room,[11] the Centers for Disease Control and Prevention and Safe Injection Practices Coalition One and Only Campaign,[29] the recommendations in the Standard Precautions section of the Centers for Disease Control and Prevention 2007 Guidelines for Isolation Precautions for Preventing the Transmission of Infectious Agents in Healthcare Settings,[30] the American Society of Anesthesiologists (ASA) Committee on Occupational Health Task Force on Infection Control Recommendations for Infection Control for the Practice of Anesthesiology (third edition),[31] American Association of Nurse Anesthetists Infection Control Guide for Certified Registered Nurse Anesthetists,[32] and Association of periOperative Registered Nurses perioperative standards and recommendations[33] are excellent resources. Pharmacists should share responsibility with ACPs and nurses for ensuring that all staff whose role may require preparation, handling, or administration of medications receive appropriate education to ensure that multiple patients do not receive medications from the same syringe, vial, or bag; single-use products are not used on multiple patients; aseptic technique is followed; and appropriate practices regarding contact precautions are in place. Anesthesia kits, trays, and carts, including ADCs and AACs, should be periodically cleaned and decontaminated. Institution-specific protocols should be followed when a patient with an infection such as *Clostridium difficile* undergoes surgery. Cleaning medication preparation areas such as the tops of anesthesia carts should also follow institutional policy. All medications should be disposed of according to institutional policy and local regulations. The pharmaceutical waste stream should also be determined in collaboration with the infection control department, as special handling may be required for waste associated with patients with contaminative diseases.

Controlled Substance Management and Surveillance

ACPs are unique in that they obtain and administer addictive substances, on a daily basis, to patients undergoing anesthesia, in order to provide analgesia (opioids, ketamine); blunt the stress response to intubation and surgical stimulation (opioids); induce general anesthesia (methohexital); and provide sedation, amnesia, and anxiolysis (benzodiazepines). Exposure and access to such addictive substances, familiarity with the pharmacology of these drugs, the relative ease of diverting small quantities for personal use, and a high-stress work environment are factors that contribute to substance use disorder (SUD) in ACPs.[34–36] Warner and colleagues[37] conducted a retrospective cohort study of physicians who began their training in U.S. anesthesiology residency programs from 1975 to 2009 to describe the incidence and outcomes of SUD among anesthesiology residents. The authors found that 0.86% of these anesthesiology residents had evidence of SUD during training, with a high risk of relapse and death. At least 11% of anesthesiology residents with evidence of SUD died of a cause directly related to SUD. The most common substance abuse category was intravenous opioids (57%), followed by alcohol (35%), marijuana or cocaine (21%), anesthetics/hypnotics (19%), and oral opioids (11%). Of the anesthetics/hypnotics, benzodiazepines were the most common substances used at the initial episode, followed by propofol, ketamine, and inhaled anesthetic agents. Although little research exists, other anesthesia care providers (e.g., CRNAs) and sedation nurses are also at risk. These providers have occupational exposure and access to highly addictive substances, can relatively easily divert small quantities for personal use, practice in remote settings, and may not fully appreciate the risks of experimenting with highly addictive substances.[38]

ASHP recently published guidelines to assist health systems in planning and implementing best practices for establishing a controlled substance diversion prevention program.[39] As with all controlled substances, anesthesia controlled substances must be:

- Managed in accordance with federal and state laws, as well as regulatory and compliance requirements.
- Accountable from the time the controlled substance is dispensed to (received by) the ACP to its final disposition (i.e., administration to patient, returned, or wasted), with amounts documented. The total amount administered, returned, and wasted must equal the total amount dispensed to (received by) the ACP. Although hand-offs of controlled substances are discouraged, a system should be in place to ensure retrievable documentation of all controlled substances handed off, should a hand-off be necessary.
- Under the direct physical control of the ACP or stored in a locked and secure location such that controlled substances are not accessible to unauthorized individuals.
- Disposed of in a manner that renders it nonretrievable—disposal systems that neutralize controlled substances on contact are preferred as these systems decrease the amount of controlled substances introduced into the environment, particularly in the water stream.

Historically, anesthesia controlled substances were dispensed to ACPs on a per-day or per-case basis. With increasing focus on diversion prevention, per-day dispensing of anesthesia controlled substances can no longer be recommended. Dispensing controlled substances on a per-case basis can be accomplished by manual dispensing from an OR pharmacy or automated dispensing from an ADC or AAC. Automated dispensing or pharmacy dispensing using an electronic controlled substances tracking tool is preferred to manual dispensing with paper records. Electronic data is more readily retrievable, allowing creation of scheduled and on-demand reports that may facilitate earlier detection of diversion. Having an AAC in every OR and procedure room (e.g., anesthetizing location) is preferred to a large ADC that services many ORs. A greater distance between the ADC and the OR room (or other point of care) can result in a provider obtaining:

1. More controlled substances than may be needed (because he or she cannot leave the OR room to obtain additional controlled substances).
2. Multiple controlled substances for multiple patients at the start of the day (due to rapid turnover of cases).
3. Controlled substances long before the start of a case without the ability to securely store them until needed.

Having an AAC at every anesthetizing location facilitates the ACP obtaining only the quantity needed at the time it is needed and allows for creation of a dedicated secure pocket or bin for storage of controlled substances when the ACP is not physically present. If controlled substances are obtained from an ADC or pharmacy and there is a need to temporarily store the controlled substances (e.g., when a case is delayed), options may include a secure (locked) drawer or box in the anesthesia cart with authorized access (e.g., badge swipe, access tracked) and a secure bin or drawer in the anesthesia cart that locks with a key. If a key is used, a procedure must be in place to track keys, secure keys, and change locks if necessary.

Although ADC and AAC manufacturers promote enhanced controlled substances accountability in the OR setting, anesthesia controlled substances discrepancies will occur with the use of this technology. In 2007, Vigoda and colleagues[40] reported reconciliation errors between the pharmacy information management system (PIMS) (e.g., dispensing and waste records from ADCs) and the AIMS (e.g., administration record) in 15% of cases. Errors occurred in both systems, with most (>75%) errors being clerical (e.g., error in recording amount wasted or amount administered). Factors that contributed to errors included the need for double documentation (ACP must document in the AIMS [amount administered] and in the PIMS [amount administered or wasted]), as well as the ACP not receiving real-time feedback. Epstein and colleagues[41] also compared PIMS and AIMS documentation and found a comparable reconciliation error rate for anesthesia controlled substances (15.8% of cases), with most errors also being clerical. Shortening the feedback time to next-day reporting decreased the reconciliation error rate to 8.8% of cases. When feedback was shortened further to near real time (same day), the error rate dropped to 5.2% of cases. Similarly, when Brenn and colleagues[42] compared AIMS and PIMS records during a 1-month audit period, the mean number of discrepancies per ACP was 5.7.

Pharmacy should reconcile all anesthesia controlled substances. Reconciliation should be timely, with prompt notification to the ACP if a discrepancy is discovered. Resolution should occur within 24 hr. When circumstances do not allow for resolution within 24 hr, the time period for resolution should not exceed 72 hr. If a discrepancy cannot be resolved, it is reported to the drug diversion compliance officer or team as well as appropriate internal anesthesia team member(s). If the loss is deemed significant following an investigation, it is reported to the Drug Enforcement Administration and the state licensing board, if required by state law. Discrepancy trend reports should be prepared and reviewed at least quarterly. A trend of poor documentation or unresolved discrepancies should be reviewed for possible diversion. Progressive discipline is enforced when a trend of unresolved discrepancies is identified, even if each loss is a small amount.[39,43]

Behaviors more specific to an addicted ACP who is diverting a drug from the workplace include:

1. Removing the contents of syringes, vials, or ampules and replacing them with saline.
2. Documenting the anesthetic was opioid-based but administered an inhaled anesthetic agent and a beta blocker.
3. Diverting waste.

An addicted ACP can be extraordinarily attentive at work and rarely put patients at risk, likely because maintaining their job, with its close proximity to their source of drugs, is so important to them. ACPs know the signs and symptoms of addiction, generally have the means to hide them, and are psychologically capable of developing sophisticated denial strategies.[44] Therefore, a comprehensive and interdisciplinary approach to diversion surveillance for anesthesia is necessary and should include the following strategies:

- *Provide controlled substances in ready-to-use concentrations and volumes.* If a ready-to-use concentration is not available (e.g., morphine, hydromorphone, remifentanil, or fentanyl for pediatric patients), pharmacy should provide such controlled substances in a ready-to-use concentration whenever possible to limit dilution by the ACP at the point of care. Providing controlled substances in ready-to-use concentrations will help to standardize dilutions, facilitate controlled substances reconciliation and analysis of waste, and reduce the likelihood of an error by the ACP when preparing a dilution of a high-risk medication. Using appropriate volume size minimizes waste and risk for diversion.
- *Pharmacy reconciliation of all anesthesia controlled substances and records.* Controlled substances removed by an ACP for a cancelled case, after case completion, or from a different location than the scheduled case must be accounted for (e.g., returned unused or documented as administration to a different patient who was cared for by that ACP as a result of an OR schedule change).
- *Regular review of atypical usage reports.* Atypical usage, such as escalating activity and excessive waste, should be regularly reviewed. Reports should compare the amount of drug (e.g., fentanyl) removed over time (per case, month, or quarter) by individual ACPs with peers for similar types of cases, as well as the amount of a drug wasted over time by individual ACPs with peers' waste for similar types of cases.[45–47] While such reports are useful screening tools, manual review of transactions and other documentation (e.g., type of anesthesia, type of surgery) is necessary to properly evaluate the likelihood of the outlying activity constituting diversion. Expert knowledge is necessary to determine reasonable ranges for various types of procedures, as well as typical activity by ACPs for handling and administration of controlled substances.[46] Building a close partnership between pharmacy and anesthesiology is critical to ensure that the screening tools, methods, and metrics are appropriate for the institution, while avoiding bias and conflict. A "one size fits all" approach cannot be used since anesthesiology departments are vastly different in the number of ACPs (<10 to >400), ACP status (full time, part time, providing services at more than one institution, trainee), type of procedure or patients cared for (specialist or generalist), and employer (institution, anesthesia group contracted to provide services to the institution, locum tenens company that provides physician staffing services).
- *Waste content is verified by the pharmacy on a random basis and when suspect.* On a random basis and when suspect (e.g., diversion is suspected, syringe returned under unusual circumstances), waste should be returned to the pharmacy to verify content. Analysis of the contents may be done with the use of a refractometer standard or a spectrophotometric devices that measure the refractive index of a substance relative to a reference standard (e.g., the dispensed product).[45,48] Many refractometers are relatively inexpensive and easy to use. Such analysis has its limitations; however, the refractive index of undiluted fentanyl is identical to that of water, and the diluent can affect the refractive reading of a diluted drug. If these limitations are not known to ACPs, an inexpensive refractometer may provide an economical first line of defense.[48] Although the cost is significantly higher, there are machines that provide a more accurate refractive index measurement to detect if the controlled substances waste does not match that of the reference standard. Such machines are small enough to house in the pharmacy, provide real-time results to reference standards, and maintain results in

a searchable database. Suspect or random syringes may be definitively analyzed internally or sent to an outside laboratory for analysis. If a controlled substance is sent to a laboratory for analysis, a clear chain of custody for the sample, as well as any required internal standard, must be maintained.

- *Staff education.* Education on SUD is required annually by Graduate Medical Education for anesthesiology residency training programs. The American Association of Nurse Anesthetists strongly recommends every ACP view the *Wearing Masks* video series and other videos on SUD in anesthesia.[49] The ASA Committee on Occupational Health posts SUD information on their website, such as key articles, a link to the *Wearing Masks* series, an SUD curriculum, and more.[50] ACPs and other healthcare workers authorized to access or handle controlled substances (e.g., OR nurses who may obtain an opioid for a surgeon to administer to the patient) should be trained and competent in controlled substances policies, procedures, and regulatory requirements.[39]

In the early 1990s and in response to several episodes of fentanyl diversion, the Department of Anesthesiology at the Mayo Clinic in Rochester, Minnesota, created a comprehensive system to reduce the incidence of diversion of anesthesia controlled substances.[51] The system included (1) ADCs in the OR, (2) secure return bins to collect waste for analysis, (3) random analysis of waste, (4) reconciliation of AIMS and PIMS records, (5) investigation of discrepancies (reconciliation errors) until resolved, and (6) frequent educational sessions for ACPs and OR staff on the risk of addiction and diversion. If diversion was suspected, all waste returned by the individual in question was assayed until diversion was confirmed or disproved. In the years following implementation of this improved and comprehensive system, the frequency of anesthesia controlled substances diversion dramatically decreased (unpublished data, Keith Berge, MD, Department of Anesthesiology, Mayo Clinic, June 7, 2012).[51]

Although provider pre-employment urine drug testing is common, random (suspicionless) drug testing is controversial. Although a majority of academic anesthesiology department chairs favor random testing, there are obstacles that require thoughtful consideration before such a program can be implemented.[52] These considerations include the logistics of the testing process itself, legal ramifications, costs, what tests to include in the panel (e.g., whether or not to limit the panel to only the drugs to which the ACP has occupational exposure), how to manage a positive or reasonably suspicious test result, risk of loss of privacy or damage to employees' reputation, and how to manage employees who refuse testing.[53–55] An article by Rice and colleagues presents possible approaches to implement random drug testing among ACPs.[55]

Preoperative and Postanesthesia Care Unit Order Review

Pharmacists have the ability to help guide practice and ensure safe medication therapy for patients in the postoperative period via prospective order review. The goal should be prospective order review of all PACU orders by pharmacists. Analgesics and antiemetics represent the majority of PACU medication orders.[56] Pharmacists should be involved in developing or reviewing PACU order sets (e.g., dose, dosing frequency, maximum dose, opioid hierarchy, rescue antiemetic dose and hierarchy) and performing medication histories to avoid unintended discontinuation or alteration of chronic medications when transitioning from the PACU to the surgical floor.

Provision of Drug Information and Education

The perioperative pharmacist should provide timely and accurate drug information proactively for known needs as well as in response to professional inquiries. The perioperative pharmacist should have ready access to electronic resources such as a drug information handbook and a clinical resource tool as well as journals and textbooks. Scientific journals are the source for practice guidelines, meta-analyses, systematic reviews, and randomized controlled trials that support recommendations. References should be current, easily accessible, and provide information in the following areas: pharmacology, pharmacokinetics, dosages, adverse effects, formulations, administration, incompatibilities, indications for use, drug interactions, and use during pregnancy and lactation. The perioperative pharmacist may also prepare a newsletter, make available articles of interest, and provide staff education. Participation in journal clubs and other educational activities (e.g., morbidity and mortality conference) is encouraged. A pharmacist should be available to answer questions that arise when the perioperative pharmacist is not available (e.g., off shifts, weekends). Ideally, a dedicated cross-coverage pharmacy team should provide services to the perioperative area. If that is not feasible, then other pharmacists should be trained in basic perioperative skills that enable them to answer questions.

Performance Improvement and Quality Assurance

Performance improvement and quality assurance are critical to providing a high level of patient care. Quality assurance is also linked to healthcare reimbursement and regulatory requirements.[57,58] An interdisciplinary approach to implement and maintain a robust quality assurance system, including medication management, is recommended for the perioperative environment. Training in methodologies to systematically improve processes and reduce waste (e.g., Six Sigma, lean principles) is helpful to ensure that the initiative's scope and stakeholders are appropriate, changes are well planned and implemented, and change is sustained.[59–61] Outlined below are activities in which participation by a pharmacist is considered essential.

Interdisciplinary Committees. The pharmacy leadership should promote, provide, and include a pharmacy representative on perioperative interdisciplinary committees charged with reviewing and improving safety, processes, culture, and productivity if medications are involved. This representative (e.g., pharmacy manager, coordinator, team lead, or designated pharmacist covering perioperative service area) should be an active participant to promote proper medication use in the perioperative area.

Medication-Use Guidelines, Protocols, and Medication-Use Evaluation. Evidence-based guidelines and protocols are important tools to guide clinical practice and appropriate use of high-cost medications. Pharmacists should lead efforts to develop such guidelines and protocols in the perioperative environment. Once approved, institutions using an AIMS with clinical decision support can create alerts or reminders to improve adherence (e.g., reminder to administer the prophylactic antibiotic if one has not been recorded or a reminder to administer prophylactic antiemetics to a patient at high risk for developing postoperative nausea and vomiting).[62–64] Medication-use guidelines, protocols, and medication-use evaluation may be conducted to determine compliance with institutional protocols or restrictions and, possibly, impact on patient outcomes. Audits should be ongoing to ensure sustainability. High-cost, high-risk, or high-use medications such as recombinant factor VII, albumin, topical hemostats, liposomal bupivacaine, and intravenous acetaminophen are examples of perioperative medications that may be selected for evaluation.

Waste Reduction. ORs generate an estimated 20% to 30% of hospital waste, primarily due to volatile anesthetics, pharmaceuticals, packing, and supplies. With a goal of greening the OR, the ASA recommends that ORs reduce, reuse, recycle, and redesign.[65–68] To identify where medication waste may be occurring, the AIMS or electronic medical record may be used to determine usage, and compounding software may be used to determine compounding productivity or volume. Good relationships between surgeons, anesthesia, OR nursing, and pharmacy staff will assist in opening communication about strategies that are likely to be successful in reducing waste. For information about hazardous pharmaceutical waste, the reader is referred to the Environmental Protection Agency website.[69]

Culture. Culture has been an increasing focus within organizations, because it plays a vital role in how employees accept and manage change. Using an interdisciplinary approach, the perioperative team should establish a culture of identifying, analyzing, resolving, and monitoring change. Although this culture should be encouraged in the workplace, it starts with education in the classroom setting. Ideally, institutions would provide formal team training in the perioperative setting that includes pharmacy staff. As previously mentioned, an important factor to improve culture is the establishment of a just culture around medication safety reporting and sharing of lessons learned. Tools exist to measure the culture of safety and should be used and shared with the affected teams.[70]

Leadership Duties and Professional Service

Depending on the health system's organizational structure and the size and scope of the OR, a pharmacy manager or supervisor may be assigned to oversee the perioperative pharmacy service. However, many perioperative pharmacy services or pharmacy satellites will use frontline staff and designate those staff pharmacists to assist with leadership tasks for pharmacy services in the perioperative area. The ASHP Statement on Leadership as a Professional Obligation asserts that all pharmacists have a professional obligation to serve as leaders in the safe and effective use of medications and encourages those practitioners to advance patient care and strengthen the pharmacy profession by embracing the responsibility to exert leadership in their practices.[71] ASHP maintains that frontline staff must display leadership each time they enter the workplace and advocates that pharmacists should take personal responsibility for leadership in the medication-use process.[71] The perioperative pharmacy management or designated perioperative pharmacist may be tasked with the role to lead as well as oversee the delivery of services by the perioperative pharmacy. The role should include responsibilities to both the main pharmacy department as well as perioperative areas. Maintaining involvement in both departments permits the perioperative pharmacist to be a liaison between groups to facilitate joint efforts.

The perioperative pharmacist leader should collaborate with healthcare professionals in all areas within operative services to develop and monitor medication-use systems that promote safe and effective medication use. By this collaboration, the practitioners can ensure that medication use in the OR is evidence based, cost effective, and in compliance with national guidelines. The perioperative pharmacist can take a lead role in ensuring these collaborations occur. To accomplish this task, the perioperative pharmacy lead should understand the OR culture and practices, work effectively with interdisciplinary teams, and recognize the medication needs of the providers and the surgical patient. In addition, the perioperative pharmacist should ensure correct handling of medication waste to meet EPA hazardous waste handling requirements.

Goals for perioperative pharmacy should be developed annually. The pharmacy lead should seek input in establishing goals for the service from other perioperative departments. The goals should be aligned with the main pharmacy department and the hospital or health system's goals.

If the perioperative pharmacist is assigned leadership responsibilities, pharmacy administration will need to provide support that will allow the pharmacist to participate in various functions, such as committee meetings, project implementations, guidelines development, financial reviews, educational endeavors, regulatory and compliance assignments, operational duties, and teaching or research efforts.

It is important for the perioperative pharmacist to stay current with new and emerging trends. Involvement within the profession through participation in local, state, and national professional organizations will be beneficial. Perioperative pharmacists should also consider involvement with other professional organizations such as ASA, Association of periOperative Registered Nurses, or the American Society of PeriAnesthesia Nurses, which may facilitate collaboration leading to further development of the perioperative pharmacy practice and the role of the pharmacist as an important member of perioperative services.

Financial Management

Financial performance of the OR pharmacy should be managed in accordance with the requirements set forth by pharmacy administration and the institution's finance department. If perioperative pharmacy services are provided through an OR pharmacy satellite, it should be determined whether the satellite will be considered a separate accounting unit or part of the overall pharmacy budget. If the OR pharmacy is a separate cost center, the OR pharmacist leader may be assigned to provide input or to oversee the following:

- Revenue and expenses (particularly expenses such as drugs, supplies, technology leases, and salary and benefits costs)[12]
- Budget development and analysis of budget variances
- Equipment requests and acquisition
- Volume projections
- Justification of new personnel according to workload productivity standards

Drug cost for anesthesia and surgery may encompass a sizeable portion of the pharmacy's drug budget. Chernin found that anesthetic drugs were 10% to 13% of the overall pharmacy department's drug budget. The author noted that pharmacy is held responsible for the budgetary effect of the cost of the anesthetic drugs as well as the patient outcomes resulting from the use of these drugs.[72] Therefore, much of the financial oversight needed for the perioperative pharmacy service will include audits and analysis of medication use to assure appropriateness and timely capture of charges and expenses.

There are several factors, such as price and use, which can drive growth in overall drug expenditures. The physician and nursing groups may be able to anticipate their future medication needs and new service development, such as adding surgery specialists, opening additional ORs, and implementing new procedures that may increase the cost of drugs. It is important to collaborate with other leaders in the OR to plan and prioritize strategies focused on cost effective use of medications (e.g., just-in-time dispensing of high-cost medications or determining the most appropriate sterile product preparation and dispensing method for select medications; in-house versus outsourced compounding; bedside prepared or commercial product use).

The perioperative pharmacist should keep apprised of the pipeline of potential new drugs used in anesthesia or surgery, and whether the new drug has the capacity to reduce length of stay, decrease use of other drugs, or offset the cost by other means. The perioperative pharmacist should assist with or directly manage addition of new perioperative medications to the formulary. Safe handling and disposal of drugs such as chemotherapy or hazardous waste should be managed according to any special handling needs.

Pharmacy benchmarking systems or best practice models that accurately assess and compare the impact of pharmacy services on patient outcomes, staffing, and costs can be valuable tools for pharmacy and organizational leadership.

Desirable Roles of the Perioperative Pharmacist

Desirable roles of the perioperative pharmacist may be considered best practices but depend on the level of practice experience of the perioperative pharmacist and the available resources. Whatever pharmacy services are able to be provided should be consistent and available to all patients in the perioperative setting. Desirable roles of the perioperative pharmacist include:

- Preoperative medication history/medication reconciliation/transitions of care
- Participation in PACU huddles/rounds
- Care of boarded patients
- Discharge prescription service
- Participation in resuscitation
- Education
- Research and other scholarly activities
- Consideration for inclusion on the Pharmacy and Therapeutics (P&T) Committee
- Quality and safety initiatives[63,73–76]

Preoperative Medication History, Medication Reconciliation, and Transitions of Care

It is important to obtain an accurate medication history (prescription and nonprescription) of the patient to identify allergies and medications the patient is currently taking or has recently stopped taking that may affect their perioperative care. The medication history may be taken while the patient is located in the preoperative unit and getting prepared for surgery or, preferentially, during a preoperative screening visit or call that occurs prior to the scheduled procedure. A preoperative medication history review by a pharmacist (or trained technician or student pharmacist with pharmacist oversight) with a mechanism for follow-up has been shown to reduce the number of missed doses of chronic medications, postoperatively.[77,78] Furthermore, patients on chronic opioids can be identified prior to surgery to allow time to develop an appropriate pre-, intra- and postoperative pain management plan.[79] With sufficient time (months) and support, patients identified as high risk for uncontrolled postoperative pain, respiratory depression, or other complications from opioids may benefit from an appropriate downward taper of their opioid dose prior to surgery.[80] One area for particular scrutiny would be any medications the patient may be on preoperatively that could interfere with neuraxial procedures, including but not limited to low-molecular-weight heparins, heparin, warfarin, or direct thrombin inhibitors. Additional populations at high risk for anticoagulation– antiplatelet drug interaction should receive pharmacist review for medication reconciliation. Familiarity with the American Society of Regional Anesthesia guidelines is necessary.[81] Prior to or at discharge, pharmacists are well positioned to perform patient counseling and medication reconciliation and assist with medication management at home during recovery.[82]

Participation in PACU Huddles and Rounds

The pharmacist has a unique opportunity to increase visibility and serve as the medication safety specialist during a critical transition period, from the OR to the PACU and from the PACU to the floor. During this transition, decisions are made regarding the postoperative pain, nausea, and surgery-related infection therapy, along with continued chronic (home) medication therapy. Studies have shown the impact on reducing preventable adverse drug events by including pharmacist participation in medical rounds in both the general and critical care environments.[83,84] Patient rounding should be explored in the postoperative setting as well. Interdisciplinary PACU rounds can provide a definitive plan of care and increase bedside education, as well as identify systems and processes that can be improved.[85] Pharmacist participation in rounding on every PACU patient may not be feasible; however, development of criteria to identify high-risk patients in PACU may be beneficial in optimizing medication usage.

Care of Boarded Patients

Patients accommodated overnight in the PACU area should ideally be treated as an inpatient and have an inpatient status from the admitting department. Medications should be dispensed according to a predetermined patient location distinct from the PACU so that pharmacy services can identify them as boarded patients separate from general PACU patients. Depending on the institution's workflow and processes, the perioperative pharmacist may or may not be assigned as the caregiver for these patients. If a profiled ADC is not physically present, medications can be centrally distributed in patient-specific packaging and delivered to a secure location in the PACU. Depending on how long a patient is boarded in PACU, pharmacy services may include medication reconciliation, order verification, pharmacokinetic monitoring, antimicrobial stewardship, anticoagulant monitoring, i.v. to oral (PO) conversion monitoring, discharge medication counseling, and cardiac arrest response. Review of high-risk patients being admitted should also include a hand-off of care.

Discharge Prescription Service

The process of discharge following surgery can often be rushed and fraught with opportunities for misinterpretation by providers, families, and patients. Additionally, obtaining prescriptions for a surgical patient after leaving the facility can be challenging for the patient and family, especially if they traveled a long distance. For outpatients, improving transitions of care from a PACU setting to home and reducing delays in PACU discharge can be accomplished by a collaborative effort between surgeons, PACU, and an outpatient pharmacy facility able to provide timely discharge medication dispensing. Ideally, discharge prescriptions should be planned for at the surgical preoperative visit or at the time of surgery to allow for the necessary processing time.[82] Identification of outpatient and short-stay (<24 hr) patients that may require a discharge prescription should be done at the beginning of the day. Communication between an outpatient pharmacy facility and the PACU can facilitate obtaining prescription insurance information, prescriptions, and a fast-track filling procedure in the pharmacy. Ideally, the majority of prescriptions are processed by the time the patient reaches Phase II of recovery.

An effort should be made to standardize medications prescribed, such as analgesics and antimicrobial agents. In addition, encouraging electronic prescribing of medications, including electronic prescribing of controlled substances (unless mandated by state law) can improve throughput. Discharge prescriptions written for medications that require prior authorization or are difficult to obtain in an outpatient setting should be discouraged. With early intervention and coordination of services, the pharmacist can assure that the patient's discharge medications are accurate, counsel the patient on their new regimen, and ensure delivery of medications at bedside prior to patient discharge from the facility. Provision of a list of nearby 24-hour pharmacies should be provided if the patient is discharged after an internal pharmacy is closed or the patient desires to have their prescriptions filled outside of the institution.

Participation in Resuscitation

It is recommended that pharmacists practicing in the perioperative setting be certified in advanced cardiac life support (ALCS) and pediatric advanced life support (PALS). At a minimum, pharmacists should have a practical knowledge of cardiopulmonary response and drugs used in resuscitation efforts. If feasible, pharmacists should assist in arrest response in individual ORs, the preoperative area, and the PACU area until the patient's condition has stabilized. Medications should be prepared either in a syringe or in an intravenous infusion with standardized concentrations. Pharmacists should be familiar with the infusion devices and drug libraries used in the perioperative areas as well as crash cart locations and content. Finally, pharmacists and other healthcare providers (including nurses) should be regularly trained to recognize and respond to other emergencies that may occur in the perioperative area, such as malignant hyperthermia and local anesthetic systemic toxicity. Dantrolene and lipid emulsion (respectively, for treatment of malignant hyperthermia and local anesthetic systemic toxicity) must be readily available in the OR and other areas where medications that may trigger these emergencies are used.[86–89] For specific recommendations, refer to the Malignant Hyperthermia Association of the United States recommendations.[87]

Education

Educational needs and opportunities can be variable and extensive in the OR. In addition to having a working knowledge of commonly used medications and the medication-use process, the perioperative pharmacist should receive specialized education about the OR environment. The perioperative pharmacist can provide education for pharmacists, technicians, students, and pharmacy residents. Topics of interest include the perioperative medication-use process, medication safety, practice guidelines, medications primarily used in the OR setting (e.g., inhaled, intravenous, and local anesthetics; intravenous opioids; neuromuscular blocking agents and reversal agents; and antiemetics), aseptic technique, regulatory requirements, drug diversion prevention and surveillance. Providing such educational topics for nurses, ACPs, and surgeons solidifies the perioperative pharmacist as a medication expert and should be offered on an ongoing basis.

Research and Other Scholarly Activities

The perioperative pharmacy should support an organization's research mission. Pharmacists are in a strong position to identify research questions, write protocols, foster resident research, assist with study randomization, provide study drug or placebo, and document study-related information. Pharmacists can be involved as the principal investigator, co- or subinvestigator with other investigators, or as the pharmacist of record for the study. Pharmacists, students, and residents should be encouraged to participate in research or other projects (e.g., process or quality improvement) as much as possible to improve efficiency, safety, or outcomes; reduce cost; and foster future collaborative endeavors.

P&T Committee

The P&T committee is responsible for managing the formulary system, as well as review and revision of medication-use policies. For medications used primarily by ACPs or intraoperatively by surgeons, the perioperative pharmacist should participate in developing, implementing, and monitoring guidelines on criteria for use and educating users in the perioperative setting on pertinent portions of medication-use policies when possible. Although patient safety issues are incorporated in the P&T committee's decision-making process, the unique medication-use process in the OR may not be fully appreciated by P&T committee members who rely on those with more expertise to incorporate appropriate safety strategies for the perioperative setting.

Quality and Safety Initiatives

In today's healthcare environment, there are many issues related to quality and safety in the perioperative setting, including external pressures, technology integration (advancements and constraints), human factors, and process improvement. Anesthesia departments often have a quality assurance committee to evaluate the current state and determine how to improve processes in the future. Pharmacists can provide valuable contributions to improvement efforts, particularly ones that involve medications (e.g., standardization of medication trays and concentrations, safe injection and administration practices, or optimal ways to provide a drug, especially when that drug is in short supply).

Competency

Pharmacists. To make effective clinical contributions, the pharmacist should become familiar with all medications used in the perioperative setting, including those used by ACPs and surgeons (e.g., contrast media, dyes, topical hemostats, irrigations). There is little focus on intraoperative medications in pharmacy school curricula, and residency programs do not consistently offer training in the perioperative arena.[90] Therefore, expertise is often acquired by self-motivated learning. Ongoing review of surgical and anesthesia literature, observation of surgery and anesthesia procedures, attendance at anesthesia and surgery conferences, presentation of assigned topics or journal clubs, and direct involvement in patient care will all contribute to the pharmacist's knowledge. In addition, the perioperative pharmacist should have a working knowledge of relevant regulatory requirements, accreditation bodies, National Patient Safety Goals, and quality initiatives.

Pharmacy Technicians. Typical activities performed by pharmacy technicians in a satellite pharmacy under the supervision of the pharmacist are drug distribution, handling of controlled substances, sterile drug preparation, drug ordering and restocking, orientation and training of new staff, and quality assurance activities. For routine accuracy-checking activities (e.g., anesthesia medication trays), a tech-check-tech process may be validated and implemented where permitted by state law. Use of barcode or radio frequency identification-based tray checking technology can add additional accuracy to the process.[91] Barcode scanning technology also allows the technician to restock ADCs and anesthesia workstations independently of a pharmacist check, where permitted by law.[92]

Pharmacy technicians assigned to the OR satellite pharmacy should become certified by passing an accredited, national exam (ASHP recommends the Pharmacy Technician Certification Exam) and should receive specialized training about the OR environment to prepare them for this role. Technician training and experience should include parenteral drug preparation, drug distribution procedures, anesthesia and OR record interpretation (if doing manual billing from anesthesia record), and controlled substances record-keeping. Specialized training should include the following areas:

1. Procedures unique to the OR environment, including special apparel (e.g. scrubs, caps, masks, foot covers), restricted movements in areas within OR suites, and infection control guidelines.
2. Roles of personnel in the OR and who may handle medications.
3. OR terminology, including abbreviations and acronyms that may be used when OR staff communicates with the pharmacy.
4. Drug classes, indications for use, and proper handling of drugs routinely used in OR (e.g., special packaging, preservative requirements for spinal and epidural drugs, infusion concentrations).
5. Controlled substances procedures.
6. Emergency medications.
7. Role in the OR and OR pharmacy.

An orientation checklist, workflow sheets, and task lists are helpful tools. As with pharmacists, an OR pharmacy technician training module would be a helpful tool to provide a consistent baseline knowledge level for technicians. If a pharmacy technician career ladder is in place in the institution, an examination evaluating this knowledge base may be useful in facilitating advancement to this specialized position.

Looking to the Future: the Perioperative Surgical Home and Enhanced Recovery After Surgery

The goal of a patient-centered medical home is to improve health and delivery of care and reduce cost. The perioperative surgical home (PSH) is a counterpart to the patient-centered medical home and is carried out through a physician-led interdisciplinary and team-based system of coordinated care that assists the patient through the surgical experience.[93] With improvements in the perioperative process, the PSH can have shared savings and incentive payments for achieving quality measures. The PSH model ensures communication with surgical patients early in the process, which facilitates reducing unrealistic expectations and ensures that patients are educated in decision-making so they can participate in the process. With less variability in perioperative care, shared decision-making, and patient-centered care, it is anticipated that a change to a PSH model would reduce duplicative or unneeded tests, delays, length of stay, and complications.[94]

Similar to the PSH, enhanced recovery after surgery (ERAS) is an evidence-based, multimodal, interdisciplinary approach to the care of the patient throughout the entire surgical experience. Components of ERAS may include carbohydrate drinks 2 hr prior to surgery (rather than overnight fasting), minimally invasive surgical approaches (rather than large incisions and open procedures), goal-directed i.v. fluid management (rather than large volumes of i.v. fluid), no drains or early removal of drains and tubes, early mobilization, and starting food and drinks on postoperative day 0 (the day of surgery). Adherence to ERAS protocols have resulted in 30% to 50% reductions in length of hospital stay, with similar reductions in complications, as well as lower costs and readmission rates when compared with traditional care of the surgical patient.[95]

With the PSH and ERAS team, the perioperative pharmacist can be involved in protocol development as well as identifying and caring for patients who may be at high risk for readmission or anticipated to have challenging postoperative pain or anticoagulation management. Pharmacists may also assist with medication reconciliation at admission, identifying high-risk drugs, polypharmacy, disease or drug interactions, and opioid-tolerant or chronic pain patients, whose postoperative pain management is often quite challenging. However, the more important impact of pharmacist involvement may be during the coordination and transition of care at discharge. Pharmacists can evaluate the discharge medications along with the prior-to-admission chronic medications and the inpatient medication list to determine appropriateness, confirm omissions and deletions, and follow up with the patient following discharge to answer questions and assess whether the patient is experiencing any difficulties with the discharge medication regimen.

Conclusion

Pharmacists responsible for services to the perioperative area should be knowledgeable in OR practice, the OR medication-use process, regulatory requirements, and medications that are administered perioperatively. By using this knowledge and working in close partnership with OR staff (e.g., ACPs, nurses, and surgeons), pharmacists are well positioned to optimize medication processes and safety in the perioperative setting. Pharmacists are also well equipped to perform or oversee medication histories and make recommendations, provide discharge medication counseling, participate in in PACU huddles and rounds, and perform other beneficial activities.

References

1. Keicher PA, McAllister JC. Comprehensive pharmaceutical services in the surgical suite and recovery room. *Am J Health-Syst Pharm.* 1985; 42:2454–62.
2. American Society of Health-System Pharmacists. ASHP technical assistance bulletin on surgery and anesthesiology pharmaceutical services. *Am J Health-Syst Pharm.* 1991; 48:319–25.
3. American Society of Health-System Pharmacists. ASHP statement on telepharmacy. *Am J Health-Syst Pharm.* 2017; 74:e236–41.
4. American Society of Health-System Pharmacists. ASHP guidelines: minimum standard for pharmacies in hospitals. *Am J Health-Syst Pharm.* 2013; 70:1619–30.
5. Food and Drug Administration. Guidance for FDA staff and industry: marketed unapproved drugs – compliance policy guide (September 2011). www.fda.gov/downloads/Drugs/GuidanceCompliance RegulatoryInformation/Guidances/UCM070290.pdf (accessed 2019 Feb 14).
6. American Association of Nurse Anesthetists. Negative impact of anesthesia drug shortages lessened through improved communication efforts, survey data reveal (May 7, 2013). https://www.aana.com/docs/default-source/fga-aana-com-web-documents-(all)/2013-drug_shortages.pdf?sfvrsn=3f5d49b1_4 (accessed 2018 May 24).
7. Anesthesia Quality Institute. Anesthesia Incident Reporting System. https://www.aqihq.org/airsintro.aspx (accessed 2019 Feb 14).
8. Murray C, Rycek W, Johnson D et al. Management of drug shortages in the perioperative setting. *Pharm Purch Prod.* 2013; 10:12.
9. American Society of Health-System Pharmacists. ASHP guidelines on managing drug product shortages in hospitals and health systems. *Am J Health-Syst Pharm.* 2018; 75:e593–601.
10. Wahr JA, Abernathy JH 3rd, Lazarra EH et al. Medication safety in the operating room: literature and expert-based recommendations. *Br J Anaesth.* 2017; 118:32–43.
11. Eichhorn JH. APSF hosts medication safety conference: consensus group defines challenges and opportunities for improved practice (2010). https://www.apsf.org/article/apsf-hosts-medication-safety-conference/ (accessed 2019 Feb 14).
12. Jelacic S, Craddick K, Nair BG et al. Relative costs of anesthesiologist prepared, hospital pharmacy prepared and outsourced anesthesia drugs. *J Clin Anesth.* 2017; 36:178–83.
13. American Society of Health-System Pharmacists. ASHP guidelines on the safe use of automated dispensing devices. *Am J Health-Syst Pharm.* 2010; 67:483–90.
14. American Society of Anesthesiologists. ASA statement on security of medications in the operating room. https://www.asahq.org/standards-and-guidelines/statement-on-security-of-medications-in-the-operating-room (accessed 2019 Feb 14).
15. Kane-Gill SL, Dasta JF, Buckley MS et al. Clinical practice guideline: safe medication use in the ICU. *Crit Care Med.* 2017; 45:e877–915.
16. Nanji KC, Patel A, Shaikh S et al. Evaluation of perioperative medication errors and adverse drug events. *Anesthesiology.* 2016; 124:25–34.
17. Lobaugh LMY, Martin LD, Schleelein LE et al. Medication errors in pediatric anesthesia: a report from the wake up safe quality improvement initiative. *Anesth Analg.* 2017; 125:936–42.
18. Cullen DJ, Bates DW, Small SD et al. The incident reporting system does not detect adverse drug events: a problem for quality improvement. *Jt Comm J Qual Improv.* 1995; 21:541–8.

19. Webster CS, Merry AF, Larsson L et al. The frequency and nature of drug administration error during anaesthesia. *Anaesth Intensive Care.* 2001; 29:494–500.
20. Merry AF, Webster CS, Hannam J et al. Multimodal system designed to reduce errors in recording and administration of drugs in anaesthesia: prospective randomized clinical evaluation. *BMJ.* 2011; 343:D55443.
21. Chen DW, Chase VJ, Burkhardt ME et al. Using human factors design principles and industrial engineering methods to improve accuracy and speed of drug selection with medication trays. *Jt Comm J Qual Patient Saf.* 2016; 42:473–7.
22. American Society of Anesthesiologists. Statement on labeling of pharmaceuticals for use in anesthesiology (October 28, 2015). https://www.asahq.org/standards-and-guidelines/statement-on-labeling-of-pharmaceuticals-for-use-in-anesthesiology (accessed 2019 Feb 14).
23. Kacmar RM, Mhyre JM. Obstetric anesthesia patient safety: practices to ensure adequate venous access and safe drug administration during transfer to the operating room for emergency cesarean delivery (October 2015). https://www.apsf.org/newsletters/html/2015/Oct/06_OBtransport.htm (accessed 2019 Feb 14).
24. Merry AF, Shipp DH, Lowinger JS. The contribution of labelling to safe medication administration in anaesthetic practice. *Best Pract Res Clin Anaesthesiol.* 2011; 25:145–59.
25. Fasting S, Gisvold SE. Adverse drug errors in anesthesia, and the impact of coloured syringe labels. *Can J Anaesth.* 2000; 47:1060–7.
26. Grigg EB, Martin LD, Ross FJ et al. Assessing the impact of the anesthesia medication template on medication errors during anesthesia: a prospective study. *Anesth Analg.* 2017; 124:1617–25.
27. Larson CM, Saine D. Medication safety officer's handbook. Bethesda, MD: American Society of Health-System Pharmacists; 2013.
28. Anesthesia Quality Institute. https://www.aqihq.org (accessed 2019 Feb 14).
29. Centers for Disease Control and Prevention. The one and only campaign. http://www.oneandonlycampaign.org/ (accessed 2019 Feb 14).
30. Siegel JD, Rhinehart E, Jackson M et al. 2007 guideline for isolation precautions: preventing transmission of infectious agents in healthcare settings. https://www.cdc.gov/niosh/docket/archive/pdfs/NIOSH-219/0219-010107-siegel.pdf (accessed 2019 Feb 14).
31. ASA Committee on Occupational Health Task Force on Infection Control. *Recommendations for infection control for the practice of anesthesiology* 3rd Ed. https://www.asahq.org/-/media/sites/asahq/files/public/resources/asa-committees/recommendations-for-infection-control-for-the-practice-of-anesthesiology.pdf (accessed 2019 Feb 14).
32. American Association of Nurse Anesthetists. Infection control guide for certified registered nurse anesthetists [archived content]. https://www.aana.com/docs/default-source/practice-aana-com-web-documents-(all)/infection-control-guide-for-crnas-archived.pdf (accessed 2019 Feb 14).
33. Conner R, ed. Perioperative standards and recommended practices. Denver, CO: Association of PeriOperative Registered Nurses; 2014.
34. Gold MS, Byars JA, Frost-Pineda K. Occupational exposure and addictions for physicians: case studies and theoretical implications. *Psychiatr Clin North Am.* 2004; 27:745–53.
35. Tetzlaff J. American Society of Anesthesiologists SUD curriculum, Committee on Occupational Health (November 2015). https://www.asahq.org/~/media/sites/asahq/files/public/resources/asa%20committees/substance-use-disorder-model-curriculum-42216.pdf (accessed 2019 Feb 14).
36. Wright EL, McGuiness T, Moneyham LD et al. Opioid abuse among nurse anesthetists and anesthesiologists. *AANA J.* 2012; 80:120–8.
37. Warner DO, Berge K, Sun H et al. Substance use disorder among anesthesiology residents, 1975–2009. *JAMA.* 2013; 310:2289–96.
38. Berge KH, Seppala MD, Lanier WL. The anesthesiology community's approach to opioid- and anesthetic-abusing personnel: time to change course. *Anesthesiology.* 2008; 109:762–4.
39. Brummond PW, Chen DF, Churchill WW et al. ASHP guidelines on preventing diversion of controlled substances. *Am J Health-Syst Pharm.* 2017; 74:325–48.
40. Vigoda MM, Gencorelli FJ, Lubarsky DA. Discrepancies in medication entries between anesthetic and pharmacy records using electronic databases. *Anesth Analg.* 2007; 105:1061–5, table of contents.
41. Epstein RH, Dexter F, Gratch DM et al. Controlled substance reconciliation accuracy improvement using near real-time drug transaction capture from automated dispensing cabinets. *Anesth Analg.* 2016; 122:1841–55.
42. Brenn BR, Kim MA, Hilman E. Development of a computerized monitoring program to identify narcotic diversion in a pediatric anesthesia practice. *Am J Health-System Pharm.* 2015; 72:1365–72.
43. United States Department of Justice. Settlement agreement between the United States and The General Hospital Corporation, d/b/a/ Massachusetts General Hospital (September 28, 2015). https://www.justice.gov/usao-ma/file/778651/download (accessed 2019 Feb 14).
44. Lefebvre LG, Kaufmann IM. The identification and management of substance use disorders in anesthesiologists. *Can J Anaesth.* 2017; 64:211–8.
45. Epstein RH, Gratch DM, Grunwald Z. Development of a scheduled drug diversion surveillance system based on an analysis of atypical drug transactions. *Anesth Analg.* 2007; 105:1053–60, table of contents.
46. Epstein RH, Gratch DM, McNulty S, Grunwald Z. Validation of a system to detect scheduled drug diversion by anesthesia care providers. *Anesth Analg.* 2011; 113:160–4.
47. Devine B, Gutierrez K, Rogers R. Drug diversion by anesthesiologists: identification through intensive auditing. *Am J Health-Syst Pharm.* 2012; 69:552–6.

48. Eagle CJ, Maltby JR, Kryski S, Hardy D. Use of refractometry to identify opioid-containing solutions. *Can J Anaesth.* 1994; 41:248–52.
49. American Association of Nurse Anesthetists. Wearing masks, the series. https://sharepoint.aana.com/resources2/health-wellness/Pages/Wearing-Masks,-The-Series.aspx (accessed 2019 Feb 14).
50. American Society of Anesthesiologists. Resources from ASA committees. https://www.asahq.org/standards-and-guidelines/resources-from-asa-committees (accessed 2019 Feb 14).
51. Berge KH, Dillon KR, Sikkink KM et al. Diversion of drugs within healthcare facilities, a multiple-victim crime: patterns of diversion, scope, consequences, detection, and prevention. *Mayo Clin Proc.* 2012; 87:674–82.
52. Booth JV, Grossman D, Moore J et al. Substance abuse among physicians: a survey of academic anesthesiology programs. *Anesth Analg.* 2002; 95:1024–30, table of contents.
53. Scott M. Legal aspects of drug testing. *ASA News.* 2005; 69:25–8.
54. Page L. Will doctors be able to escape random drug testing? *(2015).* http://www.medscape.com/viewarticle/841478 (accessed 2019 Feb 14).
55. Rice MJ, Grek SB, Swift MD et al. The need for mandatory random drug testing in anesthesia providers. *Anesth Analg.* 2017; 124:1712–6.
56. Murray C. Medication management in the perioperative setting (November 2014). https://www.pppmag.com/article/1605 (accessed 2019 May 8).
57. Burwell SM. Setting value-based payment goals–HHS efforts to improve U.S. healthcare. *N Engl J Med.* 2015; 372:897–9.
58. The Joint Commission. Crosswalk to performance improvement (January 2014). https://www.jointcommission.org/assets/1/6/Crosswalk_TJC_QAPI_ncc.pdf (accessed 2019 Feb 14).
59. Going lean in healthcare. IHI innovation series white paper. Cambridge, MA: Institute for Healthcare Improvement; 2005.
60. Shaffie S, Shabazi S. The McGraw-Hill 36-hour course: lean Six Sigma. New York: McGraw-Hill; 2012.
61. Kotter, JP. Leading change. Boston, MA: Harvard Business Review Press; 2012.
62. Cohen MM, Rose DK, Yee DA. Changing anesthesiologists' practice patterns: can it be done? *Anesthesiology.* 1996; 85:260–9.
63. Bratzler DW, Dellinger EP, Olsen KM et al. Clinical practice guidelines for antimicrobial prophylaxis in surgery. *Am J Health-Syst Pharm.* 2013; 70:195–283.
64. Kooij FO, Klok T, Hollmann MW, Kal JE. Decision support increases guideline adherence for prescribing postoperative nausea and vomiting prophylaxis. *Anesth Analg.* 2008; 106:893–8, table of contents.
65. Practice Greenhealth. Greening the operating room. https://practicegreenhealth.org/initiatives/greening-operating-room (accessed 2019 Feb 14).
66. Huncke TK, Ryan S, Hopf HW et al. Greening the operating room: reduce, reuse, recycle, and redesign. http://www.kevinmd.com/blog/2012/04/greening-operating-room.html (accessed 2019 Feb 14).
67. Gillerman RG, Browning RA. Drug use inefficiency: a hidden source of wasted healthcare dollars. *Anesth Analg.* 2000; 91:921–4.
68. Wagner DS, Naughton NN, Michel T et al. Potency and sterility of anesthetic drugs in an obstetric anesthesia. *Int J Obstet Anesth.* 2002; 11:252–4.
69. U.S. Environmental Protection Agency. Management of Pharmaceutical Hazardous Waste. https://www.epa.gov/hwgenerators/management-pharmaceutical-hazardous-waste (accessed 2019 May 8).
70. Agency for Healthcare Quality and Research. Hospital Survey on Patient Safety Culture. https://www.ahrq.gov/sops/surveys/hospital/index.html (accessed 2019 Feb 14).
71. American Society of Health-System Pharmacists. ASHP statement on leadership as a professional obligation. *Am J Health-Syst Pharm.* 2011; 68:2293–5.
72. Chernin EL. Pharmacoeconomics of inhaled anesthetic agents: considerations for the pharmacist. *Am J Health-Syst Pharm.* 2004; 61(suppl 4):S18–22.
73. American College of Surgeons, NSQIP, American Geriatrics Society. ACS NSQIP/AGS Best practice guidelines: optimal preoperative assessment of the geriatric surgical patient. https://www.facs.org/~/media/files/quality%20programs/nsqip/acsnsqipagsgeriatric2012guidelines.ashx (accessed 2019 Feb 14).
74. American College of Surgeons. ACS NSQIP Pediatric. https://www.facs.org/quality-programs/childrens-surgery/pediatric (accessed 2019 Feb 14).
75. Pai M, Douketis J. Prevention of venous thromboembolic disease in adult nonorthopedic surgical patients. https://www.uptodate.com/contents/prevention-of-venous-thromboembolic-disease-in-surgical-patients (accessed 2019 Feb 14).
76. Rosenfeld A, Tetzlaff JE. Pattern of herbal medication use in a high-risk surgical population [ASA abstract A-1184, 2002]. http://www.asaabstracts.com/strands/asaabstracts/abstract.htm?year=2002&index=13&absnum=509 (accessed 2019 Feb 14).
77. Marotti SB, Kerridge RK, Grimer MD. A randomised controlled trial of pharmacist medication histories and supplementary prescribing on medication errors in postoperative medications. *Anaesth Intensive Care.* 2011; 39:1064–70.
78. Weiner BK, Venarske J, Yu M et al. Towards the reduction of medication errors in orthopedics and spinal surgery. *Spine.* 2008; 33:104–7.
79. Douglas E. Preop med reconciliation helps improve patient safety (January 23, 2007). https://www.pharmacypracticenews.com/Operations-and-Management/Article/01-07/-Preop-Med-Reconciliation-Helps-Improve-Patient-Safety-/6407 (accessed 2019 May 8).
80. University of Michigan Health System. The University of Michigan's high-dose opioid taper initiative. http://anes-conf.med.umich.edu/opioidtaper/opioidtaper.htm (accessed 2019 Feb 14).
81. Rosenquist RW. About bloody time! Interventional spine and pain procedures in patients on antiplatelet and anticoagulant medications. *Regional Anesth Pain Med.* 2015; 40:179–81.

82. American Society of Health-System Pharmacists, American Pharmaceutical Association. ASHP-APhA medication management in care transitions best practices (February 2013). https://www.ashp.org/-/media/assets/pharmacy-practice/resource-centers/quality-improvement/learn-about-quality-improvement-medication-management-care-transitions.ashx (accessed 2018 Jun 4).
83. Kucukarslan SN, Peters M, Mlynarek M, Nafziger DA. Pharmacists on rounding teams reduce preventable adverse drug events in hospital general medicine units. *Arch Intern Med.* 2003; 163:2014–8.
84. Leape LL, Cullen DJ, Clapp MD et al. Pharmacist participation on physician rounds and adverse drug events in the intensive care unit. *JAMA.* 1999; 282:267–70.
85. Hoke N, Falk S. Interdisciplinary rounds in the postanesthesia care unit: a new perioperative paradigm. *Anesthesiol Clin.* 2012; 30:427–31.
86. Traynor K. Readiness for malignant hyperthermia can be survey stumbling block. *Am J Health-Syst Pharm.* 2016; 73:852–3.
87. Malignant Hyperthermia Association of the United States. Managing an MH Crisis. http://www.mhaus.org/healthcare-professionals/managing-a-crisis (accessed 2019 Feb 14).
88. Neal JM, Bernards CM, Butterworth JF 4th et al. ASRA practice advisory on local anesthetic systemic toxicity. *Reg Anesth Pain Med.* 2010; 35:152–61.
89. American Society of Regional Anesthesia and Pain Medicine. Checklist for treatment of local anesthetic systemic toxicity. https://www.asra.com/content/documents/checklist-for-local-anesthetic-toxicity-treatment-1-18-12.pdf (accessed 2019 Feb 14).
90. Cowart K, Sidhu A, Willis M. Description of an anesthesia/perioperative medicine rotation for post graduate year one pharmacy residents. *Pharm Pharmacol Int J.* 2016; 4:361–5.
91. Hook J, Pearlstein J, Samarth A et al. Using barcode medication administration to improve quality and safety: findings from the AHRQ Health IT Portfolio. AHRQ Publication No. 09-0023-EF. Rockville, MD: Agency for Healthcare Research and Quality; 2008.
92. ASHP statement on bar-code verification during inventory, preparation, and dispensing of medications. *Am J Health-Syst Pharm.* 2011; 68:442–5.
93. American Society of Anesthesiologists. Perioperative surgical home. https://www.asahq.org/psh (accessed 2019 Feb 14).
94. Kain ZN, Vakharia S, Garson L et al. The perioperative surgical home as a future perioperative practice model. *Anesth Analg.* 2014; 118:1126–30.
95. Ljungqvist O, Scott M, Fearon KC. Enhanced recovery after surgery: a review. *JAMA Surg.* 2016; 152:292–298.

Developed through the ASHP Section of Inpatient Care Practitioners and approved by the ASHP Board of Directors on October 30, 2018. These guidelines supersede the ASHP guidelines on surgery and anesthesiology pharmaceutical services dated November 14, 1998.

Peggy Bickham, Pharm.D., University of Illinois Hospital and Health Sciences System, Hospital Pharmacy Services, Chicago, IL.

Julie Golembiewski, Pharm.D., FASHP, University of Illinois at Chicago College of Pharmacy, Department of Pharmacy Practice, UI Health, Hospital Pharmacy and Anesthesiology, Chicago, IL.

Tricia Meyer, Pharm.D., M.S., FASHP, FTSHP, Baylor Scott & White Medical Center–Temple, Texas A&M College of Medicine, Temple, TX.

Christopher G. Murray, Pharm.D., M.S., CHI St. Luke's Health Memorial, Lufkin, TX.

Deborah Wagner, Pharm.D., FASHP, Michigan Medicine, Ann Arbor, MI.

ASHP gratefully acknowledges the following organizations and individuals for reviewing the current version of the guidelines (review does not imply endorsement): American Academy of PAs; American College of Clinical Pharmacy; American College of Physicians; American Pharmacists Association; Froedtert and the Medical College of Wisconsin; National Community Pharmacists Association; U.S. Public Health Service; Sarah Bledsoe, Pharm.D., CPHIMS; Maureen Burger, M.S.N, RN, CPHQ, FACHE; Stacy K. Cassat, Pharm.D., M.S.; Jolie M. Connell, Pharm.D., BCPS; Marsha F. Crader, Pharm.D.; Christopher W. Ellison, Pharm.D., BCPS; Leigh Fritz, Pharm.D., M.S.; Paul W. Goebel, Pharm.D., BCPS, BCCCP; Calvin J. Ice, Pharm.D., BCPS, BCCCP; David Kinard; Janet M. Kozakiewicz, Pharm.D., M.S., FASHP; Edward Lau, Pharm.D., BCPS; Ronald E. Lay, M.S., FASHP; Danielle Massee, Pharm.D., BCPS; Patrick J. McDonnell, Pharm.D., FASHP; Christopher Miller, Pharm.D., BCPS; Fred J. Pane, B.S., FASHP, FABC; Lois F. Parker, B.S., FASHP; Robert L. Poole, Pharm.D., FPPAG, FCSHP, FASHP; James R. Rinehart, M.S., FASHP, John Roefaro, Pharm.D., FASHP; Richard I. Sakai, Pharm.D., FASHP, FCSHP; Jodi L. Taylor, Pharm.D., BCPS, BCCCP; and Jody Jacobson Wedret, FASHP, FCSHP.

The authors have declared no potential conflicts of interest.

At the time of writing, Dr. Bickham was affiliated with the University of Illinois Hospital and Health Sciences System, Hospital Pharmacy Services, Chicago, IL.

Copyright © 2019, American Society of Health-System Pharmacists, Inc. All rights reserved. Contact ASHP for reprint and permissions requests. This content may not be used for commercial purposes without the express written consent of ASHP.

The bibliographic citation for this document is as follows: American Society of Health-System Pharmacists. ASHP guidelines on perioperative pharmacy services. *Am J Health-Syst Pharm.* 2019; 76:903–920.

ASHP Guidelines on Pharmacist Involvement in HIV Care

Background and Purpose

The epidemic of human immunodeficiency virus (HIV) infection in the United States has changed dramatically since its initial recognition in 1981.[1] Early in the epidemic, the incidence of HIV reached over 130,000 new cases per year, and death as a result of acquired immunodeficiency syndrome (AIDS) was an almost certain prognosis for those infected.[2] Significant advances in the strategies to prevent HIV transmission and in the medical care of patients with HIV infection led to significant reductions in both HIV transmission events and AIDS-related deaths over time. Among these advancements were an understanding of HIV infection pathophysiology, identification of HIV transmission modes, development of public health interventions targeting behavioral changes in high-risk populations, and identification of novel HIV medication targets leading to advances in HIV treatment and eventually combination antiretroviral therapy (ART). Because the application of ART can significantly suppress HIV replication, thereby restoring a patient's immune function, it has resulted in a significant decline in HIV-related mortality. As a result, patients receiving long-term therapy who maintain viral suppression can now manage their infection as a chronic illness and are likely to experience a near-normal life expectancy.[3]

Despite remarkable advances in HIV treatment and prevention, the HIV epidemic in the United States has persisted. While the annual incidence of AIDS and AIDS-related deaths initially declined after the introduction of ART in 1995, the annual numbers of new HIV infections, AIDS diagnoses, and AIDS-related deaths have remained constant since 2000.[4] From 2000 to 2011, there were 45,000–55,000 new cases of HIV infections diagnosed every year in the United States and nearly 15,000 AIDS-related deaths annually. These statistics indicate that significant challenges remain for public health officials and HIV care providers to properly address the HIV epidemic. Furthermore, while long-recognized challenges to successful HIV care remain relevant (e.g., lack of early diagnosis, inadequate linkage to and retention in care, poor adherence to ART, stigma and public perception, disparities in access to care for disenfranchised or socially marginalized populations), new challenges to successful HIV care and prevention are emerging (e.g., HIV in an aging population, the application of novel prevention methods such as preexposure prophylaxis, the optimal timing of ART initiation, management of special patient populations with HIV infection).[5-9]

As the HIV epidemic in the United States evolves and new challenges to successful care and prevention emerge, healthcare providers—including pharmacists—are expanding their roles to ensure optimal patient care.[10,11] Pharmacists have long been recognized as essential members of the HIV patient care team, and their involvement in managing HIV-infected patients has been associated with improved outcomes. Pharmacist activities such as helping the team in selecting individualized HIV treatment regimens, providing patient counseling, monitoring for treatment responses and adverse effects, evaluating regimens for potential drug–drug interactions, and identifying opportunities for regimen simplification are associated with better viral load reductions and CD4+ T-lymphocyte responses, improved ART adherence, simpler regimens, and reductions in medication errors.[12-16] To address emerging challenges, pharmacists will need to apply their traditional expertise within an interdisciplinary healthcare framework in multiple practice settings (inpatient, community, and ambulatory care) as well as identify and establish new roles in evolving areas of care, including HIV testing and diagnosis, medication therapy management, transitions of care, patient retention, acute HIV treatment, preexposure prophylaxis (PrEP), and initiation of ART in key populations, such as those with acute opportunistic infections, hepatitis coinfections, and solid organ transplantation. In developing these roles, it will be essential for pharmacists to remain highly engaged in the rapidly changing field of HIV using reliable resources such as https://aidsinfo.nih.gov—the U.S. Department of Health and Human Services (DHHS) HIV management guidelines—and others, which are listed in the **appendix**.

In 2003, ASHP published a statement on the pharmacist's role in the care of patients with HIV infection.[17] These current guidelines extend beyond the scope of that document and are intended to provide guidance for all pharmacists and other healthcare professionals involved in the care of patients with HIV. The purpose of these guidelines is to describe the ways in which pharmacists can contribute to the care of patients with HIV while working within a healthcare team. These guidelines emphasize the importance of interdisciplinary teams and collaboration among healthcare professions in order to achieve optimal patient care. Pharmacists may also find these guidelines helpful in establishing or expanding their services in an HIV practice setting. Using primary literature, therapeutic and practice guidelines, national standards, and the consensus of experts in the field of HIV pharmacy practice, these guidelines describe the available evidence for traditional pharmacist roles and identify new areas of emerging significance in which pharmacists can establish novel roles to meet the current and future challenges of the HIV epidemic in the United States. Specifically, these guidelines address in detail the involvement of pharmacists in the following 10 key aspects of HIV prevention, care, and treatment for patients:

- HIV testing
- Treatment of HIV infection
- Treatment of HIV in key patient populations
- HIV treatment failure
- Management of HIV disease state complications
- Treatment and prevention of opportunistic infections
- Prevention of HIV infection
- HIV education
- Social services and HIV infection
- Professional engagement

DOI 10.37573/9781585287048.076

Pharmacist Involvement in HIV Testing

The need for expanded HIV testing in the United States is demonstrated by the fact that one in six individuals with HIV in the United States is unaware of his or her infection and may therefore present an increased risk of transmission to others.[18] Recommendations from both the Centers for Disease Control and Prevention (CDC) and the U.S. Preventive Services Task Force (USPSTF) stress the importance of routine "opt-out" HIV testing for adults in all healthcare settings; patients are informed about and undergo testing for HIV unless they specifically decline.[19,20] Ubiquity and flexible hours make pharmacies ideal locations for HIV testing. Pharmacists, as advocates for public health, should be involved with HIV testing initiatives by recommending HIV testing, providing and/or counseling on HIV tests, and assisting healthcare providers with test interpretation.

HIV testing and early HIV diagnoses improve access to HIV treatment that prolongs life, preserves health, and prevents transmission to others. To ensure timely HIV testing, pharmacists should recommend HIV testing according to recommendations set forth by CDC and USPSTF and must be knowledgeable about the signs and symptoms of early HIV infection and the behaviors placing an individual at risk for HIV infection. CDC and DHHS maintain websites that list updated HIV testing recommendations, risk behaviors, and common symptoms of early HIV infection (www.cdc.gov/hiv and www.aids.gov, respectively). Pharmacists referring patients for testing should be knowledgeable about community HIV-testing sites. CDC maintains a list of free HIV-testing sites (hivtest.cdc.gov or 800-232-4636). Pharmacists should support routine HIV testing and help educate patients infected with HIV about how to modify their behavior to prevent disease transmission.

HIV testing may not be easily accessible for patients with limited access to healthcare. Community pharmacies are addressing this issue and improving patient access to HIV testing by offering onsite rapid HIV testing and counseling services.[21,22] Pharmacists in community and outpatient settings perform point-of-care HIV tests, provide pretest and posttest patient counseling, counsel patients with a positive result about confirmatory testing, and facilitate a linkage to care.[23] CDC is developing a toolkit for HIV testing in community pharmacies and retail clinics, and the Michigan Pharmacists Association offers an accredited certificate course for pharmacists focused on point-of-care testing in community pharmacies.[24] These training modules set forth a curriculum designed to support pharmacists in the administration of point-of-care HIV testing, including competencies in pretest and posttest patient counseling, performing the actual test, reading and interpreting the HIV test results, and identifying sites for linkage to care and confirmatory testing. When state legislation does not permit pharmacists to perform these activities, these guidelines can be used to advocate for change and improve and standardize pharmacist care nationally. Expanding HIV testing to pharmacies serves to eliminate barriers and reduce stigma by providing convenient, ubiquitous access to testing. Interest in pharmacy-based HIV testing initiatives has been documented from the perspectives of both pharmacy staff and patients.[25–28] The readiness of pharmacies to provide these services calls attention to their ideal accessibility to both urban and rural communities and to hard-to-reach populations not integrated into the formal healthcare system.

In 2012, the first point-of-care home HIV test became available for sale in community pharmacies. The OraQuick In-Home HIV Test provides results in as little as 20 minutes using a sample obtained by swabbing the test strip along the gum lines.[29] This test joined the already available over-the-counter Home Access HIV-1 Test System, which analyzes a mailed dried blood spot and provides telephone results in as little as one day. Community pharmacists should stock over-the-counter HIV test kits and be able to educate individuals about the proper method for administering the test and interpreting the results and to take action on both reactive and nonreactive test results.

In addition to recommending and providing HIV testing, clinical pharmacists can assist healthcare providers with interpreting HIV test results. HIV infection can be diagnosed by serologic assays that detect antibodies against HIV and by assays that detect HIV antigens or RNA. Reactive screening tests are always confirmed by a supplemental test. Pharmacists' expertise is useful when clinicians are faced with discordant HIV test results, especially during the period between exposure and seroconversion. Clinicians may have questions about which additional tests are necessary. New HIV diagnostic algorithms incorporating the use of fourth-generation HIV testing assays are increasingly implemented within U.S. institutions following updated recommendations from CDC.[30] Pharmacists should familiarize themselves with evolving HIV testing diagnostics; CDC maintains a website of HIV-testing recommendations (www.cdc.gov/hiv/guidelines/testing.html). At the Clinician Consultation Center, clinical pharmacists practicing in HIV medicine, and physicians are on staff to assist with healthcare provider telephone inquiries regarding HIV testing.[31,32]

HIV testing is the first step in linking persons to HIV care and prevention. Pharmacists should encourage HIV testing as part of routine care and familiarize themselves with testing methods performed at local medical facilities, at pharmacies, or at home. Pharmacist endorsement of HIV testing is important for the expansion of HIV prevention and treatment services.

Pharmacist Involvement in HIV Treatment

Patient Assessment and Laboratory Testing. As ambulatory care transitions to the patient-centered medical home model, it is becoming increasingly important for interdisciplinary healthcare teams to provide both comprehensive HIV care and primary care for HIV-positive patients. As a member of the team, a pharmacist should therefore be familiar with both HIV and primary care management guidelines (appendix) and help to ensure that laboratory testing and monitoring of patients with HIV include parameters specific to HIV as well as primary care. It is also essential that pharmacists have the ability to interpret laboratory test results and recommend appropriate treatment or additional testing when necessary in collaboration with the patient care team. Pharmacists should understand how certain laboratory test results may influence the management of HIV (e.g., the presence of baseline dyslipidemia, renal dysfunction, or hepatitis B coinfection among other conditions may influence the selection of antiretroviral agents or perhaps the timing of ART initiation). Among the laboratory tests that should be obtained at baseline in a patient with HIV are CD4+ T-lymphocyte count; viral load; HIV genotype test; hepatitis, tuberculosis, and sexually transmitted infection testing; varicella, cytomegalovirus, and toxoplasmosis serologies; complete blood count with differential; chemistry and liver panels; and fasting lipid profile.[33,34] Many of these laboratory values will require periodic assessment or ongoing monitoring, particularly the HIV viral load and CD4+ T-lymphocyte count to assess HIV disease progression or treatment response. After the initiation of ART, the HIV viral load and CD4+ T-lymphocyte count are closely monitored, though over time the frequency of monitoring may decline once a patient demonstrates a durable virological and immunologic response. For example, after receiving ART for two years and consistently achieving HIV RNA suppression and a CD4+ T-lymphocyte count of greater than 500 cells/mm^3, viral load monitoring can be extended to every six months and CD4+ T-lymphocyte count monitoring is considered optional.[35] Pharmacists should be intimately familiar with laboratory values that require periodic assessment or ongoing monitoring in HIV-positive patients and recommend that appropriate assessment and monitoring occurs. Specific laboratory testing may also be necessary before the use of specific antiretroviral agents. For example, if abacavir is considered for therapy, the patient should be tested for the presence of the human leukocyte antigen B*5701 allele to determine his or her risk for abacavir hypersensitivity; for mara-viroc, an HIV tropism assay should be performed to predict the patient's response to therapy.

Initiating and Maintaining ART. In initiating ART, current HIV management guidelines state that treatment should be offered to all patients regardless of CD4+ T-lymphocyte count to reduce the risk of HIV transmission and disease progression. Treatment is no longer based on the patient's CD4+ T-lymphocyte count but rather on the patient's willingness and interest in starting and adhering to his or her first ART regimen.[35] The pharmacist, as part of the healthcare team, should contribute to assessing a patient's willingness to initiate ART and provide a readiness assessment. This assessment should include the identification of potential adherence barriers, such as substance abuse, depression, and an unstable social or housing situation. Once potential barriers are identified, the pharmacist should help patients and providers resolve adherence barriers, providing ongoing adherence assessments and barrier management as necessary. This role includes monitoring for adverse effects after ART initiation and implementing adverse-effect management strategies with the patient and provider to improve regimen tolerability and maintain ART adherence.

In selecting an initial ART regimen, convenience, patient preference, cost, comorbidities, baseline viral load, CD4+ T-lymphocyte count, the potential for adverse effects, resistance testing, and concomitant medications must be considered.[35] Performing a thorough medication history and assessing for potential drug interactions are essential functions of the pharmacist.

Antiretroviral agents may interact with other antiretrovirals, concomitant medications, foods, nutrients, and herbal supplements. These interactions may be complex, occurring through multiple mechanisms, and may result in diminished treatment efficacy or an increased risk for toxicity. Drug interactions that are not clinically relevant, will not cause patient harm, or will not impact treatment outcomes may also occur. The pharmacist is uniquely positioned to evaluate potential drug interactions using appropriate resources and determine the clinical significance of each interaction identified. To ensure the safety and efficacy of a patient's initial ART regimen and other medications, the pharmacist should perform thorough initial and ongoing assessments of potential drug interactions, including prescription and nonprescription medicines, recreational drugs, and nutritional and herbal supplements. The results of this assessment should be communicated to the healthcare team and used to help determine the most appropriate ART regimen for the patient. When nonprescription medication, food, or nutritional supplement interactions are identified, the pharmacist should educate the patient and ensure his or her understanding of any safety and efficacy concerns that may be present.

To ensure the accurate assessment of drug interactions, the pharmacist should consult primary resources specific to HIV medications as well as the primary drug interaction literature when necessary. Because drug interaction literature is constantly expanding and may be difficult to access for efficient decision-making, the pharmacist should identify alternative resources that are current, reliable, and easily accessible and that provide an efficient assessment of drug interaction information. These sources include (but are not limited to) the DHHS HIV Treatment Guidelines for Adults and Adolescents (https://aidsinfo.nih.gov/guidelines), the UCSF HIV InSite Drug Interaction Database (http://arv.ucsf.edu), the University of Liverpool HIV Drug Interactions website and mobile application (www.hiv-druginteractions.org), and the Toronto General Hospital Immunodeficiency Clinic website (www.hivclinic.ca/main/drugs_interact.html) (appendix). Since drug interactions are considered a subset of medication errors, preventing drug interactions should lead to better patient outcomes. Patients with HIV are at high risk of medication errors, and the identification and correction of these errors by pharmacists has been instrumental in improving the care of HIV-positive patients.[36–39]

Pharmacist Involvement in HIV Treatment of Key Patient Populations

The management of HIV infection can pose unique challenges in key patient populations. These populations include women and children, patients with comorbid conditions or coinfections, patients receiving solid organ transplantation, and immigrants and refugees. These populations often have specific medical and medication needs and regularly require coordinated interdisciplinary care. Pharmacists are essential members of these interdisciplinary teams and can help to ensure optimal patient outcomes.

Women. Twenty percent of all new HIV infections annually in the United States occur in women, and nearly 25% of all persons living with HIV in the United States are women. The majority of women living with HIV and those who are newly infected in the United States are between the ages of 13 and 45, or child-bearing age.[40,41] The proper use of ART in women of child-bearing age requires several important considerations. First, it is important for pharmacists and other healthcare practitioners to identify patients who should receive preconception counseling, including all women of child-bearing age in HIV-concordant or serodiscordant relationships. To accomplish this, pharmacists should first be familiar with resources related to preconception counseling in HIV-positive women, including the DHHS Guidelines for the Treatment of HIV-Infected Pregnant Women and Prevention of Perinatal Transmission (appendix).[42] In addition, pharmacists should be engaged in the decision-making process with providers and patients regarding the use of ART to prevent HIV transmission. As part of the healthcare team, pharmacists can initiate discussions with HIV-positive patients regarding fertility, including a patient's potential desire to become pregnant or her desire to initiate or maintain contraceptive methods such as hormonal contraception. Multiple complex drug interactions exist among ART agents and commonly used oral hormonal contraceptives; therefore, it is essential for pharmacists to identity potential drug interactions and provide proper counseling to patients before initiating ART.[35] In contrast, for patients who express a desire to become pregnant or are inconsistent with contraception, the proper selection of an ART regimen that is safe during pregnancy becomes very important.

The initiation of ART is indicated for all HIV-infected pregnant women regardless of CD4+ T-lymphocyte count as a means to prevent vertical HIV transmission. Pharmacists should be knowledgeable about current treatment guidelines for the use of ART antepartum and intrapartum for the mother as well as postpartum for the infant, including the safety and efficacy of individual antiretroviral agents as well as the recommendations for preferred ART combinations.[42] When appropriate, pharmacists should report outcomes of ART exposures to the Antiviral Pregnancy Registry (www.apregistry.com), which monitors the teratogenic effects of antiretrovirals.

Pharmacists should be acutely aware of the importance of careful and frequent monitoring for ART efficacy, tolerability, and adherence for pregnant patients. They should also be aware of physiological changes that could impact the pharmacokinetics and dosing of certain ART agents, particularly in the third trimester of pregnancy.[42] Pharmacists should also consider the pregnancy-related safety of concomitant agents that are often prescribed to patients with HIV infection, including agents used for the treatment or prevention of opportunistic infections. Postpartum, pharmacists should reinforce DHHS recommendations for women to abstain from breastfeeding, even in the presence of a fully suppressive ART regimen.[42] Pharmacists should also continue to provide adherence support and encouragement for HIV-positive women dealing with the challenges associated with being a new mother.

Pediatric Patients. To make meaningful contributions to the management of established HIV infection in infants and children, pharmacists must first develop interprofessional partnerships with pediatric HIV specialty care providers. They must also have a thorough understanding of the differing immunologic and virological patterns associated with HIV infection in children and how they compare to adults and adolescents. For example, within weeks to months following acute HIV infection, very high HIV RNA levels decline rapidly in adults, whereas high HIV RNA levels persist in perinatally infected infants for prolonged periods, decreasing slowly over years after the first year of life.[43,44] The different virological pattern in infants likely reflects an immature but developing immune system's relative inability to contain viral replication compared to that of an adult. Immunologically, while declines in CD4+ T-lymphocyte counts and percentages are expected to occur in both adults and children with advancing HIV infection, absolute CD4+ T-lymphocyte counts in children younger than age five years are generally higher than their adult counterparts. However, the risk of disease progression associated with specific CD4+ T-lymphocyte counts or percentages varies with the age of the child. For any given CD4+ T-lymphocyte count or percentage, younger children, particularly those in the first year of life, face a higher risk of disease progression than other children and adults.[45–48] As a result, pharmacists and other specialty care providers must consider the age of the child in addition to HIV-specific laboratory values when determining the risk of disease progression and the need to initiate ART.

As with adults, treatment of pediatric HIV infection is a dynamic field with constant change and progression, requiring pharmacists to be knowledgeable of constantly evolving guidelines and treatment recommendations. This is particularly true for data regarding the use of specific antiretroviral agents in young children. Pharmacists must be aware of existing and emerging data describing the efficacy and safety of specific antiretroviral agents in this population. Pharmacists must also be knowledgeable about the pharmacokinetic differences that occur in children as a result of developing physiology and maturation of organs involved in the metabolism and clearance of medications.[49] These factors, in addition to developmental differences in absorption and body composition, often require that children receive higher weight-based dosing of antiretroviral agents than adults. In addition to weight, pharmacists must also be acutely aware and knowledgeable about antiretroviral agent–specific dosing recommendations that consider body surface area, age, and pubertal development staging.[50]

When treatment decisions are made, pharmacists must not only ensure proper regimen selection and dosing but take active roles in educating children (when appropriate) and caregivers about HIV infection and provide ongoing adherence counseling.[50] Adolescents face multiple barriers that can affect the initiation and maintenance of ART and other aspects of HIV care, including fear, denial, depression, substance abuse, concomitant mental illness, and lack of social and familial support.[51] Healthcare providers, including pharmacists, must work to establish trust and build strong relationships with patients and their caregivers while utilizing patient-care strategies that minimize barriers to adherence. For example, regimen fatigue can occur in young children who have been receiving ART since early childhood and can result in poor adherence, virological resistance, and the need to implement increasingly complex ART regimens.[52] Working with pediatric HIV specialty providers, pharmacists can help to reduce regimen fatigue through the provision of ongoing adherence support as well as the selection or simplification of regimens to minimize the number of required pills, volumes of prescribed liquids, frequency of doses, and presence of drug interactions or adverse effects. Pharmacists are also uniquely aware of the availability of alternative dosage formulations and delivery systems and are equipped to recommend methods to improve the palatability of crushed pills or liquid formulations to minimize treatment aversion due to offending taste.

Finally, pharmacists must be sensitive to the many psychosocial components of care that may be present in the pediatric HIV population. These include the housing status of the child and caregiver; the child's attendance at school or daycare; the presence of substance abuse, mental health issues, or other behavioral issues; and the HIV infection disclosure status of the child.[52–54] When contributing to the care of pediatric HIV patients, pharmacists may be helpful in identifying psychosocial issues that require intervention and possible referral to specialty providers, or to social services and child protective services when appropriate. These interventions can be essential to the overall health and well-being of children as well as their success in managing their HIV infection. Pharmacists may also serve as important information resources as children transition into adolescence and become sexually active. Counseling on contraceptive methods, safe sex, and preventing HIV transmission should occur regularly and should be delivered by members of the healthcare team, including the pharmacist.

Patients with Comorbid Conditions. Comorbidities are common among patients with HIV. Compared with the general population, those with HIV infection are more likely to have cardiovascular disease, hypertension, renal failure, osteoporosis, diabetes, and certain cancers. Not only do these conditions and others appear to occur more commonly in patients with HIV, they also tend to appear earlier in patients with HIV and at times progress more rapidly than in the general population, likely due to complex interactions between host risk factors, HIV infection, and ART exposure.[55] As a result, it is increasingly important for healthcare teams to not only provide effective ART to ensure viral suppression and immune reconstitution but also to provide comprehensive primary care for patients with HIV. Furthermore, due to the success of combination ART regimens in reducing AIDS-related mortality over the years, the HIV-positive population is getting older; it is estimated that more than half of all patients with HIV in the United States are over the age of 50 years.[56]

Effective management of the changing HIV population will require pharmacists and other healthcare providers specializing in HIV care to maintain proficient knowledge and clinical skills in the screening, prevention, diagnosis, treatment, and monitoring of a variety of primary care conditions. Conversely, pharmacists practicing in primary care settings will likely encounter an increasing number of patients with HIV, which will require them to develop the knowledge and skills to be increasingly proficient in the management of this infection.

Regardless of practice setting, pharmacists should be acutely aware of disease management similarities with the general population and potential differences for patients with HIV. They should also understand the potential contributions HIV infection and ART can have in the development of certain primary care disease states. For example, HIV infection and certain antiretroviral agents can contribute to dyslipidemia, insulin resistance, kidney disease, liver disease, and lipodystrophy.[57–60] They also can contribute to bone loss and an increased risk of osteoporosis and fragility fractures.[61–63] Pharmacists can play key roles in understanding the links between HIV, ART, and these disease states; educating patients and other healthcare providers; encouraging disease state screenings; implementing prevention programs; and ensuring proper disease state diagnosis and management according to available treatment guidelines. They can also assist in the selection or adjustment of HIV treatment regimens that account for a patient's baseline risk or current diagnosis of primary care conditions that can be exacerbated by certain antiretroviral agents.

Other comorbidities commonly seen in patients with HIV, such as mental health conditions and substance abuse, may require special attention by pharmacists and other healthcare professionals. Depression is among the most common mental health conditions diagnosed in patients with HIV and is one of the strongest predictors of poor patient adherence and treatment outcomes.[64] Substance abuse, including illicit drug use, and mental health conditions, including major depression, also can affect medication adherence and lead to poor patient outcomes.[65–67] The management of depression and substance abuse problems in patients with HIV is similar to that for the general population, but pharmacists must be aware of the potential for drug interactions between ART and antidepressants as well as agents used in the management of substance abuse.

It is often necessary to properly manage mental health conditions and substance abuse problems before patients are able to initiate and maintain successful ART.[68] As a result, healthcare providers, including pharmacists, need to be active in the screening processes for mental health and substance abuse problems and provide a means of linking patients as necessary to appropriate specialty care and support services. Ongoing and close collaboration with specialty services, particularly in substance abuse treatment settings, is therefore necessary, as pharmacists can identify and prevent possible drug–drug interactions between substance abuse treatment medications and ART.[69] For example, methadone is a common pharmacologic agent used for the management of opioid addiction. Because multiple cytochrome P-450 isozymes are involved in methadone metabolism, methadone is subject to several interactions with antiretroviral agents. These interactions can increase methadone concentrations and therefore toxicity or decrease methadone concentrations and trigger opioid withdrawal. Pharmacists need to educate providers about these potential interactions, assist in ART selection and dosage adjustment, and work in collaboration with substance abuse treatment programs to ensure successful HIV and substance abuse management.

Finally, many recreational drugs, including methylenedioxymethamphetamine, γ-hydroxybutyric acid, ketamine, and methamphetamine, are metabolized in part by cytochrome P-450 isozymes and can therefore interact with certain antiretroviral agents. Overdoses as a result of these interactions have been reported, and pharmacists can educate providers and identify opportunities to counsel patients as a means of prevention.[70]

Patients with Hepatitis B Coinfection. Approximately 10% of patients with HIV in the United States also have chronic hepatitis B virus (HBV) infection.[71] Compared with patients with HBV infection alone, those with HIV coinfection can have a faster progression to end-stage liver disease, cirrhosis, and hepatocellular carcinoma.[72] Pharmacists involved in HIV care should be familiar with the treatment recommendations for both infections and be acutely aware that certain medications have activity against both infections. More specifically, tenofovir, lamivudine, and emtricitabine are active against both HIV and HBV, which can be important when treatment for either infection is indicated. For example, tenofovir is a preferred agent for treating HBV infection and can be used as a single agent for management of infection. However, in a coinfected patient, initiating tenofovir alone will lead to HIV resistance. As a result, if HBV or HIV treatment is indicated in a coinfected patient, a full ART regimen should be initiated, usually with the combination of tenofovir plus emtricitabine or lamivudine as the nucleoside reverse transcriptase inhibitor backbone.[35] If tenofovir cannot be used, entecavir is often used for the management of HBV. Of note, entecavir is not an effective agent for treating HIV, but it does have some anti-HIV activity and, when used alone in coinfected patients, could lead to HIV resistance.[73] As a result, if entecavir is initiated for the management of HBV infection in an HIV patient, it must be used in addition to a fully suppressive ART regimen.

In addition to concerns regarding the proper selection of antiviral agents, pharmacists should strongly encourage patients to remain adherent to therapies, as acute HBV treatment discontinuations can cause serious hepatocellular damage due to spontaneous HBV reactivation. Pharmacists can also educate patients about avoiding hepatotoxins, such as acetaminophen, encourage patients to abstain from alcohol, and identify patients with alcohol dependence who require referrals to specialty care. Finally, pharmacists should recommend an evaluation of immunity to the hepatitis A virus (HAV) for all coinfected patients. Those not immune to HAV should receive vaccination against it.

Patients with Hepatitis C Coinfection. Nearly 25% of patients with HIV infection in the United States are also infected with hepatitis C virus (HCV).[74] Like HBV, HCV progresses more rapidly in patients with HIV, resulting in twice the risk of HCV-related death in patients with coinfection compared with patients with HCV infection alone.[75]

The initiation of ART may slow the progression of liver disease in coinfected patients, so current HIV treatment guidelines recommend considering the initiation of ART in this population regardless of CD4+ T-lymphocyte count.[35,75] However, in HIV treatment-naive patients with higher CD4+ T-lymphocyte counts (>500 cells/mm^3), some clinicians may choose to defer ART until HCV therapy is complete in order to avoid the complications of combined HIV and HCV treatment (i.e., large pill burden, drug interactions, and overlapping toxicities).[35] In patients with lower CD4+ T-lymphocyte counts, combined treatment is more likely and pharmacists can play a key role in identifying and managing treatment complications. For instance, currently available direct-acting antiviral agents for HCV have significant drug interactions with multiple antiretroviral agents, including HIV protease inhibitors, elvitegravir/cobicistat, and nonnucleoside reverse transcriptase inhibitors. Pharmacists should contribute to HIV and HCV treatment regimen selection when combined treatment is indicated in order to avoid significant interactions that can lead to treatment failure and drug toxicity. Pharmacists can also recommend self-care strategies for adverse effects and report serious adverse effects back to the prescriber.

Adherence is also essential for optimal HIV and HCV treatment outcomes. As part of an interprofessional team, pharmacists should provide counseling to ensure patients understand what are often complex regimens, including proper administration (e.g., food requirements), the importance of adherence, the benefits and goals of therapy, and the recognition and management of treatment-related adverse effects. This level of pharmacist involvement has been shown to improve overall adherence and response to therapy in patients infected with HIV or HCV and may be particularly beneficial in patients infected with both viruses.[76,77] Furthermore, because the field of HCV medicine is evolving rapidly, it is increasingly essential for pharmacists to maintain a heightened awareness of evolving HCV treatment guidelines (available at www.hcvguidelines.org) and newly available HCV medications, including those in development, and their potential impact on the management of HIV coinfection.[78] Although an increasing number of medicines available for the treatment of HCV will create opportunities to improve patient outcomes, they may also lead to additional challenges in treating coinfected patients that will require pharmacist intervention and management.

Additional roles for pharmacists in treating HIV–HCV coinfection include the evaluation of patient immunity to HAV and HBV infection and the recommendation or provision of HAV and HBV immunizations as necessary. As with patients with HBV, pharmacists should educate patients with HCV infection about avoiding hepatotoxins and encourage patients to abstain from alcohol or pursue specialized care for the treatment of alcohol abuse.

Patients Undergoing Solid Organ Transplantation. Increasing numbers of patients with HIV infection are receiving solid organ transplantation, a practice previously considered controversial or infeasible. The increasing ability to provide transplantation for patients with HIV infection is largely the result of advances in the management of HIV, having a better understanding of the effects of HIV and transplant-associated immune suppression, and accumulating clinical trial data demonstrating the viability of transplantation in the HIV population.[79,80]

Irrespective of concomitant HIV infection, the process of solid organ transplantation is complex and requires interdisciplinary collaboration. The presence of HIV infection only increases the complexity of the process by introducing additional variables to consider during screening and during pretransplantation and posttransplantation management. For example, protocols for liver and kidney transplantation often include thresholds for CD4+ T-lymphocyte count levels and usually require patients to have a sustained undetectable HIV viral load.[81] Pharmacists, in addition to other members of the healthcare team, can contribute to the screening process by reviewing criteria with patients and providing essential adherence counseling to help patients achieve CD4+ T-lymphocyte count and viral load goals.

During pretransplantation management, pharmacists should contribute to the selection and/or adjustment of antiretroviral regimens in anticipation of drug–drug interactions that can occur following transplantation. For instance, nearly all patients will receive proton pump inhibitor medications for stomach acid suppression after transplantation. As a result, ART regimens that contain medications requiring an acidic environment for adequate absorption (e.g., atazanavir and rilpivirine) may need to be avoided. In addition, pharmacists should anticipate antiretroviral drug–drug interactions with posttransplantation immunosuppressing agents. Allograft rejection has been reported to occur at a higher rate in patients with concurrent HIV infection; one of the causes may be inadequate exposure to immune-suppressing agents as a result of interactions with ART agents.[82,83] Both HIV protease inhibitors and nonnucleoside reverse-transcriptase inhibitors can cause complex interactions with commonly used immunosuppressive agents such as calcineurin inhibitors (e.g., tacrolimus, sirolimus) and cyclosporine. Pharmacists should provide close monitoring of immunosuppressive drug levels and recommend dosing adjustments as necessary to achieve stable therapeutic concentrations. Proper interdisciplinary communication should also occur between HIV specialty pharmacists, transplant pharmacy specialists, and other members of the HIV and transplantation healthcare teams. Communication will help ensure proper awareness and management of potential drug–drug interactions.

The primary indications for solid organ transplantation in patients with HIV are end-stage kidney disease due to HIV-associated nephropathy (HIVAN) and advanced liver disease due to HBV or HCV coinfection.[81] The presence of viral hepatitis adds to the complexity of both pretransplantation and posttransplantation management. Pharmacists should be acutely aware of the differences in managing these infections in transplantation patients, including the differing roles of antiviral therapy. For example, patients with HBV infection should continue to receive antiviral agents after transplantation to prevent a hepatitis flare and should also receive therapy with HBV immune globulin.[84] Patients with HCV may not require antiviral therapy initially, but recurrent infection is common and can adversely impact transplantation outcomes.[81,85,86] As a result, patients should be followed closely following transplantation to identify recurrent HCV infection and the need to initiate therapy.

During the posttransplantation stage, pharmacists should ensure that the use of medications toxic to transplanted organs is limited. They should also work closely with patients to develop strategies to maintain medication adherence to complex drug regimens. At the very least, these posttransplantation regimens will include antiretroviral agents, immunosuppressive agents, and antibiotics for opportunistic infection prophylaxis. The inclusion of the pharmacist on the transplantation team has been shown to improve patient adherence to these complex regimens and may be essential to the overall success of the patient following transplantation.[87]

Finally, pharmacists must be aware of the role of posttransplantation opportunistic infection prophylaxis. Although patients generally receive prophylaxis against *Pneumocystis jirovecii*, opportunistic infections and other AIDS-defining conditions are uncommonly reported following transplantation.[83,88] Importantly, the risk of infection may change following the administration of thymoglobulin for the treatment of acute rejection. Thymoglobulin has been associated with prolonged CD4+ T-lymphocyte declines, loss of cytotoxic antiviral T-cell responses, and development of severe bacterial infections.[89,90] To address these risks, pharmacists must have a thorough understanding of anti- rejection medications, their impact on CD4+ T-lymphocytes, and the need for increased monitoring and/or additional prophylaxis to reduce a patient's risk of severe infection.

Immigrant and Refugee Populations. In January 2010, the restriction on immigration to the United States for non-U.S. citizens living with HIV was lifted.[91] The restriction had been in place for more than 20 years, and its removal not only helped to reduce social barriers, discrimination, and stigma for immigrants and refugees with HIV, it also aligned the domestic position of the United States with its increasing efforts to combat HIV and AIDS internationally.

While there are many positive implications from the removal of the immigration restriction, there are now also challenges for U.S. healthcare professionals to ensure that immigrants and refugees living with HIV consistently receive proper care. For example, the removal of the immigration restriction also removed mandatory HIV testing as a part of the immigration process. CDC estimates that lifting the ban will allow an additional 4275 persons with HIV to enter the United States each year.[91,92] At least some of these immigrants will have missed opportunities for early HIV diagnosis and entry into care. Furthermore, although CDC recommends HIV screening for all immigrants and refugees, these patients will encounter barriers to healthcare as they enter the United States (e.g., lack of familiarity with the U.S. healthcare system) that limit not only their opportunities to receive HIV testing but also proper primary care services.[93] Pharmacists can assist in overcoming these barriers by being knowledgeable of the local medical clinics and organizations serving immigrant and refugee populations and helping to link patients into care as necessary.

As patients enter into care, additional barriers may need to be addressed before performing HIV testing. These include language differences, cultural beliefs regarding HIV and healthcare in general, and mistrust regarding confidentiality and disclosure of HIV status.[94] Pharmacists must be sensitive to these issues and help reduce barriers whenever possible. Language barriers can be addressed through the use of interpreters. Patients should receive HIV education and counseling in their primary spoken language, and interpreters should be medically knowledgeable so they can explain the complexities of HIV infection and the importance of HIV testing. Pharmacists should be sensitive to situations in which a patient declines the use of an interpreter for fear of disclosure within his or her community and seek alternative translation methods if available (family member or close friend). The delivery of information to the patient in his or her primary language and in a safe environment is paramount, as it not only helps to ensure patient understanding but can also be helpful in developing a trusting patient–provider relationship.

When providing HIV education and prevention counseling, pharmacists should also be particularly sensitive to the HIV risk profiles that may be present in immigrant populations. Specifically, foreign-born persons with HIV are more likely than patients born in the United States to be women who have acquired HIV through heterosexual contact.[95] Pharmacists should also be aware of conditions heightening HIV risk for refugees, such as sexual abuse, violence, and gender inequality.[93,96] Failure to recognize these issues may limit the patient's engagement in care as well as the pharmacist's ability to provide proper counseling and referral to social services.

When testing is performed, it is important for pharmacists and other healthcare providers to follow CDC recommendations specific to the refugee population.[93] These include specific recommendations for screening adults and adolescents as well as pregnant women and children from endemic areas. Also included are recommendations for screening patients at risk for HIV-2. Pharmacists should have an understanding of the testing for HIV-2 infection as well as groups of HIV-1 infection that are endemic in certain countries and may not be detected with assays commonly used in the United States

Finally, pharmacists, as part of an interprofessional team, should be involved in the ART selection process for HIV-positive refugees and immigrants. They should provide ongoing HIV education and adherence counseling using an interpreter as well as ongoing evaluations for potential drug–drug interactions. Patients should be assessed for coinfections endemic to their home countries and receive proper treatment, including prophylaxis therapy for opportunistic infections when necessary. Patients may encounter financial difficulty, and pharmacists should pursue available services that can assist patients in paying for their medications.

Pharmacist Involvement in the Management of HIV Treatment Failure

Once an ART regimen is initiated, it is critical to monitor the success of therapy via routine assessment of the CD4+ T-lymphocyte count and HIV RNA viral load. Pharmacists can play a key role in interpreting test results to detect possible treatment failure. Treatment failure may be defined immunologically by identifying a significant decline in CD4+ T-lymphocyte count or virologically by finding a significant quantity of virus when full viral load suppression is expected. In identifying potential treatment failure, monitoring trends in viral load is essential, as a single detectable viral load is not generally sufficient to diagnose treatment failure. These viral "blips" occur when a previously undetectable viral load becomes detectable but does not exceed 200 copies/mL and generally decreases to undetectable levels again with subsequent testing. Increasing viral loads over time or a viral load of >200 copies/mL is suggestive of treatment failure. Pharmacists can reduce the chances of unnecessary ART regimen changes in response to viral load blips by monitoring the viral load trend and understanding the definitions of virological failure. If true failure is identified, pharmacists should work with other members of the healthcare team to identify the cause of the regimen failure.

Most treatment failures are the result of nonadherence, pharmacokinetic complications, and ART resistance. Pharmacists, especially those with specialized training in adherence assessment, interventions, and motivational interviewing, can help determine which of these reasons may have contributed to valid ART failure. Many factors lead to nonadherence, including medication intolerance and adverse effects, depression, substance use, psychosocial factors, lack of social support, housing insecurity or homelessness, and patient beliefs. The pharmacist should work with the patient to assess and resolve any barriers to ART adherence. Strategies for improving adherence include utilizing an interprofessional team approach, establishing a rapport with the patient, proactively identifying adherence barriers prior to regimen initiation, assessing patients for medication intolerance and adverse effects, providing mental health and social resources for the patient, assessing adherence at every pharmacy visit, involving the patient in regimen selection, providing adherence aids such as pillboxes and calendars, and assisting the patient in setting reminders through cell phone alerts or text messages.[97] Literature has shown that virological failure has been reduced and the initial ART regimen preserved with pharmacist involvement and adherence interventions.[35]

Pharmacokinetic complications may also contribute to HIV treatment failure. Malabsorption, alterations in drug distribution, and drug–drug and drug–herbal supplement interactions may all cause subtherapeutic antiretroviral concentrations and lead to HIV resistance and ART failure. Pharmacists should be aware of and monitor for these factors and suggest treatment alternatives. Although not routinely recommended, therapeutic drug monitoring may be obtained in specific clinical situations and pharmacists may assist in the interpretation of antiretroviral drug levels.[35,98]

Once ART adherence and pharmacokinetic complications have been assessed, attention should then focus on ART resistance testing. An HIV genotype and other specific medication tests (as needed) should be obtained to determine the presence of viral mutations. Specialized pharmacists involved in HIV care should be fully versed in ordering appropriate resistance tests, including the appropriate timing of particular tests, as well as in interpreting test results. Pharmacists thus serve an important role in the review and interpretation of viral genotypes. This role requires an understanding of primary and secondary mutations, polymorphisms, and the accumulation of mutations to a critical number that will contribute to ART failure. Pharmacists should be familiar with resources available to assist with HIV resistance mutation assessment including the Stanford University HIV Drug Database and International AIDS Society-USA online repository (appendix).[99] With knowledge of the viral genotype, mutation patterns, and associated antiretroviral medications, pharmacists can be a resource for the healthcare team in determining treatment options. Pharmacists should apply the results of genotype testing as well as consider clinical guideline recommendations, ART regimen history, adverse effects, pill burden, and patient preference to provide a new ART regimen for a patient. Pharmacists should be involved in any ART regimen change, with the goals of reestablishing viral suppression and improving the CD4+ T-lymphocyte count.

Pharmacist Involvement in the Management of HIV Disease State Complications

Long-term complications of HIV infection have become an area of focus as patients with HIV live longer. Historically, research and treatment efforts have revolved around antiretroviral-related medication toxicities, and little has been known about the long-term consequences of being infected with HIV. However, recent literature has identified that chronic HIV infection can lead to end-organ toxicities, thrombotic complications, non-AIDS-defining cancers, and metabolic abnormalities.[100] Pharmacists can play a key role in the identification and treatment of these emerging complications.

The mechanism by which HIV infection causes organ toxicity remains unclear. One theory is that the virus causes a prolonged state of immune system activation that can lead to inflammation, endothelial dysfunction, and accelerated atherosclerosis, resulting in organ damage.[101] This prolonged inflammatory state may lead to the generation of free radicals and oxidative stress in various organs.[102] Another possible mechanism is via a hypercoagulable state that is seen in patients with HIV. Evidence supports a depletion of proteins C and S, leading to enhanced thrombosis and subsequent disease complications.[101,103] The extent of the contribution of the virus itself in these conditions is unknown, and the increased disease incidence may be a combination of the effects of the virus, ART, and the longevity of HIV-infected patients. Organ toxicity, via a variety of mechanisms, may be seen in virtually all organ systems, but most research has been in HIV-associated cardiovascular, renal, hepatic, and neurologic toxicities.

HIV and Cardiovascular Disease. In the cardiovascular system, HIV infection has been linked to coronary artery disease and cardiomyopathy. Cardiovascular disease is now the third-most common cause of death in HIV-infected patients in the United States, and literature has shown that patients with HIV have a greater incidence of myocardial infarction than noninfected patients.[104,105] In addition to myocardial infarction, cardiomyopathy in the form of systolic dysfunction has been seen in 10–20% and diastolic dysfunction in 48% of HIV-infected individuals.[106,107] The mechanism underlying this increase in cardiovascular disease is thought to be a combination of HIV infection, treatment with ART, and the increased lifespan of HIV-infected patients.[105] Known inflammatory markers associated with cardiovascular risk are elevated in HIV disease, leading to chronic inflammation, endothelial dysfunction, and accelerated atherosclerosis and thrombosis.[108] Additionally, adverse effects of ART, specifically protease inhibitors, include metabolic abnormalities such as hyperlipidemia and hyperglycemia that heighten the risk of cardiovascular complications.[109] Pharmacists are vitally important in assisting with the control of risk factors and improving the cardiovascular risk of patients living with HIV.

Pharmacists should be actively involved in controlling the cardiovascular risk factors of patients living with HIV. Pharmacists should recommend annual cardiovascular risk assessments that include a lipid profile, fasting glucose, glycosylated hemoglobin (HbA_{1c}), and blood pressure. Specifically, pharmacists who practice in the ambulatory care setting may advocate for complete care via pharmacist-directed outpatient clinics based on physician collaborative practice agreements. Most research on pharmacist impact has been conducted in pharmacist-managed outpatient lipid, hypertension, diabetes, and heart failure clinics. Within a collaborative practice agreement, pharmacists may conduct risk assessment screening, limited physical examinations, laboratory monitoring, medication adjustments, and patient education. While not specific to the HIV disease state, incorporation of a pharmacist into outpatient clinics has been shown to significantly reduce cardiovascular events, low-density lipoprotein cholesterol, blood pressure, and HbA and improve utilization of mortality-reducing heart failure medications.[110–114] Pharmacist patient care may be conducted by facilitating in-person clinic visits or via telephone consultations.[115] In addition, the benefits of pharmacist management of cardiovascular risk factors in the patient-centered medical home model have been demonstrated.[116,117] Pharmacists practicing in the community setting should recommend routine blood pressure monitoring at all pharmacy visits and assist in appropriate selection and training of diabetes supplies such as glucose meters and test strips.[33] Community pharmacists should perform routine medication profile review and recommend selection of safe and effective over-the-counter medications and herbal products. Pharmacists may also be proactive by recommending and overseeing the use of patient self-monitoring treatment journals documenting changes in blood pressure and glucose control. Finally, in-patient pharmacists may facilitate the increased use of medication prescriptions for cardiovascular risk reduction at hospital discharge. In all practice settings, pharmacists should be familiar with lipid, blood pressure, and blood glucose treatment goals and guidelines and should directly apply those guidelines to assist in decreasing the cardiovascular risk in HIV-infected patients. In addition, pharmacists should routinely monitor and recommend lifestyle modifications, including smoking cessation, diet modification, and exercise adherence, as these have also been shown to decrease cardiovascular risk in patients with HIV.[118–120]

In addition to controlling risk factors, pharmacists should collaborate with the healthcare team to minimize patients' exposure to direct cardiotoxic medications and other medications that have adverse effects on the lipid profile. The use of abacavir, a nucleoside reverse-transcriptase inhibitor, has been linked to a possible increased risk of myocardial infarction.[121,122] While the literature is conflicting regarding this adverse effect, pharmacists should be cognizant of this possibility and recommend alternative antiretroviral therapies as appropriate. In addition, pharmacists involved in HIV management may recommend an ART regimen that may have a less detrimental effect on the patient's lipid profile.[123]

HIV and Renal Disease. HIV infection is associated with nephropathy in the form of acute kidney injury and chronic renal failure.[124] Acute kidney injury has been found to be more common among HIV-infected patients than the general patient population and is associated with poor outcomes.[125] Acute kidney injury presents in many forms, but prerenal failure and acute tubular necrosis are the most common. Postulated mechanisms of HIV-induced acute renal failure include medication-induced toxicities, specifically nephrolithiasis with atazanavir and indinavir, Fanconi's syndrome with tenofovir, and dehydration from opportunistic infections.[125] Pharmacists are vital in the management of HIV-induced renal toxicities and should review the patient's serum creatinine level and urinary analysis results for the development of acute renal toxicity.[33] Pharmacists should readily identify contributing nephrotoxic medications that may compound nephrotoxicity and recommend possible discontinuation and therapeutic alternatives. In addition, pharmacists should be familiar with common medications used in the treatment of HIV that interfere with the tubular secretion of creatinine, such as cobicistat, rilpivirine, dolutegravir, ritonavir, and trimethoprim–sulfamethoxazole.[126] These medications, although not inherently nephrotoxic, may increase the serum creatinine level and complicate the renal assessment of patients taking these antiretroviral medications.

Patients with HIV may also have chronic forms of nephrotoxicity. Perhaps the most widely recognized form of renal failure in HIV disease is HIV-associated nephropathy (HIVAN). HIVAN is most common among patients of African descent and is a significant contributor to chronic renal failure. ART has been shown to aid in the reversal of

HIV nephropathy by suppressing viral replication in the kidneys, and pharmacists should advocate for prompt initiation of ART in these circumstances.[127,128] HIV infection may also enhance other common risk factors for chronic kidney disease, such as diabetes and hypertension. As with cardiovascular toxicity, pharmacists should assist in the management of patients' glucose and blood pressure control and recommend therapies such as angiotensin-converting enzyme inhibitors or angiotensin receptor blockers that are thought to delay the progression of kidney failure.[129,130]

For patients with renal failure, pharmacists should recommend appropriate dosage adjustments of renally eliminated medications, including antiretroviral medications and other medications on a patient's profile (appendix).[35] Active pharmacist involvement in ensuring proper doses of renally eliminated medications has been demonstrated to decrease adverse effects and result in cost savings.[131] Such dosage adjustments are especially important in patients with advanced nephropathy requiring dialysis. Pharmacists should be familiar with various dialysis modalities and their effects on medication removal. Pharmacists should then pair this knowledge with their understanding of the clearance of specific medications by renal elimination to ensure safe and effective medication regimens.

Finally, pharmacists knowledgeable about HIV may recommend ART that minimizes nephrotoxicity, taking into consideration the HIV genotype and laboratory markers of HIV disease. Alteration of a patient's ART to minimize renal involvement can lead to enhanced safety and simplification of the ART regimen. In addition, pharmacists should aim to minimize the renal toxicity of all medications prescribed, with the goal of providing a safe and effective medication profile.

HIV and Hepatic Disease. As with HIV-associated nephrotoxicity, pharmacists should be cognizant of HIV-induced hepatotoxicity. Although the majority of literature revolves around mechanisms such as medication-induced hepatotoxicity, coinfection with viral hepatitis, and alcohol injury, there is some evidence that HIV infection alone may contribute to accelerated liver damage.[132] Pharmacists should routinely monitor liver function tests to detect the presence of hepatic toxicity. If clinically significant elevations in hepatic function tests are detected, pharmacists should identify and assist in limiting all medications that may induce hepatic injury. Many classes of antiretroviral medications have been linked to hepatotoxicity, including nonnucleoside reverse-transcriptase inhibitors and protease inhibitors. Specifically, nevirapine, maraviroc, and tipranavir have boxed warnings for hepatotoxicity, and ART regimens may need to be altered for patients being treated with those medications. If toxicity progresses to advanced liver failure and cirrhosis, pharmacists need to recognize that altered drug metabolism may occur and monitor these patients for medication toxicities and possible treatment failure.[133] Pharmacists should also recommend testing for viral hepatitis, as coinfection has been known to accelerate the decline in hepatic function.[130] Pharmacists may also recognize current alcohol and illicit drug use in patients and facilitate their admission into treatment programs, if necessary.[133] In addition, recognizing that alcohol and illicit drug consumption may alter medication adherence, pharmacists should reinforce the importance of medication adherence and adopt adherence strategies that are acceptable to patients. Finally, pharmacists should recommend hepatic dosage adjustments of medications for which a need for adjustment has been identified (appendix).

HIV and Neurologic Disease. Neurotoxicity and central nervous system disorders are recognized complications of HIV infection. HIV-associated neurocognitive disorders (HAND) include certain neurologic complications of HIV infection, such as mental slowing, memory loss, motor disorders, and behavioral abnormalities.[134] These progressive symptoms lead to a decline in cognitive function that may eventually develop into HIV dementia. HAND complications occur in approximately half of patients diagnosed with HIV and represent a substantial cause of morbidity and mortality.[134–136] Although the known incidence of HAND is high, this estimate may be conservative, as HAND is often unrecognized and may be underdiagnosed. Pharmacists should be alert to symptoms of possible cognitive decline. If such symptoms are recognized, communication and facilitation with the patient's provider are recommended.

Several theories about the mechanism of HAND have been postulated, with most suggesting that the chronic inflammation state caused by HIV infection generates free radicals that inflict neuronal damage. There is no correlation between the development of HAND and HIV plasma concentration, current CD4+ T-lymphocyte count, or the presence of effective ART[134,136]; however, the development of HAND has been associated with a low CD4+ T-lymphocyte nadir.[137] This association reinforces the need for early initiation of ART to prevent low CD4+ T-lymphocyte counts and protect against the development of neurotoxicity. No other therapy has been shown to prevent or improve HAND, so pharmacists can contribute to the care of these patients by focusing on the early and effective utilization of ART.[102,138]

HAND and its complications have serious ramifications on other aspects of HIV care. Decreased neurologic function has been linked to poor patient adherence to ART and other therapies, unemployment, lack of transportation, and increased reliance on financial assistance for medications.[139] Pharmacists should work closely with their patients to create personalized medication adherence programs and provide access to medication assistance programs. Ensuring safe and effective use of medications is the pharmacists' highest priority in caring for these patients.

Other HIV-associated neurologic complications include peripheral neuropathy and ischemic stroke. Peripheral neuropathy is the most frequently reported neurologic diagnosis in HIV-positive patients and usually responds to medications typically used to treat neuropathic pain.[136] Common causes of peripheral neuropathy in HIV-infected patients include neurotoxic medications (such as didanosine), diabetes, alcohol use, and nutritional deficiencies (e.g., low vitamin B_{12} levels). Pharmacists should help to assess patients for the development and progression of peripheral neuropathy and recommend appropriate treatment options.

Hospital admissions for ischemic stroke in HIV-infected patients have increased 43% over the past decade in the United States. The higher incidence of ischemic stroke is thought to be caused by a combination of accelerated atherosclerosis and thrombosis.[101] Pharmacists should play an active role in assisting in the medication selection of acute stroke treatment. Because stroke patients often suffer from dysphagia, necessitating the use of short- and long-term enteral feeding tubes, pharmacists should be familiar with guidelines for proper administration of medications via enteral tubes (e.g., determining whether a medication may be crushed, the implications of the site of enteral medication absorption) (appendix).[140,141] After patients suffer an acute stroke episode, pharmacists should be involved in assisting in the selection of secondary prevention medications (e.g., antiplatelet and antihyperlipidemic agents) to minimize drug interactions and maximize the safety and efficacy of the patient's entire medication regimen. Pharmacists should also be aggressive in helping manage modifiable risk factors, such as hypertension, diabetes, and hyperlipidemia. The literature demonstrates that interdisciplinary teams including active pharmacist intervention improve management of ischemic stroke risk factors.[142] Pharmacists should encourage intensive management of these risk factors and other lifestyle modifications, such as smoking cessation, exercise regimens, and weight management programs.

In addition to physiological factors, medications are another important consideration in the neurologic state of the patient with HIV. Pharmacists should review the medication profile for all medications that may affect cognitive function, such as opioid narcotics and benzodiazepines. Certain antiretroviral medications, including efavirenz, have also been associated with central nervous system abnormalities. The pharmacist should be alert to and work with the healthcare team to minimize the neurologic adverse effects of medications in patients experiencing HIV-associated neurotoxicity and recommend appropriate therapeutic alternatives.

HIV and Malignancy. AIDS-associated malignancies are a well-documented complication of HIV, but HIV-infected patients also face increased incidence of other cancer types.[143] Collectively, these cancers are termed *non-AIDS-defining cancers* and include cancers such as Hodgkin's lymphoma and malignancies of the lung, kidney, anus, liver, and skin.[144,145] Guidelines for identification of these cancers overall mimic recommendations for the general population; however, some, such as cervical cancer, require more frequent monitoring, and pharmacists should recommend routine cancer screening when appropriate.

Cancer treatment in patients with HIV presents a challenge to pharmacists and practitioners, as the need to balance cancer cure must be weighed against the risk of chemotherapy-enhanced immunosuppression and resulting opportunistic infections. Given their expertise in drug–drug interaction and toxicity management, pharmacists are uniquely qualified to assist in chemotherapy and ART selection. Pharmacists should be knowledgeable in drug interactions between ART and chemotherapy agents and assist with regimen selections for both disease states that minimize toxicity while ensuring efficacy (appendix). In addition, pharmacists can aid in the initiation of appropriate opportunistic infection prophylaxis. Finally, more research is needed on the interaction between cancer, chemotherapy, HIV disease, and ART. Pharmacists should be a key component in future research teams where research is desperately needed to ensure safe and appropriate patient care.

HIV and Endocrine Disease. Patients living with HIV are also at risk for the development of traditional endocrine disorders related to HIV disease, including lipodystrophy, hypogonadism, and HIV wasting syndrome. These conditions are thought to be caused by mitochondrial toxicity and alterations in levels of growth hormone accelerated by adverse effects of antiretroviral medications, specifically protease inhibitors.[146,147] Lipodystrophy consists of an increase in visceral fat and a decrease in subcutaneous fat stores, particularly in the face and extremities.[147] Low levels of testosterone may lead to hypogonadism, sexual dysfunction, and muscle wasting in HIV-infected individuals.[148] Some patients with HIV suffer from HIV wasting syndrome due in part to increased energy expenditure that leads to a decrease in lean body mass and the total body mass index.[149] New agents are being investigated for the treatment of these disorders, and pharmacists caring for patients living with HIV should be knowledgeable about available recommended therapies.[150,151] Specifically, pharmacists may assist in testosterone formulation selection, contraindication assessment, laboratory test monitoring, and counseling on proper testosterone administration and adverse effects.[152–154] Pharmacists should also minimize ART agents that have adverse metabolic effects and recommend appropriate alternatives.[147] In addition, pharmacists should work closely with dietitians to ensure appropriate nutrition support for the complete care of the HIV-infected patient.[154] Morphological complications may have detrimental physical and psychological effects on patients, which may decrease adherence to ART. Pharmacists should be cognizant of morphological complications, recommend medical and lifestyle modifications as appropriate, and work with patients and providers to maximize treatment and adherence to HIV therapies.

In addition to traditional endocrine complications, alterations in bone metabolism have become a significant endocrine complication of HIV. HIV infection leads to earlier and more frequent loss of bone density, leading to increased incidence of osteopenia, osteoporosis, and fractures.[155] Like other chronic HIV complications, this is due to traditional risk factors, the effects of the virus itself, and the use of certain ART agents, specifically tenofovir.[156] Specific screening recommendations have been developed for patients with HIV, and pharmacists should be informed of these recommendations and take an active role in screening patients for this complication.[157] Pharmacists should also be versed on appropriate osteoporosis treatments and recommend vitamin supplementation and pharmacologic therapy when warranted. In addition, pharmacists should aid in recommending nonpharmacologic strategies for prevention of bone loss, including reducing alcohol intake, smoking cessation, and a healthy body weight.

As patients with HIV live longer, more information will emerge regarding the role of chronic HIV disease state complications. What is already evident is that proper recognition and treatment of cardiovascular, renal, hepatic, neurologic, malignant, and endocrine complications are desperately needed to fully care for HIV-infected patients. Pharmacists are integral to the medical team that must care for the whole patient, including the HIV infection itself and long-term complications of HIV disease.

Pharmacist Involvement in Management of Opportunistic Infections

Opportunistic infections contribute significantly to the morbidity and mortality of HIV-infected individuals. Although effective ART has reduced the incidence of opportunistic infections, prevention, recognition, and treatment of those infections continue to be of utmost importance in this patient population.[158] The complexity of prophylaxis and treatment of opportunistic infections in HIV-infected patients requires an interdisciplinary approach. Pharmacists can be involved in the prevention and treatment of HIV-associated opportunistic infections by providing recommendations on the initiation or discontinuation of opportunistic infection prophylaxis, the recognition and diagnosis of active opportunistic infections, treatment and dosing recommendations for active opportunistic infections, and the timing of ART initiation. Through these interventions, pharmacists play a key role in improving the medication management of individuals with HIV disease.

Pharmacists may first intervene with recommendations for when to initiate opportunistic infection prophylaxis. Medication prophylaxis for various opportunistic infections is offered to individuals with advanced HIV disease. Primary prophylaxis aims to prevent the first occurrence of an opportunistic infection; secondary prophylaxis is geared toward preventing disease recurrence.[159] The decision to initiate prophylaxis is therefore dependent on the patient's CD4+ T-lymphocyte count and the patient's history of an active opportunistic infection. Pharmacists should be familiar with and recommend specific prophylactic agents and alternative regimens for patients with medication allergies. Published guidelines are available that can help pharmacists in making recommendations regarding appropriate prophylactic medications and when to initiate primary and secondary opportunistic infection prophylaxis (appendix).[160]

The recognition of when to discontinue prophylaxis is as important as its initiation. Literature supports the safety of discontinuation of opportunistic infection prophylaxis when the CD4+ T-lymphocyte count rises above a threshold for a defined period of time while on effective ART.[159–161] Pharmacists familiar with discontinuation recommendations may intervene to discourage inappropriate continuation of drug therapy. Discontinuation of opportunistic infection prophylaxis may lead to a decrease in adverse effects and drug drug interactions, limit drug resistance, lower pill burden, increase rates of adherence, and provide cost savings.[159]

Pharmacists also play a vital role in the recognition and treatment of active opportunistic infections. Pharmacists aid in the diagnosis of opportunistic infections via symptom recognition and testing recommendations. Once a patient is diagnosed, pharmacists can contribute to the treatment of opportunistic infections by offering evidence-based recommendations on antiinfective drug selection and dosing, monitoring medication efficacy and toxicity, preventing and recognizing drug–drug and drug–nutrient interactions, and making literature-based recommendations on total treatment duration.[160]

After an opportunistic infection has been diagnosed and treatment initiated, pharmacists should be active in determining the optimal timing of ART initiation. The decision regarding ART initiation is complex and must weigh the benefits of ART against the possibility of the complication of immune reconstitution inflammatory syndrome. Although some literature has shown that early ART initiation is paramount in improving survival and decreasing AIDS progression by improved immune functioning, other studies have demonstrated that ART may not improve or may perhaps be detrimental in patients with certain types of opportunistic infections.[162–164] Current guidelines provide recommendations on when to initiate ART in patients with specific types of opportunistic infections and can help guide patients, pharmacists, and other healthcare providers in this decision-making process.[160,165] Pharmacists can assist other HIV care practitioners by providing evidence-based recommendations regarding the initiation of ART in the setting of an active opportunistic infection and contributing to the selection of an ART treatment regimen that avoids interactions with the antiinfective medication regimen.

Patients with opportunistic infections are on complex medication regimens and often require hospitalization. Pharmacists practicing in the inpatient setting play a key role in the appropriate care of these patients by preventing and resolving medication-related errors. Patients with HIV experience a high rate of medication errors due to the complexity and alteration of medication regimens, the necessity of transitions of care, and the need for their care to be provided by practitioners who may be unfamiliar with ART and HIV complications.[166] The inpatient setting provides pharmacists a unique venue to make an impact in the care of HIV-infected patients, and the literature has shown that pharmacist involvement specifically in this patient population decreases medication-related errors.[167] Pharmacists should be involved in admission and discharge medication reconciliation, provide patient discharge medication education, and assist with the transition of the patient to outpatient care.

HIV and Immunization. Immunization, as disease prevention, is important in the care of patients with HIV, as immunodeficiency creates enhanced susceptibility to infection acquisition. Pharmacists should be aware of current immunization recommendations for HIV-infected patients and work to ensure appropriate and timely routine immunization (appendix). In addition, pharmacists should be active immunization advocates by facilitating pharmacist-administered immunization programs.

The Advisory Committee on Immunization Practices publishes annual immunization recommendations for all patients, including specific recommendations for those with HIV infection. It is generally accepted that inactivated vaccines are considered safe for HIV-infected patients; some live vaccines may be administered based on a patient's CD4+ T-lymphocyte count. Patients with HIV should be immunized against infections such as influenza, pneumococcus, HAV, HBV, and tetanus/diphtheria.[168] In addition, certain immunizations may require different dosages in HIV-infected patients. Pharmacists should be aware of the immunization status of their patients and provide recommendations regarding safe and effective vaccine administration.

Effective seroprotective antibody levels after immunization are a concern in patients with HIV. Immunization is most effective at high CD4+ T-lymphocyte counts and may be delayed until the CD4+ T-lymphocyte count is above 200 cells/mm^3. There are situations, however, in which delay is not feasible, as patients with HIV may receive pneumococcal vaccination upon HIV diagnosis and an annual influenza vaccination regardless of the CD4+ T-lymphocyte count.[169] In addition, certain live vaccines are now being safely administered if the CD4+ T-lymphocyte count is near normal levels. Pharmacists should aid HIV care providers in the appropriate timing of immunizations to enhance adequate immune response while balancing the safety of vaccine administration.

After determining immunization needs and timing, pharmacists in community and clinic settings may also directly administer immunizations. Pharmacist-managed immunization programs improve access to vaccine administration and corresponding immunization rates.[170] Pharmacist vaccine administration privileges vary by type of vaccine, patient age, and immunization training requirements, so pharmacists should practice in accordance with state and local regulations. Pharmacists certified or licensed in immunization administration should take an active role in immunizing patients with HIV. Documentation of vaccine administration and communication of immunization status to prescribers and other practitioners should be completed to bridge the continuum of HIV patient care.[171]

Pharmacist Involvement in HIV Prevention

HIV prevention requires an interdisciplinary approach involving pharmacists as active members of the healthcare team. Active pharmacist participation in prevention initiatives can help prevent transmission and reduce the rate of HIV infection. Pharmacists play a key role in HIV prevention through both pharmacologic and behavioral interventions.

High viral load is a risk factor for HIV transmission.[35] By reinforcing ART adherence and subsequently lowering a patient's HIV viral load, the risk of HIV transmission can be reduced. The benefits of ART for prevention have been demonstrated in various populations, including pregnant women, HIV-serodiscordant partners, and geographic communities. Because the risk of mother-to-child transmission is strongly associated with a higher HIV viral load, the use of ART in pregnancy has dramatically reduced the incidence of perinatally transmitted HIV infections and is recommended by DHHS guidelines.[42] Decreases in HIV viral load via ART are also associated with decreased heterosexual transmission, as demonstrated in observational studies and randomized trials.[172–175] Based on these results, DHHS guidelines recommend that ART be offered to those at risk of transmitting HIV to sexual partners, including heterosexuals and other risk groups.[35] In addition to the benefits of ART for preventing HIV transmission in serodiscordant couples, data have shown that widespread use of ART may benefit entire communities via reductions in community viral load and decreased numbers of new infections.[176,177]

Medication adherence is the key to maximizing the full benefits of ART. Pharmacist involvement in improving antiretroviral medication adherence is perhaps the most well-documented preventive intervention and, as shown in a systematic review, is associated with statistically significant improvements in adherence and a positive impact on viral suppression.[178] Pharmacist involvement in direct patient care efforts focused on adherence extend well beyond required prescription counseling and may include providing practical and social support to motivate adherence, educating to enhance patient self-efficacy, regularly monitoring adherence, collaborating with other healthcare professionals, recognizing and helping to manage adverse effects, making recommendations regarding self-management, advocating for patients with insurance issues, and instructing on the use of adherence-enhancing tools.[178–180] The DHHS adult HIV guidelines provide evidence-based recommendations on assessing and monitoring adherence and outline strategies to help patients maintain high levels of adherence.[35] Identifying patients with adherence challenges requiring attention and implementing methods to enhance adherence are essential roles for all members of the treatment team, including pharmacists.

Although ART adherence is an essential component of HIV transmission prevention among HIV-infected individuals, it is also a necessary factor for prevention among HIV-exposed individuals taking PrEP or postexposure prophylaxis (PEP). PrEP is the use of antiretroviral medications by higher-risk, uninfected individuals before and during periods of risk to prevent HIV acquisition. Currently, the fixed-dose combination oral tablet of tenofovir-emtricitabine is the only FDA-approved product for PrEP; however, ongoing studies are examining the use of other antiretroviral agents in various dosage forms. When responding to patient inquiries regarding PrEP, pharmacists should be familiar with clinical practice guidelines published by CDC on the use of PrEP in high-risk populations and make informed and appropriate recommendations about PrEP safety, efficacy, acquisition, and need for routine follow-up HIV testing.[181] Pharmacists practicing in community settings that sell barrier methods or who fill prescriptions for PrEP or medications used to treat sexually transmitted infections can help identify patients who may benefit from PrEP and link them to PrEP prescribers in the community. The success of PrEP is largely dependent on high levels of medication adherence. To date, five clinical trials have demonstrated the efficacy of PrEP for HIV prevention in various patient populations, with improved efficacy for adherent individuals.[182–186] Notably, other PrEP studies have been halted early due to futility, primarily attributed to lower medication adherence.[187,188] Pharmacists have the opportunity to assist with developing PrEP protocols for newer prevention modalities, and, with appropriate training and resources, pharmacists can improve patient understanding, promote medication adherence, and enhance PrEP efficacy.[189,190] Pharmacists are well positioned to play a key role in helping patients make choices about PrEP, collaborate with prescribers to manage a patient's therapy, and advocate with other healthcare professionals regarding policy development.

PEP is the short-term use of antiretroviral medications by uninfected individuals after exposure to HIV. CDC has published guidelines for the implementation of HIV PEP after occupational and nonoccupational exposures.[191,192] Effective perinatal ART is also thought of as a form of PEP, and pharmacists are involved in the prevention of mother-to-child transmission of HIV.[193] Opportunities for pharmacist involvement in PEP vary by setting and may include developing institutional protocols, dispensing initial PEP doses, counseling patients on PEP medications, identifying drug interactions, and recommending follow-up testing. An important resource for pharmacists and other healthcare providers is the Clinician Consultation Center, which provides national expert telephone consultation, free of charge, surrounding PrEP, PEP, and perinatal HIV infection (www.nccc.ucsf.edu). The use of antiretroviral chemoprophylaxis for preventing HIV after accidental or occupational exposure and in maternal-to-fetal HIV transmission has become a widely accepted method to combat HIV, and pharmacists can effectively contribute to these initiatives.

HIV testing, in addition to ensuring early entry into care for HIV-infected individuals, is also an effective HIV prevention strategy. Pharmacists should be an entry point for early testing for HIV; they should recognize HIV risk factors and signs and symptoms of HIV/AIDS and recommend testing, whether it is provided onsite in community pharmacies or as an inhome test. Pharmacists should link individuals who test negative with effective prevention measures, including PrEP. Pharmacists should ensure that patients who test positive have access to medical care.

Decreasing circulation of contaminated syringes in and beyond the intravenous drug user (IDU) community is a central HIV prevention strategy.[194] Pharmacists can play an integral role in HIV prevention and the provision of health services to IDU populations by counseling IDUs regarding syringe access and disposal and addiction treatment programs. The literature documents pharmacist participation in providing and encouraging use of sterile syringes and injection equipment, providing patient counseling on harm-reduction strategies (e.g., substance abuse treatment, safe injection and disposal practices, safe sex practices), and supporting local syringe exchange programs.[194,195] In some areas, IDUs have the option of purchasing syringes from a pharmacy without a prescription. Such policies are controversial, however, and ultimately the decision to sell syringes without a prescription belongs to the individual pharmacist. Pharmacists should be aware of syringe replacement programs in their community and provide appropriate information to IDUs when requested. Providing HIV-related services to IDUs may not only limit HIV transmission but may also present an opportunity to expand healthcare services to a population that is historically underserved and may have limited access to other healthcare services.

Pharmacists should be knowledgeable about behavioral interventions to reduce HIV transmission, though documentation of pharmacists' delivery of behavioral interventions is still nascent. Pharmacists should provide educational messages and materials, advise patients on prevention methods (e.g., condom promotion, safer sex practices, drug-use counseling), and deliver behavioral risk-reduction counseling.

Pharmacists' unique position in society allows them to contribute to HIV prevention efforts. Pharmacist involvement includes both traditional roles (providing ART education and ensuring legal access to sterile needles and syringes) and innovative roles (developing PrEP protocols and delivering behavioral interventions). As HIV prevention becomes increasingly emphasized, pharmacists will play an important role on the healthcare team.

Pharmacist Involvement in HIV Education

Pharmacists are extensively involved in providing education to patients and providers about medication-related care, assessing the patient's readiness and ability to adhere to ART, providing initial or follow-up education on HIV-related disease and complications as well as antiretroviral medications, and evaluating adherence to a therapeutic regimen. Pharmacists perform these tasks within an interprofessional healthcare environment. As medication experts, pharmacists play a role in the education of patients, communities, and healthcare workers.

Central pharmacist roles are patient education and the provision of medication counseling to patients and communities. A recent systematic review documented the positive impact of pharmacist-conducted medication adherence education on clinical patient outcomes.[38] Education about medication indication, dose, route, frequency, potential adverse effects, and the importance of adherence should occur at every patient encounter. For returning patients, medication understanding and adherence should be reassessed not just for antiretroviral medications but for all medications. Through patient educational initiatives, pharmacists can help to ensure optimal pharmacotherapy, adherence, and successful outcomes.

Pharmacists often act as an educational liaison between the patient and the medical provider. The pharmacist's tasks can include helping with the selection of the optimal ART regimen, assisting patients in overcoming adherence issues, counseling patients, identifying and advising on potential drug–drug interactions, recognizing and managing medication adverse effects, and providing information on clinically oriented questions. Because HIV management is complex and involves coordination of multidrug therapies, pharmacists should support providers and assist prescribers and patients in attaining specific disease state goals. Pharmacists have expertise in medication dosing, adverse effects, drug–drug interactions, and medication adherence, and they serve as useful drug information sources for provider and patient inquiries.

Pharmacists practicing in HIV medicine should educate healthcare team members, provide in-service training to healthcare staff, and conduct community seminars for patients, caregivers, and the public on HIV, ART, drug interactions, and adherence. As a leader in HIV medication use, the pharmacist should train colleagues and the next generation of providers by teaching pharmacy students and residents. Trainee education could expand to other health professions, including medical students and residents; nursing students, especially those in advanced-degree programs; midlevel provider students; and allied health professions students as well as those receiving advanced training in the field of infectious diseases. Teaching may be clinical in nature (e.g., experiential rotations) or didactic training in a classroom setting.

Emphasis on the importance of keeping current with the rapidly evolving HIV field is vital for both practicing clinicians and future providers. Whatever the setting, pharmacists should continue to serve as a liaison between patients and providers to remain knowledgeable and credible within the field and to interact with colleagues in the HIV field at an interprofessional level. It is important to stay active and to be part of the exchange of information and clinical experience with other connected providers and trainees.

Pharmacist Social Services Involvement

Access to healthcare, including prescription medications, is a growing problem as the cost of healthcare rises. The cost of medications and copayments are major predictors of adherence to medication therapy regimens.[196–198] Many programs are available to assist with healthcare costs, but eligibility guidelines and application processes can be complicated. Pharmacists are well positioned to assist patients in overcoming these obstacles, making medications more accessible and reducing costs to individuals and healthcare entities.

Pharmacists are in an ideal position to educate patients, monitor adherence with therapy, and help patients work through drug-related problems. Pharmacists should monitor refills—both for availability and for timeliness—and notify the prescriber of any concerns. Pharmacists should know when prior-authorization requirements exist for medications and be able to facilitate approval to prevent delays in medication access for patients.[199] Pharmacists should ensure all antiretroviral medications and medications for opportunistic infection treatment and prophylaxis can be ordered for stock quickly and easily to minimize delays in medication access. Pharmacists can also ensure an adequate stock is available for the most common regimens. Likewise, pharmacists in all settings can play a significant role in medication reconciliation during care transitions.[200] Pharmacists should assist other healthcare providers in providing seamless care transitions (from outpatient care to institutional care, during hospitalization, and at the time of discharge) to prevent medication errors.[201] Pill burden, adverse effects, and demands on time and attention pose considerable obstacles to adherence; helping patients obtain their medications in a timely manner removes one major obstacle.

Pharmacists should assist patients at risk of nonadherence due to limited financial means. Patients often misunderstand available insurance benefits, and pharmacists can support patients by reviewing drug formularies, suggesting cost-effective options, and relaying this information to the prescriber. Pharmacists must know how to access national, state, and local resources. For patients with prescription drug insurance but difficulty affording copayments, or for patients lacking insurance, the pharmacist should confirm all medications are necessary and identify less-expensive alternatives. Many antiretroviral medication manufacturers offer prescription copayment cards that reduce a patient's out-of-pocket costs. Pharmaceutical manufacturers also offer patient assistance programs (PAPs) to ease the financial burden of medications. Eligibility criteria and enrollment requirements for PAPs vary, but they generally include documentation of limited income, lack of prescription drug coverage, and ineligibility for public assistance. Although PAP applications usually require both the prescriber's and the patient's signatures, pharmacists can assist in the application process.[197,198] Pharmacists should also be aware of pharmacies—local or mail order—that offer special generic retail pricing, which is sometimes less expensive than insurance copayments.

Pharmacists should have the knowledge to effectively help low-income patients gain access to national and state-level prescription drug programs for which they may be eligible, including Medicare Part D, Ryan White AIDS Drug Assistance Programs (ADAPs), and Medicaid. Medicare Part D is designed to offer the beneficiary a choice between prescription drug plans, and many pharmacists offer Part D plan selection assistance to help beneficiaries obtain optimal drug coverage.[202] ADAPs are available in each state, guaranteeing antiretroviral medication prescription assistance to low-income, underinsured, and uninsured HIV-infected patients. The Patient Protection and Affordable Care Act will expand health insurance program eligibility and provide opportunities for pharmacists to assist with care coordination and expand their scopes of practice.[203] Although pharmacists cannot choose prescription drug plans for patients, pharmacists should serve as a resource to help patients understand their options to ensure continued access to antiretroviral medications.

Pharmacist Professional Involvement

Although pharmacists have a role in direct HIV patient care, there are other ways pharmacists can assist the HIV patient population. Pharmacists should be active in extracurricular professional involvement, which can be achieved via organizational membership, HIV pharmacist certification, advocacy initiatives, volunteer positions, and participation in clinical research. These areas represent possible opportunities for pharmacists to supplement clinical roles.

In recent years, HIV-focused professional organizations have expanded to include pharmacist membership. State and regional AIDS education and training centers have embraced pharmacist involvement and many provide education, networking, and faculty appointments for pharmacists involved in HIV care. On a national scale, the American Academy of HIV Medicine encourages pharmacist membership and invites pharmacists to serve as active members in organizational leadership and committees. Several national HIV organizations also have pharmacist-specific registration, programming, and continuing-education credit opportunities at their educational conventions. Internationally, the Canadian HIV/AIDS Pharmacist Network strives to connect pharmacists involved in HIV care and provides educational information to its members. In addition, the International Association of Providers of AIDS Care has expanded to recognize pharmacists as part of the HIV treatment team. Pharmacists involved in HIV care should strive to be active members of professional organizations, attend organizational meetings, provide meeting lectures on HIV clinical updates, participate in the sharing of HIV information via pharmacist networks, and support enhanced pharmacist membership in these organizations (appendix).

The creation of pharmacist HIV credentialing programs highlights the importance of having pharmacists knowledgeable about and trained in the treatment of HIV disease. The American Academy of HIV Medicine HIV Pharmacist credential (AAHIVP) is offered to pharmacists who have completed certain requirements, such as evidence of direct HIV patient care, HIV continuing education, and successful completion of the AAHIVP credentialing exam.[204] Other institutions also offer specific pharmacist HIV certificate programs. Pharmacists should investigate certification opportunities, seek the knowledge and skills necessary to be certified HIV pharmacists, and lead the pharmacy profession in the care of HIV-positive patients (appendix).

Pharmacists should also be aware of local and national policy issues surrounding HIV care. The world of HIV changes rapidly, and many challenges require legislative or regulatory action. Pharmacists should be advocates for HIV patients by being familiar with current HIV legislation and national HIV programs such as the Ryan White Program. Pharmacists should also contact local and national policymakers to ensure proper education about HIV issues, be involved in HIV advisory panels, provide expert testimony, and participate in advocacy initiatives to assist in the development of laws that best serve HIV patients. Through these opportunities, pharmacists can steer policy development and actively advocate for HIV patients.

There are also many opportunities for pharmacists to volunteer for HIV-related activities. Locally, pharmacists can volunteer in their communities by participating in fundraising events such as AIDS walks, auctions, and other functions in which proceeds go to fund local HIV programs. Many communities are in need of pharmacists to serve in free medical and dental clinics, where underserved patients receive access to much-needed HIV care. Pharmacists can also choose to volunteer outside of their communities through programs such as Doctors Without Borders that focus on delivering HIV care and medications to developing countries.[205] There are numerous volunteer opportunities that benefit HIV patients outside of medical settings, and pharmacists should dedicate time to serving in these capacities.

Finally, pharmacists should play an active role in HIV clinical research. Pharmacists should be knowledgeable about ongoing clinical research trials on topic areas such as new antiretroviral medications, disease state complications, and prevention strategies that will shape the future of HIV care. Pharmacists can serve in a variety of capacities as part of HIV clinical research teams, as principal or coinvestigators, in the recruitment and obtaining the consent of trial participants, and in facilitation of clinical research trials within their practice settings.[206] Permissible scope-of-pharmacist involvement in clinical research varies by state, and pharmacists should be familiar with laws that define pharmacist activity. Pharmacists may also be involved in research by publishing case reports, serving on institutional review boards, acting as consultants in HIV clinical research trials, and serving as research mentors to other practitioners caring for patients with HIV. With over 30 antiretroviral medications available and more in the investigational pipeline, pharmacists can have an integral role in facilitating the introduction of safe and effective HIV medications and clinical research.

Pharmacist involvement in the care of the HIV patient extends beyond the bedside to include other types of professional activity. Through organizational membership, HIV pharmacist certification, advocacy initiatives, volunteer positions, and participation in clinical research, pharmacists should be true advocates in all aspects of HIV patient care. Pharmacists are a tremendous resource that should be mobilized, and each pharmacist has a responsibility to be an active proponent for the advancement of HIV care.

Conclusion

HIV medicine is a dynamic field that has evolved dramatically since its inception. It continues to evolve today, providing both opportunities for and challenges to delivering optimal patient care. These challenges and opportunities should be met with interprofessional efforts that identify and optimize the roles of all healthcare team members, including pharmacists, as a means to provide comprehensive care and improve patient outcomes. Pharmacists in particular are uniquely capable of contributing to all components of HIV care by being highly accessible to both patients and providers in a variety of healthcare settings. Their expert drug therapy knowledge and clinical skills provide an avenue for proficient clinical consultation with other healthcare providers as well as effective patient interactions through counseling and education. Furthermore, given their training and skills set, pharmacists are well positioned within the interdisciplinary healthcare team to help meet the current and future challenges of HIV medicine, including helping to deliver comprehensive primary care to an aging HIV patient population as well as working with others to identify and manage the long-term complications of HIV infection and ART. Given the ongoing evolution of HIV medicine, pharmacists must continue to evolve their roles as a part of the healthcare team to identify and meet the future needs of HIV-positive patients. This goal can be achieved through continuous assessment of the role of the HIV pharmacist, the development and maintenance of HIV specialty pharmacist training programs and expert certification, and the continued collaboration with other healthcare providers, patients, activist groups, and professional HIV medicine and pharmacy organizations.

References

1. Centers for Disease Control. Kaposi's sarcoma and pneumocystis pneumonia among homosexual men—New York City and California. *MMWR*. 1981; 30:305–8.
2. Hall HI, Song R, Rhodes P, et al. Estimation of HIV incidence in the United States. *JAMA*. 2008; 300:520–9.
3. Rodger AJ, Lodwick R, Schechter M, et al. Mortality in well controlled HIV in the continuous antiretroviral therapy arms of the SMART and ESPRIT trials compared with the general population. *AIDS*. 2013; 27:973–9.
4. Centers for Disease Control and Prevention. Estimates of new HIV infections in the United States, 2006–2009 (August 2011). www.cdc.gov/nchhstp/newsroom/docs/HIV-Infections-2006-2009.pdf (accessed 2012 Oct 16).
5. El-Sadr WM, Mayer KH, Adimora AA. The HIV epidemic in the United States: a time for action. Introduction. *J Acquir Immune Defic Syndr*. 2010; 55(suppl 2):S63.
6. Millett GA, Crowley JS, Koh H, et al. A way forward: the National HIV/AIDS Strategy and reducing HIV incidence in the United States. *J Acquir Immune Defic Syndr*. 2010; 55(suppl 2):S144–7.
7. El-Sadr WM, Mayer KH, Hodder SL. AIDS in America—forgotten but not gone. *N Engl J Med*. 2010; 362:967–70.
8. Moore RD. Epidemiology of HIV infection in the United States: implications for linkage to care. *Clin Infect Dis*. 2011; 52(suppl 2):S208–13.
9. Centers for Disease Control and Prevention. Vital signs: HIV prevention through care and treatment—United States. *MMWR*. 2011; 60:1618–23.
10. Smith M, Bates DW, Bodenheimer TS. Pharmacists belong in accountable care organizations and integrated care teams. *Health Aff*. 2013; 32:1963–70.
11. Smith M, Bates DW, Bodenheimer TS, et al. Why pharmacists belong in the medical home. *Health Aff*. 2010; 29:906–13.
12. Henderson KC, Hindman J, Johnson SC, et al. Assessing the effectiveness of pharmacy-based adherence interventions on antiretroviral adherence in persons with HIV. *AIDS Patient Care STDs*. 2011; 25:221–8.
13. Ma A, Chen DM, Chau FM, et al. Improving adherence and clinical outcomes through an HIV pharmacist's interventions. *AIDS Care*. 2010; 22:1189–94.

14. March K, Mak M, Louie SG. Effects of pharmacists' interventions on patient outcomes in an HIV primary care clinic. *Am J Health-Syst Pharm.* 2007; 64:2574–8.
15. Merchen BA, Gerzenshtein L, Scarsi KK, et al. HIV-specialized pharmacists' impact on prescribing errors in hospitalized patients on antiretroviral therapy (abstract H2-794). Presented at the 51st Interscience Conference on Antimicrobial Agents and Chemotherapy. Chicago, IL: 2011 Sep.
16. Heelon M, Skiest D, Tereso G, et al. Effect of a clinical pharmacist's intervention on duration of antiretroviral-related errors in hospitalized patients. *Am J Health-Syst Pharm.* 2007; 64:2064–8.
17. American Society of Health-System Pharmacists. ASHP statement on the pharmacist's role in the care of patients with HIV infection. *Am J Health-Syst Pharm.* 2003; 60:1998–2003.
18. Centers for Disease Control and Prevention. Monitoring selected national HIV prevention and care objectives by using HIV surveillance data—United States and 6 dependent areas—2011 (October 2013). www.cdc.gov/hiv/library/reports/surveillance (accessed 2014 Nov 24).
19. Branson BM, Handsfield HH, Lampe MA, et al. Revised recommendations for HIV testing of adults, adolescents, and pregnant women in health-care settings. *MMWR Recomm Rep.* 2006; 55:1–17.
20. Moyer VA, on behalf of the U.S. Preventive Services Task Force. Screening for HIV: U.S. Preventive Services Task Force recommendation statement. *Ann Intern Med.* 2013; 159:51–60.
21. Weidle PJ, Lecher S, Botts LW, et al. HIV testing in community pharmacies and retail clinics: a model to expand access to screening for HIV infection. *J Am Pharm Assoc.* 2014; 54:486–92.
22. Darin KM, Klepser ME, Klepser DE, et al. Pharmacist-provided rapid HIV testing in two community pharmacies. *J Am Pharm Assoc.* 2015; 55:81–8.
23. Sherman EM, Elrod S, Allen D, et al. Pharmacist testers in multidisciplinary health care team expand HIV point-of-care testing program. *J Pharm Pract.* 2014; 27:578–81.
24. Michigan Pharmacists Association. Community pharmacy-based rapid diagnostic testing certificate course and Train-the-Trainer program. www.michiganpharmacists.org/resources/pointofcare (accessed 2016 Jan 21).
25. Amesty S, Blaney S, Crawford ND, et al. Pharmacy staff characteristics associated with support for pharmacy-based HIV testing. *J Am Pharm Assoc.* 2012; 52:472–9.
26. Deas CM, McCree DH. Pharmacists and HIV/AIDS prevention: review of the literature. *J Am Pharm Assoc.* 2010; 50:411–5.
27. Lutnick A, Case P, Kral AH. Injection drug users' perspectives on placing HIV prevention and other clinical services in pharmacy settings. *J Urban Health.* 2012; 89:354–64.
28. Darin KM, Scarsi KK, Klepser DG, et al. Consumer interest in community pharmacy HIV screening services. *J Am Pharm Assoc.* 2015; 55:67–72.
29. Food and Drug Administration. FDA approves first over-the-counter home-use rapid HIV test (July 3, 2012). www.fda.gov/NewsEvents/Newsroom/PressAnnouncements/ucm310542.htm (accessed 2012 Aug 9).
30. Branson BM, Owen SM, Wesolowski LG, et al. Laboratory testing for the diagnosis of HIV infection: updated recommendations (June 27, 2014). http://stacks.cdc.gov/view/cdc/23447 (accessed 2014 Dec 4).
31. Waldura JF, Neff S, Goldschmidt RH. Teleconsultation for clinicians who provide human immunodeficiency virus care: experience of the National HIV Telephone Consultation Service. *Telemed J E Health.* 2011:17:472–7.
32. Neff S, Goldschmidt RH. State human immunodeficiency virus testing laws. *Arch Intern Med.* 2008; 168:1717–8.
33. Aberg JA, Gallant JE, Ghanem KG, et al. Primary care guidelines for the management of persons infected with HIV: 2013 update by the HIV Medicine Association of the Infectious Diseases Society of America. *Clin Infect Dis.* 2014; 58:e1–34.
34. Health Resources and Services Administration, HIV/AIDS Bureau. Guide for HIV/AIDS clinical care, 2014. http://hab.hrsa.gov/deliverhivaidscare/2014guide.pdf (accessed Jan 21).
35. Panel on Antiretroviral Guidelines for Adults and Adolescents. Guidelines for the use of antiretroviral agents in HIV-1-infected adults and adolescents. http://aidsinfo.nih.gov/ContentFiles/AdultandAdolescentGL.pdf (accessed 2016 Jan 21).
36. Yehia BR, Mehta JM, Ciuffetelli D, et al. Antiretroviral medication errors remain high but are quickly corrected among hospitalized HIV-infected adults. *Clin Infect Dis.* 2012; 55:593–9.
37. Liao TV, Rab S, Armstrong WS. Evaluation of medication errors in patients infected with human immunodeficiency virus treated with antiretroviral therapy. *Am J Health-Syst Pharm.* 2012; 69:1461–2.
38. Saberi P, Dong BJ, Johnson MO, et al. The impact of HIV clinical pharmacists on HIV treatment outcomes: a systematic review. *Patient Prefer Adherence.* 2012; 6:297–322.
39. Kauffman Y, Nair V, Herist K, et al. HIV medication therapy management services in community pharmacies. *J Am Pharm Assoc.* 2012; 52:e287–91.
40. Centers for Disease Control and Prevention. Monitoring selected national HIV prevention and care objectives by using HIV surveillance data—United States and 6 U.S. dependent areas—2010. www.cdc.gov/hiv/surveillance/resources/reports/2010supp_vol17no3/index.htm (accessed 2016 Jan 21).
41. Centers for Disease Control and Prevention. Estimated HIV incidence in the United States, 2007–2010. www.cdc.gov/hiv/pdf/statistics_hssr_vol_17_no_4.pdf (accessed Jan 21).
42. Panel on Treatment of HIV-Infected Pregnant Women and Prevention of Perinatal Transmission. Recommendations for use of antiretroviral drugs in pregnant HIV-1-infected women for maternal health and interventions to reduce perinatal HIV transmission in the

United States. http://aidsinfo.nih.gov/contentfiles/lvguidelines/PerinatalGL.pdf (accessed 2016 Jan 21).

43. Palumbo PE, Kwok S, Waters S, et al. Viral measurement by polymerase chain reaction-based assays in human immunodeficiency virus-infected infants. *J Pediatr.* 1995; 126:592–5.
44. Shearer WT, Quinn TC, LaRussa P, et al. Viral load and disease progression in infants infected with human immunodeficiency virus type 1. *N Engl J Med.* 1997; 336:1337–42.
45. HIV Paediatric Prognostic Markers Collaborative Study. Predictive value of absolute CD4 cell count for disease progression in untreated HIV-1-infected children. *AIDS.* 2006; 20:1289–94.
46. Dunn D, for the HIV Paediatric Prognostic Markers Collaborative Study Group. Short-term risk of disease progression in HIV-1-infected children receiving no antiretroviral therapy or zidovudine monotherapy: a meta-analysis. *Lancet.* 2003; 362:1605–11.
47. Dunn D, Woodburn P, Duong T, et al. Current CD4 cell count and the short-term risk of AIDS and death before the availability of effective antiretroviral therapy in HIV-infected children and adults. *J Infect Dis.* 2008; 197:398–404.
48. Boyd K, Dunn DT, Castro H, et al. Discordance between CD4 cell count and CD4 cell percentage: implications for when to start antiretroviral therapy in HIV-1 infected children. *AIDS.* 2010; 24:1213–7.
49. Kearns GL, Abdel-Rahman SM, Alander SW, et al. Developmental pharmacology—drug disposition, action, and therapy in infants and children. *N Engl J Med.* 2003; 349:1157–67.
50. Panel on Antiretroviral Therapy and Medical Management of HIV-Infected Children. Guidelines for the use of antiretroviral agents in pediatric HIV infection. http://aidsinfo.nih.gov/contentfiles/lvguidelines/pediatricguidelines.pdf (accessed 2013 May 1).
51. Murphy DA, Sarr M, Durako SJ, et al. Barriers to HAART adherence among human immunodeficiency virus-infected adolescents. *Arch Pediatr Adolesc Med.* 2003; 157:249–55.
52. Merzel C, Vandevanter N, Irvine M. Adherence to antiretroviral therapy among older children and adolescents with HIV: a qualitative study of psychosocial contexts. *AIDS Patient Care STDs.* 2008; 22:977–87.
53. Mellins CA, Brackis-Cott E, Dolezal C, et al. The role of psychosocial and family factors in adherence to antiretroviral treatment in human immunodeficiency virus-infected children. *Pediatr Infect Dis J.* 2004; 23:1035–41.
54. Malee K, Williams P, Montepiedra G, et al. Medication adherence in children and adolescents with HIV infection: associations with behavioral impairment. *AIDS Patient Care STDs.* 2011; 25:191–200.
55. Guaraldi G, Orlando G, Zona S, et al. Premature age-related comorbidities among HIV-infected persons compared with the general population. *Clin Infect Dis.* 2011; 53:1120–6.
56. Centers for Disease Control and Prevention. Fact sheet: HIV/AIDS among persons aged 50 and older. www.cdc.gov/hiv/pdf/library_factsheet_HIV_among_PersonsAged50andolder.pdf (accessed 2016 Jan 21).
57. Anuurad E, Semrad A, Berglund L. Human immunodeficiency virus and highly active antiretroviral therapy–associated metabolic disorders and risk factors for cardiovascular disease. *Metab Syndr Relat Disord.* 2009; 5:401–9.
58. Kotler DP. HIV and antiretroviral therapy: lipid abnormalities and associated cardiovascular risk in HIV-infected patients. *J Acquir Immune Defic Syndr.* 2008; 49(suppl 2):S79–85.
59. Gupta SK, Eustace JA, Winston JA, et al. Guidelines for the management of chronic kidney disease in HIV-infected patients: recommendations of the HIV Medicine Association of the Infectious Diseases Society of America. *Clin Infect Dis.* 2005; 40:1559–85.
60. Dube MP. Disorders of glucose metabolism in patients infected with human immunodeficiency virus. *Clin Infect Dis.* 2000; 31:1467–75.
61. Triant VA, Brown TT, Lee H, et al. Fracture prevalence among human immunodeficiency virus (HIV)-infected versus non-HIV-infected patients in a large U.S. health care system. *J Clin Endocrinol Metab.* 2008; 93:3499–504.
62. Young B, Dao CN, Buchacz K, et al. Increased rates of bone fracture among HIV-infected persons in the HIV Outpatient Study (HOPS) compared with the US general population, 2000-2006. *Clin Infect Dis.* 2011; 52:1061–8.
63. Bedimo R, Maalouf NM, Zhang S, et al. Osteoporotic fracture associated with cumulative exposure to tenofovir and other antiretroviral agents. *AIDS.* 2012; 26:825–31.
64. Do AN, Rosenberg ES, Sullivan PS, et al. Excess burden of depression among HIV-infected persons receiving medical care in the United States: data from the medical monitoring project and behavioral risk factor surveillance system. *PloS One.* 2014; 9:e92842.
65. Hicks PL, Mulvey KP, Chander G, et al. The impact of illicit drug use and substance abuse treatment on adherence to HAART. *AIDS Care.* 2007; 19:1134–40.
66. Cofrancesco J Jr, Scherzer R, Tien PC, et al. Illicit drug use and HIV treatment outcomes in a US cohort. *AIDS.* 2008; 22:357–65.
67. Tucker JS, Burman MA, Sherbourne CD, et al. Substance use and mental health correlates of nonadherence to antiretroviral medications in a sample of patients with human immunodeficiency virus infection. *Am J Med.* 2003; 114:573–80.
68. Morris JD, Golub ET, Mehta SH, et al. Injection drug use and patterns of highly active antiretroviral therapy use: an analysis of ALIVE, WIHS, and MACS cohorts. *AIDS Res Ther.* 2007; 4:12.
69. Gruber VA, McCance-Katz EF. Methadone, buprenorphine, and street drug interactions with antiretroviral medications. *Curr HIV/AIDS Rep.* 2010; 7:152–60.
70. Bruce RD, Altice FL, Gourevitch MN, et al. A review of pharmacokinetic drug interactions between drugs of abuse and antiretroviral medications: implications and management for clinical practice. *Exp Rev Clin Pharmacol.* 2008; 1:115–27.

71. Spradling PR, Richardson JT, Buchacz K, et al. Prevalence of chronic hepatitis B virus infection among patients in the HIV Outpatient Study, 1996–2007. *J Viral Hepat.* 2010; 17:879–86.
72. Thio CL, Seaberg EC, Skolasky R Jr, et al. HIV-1, hepatitis B virus, and risk of liver-related mortality in the Multicenter Cohort Study (MACS). *Lancet.* 2002; 360:1921–6.
73. McMahon MA, Jilek BL, Brennan TP, et al. The HBV drug entecavir - effects on HIV-1 replication and resistance. *N Engl J Med.* 2007; 356:2614–21.
74. Sulkowski MS, Mast EE, Seeff LB, et al. Hepatitis C virus infection as an opportunistic disease in persons infected with human immunodeficiency virus. *Clin Infect Dis.* 2000; 30(suppl 1):S77–84.
75. Macias J, Berenguer J, Japon MA, et al. Fast fibrosis progression between repeated liver biopsies in patients coinfected with human immunodeficiency virus/hepatitis C virus. *Hepatology.* 2009; 50:1056–63.
76. Marino EL, Alvarez-Rubio L, Miro S, et al. Pharmacist intervention in treatment of patients with genotype 1 chronic hepatitis C. *J Manag Care Pharm.* 2009; 15:147–50.
77. Rosenquist A, Best BM, Miller TA, et al. Medication therapy management services in community pharmacy: a pilot program in HIV specialty pharmacies. *J Eval Clin Pract.* 2010; 16:1142–6.
78. American Association for the Study of Liver Diseases, Infectious Diseases Society of America. HCV guidance: recommendations for testing, managing, and treating hepatitis C. www.hcvguidelines.org (accessed 2014 Dec 26).
79. Stock PG, Barin B, Murphy B, et al. Outcomes of kidney transplantation in HIV-infected recipients. *N Engl J Med.* 2010; 363:2004–14.
80. Terrault NA, Roland ME, Schiano T, et al. Outcomes of liver transplant recipients with hepatitis C and human immunodeficiency virus coinfection. *Liver Transpl.* 2012; 18:716–26.
81. Blumberg EA, Stock P, AST Infectious Diseases Community of Practice. Solid organ transplantation in the HIV-infected patient. *Am J Transplant.* 2009; 9(suppl 4):S131–5.
82. Roland ME, Barin B, Carlson L, et al. HIV-infected liver and kidney transplant recipients: 1- and 3-year outcomes. *Am J Transplant.* 2008; 8:355–65.
83. Stock P, Roland M, Hanto D, et al. Early and unexpected results in a multicenter study of kidney transplant recipients. *Am J Transplant.* 2009; 9(suppl 2):197.
84. Terrault NA, Carter JT, Carlson L, et al. Outcome of patients with hepatitis B virus and human immuno-deficiency virus infections referred for liver transplantation. *Liver Transpl.* 2006; 12:801–7.
85. De Vera ME, Vorchik I, Tom K, et al. Survival of liver transplant patients coinfected with HIV and HCV is adversely impacted by recurrent hepatitis C. *Am J Transplant.* 2006; 6:2983–93.
86. DuClos-Vallee JC, Feray JC, Sebagh M, et al. Survival and recurrence of hepatitis C after liver transplantation in patients coinfected with human immunodeficiency virus and hepatitis C virus. *Hepatology.* 2008; 47:407–17.
87. Chisholm MA, Mulloy LL, Jaqadeesan M, et al. Impact of clinical pharmacy services on renal transplant patients' compliance with immunosuppressive medications. *Clin Transplant.* 2001; 15:330–6.
88. Roland ME, Barin B, Carlson L, et al. HIV-infected liver and kidney transplant recipients: 1- and 3-year outcomes. *Am J Transplant.* 2008; 8:355–65.
89. Gasser O, Bihl F, Sanghavi S, et al. Treatment-dependent loss of polyfunctional CD8+ T-cell responses in HIV-infected kidney transplant recipients is associated with herpesvirus reactivation. *Am J Transplant.* 2009; 9:794–803.
90. Carter JT, Melcher ML, Carlson LL, et al. Thymoglobulin-associated CD4+ T-cell depletion and infection risk in HIV-infected renal transplant recipients. *Am J Transplant.* 2006; 6:753–60.
91. Centers for Disease Control and Prevention, U.S. Department of Health and Human Services. Medical examination of aliens – removal of human immuno-deficiency virus infection from definition of communicable disease of public health significance. Final rule. *Fed Regist.* 2009; 74:56547–62.
92. Winston SE, Beckwith CG. The impact of removing the immigration ban on HIV-infected persons. *AIDS Patient Care STDs.* 2011; 25:709–11.
93. Centers for Disease Control and Prevention, U.S. Department of Health and Human Services, National Center for Emerging and Zoonotic Infectious Diseases. Screening for HIV infection during the refugee domestic medical examination (April 16, 2012). www.cdc.gov/immigrantrefugeehealth/pdf/hiv-screening-domestic-medical.pdf (accessed 2016 Jan 3).
94. Akinsete OO, Sides T, Hirigoyen D, et al. Demographic, clinical, and virologic characteristics of African-born persons with HIV/AIDS in a Minnesota hospital. *AIDS Patient Care STDs.* 2007; 21:356–65.
95. Prosser AT, Tang T, Hall HI. HIV in persons born outside the United States, 2007-2010. *JAMA.* 2012; 308:601–7.
96. Tanaka Y, Kunii O, Hatano T, et al. Knowledge, attitude, and practice (KAP) of HIV prevention and HIV infection risks among Congolese refugees in Tanzania. *Health Place.* 2008; 14:434–52.
97. Thompson MA, Mugavero MJ, Amico KR, et al. Guidelines for improving entry into and retention in care and antiretroviral adherence for persons with HIV: evidence-based recommendations from an International Association of Physicians in AIDS Care panel. *Ann Intern Med.* 2012; 146:817–33.
98. Kredo T, Van der Walt JS, Siegfried N, et al. Therapeutic drug monitoring of antiretrovirals for people with HIV. *Cochrane Database Syst Rev.* 2009; 3:CD007268.
99. Liu TF, Shafer RW. Web resources for HIV type 1 genotypic-resistance test interpretation. *Clin Infect Dis.* 2006; 42:1608–18.
100. Neuhaus J, Angus B, Kowalska JD, et al. Risk of all-cause mortality associated with nonfatal AIDS and serious non-AIDS events among adults infected with HIV. *AIDS.* 2010; 24:697–706.
101. Benjamin LA, Bryer A, Emsley HC, et al. HIV infection and stroke: current perspectives and future directions. *Lancet Neurol.* 2012; 11:878–90.

102. Schifitto G, Zhang J, Evans SR, et al. A multicenter trial of selegiline transdermal system for HIV-associated cognitive impairment. *Neurology.* 2007; 69:1314–21.
103. Auerbach E, Aboulafia DM. Venous and arterial thromboembolic complications associated with HIV infection and highly active antiretroviral therapy. *Semin Thromb Hemost.* 2012; 38:830–8.
104. Friis-Moller N, Sabin CA, Weber R, et al. Combination antiretroviral therapy and the risk of myocardial infarction. *N Engl J Med.* 2003; 349:1993–2003.
105. Boccara F, Mary-Krause M, Teiger E, et al. Acute coronary syndrome in human immunodeficiency virus-infected patients: characteristics and 1 year prognosis. *Eur Heart J.* 2001; 32:41–50.
106. Dakin CL, O'Connor CA, Patsdaughter CA. HAART to heart: HIV-related cardiomyopathy and other cardiovascular complications. *AACN Clin Issues.* 2006; 17:18–29.
107. Reinsch N, Neuhasu K, Esser S, et al. Prevalence of cardiac diastolic dysfunction in HIV-infected patients: results of the HIV-HEART study. *HIV Clin Trials.* 2010; 11:156–62.
108. Calmy A, Gayet-Ageron A, Montecucco F, et al. HIV increases markers of cardiovascular risk: results from a randomized, treatment interruption trial. *AIDS.* 2009; 23:929–39.
109. El-Sadr WM, Lundgren JD, Neaton JD, et al. CD4+ count-guided interruption of antiretroviral treatment. *N Engl J Med.* 2006; 335:2283–96.
110. Bunting BA, Smith BH, Sutherland SE. The Ashville Project: clinical and economic outcomes of a community-based long-term medication therapy management program for hypertension and dyslipidemia. *J Am Pharm Assoc.* 2008; 48:23–31.
111. Till LT, Voris JC, Horst JB. Assessment of clinical pharmacist management of lipid-lowering therapy in a primary care setting. *J Manag Care Pharm.* 2003; 9:269–73.
112. Simpson SH, Majumdar SR, Tsuyuki RT, et al. Effect of adding pharmacists to primary care teams on blood pressure control in patients with type 2 diabetes: a randomized controlled trial. *Diabetes Care.* 2011; 34:20–6.
113. Morello CM, Zadvorny EB, Cording MA, et al. Development and clinical outcomes of pharmacist-managed diabetes care clinics. *Am J Health-Syst Pharm.* 2006; 63:1325–31.
114. Gerber J, Parra D, Beckey NP, et al. Optimizing drug therapy in patients with cardiovascular disease: the impact of pharmacist-managed pharmacotherapy clinics in a primary care setting. *Pharmacotherapy.* 2002; 22:738–47.
115. Doler NM, Dolder CR. Comparison of a pharmacist-managed lipid clinic: in-person versus telephone. *J Am Pharm Assoc.* 2010; 50:375–8.
116. Pape GA, Hunt JS, Butler KL, et al. Team-based care approach to cholesterol management in diabetes mellitus. *Arch Intern Med.* 2011; 17:1480–6.
117. Johnson KA, Chen S, Cheng IN, et al. The impact of clinical pharmacy services integrated into medical homes on diabetes-related clinical outcomes. *Ann Pharmacother.* 2010; 44:1877–86.
118. Petoumenos K, Worm S, Reiss P, et al. Rates of cardiovascular disease following smoking cessation in patients with HIV infection: results from the D:A:D study. *HIV Med.* 2011; 12:412–21.
119. Mutimura E, Crowther NJ, Cade TW, et al. Exercise training reduces central adiposity and improves metabolic indices in HAART-treated HIV-positive subjects in Rwanda: a randomized controlled trial. *AIDS Res Hum Retroviruses.* 2008; 24:15–23.
120. Lima EM, Gualandro DM, Yu PC, et al. Cardiovascular prevention in HIV patients: results from a successful intervention program. *Atherosclerosis.* 2009; 204:229–32.
121. Sabin CA, Worm SW, Weber R, et al. Use of nucleoside reverse transcriptase inhibitors and risk of myocardial infarction in HIV-infected patients enrolled in the D:A:D study: a multi-cohort collaboration. *Lancet.* 2008; 371:1417–26.
122. El-Sadr WM, Lundgren J, Neaton JD, et al. CD4+ count-guided interruption of antiretroviral treatment. *N Engl J Med.* 2006; 355:2283–96.
123. Friis-Moller N, Reiss P, Sabin CA, et al. Class of antiretroviral drugs and the risk of myocardial infarction. *N Engl J Med.* 2007; 356:1723–35.
124. Yongmei L, Skilpak MG, Grunfeld C, et al. Incidence and risk factors for acute kidney injury in HIV infection. *Am J Nephrol.* 2012; 35:327–34.
125. Wyatt CM. The kidney in HIV infection: beyond HIV-associated nephropathy. *Top Antivir Med.* 2012; 20:106–10.
126. Maggi P, Montinaro V, Mussino C, et al. Novel antiretroviral drugs and renal function monitoring of HIV patients. *AIDS Rev.* 2014; 16:144–51.
127. Atta MG, Gallant JE, Rahman MH, et al. Antiretroviral therapy in the treatment of HIV-associated nephropathy. *Nephrol Dial Transplant.* 2006; 21:2809–13.
128. Kalayjian RC, Franceschini N, Gupta SK, et al. Suppression of HIV-1 replication by antiretroviral therapy improves renal function in persons with low CD4 cell counts and chronic kidney disease. *AIDS.* 2008; 22:481–7.
129. Choi AI, Yongmei L, Deeks SG, et al. Association between kidney function and albuminuria with cardiovascular events in HIV-infected persons. *Circulation.* 2010; 121:651–8.
130. Appelbaum JS, McCormick WC. HIV and Aging Consensus Project executive summary: recommended treatment strategies for clinicians managing older patients with HIV (April 2013). www.aahivm.org/Upload_Module/upload/HIV%20and%20Aging/AAHIVM%20Executive%20Summary%20FINAL%202.pdf (accessed 2016 Jan 4).
131. Hassan Y, Al-Ramahi RJ, Aziz NA, et al. Impact of a renal drug dosing service on dose adjustment in hospitalized patients with chronic kidney disease. *Ann Pharmacother.* 2009; 43:1598–605.
132. Mendes-Correa MC, Andrade HF Jr, Fumica Takakura C, et al. Hepatic ultrastructural mitochondrial changes prior to antiretroviral therapy in HIV-infected patients in Brazil. *J Int Assoc Physicians AIDS Care.* 2008; 7:252–8.

133. Neuman MG, Schneider M, Nanau RM, et al. HIV-antiretroviral therapy induced liver, gastrointestinal, and pancreatic injury. *Int J Hepatol.* 2012; 2012:760706.
134. Simioni S, Cavassini M, Annoni JM, et al. Cognitive dysfunction in HIV patients despite long-standing suppression of viremia. *AIDS.* 2010; 24:1243–50.
135. Heaton RK, Clifford DB, Franklin DR Jr, et al. HIV-associated neurocognitive disorders persist in the era of potent antiretroviral therapy: CHARTER Study. *Neurology.* 2010; 75:2087–96.
136. Mateen FJ, Shinohara RT, Carone M, et al. Neurological disorders incidence in HIV+ vs HIV-men: Multicenter AIDS Cohort Study, 1996–2011. *Neurology.* 2012; 79:1873–80.
137. Ellis RJ, Badiee J, Vaida F, et al. CD4 nadir is a predictor of HIV neurocognitive impairment in the era of combination antiretroviral therapy. *AIDS.* 2011; 25:1747–51.
138. Schifitto G, Navia BA, Yiannoutsos CT, et al. Memantine and HIV-associated cognitive impairment: a neuropsychological and proton magnetic resonance spectroscopy study. *AIDS.* 2007; 21:1877–86.
139. Silva MM. Neurologic complications of HIV in the HAART era: where are we? *Braz J Infect Dis.* 2012; 16:373–8.
140. Prohaska ES, King AR. Administration of antiretroviral medication via enteral tubes. *Am J Health-Syst Pharm.* 2012; 69:2140–6.
141. Nyberg CR, Patterson BY, Williams MM. When patients cannot take pills: antiretroviral drug formulations for managing adult HIV infection. *Top Antivir Med.* 2011; 19:126–31.
142. Chiu CC, Wu SS, Lee PY, et al. Control of modifiable risk factors in ischemic stroke outpatients by pharmacist intervention: an equal allocation stratified randomized study. *J Clin Pharm Ther.* 2008; 33:529–35.
143. Patel P, Hanson DL, Sullivan PS, et al. Incidence of types of cancer among HIV-infected persons compared with the general population in the United States, 1992-2003. *Ann Intern Med.* 2008; 148:728–36.
144. Deeken JF, Tjen-A-Looi A, Rudek MA, et al. The rising challenge of non-AIDS-defining cancers in HIV-infected patients. *Clin Infect Dis.* 2012; 55:1228–35.
145. Engels EA, Biggar RJ, All HI, et al. Cancer risk in people infected with human immunodeficiency virus in the United States. *Int J Cancer.* 2008; 123:187–94.
146. Falutz J. Management of fat accumulation in patients with HIV infection. *Curr HIV/AIDS Rep.* 2011; 8:200–8.
147. Chen D, Misra A, Garg A. Lipodystropy in human immunodeficiency virus-infected patients. *J Clin Endocrinol Metab.* 2002; 87:4845–56.
148. Poretsky L, Can S, Zumoff B. Testicular dysfunction in human immunodeficiency virus-infected men. *Metabolism.* 1995; 44:946–53.
149. Kosmiski L. Energy expenditure in HIV infection. *Am J Clin Nutr.* 2011; 94(suppl):1677S–1682S.
150. Falutz J, Mamputu JC, Potvin D, et al. Effects of tesamorelin (TH9507), a growth hormone-releasing factor analog, in human immunodeficiency virus-infected patients with excess abdominal fat: a pooled analysis of two multicenter, double-blind placebo-controlled phase 3 trials with safety extension data. *J Clin Endocrinol Metab.* 2010; 95:4291–304.
151. Hadigan C, Corcoran C, Basgoz N, et al. Metformin in the treatment of HIV lipodystrophy syndrome. *JAMA.* 2000; 284:472–7.
152. Kong A, Edmonds P. Testosterone therapy in HIV wasting syndrome: systemic review and meta-analysis. *Lancet Infect Dis.* 2002; 2:692–9.
153. Sardar P, Jha A, Roy D, et al. Therapeutic effects of nandrolone and testosterone in adult male HIV patients with AIDS wasting syndrome (AWS): a randomized, double-blind, placebo-controlled trial. *HIV Clin Trials.* 2010; 11:220–9.
154. Gold J, Batterham MJ, Rekers H, et al. Effects of nandrolone decanoate compared to placebo or testosterone on HIV-associated wasting. *HIV Med.* 2006; 7:146–55.
155. Guaraldi G, Orlando G, Zona S, et al. Premature age-related comorbidities among HIV-infected persons compared with the general population. *Clin Infect Dis.* 2011; 53:1120–6.
156. Schafer JJ, Manlangit K, Squires KE. Bone health and human immunodeficiency virus infection. *Pharmacotherapy.* 2013; 33:665–82.
157. McComsey GA, Tebas P, Shane E, et al. Bone disease in HIV infection: a practical review and recommendations for HIV care providers. *Clin Infect Dis.* 2010; 51:937–46.
158. Redondo Sanchez C, Poza Cisneros G, Galera Penaranda G, et al. Changes in hospitalizations due to opportunistic infections, chronic conditions and other causes among HIV patients (1989-2011). A study in a HIV unit. *J Int AIDS Soc.* 2012; 15(suppl 4):18089.
159. Hermsen ED, Wynn HE, McNabb J. Discontinuation of prophylaxis for HIV-associated opportunistic infections in the era of highly active antiretroviral therapy. *Am J Health-Syst Pharm.* 2004; 61:245–56.
160. Panel on Opportunistic Infections in HIV-Infected Adults and Adolescents. Guidelines for the prevention and treatment of opportunistic infections in HIV-infected adults and adolescents: recommendations from the Centers for Disease Control and Prevention, the National Institutes of Health, and the HIV Medical Association of the Infectious Diseases Society of America. http://aidsinfo.nih.gov/contentfiles/lvguidelines/adult_oi.pdf (accessed 2013 May 9).
161. Foisy MM, Akai PS. Pharmaceutical care for HIV patients on directly observed therapy. *Ann Pharmacother.* 2004; 38:550–6.
162. Zolopa AR, Andersen J, Komarow L, et al. Early antiretroviral therapy reduces AIDS progression/death in individuals with acute opportunistic infections: a multicenter randomized strategy trial. *PLoS ONE.* 2009; 4:e5575.
163. Grant PM, Zolopa AR. When to start ART in the setting of acute AIDS-related opportunistic infections: the time is now! *Curr HIV/AIDS Rep.* 2012; 9:251–8.
164. Bisson GP, Molefi M, Bellamy S, et al. Early versus delayed antiretroviral therapy and cerebrospinal fluid fungal clearance in adults with HIV and cryptococcal meningitis. *Clin Infect Dis.* 2013; 53:1165–73.

165. Blanc FX, Sok T, Laureillard D, et al. Earlier versus later start of antiretroviral therapy in HIV-infected adults with tuberculosis. *N Engl J Med.* 2011; 365:1471–81.
166. Yehia BR, Mehta JM, Ciuffetelli D, et al. Antiretroviral medication errors remain high but are quickly corrected among hospitalized HIV-infected adults. *Clin Infect Dis.* 2012; 55:593–99.
167. Eginger KH, Yarborough LL, Inge LD, et al. Medication errors in HIV-infected hospitalized patients: a pharmacist's impact. *Ann Pharmacother.* 2013; 47:953–60.
168. Bridges CB, Woods L, Coyne-Beasley T, et al. Advisory Committee on Immunization Practices (ACIP) recommended immunization schedule for adults aged 19 and older—United States, 2013. *MMWR Surveill Summ.* 2013; 62:9–19.
169. Stenger M, Spach DH. Immunizations for HIV-infected adults: indications, timing and response. *Top HIV Med.* 2006; 14:154–8.
170. Higginbotham S, Stewart A, Pfalzgraf A. Impact of a pharmacist immunizer on adult immunization rates. *J Am Pharm Assoc.* 2012; 52:367–71.
171. Skelton JB. Pharmacist-provided immunization compensation and recognition: white paper summarizing APhA/AMCP stakeholder meeting. *J Am Pharm Assoc.* 2011; 51:704–12.
172. Centers for Disease Control and Prevention. HIV prevention in the United States: at a critical crossroads (August 2009). www.cdc.gov/hiv/resources/reports/pdf/hiv_prev_us.pdf (accessed 2016 Jan 21).
173. Cohen MS, Chen YQ, McCauley M, et al. Prevention of HIV-1 infection with early antiretroviral therapy. *N Engl J Med.* 2011; 365:493–505.
174. Bunnell R, Ekwaru JP, Soldberg P, et al. Changes in sexual behavior and risk of HIV transmission after antiretroviral therapy and prevention interventions in rural Uganda. *AIDS.* 2006; 20:85–92.
175. Sullivan P, Kayitenkore K, Chomba E, et al. Is the reduction of HIV transmission while prescribed antiviral therapy (ARVT) different for men and women? Results from discordant couples in Rwanda and Zambia. Presented at the 5th IAS Conference on HIV Pathogenesis, Treatment, and Prevention. Capetown, South Africa; 2009 Jul.
176. Das M, Chu PL, Santos GM, et al. Decreases in community viral load are accompanied by reductions in new HIV infections in San Francisco. *PLoS One.* 2010; 5:e11068.
177. Montaner JS, Lima VD, Barrios R, et al. Association of highly active antiretroviral therapy coverage, population viral load, and yearly new HIV diagnoses in British Columbia, Canada: a population-based study. *Lancet.* 2010; 376:532–9.
178. Saberi P, Dong BJ, Johnson MO, et al. The impact of HIV clinical pharmacists on HIV treatment outcomes: a systematic review. *Patient Prefer Adherence.* 2012; 6:297–322.
179. Cocohoba JM, Althoff KN, Cohen M, et al. Pharmacist counseling in a cohort of women with HIV and women at risk for HIV. *Patient Prefer Adherence.* 2012; 6:457–63.
180. Kibicho J, Owczarzak J. Pharmacists' strategies for promoting medication adherence among patients with HIV. *J Am Pharm Assoc.* 2011; 51:746–55.
181. Centers for Disease Control and Prevention. Preexposure prophylaxis for the prevention of HIV infection in the United States - 2014: a clinical practice guideline. www.cdc.gov/hiv/pdf/PrEPguidelines2014.pdf (accessed 2014 Dec 5).
182. Abdool Karim Q, Abdool Karim SS, Frolich JA, et al. Effectiveness and safety of tenofovir gel, an antiretroviral microbicide, for the prevention of HIV infection in women. *Science.* 2010; 329:1168–74.
183. Grant RM, Lama JR, Anderson PL, et al. Preexposure chemoprophylaxis for HIV prevention in men who have sex with men. *N Engl J Med.* 2010; 363:2587–99.
184. Baeten JM, Donnell D, Ndase P, et al. Antiretroviral prophylaxis for HIV prevention in heterosexual men and women. *N Engl J Med.* 2012; 367:399–410.
185. Thigpen MC, Kebaabetswe PM, Paxton LA, et al. Antiretroviral preexposure prophylaxis for heterosexual HIV transmission in Botswana. *N Engl J Med.* 2012; 367:423–34.
186. Choopanya K, Martin M, Suntharasamai P, et al. Antiretroviral prophylaxis for HIV infection in injecting drug users in Bangkok, Thailand (the Bangkok Tenofovir Study): a randomised, double-blind, placebo controlled phase 3 trial. *Lancet.* 2013; 381:2083–90.
187. Van Damme L, Corneli A, Ahmed K, et al. Preexposure prophylaxis for HIV infection among African women. *N Engl J Med.* 2012; 367:411–22.
188. Marrazzo J, Ramjee G, Nair G, et al. Pre-exposure prophylaxis for HIV in women: daily oral tenofovir, oral tenofovir/emtricitabine, or vaginal tenofovir gel in the VOICE Study (MTN 003). Presented at the 20th Conference on Retroviruses and Opportunistic Infections. Atlanta, GA; 2013 Mar.
189. Bruno C, Saberi P. Pharmacists as providers of HIV pre-exposure prophylaxis. *Int J Clin Pharm.* 2012; 34:803–6.
190. Shaeer KM, Sherman EM, Shafiq S, et al. Exploratory survey of Florida pharmacists' experience, knowledge, and perception of HIV pre-exposure prophylaxis. *J Am Pharm Assoc.* 2014; 54:610–7.
191. Kuhar DT, Henderson DK, Struble KM, et al. Updated US public health service guidelines for the management of occupational exposures to human immunodeficiency virus and recommendations for postexposure prophylaxis. *Infect Control Hosp Epidemiol.* 2013; 34:875–93.
192. Smith DK, Grohskopf LA, Black RJ, et al. Antiretroviral postexposure prophylaxis after sexual, injection-drug use, or other nonoccupational exposure to HIV in the United States: recommendations from the U.S. Department of Health and Human Services. *MMWR Recomm Rep.* 2005; 54:1–20.
193. Foisy M, Highes C. Role of the pharmacist in perinatal management of HIV disease. *Am J Health-Syst Pharm.* 2011; 68:2116–22.
194. Nacopoulos AG, Lewtas AJ, Ousterhout MM. Syringe exchange programs: impact on injection drug users and the role of the pharmacist from a US perspective. *J Am Pharm Assoc.* 2010; 50:148–57.
195. Janulis P. Pharmacy nonprescription syringe distribution and HIV/AIDS: a review. *J Am Pharm Assoc.* 2012; 52:787–97.

196. Sherman EM, Cocohoba JM, Neff SE, et al. Health care provider satisfaction with telephone consultations provided by pharmacists and physicians at the National HIV/AIDS clinicians' consultation center. *Ann Pharmacother.* 2011; 45:1499–505.
197. Bartlett D, Evans P, Sullivan M. Effect of a pharmacist-run call center on medication access for ambulatory care patients. *Am J Health-Syst Pharm.* 2009; 66:1666–8.
198. Sarrafizadeh M, Waite NW, Hobson E, et al. Pharmacist-facilitated enrollment in medication assistance programs in a private ambulatory care clinic. *Am J Health-Syst Pharm.* 2004; 61:1816–20.
199. Raper JL, Willig JH, Lin HY, et al. Uncompensated medical provider costs associated with prior authorization for prescription medications in an HIV clinic. *Clin Infect Dis.* 2010; 51:718–24.
200. American College of Clinical Pharmacy. Improving care transitions: current practice and future opportunities for pharmacists. *Pharmacotherapy.* 2012; 32:e326–37.
201. Li EH, Foisy MM. Antiretroviral and medication errors in hospitalized HIV-positive persons. *Ann Pharmacother.* 2014; 48:998–1010.
202. Cutler TW, Stebbins MR, Smith AR, et al. Promoting access and reducing expected out-of-pocket prescription drug costs for vulnerable Medicare beneficiaries: a pharmacist-directed model. *Med Care.* 2011; 49:343–7.
203. Matzke GR. Health care reform 2011: opportunities for pharmacists. *Ann Pharmacother.* 2012; 46:S27–32.
204. American Academy of HIV Medicine. Credentialing. www.aahivm.org/about (accessed 2016 Jan 21).
205. Traynor K. U.S. pharmacists respond to global AIDS crisis. *Am J Health-Syst Pharm.* 2005; 62:1108, 1110,1112. [Erratum, *Am J Health-Syst Pharm.* 2005; 62:1241.]
206. Okubanjo T, Gonzalez LS 3rd. Pharmacists as investigators in FDA-regulated drug trials. *Am J Health-Syst Pharm.* 2008; 65:1010–1.

Appendix—Additional Sources of Information

Website Resources

General HIV Care and Treatment Information

- U.S. Department of Health and Human Services AIDSinfo website (www.aidsinfo.nih.gov)
- Clinical Care Options HIV – in Practice (www.inpractice.com/Textbooks/HIV.aspx)

Clinical Practice Guidelines and Recommendations

- U.S. Department of Health and Human Services AIDSinfo website (www.aidsinfo.nih.gov)
- International Antiviral Society- USA (www.iasusa.org/guidelines)
- World Health Organization (www.who.int/hiv/pub/guidelines/en/)
- European AIDS Clinical Society (eacsociety.org/Guidelines.aspx)

Antiretroviral Information (Drug Interactions, Renal/Hepatic Dose Adjustments, and Crushing/Liquid Formulations)

- U.S. Department of Health and Human Services AIDSinfo website (www.aidsinfo.nih.gov)
- University of Liverpool Drug Interaction Database and Mobile Application (www.hiv-druginteractions.org/)
- Toronto General Hospital Immunodeficiency Clinic website (www.hivclinic.ca/main/drugs_interact.html and www.hivclinic.ca/main/drugs_extra.html)
- HIV Insite (hivinsite.ucsf.edu)
- Clinician Consultation Center, Antiretroviral Drug Tables (nccc.ucsf.edu/clinical-resources/hiv-aids-resources/pharmacy)
- Florida/Caribbean AIDS Education and Training Center Antiretroviral Therapy Pocket Cards (www.fcaetc.org/treatment-guidelines.php)

HIV Resistance Testing and Mutations

- HIV Drug Resistance Database – Stanford University (www.hivdb.stanford.edu)
- International Antiviral Society – USA (www.iasusa.org/resistance_mutations/mutations_figures.pdf)

Immunizations

- Centers for Disease Control and Prevention (www.cdc.gov/vaccines/schedules/hcp/index.html)

Professional Organizations

- American Academy of HIV Medicine (www.aahivm.org)
- British HIV Association (www.bhiva.org)
- HIV Medicine Association (www.hivma.org)
- International Association of Providers of AIDS Care (www.iapac.org)
- International AIDS Society (www.iasociety.org)

Information Exchange

- The Canadian HIV/AIDS Pharmacists Network (hivclinic.ca/chap)
- National AIDS Treatment Advocacy Project (natap.org)
- American College of Clinical Pharmacy, HIV Practice and Research Network (www.accp.com/about/prns.aspx)

Clinical Trials

- U.S. Department of Health and Human Services AIDSinfo website (www.aidsinfo.nih.gov)

Hotlines and Clinical Consultation

- Clinicians Consultation Center (nccc.usf.edu)
- Pre-Exposure Prophylaxis (855) 448-7737
- Post-Exposure Prophylaxis (888) 448-4911
- HIV/AIDS Management (800) 933-3413
- Perinatal HIV/AIDS (888) 448-8765

HIV Certificate and Credentialing Programs

- American Academy of HIV Medicine, HIV Pharmacist Credentialing (www.aahivm.org/about)
- University of Buffalo School of Pharmacy and Pharmaceutical Sciences (tdm.pharm.buffalo.edu/hiv_cert_main)

Continuing Education for Pharmacists

- Clinical Care Options – HIV (www.clinicaloptions.com/HIV.aspx)
- International Antiviral Society – USA (iasusa.org)
- American Academy of HIV Medicine (aahivm.org)
- AIDS Education and Training Centers (aidsetc.org)

Approved by the ASHP Board of Directors on September 17, 2015. Developed through the ASHP Section of Clinical Specialists and Scientists. These guidelines supersede the ASHP Statement on the Pharmacist's Role in HIV Care published in the October 1, 2003, issue of *AJHP*.

ASHP gratefully acknowledges the American Academy of HIV Medicine for reviewing and endorsing these guidelines. ASHP gratefully acknowledges the following organizations and individuals for reviewing these guidelines (review does not imply endorsement): American Pharmacists Association; Canadian HIV/AIDS Pharmacists Network; HIV Medicine Association; Society of Infectious Disease Pharmacists; South Carolina Society of Health-System Pharmacists; Melissa Badowski, Pharm.D., BCPS, AAHIVP; Carol J. Bickford, Ph.D., RN-BC, CPHIMS; Shanna Chan, B.Sc.Pharm., ACPR, AAHIVP; Patrick Clay, Pharm.D. FCCP, CCTI; Natalie Dayneka, B.Sc.Pharm., ACPR, Pharm.D., FCSHP; Heather Easterling, Pharm.D., M.B.A.; Devon Flynn, Pharm.D., BCPS, AAHIVP; Michelle Foisy, B.Sc.Pharm., Pharm.D., FCSHP, AAHIVP; Patricia Pecora Fulco, Pharm.D., BCPS, FASHP, AAHIVP; Barbara Giacomelli, Pharm.D., M.B.A., FASHP; Pierre Giguère, B.Sc.Pharm., M.Sc.; Christine Hughes, B.Sc.Pharm., Pharm.D, AAHIVP; Tara K. Jellison, Pharm.D., M.B.A., FASHP; Deborah V. Kelly, B.Sc. Pharm., Pharm.D, ACPR, FCSHP, AAHIVP; William Kuykendall, Pharm.D.; Kristina Lantis; J. Craig Phillips, Ph.D., LLM, RN, ARNP, PMHCNS-BC, ACRN; Carlo Quaia, B.Sc.Pharm., ACPR; James R. Rinehart, B.S.Pharm., M.S., FASHP; Linda Robinson, B.Sc.Pharm., AAHIVE; Nancy Sheehan, B.Sc.Pharm., M.Sc.; Shannon Stone, B.Sc.Pharm., ACPR; Alice Tseng, B.Sc.Pharm., Pharm.D., FCSHP, AAHIVP; Andrea Weddle, M.S.W.; Jody Jacobson Wedret, FASHP, FCSHP; and Deborah Yoong, B.Sc.Pharm., Pharm.D., ACPR.

The authors have declared no potential conflicts of interest.

At the time of writing Ian R. McNicholl, Pharm.D., FCCP, BCPS (AQ-ID), AAHIVP, worked at the UCSF Positive Health Program at San Francisco General Hospital, San Francisco, CA.

Jason J. Schafer, Pharm.D., M.P.H., BCPS, AAHIVP, Department of Pharmacy Practice, Jefferson School of Pharmacy, Thomas Jefferson University, Philadelphia, PA.

Taylor K. Gill, Pharm.D., BCPS, AAHIVP, Internal Medicine, Via Christi Hospitals Wichita, Wichita, KS.

Elizabeth M. Sherman, Pharm.D., AAHIVP, College of Pharmacy, Nova Southeastern University, Fort Lauderdale, FL, and South Broward Community Health Services, Memorial Healthcare System, Hollywood, FL.

Ian R. McNicholl, Pharm.D., FCCP, BCPS (AQ-ID), AAHIVP, Gilead Sciences, Foster City, CA.

Copyright © 2016, American Society of Health-System Pharmacists, Inc. All rights reserved. Contact ASHP for reprint and permissions requests. This content may not be used for commercial purposes without the express written consent of ASHP.

The bibliographic citation for this document is as follows: American Society of Health-System Pharmacists. ASHP guidelines on pharmacist involvement in HIV care. *Am J Health-Syst Pharm.* 2016; 73:468–94.

ASHP Guidelines on the Pharmacist's Role in Immunization

Purpose

Pharmacists can play an important role in disease prevention by advocating and administering immunizations. Such activities are consistent with the preventive aspects of pharmaceutical care and have been part of pharmacy practice for over a century.[1,2] These guidelines address the pharmacist's role in promoting and conducting proper immunization of patients in all organized health care settings. The pharmacist's role in promoting disease prevention through participation in community efforts is also discussed.

Background

Each year, an average of 90,000 Americans die of vaccine-preventable infections such as influenza, pneumococcal disease, and hepatitis B.[3,5] Most of these people visited health care providers in the year preceding their deaths but were not vaccinated.[6–11] Influenza and pneumonia, considered together, are the fifth leading cause of death for Americans 65 years of age or older.[12] Although vaccination rates for U.S. children at the time they enter school exceed 95%, nearly 25% do not complete their primary series by the age of two years.[13] Most American adults are inadequately vaccinated, particularly against pneumococcal disease, influenza, hepatitis B, tetanus, and diphtheria.[6] Tens of millions of Americans remain susceptible to potentially deadly infections despite the availability of effective vaccines.

This long-standing failure to adequately immunize the U.S population helped prompt the inclusion of immunization as a leading health indicator for Healthy People 2010.[14] The renewed focus on immunization and the potential for increased vaccination needs in response to threats of bioterrorism should stimulate pharmacists, as well as other health care providers, to reassess what they and their institutions can do to improve immunization rates in their communities. Pharmacists can contribute to this effort by administering immunizations where scope of practice allows and by promoting immunization in other ways.

Immunization Administration

As health care providers, pharmacists can administer vaccines or host other health care professionals who can administer vaccines. Pharmacists must understand the legal and professional mechanisms by which authorization to administer vaccines is granted, as well as the additional responsibilities and considerations that accompany this expanded role. The feasibility of vaccine administration by pharmacists within a particular practice site or health care system can be determined by analyzing the issues of legal authority, training, and program structure.

Legal Authority. The pharmacist's authority to administer vaccines is determined by each state's laws and regulations governing pharmacy practice. At least 36 states permit vaccine administration by pharmacists as part of the scope of pharmacy practice.[15] The American College of Physicians–American Society of Internal Medicine supports pharmacists as sources of immunization information, hosts of immunization sites, and immunizers.[16] Vaccine administration may occur pursuant to individual prescription orders or through standing orders or protocols. The Centers for Disease Control and Prevention (CDC) Advisory Committee on Immunization Practices recommends the use of standing orders to improve adult immunization rates.[17] Its recommendations encourage pharmacists, among other providers, to establish standing-order programs in long-term-care facilities, home health care agencies, hospitals, clinics, workplaces, and managed care organizations. The Centers for Medicare and Medicaid Services (CMS) no longer requires a physician order for influenza or pneumoccocal immunizations administered in participating hospitals, long-term-care facilities, or home health care agencies.[18] Development of state-specific protocols or standing-order programs can be facilitated through partnerships with state pharmacy associations, boards of pharmacy, and health departments.

Training. Although legal authority to administer vaccines may be granted through pharmacy practice acts, pharmacists must achieve competency in all aspects of vaccine administration. A comprehensive training program should address the following:

1. The epidemiology of and patient populations at risk for vaccine-preventable diseases
2. Public health goals for immunization (e.g., local, regional, state, and federal goals)
3. Vaccine safety (e.g., risk–benefit analysis)
4. Screening for contraindications and precautions of vaccination in each patient
5. Vaccine stability and transportation and storage requirements
6. Immunologic drug interactions
7. Vaccine dosing (including interpreting recommended immunization schedules and patient immunization records and determining proper dosing intervals and the feasibility of simultaneous administration of multiple vaccines)
8. Proper dose preparation and injection technique
9. Signs and symptoms of adverse reactions to vaccines, adverse reaction reporting, and emergency procedures, such as basic and advanced cardiac life support (BCLS and ACLS)
10. Documentation
11. Reporting to the primary care provider or local health department
12. Billing

Live and videotaped programming is available through some state and national pharmacy associations and offered in many college of pharmacy curricula. Information regarding immunizations can change rapidly. To maintain competency, pharmacists must have access to current immunization

DOI 10.37573/9781585287048.077

references (e.g., CDC's National Immunization Program publications, including the "Pink Book"[19]) and continuing-education programs to stay abreast of evolving guidelines and recommendations.

Program Structure. A vaccine administration program requires a solid infrastructure of appropriately trained staff, physical space, and written policies and procedures to ensure appropriate vaccine storage and handling, patient screening and education, and documentation. The structure of a vaccine administration program must also provide for storage and disposal of injection supplies, disposal of and prevention of exposure to biological hazards as dictated by the Occupational Safety and Health Administration (OSHA), and emergency procedures (e.g., BCLS and ACLS). Pharmacists should be fully immunized to protect their health and the health of their patients.[20]

Reimbursement. Immunization has repeatedly been shown to be cost-effective[21–24]; it may be the most cost-effective practice in medicine. However, third-party reimbursement policies often do not provide coverage for recommended vaccines despite this evidence. A major exception is Medicare Part B, which not only covers immunization services for its participants but also recognizes and compensates pharmacists as mass immunization providers. Enrollment as a Medicare provider is required to bill for covered services. Provider status can be obtained through local Medicare offices, which also process CMS claims for reimbursement (CMS-1500 claims). The CMS Web site (www.cms.hhs.gov) is a useful source for billing information. Pharmacists should continue to closely monitor other immunization reimbursement policies and advocate third-party coverage for immunizations as a cost-effective preventive measure. For patients without insurance coverage, requesting out-of-pocket payments from the patient remains a viable option for pharmacists to obtain compensation for their immunization services.

Immunization Promotion

Pharmacists who do not administer vaccines can promote immunization through six types of activities: (1) history and screening, (2) patient counseling, (3) documentation, (4) formulary management, (5) administrative measures, and (6) public education.[25,26] These promotional activities can also be integrated into or accompany a pharmacy-based immunization program.

History and Screening. Pharmacists can promote proper immunization by identifying patients in need of immunization. Tasks that support this objective include gathering immunization histories, encouraging use of vaccine profiles, issuing vaccination records to patients,[27–34] preventing immunologic drug interactions,[35,36] and screening patients for immunization needs.[28–33,37–39]

Immunization screening should be a component of all clinical routines, regardless of the practice setting. All health care institutions should implement consistent, systematic monitoring systems and quality indicators to ensure that all patients are assessed for immunization adequacy before they leave the facility. The health care provider designated to identify patient immunization needs should have the authority, knowledge, and responsibility to provide or arrange for the immunization service.[40] Clinics that provide treatment for a large number of patients at high risk for contracting vaccine-preventable diseases (e.g., diabetic, asthmatic, heart disease, and geriatric clinics) have a particular obligation to employ immunization screening and ensure appropriate vaccine use.

Screening for immunization needs may be organized in several ways; prototype screening forms are available.[39,41] Pharmacists should seek out leadership roles in some or all of the following forms of immunization screening.

Occurrence screening. With this type of screening, vaccine needs are identified at the time of particular events, such as hospital or nursing home admission or discharge, ambulatory care or emergency room visits, mid-decade birthdays (e.g., years 25, 35, and 45),[42,43] and any contact with a health care delivery system for patients under 8 years or over 50 years of age.

Diagnosis screening. This screening reviews the vaccine needs of patients with conditions that increase their risk of preventable infections. Diagnoses such as diabetes, asthma, heart disease, acute myocardial infarction, congestive heart failure, chronic obstructive pulmonary disease, hemophilia, thalassemia, most types of cancer, sickle cell anemia, chronic alcoholism, cirrhosis, human immunodeficiency virus infection, and certain other disorders should prompt specific attention to the patient's vaccine needs.[12,33,42] The immunization rate for patients diagnosed with community-acquired pneumonia is considered a marker for quality by some accrediting bodies. Incorporating assessment of vaccination status into an institution's critical pathways has been shown to improve vaccination rates.[44]

Procedure screening. Immunization needs are assessed on the basis of medical or surgical procedures using this type of screening. These procedures include splenectomy, heart or lung surgery, organ transplantation, antineoplastic therapy, radiation therapy, immunosuppression of other types, dialysis, and prescription of certain medications used to treat conditions that increase patients' risk of preventable infections.[45,46] When designing and implementing automated prescription databases, pharmacy managers should consider specifications that allow retrieval of lists of patients receiving drugs that suggest the need for immunization.[33,37]

Periodic mass screening. This type of screening is a comprehensive assessment of immunization adequacy in selected populations at a given time. Such screening may be conducted, for example, during autumn influenza programs or outbreaks of certain vaccine-preventable illnesses (e.g., measles and meningococcal disease).[29,32,33] Schools and other institutions can perform mass screening when registering new students or residents. Mass screening may also be appropriate in areas where no comprehensive immunization program has been conducted recently. This type of screening helps improve vaccine coverage rates at a given time, but long-term benefits are much greater when such intermittent programs are combined with ongoing comprehensive screening efforts. Several states, including South Dakota, New Jersey, and Oklahoma, have enacted laws requiring that influenza and pneumococcal vaccines be offered annually to residents of nursing homes.

Occupational screening. This screening method focuses on the immunization needs of health care personnel whose responsibilities place them at risk of exposure to certain vaccine-preventable diseases or bring them into contact with high-risk patients (i.e., patients with those conditions listed in the *Diagnosis screening* section above). Health care providers who have contact with these patients should receive an annual influenza vaccination. Health care employers frequently provide immunization screening and vaccination of employees as part of employee health programs. OSHA requires that health care employers provide hepatitis B vaccination at no cost, on a voluntary basis, to all employees at risk for occupational exposure to blood borne pathogens.[47] Depending on their risk of exposure, it may be advisable for members of the pharmacy staff to receive hepatitis B vaccination.

Screening for contraindications and precautions. After candidates for immunization have been identified, they should be screened for contraindications and precautions. A CDC-reviewed contraindication screening questionnaire is available.[48]

Patient Counseling. Patients in need of immunization should be advised of their infection risk and encouraged to accept the immunizations they need. Patient concerns about vaccine safety and efficacy should be discussed and addressed.[49,50] Health care providers can influence patients' attitudes regarding immunization.[51,52] Physicians should be informed of their patients' need for vaccination if standing orders or collaborative practice agreements are not in place. Patients who need immunizations should be vaccinated during the current health care contact unless valid contraindications exist. Delaying vaccination until a future appointment increases the risk that the patient will not be vaccinated.

Advising patients of their need for immunization can take several forms. In the ambulatory care setting, individualized or form letters can be mailed to patients, patients can be called by telephone, or an insert can be included with prescriptions informing patients of their infection risk and the availability and efficacy of vaccines.[30,33,53–55] Adhesive reminder labels can also be affixed to prescription containers for drugs used to treat conditions that may indicate the need for vaccination against influenza and pneumococcal disease (e.g., digoxin, warfarin, theophylline, and insulin[33]); these labels would be analogous to labels currently in widespread use (e.g., "Shake well" and "Take with food or milk"). Such labels might read, "You may need flu or pneumonia vaccine: Ask your doctor or pharmacist." Chart notes, consultations, messages to patients, one-on-one conversations, and similar means can be used to communicate with inpatients and institutional patients.[28,31,56]

Federal law requires that health care providers who administer diphtheria, tetanus, pertussis, measles, mumps, rubella, varicella, polio, *Haemophilus influenzae* type B, hepatitis B, and pneumococcal conjugate vaccines give the most recent version of the CDC-developed Vaccine Information Statement (VIS) to the adult or the parent or legal guardian of the child to be vaccinated.[57] VISs are available in many languages from state or local health departments or the CDC.[58] VISs are also available for other commonly used vaccines, such as influenza, pneumococcal polysaccharide, hepatitis A, meningococcal, and anthrax vaccines. Pharmacists should also ensure that informed consent is obtained in a manner that complies with state laws.[20]

Documentation. The National Childhood Vaccine Injury Act of 1986 (NCVIA) requires all health care providers who administer vaccines to maintain permanent vaccination records and to report occurrences of certain adverse events specified in the act.[57,59] The recipient's permanent medical record (or the equivalent) must state the date the vaccine was administered, the vaccine's manufacturer and lot number, and the name, address, and title of the person administering the vaccine. Pharmacists in organized health care settings may encourage compliance with this requirement by providing reminder notices each time doses of vaccines are dispensed.[60] Automated databases that allow for long-term storage of patient immunization information may provide an efficient method for maintaining and retrieving immunization records.[39] Efforts to develop electronic vaccination registries, especially for children, are under way by states collaborating with CDC.[61]

NCVIA also mandates that selected adverse effects noted after any inoculation be reported to the Vaccine Adverse Event Reporting System (www.vaers.org).[57,59,62] Because pharmacists have experience with adverse-drug-reaction reporting, they can take the lead in developing and implementing a program to meet this requirement, even if they are not responsible for administering the vaccine.

Patients should maintain personal immunization records that document all immunization experiences and function as a backup if the clinicians' immunization records are lost. Several personal immunization record forms are available. Public Health Service Form 731 (International Certificate of Vaccination), colloquially called the "yellow shot record," is used to document vaccines indicated for international travel but can also serve as a patient's personal record of vaccinations. The Immunization Action Coalition distributes a standard adult immunization record card developed in collaboration with CDC.[63] In addition, each state and the District of Columbia prints its own uniform immunization record form for pediatric immunizations, which may also be a suitable personal patient record. It has been recommended that adults carry personal immunization records in their wallets.[46]

Formulary Management. Formulary systems in organized health care settings should include vaccines, toxoids, and immune globulins available for use in preventing diseases in patients and staff. Decisions by the pharmacy and therapeutics committee (or its equivalent) on immunologic drug choices require consideration of relevant immunologic pharmaceutics, immunopharmacology, and disease epidemiology. Because of their expertise and training, pharmacists are well equipped to provide information and recommendations on which these decisions may be based.

It is the pharmacist's responsibility to develop and maintain product specifications to aid in the purchase of drugs under the formulary system.[64,65] The pharmacist should establish and maintain standards to ensure the quality, proper storage, and proper use of all pharmaceuticals dispensed. Pharmacists must choose between single dose or multidose containers of vaccines on the basis of efficiency, safety, economic, and regulatory considerations. Pharmacists in institutions should develop guidelines on the routine stocking of immunologic drugs in certain high-use patient care areas.

Proper transportation and storage are an important consideration for immunologic drugs, including vaccines, because many require storage at refrigerated or frozen temperatures. Pharmacists have an important responsibility to maintain the "cold chain" in the handling of these drugs.

Detailed references on this topic have been published.[66–73] Storage considerations include the conditions in all areas in which immunologic drugs are kept, as well as a method for ensuring that immunologic drugs received by the pharmacy have been transported under suitable conditions.

It is important that methods be established for detecting and properly disposing of outdated and partially administered immunologic agents. Live viral (e.g., varicella, yellow fever, and smallpox) and live bacterial (e.g., bacille Calmette-Guérin) vaccines should be disposed of in the same manner as other infectious biohazardous waste.

Administrative Measures. Pharmacists on key committees (e.g., infection control and risk management) in organized health care settings can promote adequate immunization delivery among staff and patients by encouraging the development of sound organizational policies on immunization. Health care organizations should develop policies and protocols that address the following:

1. Hepatitis B preexposure prophylaxis for health care workers at risk for exposure to blood products and other contaminated items.[45,74–76]
2. Hepatitis B postexposure (e.g., needle stick) prophylaxis for previously unvaccinated patients, health care personnel, and personnel who have been vaccinated but do not have a previously documented serologic response.[45,74–76]
3. Rabies preexposure and postexposure prophylaxis.[77]
4. Wound management guidelines designed to prevent tetanus and diphtheria.[78,79]
5. Valid contraindications to vaccination to ensure patient safety and minimize inappropriate exclusions from vaccination.[78,80,81]
6. Requirements for employee immunization against measles, rubella, influenza, and other diseases.[42,82]
7. Tuberculosis screening of patients and staff.[83,84]
8. Immunization of persons at high risk (e.g., patients with diabetes, asthma, heart disease, and pregnant or immunocompromised patients). Current authoritative guidelines on this subject should be consulted.[42,46,58,85,86]
9. Emergency measures in the event of vaccine-related adverse reactions. Such measures should address the availability of epinephrine and other emergency drugs, as well as BCLS and ACLS.

Public Education. Pharmacists have ample opportunities to advance the public health through immunization advocacy. Pharmacists can facilitate disease prevention strategies, because many potential victims of influenza and pneumococcal disease visit pharmacies and are seen by pharmacists daily. Pharmacists can lead local activities in observance of National Adult Immunization Week each October.[37] Working with local public health departments, state or national immunization coalitions, and other groups (e.g., state or local parent—teacher, diabetes, heart, lung, or retired persons' associations), pharmacists can promote vaccination among high-risk populations. Newsletters, posters, brochures, and seminars may be used to explain the risk of preventable infections to pharmacy staff, other health care personnel, and patients. Excellent resources are available from the Immunization Action Coalition and the National Coalition for Adult Immunization.

References

1. Hepler CD, Strand LM. Opportunities and responsibilities in pharmaceutical care. *Am J Hosp Pharm.* 1990; 47:533–43.
2. Grabenstein JD. Pharmacists and immunization: increasing involvement over a century. *Pharm Hist.* 1999; 41:137–52.
3. Prevention and control of influenza: recommendations of the Advisory Committee on Immunization Practices. *MMWR Recomm Rep.* 2002; 51(RR-3):1–31.
4. Prevention of pneumococcal disease: recommendations of the Advisory Committee on Immunization Practices (ACIP). *MMWR Recomm Rep.* 1997; 46(RR-8):1–24.
5. Thompson WW, Shay DK, Weintraub E, et al. Mortality associated with influenza and respiratory syncytial virus in the United States. *JAMA.* 2003; 289:179–86.
6. Williams WW, Hickson MA, Kane MA, et al. Immunization policies and vaccine coverage among adults. The risk for missed opportunities. *Ann Intern Med.* 1988; 108:616–25.
7. Fedson DS, Harward MP, Reid RA, et al. Hospital-based pneumococcal immunization. Epidemiologic rationale from the Shenandoah study. *JAMA.* 1990; 264:1117–22.
8. Fedson DS. Influenza and pneumococcal immunization strategies for physicians. *Chest.* 1987; 91:436–43.
9. Fedson DS. Improving the use of pneumococcal vaccine through a strategy of hospital based immunization: a review of its rationale and implications. *J Am Geriatr Soc.* 1985; 33:142–50.
10. Magnussen CR, Valenti WM, Mushlin AI. Pneumococcal vaccine strategy. Feasibility of a vaccination program directed at hospitalized and ambulatory patients. *Arch Intern Med.* 1984; 144:1755–7.
11. Vondracek TG, Pham TP, Huycke MM. A hospital-based pharmacy intervention program for pneumococcal vaccination. *Arch Intern Med.* 1998; 158:1543–7.
12. Bratzler DW, Houck PM, Jiang H, et al. Failure to vaccinate Medicare inpatients: a missed opportunity. *Arch Intern Med.* 2002; 162:2349–56.
13. Barker L, Luman E, Zhao Z, et al. National, state, and urban area vaccination coverage levels among children aged 19-35 months—United States, 2001. *MMWR. Morb Mortal Wkly Rep.* 2002; 51(30):664–6.
14. Office of Disease Prevention and Health Promotion. Healthy people 2010. www.healthypeople.gov (accessed 2003 Mar 12).
15. American Pharmaceutical Association. States where pharmacists can immunize. www.aphanet.org/pharm care/immunofact.html (accessed 2003 Mar 6).
16. Keely JL. Pharmacist scope of practice. *Ann Intern Med.* 2002; 136:79–85.
17. Use of standing orders programs to increase adult vaccination rates: recommendations of the Advisory Committee on Immunization Practices (ACIP). *MMWR Recomm Rep.* 2000; 49(RR01):15–26.
18. 42 C.F.R. §482–4.

19. Centers for Disease Control and Prevention. Epidemiology and prevention of vaccine-preventable diseases. 7th ed. Atlanta: U.S. Department of Health and Human Services; 2003.
20. Grabenstein JD. High expectations: standards and guidelines for immunization delivery. *Hosp Pharm.* 2000; 35:841–51.
21. Sisk JE, Moskowitz AJ, Whang W, et al. Cost-effectiveness of vaccination against pneumococcal bacteremia among elderly people. *JAMA.* 1997; 278:1333–9.
22. Van den Oever R, de Graeve D, Hepp B, et al. Pharmacoeconomics of immunisation: a review. *Pharmacoeconomics.* 1993; 3:286–308.
23. Nichol KL, Lind A, Margolis KL, et al. The effectiveness of vaccination against influenza in healthy, working adults. *N Engl J Med.* 1995; 333:889–93.
24. Nichol KL, Margolis KL, Wuorenma J, et al. The efficacy and cost-effectiveness of vaccination against influenza among elderly persons living in the community. *N Engl J Med.* 1994; 331:778–84.
25. Grabenstein JD. Immunizations: what's a health-system pharmacy to do? Part 1. *Hosp Pharm.* 1998; 33:742,745–50,753.
26. Grabenstein JD. Immunizations: what's a health-system pharmacy to do? Part 2. *Hosp Pharm.* 1998; 33:870–2,876–80.
27. Huff PS, Hak SH, Caiola SM. Immunizations for international travel as a pharmaceutical service. *Am J Hosp Pharm.* 1982; 39:90–3.
28. Spruill WJ, Cooper JW, Taylor WJR. Pharmacist-coordinated pneumonia and influenza vaccination program. *Am J Hosp Pharm.* 1982; 39:1904–6.
29. Grabenstein JD, Smith LJ, Carter DW, et al. Comprehensive immunization delivery in conjunction with influenza vaccination. *Arch Intern Med.* 1986; 146:1189–92.
30. Williams DM, Daugherty LJ, Aycock DG, et al. Effectiveness of improved targeting efforts for influenza immunization in an ambulatory-care setting. *Hosp Pharm.* 1987; 22:462–4.
31. Morton MR, Spruill WJ, Cooper JW. Pharmacist impact on pneumococcal vaccination rates in long-term-care facilities. *Am J Hosp Pharm.* 1988; 45:73. Letter.
32. Grabenstein JD, Smith LJ, Watson RR, et al. Immunization outreach using individual need assessments of adults at an Army hospital. *Public Health Rep.* 1990; 105:311–6.
33. Grabenstein JD, Hayton BD. Pharmacoepidemiologic program for identifying patients in need of vaccination. *Am J Hosp Pharm.* 1990; 47:1774–81.
34. Grabenstein JD. Get it in writing: documenting immunizations. *Hosp Pharm.* 1991; 26:901–4.
35. Grabenstein JD. Drug interactions involving immunologic agents. Part I. Vaccine–vaccine, vaccine–immunoglobulin, and vaccine–drug interactions. *DICP.* 1990; 24:67–81.
36. Grabenstein JD. Drug interactions involving immunologic agents. Part II. Immunodiagnostic and other immunologic drug interactions. *DICP.* 1990; 24:186–93.
37. Grabenstein JD. Pneumococcal pneumonia: don't wait, vaccinate. *Hosp Pharm.* 1990; 25:866–9.
38. Grabenstein JD, Casto DT. Recommending vaccines to your patients' individual needs. *Am Pharm.* 1991; NS31:58–67.
39. Grabenstein JD. Immunization delivery: a complete guide. St. Louis: Facts and Comparisons; 1997.
40. Fedson DS, Houck P, Bratzler D. Hospital-based influenza and pneumococcal vaccination: Sutton's law applied to prevention. *Infect Control Hosp Epidemiol.* 2000; 21:692–9.
41. Immunization Action Coalition. Do I need any vaccinations today? www.immunize.org/catg.d/4036need.htm (accessed 2003 Mar 12).
42. Guide for adult immunization. 3rd ed. Philadelphia: American College of Physicians; 1994.
43. Slobodkin D, Zielske PG, Kitlas JL, et al. Demonstration of the feasibility of emergency department immunization against influenza and pneumococcus. *Ann Emerg Med.* 1998; 32:537–43.
44. Robke JT, Woods M, Heitz S. Pharmacist impact on pneumococcal vaccination rates through incorporation of immunization assessment into critical pathways in an acute care setting. *Hosp Pharm.* 2002; 37:1050–4.
45. Hepatitis B virus: a comprehensive strategy for eliminating transmission in the United States through universal childhood vaccination. Recommendations of the Immunization Practices Advisory Committee (ACIP). *MMWR Recomm Rep.* 1991; 40 (RR-13):1–25.
46. Canadian National Advisory Committee on Immunization. Canadian immunization guide. 5th ed. Ottawa, Ont.: Ministry of National Health and Welfare; 1998.
47. 29 C.F.R. §1910.1030.
48. Immunization Action Coalition. Screening questionnaire for adult immunization. www.immunize.org/catg.d/p4065scr.pdf (accessed 2003 Mar 12).
49. Grabenstein JD, Wilson JP. Are vaccines safe? Risk contamination applied to vaccination. *Hosp Pharm.* 1999; 34:713–4,717–8,721–3,727–9.
50. Kirk JK, Grabenstein JD. Interviewing and counseling patients about immunizations. *Hosp Pharm.* 1991; 26:1006–10.
51. Nichol KL, MacDonald R, Hauge M. Factors associated with influenza and pneumococcal vaccination behavior among high-risk adults. *J Gen Intern Med.* 1996; 11:673–7.
52. Gene J, Espinola A, Cabezas C, et al. Do knowledge and attitudes about influenza and its immunization affect the likelihood of obtaining immunization? *Fam Pract Res J.* 1992; 12:61–73.
53. Grabenstein JD, Hartzema AG, Guess HA, et al. Community pharmacists as immunization advocates: a clinical pharmacoepidemiologic experiment. *Int J Pharm Pract.* 1993; 2:5–10.
54. Grabenstein JD, Guess HA, Hartzema AG. People vaccinated by pharmacists: Descriptive epidemiology. *J Am Pharm Assoc.* 2001; 41:46–52.
55. Grabenstein JD, Guess HA, Hartzema AG, et al. Effect of vaccination by community pharmacists among adult prescription recipients. *Med Care.* 2001; 39:340–8.

56. Casto DT. Prevention, management, and control of influenza: roles for the pharmacist. *Am J Med.* 1987; 82(suppl 6A):64–7.
57. Health Services & Resources Administration. Vaccine injury table. *Fed Regist.* 1997; 62:7685–90.
58. Centers for Disease Control and Prevention. Vaccine Information Statements. www.cdc.gov/nip/publications/vis (accessed 2003 Mar 27).
59. Update on adult immunization. Recommendations of the Immunization Practices Advisory Committee (ACIP). *MMWR Recomm Rep.* 1991; 40(RR-12): 1–94.
60. Grabenstein JD. Compensation for vaccine injury: balancing society's need and personal risk. *Hosp Pharm.* 1995; 30:831–2,834–6.
61. Grabenstein JD. Vaccination records must be available to be used. *J Am Pharm Assoc.* 2000; 40:113.
62. Kapit RM, Grabenstein JD. Adverse events after immunization: reports and results. *Hosp Pharm.* 1995; 30:1031–2,1035–6,1038,1041.
63. Immunization Action Coalition. Adult immunization record card. www.immunize.org/adultizcards/index.htm (accessed 2003 Mar 12).
64. American Society of Hospital Pharmacists. ASHP technical assistance bulletin on hospital drug distribution and control. *Am J Hosp Pharm.* 1980; 37:1097–103.
65. ASHP statement on the pharmacist's responsibility for distribution and control of drug products. In: Deffenbaugh JH, ed. Best practices for health-system pharmacy. Positions and guidance documents of ASHP. 2002–2003 ed. Bethesda, MD: American Society of Health-System Pharmacists; 2002:91.
66. Grabenstein JD. ImmunoFacts: vaccines and immunologic drugs. 28th ed. St Louis: Facts and Comparisons; 2002.
67. Centers for Disease Control and Prevention. Vaccine management: recommendations for handling and storage of selected biologicals. www.cdc.gov/nip/publications/vac_mgt_book.htm (accessed 2003 Mar 27).
68. Casto DT, Brunell PA. Safe handling of vaccines. *Pediatrics.* 1990; 87:108–12.
69. Ross MB. Additional stability guidelines for routinely refrigerated drug products. *Am J Hosp Pharm.* 1988; 45:1498–9. Letter.
70. Sterchele JA. Update on stability guidelines for routinely refrigerated drug products. *Am J Hosp Pharm.* 1987; 44:2698, 2701. Letter.
71. Miller LG, Loomis JH Jr. Advice of manufacturers about effects of temperature on biologicals. *Am J Hosp Pharm.* 1985; 42:843–8.
72. Vogenberg FR, Souney PF. Stability guidelines for routinely refrigerated drug products. *Am J Hosp Pharm.* 1983; 40:101–2.
73. Wolfert RR, Cox RM. Room temperature stability of drug products labeled for refrigerated storage. *Am J Hosp Pharm.* 1975; 32:585–7.
74. Update: recommendations to prevent hepatitis B virus transmission—United States. *MMWR Morb Mortal Wkly Rep.* 1995; 44:574–5.
75. Update: recommendations to prevent hepatitis B virus transmission—United States. *MMWR Morb Mortal Wkly Rep.* 1999; 48:33–4.
76. Prevention of hepatitis A through active or passive immunization: recommendations of the Advisory Committee on Immunization Practices (ACIP). *MMWR Recomm Rep.* 1999; 48(RR-12):1–37.
77. Human rabies prevention—United States, 1999. Recommendations of the Advisory Committee on Immunization Practices (ACIP). *MMWR Recomm Rep.* 1999; 48(RR-1):1–21.
78. Diphtheria, tetanus, and pertussis: recommendations for vaccine use and other preventive measures. Recommendations of the Immunization Practices Advisory Committee (ACIP). *MMWR Recomm Rep.* 1991; 40(RR-10):1–28.
79. Grabenstein JD. Stop buying tetanus toxoid (with one exception). *Hosp Pharm.* 1990; 25:361–2.
80. Pertussis vaccination: use of acellular pertussis vaccines among infants and young children. Recommendations of the Advisory Committee on Immunization Practices (ACIP). *MMWR Recomm Rep.* 1997; 46(RR-7):1–25.
81. American Academy of Pediatrics Committee on Infectious Diseases. The relationship between pertussis vaccine and brain damage: reassessment. *Pediatrics.* 1991; 88:397–400.
82. Immunization of health-care workers: recommendations of the Advisory Committee on Immunization Practices (ACIP) and the Hospital Infection Control Practices Advisory Committee (HICPAC). *MMWR Recomm Rep.* 1997; 46(RR-18):1–42.
83. Screening for tuberculosis and tuberculosis infection in high-risk populations: recommendations of the Advisory Council for the Elimination of Tuberculosis. *MMWR Recomm Rep.* 1995; 44(RR-11):19–34.
84. Anergy skin testing and tuberculosis [corrected] preventive therapy for HIV-infected persons: revised recommendations. *MMWR Recomm Rep.* 1997; 46(RR-15):1–10.
85. Health information for international travel, 2001–02. Washington, DC: Government Printing Office; 2001.
86. American College of Obstetricians and Gynecologists committee opinion. Immunization during pregnancy. *Obstet Gynecol.* 2003; 101:207–12.

These guidelines were reviewed in 2013 by the Council on Pharmacy Practice and by the Board of Directors and were found to still be appropriate.

Developed through the ASHP Council on Professional Affairs and approved by the ASHP Board of Directors on May 31, 2003.

Copyright © 2003, American Society of Hospital Pharmacists, Inc. All rights reserved. Contact ASHP for reprint and permissions requests. This content may not be used for commercial purposes without the express written consent of ASHP.

The bibliographic citation for this document is as follows: American Society of Health-System Pharmacists. ASHP guidelines on the pharmacist's role in immunization. *Am J Health-Syst Pharm.* 2003; 60:1371–7.

ASHP Guidelines on the Pharmacist's Role in Palliative and Hospice Care

Palliative care arose from the modern hospice movement and has evolved significantly over the past 50 years.[1] Numerous definitions exist to describe palliative care, all of which focus on aggressively addressing suffering. The World Health Organization and the U.S. Department of Health and Human Services both stipulate the tenets of palliative care to include a patient-centered and family-centered approach to care, with the goal of maximizing quality of life while minimizing suffering.[2] In its clinical practice guidelines, the National Consensus Project for Quality Palliative Care of the National Quality Forum (NQF) describes palliative care as "patient and family-centered care that optimizes quality of life by anticipating, preventing, and treating suffering . . . throughout the continuum of illness . . . addressing the physical, intellectual, emotional, social, and spiritual needs and to facilitate patient autonomy, access to information, and choice."[2] NQF further specifies the foundation of palliative care to include professional and family collaboration, the availability of services regardless of pursuit of curative or life-extending care, and, most importantly, the provision of care coordinated by an interdisciplinary team.[2] The continuum of care provided by palliative care pharmacists (**Figure 1**) incorporates the concepts that curative and palliative care should coexist and that hospice care is an extension of palliative care that occurs when curative care is no longer part of the patient's plan of care.[3]

The practice of palliative care, while rooted in traditional hospice and hematology and oncology programs, has changed dramatically in its delivery, competency assessment, and methods for preparing future members of the interdisciplinary team.[4,5] Previously, health professionals obtained the necessary skills and knowledge for participation in the interdisciplinary delivery of palliative care via encompassing specialty areas (e.g., internal medicine, geriatrics, oncology).[6,7] Numerous efforts to enhance professional education on palliative care largely drove its eventual recognition as a medical subspecialty in 2006.[8,9]

Specialized training programs and board certification opportunities exist today for most members of the palliative care interdisciplinary team.[10–14] As the model of palliative care has progressed, so too has each team member's potential for contribution. Despite representation within the first hospice demonstration project in the United States, participation of the pharmacist as an essential member of the interdisciplinary team has been traditionally overlooked.[15–18] Evidence of the pharmacist's contribution to the delivery of palliative care and supportive care services beyond the original role of medication dispensing and compounding has garnered growing recognition across numerous practice settings.[15–17,19–27]

Perhaps no other practice setting presents as diverse a collection of potential roles and responsibilities for the affiliated palliative and hospice care (PHC) pharmacist. Here, the PHC pharmacist may support the PHC services in an administrative role (policy and procedure, formulary management), in a consultative role (order set development, treatment algorithm development, best practices education), and in advanced clinical practice (medication therapy management services, pain and symptom management consultations, and interdisciplinary team participation).

Purpose

In 2002, ASHP published the ASHP Statement on the Pharmacist's Role in Hospice and Palliative Care.[28] These guidelines extend beyond the scope of that statement and are intended to define the role of the pharmacist engaged in the practice of PHC. Role definition will include goals for providing services that establish general principles and best practices in the care of this patient population. This document is based on literature resources, consensus of pharmacist experts in the field of PHC, therapeutic practice guidelines, and regulatory standards.[1,2,4,29]

The terms *palliative*, *end-of-life*, *hospice*, and *supportive care* are frequently, and incorrectly, used interchangeably. While these philosophies of care share similarities, each represents overlapping yet delineable points along the healthcare continuum. For the purposes of these guidelines, the term *PHC* will be used to describe the common services afforded to patients with a serious or life-limiting illness, including those enrolled in a formal hospice program.

Two levels of PHC services are described: (1) essential services, which include core processes, and (2) desirable services, which include higher levels of practice, teaching, and research. The level of service provided by the PHC pharmacist will vary based on the level of practice experience of the pharmacist as well as the level of palliative care services provided in each respective setting. Services provided by a pharmacist will therefore be unique and should be designed to best meet the needs of the institution, hospice, or other healthcare practice setting.

In concert with the palliative care team or hospice chief executive officer and medical director, the PHC pharmacist uses his or her professional judgment to individually weigh the factors that determine the extent of services provided. These factors include the population served, number of pharmacists, and time dedicated to the palliative care or hospice team. Corresponding duties required of the PHC pharmacist in other areas of the pharmacy service and the extent of time required for administrative duties and obligations should be considered. Services provided by the PHC pharmacist will vary among practices and should be designed to best meet the needs of the site and the patient.

Delineation and Description

Before the development of these guidelines, a task force was appointed by the Section Advisory Group, Pain and Palliative Care, within the Section of Ambulatory Care Pharmacists of ASHP. A comprehensive literature review was performed using PubMed, EMBASE, PsychInfo, Google Scholar, and International Pharmaceutical Abstracts to search for all relevant articles published between January 1975 and December 2014. The literature search was conducted using MeSH terms

DOI 10.37573/9781585287048.078

FIGURE 1. Continuum of curative, palliative, supportive, and hospice care in disease trajectory. Reprinted under terms of the Creative Commons Attribution License from Guo Q, Jacelon CS, Marquard JL. An evolutionary concept analysis of palliative care. *J Palliat Care Med.* 2012; 2:1–6.

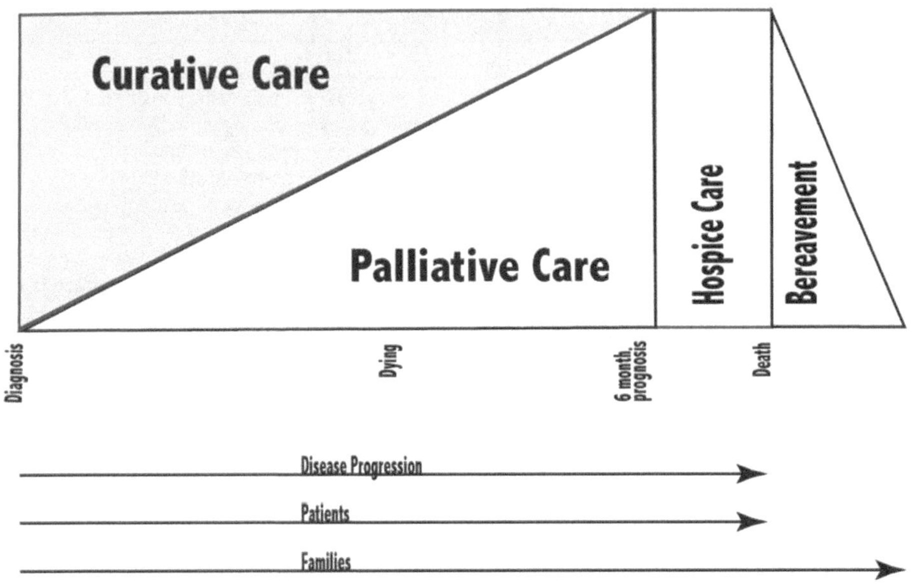

and keywords alone and in combination with other terms, including *pharmacy, pharmacist, pharmaceutical care, pharmacotherapy, medication therapy management, hospice, end of life, terminal illness, palliative care, supportive care, symptom management*, and *pain management*.

Similar to other areas of specialty or subspecialty practice within the profession of pharmacy, some level of palliative and supportive care knowledge is essential for all pharmacists providing patient care, regardless of scope or setting. The European Association for Palliative Care (EAPC) recently updated a two-part guidance document on essential competencies for healthcare and social workers involved in the delivery of palliative care.[1,4] In that guidance document, EAPC delineates recommendations for those providing general palliative care (i.e., palliative care services provided by primary care and nonpalliative care specialists) and those providing specialist palliative care (i.e., health professionals whose main activity focuses on delivery of palliative care). These guidelines also incorporate that dichotomy.

To address the heterogeneous nature of the pharmacy profession, the pharmacist's roles and activities described herein will be categorized as either essential or desirable. Essential roles and activities describe the practice of palliative and supportive care pharmacy, whereas desirable roles and activities denote delivery of palliative and supportive care services by pharmacist specialists at the highest level of advanced practice, such as leading palliative and supportive care teams, engaging in medication therapy management, teaching, and contributing to new knowledge of the field. Essential and desirable roles and activities, as outlined within these guidelines, should not be considered mutually exclusive. Recommendations will focus on the pharmacist's roles and activities within clinical practice and administration as well as practice and professional development.

Essential Clinical Roles and Activities

Essential clinical roles and activities for the PHC pharmacist may vary widely, and services may be provided either directly or indirectly to the patient, depending on the practice setting. While not an exhaustive list of potential practice sites for the PHC pharmacist, settings of PHC delivery include various hospice settings, hospitals, outpatient clinics, outpatient community pharmacies, home care or long-term care (LTC) facilities, and consulting and managed care settings. Essential clinical roles and activities of the PHC pharmacist are presented in **Table 1**, and aspects of those roles and activities that traverse the various PHC practice settings are discussed below.

Hospice Programs. The PHC pharmacist providing care within hospice must be thoroughly familiar with symptom management and reduction. Hospice services are provided in the following settings: standalone hospice inpatient units and hospice residential units, LTC facilities, and hospitals, in addition to the more traditional home care paradigm. PHC pharmacists also must be cognizant of the many regulatory requirements associated with controlled substances, medication reimbursement requirements, and commonly managed symptoms. The Centers for Medicare and Medicaid Services (CMS), as part of the Conditions of Participation, stipulate that hospices are responsible for the costs associated with all services, including medications, related to the terminal diagnosis and related conditions for which the patient was referred and that are contributing to the terminal prognosis.[30,31] (The terminal prognosis includes the terminal and related diagnoses that contribute to the terminal prognosis, to include the symptoms caused or exacerbated by the terminal diagnosis, related diagnosis or treatment of terminal and related diagnosis.) Pharmacists are often called upon to review all patient medications, both at admission and periodically, requiring a

TABLE 1.

Essential Clinical and Administrative Roles, Practice Activities, and Examples of Tasks, Skills, and Knowledge of the PHC Pharmacist[a]

Role and Specialty Practice Activity	Example(s) of Tasks, Skills, and Knowledge
Direct patient care	
• Optimize the outcomes of symptom management and palliative care patients through the expert provision of evidence-based, patient-centered medication therapy as an integral part of an interdisciplinary team • Serve as an authoritative resource on the optimal use of medications in symptom management and palliative care • Anticipate transitions of care when recommending, initiating, modifying, or discontinuing pharmacotherapy for pain and symptoms	• Conduct patient symptom assessment and drug therapy management, including comorbid conditions • Review and provide recommendations on managing ineffective, futile, and nonessential medications • Review pharmacotherapy and facilitate discussion with patients, caregivers, and families to reset therapeutic goals • Participate in hospice or palliative care planning meetings, inpatient patient care rounds, or consultations as appropriate based on setting • Document direct patient care activities appropriately • Establish collaborative pharmacist–patient and pharmacist–caregiver relationships • Provide concise, applicable, comprehensive, and timely responses to formal or informal requests for drug information • Recommend alternative routes of medication administration when traditional routes are not feasible or are impractical
Medication order review and reconciliation	
• Manage and improve the medication-use process in patient care settings	• Assist with preparation and dispensing of medications for symptom management and palliative care patients following existing standards of practice and the organization's policies and procedures • Contribute to the work of the team that secures access for drugs used in a patient's regimen, including facilitation of REMS programs • Assist in drug shortage management, including patient-focused and supply/management decisions • Employ medication adherence strategies • Perform opioid equianalgesic conversions • Conduct clinical medication regimen reviews to identify and resolve medication-related problems associated with symptom management
Education and medication counseling	
• Demonstrate excellence in the provision of medication counseling to patients, caregivers, and families	• Ensure safe and legal disposal of medication
Administrative roles	
• Ensure safe use of medications in the treatment of pain and symptoms • Medication supply chain management	• Pharmacy and therapeutics committee implementation and participation • Medication formulary and therapeutic substitution/interchange policy development and oversight • Development of medication-use policies and procedures • Support development of medication-use algorithms that follow evidence-based best practices • Perform continuous quality-improvement reviews toward medication-use compliance • Medication administration management (e.g., pumps, dosage forms, stock medication) • Safe and effective disposal of medications • Support medication contract negotiations with pharmacy vendors (e.g., PBMs, retail pharmacies, purchasing groups, wholesalers)

[a]PHC = palliative, supportive, and hospice care, REMS = risk evaluation and mitigation strategy, PBM = pharmacy benefit manager.

thorough understanding of the pathophysiology of common life-limiting illnesses and their corresponding symptoms. Recent CMS guidance documents changed the expectations for hospice medication responsibility from those under the current Medicare Part D program, and a growing role for the PHC pharmacist is anticipated, particularly in the types of services provided by a PHC pharmacist on hospice admission.[19,26,32–34] Transitions-of-care planning on admission is of paramount importance to reduce the risk of analgesic or symptom control gaps. The PHC pharmacist should be intimately involved in the medication history and reconciliation of new hospice admissions, with special attention being paid to nonprescription medications and dietary supplements. Prompt identification of high-risk or problem-prone drug therapies should occur. Medication review to assess appropriateness of continued treatment given each drug's potential benefit, burden, and ability to administer, based on each patient's prognosis, should occur, paying particular attention to the identification of nonessential and futile treatment regimens. Equally important is the communication of drug-related changes to the patient and family. CMS's Conditions of Participation mandate that the interdisciplinary group confer with an individual possessing education and training in drug management to perform this ongoing review, though CMS stops short of dictating that these services be provided by a licensed pharmacist.

Caregiver and family education should extend beyond the patient's death. Providing guidance on safe disposal of medications to avoid diversion and improper disposal is easily overlooked but could have a significant impact on the family's health and public health. The PHC pharmacist, regardless of practice setting, must be familiar with current federal and state laws regarding drug disposal as well as local options for safe disposal (e.g., drug take-back programs).

Inpatient Palliative and Supportive Care Teams. The development of institutional palliative care teams is becoming more common in U.S. hospitals and health systems. Pharmacists may be engaged in numerous capacities, ranging from decentralized, full-time, or part-time team members dedicated to the PHC team to reactive participation and consultation when requested. Pharmacists who lead PHC teams require even greater expertise.[16,33] PHC pharmacists should be involved in symptom management strategies as well as facilitating timely medication administration, monitoring and reporting adverse drug reactions, providing education to patients and their families, and monitoring for drug–drug and drug–disease interactions. Regardless of scope of practice for the PHC pharmacist, the necessary knowledge and skills remain unchanged.

Outpatient Palliative and Supportive Care Teams. A growing sector of palliative and supportive care strives to deliver PHC to patients requiring pain and symptom management in an outpatient setting. These services may be housed within oncology and other similar group practices as well as larger primary care services under the patient-centered medical home model.[22,35,36] In addition, many hospices and health systems are establishing palliative care programs to address symptom relief in patients who have yet to initiate their hospice benefit or are not yet hospice appropriate. The PHC pharmacist in this setting must be thoroughly familiar with the medications used to alleviate suffering, with state and federal controlled substances laws, and with the nuances between standard community-dwelling patients, patients residing in LTC facilities, patients residing in assisted-living facilities, and patients receiving hospice care. In the outpatient setting, the PHC pharmacist's assistance is often sought when medication formularies and cost are of concern or drug administration difficulties are encountered.[37–39] Given the inability to closely observe outpatient PHC patients, tailored monitoring plans are required, while balancing the risks and benefits of a selected drug therapy is critical (e.g., symptoms, adverse drug effects, drugs with a narrow therapeutic range, opioids). Unique challenges may be encountered in this setting, requiring assistance from the PHC pharmacist regarding the safe use of and risk mitigation for opioids (e.g., previous patient or family history of substance use disorder or drug diversion).

Consulting, Distributive, and Compounding Services. Many patients residing in LTC facilities may either be candidates for PHC or currently under the care of a hospice organization. Pharmacists serving in a consulting capacity to these LTC facilities may significantly improve symptom management. In addition, advocating for patients who may be noncommunicative is essential. Essential roles of the PHC pharmacist serving in this capacity include ensuring routine use of medications as needed for pain or other symptom management, conducting appropriate monitoring for required maintenance medications, and having a thorough understanding of the interplay between regulatory compliance and the needs of the patient (e.g., antipsychotic use for terminal agitation in an LTC facility).

Pharmacists working in distributive or compounding services supporting PHC also have an important role in the provision of care. The art and science of preparing specially compounded medication formulations support the provision of personalized care to the terminally ill. The dispensing pharmacist will utilize his or her education and knowledge to ensure that the patient and family members understand the role of prescribed medications and necessary precautions with their use.

Many state regulations require hospices to retain a consultant or employed pharmacist for oversight of all medication-use processes within a hospice inpatient facility. These pharmacists collaborate with the hospice care team in a number of activities, including medication therapy reviews, clinical consults, and medication regulatory compliance oversight and guidance.

Desirable Clinical Roles and Activities

Desirable clinical roles and activities of a PHC pharmacist represent those typically reserved for the pharmacist engaged in dedicated palliative or supportive care services. These activities will, in most cases, embody the highest levels of service provided by the pharmacist allowed by the institution's scope of practice policies and state's pharmacy practice act. Most notably, the PHC pharmacist will often participate in the direct care of patients with respect to symptom assessment, laboratory monitoring, medication management, and prescribing in states that grant prescriptive authority to pharmacists through collaborative practice agreements (CPAs). A PHC pharmacist should actively seek and engage in collaborative practice whenever allowed by the state and institution. Practicing at the top of one's professional license in this regard will facilitate provision of care to patients who otherwise may not have the opportunity for specialized services. Pharmacists will be actively involved with patient and family medication-use education to support their understanding of prescribed therapies and compliance with the plan of care. Desirable clinical roles and activities of the PHC pharmacist are described in **Table 2**, and aspects of those roles and activities that traverse the various PHC practice settings are discussed below.

Hospice Programs. The care model in many home care hospice programs, in which the patient's primary physician remains in that role, has evolved to utilize the PHC pharmacist as the hospice team member who develops specific medication recommendations through a consultative process. These PHC pharmacists are practicing as specialists in palliative care and often are familiar with palliative medication provision and can make patient-specific and cost-effective recommendations that are widely accepted by primary physicians.[34,40]

TABLE 2.

Desirable Clinical and Administrative Roles, Practice Activities, and Examples of Tasks, Skills, and Knowledge of the PHC Pharmacist[a]

Desirable Role and Specialty Practice Activity	Examples of Specific Tasks, Skills, and Knowledge
Direct patient care	
• Conduct advanced pain and symptom assessment, including comorbid conditions • Establish and maintain a collaborative practice agreement with managing medical practitioner • Initiate, modify, and discontinue medication therapy • Monitor medication therapy using patient and caregiver history and order, recommend, or interpret laboratory and test results • Develop an accountable role within the PHC interdisciplinary team • Thoroughly understand scope of practice and roles of nonpharmacist members of the PHC team • Participate in or lead family meetings • Establish goals of care and educate patient and family on medication therapy decisions (e.g., discontinuation of futile or nonessential medications) • Participate in or lead decisions on hospice or outpatient palliative care appropriateness and referral • Guide transitions of care • Assist in health-system policy as it relates to PHC • Educate patients, caregivers, and families regarding medications	• Complete thorough history and symptom analysis • Perform limited physical examination • Prescribe, order, or recommend medication therapy in the management of symptoms and pain using evidence-based medicine when available • Order or recommend and interpret labs or tests • Utilize or recommend validated, patient-specific, uni- or multidimensional assessment tools and screens (e.g., Patient Health Questionnaire, McGill Pain Questionnaire, Edmonton Symptom Assessment Scale, Beck Depression Inventory) • Coordinate seamless transitions of care from hospital to home, home to hospital, hospital to LTC facility, LTC facility to hospital, or any setting to hospice • Develop institutional, evidence-based, or guideline-driven policies, order sets, and protocols • Create competencies that support the daily practice and growth of the PHC role • Develop a collaborative practice agreement that promotes patient-centered care and supports practicing at the top of pharmacy license
Education	
• Develop health profession students' understanding of PHC • Develop practicing health professionals' understanding of PHC	• Develop didactic and experiential PHC learning experiences (e.g., lectures, rotations, residency, shadowing) • Serve as a preceptor for pharmacy students and other health students • Serve as a preceptor for PGY1 PHC rotation • Serve as a preceptor for PGY2 PHC specialty residency
Scholarship	
• Contribute to the body of knowledge of PHC via writing, speaking, or research	• Conduct and disseminate research via publication, poster presentation, and lecturing • Participate in development of clinical guidelines, guidance documents, or treatment algorithms
Administrative roles	
• Practice development and management • Interdisciplinary leadership	• Policy and procedure/guideline development (e.g., ketamine, propofol, or lidocaine infusions; palliative sedation) • Proposal of new or expanded PHC pharmacy services • Establish reimbursement structure for pharmacist services • Ensure coverage and scheduling of PHC pharmacist services • Development of postgraduate training opportunities (e.g., PGY2 pain and palliative care residencies) • Maintain a leadership role on organizational committees (e.g., chair or vice-chair the pharmacy and therapeutics committee) • Develop interprofessional continuing-education programs

[a]PHC = palliative, supportive, and hospice care, PGY1 = postgraduate year 1, PGY2 = postgraduate year 2, LTC = long-term care.

Inpatient Palliative and Supportive Care Teams. The PHC pharmacist should provide direct patient care services of varying scopes within the inpatient setting. These services may result from specialty team consultation, from individual consultation, or as part of health-system policy–directed automatic consultation (e.g., upon ordering of high-risk medications in nonadvanced care units). Typically, direct patient care services provided to inpatients by the PHC pharmacist will be directed by the pharmacy and therapeutics committee and medical staff executive committee. The individual institution or health system must direct the credentialing and privileging of PHC pharmacists in the absence of board certification availability. Other equally important functions of the inpatient PHC pharmacist include medication stewardship utilizing the principles of pharmaceutical care practice, adverse-effect anticipation and monitoring, pain and symptom management, patient and family education, discharge and transition planning, and follow-up coordination of care between multiple providers after transitions to new settings. Pharmacists may even be called on to lead a PHC team, which would require even greater expertise.[16,33]

Outpatient Palliative and Supportive Care. Lack of access to palliative care providers in ambulatory clinic settings creates an opportunity for a PHC pharmacist to provide symptom management to a variety of patient populations. The resulting improvement in quality of life and potential reduction in the number of acute visits to the physician office or emergency department for symptom-related complaints would represent the primary quality indicator for such a pharmacist. The PHC pharmacist should simultaneously be aware of the relative financial impact of medication therapies. Consideration of cost and insurance coverage at the time of medication selection is paramount in the outpatient setting. In addition, avoidance of high-cost medications when other equally effective and tolerated therapies are available reduces the likelihood of interruption to optimal symptom control should the patient transition to hospice care. When possible, having the PHC pharmacist work within a clinic focused on palliative care enhances the interdisciplinary approach to patient care. Although it is arguably an essential role of pharmacists in any practice setting, PHC pharmacists should possess the basic understanding and skills necessary to identify the risk for and current substance abuse among patients, caregivers, and family members.

While the direct patient care services of PHC pharmacists practicing in the hospice environment are not frequently described, their impact on patient care is noteworthy. CMS regulations concerning the provision of hospice services may preclude a PHC pharmacist from acting as the sole provider for a patient or directing an interdisciplinary team.

Supporting Transitions of Care. An important desirable clinical role for PHC pharmacists is the active support of patients transitioning from aggressive treatment to comfort-focused care. The PHC pharmacist is in an ideal position to assist in evaluating the changing risk:benefit ratio of medications as the patient transitions through the continuum of care. Patients experiencing a steady decline often declare for themselves when a treatment is no longer beneficial or tolerable, either orally or through the inability to continue the regimen (e.g., due to lost availability of intravenous access or ability to administer oral medications). Equally important is the ability to recognize when a given treatment has failed to demonstrate continued benefit and should be discontinued (e.g., reevaluation of lipid-lowering therapy, dementia-related medications, certain chemotherapy agents).[41] For patients with chronic illnesses who experience intermittent severe exacerbations, there may be multiple inflection points and changes between life-prolonging and symptom-focused approaches. The PHC pharmacist should assist the patient, family, caregiver, and other healthcare providers in navigating the changes in medication regimens that are necessary to provide a patient-centered, cost-effective, and (when available) evidence-based approach. Evaluation for discontinuation of medications should occur, at a minimum, during transitions of care.[42,43] The PHC pharmacist is often one of the few consistent members of the interdisciplinary team and therefore has an essential role in this process. His or her involvement allows for continuity of care during patient handoffs between healthcare providers and a historical account of the effectiveness of previous medication regimens. PHC pharmacists may also be engaged in assisting in the enrollment and discharge of PHC patients from hospice care.

Educating and Training Student Pharmacists and Other Clinicians. PHC pharmacists should be actively engaged in the education and training of students, pharmacists, and patient care clinicians of various disciplines. They possess knowledge about the rational and practical use of medications that is often not taught in didactic learning environments or in clinical or experiential training outside that specific to palliative care providers. In addition to the clinical and administrative expertise required by the inpatient PHC pharmacist, teaching staff peers, the PHC team, and health profession students should be considered part of these essential activities.

Scholarship. Ongoing evaluation of current practices and the dissemination of novel treatments or processes are critical for the continued improvement in patient care and sustainability of the PHC pharmacist. Scholarship should be pursued when possible and in any form to share best practices, research methodology, and outcomes. Clinical research in palliative care and hospice is lacking, and the PHC pharmacist should contribute to the overall body of knowledge when possible.

Essential Administrative Roles and Activities

The pharmacist's essential administrative roles and activities in PHC should incorporate basic practice activities that promote positive treatment outcomes, adverse-event avoidance, and medication cost containment.

A primary component of the PHC pharmacist's role is continuous review of medications. Continuous review of patient medication records and ongoing contact with the primary physician, as well as with the patient or caregiver, are essential to minimizing medication-related problems and expenses while improving outcomes and efficacy.

Pharmacists engaged in the development and oversight of a medication formulary will support palliative and end-of-life care programs to achieve evidence-based and cost-effective medication use, minimize delays in therapy due to drug shortages, and contain medication expenses.

Hospices and palliative care programs will often seek to develop standards to ensure consistency in the care of patients. Part of this effort is the development of policies and procedures to guarantee that activities associated with medication use are consistent across all levels of care.

Hospice. Proactive review of patient medication regimens over time can significantly reduce medication burden and costs. Ongoing rapport and dialogue must be sustained with the hospice or palliative care physician and nurse, as well as with the patient or caregiver. This dialogue is essential to establish and maintain a picture of the patient's functional status, providing the opportunity for the PHC pharmacist to identify and recommend changes in nonessential or overly burdensome medication therapy or the addition of medications for symptom management. An extensive and more comprehensive example of the medication review process occurs at hospice interdisciplinary team meetings.

The PHC pharmacist's contributions to the development of medication-use policies and procedures will serve to strengthen compliance with federal and state regulations and with best practices. All hospices are regulated by state and federal agencies, which include standards associated with medication use. In addition, 75% of hospices report accreditation with agencies such as the Joint Commission, Community Health Accreditation Program, and Accreditation Commission for Health Care.[44,45] With a working knowledge of regulatory and accreditation standards on medication use, pharmacists are well positioned to support the development and updating of medication-use policies and procedures to achieve compliance.

As a representative of a hospice organization, the PHC pharmacist is in an excellent position to support contract negotiations with pharmacy providers (e.g., local retail pharmacies, pharmacy benefit managers, purchasing groups, national pharmacy provider groups). The PHC pharmacist should also work with local pharmacy providers to ensure that appropriate medications are consistently available to the hospice and communicate regularly with them regarding prescription adjudication concerns, coverage, and other required quality and regulatory issues.

If a hospice is of sufficient size to support a dedicated pharmacy and therapeutics committee, the PHC pharmacist must be an active member and would ideally serve in a leadership capacity. The pharmacist's role would involve input into all aspects of medication-use management, ranging from decisions on approved medications prescribed under the hospice plan of care, continuous quality-improvement activities, policy development for medication use, therapeutic substitution parameters, tiered medication selection, and protocol or algorithm development.

An essential activity for PHC pharmacists is evaluating all patient medications on patient admission to a hospice program for payment under the hospice plan of care. The PHC pharmacist is equipped to address the suitability of medications, given the hospice diagnosis and related conditions contributing to the terminal prognosis. Upon the physician's certification of a terminal prognosis, the PHC pharmacist, in discussion either with the admitting nurse or during the team nurse's initial visit, will provide payment approval of medications to be covered under the hospice plan of care as well as identify and discontinue nonessential medications. For medications identified as necessary to continue and not covered under the hospice plan of care, a source of payment must be determined (e.g., patient pay, supplemental health insurance, Medicare Part D).[46] During this evaluation, the pharmacist can identify alternative, cost-effective therapies appropriate for the patient's medical conditions. This admission medication review process alone can result in significant cost savings for a hospice.[40]

Hospital and Institutional Practice. Pharmacists working in large healthcare organizations, hospitals, and other institutions have additional opportunities to shape institutional medication-use policies and procedures regarding drug-related protocols, formulary development, and algorithms by providing evidence-based recommendations that can improve the safety and efficacy of analgesics as well as other commonly used palliative care agents. Other important roles for PHC pharmacists include (1) participating in institutional committees and medication safety–reporting systems that address medication errors, adverse drug reactions, and the safety of analgesics and symptom-management agents, (2) acting as a resource and actively participating in the pharmacy and therapeutics committee or similar committees, (3) serving as an institutional resource to healthcare professionals, patients, and patients' families on the optimal use of medications in symptom management and palliative care, (4) providing continuous evaluation and review of all existing drug-related protocols and algorithms to ensure that they reflect current best practices, and (5) assisting in the development of urgency plans that address inappropriate use of emergency department services or hospital admission. In addition, it is essential that the PHC pharmacist assist the institution or health system in compliance with accreditation, legal, regulatory, and safety requirements related to the use of analgesics and other symptom-management agents. The activities discussed above provide considerable opportunities for pharmacists to be involved in establishing and supporting medication-use practice patterns that positively affect patient outcomes and the financial well-being of institutions.

Desirable Administrative Roles and Activities

Desirable administrative roles and activities include quality improvement, oversight and improvement of education, practice development and advancement, and advocacy.

Quality Improvement. As the pharmacist with a distinct skill set serving on an interdisciplinary PHC team, there is a unique opportunity to identify processes or protocols that need development or revision to improve the quality of care delivered. One avenue for achieving this goal is a leadership role on the pharmacy and therapeutics committee or similar committees. Participation in such committees is also an essential administrative role, but by practicing at a higher level the PHC pharmacist may provide services such as care set development to guide the use of complex, high-cost, or high-risk therapies (e.g., lidocaine or ketamine). Revisions to existing practices might include updating institution medication administration guidelines to allow for the use of medications or dosages that are typically restricted to an intensive treatment unit or similar setting (e.g., development of protocols for palliative sedation or refractory terminal delirium).

Quality-improvement processes related to drug delivery or medication use are also an important area of practice. Medication-use evaluation or drug utilization review may identify the need for significant practice changes (e.g., development of safe practices for the use of methadone for pain control, approval of opioid guidelines). Quality-improvement processes usually align with the development of clinical practice guidelines or algorithm development for the expert palliative care team (e.g., palliative sedation or pain emergencies). The PHC pharmacist should play a key or leading role in the interdisciplinary development of algorithms to standardize the approach to common palliative care symptoms such as agitation, anxiety, anorexia, cachexia, constipation, delirium, dyspnea, fatigue, nausea, pain, secretions, and sleep disturbances.

Education. Maintenance and improvement of different aspects of palliative care education are important to the continued sustainability of the pharmacist's role in PHC practice. The development and oversight of postgraduate year 2 (PGY2) specialty pharmacy residency programs that incorporate education and training in PHC are essential to the growth of the specialty. Another key educational component is ensuring that core PHC competency is incorporated into postgraduate year 1 (PGY1) pharmacy residencies and other specialty residencies. Integration into the curricula at colleges of pharmacy can provide student pharmacists with the basic skills and knowledge about the medication management approach for a palliative care patient, and these learning experiences should be taught by those practicing at the highest levels to encourage continued forward movement of the profession. Interprofessional education of nursing students, medical students and residents, and palliative care physician fellows through didactic and experiential teaching is another important role for the PHC pharmacist. Modeling the role of the PHC pharmacist for learners in other disciplines not only teaches them core skills in medication management of the palliative care patient but also promotes the expertise of pharmacists in the minds of future palliative care clinicians. Nurse practitioners, nurses, and physician assistants can also benefit from a pharmacist's expert knowledge through inservice or continuing-education programs hosted by the health system or area professional organizations.

A significant amount of a palliative care team's time is devoted to communicating the care plan to other providers, staff, families, and caregivers involved in the patient's care. Because of his or her knowledge of disease processes and treatment regimens, the interdisciplinary PHC team pharmacist is well positioned to provide such communication.

Practice Development, Advocacy, and Advancement

The clinical and administrative roles of the PHC pharmacist in any setting rely on sound practice development, advocacy, and engagement to promote practice advancement. Recommendations regarding practice development, advocacy, and advancement are outlined in **Appendix A** and presented below.

Practice Development. When developing the proposed role of a PHC pharmacist within an institution, health system, or hospice, the identification of the key stakeholders, examination of the infrastructure or currently offered services, and performance of a needs assessment are required. This process will provide the groundwork for the focus and potential utility of the PHC pharmacist. A commonly encountered barrier to the establishment of new services, regardless of setting, is the overcommitment of the PHC pharmacist or underestimation of the time requirement for the services proposed. The Center for the Advancement of Palliative Care provides excellent resources guiding the first steps, whether establishing an entirely new PHC service or simply adding personnel to the team. For example, if the institution's main priorities are preventing long inpatient stays, curtailing futile high-cost resource utilization, and facilitating discharges, then the focus of the proposed position should be on the inpatient setting. On the other hand, if the institution's priorities focus on preventing frequent emergency department visits or hospital admissions for pain and symptom issues that can be managed through outpatient services, then the proposal should seek to provide services within the outpatient setting.

Consideration should be given to the funding of such a position, which should be established at the beginning of such discussions. Engagement of nonclinical departments (e.g., finance) is critical. There are numerous practice models for clinical pharmacy PHC services, including drug information, drug utilization review, clinical interdisciplinary team involvement, and medication therapy management through collaborative protocols. The needs assessment also applies to evaluating what the PHC pharmacist will need for continued professional development.

After identification of the funding source for the PHC pharmacist and the anticipated level of support for the PHC service, a formal job description or policy of roles and responsibilities will need to be drafted and vetted by all potential stakeholders. A model job description on roles and responsibilities of the PHC pharmacist appears in **Appendix B**. Typical activities may include daily review of patient medications for which the PHC team has been consulted, regular consultation team and house staff educational programming, and representation on quality-improvement committees or task forces. The heterogeneity of PHC programs in today's institutions precludes a complete description for every model or setting. In some institutions, the PHC pharmacist plays an indispensable role in the development of new policies and procedures concerning such difficult topics as palliative sedation and terminal wean from mechanical ventilation.

Health systems or hospices must develop standardized policies to address the clinical credentialing and privileging of the PHC pharmacist. There are several common barriers to this undertaking. First, no profession-recognized board certification currently exists for the PHC pharmacist to demonstrate knowledge or skills above the minimum competency state licensure examinations. Second, there is a paucity of specialized training programs that prepare pharmacists interested in PHC practice. This creates a very real chasm when considering specific PHC privileges in today's climate for pharmacists seeking to enter this area of practice without an already developed and successful service or practice.

Other considerations include the PHC team design, referral-only versus automatically triggered evaluation, scope of practice for the PHC pharmacist, and documentation processes. A key element to the documentation process will be the reimbursement or billing model that is established. Reimbursement regulations are everchanging and specific for various practice settings, as described earlier. Those seeking to establish or expand PHC pharmacist services should seek out resources and guidance on best practices for sustainability, including both revenue generation and cost-avoidance tracking.

Before the development of a practice model for the PHC pharmacist, the department or team should evaluate the state-specific laws and relevant pharmacy practice act rules by which the pharmacist must abide. Depending on the practice site, the scope of practice may differ significantly. Advanced scope of practice pharmacists may often undertake greatly expanded roles in patient care under CPAs approved by a pharmacy and therapeutics committee or executive medical staff. At the time of writing, pharmacists practicing under appropriately drafted CPAs may hold Drug Enforcement Administration (DEA) practitioner registration in California, Massachusetts, Montana, New Mexico, North Carolina, North Dakota, and Washington. DEA is currently reviewing Idaho's Pharmacy Practice Act and Controlled Substances Act for possible inclusion. Pharmacists licensed in one of these states may additionally obtain fee-exempt DEA registration if employed and practicing within the U.S. Armed Forces, Department of Veterans Affairs, Indian Health Service, or federal prison system. Typically, the credentialing officer within these organizations can assist obtaining registration. A sample CPA for a PHC pharmacist is provided in **Appendix C**.

Attention should be given to creating an infrastructure to sustain pharmacy's involvement on the interdisciplinary PHC team. Integrating pharmacists into a health system's palliative care staffing matrix may be a first step to accomplishing this. Proactively budgeting for additional pharmacy positions as the number of consultations performed per year increases would also support sustainability of PHC pharmacists' presence. To justify such positions, the PHC pharmacist must be familiar with reimbursement models and opportunities to further support these positions.

Competencies and Certification. There are no recognized board certification opportunities for pharmacists with a unique expertise in the area of palliative and supportive care in the United States. Without the opportunity for board certification to verify PHC pharmacists' expertise, it is difficult to advocate for their importance to health-system administrators, payers, and other professionals. Lack of certification also complicates the credentialing and privileging process of such clinicians. The Board of Pharmacy Specialties (BPS) previously conducted a role delineation study to investigate the feasibility of recognizing pain and palliative care as a specialty within the profession of pharmacy. Although BPS did not elect to pursue pain and palliative care as a recognized specialty when combined, perhaps differentiating between the two distinct yet often overlapping clinical skill sets will provide sufficient demarcation in future consideration. BPS is also investigating opportunities for added qualifications in numerous areas, including palliative care.

There are opportunities for pharmacists to further enhance their training in palliative and supportive care. The ASHP Research and Education Foundation Pain and Palliative Care Traineeship provides a three-level program consisting of Web-based narrated lectures followed by onsite training with an established PHC pharmacist. There are various other training programs to further pharmacists' understanding of palliative and supportive care outside of formalized residency or fellowship training. Recommended journals, books, and websites for professional development of the PHC pharmacist are listed in **Appendix D**.

Development of Didactic and Experiential Education. The Strategic Planning Summit for the Advancement of Pain and Palliative Care Pharmacy, convened in 2009, produced a comprehensive consensus document on strategies to integrate standardized palliative care education in the doctor of pharmacy core curriculum, elective courses, PGY1 programs, and PGY2 palliative care specialty residencies.[29] There are currently 12 ASHP-accredited or accreditation-eligible PGY2 palliative care or pain management programs and many others with exposure or emphasis in pain or palliative care.[47] It is important that there are formal and standardized education programs available in the area of PHC for pharmacists' involvement in the field to continue to grow. In addition, there is a training opportunity for pharmacists in the one-year Interprofessional Palliative Care Fellowship Program offered by the Department of Veterans Affairs.

Advocacy. The importance of the role of a PHC pharmacist needs to be established at the national level, with individual pharmacists contributing grassroots advocacy. The Joint Commission palliative care certification requirements currently do not include a palliative care pharmacist as a core member of the interdisciplinary program team as they do for physicians, registered nurses, social workers, and chaplains. The current Joint Commission requirements state that a clinical pharmacist should be "utilized" based on patient needs. Most palliative care patients have complicated medical histories and are taking medications (mainly controlled substances with narrow therapeutic ranges) that require close clinical monitoring and attention to regulatory compliance issues, which should justify a pharmacist as an integral part of providing comprehensive care to the patient.

Advocacy efforts of the PHC pharmacist should be multitiered and involve discipline-specific professional development, practice development, and quality-improvement initiatives. Reaching out to state, regional, and national professional organizations and legislators to discuss the importance of pharmacist involvement in the PHC team must be universally practiced to continue the growth of the field. Scholarly pursuits demonstrating the effects that PHC pharmacists have on patient care are equally important.

Conclusion

PHC pharmacists bring a diversity of essential services to palliative and supportive care teams. Central to the role of the PHC pharmacist is symptom management through participation in direct patient care, providing pharmacotherapy regimens that support optimal patient outcomes. Medication therapy management and the application of transitional continuity of care are key services pharmacists provide to patients in this care setting.

Collaborative practice opportunities have strengthened the working relationship with palliative and supportive care medical practitioners, furthering PHC pharmacist practice development. In addition, PHC pharmacists may participate in advocacy, research, and scholarly activities in palliative and supportive care, furthering the growth of this area of practice. The PHC pharmacist should provide education to student pharmacists and PGY1 and PGY2 residents, as well as members of the interdisciplinary team, peers, patients, and caregivers. Activities outlined in these guidelines showcase a considerable breadth and depth of opportunities for pharmacists' involvement in the daily management and oversight of medication-use processes across all palliative and supportive care venues, positively affecting patient outcomes while maintaining fiscal responsibility.

References

1. Gamondi C, Larkin P, Payne S. Core competencies in palliative care: an EAPC white paper on palliative care education—part 1. *Eur J Palliat Care.* 2013; 20:86–91.
2. National Consensus Project for Quality Palliative Care. Clinical practice guidelines for quality palliative care, 3rd ed. www.nationalconsensusproject.org/guidelines_download2.aspx (accessed 2016 Feb 19).
3. Guo Q, Jacelon CS, Marquard JL. An evolutionary concept analysis of palliative care. *J Palliat Care Med.* 2012; 2:1–6.
4. Gamondi C, Larkin P, Payne S. Core competencies in palliative care: an EAPC white paper on palliative care education—part 2. *Eur J Palliat Care.* 2013; 20:140–5.
5. Oya H, Matoba M, Murakami S, et al. Mandatory palliative care education for surgical residents: initial focus on teaching pain management. *Jpn J Clin Oncol.* 2013; 43:170–5.
6. Daly D, Matzel SC. Building a transdisciplinary approach to palliative care in an acute care setting. *Omega.* 2013; 67:43–51.
7. Suhrie EM, Hanlon JT, Jaffe EJ, et al. Impact of a geriatric nursing home palliative care service on unnecessary medication prescribing. *Am J Geriatr Pharmacother.* 2009; 7:20–5.
8. Battley JE, Connell LC, O'Reilly S. Early specialty palliative care. *N Engl J Med.* 2014; 370:1075.
9. Berman HD. Palliative care is a specialty. *Can Fam Physician.* 2008; 54:1526.
10. Ingleton C, Gardiner C, Seymour JE, et al. Exploring education and training needs among the palliative care workforce. *BMJ Support Palliat Care.* 2013; 3:207–12.
11. Tice MA. Nurse specialists in home health nursing: the certified hospice and palliative care nurse. *Home Healthc Nurse.* 2006; 24:145–7.
12. Von Gunten CF, Sloan PA, Portenoy RK, et al. Physician board certification in hospice and palliative medicine. *J Palliat Med.* 2000; 3:441–7.
13. National Association of Social Workers. The Advanced Certified Hospice and Palliative Social Worker (ACHP-SW). www.socialworkers.org/credentials/credentials/achp.asp (accessed 2015 Jan 3).
14. Juba KM. Pharmacist credentialing in pain management and palliative care. *J Pharm Pract.* 2012; 25:517–20.
15. Dean TW. Pharmacist as a member of the palliative care team. *Can J Hosp Pharm.* 1987; 40:95–6.
16. Gilbar P, Stefaniuk K. The role of the pharmacist in palliative care: results of a survey conducted in Australia and Canada. *J Palliat Care.* 2002; 18:287–92.
17. Hanif N. Role of the palliative care unit pharmacist. *J Palliat Care.* 1991; 7:35–6.
18. O'Connor M, Pugh J, Jiwa M, et al. The palliative care interdisciplinary team: where is the community pharmacist? *J Palliat Med.* 2011; 14:7–11.
19. Atayee RS, Best BM, Daniels CE. Development of an ambulatory palliative care pharmacist practice. *J Palliat Med.* 2008; 11:1077–82.
20. Chen J, Lu XY, Wang WJ, et al. Impact of a clinical pharmacist-led guidance team on cancer pain therapy in China: a prospective multicenter cohort study. *J Pain Symptom Manage.* 2014; 48:500–9.
21. Eischens KP, Gilling SW, Okerlund RE, et al. Improving medication therapy management through collaborative hospice care in rural Minnesota. *J Am Pharm Assoc.* 2010; 50:379–83.
22. Edwards SJ, Abbott R, Edwards J, et al. Outcomes assessment of a pharmacist-directed seamless care program in an ambulatory oncology clinic. *J Pharm Pract.* 2014; 27:46–52.
23. Gagnon L, Fairchild A, Pituskin E, et al. Optimizing pain relief in a specialized outpatient palliative radiotherapy clinic: contributions of a clinical pharmacist. *J Oncol Pharm Pract.* 2012; 18:76–83.
24. Gammaitoni AR, Gallagher RM, Welz M, et al. Palliative pharmaceutical care: a randomized, pro-spective study of telephone-based prescription and medication counseling services for treating chronic pain. *Pain Med.* 2000; 1:317–31.
25. Hussainy SY, Box M, Scholes S. Piloting the role of a pharmacist in a community palliative care multidisciplinary team: an Australian experience. *BMC Palliat Care.* 2011; 10:16.
26. Ise Y, Morita T, Katayama S, et al. The activity of palliative care team pharmacists in designated cancer hospitals: a nationwide survey in Japan. *J Pain Symptom Manage.* 2014; 47:588–93.
27. Ise Y, Morita T, Maehori N, et al. Role of the community pharmacy in palliative care: a nationwide survey in Japan. *J Palliat Med.* 2010; 13:733–7.
28. Lipman AG, Arter SG, Berry JI, et al. ASHP statement on the pharmacist's role in hospice and palliative care. *Am J Health-Syst Pharm.* 2002; 59:1770–3.
29. Herndon CM, Strassels SA, Strickland JM, et al. Consensus recommendations from the strategic planning summit for pain and palliative care pharmacy practice. *J Pain Symptom Manage.* 2012; 43:925–44.
30. Centers for Medicare and Medicaid Services. Medicare and Medicaid programs: hospice conditions of parti-cipation. Final rule. *Fed Regist.* 2008; 73:32087–220.
31. Centers for Medicare and Medicaid Services. Medicare program; FY 2015 hospice wage index and payment rate update; hospice quality reporting requirements and process and appeals for Part D payment for drugs for beneficiaries enrolled in hospice. Final rule. *Fed Regist.* 2014; 79:50451–510.

32. Craig DS. Introduction: pharmacist role in pain management. *J Pharm Pract.* 2012; 25:496.
33. Lucas C, Glare PA, Sykes JV. Contribution of a liaison clinical pharmacist to an inpatient palliative care unit. *Palliat Med.* 1997; 11:209–16.
34. Wilson S, Wahler R, Brown J, et al. Impact of pharmacist intervention on clinical outcomes in the palliative care setting. *Am J Hosp Palliat Care.* 2011; 28:316–20.
35. Shah S, Dowell J, Greene S. Evaluation of clinical pharmacy services in a hematology/oncology outpatient setting. *Ann Pharmacother.* 2006; 40:1527–33.
36. Valgus JM, Faso A, Gregory KM, et al. Integration of a clinical pharmacist into the hematology-oncology clinics at an academic medical center. *Am J Health-Syst Pharm.* 2011; 68:613–9.
37. Martin CM. Exploring new opportunities in hospice pharmacy. *Consult Pharm.* 2009; 24:114–9.
38. Snapp J, Kelley D, Gutgsell TL. Creating a hospice pharmacy and therapeutics committee. *Am J Hosp Palliat Care.* 2002; 19:129–34.
39. Walker KA, Scarpaci L, McPherson ML. Fifty reasons to love your palliative care pharmacist. *Am J Hosp Palliat Care.* 2010; 27:511–3.
40. Latuga NM, Wahler RG, Monte SV. A national survey of hospice administrator and pharmacist perspectives on pharmacist services and the impact on medication requirements and cost. *Am J Hosp Palliat Care.* 2012; 29:546–54.
41. Kominek C, DiScala S. Quality improvement project of pharmacist-assisted medication reconciliation and regimen review following veteran discharge to hospice. *J Pharm Pharmacol.* 2014; 2:489–500.
42. Holmes HM, Todd A. Evidence-based deprescribing of statins in patients with advanced illness. *JAMA Intern Med.* 2015; 175:701–2.
43. Scott IA, Hilmer SN, Reeve E, et al. Reducing inappropriate polypharmacy: the process of de-prescribing. *JAMA Intern Med.* 2015; 175:827–34.
44. Levi L. New hospice accreditation manual released by ACHC. *Home Healthc Nurse.* 2003; 21:559–61.
45. Murray NS. Hospice accreditation: a useful tool for quality assurance. *Am J Hosp Care.* 1989; 6:44–6.
46. Vogenberg FR, Marcoux RM, Larrat EP. Understanding insurance coverage in the senior market: reimbursement and emerging trends. *Consult Pharm.* 2012; 27:641–9.
47. American Society of Health-System Pharmacists. ASHP residency directory, 2015. www.ashp.org/menu/Accreditation/ResidencyDirectory (accessed 2015 Jan 3).

Appendix A—Summary of Recommendations for Practice Development, Advocacy, and Advancement of the Palliative and Hospice Care (PHC) Pharmacist

- Before the development or expansion of PHC pharmacy services, a needs assessment, funding allocation, and staffing must be thoroughly evaluated
- Job descriptions or scope of practice policies, as well as institution credentialing, should be developed for all pharmacists providing PHC services
- Pharmacists providing PHC services should practice to the full capacity of institutional policies and state pharmacy practice acts up to and including collaborative practice agreements and Drug Enforcement Administration practitioner registration
- PHC pharmacists should take an active role in disseminating best practices, scholarly pursuits, and other advocacy efforts to further promote the profession within PHC
- PHC pharmacists must embrace the education of pharmacy students and residents at all levels of PHC services

Appendix B—Model Job Description or Roles and Responsibilities Document for a Palliative and Hospice Care (PHC) Pharmacist Position

Position purpose:

The PHC pharmacist is responsible for (a) representation of pharmacy services on the palliative care/hospice care team and (b) representation of the palliative care/hospice team within pharmacy services in the provision of high-quality PHC services to the patients of ________________ health system/palliative care team/hospice

Duties and responsibilities:

1. Serve as a resource to the medical, nursing, and pharmacy staff regarding the safe and effective management of medications used in the treatment of pain and other symptoms.
2. Conduct rounds on all patients with current consultations for palliative and supportive care (where applicable).
3. Attend all interdisciplinary PHC team meetings (where applicable).
4. Provide clinical consultations or recommendations to palliative care team, hospice staff, house staff, and consulting providers on symptom management, pain control, cost-effective medication therapy management, palliative sedation, and transitions of care.
5. Respond to drug information requests from providers, nurses, and administrators pertaining to palliative and supportive care medications.
6. Review all medication profiles of all patients receiving hospice or palliative and supportive care services for undertreated symptoms, untreated symptoms, or unnecessary medication therapy.
7. Oversee medication-use evaluations to optimize safe and effective medication use for patients receiving palliative and supportive care services.
8. Evaluate medical literature for evidence-based treatments.
9. Develop or implement treatment guidelines, protocols, order sets, formulary management or interchanges, relatedness, and algorithms or critical pathways.

10. Provide submission, tracking, and follow-up for Medicare Part D prior authorization for medications used by patients enrolled in the hospice benefit not related to the terminal prognosis.
11. Manage department of pharmacy financials to include expense, revenue, and budget as they pertain to palliative and supportive care services.
12. Develop and manage health-system opioid risk mitigation and monitoring strategies.
13. Participate in committees and task forces including but not limited to pain, palliative and supportive care, sedation, transitions of care, and pertinent pharmacy and therapeutics committee or subcommittees.
14. Provide on-call pharmacy PHC services when appropriate.
15. Serve as department of pharmacy services representative or palliative and supportive care services representative for site surveys or accreditation visits.
16. Compile and manage relevant data to support performance measures as pertains to palliative and supportive care.
17. Oversee quality and performance improvement activities pertaining to palliative and supportive care services.
18. Provide educational programming on palliative and supportive care services to hospice staff, providers, house staff, or department of pharmacy services staff every ____________ months/weeks.
19. Review all submitted research protocols involving patients receiving PHC services.
20. Support adherence and development of policies and procedures that adhere to state and federal regulations including Drug Enforcement Administration, ____________ Board of Pharmacy, Community Health Accreditation Program, and Medicare Conditions of Participation, where applicable.
21. Serve as preceptor for __________ introductory pharmacy practice experience pharmacy students, ___________ advanced pharmacy practice experience pharmacy students, ______________ postgraduate year one pharmacy residents, and ___________ postgraduate year two pharmacy residents.
22. Maintain necessary professional licensure or specialty certification, where appropriate, to maintain the highest level of care to patients of the ________________ health system or hospice.

Appendix C—Sample Collaborative Practice Agreement for a Pharmacist Seeking an Advanced Patient Care Practice in Palliative Care in an Outpatient Setting

I. Scope of Practice

This collaborative practice agreement (CPA) serves as a delegation/authorization of specific roles, functions, and authority by the supervising physician (PHYSICIAN) to the palliative and hospice care pharmacist (PHARMACIST) consistent with the PHARMACIST's education, training, and experience and within the scope of practice of the supervising physician.

Under these guidelines, the PHARMACIST will work with the PHYSICIAN in an active practice to deliver palliative and hospice care (PHC) services provided to patients of ____________________.

The PHARMACIST is authorized to render those services and perform those procedures outlined herein with prescriptive authority for pharmacologic categories identified in CPA attachment A and may utilize prescriptive authority as delegated in CPA attachment B.

The PHARMACIST must inform patients of his or her status and provide the name of the supervising physician. The PHARMACIST may provide service only for those patients of the supervising or alternative physician.

These written guidelines shall be reviewed and updated annually by the PHYSICIAN and PHARMACIST.

A copy of these guidelines along with the PHARMACIST's Drug Enforcement Administration (DEA) number (if applicable) shall remain on file at all sites where the PHARMACIST renders service.

The supervising physician maintains final responsibility for the PHARMACIST's performance and maintains final responsibility for the patient. Services rendered and procedures performed by the PHARMACIST are pursuant to the written guidelines that are specific to the practice setting.

The supervising physician directs and reviews the records and practice of the PHARMACIST in a timely manner to assure appropriate and safe patient care.

WE THE UNDERSIGNED AGREE TO THE TERMS AND CONDITIONS OF THESE WRITTEN GUIDELINES.

____

Supervising Physician Date

____

PHARMACIST Date

II. Functions

The PHARMACIST is authorized to perform services and procedures relative to the pain and symptom management within the scope of this palliative and supportive care practice as part of a multidisciplinary group to include physicians, nurse practitioners, physician assistants, and direct care registered nurses. The active management of patients by the PHARMACIST will be provided based on an established patient medical diagnosis and plan of care and performed under the direction and supervision of the supervising physician and include the following.

III. Patient Care Activities

The PHYSICIAN delegates authority to the PHARMACIST for the following patient care activities:

1. PHARMACIST will conduct complete medical history and medication reconciliation, with emphasis on pharmacotherapy history, symptom assessment, and identification of drug-related problems.
    a. Symptom assessment may include limited physical assessment as well as the order and interpretation of laboratory and diagnostic tests related to drug therapy management in accordance with current evidence-based recommendations.

   b. Administering drugs and biologicals.
   c. Order of routine laboratory tests to ensure safe use of prescribed medications and avoidance of misuse, abuse, or diversion.
   d. Order of 12-lead electrocardiogram in instances of ongoing monitoring of pharmacotherapy, where warranted.
   e. Refer to specialists, when appropriate, based on current evidence-based medicine or standard of care.
   f. Prescriptive authority to include initiation, modification, or discontinuation of the classes and categories of drugs in attachment A for pain or symptoms based on current labeling, accepted medical practice, the disease process and the patient's condition, and, where available, evidence-based treatment guidelines and recommendations.
   g. A pharmacist practicing collaboratively under the Pharmacy Practice Act: *State Pharmacy Law, Number xxxx.xx, xxxx.x,* and the DEA Controlled Substance Act is authorized to order controlled substances to provide patient care.
2. The pharmacist will
   a. Thoroughly assess the patient's response to the prescribed treatment plan with regular assessments and evaluations conducted to include
      i. Severity, duration, and frequency of symptoms
      ii. Therapeutic response
      iii. Adverse drug effects
      iv. Renal and liver function
   b. Patients prescribed scheduled opioids for chronic pain will have an opioid agreement on file.
   c. All prescriptions will be limited to a quantity and for a length of time as are reasonably necessary.
   d. Pharmacist provides education on medications to patient or caregiver and family.

IV. Communication and Documentation

The PHARMACIST shall, within ___ hours of seeing the patient, complete a chart or progress note with a detailed history of present illness, review of systems, physical examination (when warranted), assessment of patient response to treatment plan, and treatment plan going forward. This documentation shall be in the form of a general SOAP note entered into the permanent patient chart or electronic medical record. The referring or supervising PHYSICIAN shall review and provide signature documentation on each patient seen by the pharmacist.

The referring or supervising PHYSICIAN may override any treatment decisions or orders made by the PHARMACIST with communication made back to the PHARMACIST via notation in the patient chart.

V. Quality Assurance and Oversight

Peer and PHYSICIAN oversight review will occur in accordance with applicable state Pharmacy Practice Act rules, and set forth in the Business and Professional Code for the State of_______________________.

VI. Severability

Either party may cancel this agreement via written notification. This collaborative practice agreement is subject to the ongoing licensure, credentialing, and privileging of both the PHARMACIST and PHYSICIAN.

Pharmacist qualifications:

- Active registration to practice in the state of _____________
- DEA license registration
- Successfully completed clinical residency training (see curriculum vitae [CV])
- Demonstrated clinical experience in direct patient care delivery (see CV work history)
- Ongoing continuing education or activities related to the field of practice

VII. Effective Date

This collaborative practice agreement is entered into on the _________day of _________, 20___.

For PHARMACIST:

____

____

Signature Printed Name Date

For PHYSICIAN:

____

____

Signature Printed Name Date

CPA Attachment A

This list of medication classes and categories is not exhaustive yet provides examples of medications managed by the PHC pharmacist for patients seen at the XYZ palliative and supportive care clinic:

1. *Antidepressants,* including selective serotonin reuptake inhibitors, serotonin–norepinephrine reuptake inhibitors, tri- and tetracyclic antidepressants, and atypical antidepressants in the treatment of anorexia, anxiety, depression, insomnia, and pain
2. *Antipsychotics,*' including first-, second-, and third-generation antipsychotics in the treatment of agitation, anxiety, and delirium or other mood disorders
3. *Corticosteroids* (oral and topical) in the treatment of pain, skin lesions, swelling, ulcers, and wounds where appropriate
4. *Anticonvulsants,* including first-, second-, and third-generation anticonvulsants in the treatment of anxiety, depression, pain, and seizures
5. *Nonsteroidal antiinflammatory drugs* in the treatment of inflammation and pain
6. *Serotonin antagonists and phenothiazine derivatives* in the treatment of nausea
7. *Stimulants* in the treatment of depression, fatigue, opioid-associated sedation, and somnolence
8. *Benzodiazepines* in the treatment of anxiety, dyspnea, and pain (abuse potential by patient will be assessed and documented)
9. *Skeletal muscle relaxants* in the treatment of pain (abuse potential by patient will be assessed and documented)

10. *Opioid agonists and antagonists* in the treatment of cough, diarrhea, dyspnea, pruritus, pain, and respiratory depression (abuse potential by patient will be assessed and documented)
11. *Laxatives and stool softeners* in the treatment of constipation and straining
12. *Anticholinergic medications* in the treatment of pain and terminal secretions
13. Other adjuvant analgesics, medications, or therapies not listed above in the treatment of pain, symptoms, and medication-related adverse effects, including compounded preparations

CPA Attachment B

DELEGATION OF PRESCRIPTIVE AUTHORITY

The PHARMACIST may prescribe medications in association with the scope of services described in the written guidelines.

1. ***The PHARMACIST is authorized to write and sign orders for medications in controlled substance Schedules II, III, IV, and V and orders for general prescription medications in association with the scope of services described herein.***

Appendix D—Recommended Journals, Books, and Websites for Professional Development of the Palliative and Hospice Care Pharmacist

Professional Journals

American Journal of Hospice and Palliative Care
Annals of Palliative Medicine
BMC Palliative Care
British Medical Journal Supportive and Palliative Care
Current Opinion in Supportive and Palliative Care
International Journal of Palliative Nursing
Journal of Community and Supportive Oncology
Journal of Geriatrics and Palliative Care
Journal of Hospice and Palliative Nursing
Journal of Pain and Palliative Care Pharmacotherapy
Journal of Pain and Symptom Management
Journal of Palliative Care
Journal of Palliative Care and Medicine
Journal of Palliative Medicine
Journal of Supportive Oncology
Palliative Care
Palliative Medicine
Palliative Medicine and Care
Palliative and Supportive Care
Supportive Care in Cancer

Books

Appleton M. Good end: end-of-life concerns and conversations about hospice and palliative care. Tuscon, AZ: Wheatmark; 2015.

Bourke S, Peel ET, eds. Integrated palliative care of respiratory disease. New York: Springer; 2013.

Bruera E, Higginson I, von Gunten CF, et al, eds. Textbook of palliative medicine and supportive care. 2nd ed. Boca Raton, FL: CRC; 2014.

Emanuel LL, Librach SL, eds. Palliative care: core skills and clinical competencies. 2nd ed. New York: Saunders Elsevier; 2011.

Goldhirsch S, Chai E, Meier D, et al., eds. Geriatric palliative care. New York: Oxford Univ. Press; 2014.

Goldstein NE, Morrison RS, eds. Evidence-based practice of palliative medicine. New York: Saunders Elsevier; 2012.

Hanks G, Cherny NI, Christakis NA, eds. Oxford textbook of palliative medicine. 5th ed. New York: Oxford Univ. Press; 2015.

McPherson ML, ed. Demystifying opioid conversion calculations: a guide for effective dosing. Bethesda, MD: American Society of Health-System Pharmacists; 2009.

Pantilat SZ, Anderson W, Gonzales M, et al., eds. Hospital based palliative medicine: a practical, evidence-based approach. Hoboken, NJ; 2015.

Protus BM, Kimbrel JM, Grauer PA, eds. Palliative care consultant. Montgomery, AL: HospiScript; 2015.

Quill TE, Bower KA, Holloway RG, eds. Primer of palliative care. 6th ed. Glenview, IL: American Academy of Hospice and Palliative Medicine; 2014.

Sackheim KA. Pain management and palliative care: a comprehensive guide. New York: Springer; 2015.

Smith TJ. Geriatric palliative care: clinics in geriatric medicine. New York: Elsevier; 2015.

Strickland JM, ed. Palliative pharmacy care. Bethesda, MD: American Society of Health-System Pharmacists; 2009.

Yennurajalingam S, Bruera E, eds. Oxford American handbook of hospice and palliative medicine. New York: Oxford Univ. Press; 2011.

Websites and Other Resources

American Academy of Hospice and Palliative Medicine
www.aahpm.org

American Society of Health-System Pharmacists. Pain Management and Palliative Care PGY2 Outcomes, Goals, and Objectives. www.ashp.org/menu/Accreditation/ResidencyAccreditation

Center to Advance Palliative Care
www.capc.org

City of Hope Pain and Palliative Care Resource Center
prc.coh.org

Growthhouse.org
www.growthhouse.org

Harvard Medical School Center for Palliative Care
www.hms.harvard.edu/pallcare

International Association for Hospice and Palliative Care
www.hospicecare.com

National Hospice and Palliative Care Organization
www.nhpco.org

National Palliative Care Research Center
www.npcrc.org

Society of Palliative Care Pharmacists
www.palliativepharmacist.org

Curricular Design Resource

Consensus recommendations from the Strategic Planning Summit for Pain and Pallliative Care Pharmacy Practice. *J Pain Symptom Manage.* 2012; 43:925–44.

Approved by the ASHP Board of Directors on March 15, 2016. Developed through the ASHP Section of Ambulatory Care Pharmacists.

ASHP gratefully acknowledges the following organizations and individuals for reviewing these guidelines (review does not imply endorsement): American College of Clinical Pharmacy Pain and Palliative Care Practice Resource Network; American Pharmacists Association; New Hampshire Society of Hospital Pharmacists; Melhim Bou Alwan, M.D.; Cynthia Brucato, Pharm.D., BCACP; Mitchell Buckley, Pharm.D., FASHP, FCCP, SCCM, BCPS; Trinh T. Bui, Pharm.D.; Nina M. Cimino, Pharm.D., CPE; Steven J. Crosby, M.A., FASCP; Emily Davies, Pharm.D., CPE; Sandra DiScala, Pharm.D., BCPS; Steven Dzierba, Pharm.D., M.S., BCPS, FASHP; Abimbola Farinde, Ph.D., Pharm.D; Lauren Gashlin, Pharm.D., Jessica Erin Geiger-Hayes, Pharm.D., BCPS; Michael A. Gillette, Pharm.D., BCPS (AQ–Cardiology), BCACP; Kerry Goldrosen, Pharm.D.; Timothy J. Ives, Pharm.D., M.P.H., FCCP, FASHP, CPP; Donna Jolly, Pharm.D., BCPS; Katherine Juba, Pharm.D., BCPS; Syeda Saba A. Kareem, Pharm.D., BCOP; Allison R. King, Pharm.D.; Justin Kullgren, Pharm.D., CPE; Eric C. Kutscher, Pharm.D., BCPP, FASHP; Maritza Lew, Pharm.D., PMP; Matthew Malone, D.O.; Fred Meister, Pharm.D.; James Ponto, M.S., BCNP; Jennifer Pruskowski, Pharm.D., BCPS, CGP; Curt W. Quap, M.S. Pharm., FASHP; James R. Rinehart, M.S., FASHP; Eve M. Segal, Pharm.D.; Victoria Snyder; Dennis A. Tribble, Pharm.D., FASHP; Rebecca Wagner, Pharm.D.; Jody Jacobson Wedret, FASHP, FCSHP; Ricke J. Weickum, Pharm.D., BCOP; Traci White, Pharm.D., PhC; and Amanda R. McFee Winans, Pharm.D., BCPS. The contributions of Justine Coffey, J.D., L.L.M., to this document are gratefully acknowledged.

The authors have declared no potential conflicts of interest.

Christopher M. Herndon, Pharm.D., BCPS, CPE, FASHP, School of Pharmacy, Southern Illinois University Edwardsville, Edwardsville, IL.

Douglas Nee, Pharm.D., M.S., Hospice and Palliative Care, OptiMed, San Diego, CA.

Rabia S. Atayee, Pharm.D., BCPS, Pain and Palliative Care Service, University of California, San Diego, Skaggs School of Pharmacy and Pharmaceutical Sciences, La Jolla, CA.

David S. Craig, Pharm.D., Department of Pharmacy, H. Lee Moffitt Cancer Center & Research Institute, Tampa, FL.

Julie Lehn, Pharm.D., Palliative Medicine, Banner University Medical Center, Phoenix, AZ.

Pamela S. Moore, Pharm.D., BCPS, CPE, Pain and Palliative Care, Summa Health System, Akron, OH.

Suzanne Amato Nesbit, Pharm.D., BCPS, CPE, Department of Oncology, Center for Drug Safety and Effectiveness, Department of Pharmacy, Johns Hopkins Hospital, Baltimore, MD.

James B. Ray, Pharm.D., CPE, James A. Otterbeck OnePoint Patient Care, Department of Pharmacy Practice, University of Iowa College of Pharmacy, Iowa City, IA.

Bridget Fowler Scullion, Pharm.D., BCOP, Palliative Care, Dana-Farber Cancer Institute, Boston, MA.

Robert G. Wahler Jr., Pharm.D., CPE, School of Pharmacy and Pharmaceutical Sciences, University at Buffalo, The State University of New York, Buffalo, NY.

Julie Waldfogel, Pharm.D., CPE, Pain and Palliative Care, Department of Pharmacy, Johns Hopkins Hospital, Baltimore, MD.

Copyright © 2016, American Society of Health-System Pharmacists, Inc. All rights reserved. Contact ASHP for reprint and permissions requests. This content may not be used for commercial purposes without the express written consent of ASHP.

The bibliographic citation for this document is as follows: American Society of Health-System Pharmacists. ASHP guidelines on the pharmacist's role in palliative and hospice care. *Am J Health-Syst Pharm.* 2016; 73:1351–67.

ASHP Guidelines on the Pharmacist's Role in Providing Drug Information

Background and Rationale

The provision of drug information (DI) is among the fundamental professional responsibilities of all pharmacists. Recent practice trends, including increased provision of medication therapy management services and efforts to obtain provider status, have placed pharmacists in increasingly complex patient-care roles and necessitated a higher level of competence by all pharmacists in meeting DI needs. Drug information may be patient specific, academic (for educational purposes), or population based (to aid in the decision-making process for evaluating medication use for groups of patients). The goal of providing carefully evaluated, evidence-based recommendations to support specific medication-use practices is to enhance the quality of patient care, improve patient outcomes, and ensure the prudent use of resources. The primary focus of these guidelines is to describe contemporary DI activities, including the application of a systematic approach, appropriate documentation methods, and use of high-quality DI resources. This information is intended to assist pharmacists in providing optimal DI services in a variety of practice settings, including hospitals and health systems, outpatient care centers, managed care environments, medical communication departments, and university or academic-based drug information centers. Some of the activities described in these guidelines are the subjects of other American Society of Health-System Pharmacists (ASHP) policy and guidance documents, which should be referred to for additional information. Pharmacists providing DI should use professional judgment in assessing ASHP's policy and guidance documents and in adapting them to meet their health care organizations' and patients' needs and circumstances.

Drug Information Activities

To be an effective provider of DI, the pharmacist must exercise excellent oral and written communication skills and be able to

1. Anticipate and evaluate the DI needs of patients and health care professionals.
2. Obtain appropriate and complete background information as described under the section Systematic Approach for Responding to Drug Information Requests.
3. Use a systematic approach to address DI needs by effectively searching, retrieving, and critically evaluating the literature (i.e., assessment of study design, statistics, bias, limitations, applicability).
4. Appropriately synthesize, communicate, document, and apply pertinent information to the patient care situation.[1,2]

A variety of DI activities may be performed by pharmacists, depending on the particular practice setting and need. Every pharmacist should have the skills to perform the following DI activities[2,3]:

1. Providing DI to patients, caregivers, and health care professionals.
2. Creating and maintaining currency of a variety of print and online educational resources for patients (e.g., tip sheets, pamphlets) and health care professionals (e.g., in-service documents, newsletters) on topics such as optimal medication use, general health, or select clinical questions.
3. Educating health care professionals on safe and effective medication-use policies and processes, including development of resources to communicate this information.
4. Leading or participating in continuing education services for health care professionals.
5. Precepting and educating pharmacy students and residents.
6. Participating in quality improvement research projects and drug cost analyses.
7. Contributing to the biomedical literature and providing peer review for other contributors.

Some activities may be more appropriate for pharmacists with additional expertise and training in DI, such as those who have completed a postgraduate year two (PGY2) drug information residency. Drug information specialists often perform DI activities that overlap with other pharmacists and health care professionals. However, as a result of their advanced training and experience, DI specialists may be able to more efficiently retrieve, evaluate, and disseminate information in order to develop evidence-based recommendations and assist in patient care decisions.[2] Many DI specialists are also involved in medication-safety activities and collaborate with experts in informatics. These activities are highlighted in other ASHP statements.[4,5] Specific activities of the DI specialist may include some or all of the following[2,6–11]:

1. Providing information when there is not sufficient time for other health care professionals to appropriately research the DI question, when there is a knowledge gap, or when the question requires more thorough research.
2. Establishing and maintaining a formulary based on scientific evidence of efficacy and safety, pharmacoeconomics, and institution-specific factors.
3. Coordinating programs to support population-based medication practices that maximize patient outcomes (e.g., development of pharmacotherapeutic guidelines, medication-use evaluation criteria, and therapeutic interchange protocols).
4. Developing and participating in efforts to prevent medication errors and adverse drug events, including surveillance, ensuring institutional compliance to Risk Evaluation and Mitigation Strategies (REMS),

DOI 10.37573/9781585287048.079

and leading reporting and analysis programs (e.g., MedWatch).

5. Monitoring and assessing the clinical significance of medication safety alerts communicated by the FDA, drug manufacturers, and other sources.
6. Performing health outcome and comparative effectiveness analyses.
7. Coordinating investigational drug services, including participating on institutional review boards (IRBs), evaluating protocols, and providing DI to patients, caregivers, and health care professionals.
8. Managing drug shortages, including identifying alternative treatments, developing protocols for restrictive use, and addressing formulary concerns.
9. Developing clinical decision support tools such as order sets, dosing protocols, and order-entry alerts.
10. Maintaining DI and medication-use policy-related intranet resources.
11. Precepting or providing advanced DI education and training to interprofessional and pharmacy students and residents.
12. Coordinating selection and purchase of pharmacy and institution-wide DI resources.
13. Participating in various fee-for-service projects (e.g., formulary support, database development, training programs) for clients.
14. Planning and delivering academic detailing programs.

Although the above activities may be best suited for pharmacists with advanced DI training, many institutions lack a formal DI specialist. Therefore, other pharmacists may be involved in more in-depth DI activities, depending on their level of expertise. For example, preparing drug monographs for pharmacy and therapeutics committees was once considered almost exclusively the responsibility of the DI specialist. As pharmacy practice has evolved, the expertise and knowledge of all pharmacy practitioners have been integrated into this process.

Today, depending on the institution, pharmacists without specialized DI training may prepare monographs, assist in the design of medication-use evaluation criteria, participate in medication monitoring activities, or educate health care professionals on appropriate medication use. If available, a DI specialist may serve in an oversight role by editing and providing feedback on these projects or providing general DI support to pharmacists involved in direct patient care. Moreover, a DI specialist may be involved in implementation and follow-up of medication-use policies and formulary changes as part of a larger medication policy management program, which may include interpreting the impact of legislation, regulation, and public policy on medication utilization.

Systematic Approach for Responding to Drug Information Requests

A systematic approach for responding to DI requests was first introduced by Watanabe, et al. in 1975.[12] This approach has been modified and expanded over the years to ensure that all relevant information is considered prior to formulating a response.[1,13] The importance of gathering pertinent patient data and understanding the context of a question prior to answering a DI request is described in the literature.[14–16] Of note, a full systematic approach may not be practical for all requests, especially for urgent clinical needs in the direct patient care setting. In addition, consideration should be given to the ethical and legal aspects of responding to DI requests, including patient privacy concerns.[1]

A systematic approach may be outlined as follows.[1,13]

1. *Identify the requestor.* In order to obtain complete information and develop a response with the appropriate perspective, consider the health literacy and professional background of the requestor.
2. *Define the true question and information need.* Identify the true question and information needed by asking probing questions of the requestor. For example, "Why is the question being asked?" and "Does the question pertain to a specific patient?" may help reveal important details of the true question.[1] This kind of information helps in optimizing the search process and assessing the appropriate time frame of response need.
3. *Obtain complete background information.* Obtain more complete background information, including examining the medical record for patient data, if applicable, to individualize the response to meet the requestor's need.
4. *Categorize the question.* Classify requests as patient-specific or academic and by type of question (e.g., product availability, adverse drug event, compatibility, compounding/formulation, dosage/administration, drug interaction [drug-drug, drug-disease, drug-laboratory], drug product identification, pharmacokinetics, therapeutic use/efficacy [FDA approved vs. unlabeled indications], safety in pregnancy/nursing toxicity/poisoning) to aid in tailoring the search strategy and selecting resources.
5. *Perform a systematic search.* Perform a systematic search of appropriate tertiary, secondary, and primary resources, including electronic resources, as necessary.
6. *Analyze the information.* Evaluate, interpret, and combine information from the resources used. Other information needs should be anticipated as a result of the information gathered.
7. *Disseminate the information.* Provide an oral or written response, or both, as needed by the requestor that specifically applies the information to the particular situation. The information, its urgency, and its purpose may influence the method of response. Supporting documentation (e.g., primary literature) should be included when possible.
8. *Document.* Document the request, information resources used, the information found in each source, time spent on the response, and the response itself as appropriate for the request and the practice setting.
9. *Follow-up.* Perform a follow-up assessment to determine the utility of the information provided and whether the information resulted in changes in medication-use practices or patient outcomes.

Documentation and Quality Assessment

Numerous methods of documenting pharmacist interventions, including the provision of DI, have been described in the literature. Drug information centers are moving toward increased use of electronic documentation systems, which have helped to increase the depth and quantity of documentation, as well as provide increased efficiency and cost savings.[17-21] In addition, an electronic system can promote a standardized and systematic approach and provides a readily retrievable archive that can be used to rapidly search previously answered questions.[22,23] Documentation of DI services should incorporate elements identified through the systematic approach. The ASHP Guidelines on Documenting Pharmaceutical Care in Patient Medical Records states that "the professional actions of pharmacists that are intended to ensure safe and effective use of drugs and that may affect patient outcomes should be documented in the patient medical record."[24] Therefore, if the DI request is patient-specific, it is appropriate, but not always necessary, to document the request and response in the patient's medical record. Documentation is critical to appropriate patient care, highlights the value of pharmacist services, demonstrates accountability, provides a basis for quality assessment and performance improvement, and details an appropriate systematic approach in case a medico-legal dispute arises from a DI request. Consequently, even academic or population-based DI activities should be appropriately documented. Despite the importance of assessing the quality of drug-related information provided by pharmacists, there is currently no standardized method described in the literature. However, some DI centers have reported use of double-check systems prior to providing a response, random retrospective audits by a DI specialist or another individual, obtaining feedback from the requestor, and conducting an internal review by a committee as methods of quality assessment.[25]

Resources

It is important for pharmacists to use appropriate and credible resources. The amount of medical knowledge has grown substantially and access to information has changed dramatically over the last few decades. Traditional print resources are rapidly being replaced by electronic databases (both online and included in health information management systems), online resources, and mobile applications.[26] The internet and mobile technology have allowed for convenient and quick access to medical information. However, pharmacists should critically evaluate all resources prior to use to ensure that they are accurate, current, and unbiased.

General principles to consider when critically evaluating medical information available on the internet have been published.[27] Pharmacists should work closely with others within the organization to ensure that up-to-date resources, including representative primary (e.g., peer-reviewed original studies), secondary (e.g., indexing or abstracting services such as MEDLINE and International Pharmaceutical Abstracts), and tertiary resources (e.g., electronic databases, textbooks, review articles, clinical practice guidelines) are available to assist in answering a variety of DI requests. Pharmacists should be familiar with the features of each resource; familiarity makes searching more efficient so that more time can be devoted to analyzing, applying, and communicating the information.

The following factors should be considered when purchasing DI resources, including electronic subscriptions, for the pharmacy department or practice setting:

1. Features of the resource (e.g., frequency of updates, qualifications and affiliations of authors, year of publication, type of information, organization of material, method of delivery, cost).
2. Practice setting (e.g., type of facility and needs of health care professionals within that environment, state-specific regulatory requirements).
3. Accessibility of the resource (e.g., location of print resources, number of users allowed by subscription).

Keeping Current

Pharmacists are challenged with keeping up to date with an increasing number of new drugs and literature.[3] Drug information and literature evaluation skills are crucial for building clinical knowledge and providing evidence-based recommendations. It is the responsibility of the pharmacist to commit to lifelong learning and make an effort to keep abreast of advances both in the methods of delivering DI and the information itself. In addition to keeping up to date with clinical knowledge, it is important for pharmacists to keep current on changes in pharmacy practice as the health care system evolves. Recommendations for staying current include the following:

1. Subscribe to table of contents of or full access to relevant journals, as appropriate.
2. Subscribe to appropriate email listservers (e.g., Food and Drug Administration Drug Information Updates, National Guideline Clearinghouse, Centers for Disease Control and Prevention, Medline Plus).
3. Receive email alerts from relevant health-related websites (e.g., MedWatch, Medline Plus).
4. Bookmark important websites and check regularly for updates (e.g., Institute for Safe Medication Practices, ASHP Drug Shortages Resource Center).
5. Choose pertinent continuing education activities and methods that challenge learning.
6. Maintain active membership in local, state, and national pharmacy associations/societies.
7. Pursue board certification from the Board of Pharmacy Specialties.

Conclusion

All pharmacists are involved in the provision of DI, which includes a broad array of activities. A systematic approach should be considered for all DI requests, and pharmacists should document their services to demonstrate accountability and justify the value of pharmacist care. Increased availability of medical information, both due to increased knowledge and technological advances, has not changed the overall process of DI practice. It is important for pharmacists to select appropriate resources and keep current on new literature and new tools to address a variety of DI requests.

References

1. Malone PM, Kier KL, Stanovich JE. Drug information: a guide for pharmacists, 4th ed. New York: McGraw-Hill; 2012.
2. Bernknopf AC, Karpinski JP, McKeever AL, et al. Drug information: from education to practice. *Pharmacotherapy*. 2009; 29:331–46.
3. Wang F, Troutman WG, Seo T, et al. Drug information education in doctor of pharmacy programs. *Am J Pharm Educ*. 2006; 70(3):51.

4. American Society of Health-System Pharmacists. ASHP statement on the role of the medication safety leader. *Am J Health-Syst Pharm.* 2013; 70:448–52.
5. American Society of Health-System Pharmacists. ASHP statement on the pharmacist's role in informatics. *Am J Health-Syst Pharm.* 2007; 64:200–3.
6. American Society of Health-System Pharmacists. ASHP accreditation standards for postgraduate year one (PGY1) pharmacy residency programs. **http://www.ashp.org/DocLibrary/Accreditation/ASD-PGY1-Standard.aspx** (accessed 2013 May 9).
7. American Society of Health-System Pharmacists. ASHP accreditation standards for postgraduate year two (PGY2) pharmacy residency programs. **http://www.ashp.org/DocLibrary/Accreditation/ASD-PGY2-Standard.aspx** (accessed 2013 May 9).
8. Rosenberg JM, Schilit S, Nathan JP, et al. Update on the status of 89 drug information centers in the United States. *Am J Health-Syst Pharm.* 2009; 66:1718–22.
9. Powell L, Pepper M. Reviewing the pharmacy department's drug information activities. *Am J Health-Syst Pharm.* 2000; 57:2260–1.
10. American Society of Health-System Pharmacists. ASHP guidelines on managing drug product shortages in hospitals and health systems. *Am J Health-Syst Pharm.* 2009; 66:1399–1406.
11. Wisniewski CS, Robert S, Ball S. Collaboration between a drug information center and an academic detailing program. *Am J Health-Syst Pharm.* 2014; 71:128–33.
12. Watanabe AS, McCart G, Shimomura S, et al. Systematic approach to drug information requests. *Am J Hosp Pharm.* 1975; 32:1282–5.
13. Nathan JP. Drug information—the systematic approach: continuing education article. *J Pharm Pract.* 2013; 26:78–84.
14. Calis KA, Anderson DW, Auth DA, et al. Quality of pharmacotherapy consultations provided by drug information centers in the United States. *Pharmacotherapy.* 2000; 20:830–6.
15. Beaird SL, Coley RM, Blunt JR. Assessing the accuracy of drug information responses from drug information centers. *Ann Pharmacother.* 1994; 28:707–11.
16. Halbert MR, Kelly WN, Miller DE. Drug information centers: lack of generic equivalence. *Drug Intell Clin Pharm.* 1977; 11:728–35.
17. Wisniewski CS, Pummer TL, Krenzelok EP. Documenting drug information questions using software for poison information documentation. *Am J Health-Syst Pharm.* 2009; 66:1039–43.
18. Simonian AI. Documenting pharmacist interventions on an intranet. *Am J Health-Syst Pharm.* 2003; 60:151–5.
19. Nurgat ZA, Al-Jazairi AS, Abu-Shraie N, et al. Documenting clinical pharmacist intervention before and after the introduction of a web-based tool. *Int J Clin Pharm.* 2011; 33:200–7.
20. Abe AM. Implementation of a cloud computing system for documenting drug information consultation requests and responses. Poster presented at: ASHP Midyear Clinical Meeting; December 2012; Las Vegas, NV.
21. Brown JN. Cost savings associated with a dedicated drug information service in an academic medical center. *Hosp Pharm.* 2011; 46:680–4.
22. Erbele SM, Heck AM, Blankenship CS. Survey of computerized documentation system use in drug information centers. *Am J Health-Syst Pharm.* 2001; 58:695–7.
23. Cheng SC. Computerized tools that standardize the systematic approach to researching drug information requests. Poster presented at: ASHP Midyear Clinical Meeting; December 2006; Anaheim, CA.
24. American Society of Health-System Pharmacists. ASHP guidelines on documenting pharmaceutical care in patient medical records. *Am J Health-Syst Pharm.* 2003; 60:705–7.
25. Rosenberg JM, Koumis T, Nathan JP, et al. Current status of pharmacist-operated drug information centers in the United States. *Am J Health-Syst Pharm.* 2004; 61:2023–32.
26. Fass JA, Carvajal M, Polen H, et al. Knowledge, use, and decision-making considerations for drug information resources in community and hospital pharmacies. Poster presented at: ASHP Midyear Clinical Meeting; December 2012; Las Vegas, NV.
27. Grossman S, Zerilli T. Health and medication information resources on the World Wide Web. *J Pharm Pract.* 2013; 26:85–94.

Developed through the ASHP Council on Therapeutics and approved by the ASHP Board of Directors on April 10, 2014. These guidelines supersede the ASHP Guidelines on the Provision of Medication Information by Pharmacists dated April 24, 1996.

Shadi Ghaibi, Pharm.D., BCPS, is Pharmacist, Drug Information and Medication Safety, Intermountain Medical Center, Murray, UT. Heather Ipema, Pharm.D., BCPS, is Clinical Assistant Professor; and Michael Gabay, Pharm.D., J.D., BCPS, is Clinical Associate Professor, Pharmacy Practice, University of Illinois at Chicago, Chicago.

ASHP gratefully acknowledges contributions made to these guidelines by the following individuals: Karim Calis, Pharm.D., M.P.H., FASHP, FCCP; Erin Fox, Pharm.D.; Randy Hatton, Pharm.D., BCPS, FCCP; Corinne Johnson, Pharm.D., M.B.A.; Joe Jordan, Pharm.D.; Mandy Leonard, Pharm.D., BCPS; Michelle W. McCarthy, Pharm.D., FASHP; Genevieve Ness, Pharm.D.; Jennifer Riggins, Pharm.D.; Ryan Rodriguez, Pharm.D., BCPS; and Sheri VanOsdol, Pharm.D., BCPS.

ASHP also gratefully acknowledges the following organizations and individuals for reviewing these guidelines (review does not imply endorsement): American Pharmacists Association (APhA); Institute for Safe Medication Practices (ISMP); Joseph Aloi, Pharm.D., BCPS; Jason Babby, Pharm.D., BCPS; Linda Banares, Pharm.D., BCACP; Sara J. Beis, M.S., FASHP; John D. Bowman, B.S.Pharm., M.S., BCPS, FASHP; Susan Teil Boyer, M.S., FASHP; Jamie N. Brown, Pharm.D., BCPS; William Budris, B.S.Pharm.; Juan Hincapie Castillo, Pharm.D.; Erin S. Christensen, Pharm.D., BCPS; Jason C. Cooper, Pharm.D.; Michelle C. Corrado, Pharm.D., M.H.A.; Paul Driver, Pharm.D., BCPS, FASHP; Steven Dzierba, Pharm.D., M.S., FASHP; Lauren Ellison, Pharm.D.; Margo Farber, Pharm.D.; Leah Frantzen, Pharm.D., BCPS; Kelli Garrison, Pharm.D., BCPS; Kelly N. Glover, Pharm.D.; Conor Hanrahan, Pharm.D., BCPS; Joe Jordan, Pharm.D., BCPS; Julie P. Karpinski, Pharm.D., BCPS; Tim

Lanese, M.B.A.; Ashley Lewis, Pharm.D.; Gregory Light, Pharm.D. (candidate); Jim Lile, Pharm.D., FMPA, FASHP; Patrick M. Malone, Pharm.D., FASHP; Jeannell Mansur, Pharm.D., FASHP, FSMSO; Shannon Manzi, Pharm.D., NREMT; Linda Gore Martin, Pharm.D., M.B.A., BCPS; Theresa Mays, B.S., Pharm.D., BCOP, FASHP; Leslie McCament-Mann, Ph.D.; John F. Mitchell, Pharm.D., FASHP; Ruth W. Ndungi, Pharm.D.; Genevieve Ness, Pharm.D.; James A. Owen, Pharm.D., BCPS (APhA); Frank P. Paloucek, Pharm.D., DABAT, FASHP; Fred J. Pane, B.S.Pharm., FASHP; Lois F. Parker, B.S.; Peter Pascale, M.S.; Stephanie C. Peshek, Pharm.D., M.B.A., M.S.Ed., FASHP; James Ponto, M.S., BCNP, FASHP; William H. Puckett, M.S., M.B.A., FASHP; Curt W. Quap, M.S., FASHP; Dan Rackham, Pharm.D., BCPS; James R. Rinehart, M.S., FASHP; Martha M. Rumore, M.S., Pharm.D, J.D., FAPhA; Sam Shimomura, Pharm.D., CGP, FASHP; Sarah J. Steinhardt, Pharm.D., J.D., M.S.; Allen J. Vaida, Pharm.D., FASHP (ISMP); Kristina Ward, Pharm.D., BCPS; Jody Jacobson Wedret, FASHP, FCSHP; Tom Westerkamp, M.S.; Phipson Wu, Pharm.D., BCPS; and Kristi Yamasaki, Pharm.D.

The authors have declared no potential conflicts of interest.

Copyright © 2015, American Society of Health-System Pharmacists, Inc. All rights reserved. Contact ASHP for reprint and permissions requests. This content may not be used for commercial purposes without the express written consent of ASHP.

The bibliographic citation for this document is as follows: Ghaibi S., Ipema H., Gabay M. ASHP guidelines on the pharmacist's role in providing drug information. *Am J Health-Syst Pharm.* 2015; 72:573–7.

ASHP Guidelines on Pharmacy Services in Solid Organ Transplantation

Evidence of pharmacists' contributions to the care of organ transplant recipients has existed since the 1970s. Since then, literature describing pharmacist's impact on clinical and pharmacoeconomic outcomes has grown exponentially,[1–14] with pharmacists establishing themselves as integral members of the transplantation community and expanding their presence in multiple areas, including pharmaceutical industry, research, academia, quality improvement, and clinical settings.[15–20] Transplant pharmacists (sometimes referred to as *clinical transplant pharmacists* or *solid organ transplantation pharmacists*) have a strong presence in the areas of pharmacogenomics, innovative collaborative drug therapy management (CDTM), and prospective practice management.

The United Network for Organ Sharing (UNOS) and the Centers for Medicare & Medicaid Services (CMS), respectively, require transplantation centers document the participation of a clinical transplant pharmacist or pharmacology expert on multidisciplinary transplantation teams in order to meet accreditation standards. These regulations make transplant pharmacy the only pharmacist specialty practice in the United States to have such a requirement.[21–24] These mandates outline the responsibilities of the transplant pharmacist in preoperative and postoperative pharmaceutical management and education of transplant recipients. In response to the demand for pharmacists to meet these accreditation standards, some transplantation programs may meet the need by utilizing pharmacists without specific transplantation training or experience due to lack of fully trained personnel or funding resources.

As of 2016, there were over 30,000 solid organ transplantations performed annually in the United States, and over 500,000 have been performed since the year 2000.[25] Despite the volume of transplantations per year, there was a median of 1.4 transplant pharmacist full-time equivalents (FTE) per 100 transplantations performed, according to a national workforce survey conducted by the American Society of Transplantation across accredited U.S. transplantation programs.[26] The median number of FTE did not increase beyond 1.4 FTE even in programs with >400 transplantations per year. These data indicate that transplant pharmacy services are provided by nonspecialists in many of these programs. Currently, there is no standard of practice for the provision of transplant pharmacy services, as the CMS Conditions of Participation allow for a broad interpretation for how to best meet the needs for each patient.[27] This broad interpretation allows for a wide spectrum of transplant pharmacy services, with some centers providing a more inclusive model than others. This variability has led to recent CMS citations during program-specific surveys when the pharmacists involved in the care of transplant patients and donors were unable to provide sufficient evidence of qualifications, training, and expertise in transplantation.

Purpose

In 2011, the American Society of Transplantation (AST), Transplant Pharmacy Community of Practice, in collaboration with the American College of Clinical Pharmacy (ACCP) Immunology/Transplantation Practice and Research Network, developed a white paper that provided a blueprint for the training and qualifications of pharmacists working in transplant patient care and detailed the contributions of pharmacists serving the transplantation population.[21] These guidelines augment the previously published work by promoting understanding of the evolving role of pharmacists' contribution to the care of transplant recipients and living donors, helping define the role of the transplant pharmacist, suggesting goals for providing services to meet institution-specific needs, and describing best practices for transplant pharmacy services. These guidelines were developed based on primary literature, expert consensus on best practices, and CMS and Organ Procurement and Transplant Network (OPTN) bylaws, and are meant to aid transplant pharmacists, administrators, physicians, surgeons, allied health professionals (e.g., nurses, dietitians, financial coordinators, business managers), accreditors, surveyors, and others with a need to understand transplant pharmacy services.

Although the nature of these services are unique to each solid organ and with each institution's protocols and resources, these guidelines describe both transplant pharmacist services that meet the minimum required by regulations (as of publication) as well as optimal services. In conjunction with pharmacy, transplant surgery, and medicine administrators, each transplant pharmacist should use his or her professional judgment to individually weigh the factors that determine which services should be provided. These factors include the patient populations served, the number of pharmacists and time dedicated to services provided to the care of transplant patients, whether corresponding duties are required of transplant pharmacists in other areas of the hospital, and the extent of time dedicated to administrative, research, and quality endeavors. Finally, it should be noted that the many responsibilities described in these guidelines could not be provided by a single pharmacist. When used in these guidelines, the term *transplant pharmacist* should not be interpreted to imply that a single pharmacist could or should be expected to provide every service described.

Pharmacy Services in the Pretransplantation Phase

The pretransplantation phase includes all activities related to the assessment and evaluation of a donor or candidate's readiness for transplantation and the execution of any plans to increase a donor or candidate's success. This includes the initial assessment and any re-evaluation that may occur during the waiting list period, as described in **Appendix A.**

Pharmacologic Evaluation. At a minimum, a transplant pharmacist should be present during the multidisciplinary patient selection committee meeting. Transplant pharmacists are expected to present an objective assessment of the candidate's pharmacologic and nonpharmacologic risks pertaining to transplantation.[28,29] Although each assessment should be tailored to the individual patient, an assessment

DOI 10.37573/9781585287048.080

of anticoagulation, drug interactions, medications related to mental health, medications for chronic pain, medication allergies, hormonal contraception and replacement therapy, current use of immunosuppressants or immunomodulators, issues with drug absorption, illicit substance use or abuse, and use of herbal supplements or nutraceuticals should be completed. Although not universal, an assessment of immunologic risk as it pertains to induction therapy selection and need for desensitizing therapies during the selection meeting provides an opportunity to discuss protocol versus off-protocol decisions and may expedite the perioperative immunosuppressant selection process. The impact of current pharmacologic therapies on pretransplantation testing (i.e., false-positive drug screens, timing of vaccinations in relation to antibody titers) and peri- and post-transplantation risks should be discussed at this time.

Nonpharmacologic Evaluation. In addition, an assessment of nonpharmacologic risks and socially related risks should be presented, in conjunction with members of the multidisciplinary team, including transplant social workers and financial coordinators.[28,29] Transplant pharmacists are well-suited to identify gaps in health literacy, markers of medication nonadherence, and preexisting intolerances and adverse effects to pharmacotherapy that may affect post-transplantation immunosuppressant adherence. Along with financial coordinators, pharmacy technicians and community/specialty pharmacy partners, transplant pharmacists should be involved in conversations regarding pharmacy benefit and out-of-pocket medication costs and proactively understand the specific distribution requirements of each patient's pharmacy benefit manager.

Mitigation Plan. Along with the initial assessment, a thorough mitigation plan, when warranted, should be presented, along with any risks identified. Risks may be identified in one of two ways. The first is a basic chart review, which includes assessing the demographics of the patient (age, race, height, weight, body surface area, body mass index, distance from transplantation program, type of insurance), basic vitals, a complete medication list (including nonprescription medications, dietary supplements, and herbal remedies) and immunologic history (cause of end-stage organ disease, calculated panel reactive antibody, unacceptable antigens, deceased versus live-donor transplant). This type of review is limited in the breadth of information available and in its dependence on the accuracy of information provided. A more comprehensive face-to-face assessment includes the elements of the basic chart review and may include a health literacy assessment, an interview to elucidate barriers to adherence, accuracy of the medication history, and provision of initial medication education. Documentation of transplant pharmacy services in the pretransplantation setting must meet the regulatory requirements for individual centers based on policies developed in accordance with CMS Conditions of Participation and UNOS policy.

Pharmacy Services in the Perioperative Patient

Pharmacist involvement in the care of a patient receiving a transplant is intended to facilitate transition from the pretransplantation phase through inpatient discharge from the transplantation encounter. Transplant pharmacists work with healthcare professionals in all settings of care to ensure a seamless medication-use process, provision of transplantation medication education, and discharge planning through each transition of care.[21,22]

Direct Patient Care of the Transplant Recipient. Transplant pharmacists are charged with providing comprehensive pharmacy services to transplant recipients during the peritransplantation hospitalization.[1,2,27,29] Activities routinely performed as part of this suite of services are outlined in Appendix A. In 2015, the transplant pharmacist workforce was surveyed to enumerate several data points, including perioperative pharmacy services performed.[26] Notably, the vast majority of the surveyed pharmacists routinely performed medication and laboratory review, recommended changes to both transplantation-related and unrelated medications, performed bedside rounding as part of the multidisciplinary team, and provided medication education to the transplant recipient. As part of comprehensive pharmacy services, the transplant pharmacist serves as the medication expert, provides drug information to all members of the team (including information regarding drug-drug interactions), and participates in collaborative decision-making, especially at the bedside, for the transplant recipient.

Certain medications used for induction and maintenance therapy as well as in the treatment for rejection warrant restrictions on use per center-specific policy. The role of the transplant pharmacist may focus on the recommendation and approval of high-risk medications, such as mono- and polyclonal antibodies, intravenous immune globulin, and certain formulations of immunomodulators (e.g., intravenous calcineurin inhibitors) to ensure appropriate use, patient safety, and cost containment. Having a bedside presence facilitates the determination of optimal therapy, selection, and dosing recommendations in a timely manner. To facilitate the bedside presence, it is recommended that designated transplant pharmacists be provided handheld technology or portable computers. Other factors to consider include the integration of the transplant pharmacist's clinical duties into hospital information systems (e.g., computerized provider order entry systems) as well as the workflow and communication with decentralized, floor-, or unit-based pharmacists.

Direct Patient Care of the Living Donor. The proportion of living related and unrelated directed donation of kidney and liver allografts is increasing.[3,4] Many factors contribute to this trend, most notably, kidney paired and chain donation and the increasing success of living-donor liver transplantation. The transplant pharmacist is responsible for providing comprehensive pharmacy services to the living donor as well as the transplant recipient.[1,2,30] These services include pain management, bowel care, fluid and electrolyte management, and education on aftercare regimens. Moreover, the expertise of the transplant pharmacist is needed to modify existing medication regimens to minimize the risk to the retained kidney or liver lobe to ensure its long-term health and viability.[5,6]

Multidisciplinary Team Participation. Transplant pharmacists are required members of the multidisciplinary transplant team.[1,2,21–24,26,27,29,30] Transplant pharmacists provide valuable services to the team, as described in Appendix A. Fruitful collaboration with all members of the team should be undertaken by the transplant pharmacist. In addition to active participation in preoperative evaluation and as a member of the patient selection committee, the transplant pharmacist works closely with their primary surgical and medical colleagues as well as with consultants in the perioperative period to contribute to medical decision-making as described previously. Further collaboration with the transplantation coordinator, social worker, financial coordinator, and others should be undertaken to enhance medication access to confirm and expand on work done during the pre-transplantation phase. When appropriate, additional collaboration on scientific research with members of the team can help provide high-risk patients with novel approaches to pharmacotherapy.

Medication Access and Planning. As described by Spivey and colleagues, access to pharmacotherapy is strongly correlated with adherence behaviors, which is closely tied to allograft survival.[31] Moreover, decisions regarding medication coverage by CMS in the United States rely nearly exclusively on the Food and Drug Administration (FDA) labeled indications. Labeled indications are most common for immunomodulating agents in kidney transplantation and are absent in lung transplantation. Thus, access to critical medications for allograft and patient survival vary by organ.[32] The transplant pharmacist engages with transplant coordinators, social workers, finance coordinators, and physicians to advocate for and garner access to such critical medications through multiple avenues. Strategies to ensure access include federal and private insurance coverage, pharmaceutical manufacturer access programs, foundation grants, local government support, and others and should be undertaken by members of the transplant team in consultation with a transplant pharmacist. Importantly, transplant pharmacists can provide critical information to enhance the success of appeals both in drug information and navigating the industry. A critical practice recognized in transplantation is the bedside delivery of transplantation-related medications. Alongside retail and specialty pharmacy colleagues, transplant pharmacists are integral in the logistics of coordinating the initial supply of medications upon discharge. Bedside delivery of medications is critical for hands-on discharge education (including the use of patient-directed filling of medication pill boxes) and verification of the accuracy of dosing, dosage forms, and formulation (i.e., innovator versus generic). This crucial step in discharge planning enables identification of insurance barriers to access medications, such as the need for prior authorization, formulary management, or need for patient assistance programs.

Patient and Caregiver Education. As the medication expert, the transplant pharmacist is the most qualified person on the multidisciplinary team to provide or oversee medication-related education to the recipient and caregiver. As described previously, adherence to the post-transplantation regimen is directly related to long-term organ survival.[8,9] Appropriate education enhances medication adherence, extending allograft life. Using education level-appropriate language, the transplant pharmacist provides medication education to the recipient and caregiver and assesses the adequacy of understanding using validated scales, tests, or recall approaches such as teach-back. Strategies include multimodal interventions, which may include traditional verbal education, web- or video-based technologies, visual aids for low-literacy or illiterate patients, hands-on medication training, and applications on smart phones.

Documentation. CMS program accreditors directly examine the medical record for evidence of comprehensive pharmacy services provided to individual transplant recipients and transplant pharmacist involvement in multidisciplinary rounds.[1,2,21,22] In the perioperative period, the transplant pharmacist is required to follow their hospital's multidisciplinary care policy. Each hospital policy at minimum must detail how the transplant pharmacist is involved in the transplant phase and discharge phase of care for each transplant patient. Transplant pharmacists should be able to provide evidence of collaboration on medication-related decision-making; sufficient completion and understanding of patient and caregiver education prior to discharge; and the discharge medication regimen, goals, frequency of testing, and expected adherence ability. It is critical that there is evidence of the transplant pharmacist's involvement in the transplant and discharge phase of transplant.

Pharmacy Services in the Post-Transplantation Phase and Ambulatory Setting

Because transplantation immunosuppression is the cornerstone of allograft success, transplant pharmacists are essential in the long-term management of transplant recipients. Ideally, transplant recipients should have access to a transplant pharmacist for the duration of their allograft, and the transplant pharmacist must be part of the multidisciplinary team providing care to transplant patients, as described in Appendix A.

Direct Patient Care. Monitoring immunosuppression and allograft function, making appropriate adjustments after transplantation, and managing co-morbid disease states are integral roles of the transplant pharmacist. As transplant pharmacists transition from a retrospective, chart-review model to a role that involves prospective and real-time decision-making, participation on inpatient rounds and in the ambulatory setting is critical. Provision of direct patient care through participation in selection and adjustment of critical medication regimens, discussion and mitigation of medication-related adverse events, and facilitation of education regarding and consideration of evidence-based practices by the medical and surgical teams at the time of decision-making is an expected element of pharmacotherapy provided by a transplant pharmacist. The ideal is to be physically present during rounds and clinic visits and represent a visible, well-integrated member of the multidisciplinary team. Depending on the number of patients and their acuity, these activities may be tailored to focus on the most critically ill patients or on medications that bear a heightened risk of causing significant patient harm when they are used in error, associated with high rates of adverse effects, or the activities may be based on a triage system developed with or without clinical decision support software. Documentation of the transplant pharmacist's activities during the encounter and resultant discussion with the multidisciplinary team will be utilized to facilitate transitions of care from the inpatient to outpatient encounter as well as from each clinic visit to the next.

In addition to the management of transplantation immunosuppression, the selection and adjustment of post-operative antimicrobial prophylaxis regimens and involvement in antimicrobial stewardship is a standard role for transplant pharmacists.[33] Through transplantation- and organ-specific guidelines, centers each have their own specific antimicrobial prophylactic protocols.[2,3,33,34] After discharge, the metabolic function of patients' organs are often evolving. Patients with impaired renal function or impaired hepatic function often require close monitoring and medication dose adjustment in the ambulatory setting.

Drug-drug interactions are also a concern when starting or stopping prophylactic medications, primarily in aspergillosis prophylaxis, for which azole antifungals are the drugs of choice.[34] These medications have substantial interactions with calcineurin inhibitors and mammalian target of rapamycin (mTOR) inhibitors, and dosage adjustments must be taken into account both when azoles are started, stopped, or have dose adjustments.[34]

Medication and Adherence Education. Two critical services provided by the transplant pharmacist that help ensure the long-term success of transplantation are communicating drug therapy regimen changes to other healthcare providers and providing patients with the tools they need to understand their complicated medication regimens.[11] Access to transplantation-specific medication expertise is an integral part of patient adherence, welfare, and satisfaction, and such education enhances the transplant center's ability to provide high-quality, individualized care to each patient.[11,35,36]

Drug therapy regimen changes can be relayed in a number of ways and these methods will vary according to the established practice at a local center. A common means of communication is verbally during multidisciplinary patient care rounds and patient care discussions. Written documentation in the medical chart, computerized order entry, and use of collaborative practice protocols can also serve as communication between members of the transplantation team. Conveying medication changes to patients and their support may include use of web- and app-based medication lists, handwritten medication sheets, in-person changes made during clinic visits and phone calls.

The provision of medication education is an essential requirement in transplantation. Often, this education is provided by transplantation coordinators, nursing staff, dedicated educators, or pharmacy technicians, in addition to transplant pharmacists. If the primary education is provided by someone other than a transplant pharmacist, the transplant pharmacist should serve as the final assessor of the comprehension of the salient points of medication adherence. Although this process most often is initiated perioperatively, provision of adherence education in the post-transplantation phase is critical for maintaining the patient's adherence skills as well as real-time assessment of the patient's changing adherence needs over time. Ongoing pharmaceutical education throughout the continuum of care is a necessary service each center should provide. The transplant pharmacist has the insight and knowledge to tailor each regimen while staying in compliance with department-specific protocols. At a minimum, the transplant pharmacist should provide structured education either during the pre-evaluation or waiting-list period through discharge from the transplantation hospitalization. Essential components include provision of education focused on names, indications, adverse effects, monitoring, and goals of therapy of transplantation immunosuppression and associated antimicrobial therapy. A self-assessment checklist or competency should be demonstrated prior to discharge from hospitalization, and targeted education should be provided on an ongoing basis in the post-transplantation setting focused on areas of deficiency. Education should be provided beyond the immediate post-transplantation time period, at annual transplantation visits at a minimum, but ideally more frequently, to ensure lifelong adherence. Essential activities that transplant pharmacists should be involved with either directly or in a supervisory role include bedside delivery of transplantation medications, education on use of aids such as medication pill boxes, supervised filling of medication pill boxes, visual use of medication lists, installation of adherence mobile health technology applications, and continued aid from the transplantation team for medication refills, medication access, or delivery, as well as help navigating the health insurance marketplace.

Execution of Protocols. Transplant pharmacists play an integral role in the development and maintenance of organ-specific post-transplantation immunosuppression protocols.[21] These protocols should address not only the direct postoperative hospital stay but also include care throughout the life of the allograft. Through collaborative practice agreements and CDTM, the transplant pharmacist is involved in routine follow-up of post-transplantation care to assist in compliance with each center's protocols.

The need to deviate from protocols due to various factors is a common occurrence. The transplant pharmacist is uniquely positioned to identify adverse drug effects identified through both laboratory monitoring and direct patient interaction. Detailed monitoring of protocol deviations, either from a research standpoint or from a quality- or process-improvement initiative, helps programs identify areas of need for protocol and policy revisions. When adverse drug effects are identified, the transplant pharmacist is involved in decision-making and face-to-face patient interaction regarding planned follow-up and further monitoring of immunomodulatory medications.[20,36] Evidence of therapy management and patient education in all settings should be easily accessible within the medical record.

Transitions of Care. The transition of care from the inpatient transplantation event to the post-transplantation clinic is a critical threshold for the transplant patient to cross. The transplant pharmacist serves a critical role in discharge planning, patient education, and meeting center length-of-stay goals.[13,17,34]

The optimal model is for transplant pharmacists to have direct involvement in medication reconciliation from the inpatient encounter to the outpatient transplantation team to convey critical information and ensure patient safety. Most important are medication changes made during the discharge process, which may encompass formulation changes, dose adjustments, therapeutic substitutions made due to insurance formularies, and follow-up processes related to prior authorizations and patient assistance applications. Transplant pharmacists often serve as a resource for medication optimization, medication access, and patient advocacy.[7,8,18,19,21,26]

Management of Allograft Injury and Loss. Even with optimal adherence and medication management, patients are still at risk for acute and chronic immune-mediated allograft injury. Development of protocols for the management of cell-mediated, antibody-mediated, and chronic allograft rejection or dysfunction is an integral role of the transplant pharmacist.[21] Because rejection or dysfunction in each organ presents differently, the transplant pharmacist must be familiar with the immune-mediated complications specific to each organ type. Treatment of these immune-mediated disease states often requires administration of biological medications. These treatment modalities are high-cost, high-toxicity regimens, and should only be used when necessary. Through development and implementation of evidence-based protocols, the transplant pharmacist should lead the biological medication stewardship program within the transplant patient population.[15]

Many renal allografts are lost secondary to patient death from cardiac disease, highlighting the importance of managing comorbid conditions following transplantation. Disease states such as infections, diabetes, hypertension, hyperlipidemia, heart failure, hyperparathyroidism, and osteoporosis are common after transplantation.[6,16,18,37,38] To compound the challenge of managing these conditions, many of the medications necessary for transplantation exacerbate these disease states.

As transplantation centers grow and transplant patients live longer, the need for transplantation center providers to become medical hubs increases.[39] Through CDTM and collaborative practice agreements, many of these comorbid conditions can be managed by a transplant pharmacist along with immunosuppression. The transplant pharmacist has the ability to combine transplantation-specific medications and disease-specific best practices to optimally manage patients' pharmacotherapy.

Pharmacist Involvement in Treatment of Key Patient Populations

Transplant pharmacists participate in the care of high-risk patient populations following transplantation, as described in Appendix A. In particular, a transplant pharmacist may have great impact on the care provided to pediatric patients, given the inherent risks and unique issues associated with this population. Pediatric transplant recipients present distinctive pharmacology challenges, such as an evolving immune system, variances in pharmacokinetics, pediatric-specific disease states, growth and cosmetic considerations, coming of child-bearing age, and many more. Because of these factors, transplant pharmacists caring for pediatric patients need to be knowledgeable in pediatric dose calculations, routes of administration, and dosage forms. Pediatric patients may require dosage forms not commercially available, and transplant pharmacists serve as a resource for compounding and acquisition for outpatient use. Along with pharmacology challenges, pediatric transplant recipients also have added communication and socioeconomic barriers often unique to this population.

Transplant pharmacists also have a key role in the long-term and ambulatory care of pediatric transplant recipients. A pediatric transplant pharmacist's responsibilities include immunosuppression and opportunistic infection prophylaxis management, assessment of adherence and participation in treatment of nonadherence, reinforcement of education with parents and patients (if appropriate), growth-related medication dose adjustment, recommendations to ensure proper vaccinations, and participation in transitioning adolescents to teenage or adult care. Furthermore, this population may be exposed to immunosuppression for decades. Transplant pharmacists collaborate with providers to optimize regimens, including adjunct therapies, that consider chronic effects of immunosuppressants.

Pregnancy following transplantation is not uncommon, and it is recommended that transplant pharmacists have a key role in contraception, pre-conception, and perinatal care. These high-risk mothers should be managed by both transplantation practitioners and specialists in high-risk pregnancies.[40,41] Clinicians are challenged to find medications regimens that are safe, due to limited data regarding safety during pregnancy or breast feeding. To optimize care of patients who desire pregnancy or who are pregnant following transplantation, transplant pharmacists should work with transplant physicians to create a plan for transitioning to a safe immunosuppression regimen for pregnancy, including a monitoring plan that accounts for the changes in pharmacokinetics of immunosuppression that occur as a pregnancy progresses, and provide education to patients regarding their new regimens, including post-partum implications, such as medication safety while breast-feeding.

An important regulatory requirement transplant pharmacists fill in the care of women of childbearing age is the provision of risk evaluation and mitigation strategies and elements to assure safe use education for mycophenolic acid products.[40] As part of transplantation medication education, transplant pharmacists provide important education regarding timing of pregnancy and conversion to alternative immunosuppressive agents. Furthermore, transplant pharmacists work closely with transplant and OB/GYN teams for immunosuppressive management during preconception, conception, and post-delivery care.

The breadth and scope of healthcare conditions within the transplant population is constantly expanding, and as the population changes and medication management evolves, so too must the transplant pharmacist. Specialty populations, such as human immunodeficiency virus-positive, geriatric, bariatric, cystic fibrosis, and pediatric patients, as well as patients with multiple comorbid disease states, require knowledge of transplant immunomodulation and the ability to tailor the application of treatment best practices to the transplant-specific framework where appropriate. The experienced transplant pharmacist clinician is uniquely equipped to provide patients with the optimal care plan in these situations.

Transplant Pharmacist Administrative Responsibilities

Due to the regulatory requirements unique to transplantation programs, transplant pharmacists perform many administrative duties, as described in Appendix A. As integral members of the multidisciplinary transplantation team, transplant pharmacists have the essential skill set that allows them to develop, maintain, and govern transplantation policies and protocols, contribute to quality measures, and ensure a high level of care for all transplant recipients and donors.

Transplantation is perhaps the most highly regulated of all pharmacy specialties. It is imperative that transplant pharmacists become familiar with the requirements in all phases of transplantation based on their center's internal policies, which must be written in accordance with regulatory agencies. As members of the multidisciplinary team who have roles in all three phases of transplantation (pre-transplantation, perioperative, and post-transplantation), transplant pharmacists are suited to have a designated role in formulary management, development of collaborative practice agreements, and medication-use evaluation. Transplant pharmacists have been instrumental in analysis of center-specific protocols to ensure efficacy and safety and minimize cost to help maintain transplantation as a fiscally solvent option for centers.

It is an expectation that transplant pharmacists will facilitate quality improvement efforts related to pharmaceutical care, including but not limited to the evaluation of adverse drug events, outcomes, cost and optimization in accordance with UNOS- and CMS-prescribed Focused Quality Assessment and Performance Improvement (FQAPI) activities. Several transplant pharmacists from around the country have assumed roles within transplantation quality and facilitate the FQAPI process.[23,24] They are able to fill this unique position through their experience conducting clinical research, performing analysis of medication-related adverse events, and facilitating care during the pre-transplantation, perioperative, and post-transplantation periods. Center- and organ-specific transplantation protocol development and continuing review is paramount to ensuring quality of care. To facilitate ongoing review of center- and organ-specific protocols, transplant pharmacists use internal and external data to evaluate and optimize safety and efficacy. Several transplant pharmacist-led evaluations of induction, maintenance, and de novo immunosuppressant studies have been published.[42–45] In addition, transplant pharmacists are in a unique position to aid in development of guidelines and protocols to monitor and treat infectious diseases and the various metabolic and endocrine issues that arise following transplantation as a result of post-transplantation immunosuppression.

Transplantation-specific competencies are required as part of annual performance evaluations for transplant pharmacists caring for transplant recipients. The transplantation pharmacy community is eager to standardize pharmacist competency and knowledge in this specialty area to ensure the level of clinical expertise is similar among transplant pharmacists from center to center.

Professional Development of Pharmacists in Transplantation

Transplant pharmacists are expected to participate, lead, and manage quality improvement initiatives related to clinical practice, as described in Appendix A. Areas of involvement include transplant pharmacist professional groups on a local, state, and national level, as well as scholarly activity including research, publication, presentation of symposia, and didactic and hands-on preceptorship of pharmacy trainees. Several societies exist for the growth and professional development of transplant pharmacists. Resources include the ASHP Section of Clinical Specialists and Scientists Networking Session on Immunology/Transplantation, the ACCP Immunology/Transplantation Practice and Research Network, the AST Transplant Pharmacy Community of Practice, and the International Society for Heart and Lung Transplantation Scientific Council on Pharmacy and Pharmacology. These are pharmacist-based transplantation societies that host live educational opportunities during annual meetings, offer online webinars, publish newsletters on relevant and timely topics, and provide essential networking opportunities. In addition to the educational aspect of these societies, transplant pharmacists have opportunities for leadership positions not only within the pharmacist-based organizations but within the larger societies, including regulatory organizations such as UNOS. Transplant pharmacists have been elected to influential positions on the board of directors as well as member-at-large and committee chair positions, where they are able to share the work of the profession and provide pharmacist-specific knowledge in areas of public policy and strategic development.

The Board of Pharmacy Specialties recognized solid organ transplantation pharmacy as a specialty in 2018.[46] It is ASHP policy that "pharmacists who practice where a pharmacy specialty has been formally recognized by the profession should become board certified in the appropriate specialty area," while recognizing an obligation "to be sensitive to the needs of current practitioners as prerequisites evolve."[47]

Advancing the Education and Training of Pharmacists in SOT

ASHP supports an increase in the number of education and training opportunities in transplantation for pharmacists as well as pharmacy students, fellows, and residents. Transplant pharmacists have important roles in the education of other practitioners that aids in advancing the transplant pharmacy profession. Current college of pharmacy curricula have minimal focus on transplantation, with many pharmacy students' first exposure to the topic delayed until introductory or advance pharmacy practice experiences rotations.[48] Teaching through lectures or precepting on rotation is an important venue to introduce transplant as a specialty for young practitioners. Postgraduate training of pharmacists provides a pipeline of clinicians, educators, leaders, and scientists who are experts in this specialty and committed to quality care of the transplant patient. There are currently 42 ASHP-accredited postgraduate year 2 training programs as well as two fellowships in transplantation. A recent workforce survey indicated that of the 278 transplant centers listed in the UNOS directory, 33 centers could not participate in the survey due to not having a dedicated transplant pharmacist.[26] A primary goal of these guidelines is to promote the expansion of training of pharmacists in transplantation to allow for all transplant patients to have access to a transplant pharmacist to ensure consistency in the care provided to all transplantation recipients across all centers. **Appendix B** contains a list of recommended readings, references, and resources that complement the references and resources provided in these guidelines.

Conclusion

Every transplantation program in the United States is required to identify transplant pharmacology experts as part of multidisciplinary teams to provide safe and effective care to transplant recipients and living donors and support to maintain organ function. These services span inpatient and ambulatory direct patient care of transplant recipients and donors and are tailored to meet regulatory and compliance standards. ASHP supports the expansion of pharmacy education and postgraduate and fellowship training to include transplantation and patient- and program-specific outcomes, to develop a workforce with the necessary specialized training to deliver these required and essential pharmacy services.

References

1. Organ Procurement and Transplantation Network (OPTN). OPTN Bylaws. https://optn.transplant.hrsa.gov/governance/bylaws (accessed 2018 Aug 9).
2. Costanzo MR, Dipchand A, Starling R et al. The International Society of Heart and Lung Transplantation guidelines for the care of heart transplant recipients. *J Heart Lung Transplant.* 2010; 29:914–56.
3. Kidney Disease: Improving Global Outcomes (KDIGO) Transplant Work Group. KDIGO clinical practice guideline for the care of kidney transplant recipients. *Am J Transplant.* 2009; 9(Suppl 3): S1–155.
4. Mitchell JF. Pharmacist involvement as a member of a renal transplant team. *Am J Hosp Pharm.* 1976; 33:55–8.
5. Burckart GJ. Transplant pharmacy: 30 years of improving patient care. *Ann Pharmacother.* 2007; 41:1261–3.
6. Chisholm MA, Mulloy LL, Jagadeesan M et al. Effect of clinical pharmacy services on the blood pressure of African-American renal transplant patients. *Ethn Dis.* 2002; 12:392–7.
7. Chisholm MA, Vollenweider LJ, Mulloy LL et al. Cost-benefit analysis of a clinical pharmacist-managed medication assistance program in a renal transplant clinic. *Clin Transplant.* 2000; 14 (4 Pt 1):304–7.
8. Chisholm-Burns MA, Spivey CA, Garrett C et al. Impact of clinical pharmacy services on renal transplant recipients' adherence and outcomes. *Patient Prefer Adherence.* 2008; 2:287–92.
9. Ciminelli AM, Dupuis R, Williams D et al. Patient education role of a pharmacist on a transplant service. *Am J Health-Syst Pharm.* 2000; 57:767–8.
10. Hlubocky JM, Stuckey LJ, Schuman AD et al. Evaluation of a transplantation specialty pharmacy program. *Am J Health-Syst Pharm.* 2012; 69:340–7.
11. Klein A, Otto G, Kramer I. Impact of a pharmaceutical care program on liver transplant patients' compliance with immunosuppressive medication: a prospective, randomized, controlled trial using electronic monitoring. *Transplantation.* 2009; 87:839–47.
12. Maldonado AQ, Seiger TC, Urann CL, et al. Billing for outpatient transplant pharmacy services. *Am J Health-Syst Pharm.* 2012; 69:144–7.
13. Maldonado AQ, Weeks DL, Bitterman AN et al. Changing transplant recipient education and inpatient transplant pharmacy practices: a single-center perspective. *Am J Health-Syst Pharm.* 2013; 70:900–4.
14. Martin JE, Zavala EY. The expanding role of the transplant pharmacist in the multidisciplinary practice of transplantation. *Clin Transplant.* 2004; 18 (Suppl 12):50–4.
15. McGillicuddy JW, Taber DJ, Pilch NA et al. Clinical and economic analysis of delayed administration of antithymocyte globulin for induction therapy in kidney transplantation. *Prog Transplant.* 2013; 23:33–8.
16. Migliozzi DR, Zullo AR, Collins C et al. Achieving blood pressure control among renal transplant recipients by integrating electronic health technology and clinical pharmacy services. *Am J Health-Syst Pharm.* 2015; 72:1987–92.
17. Musgrave CR, Pilch NA, Taber DJ et al. Improving transplant patient safety through pharmacist discharge medication reconciliation. *Am J Transplant.* 2013; 13:796–801.
18. Pinelli NR, Clark LM, Carrington AC et al. Pharmacist managed diabetes and cardiovascular risk reduction clinic in kidney transplant recipients: bridging the gap in care transition. *Diabetes Res Clin Pract.* 2014; 106:e64–7.
19. Sebaaly J, Parsons LB, Pilch NA et al. Clinical and financial impact of pharmacist involvement in discharge medication reconciliation at an academic medical center: a prospective pilot study. *Hosp Pharm.* 2015; 50:505–13.
20. Staino C, Pilch N, Patel S et al. Optimizing finite resources: pharmacist chart reviews in an outpatient kidney transplant clinic. *J Am Pharm Assoc.* 2015; 55:613–20.
21. Alloway RR, Dupuis R, Gabardi S et al. Evolution of the role of the transplant pharmacist on the multidisciplinary transplant team. *Am J Transplant.* 2011; 11:1576–83.
22. Maldonado AQ, Tichy EM, Rogers CC et al. Assessing pharmacologic and nonpharmacologic risks in candidates for kidney transplantation. *Am J Health-Syst Pharm.* 2015; 72:781–93.
23. United Network for Organ Sharing (UNOS) bylaws. Effective date: February 1, 2015. https://www.unos.org/wp-content/uploads/unos/UNOS_Bylaws.pdf. (accessed 2017 Dec 28).
24. Organ Procurement and Transplantation Network (OPTN) policies. Effective date: December 12, 2017. https://optn.transplant.hrsa.gov/media/1200/optn_policies.pdf (accessed 2019 Jan 29).
25. Organ Procurement and Transplantation Network (OPTN). National data. https://optn.transplant.hrsa.gov/data/view-data-reports/national-data/# (accessed 2019 Jan 29).
26. Taber DJ, Pilch NA, Trofe-Clark J et al. A national survey assessing the current workforce of transplant pharmacists across accredited U.S. solid organ transplant programs. *Am J Transplant.* 2015; 15:2683–90.
27. Survey & Certification Group, Center for Medicaid and State Operations. Organ transplant program interpretive guidelines. https://www.cms.gov/Medicare/Provider-Enrollment-and-Certification/SurveyCertificationGenInfo/downloads/SCLetter08-25.pdf (accessed 2018 Jan 31).

28. Maldonado AQ, Tichy EM, Rogers CC et al. Assessing pharmacologic and nonpharmacologic risks in candidates for kidney transplantation. *Am J Health-Syst Pharm.* 2015; 72:781–93.
29. Dew MA, DiMartini AF, Dobbels F, et al. The 2018 ISHLT/APM/AST/ICCAC/STSW recommendations for the psychosocial evaluation of adult cardiothoracic transplant candidates and candidates for long-term mechanical circulatory support. *J Heart Lung Transplant.* 2018;37:803–823.
30. Department of Health and Human Services, Centers for Medicare & Medicaid Services. 42 CFR Parts 405, 482, 488, and 498 Medicare program; hospital conditions of participation: requirements for approval and re-approval of transplant centers to perform organ transplants; final rule. *Fed Reg.* 2007; 72:15197–279.
31. Spivey CA, Chisholm-Burns MA, Damadzadeh B. Determining the effect of immunosuppressant adherence on graft failure risk among renal transplant recipients. *Clin Transplant.* 2014; 28:96–104.
32. Potter LM, Maldonado AQ, Lentine KL. Transplant recipients are vulnerable to coverage denial under Medicare part D. *Am J Transplant.* 2018;18:1502–09.
33. Trofe-Clark J., Kaiser T, Pilch N et al. Value of solid organ transplant-trained pharmacists in transplant infectious diseases. *Curr Infect Dis Rep.* 2015; 17:475.
34. Taber DJ, Spivey JR, Tsurutis VM et al. Clinical and economic outcomes associated with medication errors in kidney transplantation. *Clin J Am Soc Nephrol.* 2014; 9:960–6.
35. Taber DJ, Pilch NA, McGillicuddy JW et al. Improved patient safety and outcomes with a comprehensive interdisciplinary improvement initiative in kidney transplant recipients. *Am J Med Qual.* 2013; 28:103–12.
36. Wang HY, Chan AL, Chen MT et al. Effects of pharmaceutical care intervention by clinical pharmacists in renal transplant clinics. *Transplant Proc.* 2008; 40:2319–23.
37. Potter LM, Tichy EM, Horwedel TA et al. Impact of the Pharmacy Practice Model Initiative on clinical pharmacy specialist practice: an alternative viewpoint. *Pharmacotherapy.* 2016; 36:e195–7.
38. Casale JP, Taber DJ, Staino C et al. Effectiveness of an evidence-based induction therapy protocol revision in adult kidney transplant recipients. *Pharmacotherapy* 2017; 37:692–9.
39. Elrod JK, Fortenberry JL Jr. Adaptive reuse in the healthcare industry: repurposing abandoned buildings to serve medical missions. *BMC Health Serv Res.* 2017; 17(Suppl 1):451.
40. McKay DB, Josephson MA. Pregnancy after kidney transplantation. *Clin J Am Soc Nephrol.* 2008; 3 (Suppl 2):S117–25.
41. Bramham K, Nelson-Piercy C, Gao H et al. Pregnancy in renal transplant recipients: a UK national cohort study. *Clin J Am Soc Nephrol.* 2013; 8:290–8.
42. Bowman LJ, Brennan DC. The role of tacrolimus in renal transplantation. *Expert Opin Pharmacother.* 2008; 9:635–43.
43. Riella LV, Gabardi S, Azzi J. Belatacept and long-term outcomes in kidney transplantation. *N Engl J Med.* 2016; 374:2599–600.
44. Lee RA, Gabardi S. Current trends in immunosuppressive therapies for renal transplant recipients. *Am J Health-Syst Pharm.* 2012; 69:1961–75.
45. Tremblay S, Alloway RR. Clinical evaluation of modified release and immediate release tacrolimus formulations. *AAPS J.* 2017; 19:1332–47.
46. Board of Pharmacy Specialties. Solid Organ Transplantation Pharmacy Recognized as New Specialty. https://www.bpsweb.org/2018/08/22/solid-organ-transplantation-pharmacy-recognized-as-new-specialty/ (accessed 2019 Mar 15).
47. American Society of Health-System Pharmacists [ASHP]. ASHP policy position 1225, Board Certi-fication for Pharmacists. https://www.ashp.org/-/media/assets/policy-guidelines/docs/policy-positions/policy-positions-human-resources.ashx (accessed 2019 Mar 15).
48. Accreditation Council for Pharmacy Education. Accreditation Standards and Key Elements for the Professional Program in Pharmacy Leading to the Doctor of Pharmacy Degree (Standards 2016). https://www.acpe-accredit.org/pdf/Standards2016FINAL.pdf (accessed 2019 Mar 15).

Appendix A—Summary of Recommendations

Pretransplantation Phase

The pretransplantation phase includes the initial assessment and any reevaluation that may occur during the waiting-list period. The transplant pharmacist assesses

- Pharmacologic risks (e.g., anticoagulation, drug interactions, medications related to mental health, medications for chronic pain, medication allergies, hormonal contraception and replacement therapy, current use of immunomodulators, issues with drug absorption, illicit substance use, use of herbal supplements).
- Immunologic risk as it pertains to induction selection and need for desensitizing therapies.
- The impact of current pharmacologic therapies on pretransplant testing and perioperative and post-transplantation risks.
- The potential for medication non-adherence.

The transplant pharmacist also assesses nonpharmacologic risks and socially related risks in conjunction with members of the multidisciplinary team, including transplant social workers and financial coordinators. The transplant pharmacist presents risks and mitigation plans as part of the multidisciplinary selection committee. The transplant pharmacist must document transplant pharmacy services provided in accordance with regulatory requirements for individual centers based on policies developed in accordance with CMS Conditions of Participation and UNOS policy.

Perioperative Phase

Transplant pharmacists work with healthcare professionals involved in all settings of the transplantation encounter to ensure a seamless medication-use process, provision of transplant medication education, and discharge planning through each transition of care. The transplant pharmacist provides

- Consultation services for medications related to induction, maintenance, and discharge immunosuppression and their potential impact on other treatments or disease-state management.
- Guidance on patient-specific medication selection, dosing, dosage adjustments during the critical period of improvement in allograft function.
- Drug information to transplantation surgeons, organ specific physicians, nurses, and other clinicians.
- Care to living donors, including pain management, bowel care, fluid and electrolyte management and education of after care.
- Provides medication education to the recipient and caregiver prior to discharge.

The transplant pharmacist must also document transplant pharmacy services provided in accordance with regulatory requirements for individual centers based on policies developed in accordance with CMS Conditions of Participation and UNOS policy.

Post-Transplantation Phase and Ambulatory Setting

Because transplantation immunosuppression is the cornerstone of allograft success, transplant pharmacists are essential in the long-term management of transplant recipients. Ideally, a transplantation recipient will have access to a transplant pharmacist for the duration of their allograft, and the transplant pharmacist will be part of the multidisciplinary team providing care to these patients. The transplant pharmacist modifies existing immunosuppression regimens according to patient-specific needs, adverse effects, and laboratory parameters, and provides ongoing medication and adherence education. The transplant pharmacist detects, monitors, and creates treatment plans for acute cellular rejection, antibody-mediated rejection, and chronic allograft vasculopathy; modifies opportunistic infection prophylaxis and treatment regimens based on renal function and tolerability; and provides guidance in detection and management of opportunistic infections.

Treatment of Key Patient Populations

The transplant pharmacist maintains specific knowledge and experience in the treatment of pediatric and pregnant patients. The transplant pharmacist also provides pharmacotherapy management for comorbid disease state management.

Administrative Responsibilities

Due to the regulatory requirements unique to transplantation programs, transplant pharmacists perform many administrative duties. Transplant pharmacists develop, maintain, and govern transplantation policies and protocols; contribute to quality measures; and ensure a high level of care for all transplant recipients and donors. The transplant pharmacist provides formulary management, engages in and maintains collaborative practice agreements, and undertakes medication-use evaluations. The transplant pharmacist facilitates quality efforts related to pharmaceutical care, including but not limited to the evaluation of adverse drug events, outcomes, cost, and optimization of safety and efficacy in accordance with UNOS- and CMS-prescribed FQAPI activities. The transplant pharmacist develops and maintains center- and organ-specific transplantation protocols and transplant-specific competencies as part of annual performance evaluations.

Professional Development

Transplant pharmacists participate, lead, and manage quality improvement initiatives related to clinical practice. The transplant pharmacist should engage in professional organizations on a local, state, and national level. The transplant pharmacist should participate and lead scholarly activities, including research, publication, presentation of symposia, and didactic and hands-on preceptorship.

Appendix B—Recommended Readings, References, and Resources

The following list represents suggested readings that should be considered in addition to the references and resources provided in the guidelines. The suggested readings are grouped into applicable categories and are then listed in alphabetical order by the primary author.

Laws, Policies, and Guidelines

1. Department of Health and Human Services, Centers for Medicare and Medicaid Services. Organ transplant interpretive guidelines update. Effective June 13, 2008.
2. Organ Procurement and Transplantation Network (OPTN) policies. Effective date: January 17, 2019. Available at: https://optn.transplant.hrsa.gov/media/1200/optn_policies.pdf (accessed 2019 Feb 26).
3. United Network for Organ Sharing (UNOS) bylaws. Effective date: February 1, 2015. Available at: https://www.unos.org/wp-content/uploads/unos/UNOS_Bylaws.pdf (accessed 2019 Feb 26).

Internet Resources

1. Shullo MA, Page RL II, Ensor CR, et al. International Society for Heart and Lung Transplantation (ISHLT) thoracic transplant pharmacy professionals core competency curriculum, first edition. Available at: https://ishlt.org/ishlt/media/ISHLT/Content%20Documents/ISHLT_Pharm_Competencies_final1.pdf (accessed 2019 Feb 26).

Primary Literature

Surveys

1. Staino C, Lewin JJ 3rd, Nesbit TW, Sullivan B, Ensor CR. Survey of transplant-related pharmacy services at large comprehensive transplant centers in the United States. *Prog Transplant.* 2013; 23:23–7.
2. Taber DJ, Pilch NA, Trofe-Clark J, Kaiser TE. A national survey assessing the current workforce of transplant pharmacists across accredited US solid organ transplant programs. *Am J Transplant.* 2015; 15:2683–90.

Practice

1. Alloway RR, Dupuis R, Gabardi S, Kaiser TE, Taber DJ, Tichy EM. Evolution of the role of the transplant pharmacist on the multidisciplinary transplant team. *Am J Transplant.* 2011; 11:1575–83.

2. Burckart GJ. Transplant pharmacy: 30 years of improving patient care. *Ann Pharmacother.* 2007; 41:1261–3.
3. Chisholm MA, Vollenweider LJ, Mulloy LL et al. Cost-benefit analysis of a clinical pharmacist-managed medication assistance program in a renal transplant clinic. *Clin Transplant.* 2000; 14:304–7.
4. Chisholm-Burns MA, Spivey CA, Garrett C et al. Impact of clinical pharmacy services on renal transplant recipients' adherence and outcomes. *Patient Prefer Adherence.* 2008; 2:287–92.
5. Klein A, Otto G, Krämer I. Impact of a pharmaceutical care program on liver transplant patients' compliance with immunosuppressive medication: a prospective, randomized, controlled trial using electronic monitoring. *Transplantation.* 2009; 87:839–47.
6. Maldonado AQ, Weeks DL, Bitterman AN et al. Changing transplant recipient education and inpatient transplant pharmacy practices: a single-center perspective. *Am J Health-Syst Pharm.* 2013; 70:900–4.
7. Maldonado AQ, Seiger TC, Urann Cl et al. Billing for outpatient transplant pharmacy services. *Am J Health-Syst Pharm.* 2012; 69:144–7.
8. Maldonado AQ, Tichy EM, Rogers CC et al. Assessing pharmacologic and nonpharmacologic risks in candidates for kidney transplantation. *Am J Health-Syst Pharm.* 2015; 72:781–93.
9. Martin JE, Zavala EY. The expanding role of the transplant pharmacist in the multidisciplinary practice of transplantation. *Clin Transplant.* 2004; 18 (Suppl 12):50–4.
10. Musgrave CR, Pilch NA, Taber DJ et al. Improving transplant patient safety through pharmacist discharge medication reconciliation. *Am J Transplant.* 2013; 13:796–801.
11. Spivey CA, Chisholm-Burns MA, Damadzadeh B, Billheimer D. Determining the effect of immunosuppressant adherence on graft failure risk among renal transplant recipients. *Clin Transplant.* 2014; 28:96–104.
12. Taber DJ, Pilch NA, McGillicuddy JW et al. Improved patient safety and outcomes with a comprehensive interdisciplinary improvement initiative in kidney transplant recipients. *Am J Med Qual.* 2013; 28:103–12.
13. Tichy EM, Pilch NA, Smith LD, Maldonado AQ, Taber DJ. Building a business plan to support a transplantation pharmacy practice model. *Am J Health-Syst Pharm.* 2014; 71:751–7.
14. Trofe-Clark J, et al. Value of solid organ transplant-trained pharmacists in transplant infectious diseases. *Curr Infect Dis Rep.* 2015; 17:475.
15. Doyle I, Maldonado AQ, Heldenbrand S et al. Nonadherence to therapy after adult solid organ transplantation: A focus on risks and mitigation strategies. *Am J Health-System Pharm.* 2016; 73:909–20.

Developed through the ASHP Section of Clinical Specialists and Scientists and approved by the ASHP Board of Directors on April 30, 2019.

Angela Q. Maldonado, Pharm.D., CPP, BCPS, FAST, Hansa Bio-Pharma, Lund, Sweden.

Reed C. Hall, Pharm.D., BCPS, University Health System, San Antonio, TX; Pharmacotherapy Division, College of Pharmacy, The University of Texas at Austin, TX.

Nicole A. Pilch, Pharm.D., MSCR, BCPS, FAST, Medical University of South Carolina, Charleston, SC.

Christopher R. Ensor, Pharm.D., BCPS, FAST, FCCP, Advent-Health Orlando, Orlando, FL.

Stephanie Anders, Pharm.D., BCPS, Transplant Pharmacy Services, Ochsner Clinic Foundation, New Orleans, LA.

Jennifer A. Gilarde, Pharm.D., Pediatric Transplant Center, Boston Children's Hospital, Boston, MA.

Eric M. Tichy, Pharm.D., M.B.A., BCPS, FCCP, FAST, Supply Chain Management, Mayo Clinic, Rochester, MN.

ASHP gratefully acknowledges the following organizations and individuals for reviewing these guidelines (review does not imply endorsement): American Association of Critical-Care Nurses (AACN); Academy of Managed Care Pharmacy (AMCP); American College of Clinical Pharmacy (ACCP) and ACCP Immunology/Transplantation Practice and Research Network; ASHP Section of Clinical Specialists and Scientists Section Advisory Group on Immunology/Transplantation; American Society of Transplantation Transplant Pharmacy Community of Practice; Childrens of Alabama (COA); Emory Healthcare (EH); Institute for Safe Medication Practices (ISMP); International Society for Heart and Lung Transplantation Scientific Council on Pharmacy and Pharmacology; Iowa Pharmacy Association (IPA); Maryland Society of Health-System Pharmacists (MSHP); Nemours-Alfred I. duPont Hospital for Children (NAIDHFC); Nicole R. Alvey, Pharm.D., BCPS (ACCP); Eve Anderson, Pharm.D., BCPS; Beth Brady, Pharm.D.; Dennis Brierton, Pharm.D., BCPS, FASHP; Jennifer Burnette, Pharm.D., BCPS; Samantha Burton, Pharm.D. (ISMP); Maya Campara, Pharm.D., BCPS; Jeanne Chen, Pharm.D., BCPS; Marie Chisholm-Burns, Pharm.D., M.P.H., M.B.A., FCCP, FASHP, FAST; Wendy Cross, Ph.D., M.Ed., B.Apps.Sc. (AdvNsg), RN, FACN, FACMHN (AACN); Barrett R. Crowther, Pharm.D., BCPS, FAST (ACCP); Brenda Denson, Pharm.D., BCPPS (COA); Travis B. Dick, Pharm.D., M.B.A., BCPS; Kathleen Doan, Pharm.D., BCPPS; Christina T. Doligalski, Pharm.D., BCPS, CPP (ACCP); James N. Fleming, Pharm.D., BCPS (ACCP); Rena Gosser, Pharm.D., BCPS; Kris Gutierrez, Pharm.D.; Laura Halder, Pharm.D.; Erik Henricksen, Pharm.D. (ACCP); Elora Hilmas, Pharm.D., BCPS (NAIDHFC); Karen Khalil, Pharm.D. (ACCP); Miae Kim, Pharm.D.; John Knorr, Pharm.D., BCPS; Erin Lush, Pharm.D., BCPS; Kathryn Clark McKinney, Pharm.D., M.S., BCPS, FACHE, FASHP; Edna Patatanian, Pharm.D.; Catherine Pennington, Pharm.D., M.S., BCPS; Kathy Pham, Pharm.D., BCPPS (ACCP); Anthony Pudlo, Pharm.D., M.B.A., BCACP (IPA); James R. Rinehart, M.S., FASHP; Amelia K. Sofjan, Pharm.D., BCPS; Aaron Steffenhagen, Pharm.D., BCPS, FASHP; Nimisha Sulejmani, Pharm.D., BCPS; Paul Szumita, Pharm.D., FASHP, FCCM, BCCCP, BCPS; Sarah Todd, Pharm.D., BCPS (EH); Molly Wascher, Pharm.D., M.B.A., BCPS (MSHP); Jody Jacobson Wedret, FASHP, FCHSP; and Tricia Lee Wilkins, Pharm.D., M.S., Ph.D. (AMCP).

Christopher R. Ensor declares having received research funding from Amgen, Inc.

Copyright © 2020, American Society of Health-System Pharmacists, Inc. All rights reserved. Contact ASHP for reprint and permissions requests. This content may not be used for commercial purposes without the express written consent of ASHP.

The bibliographic citation for this document is as follows: ASHP guidelines on pharmacy services in solid organ transplantation. *Am J Health-Syst Pharm.* 2020; 77(3):222–32.

ASHP–PPAG Guidelines for Providing Pediatric Pharmacy Services in Hospitals and Health Systems

Purpose

The purpose of these guidelines is to assist pharmacists and pharmacy departments in meeting the special needs of pediatric patients in hospitals and health systems. Pharmacists encounter numerous challenges when providing care to pediatric patients, including the limited data available on the safety and efficacy of medications; the lack of appropriate commercially available medication dosage forms and concentrations; weight-based dosing; complex calculations, especially when dilutions are required; and patients' limited capacity to communicate regarding symptoms, responses to therapy, and possible adverse drug events (ADEs).[1] In addition, pediatric pharmacy practice is associated with different operational demands and requirements than a practice focused exclusively on adults. Pediatric patients are defined as all children from neonate until adulthood. These guidelines supplement the ASHP Minimum Standard for Pharmacies in Hospitals and provide additional recommendations specific to providing pediatric pharmacy services.[2]

Organizational Models

There are various models under which hospital or health-system pharmacy departments typically provide care to pediatric patients, ranging from children's hospitals to general hospitals or health systems providing services to pediatric patients. Depending on which model is adopted, pharmacy departments will provide a different scope of services for pediatric patients. Some institutions provide acute care for pediatric patients with general needs, while others will treat critically ill or specialty patients, such as oncology or transplant patients, in addition to general pediatric patients. Although the pharmacy services provided may be distinctly different based on the type of institution and other factors, there are best practices listed within these guidelines to which all hospitals and health systems should aspire when caring for pediatric patients.

Elements of Care

The elements of pharmacy services that are critical to safe, effective, innovative, and cost-conscious medication use in hospitals and health-systems include

- Practice management
- Medication-use policy development
- Medication therapy optimization
- Drug product procurement and inventory management
- Preparing, packaging, and labeling medications
- Medication delivery
- Medication-use monitoring
- Evaluating the effectiveness of the medication-use system
- Research

Although the scope of pharmacy services will vary among sites depending on the needs of patients, the hospital or health system, and the resources available, these core elements are inextricably linked to successful outcomes. Failure to provide any of these services may compromise the quality of pediatric patient care.

Standard I. Practice Management

The pharmacy department should be organized under the direction of a qualified pharmacist competent to meet the needs of the institution's pediatric patients and be provided with sufficient physical facilities, financial resources, personnel, and equipment to meet the pharmacy care needs of the pediatric population.

A. Pharmacy and Pharmacist Services

Pharmacy Mission, Goals, and Scope of Services. The pharmacy's mission statement shall address the specific patient care needs of pediatric patients. Measured outcomes that focus on value added by pediatric pharmacy practice should focus on safety, productivity, efficiency, quality, education, research, and innovation. Pharmacists' responsibilities for the timely, safe, and accurate order processing and medication reconciliation; medication delivery; prevention of readmissions; patient education at the time of discharge; and other specialized clinical interventions and cost avoidance associated with the prevention of ADEs are vital. Implementation of lean systems management in inpatient and outpatient operations and the innovative use of healthcare technology, revenue-generating services, and specialized pediatric care should be incorporated into the pharmacy practice model.

Hours of Pharmacy Services. Adequate hours of operation for the provision of needed pharmacy services shall be maintained; when possible, 24-hour pharmacy services should be provided to the pediatric population. Essential services include clinical pharmacy services in specialized, high-risk units (e.g., pediatric intensive care unit [ICU], neonatal ICU, hematology–oncology unit, operating rooms, emergency department). Satellite pharmacies in these locations are beneficial, especially if there is evidence of significant service failures caused by central pharmacy delays or if there are location-specific barriers that could affect efficiency or safety. When 24-hour pharmacy services are not feasible, a safe and consistent alternative process shall be established, and a pharmacist with pediatric training should be available on an on-call basis. Remote medication order processing may be employed (to the extent permitted by law and regulation) to help provide pharmacy services but is not a substitute for an on-call pharmacist.[3] Pharmacists who participate in remote order processing should be trained in pediatric care or demonstrate competency in caring for pediatric patients. Automated drug dispensing equipment and computer databases are also not substitutes for the skills and knowledge of a pharmacist with pediatric training and should not be considered alternatives to 24-hour pharmacy services.[4]

DOI 10.37573/9781585287048.081

In the absence of 24-hour pharmacy services, access to a limited supply of medications shall be available only to authorized, licensed healthcare professionals for urgent medication needs. Access to such medications shall be carefully monitored and documented, and after-hours access shall be reviewed regularly to ensure appropriate use. The list of medications to be accessible and the policies and procedures to be used (including subsequent review of all activities by a pharmacist) shall be developed by a multidisciplinary committee of physicians, pharmacists, and nurses (the pharmacy and therapeutics [P&T] committee or its equivalent).[5] Access to medications should be limited to cases in which the P&T committee (or an equivalent multidisciplinary committee) determines that the urgent clinical need for the medication outweighs the potential safety risks of making the medication accessible. Medications, quantities, dosage forms, and container sizes that might increase the risk for ADEs shall also be evaluated. Routine after-hours access to the pharmacy by nonpharmacists for dispensing of medications shall not be permitted. The use of well-designed and secured cabinets, medication carts, automated dispensing devices, and other methods precludes the need for nonpharmacists to enter the pharmacy.[4,6]

Practice Standards and Guidelines. The standards and regulations of all relevant government bodies (e.g., state boards of pharmacy, departments of health, Food and Drug Administration [FDA], United States Pharmacopeia, Drug Enforcement Administration) shall be met. The practice standards and guidelines of ASHP and appropriate accrediting bodies (i.e., the Joint Commission, Institute for Safe Medication Practices [ISMP], American Osteopathic Association Healthcare Facilities Accreditation Program, Det Norske Veritas, and Centers for Medicare and Medicaid Services [CMS]) shall be viewed as applicable, and the hospital should strive to meet all applicable standards. The pharmacy department is encouraged to seek further information on pediatric healthcare services from other organizations, such as the Children's Hospital Association, Pediatric Pharmacy Advocacy Group, Children's Oncology Group, American Society for Parenteral and Enteral Nutrition, and American Academy of Pediatrics.

B. Laws and Regulations

Applicable local, state, and federal laws and regulations shall be met, and relevant documentation of compliance shall be maintained. The pharmacy should actively participate and collaborate with local and national organizations, especially those specific to pediatric patient care.[2]

C. Policies and Procedures

Policies and Procedures Manual. The institution's policies and procedures manual shall address the care of pediatric patients, and all pharmacy personnel shall follow those policies and procedures, regardless of whether a pharmacist with pediatric training is on duty.

Emergency Preparedness. The facility's business continuity plan shall include procedures for providing safe and efficient pediatric pharmacy services to patients and their adult family members in case of emergencies or disaster situations.[7,8] Adequate supplies shall be maintained for these situations, and the unique needs of the pediatric patient population must be considered when selecting these supplies. The institution's emergency preparedness team should have pediatric pharmacy representation and expertise.

Medical Emergencies. The pharmacy shall participate in hospital decisions about the contents of code carts, pediatric dosing references for emergency medication kits and trays, and the role of pharmacists in medical emergencies. Pharmacists should serve on trauma and cardiopulmonary resuscitation committees and teams, and such pharmacists should receive appropriate training and maintain appropriate certifications. Pharmacists with pediatric training should participate in neonatal and pediatric codes and be certified in basic life support, advanced cardiovascular life support, neonatal resuscitation program, or pediatric advanced life support. Health systems with rapid response teams should consider the inclusion of a pharmacist with pediatric training on such a team.

Immunization Programs. The pharmacy shall participate in the development of hospital and health-system policies and procedures concerning preventive and postexposure immunization programs for pediatric patients and hospital employees.[9] When feasible and when permitted by state law or regulations, pharmacists should participate as active immunizers for hospital and health-system–based preventive immunization programs (e.g., influenza).

D. Human Resources

Position Descriptions. Areas of responsibility within the scope of pharmacy services shall be clearly defined. Position descriptions should reflect the position's responsibilities to the specific pediatric population being served (e.g., pediatric ICU, neonatal ICU, emergency department).

Director of Pharmacy. The director of pharmacy should understand the unique needs of pediatric patients and be knowledgeable about and have experience in pediatric hospital pharmacy practice. An advanced management degree (e.g., master of business administration, master of health administration) or an administrative specialty residency is desirable.[10]

Pharmacists. Pharmacy management shall employ an adequate number of competent, licensed pharmacists in good standing with their state board to meet the specific medication-use needs of the hospital's and health system's pediatric patients.

Support Personnel. Sufficient support personnel (e.g., pharmacy technicians, inventory coordinators, business managers, other administrative personnel) shall be employed to facilitate pharmacy services. Human resources collaboration and support are necessary, and additional education for practitioners in this area may need to be considered for practice leadership. A support position shall have a written job description that includes a statement of the competencies required for that position. Support staff shall be properly trained and supervised, and professional development programs for these staff are desirable. Pharmacy technicians should have completed an ASHP-accredited pharmacy technician training program, should be certified by the Pharmacy Technician Certification Board, and shall meet the requirements of applicable laws and regulations. Pharmacy technicians working in advanced roles should have additional training and demonstrate competencies specific to the tasks to be performed for pediatric patients.

Education and Training. All personnel shall possess the education and training required to fulfill their responsibilities and shall participate in relevant continuous professional development (e.g., continuing-education programs) and activities as necessary to maintain or enhance their competence.[11] Pharmacists providing care to pediatric patients should possess the knowledge and skills necessary to make that care safe and effective for the patient population. The pharmacy department should provide adequate training for all staff members who may be called on to provide care to pediatric patients. Core competencies should be age based and include mastery of pharmacokinetic and pharmacodynamic differences, weight-based dosing and calculations, fluid and nutrition requirements, common pediatric diseases and drugs, pharmacogenomics, drug information resources, and specialized drug preparation and administration techniques for pediatric patients. Pharmacists' core competence in these areas should be established initially and then periodically reassessed based on the level of care provided.

The pharmacy director or designee should be responsible for all staff development, taking into account the specific needs of the department and the various pediatric populations served. Staff development programs should be current, frequently scheduled, and easily accessible. Online tools for continuing education and staff development can also be a convenient source for education and development.

Pharmacists seeking positions in pediatric pharmacy practice should complete postgraduate residency training to enhance their clinical skills and knowledge base in pediatric pharmacy practice. The knowledge, skills, and abilities obtained through completion of a postgraduate year 1 (PGY1) residency are essential for new graduates seeking roles as pediatric pharmacists. Specialty training through a postgraduate year 2 pediatric residency program offers a unique opportunity to focus on practice in a specific pediatric population (e.g., critical care, neonatology, hematology–oncology) and is strongly recommended for pediatric pharmacists. Pharmacists, through experience, may also demonstrate mastery of the knowledge, skills, attitudes, and abilities to care for pediatric patients (e.g., PGY1 residency in a pediatric hospital, multiple pediatric rotations during a PGY1 program).

Pharmacy directors should encourage staff to seek competency-related certifications through the Board of Pharmacy Specialties certification (e.g., board-certified pediatric pharmacy specialist) or through other pediatric pertinent certifications (e.g., asthma education, immunization). Pharmacy directors should consider incentives or recognition for pharmacists who seek additional training and certifications.

Orientation of Personnel. There shall be an established, structured procedure for orienting new personnel to the pharmacy, the hospital or health system, and their respective positions to provide care for the pediatric patient.[12] Evaluation of the effectiveness of orientation programs should be done in conjunction with the competency assessment required before a new hire can assume full responsibility for the position.

Work Schedules and Assignments. The director of pharmacy or designee shall ensure that work schedules, procedures, and assignments optimize the use of personnel and resources. Internal benchmarking may be useful to determine the best use of resources and personnel specific to pediatrics. National benchmarks may lack the understanding that workflow and workload for pediatric pharmacy are very different than for adult pharmacy practice and are not as standardized. The specialized and customized needs of pediatric patients require significantly more resources when compared with adult patients. There shall be a written departmental staffing plan that addresses how pediatric patients' needs will be met during periods of staff shortages, fluctuation in workload, inclement weather, or patient acuity. Remote medication order processing may be employed to help address staff shortages or workload fluctuations.[3]

Performance Evaluation. There shall be procedures for regularly scheduled evaluation of the performance of pharmacy personnel. The evaluation format should be consistent with that used by the hospital or health system. The competencies of the position should be well defined in the position description, short- and long-term goals should be established for each employee, and the employee's competency shall be assessed on a scheduled basis. Pediatric competencies should be routinely assessed for all pharmacists caring for pediatric patients. Pharmacists not meeting minimum standards for competency should be reassigned to other areas and not be allowed to practice until such competency is met. The pharmacy director shall ensure that an ongoing competency assessment program is in place for all staff, and each staff member should have a continuous professional development plan.

E. Facilities

Pharmacy. Adequate space, equipment, and supplies shall be available for all professional and administrative functions relating to pediatric inpatient and outpatient pharmacy services. These resources shall meet all applicable laws and regulations; shall be located in areas that facilitate the provision of services to patients, nurses, prescribers, and other healthcare providers; and shall be integrated with the hospital's or health system's communication and delivery or transportation systems.

Outpatient Pharmacy Services. Outpatient pharmacy services should be attentive to the unique medication needs of the pediatric patient. Outpatient pharmacy services should stock pediatric dosage forms (e.g., liquids, chewable tablets) and appropriate measuring devices (e.g., oral syringes) suitable for pediatric patients. All oral liquid medications for children should be dispensed with the appropriate measuring device. The pharmacy may provide flavoring services to improve the palatability of medications. In unique circumstances where medication preparation will need to be performed by the patient or caregiver (e.g., short-stability medications, reconstitution), education should be provided by the appropriate pharmacy staff member. Consideration must be given to the need for an extra medication supply with a labeled container to be taken to school, daycare, or other places where medication may be administered. For outpatient medication services (e.g., ambulatory care infusion centers, home infusion services, compounding services), issues, such as preparation and batching of medications, need to be considered. If a hospital or health system outsources for these services, selected facilities shall be able to support the care and needs of pediatric patients.

Medication Storage and Preparation Areas. There shall be suitable facilities to enable and document the receipt, storage, and preparation of medications under proper conditions of sanitation, temperature, light, moisture, ventilation, segregation, and security to ensure medication integrity and personnel safety throughout the hospital and health system.[4,13]

Compounding Areas. There shall be suitable facilities to enable the compounding, preparation, and labeling of sterile and nonsterile products, including hazardous drug products, in accordance with national and local established quality assurance procedures. The work environment shall promote orderliness and efficiency and minimize the potential for medication errors and contamination of products.[14–20] Resources necessary for compounding and testing alternative doses and dosage forms of commercially available products are essential. Preparation of pediatric doses often requires more time and actions (e.g., calculation of proper dose, dilution, preparation of patient-specific dose in the most ready-to-administer form) than preparation of standard adult doses, many of which are available in ready-to-use form from manufacturers. Resources shall be allocated to maintain the efficiency and safety of the medication-use process while meeting the additional requirements of providing pediatric doses.

Information Technology. A comprehensive pharmacy computer system shall be employed and should be integrated to the fullest extent possible with other hospital information systems and software, including computerized provider order entry (CPOE), barcode-assisted medication administration, electronic health record, and patient billing systems. To obtain patient-specific clinical information for medication therapy monitoring and other clinical functions and to facilitate the continuity of care to and from other care settings, computer resources should be used to support the following:

- Access the patient medical record.
- Document patient care activities.
- Interface with other computerized systems.
- Maintain patient medication profile records.
- Manage clerical functions.
- Manage drug product inventories.
- Manage electronic prescribing.
- Perform necessary patient billing procedures.
- Provide clinical decision support (CDS).
- Provide drug information.

Pediatric specific needs within the computer resources shall be carefully evaluated and allow for customization if warranted. Additional informatics resources may need to be considered for implementation and development of sophisticated CDS. A pharmacist with pediatric training should be involved in the development and maintenance of order sets, templates, and dose ranges used in CPOE and CDS systems. Pharmacy computer systems should be integrated with the hospital's clinical, financial, and administrative information systems. All computer systems shall include adequate safeguards to maintain the confidentiality and security of patient records, and a backup system should be available to continue essential computerized functions (e.g., those that support patient care) during equipment failure.

Drug Information. Adequate space, current resources, and information-handling and communication technology shall be available to facilitate the provision of drug information. The pharmacy department shall select and standardize its drug information resources, and a pharmacist with pediatric training shall play a leadership role in the selection of pediatric drug information resources used by other healthcare providers in the hospital. Current objective pediatric and adult drug information shall be available, including print or electronic periodicals, newsletters, best practices guidelines, and recent editions of reference books in appropriate pediatric pharmaceutical and biomedical subject areas. Specifically, information on pediatric dosages, extemporaneous formulations, drug compatibilities and stability, toxicology, drug effects, and safety during pregnancy and lactation should be readily obtainable. Literature supporting the use of drugs for unlabeled uses in pediatric patients should also be accessible.[21] Available information sources should support research on patient care issues and facilitate the provision of pharmacy care and safety in the medication-use process. Appropriate drug information resources shall be readily accessible to pharmacists located in specialized pediatric patient care areas (e.g., neonatal intensive care). This information may be accessed in conjunction with medical libraries and other available resources. Resources should have the capability to provide hard copies of drug information or counseling points focused on the pediatric population that the pharmacist can provide to the patient and caregiver.

Electronic drug information databases are preferred because they are frequently updated and can be made available to all healthcare professionals, but sufficient access to print information shall be available in case of equipment failure or downtime. Electronic databases and convenient methods of data dissemination (e.g., e-mail, handheld devices) are desirable. Electronic drug information resources shall be accessible at the point of care for all healthcare personnel.

F. Health Information Technology

Standards. The pharmacy director or designee shall maintain an understanding of current regulatory standards and best practices related to the use of health information technology (HIT), including but not limited to the Health Insurance Portability and Accountability Act, American Recovery and Reinvestment Act/Health Information Technology for Economic and Clinical Health, and CMS e-reporting requirements pertaining to medication use and pharmacy practice. Staff will comply with these regulations.

HIT Components of the Medication-Use Cycle. Pharmacy HIT should be an integrated part of the health system's clinical and financial information systems. The pharmacy executive or designee shall be an active participant in the evaluation and decision to purchase any new clinical information system by the health system.

CPOE and CDS Systems. CPOE and CDS systems should be evaluated and customized as necessary to support age-specific requirements for safe and effective medication use. Computer systems shall report patient weight and height in metric units. At a minimum, these systems shall include age-specific, weight-specific, and body surface area–specific drug dose checking; dose capping; and drug–allergy, drug–drug interaction, and drug–disease state checking. CPOE order sets and order sentences intended for use in pediatric patients should be reviewed by the pharmacy department or by the pediatric pharmacy specialist in the case of a children's hospital or pediatric services within an adult hospital or health system.

Automation. Automation, including but not limited to dispensing cabinets, carousels, and robotics, should be used and able to accommodate pediatric dosage forms, dosage amounts, and delivery rates (e.g., neonatal i.v. syringes, oral liquid dose forms). Hospitals should evaluate the use of other barcode-enabled technologies to ensure patient safety, such as medication tracking and i.v. workflow software. Use of this automation should also include a continuous quality-improvement plan to optimize the effectiveness of these technologies for pediatric patients.

Electronic Medication Administration Record. An electronic medication administration record (eMAR) should be integrated or directly interfaced with the pharmacy information system. Information systems should populate the eMAR with medication dose and volume for pediatric patients. The eMAR should include nursing notification for late doses as well as the ability to document a reason for any doses not administered. Ideally, the eMAR should be integrated with assistive technology (i.e., either barcode or radio frequency identification [RFID] technology) to provide electronic tracking and decision support around the 5 rights of medication administration.[22] Documentation of medication-specific patient parameters (e.g., corresponding pain score with administration of a pain medication) should be encouraged.

Barcode or RFID Medication Administration. A point-of-care barcode or RFID medication administration system shall be employed and integrated with the eMAR and pharmacy information system.[23] Point-of-care technology shall be carefully evaluated for use in a pediatric setting, specifically success rates for scanning labels on smaller syringe dosages and on patient armbands sized for young children and infants. Careful consideration and monitoring of nursing workarounds should be evaluated periodically and specific barriers addressed by the medication safety team or committee. In those circumstances where barcode or RFID tags are applied onsite to compounded or repackaged medications, workflows and quality assurance procedures must be in place to ensure accurate labeling.

E-prescribing. E-prescribing systems shall include age- and weight-specific drug dose checking and drug–allergy, drug–drug interaction, and drug–disease state checking. When possible, e-prescribing systems should be integrated into the organization's primary electronic medical record/CPOE system or, at a minimum, should be interfaced with the CPOE system in order to share allergy, drug interaction, and medication reconciliation history data.

Smart Infusion Pumps. The hospital shall purchase and maintain pumps that are built with a medication library (i.e., smart infusion pumps). These include large-volume bag pumps, small-volume syringe pumps, and patient-controlled analgesia pumps. Pharmacy departments should be involved in the purchasing, implementation, and maintenance of all infusion devices capable of administering medications to patients (e.g., magnetic resonance imaging compatible devices, epidural pumps). The medication library shall include standard concentrations of i.v. medications, dose limits, and warnings as appropriate. The medication library shall be maintained by a pharmacist with training in pediatrics. The library shall be maintained and checked on a regular basis, at least annually, and adjustments made as needed. Dosing alerts shall be installed as appropriate to add safeguards for high-risk medications. These alerts should use hard limits wherever possible, as they have been shown to decrease errors to a greater extent than soft limits, which can be overridden.[24] Pump usage should be closely monitored to ensure that providers of care are appropriately using the library and not overriding safeguards.

CDS Technology. The pharmacy department shall actively participate in the acquisition, development, and maintenance of CDS systems that impact pharmacy services, including membership on any committee tasked with CDS governance. Policies and procedures shall be developed to describe the CDS request lifecycle and CDS governance process. Content and execution of CDS rules shall follow industry best practice. Opportunities for CDS should be continually evaluated based on hospital event reports and published sources. The effectiveness of any CDS intervention should be evaluated postimplementation and modified as needed. The pharmacy department shall be involved in the regular review of medication-related alerts and reminders within the electronic health record to ensure that CDS content remains current and accurate to minimize the generation of nuisance alerts and to identify and correct any CDS content that may lead to confusion or risk of medication errors.[25,26]

CDS Governance. CDS rules may be locally developed or provided by the system vendor. A pediatric-specific workgroup that includes a pharmacist with pediatric training should be established for consideration of pediatric-specific workflow and needs assessment. In either case, rules should be as sensitive and specific as possible in order to minimize alert fatigue.[26] Vendor-supplied CDS rules should be evaluated and customized before implementation, and all CDS rules shall be evaluated on an ongoing basis to ensure continued relevance. At a minimum, the CDS system should provide mechanisms for drug–drug, drug–allergy, and drug–disease state interactions, as well as dose range checking and other dosing guidance. CDS should be utilized to collect quality measures data for reporting to CMS under the Meaningful Use of the Electronic Health Record Incentive Program.

CDS Development and Customization. Customization of vendor-supplied CDS or local development of CDS solutions shall follow a defined life cycle, which shall include the following stages[26]:

- Requirements gathering: review of current workflow and identification of opportunities for CDS solutions.
- Detailed specifications for the proposed CDS solution to be developed in conjunction with a pharmacy informatics or information technology expert and approved by the affected clinical end users (e.g., nursing, medical, and pharmacy staff representatives) as well as quality-control and regulatory department representatives.
- Development and testing of the proposed CDS solution.

- Education of the affected end users regarding the proposed solution and any impact it may have on current workflow.
- Implementation of the CDS solution.
- Ongoing monitoring as described above under CDS governance to identify and correct any unintended consequences of the new CDS rule.

G. Committee Involvement

A pharmacist with pediatric training shall be a member of and actively participate in hospital and health-system committees responsible for establishing and implementing medication-related policies and procedures for pediatric patients as well as those committees responsible for the provision of pediatric patient care, including the P&T, infection prevention and control, patient care, medication-use evaluation and process, medication safety, transitions-of-care, nutrition, and pain management committees (or their equivalents), as well as the institutional review board, quality-improvement committee, and information technology committee (or their equivalents).[5,27–29]

A pharmacist with pediatric training should participate in or be appointed to the hospital's P&T committee and should provide input regarding all P&T decisions and their impact on pediatric patient populations. A pediatrics subcommittee or other appropriate pediatric representation should be established if the P&T committee is focused primarily on adult patients. If such a subcommittee is not established, all P&T committee decisions should denote whether they apply to pediatric patients or only adult patients.

A pharmacist with pediatric training should be similarly involved in the development, implementation, and assessment of care plans (medication-use processes, protocols, critical pathways, disease state management programs, transitions-of-care, and clinical practice guidelines), standing orders, and order sets that involve medication therapy for pediatric patients.

Standard II. Medication-Use Policy Development

A. Policy Development

All committees that make decisions concerning pediatric medication management and use shall have at least 1 pharmacist with pediatric training as a member. These include but are not limited to the P&T, infection control, patient care, medication-use evaluation, medication safety, transitions-of-care, nutrition, pain management, and information technology committees (or their equivalents), as well as the institutional review board.[5,27–29] A pharmacist with pediatric training shall be involved in the development, implementation, and assessment of pediatric care plans (protocols, critical pathways, disease state management programs, and clinical practice guidelines), standing orders, and order sets that involve medication therapy.[30]

B. Formulary

Formulary. A well-controlled formulary of approved medications shall be maintained and regularly updated by the P&T committee (or its equivalent). The impact of and compliance with the formulary should be periodically reviewed (e.g., through drug utilization reviews), and the P&T committee should regularly review the formulary for pediatric efficacy and safety information. The P&T committee shall be responsible for developing and maintaining written criteria for drug product selection, which shall address formulary requests for medications intended for use in pediatric populations. The P&T committee shall be responsible for approving and maintaining adequate product specifications to aid in the purchase of medications and related supplies for pediatric patients. The pharmacy shall disseminate the formulary by electronic (preferred) or other means to meet the needs of all healthcare professionals.

There shall be policies and procedures for the following:

- Use of dietary supplements.
- Other alternative therapies.
- Procurement, control, and use of nonformulary medications required for pediatric patient care.[5]

Nondrug Substances. Some institutions may have nondrug substances that may be handled or distributed by the pharmacy (donor breast milk and other nutrition products). There should be policies and procedures that describe how the pharmacy shall seek and obtain documented authorization from appropriate medical staff and hospital committees before the medical use of any nondrug substance, as well as appropriate documentation for tracking and quality-control purposes (e.g., lot numbers). These policies and procedures should clearly define the pharmacy procedure for storage, preparation, and distribution of these nondrug substances. A pharmacist with pediatric training should be involved in the development and approval of these policies and procedures.

C. Drug Information

Drug Information Services. Pediatric drug information services should be provided by the pharmacist practicing in the pediatric setting by supplying information unique to the pediatric population. These services may be developed as a focused service with pharmacists solely working in this area in the health system, or drug information responsibilities may be incorporated throughout the department with several pharmacists contributing to different services. A pharmacy department may have a drug information telephone line, e-mail address, or other mode of communication (e.g., text message, discussion board) to answer questions from practitioners. A pharmacist with pediatric training should provide the pharmacy department and other healthcare professionals with information on new and investigational drugs, adverse effects of and contraindications to drug therapy, compatibility and stability information, drug shortages and alternatives, dosage computations, pharmacokinetics, pharmacogenomics, and drug interactions related to the pediatric population. The drug information service should also conduct medication-use evaluations to assist the P&T committee or its equivalent and may provide medication-use policies specific for pediatric patients (e.g., off-label use of medications, use of patient's home medications).

Drug Information Requests. The pharmacist shall provide pediatric patient–specific drug information and accurate, comprehensive information about drugs and drug therapy to health professionals, patients, and patients' caregivers as appropriate. Responses to general and patient-specific drug information requests shall be provided in an accurate and timely manner by a pharmacist, and there should be a process for documenting and ensuring the quality of responses.[31] Documentation of drug information requests and other services shall be gathered and evaluated by the pharmacy department.

Dissemination of Drug Information. Pharmacists shall keep the hospital's staff and healthcare providers informed about the use of medications in the pediatric population on an ongoing basis through appropriate publications, presentations, and programs. Pharmacists shall ensure timely dissemination of drug product information (e.g., recall notices, labeling changes, changes in product availability). Electronic communications (e.g., websites, e-mail newsletters, intranet postings) are effective due to their timeliness and accessibility.[31]

Standard III. Optimizing Medication Therapy

An important responsibility of the pharmacist is optimizing medication use. A pharmacist with pediatric training, in collaboration with medical and nursing staff, shall develop policies and procedures based on demonstrated best practices for ensuring the quality of medication therapy in pediatric patients. Clinical imperatives should be the primary determinant of medication-use decisions.

Clinical Services. Clinical services provided by the pharmacy department will vary, depending on the needs of patients, the resources available, the structure of the department, and other factors. However, the goal should be to provide all children with the same level of clinical expertise on a consistent basis. Decentralized clinical pharmacy services are warranted for standalone children's hospitals and other hospitals that support a large number of pediatric patients. Clinical pediatric pharmacy services shall be prioritized to provide the highest level of care to populations that are at highest risk, such as patients in the critical care, neonatology, hematology–oncology, and emergency departments. If perioperative or procedural services are provided in the health system, a pharmacist should also be directly assigned to those units.[32] The clinical pharmacy services provided should include but are not limited to patient care rounds, drug therapy monitoring, drug information, medication profile review, medication reconciliation, ADEs surveillance, patient education, and discharge counseling. Additional services provided by the pharmacy should include routine nursing and prescriber education, order set development, policy development, drug evaluation reviews, and other medication safety and quality initiatives for pediatric patients. Hospitals should deploy additional clinical pediatric pharmacy specialists to high-risk care areas (e.g., critical care, neonatology, hematology–oncology, transplant, and emergency departments). Documentation of pharmacy services is warranted for quality assurance. Communication of patient care recommendations is also critical for continuity of care. Documentation in the electronic medical record is preferred when feasible.

A. Creating a Relationship with the Patient

Pharmacist's Role in Direct Patient Care. Hospital and pharmacy department policies should encourage pharmacists with pediatric training to provide direct patient care in both inpatient and outpatient settings. Hospital and pharmacy department policies should encourage pharmacists with pediatric training to engage in medication therapy management, collaborative drug therapy management, immunization, medication ordering and administration, and other patient care activities to the extent permitted by law, regulations, and hospital requirements.[33]

Continuity of Care. Pharmacists should assume responsibility for continuity of care for patients' medication therapy. Pharmacists and pharmacy departments should take a leadership role in developing and implementing policies and procedures for medication therapy management for admissions, discharges, transfers, and transitions across care settings and shifts (e.g., hospital unit changes, outpatient clinics, home care).

B. Acquiring Essential Patient Data

Medication Histories. Pharmacists or their designee should obtain, prepare, or have immediate access to comprehensive medication histories for each patient, from the patient's medical record or other databases (e.g., a medication profile) or both. It is preferred that a pharmacist with pediatric training conduct a medication and vaccination history for each pediatric patient when feasible. The patient or caregiver may be interviewed, depending on the patient's level of communication. Electronic medical records should be constructed so that medication histories and other data required for medication management, including medication reconciliation, are available and easily accessible to all health professionals caring for a patient. For many pediatric patients, medication and vaccination histories may be obtained from caregivers who may or may not provide routine care for the child (e.g., grandparents, divorced parent). If available, efforts should be made to contact caregivers who provide routine care for the child and to pharmacies to gather accurate medication histories.

Standard IV. Managing Inventory

Medication Storage. Medications shall be received, stored, and prepared under proper conditions of sanitation, temperature, light, moisture, ventilation, segregation, and security to ensure medication integrity and personnel safety in accordance with all federal and state laws.[4]

Drug Shortages. There shall be policies and procedures for managing drug product shortages. The pharmacy's inventory management system should be designed to detect and mitigate subminimum inventory levels and alert the pharmacy to potential shortages. Pharmacy staff should monitor reliable sources of information regarding drug product shortages (e.g., ASHP and FDA drug shortages Web resource centers).[34,35] The pharmacy should develop strategies for identifying alternative therapies, working with suppliers, collaborating with physicians and other healthcare providers, and conducting an awareness campaign in the event of a drug product shortage.[36] Pharmacy should provide leadership in communicating specific operational changes and work with appropriate medical personnel and the P&T committee or its equivalent for specific clinical changes affecting pediatric patient care due to drug shortages.

Standard V. Preparing, Packaging, and Labeling Medications

A. Preparing Medications

Compounding. Drug formulations, dosage forms, strengths, and packaging that are not available commercially but are needed for pediatric patient care shall be prepared by appropriately trained personnel in accordance with applicable practice standards and regulations. Medications shall be ordered by the institution in standardized concentrations of commercially available and validated master formulas—ideally evidence-based and referenced—as part of an effort to reduce medication errors. The pharmacy shall follow federal and state regulations and shall provide adequate quality assurance procedures for these operations.[19,20,37] Pharmacy departments shall ensure patient safety as well as true patient need versus anticipated cost savings. Written master formulations and batch records (including product test results, as appropriate) shall be maintained, and a lot number or other method to identify each finished product with its production and control history shall be assigned to each batch.[14–20] Sterile and nonsterile compounding shall meet all applicable federal and state laws, regulations, standards, and accreditation requirements.[14,19,20]

Sterile Preparations. When possible, manufactured sterile preparations should be preferred to compounding in the pharmacy. All sterile medications shall be prepared and labeled in a suitable environment by appropriately trained personnel in accordance with established quality assurance and beyond use dating procedures.[14,19] The use of sterile medications compounded outside the pharmacy (e.g., nursing units) should be avoided to the extent possible; when they are used in urgent or emergent circumstances, there shall be procedures for aseptic preparation, quality assurance, expiration dating, and ongoing competency evaluations for compounding personnel.[14,19,38] Sterile compounding outside the pharmacy or satellite pharmacies (e.g., on nursing units) should be minimized and occur only in emergency situations.[14,19] If outsourcing of sterile compounding services is necessary, the pharmacy department shall ensure that the process provides appropriate guarantees of safety and quality assurance.[38]

B. Packaging Medications

Unit Dose Packaging. A lack of availability of commercially prepared dosage forms, combined with the documented risk of calculation errors, requires the use of comprehensive unit dose drug distribution systems and i.v. admixture services for pediatric patients. The use of standardized doses for both oral and parenteral medications where appropriate may facilitate the provision of these services. Every attempt shall be made to provide patient-specific dosing, realizing that patient-specific doses are more often required in pediatric patients. All scheduled pediatric medications should be dispensed in patient-specific unit doses.

Manipulation of medications before administration (e.g., withdrawal of doses from containers, reconstitution of powdered drug products, labeling of containers, splitting of tablets) by final users or providers should be minimized.[15] Repackaging of oral or sterile products shall meet all applicable laws, regulations, standards, and accreditation requirements.[14,18,19]

Barcoding of Unit Dose Packaging and Point-of-Care Administration. Unit dose packages should contain a barcode, and that code should be used in inventory management, dose preparation and packaging, dispensing, and administration. It is the responsibility of the pharmacy department to ensure the quality of all aspects of barcode medication administration, including scannability of barcodes and database management.[23,39]

Standard VI. Medication Delivery

A. Medication Prescribing

Prescribing. Medications shall be prescribed by individuals who have been granted appropriate clinical privileges in the hospital and are legally permitted to order medications. The pharmacy shall advocate and foster practitioners' conformance with standardized, approved, and safe terminology and abbreviations to be used throughout the hospital when prescribing medications and discourage use of nonstandard and unapproved terminology and abbreviations.[4] The metric system shall be utilized for ordering oral liquid medications for the pediatric population.[40,41]

Diagnostic or Therapeutic Purpose. Pharmacists shall have access to the patient's diagnosis or the intended therapeutic or medical purpose of medications in a timely manner. For many medications, pediatric labeling does not exist, and off-label use is common. Resources shall be available to the pharmacist to assist with identifying medication indications or uses.

Medication Orders. All patient medication orders shall be contained in the patient's medical record. A direct copy of the prescriber's order, either hard copy (including facsimile) or prescriber-entered electronic transmission (preferred method), shall be received by the pharmacist. Verbal orders shall be avoided to the extent possible. When verbal orders are necessary, they shall follow the organization's established procedures for their use and documentation. Order transmittal safeguards shall be used to ensure the security of the prescriber's order. Appropriate records of each medication order and its processing in the pharmacy shall be maintained in accordance with applicable laws and regulations.

A system shall exist to ensure that medication orders are not inappropriately continued.[4] The pharmacy department should establish, regularly review and revise, and enforce policies and procedures that ensure a prospective review of every medication order for a pediatric patient by a pharmacist trained in pediatrics. A standard definition should be established for who constitutes a pediatric patient in the institution; this definition may be based on weight, age, congenital defects, developmental delays, or a combination of these factors. All medication orders for pediatric patients shall include the patient's allergies, the patient's weight in kilograms, a weight-based dose designation (e.g., mg/kg), and a total dose, where applicable. Height, in centimeters, shall also be obtained to calculate body mass index, body surface area, and renal function. Standardization for doses to be provided in milligrams or milliliters should be evaluated closely, and the correct process for entering orders should be standardized and communicated to providers to mitigate order errors. All elements of the medication order are required. The use of abbreviations shall be limited based on specific recommendations provided by the Joint Commission on "do not use" abbreviations.[41]

Review of Medication Orders. Pediatric medication orders shall be prospectively reviewed by a pharmacist with adequate pediatric training and assessed in relation to pertinent patient and clinical information before the first dose is dispensed or made available in an automated dispensing device, except in emergent situations in which the treatment of the patient would be significantly compromised by the delay that would result from pharmacist review of the order. There shall be a procedure for retrospective review of these orders.

Any questions regarding an order shall be resolved with the prescriber before dispensing or administration. Pharmacist consultations should be documented in the patient's medical record. Information concerning changes shall be communicated to the appropriate health professionals caring for the patient.[4]

B. Medication Delivery and Administration

Drug Delivery Systems, Administration Devices, and Automated Distribution Devices. The pharmacy shall be responsible for developing policies, procedures, and quality assurance programs regarding drug delivery systems, administration devices, and automated distribution devices to ensure safety, accuracy, security, and patient confidentiality in the pediatric population. Administration technology consideration shall include standard concentrations, patient size, and administration rate. The potential for medication errors associated with such systems and devices in the pediatric population shall be thoroughly evaluated.[4,6] Pharmacy personnel shall supervise the stocking and documentation of medications in automated dispensing devices.[6] Whenever possible, automated dispensing cabinets should employ profile-based technology integrated with remote medication order-entry capabilities.

Medication Administration. Only personnel who are authorized by the hospital in accordance with applicable laws and regulations and who are appropriately trained shall be permitted to administer medications to a patient. All administered, refused, or omitted medication doses shall be recorded in the patient's medical record according to an established procedure, and all medications that have not been administered shall be returned to the pharmacy or discarded appropriately. No medication should be administered to a patient unless medical and nursing personnel have been provided with adequate information about and are familiar with its therapeutic use, method of administration, potential adverse effects, and dosage. Caregivers and patients shall be informed of these policies on admission so they do not administer home medications without the healthcare provider's knowledge and approval.

Patients who are admitted to the hospital with functional insulin pumps shall work with the physician, nurse, and pharmacist to ensure that the pump is set up appropriately. The patient and/or parent must demonstrate competence in pump use and programming and agree to communicate all insulin doses with the nurse to ensure appropriate administration and documentation. Hospitals shall have a policy to address insulin pumps and their use in the hospital setting.

Standard VII. Monitoring Medication Use

A. Reviewing Patient Responses to Medication Therapy

Medication Therapy Monitoring. Medication therapy monitoring shall be conducted by pharmacists. Medication therapy monitoring includes a proactive assessment of patient problems and an assessment of the following:

- The therapeutic appropriateness of the patient's medication regimen.
- Therapeutic duplication or omissions in the patient's medication regimen.
- The appropriateness of the dose of the medication, as well as the route, method, and frequency of administration of the medication.
- Patient adherence to the prescribed medication regimen.
- Drug–drug, drug–food, drug–dietary supplement, drug–laboratory test, and drug–disease interactions.
- Adverse drug reactions (ADRs) and other undesired effects.[42]
- Patient medication allergies and sensitivities.
- Clinical and pharmacokinetic laboratory data to evaluate the efficacy and safety of medication therapy and to anticipate toxicity and adverse effects.
- Physical signs and clinical symptoms relevant to the patient's medication therapy.
- Assessment of the effectiveness of the patient's medication therapy.

Therapeutic Drug Monitoring. Therapeutic drug monitoring services shall be provided by the pharmacy for all pediatric patients for medications that include, but are not limited to, drugs with a narrow therapeutic window (e.g., vancomycin, aminoglycosides, anticonvulsants, antirejection medications, digoxin), anticoagulation medications, and other medications associated with high rates of adverse events. Any pharmacists caring for pediatric patients must be knowledgeable of the unique pharmacokinetic differences in a pediatric patient, including alterations in absorption, distribution, metabolism, and excretion. The most important of these is the larger volume of distribution for water-soluble drugs (e.g., aminoglycosides), which can significantly affect dosing in younger patients. The pharmacist should ensure that the drug being monitored has been administered appropriately before samples are taken for the measurement of serum drug concentrations. The frequency and timing of sampling should also be coordinated to avoid excessive and traumatic sampling in pediatric patients. Documentation of pharmacokinetic services in a readily accessible format should be completed by the clinical pharmacist with pediatric training.

B. Educating and Counseling Patients and Family

Patient Education. Counseling of pediatric patients and their caregivers is an important role for the pharmacist. For younger patients or patients who lack developmental cognition, the pharmacist may have to focus education toward the caregiver; older children and adolescents will require counseling and education provided at an age-appropriate level. When language barriers exist, interpreters may help communicate with non-English-speaking patients and caregivers.

The education level and general health literacy of the patient and caregiver may also present barriers for verbal or written communication. Medication-related material developed by other services and departments as well as commercial sources should be reviewed by the pharmacy staff for accuracy, currency, literacy appropriateness, and completeness. If necessary, interpretive language services (written or oral) should be made available to patients.[43] Commercially available, pediatric-friendly patient education handouts in multiple languages are warranted in a pediatric health system.

Patients and caregivers should be counseled on medication use both in the inpatient and outpatient settings and should be provided with the following information at a minimum:

- Medication's brand and generic names
- Dosing instructions
- Methods of administration (e.g., crush, chew, apply)
- Information about potential adverse effects and drug interactions
- Proper medication storage
- Strategies to prevent accidental ingestion

Specifically, caregivers shall be instructed in the differences between milliliters and teaspoons for administration amounts. The recommended measurement to be used for liquid formulations is milliliter.[40,44] Adherence shall be emphasized for all patients and caregivers. It is helpful to provide pediatric-specific patient care handouts with dosing instructions for discharge medications and education on the proper use of a pediatric-friendly measuring device (e.g., not the household teaspoon) and the possible options for flavoring medications. During a counseling session, the pharmacist is well positioned to play a role in preventive healthcare, including immunization and poison prevention.[9]

Standard VIII. Evaluating the Effectiveness of the Medication-Use System

There shall be an ongoing, systematic program for quality assessment and improvement of pharmacy services and the medication-use system. The pediatric pharmacy services program should include routinely evaluating the literature for new technologies or successful practices that have been demonstrated to enhance safety in other organizations to determine if such technologies or practices can improve the hospital's medication-use system. This program should be integrated with the hospital's or health system's quality assessment and quality-improvement activities. Quality-improvement activities related to the selection, prescription, procurement, storage, preparation, dispensing, distribution, administration, documentation, monitoring, and use of medications for the pediatric population shall be routinely performed in cooperation with other healthcare providers. Feedback shall be provided to appropriate individuals or entities about the quality achieved.

A. Assessing Pharmacy Services and Practices

Documentation of Pharmacist-Provided Patient Care Services and Medication Therapy Outcomes. The pharmacy shall have an ongoing process for consistent documentation of all pharmacy interventions and the pediatric patient care services provided by pharmacists and patient outcomes from medication therapy.[45] This documentation can serve as objective data supporting the need to hire a full-time pharmacist with pediatric training in a particular area where focused services may not currently exist or optimization of pharmacy resources for the pediatric population is needed.

Workload and Financial Performance. A process shall exist to routinely monitor and document workload and financial performance. Metrics should encompass the full scope of patient care, including the increased workload provided by pharmacists and the pharmacy enterprise. This process should provide for the determination and analysis of hospital and systemwide costs of pediatric medication therapy. A pharmacist should be an integral part of the hospital's leadership teams (e.g., administrative, financial) and report directly to the organization's principal executive.

B. Improving the Medication-Use Process

Medication-Use Evaluation. There shall be an ongoing program for monitoring pediatric drug utilization and costs to ensure that medications are used appropriately, safely, and effectively and to increase the probability of desired patient outcomes. The P&T committee (or its equivalent) should define specific parameters for evaluation (e.g., disease state, pharmacologic category, high-use/high-cost drug products) as appropriate for the organization. Through the ongoing evaluation of pediatric medication use, areas in need of improvement in pediatric medication prescribing and management can be identified and targeted for intervention.[46,47]

Medication Safety. Medication errors are common and costly.[48] Pediatric patients are most vulnerable and are 3 times more likely to be involved in a medication error than adults.[49] Pediatric patients have unique differences in pharmacokinetic and pharmacodynamic responses to medication therapy that put them at higher risk of experiencing ADEs.[49] In addition, there is a lack of ready-to-use medication forms available from manufacturers, and commercially available products often require extensive manipulation, which may include complex calculations, to make them suitable for pediatric patients. Medication dosing is more complex, because most doses are not standardized and are dependent on weight. Infants and children also lack the developmental ability to recognize or describe unintended adverse effects or ADRs should they occur.

Pharmacists shall provide leadership to and participate in collaborative, multidisciplinary efforts to prevent, detect, and resolve drug-related problems that can result in patient harm such as root cause analysis or failure mode and effects analysis. A pharmacist with pediatric training and other appropriate hospital personnel shall establish and regularly revise policies and procedures regarding pediatric medication error and adverse-event prevention and reporting. Monitoring, detecting, review, and analysis of the hospital's and health system's medication errors and near misses should be an ongoing process in a just culture environment, and corresponding corrective actions should be documented.[50] An ongoing program for preventing, monitoring, resolving, and reporting ADEs shall be developed.[42] A pharmacist shall participate in appropriate organizational committees and work with physicians, nurses, administrators, and others to examine and improve systems to ensure that medication-use processes are safe.[47] To ensure the safety of pediatric patients, the pharmacy department shall establish, regularly review and revise, and enforce pediatric-specific requirements for medication management, including considerations for look-alike/sound-alike drugs, high-alert medications, ready-to-administer doses, turnaround times, overrides, and medication storage and labeling.

Systems shall be in place to routinely evaluate medication errors that occur, and interventions should be made to processes to prevent error recurrence. Due to the complex nature of the pediatric medication-use system, including confusing packaging and dosage forms, proactive evaluation of errors reported from other sources (e.g., ISMP, the Joint Commission, the manufacturer) shall be routinely evaluated, and necessary process changes for error prevention should be made. Self-reporting systems for ADEs used in isolation are insufficient. An additional surveillance or trigger-based system shall also be in place to more adequately monitor for and capture events.[51,52]

ADRs. ADRs are defined as unintended responses to a drug that poses harm or other negative patient outcomes.[42] Pharmacies should have a formal and comprehensive program to identify and report ADRs. Effective monitoring and evaluation of ADRs shall be focuses of such programs. ADRs should be reported through FDA's MedWatch program as a part of postmarketing data analysis in addition to internal hospital voluntary reporting mechanisms to ensure appropriate follow-up and evaluation.

Antimicrobial Stewardship and Infection Prevention and Control. There shall be policies and procedures to promote the optimal use of antimicrobial agents, reduce the transmission of infections, and educate health professionals, patients, and the public about these topics. Pharmacists should lead antimicrobial stewardship and infection prevention and control efforts through clinical endeavors focused on proper antimicrobial utilization and membership on relevant multidisciplinary work groups and committees within the health system. Efforts should be made to have a specific pharmacist with pediatric training devoted to antimicrobial stewardship and other infectious diseases programs that focus on the pediatric population.

Pharmacists should monitor patients' laboratory reports of microbial sensitivities or applicable diagnostic markers and advise prescribers if microbial resistance is suspected, evaluate trends in microbial prescribing relative to changes in microbial resistance patterns, and assist in developing prescribing patterns to help minimize the development of drug resistance.[27]

Standard IX. Research

The pharmacist should initiate, participate in, and support clinical and practice-related research appropriate to the goals, objectives, and resources of the specific hospital or health system. Pediatric patients have long been recognized as "therapeutic orphans" because of the relative absence of therapeutic trials in this patient population. The pharmacist must take into consideration that pediatric patients may not be able to provide informed consent and must have a procedure in place to address this vulnerable population. The reasons for this are numerous and include ethical issues, potential adverse publicity, possible litigation, methodological hurdles, and an inability to justify such studies for economic reasons. The advent of the Best Pharmaceuticals for Children Act of 2007[53,54] and additional pediatric formulation initiatives has greatly improved the number of resources available and the amount of research performed in children. The pharmacist with pediatric training can be directly involved in collaboration with other healthcare providers in conducting pediatric research. Examples of pediatric research topics include, but are not limited to, the following:

- Safety and efficacy of drug products in pediatric patients
- Pharmacokinetics and pharmacodynamics of new medications
- Pharmacogenomic considerations and prediction of ADEs
- Stability, safety, and efficacy of extemporaneously compounded sterile and nonsterile drug products
- Safety and efficacy of administration techniques
- Off-label use of medications
- Comparative evaluations of medications addressing treatment regimens, outcomes of therapy, and their relative costs
- Behavioral and socioeconomic adherence issues in pediatric pharmacy care
- New and existing pharmacy drug distribution systems and services for pediatric patients

Examples of direct involvement include, but are not limited to, the following:

- Serving as a member of an institutional review board.
- Maintenance, oversight, and dissemination of all information on investigational drug studies, expanded access programs, and comparative trials involving medications in the pediatric population.
- Maintenance, coordination, and oversight of policies and procedures involving investigational drug studies, expanded access programs, and comparative trials involving medications in the pediatric population.
- Primary or coinvestigator of studies or trials described above.

Conclusion

The unique challenges of the pediatric population require careful consideration for pharmacists and pharmacy departments in hospitals and health systems. Pharmacists caring for pediatric patients must be knowledgeable and competent in pediatric pharmacy. Pharmacy departments must ensure that the elements of pharmacy services meet the pediatric patient needs that are critical to safe, effective, innovative, and cost-conscious medication use in a hospital or health system.

References

1. Pediatric Pharmacy Administrative Group Committee on Pediatric Pharmacy Practice. Pediatric pharmacy practice guidelines. *Am J Hosp Pharm.* 1991; 48:2475–7.
2. American Society of Health-System Pharmacists. ASHP guidelines: minimum standard for pharmacies in hospitals. *Am J Health-Syst Pharm.* 2013; 70:1619–30.

3. American Society of Health-System Pharmacists. ASHP guidelines on remote medication order processing. *Am J Health-Syst Pharm.* 2010; 67:672–7.
4. American Society of Hospital Pharmacists. ASHP technical assistance bulletin on hospital drug distribution and control. *Am J Hosp Pharm.* 1980; 37:1097–103.
5. American Society of Health-System Pharmacists. ASHP guidelines on the pharmacy and therapeutics committee and the formulary system. *Am J Health-Syst Pharm.* 2008; 65:1272–83.
6. American Society of Health-System Pharmacists. ASHP guidelines on the safe use of automated dispensing devices. *Am J Health-Syst Pharm.* 2010; 67:483–90.
7. American Society of Health-System Pharmacists. ASHP statement on the role of health-system pharmacists in emergency preparedness. *Am J Health-Syst Pharm.* 2003; 60:1993–5.
8. American Academy of Pediatrics. Ensuring the health of children in disasters. *Pediatrics.* 2015; 136:e1407–17.
9. American Society of Health-System Pharmacists. ASHP guidelines on the pharmacist's role in immunization. *Am J Health-Syst Pharm.* 2003; 60:1371–7.
10. American Society of Health-System Pharmacists. ASHP residency accreditation. www.ashp.org/Professional-Development/Residency-Information (accessed 2018 Jan 24).
11. ASHP policy position 0916: continuing professional development. In: Hawkins B, ed. Best practices: positions and guidance documents of ASHP. 2016–2017 ed. Bethesda, MD: American Society of Health-System Pharmacists; 2016:150.
12. American Society of Health-System Pharmacists. ASHP guidelines on the recruitment, selection, and retention of pharmacy personnel. *Am J Health-Syst Pharm.* 2003; 60:587–93.
13. Centers for Medicare and Medicaid Services. CMS manual system. www.cms.gov/Regulations-and-guidance/Guidance/Transmittals/Downloads/R151SOMA.pdf (accessed 2018 Jan 24).
14. American Society of Health-System Pharmacists. ASHP guidelines on compounding sterile preparations. *Am J Health-Syst Pharm.* 2014; 71:145–66.
15. American Society of Hospital Pharmacists. ASHP technical assistance bulletin on single unit and unit dose packages of drugs. *Am J Hosp Pharm.* 1985; 42:378–9.
16. American Society of Hospital Pharmacists. ASHP technical assistance bulletin on compounding nonsterile products in pharmacies. *Am J Hosp Pharm.* 1994; 51:1441–8.
17. American Society of Health-System Pharmacists. ASHP guidelines on handling hazardous drugs. *Am J Health-Syst Pharm.* 2006; 63:1172–93.
18. American Society of Hospital Pharmacists. ASHP technical assistance bulletin on repackaging oral solids and liquids in single unit and unit dose packages. *Am J Hosp Pharm.* 1983; 40:451–2.
19. United States Pharmacopeial Convention. General chapter 797—pharmaceutical compounding: sterile preparations. www.usp.org/usp-healthcare-professionals/compounding/compounding-general-chapters/general-chapter-797 (accessed 2018 Jan 24).
20. United States Pharmacopeial Convention. General chapter 795—pharmaceutical compounding: nonsterile preparations. www.usp.org/usp-healthcare-professionals/compounding/general-chapter-795 (accessed 2018 Jan 24).
21. American Society of Hospital Pharmacists. ASHP statement on the use of medications for unlabeled uses. *Am J Hosp Pharm.* 1992; 49:2006–8.
22. 10 Golden rules for administering drugs safely. In: McGovern K. Preventing medication errors. North Wales, PA: Springhouse; 1994:2–3.
23. American Society of Health-System Pharmacists. ASHP statement on bar-code-enabled medication administration technology. *Am J Health-Syst Pharm.* 2009; 66:588–90.
24. Ohashi K, Dallcur O, Dykes PC, Bates DW. Benefits and risks of using smart pumps to reduce medication error rates: a systematic review. *Drug Saf.* 2014; 37:1011–20.
25. Osheroff JA, Teich JM, Levick D et al. Improving outcomes with clinical decision support: an implementer's guide, 2nd ed. Chicago: Healthcare Information and Management Systems Society; 2012.
26. Dumitru D, ed. The pharmacy informatics primer. Bethesda, MD: American Society of Health-System Pharmacists; 2009:48–52.
27. American Society of Health-System Pharmacists. ASHP statement on the pharmacist's role in antimicrobial stewardship and infection prevention and control. *Am J Health-Syst Pharm.* 2010; 67:575–7.
28. American Society of Health-System Pharmacists. ASHP statement on the pharmacist's role in clinical informatics. *Am J Health-Syst Pharm.* 2016; 73:410–3.
29. American Society of Health-System Pharmacists. ASHP statement on the roles and responsibilities of the pharmacy executive. *Am J Health-Syst Pharm.* 2016; 73:329–32.
30. American Society of Health-System Pharmacists. ASHP guidelines on the pharmacist's role in the development, implementation, and assessment of critical pathways. *Am J Health-Syst Pharm.* 2004; 61:939–45.
31. Ghaibi S, Ipema H, Gabay M. ASHP guidelines on the pharmacist's role in providing drug information. *Am J Health-Syst Pharm.* 2015; 72:573–7.
32. American Society of Health-System Pharmacists. ASHP guidelines on surgery and anesthesiology pharmaceutical services. *Am J Health-Syst Pharm.* 1999; 56:887–95.
33. Office of the Law Revision Counsel, United States House of Representatives. 42 U.S.C. Sec. 299b-35(c). MTM services to eligible individuals. http://uscode.house.gov/view.xhtml?req=MTM+services+to+eligible+individuals&f=treesort&fq=true&num=0&hl=true&edition=prelim&granuleId=USC-prelim-title42-section299b-35 (accessed 2018 Jan 24).

34. American Society of Health-System Pharmacists. ASHP Drug Shortages Resource Center. www.ashp.org/Drug-Shortages (accessed 2018 Jan 24).
35. Food and Drug Administration. Drug shortages. www.fda.gov/cder/drug/shortages/ (accessed 2018 Jan 24).
36. American Society of Health-System Pharmacists. ASHP guidelines on managing drug product shortages in hospitals and health systems. *Am J Health-Syst Pharm.* 2009; 66:1399–406.
37. U.S. Pharmacopeial Convention. General chapter 800—hazardous drugs handling in healthcare settings. www.usp.org/usp-healthcare-professionals/compounding/compounding-general-chapters/usp-general-chapter-hazardous-drugs-handling-healthcare-se (accessed 2018 Jan 24).
38. American Society of Health-System Pharmacists. ASHP guidelines on outsourcing sterile compounding services. *Am J Health-Syst Pharm.* 2015; 72:1664–75.
39. American Society of Health-System Pharmacists. ASHP statement on bar-code verification during inventory, preparation, and dispensing of medications. *Am J Health-Syst Pharm.* 2011; 68:442–5.
40. Institute for Safe Medication Practices. ISMP statement on use of metric measurements to prevent errors with oral liquids (October 2011). www.ismp.org/pressroom/PR20110808.pdf (accessed 2018 Jan 24).
41. Elements of performance 2 and 3 for information management standard IM.02.02.01. In: Comprehensive accreditation manual for hospitals. Oakbrook Terrace, IL: Joint Commission; 2012:IM-02-02-01.
42. American Society of Health-System Pharmacists. ASHP guidelines on adverse drug reaction monitoring and reporting. *Am J Health-Syst Pharm.* 1995; 52:417–9.
43. American Society of Health-System Pharmacists. ASHP guidelines on pharmacist-conducted patient education and counseling. *Am J Health-Syst Pharm.* 1997; 54:431–4.
44. American Academy of Pediatrics. Metric units and the preferred dosing of orally administered liquid medications. *Pediatrics.* 2015; 135:D1–5.
45. American Society of Health-System Pharmacists. ASHP guidelines on documenting pharmaceutical care in patient medical records. *Am J Health-Syst Pharm.* 2003; 60:705–7.
46. American Society of Health-System Pharmacists. ASHP guidelines on medication cost management strategies for hospitals and health systems. *Am J Health-Syst Pharm.* 2008; 65:1368–84.
47. American Society of Health-System Pharmacists. ASHP guidelines on medication-use evaluation. *Am J Health-Syst Pharm.* 1996; 53:1953–5.
48. Kohn LT, Corrigan JM, Donaldson MS, eds. To err is human: building a safer health system. Washington, DC: National Academy Press; 1999.
49. Kaushal R, Bates DW, Landrigan C, et al. Medication errors and ADEs in pediatric inpatients. *JAMA.* 2001; 285:2114–20.
50. Khatri N, Brown GD, Hicks LL. From a blame culture to a just culture in health care. *Health Care Manage Rev.* 2009; 34:312–22.
51. Takata GS, Mason W, Taketomo C, et al. Development, testing, and findings of a pediatric-focused trigger tool to identify medication-related harm in US children's hospitals. *Pediatrics.* 2008; 121:e927–35.
52. Institute for Healthcare Improvement. IHI global trigger tool for measuring adverse events. www.ihi.org/resources/pages/tools/ihiglobaltriggertool formeasuringaes.aspx (accessed 2018 Jan 24).
53. Best Pharmaceuticals for Children Act of 2007, title V, Sept. 27, 2007; 121 Stat. 876.
54. S. 650, 108th Congress: Pediatric Research Equity Act of 2003. www.govtrack.us/congress/bills/108/s650 (accessed 2018 Jan 24).

Developed through the ASHP Section of Clinical Scientists and Specialists and PPAG and approved by the ASHP Board of Directors on October 23, 2017. This document supersedes a previous version approved by the ASHP Board of Directors on April 27, 1994.

Lea S. Eiland, Pharm.D., BCPS, BCPPS, FASHP, FPPAG, Auburn University Harrison School of Pharmacy, Auburn, AL.

Kim Benner, Pharm.D., BCPS, FASHP, FPPAG, Samford University McWhorter School of Pharmacy, Birmingham, AL.

Karl F. Gumpper, M.S.M.I., BCPS, CPHIMS, FASHP, Boston Children's Hospital, Boston, MA.

Melissa K. Heigham, Pharm.D., M.H.A., BCOP, BCPPS, St. Louis Children's Hospital, St. Louis, MO.

Rachel Meyers, Pharm.D., BCPS, BCPPS, Ernest Mario School of Pharmacy, Rutgers, The State University of New Jersey, Saint Barnabas Medical Center, Piscataway, NJ.

Katherine Pham, Pharm.D., BCPPS, Children's National Medical Center, Washington, DC.

Amy L. Potts, Pharm.D., BCPS, Vanderbilt Children's Hospital Pharmacy, Nashville, TN.

The contributions of Eric Rose, Pharm.D., PMP, are acknowledged.

ASHP gratefully acknowledges the following organizations and individuals for reviewing these guidelines (review does not imply endorsement): American Pharmacists Association; Ascension; ISMP; Kentucky Society of Health System Pharmacists; National Healthcareer Association; Valley Children's Hospital; James L. Besier, Ph.D., M.S., B.S.Pharm., FASHP; Carly Brown, Pharm.D., BCPS; Derek R. Burns, Pharm.D., BCPS; Christopher T. Campbell, Pharm.D.; Mary Petrea Cober, Pharm.D., BCNSP, BCPPS; Justin W. Cole, Pharm.D., BCPS; Michele Corriveau, B.S.Pharm.; Jeffrey Goff, M.S.; Charlene Hope, Pharm.D., M.S., BCPS; Peter Johnson, Pharm.D., BCPS, BCPPS, FPAG; Julie Kasap, Pharm.D., BCPPS; Susannah E. Koontz, Pharm.D., BCOP, FHOPA; Ken Kurek, Pharm.D.; Carlton K. K. Lee, Pharm.D., M.P.H., FASHP, FPPAG; Nancy C. MacDonald, Pharm.D., BCPS; Shannon Manzi, Pharm.D., FPPAG; Patrick McDonnell, Pharm.D., FASHP; Julie Neuman, Pharm.D.; Penny Ngo, Pharm.D.; Barbara Petroff, M.S., FASHP; James Ponto, M.S., BCNP, FASHP; Robert Poole, Pharm.D., FPPAG, FCSHP, FASHP; James R. Rinehart, M.S., FASHP; LCDR Teisha A. Robertson, Pharm.D., M.B.A.; Colleen Smith, Pharm.D., BCPPS, FCCM; Christine Steffensen, Pharm.D., M.A., BCPPS; James Stevenson, Pharm.D., FASHP; Sharon Ternullo, Pharm.D., DABAT; Courtney Terry, Pharm.D., BCPS; Carol G. Vetterly, Pharm.D., BCPS, BCPPS; Jody Jacobson Wedret, B.S.Pharm., FASHP, FCSHP; Wyn Wheeler, Pharm.D., BCPPS, FCCM; and Ed Wong, Pharm.D.

The authors have declared no potential conflicts of interest.

At the time of writing, Dr. Pharm was affiliated with the Pew Charitable Trust, Washington, DC.

Copyright © 2018, American Society of Health-System Pharmacists, Inc., and the Pediatric Pharmacy Advocacy Group. All rights reserved. Contact ASHP for reprint and permissions requests. This content may not be used for commercial purposes without the express written consent of ASHP.

The bibliographic citation for this document is as follows: American Society of Health-System Pharmacists. ASHP–PPAG guidelines for providing pediatric pharmacy services in hospitals and health systems. *Am J Health-Syst Pharm.* 2018; 75:1151–65.

ASHP-HOPA Guidelines on the Roles and Responsibilities of the Pharmacy Technician in Ambulatory Oncology Pharmacy

The roles and responsibilities of the pharmacy technician in ambulatory oncology practice have evolved considerably over the past several decades. Historically, technician roles consisted mainly of compounding and technical activities, but technicians in the ambulatory oncology setting currently serve in a variety of advanced roles.[1] A number of recent changes and initiatives, including the expansion of pharmacy services, an increase in the utilization of oral anticancer medications, greater focus on quality improvement, and the growing role of technology in pharmacy operations, have expanded the scope of the technician's role and created the need for advanced, well-trained technicians to support these functions.[2] Pharmacy technicians provide integral support to pharmacy staff, allowing for streamlined workflow and increased operational and technological oversight of pharmacy functions while maintaining high-quality patient care. The Hematology/Oncology Pharmacy Association (HOPA) and the American Society of Health-System Pharmacists (ASHP) have partnered to define the roles and responsibilities of pharmacy technicians in the ambulatory oncology setting to promote standardization and further advancement and expansion of ambulatory oncology pharmacy practice.

The ambulatory oncology setting is a complex care environment with a variety of models for the role of the pharmacy technician, and there is minimal guidance and evidence-based literature to support a particular practice model. For the purposes of these guidelines, the ambulatory setting is defined as an outpatient patient care setting, including community-based and academia-affiliated settings. Because the vast majority of cancer care is delivered in the ambulatory setting,[3] it is particularly important to establish guidelines to promote pharmacy technicians as a readily available resource, with the goal of optimizing the delivery of pharmacy services in this environment.

Nationwide variations in the regulatory aspects of drug preparation and dispensing demonstrate a need for the universal adoption of standardized guidelines. In addition, rapidly changing practice standards, such as the anticipated impact of United States Pharmacopeia (*USP*) chapter 800[4] on the handling of hazardous drugs, further emphasize the necessity of standardized recommendations. Nevertheless, although these guidelines are generally applicable, pharmacists and other healthcare professionals responsible for the selection, preparation, dispensing, and administration of drugs are urged to exercise professional judgment in interpreting and applying these guidelines to their specific circumstances, especially regarding compliance with applicable laws and regulations concerning the delegation of responsibilities to pharmacy technicians. Users of these guidelines are cautioned that the information provided is current as of publication and are urged to consult current editions of original sources (e.g., laws; regulations; applicable standards, including *USP* compendial standards) to ensure patient safety as well as legal and regulatory compliance.

The focus of these guidelines is to define the role and scope of the pharmacy technician in an ambulatory oncology pharmacy setting; however, the principles of this document may be applied to other areas in which technicians contribute to pharmacy practice. It is intended to supplement documents such as the "ASHP Statement on the Roles of Pharmacy Technicians"[5] and ASHP's summary of the 2017 Pharmacy Technician Stakeholder Consensus Conference,[6] which broadly covers the roles of technicians in all settings of pharmacy practice. The current document provides recommendations regarding a number of areas of technician practice within the ambulatory oncology setting, including education and training; medication compounding, dispensing, and distribution; patient care services; revenue cycle optimization; supply chain management; technology and informatics; and quality improvement.

Education and Training

Education and training recommendations for pharmacy technicians have increased with the advancement of pharmacy technician roles. ASHP has advocated for advanced technician roles within the ASHP Practice Advancement Initiative. The components of this initiative address the need for pharmacy technicians to have appropriate training and credentials for medication preparation and distribution and for the performance of other functions not necessarily requiring a pharmacist's professional judgment.[7] Other countries, such as Canada, have a standardized accreditation process for pharmacy technician programs; only individuals completing the prescribed process are allowed to practice as technicians.[8] While similar standardization of technician competency certification has been advocated for in the United States by pharmacy organization leadership, efforts are still in progress.[6,9] ASHP and the Accreditation Council for Pharmacy Education established the Pharmacy Technician Accreditation Commission (PTAC) to advance the quality of technician education and training programs.[10]

The Pharmacy Technician Certification Board (PTCB) was created in 1995 with the goal of certifying technicians to support pharmacists and patient care efforts in all practice settings.[11,12] Technicians become certified by achieving a passing score on the Pharmacy Technician Certification Exam. However, certification is not regulated or standardized in the United States. As of 2015, 45 states registered or licensed pharmacy technicians; in 23 states, it may be necessary for technicians to be certified by PTCB to become licensed through the state board of pharmacy.[13] Results from a cross-sectional study revealed that there are currently over 698 pharmacy technician training programs in the United States.[12] Of 216 programs that provided complete data, 29.6% were accredited by ASHP, 65.3% were affiliated with PTCB, and 24.5% were both accredited by ASHP and affiliated with PTCB.[12] Clearly, there is a need for standardized,

DOI 10.37573/9781585287048.082

accredited training of technicians; PTAC was created to address this deficiency.[10]

Given the complexity of the ambulatory oncology setting and varied roles of pharmacy technicians in the workplace, data regarding education and training are sparse. A survey specific to oncology pharmacy services was distributed to 41 U.S. institutions designated by the National Cancer Institute to assess their progress toward transforming pharmacy practice as recommended by the ASHP Practice Advancement Initiative.[7] Results from half of the surveyed institutions indicated the existence of roles for technicians in the distribution and performance of other functions not necessarily requiring a pharmacist's professional judgment. Only 39% indicated that technician preparation and distribution tasks were assigned in a manner that allowed pharmacists to provide more direct patient care.[7] Standardized, accredited training of technicians in the manner proposed by PTAC will help ensure safe practices to patients and stakeholders and move the profession forward for pharmacists and technicians.

The **appendix** summarizes ASHP-HOPA recommendations regarding education and training, including general and specialized training and certification, proof of competency, and compliance.

Medication Compounding, Dispensing, and Distribution

Throughout the years, pharmacy technicians have played an essential role in the preparation, compounding, dispensing, and distribution of sterile and nonsterile hazardous medications in the ambulatory oncology setting. Pharmacy technicians are often vital to other pharmacy roles such as inventory management and oversight of automated dispensing machines. It is critical that technicians receive adequate education and training to follow safe practices ensuring patients receive quality medications and technicians, patients, and the public are protected from hazardous medication exposure. To ensure these safe practices are carried out, healthcare organizations must engage pharmacy technicians to incorporate safe medication preparation, handling, and distribution processes for hazardous medications, including disposal and documentation. The 2004 National Institute for Occupational Safety and Health (NIOSH) Alert initially warned healthcare workers about the risks of working with hazardous drugs and recommended methods and equipment for protecting their health.[20] Subsequent NIOSH updates have continued to encourage the identification and safe handling procedures of hazardous medications.[25–27] *USP* chapter 797 has established standards for preparing medications, including some standards on safely handling hazardous medications.[28] *USP* chapter 800 further provides additional standards for frontline workers who handle hazardous medications.[4] The "ASHP Guidelines on Handling Hazardous Drugs" provides guidance based on sources.[21] Engaging pharmacy technicians to help operationalize workflow while adhering to regulations will help optimize processes for medication compounding, dispensing, and distribution.

The appendix summarizes ASHP-HOPA recommendations regarding pharmacy technicians' roles in medication compounding, dispensing, and distribution in ambulatory oncology settings, including drug preparation, handling of hazardous waste, documentation, and pump management.

Patient Care Services

Patients being treated in ambulatory oncology settings face many challenges related to the safe and effective use of medications. Pharmacy technicians have the skills and knowledge to help patients navigate many of these challenges. Patients who are receiving chemotherapy (i.v. or oral) are at high risk for experiencing medication errors and interactions; thus, it is important that an accurate medication history is recorded and subsequent reconciliation is performed.[29] Pharmacy technicians can assist in the collection of medication histories, including serving in a lead role for conducting patient interviews.[5,30–33] During this interview, technicians should follow a standardized script to ensure that appropriate information is obtained. In addition, technicians can have an integral role in monitoring patients initiated or maintained on oral anticancer medications, using a standardized script to uncover toxicities that may benefit from pharmacist intervention and reinforcing the importance of adherence to medication regimens.

An additional barrier encountered by patients when obtaining oncology medications revolves around Food and Drug Administration (FDA) risk evaluation and mitigation strategy (REMS) programs. Each REMS program has a defined set of requirements; pharmacy technicians can assist with navigating the requirements and coordinating completion, such as ensuring distribution of medication guides and providing contact information and schedules for patient follow-up.

Finally, pharmacy technicians' responsibility for many investigational medication procedures has become routine throughout healthcare. These individuals assist in the management of clinical investigational drug inventories, provide technical direction and assistance with clinical trial protocols, maintain information and record keeping required by study protocols, prepare investigational products for dispensing, and perform education and training of pharmacy team members pursuant to study protocol requirements.[34]

The appendix summarizes ASHP-HOPA recommendations regarding pharmacy technicians' roles in providing patient care services in ambulatory oncology settings, including medication histories and reconciliation, oral anticancer medication patient outreach, REMS program requirements, and investigational drug management.

Revenue Cycle Optimization

Revenue cycle optimization has become a critical focus for the pharmacy enterprise. Pharmacy technicians, especially those with a background in finances and auditing, play a key role in the management of the business of pharmacy.[5] Key aspects to ambulatory oncology pharmacy include prior authorization of clinic-administered medications and specialty pharmacy medications, validation of drug claims through revenue work queues (e.g., JW modifiers, Healthcare Common Procedure Coding System codes), and management of denied claims.

Healthcare organizations have undertaken efforts to optimize product selection when compounding infusion medications (e.g., dose vial rounding, maximizing vial selection) and minimizing waste for expensive chemotherapy and biologics. A pharmacy technician, under the supervision of a pharmacist, can work to minimize medication waste by participating on an interdisciplinary waste management team, monitoring compliance with policies and procedures, and optimizing drug use through scheduling coordination.[35] Technicians may oversee inventory management to avoid the use of products after their expiration dates, coordinate product replacement acquisition, and reverse distribution processes to minimize financial loss from unavoidable waste. As of January 1, 2017, claims for certain discarded drug or biologic amounts not administered to any patient have to be submitted using the JW modifier.[36] This creates an ongoing regulatory compliance issue, which would be an important function assigned to pharmacy technicians to ensure compliance from the point of dispensation to charge.[37]

The process for obtaining expensive medications used to treat cancer patients has become increasingly complicated. As new oncology medications are approved, many require users to navigate the requirements of a limited distribution network, which can create barriers to medication access for patients and healthcare organizations. Pharmacy technicians, under the supervision of a pharmacist, can review financial claim requests and manage records to ensure that financial approval, including any necessary prior authorization, is obtained in advance of medication administration.[38] Technician involvement in these activities may improve patient care fragmentation, enhance advocacy and logistics support for patients and providers, and enhance top-of-license activities for other healthcare providers. For patients who cannot afford specific medications, pharmacy technicians can lead efforts to connect patients with financial assistance programs or receive medications from manufacturers.[5]

Finally, pharmacy technicians can play a key role in off-label medication use. Those practicing in the ambulatory oncology setting recognize the dynamic nature between clinical literature, the use of medications in off-label prescribing, and the timeline for guideline updating. Technicians are instrumental in completing paperwork and tracking drug replacement acquired for off-label indications, providing billing support, and managing inventory across various access channels (e.g., traditional wholesaler, manufacturer, limited distribution network).

The appendix summarizes ASHP-HOPA recommendations regarding pharmacy technicians' roles in revenue cycle optimization in ambulatory oncology settings, including therapy authorization, patient financial assistance, and minimization of medication waste.

Supply Chain Management

Pharmacy technicians play a pivotal role in supply chain management of oncology and supportive care medications and supplies necessary to compound these drugs. Supply chain management responsibilities that may be led by pharmacy technicians include purchasing or procurement, inventory control, and drug shortage management.[5,39]

Current chemotherapy medications often require complicated purchasing approaches, including navigation of complicated vendor, group purchasing organization, and manufacturer contracts across the outpatient and inpatient settings. Drug distribution models are often supported by pharmacy technicians responsible for purchasing products within cancer centers, including navigating potential challenges of high costs and accessibility.[2]

In addition to purchasing, technicians play a crucial role in inventory control with the storage and tracking of therapies for oncology treatment. An important inventory control consideration is product expiration dating; technicians should ensure that no expired product is stocked. Strategies to minimize expired products include calculation of inventory par levels based on medication turnover rates and consideration of length of product dating when ordering.[40] In addition to expiration dating, pharmacy technicians should promote adequate medication turnover by forecasting anticipated use and setting par levels accordingly. Lastly, when receiving any product, technicians should ensure that any products requiring special storage conditions, such as freezing or refrigeration, should be identified and stored properly.

Finally, pharmacy technicians play a critical role in the management of drug shortages.[39] Drug shortages are increasingly common, particularly with high-cost oncology medications.[41,42] A 2011 survey revealed that both pharmacists and pharmacy technicians spend an average of 8–9 hours per week handling issues related to drug shortages.[43] Pharmacy technicians can help manage organizational approaches to shortages, including managing purchasing workflows and investigating alternative procurement strategies using ASHP and FDA resources.[44]

The appendix summarizes ASHP-HOPA recommendations regarding pharmacy technicians' roles in supply chain management in ambulatory oncology settings, including purchasing, managing inventory control, and responding to drug shortages.

Technology and Informatics

Informatics is a growing space within the national workforce and in pharmacy practice. In addition, pharmacy services have continued to see the increased utilization of technology, both software and hardware, throughout the pharmacy enterprise. Specialty-trained pharmacy technicians can assume roles in pharmacy informatics.[23] Domains may include automation and technology systems management, supervision of projects, policy and governance, customer service, charge integrity, reporting interface/database management, automation management, new technology assessment, workflow optimization, and end-user training and education.[23] These roles will be vital in the implementation and maintenance of technology systems management in the oncology setting. Examples include i.v. workflow systems and interface/database management between the electronic health record and pharmacy automation.

Outside of large municipalities, healthcare organizations continue to struggle with sustainability and access to pharmacy services. As onsite pharmacy services might not be cost-effective for all entities, telepharmacy has become an important cost-effective alternative to allow the provision of some onsite pharmacy services. With the advent of technology and workflow solutions, pharmacy technicians now have the ability to prepare i.v. medications following *USP* guidelines pursuant to medication orders under the supervision of a remote pharmacist.

The appendix summarizes ASHP-HOPA recommendations regarding pharmacy technicians' roles in technology and informatics in ambulatory oncology settings, including automation and technology systems management and telepharmacy services.

Quality Improvement

Healthcare delivery is a complex process involving many integrated and interdependent steps, each of which has the potential to fail. In all healthcare organizations, continuous monitoring of medical care processes, including medication management, is critical to the identification and prevention of errors. Pharmacists have often been one of the key point members of this process, but, with expanding roles, pharmacy technicians are also positioned to address quality review, improvement implementation, quality-assurance evaluations, and metrics implementation.[5]

In the oncology pharmacy setting, a variety of equipment is used for many different processes.[21] Environmental monitoring is critical for compliance with *USP* chapters 797 and 800 for sterile i.v. compounding.[4,28] Oncology pharmacy technicians are often at the forefront of monitoring and evaluating compliance of pharmacy equipment used in the oncology setting. This responsibility includes monitoring engineering controls, environmental monitoring, monitoring the quality of sterile preparations, and equipment monitoring. Policies and procedures for the evaluation, selection, use, calibration, monitoring, and maintenance of these systems will be followed by pharmacy technicians based on applicable regulations and state board of pharmacy laws.[45–47]

The appendix summarizes ASHP-HOPA recommendations regarding pharmacy technicians' roles in quality improvement in ambulatory oncology settings, including error-prevention strategies and the monitoring of equipment and storage facility temperatures.

Conclusion

The role of pharmacy technicians in the ambulatory oncology setting has grown considerably in recent years to support increased operational needs, especially with implementation of *USP* chapters 797 and 800, as well as the growing need for pharmacy involvement with patient and caregiver services. To support technicians in this advanced role, education and training should include a structured pharmacy technician training program, certification by PTCB, and completion of formal oncology-specific job training. As the oncology environment has increased in complexity, the role of the pharmacy technician has expanded beyond traditional needs with medication compounding, dispensing, and distribution. Technicians can contribute to ambulatory oncology pharmacy practice through involvement in additional areas of pharmacy practice, including patient and caregiver education and services, financial aspects such as revenue cycle, technology and informatics, quality improvement, and inventory management. Activities outlined in these guidelines highlight the expanding technician role in the ambulatory oncology setting and depth of opportunity for technicians' contributions to the medication-use process.

References

1. Council on Credentialing in Pharmacy. 2002 white paper on pharmacy technicians: needed changes can no longer wait. *J Manag Care Pharm.* 2003; 9:72–83.
2. Friesner DL, Scott DM. Identifying characteristics that allow pharmacy technicians to assume unconventional roles in the pharmacy. *J Am Pharm Assoc.* 2010; 50:686–97.
3. Association of National Account Care Executives. Cancer care migrates to outpatient setting (May 16, 2011). www.jhconline.com/cancer-care-migrates-to-outpatient-setting-2.html (accessed 2017 Jun 23).
4. Hazardous drugs—handling in healthcare settings (general chapter 800). In: The United States pharmacopeia, 39th rev., and The national formulary, 34th ed. First supplement. Rockville, MD: United States Pharmacopeial Convention; 2016.
5. Schultz JM, Jeter CK, Martin NM, et al. ASHP statement on the roles of pharmacy technicians. *Am J Health-Syst Pharm.* 2016; 73:928–30.
6. Zellmer WA, McAllister EB, Silvester JA, et al. Toward uniform standards for pharmacy technicians: summary of the 2017 Pharmacy Technician Stakeholder Consensus Conference. *Am J Health-Syst Pharm.* 2017; 74:e377–91.
7. Smith MB, Gumpper KF, Riebandt G, Handel EM. Implementation of the pharmacy practice model initiative within comprehensive cancer centers. *Am J Health Syst Pharm.* 2014; 71:1647–60.
8. The Canadian Council for Accreditation of Pharmacy Programs. CCAPP standards for accreditation of pharmacy technician programs in Canada (revised August 2015). http://ccapp-accredit.ca/pharmacy-technician-programs/ (accessed 2017 Jul 5).
9. Manasse HR, Menighan TE. Single standard for education, training, and certification of pharmacy technicians. *Am J Health-Syst Pharm.* 2010; 67:348–9.
10. American Society of Health-System Pharmacists. ASHP and ACPE update pharmacy technician accreditation standards (December 10, 2015). www.pharmacist.com/article/ashp-and-acpe-update-pharmacy-technician-accreditation-standards (accessed 2018 May 23).
11. Anderson DC, Draime JA, Anderson TS. Description and comparison of pharmacy technician training programs in the United States. *J Am Pharm Assoc.* 2016; 56:231–6.
12. Pharmacy Technician Certification Board. Mission statement. www.ptcb.org/about-ptcb#.V2v8HvkrLcs (accessed 2017 Jul 5).
13. Pharmacy Technician Certification Board. Pharmacy technician state regulations. www.ptcb.org/resources/cpht-toolkit/state-regulations#.V2v-iPkrLct (accessed 2017 Jul 5).
14. Ballington DA, Green DA, eds. Pharmacy calculations for technicians, 5th ed. St Paul, MN: Paradigm; 2014.
15. Chabner DE. Medical terminology: a short course, 7th ed. Cambridge, MA: Elsevier; 2015.
16. Wallace L. Basics of aseptic compounding technique video training program. Bethesda, MD: American Society of Health-System Pharmacists; 2006.
17. Buchanan EC, Schneider PJ. Compounding sterile preparations. Bethesda, MD: American Society of Health-System Pharmacists; 2009.
18. Therapeutic Research Center. *Pharmacy Technician's Letter.* https://pharmacytech.therapeuticresearch.com/home/experience/PTL (accessed 2017 Jun 23).
19. American Society of Health-System Pharmacists. PharmacyTechCE. www.pharmacytechce.org/ (accessed 2017 Jun 23).

20. National Institute for Occupational Safety and Health. NIOSH alert: preventing occupational exposure to antineoplastic and other hazardous drugs in health care settings. www.cdc.gov/niosh/docs/2004-165/ (accessed 2017 Jun 20).
21. American Society of Health System Pharmacists. ASHP guidelines on handling hazardous drugs. *Am J Health-Syst Pharm.* 2006; 63:1172–93.
22. Goodin S, Griffith N, Chen B, et al. Safe handling of oral chemotherapeutic agents in clinical practice: recommendations from an international pharmacy panel. *J Oncol Pract.* 2011; 7:7–12.
23. American Society of Health-System Pharmacists. ASHP statement on the pharmacy technician's role in pharmacy informatics. *Am J Health-Syst Pharm.* 2014; 71:247–50.
24. Alexander E, Butler CD, Darr A, et al. ASHP statement on telepharmacy. *Am J Health-Syst Pharm.* 2017; 74:e236–41.
25. Centers for Disease Control and Prevention. NIOSH list of antineoplastic and other hazardous drugs in healthcare settings 2014: proposed additions and deletions to the NIOSH hazardous drug list (June 3, 2013). www.cdc.gov/niosh/docket/review/docket233/pdf/CDC-2013-0007.pdf (accessed 2017 Mar 30).
26. National Institute for Occupational Safety and Health. NIOSH list of antineoplastic and other hazardous drugs in healthcare settings, 2014. www.cdc.gov/niosh/docs/2014-138/default.html (accessed 2017 Mar 30).
27. National Institute for Occupational Safety and Health. NIOSH list of antineoplastic and other hazardous drugs in healthcare settings, 2016. www.cdc.gov/niosh/docs/2016-161/default.html (accessed 2017 Mar 30).
28. Pharmaceutical compounding—sterile preparations (general chapter 797). In: United States pharmacopeia, 31st rev., and The national formulary, 26th ed. Rockville, MD: United States Pharmacopeial Convention; 2008.
29. Weingart S, Cleary A, Seger A, et al. Medication reconciliation in ambulatory oncology. *Jt Comm J Qual Patient Saf.* 2007; 33:750–8.
30. Irwin AN, Ham YY, Gerrity TM. Expanded roles for pharmacy technicians in the medication reconciliation process: a qualitative review. *Hosp Pharm.* 2017; 52:44–53.
31. Vega T, Sierra-Sanchez J, Martinez-Bautista M, et al. Medication reconciliation in oncological patients: a randomized clinical trial. *J Manag Care Spec Pharm.* 2016; 22:734–40.
32. Michels RD, Meisel SB. Program using pharmacy technicians to obtain medication histories. *Am J Health-Syst Pharm.* 2003; 60:1982–6.
33. Van den Bemt PM, van den Broek S, van Nunen AK, et al. Medication reconciliation performed by pharmacy technicians at the time of preoperative screening. *Ann Pharmacother.* 2009; 43:868–74.
34. Hematology/Oncology Pharmacy Association. HOPA investigational drug service best practice standards (2014). www.hoparx.org/images/hopa/resource-library/professional-tools/HOPA16_IDS_Guidelines.pdf (accessed 2017 Jun 20).
35. Fasola G, Aprile G, Marini L, et al. Drug minimization as an effective strategy of cost-containment in oncology. *BMC Health Serv Res.* 2014; 14:57.
36. Rinkle VA. CMS requires modifier-JW starting July 1. https://revenuecycleadvisor.com/news-analysis/cms-requires-modifier-jw-starting-july-1 (accessed 2017 Jun 20).
37. Centers for Medicare and Medicaid Services. Medicare program JW modifier: drug/biological amount discarded/not administered to any patient: frequently asked questions. www.cms.gov/medicare/medicare-fee-for-service-payment/hospitaloutpatientpps/downloads/jw-modifier-faqs.pdf (accessed 2017 Jun 20).
38. ASHP Practice Advancement Initiative. Advanced pharmacy technician role: ambulatory medication prior authorization coordinator. www.ashpmedia.org/pai/docs/Case-Study-Ambulatory-Medication-Prior-Authorization-Coordinator-Advanced-Technician-Role.pdf (accessed 2017 Jun 20).
39. Mangan MN, Powers MF. Drug shortages and the role of the pharmacy technician: a review. *J Pharm Tech.* 2011; 27:247–50.
40. Montesarchio V, Grimaldi AM, Fox BA, et al. Lean oncology: a new model for oncologists. *J Transl Med.* 2012; 10:74.
41. Kantarjian H. Chemotherapy drug shortages in the United States revisited. *J Oncol Pract.* 2014; 5:329–31.
42. McBride A, Holle LM, Westendorf C, et al. National survey on the effect of oncology drug shortages on cancer care. *Am J Health-Syst Pharm.* 2013; 70:609–17.
43. Kaakeh R, Sweet BV, Reilly C, et al. Impact of drug shortages on U.S. health systems. *Am J Health-Syst Pharm.* 2011; 68:1811–9.
44. Fox ER, Birt A, James KB, et al. ASHP guidelines on managing drug product shortages in hospitals and health systems. *Am J Health-Syst Pharm.* 2009; 66:1399–406.
45. American Society of Health-System Pharmacists. ASHP guidelines on the safe use of automated compounding devices for the preparation of parenteral nutrition admixtures. *Am J Health-Syst Pharm.* 2000; 57:1343–8.
46. American Society of Health-System Pharmacists. ASHP guidelines on pharmacy planning for implementation of computerized provider order entry systems in hospitals and health systems. *Am J Health-Syst Pharm.* 2011; 68:e9–31.
47. American Society of Health-System Pharmacists. ASHP guidelines on the safe use of automated dispensing devices. *Am J Health-Syst Pharm.* 2010; 67:483–90.

Appendix—ASHP-HOPA Recommendations for Pharmacy Technician Roles In Ambulatory Oncology Settings[a]

Education and Training

General Training and Certification

1. All pharmacy technicians shall complete a pharmacy technician training program accredited by ASHP and the Accreditation Council for Pharmacy Education and earn and maintain PTCB certification.[12,13]
2. Technicians may attain the necessary knowledge base in a variety of ways, ranging from on-the-job training to online or publication-based training, employer-based structured didactic learning, and formalized study with programs that may or may not have proper professional accreditation status.
3. The importance of specialized training, including in the oncology setting, should be emphasized within these applicable training programs.
4. Education and training requirements must reflect the responsibilities the technicians will have in their daily activities.

Specialized Training and Certification

1. Technicians in the ambulatory oncology setting should receive training through a formalized process through either an internal or an external pharmacy technician education program.
2. An ideal, well-rounded technician training program should include elements of didactic and experiential education.
   a. Oncology-specific training shall be a component of the program.
   b. Technician competencies relevant for ambulatory oncology include mastery of pharmacy calculations and medical and pharmacy terminology.[14,15]
   c. Essential components of training for compounding roles are practicum experiences that address techniques in aseptic compounding and handling of hazardous drugs.
   d. Technician should gain these experiences during training and receive evaluations that include feedback on technique.[16,17]
   e. Pharmacy technicians shall undergo site-specific training to the specific roles and responsibilities that they will perform.
   f. Technicians and personnel involved in designing training programs should review updated resources related to compounding from regulatory bodies as regulations surrounding compounding continue to evolve as well as resources from ASHP, HOPA, and other authoritative organizations.
3. If PTCB designates for specialty certification any relevant practice area (e.g., compounding or oncology), technicians should successfully complete the appropriate certifications before practicing in that specialty area.

Proof of Competency

Employers of pharmacy technicians should maintain pharmacy-technician-specific proof of initial and ongoing (e.g., annual) competency to ensure to stakeholders and the public that the technicians are practicing to the best of their abilities.

   a. Some resources for general continuing education include *Pharmacy Technician's Letter*[18] and pharmacy technician continuing education provided by ASHP.[19]
   b. Quality measures should be employed to assess the accuracy of the pharmacy technician's performance.

Compliance

In a manner similar to pharmacists, pharmacy technicians must comply with state licensure and registration regulations and requirements, including those regarding education, training, and certification. It is the technician's responsibility to be familiar with and meet state requirements. PTCB has resources to assist with keeping track of these requirements.[13]

Medication Compounding, Dispensing, and Distribution

Drug Preparation

1. I.V. anticancer medications
   a. Pharmacy technicians should share responsibility for ensuring safe preparation and dispensing of i.v. anticancer medications.
   b. Technicians should practice correct usage of PPE, including compliance with regulatory requirements mandating PPE be donned across all aspects of hazardous drug handling.[4]
   c. Pharmacy technicians should play a role in embracing CSTDs for preparation of anticancer medications, including involvement in the evaluation process and familiarity with regulatory standards.[4]
2. Oral anticancer medications
   a. Technicians shall dispense oral anticancer medications according to best practice recommendations, including those of ASHP, NIOSH, and *USP* chapter 800, including use of disposable gloves and restricting product manipulation to performance within a PEC involving use of PPE.[4,20–22]
   b. Technicians shall be familiar with storage requirements, including separation of hazardous drugs from nonhazardous drugs, recommended by ASHP, NIOSH, and *USP* chapter 800.[4,20,21]
   c. Technicians should decontaminate or wash nondisposable materials as appropriate, including counting trays and tools exposed to oral anticancer medications thoroughly after use.[22]

Handling of Hazardous Waste

1. Pharmacy technicians shall be fully trained in the storage, handling, and disposal of hazardous drugs per employer, state, and national guidelines; this training

shall occur before preparing or handling hazardous preparations, and the effectiveness of the training should be verified by testing specific techniques.

   a. All training should be documented, and competency should be reassessed and documented at least every 12 months.[4]

2. Technicians should be trained on hazardous drug exposure and spill control, including treatment of individuals accidently exposed to hazardous medications and on the disposal of hazardous medications.[4,21,22]

   a. It is recommended that annual spill simulation exercises be conducted.[22]

Documentation

1. An updated list of hazardous medications should be readily accessible to all healthcare personnel involved in handling of hazardous medications.[22]
2. If exposed to a hazardous drug spill, personnel should complete an incident report or exposure form and report to the designated emergency service for initial evaluation.[4]
3. Activities that shall be documented include but are not limited to the acquisition, preparation, and dispensing of a compounded hazardous drug, personnel training, and the use and maintenance of equipment and supplies.[4]

Pump Management

1. Pharmacy technicians should assist in identifying pump libraries ensuring safe administration of chemotherapy in conjunction with pharmacists and nursing ensuring accuracy of pump libraries.
2. Pharmacy technicians may aid in CADD pump preparation upon demonstration of competency.

Patient Care Services

Medication Histories and Reconciliation

1. Pharmacy technicians should be involved in obtaining accurate medication histories for patients with cancer using a standardized script.
2. Medication history training should include patient interview skills and specific criteria to triage for pharmacist intervention.
3. Pharmacy technicians may participate in medication reconciliation processes under appropriate supervision to expand the healthcare organization's capacity to offer these services.

Oral Anticancer Medication Patient Outreach

1. Pharmacy technicians can be involved in monitoring adherence and toxicity of patients initiated and/or maintained on oral anticancer medications by using a standardized script.
2. Technicians should review medication adherence when completing medication histories; feedback regarding ways to improve adherence should be raised with pharmacist and remainder of healthcare team.

REMS Program Requirements

Pharmacy technicians should assist in compliance with REMS program requirements.

Investigational Drug Management

Pharmacy technicians should support multiple aspects of investigational drug management, including inventory, information and record keeping, and preparation of investigational products for dispensing.

Revenue Cycle Optimization

Therapy Authorization

1. Pharmacy technicians should be engaged in specific aspects of the revenue cycle, including authorization of high-cost medications, off-label medication workflows, and billing work queues.
2. Technicians should review financial review requests and manage records to ensure financial approval prior to therapy initiation.

Patient Financial Assistance

1. Pharmacy technicians may assist in discussing with patients out-of-pocket expenses associated with chemotherapy medications.
2. Pharmacy technicians may lead efforts to assist patients with securing copayment assistance or referring them to an appropriate financial counselor.
   a. Assistance may include completion of required paperwork and financial information.
   b. Pharmacy technicians may assist with enrollment for foundation assistance.

Minimizing Medication Waste

Pharmacy technicians should minimize medication waste through monitoring compliance with policies and procedures including dose rounding and optimizing drug use through schedule coordination.

Supply Chain Management

Purchasing

1. Pharmacy technicians should assist with navigation of complicated vendor, group purchasing organization, and manufacturer contracts.
2. Technicians may carry out daily purchasing activities under pharmacist supervision.

Inventory Control Management

1. Pharmacy technicians should promote inventory control strategies, including minimization of expired product, promotion of adequate medication turnover, and alignment with product-line purchasing, to ensure inventory control management of high-cost items while reducing overall stock supplies.
2. When receiving products, pharmacy technicians should employ special precautions for hazardous substances and ensure fidelity of drug product specific shipping and handling requirements.

Drug Shortages

Pharmacy technicians should contribute to drug shortage management, including managing purchasing strategies and investigating procurement of alternative products.

Technology and Informatics

Automation and Technology Systems Management

Pharmacy technicians should work under the supervision of a pharmacist to leverage information technology resources to improve the quality and efficiency of the healthcare organization, including:

- **a.** Management of applicable interfaces between electronic health record and pharmacy automation.
- **b.** Placement, configuration, monitoring, maintenance, and troubleshooting of automation and technology systems.
- **c.** Preparation of reports from clinical and automation systems to facilitate organizational, departmental, and individual decision-making.
- **d.** End-user training and education.
- **e.** Providing users and staff with consultative support.[23]

Remote Telepharmacy Services

Pharmacy technicians may function in important roles at remote sites through telepharmacy services, including preparation of i.v. medications, under the supervision of a pharmacist.[24]

Quality Improvement

Error Prevention Strategies

Oncology pharmacy technicians should be included in quality-improvement projects to address metrics for workflow evaluation for oncology care.

Equipment and Storage Facility Temperature Monitoring

Pharmacy technicians should evaluate monitoring for equipment and storage facilities based on current standard operating protocols for continued fidelity checks of equipment for medication storage, compounding, and delivery.

[a]PPE = personal protective equipment, CSTD = closed-system transfer device, PEC = primary engineering control, CADD = continuous ambulatory delivery device.

Approved by the ASHP Board of Directors on April 30, 2018, and by the HOPA Board of Directors on February 21, 2018. Developed through a joint panel of the ASHP Section of Inpatient Care Practitioners Section Advisory Group on Advancing Pharmacy Practice with Technicians and the HOPA Ambulatory Oncology Pharmacy Task Force.

Jason Bergsbaken, Pharm.D., BCOP, Regional Oncology Services, UW Health, Madison, WI.

Danielle Roman, Pharm.D., BCOP, Clinical Pharmacy Services, Allegheny Health Network Cancer Institute, Pittsburgh, PA.

Marc A. Earl, Pharm.D., BCOP, Cleveland Clinic, Cleveland, OH.

Ali McBride, Pharm.D., M.S., BCOP, FazPA, Hematology/Oncology, University of Arizona Cancer Center, Tucson, AZ, and Clinical Assistant Professor, University of Arizona College of Pharmacy, Tucson, AZ.

Jacqueline L. Olin, M.S., Pharm.D., BCPS, CDE, FASHP, FCCP, Wingate University School of Pharmacy, Wingate, NC.

Adam Peele, Pharm.D., M.H.A., BCPS, BCOP, Cone Health, Greensboro, NC.

Jeffrey S. Reichard, Pharm.D., M.S., BCPS, Novant Health, Winston-Salem, NC.

ASHP gratefully acknowledges the following organizations and individuals for reviewing these guidelines (review does not imply endorsement): American Association of Pharmacy Technicians; Institute for Safe Medication Practices; United States Public Health Service, Indian Health Service; Sally Y. Barbour, Pharm.D., BCOP, CPP, FHOPA; CDR Anne Marie Bott, Pharm.D., BCOP, BCPS, NCPS; Bryna Ewachiw, Pharm.D., BCOP; Katie Burenheide Foster, Pharm.D., M.S., FCCM; Marco Martino, Pharm.D., M.B.A., BCPS, BCOP; Judy Neville, CPhT; Edna Patatanian, Pharm.D.; James R. Rinehart, M.S., FASHP; Richard I. Sakai, Pharm.D., FASHP, FCSHP; CDR Ashley Schaber, Pharm.D., M.B.A., BCPS, NCPS; Allen J. Vaida, Pharm.D., FASHP; and Suzanne M. Walton, Pharm.D., BCPS, BCOP.

The authors have declared no potential conflicts of interest.

Copyright © 2018, American Society of Health-System Pharmacists, Inc., and Hematology/Oncology Pharmacy Association. All rights reserved. Contact ASHP for reprint and permissions requests. This content may not be used for commercial purposes without the express written consent of ASHP.

The bibliographic citation for this document is as follows: American Society of Health-System Pharmacists. ASHP-HOPA guidelines on the roles and responsibilities of the pharmacy technician in ambulatory oncology pharmacy. *Am J Health-Syst Pharm.* 2018; 75 (17):1304–11.

Position Paper on Critical Care Pharmacy Services: 2020 Update

Ishaq Lat, PharmD, FCCM, FCCP[1]; Christopher Paciullo, PharmD, FCCM, FCCP, BCCCP[2]; Mitchell J. Daley, PharmD, FCCM, BCPS[3,4]; Robert MacLaren, PharmD, MPH, FCCM, FCCP[5]; Scott Bolesta, PharmD, FCCM, FCCP, BCPS[6]; Jennifer McCann, PharmD, BCCCP[7]; Joanna L. Stollings, PharmD, FCCM, FCCP, BCCCP, BCPS[8,9]; Kendall Gross, PharmD, BCPS, BCCCP[10]; Sarah A. Foos, PharmD, BCCCP[11]; Russel J. Roberts, PharmD, FCCM, BCCCP, BCPS[12]; Nicole M. Acquisto, PharmD, FCCP, BCCCP[13,14]; Scott Taylor, PharmD, MS, BCPS[15]; Michael Bentley, PharmD, FCCM, FCCP[16,17]; Judith Jacobi, PharmD, MCCM, FCCP, BCCCP[18]; Tricia A. Meyer, PharmD, MS, FASHP, FTSHP[19,20]

1 Department of Pharmacy Services, Shirley Ryan Ability Lab, Chicago, IL.
2 Shields Health Solutions, Stoughton, MA.
3 Dell Seton Medical Center at the University of Texas, Austin, TX.
4 Dell Medical School at the University of Texas, Austin, TX.
5 Department of Pharmacy Practice, Skaggs School of Pharmacy, University of Colorado, Aurora, CO.
6 Department of Pharmacy Practice, Nesbitt School of Pharmacy, Wilkes University, Wilkes-Barre, PA.
7 Department of Pharmacy Practice, School of Pharmacy and Health Sciences, Butler University, Indianapolis, IN.
8 Department of Pharmaceutical Services, Vanderbilt University Medical Center, Nashville, TN.
9 Critical Illness, Brain Dysfunction, and Survivorship (CIBS) Center, Nashville, TN.
10 Department of Pharmacy, UCSF Health, San Francisco, CA.
11 Department of Pharmacy Services, OhioHealth Doctors Hospital, Columbus, OH.
12 Department of Pharmacy, Massachusetts General Hospital, Boston, MA.
13 Department of Pharmacy, University of Rochester Medical Center, Rochester, NY.
14 Department of Emergency Medicine, University of Rochester Medical Center, Rochester, NY.
15 Steward Health Care, Dallas, TX.
16 Virginia Tech Carilion School of Medicine, Roanoke, VA.
17 AstraZeneca Pharmaceuticals, Wilmington, DE.
18 Visante Inc., St. Paul, MN.
19 Baylor Scott and White Health-Temple Region, Temple, TX.
20 Department of Anesthesiology, Texas A&M College of Medicine, Temple, TX.

For information regarding this article, e-mail: ilat@sralab.org

Supplemental digital content is available for online versions of this article. Direct URL citations appear in the printed text and are provided in the HTML and PDF versions of this article on the journal's website (http://journals.lww.com/ccmjournal); that supplemental content is included as **Tables 1-3** in this prepress version.

This article is being co-published by *Critical Care Medicine, American Journal of Health System Pharmacy*, and the *Journal of the American College of Clinical Pharmacy*.

Copyright © 2020, American Society of Health-System Pharmacists, Inc. All rights reserved. Contact ASHP for reprint and permissions requests. This content may not be used for commercial purposes without the express written consent of ASHP.

Key Words: collaborative medication management; credentialing; critical care; pharmacy; professional development

Disclosures: Mrs. Foos received reimbursement for travel to meetings. Mr. Bentley has disclosed that he is a currently employee of Astra Zeneca. Mrs. Jacobi received funding from Merck (advisory board) and Visante (consulting), and she is on the Board of Pharmacy Specialists. Mrs. Meyer received funding from Acacia and Neumentum.

The remaining authors have disclosed that they do not have any potential conflicts of interest.

Objectives: To provide a multiorganizational statement to update recommendations for critical care pharmacy practice and make recommendations for future practice. A position paper outlining critical care pharmacist activities was last published in 2000. Since that time, significant changes in healthcare and critical care have occurred.

Design: The Society of Critical Care Medicine, American College of Clinical Pharmacy Critical Care Practice and Research Network, and the American Society of Health-System Pharmacists convened a joint task force of 15 pharmacists representing a broad cross-section of critical care pharmacy practice and pharmacy administration, inclusive of geography, critical care practice setting, and roles. The Task Force chairs reviewed and organized primary literature, outlined topic domains, and prepared the methodology for group review and consensus. A modified Delphi method was used until consensus (> 66% agreement) was reached for each practice recommendation. Previous position statement recommendations were reviewed and voted to either retain, revise, or retire. Recommendations were categorized by level of ICU service to be applicable by setting and grouped into five domains: patient care, quality improvement, research and scholarship, training and education, and professional development.

Main Results: There are 82 recommendation statements: 44 original recommendations and 38 new recommendation statements. Thirty-four recommendations represent the domain of patient care, primarily relating to critical care pharmacist duties and pharmacy services. In the quality improvement domain, 21 recommendations address the role of the critical care pharmacist in patient and medication safety, clinical quality programs, and analytics. Nine recommendations were made in the domain of research and scholarship. Ten recommendations were made in the domain of training and education and eight recommendations regarding professional development.

Conclusions: Critical care pharmacists are essential members of the multiprofessional critical care team. The statements recommended by this taskforce delineate the activities of a critical care pharmacist and the scope of pharmacy services within the ICU. Effort should be made from all stakeholders to implement the recommendations provided, with continuous effort toward improving the delivery of care for critically ill patients.

Since the formation of the first ICU in the 1930s to present day, the field of critical care medicine has evolved and increased in complexity.[1] In parallel, clinical pharmacy practice advanced from a dispensary role to one primarily of

DOI 10.37573/9781585287048.083

medication management. In the 1940s, pharmacists began attending interprofessional rounds and became more involved in the clinical aspects of care.[2] In the intervening decades, critical care pharmacy developed into a distinct subspecialty within pharmacy practice, with specialized training and credentials. As the subspecialty evolved so too did the need for practice standards. The first position paper on critical care pharmacy services was published in 2000 and described pharmacy services that were foundational, desirable, and optimal.[3] A subsequent survey of 1,034 ICUs to evaluate critical care pharmacy services found lower level services were commonly provided but desirable or optimal activities were inconsistent.[4] Rapid progress in the field of pharmacotherapy, improvement in the application of technology, workforce trends, and evolution of healthcare delivery necessitate a continual assessment of practice standards in an effort to best serve patients. Since that first position paper, critical care medicine has continued to progress to the extent that the recommendation statements from the original position paper may no longer apply or need revision to be relevant for the current practice environment.

The purpose of this position paper is to delineate the activities of a critical care pharmacist and the scope of pharmacy services within the ICU. Critical care pharmacist activities and pharmacy services are categorized by the level of critical care services offered. We aim to provide recommendations on pharmacy practice for the current critical care environment. With an increasing emphasis placed on value in healthcare, a secondary objective of this position paper is to provide the means to demonstrate the value of a critical care pharmacist by describing activities that can be used by pharmacy administrators and hospital executives to measure and report. Finally, this position paper intends to serve as a guideline for critical care pharmacy practice for the coming decade.

The task force determined that guideline recommendations should be inclusive of pharmacy services across the continuum of critical illness. Therefore, the position paper addresses activities of the individual critical care pharmacist and those best served by pharmacy administrators. These individuals and members of the multiprofessional team should design comprehensive pharmacy services that meet the pharmacotherapy needs of the critically ill patient. The success of the multiprofessional critical care team is contingent on the support of administrators and executives. This model relies on collaborative engagement in care delivery designed to best serve patients, while promoting the needs of patients and staff to improve institutional performance.

Methods

A task force was created in January 2015 to review, and revise, the existing position paper on critical care pharmacy services. The Society of Critical Care Medicine (SCCM), American College of Clinical Pharmacy (ACCP) Critical Care Practice and Research Network, and the American Society of Health-System Pharmacists (ASHP) were contacted to support this work. The task force included 15 members representing a broad cross-section of critical care pharmacy practice (hospital, academia, administration, urban, rural, and clinical practice setting) and the membership of SCCM, ACCP, and ASHP. Task force members convened in-person at the SCCM Annual Congress in February 2016 and subsequently held a series of conference calls to vote on statements using a modified Delphi method, refine verbiage, and generate the article text.

There are three notable modifications in this article that differ from the previous recommendations.[3] The first is a simplification from three levels of recommendations (fundamental, desirable, and optimal) to two (foundational and desirable). The task force felt this was necessary to improve interpretation and implementation of these recommendations. Consistent with the original position paper, foundational activities are those services or activities deemed essential to critical care practice. Therefore, foundational services should be interpreted not as the minimum level of service or activities, but rather, those activities that serve as the core of critical care pharmacy services and provide the underpinning of care from which to expand pharmacy services. Additionally, desirable services or activities are those deemed to be "value added"; they are not as essential but extend the scope of practice toward a higher level. The second modification to this position paper was to use existing guidance for delivery of critical care services and assign recommendations to each level of ICU service.[5] Level I critical care services are defined as ICUs that provide complete care for a wide range of disorders requiring intensive care, deliver comprehensive support services, and generally fulfill an academic mission. Level II critical care services provide comprehensive care but may not have the resources to care for specific populations and may not have an academic mission. Level III critical care services provide initial stabilization of critically ill patients, but do not offer comprehensive critical care. In recognition of the varying levels of critical care services, some activities are not possible, or needed, at all types of healthcare systems. Similarly, pharmacy departments for institutions with some level II and likely all level III ICUs are not staffed with the same number of personnel. In this way, the task force sought to provide recommendations that were specific to the level of resources available at each institution and are immediately relevant to practitioners, administrators, and executives. Throughout the article, the terms "critical care pharmacist," "pharmacist," and "designee" are used. The "critical care pharmacist" is intended to denote the pharmacist who is specialty trained and dedicated as a resource to delivering critical care pharmacy services. The "pharmacist" is intended to denote a generalist pharmacist who provides prospective order review and clinical services within their scope and expertise when a critical care pharmacist is not present. In those instances where the services of a "critical care pharmacist" may not be available, the statement would default to "pharmacist." The "designee" is intended to denote a pharmacy resident or student pharmacist completing a practice experience under the supervision of the critical care pharmacist or pharmacist. It is not intended to suggest that such activities can or should be carried out solely by designees without a supervising pharmacist.

The task force identified five domains to describe critical care pharmacy services: 1) patient care; 2) quality improvement; 3) research and scholarship; 4) training and education; and 5) professional development. The task force co-chairs (I.L., C.P.) completed an initial literature review using PubMed with relevant search terms ("critical care," "pharmacy," and "pharmacotherapy"), collated references by section, and provided them to the task force to review. The literature review was broad and inclusive as the purpose was to ensure that all task force members were aware of current critical care pharmacy practices. The body of literature was expanded by members of the task force. Due to the lack of strong evidence, the task force sought to make recommendations using a modified Delphi method. All task force members were considered pharmacy experts and the co-chairs acted as facilitators, circulating anonymized responses and comments after each round of voting. There were no predefined stopping criteria. Voting continued until consensus was reached on a specific guideline statement, or it was retired. Experts rated statements on a 1–9 Likert scale, with a score of 1 indicating strong disagreement and 9 indicating strong agreement, with incremental levels of agreement in between. The scores were then grouped into tertiles, with the score range of 1–3 indicating disagreement, 4–6 indicating neutral, and 7–9 indicating agreement. Consensus was defined as greater than 66% of task force members agreeing on each statement and recommendation level according to the level of critical care services (I, II, or III). Task force co-chairs initiated the first phase of voting by circulating previously published guideline statements to determine if existing recommendation statements required revision or no longer applied in the current healthcare environment and, therefore, should be retired (**Table 1**). If a consensus was reached on the need for revision, the task force chairs revised statements and proposed additional rounds of voting until consensus was reached by the task force. If consensus was

TABLE 1.
Round 1 Task Force Panel Voting

Activity	Ratings 1–3	Ratings 4–6	Ratings 7–9
The pharmacist's time is dedicated to critical care patients, with few commitments outside the ICU area.	0	0	15
The pharmacist prospectively evaluates all drug therapy for appropriate indication, dose, drug interactions, drug allergies, and monitors the patient's pharmacotherapeutic regimen for effectiveness and ADEs, and intervenes as needed.	0	0	15
In conjunction with the clinical dietitian, the pharmacist evaluates all orders for parenteral nutrition and recommends modifications as indicated to optimize the nutritional regimen.	0	8	7
The pharmacist identifies and assists in the management and prevention of ADE; the pharmacist develops process improvements to reduce medication errors and preventable ADEs.	0	0	15
The pharmacist uses the medical record as one means to communicate with other healthcare professionals, and to document specific pharmacotherapeutic recommendations.	1	1	13
The pharmacist provides pharmacokinetic monitoring when a targeted drug is prescribed.	0	0	15
The pharmacist provides drug information and IV compatibility information to the ICU team and uses the regional poison information center when indicated.	1	1	13
The pharmacist maintains current tertiary drug references.[a]	3	2	10
The pharmacist provides drug therapy-related education to ICU team members.	0	0	15
The pharmacist participates in reporting ADEs to institutional committees and to the Food and Drug Administration Medwatch program.	0	1	14
The pharmacist documents clinical activities that include, but are not limited to, disease state management, general pharmacotherapeutic monitoring, pharmacokinetic monitoring, ADEs, education, and other patient care activities.	0	1	14
The pharmacist acts as a liaison among pharmacy, nursing, and the medical staff to educate health professionals regarding current drug-related policies, procedures, guidelines, and pathways.	0	1	14
The pharmacist contributes to the hospital newsletter and drug monographs, on issues related to medication use in the ICU.	1	4	10
The pharmacist implements and maintains departmental policies and procedures related to safe and effective use of medications in the ICU.	0	3	12
The pharmacist collaborates with nursing, medical staff, and hospital administration to prepare the ICU for the Joint Commission on the Accreditation of Healthcare Organizations survey and responds to any deficiencies identified.	0	3	12
The pharmacist provides consultation to hospital committees such as Pharmacy and Therapeutics, when critical care pharmacotherapy issues are discussed.	0	1	14
The pharmacist identifies how drug costs may be minimized through appropriate use of drugs in the ICU and through implementation of cost containment measures.	0	2	13
The pharmacist participates in quality assurance programs to enhance pharmaceutical care.	0	1	14
The pharmacist regularly makes rounds as a member of the multidisciplinary critical care team (if available) to provide pharmacotherapeutic management for all ICU patients.	0	3	12

TABLE 1. *(continued)*

Activity	Ratings 1–3	Ratings 4–6	Ratings 7–9
The pharmacist maintains knowledge of current primary references pertinent to critical care pharmacotherapy.	0	0	15
The pharmacist reviews the medication history to determine which maintenance medications should be continued during the acute illness. a. The pharmacist clarifies previously effective doses and dosage regimens. b. For all suspected drug-related ICU admissions, the pharmacist assesses the patient medication history for causality and documents any findings that will impact patient management in the medical record.	0	2	13
In collaboration with the clinical dietitian, the pharmacist provides formal nutrition consultation on request and responds within 24 hr.	3	7	5
The advanced cardiac life support-certified (or pediatric advanced life support certified for pediatrics) pharmacist responds to all resuscitation events in the hospital 7 d/wk, 24 hr/d.	0	1	14
The pharmacist provides didactic lectures to health professional students in critical care pharmacology and therapeutics, where applicable.	0	5	10
The pharmacist participates in training pharmacy students, residents, and fellows through experiential critical care rotations, where applicable.	0	2	13
The pharmacist coordinates the development and implementation of drug therapy protocols and/or critical care pathways to maximize benefits of drug therapy.	0	0	15
The pharmacist uses a documentation program that attaches both a clinical significance and economic value to clinical interventions.	1	4	10
The pharmacist is actively involved in critical care pharmacotherapy research by assisting in the screening and enrollment of patients, and by serving as a study coordinator or contact person, where applicable.	2	8	5
The pharmacist participates in research design and data analysis, where applicable.	0	4	11
The pharmacist contributes to the pharmacy and medical literature (e.g., case reports, letters to the editor, and therapeutic, pharmacokinetic, and pharmacoeconomic reports).	0	4	11
The pharmacist is involved in non-patient care activities, including multidisciplinary committees and educational inservices.	0	2	13
The pharmacist assists physicians in discussions with patients and/or family members to help make informed decisions regarding treatment options.	1	8	6
The pharmacist provides formal accredited educational sessions (such as medical grand rounds or intensive care rounds) for medical staff, students, and residents.	0	4	11
The pharmacist participates in teaching advanced cardiac life support.	3	9	3
The pharmacist develops residencies and/or fellowships in critical care pharmacy practice.	0	3	12
The pharmacist develops and implements pharmacist and pharmacy technician training programs for personnel working in the ICU.	1	6	8
The pharmacist identifies and educates lay groups and medical personnel in the community about the role of pharmacists as part of the multidisciplinary healthcare team in the ICU.	2	8	5
The pharmacist independently investigates or collaborates with other critical care practitioners to evaluate the impact of guidelines and/or protocols used in the ICU for drug administration and management of common disease states.	0	2	13
The pharmacist uses pharmacoeconomic analyses to prospectively evaluate existing/new pharmacy services and the place of new drugs in critical care pharmacotherapy.	0	6	9
The pharmacist is proactive in designing, prioritizing, and promoting new pharmacy programs and services.	0	1	14
The pharmacist secures funds for conducting research.	3	11	1
The pharmacist reports results of clinical research and pharmacoeconomic analyses to the pharmacy and medical community at regional and national meetings.	1	3	11
The pharmacist publishes in peer-reviewed pharmacy and medical literature as a result of any of the following activities: a. clinical research or other original research that qualitatively and quantitatively evaluates drug therapy and the provision of pharmacy service; b. investigator-initiated grants and contracts; and c. pharmacoeconomic and outcomes research	0	2	13

Continued on next page

TABLE 1. *(continued)*

Activity	Ratings 1–3	Ratings 4–6	Ratings 7–9
Medication use systems have the ability to: a. create and maintain patient medication profiles; b. interface with patient laboratory data; c. alert users to drug allergies; d. alert users to maximum dose limits; and e. alert users to drug-drug and drug-food/nutrient interactions.	0	2	13
If manual medication administration records are the only available medication administration record document, quality assurance systems are in place to verify the accuracy of this process.[a]	2	2	11
A "ready to administer" (unit-dose) drug distribution system is available in the ICU with no more than a 24-hr supply for each patient.[a]	0	3	12
Large- and small-volume parenteral products are prepared in the pharmacy and delivered at regularly scheduled time intervals to the patient care area 7 d/wk.[a]	0	2	13
Pharmacy space and facilities in the ICU are regularly assessed to determine whether efficiency can be improved, where applicable.	0	4	11
Procurement, storage, inventory, and distribution of investigational drugs, where applicable, are under the supervision of a pharmacist.[a]	0	1	14
The pharmacy department is represented on the Institutional Review Board and/or Scientific Review Board, as applicable.	0	2	13
The hospital information management system is computerized, is able to comply with those requirements listed for medication use processes, and has the ability to: a. alert users to disease state-drug interactions; b. provide IV admixture information (compatibility, stability, preparation, etc); c. provide online drug and poison information; and d. document clinical pharmacy patient care interventions.	0	2	13
Computerized medication administration records are generated. Manual medication administration records are only used in emergencies.[a]	0	1	14
An ICU satellite pharmacy with unit-dose drug distribution and IV admixture capabilities is open a minimum of 40 hr/wk.[a]	4	7	4
The computerized hospital information management system serving the ICU has the following additional capabilities: a. direct physician medication order entry at the patient bedside; and b. interface with bedside clinical information system.	0	2	13
An ICU satellite pharmacy with unit-dose drug distribution and IV admixture capabilities is open 24 hr/d, 7 d/wk.[a]	5	8	2

ADE = adverse drug event.

[a]Denotes retired statement.

reached determining retirement of a previously published statement with greater than 66% of the Task Force voting to "retire," the statement was excluded from new guidelines. Reasons for retiring a statement were primarily based on the consensus that the statement no longer applied to the current practice environment either due to regulatory requirements or technologic advancement. Once previous recommendation statements were either retired or revised, co-chairs moved to phase 2 by soliciting new guideline recommendations from panel experts. New recommendations were grouped by domain. If two or more new recommendation statements submitted by task force members were similar, the phrasing of these statements was revised by the facilitators for another round of voting. Consensus was reached on all statements following the second round of voting (**Table 2**). In the third round, recommendation statements were approved as "foundational" or "desirable" and assigned level of critical care services (**Table 3**). Each domain was then organized into written statement recommendations followed by brief discussion, supported by evidence, when available, from additional literature searches. The deliberations and voting from the Task Force resulted in 82 recommendation statements and eight recommendation statements from the previous position paper.

Patient Care

Recommendations

1. The critical care pharmacist regularly makes rounds as a member of the interdisciplinary critical care team to provide comprehensive medication management (CMM) for all ICU patients.

   Level I: Foundational

   Level II: Foundational

   Level III: Desirable

TABLE 2.
Round 2 Voting, with New Recommendation Statements

Activity	Ratings 1–3	Ratings 4–6	Ratings 7–9
The pharmacist's time is dedicated to critical care patients, with few commitments outside the ICU area.	0	0	15
The pharmacist prospectively evaluates all drug therapy for appropriate indication, dose, drug interactions, drug allergies, and monitors the patient's pharmacotherapeutic regimen for effectiveness and ADEs, and intervenes as needed.	0	0	15
In conjunction with the clinical dietitian, the pharmacist evaluates all orders for parenteral nutrition and recommends modifications as indicated to optimize the nutritional regimen.	0	8	7
The pharmacist identifies and assists in the management and prevention of ADE; the pharmacist develops process improvements to reduce medication errors and preventable ADEs.	0	0	15
The pharmacist uses the medical record as one means to communicate with other healthcare professionals, and to document specific pharmacotherapeutic recommendations.	1	1	13
The pharmacist provides pharmacokinetic monitoring when a targeted drug is prescribed.	0	0	15
The pharmacist provides drug information and IV compatibility information to the ICU team and uses the regional poison information center when indicated.	1	1	13
The pharmacist provides drug therapy-related education to ICU team members.	0	0	15
The pharmacist participates in reporting ADEs to institutional committees and to the Food and Drug Administration Medwatch program.	0	1	14
The pharmacist acts as a liaison among pharmacy, nursing, and the medical staff to educate health professionals regarding current drug-related policies, procedures, guidelines, and pathways.	0	1	14
The pharmacist contributes to the hospital newsletter and drug monographs, on issues related to medication use in the ICU.	1	4	10
The pharmacist implements and maintains departmental policies and procedures related to safe and effective use of medications in the ICU.	0	3	12
The pharmacist collaborates with nursing, medical staff, and hospital administration to prepare the ICU for the Joint Commission on the Accreditation of Healthcare Organizations survey and responds to any deficiencies identified.	0	3	12
The pharmacist provides consultation to hospital committees, such as Pharmacy and Therapeutics, when critical care pharmacotherapy issues are discussed.	0	1	14
The pharmacist identifies how drug costs may be minimized through appropriate use of drugs in the ICU and through implementation of cost containment measures.	0	2	13
The pharmacist participates in quality assurance programs to enhance pharmaceutical care.	0	1	14
The pharmacist regularly makes rounds as a member of the multidisciplinary critical care team (if available) to provide pharmacotherapeutic management for all ICU patients.	0	3	12
The pharmacist maintains knowledge of current primary references pertinent to critical care pharmacotherapy.	0	0	15
The pharmacist reviews the medication history to determine which maintenance medications should be continued during the acute illness. a. The pharmacist clarifies previously effective doses and dosage regimens. b. For all suspected drug-related ICU admissions, the pharmacist assesses the patient medication history for causality and documents any findings that will impact patient management in the medical record.	0	2	13
In collaboration with the clinical dietitian, the pharmacist provides formal nutrition consultation on request and responds within 24 hr.	3	7	5
The ACLs-certified (or PALS certified for pediatrics) pharmacist responds to all resuscitation events in the hospital 7 d/wk, 24 hr/d.	0	1	14
The pharmacist provides didactic lectures to health professional students in critical care pharmacology and therapeutics, where applicable.	0	5	10
The pharmacist participates in training pharmacy students, residents, and fellows through experiential critical care rotations, where applicable.	0	2	13
The pharmacist coordinates the development and implementation of drug therapy protocols and/or critical care pathways to maximize benefits of drug therapy.	0	0	15
The pharmacist uses a documentation program that attaches both a clinical significance and an economic value to clinical interventions.	1	4	10

Continued on next page

TABLE 2. *(continued)*

Activity	Ratings 1–3	Ratings 4–6	Ratings 7–9
The pharmacist is actively involved in critical care pharmacotherapy research by assisting in the screening and enrollment of patients, and by serving as a study coordinator or contact person, where applicable.	2	8	5
The pharmacist participates in research design and data analysis, where applicable.	0	4	11
The pharmacist contributes to the pharmacy and medical literature (e.g., case reports, letters to the editor, and therapeutic, pharmacokinetic, and pharmacoeconomic reports).	0	4	11
The pharmacist is involved in non-patient care activities, including multidisciplinary committees and educational inservices.	0	2	13
The pharmacist assists physicians in discussions with patients and/or family members to help make informed decisions regarding treatment options.	1	8	6
The pharmacist provides formal accredited educational sessions (such as medical grand rounds or intensive care rounds) for medical staff, students, and residents.	0	4	11
The pharmacist participates in teaching ACLS.	3	9	3
The pharmacist develops residencies and/or fellowships in critical care pharmacy practice.	0	3	12
The pharmacist develops and implements pharmacist and pharmacy technician training programs for personnel working in the ICU.	1	6	8
The pharmacist identifies and educates lay groups and medical personnel in the community about the role of pharmacists as part of the multidisciplinary healthcare team in the ICU.	2	8	5
The pharmacist independently investigates or collaborates with other critical care practitioners to evaluate the impact of guidelines and/or protocols used in the ICU for drug administration and management of common disease states.	0	2	13
The pharmacist uses pharmacoeconomic analyses to prospectively evaluate existing/new pharmacy services and the place of new drugs in critical care pharmacotherapy.	0	6	9
The pharmacist is proactive in designing, prioritizing, and promoting new pharmacy programs and services.	0	1	14
The pharmacist secures funds for conducting research.	3	11	1
The pharmacist reports results of clinical research and pharmacoeconomic analyses to the pharmacy and medical community at regional and national meetings.	1	3	11
The pharmacist publishes in peer-reviewed pharmacy and medical literature as a result of any of the following activities: a. clinical research or other original research that qualitatively and quantitatively evaluates drug therapy and the provision of pharmacy service; b. investigator-initiated grants and contracts; and c. pharmacoeconomic and outcomes research.	0	2	13
Medication use systems have the ability to: a. create and maintain patient medication profiles; b. interface with patient laboratory data; c. alert users to drug allergies; d. alert users to maximum dose limits; and e. alert users to drug-drug and drug-food/nutrient interactions.	0	2	13
Pharmacy space and facilities in the ICU are regularly assessed to determine whether efficiency can be improved, where applicable.	0	4	11
The pharmacy department is represented on the Institutional Review Board and/or Scientific Review Board, as applicable.	0	2	13
The hospital information management system is computerized, is able to comply with those requirements listed for medication use processes, and has the ability to: a. alert users to disease state-drug interactions; b. provide IV admixture information (compatibility, stability, preparation, etc); c. provide online drug and poison information; and d. document clinical pharmacy patient care interventions.	0	2	13
The computerized hospital information management system serving the ICU has the following additional capabilities: a. direct physician medication order entry at the patient bedside; and b. interface with bedside clinical information system.	0	2	13
Pharmacotherapeutic, pharmacokinetic, and nutrition consultation are available 24 hr/d, 7 d/wk.[a]	1	4	10

TABLE 2. *(continued)*

Activity	Ratings 1–3	Ratings 4–6	Ratings 7–9
Pharmacists practicing extensively in critical care will seek board certification in critical care when eligible.[a]	1	1	13
Critical care pharmacy trainees should be evaluated on educational outcomes and documented quantitative experiences to demonstrate competence for a given subject.[a]	0	1	14
The pharmacist maintains certification in ACLS, or PALS, and emergency neurologic life support, as applicable.[a]	0	0	15
Decentralized clinical pharmacy services in the ICU should include routine and consistent patient care coverage, inclusive of: day, evening, and weekend coverage.[a]	0	0	15
Critical care pharmacist will have the majority of their clinical activity focused in the care of the critically ill population.[a]	0	0	15
Critical care pharmacy services are developed as "teams", with multiple critical care pharmacists available, to deliver consistent and quality pharmaceutical care.[a]	0	2	13
The ICU pharmacist-to-patient ratio is defined based on patient acuity and complexity in addition to the scope of clinical and operational services provided.[a]	0	2	13
The critical care pharmacist should be involved in continual evaluation of the availability of critical medications through optimization of automated dispensing cabinets.[a]	0	2	13
Pharmacy administrators should seek ways to enhance career and professional development for critical care pharmacists within health systems.[a]	0	1	14
Pharmacy administrators should seek to provide protected time for critical care pharmacists to facilitate education, administrative, research, and scholarly activities.[a]	0	1	14
In the absence of onsite critical care pharmacist, comprehensive medication management may be supplemented through telemedicine.[a]	0	3	12
The pharmacist performs medication reconciliation for ICU patients at the time of ICU admission, transfer from the ICU to the ward, or discharge to home or facility.[a]	0	1	14
Pharmacists document pertinent pharmaceutical care problems and progress notes daily.[a]	1	2	13
The critical care pharmacist educates patients and/or patient's family members regarding medication therapies used to treat patients during and after acute illness, as appropriate.[a]	0	2	13
The pharmacist responds, or coordinates, pharmacist response to all resuscitation and timedependent emergencies in the hospital, including, but not limited to cardiac arrest, rapid response, trauma response, hemorrhagic shock, sepsis response, and acute neurologic life support.[a]	0	2	13
The pharmacist performs independent patient assessment (e.g., pain/ analgesia/delirium, nutrition).[a]	0	2	13
The pharmacist provides clinical consultation to the caregiver team, both within and outside the ICU, for pharmacotherapeutic issues related to critical illness.[a]	0	0	15
The pharmacist collaborates with other pharmacists (e.g., emergency medicine, infectious diseases, transplant, oncology), as needed, to address patient and disease-specific therapeutic issues.[a]	0	0	15
The pharmacist provides routine stewardship activities targeted at anti-infectives and other medications, including those that may be high risk and/or high cost and inappropriate utilization (factor products, anticoagulants, sedatives, acid-suppressive therapies, etc.).[a]	0	0	15
The pharmacist should collaborate with the medical staff to prevent potentially inappropriate drug therapy.[a]	2	0	13
Safety technology is implemented, inclusive of bedside barcode scanning, clinical decision support systems, and intelligent IV infusion devices in the routine care of critically ill patients.[a]	0	0	15
Critical care pharmacists should be involved in identifying local quality metrics for continuous quality improvement (e.g., risk-adjusted mortality, medication errors per medications ordered/dispensed, mechanical ventilation duration, delirium, mobilization).[a]	1	0	14
Real-time dashboard, or analytics monitoring, of quality metrics and drug utilization are available for the pharmacist to review for patient care and research.[a]	0	1	14
The critical care pharmacist serves as the medication safety leader for critically ill patients by identifying potential ADEs, resolving existing ADEs, and improving medication use practices.[a]	0	0	15

Continued on next page

TABLE 2. *(continued)*

Activity	Ratings 1–3	Ratings 4–6	Ratings 7–9
The critical care pharmacist shares responsibility in hospital performance for quality and process measure compliance, such as core measures and other hospital metrics (i.e., *Clostridium difficile* rates, vaccinations, patient satisfaction), as it relates to critical care patients.[a]	0	0	15
Pharmacy administrators evaluate clinical programs/services for stakeholder satisfaction, significance, and economic value.[a]	1	2	12
The critical care pharmacist prepares and presents drug therapy monographs and formulary reviews to the Pharmacy and Therapeutics committee for medications used in the care of critically ill patients.[a]	0	1	14
The critical care pharmacist leads, or provides, consultation to the hospital committees when critical care pharmacotherapy issues are discussed.[a]	0	0	15
The pharmacist should participate in planning and implementation of processes for disaster, or mass causalities, scenarios as applicable to the critically ill patient.[a]	0	0	15
The critical care pharmacist should be involved as a team member in the design process for building a new or remodeling critical care area.[a]	0	3	12
Critical care pharmacists are actively involved in collaborating in multicenter research projects.[a]	0	4	11
The critical care pharmacist participates as a key investigator for critical care research.[a]	0	4	11
The pharmacist contributes to the medical literature as a peer reviewer.[a]	0	4	11
The critical care pharmacist should be a member of professional critical care professional organizations, in addition to pharmacy organizations.[a]	1	1	13
The pharmacist participates in the education of pharmacy students, residents, and/or fellows by serving as a project advisor.[a]	0	3	12
The critical care pharmacist leads efforts to provide an interdisciplinary experience for experiential rotation exposure to students.[a]	0	4	11
The pharmacist has an active role in interdisciplinary simulation activities, where available.[a]	0	4	11
The pharmacist provides formal accredited education sessions at local, regional, state, and national meetings.[a]	0	2	13

ACLS = advanced cardiac life support, ADE = adverse drug event, PALS = pediatric advanced life support.

[a]Denotes a recommendation statement.

TABLE 3.
Recommendation Statements Approved as "Foundational" or "Desirable" and Assigned a Level of Critical Care Services

Patient Care

Statement	Level I	Level II	Level III
1. The critical care pharmacist regularly makes rounds as a member of the interdisciplinary critical care team to provide comprehensive medication management (CMM) for all ICU patients.	F	F	D
2. As part of the interdisciplinary team, the critical care pharmacist assists healthcare professionals in discussions with patients and/or family members to help make informed decisions regarding pharmacotherapy options.	F	F	D
3. The critical care pharmacist provides pertinent, comprehensive drug information to the critical care team.	F	F	F
4. The critical care pharmacist provides drug therapy related education to critical care team members.	F	F	D
5. The pharmacist should collaborate with the healthcare team to prevent potentially inappropriate drug therapy.	F	F	F
6. The critical care pharmacist provides clinical consultation to the care team, both within and outside the ICU, for pharmacotherapeutic issues related to critical illness.	F	F	F
7. Medication related consults (i.e. pharmacotherapeutic, pharmacokinetic, and nutrition patient counseling) are available 24 hours/day, 7 days/week to all critically ill patients.	F	D	D
8. The critical care pharmacist provides pharmacokinetic monitoring and therapeutic adjustments when a targeted drug is prescribed.	F	F	F

TABLE 3. *(continued)*

Statement	Level I	Level II	Level III
9. The critical care pharmacist reviews the medication history to determine which maintenance medications should be continued during the acute illness.	F	F	D
10. The pharmacist assists with medication reconciliation for ICU patients at the time of ICU admission, transfer from the ICU to the ward, or discharge to home or facility.	F	F	F
11. When reviewing orders for verification, the critical care pharmacist prospectively evaluates all drug therapy for appropriate indication, dose, drug interactions, drug allergies, and monitors the patient's pharmacotherapeutic regimen for effectiveness and adverse drug events (ADEs), and intervenes as needed.	F	F	F
12. The critical care pharmacist educates patients and/or patients' care givers regarding medication therapies used to treat patients during and after acute illness, as appropriate.	F	F	D
13. The pharmacist performs independent patient assessment (e.g. pain/agitation/delirium, nutrition).	F	D	D
14. A pharmacist certified in advanced cardiac life support (or pediatric advanced life support) responds to all resuscitation events in the hospital 24 hours/day, 7 days/week.	F	F	D
15. The pharmacist responds, or coordinates pharmacist response to all resuscitation and timedependent emergencies in the hospital including, but not limited to cardiac arrest, rapid response, trauma response, hemorrhagic shock, sepsis response, and acute neurologic life support.	F	F	D
16. The pharmacist provides routine stewardship activities targeted at anti-infectives and other medications, including those that may be high risk for adverse events, high cost concerns, and inappropriate utilization (e.g. factor products, anticoagulants, sedatives, acid-suppressive therapies).	F	F	F
17. The critical care pharmacist collaborates with other pharmacists (e.g. emergency medicine, infectious diseases, transplant, oncology, etc.), as needed, to address patient and diseasespecific therapeutic issues.	F	F	F
18. In conjunction with the clinical dietitian, the critical care pharmacist reviews the nutrition therapy plan and recommends modifications as indicated to optimize the nutritional regimen.	F	D	D
19. The critical care pharmacist utilizes the medical record as one means to communicate with other healthcare professionals, and/or to document specific pharmacotherapeutic recommendations or activities.	F	F	F
20. The critical care pharmacist uses appropriate documentation tools to demonstrate their impact on patient care and economic value.	F	F	F
21. Critical care pharmacists document pertinent pharmaceutical care problems and progress notes daily.	D	D	D
22. The critical care pharmacist documents clinical activities that include, but are not limited to, disease state management, general pharmacotherapeutic monitoring, pharmacokinetic monitoring, ADEs, education and other patient care activities.	F	F	F
23. The critical care pharmacist acts as a liaison between the pharmacy department and the interdisciplinary team to educate health professionals regarding current drug-related policies, procedures, guidelines, and pathways.	F	F	F
24. The critical care pharmacist uses pharmacoeconomic analyses in conjunction with the interdisciplinary team to evaluate existing/new pharmacy services and the place of new drugs in critical care pharmacotherapy.	F	F	D
25. The critical care pharmacist is proactive in designing, prioritizing, and promoting new clinical pharmacy programs and services.	F	F	D
26. Pharmacy administrators evaluate clinical programs/services for stakeholder satisfaction, significance, and economic value.	F	F	F
27. The critical care pharmacist prepares and presents drug therapy monographs and formulary reviews to the Pharmacy and Therapeutics committee for medications used in the care of critically ill patients.	D	D	D
28. The pharmacist should participate in planning and implementation of processes for disaster, or mass causalities, scenarios as applicable to the critically ill patient.	F	F	D
29. The majority of the critical care pharmacist's time is dedicated to critical care services, with few commitments, outside of critical care activities.	F	F	D
30. Critical care pharmacists will have the majority of their clinical activity focused in the care of the critically ill population.	F	F	D

Continued on next page

TABLE 3. *(continued)*

Statement	Level I	Level II	Level III
31. Decentralized clinical pharmacy services in the ICU should include routine and consistent patient care coverage, inclusive of day, evening, and weekend coverage.	F	F	D
32. Critical care pharmacy services are developed as "teams", with multiple critical care pharmacists available, to deliver consistent and quality pharmaceutical care.	F	F	D
33. In the absence of an onsite critical care pharmacist, CMM may be supplemented through telemedicine.	D	D	D
34. The ICU pharmacist-to-patient ratio is defined based on patient acuity and complexity in addition to the scope of clinical and operational services provided.	F	F	D

Quality Improvement

Statement	Level I	Level II	Level III
1. The critical care pharmacist serves as the medication safety leader for critically ill patients by identifying potential ADEs, resolving existing ADEs, and improving medication use practices.	F	F	F
2. The critical care pharmacist assists with the management of ADEs and develops process improvements to reduce and/or prevent medication errors.	F	F	F
3. The critical care pharmacist participates in reporting ADEs to institutional committees and national programs (e.g. the Food and Drug Administration (FDA) Medwatch program).	F	F	F
4. The critical care pharmacist is involved in continual evaluation of the availability of critical medications through optimization of automated dispensing cabinets.	F	F	F
5. The critical care pharmacist should be involved as a team member in the design process for building a new or remodeling critical care area.	D	D	D
6. The critical care pharmacist implements and maintains departmental policies and procedures related to safe and effective use of medications in the ICU.	F	F	F
7. The critical care pharmacist coordinates the development and implementation of ICU- focused drug therapy protocols, guidelines, order sets, and/or care pathways to maximize benefits of pharmacotherapy.	F	F	D
8. The pharmacist independently investigates or collaborates with other critical care healthcare team members to evaluate the impact of drug therapy protocols, guidelines, order sets, and/or care pathways used in the ICU (e.g. drug administration, disease state management algorithms).	F	D	D
9. The critical care pharmacist leads or provides consultation to hospital committees when critical care pharmacotherapy issues are discussed.	F	F	D
10. The critical care pharmacist serves on and provides consultation to hospital committees when critical care pharmacotherapy issues are discussed.	F	F	F
11. The critical care pharmacist contributes to the hospital newsletter and drug monographs, on issues related to medication use in the ICU.	F	F	D
12. The critical care pharmacist identifies and evaluates drug cost minimization opportunities and implements cost containment measures.	F	F	D
13. Critical care pharmacist is involved in identifying local quality metrics for continuous quality improvement (e.g. risk-adjusted mortality, medication errors per medications or- dered/ dispensed, mechanical ventilation duration, delirium, mobilization).	F	D	D
14. The critical care pharmacist participates in quality assurance programs to enhance CMM, minimize costs, provide ongoing evaluation of current processes, and identify the need for new programs/processes.	F	F	D
15. The critical care pharmacist shares responsibility for hospital performance for quality and process measure compliance, such as core measures and other hospital metrics (e.g. *C. difficile* infection rates, vaccinations, patient satisfaction surveys), as it relates to critical care patients.	F	F	D
16. The critical care pharmacist collaborates with medical staff, nursing, other members of the healthcare team, and hospital administration to prepare the ICU for healthcare accreditation and to address any deficiencies identified.	F	F	D
17. Pharmacy space and facilities in the ICU are regularly assessed to determine whether efficiency can be improved, where applicable.	F	D	D
18. Real time dashboard, or analytics monitoring, of quality metrics and drug utilization are available for the pharmacist to review for patient care and research.	D	D	D
19. Safety technology is implemented, inclusive of bedside barcode scanning, clinical decision support systems and intelligent intravenous infusion devices in the routine care of critically ill patients.	F	F	F

TABLE 3. *(continued)*

Statement	Level I	Level II	Level III
20. Medication use systems have the ability to: i. Create and maintain patient medication profiles ii. Interface with patient laboratory data and other relevant test results iii. Interface with patient charts (medication profiles) from other health-systems and outpatient clinics iv. Alert users to drug allergies v. Alert users to medication maximum dose limits vi. Alert users to medications prior to admission vii. Alert users to diagnoses viii. Alert users to drug-drug and drug-food/nutrient interactions ix. Alert users to formulary and non-formulary medications as well as approved substitutions x. Alert users to pertinent medication shortages xi. Provide live, real time data that can be incorporated in pharmacotherapy decision making	F	F	F
21. The hospital information management system is computerized, is able to comply with those requirements listed for medication use processes, and has the ability to: i. Allow direct provider order entry ii. Interface with bedside clinical information systems in real-time iii. Alert users to disease state-drug and drug-drug interactions iv. Provide intravenous admixture information (e.g. compatibility, stability, preparation) v. Provide medication information via references or internal guidelines/documents vi. Allow documentation of pharmacy patient care interventions vii. Provide benchmarking and quality data viii. Access to policies and procedures related to medications ix. Interface with mobile devices x. Provide patient-specific treatment algorithms	F	F	F

Research/ Scholarship

Statement	Level I	Level II	Level III
1. The pharmacist is actively involved in critical care pharmacotherapy research including, but not limited to, developing and reviewing study proposals, screening and/or enrollment of patients, publication of study results, and serving as a Principal Investigator, coinvestigator, study coordinator or contact person, where applicable.	D	D	D
2. The pharmacist contributes to the pharmacy and medical literature (e.g., case reports, letters to the editor, and therapeutic, pharmacokinetic, and pharmacoeconomic reports).	D	D	D
3. The pharmacist reports research results to the pharmacy and medical community at regional, national, and international meetings.	D	D	D
4. The pharmacist participates in research design and data analysis.	D	D	D
5. The pharmacist secures funds for conducting research.	D	D	D
6. The critical care pharmacist participates as a key investigator for critical care research.	F	D	D
7. Critical care pharmacists are actively involved in collaborating in multicenter research projects.	D	D	D
8. The profession of pharmacy is represented on the Institutional Review Board and/or Scientific Review Board, as applicable.	F	D	D
9. The pharmacist contributes to the medical literature as a peer reviewer.	D	D	D

Training/ Education

Statement	Level I	Level II	Level III
1. The critical care pharmacist provides an interprofessional experience in training and mentoring pharmacy students, residents, and fellows through experiential critical care rotations.	F	F	D
2. The critical care pharmacist supports postgraduate residencies and/or fellowship training in critical care pharmacy practice.	F	F	D
3. Critical care pharmacy trainees should be evaluated on educational outcomes and documented experiences in order to demonstrate competence for a given subject.	F	F	F
4. The pharmacist participates in the education of pharmacy students, residents and/or fellows by serving as a project advisor.	D	D	D

Continued on next page

TABLE 3. *(continued)*

Statement	Level I	Level II	Level III
5. The critical care pharmacist provides education to health professional students and trainees pertinent to critical care pharmacotherapy.	F	F	D
6. The critical care pharmacist provides formal accredited interprofessional educational sessions (such as medical grand rounds or intensive care rounds).	D	D	D
7. The pharmacist has an active role in interdisciplinary simulation activities.	D	D	D
8. The critical care pharmacist is a certified instructor and provides certification classes to other healthcare providers (ACLS, PALS, ENLS, as applicable).	D	D	D
9. The pharmacist develops and implements training programs for personnel working in the ICU.	F	D	D
10. The pharmacist identifies and educates medical and community groups about the role of pharmacists as part of the interdisciplinary healthcare team in the ICU.	D	D	D

Professional Development

Statement	Level I	Level II	Level III
1. The pharmacist maintains a mastery of knowledge related to current resources and primary literature pertinent to critical care pharmacotherapy.	F	F	D
2. The pharmacist maintains certification in available life-support courses (e.g. advanced cardiac life support [ACLS], pediatric advanced life support [PALS], emergency neurological life support [ENLS], advanced trauma life support [ATLS - audit], advanced burn life support [ABLS]), as applicable to practice.	F	F	D
3. Pharmacists practicing extensively in critical care will seek board certification in critical care pharmacy when eligible.	F	F	D
4. The pharmacist is involved in non-patient care activities including interdisciplinary committees and educational lectures.	F	F	D
5. The pharmacist provides formal accredited educational sessions at local, regional, state, and national meetings.	F	F	D
6. The critical care pharmacist is a member of a professional critical care organization, in addition to pharmacy organizations.	F	F	D
7. Pharmacy administrators should provide protected time for critical care pharmacists to facilitate education, administrative, research and scholarly activities.	F	D	D
8. Pharmacy administrators should create mechanisms for critical care pharmacists to develop their career and professional role within a health-system.	F	F	D

F=Foundational, D=Desirable

2. As part of the interdisciplinary team, the critical care pharmacist assists healthcare professionals in discussions with patients and/or family members to help make informed decisions regarding pharmacotherapy options.

   Level I: Foundational

   Level II: Foundational

   Level III: Desirable

3. The critical care pharmacist provides pertinent, comprehensive drug information to the critical care team.

   Level I: Foundational

   Level II: Foundational

   Level III: Foundational

4. The critical care pharmacist provides drug therapy–related education to critical care team members.

   Level I: Foundational

   Level II: Foundational

   Level III: Desirable

5. The pharmacist collaborates with the healthcare team to prevent potentially inappropriate drug therapy.

   Level I: Foundational

   Level II: Foundational

   Level III: Foundational

6. The critical care pharmacist provides clinical consultation to the care team, both within and outside the ICU, for pharmacotherapeutic issues related to critical illness.

   Level I: Foundational

   Level II: Foundational

   Level III: Foundational

7. Medication-related consults (i.e., pharmacotherapeutic and pharmacokinetic) are available 24 hr/d, 7 d/wk to all critically ill patients.

   Level I: Foundational

   Level II: Desirable

   Level III: Desirable

8. The critical care pharmacist provides pharmacokinetic monitoring and therapeutic adjustments when a targeted drug is prescribed.

   Level I: Foundational

   Level II: Foundational

   Level III: Foundational

9. The critical care pharmacist reviews the medication history to determine which maintenance medications should be continued during the acute illness.

   Level I: Foundational

   Level II: Foundational

   Level III: Desirable

10. The pharmacist assists with medication reconciliation for ICU patients at the time of ICU admission, transfer from the ICU to the ward, or discharge to home or facility.

    Level I: Foundational

    Level II: Foundational

    Level III: Foundational

11. When reviewing orders for verification, the critical care pharmacist prospectively evaluates all drug therapy for appropriate indication, dose, drug interactions, drug allergies, and monitors the patient's pharmacotherapeutic regimen for effectiveness and adverse drug events (ADEs), and intervenes as needed.

    Level I: Foundational

    Level II: Foundational

    Level III: Foundational

12. The critical care pharmacist educates patients and/or patients' care givers regarding medication therapies used to treat patients during and after acute illness, as appropriate.

    Level I: Foundational

    Level II: Foundational.

    Level III: Desirable

13. The pharmacist performs independent patient assessment (e.g., pain/agitation/delirium, nutrition).

    Level I: Foundational

    Level II: Desirable

    Level III: Desirable

14. A pharmacist certified in advanced cardiac life support (ACLS; or pediatric advanced life support [PALS]) responds to all resuscitation events in the hospital 24 hr/d, 7 d/wk.

    Level I: Foundational

    Level II: Foundational

    Level III: Desirable

15. The pharmacist responds, or coordinates pharmacist response to all resuscitation and time-dependent emergencies in the hospital, including, but not limited to cardiac arrest, rapid response, trauma response, hemorrhagic shock, sepsis response, and acute neurologic life support.

    Level I: Foundational

    Level II: Foundational

    Level III: Desirable

16. The pharmacist provides routine stewardship activities targeted at anti-infectives and other medications, including those that may be high risk for adverse events, high-cost concerns, and inappropriate utilization (e.g., factor products, anticoagulants, sedatives, acid-suppressive therapies).

    Level I: Foundational

    Level II: Foundational

    Level III: Foundational

17. The critical care pharmacist collaborates with other pharmacists (e.g., emergency medicine, infectious diseases, transplant, oncology), as needed, to address patient- and disease-specific therapeutic issues.

    Level I: Foundational

    Level II: Foundational

    Level III: Foundational

18. In conjunction with the clinical dietitian, the critical care pharmacist reviews the nutrition therapy plan and recommends modifications as indicated to optimize the nutritional regimen.

    Level I: Foundational

    Level II: Desirable

    Level III: Desirable

19. The critical care pharmacist uses the medical record as one means to communicate with other healthcare professionals, and/or to document specific pharmacotherapeutic recommendations or activities.

    Level I: Foundational

    Level II: Foundational

    Level III: Foundational

20. The critical care pharmacist uses appropriate documentation tools to demonstrate their impact on patient care and economic value.

    Level I: Foundational

    Level II: Foundational

    Level III: Foundational

21. Critical care pharmacists document pertinent collaborative medication management problems and progress notes daily.

    Level I: Desirable

    Level II: Desirable

    Level III: Desirable

22. The critical care pharmacist documents clinical activities that include, but are not limited to, disease state management, general pharmacotherapeutic monitoring, pharmacokinetic monitoring, ADEs, education, and other patient care activities.

    Level I: Foundational

    Level II: Foundational

    Level III: Foundational

23. The critical care pharmacist acts as a liaison between the pharmacy department and the interdisciplinary team to educate health professionals regarding current drug-related policies, procedures, guidelines, and pathways.

    Level I: Foundational

    Level II: Foundational

    Level III: Foundational

24. The critical care pharmacist uses pharmacoeconomic analyses in conjunction with the interdisciplinary team

to evaluate existing/new pharmacy services and the place of new drugs in critical care pharmacotherapy.

Level I: Foundational

Level II: Foundational

Level III: Desirable

25. The critical care pharmacist is proactive in designing, prioritizing, and promoting new clinical pharmacy programs and services.

Level I: Foundational

Level II: Foundational

Level III: Desirable

26. Pharmacy administrators evaluate clinical programs/services for stakeholder satisfaction, significance, and economic value.

Level I: Foundational

Level II: Foundational

Level III: Foundational

27. The critical care pharmacist prepares and presents drug therapy monographs and formulary reviews to the Pharmacy and Therapeutics committee for medications used in the care of critically ill patients.

Level I: Desirable

Level II: Desirable

Level III: Desirable

28. The pharmacist should participate in planning and implementation of processes for disaster, or mass causalities, scenarios as applicable to the critically ill patient.

Level I: Foundational

Level II: Foundational

Level III: Desirable

29. The majority of the critical care pharmacist's time is dedicated to critical care services, with few commitments, outside of critical care activities.

Level I: Foundational

Level II: Foundational

Level III: Desirable

30. Critical care pharmacists will have the majority of their clinical activity focused in the care of the critically ill population.

Level I: Foundational

Level II: Foundational

Level III: Desirable

31. Decentralized clinical pharmacy services in the ICU should include routine and consistent patient care coverage, inclusive of day, evening, and weekend coverage.

Level I: Foundational

Level II: Foundational

Level III: Desirable

32. Critical care pharmacy services are developed as "teams," with multiple critical care pharmacists available, to deliver consistent and quality collaborative medication management.

Level I: Foundational

Level II: Foundational

Level III: Desirable

33. In the absence of an onsite critical care pharmacist, CMM may be supplemented through telemedicine.

Level I: Desirable

Level II: Desirable

Level III: Desirable

34. The ICU pharmacist-to-patient ratio is defined based on patient acuity and complexity in addition to the scope of clinical and operational services provided.

Level I: Foundational

Level II: Foundational

Level III: Desirable

Discussion. The value of the critical care clinical pharmacist-to-patient care is well established.[6–9] Medication management is the most frequent decision category on patient care rounds; therefore, pharmacists on rounds have the opportunity to facilitate CMM and prevent ADEs.[10] An ADE is defined as an injury resulting from the use of a drug and can result in a wide range of consequences. A landmark trial justified the presence of a critical care pharmacist on rounds by reducing rates of preventable ADEs by 66% with a 99% acceptance rate for medication management recommendations.[11] An observational multicenter study in the United Kingdom identified approximately one of every six medication orders in the ICU required an intervention from a pharmacist, with two thirds rated as moderate to high impact.[12] Specifically, available evidence suggests enhanced patient safety and clinical outcomes with involvement of a pharmacist in the management of the following therapeutic domains: antimicrobial therapy, anticoagulation, pharmacokinetic dosing, pain/agitation/delirium, and emergency response.[13–31] Application of activities generally considered foundational has been shown to reduce overall hospital mortality across 885 hospitals.[32] Evolving evidence continues to support the benefit of a critical care pharmacist internationally with a broadening scope of practice in adult/PICUs and within various subspecialty critical care practices or post-ICU care clinics.[9,12,33–38] In the era of value-based care with rapidly rising medication costs, the economic impact of the critical care pharmacist has also been described.[11,19,22,39–41] It has been estimated that the return on investment of a critical care pharmacist approaches 25:1 in patients with infection.[19] Decentralized critical care pharmacists may achieve cost avoidance in excess of $200,000 per year when compared with centralized practice models.[40] A more conservative estimate of benefit up to $5 per $1 in labor costs would still represent a substantial benefit, considering the high cost of medications in critical care, averaging 31% of a hospital's total drug cost.[42,43] Evolving literature over the last several decades has demonstrated the clinical and pharmacoeconomic impact the critical care pharmacist has when providing direct patient care. As a result, the critical care pharmacist is recognized as an essential member of the interdisciplinary team by pharmacy and interprofessional organizations.[3,5,44–48]

Many services that were deemed "desirable" in the recommendations published in 2000 are now considered foundational activities, reflecting the progression of the profession in general and the growing body of literature that supports the role of a critical care pharmacist to positively affect therapy. Active participation of a critical care pharmacist in patient care rounds and within an interprofessional team is foundational at level I and II institutions (statement 1). Participation in rounds facilitates provision of CMM through review of medication orders for appropriateness and safety (statements 9–11), allows collaboration and communication of recommendations regarding the therapy plan (statements 5, 6, 17–21), and provides drug information (statements 2, 3, 12) and education to the interdisciplinary critical care team (statement 4, 23). Institutions with level III critical care services may not have formal rounds, but the critical care pharmacist or pharmacist should strive to review individual patient care plans and make recommendations, provide drug information, and educate the critical care staff.

Given that critical care pharmacists have demonstrated improvements in clinical and economic outcomes, it is essential that they are optimally deployed to maximize their benefit for the care of critically ill patients, such as the management of drugs with therapeutic monitoring to achieve pharmacologic endpoints (statements 7, 8, 13–16).[6–9,11,19,22,39,40,47] The critical care pharmacist thoroughly reviews individual patient pharmacotherapy needs, inclusive of prior to critical illness and postdischarge, and communicates recommendations to the critical care team to facilitate transitions of care (statements 9 and 10). The role of the critical care pharmacist continues to evolve since its transition from a pure dispensing role to clinical or hybrid clinical-operational roles, including involvement in multidisciplinary rounds, CMM, medication safety, quality improvement, protocol development, transitions of care, emergency response/resuscitation, patient and family communication, education, management of drug shortages and recalls, research, disaster preparedness, and prescribing once a diagnosis is made (statements 22, 24, 25, 27, 28).[3,8,10,47,49–58]

The ASHP Practice Advancement Initiative (PAI) recommends institutions to determine drug therapy management services for consistent delivery by pharmacists, devote resources to the provision of those services, and assign pharmacists to patient care units.[47] At the very least, it is deemed foundational at level I and II institutions that the majority of a critical care pharmacist's time is dedicated to the ICU and focused on clinical activities, and that the staffing model provides consistent critical care pharmacist coverage (statements 29, 30). Recent surveys report that only 43.5–62.2% of ICUs have pharmacists assigned to care for ICU patients along with significant variability in clinical activities, institutional type, and ICU bed allocation.[4,59] Ideally, critical care pharmacist coverage would be available 24 hr/d, 7 d/wk (statement 31). However, since economic and personnel constraints limit many institutions, it is recommended that institutions prioritize critical care pharmacy services to patients with the highest acuity and extend daily coverage to evening hours at a minimum.[60,61]

One approach to facilitate consistent coverage (foundational activity at level I and II institutions) is to develop teams of critical care pharmacists (statement 32).[3,60] As critical care pharmacy services expand to include the development of critical care pharmacist teams, it may be prudent to create critical care team leadership positions. The team leader can ensure establishment of cohesive and best practice pharmacy services, mentor the team of pharmacists, and lead the critical care pharmacy team in creation of clinical programs and development of team goals to optimize critical care pharmacy services. Pharmacy services may be designed to align with subspecialty critical care services in hospitals (e.g., medical, surgical, neuro, cardiac, trauma, burn) necessitating pharmacists with differing daily responsibilities to provide patient-centered care. Academic critical care pharmacists especially benefit from a team of pharmacists and designees to maintain consistent services. Additionally, resource-limited ICUs may choose to supplement coverage with critical care pharmacist participation through telemedicine services (statement 33). Recent reports have highlighted critical care pharmacist involvement in telepharmacy services and demonstrated that their involvement contributes to improved scores on process measures.[29,62,63] Establishing appropriate ICU pharmacist-to-patient ratios is foundational at level I and II institutions (statement 34). Bond and Raehl[32] described an association between clinical pharmacist-to-occupied bed ratio and lower mortality, but limited data are available to guide optimal ratios. Critical care pharmacist-to-patient ratios have been suggested in literature, although evidence is sparse and further research is needed.[8,64] Determinations regarding coverage and service design should be based on patient acuity and complexity and the scope of pharmacist services to ensure that critical care pharmacists are allocated time to perform the full range of patient care and other services associated with improved outcomes.

Although a single model will not meet the needs of all critical care practice settings, key components of ideal practice models outlined in the PAI and the literature can apply across practice settings.[10,47,48,53,54,61,65–70] It is recommended that each site determines how to best incorporate these recommendations such that every ICU patient receives CMM by a critical care pharmacist (statement 26).

Quality Improvement

Recommendations

1. The critical care pharmacist serves as the medication safety leader for critically ill patients by identifying potential ADEs, resolving existing ADEs, and improving medication use practices.

   Level I: Foundational

   Level II: Foundational

   Level III: Foundational
2. The critical care pharmacist assists with the management of ADEs and develops process improvements to reduce and/or prevent medication errors.

   Level I: Foundational

   Level II: Foundational

   Level III: Foundational
3. The critical care pharmacist participates in reporting ADEs to institutional committees and national programs (e.g., the Food and Drug Administration Medwatch program).

   Level I: Foundational

   Level II: Foundational

   Level III: Foundational

4. The critical care pharmacist is involved in continual evaluation of the availability of critical medications through optimization of automated dispensing cabinets.

    Level I: Foundational

    Level II: Foundational

    Level III: Foundational

5. The critical care pharmacist should be involved as a team member in the design process for building a new or remodeling critical care area.

    Level I: Desirable

    Level II: Desirable

    Level III: Desirable

6. The critical care pharmacist implements and maintains departmental policies and procedures related to safe and effective use of medications in the ICU.

    Level I: Foundational

    Level II: Foundational

    Level III: Foundational

7. The critical care pharmacist coordinates the development and implementation of ICU-focused drug therapy protocols, guidelines, order sets, and/or care pathways to maximize benefits of pharmacotherapy.

    Level I: Foundational

    Level II: Foundational

    Level III: Desirable

8. The pharmacist independently investigates or collaborates with other critical care healthcare team members to evaluate the impact of drug therapy protocols, guidelines, order sets, and/or care pathways used in the ICU (e.g., drug administration, disease state management algorithms).

    Level I: Foundational

    Level II: Desirable

    Level III: Desirable

9. The critical care pharmacist leads or provides consultation to hospital committees when critical care pharmacotherapy issues are discussed.

    Level I: Foundational

    Level II: Foundational

    Level III: Desirable

10. The critical care pharmacist serves on and provides consultation to hospital committees when critical care pharmacotherapy issues are discussed.

    Level I: Foundational

    Level II: Foundational

    Level III: Foundational

11. The critical care pharmacist contributes to the hospital newsletter and drug monographs, on issues related to medication use in the ICU.

    Level I: Foundational

    Level II: Foundational

    Level III: Desirable

12. The critical care pharmacist identifies and evaluates drug cost minimization opportunities and implements cost containment measures.

    Level I: Foundational

    Level II: Foundational

    Level III: Desirable

13. The critical care pharmacist is involved in identifying local quality metrics for continuous quality improvement (e.g., risk-adjusted mortality, medication errors per medications ordered/dispensed, mechanical ventilation duration, delirium, mobilization).

    Level I: Foundational

    Level II: Desirable

    Level III: Desirable

14. The critical care pharmacist participates in quality assurance programs to enhance collaborative medication management, minimize costs, provide ongoing evaluation of current processes, and identify the need for new programs/processes.

    Level I: Foundational

    Level II: Foundational

    Level III: Desirable

15. The critical care pharmacist shares responsibility for hospital performance for quality and process measure compliance, such as core measures and other hospital metrics (e.g., *Clostridium difficile* infection rates, vaccinations, patient satisfaction surveys), as it relates to critical care patients.

    Level I: Foundational

    Level II: Foundational

    Level III: Desirable

16. The critical care pharmacist collaborates with medical staff, nursing, other members of the healthcare team, and hospital administration to prepare the ICU for accreditation and to address any deficiencies identified.

    Level I: Foundational

    Level II: Foundational

    Level III: Desirable

17. Pharmacy space and facilities in the ICU are regularly assessed to determine whether efficiency can be improved, where applicable.

    Level I: Foundational

    Level II: Desirable

    Level III: Desirable

18. Real-time dashboard, or analytics monitoring, of quality metrics and drug utilization are available for the pharmacist to review for patient care and research.

    Level I: Desirable

    Level II: Desirable

    Level III: Desirable

19. Safety technology is implemented, inclusive of bedside barcode scanning, clinical decision support systems, and intelligent IV infusion devices in the routine care of critically ill patients.

    Level I: Foundational

    Level II: Foundational

    Level III: Foundational

20. Medication use systems have the ability to:

    i. create and maintain patient medication profiles;

    ii. interface with patient laboratory data and other relevant test results;

    iii. interface with patient charts (medication profiles) from other health systems and outpatient clinics;

iv. alert users to drug allergies;
v. alert users to medication maximum dose limits;
vi. alert users to medications prior to admission;
vii. alert users to diagnoses;
viii. alert users to drug-drug and drug-food/nutrient interactions;
ix. alert users to formulary and nonformulary medications as well as approved substitutions;
x. alert users to pertinent medication shortages; and
xi. provide live, real-time data that can be incorporated in pharmacotherapy decision-making.

Level I: Foundational

Level II: Foundational

Level III: Foundational

21. The hospital information management system is computerized, is able to comply with those requirements listed for medication use processes, and has the ability to:

i. allow direct provider order entry;
ii. interface with bedside clinical information systems in real time;
iii. alert users to disease state-drug and drug-drug interactions;
iv. provide IV admixture information (e.g., compatibility, stability, preparation);
v. provide medication information via references or internal guidelines/documents;
vi. allow documentation of pharmacy patient care interventions;
vii. provide benchmarking and quality data;
viii. access to policies and procedures related to medications;
ix. interface with mobile devices; and
x. provide patient-specific treatment algorithms.

Level I: Foundational

Level II: Foundational

Level III: Foundational

Discussion. As many as 98,000 people die in hospitals each year due to preventable medical errors.[71] In the ICU, medication errors represent the most common type of medical error and often lead to ADEs.[72,73] When compared with non-ICUs, the rate of preventable and potential ADEs occur twice as often in critical care settings.[74] More worrisome is that for every fifth dose of administered medications, one preventable error will occur, most commonly due to dose omission, incorrect dose, incorrect drug or technique, or interaction.[75] Only recently, guidelines for the safe use of medication in the ICU have been introduced.[76] Our recommendation regarding implementation of barcode medication administration provides the same intent as these guidelines while noting the weak nature of the existing evidence.

Optimizing safe medication use requires involvement of the critical care pharmacist throughout the entire medication use process (statements 2, 3, 6). Whether by rounding with the ICU team or developing ICU-focused policies and procedures, protocols, guidelines, order sets, and pathways, these functions are considered foundational for critical care pharmacists (statements 7, 8, 20). Other areas of pharmacist involvement include the implementation and maintenance of safe medication technologies (e.g., bedside barcode scanning, computerized prescriber order entry, and intelligent IV infusion devices), clinical decision support, and surveillance programs (statements 19, 21).[77–79] Given that most errors in the ICU are medication related, pharmacists are uniquely positioned to lead the healthcare team in preventing, identifying, and investigate the cause of errors and make recommendations to prevent future events from occurring (statements 1, 9–11).

Stemming from involvement in institutional committees and from the pharmacist's role on the interprofessional team, critical care pharmacists have become involved in quality improvement initiatives, assisted in determining and meeting various quality metrics and performance measures, and promoted adherence to guidelines and protocols (statements 4, 8, 13, 18). Numerous studies have demonstrated the critical care pharmacist's role in implementation and maintenance of compliance with various quality improvement initiatives.[25,26,30,80–84] Additionally, pharmacists have promoted appropriate utilization of stress ulcer prophylaxis,[85,86] adherence to a vasopressin protocol,[87] reduction of door to needle time for tissue plasminogen activator,[88] reduction in ADEs,[11] reducing the risk of QTc interval prolongation,[89] improvement in patient safety,[90] and a decrease in drug-drug interactions.[91] Similarly, committee involvement and clinical practice experience enable critical care pharmacists to facilitate rapid access to critical medications for emergency scenarios (statements 5, 16, 17).[5,92] Pharmacist participation in accreditation surveys is necessary to fulfill certain regulatory standards (statement 15).

One of the principle responsibilities of critical care pharmacists regarding quality improvement is assurance of high-quality cost-effective care (statements 12–14). The American College of Critical Care Medicine critical care services and personnel guidelines recommend pharmacists implement and maintain policies and procedures regarding safe and effective medication use.[5] It has been found that critical care pharmacists reduce medication cost while maintaining appropriate treatment.[19,22,38,87,93–96] Critical care pharmacists are equipped with select knowledge and skills useful in determining the most cost-effective use of medications in the ICU, while still maintaining quality of care and patient outcomes.[97]

Research/Scholarship

Recommendations

1. The pharmacist is actively involved in critical care pharmacotherapy research, including, but not limited to, developing and reviewing study proposals, screening and/or enrollment of patients, publication of study results, and serving as a Principal Investigator, co-investigator, study coordinator, or contact person, where applicable.

   Level I: Desirable

   Level II: Desirable

   Level III: Desirable

2. The pharmacist contributes to the pharmacy and medical literature (e.g., case reports, letters to the editor, and therapeutic, pharmacokinetic, and pharmacoeconomic reports).

   Level I: Desirable

   Level II: Desirable

   Level III: Desirable

3. The pharmacist reports research results to the pharmacy and medical community at regional, national, and international meetings.
   Level I: Desirable
   Level II: Desirable
   Level III: Desirable
4. The pharmacist participates in research design and data analysis.
   Level I: Desirable
   Level II: Desirable
   Level III: Desirable
5. The pharmacist secures funds for conducting research.
   Level I: Desirable
   Level II: Desirable
   Level III: Desirable
6. The critical care pharmacist participates as a key investigator for critical care research.
   Level I: Foundational
   Level II: Desirable
   Level III: Desirable
7. Critical care pharmacists are actively involved in collaborating in multicenter research projects.
   Level I: Desirable
   Level II: Desirable
   Level III: Desirable
8. The profession of pharmacy is represented on the Institutional Review Board and/or Scientific Review Board, as applicable.
   Level I: Foundational
   Level II: Desirable
   Level III: Desirable
9. The pharmacist contributes to the medical literature as a peer reviewer.
   Level I: Desirable
   Level II: Desirable
   Level III: Desirable

Discussion. In contrast to many of the clinical pharmacy services that are rated by the taskforce as foundational, those involving research/scholarship are considered desirable across all ICU levels of services for eight of nine statements. This suggests that the scope of activities provided by the pharmacist should extend beyond clinical services, many of which are now engrained in patient care, to functions that include research/scholarship, especially at level I ICUs.[7] The two research/scholarship functions that are rated as "foundational" are representation of the pharmacist on the Institutional/Scientific Review Board and participation of the pharmacist as a key investigator, both only at level I ICUs (statements 6 and 8). The only function related to research/scholarship that was rated as "foundational" in the position paper published in 2000 was the representation of a pharmacist on the Institutional/Scientific Review Board.[3] It should be noted that unlike the 2000 paper, the current taskforce did not address the role of the pharmacist in providing Investigational Drug Services, as these functions are carried out in accordance with the Good Clinical Practice Guidelines as mandated by the Code of Federal Regulations and should be "foundational" activities at all institutions.[98]

Many pharmacists already actively engage in research/scholarship, so it is not surprising that the taskforce recognized the pharmacist as a key investigator as a foundational service, albeit only at level I ICUs. The term "key investigator" in this sense is meant to describe the investigator who conceived the project and is responsible for its completion. In many cases, project results may never be disseminated beyond the home institution, so presenting at scientific meetings or contributing to the medical literature are considered "desirable" activities. The results of a survey of ICU pharmacy functions conducted over a decade ago showed nearly half (45.5%) of pharmacists engage in research in high-level roles.[4] However, many of the pharmacists responding to this survey practiced in level I ICUs, so it is not evident that these services are commonly provided across all ICUs. Many granting agencies and research practices promote multidisciplinary involvement in research/scholarship. Therefore, it is highly likely in the future that the level and scope of pharmacy services related to research/scholarship will continue to expand to the extent that many more activities will become foundational across all ICUs.

It is expected that demand by other healthcare disciplines for pharmacists to directly engage in functions involving research/scholarship will increase as pharmacists possess unique knowledge and skills about study design, data analyses, and pharmacotherapy application in research.[99] The results of another survey of ICU providers and pharmacists showed nonpharmacist providers consistently valued the clinical and financial impact of all pharmacy services, including those involving research/scholarship.[100] It will be incumbent on the profession of pharmacy to ensure that critical care pharmacists are appropriately trained to deliver the functions of research/scholarship across all ICUs.

Training/Education

Recommendations

1. The critical care pharmacist provides an interprofessional experience in training and mentoring pharmacy students, residents, and fellows through experiential critical care rotations.
   Level I: Foundational
   Level II: Foundational
   Level III: Desirable
2. The critical care pharmacist supports postgraduate residencies and/or fellowship training in critical care pharmacy practice.
   Level I: Foundational
   Level II: Foundational
   Level III: Desirable
3. Critical care pharmacy trainees should be evaluated on educational outcomes and documented experiences to demonstrate competence for a given subject.
   Level I: Foundational
   Level II: Foundational
   Level III: Foundational

4. The pharmacist participates in the education of pharmacy students, residents, and/or fellows by serving as a project advisor.

   Level I: Desirable

   Level II: Desirable

   Level III: Desirable

5. The critical care pharmacist provides education to health professional students and trainees pertinent to critical care pharmacotherapy.

   Level I: Foundational

   Level II: Foundational

   Level III: Desirable

6. The critical care pharmacist provides formal accredited interprofessional educational sessions (such as medical grand rounds or intensive care rounds).

   Level I: Desirable

   Level II: Desirable

   Level III: Desirable

7. The pharmacist has an active role in interdisciplinary simulation activities.

   Level I: Desirable

   Level II: Desirable

   Level III: Desirable

8. The critical care pharmacist is a certified instructor and provides certification classes to other healthcare providers (ACLS, PALS, emergency neurologic life support [ENLS], as applicable).

   Level I: Desirable

   Level II: Desirable

   Level III: Desirable

9. The pharmacist develops and implements training programs for personnel working in the ICU.

   Level I: Foundational

   Level II: Desirable

   Level III: Desirable

10. The pharmacist identifies and educates medical and community groups about the role of pharmacists as part of the interdisciplinary healthcare team in the ICU.

    Level I: Desirable

    Level II: Desirable

    Level III: Desirable

Discussion. An interdisciplinary, collaborative approach to patient care is necessary as the complexity of healthcare expands, especially in the critical care population. Consequently, education of healthcare professions should be interprofessional to foster interactions that enhance the practice of each individual discipline within the team (statements 1, 4). The ACCP position statement on interprofessional education and practice supports interprofessional learning and skills development, an understanding of respective disciplinary roles, mutual respect, and a sustained commitment to interprofessional learning and patient care.[101] Therefore, the critical care pharmacist should be deeply involved in interprofessional training and these activities are considered foundational for critical care pharmacists practicing in level I ICUs and foundational or desirable for level II and III ICUs (statements 1–4, 8). Direct patient care experience for trainees provides invaluable opportunity to develop and refine problem-solving abilities, accountability, efficiency, build confidence, understand clinical disease and pharmacotherapy, and to mature professionally. Practical skills training is foundational, as opposed to didactic education (statement 4, 5, 10).[102] Trainees can facilitate expansion of clinical services or support clinical programs in areas that are underserved, and critical care pharmacist participation in training programs is considered foundational for level I and II ICUs (statement 3). The fact that many of these educational services are deemed "foundational" represents advancements in practice as all educational and training activities were considered desirable or optimal services in the recommendations published in 2000.[3]

The critical care pharmacist should provide interprofessional experiences to trainees but also create and deliver education to all members of the team. As highlighted in the statements (statements 6–9), this may include the interdisciplinary critical care team, other community healthcare members, or through certification classes or simulation activities. These activities are considered desirable, in addition to the core foundational activities recommended above. The ACCP white paper on interprofessional education provides environment specific models, assessment methods, and important implications and barriers to the application of interprofessional education for the clinical pharmacist.[103]

Finally, to accomplish the vision of ACCP and ASHP that all entry-level hospital pharmacists will complete postgraduate residency training, or have sufficient hospital experience, prior to entering practice, the critical care pharmacist should develop opportunities and support the infrastructure of first- and second-year residency programs and fellowships (statement 3).[104,105]

Professional Development

Recommendations

1. The pharmacist maintains a mastery of knowledge related to current resources and primary literature pertinent to critical care pharmacotherapy.

   Level I: Foundational

   Level II: Foundational

   Level III: Desirable

2. The pharmacist maintains certification in available life-support courses (e.g., ACLS, PALS, ENLS, advanced trauma life support [ATLS—audit], and advanced burn life support [ABLS]), as applicable to practice.

   Level I: Foundational

   Level II: Foundational

   Level III: Desirable

3. Pharmacists practicing extensively in critical care will seek board certification in critical care pharmacy when eligible.

   Level I: Foundational

   Level II: Foundational

   Level III: Desirable

4. The pharmacist is involved in non–patient care activities, including interdisciplinary committees and educational lectures.
   Level I: Foundational
   Level II: Foundational
   Level III: Desirable
5. The pharmacist provides formal accredited educational sessions at local, regional, state, and national meetings.
   Level I: Foundational
   Level II: Foundational
   Level III: Desirable
6. The critical care pharmacist is a member of a professional critical care organization, in addition to pharmacy organizations.
   Level I: Foundational
   Level II: Foundational
   Level III: Desirable
7. Pharmacy administrators should provide protected time for critical care pharmacists to facilitate education, administrative, research, and scholarly activities.
   Level I: Foundational
   Level II: Desirable
   Level III: Desirable
8. Pharmacy administrators should create mechanisms for critical care pharmacists to develop their career and professional role within a health system.
   Level I: Foundational
   Level II: Foundational
   Level III: Desirable

Discussion. To provide CMM to their patients, critical care pharmacists require appropriate preparation (statement 1). The goals and objectives of a postgraduate year 2 critical care pharmacy residency are a starting point, along with basic credentials such as the life-support certifications (e.g., ACLS, PALS, ENLS, ATLS, and ABLS) for any practitioner who participates in resuscitation activities (statements 2–3). Required competency of a clinical pharmacist has been defined and includes six essential domains, including board certification.[106] Thus, board certification in critical care pharmacotherapy is a foundational credential for critical care pharmacists in level I and II settings, and board certification in general pharmacotherapy is a desirable competency for any pharmacist practicing direct patient care in the hospital (statement 3). Board certification ensures high-quality–continuing education, provides a recognized minimum credential for direct patient care, and is becoming a required credential in hospitals.[107] Board certification may increase pharmacist credibility within the critical care team, as a parallel to the medical model. The Board of Pharmacy Specialties credential of Board Certified Critical Care Pharmacist is most applicable. However, alternative or additional board certifications may be appropriate for a critical care pharmacist practicing in subspecialized areas (e.g., pediatrics, nutritional support).

Employers benefit from highly competent staff and should facilitate the development process and create privileging standards and rewards.[107] A career recognition process with medical staff/hospital privileging creates a standardized platform for "top of the license" practice and allows for prescribing and other practice benefits in a variety of practice settings.[51] Pharmacy department leaders will need to demonstrate strong leadership and advocacy to achieve a credentialing and privileging process. A standard template for evaluation of the many practice-related, educational, and scholarly activities of a clinical pharmacist should be implemented.[108] Professionalism and scholarly activity can be further encouraged through the provision of protected time to attend meetings and participate in scholarly activities as a component of critical care pharmacist career development and is a foundational need in level I settings (statements 4–8). Ensuring ongoing competence and professional development is essential to ensure ongoing high-quality practice and is foundational in level I and II settings. Membership in critical care organizations creates opportunities for foundational, high-level professional education (statement 6).

The completion of tasks related to professional development will increase visibility of the pharmacist and their employer and facilitates peer recognition both within and outside of pharmacy (statement 5, 7–8). Activities can include scholarly efforts such as conducting research and publishing in respected journals. The pharmacist should be actively engaged in providing pharmacy and interdisciplinary education, further establishing one's self as the medication expert at the local, regional, state, national, and international level. Active membership and involvement in critical care organizations and pharmacy-specific organizations are important and foundational for level I and II and can provide opportunities for education, appointment or election to offices, committee participation, and nominations for various awards and fellowship status. Although recognition enhances the image of the individual pharmacist, the opportunity to network and work to support the profession can enhance their effectiveness as a practitioner.

Summary

Through multiorganizational collaboration among the SCCM, American Society of Health-System Pharmacists, and ACCP, this article provides an updated roadmap for establishing and refining critical care pharmacy services in the form of 82 statement recommendations. Informed by task force members from various critical care and administrative practice settings, these guidelines address the various domains of critical care pharmacy practice. Guideline recommendation statements were generated through a rigorous process of literature evaluation and debate.

Technology, regulation, and the services and role of pharmacists continue to evolve within the healthcare setting. Critical care pharmacists have been leaders in defining their roles and provided the framework for these statements. Although this is a potential limitation of this document, and may appear self-serving, it also creates a framework to stimulate self-reflection. This document is an important tool that critical care practitioners and administrators should use to evaluate progress toward the highest levels of activity within the realms of patient care, quality improvement, research and scholarship, training and education, and professional development. Although limited resources may impact optimal implementation within any setting, these statements can serve as a roadmap to the highest level of care. It is hoped that practitioners will continue to document their roles and impact on patient outcome to make this an ongoing process.

References

1. Vincent JL: Critical care—where have we been and where are we going? *Crit Care* 2013; 17(Suppl 1):S2.
2. Harvey AK Whitney J, Nahata MC, et al: Francke's legacy—40 years of clinical pharmacy. *Ann Pharmacother* 2008; 42:121–126.
3. Rudis MI, Brandl KM: Position paper on critical care pharmacy services. Society of Critical Care Medicine and American College of Clinical Pharmacy Task Force on critical care pharmacy services. *Crit Care Med* 2000; 28:3746–3750.
4. Maclaren R, Devlin JW, Martin SJ, et al: Critical care pharmacy services in United States hospitals. *Ann Pharmacother* 2006; 40:612–618.
5. Haupt MT, Bekes CE, Brilli RJ, et al; Task Force of the American College of Critical Care Medicine, Society of Critical Care Medicine: Guidelines on critical care services and personnel: Recommendations based on a system of categorization of three levels of care. *Crit Care Med* 2003; 31:2677–2683.
6. Dager W, Bolesta S, Brophy G, et al: An opinion paper outlining recommendations for training, credentialing, and documenting and justifying critical care pharmacy services. *Pharmacotherapy* 2011; 31.
7. Preslaski CR, Lat I, MacLaren R, et al: Pharmacist contributions as members of the multidisciplinary ICU team. *Chest* 2013; 144:1687–1695.
8. Horn E, Jacobi J: The critical care clinical pharmacist: Evolution of an essential team member. *Crit Care Med* 2006; 34:S46–S51.
9. McKenzie MS, Auriemma CL, Olenik J, et al: An observational study of decision making by medical intensivists. *Crit Care Med* 2015; 43:1660–1668.
10. Bauer SR, Kane-Gill SL: Outcome assessment of critical care pharmacist services. *Hosp Pharm* 2016; 51:507–513.
11. Leape LL, Cullen DJ, Clapp MD, et al: Pharmacist participation on physician rounds and adverse drug events in the intensive care unit. *JAMA* 1999; 282:267–270.
12. Shulman R, McKenzie CA, Landa J, et al; PROTECTED-UK Group: Pharmacist's review and outcomes: Treatment-enhancing contributions tallied, evaluated, and documented (PROTECTED-UK). *J Crit Care* 2015; 30:808–813.
13. Carver PL, Lin SW, DePestel DD, et al: Impact of mecA gene testing and intervention by infectious disease clinical pharmacists on time to optimal antimicrobial therapy for Staphylococcus aureus bacteremia at a university hospital. *J Clin Microbiol* 2008; 46:2381–2383.
14. Gentry CA, Greenfield RA, Slater LN, et al: Outcomes of an antimicrobial control program in a teaching hospital. *Am J Health Syst Pharm* 2000; 57:268–274.
15. Bond CA, Raehl CL: Clinical and economic outcomes of pharmacist-managed antimicrobial prophylaxis in surgical patients. *Am J Health Syst Pharm* 2007; 64:1935–1942.
16. Bond CA, Raehl CL: Clinical and economic outcomes of pharmacist-managed aminoglycoside or vancomycin therapy. *Am J Health Syst Pharm* 2005; 62:1596–1605.
17. Wade WE, McCall CY: Pharmacist-managed aminoglycoside therapy in combination with a beta-lactam agent in the treatment of nosocomial pneumonia in critically ill patients. *Pharmacotherapy* 1995; 15:216–219.
18. Streetman DS, Nafziger AN, Destache CJ, et al: Individualized pharmacokinetic monitoring results in less aminoglycoside-associated nephrotoxicity and fewer associated costs. *Pharmacotherapy* 2001; 21:443–451.
19. MacLaren R, Bond CA, Martin SJ, et al: Clinical and economic outcomes of involving pharmacists in the direct care of critically ill patients with infections. *Crit Care Med* 2008; 36:3184–3189.
20. Petitta A: Assessing the value of pharmacists' health-systemwide services: Clinical pathways and treatment guidelines. *Pharmacotherapy* 2000; 20:327S–332S.
21. To L, Schillig JM, DeSmet BD, et al: Impact of a pharmacist-directed anticoagulation service on the quality and safety of heparin-induced thrombocytopenia management. *Ann Pharmacother* 2011; 45:195–200.
22. MacLaren R, Bond CA: Effects of pharmacist participation in intensive care units on clinical and economic outcomes of critically ill patients with thromboembolic or infarction-related events. *Pharmacotherapy* 2009; 29:761–768.
23. Bond CA, Raehl CL: Pharmacist-provided anticoagulation management in United States hospitals: Death rates, length of stay, Medicare charges, bleeding complications, and transfusions. *Pharmacotherapy* 2004; 24:953–963.
24. Dager WE, Branch JM, King JH, et al: Optimization of inpatient warfarin therapy: Impact of daily consultation by a pharmacist-managed anticoagulation service. *Ann Pharmacother* 2000; 34:567–572.
25. MacLaren R, Plamondon JM, Ramsay KB, et al: A prospective evaluation of empiric versus protocol-based sedation and analgesia. *Pharmacotherapy* 2000; 20:662–672.
26. Marshall J, Finn CA, Theodore AC: Impact of a clinical pharmacist-enforced intensive care unit sedation protocol on duration of mechanical ventilation and hospital stay. *Crit Care Med* 2008; 36:427–433.
27. Devlin JW, Nasraway SA Jr: Reversing oversedation in the intensive care unit: The role of pharmacists in energizing guideline efforts and overcoming protocol fatigue. *Crit Care Med* 2008; 36:626–628.
28. Devlin JW, Holbrook AM, Fuller HD: The effect of ICU sedation guidelines and pharmacist interventions on clinical outcomes and drug cost. *Ann Pharmacother* 1997; 31:689–695.
29. Forni A, Skehan N, Hartman CA, et al: Evaluation of the impact of a tele-ICU pharmacist on the management of sedation in critically ill mechanically ventilated patients. *Ann Pharmacother* 2010; 44:432–438.
30. Louzon P, Jennings H, Ali M, et al: Impact of pharmacist management of pain, agitation, and delirium in the intensive care unit through participation in multidisciplinary bundle rounds. *Am J Health Syst Pharm* 2017; 74:253–262.
31. Draper HM, Eppert JA: Association of pharmacist presence on compliance with advanced cardiac life support guidelines during in-hospital cardiac arrest. *Ann Pharmacother* 2008; 42:469–474.

32. Bond CA, Raehl CL: Clinical pharmacy services, pharmacy staffing, and hospital mortality rates. *Pharmacotherapy* 2007; 27:481–493.
33. Tripathi S, Crabtree HM, Fryer KR, et al: Impact of clinical pharmacist on the pediatric intensive care practice: An 11-year tertiary center experience. *J Pediatr Pharmacol Ther* 2015; 20:290–298.
34. Beardsley JR, Jones CM, Williamson J, et al: Pharmacist involvement in a multidisciplinary initiative to reduce sepsis-related mortality. *Am J Health Syst Pharm* 2016; 73:143–149.
35. Michalets E, Creger J, Shillinglaw WR: Outcomes of expanded use of clinical pharmacist practitioners in addition to team-based care in a community health system intensive care unit. *Am J Health Syst Pharm* 2015; 72:47–53.
36. Jiang SP, Chen J, Zhang XG, et al: Implementation of pharmacists' interventions and assessment of medication errors in an intensive care unit of a Chinese tertiary hospital. *Ther Clin Risk Manag* 2014; 10:861–866.
37. Fideles GM, de Alcântara-Neto JM, Peixoto Júnior AA, et al: Pharmacist recommendations in an intensive care unit: Three-year clinical activities. *Rev Bras Ter Intensiva* 2015; 27:149–154.
38. Montazeri M, Cook DJ: Impact of a clinical pharmacist in a multidisciplinary intensive care unit. *Crit Care Med* 1994; 22:1044–1048.
39. Stollings JL, Caylor MM: Postintensive care syndrome and the role of a follow-up clinic. *Am J Health Syst Pharm* 2015; 72:1315–1323.
40. Kopp BJ, Mrsan M, Erstad BL, et al: Cost implications of and potential adverse events prevented by interventions of a critical care pharmacist. *Am J Health Syst Pharm* 2007; 64:2483–2487.
41. Hammond DA, Flowers HJ, Meena N, et al: Cost avoidance associated with clinical pharmacist presence in a medical intensive care unit. *J Am Coll Clin Pharm* 2019; 2:610–615.
42. Haas CE, Vermeulen LC: Caution warranted when torturing data until they confess. *J Am Coll Clin Pharm* 2019; 2:606–607.
43. Altawalbeh SM, Saul MI, Seybert AL, et al: Intensive care unit drug costs in the context of total hospital drug expenditures with suggestions for targeted cost containment efforts. *J Crit Care* 2018; 44:77–81.
44. Brilli RJ, Spevetz A, Branson RD, et al; American College of Critical Care Medicine Task Force on Models of Critical Care Delivery. The American College of Critical Care Medicine Guidelines for the Definition of an Intensivist and the Practice of Critical Care Medicine: Critical care delivery in the intensive care unit: Defining clinical roles and the best practice model. *Crit Care Med* 2001; 29:2007–2019.
45. Dellit TH, Owens RC, McGowan JE Jr, et al; Infectious Diseases Society of America; Society for Healthcare Epidemiology of America: Infectious Diseases Society of America and the Society for Healthcare Epidemiology of America guidelines for developing an institutional program to enhance antimicrobial stewardship. *Clin Infect Dis* 2007; 44:159–177.
46. Doherty RB, Crowley RA; Health and Public Policy Committee of the American College of Physicians: Principles supporting dynamic clinical care teams: An American College of Physicians position paper. *Ann Intern Med* 2013; 159:620–626.
47. The consensus of the pharmacy practice model summit. *Am J Health Syst Pharm* 2011; 68:1148–1152.
48. American College of Clinical Pharmacy: Standards of practice for clinical pharmacists. *Pharmacotherapy* 2014; 34:794–797.
49. International Pharmaceutical Federation: The Role of the Pharmacist in Crisis Management: Including Manmade and Natural Disasters and Pandemics. 2005:1–4. Available at: http://www.fip.org/www/uploads/database_file.php?id=208&table_id.
50. ASHP statement on the role of health-system pharmacists in emergency preparedness. *Am J Health Syst Pharm* 2003; 60:1993–1995.
51. Jordan TA, Hennenfent JA, Lewin JJ 3rd, et al: Elevating pharmacists' scope of practice through a health-system clinical privileging process. *Am J Health Syst Pharm* 2016; 73:1395–1405.
52. Abramowitz PW, Thompson KK, Cobaugh DJ: The time has come: Increased prescribing authority for pharmacists. *Am J Health Syst Pharm* 2016; 73:1386–1387.
53. Shane R: Critical requirements for health-system pharmacy practice models that achieve optimal use of medicines. *Am J Health Syst Pharm* 2011; 68:1101–1111.
54. Jacobi J, Ray S, Danelich I, et al: Impact of the pharmacy practice model initiative on clinical pharmacy specialist practice. *Pharmacotherapy* 2016; 36:e40–e49.
55. Feih J, Peppard WJ, Katz M: Pharmacist involvement on a rapid response team. *Am J Health Syst Pharm* 2017; 74:S10–S16.
56. Bauer SR, Abraham PE, Barletta JF, et al: Development of the Critical Care Pharmacotherapy Trials Network. *Am J Health Syst Pharm* 2017; 74:287–293.
57. Alkhalili M, Ma J, Grenier S: Defining roles for pharmacy personnel in disaster response and emergency preparedness. *Disaster Med Public Health Prep* 2017; 11:496–504.
58. Pincock LL, Montello MJ, Tarosky MJ, et al: Pharmacist readiness roles for emergency preparedness. *Am J Health Syst Pharm* 2011; 68:620–623.
59. Pedersen CA, Schneider PJ, Scheckelhoff DJ: ASHP national survey of pharmacy practice in hospital settings: Dispensing and administration–2011. *Am J Health Syst Pharm* 2012; 69:768–785.
60. Erstad BL: A primer on critical care pharmacy services. *Ann Pharmacother* 2008; 42:1871–1881.
61. Granko RP, Poppe LB, Savage SW, et al: Method to determine allocation of clinical pharmacist resources. *Am J Health Syst Pharm* 2012; 69:1398–1404.
62. Hassan E, Depietro M, Zubrow M, et al: Effect of sedation tapering as part of multiprofessional pain, agitation and delirium program on ICU outcomes. In: American Society of Health System Pharmacists 47th Annual Midyear Clinical Meeting. Las Vegas, NV, 2012, pp A5–A050.

63. Meidl TM, Woller TW, Iglar AM, et al: Implementation of pharmacy services in a telemedicine intensive care unit. *Am J Health Syst Pharm* 2008; 65:1464–1469.
64. SHPA Committee of Specialty Practice in Critical Care: SHPA standards of practice for critical care pharmacy practice. *J Pharm Pract Res* 2008; 38:58–60.
65. Mason KC: Cutting-edge practice model: An integrated model within a large academic medical center. *Am J Health Syst Pharm* 2011; 68:1112.
66. Geiger BL: Cutting-edge practice model: Experience in a veterans affairs hospital. *Am J Health Syst Pharm* 2011; 68:1112–1113.
67. Berry R: Cutting-edge practice model: Experience in a small community hospital. *Am J Health Syst Pharm* 2011; 68:1113.
68. Pickette SG: Cutting-edge practice model: Experience in a community hospital system. *Am J Health Syst Pharm* 2011; 68:1114.
69. Berensen NM: Cutting-edge practice model: A mixed integrated and clinical specialist model in a large health system. *Am J Health Syst Pharm* 2011; 68:1114–1115.
70. Kucukarslan SN, Corpus K, Mehta N, et al: Evaluation of a dedicated pharmacist staffing model in the medical intensive care unit. *Hosp Pharm* 2013; 48:922–930.
71. Kohn LT, Corrigan JM, Molla S: To err is human. *Medicine (Baltimore)* 1999; 126:312.
72. Hale GM, Kane-Gill SL, Groetzinger L, et al: An evaluation of adverse drug reactions associated with antipsychotic use for the treatment of delirium in the intensive care unit. *J Pharm Pract* 2016; 29:355–360.
73. Smithburger PL, Buckley MS, Culver MA, et al: A multicenter evaluation of off-label medication use and associated adverse drug reactions in adult medical ICUs. *Crit Care Med* 2015; 43:1612–1621.
74. Cullen DJ, Sweitzer BJ, Bates DW, et al: Preventable adverse drug events in hospitalized patients: A comparative study of intensive care and general care units. *Crit Care Med* 1997; 25:1289–1297.
75. Kopp BJ, Erstad BL, Allen ME, et al: Medication errors and adverse drug events in an intensive care unit: Direct observation approach for detection. *Crit Care Med* 2006; 34:415–425.
76. Kane-Gill SL, Dasta JF, Buckley MS, et al: Clinical practice guideline: Safe medication use in the ICU. *Crit Care Med* 2017; 45:e877–e915.
77. Smithburger PL, Buckley MS, Bejian S, et al: A critical evaluation of clinical decision support for the detection of drug-drug interactions. *Expert Opin Drug Saf* 2011; 10:871–882.
78. DiPoto JP, Buckley MS, Kane-Gill SL: Evaluation of an automated surveillance system using trigger alerts to prevent adverse drug events in the intensive care unit and general ward. *Drug Saf* 2015; 38:311–317.
79. Bickham P, Golembiewski J, Meyer T, et al: ASHP guidelines on perioperative pharmacy services. *Am J Health Syst Pharm* 2019; 76:903–820.
80. Devlin JW, Marquis F, Riker RR, et al: Combined didactic and scenario-based education improves the ability of intensive care unit staff to recognize delirium at the bedside. *Crit Care* 2008; 12:R19.
81. Stollings JL, Foss JJ, Ely EW, et al: Pharmacist leadership in ICU quality improvement: Coordinating spontaneous awakening and breathing trials. *Ann Pharmacother* 2015; 49:883–891.
82. Gesin G, Russell BB, Lin AP, et al: Impact of a delirium screening tool and multifaceted education on nurses' knowledge of delirium and ability to evaluate it correctly. *Am J Crit Care* 2012; 21:e1–e11.
83. Swan JT: Decreasing inappropriate unable-to-assess ratings for the confusion assessment method for the intensive care unit. *Am J Crit Care* 2014; 23:60–69.
84. Marino J, Bucher D, Beach M, et al: Implementation of an intensive care unit delirium protocol: An interdisciplinary quality improvement project. *Dimens Crit Care Nurs* 2015; 34:273–284.
85. Tasaka CL, Burg C, VanOsdol SJ, et al: An interprofessional approach to reducing the overutilization of stress ulcer prophylaxis in adult medical and surgical intensive care units. *Ann Pharmacother* 2014; 48:462–469.
86. Buckley MS, Park AS, Anderson CS, et al: Impact of a clinical pharmacist stress ulcer prophylaxis management program on inappropriate use in hospitalized patients. *Am J Med* 2015; 128:905–913.
87. Wu JY, Stollings JL, Wheeler AP, et al: Efficacy and outcomes after vasopressin guideline implementation in septic shock. *Ann Pharmacother* 2017; 51:13–20.
88. Rech MA, Bennett S, Donahey E: Pharmacist participation in acute ischemic stroke decreases door-to-needle time to recombinant tissue plasminogen activator. *Ann Pharmacother* 2017; 51:1084–1089.
89. Ng TM, Bell AM, Hong C, et al: Pharmacist monitoring of QTc interval-prolonging medications in critically ill medical patients: A pilot study. *Ann Pharmacother* 2008; 42:475–482.
90. Buckley MS, Harinstein LM, Clark KB, et al: Impact of a clinical pharmacy admission medication reconciliation program on medication errors in "high-risk" patients. *Ann Pharmacother* 2013; 47:1599–1610.
91. Rivkin A, Yin H: Evaluation of the role of the critical care pharmacist in identifying and avoiding or minimizing significant drug-drug interactions in medical intensive care patients. *J Crit Care* 2011; 26:104. e1–104.e6.
92. Chapuis C, Roustit M, Bal G, et al: Automated drug dispensing system reduces medication errors in an intensive care setting. *Crit Care Med* 2010; 38:2275–2281.
93. Claus BO, Robays H, Decruyenaere J, et al: Expected net benefit of clinical pharmacy in intensive care medicine: A randomized interventional comparative trial with matched before-and-after groups. *J Eval Clin Pract* 2014; 20:1172–1179.
94. Weant KA, Armitstead JA, Ladha AM, et al: Cost effectiveness of a clinical pharmacist on a neurosurgical team. *Neurosurgery* 2009; 65:946–950.
95. Kane SL, Weber RJ, Dasta JF: The impact of critical care pharmacists on enhancing patient outcomes. *Intensive Care Med* 2003; 29:691–698.
96. Hamblin S, Rumbaugh K, Miller R: Prevention of adverse drug events and cost savings associated with PharmD interventions in an academic level I trauma center: An evidence-based approach. *J Trauma Acute Care Surg* 2012; 73:1484–1490.

97. Flannery AH, Pandya K, Laine ME, et al: Managing the rising costs and high drug expenditures in critical care pharmacy practice. *Pharmacotherapy* 2017; 37:54–64.
98. American Society of Health-System Pharmacists: ASHP guidelines on clinical drug research. *Am J Health Syst Pharm* 1998; 55:369–376.
99. American Society of Hospital Pharmacists: ASHP statement on pharmaceutical research in organized health-care settings. *Am J Hosp Pharm* 1991; 48:1781.
100. MacLaren R, Brett McQueen R, Campbell J: Clinical and financial impact of pharmacy services in the intensive care unit: Pharmacist and prescriber perceptions. *Pharmacotherapy* 2013; 33:401–410.
101. American College of Clinical Pharmacy: Interprofessional education and practice. *Pharmacotherapy* 2009; 29:880–881.
102. Rathbun RC, Hester EK, Arnold LM, et al: Importance of direct patient care in advanced pharmacy practice experiences. *Pharmacotherapy* 2012; 32:e88–e97.
103. Lee R, Ii P, Hume AL, et al: Interprofessional education: Principles and application. A framework for clinical pharmacy. *Pharmacotherapy* 2009; 29:145e–164e.
104. Murphy JE, Nappi JM, Bosso JA, et al; American College of Clinical Pharmacy: American College of Clinical Pharmacy's vision of the future: Postgraduate pharmacy residency training as a prerequisite for direct patient care practice. *Pharmacotherapy* 2006; 26:722–733.
105. American Society of Health-System Pharmacists: ASHP long-range vision for the pharmacy work force in hospitals and health systems: Ensuring the best use of medicines in hospitals and health systems. *Am J Health Syst Pharm* 2007; 64:1320–1330.
106. Saseen JJ, Ripley TL, Bondi D, et al: ACCP clinical pharmacist competencies. *Pharmacotherapy* 2017; 37:630–636.
107. Hager DR, Hartkopf KJ, Koth SM, et al: Creation of a certification requirement for pharmacists in direct patient care roles. *Am J Health Syst Pharm* 2017; 74:1584–1589.
108. Lee M, Badowski ME, Acquisto NM, et al: ACCP template for evaluating a clinical pharmacist. *Pharmacotherapy* 2017; 37:e21–e29.

Pharmaceutical Industry

DOI 10.37573/9781585287048

Drug Products, Labeling, and Packaging

2221

TAMPER-EVIDENT PACKAGING ON MULTIDOSE PRODUCTS

Source: Council on Pharmacy Practice

To support the standardization and requirement of tamper-evident packaging on all multidose prescription and nonprescription products; further,

To encourage proper safety controls be in place to prevent harm and ensure proper disposal of multidose products.

This policy supersedes ASHP policy 9211.

Rationale

Multidose products provide more than one dose of a medication. Medications available in multidose forms include but are not limited to topical creams, gels, and ointments, inhalers, and solutions. Tamper-evident packaging is needed to ensure the viability and safety of medications in multidose containers. The Food and Drug Administration defines a tamper-evident package as "one having one or more indicators or barriers to entry which, if breached or missing, can reasonably be expected to provide visible evidence to consumers that tampering occurred." In addition, when multidose products are disposed of, best practices in medication waste disposal need to be employed to prevent harm or diversion.

2244

PEDIATRIC DOSAGE FORMS

Source: Council on Therapeutics

To support research on and development of pediatric-specific drug formulations; further,

To encourage manufacturers to develop formulations suitable for pediatric administration during research that includes pediatric patients; further,

To encourage manufacturers of off-patent medications that are used in pediatric patients to develop formulations suitable for pediatric administration; further,

To advocate that manufacturers comparably price a newly developed pediatric-specific commercial product to that of its extemporaneously prepared formulation; further,

To educate prescribers and caregivers regarding the nuances of pediatric drug administration to ensure the availability of an appropriate dosage form is considered when selecting and administering safe and effective therapies for a pediatric patient.

This policy supersedes ASHP policy 9707.

Rationale

Pediatric patients are at high risk for medication errors because so few formulations are created for them. Challenges to pediatric dosage development include insufficient background information on the drug molecule in the target population, issues with safety and tolerability of excipients, taste-masking issues, technology requirements, the risks involved in clinical trials, small market size and low profitability, and lack of regulatory clarity.

To ensure that the proper dose is administered, different routes of administration, dosage forms, and strengths may be required. Because many existing formulations are not suitable for children, many hospitals and health systems will use components to extemporaneously prepare a formulation that provides a measurable, stable, and consistent delivery of a needed medication. The concentration and availability of these formulations, most often in the form of suspensions and solutions, may also vary in storage requirements, bioavailability, and palatability, all which can affect patient tolerability and adherence.

Furthermore, since many medications are needed for a relatively small patient population, often only a few commercial products are manufactured, resulting in the need for compounding. As a result, research is often stymied in the pediatric patient population as well, since compounding a medication may introduce variables that may affect results in unpredictable ways.

Boards of pharmacy have also recognized the safety issues surrounding variability in stability and concentrations of the same drug, and many have laws in place that prohibit the extemporaneous compounding of drugs in concentrations that are commercially available.

As pediatric patients have different tolerability to excipients, organ development, taste preferences, and swallowing abilities as they age, it is essential that pharmacists are a part of the team that determines a medication regimen. It is also important that caregivers are taught to properly measure, store, and administer pediatric formulations as a part of patient care.

2253

UNIT DOSE PACKAGING AVAILABILITY

Source: Council on Pharmacy Management

To advocate that pharmaceutical manufacturers provide all medications used in health systems in unit dose packages or, when applicable, in packaging that optimizes medication safety, improves operational efficiency, and reduces medication waste; further,

To urge the Food and Drug Administration to support this goal in the interest of public health and healthcare worker and patient safety.

This policy supersedes ASHP policy 1801.

Rationale

The benefits of unit dose drug administration were well established in the 1960s. Despite these benefits, some drugs are not available from manufacturers in unit dose packages. One reason sometimes cited for this lack of availability is that because unit dose packages make up a relatively small portion of business for many manufacturers, some manufacturers are making a business decision to discontinue this form of packaging. When manufacturers do not provide drugs in unit dose form, the pharmacy must repackage them, introducing opportunities for error. Although it may not be practical for FDA to mandate unit dose packaging to optimize medication and patient safety; improve operational efficiency; and support the interest of public health, FDA could encourage such packaging in other ways, such as by developing packaging guidelines for the pharmaceutical industry. In cases in which unit dose packaging is not practical, manufacturers should at a minimum provide package sizes that reduce medication waste.

DOI 10.37573/9781585287048.084

2146

EXPIRATION DATING OF PHARMACEUTICAL PRODUCTS

Source: Council on Pharmacy Practice

To support and actively promote the maximal extension of expiration dates of commercially available pharmaceutical products as a means of increasing access to drugs, such as medications in shortage or used for medical countermeasures, and reducing healthcare costs; further,

To advocate that the Food and Drug Administration implement procedures for pharmaceutical manufacturers to readily update expiration dates to reflect current evidence regarding the maximum length of drug potency and safety, using technology solutions when available; further,

To advocate that regulators and accreditation agencies recognize authoritative data on extended expiration dates for commercially available pharmaceutical products.

This policy supersedes ASHP policy 1712.

Rationale

Extending the expiration date of commercially available pharmaceutical products for as long as possible, while maintaining drug potency and safety, reduces healthcare costs and increases access. This is especially important with medications in short supply or those used as medical countermeasures (i.e., FDA-regulated products [biologics, drugs, devices] that may be used in the event of a potential public health emergency stemming from a terrorist attack with a biological, chemical, or radiological/nuclear material, or a naturally occurring emerging disease). ASHP encourages pre- and post-marketing research on expiration dates and the use of the most current authoritative data on expiration dates in drug product management. However, the current process for updating expiration dates in drug product labeling presents barriers to timely revision and should be streamlined to allow for timely updates. Technology solutions should be leveraged when possible to determine and communicate about expiration date extensions. Until such a process is implemented, regulators and accreditation agencies should permit healthcare organizations to rely on authoritative data when determining appropriate extended expiration dates for commercially available pharmaceutical products.

2002

EXCIPIENTS IN DRUG PRODUCTS

Source: Council on Therapeutics

To advocate that manufacturers remove unnecessary, potentially allergenic excipients from all drug products; further,

To encourage manufacturers to publicly disclose all excipients in drug products; further,

To advocate that the Food and Drug Administration require manufacturers to declare the name and derivative source of all excipients in drug products on the official label; further,

To advocate that vendors of medication-related databases incorporate, expand, and maintain interoperable information about excipients; further,

To promote research that evaluates the safety of excipients to guide clinical practice and to support the reporting and dissemination of this information via published literature, registries, and other mechanisms; further,

To foster education on the potential adverse events that may be caused by excipients; further,

To encourage documentation of allergic reactions or intolerances to or restrictions on specific excipients in the health record.

This policy supersedes ASHP policy 1528.

Rationale

Excipients are intended to be inactive ingredients that assist in delivering a pharmaceutically elegant medication. Ideally, excipients should have a specific purpose, including serving as a binder, disintegrant, solubilizer, preservative, or for pH adjustment for the proper performance of the dosage form. The properties of the final dosage form (e.g., stability) are, for the most part, highly dependent on the excipients chosen, their concentrations, and interaction with both the active compound and each other. Poor aqueous solubility and rate of dissolution are often the two critical factors that affect the formulation and development process and as a result, some formulations of medications may include high percentages of excipients to ensure the active ingredients are able to be delivered. However, some excipients are added to formulations to enhance color or texture and are not necessary for a stable and soluble product.

In some patients, however, excipients may cause adverse events or aggravate medical conditions. Examples include patients with a red-dye allergy reacting to a suspension containing red dye, fillers that have a high carbohydrate content breaking ketosis in patients who are on a ketogenic diet for seizure management, exacerbation of kidney dysfunction in patients receiving a parenteral solution containing cyclodextrins, or metabolic ketoacidosis requiring dialysis in patients who are receiving high amounts of propylene glycol. Additionally, these adverse effects are not always well known or studied.

Inclusion of excipients in drug product labeling, including their derivative source would allow substitution of a nonallergenic alternative, modification of therapy (such as giving a tablet instead of a dextrose containing suspension), closer monitoring of organ function, or ordering pertinent lab values that may alert practitioners to toxicities associated with excipients as opposed to the active drug.

Additionally, many patients and providers are unaware of the potential impact that excipients may have when selecting therapies and monitoring for adverse events. Currently, the FDA only provides guidance on excipient safety for new products but does not require it unless specific regulatory or statutory requirements are cited. These guidance documents do not establish legally enforceable responsibilities nor do they require the manufacturer to disclose these excipients unless specifically requested by the FDA. Conversely, the European Union requires manufacturers to declare excipients on labelling if the medicinal product is an injectable, topical, or an eye preparation, as well as requiring excipients known to have a recognized action or effect to be declared on the labelling of all other medicinal products.

Education of manufacturers, pharmacists and other healthcare professionals, and patients regarding the use and potential adverse effects of excipients will be required. Medication-related databases will need to be configured and continuously updated to include information about drug product excipients, and electronic health record systems will need to permit documentation of allergies and medical conditions related to excipients.

1812

AVAILABILITY AND USE OF APPROPRIATE VIAL SIZES

Source: Council on Pharmacy Practice

To advocate that pharmaceutical manufacturers provide drug products in vial sizes that reduce pharmaceutical waste and enhance safety; further,

To collaborate with regulators, manufacturers, and other healthcare providers to develop best practices on the safe and appropriate use of single-dose, single-use, and multiple-dose vials.

This policy was reviewed in 2023 by the Council on Pharmacy Practice and by the Board of Directors and was found to still be appropriate.

Rationale

A 20 study estimated that the U.S. may spend close to $2 billion on oncology drug products that are discarded because they come in vials in which the volume of drug product exceeds what is needed for most doses. Since that landmark study, policymakers, healthcare providers, and payers have been calling for action on vial sizes. The Centers for Medicare & Medicaid Services (CMS) has begun to require that billing for Part B drug products distinguish between claims for those received by a patient and those for discarded drug product, and the Office of the Inspector General (OIG) of the Department of Health and Human Services has initiated a study to determine the cost of such waste. Considerable savings could be gained if vial sizes more closely matched doses, and one of the goals of the OIG study is to determine how much could be saved by using vial sizes available overseas that more closely match doses. As one analysis has pointed out, pharmacoeconomic analyses done in the U.S. typically do not incorporate leftover drug product in cost calculations, which may inflate cost-effectiveness ratios, and drug manufacturers may be exploiting that omission. In contrast, the United Kingdom National Institute for Clinical Excellence requires manufacturers to include the cost of leftover drug in manufacturers' submissions, and vials of two cancer drugs studied (bortezomib and pembrolizumab) contain 1 mg and 50 mg, respectively, in the U.K., and 3.5 mg and 100 mg in the U.S. Further, the availability of different vial sizes can enhance patient and worker safety. Vial sizes that more closely match doses can minimize preparation time and steps, reducing employee fatigue and the number of opportunities for error.

ASHP advocates that pharmaceutical manufacturers provide drug products in vial sizes that reduce drug waste (e.g., multiple-dose vials or single-dose vials of differing doses), and that regulators, manufacturers, and healthcare providers cooperate to develop and implement best practices for drug vial optimization.

1821

ENSURING EFFECTIVENESS, SAFETY, AND ACCESS TO ORPHAN DRUG PRODUCTS

Source: Council on Therapeutics

To encourage continued awareness of, research on, and development of orphan drug products; further,

To advocate for the use of innovative strategies and incentives to expand the breadth of rare diseases addressed by this program; further,

To encourage postmarketing research to support the safe and effective use of orphan drug products for approved and off-label indications; further,

To advocate that health policymakers, payers, and pharmaceutical manufacturers ensure continuity of care and patient access to orphan drug products; further,

To advocate federal review to evaluate whether orphan drug designation is being used inappropriately to receive FDA approval, extend patents, decrease competition, or limit discounts, thereby reducing patient access.

This policy supersedes ASHP policy 1413.

Rationale

The U.S. Orphan Drug Act of 1983 and similar programs in other countries have greatly expanded the number of therapies available to treat rare diseases through the use of financial and other incentives that encourage drug manufacturers to develop medications for limited patient populations. Despite the overall success of orphan drug programs, concerns have been raised about the breadth of drugs approved through these mechanisms. Although there are more than 7,000 designated orphan diseases in the United States, oncology drugs represent approximately 33 percent of all orphan drug approvals. ASHP believes that there is a significant need to develop a more comprehensive approach to orphan drug development in order to encourage drug manufacturers to expand the breadth of rare conditions treated by these therapies.

Once an orphan drug is approved, it may be used without restrictions, and these therapies are frequently used to treat patients and conditions that were not assessed during pre-approval clinical studies. While this use can spur innovation and lead to advances in the treatment of common diseases, ASHP believes that this use is also associated with the potential for increased patient harm, given the small patient populations and other characteristics common to studies used to support orphan drug approval. Research is necessary to evaluate the safety and effectiveness of these therapies under real-use conditions. In addition to manufacturer-conducted research, ASHP encourages private and public sector research in order to provide sufficient evidence to support off-label use.

ASHP is concerned about the high cost of these therapies, which contributes to increased healthcare costs and potentially decreases patient access, especially among those who are under- or uninsured. Further, some orphan drugs have later been discontinued by the drug manufacturer—an occurrence that often leaves patients with rare conditions without a treatment alternative. It is essential that stakeholders (e.g., health policymakers, payers, and pharmaceutical manufacturers) continue efforts to provide patient access to these therapies, including developing strategies to ensure that the cost of these therapies does not create an unreasonable barrier to patient access.

There are additional challenges regarding patient access to orphan drugs. There is a need for more emphasis on increasing patient access and addressing 340B issues, especially with critical access facilities. Orphan drug development and marketing in the U.S. is concentrated in a few therapeutic areas. Despite the increase in the number of orphan drugs approved by the Food and Drug Administration (FDA), the unmet needs of patients with rare diseases provide evidence that the current incentives are not efficiently stimulating orphan drug development. There is need to balance economic incentives to stimulate the development and marketing of orphan drugs without jeopardizing patients' access to treatment.

Finally, one study (Sarpatwari A, Beall RF, Abdurrob A et al. Evaluating The Impact Of The Orphan Drug Act's Seven-Year Market Exclusivity Period. *Health Aff.* 2018; 37:732–7. doi:10.1377/hlthaff.2017.1179) concluded that the orphan drug incentive of 7-year exclusivity only benefits about 33% of orphan drugs. The remainder have 20-year patent exclusivity that outlives the orphan drug incentive. Despite this discrepancy, the number of orphan drugs still grows every year, which may stem from manufacturers' unfettered freedom to price these new drugs as they see fit. ASHP encourages federal review of current incentives to evaluate whether orphan drug designation is being used inappropriately to receive FDA approval, extend patents, decrease competition, or limit discounts, which can raise prices and reduce patient access.

1711

READY-TO-ADMINISTER PACKAGING FOR HAZARDOUS DRUG PRODUCTS INTENDED FOR HOME USE

Source: Council on Pharmacy Practice

To advocate that pharmaceutical manufacturers provide hazardous drug products intended for home use in ready-to-administer packaging; further,

To advocate that regulators (e.g., the Food and Drug Administration) have the authority to impose requirements on pharmaceutical manufacturers to provide hazardous drug products intended for home use in ready-to-administer packaging; further,

To advocate that when hazardous drug products intended for home use are not available from manufacturers in ready-to-administer packaging, pharmacies repackage those drug products to minimize the risk of exposure; further,

To advocate that hazardous drug products intended for home use be labeled to warn that special handling is required for safety; further,

To advocate that pharmacists provide education to patients and caregivers regarding safe handling and appropriate disposal of hazardous drug products intended for home use.

This policy was reviewed in 2022 by the Council on Pharmacy Practice and by the Board of Directors and was found to still be appropriate.

Rationale

Home use of oral chemotherapy increases patient convenience and lowers healthcare costs, but it presents unique safety risks. In a hospital or clinic setting, healthcare professionals manage the risks posed by hazardous drugs, defined as any drug identified by at least one of the following six criteria: carcinogenicity, teratogenicity or developmental toxicity, reproductive toxicity in humans, organ toxicity at low doses in humans or animals, genotoxicity, and new drugs that mimic existing hazardous drugs in structure or toxicity (NIOSH Alert: Preventing Occupational Exposure to Antineoplastic and Other Hazardous Drugs in Health Care Settings). In the home environment, however, patients and caregivers must be prepared to fill that role. Ready-to-administer packaging of hazardous drugs minimizes patient, caregiver, and family exposure to hazardous drugs, promotes patient adherence, and enhances safe medication use. Ready-to-administer packaging is defined as packaging that provides the product in a way that requires no manipulation before the patient or caregiver can administer the medication. In contrast, ready-to-use packaging may require a small amount of manipulation (e.g., reconstitution). These definitions are consistent with United States Pharmacopeia and Institute for Safe Medication Practices terminology. ASHP advocates that pharmaceutical manufacturers provide hazardous drug products intended for home use in ready-to-administer packaging, and that regulators have the authority to require manufacturers to (1) provide hazardous drug products intended for home use in ready-to-administer packaging, and (2) label hazardous drug products intended for home use to warn that special handling is required to ensure safety. ASHP further advocates that when hazardous drug products intended for home use are not available in ready-to-administer packaging, pharmacies repackage those drug products to minimize exposure risk for caregivers and others in the patient's household. For example, intravenous drug products should be dispensed in a container designed so the patient or caregiver does not have to puncture a vial; tablets are split or crushed prior to dispensing; compounding of liquid medications is done by the pharmacy, if stability information for the drug product supports advanced compounding and transport; and all liquid medications are dispensed with a dispensing cap that can accommodate attachment of an oral syringe. Finally, ASHP advocates that patients and caregivers be provided education regarding safe handling of hazardous drug products from a qualified healthcare professional, preferably a pharmacist experienced in managing the risks of hazardous drug products.

1615

PROTECTING WORKERS FROM EXPOSURE TO HAZARDOUS DRUGS

Source: Council on Pharmacy Management

To advocate that pharmaceutical manufacturers eliminate surface contamination on packages and vials of hazardous drugs; further,

To inform pharmacists and other personnel of the potential presence of surface contamination on the packages and vials of hazardous drugs; further,

To advocate that the Food and Drug Administration require standardized labeling and package design for hazardous drugs that would alert handlers to the potential presence of surface contamination; further,

To encourage healthcare organizations, wholesalers, and other trading partners in the drug supply chain to adhere to published standards and regulations, such as ASHP guidelines and United States Pharmacopeia Chapter 800, to protect workers from undue exposure to hazardous drugs.

This policy was reviewed in 2021 by the Council on Pharmacy Management and by the Board of Directors and was found to still be appropriate.

Rationale

The outer surfaces of vials of hazardous drugs have been shown to be contaminated with hazardous substances, and pharmacy and other personnel handling those vials may unknowingly be exposed. ASHP advocates that individuals involved in drug distribution, receiving, and inventory control adhere to safe handling guidelines, including ASHP guidelines and United States Pharmacopeia Chapter 800, to avoid undue exposure to hazardous substances but recognizes the limits of these best practices. Pharmaceutical manufacturers have a responsibility to provide vials that are devoid of surface contamination due to inadequate vial-cleaning procedures, and can reduce contamination by using decontamination equipment and protective sleeves during the manufacturing process.

The purpose of United States Pharmacopeia (USP) Chapter 800 is to establish standards for protecting personnel and the environment when handling hazardous drugs. Each year, approximately 8 million U.S. healthcare workers are potentially exposed to hazardous drugs, according to the Centers for Disease Control and Prevention. USP Chapter 800 includes definitions, processes, and worker responsibilities that enhance understanding of risk and limit exposure. To support workers in protecting their patients, themselves, and the environment, the FDA and manufacturers will need to develop new production and processing standards to mitigate exposures, including labeling and package design that alerts handlers to the possibility of contamination.

1535

NONPROPRIETARY NAMING OF BIOLOGICAL PRODUCTS

Source: Council on Public Policy

To advocate that originator biological products, related biological products, and biosimilar products share the same global nonproprietary name as defined by the United States Adopted Name Council, the World Health Organization Programme on International Nonproprietary Names, and United States Pharmacopeial Convention; further,

To oppose unique nonproprietary naming for originator biological products, related biological products, and biosimilar products.

This policy was reviewed in 2020 by the Council on Public Policy and by the Board of Directors and was found to still be appropriate.

Rationale

As biosimilar products obtain approval for use in patients in the U.S., discussion continues among stakeholders over what type of naming process should be applied. A number of stakeholder groups have adopted policy regarding biologic and biosimilar naming, including FDA, National Council for Prescription Drug Programs, (NCPDP), United States Pharmacopoeia (USP), United States Adopted Name (USAN) Council, World Health Organization (WHO), American Medical Association (AMA), and other national pharmacy groups.

The recognized authorities for applying standardized principles of drug and biologic naming include the WHO Programme on International Nonproprietary Names (INN), USAN Council, and USP. These authorities have developed a harmonized biosimilar naming approach based on applying a shared nonproprietary name for originator biological products, related biological products, and biosimilar products. Under their authority, these products essentially share the same nonproprietary name (e.g., "filgrastim" for Neupogen, Zarxio, and Granix), but can be individually identified through their unique National Drug Code (NDC), other unique codified identifiers, and trade names. Thus, well-accepted and widely used existing mechanisms for distinguishing individual products obviate the need for deviation from these existing authoritative approaches by adding a prefix or suffix to the nonproprietary name. Other national pharmacy organizations (e.g., American Pharmacists Association [APhA], Academy of Managed Care Pharmacists [AMCP], National Association of Chain Drug Stores [NACDS], and National Community Pharmacists Association [NCPA]) as well as NCPDP support application of the identical nonproprietary name to these products.

FDA has proposed a nonproprietary naming process that deviates from the existing standardized approach that has been applied by international authorities such as INN and USAN. Under FDA's proposal, a unique, randomly generated suffix composed of four lowercase letters, or a suffix relating to the license holder of the product (which could change over time), would be applied to originator biological products, related biological products, and biosimilar products.

In its proposed rule for the biologics to which this naming method would initially be applied, FDA has recommended changing the official names for biologics with globally adopted INNs and USANs as outlined below.

INN/USAN Name	Proposed FDA Name(s)	Former FDA Placeholder Name
filgrastim	filgrastim-bflm filgrastim-vkzt filgrastim-jcwp	filgrastim-sndz tbo-filgrastim
epoetin alfa	epoetin alfa-cgkn	
pegfilgrastim	pegfilgrastim-ljfd	
infliximab	infliximab-hjmt	

These would be just the first name changes that FDA would implement. The proposed plan would then retrospectively change the names of a broad group of existing products to include unique, randomly generated, four-letter suffixes. Such a naming regime would require extensive education and reprogramming present a risk for medication errors.

Although FDA's proposed naming process differs from the internationally recognized naming processes supported by WHO, USAN, NCPDP, USP, and others, it appears similar to WHO's current proposal for four-consonant biological qualifiers that can be employed by countries not having other effective means of tracking specific drug products (e.g., with NDCs or other codified identifiers). Thus, it would result in the existence of two different four-letter modifications of the INN for the same product—the one assigned independently by FDA and the one assigned by WHO. For example, under this scenario, FDA would assign the nonproprietary name "epoetin alfa-cgkn" to the product INN would maintain under the long-established nonproprietary name "epoetin alfa," but the FDA guidance would allow a qualified name such as "epoetin alfa-xktz."

FDA cites safety concerns and the ability to track these products precisely to the patients receiving them as justifications for the proposed naming standard. However, stakeholders such as NCPDP have recently commented in opposition to FDA's proposed naming standard, arguing that FDA's random, no-vowel suffix could create confusion among clinicians and a potential safety issue if unrecognizable names are used.

0920

STANDARDIZED CLINICAL DRUG NOMENCLATURE

Source: Council on Pharmacy Management

To encourage federal agencies, the pharmaceutical industry, pharmacy and medical software providers, and purveyors of clinical data repositories and drug databases to explore the potential benefits of supplementing or modifying the National Drug Code with a coding system that can be used effectively to support patient care, research, and financial management; further,

To encourage that such a coding system encompass prescription drug products, nonprescription medications, and dietary supplements and include both active and inactive ingredients.

This policy was reviewed in 2019 by the Council on Pharmacy Management and by the Board of Directors and was found to still be appropriate.

Rationale

Clinical decision support systems (CDSS) in computerized provider order entry (CPOE) and pharmacy information systems have been widely used for screening drug interactions and patient allergies. For this screening to be effective, a baseline coding structure for medications must be available, and the coding system needs to include prescription and nonprescription medications, dietary supplements, and drug excipients.

The National Committee on Vital and Health Statistics (NCVHS) has recommended regulatory changes to give the Food and Drug Administration (FDA) full control over the National Drug Code (NDC). Currently, FDA controls only a portion, and manufacturers control the remainder. FDA has made recommendations for uniform standards to enable electronic prescribing (e-prescribing) in ambulatory care. During the past several years, NCVHS has focused considerable attention on the feasibility and desirability of standards to support e-prescribing and the need for standard terminology for clinical drugs to facilitate automated drug-use review and decision support for patient safety. In previous reports, NCVHS documented NDC shortcomings, most notably concern about perceived weaknesses of the current NDC database and linkage of the NDC to RxNorm concepts. NCVHS expressed the need for harmonization of terminologies to eliminate incompatibilities that impair drug utilization studies and may negatively affect patient safety. RxNorm, a standardized nomenclature for clinical drugs, is produced by the National Library of Medicine. In RxNorm, the name of a clinical drug combines its ingredients, strengths, and form. RxNorm has limitations, however; it does not identify a product's excipients or include herbal products or nonprescription medications.

0720

STANDARDIZING PREFIXES AND SUFFIXES IN DRUG PRODUCT NAMES

Source: Council on Public Policy

To collaborate with others, including the United States Pharmacopeia and the Food and Drug Administration, in standardizing and defining the meaning of prefixes and suffixes for prescription and nonprescription drugs to prevent medication errors and ensure patient safety.

This policy was reviewed in 2022 by the Council on Public Policy and by the Board of Directors and was found to still be appropriate.

0402

READY-TO-USE PACKAGING FOR ALL SETTINGS

Source: Council on Professional Affairs

To advocate that pharmaceutical manufacturers provide all medications used in ambulatory care settings in unit-of-use packages; further,

To urge the Food and Drug Administration to support this goal; further,

To encourage pharmacists to adopt unit-of-use packaging for dispensing prescription medications to ambulatory patients; further,

To support continued research on the safety benefits and patient adherence associated with unit-of-use packaging and other dispensing technologies.

(*Note:* A unit-of-use package is a container–closure system designed to hold a specific quantity of a drug product for a specific use and intended to be dispensed to a patient without any modification except for the addition of appropriate labeling.)

This policy was reviewed in 2021 by the Council on Pharmacy Practice and by the Board of Directors and was found to still be appropriate.

0002

DRUG SHORTAGES

Source: Council on Administrative Affairs

To declare that pharmaceutical manufacturers, distributors, group purchasing organizations, and regulatory bodies, when making decisions that may create drug product shortages, should strive to prevent those decisions from compromising the quality and safety of patient care.

This policy was reviewed in 2023 by the Council on Pharmacy Practice and by the Board of Directors and was found to still be appropriate.

Rationale

Drug product shortages continue to be a critical issue because of their frequency, duration, and widespread nature. Although the effects of drug product shortages on patient care and pharmacy services are complex and have not been comprehensively described, the negative effects include increases in (1) patient safety risks, (2) drug expenditures due to higher prices paid for noncontract or alternative product supplies, (3) physician dissatisfaction and patient dissatisfaction, and (4) staff time spent resolving shortage problems. Pharmacy managers are hampered in addressing shortages by the lack of any advance notice of shortages from manufacturers, group purchasing organizations (GPOs), distributors, or the Food and Drug Administration (FDA); limited information regarding the estimated duration of shortages; and limited information on the reasons behind the shortages. Further, managers lack immediate information on what options are available (i.e., alternative sources of products or appropriate therapeutic alternatives) to ameliorate the problem on both a short- and long-term basis. In addition, the concerted effort to decrease inventories across the drug supply chain leave little buffer when drug product shortages occur.

Drug shortages occur for a variety of reasons, including manufacturer noncompliance with FDA's Current Good Manufacturing Practices, natural disasters that damage production plants, shortages of raw materials, increases in unlabeled uses, consolidation within the industry, predetermined production quotas, and market shifts driven by large purchasers and payers. A significant factor affecting product supply is business-related decisions made by the key players in the drug supply chain. These decisions, and the limited information pharmacists are able to retrieve regarding shortages, has harmed the trust between pharmacists and the pharmaceutical supply industry. ASHP believes that these key players, including pharmaceutical manufacturers, GPOs, distributors, and regulatory bodies must consider the impact that their decisions affecting supply and demand of a product have on the quality or safety of patient care.

9608

USE OF COLOR TO IDENTIFY DRUG PRODUCTS

Source: Council on Professional Affairs

To support the reading of drug product labels as the most important means of identifying drug products; further,

To oppose reliance on color by health professionals and others to identify drug products; further,

To oppose actions by manufacturers of drug products and others to promulgate reliance on color to identify drug products.

This policy was reviewed in 2019 by the Council on Pharmacy Practice and by the Board of Directors and was found to still be appropriate.

9011

DRUG NOMENCLATURE

Source: House of Delegates Resolution

To work with the FDA, USP, and pharmaceutical industry to assure that drug products are named in a manner that clearly and without confusion permits identification of ingredients' strengths and changes.

This policy was reviewed in 2019 by the Council on Public Policy and by the Board of Directors and was found to still be appropriate.

Marketing

2210

DRUG SAMPLES

Source: Council on Public Policy

To oppose drug sampling or similar drug marketing programs that circumvent appropriate pharmacy oversight or control.

This policy supersedes ASHP policy 9702.

Rationale

Drug marketing or sampling programs that involve physical samples can create a number of drug supply and patient risks if they are not subject to strict pharmacy control. However, "virtual" programs that allow pharmacy management of the supply (e.g., situations where a limited amount of drug is dispensed from the pharmacy's supply) are not problematic if proper controls are in place. Specifically, workable drug sampling programs must (1) provide the elements of pharmaceutical care, (2) result in careful drug control, ensuring patients receive only properly labeled and packaged, unexpired, and recorded drugs, (3) provide access to prescription drugs only through authorized, trained personnel, (4) discourage inappropriate prescribing habits, or (5) do not increase the cost of treatment for all patients.

1806

MANUFACTURER-SPONSORED PATIENT ASSISTANCE PROGRAMS

Source: Council on Pharmacy Management

To advocate that pharmaceutical manufacturers extend their patient assistance programs (PAPs) to serve the needs of both uninsured and underinsured patients, regardless of distribution channels; further,

To advocate expansion of PAPs to inpatient settings; further,

To advocate that pharmaceutical manufacturers and PAP administrators enhance the efficiency of PAPs by standardizing application criteria, processes, and forms; further,

To advocate that pharmaceutical manufacturers and PAP administrators enhance access to and visibility of PAPs to pharmacy personnel and other healthcare providers; further,

To encourage pharmacy personnel, other healthcare providers, and pharmaceutical manufacturers to work cooperatively to ensure PAPs include the essential elements of pharmacist patient care, are patient-centered, and are transparent; further,

To develop education for pharmacy personnel and other healthcare providers on the risks and benefits of PAPs.

This policy supersedes ASHP policy 1420.

This policy was reviewed in 2023 by the Council on Pharmacy Management and by the Board of Directors and was found to still be appropriate.

Rationale

ASHP recognizes the value of patient assistance programs (PAPs) in improving continuity of care while controlling costs and advocates expanded use of these programs for uninsured and underinsured patients in ambulatory and inpatient care settings. Some organizations have demonstrated success in achieving the benefits of these programs through dedicated resources and a mastery of the many programs available. Simplification of these programs (similar eligibility criteria, a common data format) would reduce the resources required to participate and improve access and utilization. Other barriers for enrolling patients in PAPs include annual out-of-pocket spend requirements to re-enroll, confusing forms, and inability to renew in advance of new year. ASHP notes that while the number of PAPs in ambulatory care settings has increased, there has been little growth in programs for inpatients. Hospitals must then absorb the costs of patient care, which results in fewer resources in the overall healthcare system. ASHP believes that expansion of PAPs to indigent inpatients would significantly offset some of the costs to hospitals and ultimately improve care. In addition, interprofessional cooperation will be needed to support patients in accessing drug products when the PAP doesn't cover the cost of the drug product due to high deductibles or co-pays. To ensure that these programs achieve their objectives, ASHP advocates that development of these programs ensure that they contain the elements of pharmacist patient care to enhance access to and visibility of PAPs.

1714

RESTRICTED DRUG DISTRIBUTION

Source: Council on Public Policy

To oppose restricted drug distribution systems that (1) limit patient access to medications; (2) undermine continuity of care; (3) impede population health management; (4) adversely impact patient outcomes; (5) erode patients' relationships with their healthcare providers, including pharmacists; (6) are not supported by publicly available evidence that they are the least restrictive means to improve patient safety; (7) interfere with the professional practice of healthcare providers; or (8) are created for any reason other than patient safety.

This policy was reviewed in 2022 by the Council on Public Policy and by the Board of Directors and was found to still be appropriate.

Rationale

Restricted drug distribution systems (RDDSes) that are not created solely for patient safety reasons (e.g., those that misuse risk evaluation and mitigation strategies [REMS] programs for the purposes of limiting distribution) significantly restrict patient access to medications. These systems were justified as a means to closely monitor patient use of medications that could potentially pose a safety risk. They were never intended to allow drug manufacturers to reduce pharmacists' access to medications through limited distribution networks. Using restricted distribution as a tool to gain marketplace advantage rather than for patient safety undermines the justification for such limited systems. Similarly, the use of insurer-imposed restrictions to artificially limit drug distribution creates access problems for patients and administrative issues for providers. However, hospital- and health system-owned or -operated specialty pharmacies do

DOI 10.37573/9781585287048.085

not result in the same access concerns, as they generally reduce prior approval burdens and ensure patient access to medications.

ASHP opposes the use of RDDSes (e.g., the misuse of REMS and insurer-forced limited distribution) for anything other than patient safety and encourages the FDA or other appropriate authorities to investigate whether REMS-related RDDSes are being used in a manner inconsistent with the original intent. In addition, both REMS-related and insurer-forced RDDSes may compromise continuity of care or interfere with pharmacists' accountability for care to certain patient populations, such as when an RDDS prevents a patient's pharmacist from obtaining it. Some investigational drugs approved for marketing under an RDDS are no longer available for qualifying patients on admission through the institution, despite the institution having a history of managing the drug while it was investigational. Such circumstances force the patient to seek care elsewhere or require them and their healthcare providers to unnecessarily utilize additional resources to provide care. In addition, healthcare organizations, responsible for the total care of the patient, including maintaining the patient's medical records, may lose the established patient-care relationship when a patient must go to a specialty pharmacy for a drug the healthcare organization cannot access. RDDSes fragment the healthcare delivery system at a time when public and private payers are increasing incentives to integrate patient care.

1620

MANUFACTURER PROMOTION OF OFF-LABEL USES

Source: Council on Public Policy

To advocate for authority for the Food and Drug Administration (FDA) to regulate the promotion and dissemination of information about off-label uses of medications and medication-containing devices by manufacturers and their representatives; further,

To advocate that such off-label promotion and marketing be limited to the FDA-regulated dissemination of unbiased, truthful, and scientifically accurate information based on peer-reviewed literature not included in the New Drug Approval process.

This policy was reviewed in 2021 by the Council on Public Policy and by the Board of Directors and was found to still be appropriate.

Rationale

Congress is considering significant changes in the way drugs are developed, approved, and marketed in the United States. A provision in the House-passed 21st Century Cures bill (H.R. 6) would allow pharmaceutical manufacturers to promote off-label uses of their products to clinicians and formulary committees. This change has raised concerns about the accuracy and sources of such information. Sources of such information, if unreliable, could put patient safety at risk. Despite these concerns about promotion of off-label uses by manufacturers and their drug representatives, ASHP has suggested an amendment that would require Food and Drug Administration (FDA) oversight of such promotion and require promotional materials to be unbiased, truthful, scientifically accurate, and based upon peer-reviewed literature not included in the approved labeling of the drug. Materials would therefore require approval by the proper authority (FDA), meet certain requirements, and be truthful and scientifically accurate. This policy is not intended to curtail the ability of clinicians to use, or discuss the use of, products off-label.

1624

BAN ON DIRECT-TO-CONSUMER ADVERTISING FOR PRESCRIPTION DRUGS AND MEDICATION-CONTAINING DEVICES

Source: Council on Public Policy

To advocate that Congress ban direct-to-consumer advertising for prescription drugs and medication-containing devices.

This policy supersedes ASHP policy 1119.

Rationale

Direct-to-consumer advertising (DTCA) of prescription drugs and drug-containing implantable medical devices has both positive and negative potential effects. The positive potential effects include broader public awareness and use of therapies, increased patient engagement in their healthcare, and better return on investment in drug and medical device research. These potential benefits need to be weighed against the potential negative effects, however, which include higher drug and device costs, inappropriate prescribing of more costly new drugs or devices without any justifying improvement in patient outcomes, and increased adverse effects. In 2015, the American Medical Association (AMA) adopted a policy calling for a ban on DTCA of prescription drugs and implantable medical devices due to its impacts on drug prices and physician prescribing practices.

Public health researchers have characterized the U.S. experience with direct-to-consumer advertising (DTCA) of prescription drugs since 1997 as "a large and expensive uncontrolled experiment in population health, which to date shows decidedly mixed effects."[1] Those researchers and others[2–5] have identified major impacts of DTCA on public health, including an increase in inappropriate prescribing and adverse effects, medicalization of symptoms previously not defined as illness, and increased costs due to inappropriate prescribing.

The impact of DTCA on the prescriber-patient relationship is hard to quantify. In some surveys, physicians have indicated that they fulfilled questionable DTCA-prompted patient requests for prescriptions.[1] A Food and Drug Administration (FDA) survey found that "many physicians felt some pressure to prescribe something" when patients mentioned a drug they learned about through DTCA.[2] Studies of claims data support the conclusion that DTCA led to inappropriate prescribing of COX-2 inhibitors and proton pump inhibitors, and experimental evidence suggests that DTCA could induce clinically questionable prescribing of antidepressants for adjustment disorder.[1] Although the connection cannot be proved, it has been suggested that the increasing reliance of physician payments on patient satisfaction surveys could present an economic risk to prescribers who deny patient requests. Studies show that DTCA increases prescribing volume and patient demand, and shifts prescribing.[3] DTCA's effects include overuse of prescription drugs,[4] a shift to less appropriate prescribing,[3] and switches to less cost-effective treatment.[3] In addition, differential effects by patient price sensitivity have been implicated in sustained sales despite a price increase.[3] Researchers have concluded that the overall effects of DTCA on physician–patient communication are unclear,[1] and that the effects of DTCA on improving the quality of care are mixed1 or lacking in evidence.[3]

The educational value of DTCA has also been questioned. Consumers of DTCA recall more benefit than risk information.[1] Critics of the educational value of DTCA also note that DCTA could exacerbate health disparities due to differing levels of health literacy and lack of incentive to advertise to low-income populations.[1] Researchers have questioned whether purported improvements in adherence, based mainly on negative trials, stand up to scrutiny.[3]

ASHP recognizes that banning a constitutionally protected right to free speech, even commercial speech, must be reinforced by evidence that indicates the banned speech negatively impacts society. In the case of DCTA, those negative impacts, including intrusion on the patient-prescriber relationship and increased healthcare costs, are evident and overwhelming. Given the outsized role prescription drug products have as a cost driver to the healthcare system, the detrimental effects of DCTA, and the limited potential benefits, ASHP has concluded that a ban on DTCA of prescription drugs and drug-containing implantable medical devices is warranted.

1. Frosch DL, Grande D, Tarn DM, et al. A decade of controversy: Balancing policy with evidence in the regulation of prescription drug advertising. *Am J Publ Health* 2010; 100:24–32. Available at: http://www.ncbi.nlm.nih.gov/pmc/articles/PMC2791253/ (accessed 2016 Jun 22).
2. http://www.fda.gov/Drugs/ResourcesForYou/Consumers/ucm143562.htm
3. Mintzes B. Advertising of prescription-only medicines to the public: Does evidence of benefit counterbalance harm? *Annu Rev Publ Health* 2012; 33:259–77. DOI: 10.1146/annurev-publhealth-031811-124540.
4. Donohue JM, Cevasco M, Rosenthal MB. *N Engl J Med.* 2007; 357:673–81. DOI: 10.1056/NEJMsa070502. Available at www.nejm.org/doi/full/10.1056/NEJMsa070502 (accessed 2016 Jun 22).
5. Dhaval D, Henry S. Impact of direct-to-consumer advertising on pharmaceutical prices and demand. *Southern Econ J.* 2012; 79: 97–126.

1521

IDENTIFICATION OF PRESCRIPTION DRUG COVERAGE AND ELIGIBILITY FOR PATIENT ASSISTANCE PROGRAMS

Source: Council on Pharmacy Management

To advocate that pharmacists or pharmacy technicians ensure that the use of patient assistance programs is optimized and documented to promote continuity of care and patient access to needed medications; further,

To advocate that patient assistance programs should incorporate the pharmacist-patient relationship, including evaluation by a pharmacist as part of comprehensive medication management; further,

To support the principle that medications provided through manufacturer patient assistance programs should be stored, packaged, labeled, dispensed, and recorded using systems that ensure the same level of safety as prescription-based programs that incorporate a pharmacist-patient relationship.

This policy was reviewed in 2020 by the Council on Pharmacy Management and by the Board of Directors and was found to still be appropriate.

Rationale

Ensuring patients' medication histories are accurate and continuity of medication therapies is a critical role for pharmacists to monitor and document as patients transition through the healthcare system. Additionally, pharmacists have an important role in ensuring patients have means to access their medications, both upon hospital admission and discharge. With the numerous channels patients use to obtain their medications, it has become increasingly difficult to verify this information and in some cases obtain the medications needed to care for a patient.

Patient assistance programs (PAPs) present a unique challenge for healthcare providers. Documentation of the utilization of a PAP by a patient is important information for providers accessing the patient electronic health record, and improving that documentation should be a priority for healthcare providers. Additionally, pharmacists need to provide leadership in facilitating the utilization of PAPs to ensure continuity of care, the patient's ability to access needed medications when appropriate, and a comprehensive pharmacist-patient relationship.

ASHP Guidelines for Pharmacists on the Activities of Vendors' Representatives in Organized Health Care Systems

For purposes of this document, vendors' representatives are defined as agents who promote products and provide information and services to health care providers on behalf of manufacturers and suppliers. The narrow focus of this document is on those vendors who serve and interact with settings with respect to drug products, drug-related devices, and other equipment, supplies, and services purchased by pharmacies.

Each individual setting should develop its own specific policies and procedures relating to the activities of vendors' representatives. Such policies and procedures should supplement and complement applicable federal, state, and local laws and regulations (for example, statutes that address prescription drug-product sampling). The ASHP Guidelines on Pharmacists' Relationships with Industry, the ASHP Guidelines for Selecting Pharmaceutical Manufacturers and Suppliers, and setting-specific conflict-of-interest policies may be helpful in the development of policies and procedures.[1,2] The policies and procedures should be developed by the setting's pharmacy and therapeutics committee (or equivalent body) and approved by higher authorities in the setting as required. Depending on the individual setting, policies and procedures may be useful in the following areas.

1. *A defined scope of applicability.* The vendors' representatives to which any policies and procedures apply should be defined by the individual setting. For example, if the policies and procedures are applicable only to drug-product vendors' representatives and not to those promoting medical–surgical supplies, packaging equipment, or drug administration devices, this should be clearly stated.
2. *Orientation of representatives.* In some individual settings, vendors' representatives receive an orientation packet upon their initial visit to the setting. Such a packet might contain a copy of the setting's policies and procedures, a medical staff directory, and the formulary. Some settings provide a formal orientation program that includes meeting key individuals and touring the setting.
3. *Directory.* In some individual settings, a file of current vendor-contact information is maintained in the pharmacy. A form for recording such information might include the following:
   - The vendor's name and address.
   - The name, address, telephone number, and answering service number (if any), and drug-product assignment (purview) of each representative.
   - The name, address, and telephone number of the representative's manager.
   - The names, telephone numbers, and emergency telephone numbers of the vendor's directors of distribution, sales, and product information (titles may vary).
   - The names and telephone numbers of the vendor's medical director and research director (titles may vary).
4. *Availability of vendor-contact information to professionals in the setting.* In some individual settings, the pharmacy department provides the setting's professional staff with the information in item 3, upon request.
5. *Registration while on premises.* In some individual settings, vendors' representatives register with the pharmacy department or other designated department upon each visit to the setting. At such time, the vendors' representatives document the time, purpose, and location of their appointments. In many settings, during the registration process, the representative is provided with a dated name badge to be prominently worn along with the representative's current vendor-supplied name tag (if any).
6. *Locations permitted.* In some individual settings, restriction (if any) from patient care and pharmacy storage and work areas in the setting are specified in the policies and procedures. Meetings with professional staff are conducted in areas convenient to staff and generally in non-patient-care areas.
7. *Appointments and purposes.* In some individual settings, representatives are encouraged to schedule appointments with appropriate pharmacy department staff to
   - Provide information useful for product evaluation. Representatives might be asked to include balanced scientific literature (journal reprints, for example) on drug-product safety and efficacy, as well as documentation of likely cost benefits.
   - Provide timely information on the vendor's products and services.
   - Facilitate procurement and crediting transactions.
   - Obtain and provide information necessary to support the setting's formulary system.
   - Facilitate informational activities for the pharmacy staff and other health care professionals with respect to the vendor's products.
8. *Exhibits.* In some individual settings, the pharmacy department provides opportunities for vendors' representatives to distribute informational material by arranging for organized, scheduled exhibits. Policies and procedures about the times, places, content, and conduct of such events are established.
9. *Dissemination of promotional materials.* In some individual settings, there are policies and procedures about the dissemination (by vendors' representatives) of information on formulary and nonformulary products, including the designation of appropriate categories of recipients of the information (e.g., attending physicians, department chairmen, house staff physicians).

DOI 10.37573/9781585287048.086

Representatives may be asked to promptly provide the pharmacy department with copies of all informational and promotional materials disseminated in the setting. The Food and Drug Administration (FDA) prohibits the advertising and promotion of drug products for uses not reflected in FDA-approved product labeling ("unlabeled uses").[3] Pharmacists and other health care professionals should be aware of these laws and regulations when evaluating the content of promotional materials.

10. *Samples.* In some individual settings, there are policies and procedures with respect to product samples. ASHP urges that the use of drug samples within the institution be eliminated to the extent possible.[4,5]

11. *Noncompliance.* In some individual settings, policies and procedures exist to address noncompliance with the policies and procedures by either vendors' representatives or professional staff.

Each setting should have policies and procedures concerning research to be conducted on its premises. Pharmacists and vendors' representatives should clearly differentiate research from sales and promotional activities, applying appropriate policies and procedures accordingly.[6] Generally, scientific research involving drug products is coordinated through research departments of product manufacturers rather than through sales and promotional representatives.

References

1. American Society of Hospital Pharmacists. ASHP guidelines on pharmacists' relationships with industry. *Am J Hosp Pharm.* 1992; 49:154.
2. American Society of Hospital Pharmacists. ASHP guidelines for selecting pharmaceutical manufacturers and suppliers. *Am J Hosp Pharm.* 1991; 48:523–4.
3. American Society of Hospital Pharmacists. ASHP statement on the use of medications for unlabeled uses. *Am J Hosp Pharm.* 1992; 49:927–8.
4. American Society of Hospital Pharmacists. ASHP guidelines: minimum standard for pharmacies in institutions. *Am J Hosp Pharm.* 1985; 42:372–5.
5. Greenberg RB. The Prescription Drug Marketing Act of 1987. *Am J Hosp Pharm.* 1988; 45:2118–26.
6. American Society of Hospital Pharmacists. ASHP guidelines for pharmaceutical research in organized health-care settings. *Am J Hosp Pharm.* 1989; 46:129–30.

This guideline was reviewed in 1998 by the Council on Professional Affairs and by the ASHP Board of Directors and was found to still be appropriate.

Approved by the ASHP Board of Directors, November 17, 1993. Developed by the Council on Professional Affairs.

Copyright © 1994, American Society of Hospital Pharmacists, Inc. All rights reserved. Contact ASHP for reprint and permissions requests. This content may not be used for commercial purposes without the express written consent of ASHP.

The bibliographic citation for this document is as follows: American Society of Hospital Pharmacists. ASHP guidelines for pharmacists on the activities of vendors' representatives in organized health care systems. *Am J Hosp Pharm.* 1994; 51:520–1.

Pharmacy Management

DOI 10.37573/9781585287048

Pharmacy Management

2311

PHARMACY ACCREDITATIONS, CERTIFICATIONS, AND LICENSES

Source: Council on Pharmacy Management

To advocate that healthcare accreditation, certification, and licensing organizations adopt consistent standards for the medication-use process, based on established evidence-based principles of patient safety and quality of care; further,

To advocate that health-system administrators allocate the resources required to support medication-use compliance and regulatory demands.

This policy supersedes ASHP policy 1810.

Rationale

Pharmacy leaders have years of experience managing the demands and challenges of ensuring that pharmacy services meet the standards of accreditation organizations. In the past, this responsibility was predominantly achieved through accreditation by The Joint Commission (TJC) and compliance with state laws and Board of Pharmacy regulations, as well as with federal requirements (e.g., those of the Drug Enforcement Administration). The number of accreditation standards pharmacy leaders needed to be knowledgeable about was limited. Healthcare organizations with ambulatory care services (e.g., home infusion, specialty pharmacy) have had to manage the additional accreditation process for these business units. Recent changes in healthcare have increased this challenge for pharmacy leaders: (1) TJC is no longer the only accreditor for hospitals and health systems; (2) healthcare organizations are developing or acquiring new business units that have their own accreditation processes that need to be integrated into existing ones; and (3) new accreditation, certification, or licensure processes have been created for services and businesses that fall under the responsibility of pharmacy leaders.

The expansion of healthcare organizations and the growth of the pharmacy enterprise are creating a new environment with multiple accreditors and regulators, presenting pharmacy leaders with the growing challenge of compliance with overlapping accreditation, certification, and regulatory standards. Examples include the Michigan Board of Pharmacy requirement to obtain certification to conduct compounding and the California Board of Pharmacy requirement that each IV hood have its own pharmacy license. In addition, community pharmacy accreditation processes and standards are being implemented that pharmacy leaders need to consider as well.

ASHP recognizes the difference between certifications that are the sole responsibility of and have a direct impact on a pharmacy and certifications of a healthcare organization's service line (e.g., stroke or transplant services) that are the responsibility of the organization but have medication management components that need to be addressed by the pharmacy. Pharmacists and pharmacy departments are being challenged by a growing number of required accreditations, certifications, and licensures, which result in increased need for pharmacist-in-charge designations, workforce fatigue, and direct and indirect costs. Health-system administrators need to recognize this changing environment and allocate the resources required to support medication-use compliance and regulatory demands.

2218

PHARMACY EXECUTIVE OVERSIGHT OF AREAS OUTSIDE PHARMACY

Source: Council on Pharmacy Management

To advocate for opportunities for pharmacy leaders to assume healthcare executive leadership roles outside the pharmacy department; further,

To urge pharmacy leaders to seek out formal and informal opportunities to provide such leadership; further,

To encourage pharmacy leaders to use tools, resources, and credentialing identified by national pharmacy and professional healthcare organizations to demonstrate competence and readiness for healthcare executive leadership; further,

To encourage pharmacy leaders to support development of leaders with a broader scope of executive responsibilities by balancing generalization and service-line specialization in their career development and the career development of rising pharmacy leaders; further,

To advocate for healthcare organization structures that provide pharmacy leaders with opportunities to assume leadership responsibilities outside the pharmacy department; further,

To promote continuing professional development opportunities in executive leadership to provide pharmacy leaders with evidence of a commitment to lifelong learning and leadership excellence.

Rationale

In health systems, pharmacy operations often span multiple practice settings, and pharmacists contribute to many different interdisciplinary teams. ASHP's Statement on the Roles and Responsibilities of the Pharmacy Executive notes there is need for a "strategic and innovative pharmacy executive who plans and oversees the design and operation of the entire and complex medication-use process throughout the system." As each health system is unique in the size and range of services offered to patients, there is significant variability of the scope for the pharmacy executive's position. The role of the pharmacy executive, as it originated, was to provide cohesive oversight of the entirety of the medication-use process, including medication-use policy considerations. However, as practice has evolved, medication use and pharmaceutical management has as well. Recent areas of expansion related to medication management in health systems include drug shortages, medication safety and quality, 340B Drug Pricing Program oversight, investigational drugs, and patient assistance support. Some areas for which health systems have sought pharmacy executive oversight that are less directly related to medication management include compliance and regulatory assurance, transitions of care, supply chain, laboratory operations, and dietary services. Pharmacy executives also manage relationships with stakeholders, evaluate quality and outcome metrics, support medication access, and provide leadership in optimizing reimbursement.

Health-system pharmacy leaders possess skills that have often made them candidates for positions outside pharmacy.

DOI 10.37573/9781585287048.087

As senior leadership teams become smaller to reduce labor costs, pharmacy leaders may be asked to take on additional responsibilities. Over 70% of the 2020 ASHP Foundation Pharmacy Forecast panelists indicated this will be a likely occurrence in many organizations within five years. Adding to a pharmacy leader's portfolio of responsibility creates opportunities for sharing experience and resources across multiple departments. Placing multiple departments under the leadership of one executive also makes it easier to reduce silo budgeting by identifying and implementing interventions that may increase cost in one department while reducing cost to a greater degree in another. Pharmacy leaders who accept responsibility for other service lines must exploit the strengths of their other departments, drive collaboration across all areas they lead, and avoid undermining authority entrusted to subordinate service-line leaders.

Pharmacy executive leaders should strive to demonstrate a commitment to achieving and maintaining excellence in pharmacy and healthcare leadership to communicate value to colleagues, healthcare administrators, and the public. This goal could be achieved by seeking national recognition of core competencies (e.g., leading people and processes, professionalism, financials) identified by national pharmacy and professional healthcare organizations (e.g., American College of Healthcare Executives fellowship program, 360 evaluations, career coaching, professional leadership certificates, ASHP Certified Pharmacy Executive Leader credential). Pharmacy executive leaders should continually seek opportunities for professional development to demonstrate their competence, leadership, and commitment to the profession and to enhance their essential executive knowledge, skills, and abilities in order to facilitate team success.

A key driver enabling a pharmacy executive leader the ability to devote the time and energy for expanded roles includes striking a balance with service-line personnel breadth and depth. This balance is of particular importance when establishing a talent pipeline of capable leaders that will keep the service lines running with little to no interruption. In some health systems, pharmacists hold roles such as chief executive officer, chief operating officer, and senior vice president. Some institutions include oversight of additional service lines within the purview of their highest-ranking pharmacist administrator, such as combining "Pharmaceutical and Nutrition Care," or appointing a pharmacist to manage all "intravenous admixture services."

To achieve maximum performance in an expanded leadership role, the conditions for success must exist. Organizational structure (e.g., hierarchal, matrix, divisional) aligns and defines the relationships of parts of an organization, and the structure chosen affects an organization's success in carrying out its strategy, goals, and objectives. Leadership should understand the characteristics, benefits, and limitations of various structures in aligning organizational structure with the enterprise's business strategy.

2228

ROLE OF THE PHARMACIST IN SERVICE-LINE DEVELOPMENT AND MANAGEMENT

Source: Council on Pharmacy Management

To recognize pharmacists bring unique clinical, operational, and financial expertise to help organizations develop and manage high-value health-system service lines; further,

To support the role of pharmacy leadership in the development and management of high-value health-system service lines.

Rationale

To drive success in the current market, health systems, especially those within integrated delivery networks, must optimize growth by applying strong tactics to acquire and retain patients. Service-line development is structuring patient-centered care in clinically specific areas across the healthcare system. Service-line design groups patients into specific areas of need, improving care coordination and accountability and allowing for a nimble response to changes (e.g., in the allocation of resources).

Pharmacists bring clinical, operational, and financial expertise to help organizations (1) optimize resources, (2) ensure safe medication use and patient-centric system design, (3) drive patient and provider satisfaction, (4) improve patient outcomes, and (5) achieve financial growth when part of critical decision-making for setting an organization's overall service-line growth and management strategy. For example, pharmacists working as part of a specialty pharmacy can leverage their expertise to assess a certain population within a service line, with the goal of improving care and patient safety while promoting use of cost-effective treatments. Most specialty pharmacies allow pharmacists to oversee financial, operational, and clinical services, which has led to growth in patient access and revenue for health systems. Health systems can reap many benefits from expanding service lines, including increased patient volumes, improved health outcomes, boosted market share, and improved patient and provider satisfaction. By focusing on developing high-value service lines, health systems have the opportunity to achieve financial growth and significant return on investment. Growing high-value service lines is one of the most effective ways in which hospitals and health systems can add value to the healthcare system. Growing service lines requires careful strategic planning, and success hinges on an organization's proficiency in (1) understanding and predicting patient needs; (2) acquiring commercial health plans; (3) using an omnichannel approach; (4) focusing on provider referrals; (5) safe medication use and patient-centric system design (e.g., medication stewardship, formulary alignment, medication-use policies); and (6) ensuring the C-suite is fully committed to the service-line development strategy. High-value service lines exemplify exceptional performance in many ways, including attracting the most patients and providers, driving the most revenue, achieving the highest care success rates, and presenting the greatest growth potential. Healthcare organizations identify their high-value service lines by analyzing financial data, external market factors (e.g., value-based contracts), and other relevant economic conditions. Data analytics and effective patient communication are important when healthcare organizations are working to grow service lines. High-value service lines may differ among hospitals, depending on the patients and markets they serve. During times of scarce capital and growing demand for services, service-line analysis becomes a high-priority task for hospital and health-system decision-makers. Leaders must face hard questions when it comes to identifying the areas of operations critical to an institution's long-term financial viability and should ensure those service lines get the investment and management attention they need. Service-line analysis may also mean eliminating low-volume and/or unprofitable service lines that drain resources. Before hospital leaders decide to discontinue a given service line, they should consider whether the line has been properly managed. Many hospitals may have inadvertently harmed service-line management by not investing sufficiently in the resources needed for success.

In today's environment, successful service-line development efforts need input from pharmacy leaders from the outset of discussions through implementation and management. Engagement in every step of service-line development and management assures long-term success as strategic direction is set. Success as a pharmacy leader is predicated on building and maintaining relationships with diverse groups of people in order to be part of setting the overall strategy for an organization. This relationship-building may include partnering with nontraditional healthcare participants to develop new strategies for care. As healthcare markets continue to shift away from volume and toward value, appealing to patients by building high-value service lines designed to meet patients' unique needs will become increasingly important.

2028

PHARMACIST'S ROLE IN HEALTH INSURANCE BENEFIT DESIGN

Source: Council on Pharmacy Management

To advocate that pharmacy practice leaders collaborate with internal and external partners who design, negotiate, and select their own organization's health plans and pharmacy benefit management contracts to preserve patient continuity of care and the integrity of the health-system pharmacy enterprise; further,

To provide education and resources for all partners on the health plan development process, analysis of pharmacy benefit design, contemporary formulary review processes, and application of medication safety principles on formulary decision-making.

Rationale

Pharmacy leadership should be directly involved in the selection of the health system's pharmacy benefit manager (PBM) servicing their employee's health plan, and the terms of that contract with that PBM. Employers typically look to balance value for the employee while attempting to control costs. As health systems evaluate and select plans, there may not always be due consideration given to the potential impacts on patient continuity of care and on that health system's pharmacy enterprise and financial solvency in servicing employees' prescriptions through the selected PBM. Aside from the safety and continuity of care implications to the patient if the health system's pharmacy is excluded from the employees' network, organizations may unknowingly undermine utilization of their outpatient cancer and infusion programs. Three PBMs control the majority of the PBM market, exerting heavy influence in costs, pharmacy participation, formulary, and prior authorization criteria. By including pharmacy leadership to help make a well-informed decision about selecting a servicing PBM for a health system, and the contract terms associated with that PBM (i.e., clinical and financial aspects), some of these unintended consequences could be avoided.

1914

SAFE MEDICATION PREPARATION, COMPOUNDING, AND ADMINISTRATION IN ALL SITES OF CARE

Source: Council on Pharmacy Management

To advocate that all sites of care be required to meet the same regulatory standards for medication preparation, compounding, and administration to ensure safety and quality.

Rationale

As pharmacy costs become increasingly relevant in managing the overall cost of healthcare, third-party payers have increased their attention to sites of care, increasing the pressure to manage this trend. Integrated pharmacy benefit models are working to funnel patients to lower-cost settings and deliver more comprehensive care by leveraging big data.

Consolidation in the pharmacy benefit management sector has resulted in just three major companies. To protect and further grow their margins and fend off disruptive entrants, the big three are reinventing themselves within vertically integrated conglomerates, allowing them to tap into other parts of the healthcare value chain. Patients are increasingly receiving care at nonhospital sites of care, where they can receive the care they need at a lower cost, rather than through traditional venues, such as hospital outpatient infusion centers. In addition to these alternative sites being less expensive for payers and purchasers, patients who seek care from alternative sites often have lower out-of-pocket costs and may perceive these sites as more convenient than traditional sites of care (e.g., emergency departments, hospital-based clinics). This trend has led to lower hospital outpatient revenues. Vertical integration of the healthcare value chain has given payers more control over healthcare costs and has better positioned them to link directly with providers and negotiate value-based contracts. Vertically integrated systems may allow payers to steer patients toward lower cost-of-care options (e.g., providers, pharmacies). In the ASHP Foundation Pharmacy Forecast 2018, 44% of panelists predicted at least 25% of health systems will discontinue or abandon plans to begin drug dispensing services (e.g., distribution of specialty or infusion products) because of insufficient financial margins.

One of the challenges that confronts health systems is the level of infrastructure investment required to adequately address regulatory and accreditation requirements focused on quality and safety (e.g., United States Pharmacopeia Chapters 797 and 800, state boards of pharmacy regulations, and the standards of accreditors such as The Joint Commission and Det Norske Veritas Healthcare). Physician offices, dialysis centers, stand-alone cancer care centers, freestanding neighborhood hospitals, and other nonhospital sites of care are commonly devoid of this same level of regulatory and accreditation scrutiny.

1915

PHARMACY DEPARTMENT BUSINESS PARTNERSHIPS

Source: Council on Pharmacy Management

To recognize that a key objective of pharmacy departments is to provide medication management services across the continuum of patient care, and that pharmacy leaders should proactively evaluate potential business partnerships against this objective; further,

To recognize that hospitals and health-system pharmacy leaders must ensure that business partners meet all applicable patient safety and accountability standards; further,

To provide education and tools for pharmacy leaders to aid in the evaluation of and development of business partnerships; further,

To educate health-system administrators on the importance of pharmacy leadership in evaluating and developing pharmacy-related business partnerships; further,

To encourage health-system pharmacy leaders to consider evolving healthcare financing systems when evaluating and developing business partnerships.

This policy supersedes ASHP policy 1416.

Rationale

Hospitals and health-system pharmacy leaders have to increasingly assess and engage with external business partners in order to facilitate continuity of care for their patients and optimize outcomes. Hospitals and health-system leaders must be positioned to provide the most comprehensive care for their patient populations. As these external entities expand their market share and become more engaged across the healthcare continuum, a significant number of hospitals and health systems are dealing with how to best evaluate potential business partnerships. In some cases hospital or health-system pharmacy leaders are seeking to create a network of pharmacy locations and services for their patients that the health system cannot build itself. In other cases hospital and health-system pharmacy leaders need to engage with external business partners to provide services they cannot provide or to improve the efficiency of services provided by the hospital or health system. Additionally, a number of business entities see changes in value-based purchasing and readmission payment as an opportunity to contract with health systems. Finally, there are also business partners (e.g., data management, automation, compounding, and consulting organizations) that pharmacy leaders need to engage with in order to manage their pharmacy enterprise. These changes have posed a political, logistical, and professional challenge for pharmacy leaders.

1522

DISPOSITION OF ILLICIT SUBSTANCES

Source: Council on Pharmacy Management

To advocate that healthcare organizations be required to develop procedures for the disposition of illicit substances brought into a facility that ensure compliance with applicable laws and accreditation standards; further,

To advocate that healthcare organizations be required to include pharmacy leaders in formulating such procedures.

This policy was reviewed in 2020 by the Council on Pharmacy Management and by the Board of Directors and was found to still be appropriate.

Rationale

Hospitals and health systems often treat patients that have in their possession illicit substances (e.g., Schedule I drugs, or other illegal or illegally possessed substances), which requires the facility to make decisions about how to secure the substances, ensure the appropriate chain of custody, and document possession in the patient's medical record, as well as decide whether to inform law enforcement. Such decisions benefit from the organization's legal counsel making a determination for the organization, in consultation with pharmacy leaders who can help interpret the pharmacist-in-charge's legal requirements and related accreditation standards.

1417

INTEGRATION OF PHARMACY SERVICES IN MULTIFACILITY HEALTH SYSTEMS

Source: Council on Pharmacy Management

To advocate that pharmacists are responsible for organizational efforts to standardize and integrate pharmacy services throughout the entire pharmacy enterprise in multifacility health systems and integrated delivery networks; further,

To educate health-system administrators about the importance of pharmacy leadership in setting system-wide policy regarding the safe and effective use of medications; further,

To advocate for the regulations and resources needed to support efforts to achieve optimal patient health outcomes in multifacility organizations.

This policy was reviewed in 2019 by the Council on Pharmacy Management and by the Board of Directors and was found to still be appropriate.

Rationale

Data from a 2011 American Hospital Association annual survey of hospitals indicate that at the time of the survey, 4432 of 5724 hospitals were part of either a system or a network, reflecting the evolution of the health care enterprise from single hospitals to integrated systems and networks. Multiple hospitals organized and owned by the same system have been in the United States marketplace for decades, but the rapidly changing marketplace in the past 2–3 years seems to foreshadow a future in which every hospital in the country will be part of a system. These systems have become increasingly complex as they also delve into non-hospital based businesses and seek to standardize and gain economies of scale across the organization.

These new organizations and the recognition of the importance of medication management to the overall health of these organizations have led to new roles and new challenges for pharmacy leaders. The pharmacy enterprise of the future will be more sophisticated and corporate in its nature. Pharmacy leaders both at the local hospital and at the corporate level have to more so than ever look at their pharmacy services in the context of the overall goals and needs of the organization or health system and determine the most efficient and effective means to provide these services. Leadership of the pharmacy must evolve from a department leader in a single facility to an effective corporate leader of medication use across a wide array of business units, care settings, and organizations. Centralization of medication management services is no longer confined to drug distribution but also includes human resources management, integrity of the electronic health record and related patient-care information, and oversight of various business partners. Pharmacy leaders within these evolving health systems will have many challenges, ranging from communication among the pharmacy management team, decisions on pharmacy infrastructure purchases and contracting, identification of critical services and standardization, succession planning and workforce development, supply chain management, human resource coordination, and strategic planning across diverse hospitals within the system. Further challenging health system pharmacy leaders are coordinating pharmacy services across larger geographical regions.

The nature and culture of decision making will be changed as some decisions become more centralized and corporatized and new practice models are developed to capitalize and adapt to the changing market place. Especially as merged systems extend beyond local and regional markets, health care will likely become even more business-like in its decision-making and fewer decisions will be made at the local facility level. The pharmacy enterprise will need to adapt to this changing environment. Many important decisions that influence medication-use policy will be made at the level of corporate leadership, and it will be critical that pharmacists provide leadership in this corporate decision-making. The ability to demonstrate the financial impact of pharmacy services will be critical and the development and implementation of effective drug-use policy across the enterprise will be crucial to success.

Along with increasing consolidation and integration of health systems, the business model for health care is also evolving. Pharmacy leaders will need to become familiar with changing business imperatives and align the pharmacy business plan with that of the health system. Planning must integrate at both the strategic and tactical level. Pharmacy needs to be envisioned as a service rather than a department. These changes have resulted in the need to evaluate best practices, legal and regulatory requirements, and leadership structure.

0901

WORKLOAD MONITORING AND REPORTING

Source: House of Delegates Resolution

To strongly discourage the use of pharmacy workload and productivity measurement systems ("pharmacy benchmarking systems") that are based solely upon dispensing functions (e.g., doses dispensed or billed) or a variant of patient days, because such measures do not accurately assess pharmacy workload, staffing effectiveness, clinical practice contributions to patient care, or impacts on costs of care, and therefore these measurement systems are not valid and should not be used; further,

To advocate the development and implementation of pharmacy benchmarking systems that accurately assess the impact of pharmacy services on patient outcomes and total costs of care; further,

To define pharmacy workload as all activities related to providing pharmacy patient care services; further,

To continue communications with health-system administrators, consulting firms, and professional associations regarding the value of pharmacists' services and the importance of using valid, comprehensive, and evidence-based measures of pharmacy workload and productivity; further,

To encourage practitioners and vendors to develop and use a standard protocol for collecting and reporting pharmacy workload data and patient outcomes; further,

To advocate to health-system administrators, consulting firms, and vendors of performance-measurement services firms the development and implementation of pharmacy benchmarking systems that accurately assess the impact of pharmacy services on patient outcomes and total costs of care.

This policy was reviewed in 2019 by the Council on Pharmacy Management and by the Board of Directors and was found to still be appropriate.

Rationale

Although the practice of health-system pharmacy has evolved and changed significantly over the past two decades, benchmarking systems used to gauge the value and productivity of health-system pharmacy have remained largely unchanged. Productivity measures based solely on dispensing functions or a variant of patient days are not valid tools to assess current health-system pharmacy practice. These outdated measures do not reflect ASHP's aspirations for health-system pharmacy (e.g., ASHP best practices and the 2015 Initiative) or evolving Joint Commission requirements. Use of these inappropriate productivity recommendations may result in inadequate staffing, which increases stress on pharmacy leadership, discourages pharmacists from becoming pharmacy directors, and contributes to the leadership gap in health-system pharmacy.

Alternative benchmarking systems that more accurately reflect true health-system pharmacy productivity have been developed. The ASHP Section of Pharmacy Practice Managers has made recommendations for the effective use of workload and productivity systems in health-system pharmacy that elaborates the types of metrics that should be used.

0918

PHARMACIST LEADERSHIP OF THE PHARMACY DEPARTMENT

Source: Council on Pharmacy Management

To affirm the importance of an organizational structure in hospitals and health systems that places administrative, clinical, and operational responsibility for the pharmacy department under a pharmacist leader; further,

To affirm the role of the pharmacist leader in oversight and supervision of all pharmacy personnel; further,

To recognize the supporting role of nonpharmacists in leadership and management roles within pharmacy departments.

This policy was reviewed in 2019 by the Council on Pharmacy Management and by the Board of Directors and was found to still be appropriate.

Rationale

The ASHP Long Range Vision for the Pharmacy Work Force in Hospitals and Health Systems sees a growing role for nonpharmacists in management and leadership positions in hospitals and health systems. Many factors are fueling this expansion, including a shortage of pharmacists, pharmacists' salaries, and the growing complexity of the pharmacy enterprise. There are many functions in the pharmacy department that can be led or managed by nonpharmacists, including management of technological, business, or financial matters. Although nonpharmacists fill many important supporting leadership and management roles within pharmacy departments, a pharmacist should lead the pharmacy enterprise, supervise and manage all pharmacy personnel, and be responsible for the administrative, clinical, and operational functions of pharmacy departments in hospitals and health systems. Use of specialized nonpharmacist expertise will vary, depending on the size and complexity of the pharmacy enterprise. These roles will be more prevalent in large facilities and less so in small or rural facilities, where there is likely to be less specialization in pharmacy functions.

0504

PHARMACY STAFF FATIGUE AND MEDICATION ERRORS

Source: Council on Administrative Affairs

To encourage pharmacy managers to consider workload fatigue, length of shifts, and similar performance-altering factors when scheduling pharmacy staff, in order to ensure safe pharmacy practices; further,

To oppose state or federal laws or regulations that mandate or restrict work hours for pharmacy staff; further,

To support research on the effects of shift length, fatigue, and other factors on the safe practice of pharmacy.

This policy was reviewed in 2020 by the Council on Pharmacy Management and by the Board of Directors and was found to still be appropriate.

ASHP Statement on the Roles and Responsibilities of the Pharmacy Executive

Position

Leading hospitals and health systems must have a strategic and innovative pharmacy executive who plans and oversees the design and operation of the entire and complex medication-use process throughout the system. It is essential that this leader report to an executive who can help the leader execute the practice models of tomorrow that include business outside normal hospital practice. As the most knowledgeable leader of the medication-use process, this leader (may be referred to as the "chief pharmacy officer" but hereafter "the pharmacy executive") proactively aligns pharmacy goals with strategic organizational initiatives to advocate for pharmacy practice advancement and improved patient care. The intrinsic value a pharmacy executive brings to the organization's enterprise and executive leadership includes the following:

- Ensuring the enterprise's strategic planning leverages pharmacy services across the continuum of care to improve health outcomes.
- Ensuring pharmaceuticals and pharmaceutical benefit designs focus on total health through the formulary, with procurement driven by clinical efficacy.
- Collaborating with healthcare executives within and external to the health system to foster and build cross-functional relationships and to align interdisciplinary services with initiatives such as quality metrics and financial performance.
- Advancing patient care services through the promotion of pharmacy best practices by the creation and adoption of emerging technologies and innovative services.
- Ensuring the pharmacy workforce is provided an environment that is free of discrimination and harassment and supportive of diversity, equity, and inclusion.

Background

Significant changes in pharmacy practice, healthcare, and health-system management over the past 20 years have dramatically transformed the traditional role of the pharmacy director.[1] More widespread use of the title "chief pharmacy officer" was first proposed in 2000 in an attempt to meet these new transformations and to enhance the contribution pharmacy makes to patient care by creating organizational parity between the pharmacy executive and other executive officers (e.g., chief nursing, medical, and information officers).[2]

Responsibilities and Value of the Pharmacy Executive

The pharmacy executive assesses the ever-changing healthcare environment for emerging trends and identifies opportunities to leverage the pharmacy team's expertise to improve the value of care across the healthcare continuum. Success as a pharmacy executive is predicated on building and maintaining relationships with diverse groups of people in order to be part of setting the overall strategy for the organization. Navigating solid and dotted-line reporting relationships, such as in a matrixed organizational structure, requires the pharmacy executive to exercise a wider range of influence and persuasiveness rather than relying on traditional hierarchy and formal control to accomplish objectives. As it relates to patient care and clinical services, the pharmacy executive leads all pharmacists and pharmacy staff across the organization. The pharmacy executive ensures that pharmacists are optimally positioned and resourced to improve the quality, safety, and efficiency of medication management and patient outcomes in the most cost-effective manner. The pharmacy executive leads the pharmacy's financial performance within the context of the broader health system through the evaluation of medication expenditure patterns and reimbursement trends, including value-based reimbursement and purchasing. As reimbursement and revenue capture become increasingly complex, the pharmacy executive can provide leadership across multiple disciplines (e.g., finance, nursing, medicine, pharmacy) to optimize reimbursement from involved government and commercial payment programs and meet metrics for value-based contract requirements.[3,4] She or he is also responsible for medication access in their organization to ensure patients have the most effective and affordable medications.

In performing these responsibilities, the pharmacy executive must bring continuous and evergreen value to the pharmacy team, the health system's executive team, and the organization as a whole. The pharmacy executive establishes key relationships with both internal multidisciplinary executives and external vendors, group purchasing organizations, and manufacturers to elevate services and optimize the pharmaceutical supply chain, respectively. In addition to optimizing the supply chain, the pharmacy executive plays a key role in developing a vision for information and technology solutions in the medication-use process and must work collaboratively with the chief information officer to advance pharmacy informatics and technology. During all phases of a public health emergency or disaster event, pharmacy executive presence in a hospital or health system's emergency operations center is pivotal for proactive planning and maintaining secure, functional, and resilient health and public health critical infrastructure. The pharmacy executive is integral in advancing pharmacy services in the midst of rising competitors, ensuring the vitality of the organization as healthcare transforms.[5–7] She or he must maintain a focused effort to acquire, share, and reinvest in their own self-development and the development of the leadership team striving for the continuous pursuit of practice advancement.

The pharmacy executive must commit to ensuring a culture in which all individuals are treated with respect and civility and that is conducive to the highest levels of patient care for the organization's workforce. This commitment includes leading a workplace that fosters diversity, equity, and inclusion, with zero tolerance for discrimination and harassment. Ensuring the pharmacy workforce is

DOI 10.37573/9781585287048.088

working in a safe environment and one that is supportive of growth, wellness, and resilience is a critical factor in organizational success in meeting its patient care mission, ensuring employee retention, providing training and recruitment, and ensuring an ability to advance pharmacy practice.

Experience and Education of the Pharmacy Executive

The pharmacy executive is a professionally competent, legally licensed pharmacist with a broad level of experience in health-system pharmacy practice and management and with a strategic vision for the profession. Additional qualifications may include an advanced management degree; a clearly evident successful record of leading people, operations, finance, and clinical services; and completion of a pharmacy residency program accredited by ASHP (e.g., health-system pharmacy administration and leadership residency).

What distinguishes the pharmacy executive from the established director of pharmacy position is the increased breadth and depth of the involvement in the health system's strategic planning and decision-making processes at the most senior levels. The pharmacy executive has experience in leading the medication-use process, including optimizing the pharmaceutical supply chain, making evidence-based systematic clinical decisions, supporting medication-management systems and policies, implementing technology to elevate patient care, and optimizing financial performance. The pharmacy executive, therefore, provides pharmacy's unique clinical and business perspectives in decisions related to changes in the medication-management system.8-10 To support these changes, the pharmacy executive leverages technology to develop the most cost-effective labor model.

Reporting Structure

The pharmacy executive has a market-competitive title internally consistent with others reporting at that organizational level, reports directly to the organization's principal executive (e.g., chief executive officer [CEO], chief operating officer [COO]), participates as a member of the medical executive committee, and routinely engages with the health system's executive leadership as well as the board of directors. By working collaboratively with others at this most senior executive level, the pharmacy executive ensures that health-system pharmacy services are optimally positioned to most effectively contribute to the organization's strategic initiatives and address systemwide opportunities. A structure in which pharmacy leadership reports directly to the principal executive rather than through layers of management allows the pharmacy executive to engage in critical decision-making and be more effective and influential in helping the health system anticipate and address rapid change.

Conclusion

Optimal patient care, quality health outcomes, and pharmacy practice advancement require that progressive hospitals and health systems have an educated pharmacy executive responsible for the strategic planning, design, operation, and improvement of the organization's pharmacy services across the care continuum. Because of these expected contributions, the pharmacy executive must be properly positioned within the health system's senior executive management team to ensure that health-system pharmacy services are best leveraged to meet the ever-changing demands of the future of healthcare delivery.

References

1. Nold EG, Sander WT. Role of the director of pharmacy: the first six months. *Am J Health-Syst Pharm.* 2004;61:2297–2310.
2. Godwin HN. Achieving best practices in health-system pharmacy: eliminating the "practice gap." *Am J Health-Syst Pharm.* 2000;57:2212–2213.
3. Anderson RW. Health-system pharmacy: new practice framework and leadership model. *Am J Health-Syst Pharm.* 2002;59:1163–1172.
4. Mitchell CL, Anderson ER, Braun L. Billing for inpatient hospital care. *Am J Health-Syst Pharm.* 2003;60(suppl 6):S8-S11.
5. ASHP Practice Advancement Initiative 2030: new recommendations for advancing pharmacy practice in health systems. *Am J Health-Syst Pharm.* 2020;77:113–121.
6. Knoer S. Stewardship of the pharmacy enterprise. *Am J Health-Syst Pharm.* 2014;71:1204–1209.
7. ASHP Research and Education Foundation. Pharmacy forecast reports. Accessed June 23, 2021. https://www.ashpfoundation.org/Research/Pharmacy-Forecast
8. Ivey MF. Rationale for having a chief pharmacy officer in a health care organization. *Am J Health-Syst Pharm.* 2005;62:975–978.
9. American Society of Health-System Pharmacists. ASHP long-range vision for the pharmacy work force in hospitals and health systems. *Am J Health-Syst Pharm.* 2020;77:386–400.
10. Rough S, Shane R, Armitstead JA, et al. The high-value pharmacy enterprise framework: advancing pharmacy practice in health systems through a consensus-based, strategic approach. *Am J Health-Syst Pharm.* 2021;78:498–510.

Developed through the ASHP Council on Pharmacy Management and approved by the ASHP Board of Directors on February 2, 2021, and by the ASHP House of Delegates on June 6, 2021. This statement supersedes a previous version dated June 7, 2015.

ASHP acknowledges the contributions of the drafters of previous versions of this statement: Karl Kappeler, MS, FASHP; Michael Nnadi, PharmD, MHS; Sam Calabrese, MBA, FASHP; Debra Cowan, PharmD, FASHP; Bonnie Kirshenbaum, MS, FASHP, FCSHP; John Lewin, PharmD, MBA; Christine Marchese, PharmD; Tricia Meyer, PharmD, MS, FASHP; Brandon Ordway, PharmD, MS; Roger Woolf, PharmD; Rusol Karralli, PharmD, MS; and Kelly Sennett, BS.

The authors have declared no potential conflicts of interest.

Lindsey B Amerine, PharmD, MS, BCPS, FASHP, UNC Health, Chapel Hill, NC, and University of North Carolina Eshelman School of Pharmacy, Chapel Hill, NC.

Robert P Granko, PharmD, MBA, FASHP, Moses H. Cone Memorial Hospital - Cone Health, Greensboro, NC, and University of North Carolina Eshelman School of Pharmacy, Chapel Hill, NC.

Philip W Brummond, PharmD, MS, FASHP, Froedtert and the Medical College of Wisconsin, Milwaukee, WI.

Samuel V Calabrese, BSPharm, MBA, FASHP, Cleveland Clinic, Cleveland, OH.

Kristine K Gullickson, PharmD, MBA, FASHP, FMSHP, DPLA, Allina Health, Abbott Northwestern Hospital, Minneapolis, MN.

Lindsey R Kelley, PharmD, MS, FASHP, University of Michigan Health, Michigan Medicine, Ann Arbor, MI.

Jeffrey D Little, PharmD, MPH, BCPS, FACHE, FASHP, Saint Luke's Hospital, Kansas City, MO.

Mark Sullivan, PharmD, MBA, BCPS, FASHP, Vanderbilt University Hospital & Clinics, Nashville, TN.

Copyright © 2022, American Society of Health-System Pharmacists, Inc. All rights reserved. Contact ASHP for reprint and permissions requests. This content may not be used for commercial purposes without the express written consent of ASHP.

The bibliographic citation for this document is as follows: American Society of Health-System Pharmacists. ASHP statement on the roles and responsibilities of the pharmacy executive. *Am J Health-Syst Pharm*. 2022; 79:497–499.

ASHP Statement on Standards-Based Pharmacy Practice in Hospitals and Health Systems

Position

Pharmacy practice leaders in hospitals and health systems have a distinguished history of advancing health-system pharmacy practice beyond the minimum required by law, regulation, and accreditation. The American Society of Health-System Pharmacists (ASHP) supports those efforts by developing and disseminating a comprehensive body of evidence-based, peer-reviewed descriptions of best practices in health-system pharmacy. ASHP believes that pharmacists who practice in hospitals and health systems ("health-system pharmacists") and pharmacy leaders in health systems can continuously improve the delivery of patient care by regularly assessing compliance with ASHP best practices, identifying gaps in practice, establishing practice improvement priorities appropriate for their unique circumstances, and working to close the targeted gaps.

Purpose

The purpose of this statement is to promote understanding of how health-system pharmacists use ASHP best practices to develop and promote in health systems a standard of practice that exceeds what is required by law, regulation, or accreditation.

Standards-Based Pharmacy Practice

A standard is "a statement that defines the performance expectations, structures, or processes that must be in place for an organization to provide safe and high quality care, treatment, and service."1 In health care, practice standards serve as guideposts for a profession and as a way of communicating to peers, patients, policymakers, other professionals, and the public the roles and responsibilities of members of the profession. Practice standards also provide a benchmark for evaluating the quality of services and patient care.

Health-system pharmacists, like other health care professionals, practice under a number of mandated standards. These standards include state board of pharmacy regulations, public health requirements, Drug Enforcement Administration regulations, Joint Commission accreditation standards, Centers for Medicare and Medicaid Services conditions of participation, and the standards of other accrediting bodies and professional associations. Individual health care organizations also develop their own interdisciplinary practice policies and standards of care related to medication use, with health-system pharmacists serving as key participants in their development.

ASHP members have invested decades of effort in developing and maintaining an extensive body of policy positions, statements, and guidelines (hereinafter "ASHP best practices") that serve as a guide for effective, high-quality pharmacy practice in hospitals and health systems.[2] This comprehensive set of policies is unique in pharmacy.

ASHP best practices reinforce health-system pharmacists' established roles in health care and encourage development of responsibilities that answer the growing need and public demand for expanded involvement of pharmacists in patient care. ASHP best practices are based on professional and scientific literature and are developed with input from ASHP members, the public, regulatory bodies, other professional associations, and representatives of other health care disciplines. Peer groups of ASHP expert members systematically review ASHP best practices and compare them with the existing literature, the changing expectations of society, and changes in the professional and ethical challenges faced by health-system pharmacists. A compilation of these documents is published annually as *Best Practices for Hospital and Health-System Pharmacy* and made available to the public (www.ashp.org/bestpractices).

Most ASHP best practices represent the professional beliefs and aspirations of pharmacists practicing in health systems, based on evidence and expert opinion. Only select ASHP guidelines describe a minimum level of practice that all hospital pharmacy departments should consistently provide; these guidelines are designated as ASHP minimum standards.[3–6] Institutions that offer ASHP-accredited residencies are required to meet ASHP best practices to ensure the quality of the educational experience.

ASHP best practices represent a commitment by ASHP members to advancing the standard of pharmacy practice. ASHP believes that all health-system pharmacists have a role to play in raising health-system pharmacy practice to a level consistent with the best practices that have been developed and have gained acceptance by a peer-reviewed, consensus-based process. Practicing pharmacists and pharmacy leaders in health systems should use their professional judgment to regularly assess compliance with ASHP best practices, identify gaps in practice in their settings, establish practice improvement priorities appropriate for their unique circumstances, and work to close those practice gaps to ensure continuous improvement in the delivery of patient care.

Conclusion

Health-system pharmacy practice leaders have a long tradition of striving to advance practice beyond the minimum required by law, regulation, and accreditation. ASHP best practices embody those aspirations and provide health-system pharmacists with a means to continuously improve the delivery of patient care.

References

1. Comprehensive accreditation manual for hospitals. Oakbrook Terrace, IL: Joint Commission; 2007:GL-22.
2. Zellmer WA. Overview of the history of hospital pharmacy in the United States. In: Brown TR, ed. Handbook of institutional pharmacy practice. 4th ed. Bethesda, MD: American Society of Health-System Pharmacists; 2006:19–32.

DOI 10.37573/9781585287048.089

3. American Society of Health-System Pharmacists. ASHP guidelines: minimum standard for pharmacies in hospitals. *Am J Health-Syst Pharm.* 2013; 70:1619–30.
4. American Society of Health-System Pharmacists. ASHP guidelines on home infusion pharmacy services. *Am J Health-Syst Pharm.* 2014; 71:325–41.
5. American Society of Health-System Pharmacists. ASHP guidelines: minimum standard for ambulatory care pharmacy practice. *Am J Health-Syst Pharm.* 2015; 72:1221–36.
6. American Society of Health-System Pharmacists. ASHP–PPAG guidelines for providing pediatric pharmacy services in hospitals and health systems. *Am J Health-Syst Pharm.* 2018; 75:1151–65.

This statement was reviewed in 2023 by the Council on Pharmacy Management and by the Board of Directors and was found to still be appropriate.

Developed through the ASHP Council on Pharmacy Management and approved by the ASHP Board of Directors on March 7, 2008, and by the ASHP House of Delegates on June 10, 2008.

Scott Mark, Pharm.D., M.S., M.Ed., CHE, FASHP, FABC, is gratefully acknowledged for drafting this statement.

Copyright © 2009, American Society of Health-System Pharmacists, Inc. All rights reserved. All rights reserved. Contact ASHP for reprint and permissions requests. This content may not be used for commercial purposes without the express written consent of ASHP.

The bibliographic citation for this document is as follows: American Society of Health-System Pharmacists. ASHP statement on standards-based pharmacy practice in hospitals and health systems. *Am J Health-Syst Pharm.* 2009; 66:409–10.

ASHP Guidelines on Medication Cost Management Strategies for Hospitals and Health Systems

Because medication costs comprise the majority of health-system pharmacy budgets and continue to increase faster than other health care expenditures,[1] drug costs are a constant target for cost containment initiatives. The purpose of these guidelines is to provide guidance on medication-cost-management strategies.

These guidelines recommend techniques to manage drug costs in hospitals and health systems. The guidelines focus on drug use in inpatient settings and hospital clinics, where health-system pharmacies typically have responsibility for purchasing and distributing drugs. Strategies for other settings, such as managed care and ambulatory care settings, and strategies for revenue optimization are beyond the scope of this document. Although revenue optimization and medication cost management are complementary approaches to improving the financial performance of pharmacy departments, revenue optimization is best addressed through literature specific to that topic[2,3] and is not extensively reviewed in this document.

These guidelines examine methods for nonlabor pharmaceutical cost containment, focusing primarily on variable costs (costs dependent on patient volume) and direct drug costs. Fixed and indirect costs, such as labor to prepare or administer medication, nonpharmaceutical materials, and overhead, are also beyond the scope of these guidelines. There is also not an attempt to consider the impact of drug costs and drug-cost-management strategies on other hospital departments (e.g., laboratory, respiratory care) or on the total health care costs once the patient leaves the acute care setting. Although not discussed here, these shifts in drug costs are important to consider as drug therapies influence other health care costs, and pharmacists should lead efforts to promote the value medications provide across the hospital and health care system.

A broad range of drug-cost-management strategies exist throughout hospitals and health systems. Some approaches are relatively straightforward and can be implemented within the pharmacy. Other approaches are more complex and require high-level strategic planning and extensive collaboration throughout the hospital. Successful drug cost management requires systematic attention to and integration of both approaches. Because of the different nature of various drug-cost-management activities, these guidelines present information at different levels of complexity appropriate to the approach being described.

When selecting and implementing drug-cost-management strategies, it is essential that pharmacists remain mindful of patient safety and the quality of patient care.

Drug-cost-containment initiatives must never compromise the department's ability to provide the best possible care to patients. In many cases, it is prudent and necessary to monitor and evaluate the safety and outcomes of drug-cost-management projects. Fortunately, many drug-cost-containment strategies have little or no potential for detrimental effects on patient care, and efforts to improve the quality of drug use often coincide with cost-containment initiatives.

Trends in Medication Expenditures

Senior hospital administrators have recognized the importance of drug costs to the fiscal status of health systems. For example, a health care consultancy reported that in 1996, "managing hospital drug utilization and expenditures" was not ranked in the top 20 concerns for hospital CEOs.[4] When the survey was repeated in 2000; however, hospital CEOs ranked drug costs as their seventh most important concern. The 2000 survey also reported that among hospitals' greatest financial challenges, drug and technology costs were second only to decreased reimbursement, and hospital CEOs said that drugs offered the single greatest opportunity for cost savings.[4] Although somewhat dated, these data illustrate that drug-expenditure management presents health systems with an important challenge that is recognized by senior hospital administration.

Four primary factors drive growth in overall drug expenditures: price, utilization, mix, and innovation.[1]

Price inflation is an increase in the unit price of existing medications. Utilization is an increase in use of a drug, such as an increase in number of users, days of therapy, or dose per day of therapy. Mix changes when newer, more expensive therapies are used in place of older, less expensive but equally effective drugs. Finally, a blend of the utilization and mix factors increases drug expenditures when expensive, new medications become available to treat conditions previously untreatable with drug therapy (i.e., innovative therapy).

The United States spent over $250 billion dollars on prescription drugs in 2005, but total drug costs represent a relatively small portion of total U.S. health care spending (approximately 11%).[5] However, double-digit increases in prescription drug expenditures have been common (e.g., 15% in 2000, 18% in 2001, 12% in 2002, 11% in 2003, and 9% in 2004).[1,4,6] The rate of drug-expenditure growth has frequently been higher than inflation, increases in wages, and other health care spending, including spending for hospitals, physician services, and total health care expenditures. However, with the exception of 26% growth in 2001, the recent rate of growth in hospital drug expenditures has been less than the growth of total drug expenditures. Hospital drug expenditures grew 4.9% in 2000, 26% in 2001, 9.7% in 2002, 6.3% in 2003, 7.9% in 2004, and 5.7% in 2005.[1,5–7] However, the rate of growth in clinic drug expenditures has consistently exceeded the growth of total drug expenditures. Clinic drug expenditures grew 24.6% in 2000, 23% in 2001, 21.3% in 2002, 22.2% in 2003, 13.5% in 2004, and 12.4% in 2005.[1,5,7]

While the rate of increase in prescription drug expenditures moderated somewhat between 2004 and 2006, drug-expenditure growth remains substantial. Long-range forecasts suggest that the rate of increase in total prescription drug expenditures will continue to exceed the rate of increase for

DOI 10.37573/9781585287048.090

total health care expenditures through 2014. Because drug expenditures are the largest component of every health-system pharmacy's operating budget and often a meaningful portion of the entire hospital operating budget, drug expenses attract significant attention from hospital leaders. For these reasons, it is apparent that drug-expenditure-management will remain an area of focus and responsibility for health-system pharmacists for the foreseeable future.[8]

Systematic Approach to Medication-Cost-Management Measures

A systematic approach to planning and prioritizing specific drug cost management strategies is essential when implementing initiatives that will influence drug expenditures in a health system. Annual financial planning (i.e., budgeting) is the most common planning approach, and specific drug-cost-management strategies should be considered a part of the budgeting process. However, longer-term strategic and programmatic planning activities also have an important role in managing drug expenditures.

A systematic approach to drug-cost containment requires specific and detailed data on both health-system drug purchases and actual drug-use patterns. Data must underlie all types of planning to manage medication expenditures. Systems should be established to have ready access to the data and continually review and monitor these data.

It is essential to interact and collaborate consistently with physician leaders from various specialties to successfully plan, prioritize, and implement medication-cost management efforts. Physician involvement must be sought during the annual financial planning process and when doing strategic or programmatic planning related to drug expenditures. Appropriate physician representatives must also be engaged in specific drug-cost-management initiatives. During the annual financial planning process, physicians can provide important information related to drug costs, such as anticipated use of key drugs in the pipeline, programmatic or new service implementation, anticipated recruitment of specialists who may require high-cost agents, projections for use of high-priority drugs, and insights for drug cost containment. Pharmacy leaders can also use this opportunity to update physicians on the pharmacy department's recent accomplishments and goals for the future.

Drug Budgeting. Although a complete discussion of the drug-budgeting process is beyond the scope of this document, several important suggestions are provided below. A general approach to systematically developing the annual drug budget is outlined in **Table 1.**[7] At the beginning of each calendar year, the *American Journal of Health-System Pharmacy* publishes a projection of drug expenditures for that year.[1,5–7]

Annual drug budgeting is a challenging exercise. Unanticipated situations that result in extreme increases in drug expenditures will likely occur and the pharmacy director should be prepared to explain those situations. Better data and more experience will improve a department's ability to forecast institutional drug expenditures. Regardless of the drug budget's accuracy in forecasting the institution's drug expenditures, a well-planned drug budget should help the department understand drug use patterns and identify opportu-nities for drug cost management. Specific reports that can be helpful in understanding drug use will be described below.

TABLE 1.
Steps for Developing Annual Drug Budget[7]

Collect and review data (e.g., drug purchase data, drug utilization data, workload and productivity data, other financial statements).
Develop budget for high-priority agents (top 50–60 drugs).
Identify relevant new drugs and build new agent budget.
Budget for nonformulary drugs and lower-priority drugs.
Establish a drug cost containment plan (identify drugs going off patent, opportunities for therapeutic interchange or protocol development).
Finalize and present the total drug budget.
Continue the budgeting process throughout the year through constant vigilance and monitoring of drug use.

During the annual financial planning process, it is important to identify and focus on key drug expenditures. The Pareto Principle, or 80/20 rule, applies to drug budgeting and states that in nearly all cases, a few vital factors are important and many are trivial. A relatively small number of drugs (50–60) typically account for 80% of most hospital drug budgets. Therefore, budgeting and cost-containment efforts should focus on those drugs, and the cost-management plan should especially concentrate on those top drugs for which it is feasible to influence prescribing patterns. Much of this document focuses on the need to develop a cost-containment plan after initial estimates of drug costs are completed (Table 1).

Medication-cost-management projects should be carefully selected and prioritized as part of an ongoing financial planning process. Because drug-cost containment strategies must be customized to each health system's unique characteristics, a global assessment of the pharmacy department and the hospital must be conducted to identify opportunities for drug-cost-management. This assessment must go beyond a qualitative assessment of opportunities and must include retrieval and analysis of both drug purchase and drug-utilization data. Pharmacy departments may need to obtain and develop resources, such as personnel and software, to analyze these data.

Despite the need to customize the strategy and tactics to fit the needs of different hospitals and health systems, a systematic approach to identifying, prioritizing, and implementing medication-cost containment initiatives is necessary and can be applied in any setting. A clearly defined list of cost-containment targets should be established during each financial planning cycle. To be successful, the number of initiatives should be manageable and should focus on the institution's top expenditures. In many situations, multiple approaches for cost containment will be necessary.

The foundation for effective cost-management strategies, and the first stage of the systematic approach, begins with determining current costs of medications, both as ongoing expenses and those held as assets in inventory. Understanding and tracking key medication-cost indicators on an ongoing basis is necessary to determine the opportunities for medication-cost reduction. Examples of these indicators may include:

- Medication inventory per adjusted patient day
- Medication inventory turnover rate

- Contract coverage percentage
- Contract compliance percentage
- Intravenous-to-oral dosage ratio
- Volume-adjusted total medication costs (e.g., cost per adjusted patient day, discharge, etc.)
- Volume-adjusted drug category costs (e.g., antibiotics, anesthesia-related drugs, etc.)
- Descending-order total purchase histories, tracked over time

In addition, the use of external benchmarks may provide assistance in identifying medication-cost-reduction opportunities. External benchmarks may be available as a component of services provided by consulting organizations, the pharmacy's drug wholesaler or group-purchasing organization (GPO), or from professional published data. Benchmark data should be used with care; however, because there may be important limitations to the applicability of the data to a specific site. For example, difficulties may exist in adjusting the data for the specific pharmacy practice, such as models and intensity of services, and in finding an appropriate peer group.[9]

After cost-management opportunities are identified, they need to be quantified. Dollar values should be assigned to each opportunity, including inventory reduction, improvement in inventory turns, improving contract compliance, therapeutic interchange of various agents, and others. A specific goal and action plan should be set for each drug-cost-management target. For example, one goal might be to reduce expenditures for a drug class by 8% by establishing a contract for a new, preferred agent and implementing a therapeutic interchange program to shift use to the new agent. Alternatively, the goal might be to slow the rate of increase in use of a particular drug or drug class (e.g., based on current patterns, use of this drug class is expected to grow 15% in the next fiscal year, but the goal of interventions is to limit the rate of increase to 10%). Monitoring is essential, so drug cost containment targets should be consistently measured and evaluated. Identifying and quantifying the opportunities must be completed before prioritization and in-depth evaluation begins.

Assessment and Prioritization. Once opportunities for cost management have been identified and quantified, assessment and prioritization can occur. There are many methods of prioritization, but most of them contain two key elements: determining the potential benefit and estimating the relative ease or difficulty of attaining the benefit. Even though potential benefit may be clear-cut, the degree of difficulty is often hard to establish. Important points to consider when determining the relative degree of difficulty and likelihood of achieving benefits from a given drug-cost-management opportunity include (1) the amount of time pressure (the time available until the cost reductions occur), (2) key stakeholder (e.g., nurse, physician) sensitivity and willingness to collaborate, (3) extent of leadership support for the initiative, (4) resources required, and (5) existing level of expertise within the organization for the specific cost-management opportunity.

Drug-cost management strategies that are under the direct and exclusive purview of the pharmacy department (e.g., purchasing, inventory management, and waste reduction approaches) are generally easier to implement and provide more immediate benefits. These activities, however, often provide smaller or one-time financial benefits. Utilization management tactics (e.g., clinical practice guidelines and therapeutic interchange) generally provide greater financial benefits, but these efforts have correspondingly higher degrees of difficulty and complexity.

Because of the relative ease of implementation, cost-containment opportunities in areas that are primarily under the department's control will usually be pursued first. After these initiatives are underway, more complex techniques that require collaboration with the medical staff and others should be pursued.

These guidelines are structured so that the cost-management techniques are presented in the order in which health systems often implement them. Components of a cost-management program are listed in **Table 2**. An appendix that lists specific cost management opportunities is also provided. It is important to note that although these guidelines are separated into sections on purchasing and inventory management and medication-use management, both activities are integral and indivisible to drug-cost management planning and the practice of pharmacy in hospitals and health systems.

TABLE 2.
Components of a Cost-Management Program[a]

Pharmacy-Directed Activities
Purchasing
GPO contracts
Facility contracts
Wholesaler contracts
Inventory management
Wholesaler ordering programs
Storage
Waste reduction
I.V. product waste
Returns
Interdisciplinary Activities
Medication utilization program
Clinical pharmacy services
Assessment of drug costs
Medical staff support
Formulary management
Therapeutic interchange
Guideline (protocol) development
Pharmacist interventions
Plan implementation and analysis
Reimbursement & Charging
Reimbursement
340B programs
CMS (DRG class)
Commercial insurance (payer mix)
Outpatient infusion center
Charging
Coding and processing
Indigent care programs

[a]GPO = group purchasing organization, CMS = Centers for Medicare and Medicaid Services, DRG = diagnosis-related group.

Purchasing and Inventory Management

When selecting drug-cost-containment initiatives, purchasing and inventory management procedures should be considered first.

Drug Product Costs and Procurement. At the most fundamental level, drug costs are a function of unit costs and utilization. Drug-unit costs are a function of acquisition costs (contracted or non-contracted), the external (in-bound) distribution fee, inventory management costs, and internal distribution costs.

Contracting. There are three main avenues for purchasing pharmaceuticals at discounted rates: GPO contracts, facility contracts, and wholesaler own-use contracts. All facilities should seek to maximize savings available from use of generic products, and some may have other considerations, such as use of 340B or indigent care programs.

GPO contracts. GPOs utilize the aggregate purchasing power of many facilities in negotiating pricing agreements with manufacturers. Most hospitals are members of a GPO. While there are GPOs that focus exclusively on drugs, the majority of GPOs offer contracts for medical and surgical supplies, food, and other support products and services in addition to pharmaceuticals. Most GPOs make their contract portfolio available to members via hard copy, and some GPOs have contract portfolios available on secure internet sites. Considerations in contracting with a GPO are listed in **Table 3**. It is also important to have routine surveillance, preferably an automated service, that ensures that contract prices are applied to all purchases.

GPOs are funded by one of two means. First, most, if not all, GPOs collect a contract administrative fee (CAF) from the manufacturers or distributors with which they contract. The CAF is rarely greater than 3% of the dollar volume of product purchased through the contract. Some GPOs return a portion or all of the CAF to its members. If any or all of the CAF for a particular drug product is returned to the facility by the GPO, it should be taken into account when calculating the net cost of the drug. The second method by which GPOs are funded is direct payment of fees by members to the GPO. In this arrangement, all of the CAF is returned to the facility.

Contracts through GPOs consider not only the unit cost of the pharmaceutical but also include the allowable distribution methods for the pharmaceutical, payment terms, returns policies, and supplier performance requirements. Many GPO contracts, especially those for multi-source generics, include simple line-item pricing, which only requires the purchaser to buy and pay for the product. Other contracts are more complicated, with incentive rebates for all purchases or rebates for achieving volume or market share targets.

Typically, market share agreements are utilized when two or more products can be used to treat the same disease and no generic equivalent exists. The incentive, such as a rebate, a lock-in of a current discount, or achievement of a higher discount, is contingent upon attaining a given market share for a particular product in the institution's market basket. To achieve the greatest financial advantage from the contract (lowest net drug cost), the pharmacy must work with the medical staff. This process requires a careful evaluation of comparative efficacy and safety of the product and its alternatives.

Some GPOs have multiple products on contract within categories of pharmaceuticals, allowing the facility to receive discounted pricing on similar agents when prescribing practices are not standardized to one agent. More aggressive GPOs will sometimes contract for a single agent within a particular class (e.g., for one fluoroquinolone or one liposomal amphotericin B product to the exclusion of others) in order to gain the maximum value for its members.

Successful use of GPO contracts requires a constructive and collaborative relationship between the member, the GPO, the manufacturer, and the distributor (i.e., wholesaler). Potential advantages of GPO contracts are listed in **Table 4**.

In addition to the contracting portfolio, GPOs offer services such as lost savings and compliance reports, rebate and contract administrative fee reports, clinical utilization management programs, and letters of commitment.

Lost savings and compliance reports. These reports provide data and analysis of missed savings opportunities in the user's purchase history (e.g., items purchased off-contract when a generically equivalent alternative item was on-contract). These reports may also indicate the compliance level, or the amount of purchases on-contract versus the amount of purchases that could have been made on-contract (drugs purchased on-contract plus the value of drugs purchased off-contract when alternatives were on-contract). These reports should be reviewed monthly to determine if purchasing practices are effective.

Rebate and contract administration fee report. These reports tally the amount of rebates and contract administration fees generated by the facility's purchases of specific

TABLE 3.
Considerations in Group Purchasing Organization (GPO) Contracting

Fees (e.g., contract administrative fee)
Allowable distribution methods
Payment terms
Return policies
Supplier performance requirements
Rebates
Market-share agreements
Single-agent contracts
GPO services (e.g., lost savings and compliance reports, rebate and contract administration fee reports, clinical utilization management programs)
Letters of commitment

TABLE 4.
Potential Advantages of Group Purchasing Organization Contracts[10,11]

Standardization of products
Reduction of contract labor costs for institutions
Enhancement of member institution's purchasing program
Enhancement of information sharing
Enhancement of purchasing expertise
Protracted periods of price protection
Coordination of contracting and budgeting process
Reduction of duplication of purchasing efforts among institutions
Assistance identifying alternative or secondary products during drug shortage

products under contact. When evaluating the costs of two or more equivalent products, it is important to include any applicable rebates to arrive at net cost.

Clinical utilization management programs. These programs assist facilities in managing the utilization of various drug products and classes, often through evaluation and comparison of product efficacy, safety, and cost, as well as therapeutic interchange programs.

Letters of commitment. Letters of commitment (LOC) available through GPOs should be evaluated and taken advantage of when appropriate. The LOCs usually contain requirements for the pharmacy to do one or more of the following in order to gain lower pricing or rebates:

- Declare that a particular drug is on formulary.
- Declare that a particular drug will be on formulary and will not be restricted.
- Achieve a target periodic volume.
- Achieve a target market share relative to competitive drugs for a given period of time.

The LOC may not require significantly more purchasing of the drug. If LOC requirements do not conflict with formulary and utilization management strategies, the LOC should be signed if there is a reasonable chance of meeting the requirements.

Facility contracts. The alternative to GPO contracting is individual contracting. This type of contracting may be done at the facility or the health-system level. In some cases, equal or better pricing than GPOs can be obtained by individual facilities when contracting, especially large facilities or integrated delivery networks (IDNs). Opportunities for better pricing through individual contracting may exist for specialized health systems (e.g., those focused on oncology or transplantation), that purchase a large volume of a selected drug and are able to commit to maintaining a market share for the drug.

It is important to carefully evaluate the benefits of individual contracting and its influence on the collective bargaining power of the GPO. Continual use of individual contracts that are in contravention to GPO contracts, in theory, will eventually erode the GPO's ability to consistently contract aggressively for its members. Because of larger GPO volume, manufacturers often will not offer the same pricing or other terms to individual facilities or IDNs that they offer to GPOs. Another factor to consider with individual contracting is that a facility may require contracts to be reviewed by attorneys, whereas the GPO acts as the contracting agent of the facility, obviating the need for legal review of each contract by the facility's counsel. Finally, the amount of time required to negotiate, write, and maintain an individual contract should be weighed against the incremental value gained over what a GPO contract would offer. In many situations, it may be more efficient and productive to voice contract concerns to GPO representatives and become involved in GPO committees rather than write multiple, individual contracts outside the GPO.

Some drug contracts, especially for sole-source awards to generic manufacturers, call for the manufacturer to reimburse the pharmacy for the difference in cost when the pharmacy must purchase a product off-contract because the manufacturer was not able to supply the contracted product. The manufacturer-unable-to-supply reimbursement process is time-consuming and the requirements can be rigid, but submitting reimbursement to manufacturers under these provisions can return additional funds to the pharmacy.

Wholesaler own-use contracts. Wholesalers are also able to take advantage of special pricing on certain branded and generic drugs and offer those products to their customers in the wholesaler's proprietary contract portfolio. This creates margin for the wholesalers that can be used to fund distribution discounts. Wholesalers also take advantage of cash discounts and quick-payment terms from manufacturers to increase their margin and to offer discounts to customers.

Generic Drug Savings Maximization. The expiration of patents on widely used branded drugs can result in large reductions in drug expenditures. It is important to be mindful of the opportunities presented by the first-time introduction of generics on high-spend branded drugs, both in budgeting and implementing rapid and effective uptake of generics when they are introduced.

Budgeting. There are several sources for monitoring patent expiration dates (off-patent dates) for branded drugs, including www.drugpatentwatch.com and the GPO. The GPO may also be able to estimate the potential initial savings from contracting for generic drugs that are first-time introductions. It is also important to determine when the first-time generic product will be available from multiple manufacturers. The initial savings differential between the branded and generic versions may be small because a single generic manufacturer often has a period of exclusivity before the generic drug becomes available from multiple sources. In some cases the savings may be so insignificant that health systems will choose to remain with the branded drug for safety reasons and consistency in product supply. Changing products several times within a short period of time could confuse caregivers, so pharmacy managers should weigh the benefits and risks of making such changes.

Operational considerations. Swift uptake of the generic product is necessary to maximize the savings after a branded drug comes off-patent and multiple generic versions are available. The following steps should be taken during any product conversion, but they are particularly important when converting from a brand name product to a first-time generic equivalent product.

- Contracting. Be sure that the health system has access to contract pricing on a generic product on the first date that the drug is available as a multisource item. The contract pricing will usually be through the health system's GPO, but in some cases, the health system may write its own contract for the generic product.
- Contract Price Loading. The contract pricing for the product must be loaded at the wholesaler with enough notice to become effective. Up to 30 days notice may be required before the contract pricing becomes effective through the wholesaler. Although the manufacturer or GPO typically send the contract information to the wholesalers, when the hospital or health system directly contracts for the generic drug, the contract information should be sent directly to the wholesaler by the hospital or health system.
- Demand Matching. Work with the wholesaler to ensure that there will be a sufficient supply of the generic product at the local wholesaler distribution center to match current purchases of the branded product, a process called demand matching. Wholesalers will need at least

30 days notice on demand matching to ensure sufficient stock of the generic product on the off-patent date. Working with the wholesaler on demand matching also improves overall supply chain management by allowing the wholesaler to draw down inventory of products that will be in less demand.

- Autosubstitution. Some wholesalers allow pharmacies to institute autosubstitution rules in the wholesaler ordering system to substitute a preferred generic product for a branded product or non-preferred generic products. This process maximizes savings and contract compliance. Care must be exercised in creating auto-substitution rules to ensure correct product-to-product substitution in chemical entity, dosage form, package size, package form (unit dose, bulk oral, liquid), and so forth, especially in cases in which a brand-name drug goes off-patent. Autosubstitution rules may also be implemented in the wholesaler ordering system for medication safety reasons (e.g., reduction of sound-alike and look-alike drugs) in addition to savings optimization or contract compliance.

Other Considerations. Pharmacy managers should explore whether the hospital can obtain pharmaceuticals at advantageous pricing using 340B (disproportionate share) programs. Because hospitals and health systems must meet specific criteria to be designated as a 340B facility, pharmacy managers should collaborate with the chief financial officer and financial services department to determine if they can access 340B pricing for pharmaceuticals. Detailed descriptions of the qualifications and benefits of 340B programs are also available through the Health Resources and Services Administration Office of Pharmacy Affairs www.hrsa.gov/opa/; the Pharmacy Services Support Center, pssc.aphanet.org/; the Safety Net Hospitals for Pharmaceutical Access, safetynetrx .org; and ASHP 340B Information Site www.ashp.org/s_ashp/cat1c.asp?CID=3813&DID=6225.

Pharmaceutical manufacturers also continue to offer indigent patient care programs for select drugs for qualified patients on an individual basis. Although substantial savings can be realized through replacement drugs at no charge, the process can be arduous and complex. There are independent consulting services that specialize in assisting with coordination of the program for hospitals and typically require payment as a percentage of the savings. Patients eligible for Medicaid and other regional or local low-income health insurance do not usually qualify for the indigent care programs sponsored by the pharmaceutical industry.

Wholesalers and Distribution Fees. Most hospital pharmacies purchase 80% or more (by dollar volume) of their pharmaceutical needs from a drug distributor (wholesaler). Hospital pharmacies can lower their costs by ensuring that the distribution fee mark-up is as low as possible. To understand the cost that wholesalers charge for drugs, and the distribution fee charged to hospital pharmacies, it is necessary to understand wholesalers' revenue streams and expense drivers.

The adoption of the prime-vendor system, in which a pharmacy procures a very large portion of its pharmaceutical needs from one supplier, has led to great efficiencies in the pharmaceutical supply chain. Through these efficiencies, wholesalers are able to offer low incremental fees to their customers for distribution of pharmaceuticals. In many cases, they are able to offer discounts to the contracted price of the drug or "cost-minus" discounts to the wholesale acquisition cost of the drug if it is not contracted.

Through automated inventory, stock replacement, and order fulfillment, wholesalers have streamlined the delivery process and lowered pharmaceutical costs in the supply chain. In the past, wholesalers increased their margins through speculative buying, which is buying pharmaceuticals in large quantities and holding them past the date of future manufacturer price increases. The products would then be sold to customers at the higher price. These practices have reportedly decreased since 2004.[12] However, at the same time that speculative buying decreased, the wholesale drug industry instituted inventory management agreements with manufacturers, who in return for agreements regarding product supply and demand, pay the wholesalers a negotiated fee based on the percentage of the volume that the wholesalers purchase from them. These methods of creating margin through increasing revenue and decreasing expenses can be translated into a cost-minus fee structure for the hospital that is purchasing from the wholesalers.

Individual hospital factors that influence wholesaler fee structure. Several characteristics of individual hospital-pharmacy purchasing can affect a wholesaler's revenue and expenses and result in higher or lower distribution fees. To some degree, a higher purchasing volume results in a lower distribution fee. However, other factors, including deliveries per week, dollars per drop, dollars per line extension, numbers of delivery sites per location, payment terms, and special services, must also be considered. These factors should be considered collectively and not in isolation. In addition, most major wholesalers have supply, automation, and other service and equipment divisions, and an institutional contract with multiple divisions can provide additional savings.

Deliveries per week. The fewer deliveries from the wholesaler per week, the lower the expenses for the wholesaler, which can reduce the wholesaler distribution fee to the pharmacy. Some large hospitals have up to 11 deliveries per week, but other large hospitals are able to manage inventory so that patient care can be well-maintained with only 5. Inventory and patient care can be well maintained at less than five deliveries per week at small hospitals. Fewer deliveries may require additional purchasing discipline, but some wholesalers have programs to help pharmacies improve their purchasing practices.

Dollars per drop. This factor is important to wholesalers because the higher the number of delivery locations (drops), the higher the wholesalers' cost, and vice versa. For a given dollar value of pharmaceuticals purchased, a wholesaler's expenses are lower, and margin is higher, for a lower number of delivery points. This margin can be translated into lower distribution fees for the pharmacies, particularly for IDNs of multiple pharmacies.

Dollars per line extension. For each line of products on an invoice that a wholesaler fills and delivers to a pharmacy, there is an associated cost. The dollars per line extension is the total dollars purchased by a pharmacy over a given period of time divided by the number of lines of products ordered over the same period of time. Pharmacies with higher dollars per line extension purchased can sometimes have lower distribution costs than pharmacies with lower dollars per line extension because it costs relatively less for the wholesaler to service the pharmacy with the higher dollars per line extension.

Secondary wholesalers. Secondary wholesaler relationships should be avoided if inventory levels meet patient care needs. Purchases from secondary wholesalers usually carry a much higher distribution fee. Such purchases also result in a higher primary wholesaler distribution fee because there are decreases for the pharmacy in its dollars per drop, dollars per line extension, and total volume. Wholesalers are increasingly requiring pharmacies to meet a minimum monthly volume to maintain an account, and the costs of maintaining the minimum volume at a significantly higher distribution fee can be prohibitive.

Expanding the use of the wholesaler within the health system may offer additional opportunities for cost savings. Hospital departments such as radiology, the clinical laboratory, interventional cardiology, and anesthesiology may procure pharmaceuticals directly from the manufacturer through the purchasing or materials management departments. Utilizing the pharmaceutical wholesaler for these products through a separate purchasing account does not change the process of procurement or distribution but reduces the unit cost through application of the wholesaler discount. Because some of these products may be relatively costly (e.g., contrast agents, blood factors, or anesthetic gases), there is a potential for additional savings if these purchases push the hospital into a higher tier of the wholesaler cost structure. Pharmacy directors should communicate with other department managers to determine how pharmaceuticals are purchased, and it is usually best if all drug purchases are managed by the pharmacy.

Payment method and frequency. Payment method and frequency can also affect the distribution fee. Many wholesalers offer a lower distribution fee to hospitals that pay by electronic fund transfer (EFT). Pharmacy managers should work with their accounts-payable departments to establish EFT, which is usually a more efficient method of payment for both the hospital and the wholesaler. In addition, the more frequent the payment, the lower the wholesaler distribution fee will generally be. Since 2004, the amount of speculative buying has waned and large discounts for more frequent payments have decreased. However, many wholesalers offer terms based on prepayment, or placing funds on deposit with the wholesaler, and then paying invoices on a go-forward basis. The advantage in lower distribution fee is clear, but this gain must be balanced against the time value of money for having the funds on deposit with the wholesaler rather than drawing a return for the health system.

Most GPOs have wholesaler-distribution agreements for use by their members. However, because of higher-than-average dollars per drop, dollars per line extension, and discipline in number of deliveries per week, large hospitals and health systems can often get better pricing and terms by dealing directly with wholesalers rather than through GPO wholesaler agreements.

Other wholesaler tools. Most wholesalers provide pharmacies with access to computer software or Web-based solutions for product ordering, reporting, and inventory management. The programs will allow the buyer to check for lower-priced alternatives and contract compliance prior to placing orders. Pharmacy managers should work with their wholesaler representatives to be sure that these features are available and utilized.

Some wholesalers produce contract compliance reports. These reports can be used to gauge the effectiveness of purchasing practices. Pharmacy managers should check with their wholesalers to determine if these reports are available. If they are, they should be reviewed monthly for opportunities to improve contract purchasing.

Some wholesalers have automatic substitution programs to assist pharmacy buyers in selecting the correct product when multiple generic alternatives exist. These programs allow the pharmacy manager to direct purchases of less-preferred products (as determined by the pharmacy management) to more-preferred items. For example, if one brand of unit dose acetaminophen 325-mg tablet is on contract as a sole-source award, the autosubstitution program can allow for inadvertent orders for noncontract unit dose acetaminophen 325-mg tablets to be substituted with the preferred version. Such programs may not be available from all wholesalers, and they should receive careful consideration before being implemented.

Inventory Management. Inventory management is a balancing act. It involves meeting patient and internal customer needs while committing the least amount of dollars possible to drugs on the shelves or in automated cabinets. The rate of inventory turnover (defined as total annual drug expenses divided by the dollar value of the inventory assessed on an annual basis) is dependent on many factors. Typically, the pharmacies of smaller hospitals will have a lower drug inventory turnover (8–10 turns per year) than the pharmacies of larger hospitals (12–18 turns per year or higher) and some specialty hospitals.

Many wholesalers' ordering programs provide systematic methods for asset management (i.e., inventory value optimization and increasing turnover). Wholesaler representatives can assist in the initial setup of these programs. Inventory items should be divided into high-, medium-, and low-value products, and the minimum and maximum inventory levels for at least the high- and medium-value products should be established. At the same time, reorder points and reorder quantities should be established for at least the high- and medium-value products. Systematic use of these programs can decrease the time required for the ordering process and increase inventory turns. The minimum and maximum levels, as well as the reorder points and reorder quantities, should be reviewed on a routine schedule and revised when necessary.

When seeking to increase inventory turns, storage in the central pharmacy and automated dispensing cabinets should also be considered. Configuring pharmacy storage locations so that each drug product has only one storage location in the central pharmacy sometimes helps to free capital by reducing inventory. Automated cabinet inventories should be regularly reviewed for appropriate turnover. Most cabinet systems have report capabilities to optimize both the products and the quantities that should be in a particular cabinet based on the dispensing philosophy devised by pharmacy and nursing departments. Cabinet manufacturers have product specialists that consult with pharmacy management to optimize use of the cabinets.

I.V. product waste. Many pharmacies waste a significant quantity of drugs, particularly unused IV solutions, and many do not have an accurate valuation of the amount of

TABLE 5.
Strategies for Reducing I.V. Product Waste

Establish policies that are based on the most recent literature for maximum i.v. bag hang-times and i.v. set change frequency.
Institute an i.v.-to-oral switch program for both cost reduction and patient care benefits.
Periodically audit the amount of i.v. admixtures being wasted and log the date and time of waste, date and time of preparation, the i.v. fluid type and drug admixed, quantity of products, and the cost of the products. Review the log and determine the most common occurrences.
Reduce i.v. batch sizes (creating more, smaller batches) and reduce the amount of time between preparation of the i.v. dose and the actual administration time.
Routinely monitor the status of i.v. drips that are adjusted.
Routinely return all unused i.v. admixtures to the i.v. preparation area as soon as possible.
Consider the use of manufacturer premixed products where advantageous, both economically and for patient care.
Compare the quality, economic, and regulatory (e.g., *USP* chapter 797) differences within your practice site between different administration methods such as i.v. syringe infusion, i.v. intermittent infusion (i.v. piggyback), and volumetric drip chambers.
Establish standard concentrations, dosages, and base solutions for i.v. admixtures.
Ensure that there is an efficient process for communicating changes in i.v. admixtures (e.g., rate, fluid, dosage) or discontinuation.
Reduce total parenteral nutrition use by employing enteral nutrition when possible, and establish standardized total parenteral nutrient base solutions, hang times, and related policies and procedures.

waste because it is only sporadically monitored. **Table 5** lists strategies for reduction of IV product waste.

Returns. Most pharmacies use a third party (reverse distributors or returns companies) to process wasted and expired drugs. However, not all pharmacies completely track and trend the drugs that are most commonly wasted, the dollar value of the expired and wasted drugs, or whether credits were received. The pharmacy manager and pharmacy buyer should work together to utilize reports from the reverse distributor to determine the opportunities for reducing the amount of expired and wasted drugs and insuring that all credits due to the pharmacy from the manufacturers are received.

Medication Utilization Management

Planning and Developing a Medication Utilization Management Program. An effective plan for medication utilization management must provide the health system with a road map for continuous improvement in pharmaceutical expense management, with specific goals and outcome measures of success. It is important to acknowledge that although one purpose of medication-utilization-management is to add economic value, the quality and safety of patient care are foremost in the mission of pharmacy services and should never be compromised for cost. Medication-utilization-management must integrate evidence-based science with the standards of medical practice within the health system.

Before embarking on a comprehensive medication-utilization-management plan, goals must be established, a reporting structure delineated, roles identified, measurement tools developed, and implementation procedures established. The successful plan is dependent on many levels of commitment, including commitment to administrative and clinical pharmacy management, the medical staff, and senior health-system management. The director of pharmacy provides leadership by facilitating the efforts of the medical staff, setting priorities for the clinical pharmacy staff, and cultivating the support of senior leadership. Clinical pharmacists with advanced training and education must have dedicated time to develop and implement the cost management initiatives. They must also be empowered to monitor the program and educate other staff to participate in therapeutic interchange, medication utilization review, and other interventions while encouraging the infusion of fresh ideas for pharmaceutical cost management.

Role of Clinical Pharmacy Services in Drug Cost Management. Clinical pharmacy services, activities in which pharmacists provide direct patient care, are an important foundation for a successful medication-utilization-management program that is focused on managing drug costs. Clinical pharmacy services have demonstrated an overall positive financial impact. In a systematic review of original assessments of clinical pharmacy services from 1988 to 1995, Schumock et al.[13] reported that 89% of 104 studies reviewed reported positive financial results. In the seven studies of clinical pharmacy services where sufficient information was available to calculate a benefit-to-cost ratio, the median benefit-to-cost ratio was 4.09:1. Therefore, in these studies, every dollar invested in clinical pharmacy services returned four dollars. The systematic review was updated in 2003 to review published assessments of clinical pharmacy services from 1995 to 2000, and once again, the value of clinical pharmacy services was demonstrated.[14] For this five-year period, benefit-to-cost ratios could be determined from 16 studies, and when these studies were combined, the median benefit:cost ratio was 4.68:1.

Some specific types of clinical pharmacy services have also been associated with decreased drug costs. Bond et al.[15] have used an extensive database of the outcomes of clinical pharmacy services to show that drug information services, medication admission histories, and drug protocol management are associated with lower drug costs.

In addition, clinical pharmacists' active involvement is crucial to the success of many drug-cost-management ini-tiatives. Many of the drug-cost-containment techniques can only be successful with diligent and often daily support from clinical pharmacists. For example, successful implementation of a clinical practice guideline as a drug-cost-management technique will require the expertise of the department's clinical pharmacists to develop the guideline, and will also require the pharmacy staff's consistent enforcement of the guideline in their interactions with prescribers. Similarly, it will often be the clinical pharmacist's responsibility to routinely carry out the hospital's therapeutic interchange policies.

Assessment of Drug Costs

A successful pharmaceutical-cost-management program must be data driven. GPOs, wholesalers, distributors, pharmaceutical manufacturers, and supply-chain divisions of multi-hospital systems need to track costs in a variety of ways. Advances in information technology have made drug usage data more accessible and sophisticated, and effort should be spent to manage and analyze these data. Pharmacy management must also take advantage of the data available in its own facility through the materials management department, purchasing department, and finance department. Internal and external data sources are the foundation for the decision-making process for medication-utilization-management and must be examined closely prior to setting goals for cost-management initiatives.

Because each health system has a unique mix of patients, services, and centers of excellence, the drug-cost-assessment process must be customized to create a priority list of initiatives that will provide the greatest value. Key reports that should be considered are listed in **Table 6**. Once the formulas for denominator data are established as consistent across many facilities, a multihospital health system can effectively benchmark drug costs.

Medical Staff Support. Any program that involves altering prescribing patterns to improve the cost-effectiveness of drug therapy requires the support and engagement of the medical staff. Although health systems have the ability to negotiate discounted unit prices for pharmaceuticals, the efforts of the GPOs and the increased availability of generics have leveled the expense of many high-cost drug products used in hospitals. Cost-management programs have therefore become increasingly dependent on the hospital's ability to manage utilization and prescribing, which will ultimately influence market share and drug pricing. Several effective strategies that can harness physician knowledge, cultivate a collaborative relationship, and facilitate ownership of the process by the medical staff are described in **Table 7**.

Once the medical staff is engaged and there is a commitment from senior management for the medication-utilization-management program, a detailed procedure for initiative generation can be established. Key steps include the following:

- Designating clinical sub-groups based on categories of the initiatives.
- Identifying the lead physicians, clinical pharmacists, and other key practitioners for each group.
- Using evidence-based studies and the drug assessment data to make decisions.
- Defining the types and categories of the initiatives.
- Creating a dashboard and a clear and concise reporting format for communicating progress.
- Facilitating the infusion of ideas through brainstorming and other effective meeting and group techniques.
- Defining measurable outcomes and benchmarks for evaluation.

TABLE 6.
Key Reports to Consider in Assessing Drug Costs

Report	Considerations
Wholesaler purchasing reports	For 80/20 analysis, by therapeutic class, and of top 200 drugs; drugs with multiple strengths and sizes need to be aggregated; wholesalers can also provide monthly trending reports and benchmarks from their customers.
Direct (nonwholesaler) purchase reports	Available from the purchasing or finance departments.
Interdepartmental purchasing reports	Available from materials management or other departments that have internal transfers.
Cost (total drug costs or specific drugs) per medical service or hospital area	Drug-utilization data will be needed to produce this report.
Cost per drug-related group reports	Available from internal sources (ideally) or fee-based external vendors; distinction must be made between using cost or charge data.
Cost per occupied bed, adjusted patient day, admission, discharge, or case mix index adjusted patient day	Adjusted patient days are calculated with a standard financial formula that modifies patient days with a ratio of outpatient to inpatient revenue to correct for volume changes and severity of illness.[16] External and internal benchmarking is dependent on these kinds of reports.
Pharmacy-adjusted patient days	Calculated using the same ratio of outpatient to inpatient revenue but for drugs only, and may also add specificity and value to comparative data.
Cost per case, procedure, or admission (e.g., surgical case, cardiac procedure, dialysis admission)	These are important based on the patient mix and the drugs that comprise the greatest costs within the health system. Physician participation in the dissemination of the data is essential.

Formulary Management. The guiding principles of a sound formulary management system are well described in two documents,[17,18] and are concisely summarized in the following statement: a well-managed formulary system ensures a close relationship between the organization's medication-use policies, the therapies offered by the organization, and the medication routinely stocked by the pharmacy.[18] Although the primary goal of a formulary system is to promote safe and effective drug therapy, it can be a valuable cost management tool and has inherent medical staff support through the actions of the pharmacy and therapeutics (P&T) committee. The medication-utilization-management program is highly dependent on an effective formulary system. Key aspects of formulary management in cost-management efforts are described in **Table 8**. Once again, the efforts of clinical pharmacists are crucial to successful implementation of the formulary system.

Methods of Pharmaceutical Cost Management. Pharmaceutical cost-management initiatives are typically categorized by therapeutic class or

TABLE 7.
Strategies to Involve Medical Staff in Cost-Management Efforts

- Enlist the pharmacy and therapeutic (P&T) committee to review medication-utilization management issues as a standing agenda item.
- Identify the centers of excellence and work with individual chiefs of service to gain support.
- Meet with key medical staff departments and divisions, including infectious diseases, anesthesiology, cardiology, and oncology, as well as intensivists, hospitalists, and interventionalists as appropriate.
- Develop prescriber reports on the targeted high-cost drugs and discuss methods for cost reduction.
- Provide continuous feedback to the P&T committee and individual departments and divisions on cost management successes.
- Provide hospitalwide expenditure data on the top 50 items to the P&T committee.
- Utilize evidence-based research to propose changes in medication utilization.
- Identify physician champions for specific initiatives.
- Create a consistent procedure for developing prescribing guidelines, protocols, care paths, and preprinted orders.

TABLE 8.
Key Aspects of Formulary Management in Cost-Management Efforts

- Policy for formulary drug addition and deletion through evidence-based product selection, including efficacy, safety, and pharmacoeconomic assessments
- Policy for the use and monitoring of non-formulary medications
- Policy for medication-use evaluation
- Limitation on combination, sustained-release, and long-acting products
- Policy for therapeutic interchange and prescribing guidelines
- Reduction of drugs in the same therapeutic group or class
- Periodic house cleaning to reduce under-used and discontinued line items
- Policy for drug restriction
- Procedure for consistently monitoring the use of new agents particularly if there are specific guidelines for use
- System to provide the formulary electronically with timely updated information
- Off-label or ad hoc use of medications
- Restricted use (by indication, prescriber, patient care area, patient)
- Dose adjustment or discontinuation based on clinical triggers or end points
- Injectable to oral conversion
- Therapeutic equivalence

group or by method of implementa-tion. The latter is usually subdivided into three or four different types: therapeutic interchange (therapeutic substitution), guideline (protocol) development, and pharmacist interventions (clinical and operational), such as parenteral-to-oral conversions, renal-dose adjustments, drug restrictions, repackaging, dosage-form changes, waste reduction, and others. Although the terms are sometimes used interchangeably, therapeutic group refers to a broad classification (e.g., anesthetic agents, anti-infectives, or chemotherapeutic agents), whereas therapeutic class is a narrower designation (e.g., beta-lactam antibiotics, volatile anesthetic gases, serotonin antagonists). If the decision is made to use therapeutic class, then each of the methods of implementation are used as appropriate within the medication categories. An example would be selecting third-generation cephalosporins utilizing a therapeutic interchange for cefotaxime and ceftriaxone (therapeutic interchange method). Third-generation cephalosporins may also be the preferred class of antibiotics within a pneumonia protocol (guidelines method). Examples of using the implementation method rather than the therapeutic class would be to select several drug classes for therapeutic interchange, some for guideline development, and some for other intervention types.

Therapeutic interchange. ASHP defines therapeutic interchange (TI) as "an authorized exchange of therapeutic alternatives in accordance with previously established and approved written guidelines or protocols within a formulary system."[17] This definition stipulates that the interchange is between two or more drugs that are not generic equivalents. Although FDA defines the term *therapeutic equivalent* to include generically equivalent products, therapeutic interchange or substitution in the hospital setting generally refers to drugs that are not generically identical.

The American College of Clinical Pharmacy (ACCP) Guidelines for Therapeutic Interchange[19] contain a more re-cent definition of TI:

> Therapeutic interchange is defined as the dispensing of a drug that is therapeutically equivalent to but chemically different from the drug originally prescribed. Although usually of the same pharmacological class, drugs appropriate for therapeutic interchange may differ in chemistry or pharmacokinetic properties, and may possess different mechanism of action, adverse-reaction, toxicity, and drug interaction profiles. In most cases, the interchanged drugs have close similarity in efficacy and safety profiles.

The ACCP guidelines also describe a comprehensive five-part process for health-system TI implementation, with an emphasis on patient safety; an extensive review of drug classes appropriate for therapeutic interchange, including specific evidence-based examples; discussion of legal and regulatory issues; viewpoints of other professional organizations, including the American Medical Association, the American College of Physicians, and the Pharmaceutical Research and Manufacturers of America; and medical and pharmaceutical literature references.

The health system, through the action of the P&T committee, must decide on the general policy for a TI program, particularly regarding the authority and autonomy of the pharmacy staff. The committee may define TI as an automatic conversion by the pharmacist, may require contact with the prescriber before the change can occur, or may employ a combination of both. The prescriber may be informed orally before the drug is dispensed or through written communication in the medical record. Most commonly, TI implies pharmacist autonomy once the P&T committee has sanctioned the policy, but there may be exceptions based on the level of clinical judgment required. A survey of the prevalence of TI conducted in 2002 revealed that the vast majority (88%) of hospitals use TI programs, and most of those did not require the pharmacist to contact the prescriber before making the conversion.[20]

Categories of drugs that offer modest savings with minimal challenge include various non-prescription groups, such as antacids, vitamins, nonsteroidal antiinflammatory drugs, topical products, and cold and cough remedies. To make significant gains in pharmaceutical cost savings, the health system must consider the drug classes that comprise the greatest proportion of drug expenditures, such as colony-stimulating factors, antiinfectives, cardiac agents, and drugs used in critical care settings. An abundance of literature supports the success of TI programs, both in terms of quality patient outcomes and economic benefit. Based on the literature, therapeutic classes offering the most opportunity for success with the medical staff, as well as significant cost savings, include histamine-2 antagonists, fluoroquinolones, hydroxymethylglutaryl–coenzyme A reductase inhibitors, serotonin antagonists, colony-stimulating factors, low molecular weight heparins, and proton pump inhibitors.[20–27] Although it is not the intent of these guidelines to delineate an exhaustive list of all potential TI opportunities, the appendix contains examples of the TIs that have proven successful.

Most of the evaluative studies on TI initiatives focus on the economic value and quality improvement related to standardization and formulary management. As the popularity of TI programs increases in the acute care, managed care, and ambulatory settings, an associated risk may also increase due to substitutions along the continuum of care and patient confusion regarding drug classes and duplicative therapy.[28,29] The Joint Commission standard requiring medication reconciliation can be partially traced to anecdotal reports of the potential for medication errors as a result of TI programs in various health care settings.[29] Pharmacists can play a vital role in supporting medication-reconciliation activities through medication history assessments and discharge counseling.[30,31]

Guidelines. A variety of terms are used to describe these tools, including prescribing guidelines, therapeutic position statements, therapeutic guidelines, clinical practice guidelines, protocols, or pathways. There may be subtle differences beween these tools, but they all seek to enhance patient safety, reduce variation in medical practice, and increase standardization.

Guidelines can focus on a disease state, a thera-peutic class, or a specific drug.[32] Published guidelines are available for many drugs and drug classes.[33,34] The Agency for Health Care Research and Quality maintains an extensive online collection of published guidelines at www.guideline.gov. A 2004 ASHP survey found that 83% of U.S. hospitals use guidelines that include medications.[35] Successful implementation of such general guidelines often requires customization to meet the needs of individual health systems, however. For example, local guidelines should be developed that reflect the best available evidence, incorporate the opinions of local prescriber experts when necessary, and are applicable within the context of the individual health system.

Guidelines are also an important step leading to rules-based computerized prescriber order entry (CPOE), which is recommended by NQF in its 2006 Safe Practices.[36] CPOE facilitates guideline adherence during the ordering process.

Steps to implementing an effective pharmaceutical cost-containment program using drug-specific or drug class guidelines mirror those for TI and include:

- Utilization of evidence-based criteria.
- Adoption of published, evidence-based, and peer-reviewed guidelines from national organizations.
- Solicitation of thought leaders and clinical experts (e.g., physician specialists, chiefs of service, chief medical officers).
- Review and approval of the P&T committee.
- Education of clinical staff.
- Ongoing support from front line clinical pharmacist staff.
- Use of quantifiable measures.
- Utilization of medication-use evaluation (MUE) to determine compliance.

The last step is an important distinction between TI and guidelines because what is approved by the medical staff and what is done in practice may differ. Conducting periodic MUEs with the approved criteria can determine the thoroughness and consistency of the guidelines and ultimately the success of this component of cost management. It should also be emphasized that although guidelines can be used to reduce drug costs, improving quality of care may require more spending rather than less.

When guidelines reduce inappropriate prescribing, drug costs will also be reduced. Due to the complex uses of some drugs and drug classes, such as low-molecular-weight heparins, guidelines may be more practical and effective in managing drug costs than TI and other approaches.[37] Drotrecogin alfa was one costly agent for which guidelines became the standard of care in most acute care settings.[38–40] Other successful guideline efforts have been demonstrated with a number of drugs and drug classes, such as third-generation cephalosporins,[41] statins,[42] antifungals,[43,44] albumin,[45] and serotonin-receptor antagonists.[46] Drug shortages can also be an impetus for the development and implementation of guidelines, as was the case with the use of parenteral pantoprazole, which may be used inappropriately and at a much higher cost in place of histamine-2 antagonists for stress ulcer prophylaxis.[47] Although volatile anesthetic agents are often a top-20 item in the pharmaceutical budget and offer a unique challenge for guidelines or TI implementation, accurate evaluation of cost savings can be accomplished by using the hourly cost to maintain a minimum alveolar concentration.[48]

Implementation of Medication Utilization Management Initiatives. Careful thought and attention to the implementation is required to successfully influence drug expenditures through medication utilization initiatives, and multifaceted interventions are often necessary. The active involvement and support of clinical pharmacists and the medical staff are crucial to effective implementation of these initiatives. It is necessary to seek out ways to integrate or hard-wire initiatives such as guidelines and TI into the care provided at the bedside. For example, passive guideline dissemination (e.g., simply posting to the hospital's intranet site) is rarely successful. Protocols, order sets, and pathways that reflect the evidence in the guideline should be used to integrate the guideline into daily patient care. The growing use of CPOE systems and other technologies can also be leveraged to implement medication-utilization-management endeavors. CPOE can be used to guide prescribing in such straightforward ways as leading prescribers to select formulary products or recommended dosing frequencies.[49] CPOE can also promote efficient medication use through more complex scenarios such as prompting therapeutic interchanges or requiring prescribers to follow interactive prescribing guidelines. For example, one institution established guidelines for activated protein C use and utilized an interactive computer order entry algorithm to implement the guideline.[50]

Data Analysis. To ensure the validity of the medication-utilization-management program, regardless of the method of implementation, the estimated and actual cost savings calculations must be grounded in accurate and consistent data analysis. Unfortunately, there is no standard regarding a method to determine the pharmaceutical cost savings with programs such as TI. Hospitals have struggled for years to balance practical considerations while striving for accuracy and completeness.[20] Hospitals have to decide early in the process whether to consider indirect costs such as devices and other non-pharmaceuticals, price changes during the review period, general drug price inflation, volume changes, and labor costs.

Equivalent doses for all drug alternatives for each TI must be established based on scientific evidence and current practice standards, which may not be the same as FDA-approved manufacturers' recommendations. Most of the references cited for TI above list the therapeutic equivalence for the drugs in a specific class. *Days of therapy* is the common method to compare equivalent costs of drug therapy within a therapeutic class, particularly for antibiotics and other classes that include scheduled drugs that are dosed multiple times per day. For classes that include drugs with extended half-lives and durations of action, weeks of therapy or cost per course of therapy may be more appropriate. Examples include colony-stimulating factors (e.g., epoetin versus darbopoetin and filgrastim versus pegfilgrastim). Correcting for equivalent strengths, sizes, and units of packaging is another important step in cost-savings calculations, particularly for liquid and parenteral products. The number of standard doses available from a container of liquid medication or a large volume parenteral medication varies based on the size of the container. Medical staff input is important in determining equivalent doses, particularly if there is a divergence between manufacturer's recommendations and published literature on dosing.

Once the methodology of data analysis is established, a drug savings matrix should be developed. This becomes the primary monitoring document that tracks the progress of each initiative based on the changes in utilization. Purchase data is the typical source for maintaining the cost savings matrix, but it is essential to adjust and scrub the data before matrix input. It is important to maintain a consistent common denominator. Utilization increases in certain targeted drugs may be due to patient volume and may be appropriate. Correcting for volume with denominator data and using effective MUE programs will assist with determining actual cost increases. The elements of a standard drug-savings matrix spreadsheet include the initiatives (TI and guidelines), savings targets, baseline purchase dollars corrected for volume, current purchase dollars (after implementation) corrected for volume, and actual savings monthly and year-to-date. It is important to be accurate and include both wholesaler and direct purchases, rebates, and wholesaler discounts.

To maintain commitment to and focus on the process, it is paramount to provide consistent feedback regarding the changes in the cost savings matrix to the P & T committee. Some health systems also establish a reporting structure to another oversight committee, such as a value analysis group or similar body that has overall responsibility for non-labor cost management.

Conclusion

Medication costs continue to rise and will continue to be a target for cost management. Drug costs make up a majority of health-system pharmacy budgets, and budgeting for these expenses is an important function, but longer-term programmatic and policy planning is also essential for successful cost management. An effective plan for medication utilization management must provide the health system with a road map for continuous improvement in pharmaceutical expense containment with specific goals and outcome measures of success. Gathering the data to understand drug expenditures and drug-use patterns is a prerequisite for cost-savings efforts, and constant vigilance and monitoring of these data are required.

A relatively small number of drugs usually makes up the majority of the drug budget. Cost-management efforts focused on these drugs will generally offer the best return. Cost-management strategies that fall completely under the pharmacy department's control (e.g., purchasing and inventory strategies) will be easiest to implement and should be pursued first. Strategies that require an interdisciplinary effort (e.g., use of protocols or guidelines, therapeutic interchange, IV-to-PO switches) can be led by pharmacists with the proper clinical background. Clinical pharmacy services, such as participation in rounds, pharmacokinetic monitoring, and renal dose adjustment, can also reduce drug expenses.

Cost management efforts should be coordinated. The programs should contain a clearly defined and manageable list of cost containment targets with a goal and specific targets for each initiative. Results should be measured and evaluated, and this information should be shared with the interdisciplinary team involved in the effort as well as with health-system administration.

When selecting and implementing drug-cost-management strategies, pharmacists must keep patient safety and the quality of patient care in mind. Cost-management initiatives must never compromise the pharmacy department's ability to provide the best possible care. Fortunately, there are many drug-cost-management opportunities that have little or no potential for detrimental effects on patient care, and efforts to improve appropriate use of a drug or drug class often also offer opportunities for cost containment.

References

1. Hoffman JM, Shah ND, Vermeulen LC, et al. Projecting future drug expenditures—2006. *Am J Health-Syst Pharm.* 2006; 63:123–38.
2. Vogenberg FR, ed. Understanding pharmacy reimbursement. Bethesda, MD: American Society of Health-System Pharmacists; 2005:17–42.
3. ASHP Practice Resource Center for Pharmaceutical Reimbursement. www.ashp.org/s_ashp/cat1c.asp?CID=490&DID=532 (accessed 2007 Sep 10).
4. Clinical Initiative Center interviews. The Advisory Board Company. Washington, DC 2000:20–1.

5. Hoffman JM, Shah ND, Vermeulen LC, et al. Projecting future drug expenditures—2007. *Am J Health-Syst Pharm.* 2007; 64:298–314.
6. Hoffman JM, Shah ND, Vermeulen LC, et al. Projecting future drug expenditures 2004. *Am J Health-Syst Pharm.* 2004; 61:145–58.
7. Hoffman JM, Shah ND, Vermeulen LC, et al. Projecting future drug expenditures 2005. *Am J Health-Syst Pharm.* 2005; 62:149–67.
8. Heffler S, Smith S, Keehan S, et al. U.S. health spending projections for 2004–2014. *Health Aff (Millwood).* 2005; W5:74-WS-85.
9. Rough S, Saenz R. Benchmarking and productivity monitoring: practical strategies for pharmacy managers. www.ashp.org/s_ashp/docs/files/2004 LeadershipSummary.pdf (accessed 2007 Sep 10).
10. May BE, Herrick JD. Evaluation of drug-procurement alternatives. *Am J Hosp Pharm.* 1984; 41:1373–8.
11. Wetrich JG. Group purchasing: an overview. *Am J Hosp Pharm.* 1987; 44:1581–92.
12. Yost RD. New economics of the pharmaceutical supply chain. *Am J Health-Syst Pharm.* 2005; 62:525–6.
13. Schumock GT, Meek PD, Ploetz PA, et al. Economic evaluations of clinical pharmacy services—1988–1995. *Pharmacotherapy.* 1996; 16:1188–208.
14. Schumock GT, Butler MG, Meek PD, et al. Evidence of the economic benefit of clinical pharmacy services: 1996–2000. *Pharmacotherapy.* 2003; 23:113–32.
15. Bond CA, Raehl CL, Patry RL. Evidence-based core clinical pharmacy services in United States hospitals in 2020: services and staffing. *Pharmacotherapy.* 2004; 24:427–40.
16. Bond CA, Raehl CL. Clinical and economic outcomes of pharmacist-managed aminoglycoside or vancomycin therapy. *Am J Health-Syst Pharm.* 2005; 62:1596–605.
17. Coalition Working Group. Principles of a sound drug formulary system. In: Hawkins BH, ed. Best practices for hospital & health-system pharmacy. Bethesda, MD: American Society of Health-System Pharmacists; 2005:125–8.
18. American Society of Hospital Pharmacists. ASHP guidelines on formulary system management. *Am J Hosp Pharm.* 1992; 49:648–52.
19. Gray T, Bertch K, Galt K, et al. Guidelines for therapeutic interchange - 2004. *Pharmacotherapy.* 2005; 25:1666–80.
20. Schachtner JM, Guharoy R, Medicis JJ, et al. Prevalence and cost savings of therapeutic interchange among U.S. hospitals. *Am J Health-Syst Pharm.* 2002; 59:529–33.
21. Goldwater SH, Milkovich G, Morrison AJ Jr, et al. Comparison of therapeutic interchange with standard educational tools for influencing fluoroquinolone prescribing. *Am J Health-Syst Pharm.* 2001; 58:1740–5.
22. Grace KA, Swiecki J, Hyatt R, et al. Implementation of a therapeutic-interchange clinic for HMG-CoA reductase inhibitors. *Am J Health-Syst Pharm.* 2002; 59:1077–82.
23. Steiner MA, Yorgason RZ, Vermeulen LC, et al. Patient outcomes after therapeutic interchange of dolasetron for granisetron. *Am J Health-Syst Pharm.* 2003; 60: 1023–8.
24. Stull DM, Bilmes R, Kim H, et al. Comparison of sargramostim and filgrastim in the treatment of chemotherapy-induced neutropenia. *Am J Health-Syst Pharm.* 2005; 62:83–7.
25. Bollinger KA, Vermeulen LC, Davis SN, et al. Comparative effectiveness of low-molecular-weight heparins after therapeutic interchange. *Am J Health-Syst Pharm.* 2000; 57:368–72.
26. Nelson WW, Vermeulen LC, Geurkink EA, et al. Clinical and humanistic outcomes in patients with gastroesophageal reflux disease converted from ome-prazole to lansoprazole. *Arch Intern Med.* 2000; 160:2491–6.
27. Sodorff MM, Galt KA, Galt MA, et al. Patient perceptions of a proton pump inhibitor therapeutic interchange program across the continuum of care. *Pharmacotherapy.* 2002; 22:500–12.
28. Carroll NV. Formularies and therapeutic interchange: the health care setting makes a difference. *Am J Health-Syst Pharm.* 1999; 56:467–72.
29. Rodehaver C, Fearing D. Medication reconciliation in acute care: ensuring an accurate drug regimen on admission and discharge. *Jt Comm J Qual Patient Saf.* 2005; 31:406–13.
30. Gleason KM, Groszek JM, Sullivan C, et al. Reconciliation of discrepancies in medication histories and admission orders of newly hospitalized patients. *Am J Health-Syst Pharm.* 2004; 61:1689–95.
31. Saunders SM, Tierney JA, Forde JM, et al. Implementing a pharmacist-provided discharge counseling service. *Am J Health-Syst Pharm.* 2003; 60:1101,6,9.
32. American Society of Health-System Pharmacists. ASHP guidelines on the pharmacist's role in the development, implementation, and assessment of critical pathways. *Am J Health-Syst Pharm.* 2004; 61:939–45.
33. American Society of Health-System Pharmacists therapeutic position statements. www.ashp.org/s_ashp /cat1c.asp?CID=516&DID=558 (accessed 2007 Sep 10).
34. American Society of Health-System Pharmacists therapeutic guidelines. www.ashp.org/s_ashp/cat1c. asp?CID=516&DID=559 (accessed 2007 Sep 10).
35. Pedersen CA, Schneider PJ, Scheckelhoff DJ. ASHP national survey of pharmacy practice in hospital settings: prescribing and transcribing—2004. *Am J Health-Syst Pharm.* 2005; 62:378–90.
36. Safe practices for better healthcare: 2006 Update: A Consensus Report. Washington, DC: National Quality Forum (NQF). 2006:22.
37. Schumock GT, Nutescu EA, Walton SM, et al. Survey of hospital policies regarding low-molecular-weight heparins. *Am J Health-Syst Pharm.* 2002; 59:534–8.
38. Bernard GR, Vincent JL, Laterre PF, et al. Efficacy and safety of recombinant human activated protein C for severe sepsis. *N Engl J Med.* 2001; 344:699–709.
39. Matthay MA. Severe sepsis—a new treatment with both anticoagulant and antiinflammatory properties. *N Engl J Med.* 2001; 344:759–62.
40. Thompson CA. High-cost sepsis drug forces pharmacists to weigh patients' future. *Am J Health-Syst Pharm.* 2002; 59:692,697. News.

41. Dranitsaris G, Spizzirri D, Pitre M, et al. A randomized trial to measure the optimal role of the pharmacist in promoting evidence-based antibiotic use in acute care hospitals. *Int J Technol Assess Health Care.* 2001; 17:171–80.
42. Fugit RV, Resch ND. Conversion of patients from simvastatin to lovastatin in an outpatient pharmacy clinic. *Am J Health-Syst Pharm.* 2000; 57:1703–8.
43. Mazzola JL, Belliveau PP, Cheeseman SH. Guidelines for liposomal amphotericin B. *Am J Health-Syst Pharm.* 2003; 60:1480–1.
44. Bower AN, Tang HM, Guglielmo BJ. Compliance in two medical centers with criteria for use of caspofungin and lipid-based amphotericin B. *Am J Health-Syst Pharm.* 2004; 61:915–20.
45. Vermeulen LC Jr, Ratko TA, Erstad BL, et al. A paradigm for consensus. The University Hospital Consortium guidelines for the use of albumin, nonprotein colloid, and crystalloid solutions. *Arch Intern Med.* 1995; 155:373–9.
46. Lucarelli CD. Formulary management strategies for type 3 serotonin receptor antagonists. *Am J Health-Syst. Pharm.* 2003; 60:(10, suppl)S4–S11.
47. Devlin JW. Proton pump inhibitors for acid suppression in the intensive care unit: formulary considerations. *Am J Health-Syst Pharm.* 2005; 62:(10, suppl 2):24–30.
48. Chernin EL. Pharmacoeconomics of inhaled anesthetic agents: considerations for the pharmacist. *Am J Health-Syst Pharm.* 2004; 61:(suppl 4)S18–S22.
49. Teich JM, Merchia PR, Schmiz JL, et al. Effects of computerized physician order entry on prescribing practices. *Arch Intern Med.* 2000; 160:2741–7.
50. Fischer MA, Lilly CM, Churchill WW, et al. An algorithmic computerised order entry approach to assist in the prescribing of new therapeutic agents: case study of activated protein C at an academic medical centre. *Drug Saf.* 2004; 27:1253–61.

Appendix—Therapeutic Interchanges, Prescribing Guidelines, and Other Interventions

Therapeutic Interchanges

The following are some examples of drugs and drug classes for which health systems have successfully implemented therapeutic interchange protocols:

- Angiotensin-converting-enzyme inhibitors
- Adenosine–dipyridamole for cardiac stress test
- Amphotericin, lipid-based
- Angiotensin-receptor blockers
- Benzodiazepine hypnotics
- Beta-lactamase inhibitor antibiotics
- Cephalosporins: first- (oral), second-, and third-generation
- Cholesterol-lowering agents
- Colony-stimulating factors (filgrastim and sargramostim, darbopoetin and epoetin alfa)
- Fluroquinolones
- Glycoprotein IIb/IIIa inhibitors
- Hepatitis B vaccine, pediatric strength
- Histamine H_2-receptor antagonists
- Inhaled and intranasal corticosteroids
- I.V. immune globulin
- Insulins – various, including insulin aspart and insulin lispro
- Iron products, injectable
- Low-molecular-weight heparins
- Narcotic analgesics (fentanyl group) in anesthesia
- Neuromuscular blocking agents
- Nonbenzodiazepine hypnotics
- Proton-pump inhibitors
- Respiratory agents (tiotropium interchanged with albuterol–ipratropium [Combivent, Boehringer Ingelheim], albuterol–ipratropium [Duoneb, Day] interchanged with individual drugs)
- Respiratory spacers
- Selective serotonin-reuptake inhibitors
- Serotonin-receptor antagonists
- Surfactants for newborns
- Thrombolytics
- Viscoelastic agents

Generic Substitutions

Generic products should be used routinely with few exceptions. The following are particularly important for cost savings:

- Amiodarone
- Fluconazole injection
- Megestrol
- Milrinone
- Pamidronate
- Propofol

Prescribing Guidelines

The following are some examples of drugs, drug classes, and diseases for which health-systems have developed prescribing guidelines, protocols, or pathways in collaboration with the medical staff and nursing staff.

- Albumin
- Anesthesia gas, low flow and guidelines for selection
- Antibiotic surgical prophylaxis
- Antibiogram and antibiotic guidelines
- Antifungal (injectable) agents (voriconazole, itraconazole, caspofungin)
- Aprotinin dosing
- Carbapenems
- Chemotherapy-induced nausea and vomiting
- Colony-stimulating factor guidelines/monitoring
- Drotrecogin alfa
- Fosphenytoin
- Heparin-induced thrombocytopenia
- Intensive care unit sedation protocol
- I.V. immune globulin
- Levalbuterol
- Nesiritide
- Octreotide
- Pneumonia protocol
- Postoperative nausea and vomiting
- Proton-pump inhibitors (i.v.)
- Venous thromboembolism, use of anticoagulants in acute coronary syndrome
- Ziprasidone injection

Interventions—Other

Other initiatives or activities that pharmacists can collaborate with the medical staff to reduce drug costs.

Cost per case in anesthesia
Antibiotic monitoring, laboratory reporting of sensitivities
Antibiotic restrictions
Eptifibatide waste reduction
Epoetin alfa waste reduction, prepare syringes
Pegfilgrastim is used in outpatients only

Approved by the ASHP Board of Directors on January 17, 2008. These guidelines supersede the ASHP Technical Assistance Bulletin on Assessing Cost-Containment Strategies dated September 27, 1991. Developed through the ASHP Council on Pharmacy Management.

ASHP gratefully acknowledges the expert panel that developed these guidelines: Michael Rubino, M.S., FASHP; James M. Hoffman, Pharm.D., M.S., BCPS; Larry J. Koesterer, M.B.A.; and Robert G. Swendrzynski, M.S.

Copyright © 2008, American Society of Health-System Pharmacists, Inc. All rights reserved. Contact ASHP for reprint and permissions requests. This content may not be used for commercial purposes without the express written consent of ASHP.

The bibliographic citation for this article is as follows: American Society of Health-System Pharmacists. ASHP guidelines on medication cost management strategies for hospitals and health systems. *Am J Health-Syst Pharm*. 2008; 65:1368–84.

ASHP Guidelines on Outsourcing Pharmaceutical Services

Purpose

Health-system pharmacy, as an essential component in health care organizations, is challenged by changes in the structure and financing of health care to reduce costs and improve performance. One option being used to achieve these goals is outsourcing. Outsourcing is a formal arrangement by which a health care organization contracts with an outside company to obtain selected pharmaceutical services or comprehensive management of the organization's pharmacy. Through this arrangement, the organization negotiates a contract with a company to access its expertise, technologies, and resources.

ASHP believes that the organization's pharmacist-in-charge (e.g., a pharmacy director) must take complete responsibility for patient outcomes from all medication-related activities performed at or for the organization's work sites, whether they are carried out by the organization's or contractor's onsite staff or by the contractor off site. This responsibility should be explicitly stated in all outsourcing contracts.

Health care organizations considering outsourcing pharmaceutical services should have a clear understanding of what they want to accomplish. Consideration should include, at the least, an internal needs assessment, a cost analysis, and a careful review of possible contractors. The organization should examine the potential long-term consequences of outsourcing as well as the short term outcomes expected during a contract's performance period.

The purpose of these guidelines is to provide an overview of factors and processes for health care organizations to consider when exploring outsourcing. The ideas presented in this document could be used for strategic planning with the organization's decision-makers, for drafting contract provisions, for comparing prospective contractors, for preparing for contract negotiations, or for evaluating a contractor's performance. These guidelines may be applied, for example, to independent and networked acute care hospitals, ambulatory care clinics, and home care providers.

This document includes ideas about reasons for outsourcing and reasons for not outsourcing, services available from contractors, the outsourcing process and outsourcing arrangements, and evaluation of contractor performance. The appendix provides a topical list of contract provisions, some of which relate to specific pharmaceutical services, pharmacy practices, or administrative functions that may be the subject of other ASHP practice standards. Organizations should refer to pertinent ASHP practice standards for additional information on which to base their contract provisions, agreements, and decisions. This document addresses representative outsourcing options and contract agreements and is not intended to cover all situations. Managers of pharmacy and health care organizations should use their professional judgment about applicability to their own needs and circumstances.

Environment

Various environmental influences and market forces that may contribute to outsourcing being considered as an option include the following.

DOI 10.37573/9781585287048.091

Organizational and Operational

- Re-engineering and downsizing initiatives
- Consolidation and integration of health systems and departments within health systems
- Elimination of or reduction in the size of traditional departments
- Reorganization around patient-focused care
- Implementation of automated pharmacy systems and the attendant need to reorganize medication distribution functions

Staffing

- Shortage of nurses and other health care professionals
- Shortage of pharmacists with specific experience and capabilities

Financial and Cost-Control

- Restricted budgets
- Increased operating costs
- Increased drug costs
- Increased emphasis on measuring performance in terms of staffing and costs instead of clinical outcomes

Quality

- Increased expectations of and pressures from accreditation organizations and consumer groups to improve the quality of patient care

Governmental and Regulatory

- Increased numbers of individuals dependent on federal, state, and local governments for health care
- Reduced ability of federal, state, and local governments to finance health care
- Increased government controls on reimbursement for health care

Competitive

- Increased competition among health care organizations
- Increased competition among suppliers of pharmaceutical products and related services

Purposes of Outsourcing

Health care organizations that conduct in-depth assessments may decide that outsourcing either is or is not a good option for meeting their needs. Reasons for their decision will vary according to a variety of factors.

Reasons Health Care Organizations Outsource Pharmaceutical Services. Organizations tend to outsource pharmaceutical services when guided by a careful assessment of their capabilities of providing services themselves, when unsuccessful in using their own resources to provide services, or, in some cases, when influenced by a consultant. Contracting with an outsourcing firm may produce one or more of the following results.

Organizational and Operational

- Ease the consolidation of pharmaceutical services in integrated health systems
- Resolve operational inefficiencies (e.g., by improving medication distribution systems, designing new pharmacy workspaces, reducing medication dispensing and administration errors, and improving computer and information systems)
  - Enable the organization to acquire additional resources and expertise to carry out other changes (e.g., reallocation of existing staff to pharmaceutical care roles in patient care areas)
  - Provide educational programs for patients and their families and for health care staff

Staffing

- Help the organization to staff hard-to-fill pharmacy positions
- Allow the organization to reach optimal staffing levels for achieving productivity targets

Financial and Cost-Control

- Control or reduce the cost of the organization's services
- Control or reduce labor costs (e.g., by shifting the cost of employees, benefits, and liabilities to a contractor)
- Enable the organization to acquire a contractor who will share the risks associated with operating the pharmaceutical services
- Avoid the cost of purchasing and maintaining pharmacy equipment
- Avoid the cost of physical remodeling (e.g., by using an offsite contractor to provide specific services for which remodeling would be required)
- Increase the organization's financial operating margin (e.g., by allowing the organization to purchase drugs in bulk quantities, use group purchasing contracts, decrease lost charges, improve billing accuracy, decrease drug diversion and pilferage, improve drug formularies, and transfer drug inventory, equipment, and supply activities to a contractor)

Quality

- Enable the organization to maintain or improve the quality of patient care (e.g., by expanding clinical services and pharmaceutical care, establishing new services, obtaining specialized expertise in pharmaceutical care)
- Provide support for the medical and nursing staffs and improve physician–nursing–pharmacy collaboration

Governmental and Regulatory

- Correct regulatory and accreditation problems relating to pharmaceutical services
- Ensure continuing compliance with accreditation and certification standards

Competitive

- Enhance the organization's image
- Allow the organization to gain an edge on competitors through improvements in service, quality, or price

Reasons Health Care Organizations Do Not Outsource Pharmaceutical Services. An organization's choice to continue providing its own pharmaceutical services may be based on one or more of the following reasons.

Organizational and Operational

- A belief that pharmaceutical services are well managed and are provided as effectively as or better than they could be by a contractor
- Negative experiences with outsourcing contractors (pharmacy or nonpharmacy) or awareness of other organizations' negative experiences with such contractors
- Concern that the decision to outsource pharmaceutical services can be reversed only with great difficulty
- A belief that the organization's needs are currently met cost-effectively and that changes are therefore unnecessary
- Concern about losing short-term and long-term control over decisions about pharmaceutical services
- Concern about reduced involvement of pharmacy leadership in organizationwide initiatives (e.g., development and implementation of information systems, clinical care plans or pathways, and disease management)

Staffing

- Concern that staff will be reduced to unacceptable levels
- Concern about potentially alienating relationships between pharmacists and other health care staff

Financial and Cost-Control

- An assessment that outsourcing would increase rather than decrease costs
- Concern that high-cost drugs might be excluded from contract agreements
- Concern that the organization may not be able to recapitalize pharmaceutical services if outsourcing is unsuccessful

Quality

- Concern that conflicting values and priorities of the outsourcing contractor and the organization will reduce quality
- Concern that clinical quality could be reduced as a result of a loss of continuity of pharmacy staffing and relationships with medical and nursing staffs

Professional Responsibility

- Concern that outsourcing will confuse or dilute the onsite pharmacists' ultimate professional authority and responsibility for all medication-related activities and outcomes at the site

Pharmaceutical Services Provided by Contractors

Some contractors manage and provide comprehensive pharmaceutical services. Other contracors focus more on providing specialty services or carrying out specific tasks (e.g., drug information services, offsite preparation of sterile products). The needs of the health care organization should guide the identification of potential contractors with the appropriate expertise and capabilities. Examples of services that may be available from contractors follow. (This list is likely to grow over time.)

Organizational and Operational

- Development of pharmacy policies, procedures, and processes
- Pharmacy record-keeping systems
- Productivity reviews
- Feasibility studies on expanding services (e.g., outpatient dispensing and home infusion)
- Unit dose medication distribution
- Pharmacy-based or offsite preparation of sterile products
- Pharmacokinetic monitoring and dosage determinations
- Medication therapy monitoring (e.g., for appropriate and effective use)
- Investigational drug programs
- Patient profile reviews
- Medication therapy-related consultation with physicians, nurses, and other health care professionals
- Assessment of patients' nutritional needs
- Guidance in purchasing and implementing automated pharmacy equipment
- Educational programs for patients, families, and caregivers
- Drug information services
- Packaging and repackaging of pharmaceuticals

Staffing

- Competency assessment and performance review
- Management, operational, and clinical training
- Recruitment and retention assistance

Financial and Cost-Control

- Billing
- Inventory control
- Formulary management

Quality

- Performance improvement (including improvement of medication use and reduction of medication errors)
- Quality assurance

Outsourcing Process

After the health care organization has completed an internal assessment of its needs and capabilities and decided to explore outsourcing, it should identify and contact reputable and experienced contractors. Some organizations simply identify prospective contractors and ask them to submit a proposal. A more thorough approach is to require prospective contractors to respond to a request for proposals (RFP). Although a formal RFP (and the contractor's formal proposal based on the RFP) may not be necessary, the information found in typical RFPs and proposals may be helpful for making a decision about outsourcing.

Contents of RFPs. RFPs often include the following information.

- A description of the organization (including statistical information)
- The organization's financial status (e.g., a current balance sheet and audited financial statement, the pharmacy's financial status)
- A description of the process the organization will use to select the contractor
- The organization's standard terms and conditions for contracting for services
- The names and telephone numbers of individuals in the organization who are involved in the outsourcing decision (the director of pharmacy should be included)
- A description of the specific outsourced services required of the contractor (e.g., pharmacy workspace design, intravenous admixture preparation, and implementation of an automated pharmacy system) and performance-measurement criteria or targets
- The date(s) on which the contractor can inspect the facility and the pharmacy
- The number of copies of the proposal to submit
- The name and address of the individual to whom the proposal is to be delivered
- Acceptable method(s) for delivery of the proposal (e.g., mail, delivery service, courier)
- A statement that the organization reserves the right to cancel its solicitation for services and reject any and all proposals
- A deadline date and time for receipt of the proposal
- The date on which the contractor would be expected to initiate services
- The date by which the selected contractor must provide a written contract
- Other requirements related to the proposal (e.g., that it be typewritten, that it include reference to an RFP number [if any], that it be signed by an officer of the firm who is authorized to contract)

Contents of Proposals. RFPs often require contractors to submit the following information with their proposals.

- A brief history of the contractor, including its mission, vision, and values
- The location of the contractor's offices and other facilities that would provide services to the organization
- The names, addresses, telephone numbers, and résumés or background information on the individual(s) who will provide the services
- Evidence that the contractor can provide qualified staff who are licensed or eligible for licensure by federal, state, and local agencies and a history of turnover in management, pharmacist, and support staff
- A history of the results of Joint Commission on Accreditation of Healthcare Organizations (JCAHO), Health Care Financing Administration, National Committee for Quality Assurance, state, or other accreditation or regulatory surveys conducted in the contractor's sites
- Proof of professional liability, general liability, and workers'-compensation insurance coverage (including the name, address, and telephone number of the insurance company) and a history of claims filed against the contractor

- Minimum-experience requirements (e.g., years of experience in providing outsourced pharmacy-management services, total number of clients served, current number of clients)
- A list of the requested services that the contractor can provide
- A list of the requested services that the contractor cannot provide and the reasons for the contractor's inability to provide them
- Evidence of organizational and staff experience and competence (including nature and extent) in the services the contractor can provide (e.g., pharmaceutical care, specialty clinical practice, antineoplastic medication preparation, enteral and parenteral nutrition solution preparation), as pertinent
- A copy of a standard or proposed contract
- A list of all fees and charges that would be billed under the contract and the detailed methods for their calculation, as well as a billing schedule
- A description of reports that the contractor will be expected to submit to the organization
- Information relating to the contractor's financial status and stability (e.g., balance sheets and audited financial statements for the past three years, bank references, lists of principal equity owners)
- The names, addresses, and telephone numbers of current clients receiving similar services
- The names, addresses, and telephone numbers of other clients served within the past two years and the reasons for all, if any, terminations of services
- Written references and copies of annual performance-improvement reports from clients of a similar size with similar types of patients

Visits to Contractors and Their Clients. Contractors should allow the organization's representatives to visit their corporate offices and production facilities and to tour pharmacies in the facilities of other clients. The contractor should provide ample opportunity for the organization's representatives to confer with the contractor's corporate and pharmacy staff.

Evaluating Proposals. A decision to outsource pharmaceutical services should be collaborative and should involve, as appropriate, the governing board, the chief executive officer (CEO), the chief financial officer (CFO), the chief operating officer (COO), the chief of the medical staff, the chair of the pharmacy and therapeutics committee, the director of nursing (DON), the director of pharmacy, and department heads, for example. The organization should scrutinize the following factors when evaluating proposals.

- Services offered versus services requested (including the contractor's ability to enhance current services)
- Professional experience (e.g., years of service; number, size, and types of clients; knowledge of the client's business)
- Financial stability (e.g., ability to absorb start-up expenses and to commit the resources needed to effect change)
- References and reputation (e.g., client-satisfaction reports, reputation in the health care industry, commitment to improving patient care)
- Technology or automated pharmacy systems (e.g., up-to-date hardware, proprietary software, the capability to interface with the organization's information systems)
- Education and training (e.g., internal and external continuing-education programs, educational allowances for professional and technical staff)
- Additional qualities (e.g., high employee morale, confidentiality, creativity, sensitivity to minorities and the community, willingness to share risks and rewards)
- Cost aspects of services (e.g., cost-effectiveness, ability to affect economies of scale)

The organization should assign an evaluation rating to each proposal. Ratings should be weighted appropriately with respect to professional services, experience, references, and cost of services. The organization should base its decision to outsource pharmaceutical services on its assessment of the contractor's ability to meet the organization's needs and fulfill the terms of the contract.

Negotiating the Contract. The organization should carefully review the proposal and clarify the provisions of the contract. Assistance from the organization's risk-management and legal counsel may be necessary. Negotiations can ensure a contract that best meets the needs of the organization and the contractor.

Signing the Contract. In some organizations the director of pharmacy may be authorized to sign contracts for outsourced services. If this is not the case, the director of pharmacy should be fully involved in negotiating the contract and advising the authorized signer(s).

Outsourcing Arrangement

The health care organization and the contractor should agree on the outsourcing arrangement that best meets their needs. Several outsourcing options are available to health care organizations. Variations and combinations of these options are common. The contract should clearly describe the outsourcing arrangement. Examples of outsourcing arrangements include the following.

Consulting. The contractor acts as a pharmacy consultant to the organization. Some consulting arrangements are limited to an assessment of all pharmaceutical services or to specific aspects of pharmaceutical services (e.g., clinical pharmacy services, productivity, compliance with JCAHO standards). Other consulting arrangements may include advising the pharmacy and helping it to improve its services.

Onsite Advisor. The contractor provides a full-time onsite advisor to the organization's director of pharmacy. The advisor works with the director of pharmacy and others, as needed, to carry out programs that will fulfill the contract provisions.

Management of Specific Pharmaceutical Services. The contractor provides one or more specific services (e.g., i.v. admixture preparation, drug information, stock replenishment, medication distribution). Services may be provided onsite or at an offsite location.

Comprehensive Management. The contractor assumes complete responsibility for operating the pharmacy and may provide some or all of the pharmacy staff.

Contract Provisions

A contract that meets the needs of the health care organization and of the contractor is the foundation for a successful relationship. Contracts should include provisions of the outsourcing arrangement that describe agreements between the organization and the contractor concerning their respective responsibilities. These provisions will vary depending on the kind and scope of services outsourced. For example, contractors who prepare sterile products at an offsite location will not require onsite pharmacy space and utilities. Also, the assignment of responsibilities may vary. A contract may specify that the organization will purchase all drugs. Conversely, another contract may assign this responsibility to the contractor. See the appendix for examples of contract provisions.

Evaluation of Contractor's Performance

Health care organizations should evaluate and document their contractor's performance and assess their contractor's compliance with the terms of the contract. Objective and subjective evaluations should be regular (e.g., quarterly or annually). Evaluations should address all measurable standards of performance that are specified in the contract. Evaluations should be multidisciplinary and should involve, for example, the CEO, CFO, COO, DON, and medical staff representatives, as appropriate. An evaluation may include an assessment of how well the contractor performed the following functions.

- Improved the quality of patient care
- Responded to the organization's needs
- Helped the organization to achieve its financial and patient-outcome goals
- Evaluated the productivity and performance of pharmacy staff
- Provided continuing education for pharmacy staff
- Implemented and improved pharmacy clinical programs
- Improved pharmacy processes (e.g., medication dispensing and delivery)
- Reduced and controlled pharmacy costs without compromising patient care
- Worked and communicated effectively with the organization's staff and resolved interdepartmental problems
- Participated effectively in the organization's performance-improvement program

Suggested Reading

- Curtis FR, Stai HC. Contract pharmacy services. In: Brown TR, ed. Handbook of institutional pharmacy practice, 3rd ed. Bethesda, MD: American Society of Hospital Pharmacists; 1992: 299–306.
- Talley CR. Outsourcing drug distribution. *Am J Health-Syst Pharm.* 1997; 54:37. Editorial.
- Schneider PJ. Outsourcing: a key to professional survival. *Am J Health-Syst Pharm.* 1997; 54:41–3.
- Lazarus HL. Outsourcing: a success story. *Am J Health-Syst Pharm.* 1997; 54:43–4.
- Puckett WH. Outsourcing: taking the first step. *Am J Health-Syst Pharm.* 1997; 54:45–8.
- Kolar GR. Outsourcing: route to a new pharmacy practice model. *Am J Health-Syst Pharm.* 1997; 54:48–52.
- Eckel FM. Outsourcing: at odds with pharmacy's professional foundation. *Am J Health-Syst Pharm.* 1997; 54:52–5.
- Gates DM, Smolarek RT, Stevenson JG. Outsourcing the preparation of parenteral nutrient solutions. *Am J Health-Syst Pharm.* 1996; 53:2176–8.
- Burruss RA, Carroll NV, Schraa C, et al. Outsourcing inpatient IV compounding: expense and medication error implications. *Pharm Pract Manage Q.* 1996; 16(3):52–9.
- McAllister JC III. Collaborating with re-engineering consultants: maintaining resources for the future. *Am J Health-Syst Pharm.* 1995; 52:2676–80.
- Anderson RJ. Clinical service contracts between hospital pharmacy departments and colleges of pharmacy. *Am J Hosp Pharm.* 1991; 48:1994–7.
- Murphy JE, Ward ES, Job ML. Implementing and maintaining a private pharmacokinetics practice. *Am J Hosp Pharm.* 1990; 47:591–7.
- Souhrada L. Contract management. *Hospitals.* 1990; 64(8):66–8.
- Wagner M. Basic pitfalls can undermine hospital-service firm relationship. *Mod Healthc.* 1993; 23(8):32.
- Wagner M. Contract-managed pharmacy departments are just the prescription at some hospitals. *Mod Healthc.* 1988; 18(8):36–40.

Appendix—Contract Provisions

The following are examples of contract provisions that, among others, the organization and contractor might adapt as needed and include in a contract, depending on the scope of services being considered. In addition, a contract would include provisions about the specific pharmaceutical services to be provided by the contractor. The language in contract provisions should be adapted to meet the needs of the health care organization and to comply with the organization's contracting policies and applicable laws and regulations.

Accreditation and certification: A contract may include a requirement that services meet or exceed applicable accreditation and certification standards. These include, but are not limited to, the standards (or requirements) of the following organizations.

- Joint Commission on Accreditation of Health-care Organizations
- American Osteopathic Association
- Health Care Financing Administration
- National Committee for Quality Assurance

After-hours pharmaceutical services when 24-hour services are not provided: The contractor may agree, for example, to provide an after-hours stock of drug products for authorized staff to use in filling urgent medication orders. In addition, the contractor may agree to ensure that a pharmacist is on call or available to return to the facility to provide pharmaceutical services.

Automation: A contract may outline responsibilities for the purchase or lease and the use of automated medication storage and distribution equipment and software associated with the equipment.

Choice of law: There may be a statement that the contract is governed by the laws of the state in which patient care is provided.

Compensation for contractor's services: There may be compensation arrangements, which vary greatly but are often based on one or more of the following principles.

- Management fee(s)
- Fee per item dispensed or service performed
- Fixed fee per patient per patient day, admission, discharge, adjusted patient day, adjusted admission, or adjusted discharge

Besides agreeing on a compensation arrangement, the organization and the contractor may agree on ways for the contractor to share the financial risk of contract performance with the organization; these might include guarantees or incentives for meeting targets and penalties for underperformance.

Computer equipment and information systems: A contract may outline responsibilities for the purchase, ownership, and maintenance of computer equipment and related software. Agreements might extend to personal computers used by pharmacy staff. There should be clear agreement about access to and use of data generated by the information system.

Confidentiality: There may be a requirement that information not generally available to the public (e.g., financial statements, medical records, market information) be kept confidential. Both parties must agree to safeguard access to computer databases and patient records to ensure that the patient's rights to privacy and confidentiality is protected. Use of the information should be limited solely to purposes specified in the contract.

Contractor reports: The content and regularity of performance reports that the contractor will submit to the organization may be specified.

Controlled substances: Responsibilities may be assigned for the procurement and security of controlled substances in compliance with Drug Enforcement Admi-nistration (DEA) and state regulations. For example, the organization may be required to

- Register with the DEA and any state equivalent for each site involved
- Assume complete responsibility for record keeping and security of controlled substances throughout the facility
- Ask the contractor to maintain proper records and provide adequate security for controlled substances as required by federal, state, and local laws and regulations and
- Verify that the contractor maintains proper records and provides adequate security for controlled substances

It may be necessary for the organization to grant power of attorney to the contractor to order and purchase controlled substances.

Similarly, the contractor may be required to

- Ensure that all registrations are current
- Order and maintain an adequate stock of controlled substances
- Ensure compliance with record-keeping and security requirements
- Inform the organization of problems with compliance

Cost control: A contract may include objectives, methods, and performance measures for controlling costs.

Cytotoxic and hazardous drug products: Responsibilities for ensuring the safety of the organization's staff and patients during the preparation and distribution of cytotoxic and hazardous drug products may be assigned. Either the organization or the contractor should provide a hazardous-materials handling program, including staff training, that meets Occupational Safety and Health Administration (OSHA) requirements.

Drug inventory disposition upon termination of the contract: A provision for the disposition of the drug inventory is based on inventory ownership. In cases in which the drug inventory may be purchased by either party, a mutually acceptable, independent appraiser could decide the purchase price. Legal advice may be needed to ensure that purchases comply with the Prescription Drug Marketing Act and other applicable laws and regulations.

Drug inventory ownership: If the contractor purchases the organization's inventory, a mutually acceptable, independent appraiser could decide the purchase price. Expired and other unusable drugs should be excluded from the purchase. The contractor could agree to obtain credit for the organization for expired and other unusable drugs if credit is obtainable. Legal advice may be needed to ensure that purchases comply with the Prescription Drug Marketing Act and other applicable laws and regulations.

Drug ordering: A contract may assign responsibilities for selecting vendors and purchasing drug supplies for the organization. The contract should specify that all drugs used must be subject to approval by the organization's pharmacy and therapeutics (P&T) committee or its equivalent. The organization should understand how purchasing discounts are accounted for, recorded, and distributed. The impact of removing pharmacy items from group purchasing programs should be clear also.

Early termination: There may be conditions for early termination of the contract.

Extension of period of performance: Conditions for extending the period of performance may be included in the contract.

Forms: Responsibilities for the design, approval, purchase, and storage of forms may be assigned.

Formulary system: A contract may assign responsibilities for evaluation of medications, collaboration with the P&T committee, and provision of formulary-related information services.

Hours of pharmacy operation: A contract may specify hours of operation that meet or exceed legal requirements and that are sufficient to serve patients' needs.

Laws, rules, and regulations: Requirements for services to meet or exceed federal, state, and local laws, rules, and regulations may be specified. These include but are not limited to those of FDA, DEA, OSHA, and the state board of pharmacy. The pharmacy should maintain (e.g., display, file) the appropriate licenses, permits, and records of equipment maintenance and certification. Any contractor required to be licensed as a manufacturer must be so licensed. The organization may agree to allow the contractor to act on the organization's behalf in communicating with the state board of pharmacy and other regulatory agencies.

Liability insurance: Responsibilities for maintaining liability insurance coverage for the acts of employees may be assigned. The contract might specify, for example, that the contractor must maintain adequate liability insurance coverage for the acts of its employees.

Nondiscrimination: There might be a requirement that the contractor abide by all laws and regulations relating to discrimination in appointments, promotions, and terminations.

Ownership of equipment, fixtures, and supplies: A contract may specify ownership of equipment, fixtures, and supplies and responsibilities for ensuring that equipment is maintained and certified according to applicable practice standards, laws, and regulations.

Performance improvement: Responsibilities for establishing any performance-improvement programs and integrating them with the organization's performance-improvement activities may be included. Performance-improvement programs might be appropriate, for example, for the ordering, dispensing, and administering of medications and for the monitoring of medication effects and misadventures, including adverse drug reactions and adverse drug events.

Period of performance: The contract might specify the period for which the contractor will provide services to the organization.

Pharmacy staff education and training: Responsibilities for required ongoing staff education and training may be specified. For example, there might be an agreement that the contractor's staff will participate in the organi-zation's education and training programs. In addition, the contractor may agree to provide specific training to ensure that all pharmacy personnel can perform any duties imposed by contractor-implemented functions.

Pharmacy staff employment: There may be a provision for the employment of pharmacists and technical and support personnel; this may specify those who will be employed by the organization and those who will be employed by the contractor. Whether employed by the organization or by the contractor, all staff should be competent and legally qualified. The organization should retain the right to assess, accept, or reject the performance of any of the contractor's staff who are used at the organization's work sites.

Pharmacy staff expenses: Responsibilities for any personnel expenses may be assigned. A contract might specify, for example, that the organization will be responsible for the salary, wages, and benefits of its employees whereas the contractor will be responsible for such expenses for its own employees. The contract might also allocate expenses for parking, meal discounts, and similar privileges for employees.

Pharmacy staff levels: There may be a requirement that the staffing levels for the contracted services be sufficient to meet the organization's needs.

Pharmacy staff orientation: A contract may assign responsibilities for orientation of all new pharmacy staff members to the organization and to the pharmacy, according to the organization's requirements.

Pharmacy staff performance: Responsibilities for pharmacy staff competency assessments and performance evaluations and for ensuring that assessments and evaluations are based on criteria in the individual's job description may be assigned.

Policies and procedures: Responsibilities may be assigned for developing policies and procedures covering the outsourced services, all of which should comply with applicable laws, regulations, and accreditation or certification standards. The contract should specify that the policies and procedures must not conflict with those of the organization.

Purchasing and accounts payable: Responsibilities for maintaining the pharmacy's purchasing and accounts-payable functions, including ordering drugs, monitoring costs, and authorizing payment to vendors, might be specified.

Record maintenance: A contract may assign responsibilities for maintaining and storing records. The contract should specify that all pertinent records must be kept for the time required by law and by the organization.

Space: Responsibilities for space required by the contractor to provide onsite services might be outlined. The organization should agree to provide space for the provision of onsite contractor services that is acceptable to the contractor and within the guidelines of the agencies that regulate the practice of pharmacy. Organizations might agree to provide the following facilities, depending on the contract's scope of services.

- Adequate square footage
- Space for preparing, compounding, packaging, and storing drugs under proper conditions
- Space for receiving and storing intravenous fluids and supplies
- Refrigerators and freezers
- Adequate space for maintaining and storing pharmacy records
- Laminar-airflow hoods and biological safety cabinets (if needed)

Sterile products: A contract might include requirements for the quality of sterile products provided by the contractor. The contractor should ensure that sterile products (e.g., large-volume intravenous admixtures, total parenteral nutrient solutions) are prepared and labeled in a suitable environment by trained and competent employees. The contractor should provide quality-control information periodically and on demand. For services that involve deliveries, the contract should specify order cutoff and delivery times, any penalties for late deliveries, and arrangements for after-hours or emergency services and deliveries.

Successors: The rights of each party in the event that the organization or contractor merges or transfers its business or assets to a successor may be included in a contract.

Utilities: A contract may assign responsibility for utilities required by the contractor to provide onsite services. These utilities may include the following, as appropriate.

- Electrical service
- Water
- Heating and air conditioning
- Plumbing
- Janitorial services
- Internal and external telephone services (allowance might be made for a private external telephone line for the contractor)
- Security
- Waste disposal

These guidelines were reviewed in 2013 by the Council on Pharmacy Management and by the Board of Directors and were found to still be appropriate.

Approved by the ASHP Board of Directors, April 22, 1998. Developed through the Council on Administrative Affairs.

Copyright © 1998, American Society of Health-System Pharmacists, Inc. All rights reserved. Contact ASHP for reprint and permissions requests. This content may not be used for commercial purposes without the express written consent of ASHP.

The bibliographic citation for this document is as follows: American Society of Health-System Pharmacists. ASHP guidelines on outsourcing pharmaceutical services. *Am J Health-Syst Pharm.* 1998; 55:1611–7.

ASHP Guidelines on Outsourcing Sterile Compounding Services

Purpose

The purpose of these guidelines is to provide an overview of factors and processes for healthcare organizations to consider when contracting with compounding pharmacies or outsourcing facilities to obtain sterile compounding services. These guidelines describe services available from compounding pharmacies or outsourcing facilities, reasons for outsourcing and reasons for not outsourcing, the outsourcing process and outsourcing arrangements, and recommendations for evaluating a contractor's performance. The guidelines also provide a topical list of contract provisions, some of which relate to practices that are the subject of other ASHP guidelines. Organizations should refer to pertinent ASHP guidelines for additional information on which to base their contract provisions, agreements, and decisions.[1–3] The concepts presented in this document could be used for strategic planning with the organization's decision-makers, assisting in assessing the quality of compounded sterile preparations or products, drafting contract provisions, comparing prospective contractors, preparing for contract negotiations, and evaluating contractor performance.

This document addresses representative outsourcing options and contract agreements and is not intended to cover all situations. Managers of pharmacy and healthcare organizations should use their professional judgment about applicability to their own needs and circumstances.

Services Provided by Vendors of Outsourced Sterile Compounding Services

The Drug Quality and Security Act (DQSA) of 2013 dramatically changed federal regulation of pharmacy compounding.[4] The DQSA amended the federal Food, Drug, and Cosmetic (FD&C) Act, carving out a safe harbor for traditional, prescription-based compounding pharmacies (called "503A compounding pharmacies" for the section of the FD&C Act that regulates them, or, more simply, "compounding pharmacies") and creating a new category of drug establishment, Human Drug Compounding Outsourcing Facilities. These facilities (frequently referred to as "registered 503B outsourcing facilities" for the section of the FD&C Act that regulates them, or, more simply, "outsourcing facilities") are permitted to engage in the manufacture and interstate shipment of larger quantities of compounded sterile drug products without prescriptions or medication orders. (For the purposes of these guidelines, both types of entities are referred to as "vendors of outsourced sterile compounding services" or, simply, "vendors.") The regulatory changes spawned by the DQSA have significant implications for compounding pharmacies, outsourcing facilities, and their customers. Healthcare organizations considering outsourcing sterile compounding services need to have a clear understanding of how these two distinct types of entities are regulated (**Table 1**).

Compounding Pharmacies. Section 503A clarified the FD&C Act for activities described as traditional patient-specific compounding (sometimes now called "503A compounding"). Healthcare organization pharmacies fall into this category, as do other pharmacies that fill prescriptions or medication orders within a prescriber–pharmacist–patient professional relationship. All 503A compounding pharmacies, except those in federal facilities, are regulated by state boards of pharmacy; however, they may also be subject to Food and Drug Administration (FDA) inspection under the agency's authority to enforce section 503A of the FD&C Act. The agency's expectations for compliance are specified in the FDA *Compliance Policy Guide* (CPG) *on Pharmacy Compounding of Human Drug Products Under Section 503A of the Federal Food, Drug, and Cosmetic Act*.[5] In addition to current regulatory requirements, such as prescriptions or medication orders for compounded preparations and compliance with applicable *United States Pharmacopeia* (*USP*) chapters on compounding (i.e., *USP* chapters 795 and 797),[8,9] inspectors may look for implementation of additional CPG recommendations. The services provided by compounding pharmacies are limited by the existing requirement for individual prescriptions or medication orders and may be further limited by forthcoming regulation of distribution across state lines,[7] state and federal restrictions on office-use preparations, and other limitations of section 503A.

Outsourcing Facilities. Section 503B outsourcing facilities are not required by federal regulation to be licensed pharmacies or to fill prescriptions or medication orders; however, a licensed pharmacist must supervise compounding. Outsourcing facilities are federally regulated by FDA, which has established guidance documents for the industry that will be updated as necessary. Outsourcing facilities must comply with applicable Current Good Manufacturing Practices (CGMPs) established under section 503B by FDA,[6] which differ from those for manufacturers. States may establish additional requirements with which outsourcing facilities must comply. All outsourcing facilities are inspected by FDA. The frequency of reinspections is determined by a risk-based schedule. Inspection findings are documented on form FDA-483, Inspectional Observations. A form FDA-483 is used to notify the entity of any concerns or potential violations and provide an opportunity for correction before enforcement action.[10] The compounding facility may work with inspectors to resolve issues during the inspection or respond in writing with a corrective action plan, usually within 15 days. The contents of these forms are publicly available.[11] However, findings in FDA-483 reports do not represent a final determination of noncompliance, nor is information available indicating that the findings have been satisfactorily resolved.

Healthcare organization pharmacy leaders must be aware of the quality standards that should be expected from outsourcing facilities.[12,13] In a letter sent to hospitals in January 2014, FDA encouraged healthcare organizations to purchase compounded sterile drugs from FDA-registered outsourcing facilities.[14] Although FDA usually inspects an outsourcing facility soon after registration (unless the facility has been

DOI 10.37573/9781585287048.092

TABLE 1.

Differences Between Compounding Pharmacies and Outsourcing Facilities[a]

Variable	Section 503A Compounding Pharmacies	Section 503B Registered Outsourcing Facilities
Regulatory authority	State boards of pharmacy	FDA, according to guidelines established by federal legislation; states may add requirements
Applicable standards	*USP* compounding standards; FDA Compliance Policy Guide on Pharmacy Compounding of Human Drug Products Under Section 503A of the Federal Food, Drug, and Cosmetic Act[5]	Applicable section 503B-specific FDA Current Good Manufacturing Practice[6]; subject to additional state requirements
FDA inspection	Subject to FDA inspection under authority to enforce section 503A	Subject to risk-based FDA inspection and enforcement procedures
State inspection	Subject to state board of pharmacy inspection	May be subject to state inspection if state law imposes additional requirements
Limitations on services	• May only dispense pursuant to an individual prescription or medication order for an identified patient • Anticipatory compounding of "limited quantities" is permitted, but a prescription or medication order is required before dispensing[5] • FDA limitations on interstate distribution, either 5% or 30%, depending on whether the state has entered into an MOU with FDA[b] • May not compound › Drugs that present demonstrable difficulties for compounding › Copies of FDA-approved products › Drugs using certain prohibited bulk substances	• Not required to be a licensed pharmacy or obtain prescriptions for specific patients • May compound and maintain inventory of compounded products in anticipation of customer orders • No federal limit on interstate commerce; some state regulations may apply • Compounding from bulk APIs only allowed for drugs on approved list • May compound copies of FDA-approved products from bulk substances if on FDA shortage list
Office-use compounding	Not yet addressed in FDA guidance[5]	Permitted, resale prohibited but "resale" does not include administration or dispensing by the purchaser[4]
Labeling requirements	As mandated by state law and regulation	Must include "Office use," "This is a compounded drug," and "Not for resale"

[a]FDA = Food and Drug Administration, *USP* = *United States Pharmacopeia*, MOU = memorandum of understanding, API = active pharmaceutical ingredient.

[b]At the time of writing, FDA had not issued final guidance on interstate distribution by section 503A facilities but had proposed a 30% limit on interstate distribution of compounded sterile preparations by section 503A compounding pharmacies in states that had entered into an MOU with FDA and a 5% limit in states that had not entered into an MOU.[7]

inspected previously), pharmacy leaders should be aware that registration does not necessarily mean that a particular outsourcing facility has been inspected and found to meet FDA standards. FDA's website listing registered outsourcing (503B) facilities provides dates of the initial and most recent registration as an outsourcing facility; the end date of the last FDA inspection related to compounding; whether an FDA-483 was issued; whether FDA action was taken, if any, based on the last inspection; and whether the outsourcing facility intends to compound sterile drugs from nonsterile bulk active pharmaceutical ingredients (APIs).[15] Pharmacy leaders should bear in mind that FDA or state inspections only reflect conditions at one particular time and should consider a facility's history as well as its most recent results.

Environmental Influences Affecting Outsourcing Decision

There are various environmental influences and market forces that may contribute to a facility's decision to consider outsourcing sterile compounding services. A list of some of those considerations follows.

Organizational and Operational

- Elimination of or reduction in the size of traditional pharmacy departments, re-engineering, and downsizing initiatives.
- Limited available physical or technological resources (e.g., sterile compounding area, inventory storage area, engineering controls) to provide the specific desired services.
- Consolidation and integration of health systems and departments within health systems, including pressure to provide pharmacy services to acquired entities (e.g., physician practices).
- Implementation of automated pharmacy systems and the attendant need to reorganize medication preparation and distribution functions.
- Inability to cost-effectively perform in-house testing to establish extended beyond-use dating for sterile preparations.
- Federal restriction under section 503A of the DQSA on the distribution of compounded sterile preparations from a central site in the healthcare organization to other campuses of the same system.[a]

Staffing

- Shortage of pharmacy personnel with specific experience and capabilities, especially regarding sterile preparation.
- Lack of resources, experience, or investment to effectively train staff on sterile compounding and aseptic technique.

Financial and Cost Control

- Restricted budgets.
- Increased operating costs.
- Increased drug costs.
- Increased emphasis on measuring performance in terms of staffing and costs.

Drug Shortages

- Unavailability of medications or specific dosage forms.
- Conservation of limited supplies of available medications.

Quality Assurance

- Increased expectations of and pressures from payers, regulatory agencies, accreditation organizations, and consumer groups to improve the quality of patient care, reduce the incidence of hospital infections, and demonstrate compliance with applicable standards and regulations.

Governmental and Regulatory

- Increased federal and state interest in standards for sterile compounding (i.e., *USP* chapter 797[9]).

Competitive

- Increased competition among healthcare organizations.
- Increased competition among suppliers of pharmaceutical products and related services.

Purposes of Outsourcing

Healthcare organizations should conduct an in-depth assessment to decide whether outsourcing is a good option for meeting their needs. Reasons for their decision will vary according to a variety of factors, some of which are outlined below. As with use of other contracted services, hospital leadership must be included in the decision-making process for outsourcing. A decision to outsource sterile compounding services should be collaborative and may involve, as appropriate, the governing board, chief executive officer (CEO), chief financial officer (CFO), chief operating officer (COO), chief of the medical staff, chair of the pharmacy and therapeutics (P&T) committee, director of pharmacy, director of nursing, legal counsel, medication safety officer, risk management director, and department heads.

Reasons Healthcare Organizations Outsource Sterile Compounding Services. Organizations tend to outsource sterile compounding services when guided by a careful assessment of their capabilities of providing services themselves, when unsuccessful in using their own resources to provide those services, or, in some cases, on the advice from a qualified consultant. Contracting with a compounding pharmacy or outsourcing facility may produce one or more of the following results.

Organizational and Operational

- Resolve operational inefficiencies (e.g., batch compounding, staff scheduling, high-demand periods).
- Provide compounded sterile preparations outside the scope of those routinely provided (e.g., complex or rarely compounded sterile preparations).
- Enable the organization to reallocate resources and expertise to carry out other priorities (e.g., reassignment of existing staff to roles in patient care areas).

Staffing

- Allow organizations to acquire quality compounded sterile preparations or products without hiring for hard-to-fill pharmacy positions and to concentrate on other staffing priorities.
- Allow the organization to reach optimal staffing levels for achieving quality and productivity targets.

Financial and Cost Control

- Control or reduce the cost of the organization's services (e.g., by shifting costs associated with sterile compounding services from fixed to variable).
- Control or reduce labor costs (e.g., by shifting responsibility for employees, benefits, and liabilities to a compounding pharmacy or outsourcing facility).
- Enable the organization to acquire a business partner to share the risks and other associated liability by delineating and contracting for the responsibilities associated with operating sterile compounding services.
- Minimize the cost of facility remodeling or maintenance (e.g., to meet *USP* chapter 797[9] or chapter 800[16] requirements).

Quality Assurance

- Provide consistent and high-quality pharmacy and sterile compounding services, including documented or extended beyond-use dating[b] and batch-level sterility, potency, and endotoxin testing.
- Enable the organization to maintain or improve the quality of patient care (e.g., by expanding clinical services or establishing new services).
- Enhance patient safety by providing more medications in a dose-specific, ready-to-administer form.
- Provide support for the medical and nursing staffs and improve prescriber–nursing–pharmacy collaboration.
- Improve organizational procedures by learning from contractors' experience and knowledge, especially with technologies used to improve safety (e.g., labeling, barcoding, or tamper-evident technologies).

Governmental and Regulatory

- Assist and ensure compliance with legal, regulatory, certification, and accreditation requirements.

Reasons Healthcare Organizations Do Not Outsource Sterile Compounding Services. An organization's choice to continue providing its own sterile compounding services may be based on one or more of the following reasons.

Organizational and Operational

- The organization demonstrates that its sterile compounding services meet the requirements and standards of *USP* chapter 797[9]; comply with applicable local, state, and federal regulations; are cost-effective, well managed, and provided as efficiently as or better than services that could be provided by a compounding pharmacy or an outsourcing facility.
- Negative experiences with outsourcing other clinical services, or awareness of other organizations' negative experiences with such outsourcing.
- Concern about time delays in receiving compounded sterile preparations or products, especially ones that are needed urgently or have poor stability or short beyond-use dates (BUDs).
- Concern that the contractor may experience interruptions in service, perhaps with little notice, due to quality-control issues not related to services provided to the organization.
- Concern that the decision to outsource sterile compounding services can be reversed only with great difficulty.
- Concern about losing short- and long-term control over decisions regarding or expertise in sterile compounding services.

Staffing

- Concern that staff will be reduced to unacceptable levels.

Financial and Cost Control

- An assessment that outsourcing would increase rather than decrease costs.
- Concern that high-cost drugs might be excluded from contract agreements.
- Concern that the organization may not be able to recapitalize sterile compounding services if outsourcing is unsuccessful.

Quality Assurance

- Concern that conflicting values and priorities of the contractor and the organization will reduce quality.
- Loss of direct control over quality-assurance procedures for the compounding process.
- Concern about the qualifications or competencies of contractors' pharmacy staff.

Governmental and Regulatory

- Legal, regulatory, certification, and accreditation requirements may hinder operational efficiencies.

Outsourcing Process

The needs of the healthcare organization should guide the identification of potential vendors of outsourced sterile compounding services with the appropriate expertise and capabilities. Among the services that may be available from such vendors are the preparation of implantable and external pump cartridges; total parenteral nutrition; cardiovascular solutions; anesthesia syringes and solutions; dialysis, irrigation, or cardioplegia solutions; continuous renal replacement therapy, hydration, and oxytocin solutions; antibiotics; ophthalmic injectables and solutions; chemotherapy preparations; and analgesic preparations (patient-controlled analgesia, epidural, or regional nerve-block devices).

After the healthcare organization has completed an internal assessment of its needs and capabilities and decided to explore outsourcing, it should identify and contact vendors of outsourced sterile compounding services.

Organizations that are part of a larger network (e.g., an integrated delivery network) may explore options that are available to them through the network or from other organizations in the network. A health system may be exempt from registering as a 503B entity if it compounds medications for the health system's own patients in response to a prescription or medication order or in a "limited quantity" in anticipation of such prescriptions or orders, based on a history of such prescriptions or orders, as long as the pharmacy complies with state laws.[5] This exemption is expected to be clarified by FDA in the future.[13]

Many organizations begin to identify prospective contractors through a request for information (RFI). The RFI should provide

- A short history of the prospective contractor, including number of years in business, number and location of facilities, approximate number of customers served, and approximate volume of compounded sterile products or preparations delivered per month or year.
- The prospective contractor's regulatory status (i.e., compounding pharmacy or registered outsourcing facility) and applicable licensure or registration information (e.g., pharmacy license number).
- Whether the prospective contractor compounds sterile preparations or products from nonsterile bulk APIs (for registered outsourcing facilities, this information is available on FDA Registered Outsourcing Facilities website).[15]
- Description of products and services typically available (e.g., customer support, website), value-added services available (e.g., clinical support), and typical ordering process and turnaround times.
- Representative prices for specified compounded sterile products or preparations and services at an annual unit demand.
- Whether the prospective contractor has any contracts with group purchasing organizations.
- A description of the prospective contractor's backup facility capabilities and business continuity and disaster recovery plans.
- Whether the prospective contractor has ever been the subject of an enforcement or accreditation action.

After prospective contractors have been identified through RFIs, many organizations require them to respond to a more detailed request for proposal (RFP). Although a formal RFP (and the contractor's formal proposal based on the RFP) may not always be necessary, the information found in typical RFPs and prospective contractor responses or proposals is often helpful in making a systematic decision about outsourcing.

Contents of RFPs. RFPs often include the following information:

- A description of the demographics of the organization making the RFP (e.g., number of hospitals, bed sizes, typical census).
- A description of the process the organization will use to select the contractor.
- The organization's standard terms and conditions for contracting for services or, if available, a sample contract from the organization.
- The names and telephone numbers of individuals in the organization who are involved in the outsourcing decision (the organization's director of pharmacy should be included).
- A description of the specific services required of the contractor (e.g., desired drugs, strengths, concentrations, diluents, container systems, annual demand) and performance-measurement criteria or targets. Special packaging, handling, and delivery procedures for hazardous drugs should be included.
- A request for documentation of follow-up and correction of any enforcement or accreditation findings.
- The dates on which the organization's representatives can inspect the contractor's facility, with reasonable notice. (Inspections by the organization's representatives will be more important when contracting with vendors that are not regularly inspected by FDA or state inspectors.)
- The number of copies of the proposal to submit.
- The name and address of the individual to whom the proposal is to be delivered.
- Acceptable methods for delivery of the proposal (e.g., e-mail, mail, delivery service, courier).
- A statement that the organization reserves the right to cancel its solicitation for services and reject any and all proposals for any reason or for no reason.
- A deadline date and time for receipt of the proposal.
- The date on which the contractor would be expected to initiate services.
- The date by which the selected contractor must provide a written contract.
- Other requirements related to the proposal (e.g., that it be in a specific file format, include reference to an RFP number [if any], or be signed by an officer of the firm who is authorized to contract or his or her designee).

Contents of Responses or Proposals. RFPs should require prospective contractors to submit the following information with their responses or proposals:

- A brief history of the contractor, including its mission, vision, and values.
- A history of the results of all regulatory or accreditation surveys conducted of the contractor's sites, including copies of significant regulatory actions.
- The location of the contractor's offices and other facilities that would provide services to the organization.
- The contractor's regular business hours or hours of operation and emergency and after-hours contact information.
- The names, addresses, telephone numbers, and resumés or background information on individuals who will provide the services.
- Assurance that all pharmacists employed at the compounding facility are licensed as required and that all technicians involved in the compounding process are registered (if required by the state or by the healthcare organization's policy).
- Evidence of the following documentation regarding the contractor:
    - ► Proof and description of coverage of current liability insurance.
    - ► Current accreditation or certification certificates, if applicable.
    - ► State pharmacy licensure or other appropriate licenses.
    - ► Registration with FDA as an outsourcing facility, which can be obtained on FDA's registered outsourcing facilities webpage.[15]
    - ► Proof of FDA registration as a device manufacturer, if applicable.
    - ► Current Drug Enforcement Administration (DEA) registration, consistent with federal and state regulations.
    - ► Licensure of pharmacists employed and verification that they are in good standing, are on file, and available for review.
    - ► Registration of pharmacy technicians employed and verification that they are in good standing, are on file, and available for review, if applicable.
    - ► Pharmacist and pharmacy technician notarized statements stating that they have never been convicted of a drug-related misdemeanor or felony or proof of background check, are on file, and available for review.
    - ► Pharmacist and pharmacy technician training manual are on file and available for review.
    - ► Standard operating procedures manual are on file and available for review.
    - ► Certificates of analysis for nonsterile ingredients used in compounding are on file and available for review, if applicable.
    - ► Policies and procedures for stability testing are on file and available for review.
    - ► Policies and procedures for sterility assurance testing are on file and available for review.
    - ► Policies and procedures for pyrogen testing are on file and available for review, if applicable.
    - ► Examples of batch reports for products being considered for outsourcing are on file and available for review.
    - ► Examples of the quality-control and quality-assurance reports.
    - ► Stability documents and clinical references, as well as any materials that are used to determine BUDs on file and available for review. (Because studies used to establish BUDs are sometimes considered proprietary, compounding service providers may require a nondisclosure agreement.)

- Proof of professional liability, general liability, and workers' compensation insurance coverage (including the name, address, and telephone number of the insurance company).
- Experience (e.g., years of experience in providing sterile compounding services, total number of clients served, current number of clients).
- A list of the requested services that the contractor can provide and the normal terms of service, including but not limited to normal delivery cycles, availability and cost of emergency preparation and delivery, remedies for failure to perform to the contract, specific goods and services to be provided, and the infrastructure available at the compounding site for electronic ordering.
- A list of the requested sterile compounding services that the contractor cannot provide and the reasons for its inability to provide them.
- Expectation statements to assist in meeting the Centers for Medicare and Medicaid Services (CMS) requirements[17] and accreditation organization standards[18–23] related to contracted services, if applicable.
- A copy of a standard or proposed contract.
- A list of all fees and charges, including shipping, handling, and delivery charges, and any fees associated with order changes that would be billed under the contract and the billing methodology for their calculation.
- A billing schedule and a copy of a sample bill for each of the preparations compounded by the contractor.
- A description of a routine delivery schedule (e.g., daily by a specified time) and options for nonroutine delivery (e.g., later the same day, after-hours, weekends, holidays, during emergencies).
- Examples of reports that the contractor will be expected to submit to the organization.
- The process for requesting new preparations from the contractor.
- The contractor's policy on unannounced inspections by its customers.
- The names, addresses, and telephone numbers of
    - Current clients of a similar size or those receiving similar types of compounded preparations or products, with written references and copies of annual performance-improvement reports, if possible.
    - Reference accounts currently served.

Additional information to obtain from the prospective contractor but not necessarily contained in the proposal may include

- Whether the contractor has had product liability lawsuits filed against it for preparations it compounded. If so, the contractor should be asked to provide a description of the lawsuits filed, the file date of the lawsuits, and the outcome, though such information is sometimes sealed as part of a settlement or decision and may not be disclosable.
- A description of the contractor's formal procedures for conducting recalls and whether there have ever been recalls of any of its compounded preparations. If the contractor has ever recalled any of its compounded preparations, it should be asked to provide the dates of recall, a description of the preparations recalled, and the reasons for the recall. Outsourcing facilities must comply with the specific requirements of FDA for 503B entities, which include having procedures for putting into place corrective and preventive actions.[6]
- Information related to the delivery process and backup planning when severe or catastrophic events happen (e.g., severe weather).

Visits to Contractors and Their Clients. Outsourcing facilities and compounding pharmacies should allow the organization's representatives to visit their corporate offices and compounding facilities. The contractor should provide ample opportunity for the organization's representatives to confer with the contractor's corporate, pharmacy, and compounding staff. During the evaluation phase, the organization's representative should expect to give notice of a visit, but after a contract has been signed the contractor should allow unannounced inspections, provided that the visit will be conducted in a manner that does not interfere with daily activity or compromise the state of microbial control.

For outsourcing facilities, the FDA inspection report and documentation of follow-up and correction of any enforcement or accreditation findings should be reviewed in advance of the visit. For compounding pharmacies, the healthcare organization should, in addition to requesting any FDA or state inspection reports and any applicable accreditation reports, assess the contractor's compliance with *USP* chapter 797 using a standard tool, such as the ASHP Research and Education Foundation's contractor assessment tool for outsourcing sterile products preparation.[24]

Evaluating Proposals. A decision to outsource sterile compounding services should be collaborative and may involve, as appropriate, the organization's governing board, CEO, CFO, COO, chief of the medical staff, chair of the P&T committee, director of pharmacy, director of nursing, legal counsel, medication safety officer, risk management director, and department heads, for example. The organization should scrutinize the following factors when evaluating proposals:

- Services offered versus services requested (including the contractor's potential to enhance currently offered sterile compounding services or customize to the organization's needs).
- Professional experience (e.g., years of service; number, size, and types of clients; knowledge of the organization's operations).
- Quality management program, specifically as it relates to facility cleaning and validation, environmental monitoring, staff training, and competency assessment.
- Financial stability (e.g., ability to absorb startup expenses and to commit the resources needed to initiate service).
- References and reputation.
- Information systems and other technological infrastructure (e.g., the capability to interface with the organization's information and drug delivery systems, such as infusion pumps or barcode-assisted medication administration systems).
- Demonstrated commitment to continually integrating technology and knowledge to improve patient safety.

- Education and training of the contractor's staff (e.g., internal and external continuing-education programs, educational allowances for professional and technical staff).
- The organization's and the contractor's policies on specific compounding practices (e.g., references with real-time stability data supporting beyond-use dating, compliance with standards and regulations, use of USP–National Formulary-grade ingredients or FDA-approved products in accordance with the organization's intended use).
- Risk-assessment program to ensure that medication errors are not introduced by new or increased outsourced compounding activities and that the medications dispensed are compatible with the client's medication administration devices (e.g., automated distribution devices, barcode labeling, smart pumps).
- Knowledge of the regulatory requirements and accreditation standards that the organization must meet and willingness to assist the organization in meeting these standards.
- Inventory and supply chain issues (e.g., the organization's and contractor's back-order policies, the contractor's ability to produce drug products in shortage through validated compounding procedures).
- Emergency-preparedness implications (e.g., the abilities of the organization and the contractor to deliver services in the event of a disaster).
- Additional qualities (e.g., high employee morale, confidentiality, creativity, dedication to the community, collaborative spirit).
- Cost aspects of services (e.g., cost-effectiveness, ability to achieve economies of scale).

The contractor should, at a minimum, be able to

- Provide assurance that each compounded sterile preparation or product meets applicable state and federal labeling requirements and is sterile and free of endotoxins (when required) and unintended particulate matter, according to professionally established and accepted quality-monitoring data.
- If the contractor is extending beyond-use dates longer than defined in *USP* chapter 797,[9] confirm the validity of those beyond-use dates with stability and strength,[25] sterility, and endotoxin testing that is available for review.
- If the contractor is compounding high-risk preparations or products, provide documentation of the end product–testing processes used to determine that the preparations or products are sterile, free of endotoxins and unintended particulate matter, and (for preparations or products made from bulk APIs) meet the strength requirements of the drug.
- Deliver appropriate preparations or products in tamper-resistant packaging and in containers that will maintain the sterility and stability of the drugs. All products must be shipped under proper storage temperatures and (when required) protection from light.

The organization should assign an evaluation rating to each proposal. Ratings should be weighted appropriately with respect to services, experience, references, and cost. The organization should base its decision to outsource sterile compounding services on its assessment of the contractor's ability to meet the organization's needs and fulfill the terms of the contract.

Outsourcing Arrangement. The healthcare organization and the contractor should agree on the outsourcing arrangement that best meets their needs. The contract should clearly describe all aspects of the outsourcing arrangement. The healthcare organization's pharmacy should

- Ensure that the proper body of the healthcare organization (e.g., the organization's P&T committee) has developed a formal process to identify which preparations will (and which preparations will not) be prepared by the contractor, based on the organization's assessment of the therapeutic needs of patients and logistical considerations associated with outsourcing.
- Establish the components of the medication orders or prescriptions for preparations that will be compounded by an outside facility.
- Determine whether patient consent must be obtained for use of preparations compounded outside the healthcare organization's pharmacy, consistent with state board of pharmacy regulations and prevailing law.
- Determine a method for identifying patients receiving the contractor's preparations or products.
- Ensure that the contract and the contractor's facility have been reviewed by all the necessary bodies in the pharmacy's healthcare organization (e.g., the organization's risk management team, legal counsel, P&T and infection control committees, epidemiology department).
- Determine how to handle situations in which a patient presents with a compounded medication that is not available from the healthcare organization's pharmacy or the contractor under the existing contract (e.g., medication in an implantable device, i.v. push medication, i.v. infusion) and that has not been previously considered by the P&T committee. Considerations include what the process will be for:
    - Having the P&T committee consider outsourcing the compounding of such medications to another contractor with which the healthcare organization has an agreement.
    - Acquiring certain compounded medications if the contractor already under contract cannot or will not prepare them and how the associated liability risks will be addressed (e.g., how the healthcare organization's pharmacy will negotiate an agreement with another contractor from which the preparation or product is available) until the P&T committee decision is obtained regarding such medications.

Negotiating the Contract. The healthcare organization should carefully review the proposal and clarify the provisions of the contract. Active participation by the healthcare organization's risk management team and legal counsel is highly recommended. Negotiations can ensure a contract that best meets the needs of the healthcare organization and the contractor. ASHP believes that the healthcare organization's pharmacist-in-charge (e.g., a pharmacy director) must take responsibility for patient outcomes from all medication-related activities performed at or for the organization's work sites, whether they are carried out by the organization's staff or by contractors. This responsibility should be explicitly stated in all outsourcing contracts.

The signed contract between the parties should at a minimum

- Describe the term length of the contract and the processes for the contractor's billing to the healthcare organization, including methods of determining the charge for the compounded items, payment terms, and processes for resolution of disputed invoices.
- Contain a confidentiality clause and a Health Insurance Portability and Accountability Act business associate agreement, if applicable.
- Establish the pharmacy's right to unannounced inspections of the premises where compounding occurs, including the right to inspect quality-control reports, provided that the visit will be conducted in a manner that does not interfere with daily activity or compromise the microbial state of control.
- Describe the method of communicating the medication order or prescription from the healthcare organization's pharmacy to the contractor (e.g., telephone, fax, computer transmission, hard copy, controlled-substance ordering system).
- Protect both parties from liabilities created by errors made by the other party and delineate the obligations of both parties.[26]
- Establish recall procedures that comply with hospital policy mandates and prevailing law should a preparation or product need to be recalled by the contractor.
- Address documentation, regulatory and accreditation compliance, sterile compounding process, and compounded preparation or product considerations.
- Describe the pertinent situations and processes for the return, credit, or destruction of compounded preparations or products with the contractor.
- Describe any requirements regarding the submission of quality reports by the contractor.
- Describe the procedures for resolving preparation or delivery issues encountered by the organization or the contractor.
- Describe the expectations to be met by the contractor. These expectations must comply with CMS Hospital Conditions of Participation for Contracted Services requirements,[17] which state (in part) that "The governing body must ensure that a contractor of services . . . furnishes services that permit the hospital to comply with all applicable conditions of participation and standards for the contracted services." Hospital accreditation organizations (Joint Commission,[18] DNV GL Healthcare,[19] the Healthcare Facilities Accreditation Program,[20] and the Center for Improvement in Healthcare Quality[21]) and other accreditation organizations (e.g., Accreditation Commission for Health Care's Pharmacy Compounding Accreditation Board,[22] National Association of Boards of Pharmacy Verified Pharmacy Program[23]) have additional standards that must be addressed.

Both operational and quality expectations should be defined by the organization, such as expectations that

- Delineate routine sterile compounding turnaround times (e.g., from receipt of the request, medication order, or prescription by the contractor to delivery to the healthcare organization) and describe acceptable deviations from the agreed-upon schedules (e.g., raw product availability problems, unique end-product testing requirements, compounded preparation stability characteristics, nonroutine and emergency delivery requests).
- Describe the specific drugs provided, documentation flow, delivery methods, security considerations, and time frames for the provision of controlled substances by the contractor.
- Describe any special processes, documentation flow, delivery methods, security considerations, and time frames for the provision of hazardous drugs by the contractor.
- Describe the frequency of quality statements provided to the healthcare organization, such as quarterly summaries of facility, personnel, and environmental monitoring.

Signing the Contract. In some organizations, the director of pharmacy may be authorized to sign contracts for outsourced services. If this is not the case, the director of pharmacy must be fully involved in negotiating the contract and advising the authorized signers.

Contract Provisions

A contract that meets the needs of the healthcare organization and of the contractor is the foundation for a successful relationship. Contracts should specifically describe the respective responsibilities of the organization and the contractor. See the appendix for examples of contract provisions.

Evaluation of the Contractor's Performance

The healthcare organization must evaluate and document the contractor's performance and assess the contractor's compliance with the terms of the contract. The contractor should regularly submit quality reports, and the organization must regularly perform objective and subjective evaluations (e.g., quarterly, annually). Evaluations should address all measurable standards of performance specified in the contract. Evaluations should be led by the director of pharmacy, be multidisciplinary, and should involve, for example, the CEO, CFO, COO, director of nursing, and medical staff representatives, as appropriate. An evaluation may include an assessment of how well the contractor has

- Helped improve the quality of patient care.
- Responded to the organization's needs (e.g., invoicing, process adjustment).
- Met its contractual obligations, including timely and complete deliveries of products.
- Provided clear and concise quality metric data ensuring compliance with state and federal regulations and patient-safety standards.

- Helped the organization achieve its financial and patient-outcome goals.
- Improved the productivity and performance of pharmacy staff.
- Improved medication management processes (e.g., medication dispensing and delivery).
- Reduced and controlled medication costs without compromising patient care.
- Worked and communicated effectively with the organization's staff and resolved problems.

Handling Performance or Quality Issues

The contractor should provide the healthcare organization with information at least quarterly on its compliance with contract requirements and other information needed for the organization's quality-assurance programs. A mechanism should be in place for resolving preparation or delivery issues (e.g., delivery to the wrong location, late deliveries).

Conclusion

These guidelines offer an overview of factors and processes for healthcare organizations to consider when exploring the outsourcing of pharmacy sterile compounding. Such considerations include an internal needs assessment, a cost analysis, a careful review of prospective outsourcing facilities and compounding pharmacies, and an examination of the potential long-term consequences of outsourcing as well as the short-term outcomes expected during a contract's performance period. The ideas presented can be used for strategic planning, drafting of initial contract provisions, comparing prospective contractors, preparing for contract negotiations, or evaluating a contractor's performance. These guidelines are intended to address representative outsourcing options and contract agreements and may not be applicable to all situations. Managers of pharmacy and healthcare organizations should exercise professional judgment about applicability to their own needs and circumstances.

---

[a]At the time of writing, FDA had not issued final guidance on interstate distribution by 503A facilities.[7]

[b]Draft CGMP limits on BUDs for 503B outsourcing facilities may present challenges to those purchasing them. For sterile preserved drugs, the longest permissible BUD is 30 days beyond completion of a sterility test. If a sterility test is completed before release, the BUD must not exceed 14 days (at USP controlled room temperature or refrigerated) beyond completion of the test (e.g., for a 14-day sterility test, the BUD could not exceed 28 days). For terminally sterilized products without a sterility test, the BUD cannot exceed 14 days. And for aseptically processed products without a sterility test, the BUD cannot exceed 24 hours at USP controlled room temperature or 3 days refrigerated. BUDs for frozen products are considerably longer.[6]

References

1. American Society of Health-System Pharmacists. ASHP guidelines on outsourcing pharmaceutical services. *Am J Health-Syst Pharm.* 1998; 55:1611–7.
2. American Society of Health-System Pharmacists. ASHP guidelines on compounding sterile preparations. *Am J Health-Syst Pharm.* 2014; 71:145–66.
3. American Society of Hospital Pharmacists. ASHP guidelines for selecting pharmaceutical manufacturers and suppliers. *Am J Hosp Pharm.* 1991; 48:523–4.
4. Drug Quality and Security Act (November 27, 2013). www.govtrack.us/congress/bills/113/hr3204/text (accessed 2015 Jan 20).
5. Food and Drug Administration. FDA guidance on pharmacy compounding of human drug products under section 503A of the Federal Food, Drug, and Cosmetic Act (July 2014). www.fda.gov/downloads/Drugs/GuidanceComplianceRegulatoryInformation/Guidances/UCM377052.pdf (accessed 2015 Jan 20).
6. Food and Drug Administration. FDA guidance for industry: Current Good Manufacturing Practice—interim guidance for human drug compounding outsourcing facilities under section 503B of the FD&C Act (July 2014). www.fda.gov/downloads/drugs/guidancecomplianceregulatoryinformation/guidances/ucm403496.pdf (accessed 2015 Jan 20).
7. Food and Drug Administration. FDA draft memorandum of understanding addressing certain distributions of compounded human drug products (February 12, 2015). www.fda.gov/downloads/Drugs/Guidance-ComplianceRegulatoryInformation/Pharmacy-Compounding/UCM434233.pdf (accessed 2015 Feb 24).
8. General chapter 795: pharmaceutical compounding—nonsterile preparations. In: The United States pharmacopeia, 38th rev., and The national formulary, 33rd ed. Rockville, MD: United States Pharmacopeial Convention; 2014:560–7.
9. General chapter 797: pharmaceutical compounding—sterile preparations. In: The United States pharmacopeia, 38th rev., and The national formulary, 33rd ed. Rockville, MD: United States Pharmacopeial Convention; 2014:567–611.
10. Food and Drug Administration. FDA inspections, compliance, enforcement, and criminal investigations: FDA Form 483—frequently asked questions. www.fda.gov/ICECI/Inspections/ucm256377.htm (accessed 2015 Feb 24).
11. Food and Drug Administration. FDA pharmacy inspections and related records. www.fda.gov/AboutFDA/CentersOffices/OfficeofGlobalRegulatoryOperationsandPolicy/ORA/ORAElectronicReadingRoom/ucm431393.htm (accessed 2015 Apr 1).
12. Kastango E, Douglass K. Quality standards for large scale sterile compounding facilities (May 2014). www.clinicaliq.com/images/stories/clinicaliq_compounding%20quality%20standards.pdf (accessed 2015 Jan 20).
13. Kastango ES. Impact of the US Drug Quality and Security Act. www.pppmag.com/article_print.php?articleid=1595 (accessed 2015 Feb 24).
14. Food and Drug Administration. Letter to hospital/purchaser from Margaret A. Hamburg, M.D., Commissioner of Food and Drugs (January 8, 2014). www.fda.gov/downloads/drugs/guidancecomplianceregulatoryinformation/pharmacycompounding/ucm380599.pdf (accessed 2015 Jan 20).
15. Food and Drug Administration. Registered outsourcing facilities. www.fda.gov/drugs/guidancecomplianceregulatoryinformation/pharmacycompounding/ucm378645.htm (accessed 2015 Mar 16).

16. United States Pharmacopeial Convention. General chapter 800 hazardous drugs—handling in healthcare settings. www.usp.org/usp-nf/notices/general-chapter-hazardous-drugs-handling-healthcare-settings (accessed 2015 Feb 24).
17. Centers for Medicare and Medicaid Services. Conditions of participation for hospitals, §482.12 (e), (e)(1), and (e)(2). http://cms.hhs.gov/Regulations-and-Guidance/Guidance/Manuals/downloads/som107ap_a_hospitals.pdf (accessed 2015 Jan 20).
18. Joint Commission. Standard LD.04.03.09.Comprehensive accreditation manual for hospitals (update 2, November 2014). Oakbrook Terrace, IL: Joint Commission Resources; 2014.
19. National Integrated Accreditation for Healthcare Organizations (NIAHO) interpretive guidelines and surveyor guidance–version 11. Milford, OH: DNV GL Healthcare USA; 2014:20–1.
20. Accreditation requirements 01.00.29, 01.00.30, and 01.01.13. 2012 accreditation requirements for acute care facilities. Chicago: American Osteopathic Association, Healthcare Facilities Accreditation Program; 2012.
21. Accreditation standards for acute care hospitals (October 2014) Round Rock, TX: Center for Improvement in Healthcare Quality; 2014:3.
22. Pharmacy Compounding Accreditation Board, Accreditation Commission for Health Care. Pharmacy accreditation. www.achc.org/programs/pharmacy (accessed 2014 Jul 24).
23. National Association of Boards of Pharmacy. Verified Pharmacy Program. www.nabp.net/programs/licensure/verified-pharmacy-program (accessed 2015 Apr 1).
24. ASHP Research and Education Foundation. Outsourc-ing sterile products preparation: contractor assessment tool, 2011. www.ashpfoundation.org/MainMenuCategories/PracticeTools/SterileProductsTool/SterileProductsAssessmentTool.aspx (accessed 2015 Jan 20).
25. Allen LV, Bassani GS, Elder EJ, et al. Strength and stability testing for compounded preparations. www.usp.org/sites/default/files/usp_pdf/EN/2014-01-13_strength_versus_stability_testing_for_compounded_preparations_3.pdf (accessed 2015 Apr 1).
26. Food and Drug Administration. FDA draft guidance for industry: adverse event reporting for outsourcing facilities under section 503B of the Federal Food, Drug, and Cosmetic Act. www.fda.gov/downloads/Drugs/GuidanceComplianceRegulatoryInformation/Guidances/UCM434188.pdf (accessed 2015 Apr 1).

Suggested Readings

- Allen LV. Quality assurance in pharmaceutical compounding, part 2: documentation and verification. *Int J Pharm Compound.* 2012; 16:230–4.
- Donnelly AJ, Kienle PC, Lake RT et al. The Drug Quality and Security Act: a new reality for the practice of outsourcing compounded sterile preparations. *Pharm Pract News.* 2014; 41(suppl):1–8.
- Douglass K, Kastango ES. Consolidation of pharmacy compounding services: an alternative to outsourcing. *Int J Pharm Compound.* 2001; 5:140–4.
- Eberts MW, Cecere DA, Mark S. Ensuring the safety of sterile admixtures prepared outside of the institution. *Hosp Pharm.* 2013; 48:248–52.
- Fiebert L. Adjusting to the new world of outsourced compounding. www.pppmag.com/download.php?file=documents/V11N7/pdfs/ppp_1407_outsourcedcompounding.pdf (accessed 2014 Nov 28).
- Gates DM, Smolarek RT, Stevenson JG. Outsourcing the preparation of parenteral nutrient solutions. *Am J Health-Syst Pharm.* 1996; 53:2176–8.
- Kastango ES. Sterile-product preparations: mix or buy? *Int J Pharm Compound.* 2001; 5:59–63.
- Kastango ES. Impact of the US Drug Quality and Security Act. www.pppmag.com/article_print.php?articleid=1595 (accessed 2015 Feb 24).
- Kastango E, Douglass K. Quality standards for large scale sterile compounding facilities (May 2014). www.clinicaliq.com/images/stories/clinicaliq_compounding%20quality%20standards.pdf (accessed 2015 Jan 20).
- Myers CE. History of sterile compounding in U.S. hospitals: learning from the tragic lessons of the past. *Am J Health-Syst Pharm.* 2013; 70:1414–27.
- Ponto JA. Outsourcing radiopharmaceutical services. *Am J Health-Syst Pharm.* 1998; 55:2537.
- Souhrada L. Contract management. *Hospitals.* 1990; 64:66–8.
- Timko RJ, Crooker PE. Pharmaceutical compounding or pharmaceutical manufacturing: a regulatory perspective. *Int J Pharm Compound.* 2014; 18:101–11.
- Wagner M. Basic pitfalls can undermine hospital-service firm relationship. *Mod Healthcare.* 1993; 23:32.

Appendix—Contract Provisions

The following are examples of contract provisions that, among others, the organization and a contractor might adapt as needed and include in a contract, depending on the scope of services being considered. In addition, a contract would include provisions about the specific compounding services to be provided by the contractor. The language in contract provisions should always be adapted to meet the specific needs of the healthcare organization and to comply with the organization's contracting policies and applicable laws and regulations.

In reviewing the following list of suggested contract provisions, attention should be paid to the fact that listed provisions are not intended and should not be considered all-inclusive and do not constitute legal advice but rather are provided solely to convey general information related to legal issues commonly addressed in contracts for the outsourcing of sterile compounding services. The purpose of enumerating the following possible contract provisions is to provide a general understanding of the types of provisions that may be included in a contract. Because laws vary from jurisdiction to jurisdiction and are subject to varying interpretations, healthcare organizations considering outsourcing sterile compounding services should consult with professional legal counsel in their relevant jurisdictions regarding the drafting of contracts.

Accreditation and certification: A contract should include a requirement that services meet or exceed applicable accreditation and certification standards. These include, but are not limited to, the standards (or requirements) of the following organizations:

- Centers for Medicare and Medicaid Services[17]
- Joint Commission[18]
- DNV GL Healthcare[19]
- American Osteopathic Association[20]
- Center for Improvement in Healthcare Quality[21]
- Pharmacy Compounding Accreditation Board[22]
- National Association of Boards of Pharmacy Verified Pharmacy Program[23]

After-hours access: This section describes the process and extent of access to off-site contractor resources after normal business hours.

Choice of law: The contract should state by which state law the contract is governed.

Confidential information: This section describes what information is considered confidential and actions that are required to prevent unauthorized distribution of such information. Both parties must agree to safeguard access to computer databases and patient records to ensure that the patients' rights to privacy and confidentiality are protected. Use of the information should be limited solely to purposes specified in the contract.

Contractor: The outsourcing facility or compounding pharmacy contracted by the healthcare organization to provide sterile compounding services.

Contractor indemnification: This section describes in detail the indemnities the contractor owes the healthcare organization, such as

> Contractor shall indemnify and defend customer and its affiliates, and each of their respective officers, directors, trustees, employees, agents, and representatives (collectively, the "customer indemnities") and hold them harmless from and against any and all losses on account of any claims asserted by a third party in connection with, arising from, or related to (a) any of the acts or omissions related to the services and/or products provided pursuant to this contract attached hereto, (b) breach of contractor's representations and warranties, (c) injuries to persons, including death, or damage to property caused by contractor's agents, servants, or employees, or in any way attributable to contractor's performance of this contract, and (d) any breach of any laws or regulations in connection with contractor's performance of services or provision of products pursuant to the contract.

Contractor reports: The content and regularity of performance reports that the contractor will submit to the organization may be specified.

Contractor's performance responsibilities: The contractor's responsibilities and commitments associated with proper federal (if necessary) and state licensure and regulatory requirements for all the preparations or products it compounds are outlined in this section (e.g., labeling). It further describes the contractor's responsibilities to operate in accordance with applicable Current Good Manufacturing Practices, *United States Pharmacopeia* (*USP*) compounding standards, Drug Enforcement Administration (DEA) requirements (as applicable), and company standard operating procedures.

Customer responsibilities: This section describes the healthcare organization pharmacy's responsibilities for affirming that it has all required state, local, and federal licenses associated with the receipt of services being provided by the contractor. It may also describe the healthcare organization's responsibilities for determining clinical appropriateness of any compounded preparation or product it purchases from the contractor as well as the procedures to be used to ensure the traceability of compounded preparations or products.

Extension of period of performance: Conditions for extending the period of performance should be included in the contract.

Force majeure: This section describes when neither party shall be liable for nonperformance or delays related to causes that are beyond one's reasonable control.

Forms: Responsibilities for the design, approval, purchase, and storage of forms may be assigned.

General provisions: This section outlines a myriad of other contractual items, such as contract assignment, process for adding or changing compounding services, reference to other agreements, and reference to other applicable terms outside the services agreement.

Hazardous drug preparations or products: Responsibilities for ensuring the safety of the organization's staff and patients during delivery and distribution of hazardous drug preparations or products may be assigned. Either the organization or the contractor must provide a hazardous materials handling program, including staff training, that meets ASHP guidelines, Occupational Safety and Health Administration (OSHA) requirements, and *USP* compounding standards.

Indemnification: This section describes specific conditions under which, and responsibilities for which, both parties will hold each other harmless for, and potentially defend, the actions of the other.

Information transfer: This section describes the mechanisms by which the organization transfers orders and other information to the contractor.

Laws, rules, and regulations: Requirements for services to meet or exceed federal, state, and local laws, rules, and regulations may be specified. These include but are not limited to those of the Food and Drug Administration, DEA, OSHA, USP, and the state board of pharmacy. The contractor should maintain (e.g., display, file) the appropriate licenses, permits, and records of equipment maintenance and certification. Any contractor required to be registered as an outsourcing facility must be so registered.

Liability insurance: This section describes the responsibility for maintaining liability insurance coverage. The contract might specify, for example, the specific level and types of liability insurance coverage that the healthcare organization and the contractor must maintain.

Payment terms: This section describes the agreed-upon number of days from receipt of an invoice by the healthcare organization's pharmacy until payment is due to the contractor.

Period of performance: This section specifies the period for which the contractor will provide services to the organization.

Policies and procedures: This section describes the required written policies and procedures covering the outsourced services, all of which should comply with applicable laws, regulations, and accreditation or certification standards. The contract should specify that the policies and procedures must not conflict with those of the organization.

Pricing: The price of each service the hospital pharmacy is interested in purchasing from the contractor, along with conditions and methodology for price increases, is described in this section, which may be an addendum to the contract. Shipping, handling, and delivery charges for both routine and nonroutine deliveries should also be detailed.

Purchase volume requirements: This section establishes a mutual understanding of annual purchase volume commitments between the healthcare organization's pharmacy and the contractor.

Record maintenance: The contract should specify that all pertinent records must be kept for the time required by law and by the organization and describe how, where, and by whom the records will be maintained.

Staff education and training: Responsibilities for required ongoing staff training may be specified. For example, there might be a clause in the contract that the contractor's staff will participate in some of the organization's education and training programs. In addition, the contractor may agree to provide specific training to ensure that all contractor and healthcare organization personnel can perform the duties created by the contractor's services.

Successors: The rights of each party in the event that the healthcare organization or contractor merges or transfers its business or assets to a successor are described in this section.

Term of agreement: This section communicates the length of time the agreement is in effect between the healthcare organization and the contractor, including renewals.

Termination: This section describes how and when the contract will end or be terminated, including early termination. It should also address any penalties that may be appropriate or when the contract may be ended without penalty.

Developed through the ASHP Council on Pharmacy Management and approved by the ASHP Board of Directors on June 6, 2015. These guidelines supersede the ASHP Guidelines on Outsourcing Sterile Compounding Services dated January 14, 2010.

The revision of this document was led by Patricia C. Kienle, M.P.A., FASHP. The contributions of Bona E. Benjamin, B.S.Pharm., to this document are gratefully acknowledged.

The following individuals are gratefully acknowledged for reviewing draft versions of these guidelines (review does not imply endorsement): Darrell Chan, Pharm.D.; Michael Cunningham, Pharm.D.; Kate Douglass, M.S., RN, APN, CRNI; Bernadette Henrichs, Ph.D., CRNA, CCRN; Eric Kastango, M.B.A., FASHP; Michael Koch, M.B.A.; Rich Kruzynski, B.S.Pharm., M.B.A.; Kathy Parrinello, Ph.D., RN; James R. Rinehardt, M.S., FASHP; Douglas Smith, Pharm.D.; Ross W. Thompson, M.S., B.S.Pharm.; and Tom Woller, M.S., FASHP.

The drafters have declared no potential conflicts of interest.

Copyright © 2015, American Society of Health-System Pharmacists, Inc. All rights reserved. Contact ASHP for reprint and permissions requests. This content may not be used for commercial purposes without the express written consent of ASHP.

The bibliographic citation for this document is as follows: American Society of Health-System Pharmacists. ASHP guidelines on outsourcing sterile compounding services. *Am J Health-Syst Pharm.* 2015; 72:1664–75.

Compensation and Reimbursement

2331

SUSTAINABLE BILLING, REIMBURSEMENT, AND PAYMENT MODELS

Source: House of Delegates

To advocate for reimbursement, pay parity, and financially sustainable models related to cognitive services of pharmacist-accountable services, regardless of site of care; further,

To educate the pharmacy workforce and stakeholders about financially sustainable models of care; further,

To advocate that compensation for healthcare services be commensurate with the level of care provided, based on the needs of the patient; further,

To advocate for the development of consistent, transparent billing, reimbursement, and alternative payment model policies and practices by both government and commercial payers.

Rationale

The National Academy of Sciences recommends that payers, including Centers for Medicare & Medicaid Services (CMS), commercial insurers, and self-insured employers shift payment for healthcare services toward a hybrid model that includes fee-for-service and capitated payments, and that these models pay prospectively for interprofessional, integrated, team-based care. Due to lack of federal provider status for pharmacists and subsequent inability to directly bill Medicare as care providers, organizations and practices have become creative in maintaining financial sustainability of pharmacist services. Financial sustainability for services provided by pharmacists has been achieved using a variety of models. Some settings utilize indirect funding, while others take advantage of some of the limited direct insurance billing opportunities to fund pharmacist patient care. Direct billing opportunities vary based on the setting (e.g., hospital-based versus physician-based practices) as well as state-specific laws and regulations. Medicare, Medicaid, and commercial health plans may reimburse pharmacists for certain services, while some will require direct contracting with the health plan. Several states have passed pharmacist state provider status laws or reimbursement parity laws allowing for reimbursement for direct patient care pharmacist services by state Medicaid or commercial plans.

2232

REVENUE CYCLE MANAGEMENT AND REIMBURSEMENT AND PHARMACIST COMPENSATION FOR DRUG PRODUCT DISPENSING

Source: Council on Pharmacy Management

To encourage the pharmacy workforce to serve as leaders in the development and implementation of strategies to optimize medication-related revenue cycle compliance, which includes verification of prior authorization, patient portion of payment, billing, reimbursement, and financial documentation for the healthcare enterprise; further,

To advocate for the development of consistent, transparent billing and reimbursement policies and practices by both government and private payers; further,

To collaborate with payers in developing optimal methods of reimbursing pharmacies and pharmacists for the costs of drug products dispensed, pharmacy and pharmacist services, and associated overhead; further,

To educate the pharmacy workforce and stakeholders about those methods; further,

To advocate that information technology (IT) vendors enhance the capacity and capability of IT systems to support and facilitate medication-related purchasing, billing, and audit functions; further,

To investigate and publish best practices in medication-related revenue cycle compliance and management.

This policy supersedes ASHP policies 1710 and 1807.

Rationale

Pharmacy has an increasingly important role in optimizing revenue capture and avoiding revenue erosion resulting from improper billing or inadequate documentation of medication-related charges. Pharmacy needs to be involved in aspects of medication-related billing, including not just pharmacy drug charges and billing but also contracting and negotiating for carve-outs. Pharmacy leaders need to actively engage senior leadership and collaborate with various departments to ensure organizational success in revenue cycle management.

Recently, organizations have experienced increasing compliance pressures. This pressure comes from many sectors, including Centers for Medicare & Medicaid Services (CMS) programs plus state-specific requirements, third-party payers, and financial intermediaries. These policies impact organizations in two ways: increased requirements before the insurers will pay for a claim, and increased audit pressure to be sure the organizations are billing accurately. The frequency and nature of audits has also been changing. Insurers have increased the use of audits to control costs. Government agencies have also increased the use of audits. CMS has implemented Recovery Audit Contractor (RAC) audits, and the Office of the Inspector General is also auditing organizations. Results of the audits can have significant financial impact on the organization when money needs to be returned based on improper billing or lack of documentation.

Historically, pharmacy departments have great strength in managing supply chain issues. Drug expenditures are typically a significant portion of any hospital's budget, and the pharmacy department is a key leader in managing these expenses. However, pharmacy departments are involved in broader revenue cycle management in variable ways. In some organizations, the billing or patient accounting departments, or in some cases a contracted third-party vendor, handle all billing issues with various degrees of pharmacy department involvement. Accurate billing requires integration of the organization's clinical services, pharmacy, billing, and chargemaster functions. The required elements for proper billing may reside in several systems. As coverage decisions

DOI 10.37573/9781585287048.093

become more complex, pharmacy expertise is increasingly required in the clinical coverage decisions and information integration in order to be successfully reimbursed for services. For the healthcare enterprise to successfully manage compliance and optimize revenue capture there must be effective collaboration among various departments. Pharmacy knowledge and leadership is increasingly required to ensure organizational success in revenue cycle management.

In well-intentioned efforts to reduce healthcare costs, public and private payers often seek to minimize the reimbursement to pharmacies for drug products. Historically, those reimbursements have sometimes exceeded the simple cost of the drug product to reimburse pharmacies for associated costs (e.g., storage, compounding, preparation, dispensing). Each insurer has different requirements for coverage determinations, and coverage decisions have become more complex. More drugs now require prior authorization processes. In some cases, even if the prior authorization process has been used, the charge is denied. Medicare has implemented requirements for self-administered drugs (SADs), and diabetic supplies are now handled under durable medical equipment (DME) requirements, which may require different data elements before a bill is processed. Medicaid requires the National Drug Code (NDC) prior to payment, and billing requirements for Medicare and Medicaid programs are not harmonized.

Healthcare Common Procedure Coding System (HCPCS) codes also need to be attached where indicated. It is challenging to keep up with all the changes. International Classification of Disease 10 (ICD-10) codes further complicate required coding.

Current IT solutions are inadequate and do not effectively facilitate effective billing. Current systems are often not designed to capture all necessary information required to properly document and bill. Even when necessary data is captured, it often resides in different departmental computer systems that are not integrated and designed to share data. There is a need for better IT solutions to facilitate both billing and audits. Greater consistency in billing and reimbursement practices would facilitate greater compliance and enable the development of effective technology solutions to improve billing and reimbursement processes.

Since pharmacy leaders have had variable levels of engagement in revenue cycle management, there is a need for education, tools, and resources related to best practices. Because cost-management efforts are likely to continue to reduce pharmacy reimbursement, other means of compensating pharmacies for those expenses will need to be found, and pharmacists and other stakeholders will require education about those reimbursement methods. In addition, pharmacists and pharmacies need to be reimbursed for professional services associated with management of medications and related patient care. Some pharmacy departments have created a business manager position in part to deal with these issues. This position is often not a pharmacist, but a staff member with business training. New roles for pharmacy technicians have also emerged in this area. ASHP and the Section of Pharmacy Practice Leaders are committed to developing and sharing best practices and providing education to support pharmacists in optimizing reimbursement and pharmacist compensation for drug product dispensing and pharmacy's role in revenue cycle compliance.

2233

VALUE-BASED PURCHASING

Source: Council on Pharmacy Management

To support value-based purchasing reimbursement models when they are appropriately structured to improve healthcare quality, patient satisfaction, and clinical outcomes, and encourage medication error reporting and quality improvement; further,

To affirm the role of pharmacists in actively leading the design and interdisciplinary implementation of medication-related value-based purchasing initiatives; further,

To support pharmacy workforce efforts to ensure safe and appropriate medication use by using data and technology for continuous quality improvement in pharmacy-designed, medication-related value-based purchasing initiatives; further,

To advocate that the Centers for Medicare & Medicaid Services and others guide the development of a common portfolio of measures for potential alignment across regulated programs, federal programs and agencies, and the private sector.

This policy supersedes ASHP policy 1209.

Rationale

Value-based purchasing is one aspect of a portfolio of healthcare reform incentives based on pay-for-performance principles. The Hospital VBP Program adjusts payments to hospitals under the Inpatient Prospective Payment System (IPPS) based on the quality of care they deliver. In April 2021, the Centers for Medicare & Medicaid Services (CMS) announced efforts to (1) readdress 2020 policies during the duration of COVID-19 public health emergency (PHE) and (2) close healthcare equity gaps and provide greater accessibility to care, requesting comments regarding the modernization of the quality measurement enterprise to digital quality measurement. In response to the pandemic, CMS established the New COVID-19 Treatments Add-on Payment (NCTAP) for eligible discharges during the PHE. To enhance the medical workforce in rural and underserved communities, CMS is proposing to distribute 1,000 additional physician residency slots to qualifying hospitals, phasing in 200 slots per year over five years. To address the future of digital quality measurement, CMS is currently reviewing proposals and holding discussions through 2022.

CMS was seeking comment on plans to modernize its quality measurement enterprise by:

- Clarifying the definition of digital quality measures
- Using the Fast Healthcare Interoperability Resources (FHIR) Standard for electronic clinical quality measures that are currently in the various quality programs
- Standardizing data required for quality measures for collection via FHIR-based application programming interfaces
- Leveraging technological opportunities to facilitate digital quality measurement
- Better supporting data aggregation
- Developing a common portfolio of measures for potential alignment across CMS regulated programs, federal programs and agencies, and the private sector

ASHP recognizes the pharmacist's leadership role while explicitly acknowledging the interdisciplinary nature of initiatives designed to achieve value-based purchasing measures. Often, however, active membership on the design team does not include pharmacy. Because there needs to be thoughtful consideration of what pharmacy can reasonably control within an organization in terms of achievable tactics to improve a specific goal, pharmacy leaders need to engage their entire departments in these efforts to ensure that there is a concerted approach toward improving patient care. Finally, as value-based purchasing program proliferate, CMS and other stakeholder organizations need to guide the development of a common portfolio of measures for potential alignment across regulated programs, federal programs and agencies, and the private sector.

2020

CARE-COMMENSURATE REIMBURSEMENT

Source: Council on Public Policy

To advocate that reimbursement for healthcare services be commensurate with the level of care provided, based on the needs of the patient.

Rationale

As a means to reduce costs for federal programs, the Centers for Medicare & Medicaid Services (CMS) has been aggressively expanding efforts to reduce reimbursement at certain sites of care. Specifically, CMS has cut reimbursement for care services provided at hospital outpatient departments to match the rate paid physicians' offices. CMS refers to this policy as "site-neutral payment." On the basis of site neutrality, CMS also extended cuts to hospital reimbursement for drugs purchased under the 340B drug discount program to hospital outpatient departments. Private payers have also sought to impose site-neutral payment policies.

Reimbursement for services should reflect unique factors associated with a site of care. Hospital outpatient departments are held to higher quality standards with more oversight than what is often required for alternate sites of care. In addition to the Medicare Conditions of Participation, hospital outpatient departments must meet accreditation, United States Pharmacopeia (USP), and even Food and Drug Administration requirements. These standards result in high-quality patient care, but at a higher cost than what can be accomplished without the oversight.

Patients may also derive benefits from receiving care at a hospital outpatient department. Hospital care delivery models are crafted to ensure that patients receive the highest quality care possible. For hospitals that belong to an accountable care organization or are otherwise part of an integrated network, seeing patients at the outpatient department allows providers to better coordinate care, resulting in improved patient outcomes. Care provided in this setting is often highly complex and complementary to acute care that the patient receives from the hospital. Drastic cuts to hospital outpatient reimbursement could endanger the long-term viability of these care delivery models—if services are cut or outpatient departments are closed, patient access will suffer.

1814

DIRECT AND INDIRECT REMUNERATION FEES

Source: Council on Public Policy

To advocate that payers and pharmacy benefit managers be prohibited from recovering direct and indirect remuneration fees from pharmacies on adjudicated dispensing claims; further,

To oppose the application of plan-level quality measures on specific providers, such as participating pharmacies.

This policy was reviewed in 2023 by the Council on Public Policy and by the Board of Directors and was found to still be appropriate.

Rationale

Direct and indirect remuneration (DIR) fees are a growing concern among pharmacies that dispense medications in a retail pharmacy or outpatient clinic setting. Created under the Medicare Part D Program, DIR fees were originally intended as a way for the Centers for Medicare & Medicaid Services (CMS) to account for the true cost of the drug dispensed, including manufacturer rebates and pharmacy concessions. Often these rebates and concessions were unknown until the drug was dispensed and the claim adjudicated. Recently, a concerning trend has emerged in which pharmacy benefit managers (PBMs) charge DIR fees to pharmacy providers, applying their own plan performance measures as a way to assess fees on pharmacies dispensing covered Part D drugs. These fees are problematic for the following reasons:

- The fees are arbitrary and appear to result from an unintended application of measures meant for total plan performance as opposed to pharmacy-level metrics.
- The quality measures applied tend to be based on maintenance medications such as blood pressure or medications used to treat diabetes. These measures were never intended to be applied to specialty medications, or other specialized disease states such as oncology, yet PBMs assess DIR fees against the gross reimbursement for all prescriptions received by pharmacy providers, not just maintenance medications.
- PBMs are not required to define, justify, or explain to providers or to CMS the rationale or process for imposing their DIR fees.

Pharmacies providing specialty medications have been especially hard hit by DIR fees, due to the fee structure. DIR fees can be a flat rate (a fixed amount per dollar per claim) or a percentage (typically 3-9%) of the total reimbursement per claim. When the percentage-based structure is applied, the fees increase markedly for specialty drugs, which are typically much more expensive than maintenance medications.

Even more disturbing is that the fees are assessed retroactively, sometimes months after the claim has been adjudicated, providing no recourse for the pharmacy impacted by the assessment. Questions also remain as to whether Part D plan sponsors have the authority to assess DIR fees on pharmacies. There are no references to DIR fees collected on pharmacies in either the Medicare Modernization Act or corresponding CMS regulations.

DIR fees have led to higher cost-sharing responsibilities for Medicare beneficiaries, causing more of them to enter the Part D "donut hole" in which they are solely responsible for the cost of a drug. Because of higher costs, adherence rates tend to be lower among beneficiaries in the donut hole. These higher costs are a perverse result contrary to the very reason DIR fees were created—passing savings onto beneficiaries.

Pharmacies are not alone in their concern. In January 2017, CMS published a fact sheet expressing concern over DIR fees and cited them as contributing to increased drug costs, beneficiary out-of-pocket spending, and Medicare spending overall. ASHP supports legislation that would address the problem of DIR fees. For example, H.R. 1038/S.413, the Improving Transparency and Accuracy in Medicare Part D Drug Spending Act, would prohibit Medicare Part D plan sponsors from retroactively reducing payment on clean claims submitted by pharmacies under Medicare Part D.

1301

PAYER PROCESSES FOR PAYMENT AUTHORIZATION AND COVERAGE VERIFICATION

Source: Council on Pharmacy Management

To advocate that public and private payers collaborate with each other and with health care providers to create standardized and efficient processes for authorizing payment or verifying coverage for care; further,

To advocate that payment authorization and coverage verification processes (1) facilitate communication among patients, providers, and payers prior to therapy; (2) provide timely payment or coverage decisions; (3) facilitate access to information that allows the pharmacist to provide prescribed medications and medication therapy management to the patient; and (4) foster continuity in patient care.

This policy was reviewed in 2023 by the Council on Pharmacy Management and by the Board of Directors and was found to still be appropriate.

Rationale

Patients and health care providers are required to navigate an array of payment requirements from private and public payers. Private insurers enforce their own prior authorization procedures, state Medicaid programs have their individual program requirements, and Medicare has its local and national coverage determinations. These payment authorization and verification processes vary considerably from payer to payer and are time consuming and needlessly complex. The required data, forms of documentation required, submission processes, coverage verification procedures, and delivery of approval vary widely among payers. These processes are often not integrated into the patient-care process and require manual documentation and submission. The lack of timely review and approval may delay patient care. Payment authorization and verification processes should effectively facilitate communication among both patients and providers, should be standardized and automated, and should result in timely decisions that do not disrupt patient care.

0206

REIMBURSEMENT FOR UNLABELED USES OF FDA-APPROVED DRUG PRODUCTS

Source: Council on Administrative Affairs

To support third-party reimbursement for FDA-approved drug products appropriately prescribed for unlabeled uses.

This policy was reviewed in 2022 by the Council on Pharmacy Management and by the Board of Directors and was found to still be appropriate.

Rationale

Off-label use of drug products includes any use of a drug product for a diagnosis, combination with other medications, dosage, frequency, route of administration, place in therapy, or patient population that is not specifically approved by the U.S. Food and Drug Administration (FDA) and contained in the drug labeling. Drug products' labeling often fails to represent the most current therapeutic information, because making changes to FDA labeling is a time-consuming and expensive process and medical knowledge is constantly expanding based on evolving evidence.

Once a drug is FDA-approved for a specific indication, it can legally be used for any indication, and off-label prescribing is common. Researchers have conservatively estimated that it accounts for 10–20% of all prescriptions, but the practice is much more common in specific patient populations (e.g., children, geriatric patients, and patients with life-threatening or terminal conditions).

In many clinical situations, off-label use represents a therapeutic approach that has been extensively studied, is supported by the medical literature, and is most appropriate for the patient. Failure to recognize these circumstances or, more importantly, regarding such uses as unapproved or experimental, may restrict patient access to effective drug therapies. Some degree of flexibility must be maintained to optimize patient outcomes and allow for individualized care. While the ultimate responsibility for the safety and efficacy of off-label use resides with the prescriber, hospital and health-system pharmacy and therapeutics committees often develop policies and procedures for managing off-label medication use, with the goal of providing access to the most appropriate, effective treatment for each patient. Although a distinction must be made between evidence-based and inappropriate off-label use, the clinical judgment of healthcare practitioners and experts, as reflected in peer-reviewed publications, clinical practice guidelines, and approved compendia, provides better guidance than FDA labeling alone.

Human Resources

2209

DRUG TESTING AS PART OF DIVERSION PREVENTION PROGRAMS

Source: Council on Public Policy

To advocate for the use of pre-employment and random or for-cause drug testing during employment based on defined criteria and with appropriate testing validation procedures; further,

To support employer- or government-sponsored drug diversion prevention programs that include a policy and process that promote the recovery of impaired individuals; further,

To advocate that employers use validated testing panels that have demonstrated effectiveness detecting commonly abused or illegally used substances.

This policy supersedes ASHP policy 1717.

Rationale

Controlled substance diversion and abuse has reached the attention at the highest levels in the U.S., with even the White House weighing in on the crisis. In the past 4–5 years, the Drug Enforcement Administration has levied large fines on chain drugstores, drug wholesalers, and even major hospitals. Pharmacy managers and pharmacists-in-charge have increasing responsibility of ensuring controlled substance management and storage across large healthcare organizations. There is an increased risk to organizations as acquisitions of physician office practices, clinics, and other nonhospital-based business units continue, and many challenges exist for healthcare institutions in managing controlled substances.

ASHP recognizes that drug testing job applicants and employees whose responsibilities may bring them into contact with controlled substances is an essential element of diversion prevention programs and promotes worker well-being. Pre-employment and random or for-cause drug testing should be performed based on defined criteria, with appropriate testing validation procedures, and have demonstrated effectiveness detecting commonly abused or illegally used substances. In addition, drug testing should be supported by an employee addiction recovery program, as outlined in the ASHP Statement on the Pharmacist's Role in Substance Abuse Prevention, Education, and Assistance.

2217

WORKFORCE DIVERSITY

Source: Council on Education and Workforce Development

To affirm that a diverse and inclusive workforce contributes to improved health equity and health outcomes; further,

To advocate for the development and retention of a workforce whose background, perspectives, and experiences reflect the diverse patients for whom care is provided; further,

To advocate that institutions incorporate diversity, equity, and inclusion initiatives into daily practices and strategic plans.

This policy supersedes ASHP policy 1705.

Rationale

As the U.S. becomes more heterogeneous, the pharmacy workforce should reflect and respond to this increasingly diverse patient base. An inclusive pharmacy workforce is best able to positively impact the health and wellness of patients for whom care is provided. According to the Institute of Medicine, increasing diversity among healthcare providers is associated with improved access to care for racial and ethnic minority patients, greater patient choice and satisfaction, and better educational experiences for health professions students (Smedley BD, Butler AS, Bristow LR, eds. In the nation's compelling interest: ensuring diversity in the health-care workforce. Washington, DC: National Academies Press; 2004). Diversity in the pharmacy workforce includes, but is not limited to, the categories of sexual identity and gender expression, age, national origin, socioeconomic origin, ethnicity, culture, gender, race, religion, and physical, sensory, or mental disability. A diverse pharmacy workforce will provide the best care for all patients. Recognizing the positive impact of diversity, equity, and inclusion (DEI) on patient outcomes, it is important for the pharmacy workforce to incorporate DEI initiatives in strategic plans, communications, and hiring and retention practices across the pharmacy enterprise.

2234

FINANCIAL MANAGEMENT SKILLS

Source: Council on Pharmacy Management

To foster the systematic and ongoing development of management skills for the pharmacy workforce in the areas of (1) health-system economics, (2) business plan development, (3) financial analysis, (4) metrics for clinical and distributive services, (5) pharmacoeconomic analysis, (6) diversified pharmacy services, (7) compensation for pharmacists' patient-care services, and (8) revenue cycle compliance and management; further,

To encourage colleges of pharmacy to incorporate these management areas in course work, electives (e.g., financial and managerial accounting), and experiential education; further,

To promote the growth of dual PharmD/MBA degree programs, postgraduate training, and other degree programs focused on financial management, and similar certificates or concentrations; further,

To encourage financial management skills development in pharmacy residency training programs; further,

To provide education for new practitioners and student pharmacists on foundational skills for business administration and personal financial management; further,

To promote education on financial management for other members of the pharmacy workforce (e.g., pharmacy technicians, data scientists, inventory specialists, department business managers).

This policy supersedes ASHP policy 1207.

Rationale

Revenue cycle compliance and management represent an increasingly important aspect of the business operations of

DOI 10.37573/9781585287048.094

hospitals and health systems. Pharmacy leaders must exert leadership in managing medication-related revenue cycle compliance in order to ensure financial success of the healthcare enterprise. The development of foundational skills in financial literacy and business management is critical for many members of the pharmacy workforce (e.g., residents, new practitioners, student pharmacists, pharmacy technicians, and support staff such as data scientists, inventory specialists, or department business managers) to gain perspectives on contemporary management techniques and fiscal solvency. Some ways to achieve this are through (1) college of pharmacy curriculum (e.g., dual Pharm.D./M.B.A. degree or similar programs) or experiential program requirements; (2) degree programs with a concentration in financial management; (3) during residency training as incorporated projects; or (4) as a certificate program for student pharmacists, residents, and new practitioners. Pharmacy leaders must also develop and maintain knowledge in this area to sharpen skills in planning, forecasting, decision-making, and implementation.

2237

UNIVERSAL VACCINATION FOR VACCINE-PREVENTABLE DISEASES IN THE HEALTHCARE WORKFORCE

Source: Council on Pharmacy Practice

To support policies and mandates that promote universal vaccination for preventable infectious diseases among healthcare workers, including all members of the pharmacy workforce, as a safeguard to patient and public health; further,

To encourage the use of evidence-based risk assessments to determine inclusions in and exemptions from mandatory vaccine requirements; further,

To support employers in establishing and implementing mandatory vaccine requirements for healthcare workers if evidence-based risk assessments determine they are safe and promote patient and public health; further,

To urge healthcare organizations to have policies that address additional infection prevention practices required for exempted healthcare workers; further,

To develop tools, education, and other resources to promote vaccine confidence, increase vaccination rates, and minimize vaccine-preventable diseases among healthcare workers.

This policy supersedes ASHP policies 2138 and 2140.

Rationale

Vaccine-preventable diseases (VPDs) pose a threat to vulnerable patients, the healthcare workforce, and public health. Vaccines are effective in protecting the healthcare workforce and the patients they care for and with whom they interact.

Voluntary vaccination of healthcare workers (HCWs), supported by employer-offered strategies, increases vaccination rates to some extent. For example, the Centers for Disease Control and Prevention (CDC) estimates that in the 2019-2020 season, approximately 80% of healthcare workers were vaccinated against influenza, with rates over 90% among hospital employees, despite the fact that only approximately 70% of hospitals require an annual influenza vaccination and the CDC has recommended influenza vaccinations for HCWs since 1981.

Mandatory vaccination requirements, in contrast, carry heavier weight and can result in near-universal vaccination rates (Schumacher S et al. Increasing influenza vaccination coverage in healthcare workers: a review on campaign strategies and their effect. *Infection*. 2021; 49: 387–99. **https://doi.org/10.1007/s15010-020-01555-9**). The effectiveness of the mandatory approach has led to HCW vaccination requirements from the Occupational Safety and Health Administration, recommendations from the Centers for Disease Control and Prevention (CDC), policy endorsements from numerous professional organizations, and quality measures for federal and commercial payer reporting programs. For example, the CDC Advisory Committee on Immunization Practices proposes recommendations for the immunization of healthcare workforce based on (1) those diseases for which routine vaccination or documentation of immunity is recommended for healthcare personnel because of risks to them in their work settings and, should healthcare personnel become infected, to the patients they serve; and (2) those diseases for which vaccination of healthcare personnel might be indicated in certain circumstances. The current list of VPDs in which healthcare personnel are considered to be at substantial risk for acquiring or transmitting and in which vaccination is recommended includes hepatitis B, influenza, measles, mumps, rubella, pertussis, and varicella. In the future, this list may include vaccination against SARS-CoV-2.

In its recommendations, the CDC considers HCWs to include (but not be limited to) physicians, nurses, nursing assistants, therapists, technicians, emergency medical service personnel, dental personnel, pharmacists, laboratory personnel, autopsy personnel, students and trainees, contractual staff not employed by the healthcare facility, and persons (e.g., clerical, dietary, housekeeping, laundry, security, maintenance, administrative, billing, and volunteers) not directly involved in patient care but potentially exposed to infectious agents that can be transmitted to and from HCWs and patients.

The vaccination-related policies of various healthcare professional organizations contain similar themes. These policies recognize that mandatory vaccination policies improve vaccination rates, protecting patients and the healthcare workforce; acknowledge the limited circumstances that may preclude an HCW from being vaccinated (e.g., medical contraindications and legally required religious exemptions); express support for following evidence-based practices in determining which vaccines should be mandatory; and support education of the healthcare workforce on the benefits of vaccination.

2103

PROFESSIONAL DEVELOPMENT AS A RETENTION TOOL

Source: Council on Education and Workforce Development

To recognize that pharmacy workforce development is an essential component of staff recruitment, retention, and wellbeing; further,

To recognize that pharmacy workforce development encompasses more than formal education programs and includes informal learning among colleagues, mentoring, participation in activities of professional organizations, and other types of learning; further,

To encourage healthcare executives to support pharmacy workforce development programs, including leadership succession planning, as an important benefit that aids in recruiting and retaining qualified staff; further,

To support healthcare executives with pharmacy workforce development by providing educational programs, services, and resources.

This policy supersedes ASHP policy 0112.

Rationale

Workforce development can take many forms, including formal education, informal mentoring, participation in certification programs, career ladder implementation, and expanded experiences. The need for job growth and career advancement is an important motivator for job satisfaction among those entering the workforce, such as student pharmacists and residents. Evidence suggests that staff development programs are associated with increased pharmacist retention. There is also a growing need to provide education on topics, such as clinical management, that are not taught in education and training programs and nurture the workforce to provide continuous succession planning.

2129

PROFESSIONAL IDENTITY FORMATION

Source: Council on Education and Workforce Development

To encourage the pharmacy workforce and pharmacy education and training programs to foster professional identity formation, described as the process of developing a commitment to: (1) high professional standards of pharmacy practice, (2) high personal standards of integrity and competence, (3) service to humanity, (4) a just and inclusive healthcare system and society, (5) analytical thinking and ethical reasoning, (6) continuing professional development, (7) acquisition of personal leadership skills, (8) development of effective interpersonal skills, (9) maintenance of personal well-being and resiliency, and (10) membership and participation in professional organizations.

This policy supersedes ASHP policy 1113.

Rationale

The terms "professionalism" and "professional identity" are sometimes mistakenly used interchangeably. Professionalism is defined by behaviors that are often outwardly visible (e.g., credentialing, continuing education, efforts to advance the profession). In contrast, professional identity formation (PIF) is defined as the process of internalizing a profession's core values and beliefs. PIF incorporates the three domains of thinking, feeling, and acting. PIF in pharmacy may be described as the process of developing a commitment to the 10 listed characteristics.

Pharmacy professionals and educators have a direct or indirect responsibility to support the growth and success of others in the pharmacy workforce through mentorship and modelling. As pharmacy professionals interact with learners, new practitioners, and even seasoned colleagues, they have the ability to model professional behavior, integrity, ethical standards, and service to the community. Pharmacy professionals who serve in formal or informal leadership roles are in a unique position to mentor others in leadership skills. Pharmacy professionals should mentor others in the various career paths they may pursue as well as encourage them to elevate their practice level and education.

Some of the barriers to PIF include mentors and preceptors being pressured into a role rather than being allowed to decide whether they choose to do so voluntarily, increased pharmacy workload, and staff burnout. Developing student professionalism (sometimes referred to as "professional socialization") has been part of pharmacy education for decades, but a broader focus on PIF more generally will better serve the profession of pharmacy during a time of practice transformation than the current approach to teaching professionalism. Colleges of pharmacy, other providers of education and training programs, and employers could promote PIF by providing mentorship programs and other resources.

2130

CAREER OPPORTUNITIES FOR PHARMACY TECHNICIANS

Source: Council on Education and Workforce Development

To promote pharmacy technicians as valuable contributors to healthcare delivery; further,

To advocate that pharmacy technicians complete an education and training program accredited by ASHP and the Accreditation Council for Pharmacy Education (ACPE), and maintain Pharmacy Technician Certification Board certification; further,

To advocate that pharmacy technicians complete ACPE-approved certificate programs that provide training for their current or anticipated roles; further,

To develop and disseminate information about career and training opportunities that enhance the recruitment and retention of qualified pharmacy technicians; further,

To encourage employers to offer career advancement opportunities (e.g., career ladders) for pharmacy technicians; further,

To urge compensation for pharmacy technicians commensurate with advanced roles and responsibilities.

This policy supersedes ASHP policy 1610.

Rationale

As the responsibilities of pharmacy technicians expand and their role as a vital member of the healthcare team is recognized, it is imperative that pharmacy technicians be well trained and competent to perform those responsibilities. Pharmacists cannot provide quality patient care without the support of competent pharmacy technicians. To support pharmacists and promote retention, it is important that pharmacy technician positions be viewed as a career and not just a job. Pharmacy technicians should be provided opportunities for life-long advancement and compensated appropriately for advanced roles that they assume. There is current ASHP policy 1912 that addresses the Pharmacy Technician Training and Certification, which advocates for the education, training, and certification for new pharmacy technicians. This covers a need for the on-going professional development and career advancement for pharmacy technicians.

2131

ZERO TOLERANCE OF HARASSMENT, DISCRIMINATION, AND MALICIOUS BEHAVIORS

Source: Council on Education and Workforce Development

To assert that the pharmacy workforce has a right to expect and responsibility to ensure a profession in which all individuals are treated with respect and civility, with zero tolerance for all forms of harassment, discrimination, and malicious behaviors; further,

To commit to a culture of responsibility and accountability within the profession, and promote anti-retaliation policies and timely follow-up; further,

To foster the development of tools, education, and other resources to ensure such a culture.

Rationale

The Code of Ethics for Pharmacists states that "A pharmacist acts with honesty and integrity in professional relationships." The ASHP Statement on Professionalism includes among the elements of professionalism pride in and service to the profession, conscience and trustworthiness, and ethically sound decision-making. All forms of discrimination (e.g., race, color, sex, national origin, religious, sexual orientation/identity, age, disability), harassment (including sexual harassment), and malicious behaviors such as bullying, intimidation, or exploitation go against the core beliefs of the profession. All members of the pharmacy workforce have a professional responsibility to create and sustain a culture of responsibility and accountability within the profession in which all individuals are treated with respect and civility, with zero tolerance of harassment and discrimination.

A culture of responsibility and accountability requires that employers and organizations establish mechanisms for retaliation-free reporting of harassment and discrimination, and that such reports receive timely follow-up. For such a culture to thrive, the pharmacy workforce must recognize its professional obligation to not only follow institutional policies regarding prevention, reporting, and consequences for such behaviors but to seek out ways to improve the effectiveness of those policies and procedures. This culture of responsibility and accountability includes the workplace and learning environments but extends even to such personal but quasi-public conduct as interactions on social media. As stated in the ASHP Statement on the Use of Social Media by Pharmacy Professionals, the "higher standards of conduct expected of professionals, even in personal behavior" imply that "[p]ostings on social media should be subject to the same professional standards and ethical considerations as other personal or public interactions."

As stated in the ASHP Statement on Professionalism, "[o]ne of the fundamental services of a professional is recruiting, nurturing, and securing new practitioners to that profession's ideals and mission." Formal and informal mentorship relationships are fundamental to the growth and health of any profession, and abuses of those positions of trust are especially injurious to victims and the profession. These relationships should be subjected to the strictest scrutiny and oversight to ensure they are held to the highest standards of conduct.

To further the goal of creating and sustaining a culture of responsibility and accountability regarding harassment and discrimination, ASHP commits to developing tools, education, and other resources to help members, employers, and other organizations address these important issues.

2133

OPTIMAL PHARMACY STAFFING

Source: Council on Pharmacy Management

To encourage pharmacy leaders to work in collaboration with physicians, nurses, health-system administrators, and others to outline key pharmacist services that are essential to safe and effective patient care and employee engagement; further,

To encourage pharmacy leaders to be innovative in their approach and to factor into their thinking the potential benefits and risks of flexible staffing models, telehealth practices, legal requirements, accreditation standards, professional standards of practice, and the resources and technology available in individual settings; further,

To encourage pharmacy leaders to develop contingency plans for changes in staffing models to accommodate rapid changes in the healthcare environment and the needs of patients and staff; further,

To encourage pharmacy leaders to develop key performance indicators to support safe staffing models.

This policy supersedes ASHP policy 2034.

Rationale

The advancement of the pharmacy profession over the past decade has prepared and positioned pharmacists to care for complex patients and adapt to the dynamic and rapidly progressive field of medicine. Throughout the years, an increased involvement of pharmacists in specialty areas such as transplant, critical care, oncology, and pain and palliative care has been observed. Therefore, it is imperative that such advancement is considered when developing staffing models, in order to ensure the pharmacy workforce is appropriately allocated for the provision of consistent, safe, and high-quality patient care.

The complexity of patient care will continue to increase, and with that, so will the expected responsibilities, opportunities, and skills of the pharmacy workforce. Consequently, pharmacists engaged in direct patient care are encouraged to pursue and maintain their training and credentialing in order to continue to enhance their competency, skills, and participation in innovative practice. The expansion and dynamic nature of the pharmacy profession requires new approaches to explore flexible staffing models to avoid a stagnant practice, encourage continual advancement, and accommodate the evolving priorities of the pharmacy workforce.

The development and implementation of flexible staffing models can enable pharmacists to engage in further professional development and career advancement (e.g., training in areas of specialization, degree programs) and enjoy a more stable work-life integration experience. Recently, more attention has been drawn to burnout, resilience, and job satisfaction among the pharmacy workforce. Research has shown that pharmacists are reporting increased job stress over the previous years and that approximately 53% of pharmacists are reporting a high degree of burnout, which can consequently threaten patient safety. Therefore, there is an imperative to develop staffing models to meet staff members' changing priorities and provide additional flexibility in the workplace. Implementation of flexible staffing models could improve performance and promote employee engagement in the workplace. Pharmacy leaders should be committed to maintaining high-quality and consistent patient care services and to also promote models that balance patient care with staff priorities.

Various options to consider when exploring flexible staffing models include telehealth practices, remote order review and verification (i.e., telecommuting), and productivity measures to ensure patient census is well distributed among pharmacists in charge of providing clinical services. Another concept related to flexible staffing models is leveraging pharmacy technicians' roles to support pharmacist engagement in direct patient care activities. Some institutions have explored data-driven, staffing-to-demand models based on real-time patient-volume metrics. The concept is to allocate staff to tasks based on the current workload, which is evaluated daily. Other institutions are also utilizing metrics such as number of doses dispensed at a certain point in time and volume of order verification throughout the day in order to divide patient care units evenly among pharmacists that perform order verification or provide clinical services. Flexible staffing models should support the following principles:

- Sufficient qualified staff must exist to ensure safe and effective patient care.
- During periods of staff shortages, pharmacists must exert leadership in directing resources to services that are the most essential to safe and effective patient care.
- Within their own organizations, pharmacists should develop contingency plans to be implemented in the event of insufficient staff—actions that will preserve services that are the most essential to safe and effective patient care and will, as necessary, curtail other services.
- Among the essential services for safe and effective patient care is pharmacist review of new medication orders before the administration of first doses; in settings where patient acuity requires that reviews of new medication orders be conducted at any hour and similar medication-use decisions be made at any hour, there must be 24-hour access to a pharmacist.

The COVID-19 pandemic and the ensuing reduction in elective procedures, routine visits, and admissions amplified the emphasis on flexing staff to volume. To support fiscal solvency during and in the aftermath of the pandemic, organizations had to quickly pivot and align staff to accommodate shifts in volume, resulting in redesigned staffing models to optimize scheduling. These models have included a mix of onsite and remote offering of services to perform synchronous and asynchronous work in a more efficient manner, as well as staff furloughs. Flexing pharmacy staffing models have been previously described, such as pharmacy staffing-to-demand models; alternative work schedules; and productivity monitoring to guide hiring and staffing decisions.

Other healthcare disciplines (e.g., nursing) have historically utilized flexible staffing models to optimize services, reduce the risk of adverse events, and improve patient outcomes. The different models explored by nursing include patient ratio, key performance indicators, patient acuity, collaborative staffing, and supplemental staffing models. There is limited literature on the use of flexible staffing models, but the concept is being explored by various health-system pharmacy departments.

2011

CREDENTIALING AND PRIVILEGING BY REGULATORS, PAYERS, AND PROVIDERS OF COLLABORATIVE PRACTICE

Source: Council on Public Policy

To recommend the use of credentialing and privileging in a manner consistent with other healthcare professionals to assess a pharmacist's competence to engage in patient care services.

This policy supersedes ASHP policy 1907.

Rationale

Credentialing and privileging processes are key to ensuring clinician competence to provide safe and effective patient care. They are also critical elements to securing reimbursement for healthcare services. ASHP opposes the development of credentialing or privileging processes by government agencies or payers without significant pharmacist input. We recognize that state laws, state boards of pharmacy, and payers will each approach credentialing and privileging differently, making a consistent process extremely beneficial. When possible, pharmacists should be included as providers in medical staff bylaws.

1916

INTIMIDATING OR DISRUPTIVE BEHAVIOR

Source: Council on Pharmacy Management

To affirm the professional responsibility of the pharmacist to ensure patient and workplace safety by communicating with other healthcare personnel to clarify and improve medication management; further,

To advocate that hospitals and health systems adopt zero-tolerance policies for intimidating or disruptive behaviors in their institutions; further,

To encourage hospitals and health systems to develop and implement education and training programs for all healthcare personnel to encourage effective communication, set expectations for standards of conduct, promote use of de-escalation techniques, and discourage intimidating or disruptive behaviors; further,

To encourage colleges of pharmacy and residency training programs to incorporate training in communications and managing intimidating or disruptive behaviors; further,

To collaborate with other organizations to advocate codes of conduct that do not allow intimidating or disruptive behavior in hospitals and health systems; further,

To encourage hospitals and health systems to adopt processes for identification and reporting of intimidating or disruptive behaviors to evaluate and mitigate unacceptable behaviors in a timely and effective manner.

This policy supersedes ASHP policy 0919.

Rationale

Intimidating or disruptive behaviors can lead to medical errors, contribute to poor patient satisfaction, increase costs, and cause staff turnover. Such behaviors range from passive behaviors such as providers refusing to answer questions or return pages to use of condescending language to overt actions such as verbal outbursts or physical threats. The Institute for Safe Medication Practices conducted a national survey regarding intimidation in the workplace in 2003 and conducted a follow-up survey in 2013 for comparison.

There has been no reduction between 2003 and 2013 in the percentage of respondents who were aware of a medication error during the year in which disrespectful behavior played a role. In addition, healthcare workers face an increased risk of work-related assaults resulting primarily from intimidating or disruptive behavior of patients and their caregivers or family members. Disruptive behavior, including interference with treatment plans, vulgar language, and threatening statements, can impede a healthcare worker's ability to provide safe and effective care. While such behavior is often overlooked, underreported, or considered to be part of the job, it can also lead to more serious confrontations. Unfortunately, there is no clear way to identify patients or family members who will be disruptive to healthcare personnel, so every patient and family member must be treated with the same level of caution.

According to the Bureau of Labor Statistics and National Crime Victimization Survey, more assaults occur in the healthcare and social services industries than in any other industry. For healthcare workers, assaults comprise 10-11% of workplace injuries involving days away from work, compared with 3% of injuries of all private sector employees. Further, it has been identified that workplace violence can harm a person's intrinsic sense of self-worth and confidence, which can result in physical symptoms including headaches, anxiety, and depression. The American Nurses Association and the American Medical Association have taken positions concerning violence against healthcare workers and are actively promoting solutions to address the issue.

ASHP believes organizations should develop training programs to discourage disruptive behaviors and to train employees in handling disruptive situations, including de-escalation techniques, and colleges of pharmacy and residency training programs should also provide such training. These organizational efforts will help with compliance with The Joint Commission leadership standard on disruptive behavior (LD.03.01.01), which suggests that healthcare organizations should "educate all team members—both physicians and non-physician staff—on appropriate professional behavior defined by the organization's code of conduct. The code and education should emphasize respect. Include training in basic business etiquette (particularly phone skills) and people skills."

1828

PROMOTING THE IMAGE OF PHARMACISTS AND PHARMACY TECHNICIANS

Source: Council on Education and Workforce Development

To promote the professional image of pharmacists and pharmacy technicians who work in all settings of health systems to the general public, public policymakers, payers, other healthcare professionals, and healthcare organization decision-makers.

This policy supersedes ASHP policy 0703.

Rationale

The success of ASHP's advocacy efforts relies on public perception of the pharmacists, student pharmacists, and pharmacy technicians we represent. Promoting the image of pharmacy, which consistently ranks among the most trusted professions, is an ongoing priority for ASHP. In addition, as stated in the ASHP Statement on Professionalism, one of the fundamental services of a professional is recruiting, nurturing, and securing new practitioners to that profession's ideals and mission. The recruitment of pharmacists and pharmacy technicians begins in high school or even earlier, when students are exploring potential careers. ASHP is committed to highlighting opportunities for pharmacy careers in all health-system settings to maintain a pool of quality candidates for those careers.

1415

CREDENTIALING, PRIVILEGING, AND COMPETENCY ASSESSMENT

Source: Council on Education and Workforce Development

To support the use of post-licensure credentialing, privileging, and competency assessment to practice pharmacy as a direct patient-care practitioner; further,

To advocate that all post-licensure pharmacy credentialing programs meet the guiding principles established by the Council on Credentialing in Pharmacy; further,

To recognize that pharmacists are responsible for maintaining competency to practice in direct patient care.

This policy was reviewed in 2019 by the Council on Education and Workforce Development and by the Board of Directors and was found to still be appropriate.

Rationale

Pharmacists engaged in direct patient care should possess the education, training, and experience necessary to function effectively, efficiently, and responsibly in that role. As their role in direct patient care has increased, pharmacists have recognized that they are independently responsible for maintaining their credentials and competencies. Currently, no specific objective measures are available for determining competence to provide direct patient care, however. Until such measures are available, pharmacists can establish their competence through post-licensure education, training, and certification, and health care organizations can ensure that practitioners with the right skills are matched to the scope of practice expected through competency assessment and their credentialing and privileging processes.

Although many avenues of credentialing and competency assessment currently exist, hospital and health-system credentialing and privileging of pharmacists is a relatively recent phenomenon. ASHP and the Council on Credentialing in Pharmacy (CCP) are in agreement that pharmacists should be expected to participate in credentialing and privileging processes to ensure they have attained and maintain competency to provide the scope of services and quality of care that are required in their practices (Council on Credentialing in Pharmacy Guiding Principles for Post-Licensure Credentialing of Pharmacists, February 2011.) To ensure the quality of post-licensure credentialing programs, they should be required to adhere to the guiding principles developed by CCP.

Note that several definitions are integral to proper understanding of this policy (definitions taken from the Council on Credentialing in Pharmacy, Credentialing in Pharmacy: A Resource Paper, except as noted):

Credential: documented evidence of professional qualifications.

Credentialing: (1) the process of granting a credential, and (2) the process by which an organization obtains, verifies, and accesses and individual's qualifications to provide patient care services.

Privileging: the process by which an oversight body of a health care organization or other appropriate provider body, having reviewed an individual health care provider's credentials and performance and found them satisfactory, authorizes that individual to perform a specific scope of patient care services within that setting.

Competence: The ability of the individual to perform his/her duties accurately, make correct judgments, and interact appropriately with patients and colleagues.

Competency: A distinct knowledge, skill, attitude, or value that is essential to the practice of a profession.

Direct patient care: involves the pharmacist's direct observation of the patient and his or her (i.e., the pharmacist's) contributions to the selection, modification, and monitoring of patient-specific drug therapy. This is often accomplished within an interprofessional team or through collaborative practice with another health care provider. (American College of Clinical Pharmacy definition, as endorsed in: Council on Credentialing in Pharmacy. Scope of contemporary pharmacy practice: roles, responsibilities, and functions of pharmacists and pharmacy technicians.)

1225

BOARD CERTIFICATION FOR PHARMACISTS

Source: Section of Clinical Specialists and Scientists

To support the principle that pharmacists who practice where a pharmacy specialty has been formally recognized by the profession should become board certified in the appropriate specialty area; further,

To recognize the Board of Pharmacy Specialties (BPS) as an appropriate organization through which specialties are formally recognized and specialty pharmacy certification should occur; further,

To advocate prioritization for recognition of new specialties in those areas where sufficient numbers of postgraduate year two residency training programs are established and where adequate numbers of pharmacists are completing accredited training programs to prepare them to practice in the specialty area; further,

To advocate for standardization of credentialing eligibility and recertification requirements to include consistent requirements for advanced postgraduate residency training; further,

To promote a future vision encouraging accredited training as an eventual prerequisite for board certification; further,

To encourage BPS to be sensitive to the needs of current practitioners as prerequisites evolve; further,

To actively encourage and support the development of effective training and recertification programs that prepare specialists for certification examination and ensure the maintenance of core competencies in their area of specialization.

This policy was reviewed in 2022 by the Council on Education and Workforce Development and by the Board of Directors and was found to still be appropriate.

Rationale

As medication therapies become more complex, the need for specialized expertise increases. Some areas of health care practice evolve to the point where certification, based on formal accredited training and psychometrically valid examination, is needed to assure the public and other health care professionals of a level of competence, quality, and consistency among specialists practicing in that field. Certification, as defined by Council on Credentialing in Pharmacy, is the process by which a nongovernmental agency or an association grants recognition to an individual who has met certain predetermined qualifications specified by that organization. Formal recognition of pharmacy specialties demonstrates the unique knowledge, skills, and abilities of pharmacists in well-defined areas of practice and provides the assurance the public and other health care professionals need.

ASHP has long recognized the value of specialty certification. ASHP has been involved in multiple petitions to the Board of Pharmacy Specialties (BPS) requesting recognition of new pharmacy specialties. The ASHP Long Range Vision for Pharmacy Work Force in Hospitals and Health Systems states that pharmacists who provide services in an area where specialty certification exists should be certified in that specialty, and the ASHP Supplemental Standards for Postgraduate Training require such certification of residency program directors only.

It is also important to distinguish the recognition of specialties within the practice of pharmacy from other multidisciplinary certifications. Although some similarities exist in the nature of such programs, they also do not represent the recognition of a unique area of specialization and the development of processes recognized by the pharmacy profession to ensure the quality of specialty practice.

The profession should be more strategic in its efforts to grow and mature new specialties. A methodical specialty development process would prioritize recognition of areas of practice for which a sufficient number of high-quality training programs exist and would promote development of training programs in emerging areas of pharmacy specialization in advance of specialty recognition.

Eligibility requirements for Board certification vary widely among currently recognized specialties. Although it may not currently be possible to require residency training as a prerequisite for all BPS specialty certification applicants, over time postgraduate year two residency training should become the preferred prerequisite to establish consistent requirements across specialties and provide a stronger linkage between training and certification. ASHP policy currently supports the principle that accredited training is an important prerequisite for pharmacy technicians prior to certification by the Pharmacy Technician Certification Board. This same principle that accredited training should precede certification should also apply to specialists in our profession. It will be important for BPS to plan for this future vision and evolve requirements in a manner that is sensitive to the needs of existing practitioners.

0810

EDUCATION, PREVENTION, AND ENFORCEMENT CONCERNING WORKPLACE VIOLENCE

Source: Council on Public Policy

To advocate that federal, state, and local governments recognize the risks and consequences of workplace violence in the pharmacy community and enact appropriate criminal penalties; further,

To collaborate with federal, state, and local law enforcement and other government authorities on methods for early detection and prevention of workplace violence; further,

To encourage all workplace environments to develop and implement a policy for pharmacy personnel that (1) educates about prevention and deterrence of workplace violence, (2) identifies escalating situations that can lead to violence and instructs employees on protection and self-defense, and (3) provides continued support and care to heal personnel who were directly or indirectly involved in an incident of workplace violence; further,

To encourage the health care community to develop and maintain a communication network to share information about incidents of potential and real workplace violence.

This policy was reviewed in 2018 by the Council on Public Policy and by the Board of Directors and was found to still be appropriate.

0812

APPROPRIATE STAFFING LEVELS

Source: Council on Public Policy

To advocate that pharmacists at each practice site base the site's pharmacist and technician staffing levels on patient safety considerations, taking into account factors such as (1) acuity of care, (2) breadth of services, (3) historical safety data, and (4) results of research on the relationship between staffing patterns and patient safety; further,

To advocate that regulatory bodies not mandate specific, uniform pharmacy personnel ratios but rather ensure that site-specific staffing levels optimize patient safety; further,

To encourage additional research on the relationship between pharmacy staffing patterns and patient safety.

This policy was reviewed in 2023 by the Council on Public Policy and by the Board of Directors and was found to still be appropriate.

Rationale

The purpose of any staffing level should be to ensure quality patient care as well as patient and provider safety. Factors to be considered in developing an appropriate staffing level include acuity of care, breadth of services, historical safety data, and results of research on the relationship between staffing patterns and patient safety. Given the complexity of determining appropriate staffing, regulatory bodies should not mandate a specific staffing ratio in general or for specific practice settings. Rather, pharmacy leaders should exercise their professional judgment to determine the appropriate staffing level for achieving quality patient care. Such a model allows flexibility to base staffing levels on factors specific to each site. ASHP acknowledges the need for additional research on staffing models to support staffing levels that provide safe and effective patient care to aid pharmacy leaders in making such determinations.

ASHP recognizes the legitimate need for boards of pharmacy to assure minimum standards of practice to protect the public health. The ASHP Guidelines: **Minimum Standard for Pharmacies in Hospitals** states, "The pharmacy shall employ an adequate number of competent, legally qualified pharmacists to meet the specific medication-use needs of the hospital's patients" and "sufficient support personnel (e.g., pharmacy technicians and clerical or secretarial personnel) shall be employed to facilitate pharmacy services." Pharmacy leaders are the healthcare professionals best suited to making those determinations.

0218

PHARMACIST RECRUITMENT AND RETENTION

Source: Council on Legal and Public Affairs

To support federal and state incentive programs for new pharmacy graduates to practice in underserved areas; further,

To provide information and educational programming on strategies used by employers for successful recruitment and retention of pharmacists and pharmacy technicians; further,

To conduct regular surveys on trends in the health-system pharmacy work force, including retention rates for pharmacists and pharmacy technicians.

This policy was reviewed in 2017 by the Council on Public Policy and by the Board of Directors and was found to still be appropriate.

9108

EMPLOYEE TESTING

Source: Council on Legal and Public Affairs

To oppose the use of truth-verification testing such as polygraphs as routine employment practices because of the possible interference with the rights of individuals; further,

To recognize the limited use of such testing during employment where such testing may protect the rights of individuals against false witness.

This policy was reviewed in 2017 by the Council on Public Policy and by the Board of Directors and was found to still be appropriate.

ASHP Guidelines on the Recruitment, Selection, and Retention of Pharmacy Personnel

Purpose

These guidelines are intended to assist pharmacy managers in the recruitment, selection, and retention of qualified employees. The pharmacy manager working in an organized health care system will usually have to work with the system's human resources department and within the framework of the specific recruitment, selection, and hiring policies of the organization.

Recruitment

Position Descriptions. Well-developed job descriptions are extremely important in addressing many personnel issues. They are often used to establish salary ranges, define performance expectations, and write performance evaluations, but they can also be crucial tools in a successful recruitment effort.[1] The position description should contain detailed information on the knowledge, skills, experience, and abilities that an acceptable candidate should possess. The following information may be included in a position description:

- Position title and position control number (if applicable)
- Duties, essential job functions, and responsibilities of the position
- Education, training, experience, and licensure required
- Knowledge, skills, and abilities required to perform assigned duties
- Reporting relationships
- Pay grade and salary range (optional)
- Education and training required to maintain competence
- Other specifications of the position that may be required to meet legal requirements (e.g., the Americans with Disabilities Act) or the objectives of the organization (e.g., residency or certification requirements)

[*Note:* A variety of sample job descriptions can be found in Section 7.3 of the *Pharmacy Management Toolkit: Tools of the Trade for Pharmacy Managers and Directors* (CD-ROM) and in module 1 of *Competence Assessment Tools for Health-System Pharmacies* (online and print versions), both available from ASHP.]

A revised position description should be reviewed with staff members currently in that position and with the supervisor of that position. In many workplaces, human resources departments maintain a file of position descriptions and may require approval of all position descriptions in the organization. Procedures specific to the workplace should be followed. Staff with legal expertise should review revised position descriptions to determine compliance with organizational and legal requirements.

Recruitment Sources. Recruitment processes will depend on the type of position being filled. Strategies for filling a support staff position may not be appropriate when searching for a management candidate and vice versa. A recruitment plan should be developed for each position being filled. This plan should incorporate strategies that have worked in the past while allowing for innovative ideas. Organizations that recruit frequently or have very limited candidate pools should consider a continuous recruitment plan so that a list of prospective candidates is available even before an opening occurs.

Recruitment of individuals from within the department or the organization (e.g., from another department) creates internal growth opportunities and may result in greater employee retention and staff loyalty. Internal recruitment may also be less disruptive and expensive. To facilitate internal recruitment, notice of a vacant position can be posted within the organization before the information is made available to outsiders. Posting can be accomplished by various means, including memoranda, e-mail, voice mail, newsletters, announcements at staff meetings, and bulletin boards.

Recruitment of outside candidates expands the number of potential candidates and the experience available to the organization. It brings in new talent and discourages a reliance on seniority as the primary basis for promotion. Budgetary constraints and the urgency to fill a position may affect the recruitment method selected for external candidates. When recruitment of individuals outside the organization becomes necessary, the following methods should be considered:

- Advertisements in professional journals, newspapers, state professional society newsletters, and electronic bulletin boards
- Personnel placement services provided by national or state professional societies
- Oral and written recommendations from colleagues. Some organizations offer a "finder's fee" for hires that result from an employee referral
- Personal discussion or correspondence with potential candidates
- Recruitment visits to colleges of pharmacy or to facilities that conduct technician-training programs
- Professional recruiting firms, which typically charge the organization a percentage of the position's annual salary. In addition, recruitment advertising companies offer access to a list of job seekers for a fee
- Familiarizing students with the organization by offering summer jobs or participating in college of pharmacy experiential rotations
- Tuition assistance programs for students in exchange for future work commitments
- A "prospect list" of individuals applying for previous job openings, which can often be supplied by the human resources department
- Internet-job-site postings
- Community job fairs and local or state welfare- to-work programs
- Organization-sponsored events such as continuing-education sessions, award presentations, or community outreach programs

DOI 10.37573/9781585287048.095

The ability to recruit qualified candidates will depend on a multitude of factors, including the financial stability and location of the organization, the area's cost of living, the organization's compensation program (including salary, fringe benefits, and raise structure), the position's schedule and reporting structure, opportunities for professional growth and advancement, and the reputation and scope of pharmaceutical services offered. Only some of these factors are within the pharmacy manager's control.

Preinterview Information. The applicant's correspondence, resumé or curriculum vitae, letters of recommendation, academic records, and completed application form (if any) should be carefully evaluated on the basis of the position description to determine the suitability of the candidate for an interview.

There are certain legal restrictions on the type of information that may be requested from candidates on an application form. In general, an application form may request only information that relates directly to the evaluation of the applicant's ability to perform the job for which he or she is applying. If an application form different from that of the organization is used, it is advisable to have the human resources and legal departments review it before distribution to potential candidates.

Selection

Initial Screening Interview. An initial screening interview may be necessary if several qualified candidates have been identified. The screening interview is generally a brief interview conducted by the human resources department or the direct supervisor for the position; it offers a quick assessment of the suitability of the candidate for the position. This interview is often conducted by telephone, especially if the candidate lives far away. The screening interview should be documented and included in the applicant's file.

The Interview Process. A successful interview process is one that matches the best available candidate with a specific position. The process should allow the interviewers to predict the future performance of candidates as accurately as possible. One style of interview is the individual interview—one interviewer and one interviewee. Individual interviews offer the advantages of simplicity, ease of scheduling, and consistency of perspective. Because they are less intimidating to the candidate than group interviews, individual interviews may allow the interviewer to more accurately evaluate the applicant and provide the applicant with more opportunities to ask questions. The disadvantage of an individual interview is that it does not allow for multiple viewpoints and therefore increases the chance that something will be overlooked.

Another style, team interviewing, involves a group of interviewers. Members of the team may interview the candidate individually and then pool their results or they may interview the candidate as a group. The well-prepared team approach offers multiple perspectives within a standardized evaluation scheme. Its disadvantages are extra time consumed to train the team and conduct interviews and the intimidating effect it may have on candidates. Its advantage is that it incorporates more individuals into the process of analyzing a candidate's qualifications.[2] Team interviews foster the ideal of teamwork, and the involved employees share responsibility for the success or failure of the person hired. They also provide an opportunity to observe the candidate's ability to interact with groups, which may be important if the position will require that type of activity.

The composition of the interview team will depend on the position being filled. The team should include people with a common interest in the outcome of the selection process and people who have been in the organization long enough to share with the applicant some history of the organization and the department.[2]

Characteristics of an effective interview process include the following:

- Prior to the interview, the manager should provide the following to the candidate: information about the health-system institution, department, city, and state (if the applicant is not from the area); an agenda for the interview; the position description; travel directions to the facility; and clarification of expenses that will be incurred or reimbursed.
- The interview should be carefully planned. Consider the availability of those who need to participate in the process and allow adequate time for each event, including a tour of the facility (if needed).
- Interviewers should be well prepared. Preinterview information submitted by the candidate should be distributed to and reviewed by participants in advance of an interview.
- Carefully planned, open-ended questions should be developed in advance. Literature can be consulted to obtain sample questions and questions that are inadvisable or prohibited by law.[2-5] Human resources departments can usually assist in developing questions. (Refer to the appendix for sample questions.)
- To the extent possible, a core group of questions should be asked of all candidates as a means of comparing them. This does not negate the need to investigate different areas for each candidate or to pursue specific questions that surface during the interview.
- Questions should focus on predetermined criteria for the position and the qualifications of the candidates. The goal is to match the best candidate with the vacant position. Questions should focus on past performance, which is often a good indicator of future performance. In addition to questions regarding professional competency, the interview should contain questions that will help determine whether the applicant's attitudes and behaviors will be suitable for the job. Behavior-based selection criteria should be used when possible.
- The interviewer should give the candidate a realistic view of the position, including both favorable and unfavorable information. If the candidate is "oversold" on the position, dissatisfaction may set in when the truth becomes apparent.
- Performance standards and methods used for evaluation should be fully explained, and opportunities for professional growth should be presented.
- A description of employee benefits (e.g., medical insurance, vacation, sick leave, retirement benefits, and holidays) should be provided, either by the manager or by the human resources department.

- The initial salary and salary range for the position should be discussed with the candidate.
- The employee work schedule should be reviewed with the candidate.
- Any additional services or covered expenses the department offers should be outlined. Examples of these services of covered expenses include serving as a provider of continuing-education programs, travel expenses and time off for continuing-education programs, payment of professional membership fees, and any other benefits that would attract the candidate to the position.
- A tour of the department should be provided.
- If the candidate is not from the area, a tour of the region should be given. Employees of the department or a real estate agency may show a candidate the area and describe the housing market and local schools.
- A follow-up letter is sent to the candidate after the interview to express thanks for interest in the position and the organization and to advise the candidate of the next steps. Timely and well-organized communication between recruiters and candidates is essential to a successful recruitment effort.

Each interview should be documented to keep track of each candidate's responses and to avoid confusion later. Documentation could include interview questions and the candidate's responses or simply a rating of the candidate's responses to specific questions. One person may be designated to collect and collate comments from a group interview. Documentation should occur immediately after the interview.[2] When considering a potential employee, the interviewer should examine punctuality, completeness and accuracy of the resumé or curriculum vitae, communication skills, compensation expectations, skills and knowledge pertinent to the position, and optimal fit with coworkers. The recruitment team should agree in advance on a systematic method for selecting the successful candidate.

Background Verification. The accuracy of information provided by the candidate should be verified by the human resources department. Information may be obtained from the following sources:

- Personal reference letters provided by the applicant
- Letters of reference provided by previous employers or preceptors (with the applicant's permission)
- State board of pharmacy records
- Academic records
- Legal background searches (when permitted by law and/or by the applicant)

Job Offer. The job offer should be made as quickly as possible after the interview process is completed. Offers should be made to candidates with enthusiasm and should include a deadline for response. Information about candidate selection should be kept confidential until the offer has been accepted. The organization may have specific policies and procedures regarding job offers.[2]

The salary offered to a candidate will usually be competitive with salaries for similar jobs in other organizations in the same market and compatible with the organization's existing salary structure. The market may vary, depending on the position. For example, the market for a pharmacy technician may be local, whereas the market for a pharmacist or pharmacy manager may be regional or national. To preserve equity within the organization, the salary offered to a candidate generally should be consistent with salaries of staff currently in that position. When exceptions are considered, it may become necessary to reassess the compensation of existing staff.

In addition to salary, other commitments made to a candidate should be expressed in writing as part of the formal job offer. These may include the following:

- Date on which employment will begin
- Supervisor's name and position
- Position description
- Performance standards and evaluation system
- Next performance review date
- Next compensation increase date
- Expected work schedule and whether it is subject to change depending on future needs of the department
- Employee benefits (e.g., insurance, vacation, tuition assistance, sick leave, holidays, and retirement and pension benefits)
- Miscellaneous commitments (e.g., employment bonus, relocation expenses, licensure reimbursement, payment for professional association memberships, and payment for attendance at professional education programs)
- Potential drug screening (as applicable and in keeping with the law) or employee physical examination and the dates of these activities

Retention

Staff turnover is costly. The time required to recruit and train new employees has been shown to cause a temporary loss of productivity in the workplace.[6] Staff turnover also has a negative impact on staff morale, which may further reduce productivity and increase turnover. Because individuals have varied needs and wants that may change over time, there is no consistent formula for managers to apply to ensure employee retention.[7–9] Each organization's experience will depend on such factors as the age of employees, the employees' stages in life and career, the organizational structure, the work environment, and the work itself.

Retention may compete with recruitment. For example, creating staff positions with exclusively morning shifts may help retention but hurt recruitment, because fewer candidates are interested in evening shifts. When competing issues arise, pharmacy managers must balance them with the short- and long-term departmental goals and the current demand for employment.

Each organization should identify and assess retention factors by examining the unique aspects of the respective department and organization. For example, a committee broadly representing the organization could be established to determine major retention factors. On the basis of this assessment, a retention plan should be developed. The plan should be reviewed periodically as the needs of employees change; employee surveys may help determine these. The following factors may be considered in analyzing staff retention:

- *Training period.* The department should devote sufficient time and attention to training. Prepare for the new employee's first day by providing him or her with key material in advance and by developing an organized training schedule. Introduce the new employee to key people on the first day and have everyone in the department introduce themselves during the orientation period. Commu-nicate with the new employee regularly during the training period and throughout the first three months.[10] Sufficient training time ensures that the new employee is comfortable in the new work environment and decreases the likelihood that he or she will become frustrated in the new position. Some organizations have developed a structured mentoring program in which a new employee is paired with a senior employee during the training period.

- *Intent to stay.* In several studies, this factor was the best predictor of staff retention.[11] Employees can simply be asked whether they intend to stay. Replies will reflect employee perceptions and should be considered in light of behavior (i.e., the actual turnover rate). Replies also may be influenced by the employees' fear of reprisal.
- *Job satisfaction.* Job satisfaction is a measure of the degree to which individuals like their jobs, their work environment, and relationships with their coworkers. Job satisfaction is important to retention, although the relationship may be direct or indirect. Employees can be asked how satisfied they are with their jobs; there are many survey instruments to assist pharmacy managers and directors in performing this task.[12] Job dissatisfaction does not necessarily lead to staff turnover if other factors are more important to the individual.[13,14]
- *Pay and benefits.* These refer to the remuneration for work performed and the organization's overall benefit plan. Pay may be hourly (a wage) or salaried and may include overtime premiums or bonuses and incentive plans. A benefit plan may include life, medical, dental, disability, and liability insurance; tuition payments; retirement packages; paid organizational membership dues; sick leave; paid vacation; child care; and prescription benefits. The value of specific benefits to an employee will likely change over time. Many organizations offer a benefits plan that gives the employee the option of choosing benefits individually suited to stages in his or her life and career.
- *Performance management.* Performance appraisal is a periodic assessment of an employee's performance throughout the year. Performance appraisal is only one step in a performance management process that includes appraisal, ongoing feedback, goal setting, and development. This process is important to the success of the manager, the employee, and the organization. The goal of performance management is to share information that will help the employee grow, both personally and professionally, and improve the organization. Periodic discussions with the employee are necessary to provide and receive feedback and to avoid surprises at the time of the scheduled performance appraisal.[15] Direct observation and evaluation by supervisors and coworkers can contribute to a meaningful appraisal.
- *Recognition and awards.* Employees often feel that recognition is lacking in the workplace.[7–10] New supervisors or managers should receive training in employee recognition, which includes both formal and informal feedback mechanisms, from structured employee of the month (or year) programs to a simple thank-you given in private or at a department meeting. Managers should identify how employees want to be recognized, through employee surveys or informal discussions.[10] Methods of employee recognition include
  - Thank-you notes
  - Commendations
  - Acknowledgment at department meetings
  - Organization-wide events during National Pharmacy Week
  - Employee of the month, quarter, or year
  - Support for attendance at a professional meeting
  - Small awards such as movie tickets or gift certificates for coffee[16]
- *Promotion opportunities.* These may be in the form of formal promotions, career advancement programs, training opportunities, or special project or committee appointments. Flat organizational structures provide fewer formal opportunities for staff promotion. Employees who have made personal investments in the organization—through expanded responsibilities associated with promotion—may have stronger feelings of loyalty that translate into increased retention. Succession planning is a key organizational strategy that ensures the availability of future leaders.
- *Job design.* This refers to the general tasks that an employee performs—the content of the work. Job design includes autonomy, the complexity of tasks, and the support and tools provided to the employee. Studies have found that job content is more highly correlated with retention as the level of an employee's education increases.[11] Motivational theories suggest that the job itself can motivate intrinsically and that success in the job can lead to increased employee satisfaction.
- *Peer relations.* This refers to working relationships with peers, nurses, physicians, and technical support staff. Peer relations are often rated highly as a reason for staying with an organization. It is difficult to predict during the interview process how a candidate's peer relations will develop, but past behaviors and discussion of hypothetical scenarios can provide some insight.
- *Kinship responsibilities.* This refers to family considerations, such as child care needs, spouse-employment transfers, and care for elderly relatives. Child and elder care needs are important for working parents. These considerations are also difficult to screen for during the interview process, and they will change over time. Legal restrictions prevent recruiters from asking some questions; the organization's human resources department should be able to offer advice on this issue.
- *Opportunity.* This refers to other options in the job market. Obviously, tight job markets (a relative lack of alternative positions) increase retention, whereas open job markets (those with many other open positions) may increase turnover. Managers should always be attentive to retaining good employees, but in open job markets they need to be especially attentive.
- *Staff-development opportunities.* This refers to job training, educational opportunities, and tuition reimbursement or other educational and personal growth opportunities for staff. Training and educational

opportunities can affect recognition and awards, promotion opportunities, job design, and peer relations, so they can have a big impact on employee retention.

- *Management style.* This refers to the organizational structure and prevalent management style in the organization (e.g., on the spectrum from autocratic to participatory). The accessibility of management staff may be a factor as well as the extent to which staff input is encouraged. Each employee will prefer a particular management style; no one style will work equally well for all employees. Managers must be sensitive to the management styles that are effective for their staff.
- *Employee coaching.* This refers to the manager's mentorship role. Managers should provide feedback to employees regarding performance, teach specific job-related skills, hold formal and informal career discussions with employees, help employees achieve greater self-awareness, advise employees on how best to prepare for career options, and assist employees in preparing a yearly career-development plan.[10] In addition, it is important that managers recognize and acknowledge the employee's contributions to the health system.
- *Management survey.* This refers to the organization's commitment to identifying opportunities for improving management. Such opportunities can be identified by surveying employees about their manager's performance. The survey should be conducted by each manager's supervisor. Managers should also complete the survey to see how their rating compares with that of their staff. Action plans should be established on the basis of the survey results.[10] Such "360-degree" surveys should be managed with caution, however; they may create animosity and foster unhealthy relationships between management and staff.
- *Physical working conditions.* This refers to the physical characteristics and safety of the workplace, such as space, equipment, noise levels, parking accommodations, and cleanliness.
- *Scheduling.* This refers to opportunities for varied scheduling, vacation time, shift rotation, job sharing, flexible hours, and part-time work.
- *Motivation.* Extrinsic motivators for change (such as salary, promotion, and recognition) can affect behavior, but they cannot change values and attitudes.[17] In the workplace, change occurs most readily when people are motivated by the desire to bring their professional activities in line with their personal and professional values and beliefs. Living vision and value statements offer employees an opportunity to shape an inspiring organizational culture. Although each employee's motivations will be different, some theories of motivation can help managers understand what contributes to job satisfaction. Maslow's[14] hierarchy of needs, for example, states that employees will be happiest when they are working toward self-actualization, which requires that their more basic needs for security, esteem, belonging, and knowledge be satisfied first. Herzberg et al.'s[18] motivation/hygiene theory explains that employees cannot be motivated by the "hygiene" aspects of their work (organization policies, supervision, salary, peer relations, and working conditions), but that dissatisfaction with those aspects can interfere with motivating factors (the work itself, responsibility, achievement, recognition, and advancement).
- *Exit interview.* An interview should be scheduled with a director of the department, the human resources department, and the exiting employee. The director should ask in-depth questions to identify why the employee is leaving. The exit interview should explore the employee's opinion of the company, department, his or her direct manager as well as any other issues the employee may have for leaving. Pharmacy managers should validate and share this information with the appropriate management staff to decrease the likelihood that another employee may leave for a similar reason.[14]

References

1. Poremba AC. Determining the department's staffing: writing job descriptions. In: Pharmacy management toolkit: tools of the trade for pharmacy managers and directors [CD-ROM]. Bethesda, MD: American Society of Health-System Pharmacists; 2001.
2. Nimmo CM, ed. Human resources management. ACCRUE level II. Bethesda, MD: American Society of Hospital Pharmacists; 1991.
3. Yate M. Hiring the best. 3rd ed. Holbrook, MA: Adams; 1990.
4. Wilson R. Conducting better job interviews. Haup-pauge, NY: Barrons; 1991.
5. Smart B. The smart interviewer. New York: Wiley; 1989.
6. Donovan L. The shortage. *RN.* 1980; 8:21–7.
7. Smith SN, Stewart JE, Grussing PG. Factors influencing the rate of job turnover among hospital pharmacists. *Am J Hosp Pharm.* 1986; 43:1936–41.
8. Porter LW, Stears RM. Organizational work and personal factors in employee turnover and absenteeism. *Psychol Bull.* 1973; 80:151–76.
9. Loveridge CE. Contingency theory: explaining staff nurse retention. *J Nurs Adm.* 1988; 18:22–5.
10. Branham FL. Keeping the people who keep you in business. 1st ed. New York: Amacon; 2001.
11. Cavanagh SJ. Predictions of nursing staff turnover. *J Adv Nurs.* 1990; 15:373–80.
12. Section 7.5: employee satisfaction. In: Pharmacy management toolkit: tools of the trade for pharmacy managers and directors [CD-ROM]. Bethesda, MD: American Society of Health-System Pharmacists; 2001.
13. Johns G. Organizational behavior: understanding life at work. Glenview, IL: Scott, Foresman; 1983.
14. Maslow AH. Motivation and personality. 2nd ed. New York: Harper & Rowe; 1970.
15. Chrymko MM. How to do a performance appraisal. *Am J Hosp Pharm.* 1991; 48:2600–1.
16. Nelson B. 1001 ways to reward employees. New York: Workman Publishing; 1994.
17. Nimmo CM, Holland RW. The practice change model: an innovative pharmacy-specific approach to motivating staff change. In: Pharmacy management toolkit: tools of the trade for pharmacy managers and

directors [CD-ROM]. Bethesda, MD: American Society of Health-System Pharmacists; 2001.
18. Herzberg F, Mausner B, Snyderman BB. The motivation to work. 2nd ed. New York: Wiley; 1959.

Appendix—Sample Questions to Ask of Job Candidates[2]

Questions for Experienced Pharmacists and Technicians

- How did you become interested in pharmacy?
- What skills or traits do you think a pharmacist needs to be successful?
- What is the single greatest contribution you have made in your present (or most recent) position?
- What is something you have recommended or tried in your present (or most recent) position that did not work? Why didn't it?
- How are you evaluated in your present (most recent) job?
- What would your present (most recent) employer say are your strong points? Your weak points?
- Why did you (do you want to) leave your last (present) job?
- Do you prefer working on a team or alone? Why?
- What part of the job did you like the best and least?

Questions for Recent College of Pharmacy Graduates

- What was your most rewarding college experience?
- Why did you want to study pharmacy?
- What would you change about your college experience if you could?
- Do you think your grades accurately reflect your academic achievements?
- What subjects did you like most and least? Why?

General Questions

- What qualities are you looking for in your next supervisor?
- What supervisory style do you think you have?
- What are your long-term career goals?
- How does this position fit in with your long-term career goals?
- What are you looking for in your next position that has been lacking in previous positions?

Subjects About Which You May Not Ask

- Race
- National origin
- Religion
- Age
- Marital or family status
- Child care arrangements or childbearing plans
- Arrest records (although convictions related to drug use would be appropriate)
- Credit rating and other financial information (unless the position involves financial responsibilities)
- Military discharge status, unless resulting from a military conviction
- General information that would point out handicaps or health problems unrelated to job performance

---

Approved by the ASHP Board of Directors, September 27, 2002. Revised by the ASHP Council on Administrative Affairs. Supersedes the ASHP Technical Assistance Bulletin on the Recruitment, Selection, and Retention of Pharmacy Personnel dated April 27, 1994.

Copyright © 2003, American Society of Health-System Pharmacists, Inc. All rights reserved. Contact ASHP for reprint and permissions requests. This content may not be used for commercial purposes without the express written consent of ASHP.

The bibliographic citation for this document is as follows: American Society of Health-System Pharmacists. ASHP guidelines on the recruitment, selection, and retention of pharmacy personnel. *Am J Health-Syst Pharm.* 2003; 60:587–93.

ASHP Long-Range Vision for the Pharmacy Workforce in Hospitals and Health Systems

Ensuring Medication Use Is Optimal, Safe, and Effective in Acute and Ambulatory Care Settings

Purpose

Medication use for maintaining and restoring health is an interprofessional endeavor with the patient as the central focus and pharmacy personnel in positions of leadership and authority. The American Society of Health-System Pharmacists (ASHP) Vision for the Pharmacy Workforce in Hospitals and Health Systems seeks to prepare, engage, and leverage the pharmacy workforce to optimize health. With a 2030 outlook, this vision document positions the pharmacy workforce as the medication-use experts accountable for comprehensive medication management (CMM) and medication management services (MMS) in a constantly evolving healthcare environment.

Achieving the Long-Range Vision

Pharmacists are accountable for optimizing medication use to improve patient outcomes. By way of this document, ASHP expresses an aspirational and achievable vision for pharmacy personnel responsible and accountable for CMM and MMS in hospitals and health systems. Considering anticipated changes to the healthcare landscape, the vision will establish an intention to ensure a prepared and thriving pharmacy workforce through education, training, and professional development. ASHP will focus future resources, initiatives, and advocacy efforts in the areas consistent with this vision.

Introduction

Pharmacists of the future will have strengths in complex decision-making (e.g., defining problems, assessing options, and implementing solutions) and relational (e.g., reliable, empathetic, influential) competencies. Navigating the constantly evolving healthcare landscape will require advanced clinical knowledge, business and financial acumen, information systems aptitude, high reliability, and efficiency capacity. Also required will be maintenance of the human dimension that is essential for creating and sustaining meaningful connections with patients, colleagues, and other stakeholders. This vision document attempts to raise awareness of all these requirements. It builds upon content provided in the 2007 publication "ASHP Long-Range Vision for the Pharmacy Work Force in Hospitals and Health Systems: Ensuring the Best Use of Medicines in Hospitals and Health Systems," which informed decisions related to the pharmacy workforce for over 10 years.[1]

This vision document also seeks to complement other resources developed to guide the pharmacy profession, particularly within hospitals and health systems. These resources include but are not limited to the ASHP Foundation Pharmacy Forecast, the Joint Commission of Pharmacy Practitioners Future Vision of Pharmacy Practice, the ASHP Practice Advancement Initiative, and ASHP's national surveys of pharmacy practice in hospital settings.[2–4] The document:

- Affirms a constantly evolving and persistently complex healthcare delivery model that implores pharmacy practice to advance and align to meet patient care needs and marketplace forces;
- Expresses ASHP's commitment to support and build workforce capacity in hospitals and health systems to meet the challenges and demands related to optimizing the use of medications;
- Provides a guide for ASHP's strategic plan, policies, education, publications, resources, and other activities to support the development of pharmacists, student pharmacists, and pharmacy technicians for practice readiness essential to work in hospitals and health systems; and
- Informs advocacy efforts to influence and shape public policy decisions developed by policymakers, external standards groups, hospital and health-system administrators and directors, and healthcare educators to ensure that the pharmacy workforce is engaged, relevant, and utilized to its highest ability.

Drivers of Change in Hospitals and Health Systems

Changes to the healthcare system will shape and influence the direction of pharmacy practice and needs of the pharmacy workforce in hospitals and health systems. With a keen focus on the overall healthcare landscape, pharmacy leaders will demonstrate the value of CMM and MMS as leverage to influence decisions related to the strategic direction of their institutions. Leadership that is visionary, strategic, resilient, and relational will be essential for hospital and health-system pharmacy in times of change, both anticipated and unforeseen.

Pharmacy department goals will continue to align with the goals of the institution and the patients they serve while existing in and adapting to ambiguity, chaos, and increasing rates of healthcare changes. The foundational functions that the pharmacy workforce in hospitals and health systems will continue to provide are consistent with those listed in the previous long-range vision report (**Table 1**).[1] Flexible and innovative pharmacy departments, prepared to embrace roles and responsibilities that do not yet exist and may be beyond the scope of medication distribution, will be most effective.

Innovations in supply chain synergies, pharmacy shared services, specialty pharmacy, stewardship over medication therapies, specialization in clinical pharmacy, collaborative

DOI 10.37573/9781585287048.096

Vision at a Glance					
The American Society of Health-System Pharmacists (ASHP) Vision for the Pharmacy Workforce in Hospitals and Health Systems seeks to prepare, engage, and leverage the pharmacy workforce to optimize patient health. With a 2030 outlook, this vision positions the pharmacy workforce as the medication-use experts accountable for medication management services in a constantly evolving healthcare environment.					
Vision for Pharmacists					
Pharmacy Education	**Residency Training**	**Certifications**	**Credentialing & Privileging**	**Ongoing Professional Development**	**Leadership**
Pharmacy education will evolve to prepare graduates for future practice by individualized learning tracks, engagement in active learning models, dual degrees, and interprofessional activities.	Residency training will evolve to include more education around leadership, resiliency, inter-professional care delivery, population health, technology and data expertise, and soft skills.	Minimum credentials for new practitioners will expand to include board certification, specialized certificates or certifications, and PGY1 and/or PGY2 residency training along with state licensure.	The role of credentialing and privileging will gradually evolve as pharmacists continue to expand their roles and scope of practice to include more direct patient care, leading to greater recognition by the public and hospital and health system leaders.	Professional development will be focused on developing application-based skills, credentialing and privileging, obtaining board certification and professional certificates, and engaging with ASHP.	Pharmacy leadership will adapt to changes in healthcare delivery and financing by focusing on demonstration of value, stronger matrixed relationships, datadriven decisions, succession planning, and management of the multigenerational workforce.
Certificate programs will play an important role in providing focused education and training to pharmacists, student pharmacists, and pharmacy technicians to enhance and demonstrate specific skill sets.	Residents will extend patient care and experiential education efforts in hospitals and health systems through the use of the layered learning practice model.	New board certification and professional certificate programs will adapt to the evolution of the profession of pharmacy in its entirety.	Formal credentialing and privileging of pharmacists will become an organizational requirement for hospitals and health systems and a requirement in Medicare Conditions of Participation.	Pharmacists will continue to retool and reinvent themselves to stay relevant with advances in therapeutics and technology through continuing professional development.	Pharmacy leaders gain visibility and credibility as leaders among other executive leaders in managing medication expenditures and utilization.

Vision for Pharmacy Technicians		
Pharmacy Technician Roles	**Pharmacy Technician Education**	**Pharmacy Technician Certification**
Pharmacy technicians, from a standardized foundation of education and training, will expand into advanced roles, clinical roles, and quality improvement roles. New credentials will allow pharmacy technicians to interact with the public to a higher degree and complement the evolution of pharmacist roles.	Minimum credentials for entry-level pharmacy technicians will expand to include a 2-year degree, ASHP/Accreditation Council for Pharmacy Education-accredited technician training, Pharmacy Technician Certification Board certification, and state licensure.	For advanced-level pharmacy technicians, minimum credentials will also include advanced certification in an area of specialty based on practice setting and professional certificates pertaining to area of specialty.
Vision for Contributory Pharmacy Staff	**Vision for Well-being and Resilience**	**Vision for a Diverse and Inclusive Work Environment**
Contributory pharmacy staff will supplement pharmacy departments with expertise in finance, analytics, business management, quality assurance, informatics, prior authorization, and supply chain management.	Pharmacy staff will support individual efforts to develop and demonstrate coping skills and create systems to address risk factors known to cause burnout in healthcare, such as excessive workload, lack of autonomy, lack of reward, lack of community, and job–individual incongruence.	Pharmacy departments in hospitals and health systems will embrace and rely on differing demographics in the pharmacy workforce, striving to achieve equity and diversity in all clinical, technical, and leadership roles.

TABLE 1.
Pharmacy Functions In Hospitals and Health Systems Expected to Continue

- Leading the interprofessional and collaborative development of medication-use policies and procedures within the setting, including pharmacy and therapeutics committee policies and therapeutic protocols
- Reviewing patients' medication orders for safety and effectiveness
- Collaboratively managing medication therapy for individual patients
- Educating patients and caregivers about medications and their use
- Leading continuous improvements in the quality of medication-use processes
- Acquiring quality medication products from trusted supply sources
- Preparing medications in the doses and dosage forms needed
- Distributing medications to inpatients and outpatients
- Integrating the work of staff in clinical and other functions to ensure coordinated attention to safe, effective, and appropriate care
- Functioning as a gatekeeper with respect to the quality of medication information available to caregivers throughout the setting as a means to support relevant and timely evidence-based care
- Influencing medication administration policies and procedures and the use of related devices
- Conducting quality reviews of medication utilization in the hospital or health system's population of patients
- Leading and influencing decisions about medication-related informatics, other technology (including medication administration devices), medication administration, and automated medication-use processes

practice, and reliance on technicians will spread beyond early adopters and become standards of practice in hospitals and health systems. Strategies and the pace in which pharmacy practice advances will depend on institutional size and access to resources. Combining the skill set of pharmacy technicians with the potential of technology and automation will expedite the medication preparation and dispensing process, further enabling the pharmacist to be directly engaged in medication-use decisions in hospitals and health systems. Medications may not be dispensed or delivered at the same location as where care is provided; however, ensuring a safe and secure medication supply chain and distribution system will remain under the authority of pharmacy departments.

Anticipated Domains of Change. This section outlines some anticipated domains of change that will impact healthcare in hospitals and health systems and, therefore, the opportunities for the future pharmacy workforce. The following topics are recognized as broad yet interconnected and dynamic forces behind perpetual change in healthcare. They are categorized as trends, risks, and opportunities and will be discussed briefly; however, each domain deserves consideration and understanding by leaders.

Trends. Important drivers of change will include the following trends:

- Patient-centered care—The U.S. National Quality Strategy emphasizes patient-centered care as a priority and seeks to "ensure that each person and family is engaged as partners" in care decisions.[5] Patients will increasingly prioritize personalization of care as a healthcare expectation, and patient engagement will be a dominant focus in healthcare delivery.[6]
- Social determinants of health (SDH)—Globally, there will be a shift from improving healthcare to achievement of health and from prioritizing hospital and health-system care delivery to placing more emphasis on care for the community.[7] SDH influences health outcomes to a greater extent than medical care.[8–10] In light of this influence, hospitals and health systems will seek to better understand the contexts of a patient's SDH and integrate SDH considerations into patient care decisions.[11]
- The continuous care model—Patient care delivery models are shifting from episodic to longitudinal. Continuous care models, staffed by interprofessional care teams, enabled by interoperable health information systems, and reimbursed by healthcare payers reduce care fragmentation and manage the health of patients between hospitals, rehabilitation centers, nursing facilities, ambulatory care clinics, and community settings.
- Technology and information systems—Technology advancements for use by hospitals and health systems will support operational and clinical improvements. The merging of talent and technology will support logistics and operations, accelerate telehealth care delivery, reinvent the infrastructure for health information exchange, and enable clinical decision support (CDS) and learning healthcare systems.[12]

Risks. Important risks include the following:

- Marketplace and organizational dynamism—Horizontal and vertical integration in the healthcare market will enable organizations to increase economies of scale and scope, standardization of processes, and coordination of services delivered, thereby increasing market share and strengthening pursuits to invest in supply chains, capital, technology, and therapies.[13] Undertaken in an effort to lower costs over time, mergers and acquisitions introduce risks such as fragmenting of care delivery, organizational culture, and the medication distribution system, requiring careful alignment to achieve success.
- Health policy and regulatory complexity—The drive to improve patient care quality and safety has resulted in myriad policy, reimbursement, accreditation, and regulatory demands on hospitals and health systems. This complexity is expected to continue and challenge innovation and efficiency.[14]
- Finance and cost decisions—U.S. healthcare spending is projected to grow faster than our economy, reaching 25% of the gross domestic product by 2037.[15] Expensive and complex emerging technologies will require difficult cost-of-care decisions. Added to these factors are expenditures and utilization increases associated with an aging population and lifestyle diseases that become public health issues, such as diabetes and the current opioid crisis. Pharmacy departments will be forced to cope with increased budget pressures and financial

stress due to increases in medication costs and medication supply fragmentation.[16]

Opportunities. Important opportunities will include the following:

- Machine learning and artificial intelligence (AI)—Combined with CDS, machine learning and AI will allow pharmacists and other clinicians in hospitals and health systems to focus less on retrospective data to guide decisions about patient care and more on prospective planning and personalized care for patients.[2] The field of AI offers promise in achieving care delivery efficiencies, risk mitigation, and cost savings.[17,18]
- Clinical and therapeutic technology innovations—Advances in diagnosis and treatment support the management and curing of disease. Clinical and therapeutic technological innovation creates an opportunity for pharmacist expertise in addressing cost-effectiveness and ethical considerations prior to use in patients.[19,20]
- Precision medicine and pharmacogenomics—Personalized medicine and reliance on pharmacogenomics for tailoring medication-use decisions and targeting therapies promise significant improvement in patient care delivery and outcomes.[21–23] Infrastructure to support optimal use and application in hospitals and health systems will be required and offers enormous potential for pharmacist involvement (e.g., product procurement, test interpretation, patient identification, therapeutic decisions, reimbursement considerations, ordering, and documentation).[24–26]
- Professional scope of practice transformation—Highly matrixed organizations demand collaboration. The totally self-sufficient clinician no longer exists; interprofessional collaborative practice will continue to expand.[27,28]

These are just a few trends, risks, and opportunities expected to impact hospitals and health systems by 2030. **Table 2** lists additional trends and opportunities identified by ASHP members and expected to influence pharmacy innovation. With astute awareness and strategic focus, the pharmacy workforce will be positioned to minimize risks and maximize opportunities to optimize patient health and secure hospital and health system viability.

TABLE 2.
Trends and Opportunities Expected to Impact the Pharmacy Workforce by 2030

- Advances in technology and artificial intelligence will fundamentally change traditional roles of pharmacists and pharmacy technicians, innovation will require new and different expertise, and traditional regulatory constructs will be challenged.
- Pharmacy personnel will integrate closed-loop analytics (quality, data management, outcomes, predictive analytics, and compliance), cost-effectiveness, and ethics into medication management decisions.
- Pharmacists will move into the virtual space and be more present in the day-to-day lives of patients through use and development of technology, including on-demand consultations and tele-rounding.
- Pharmacists will lead and influence decisions about medication-related informatics, adoption of novel technologies (e.g., clinical decision support tools), medication administration, and automated medication-use processes.
- Artificial intelligence and clinical decision support, with the design support of pharmacists, will allow pharmacists and other clinicians to focus less on retrospective data to guide decisions about patient care and more on prospective planning and personalized care for patients.
- Pharmacists will be the primary drivers of their destiny by demonstrating their value, securing compensation, and advocating for expanded roles in the pharmacy workforce (both within the health system and externally through payer negotiations).
- Pharmacy leaders will engage in advocacy and relationship building with appropriate regulatory bodies to successfully navigate the evolving regulatory reform.
- Strategic communication is critical to improve provider confidence and acceptance of pharmacists in direct patient care roles, to improve payer recognition, and to influence medication-related legislative and regulatory efforts.
- Pharmacists' patient care responsibilities will expand to direct, coordinated, and comprehensive care roles related to medication therapy, including diagnostics, prescribing authority, and well visits.
- Efforts to obtain a position of influence as an advanced practitioner, accountable for medication management services, processes, and outcomes (i.e., clinical, financial, safety outcomes), and complementarily positioned to be a necessary and integral part of the interprofessional direct patient care team will be realized.

Ensuring an Engaged and Empowered Workforce

An engaged and empowered workforce is key to a high-performing workforce.[29] Strategic decisions related to ensuring an engaged, empowered, prepared, and sustainable workforce must address topics related to education, professional development, capacity building, performance, and professional culture. This section considers those topics for pharmacists, pharmacy technicians, and other pharmacy department contributory staff in hospitals and health systems. It ends with considerations for achieving a resilient workforce and an equitable organizational culture.

Pharmacy Education. Increases in demand for and specialization of MMS in hospitals and health systems will be addressed in pharmacy education.[30] Pharmacy education will evolve to include both informative and transformative instruction, preparing graduates for future practice and to serve as change agents for the profession.[31] To achieve this end and align with anticipated changes in healthcare, the profile of student pharmacist applicants will change, placing increased emphasis on strategic thinking, problem solving, critical reasoning, executive decision-making, information retrieval skills, professionalism, and emotional intelligence.

Curricula content will continue to prepare students to be experts in medications and therapeutics. Students will exhibit essential skills in analysis and evaluation of new therapies and advances in technology. Direct patient care skills in assessment and monitoring will be engrained. In addition, curricula content will have greater emphasis on informatics

Vision for Pharmacists

Pharmacy education will evolve to prepare graduates for future practice by individualized learning tracks, engagement in active learning models, dual degrees, and interprofessional activities.

- *Certificate programs will play an important role in providing focused education and training to pharmacists, student pharmacists, and pharmacy technicians to enhance and demonstrate specific skill sets.*
- *Residency training will evolve to include more education around leadership, resiliency, interprofessional care delivery, population health, technology and data expertise, and soft skills.*
- *Residents will extend patient care and experiential education efforts in hospitals and health systems through the use of the layered learning practice model.*
- *Minimum credentials for new practitioners will expand to include board certification, specialized certificates or certifications, and postgraduate year 1 (PGY1) and/or postgraduate year 2 (PGY2) residency training along with state licensure.*
- *New board certification and professional certificate programs will adapt to the evolution of the profession of pharmacy in its entirety.*
- *The role of credentialing and privileging will gradually evolve as pharmacists continue to expand their roles and scope of practice to include more direct patient care, leading to greater recognition by the public and hospital and health-system leaders.*
- *Formal credentialing and privileging of pharmacists will become an organizational requirement for hospitals and health systems and a requirement in Medicare Conditions of Participation.*
- *Professional development will be focused on developing application-based skills, credentialing and privileging, obtaining board certification and professional certificates, and engaging with ASHP.*
- *Pharmacists will continue to retool and reinvent themselves to stay relevant with advances in therapeutics and technology through continuing professional development.*
- *Pharmacy leadership will adapt to changes in healthcare delivery and financing by focusing on demonstration of value, stronger matrixed relationships, data-driven decisions, succession planning, and management of the multigenerational workforce.*
- *Pharmacy leaders gain visibility and credibility as leaders among other executive leaders in managing medication expenditures and utilization.*

and use of mega data analytics. Pharmacy students will be experts in merging their clinical skills with optimization of technology.

As pharmacy students and colleges of pharmacy seek to differentiate themselves, opportunities to specialize and gain advanced knowledge through advanced training will become mainstream. For example, in addition to the core doctor of pharmacy degree curriculum, colleges of pharmacy will provide certificate and dual-degree programs. Examples of potential certificates include informatics, data science and healthcare analytics, virtual care, rural and home health, operational management, human factors design, entrepreneurship, stewardship leadership, and precision medicine. Dual-degree emphases will include public health, population health, law and public policy, health and business administration, leadership, social sciences research, industrial engineering, clinical research, medicine, and pharmacoeconomics.

Pharmacy curricula will continue to incorporate interprofessional education (IPE) into didactic and experiential training to prepare learners for future team-based care delivery. Accrediting and standard-setting bodies for health professional education and clinical learning environments will continue to require IPE, and the financing and logistics for delivering IPE will ensure that it becomes commonplace.[32,33–35] Importantly, integration with IPE will instill and reinforce pharmacists' value with other disciplines. Pharmacy education will be jointly developed and delivered by faculty and practice communities, as research shows that adult learners acquire knowledge and skills best in experiential settings.[36–39] Add to this argument the mounting evidence in support of the layered learning practice model (LLPM) in improving learning, patient outcomes, and extending pharmacy services.[40–43] As they embark on their careers, residents will transition into preceptor roles, further cementing and creating permanence of experiential education and the LLPM by incorporating learners as pharmacist extenders. As this occurs, technology availability will disrupt and destructure the traditional didactic experience and learning will be offered at alternative sites, creating more opportunities for pharmacy education to be jointly conducted by colleges of pharmacy and practice communities.

Residency Training. Completion of an ASHP-accredited PGY1 or PGY1 and PGY2 residency will be a requirement for all recent pharmacy school graduates seeking employment in hospitals and health systems. Competency areas addressed during PGY1 residencies will continue to build upon the generalist level of education received in undergraduate curriculums and aim to ensure practice readiness to provide direct patient care in the hospital and health-system setting.[44] Most PGY2 residencies focus on clinical topics in specialized areas of practice, typically granting a higher likelihood of securing a clinical specialist position in a graduate's preferred specialty area.[45,46] In addition, nontraditional residencies, such as those with an emphasis on pharmacy operation and administration, supply chains and distribution, informatics, public policy, managed care, health services research, population health, and management, will evolve.

Growth in both PGY1 and PGY2 residencies will be necessary to meet pharmacy graduate demand and employer needs. Expansion of residency programs and increased residency matching will allow for further incorporation of the LLPM to resemble that of the medical training model and transform pharmacy workforce efficiency, capacity, and impact. This evolution will be necessary to accommodate the anticipated increase in residents and residency offerings and overall pharmacy service expansion. Preceptor responsibilities, ratios, and planning are likely to be redesigned to adapt.[47] Residency recruiting will reflect the patient population being served. Recruiting for retention after residency completion will be prioritized to meet patient access needs in underserved and/or impoverished communities. Residency training will build upon soft skill development initiated in undergraduate curriculums in areas such as emotional intelligence, problem solving and executive decision-making, negotiation and communication, professionalism, and leadership. In addition, residents will be adept at interprofessional care delivery, population health, consideration of SDH, and use of technology and data. Within residency programs, there will be increased availability of specialization and opportunities to pursue advanced degrees, certificates, and certifications. As care shifts more from acute and episodic to preventative and continuous, there will be more residency programs offered in non–acute care environments such as ambulatory care practices, rehabilitation centers, long-term care facilities, and community settings.

Certifications and Credentials. Statistics show that the average person will change jobs 5–7 times during his or her working life and that approximately 30% of the labor workforce changes jobs every 12 months.[48] This transience requires a commitment and capacity to reinvent oneself.[49] Board certification and professional certificate programs will adapt to the evolution of pharmacy in hospitals and health systems and provide a mechanism for practitioner reinvention.

Obtaining and maintaining specialty credentials will improve the quality of the pharmacist workforce.[50] With rigor and integrity, the Board of Pharmacy Specialties (BPS) will continue to serve as the pharmacy professions' board certification body. Pharmacists in hospitals and health systems will be expected to be board certified in the area(s) in which they practice. Board certification will ensure competence to employers and demonstrate expertise to other healthcare providers and administrators, regulatory bodies, and patients.

Board certification and the achievement of various certificates are not the same (see definitions). In addition to board certification, certificate programs will play an important role in providing focused education and training to pharmacists and other pharmacy personnel to increase knowledge and competency in specific topics or skill sets. Certificates can be used as a means to close an educational gap not covered in education or residency training, hone an area of expertise, or maintain a credential. Many of these certificate programs will confer interprofessional certificates in the management of certain disease states (e.g., diabetes or pain management), specific patient population (e.g., geriatric medicine patients), or task areas (e.g., healthcare quality or patient safety).

As the healthcare landscape evolves and pharmacists' learning needs adjust accordingly, new board certifications and certificate programs will be developed. ASHP emphasizes the need for board certification and certificate programs that are robust in nature, assessment based, and developed with expertise in content and instructional design.

In summary, pharmacist education and training is a crucial component of an engaged and thriving hospital and health-system pharmacy workforce. The following are achievements and credentials that all new pharmacist practitioners will be expected to achieve in order to practice in a hospital or health system (**Figure 1**):

- Doctor of pharmacy or other undergraduate degree in pharmacy, conferred by a college of pharmacy accredited by the Accreditation Council for Pharmacy Education (ACPE);
- State licensure to practice pharmacy;
- Completion of an ASHP-accredited pharmacy residency program;
- Graduate degrees where specialized knowledge is required;
- Achieving and sustaining board certification by BPS where board certification exists for the topic area of the pharmacist's work; and
- Completion of skills or knowledge certificates applicable to the pharmacist's work.

FIGURE 1. Entry-level and ongoing education and credentials required for pharmacists seeking employment in hospitals and health systems. PGY1 = postgraduate year 1, PGY2 = postgraduate year 2, BPS = Board of Pharmacy Specialties.

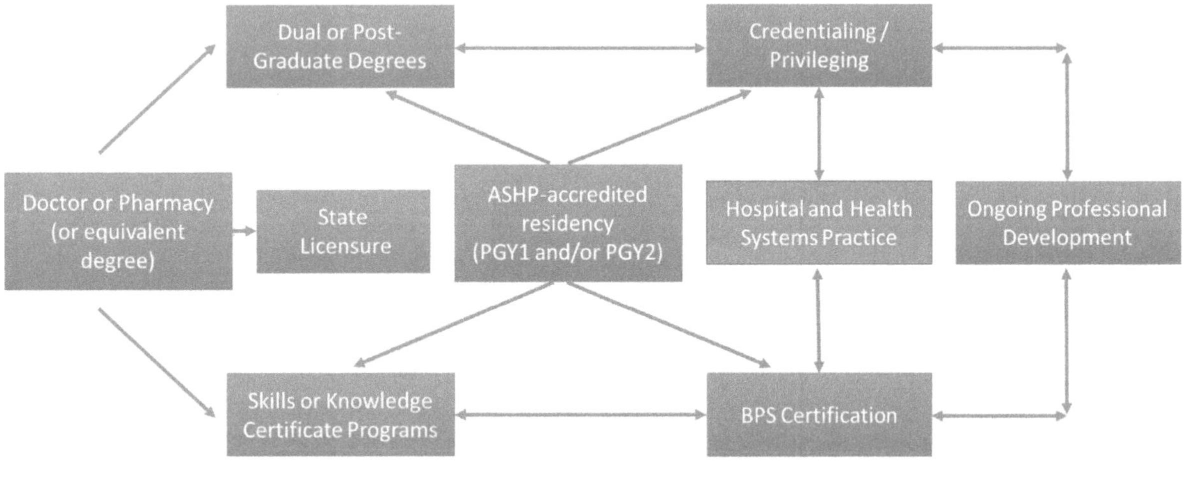

Credentialing and Privileging. Formal credentialing and privileging of pharmacists will become an organizational requirement for hospitals and health systems and a requirement in Medicare Conditions of Participation (CoP). Credentialing involves evaluating the provider's licensure, current competency, education, training, and ability in order to determine the practitioner's qualifications to perform the clinical activities he or she seeks to provide.[51] Hospitals and health systems will continue to be required to meet CoP credentialing criteria for character, competence, training, experience, and judgment. Some hospitals and health systems will create additional, more rigid expectations.[52] In addition to credentialing pharmacy personnel as they begin employment, hospitals and health systems will be responsible for ongoing verification and appraisals of pharmacy personnel as their employment assignments continue. Clinical privileging of pharmacists, granted by hospitals, health systems, and payers and within state scope of practice laws and regulations, will also increase.

Ongoing Competency and Continuing Professional Development. Continuing pharmacy education (CPE) provides a mechanism for disseminating new knowledge to pharmacists and meeting employer and licensing requirements. Completion of traditional CPE activities will continue to be an essential approach to ensuring professional competency in hospitals and health systems.

Continuing professional development (CPD) provides a framework for lifelong learning; it will continue to be a model to maintain, demonstrate, and document professional competency.[53] Hospital and health-system pharmacy departments will establish CPD requirements for pharmacy staff to plan for and sustain professional development and advancement.[54] The CPD requirements parallel those of a learning health system, defined in a 2007 report by the Institute of Medicine (since renamed the National Academy of Medicine) as a system in which "science, informatics, incentives, and culture are aligned for continuous improvement and innovation, with best practices seamlessly embedded in the delivery process and new knowledge captured as an integral by-product of the delivery experience."[55] Leveraging electronic health record functionality and access to data, hospitals and health systems will systematically gather and create evidence to inform CDS and facilitate adoption of best practices while creating instant and relevant learning opportunities, thereby cultivating a learning health system.[55]

Leadership. All pharmacists in hospitals and health systems are obligated to serve as leaders in the safe and effective use of medications.[56] Effective leadership skills will be critical for any pharmacist position, regardless of a formal leadership or management role.[74] Pharmacists will be recognized as leaders by the patients they serve, their pharmacy and interprofessional colleagues, and administrators.[57] Pharmacy departments in hospitals and health systems will continue to be led by pharmacist executives who empower managers and clinical leaders to excel in their assigned roles and responsibilities. Some pharmacist leaders also will be positioned to lead in executive roles outside of the pharmacy department. Those with formal leadership and management roles will work to close gaps between the vision for their department and its current performance.[58] Pharmacists leading at the hospital and health system executive and department levels will prepare and engage staff to influence medication-related decisions across the continuum of care and the healthcare enterprise. Numerous publications and resources outline the necessary traits and responsibilities of the pharmacy executive to provide leadership over all aspects of the medication management system.[59-62] Pharmacy executives will be expected to demonstrate the value of MMS and may have management responsibility for nonpharmacy service lines and business units in hospitals and health systems.[2]

Development of leadership skills for frontline leaders and executives will continue to be multimodal. From formal education to real-world experience, development and refinement of such skills will facilitate succession planning and prevent pharmacy leadership deficits in hospital and health-system pharmacy departments. Leaders will follow the same educational and training pathways outlined earlier and supplement them with formal and informal leadership skill development opportunities.

Vision for Pharmacy Technicians

- *Pharmacy technicians, from a standardized foundation of education and training, will expand into advanced roles, clinical roles, and quality improvement roles.*
- *Minimum credentials for entry-level pharmacy technicians will expand to include a 2-year degree, ASHP/ACPE-accredited technician training, PTCB certification, and state licensure. These new credentials will allow pharmacy technicians to interact with the public to a higher degree and complement the evolution of pharmacist roles.*
- *For advanced-level pharmacy technicians, minimum credentials will also include advanced certification in an area of specialty based on practice setting and professional certificates pertaining to area of specialty.*

Technician Roles. Pharmacy technicians will contribute to the success of hospitals and health systems by assisting pharmacists in efforts to improve patient safety and patient outcomes with medication use, create efficiencies in pharmacy department workflows, and enable overall pharmacy practice advancement. Pharmacy technicians, from a standardized foundation of education and training, will have advanced operational, clinical support, and quality improvement roles:

- Operational roles will include functions related to technology management, inventory control, distribution and logistics management, sterile and nonsterile compounding, and dispensing.
- Clinical support roles will be patient-focused, including involvement in medication histories, delivery and administration, immunization services, medication stewardship support, patient access to medication, patient counseling, home visits and delivery, and research support.
- Quality improvement roles will include optimizing prior authorization and insurance issues, real-time productivity management, revenue cycle integrity, patient

and medication safety projects, emergency preparedness and response, and performance measurement benchmarking.

Supervisory pharmacy technicians responsible for medication preparation and distribution will be licensed and have formal certificate (or higher) training in quality assurance and will routinely engage in quality assessments and system modifications with respect to the safety of those processes.

Nonclinical decision-making activities of pharmacy technicians will continue to evolve, including resolution of missing medication doses, use of automation and technology, automated dispensing cabinet barcode-scanned fills, purchasing and procurement, distribution, and inventory management. Pharmacy technicians will be accountable for the majority of tasks regarding medication preparation and distribution, without direct or immediate supervision by pharmacists. Independent product validation and verification will continue to expand through barcode (or similar technology) checking and tech-check-tech processes.

Advancement and maturation of all these activities have been incremental to date due to variation among state laws and regulations, lack of public awareness of the technician role, and disparate expectations and responsibilities among different pharmacy practice locations.[63] Achieving profession-wide common ground in defining pharmacy technicians, agreeing on pharmacy technician education, identifying entry-level knowledge, skills, and abilities, requiring pharmacy technician certification, minimizing variability in state laws and rules, and advancing pharmacy technician career pathways will eventually gain uniform acceptance and agreement.[64] Until that occurs, however, it is likely that regulatory or organizational allowances for pharmacy technician utilization in those settings will expand first in hospital and health-system settings. To enable significant gains in formalization of pharmacy technician role delineation, ASHP will continue to work toward consensus within the profession.[39,64,65] Profession-wide adoption of uniform state requirements for registration and certification of pharmacy technicians will be the foremost goal. As the pharmacy technician profile shifts and creates supply and demand challenges in the labor market, there may be differing requirements depending on practice sector (i.e., community, long-term care, or hospital and health system) and tiered requirements for entry-level and advanced roles. In that evolution, entry requirements for pharmacy technicians seeking employment in hospitals and health systems will include (**Figure 2**):

- Completion of ASHP/ACPE-accredited technician education and training, with or without a 2-year degree;
- Pharmacy Technician Certification Board (PTCB) certification; and
- State registration and state licensure.

Some advanced work roles will require completion of a 2-year degree, PTCB certification, completion of requirements for conferral of the PTCB Advanced Certified Pharmacy Technician credential, and an appropriate certificate program whose focus will depend on work assignments, such as medication history taking, technician product verification, remote dispensing, basic and advanced compounding, hazardous medication handling, inventory management (including controlled substance diversion prevention), billing and reimbursement, handling of hazardous medications, informatics, medication safety, and systems improvement.[65]

Technician Education. Direct experience and pharmacy technician apprenticeship approaches will continue to be important in pharmacy technician training. To elevate the knowledge base and skill set of pharmacy technicians and create consistent competency expectations in acute and ambulatory care settings, uniform education requirements eventually will be realized and accepted profession-wide. Standardizing pharmacy technician education and training requirements through accredited education programs mirrors the approach of other technical healthcare occupations such as laboratory technician, dental assistant, and physical therapy assistant. Training and education will have to ensure competencies needed for anticipated increases in responsibility as well as the development of interpersonal skills to foster trusted relationships with patients and interprofessional colleagues.

In collaboration with the Pharmacy Technician Accreditation Commission (PTAC), an effort between ASHP and ACPE to accredit pharmacy technician education programs and advance the pharmacy technician career path in hospitals and health systems is underway. Development of internal

FIGURE 2. Entry-level and ongoing education and credentials required for pharmacy technicians seeking employment in hospitals and health systems. ACPE = Accreditation Council for Pharmacy Education, PTCB = Pharmacy Technician Certification Board.

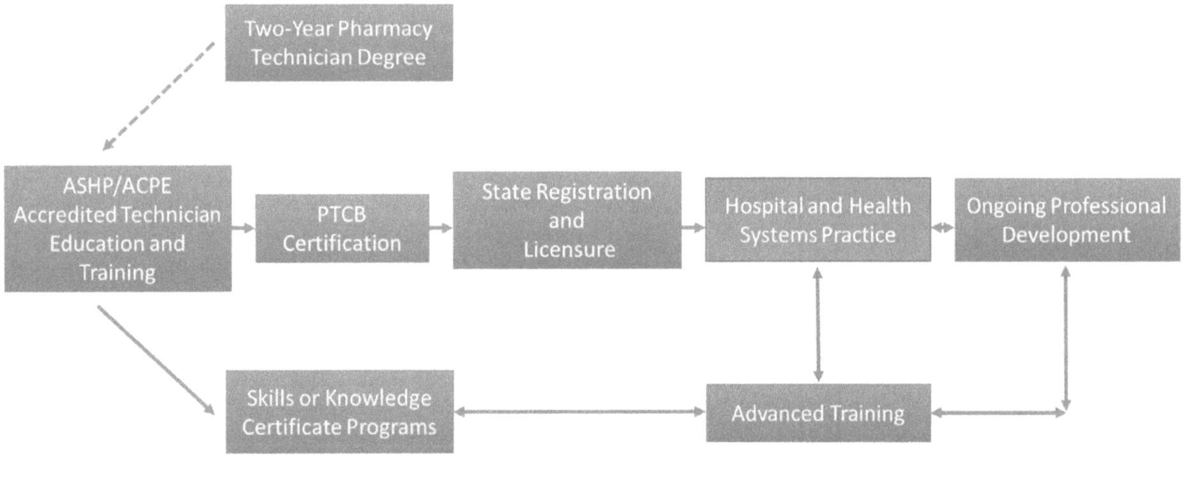

accredited pharmacy technician training programs and distance education programs will increase access to didactic and simulation course work, while experiential site offerings will develop greater capacity to absorb ncreased technician labor supply.

Technician Certification. Similar to certification for pharmacists, certification for pharmacy technicians is a credential earned by demonstrating attainment of specific skills or knowledge. PTCB reports that certified pharmacy technicians tend to have higher earnings, more promotion opportunities, enhanced self-worth, improved job satisfaction, and increased knowledge.[66] In acute and ambulatory care settings, PTCB certification will be a requirement for promotion and advanced roles for pharmacy technicians in hospitals and health systems. Requiring successful completion of the PTCB Pharmacy Technician Certification Exam will foster growth in generalized knowledge and skills in the pharmacy technician staff, while specialty certifications in a particular area, such as sterile compounding, will begin to grow in offerings and completion.

Similar to CPE expectations for pharmacists, certified pharmacy technicians will continue to be expected to complete CPE activity hours within a routinely specified time interval. ASHP will continue to support pharmacy technician CPE that meets ACPE accreditation requirements that promote problem solving and critical thinking applicable to the safe and effective practice of pharmacy.[66] Pharmacy departments will promote access to accredited CPE programs for pharmacy technicians as a means to maintain ongoing competency, support professional development, and pursue opportunities for promotion.

Vision for Contributory Pharmacy Staff

- *Contributory pharmacy staff will supplement pharmacy departments with expertise in finance, analytics, business management, quality assurance, informatics, prior authorization, and supply chain management.*

Within hospital and health-system pharmacy departments are staff that are essential to the responsibilities, operations, and objectives of the organization; however, they are not classified as a pharmacist or pharmacy technician. Contributory pharmacy staff will supplement pharmacy departments with expertise in finance, analytics, business management, quality assurance, informatics, prior authorization, and supply chain management. These staff members will be integrated into the activities of the department and be encouraged and enabled to function at the top of their education and expertise.

Vision for Well-Being and Resilience

- *Pharmacy staff will support individual efforts to develop and demonstrate coping skills and create systems to address risk factors known to cause burnout in healthcare, such as excessive workload, lack of autonomy, lack of reward, lack of community, and job—individual incongruence.*

Patient safety and quality of care are compromised when the healthcare workforce is experiencing burnout.[67,68] Well-being and resilience in the workforce promotes patient safety, patient–clinician relationships, and high-functioning care teams.[69] Evidence supports the well-being of care teams as a critical component of ensuring patient-centered care, optimal health of communities, and lower healthcare cost.[70] Healthcare well-being and resiliency will be acknowledged as a shared responsibility between individual pharmacy personnel and organizations. Interventions to improve and maintain it in hospitals and health systems will be aimed at supporting the individual and improving the system in which he or she works.[69,71] The pharmacy workforce will be expected to have resiliency in coping with ambiguity and uncertainty while operating in a work environment known to introduce unique stressors throughout education, training, and careers.[2,71] Pharmacy staff in hospitals and health systems will support development and demonstration of coping skills and will create approaches to address risk factors known to cause burnout in healthcare organizations, such as excessive workload, lack of autonomy, lack of reward, lack of community, and job–individual incongruence.[72]

Vision for a Diverse and Inclusive Work Environment

- *Pharmacy departments in hospitals and health systems will embrace and rely on differing demographics in the pharmacy workforce, striving to achieve equity and diversity in all clinical, technical, and leadership roles.*

The healthcare workforce as a whole continues to grow at a steady rate, and roles are constantly changing and being created. Ensuring equity in hiring, training, and promoting talent in hospital and health-system pharmacy departments will help optimize patient health outcomes and strengthen the workforce. ASHP affirms this in policy stating that a diverse and inclusive workforce contributes to health equity and health outcomes.[73,74] Just as healthcare providers and team members are obligated to mitigate biases in the delivery of patient care, so too must biases be mitigated in the culture of the workplace. Considerations in diversity include race and ethnicity, gender, gender identity, religious and cultural beliefs, and any other generational or experiential differences. Pharmacy departments in hospitals and health systems will embrace and rely on differing demographics in the pharmacy workforce, striving to achieve equity and diversity in all clinical, technical, and leadership roles. They will adopt zero tolerance policies for discrimination and biases to ensure an inclusive environment and culture, which will improve the practice of respect across the care continuum and the pharmacy workforce.[75]

Conflict among pharmacy personnel within hospitals and health systems and across the pharmacy profession as a whole compromises patient care and is divisive.[76] As the pharmacy workforce evolves and advances, it is essential to reinforce inter- and intraprofessional sensitivity and proactively address conflicts that may result from the diverse roles and contributions across the continuum of care, from acute care settings to community settings.[77] Different roles and practice settings may call for varying levels of education, certification, and specialization. These differences must be embraced and valued. By adopting and maintaining a patient-first mindset, inter- and intraprofessional collaboration can flourish.[78]

Conclusion

Creating a vision for the pharmacy workforce in hospitals and health systems must account for the complexity of the healthcare landscape and anticipated changes to pharmacy practice. This document outlines some key influencers of change in healthcare and provides predictions envisioned for ensuring a prepared and engaged pharmacy workforce.

Glossary

Accreditation: Process by which a private association, organization, or government agency, after initial and periodic evaluations, grants recognition to an organization, site, or program that has met certain established criteria.

Ambulatory care pharmacy practice: Provision of integrated, accessible healthcare services, including telehealth, by pharmacists who are accountable for addressing medication needs, developing sustained partnerships with patients, and practicing in the context of family and community. This is provided through direct patient care and medication management for ambulatory patients, creation and maintenance of long-term relationships, coordination of care, patient advocacy, wellness and health promotion, triage and referral, and patient education and self-management. The ambulatory care pharmacist may work in both an institutional and community-based clinic involved in direct care of a diverse patient population.

Certificate: Document issued to an individual after the successful achievement of a predetermined level of performance in an educational or training program.[79]

Certificate program: Structured, systematic education and continuing education experience that is generally smaller in magnitude and shorter in duration than a degree program and that is designed to instill, expand, or enhance practice competencies through the systematic acquisition of specific knowledge, skills, attitudes, and performance behaviors.[80]

Certification: Voluntary process by which a nongovernmental agency or an association grants recognition to an individual who has met certain predetermined qualifications specified by that organization. This formal recognition is granted to designate to the public that the individual has attained the requisite level of knowledge, skill, and experience in a well-defined, often specialized, area of the total discipline. Certification usually requires initial assessment and periodic reassessments of the individual's knowledge, skills, and experience.

Comprehensive medication management: The standard of care that ensures each patient's medications (whether they are prescription, nonprescription, alternative, traditional, vitamins, or nutritional supplements) are individually assessed to determine each medication is appropriate for the patient, effective for the medical condition, safe given the comorbidities and other medications being taken, and able to be taken by the patient as intended.[81]

Continuing professional development: Self-directed, ongoing, systematic, and outcomes-focused approach to lifelong learning that is applied into practice.[82]

Credential: Documented evidence of qualifications. Pharmacist credentials include diplomas, licenses, certificates, and certifications. For pharmacy technicians, CPhT indicates certification by the Pharmacy Technician Certification Board. Credentials are reflected in a variety of abbreviations that pharmacists place after their names (e.g., Pharm.D. for "doctor of pharmacy," an earned academic degree; RPh for "registered pharmacist," which indicates state licensure; and acronyms such as BCNSP for "Board- Certified Nutrition Support Pharmacist," which indicates that an individual has demonstrated advanced knowledge or skill in a specialized area of pharmacy).

Credentialing: Process by which an organization or institution obtains, verifies, and assesses a pharmacist's or pharmacy technician's qualifications to provide patient care services.

Interprofessional collaborative practice: Occurs when a number of health workers from different professional backgrounds work with patients, their families, caregivers, and communities to provide comprehensive service and deliver the highest practicable quality of care; accepted as an essential function of the care team.[27]

Interprofessional education: When members from 2 or more professions learn with, from, and about each other to enable effective collaboration and improve health outcomes.[27,83]

Layered learning practice model: A model of education in the clinical learning environment in which introductory and advanced experiential pharmacy students and residents are integrated into the care team.[84]

Licensure: The process by which an agency of government grants permission to an individual to engage in a given occupation upon finding that the applicant has attained the minimal degree of competency necessary to ensure that the public health, safety, and welfare will be reasonably well protected.

Medication management services: A spectrum of patient-centered, pharmacist-provided, collaborative services that focus on medication appropriateness, effectiveness, safety, and adherence with the goal of improving health outcomes.[85]

Privileging: The process used by healthcare organizations to grant to a specific practitioner the authorization to provide specific patient-care services.[79]

Resilience: The set of individual, organizational, and cultural skills, behaviors, and attitudes that contribute to personal physical, emotional, and social well-being, including the prevention of burnout. These can include self-care strategies, safety nets for crises, organizational support, peer support, financial management, life-needs support, and other forms of health promotion.[86]

Social determinants of health: Factors that contribute to a person's current state of health that may be biological, socioeconomic, psychosocial, or behavioral.[87]

Well-being: An integrative concept that characterizes quality of life with respect to an individual's health and work-related environmental, organizational, and psychosocial factors. It is the experience of positive perceptions and the presence of constructive conditions at work and in other areas of life that enables workers to thrive and achieve their full potential.[88,89]

Workforce: People engaged in a specific activity or enterprise.[90]

References

1. American Society of Health-System Pharmacists. ASHP long-range vision for the pharmacy work force in hospitals and health systems. *Am J Health-Syst Pharm.* 2007; 64:1320–30.
2. Vermeulen LC, Kolesar JM, Crismon ML et al. ASHP Foundation pharmacy forecast 2018: Strategic planning advice for pharmacy departments in hospitals and health systems. *Am J Health-Syst Pharm.* 2018; 75(2):23–54.
3. Joint Commission of Pharmacy Practitioners. JCPP vision for pharmacists' practice (May 2014). https://jcpp.net/wp-content/uploads/2016/02/JCPP_Vision-Complement_approved-May-29-2014-Final.docx (accessed 2018 Jun 20).
4. American Society of Health-Systems Pharmacists. ASHP national surveys of pharmacy practice in hospital settings. http://www.ajhp.org/cc/ashp-nationalsurveys-of-pharmacy-practice-in-hospital-settings%20?sso-checked=true (accessed 2018 Jun 20).
5. Agency for Healthcare Research and Quality. About the National Quality Strategy. https://www.ahrq.gov/workingforquality/about/index.html (accessed 2018 Jun 20).
6. Deloitte. 2016 consumer priorities in health care survey. https://www2.deloitte.com/content/dam/Deloitte/us/Documents/life-sciences-health-care/us-lshc-deloitte-2016-consumer-priorities-in-health-care-survey.pdf (accessed 2018 Jun 20).
7. Deloitte. 2018 global health care outlook: The evolution of smart health care. https://www2.deloitte.com/content/dam/Deloitte/global/Documents/Life-Sciences-Health-Care/gx-lshc-hc-outlook-2018.pdf (accessed 2018 Jun 19).
8. Office of Disease Prevention and Health Promotion. HealthyPeople: social determinants of health. https://www.healthypeople.gov/2020/topics-objectives/topic/social-determinants-of-health (accessed 2018 Jun 21).
9. Henry J Kaiser Family Foundation. Beyond health care: the role of social determinants in promoting health and health equity (May 2018). https://www.kff.org/disparities-policy/issue-brief/beyond-health-care-therole-of-social-determinants-in-promoting-health-andhealth-equity/ (accessed 2018 Jun 21).
10. Woolf SH, Johnson RE, Phillips RL Jr, Philipsen M. Giving everyone the health of the educated: an examination of whether social change would save more lives than medical advances. *Am J Public Health.* 2007; 97(4):679–83.
11. DeVoe JE, Bazemore AW, Cottrell EK. Perspectives in primary care: a conceptual framework and path for integrating social determinants of health into primary care practice. *Ann Fam Med.* 2016; 14(2):104–8.
12. Johnson TJ, Brownlee MJ. Development and innovation of system resources to optimize patient care. *Am J Health-Syst Pharm.* 2018; 75(7):465–72.
13. Robinson JC. Biomedical innovation in the era of health care spending constraints. *Health Aff.* 2015; 34:203–9.
14. Frakt A, Carroll A. In defense of health-care regulation (June 3, 2011). https://www.washingtonpost.com/blogs/ezra-klein/post/indefense-of-health-care-regulation/2011/06/03/AGttq8HH_blog.html?noredirect=on&utm_term=.3a66e0a29ca3&wprss=ezra-klein (accessed 2019 Jun 30).
15. Emanuel E, Tanden M, Altman S et al. A systemic approach to containing health care spending. *N Engl J Med.* 2012; 367:949–54.
16. American Hospital Association, Federation of American Hospitals, and American Society of Health-System Pharmacists. *Recent trends in hospital drug spending and manufacturer shortages.* Chicago, IL: NORC at the University of Chicago; 2019 Jan.
17. Accenture. Artificial intelligence (AI): healthcare's new nervous system. https://www.accenture.com/us-en/insight-artificial-intelligence-healthcare (accessed 2018 Jun 21).
18. Kalis B, Collier M, Fu R. 10 Promising AI applications in health care (May 10, 2018). https://hbr.org/2018/05/10-promising-ai-applications-in-healthcare (accessed 2018 Jun 21).
19. Congressional Budget Office. A CBO study: the long-term outlook for health care spending (November 2007). https://www.cbo.gov/sites/default/files/cbofiles/ftpdocs/87xx/doc8758/11-13-lt-health.pdf (accessed 2018 Jun 21).
20. Dunn A, Witmire B, Batch A et al. High spending growth rates for key diseases in 2000—14 were driven by technology and demographic factors. *Health Aff.* 2018; 37(6):915–24.
21. White House. The Precision Medicine Initiative. https://obamawhitehouse.archives.gov/node/333101 (accessed 2018 Aug 10).
22. Schwaederle M, Zhao M, Lee JJ et al. Association of biomarker-based treatment strategies with response rates and progression-free survival in refractory malignant neoplasms: a meta-analysis. *JAMA Oncol.* 2016; 2:1452–9.
23. Miller KL, Lanthier M. Regulatory watch: innovation in biologic new molecular entities: 1986–2014. *Nat Rev Drug Discov.* 2015; 14:83.
24. McDonagh EM, Whirl-Carrillo M, Garten Y et al. From pharmacogenomic knowledge acquisition to clinical applications: the PharmGKB as a clinical pharmacogenomics biomarker resource. *Biomark Med.* 2011; 5:795–806.
25. O'Donnell PH, Bush A, Spitz J et al. The 1200 Patients Project: creating a new medical model system for clinical implementation of pharmacogenomics. *Clin Pharmacol Ther.* 2012; 92:446–9.
26. Caudle KE, Klein TE, Hoffman JM et al. Incorporation of pharmacogenomics into routine clinical practice: the Clinical Pharmacogenomics Implementation

Consortium (CPIC) guideline development process. *Curr Drug Metab.* 2014; 15(2):209–17.

27. Health Professions Networks Nursing & Midwifery Human Resources for Health, World Health Organization. Framework for action on interprofessional education & collaborative practice (2010). https://apps.who.int/iris/bitstream/handle/10665/70185/WHO_HRH_HPN_10.3_eng.pdf;jsessionid=2ED69B4D11D5D3A9E309A86A35CE93D4?sequence=1 (accessed 2018 Jun 18).
28. Berwick DM. Era 3 for medicine and health care. *JAMA.* 2016; 315(13):1329–30.
29. Kruse K. What is employee engagement? https://www.forbes.com/sites/kevinkruse/2012/06/22/employeeengagement-what-and-why/#2f96ddd37f37 (accessed 2018 Aug 14).
30. World Health Organization. Global strategy on human resources for health: workforce 2030. http://www.who.int/hrh/resources/globstrathrh-2030/en/ (accessed 2018 Aug 10).
31. Frenk J, Chen L, Bhutta ZA et al. Health professionals for a new century: transforming education to strengthen health systems in an interdependent world. *Lancet.* 2010; 376(9756):1923–58.
32. Greiner AC, Knebel E, eds., for the Institute of Medicine Committee on the Health Professions Education Summit. *Health professions education: a bridge to quality.* Washington, DC: National Academies Press; 2003.
33. Ward A, Berensen N, Daniels R. Creating a learning organization to help meet the needs of multihospital systems. *Am J Health-Syst Pharm.* 2018; 75(7):473–81.
34. Accreditation Council for Pharmacy Education. Accreditation standards and key elements for the professional program in pharmacy leading to the doctor of pharmacy degree. https://www.acpe-accredit.org/pdf/Standards2016FINAL.pdf (accessed 2018 Jun 23).
35. Turner C. Shared responsibility for the education of pharmacy students. *Am J Health-Syst Pharm.* 2018; 75(4):223–9.
36. Blouin RA, Riffee WH, Robinson ET et al. Roles of innovation in education delivery. *Am J Pharm Educ.* 2009; 73(8):article 154.
37. Speedie MK, Baldwin JN, Carter RA et al. Cultivating "habits of mind" in the scholarly pharmacy clinician: report of the 2011–12 Argus Commission. *Am J Pharm Educ.* 2012; 76(6):article S3.
38. Catizone C, Maine L, Menighan T. Continuing our collaboration to create practice-ready, team oriented patient care pharmacists. *Am J Pharm Educ.* 2013; 77:article 43.
39. The consensus of the pharmacy practice model summit. *Am J Health-Syst Pharm.* 2011; 68(12):1148–52.
40. Bates JS, Buie LW, Amerine LB et al. Expanding care through a layered learning practice model. *Am J Health-Syst Pharm.* 2016; 73(22):1869–75.
41. Pinelli NR, McLaughlin JE, Khanova J et al. Identifying the presence of cognitive apprenticeship in the layered learning practice model. *Am J Pharm Educ.* 2018; 82(1):article 6155.
42. Dornan T, Littlewood S, Margolis SA et al. How can experience in clinical and community settings contribute to early medical education? A BEME systematic review. *Med Teach.* 2006; 28:3–18.
43. Homested FA, Chen DF, Knoer SJ. Building value: expanding ambulatory care in the pharmacy enterprise. *Am J Health-Syst Pharm.* 2016; 73(10):635–41.
44. American Society of Health-System Pharmacists. Required competency areas, goals, and objectives for postgraduate year one (PGY1) pharmacy residencies. https://www.ashp.org/-/media/assets/professionaldevelopment/residencies/docs/required-competencyareas-goals-objectives (accessed 2018 Jun 26).
45. Bishop BM, Silvester JA, Martin CY, Bush CG. National survey of pharmacy residents nearing completion of the 2014–2015 residency year. *Am J Health-Syst Pharm.* 2017; 74(11):843–52.
46. American Society of Health-System Pharmacists. ASHP accreditation standard for postgraduate year two (PGY2) pharmacy residency programs. https://www.ashp.org/-/media/assets/professional-development/residencies/docs/pgy2-residency-accreditation-standard-June2017.ashx?la=en&hash=6AB9A9CCAC47929779FB5B9240D4490B2250FCD6 (accessed 2018 Jun 22).
47. Loy BM, Yang S, Moss JM et al. Application of the layered learning practice model in an academic medical center. *Hosp Pharm.* 2017; 52(4):266–72.
48. Bureau of Labor Statistics. Number of jobs held, labor market activity, and earnings growth among the youngest baby boomers: results from a longitudinal survey. https://www.bls.gov/news.release/pdf/nlsoy.pdf (accessed 2018 Jun 23).
49. Altucher J. *Reinvent yourself.* Jupiter, FL: Choose Yourself Media; 2017:378.
50. Schneider PJ, Pedersen CA, Scheckelhoff DJ. ASHP national survey of pharmacy practice in hospital settings: dispensing and administration—2017. *Am J Health-Syst Pharm.* 2018; 75(16):1203–26.
51. Matzke K, ed. *2010 credentials verification desk reference.* Middleton, MA: Credentialing Resource Center; 2010.
52. 42 CFR 482.12 (a)(6).
53. Rouse MJ. Continuing professional development in pharmacy. *Am J Health-Syst Pharm.* 2004; 61(19):2069–76.
54. Hager D, Chmielewski E, Porter AL et al. Interprofessional development and implementation of a pharmacist professional advancement and recognition program. *Am J Health-Syst Pharm.* 2017; 74(22):1895–1902.
55. Institute of Medicine (US) Roundtable on Evidence-Based Medicine; Olsen LA, Aisner D, McGinnis JM, eds. *The learning healthcare system: workshop summary.* Washington, DC: National Academies Press; 2007.
56. American Society of Health-System Pharmacists. ASHP statement on leadership as a professional obligation. *Am J Health-Syst Pharm.* 2011; 68:2293–5.
57. Bush PW. Inaugural address of the incoming president: caring for patients and frontline pharmacy staff. *Am J Health-Syst Pharm.* 2017; 74(16): 1267–70.

58. Zellmer WA. Pharmacy vision and leadership: revisiting the fundamentals. *Pharmacotherapy*. 2008; 28(12):1437–42.
59. American Society of Health-System Pharmacists. ASHP statement on the roles and responsibilities of the pharmacy executive. *Am J Health-Syst Pharm*. 2016; 73:329–32.
60. Boyd AM, Clark JS, Kent SS. Strategic thinking in pharmacy. *Am J Health-Syst Pharm*. 2017; 74(14):103–8.
61. Knoer S. Stewardship of the pharmacy enterprise. *Am J Health-Syst Pharm*. 2014; 71(14):1204–9.
62. Ivey MF. Rationale for having a chief pharmacy officer in a health care organization. *Am J Health-Syst Pharm*. 2005; 62(9):975–8.
63. Zellmer WA, McAllister EB, Silvester JA, Vlasses PH. Toward uniform standards for pharmacy technicians: summary of the 2017 Pharmacy Technician Stakeholder Consensus Conference. *Am J Health-Syst Pharm*. 2017; 74:1321–32.
64. Abramowitz PW, Cobaugh DJ. Education and certification of pharmacy technicians: a noble decision is long overdue. *Am J Health-Syst Pharm*. 2017; 74(17):1303–4.
65. Pharmacy Technician Certification Board. PTCB developing advanced CPhT credential. https://www.ptcb.org/about-ptcb/news-room/news-landing/2019/03/19/ptcb-developing-advanced-cpht-credential (accessed 2019 Mar 22)
66. Pharmacy Technician Certification Board. https://www.ptcb.org/who-we-serve#.WzVf3uSWzcs (accessed 2018 Jun 28).
67. Hall LH, Johnson J, Watt I et al. Healthcare staff wellbeing, burnout, and patient safety: a systematic review. *PLoS ONE*. 2016; 11(7):e0159015.
68. Mossburg SE, Himmelfarb CD. The association between professional burnout and engagement with patient safety culture and outcomes: a systematic review. *J Patient Saf.* Epub ahead of print. 2018 Jun 25.
69. Dzau VJ, Kirch DG, Nasca TJ. To care is human—collectively confronting the clinician-burnout crisis. *N Engl J Med*. 2018; 378(4):312–4.
70. Bodenheimer T, Sinsky C. From triple aim to quadruple aim: care of the patient requires care of the provider. *Ann Fam Med*. 2014; 12(6):573–6.
71. American Society of Health-System Pharmacists Council on Education and Workforce Development. ASHP policy 1825. Clinician well-being and resilience (2018). https://www.ashp.org/-/media/assets/policyguidelines/docs/browse-by-document-type-policypositions-1982-2018-with-rationales-pdf.pdf (accessed 2019 Oct 18).
72. Bridgeman PJ, Bridgeman MB, Barone J. Burnout syndrome among healthcare professionals. *Am J Health-Syst Pharm*. 2017; 74(3):147–52.
73. American Society of Health-System Pharmacists Council on Education and Workforce Development. ASHP policy 1705. Workforce diversity (2018). https://www.ashp.org/-/media/assets/policy-uidelines/docs/browse-by-document-type-policy-positions-1982-2018-with-rationales-pdf.pdf (accessed 2019 Oct 18).
74. American Society of Health-System Pharmacists. ASHP statement on racial and ethnic disparities in health care. *Am J Health-Syst Pharm*. 2008; 65:728–33.
75. Sokol-Hessner L, Henry Folcarelli P, Annas CL, et al. A road map for advancing the practice of respect in health care: the results of an interdisciplinary modified Delphi consensus study. *Jt Comm J Qual Patient Saf.* 2018; 44(8):463–76.
76. Gregory PA, Austin Z. Conflict in community pharmacy practice: the experience of pharmacists, technicians, and assistants. *Can Pharm J*. 2017; 150(1):32–41.
77. Alsharif NZ. Intraprofessional sensitivity: a must for the academy and the profession. *Am J Pharm Educ*. 2013; 77(3):article 42.
78. Gobis B, Yu A, Reardon J et al. Prioritizing intraprofessional collaboration for optimal patient care: a call to action. *Can Pharm J*. 2018; 151(3):170–5.
79. Council on Credentialing in Pharmacy. Credentialing and privileging of pharmacists: a resource paper from the Council on Credentialing in Pharmacy. *Am J Health-Syst Pharm*. 2014; 71:1891–1900.
80. Council on Credentialing in Pharmacy. Credentialing in pharmacy: a resource paper (November 2010). http://www.pharmacycredentialing.org/Files/CCP-WhitePaper2010.pdf (accessed 2019 Oct 18).
81. Patient-Centered Primary Care Collaborative Medication Management Task Force Collaborative. The patient-centered medical home: integrating comprehensive medication management to optimize patient outcomes resource guide, 2nd edition (2012). https://www.pcpcc.org/sites/default/files/media/medmanagement.pdf (accessed 2019 Dec 3).
82. Accreditation Council for Pharmacy Education. Continuing professional development. https://www.acpe-accredit.org/continuing-professional-development/ (accessed 2018 August 22).
83. Joint Accreditation for Interprofessional Continuing Education. About joint accreditation. http://www.jointaccreditation.org/about-joint-accreditation (accessed 2018 August 22).
84. Pinelli NR, Eckel SF, Vu MB et al. The layered learning practice model: lessons learned from implementation. *Am J Health-Syst Pharm*. 2016; 73(24):2077–82.
85. Joint Commission of Pharmacy Practitioners. Medication Management Services (MMS) Definition and Key Points. (2018) https://jcpp.net/wp-content/uploads/2018/05/Medication-Management-Services-Definition-and-Key-Points-Version-1.pdf
86. Trockel M, Hamidi M, Murphy ML et al., for Stanford Medicine. 2016 physician wellness survey full report. https://wellmd.stanford.edu/content/dam/sm/wellmd/documents/Full-2016-Physician-Wellness-Survey-Report-16-Aug-2017-Final-rd.pdf (accessed 2019 Oct 18).
87. HealthyPeople.gov. Social determinants of health. https://www.healthypeople.gov/2020/topics-objectives/topic/social-determinants-of-health (accessed 2019 Mar 13).

88. Centers for Disease Control and Prevention. The National Institute for Occupational Safety and Health: total worker health (2016). https://www.cdc.gov/niosh/twh/letsgetstarted.html (accessed 2018 Jul 9).
89. Harvard T.H. Chan School of Public Health. SafeWell practice guidelines: an integrated approach to worker health (2013). http://centerforworkhealth.sph.harvard.edu/resources/safewell-resources (accessed 2018 Jul 9).
90. Merriam-Webster Dictionary. Workforce [definition]. https://www.merriam-webster.com/dictionary/workforce (accessed 2019 Mar 12).

Approved by the ASHP Board of Directors, May 15, 2019. Revised by the ASHP Council on Education and Workforce Development. Supersedes the ASHP Long-Range Vision for the Pharmacy Work Force in Hospitals and Health Systems dated January 11, 2007.

The following are acknowledged for reviewing the draft vision documents: Scott V. Anderson, Pharm.D., M.S., University of Virginia Health System; CDR Anne Marie Bott, Pharm.D., BCPS, BCOP, Alaska Native Medical Center; Jackie Boyle, Pharm.D, M.S., M.B.A., BCPS, BCACP, NEOMED School of Pharmacy; Ryan Burke, Pharmacy Technician Certification Board; Ashley Chen, Pharm.D., Ruohola-Baker Research Lab; Daan Chen, Pharm.D., FCI La Tuna; Lourdes M. Cuellar, M.S., TIRR Memorial Hermann; Brook Smith DesRivieres, Pharm.D., M.S., Ascension Wisconsin; Jean Douglas, B.S.Pharm., Pharm.D., RPh, FASHP, High Point University School of Pharmacy; Lea S. Eiland, Pharm.D., BCPS, BCPPS, FASHP, FPPAG, Auburn University; Rena Gosser, Pharm.D., BCPS, University of Washington Medicine; Roy Guharoy, Pharm.D., M.B.A., Baptist Health; David Hager, Pharm.D., BCPS, UW Health; John Hertig, Pharm.D., M.S., Butler University; Eric C. Kutscher, Pharm.D., M.B.A., BCPP, FASHP, University of Arizona; LCDR Michelle Locke, Pharm.D., NCPS, Alaska Native Medical Center; Robert Macky, Pharm.D., FCC Butner; Katie Clark McKinney, Pharm.D., M.S., BCPS, FACHE, FASHP, UC Health–University of Cincinnati Medical Center; Ryan Mills, Pharm.D., M.B.A., M.H.A., BCPS, Novant Health; Zachary Obert, Pharm.D., UC Health–University of Cincinnati Medical Center and University of Cincinnati James L. Winkle College of Pharmacy; Daniel Pons, Pharm.D., LMH Health; James R Rinehart, RPh, M.S., FASHP, Winovation Associates LLC; CDR Ashley Schaber, Pharm.D., M.B.A., BCPS, Alaska Native Medical Center; Rebecca Taylor, Pharm.D., M.B.A., BCPS, Cleveland Clinic; Taylor MacKinnon, Pharm.D., UW Health; Kathy Pham, Pharm.D., American College of Clinical Pharmacy; Laura Traynor, Pharm.D, BCPS, AE-C, Concordia University Wisconsin School of Pharmacy; Dennis Tribble, Pharm.D., FASHP, BD; Allen Vaida, Pharm.D., FASHP, Institute for Safe Medication Practices; Elizabeth Wade, Pharm.D., BCPS, Concord Hospital; Molly Wascher, Pharm.D., M.B.A., BCPS, Maryland Society of Health-System Pharmacists; Tricia Lee (Wilkins) Rolle, Pharm.D., Ph.D., Academy of Managed Care Pharmacy; Roger Woolf, Pharm.D., FASHP, Virginia Mason Medical Center.

Copyright © 2020, American Society of Health-System Pharmacists, Inc. All rights reserved. Contact ASHP for reprint and permissions requests. This content may not be used for commercial purposes without the express written consent of ASHP.

The bibliographic citation for this document is as follows: American Society of Health-System Pharmacists. ASHP long-range vision for the pharmacy workforce in hospitals and health systems: Ensuring medication use is optimal, safe, and effective in acute and ambulatory care settings. *Am J Health-Syst Pharm.* 2020; 77:386–400.

Practice Settings

DOI 10.37573/9781585287048

Practice Settings

2219

HOSPITAL-AT-HOME CARE

Source: Council on Pharmacy Practice

To affirm that patients treated in the hospital-at-home (HAH) setting are entitled to the same level of care as those treated in an inpatient hospital setting; further,

To support HAH care models that provide high-quality, patient-centered pharmacist care, including but not limited to: (1) clinical pharmacy services that are fully integrated with the care team; (2) a medication distribution model that is fully integrated with the providing organization's distribution model and in which the organization's pharmacy leader retains authority over the medication-use process; (3) information technology (IT) systems that are integrated or interoperable with the organization's IT systems and that allow patient access to pharmacy services, optimize medication management, and promote patient safety; and (4) ensuring the safety of the pharmacy workforce throughout the HAH care delivery process; further,

To advocate that pharmacists be included in the planning, implementation, and maintenance of HAH programs; further,

To advocate for legislation and regulations that would promote safe and effective medication use in the HAH care setting, and for adequate reimbursement for pharmacy services, including clinical pharmacy services, provided in the HAH care setting; further,

To provide education, training, and resources to empower the pharmacy workforce to care for patients in HAH care settings and to support the organizations providing that care; further,

To encourage research on HAH care models.

Rationale

Hospital-at-home (HAH) care is a patient care model that provides acute-level care to patients in their own homes. The first described HAH program was originally developed by the Johns Hopkins Schools of Medicine and Public Health over 25 years ago, and the HAH care model has seen broader adoption by other hospitals and health systems in recent years. HAH care models have been shown to improve clinical outcomes, reduce length of stay, provide higher patient satisfaction, and reduce costs and medical complications.

The COVID-19 pandemic forced hospitals and health systems to explore new and innovative care models, with a heightened focus on remote care. In March 2020, the Centers for Medicare & Medicaid Services (CMS) announced its Hospitals Without Walls program, which resulted in broader regulatory flexibility in providing services beyond hospital walls. This program was expanded in November 2020 to include the Acute Hospital Care at Home program, which allows eligible patients to be treated for acute illnesses in the comfort of their homes. CMS has outlined more than 60 acute conditions such as heart failure, asthma, pneumonia, and chronic obstructive pulmonary disease (COPD) that can be safely managed from a patient's home with proper monitoring and treatment protocols. As of June 4, 2021, there were 59 health systems and 133 hospitals in 32 different states participating in the Acute Hospital Care at Home program.

DOI 10.37573/9781585287048.097

Medication management is a mainstay for most, if not all, of the conditions treated under HAH programs. Pharmacy practice leadership and expertise is therefore needed to ensure patient safety and quality outcomes. Patients treated in HAH programs are entitled to the same level of high-quality, patient-centered pharmacist care as those treated in an inpatient hospital setting. ASHP supports HAH care models that provide high-quality, patient-centered pharmacist care. Patients receiving HAH care should have access to clinical pharmacy services that are fully integrated with the services provided by rest of the patient's care team. To ensure optimal medication use, the HAH program should use a medication distribution model that is fully integrated with the providing organization's distribution model, and the organization's pharmacy leader should retain authority over the entire HAH medication-use process to promote integration with the organization's pharmacy enterprise. The HAH program should use information technology (IT) systems that are integrated or interoperable with the organization's IT systems to allow patients to access pharmacy services, the pharmacy workforce to optimize medication management, and the organization to promote patient safety. Finally, HAH programs should ensure the safety of the healthcare workers delivering care, including members of the pharmacy workforce.

The pharmacy workforce needs to be included in the planning, implementation, and maintenance of HAH programs. Early in the planning process, pharmacy departments can evaluate and determine (1) the in-person, virtual, and electronic patient assessment role for pharmacists in the HAH program to determine staffing requirements; (2) how medications will be provided and stored for patients, especially controlled substances and medications with strict storage requirements (e.g., temperature-sensitive medications); (3) formulary considerations and payer design; (4) state and federal regulations and licensure interpretations to support the practice and supply chain model requirements necessary for HAH programs; (5) how medication administration will be documented (e.g., through bar-code-enabled medication administration), including waste management; (6) electronic healthcare record platform capabilities required to support the HAH program, including an assessment of ancillary information systems or platforms that will need to be integrated with the organizations IT systems to support medication-use documentation and pharmacist consultations; and (8) differences between HAH and home infusion models, and when to deploy the appropriate model.

Pharmacy departments should proactively assess the pharmacy clinical services needed to care for patients in the HAH program and determine the competencies and training to meet expected demands. Examples would include determining how drug information questions will be channeled and how care transitions will be managed (e.g., follow-up appointments for chronic care management, transitions to palliative care). The pharmacy department will need to develop processes to integrate telehealth services for patients to receive pharmacist care (e.g., education). Other considerations include patient choice and healthcare disparities, which may impact the ability to meet the criteria to receive HAH care.

Changes in law, regulations, and standards will be required to support HAH care models, particularly because some elements of the HAH care model were supported by temporary regulatory flexibilities granted to address the COVID-19 public health emergency. Specifically, the continued adoption and expansion of the HAH model will require the creation of sustainable reimbursement models for pharmacist-provided HAH services. Additionally, regulatory changes, particularly from CMS may be needed to ensure that pharmacists can administer medications in the home setting.

To prepare the pharmacy workforce to meet the needs of patients in HAH programs and the organizations managing them, ASHP will need to provide education, training, and resources to prepare the pharmacy workforce for these new and evolving roles, including the development of best practices, residency standards, and workforce competencies. To achieve these goals, ASHP will need to collaborate with interprofessional organizations such as the Hospital at Home Users Group (https://hahusersgroup.org/), a collaborative of HAH programs around the U.S. and Canada that fosters the development and dissemination of resources and best practices to expand the reach of HAH programs, drive practice advancement, and inform regulatory and reimbursement policies to spread the HAH model of care. To provide a basis for these efforts, ASHP will also need to encourage research on the HAH model of care.

2010

USE OF TWO PATIENT IDENTIFIERS IN THE OUTPATIENT SETTING

Source: Council on Pharmacy Practice

To encourage the use of two identifiers to confirm patient identity when transferring filled prescriptions to the possession of the patient or patient's agent for outpatient use.

This policy supersedes ASHP policy 1024.

Rationale

Errors caused by dispensing medications to the wrong patient are largely preventable. Although two patient identifiers are routinely used when medications are administered in inpatient settings, similar practices are not employed when dispensing medications for outpatient use. ASHP supports consistent use of two patient identifiers and believes that this safety strategy should be used to confirm patient identity at the time patients or their agents pick up filled prescriptions for outpatient use.

1623

HOME INTRAVENOUS THERAPY

Source: Council on Public Policy

To support the continuation of a home intravenous therapy benefit under federal and private health insurance plans and expansion of the home infusion benefit under Medicare at an appropriate level of reimbursement for pharmacists' patient care services provided, medications, supplies, and equipment.

This policy was reviewed in 2021 by the Council on Public Policy and by the Board of Directors and was found to still be appropriate.

Rationale

The Medicare Modernization Act of 2003 created an outpatient prescription drug benefit for Medicare beneficiaries, Medicare Part D. The new benefit provided prescription drug coverage for Medicare beneficiaries by private health plans and pharmacy benefit managers (PBMs).

Although the law requires certain basic coverage packages across the plan continuum, it provides no coverage for services and supplies used in home infusion. The result is that the drug products used in home infusion may be covered, but the supplies (e.g., IV bags, tubing) and services related to providing and administering the drug products are not.

The 21st Century Cures Act of 2016 redefined coverage for home infusion services, establishing a new benefit in Medicare Part B that covers professional services associated with home infusion. However, the benefit does not take effect until 2021, and the current benefit reimbursement is far lower than the value of the services. Although there is a transitional gap program to slightly buffer providers from the low reimbursement rates, the cuts have taken a toll on home infusion providers, making it essential that Centers for Medicare & Medicaid Services implement the higher reimbursement rate for 2021. ASHP also remains concerned that under the new Cures Act benefit, reimbursement is made only to the pharmacy, not the pharmacist. Continued advocacy is needed to allow pharmacists to bill directly for the benefit.

ASHP Guidelines on Evaluating and Using Home or Alternate-Site Infusion Service Providers

These guidelines describe the roles of home or alternate-site infusion service providers and pharmacies (hereinafter "home infusion service providers" and "home infusion pharmacies") and provide guidance on how to successfully work with a home infusion service provider in continuing care that has been initiated in a health system or other facility. For the purposes of these guidelines, a *home infusion service provider* is defined as an organization that continues or completes a patient's parenteral medication in the home or alternate site after the patient is released from a hospital or other facility. A home infusion service provider may offer nursing or other services in addition to pharmacist care. A *home infusion pharmacy* is defined as a licensed pharmacy that prepares and dispenses parenteral sterile medications directly to a patient, pursuant to a valid individual prescription and in individualized doses.

Roles of Home Infusion Service Providers

The typical role of a home infusion service provider is to continue or complete a patient's parenteral medication course of therapy in the home or in an alternate site (e.g., infusion suite) after the patient is released from the hospital or other facility. Regardless of the business model of the home infusion service provider (e.g., owned by a health system or a private company), the referring entity and the home infusion service provider maintain a relationship as direct healthcare providers with responsibility for patient care. After accepting a referral, the home infusion service provider is in direct contact with the patient for whom the medication is dispensed and shares responsibility with the prescriber for the clinical outcome of that patient's care.[1,2]

Where recommended due to patient safety concerns or insurance requirements, the parenteral medication may be infused in an infusion suite that is associated with the home infusion service provider, rather than at the patient's residence. Home infusion service providers may employ their own infusion nurses or they may contract with a home health agency (HHA) to provide home nursing care to a patient. Office-based prescribers may also coordinate home infusion services with a home infusion service provider when parenteral medications are prescribed but hospitalization is not needed, which often results in lower healthcare costs.[3]

Roles of the Home Infusion Pharmacy

A home infusion pharmacy prepares and dispenses parenteral sterile medications directly to a patient, pursuant to a valid individual prescription and in individualized doses. These medications include many of the same sterile medications that are prepared in a hospital's inpatient pharmacy, including i.v. antibiotics, antifungals, hydration fluids, parenteral nutrition, chemotherapy, and pain medications. Some home infusion pharmacies also supply i.v. and subcutaneous immune globulins, antihemophilic factor products, and other parenteral medications for chronic conditions. Unlike a hospital pharmacy that dispenses i.v. medications to inpatients on a daily basis, home infusion pharmacies typically dispense on a weekly basis (subject to the stability and sterility parameters of the preparations dispensed).

Home infusion pharmacies differ in many respects from 503B-registered outsourcing facilities.[4,5] A 503B-registered outsourcing facility manufactures multiple containers of a specific medication in batches and predetermined concentrations and sells these compounded sterile products under contract to end users (hospitals, health systems, or physicians' offices). This manufacturing does not occur pursuant to an individual patient prescription, and the 503B-registered outsourcing facility has no direct relationship with the patient to whom the medication is administered. (More information on this topic can be found in ASHP Guidelines on Outsourcing Sterile Compounding Services.[5]) While some home infusion pharmacies may provide both home infusion and compounding pharmacy services, it is important to evaluate these distinct lines of service individually within the correct parameters.

Working with Home Infusion Service Providers

Parenteral medication administration is more complicated than other routes of medication delivery because aseptic technique must be used to prepare and administer each dose. In addition, many parenteral medications require the use of a pump or a rate-controlled delivery system for safe administration. Arranging postdischarge home infusion therapy requires planning to achieve a successful transition of care. Patients who are discharged with orders for parenteral medications to be administered at the home setting or alternate site of service usually require both home health nursing and home infusion pharmacy services. The pharmacy and nursing services may be provided by a single company or by separate providers. Hospitals and health systems should identify high-quality providers of home infusion services before patient discharge and engage in other advanced planning, including communication with the provider, so that the process of discharging a patient with parenteral medications is seamless and supports the patient's clinical goals.

Identifying High-Quality Home Infusion Service Providers. Most hospital discharge planning departments provide patients with a list of home infusion service providers to allow patients freedom in choosing a provider, which is a requirement of any government payer. A checklist that can be used when researching providers of home infusion services is provided in the appendix. Factors that will affect the selection of preferred providers of home infusion services include the following:

1. Whether the home infusion service provider's nursing services are provided by its own employees or through a separate HHA.
   a. If HHAs are used, does the home infusion service provider offer seamless integration of home infusion therapy so that one call coordinates both

DOI 10.37573/9781585287048.098

pharmacy and nursing services? If the patient needs home nursing and has Medicare or Medicaid as the primary insurance payer, an HHA with the appropriate Medicare or Medicaid nursing licenses must be used.[6] Does the home infusion service provider have relationships with Medicare-certified HHAs?

   b. If the home infusion service provider coordinates with an HHA, does the provider maintain a preferred provider list of HHAs? How is that list determined? Accreditation or Medicare certification should be required for all providers of home infusion nursing.
   c. Is the home infusion service provider willing to work with HHAs that the referral source prefers to use?

2. Whether the home infusion service provider is accredited and licensed. Accreditation should be required for a preferred home infusion service provider. Accreditation standards for home infusion (e.g., those of the Accreditation Commission for Health Care,[7] Community Health Accreditation Program,[8] Center for Pharmacy Practice Accreditation,[9] Healthcare Quality Association on Accreditation,[10] National Association of Boards of Pharmacy,[11] The Compliance Team,[12] or the Joint Commission[13]) are very similar to those applied to hospitals and ensure that the organization has undergone peer review and operates with best practices to safeguard patients. To ensure licensing and accreditation, the healthcare organization should
   a. Request a copy of the home infusion service provider's pharmacy and Drug Enforcement Administration licenses.
   b. Request a copy of the accreditation certificate and note the expiration date.
3. Whether the home infusion service provider complies with appropriate compounding standards and regulations. To ensure compliance, the healthcare organization should
   a. Request an attestation from the home infusion pharmacy stating that it complies with applicable state regulations and follows *United States Pharmacopeia* (*USP*) chapter 797 standards for compounding sterile preparations,[1] and request a recent copy of the pharmacy's *USP* chapter 797 gap analysis, if available.
4. The provider's service area and normal hours of operation for pharmacy and nursing services.
   a. For home infusion pharmacy services, the following questions may be pertinent to the selection of a provider:
      i. Does the pharmacy hold any out-of-state pharmacy licenses (if there is a need to serve patient populations from multiple states)?
      ii. Does the pharmacy have the capability to ship medications?
      iii. Does the pharmacy have the capability to make local deliveries?
   b. For home infusion nursing services, the following questions may be pertinent to the selection of a provider:
      i. Is the area of service restricted to certain areas (e.g., counties)?
      ii. Where applicable, is nursing service provided across state boundaries?
      iii. What are the specific geographic boundaries of the nursing service area?
      iv. What are the state requirements concerning licensed or nonlicensed agencies?
5. Whether the home infusion service provider offers 24–7 patient services. If not, how does a patient reach a clinician after regular business hours?
6. Whether the infusion provider offers specialized pharmacy or nursing services (e.g., nutrition support, particular expertise such as pediatric or neonatal, hemophilia, heart failure, or oncology) or advanced infusion skills certification (e.g., certified registered nurse infusion or oncology certification).
7. Referral and transition-of-care process support by the home infusion service provider.
   a. How is patient training performed, and who conducts the training?
   b. Can the home infusion service provider provide a nurse to start the patient's medication in the hospital at the time of discharge for therapies that cannot be interrupted (e.g., pain management, inotropes)?
   c. What is the expected turnaround time from the point of referral to delivery of patient medications and the first home nursing visit?
8. Whether the home infusion service provider can demonstrate success (e.g., patient data showing positive clinical outcomes or positive patient satisfaction survey results).

Transitioning the Infusion Patient from Hospital to Home. The hospital or health system should implement processes that support a successful transition of care for all discharged patients, but preplanning for patients to be discharged with home infusion services is critically important for ensuring a smooth transition of care.[2,14–16] Advanced home infusion discharge planning includes the following:

- Gathering all of the information needed by the home infusion service provider.
- Checking that the home infusion services are covered by the payer and that the home infusion service provider has a contract with the payer. Therapies covered by Medicare must often meet Medicare criteria, which can include specific laboratory tests or invasive monitoring (e.g., inotropes, parenteral nutrition). It must be determined in advance of discharge that the patient's ordered home infusion therapy will be covered by Medicare or other insurance, and any co-payment or out-of-pocket expenses must be communicated to the patient in advance.
- Arranging prior authorization, if required by the payer; prior authorization may require several business days.

- Avoiding a weekend or holiday discharge, unless planned sufficiently in advance that the insurance has been verified and home nursing has been arranged. A weekend or holiday discharge can be accommodated but is not recommended. Most insurance companies are closed on the weekend, and a patient's benefits cannot be determined until the next business day. Such a discharge could result in significant out-of-pocket costs for the patient. In addition, the home health nursing schedule may not permit opening a new case on a weekend.
- Allowing time for placement of a peripherally inserted central catheter (PICC) and PICC catheter tip evaluation before discharge, if necessary.
- Ensuring that a home infusion nurse is available for the first home visit. This visit may last more than two hours and includes a full nursing assessment; it may also include teaching the patient or caregiver how to prepare the medication, administer the medication (including the use of a pump or other medication delivery system), properly store the medication, and care for a vascular access device.
- Allowing time for the home infusion pharmacy to dispense the patient's medication, which includes pharmacist review of the patient's medication list, a check for drug interactions, clarification of any prescription information that is unclear or missing, time for compounding the medication, and time to arrange for the delivery of medications and supplies to the patient. Obtaining a complete and valid prescription from the prescriber who will be treating the patient can require extra time. A valid prescription includes orders for the medication, the number of doses or length of therapy, flushes for catheter care, nursing orders (if applicable), and laboratory test orders.
- Planning extra time to discharge patients who will require a continuous infusion of controlled substances or an inotrope. Typically, these patients need to have their home medication infusion initiated in the hospital at the time of discharge.

Transitional Care Program. A transitional care program for home infusion patients may be offered by the home infusion service provider. This type of program can help identify risk factors that could jeopardize the success of a planned discharge on home infusion therapy, so that any anticipated extra challenges (e.g., lack of a caregiver in the home, orders for more than one parenteral medication) can be mitigated before discharge.

Some home infusion service providers offer clinical liaison nurses who will meet with patients before hospital discharge to explain the patient's home infusion therapy and how those services will be provided. This service may also include initiation of the home infusion teaching process so that the patient or caregiver can become familiar with the home infusion therapy in advance. A clinical liaison nurse employed by a home infusion service provider must have the hospital or health-system's permission to meet with hospitalized patients. Where permitted by the hospital and required by the therapy (e.g., continuous parenteral pain management or inotropic therapy), a clinical nurse liaison may also be available at the time of discharge to initiate the home infusion service, including starting the first dose, which would avoid an interruption in the therapy as the patient transitions from the hospital to the home.

Communication with the Home Infusion Service Provider. Communication between the hospital or health system and the home infusion service provider is essential for maintaining a positive working relationship that will ultimately benefit both patients and providers. It is important for hospital or health-system discharge planners, social workers, and prescribers to understand the information needed by an accredited home infusion service provider. The home infusion pharmacist should be provided with the patient's history and physical summary, a copy of the most recent laboratory test results, an accurate medication list, a document validating appropriate placement of a central venous access device, and complete orders for the infusion medications. The provider who receives the referral information, whether it is the home infusion pharmacy or an HHA, is responsible for communicating the patient's information to any other partners in the patient's home care.

A major challenge to home infusion service providers can arise when home infusion therapy is ordered without a clear plan for prescriber oversight after discharge (e.g., when there is a communication gap between the hospitalist physician who managed the patient's care during hospitalization and the patient's primary care or specialist physician at the point of discharge). If there is no firm arrangement for a prescriber to be responsible for the patient's infusion therapy after discharge and complications arise, the infusion pharmacist or nurse has no option but to refer the patient to the emergency department for a potential readmission. Hospitals and health systems can avoid such an outcome by implementing good advance discharge planning.

Conclusion

Home infusion therapy plays a crucial role in the provision of healthcare, including the provision of cost-effective care outside of an institutional setting. Choosing a home infusion service provider with high-quality standards can make a difference in whether a patient has a positive or negative response to treatment. In addition, a smooth transition of care based on advanced planning will improve outcomes and control costs.

References

1. Pharmaceutical compounding—sterile preparations (general information chapter 797). In: The United States pharmacopeia, 27th rev., and The national formulary, 22nd ed. Rockville, MD: United States Pharmacopeial Convention; 2004:2350–70.
2. Nigro SC, Garwood CL, Berlie H, et al. Clinical pharmacists are key members of the patient-centered medical home: an opinion statement of the Ambulatory Care Practice and Research Network of the American College of Clinical Pharmacy. *Pharmacotherapy.* 2014; 34:96–108.
3. Kennedy S. Home infusion therapy: safety, efficacy and cost-savings. http://psqh.com/home-infusion-therapy-safety-efficacy-and-cost-savings (accessed 2014 Nov 18).

4. American Society of Health-System Pharmacists. ASHP guidelines on home infusion pharmacy services. *Am J Health-Syst Pharm.* 2014; 71:325–41.
5. American Society of Health-System Pharmacists. ASHP guidelines on outsourcing sterile compounding services. *Am J Health-Syst Pharm.* 2015; 72:1664–75.
6. Centers for Medicare and Medicaid Services. Survey & certification—certification and compliance. www.cms.gov/Medicare/Provider-Enrollment-and-Certification/CertificationandComplianc/index.html (accessed 2014 Nov 5).
7. Accreditation Commission for Health Care. Home health accreditation. www.achc.org/programs/home-health (accessed 2016 Mar 9).
8. Community Health Accreditation Program. Pharmacy. www.chapinc.org/services-we-accredit/pharmacy.aspx (accessed 2016 Mar 9).
9. Center for Pharmacy Practice Accreditation. Community pharmacy practice accreditations. www.pharmacypracticeaccredit.org/practices (accessed 2016 Mar 9).
10. Healthcare Quality Association on Accreditation. Infusion pharmacy accreditation. www.hqaa.org (accessed 2016 Mar 9).
11. National Association of Boards of Pharmacy. DMEPOS accreditation program. www.nabp.net/programs/accreditation/dmepos (accessed 2016 Mar 9).
12. The Compliance Team. Exemplary provider accreditation program. www.thecomplianceteam.org (accessed 2016 Mar 9).
13. Joint Commission. Home care accreditation program. www.jointcommission.org/accreditation/home_care_accreditation.aspx (accessed 2016 Mar 9).
14. Hume AL, Kirwin J, Bieber HL, et al. Improving care transitions: current practice and future opportunities for pharmacists. *Pharmacotherapy.* 2012; 32:e326–37.
15. Tucker A, Ybarra J, Bingham A, et al. American Society for Parenteral and Enteral Nutrition (A.S.P.E.N.) standards of practice for nutrition support pharmacists. *Nutr Clin Pract.* 2015; 30:139–46.
16. Labson MC, Prosser BS, Tharp J. Establishing a culture of safety in the prevention of medication errors. Paper presented at the National Home Infusion Association, 2015 Annual Conference and Exposition. Phoenix, AZ; 2015 Mar.

Appendix—Checklist for Evaluating a Home Infusion Service Provider

Criterion	Yes	No
Does the provider service the area where the patient lives?		
Is the provider licensed by the State Board of Pharmacy?		
Is the provider accredited?		
Is the provider *United States Pharmacopeia* chapter 797 compliant?		
Does the provider have its own nursing staff?		
Is the provider willing to work with preferred nursing agencies?		
Are the provider's normal hours of operation sufficient to fulfill all requirements and needs?		
Does the provider provide 24-7 coverage for nursing?		
Does the provider provide 24-7 coverage for pharmacy?		
Does the provider have a nutrition support team? (if applicable)		
Does the provider have pediatric expertise? (if applicable)		
Does the provider have any other areas of expertise needed?		
Does the provider have clinical liaisons? (if applicable)		
Will the provider come to the hospital to initiate therapy if needed?		
Can the provider meet the expected turnaround time needed?		
Can the provider accept the patient's insurance?		
Does the provider have evidence of positive outcomes?		
Does the provider provide timely feedback?		
Will the provider accept after-hours referrals?		
Can the provider accept patients who do not speak English? (if applicable)		
Can the provider accept electronic prescriptions?		
Has the patient been a patient with this provider in the past?		

Approved by the ASHP Board of Directors on November 30, 2015, and developed through the ASHP Section of Ambulatory Care Practitioners Advisory Group on Home Infusion.

The authors have declared no potential conflicts of interest.

Barbara Petroff, M.S., FASHP, Soleo Health, Novi, MI.

Cathy Johnson, B.S.Pharm., Bioscrip, Cincinnati, OH.

ASHP gratefully acknowledges the following organizations and individuals for reviewing these guidelines (review does not imply endorsement): American Pharmacists Association; Idaho Society of Health-System Pharmacists; Infusion Nurses Society; New Hampshire Society of Health-System Pharmacists; Tolulope Akinbo, Pharm.D., M.P.H.; Megan Brafford, Pharm.D., BCOP; Clyde Buchanan, M.S., FASHP; John S. Clark, Pharm.D., M.S., BCPS; Debra Cowan, Pharm.D., FASHP; Travis B. Dick, Pharm.D., M.B.A., BCPS; Kaci Elmore, RN; Michael Fadeyi, B.S., M.S.; Steven Gray, Pharm.D., J.D.; Kathleen M. Gura, Pharm.D., BCSNP, FASHP, FPPAG, FASPEN; Lois F. Parker, B.S.Pharm.; James Ponto, B.S.Pharm., M.S., BCNP, FASHP; James R. Rinehart, M.S., FASHP; Brandon Shank, Pharm.D., BCOP; Marc Stranz, Pharm.D.; Paul Wittmer, M.B.A.; and Jody Jacobson Wedret, FASHP, FCSHP.

Copyright © 2016, American Society of Health-System Pharmacists, Inc. All rights reserved. Contact ASHP for reprint and permissions requests. This content may not be used for commercial purposes without the express written consent of ASHP.

The bibliographic citation for this document is as follows: American Society of Health-System Pharmacists. ASHP guidelines on evaluating and using home or alternate-site infusion service providers. *Am J Health-Syst Pharm*. 2016; 73:922–6.

ASHP Guidelines on Home Infusion Pharmacy Services

Background and Purpose

Background. Home infusion services are provided by a variety of organizations, including hospitals, community pharmacies, home health agencies, hospices, and specialized infusion companies. Patients receive care in non-inpatient settings, such as their homes and ambulatory infusion centers, or in alternative-site settings, such as skilled-nursing facilities. Home infusion pharmacies may provide one or more of several service lines:

- Infusion therapies (e.g., intravenous, subcutaneous, intrathecal, epidural)
- Specialty pharmacy services
- Ambulatory infusion center services
- Home health nursing
- Private duty nursing
- Respiratory equipment and clinical respiratory services;
- Hospice services
- Home medical equipment and supplies (with or without oxygen service)
- Enteral products and supplies

It should be noted that different aspects of home infusion can be provided by different organizations. When services are shared among providers, pharmacists have a professional responsibility to ensure that all patient care responsibilities are defined, understood, agreed upon, coordinated, and documented in advance by all providers. These guidelines apply to the provision of home infusion services by pharmacists practicing in all health care settings.

Purpose. The purposes of these guidelines are to define the role of the pharmacist in providing home infusion care to patients and to outline minimum requirements (indicated by use of the word "shall") and best practices for the operation and management of services provided by pharmacies in the home or alternative-site setting. In broad terms, home infusion includes the provision of specialized, complex pharmaceutical products; development and execution of plans to manage the medication therapy of patients; and clinical assessment and monitoring of patients in their homes. These services generally include home infusion therapy; other injectable drug therapy; parenteral and enteral nutrition therapy; and occasionally preparation of other sterile preparations, compounds, or products. As the number and types of therapies administered in the home and alternative sites expand, the resources and support required to provide these therapies will expand as well. Specific and unique pharmacist education and training in drug product admixtures and administration techniques, equipment operation and maintenance, patient monitoring, and patient and family education are required to ensure successful outcomes. These guidelines outline the pharmacist's role in providing these services and products. They are not intended to apply to home health or previously mentioned services that do not involve the provision of home infusion pharmacy services.

Many of the activities included in these guidelines are the subjects of other American Society of Health-System Pharmacists (ASHP) policy and guidance documents, which should be referred to for additional information. Pharmacists practicing in home infusion should use professional judgment in assessing ASHP's policy and guidance documents and in adapting them to meet their health care organizations' and patients' needs and circumstances.

To ensure the safe, appropriate, and effective use of medications in the home, home infusion pharmacies should develop comprehensive services to address factors unique to home infusion. Caregivers such as family members, who often have no health care experience, should be trained if deemed safe and appropriate to properly administer, store, and dispose of medications supplies and biohazard waste; operate medication administration devices; and monitor patients as necessary. Many medications must be aseptically compounded, often in quantities sufficient for a week's use, and delivered under conditions that will ensure that product potency and purity are maintained. Vascular access for infused therapies should be maintained for the intended duration of treatment, which may range from days to years. Medication administration devices should be selected and maintained to accurately and safely administer a variety of therapeutic regimens. Potential complications should be anticipated, and a proactive individualized plan of care should be established for monitoring, detecting, and managing complications, including those related to equipment, enteral and parenteral access, compliance, response to therapy, and patient and family education. Economic considerations should be taken into account so that care is provided in the most cost-effective manner. Home infusion pharmacies should have an effective organizational structure with the flexibility to meet the changing needs of patients, as well as to keep pace with the rapid growth of the industry and changes in health systems. As health care providers in the home setting, pharmacists must be concerned with the outcomes of therapy and not just the provision of services. Effective management is necessary to ensure that quality outcomes of therapy are achieved. While the scope of pharmacy services is likely to vary from site to site, depending upon the needs of the patients served, these criteria are strongly linked to patient outcomes; neglect of any one area may compromise quality.

Practice Management

Mission and Goals of the Home Infusion Organization. The pharmacy or its affiliated organization shall have a written mission statement that reflects patient safety, quality of care, and operational responsibilities. The statement should be consistent with the mission of the parent home infusion organization and/or health system, if applicable. The development and prioritization of goals, objectives, and work plans shall be consistent with the pharmacy's mission statement. The mission should be understood by employees,

DOI 10.37573/9781585287048.099

contract staff, and other participants (e.g., students and residents) in the pharmacy's activities.

Laws and Regulations. The home infusion pharmacy shall comply with all applicable local, state, and federal laws and regulations. Laws and regulations change frequently, so it is imperative to remain up to date on these changes so that the pharmacy remains in compliance. The pharmacy shall maintain written or computerized documentation of compliance regarding procurement, storage, and distribution of drug products, patient information, and related safety regulations from applicable state boards of pharmacy, the federal Food and Drug Administration (FDA), the United States Pharmacopeia (USP), the Drug Enforcement Administration (DEA), the Centers for Medicare & Medicaid Services (CMS), the Occupational Safety and Health Administration (OSHA), the National Institute for Occupational Safety and Health (NIOSH), and the Environmental Protection Agency (EPA), among others. Pharmacy management of patient information shall conform to the Health Insurance Portability and Accountability Act of 1996[1] (HIPAA) and to the parent organization's policies and procedures. Pharmacies that participate in Medicare Part D plans shall comply with government regulations for Medicare Part D, which may include annual compliance training regarding Medicare fraud and abuse. Appropriate business licenses, permits, and tax stamps should also be available.

Licensure. Professional staff shall maintain pharmacist licensure applicable to their practice. Policies and procedures should be available to ensure that health care providers meet applicable state licensure and home infusion organization authorization, if required, for prescribing medications.

Many states require pharmacies with out-of-state pharmacy licenses to also have a pharmacist licensed in the state of the prescription recipient. Pharmacies dispensing drugs across state lines shall comply with out-of-state licensure requirements, as well as other state and federal interstate laws and regulations. The pharmacy director shall have a process in place for validating current licensure of all professional staff, and the source(s) of this validation shall also be verified. In locations in which pharmacy technicians are required to be registered and/or certified, such registration and/or certification shall be validated annually or as required by law or regulation.

Accreditation. Accreditation provides patients, referral sources, and payers the assurance that the pharmacy meets a basic level of quality in patient care. Accreditation may be required by some payers and is recommended for the home infusion pharmacy. Accrediting bodies may include the Joint Commission, Community Health Accreditation Program (CHAP), Pharmacy Compounding Accreditation Board (PCAB), Healthcare Quality Association on Accreditation (HQAA), Accreditation Commission for Healthcare (ACHC), and Medicare.

Practice Standards and Guidelines. Appropriate practice standards and guidelines of professional pharmacy organizations such as ASHP should be assessed and utilized as appropriate to the scope of pharmacy services provided. The standards of other professional clinical organizations, such as the American Society for Parenteral and Enteral Nutrition (A.S.P.E.N.), the Infusion Nurses Society (INS), the Infectious Diseases Society of America (IDSA), and the Oncology Nursing Society (ONS), should also be assessed and used when applicable to the home infusion organization, its scope of services, and the population served. Such practice standards and guidelines should be adapted into the organization's policies and procedures when appropriate.

Policies and Procedures Manual. A policies and procedures manual governing the scope of the home infusion pharmacy services (e.g., administrative, operational, clinical, quality performance and/or improvement, infection control, drug preparation and dispensing, equipment maintenance) shall be properly maintained and available. The manual should be reviewed and revised annually or whenever necessary to reflect changes in procedures specific to the sites where the pharmacy's products and services are provided. All personnel should be familiar with the contents of the manual. Appropriate mechanisms should be established to ensure compliance with the policies and procedures.

Human Resources

The responsibilities and related competencies for home infusion pharmacy employees should be clearly defined in written position descriptions for all job categories.

Director of Home Infusion Pharmacy Services. Effective leadership and practice management skills are necessary for pharmacists' delivery of care that meets the needs of patients and the health system and results in continuous improvement in patient outcomes. These guidelines use the term *director of home infusion pharmacy services* (or, more simply, *director*) to indicate the person responsible for managing those services. Depending on the health system's organizational structure and other factors, designations such as manager or pharmacist-in-charge may also be used.

The director of the home infusion pharmacy services must work in collaboration with appropriate health-system leaders to create a long-term vision for the home infusion pharmacy department that is consistent with that of the health system. Depending on the size and scope of the setting, these functional responsibilities may be assigned to a single person or a team. It is the responsibility of the director to monitor the status of the goals set forth in the department's vision, provide feedback to the pharmacy team as necessary, and support the team's implementation of the core functions of the pharmacy practice.

Home infusion pharmacy services should be managed by a professionally competent, legally qualified pharmacist. In addition to the requirements for a staff pharmacist, the director shall be thoroughly knowledgeable about home infusion pharmacy practice and management. Completion of a pharmacy residency program and/or home infusion experience is desirable.

The director shall be responsible for

- Establishing the mission, vision, goals, and scope of services of the pharmacy on the basis of the needs of the patients served, the needs of the health system, and developments and trends in health care.
- Developing, implementing, evaluating, and updating plans and activities to fulfill the mission, vision, goals, and scope of services of the pharmacy.

- Ensuring the development and implementation of policies and procedures that provide safe and effective medication use for the patients served by the institution.
- Mobilizing and managing the resources, both human and financial, necessary for the optimal provision of pharmacy services.
- Overseeing contracts (for example vendors, home health agencies, payers, etc.).
- Ensuring that pharmacy services are delivered in compliance with applicable state and federal laws and regulations, as well as national practice standards.
- Ensuring all technology and automation used throughout the medication use process is implemented, maintained, and utilized to promote patient safety.

A part-time or contract director shall have the same obligations and responsibilities as a full-time director. The director, in carrying out these responsibilities, should supervise an adequate number of competent, qualified personnel.

Home Infusion Pharmacists. Pharmacists who provide home infusion services shall have an active license to practice pharmacy issued by the applicable state board of pharmacy and other credentials as required by local, state, or federal laws and regulations. Some states require special licensure or training for preparing sterile preparations. Pharmacists dispensing medications to patients who reside in other states may also be subject to laws and regulations in those states; additional licensure may be required. The pharmacist should be knowledgeable about all applicable federal and state laws and regulations. The pharmacist is responsible for:

- Day-to-day supervision of dispensing sterile preparations and delivery activities.
- Drug information provided to nurses, physicians, pa-tients, and caregivers.
- Clinical monitoring, care planning, and assessment of home infusion patients.
- Maintaining a professional image and demeanor in both appearance and actions.
- Maximizing work efficiency and patient safety through the use of technology.
- Maintaining confidentiality of patient and proprietary information.
- Utilizing support personnel effectively.

Technicians and Other Support or Clinical Staff. Sufficient support personnel (pharmacy technicians, clinical staff [e.g., nurses, dietitians, respiratory therapists], and customer service, procurement, delivery, clerical, and administrative personnel) should be available to facilitate the delivery of home infusion pharmacist care and services. Pharmacy technicians should have completed an accredited pharmacy technician training program and be certified by the Pharmacy Technician Certification Board (PTCB). The pharmacy should hire pharmacy technician trainees without those qualifications only if those individuals (1) are required to both successfully complete an accredited pharmacy technician training program and successfully complete PTCB certification within 12 months of employment or as required by law or regulation, and (2) are limited to positions with lesser responsibilities until they successfully complete such training and certification. The pharmacy should require ongoing PTCB certification as a condition of continued employment. Appropriate supervisory controls should be maintained and documented, consistent with federal and state laws and regulations. In states in which registration of pharmacy technicians and/or special licensure or training is required for specific responsibilities (e.g., preparing sterile preparations), the pharmacy shall ensure that such requirements are met.

Pharmacy technicians are responsible for compounding sterile and nonsterile preparations in a manner to ensure patient safety, managing drug inventory, contacting patients about scheduled deliveries, and other duties as assigned. Customer service staff may be tasked with contacting patients about scheduled deliveries, communication with customers (e.g., other suppliers, patients, families, referral sources), and other duties as assigned. Drivers and/or warehouse managers may be responsible for delivery of medication to the patient, processing of initial paperwork to be signed, storage of medication in the home, observation of quantities of medications and supplies left in the home, and/or communication with the pharmacist if there are any questions or concerns. Intake personnel, insurance verification staff, and/or billers take referrals, determine insurance coverage, obtain authorizations or precertifications and renew them as needed, bill payers for services provided, and follow up on rejected claims.

Staffing, Work Schedules, and Assignments. The director should ensure that work schedules, procedures, and assignments make the best use of pharmacy personnel and other resources. Resources should be sufficient to ensure patient safety. Flex time, weekend options, exempt and nonexempt status, shift differentials, and on-call pay and responsibilities should all be considered when creating a staffing plan.

Recruitment and Selection of Personnel. Personnel should be recruited and selected on the basis of the requirements stated in the established job description, the candidates' job-related qualifications, and their prior performance. The pharmacy director should assist in identifying the relevant professional and technical qualifications for each job description and should participate in candidate interviews and final selection. The organization should have a human resources manual stating the requirements for reference checks, criminal background checks, and primary source verification of professional licenses. In addition, it should be organization policy that the Office of the Inspector General (OIG) List of Excluded Individuals/Entitites[2] is checked to ensure that potential candidates for employment have not been excluded from federally funded health care programs. Employees' professional licenses and the OIG List of Excluded Individuals/Entities should be verified at least annually.

Recruitment for home infusion pharmacy positions can be a challenge, especially when the pharmacist labor market is tight. Home infusion pharmacy practice is a unique practice setting with which many pharmacists are not familiar, especially new graduates. Infusion pharmacy practice training in college of pharmacy curricula varies, so recruiting staff with home infusion experience may not be possible. Creative recruitment techniques, such as hiring part-time pharmacists to cover open positions and offering on-site training, may help recruitment.

Orientation and Training. All employees shall be oriented to the type(s) of care and services provided by the organization. There should be an established procedure for orienting new personnel to the pharmacy, the parent organization, the health system(s) that the home infusion pharmacy serves, respective staff positions, and the patient populations served. All employees should understand the roles and responsibilities of others in the organization and should be oriented and demonstrate proficiency on equipment they are expected to operate or support as part of their duties. Employees should be knowledgeable about the supplies and equipment that are delivered to the patient. All personnel should possess the education and training needed to fulfill their responsibilities, including specific knowledge related to home infusion. All personnel should participate in continuing education programs and activities relevant to home infusion practice as necessary to maintain or enhance their competence.[3]

A home infusion organization is responsible for helping teach employees, patients, family members, and caregivers about standard safety precautions. The pharmacist should ensure that the home infusion organization provides appropriate education for its employees and patients, including education about appropriate disposal and handling of medical waste, procedures for preventing and managing needle and sharps stick injuries,[4] handling of cytotoxic and hazardous medications,[5] and material safety data sheets (MSDSes).[6] The pharmacist should be a key resource in the development of such educational programs. The pharmacist should assume an active role in the home infusion organization's infection-control activities.

Pharmacists should receive training as necessary to ensure that they possess the knowledge and skills required for the provision of home infusion services. They should participate in ongoing continuing education activities to update and enhance their knowledge and skills related to home infusion. Pharmacists should also participate in an ongoing competence assessment program as part of an overall staff development program. A valid assessment of competence should consider the pharmacist's responsibilities and the types and ages of patients served. The assessment should be conducted and documented on an ongoing basis for all pharmacists. When appropriate, pharmacists should assist in training and in continuing education programs for other home infusion providers.

Performance Evaluation, Contribution Management, and Competency Assessment. Policies and procedures should define the ongoing performance evaluations, contribution management, and competency assessments of home infusion pharmacy personnel. All home infusion pharmacy personnel should receive regular and timely evaluations. Performance should be evaluated on the basis of position description requirements and expected competencies. ASHP guidelines[7] and *USP* Chapter 797[8] describe requirements for initial and ongoing assessment of compounding knowledge and skills. Competency assessments should include practical skills (e.g., aseptic technique challenge), clinical competencies (e.g., assessing patients, developing a plan to manage patient care, and executing the plan), equipment competencies, and patient teaching competencies, if appropriate (i.e., if the employee will be instructing patients). Monitoring clinical outcomes is a critical part of the home infusion pharmacist's roles.

Financial Management

Budget Management. The home infusion pharmacy should have a budget that is consistent with the health system's financial management process and supports the scope of and demand for pharmacy services. Oversight of workload and financial performance should be managed in accordance with the health system's requirements. Management should provide for the determination and analysis of pharmacy service costs, the determination and analysis of capital equipment costs, and the determination and analysis of new project growth.

The pharmacy budget processes should enable the analysis of pharmacy services by unit of service and other parameters appropriate to the organization (e.g., organization-wide costs by medication therapy, clinical service, specific disease management categories, and patient third-party enrollment). The director should have an integral part in the organization's financial management process.

Health-System Integration. Other functional units within the health system should factor the cost of pharmacy services being provided by the home infusion pharmacy into their departmental budget when appropriate.

Third-Party Contract Review. In conjunction with the organization's legal department, the pharmacy director's team should review third-party payer contracts to ensure that reimbursement is appropriate for services being rendered and that terms of the contracts are in the best interests of the patient and the health system. The pharmacy should contract with third-party payers that are relevant to the pharmacy's patient population.

Drug and Supply Expenditures. Specific policies and procedures for managing drug expenditures should address such methods as competitive bidding, group purchasing, utilization review programs, inventory management, and cost-effective patient services.

Manufacturers and Suppliers. Criteria for selecting drug product manufacturers and suppliers should be established by the pharmacy to ensure the quality of drug products and the best prices, and that vendors are able to supply products in the volume required.

Reimbursement. The director of the pharmacy or home infusion organization should be knowledgeable about reimbursements for home infusion pharmaceutical services, medications, supplies, durable medical equipment, and, if applicable, nursing services. Processes should exist for routine verification of patient reimbursement benefits and for counseling patients about their anticipated financial responsibility for planned therapies. A process should also exist for responding to service requests from medically indigent patients.

The director of the pharmacy or home infusion organization should also be responsible for policies regarding drug procurement, drug expenditures, inventory management, determination and analysis of pharmacy service costs, capital equipment acquisition, budgeting (including analysis of budgetary variances, patient revenue projections, and justification of personnel commensurate with workload productivity), and payer audits.

Medication Use and Drug Information Services

Medication-Use Policy Development. Medication-use policy decisions should be founded on the evidence-based clinical, ethical, legal, social, philosophical, quality-of-life, safety, and economic factors that result in optimal patient care. Committees within the organization (e.g., pharmacy and therapeutics, infection control) that make decisions concerning medication use should include the active and direct involvement of physicians, pharmacists, and other appropriate health care professionals. The pharmacy should actively participate on committees whose decisions could affect the quality, safety, effectiveness, or cost of pharmacy services or the medication-use process.

Medication Therapy Decisions. The pharmacist's prerogatives to initiate, monitor, and modify medication therapy for individual patients, consistent with laws, regulations, home infusion organization policy, and clinical protocols, should be clearly delineated and approved by the home infusion organization's authorized leadership.

Formulary. An independent home infusion provider does not have to abide by a formulary; drugs are dispensed according to the orders of the physicians in its service area. A hospital- or health-system-based infusion pharmacy may have to abide by the same formulary restrictions as the rest of the hospital or health system. The home infusion pharmacist should have a mechanism for providing input to the formulary committee.[9] The pharmacy should have access to specialty medications distributed through closed network systems when needed to support consistent delivery of patient care and medication reconciliation.

Selection of Medications. Policies and procedures addressing the selection of medications should be available. These policies should be based on clinical appropriateness and USP standards. For bulk powders, USP or chemical standards for purity should be applied. Selection criteria should also include safety (including clinical and labeling safety such as manufacturer use of "tall man" lettering), efficacy, and ability to detect counterfeit medications.

Drug Information. The home infusion pharmacist should provide accurate, comprehensive, and patient-specific drug information to patients, caregivers, other pharmacists, physicians, nurses, and other health care providers as appropriate, both proactively and in response to requests associated with the delivery of pharmacy patient care, educational programs, and publications. Pharmacists should provide concise, applicable, and timely responses to requests for drug information from health care providers and home infusion patients. Responses to general and patient-specific drug information requests should be accurate and prompt. Drug information requests and responses should be documented and monitored for accuracy and timeliness as part of performance improvement activities. Policies and procedures should be in place for reviewing responses to requests for drug information for the purpose of performance improvement and education.

Adequate information about a medication's therapeutic use, dosage, potential adverse effects, and safe administration in the home, including storage and stability requirements, should be supplied before the medication is administered. Information about the stability of drugs for home infusion should address administration via a variety of alternative delivery devices, such as portable infusion pumps, syringe pumps, implantable infusion devices, elastomeric infusion pumps, and common peripheral and central-line administration devices.

Adequate space, resources, and information handling and communication technology shall be available to facilitate the provision of drug and related information to patients, caregivers, health care providers, multidisciplinary team members, and referring physicians. The director shall identify a core library (hard copy or electronic) appropriate for a home infusion pharmacy practice setting and ensure that those resources are readily available to users. Drug information sources should include current professional and scientific periodicals, Web-based research tools (e.g., AHFS-DI, MicroMedex, Lexi-Comp Online), the latest editions of drug compendia and textbooks in appropriate pharmaceutical and biomedical subject areas, and any references required by state boards of pharmacy. Availability of drug information on electronic media is desirable. Information may be accessed and provided in conjunction with medical libraries and other resources.

Available information sources should support research on patient care issues, facilitate provision of patient care, and promote safety in the medication-use process. When possible, a pharmacist should have a role within the health system for addressing complex drug information questions presented by professional staff (e.g., pharmacists, nurses, physicians).

If applicable, pharmacists should have access to information on all investigational studies and similar research projects involving medications and medication-related devices used by the organization. Pharmacists should, following the organization's procedures, provide pertinent written information (to the extent known) about the safe and proper use of investigational drugs, including possible adverse effects, to family members, nurses, pharmacists, physicians, and other health care providers involved in the care of patients admitted to the investigational drug protocols. Pharmacist representation on the health system's institutional review board is preferred.[10,11]

Education and Mentoring of Staff, Students, and Providers. The home infusion pharmacy staff should provide in-service education to physicians, nurses, pharmacy technicians, and other practitioners on home infusion pharmacy-related issues. They should also provide, to the extent possible in their organizations, student experiential education, externship, and internship training, as well as postgraduate residency training. Home infusion pharmacy staff also have a responsibility to keep the home infusion organization's staff informed about the use of medications on an ongoing basis through appropriate consultations, publications, and presentations. Pharmacists should ensure the timely dissemination of drug product recall notices, safety alerts, market withdrawals, and labeling changes.

Administration Devices, Delivery Systems, and Automated Dispensing Devices. Home infusion pharmacists should provide leadership and advice in organizational and clinical decisions about the selection of drug delivery systems, administration devices, and automated compounding and dispensing devices, and should participate in the evaluation, use, and monitoring of these systems and devices.[12] The potential for medication errors associated with such systems and devices should be thoroughly evaluated. Policies and procedures should be available for the certification (calibration) and maintenance of equipment and devices. Equipment should be adequately maintained and certified in compliance with applicable standards, laws, and regulations. Equipment maintenance and certification should be documented.

Preventive and Postexposure Immunization Programs. The pharmacy should participate in the development of policies and procedures concerning preventive and postexposure programs for infectious diseases (including, but not limited to, human immunodeficiency virus infection, tuberculosis, and hepatitis) for patients and employees.

Substance Abuse Programs. The pharmacy should assist in the development of, and participate in, substance abuse prevention, education, and employee and patient assistance programs.[13]

Development of Patient Care Services. The home infusion pharmacy services team should be involved in the development, implementation, and evaluation of new or changing patient care services within the organization, such as the development of new clinic sites or new service areas or lines. In reviewing the potential for new services, both the value added to patient care by the new service and the financial and logistical implications of the new service should be considered. These efforts should promote the continuity of pharmacist patient care across the continuum of care, practice settings, and geographically dispersed facilities.

Committee Involvement. The director and other pharmacy staff should contribute to the organization's goals through effectively participating in or leading committees and informal work groups. The pharmacist should be involved in the home infusion organization's initiatives to develop model clinical protocols and assessments that develop pharmacist care plans, pathways, or disease management guidelines to ensure that pharmacist care elements are included.[14] Clinical protocols should be used whenever appropriate to maximize the safety of medication use in the home.

A pharmacist should be a member of and actively participate on committees responsible for establishing policies and procedures for medication use, patient care, and performance improvement, among other things.[9] Pharmacists should also participate in the activities of similar committees of a parent home infusion organization or health system, as applicable.

The director or a designee should be a member of the home infusion organization's or health system's institutional review board, if applicable.

Drug Procurement and Management

The home infusion pharmacy should be responsible for the proper acquisition, compounding, dispensing, storage, delivery, and administration of all drug products used in the treatment of the organization's patients, as well as the proper use of related equipment and supplies. Policies and procedures governing medication procurement and management should be developed by the pharmacy in collaboration with other appropriate organization staff and committees.

Selection of Medications and Management of Supplies and Inventory. Policies and procedures governing selection of medications and management of supplies and inventory should be developed by the pharmacy director in collaboration with other appropriate home infusion organization staff members.

Procurement through Wholesalers, Manufacturers, or Group Purchasing Organizations. Each pharmacy should have a primary drug wholesaler for routine stock orders and a local source (e.g., a local hospital) for obtaining medications it does not have in stock. Group purchasing organizations (GPOs) may be used to control purchasing costs for drugs and supplies. Policies and procedures should address procurement and management of medications that must be obtained directly from the manufacturer or a limited set of distributors to ensure safe and proper pedigree of pharmaceutical products.[15,16]

Storage and Stock Levels. Each pharmacy should determine the appropriate level of stock required to serve the local patient population and manage its physical inventory for maximum cost control and operational efficiency.

Returns, Recalls, and Backorders. Procedures should be in place for responding to drug and device product returns, recalls, and backorders; for identifying patients who received or used a recalled product; and for removing the drug or device product from the pharmacy or home when the recall is at the user level. All stocks of medications stored in the home infusion pharmacy or in the organization's facilities should be inspected routinely to ensure the absence of recalled, outdated, unusable, or mislabeled products. Inspections should include identification of storage conditions that could compromise medication integrity, storage arrangements that might contribute to medication errors, and storage locations that might be vulnerable to drug diversion efforts.

Drug Shortages. There shall be policies and procedures for managing drug product shortages. The pharmacy's inventory management system should be designed to detect subminimum inventory levels and alert the pharmacy to potential shortages, and pharmacy staff should monitor reliable sources of information regarding drug product shortages (e.g., the ASHP[17] and FDA[18] drug shortages web resource centers). The pharmacy should develop strategies for identifying alternative therapies, working with suppliers, collaborating with physicians and other health care providers, and conducting an awareness campaign in the event of a drug product shortage.[19]

Compounding. The home infusion pharmacist is responsible for assuring appropriate techniques are used for preparing and dispensing medications, following the home infusion pharmacy's policies and procedures and accepted standards of practice. Double checks are a good practice in many steps of the pharmacy dispensing process. The pharmacy should have a process by which all high-risk calculations are checked for accuracy by a second clinician. Pediatric medications (e.g., doses), parenteral nutrition (PN), chemotherapy, pain management, and inotropes are examples of high-risk therapies. It is also good practice that the pharmacist who processed a new order should not be the same person who checks the order for accuracy and completeness. In addition to double checks on calculations, there should be visual double checks on all medications listed as high-alert medications by the Institute for Safe Medication Practices (ISMP) (e.g., heparin, insulin, chemotherapy agents, PN additives).[20]

Compounding Sterile Preparations. Compounding of sterile preparations should comply with applicable practice standards, accreditation standards, and pertinent state and federal laws and regulations. If these services are being provided by another pharmacy, the pharmacist should have reasonable assurance that these standards are being met by the pharmacy providing the service.[21]

Home infusion pharmacists are responsible for ensuring the quality of sterile preparations intended for use in the home. Guidance is available from various sources for developing an adequately designed and equipped facility, training and validating employees, validating and documenting compounding procedures, practicing aseptic technique, monitoring the work environment, maintaining the facility and equipment, ensuring the quality of prepared preparations, and developing policies and procedures.[7,8]

Stability and Compatibility Issues. Home infusion pharmacies are often required to assign extended beyond-use dates to sterile preparations so that a multiple-day supply of medications can be dispensed and delivered. However, pharmacists should take into account circumstances that may affect the medication's potency and stability, including:

- Delivery of sterile preparations to the home, either by the pharmacy's own vehicles or by a common carrier.
- Storage of sterile preparations in the home before use.
- Manipulation of sterile preparations in the home environment to add ingredients (such as vitamins) and to set up tubing and filters for administration.
- Administration of preparations at temperatures that are warmer than controlled room temperature because of administration in outdoor or non-air-conditioned environments or the use of ambulatory infusion pumps worn close to the body.

The home infusion pharmacist should consult *USP* Chapter 797[8] and other appropriate resources to establish an appropriate beyond-use date. Applying published stability data can introduce inaccuracies if the intended conditions of use differ greatly from the reported conditions. Pharmacists should maintain a record of the resources used for establishing beyond-use dates. A table or chart of accepted beyond-use dates, formulations, and conditions of use for commonly prepared preparations may be helpful in ensuring that assigned dates are consistent and appropriate. Patients should be trained to check preparations for current beyond-use dates prior to their use.

Labeling. Medications for home use should be labeled so that patients and caregivers can easily understand instructions for drug storage, preparation, and administration. Auxiliary labels should be used as necessary. When manipulation of medications is required before administration, labeling should clearly state current contents and the steps for measuring, reconstituting, or adding other ingredients. Labels for compounded medications should state the total content of the medication or nutrient per container so that it can be clearly known in case the patient is transferred to another treatment setting. If medications are to be administered with an infusion device, pump settings should be included on the label. All labels shall conform to the requirements of the law. Home infusion pharmacies should adopt the list of prohibited abbreviations as another safety precaution to ensure that patients and caregivers receive clear instructions for drug use.

Packaging and Delivery. Policies and procedures should be available to ensure product integrity and temperature control during home delivery or patient pickup of supplies and drugs. The pharmacist should ensure that the delivery of medications and supplies to the patient occurs in a timely manner to avoid interruptions in drug therapy. Furthermore, the pharmacist should ensure that storage conditions during delivery and while in the patient's home are consistent with the recommendations for storing the product and beyond-use dating. The temperature of home refrigerators or freezers in which medications are stored should be within acceptable limits and should be monitored by the patient or caregiver. The pharmacist should ensure that an adequate inventory of medications and ancillary supplies is available in the patient's home. It may be appropriate to provide additional inventory for unforeseen circumstances in which extra doses or supplies may be required (e.g., waste, breakage, and emergencies). The pharmacist is responsible for providing sufficient quantities of medications and supplies to the patient, so that the ordered dosing regimen is maintained in the home setting without missed doses due to lack of drugs or supplies. Delivery to the patient should also include inventory management to avoid excessive accumulation of supplies and drugs. Excesses may indicate poor compliance, inadequate patient training, failure to assess patient needs, or ineffective inventory management by the patient. When common carriers are used, the pharmacy is responsible for ensuring that the carrier can provide timely delivery, proper handling, and external temperature control. Delivery personnel should know the shipping requirements for each package. If products are packaged so that product labels containing storage instructions are concealed, an exterior label specifying the storage conditions shall be used. To protect patient confidentiality, prescription labels with medication names and directions should not be used to label boxes. Box labels should include only the patient's name and address, the storage requirements, and delivery instructions. Additional precautions (i.e., double bagging, using at least one leak-proof container, and cushioning) should be used to safeguard hazardous products from breaking and leaking. The delivery person, patient, and caregiver shall be trained to recognize and manage accidental spills. Packages containing hazardous products should have appropriate precautionary labels.

Products should be delivered in appropriate packaging to ensure that labeled storage requirements are met during transit under the expected environmental conditions. The pharmacy should develop and follow written procedures for packaging; these procedures should include privacy-protection considerations. Product confirmation after delivery should be used to ensure that the packaging procedures and materials used were effective in maintaining product integrity and temperature control during transit. The stability of refrigerated products at room temperature should be taken into account in the development of packaging procedures. A few refrigerated products have extended stability at room temperature and may be safely delivered without refrigerated packaging. Products that are stable for 24 hours or less at room temperature should always be delivered in temperature-controlled packaging (coolers, ice packs, etc.).

Hazardous Drugs. Policies and procedures for the definition, storing, handling, and disposing of hazardous drug products should be available to ensure patient and employee safety in compliance with applicable local, state, and federal laws and regulations. Receipt, storage, and disposal of hazardous substances shall comply with all applicable federal, state, and local laws and regulations, including the Resource Conservation and Recovery Act (RCRA), as well as applicable guidance (e.g., ASHP guidelines,[22] *USP* Chapter 797[8]). Hazardous drug products should be stored in a negative pressure compounding room whenever possible. Additional storage precautions may include placement on a lower shelf or containment in a resealable plastic bag. Employees should be specially trained, and their handling and disposal of these products should be monitored. Spill kits should be available in locations where hazardous drugs are handled, and all personnel who handle these agents should be trained on using the kits.[4,22]

Controlled Substances. Policies and procedures for the storage, distribution, use, and accountability of controlled substances should be available to ensure appropriate use and to prevent diversion in compliance with applicable local, state, and federal laws and regulations. Controlled substances shall be kept in a secure and locked storage area that meets the requirements of state law. Pharmacists should be aware of the ways drugs can be diverted. Employees should be carefully screened before hire. Processes should be in place to minimize the risk of drug diversion and allow detection should diversion occur. Policies or procedures for activities such as ordering, receiving product, and conducting inventories should assure proper supervision and limit opportunities for a single individual to control the entire process.

Drug Samples. The use of drug samples should be eliminated to the fullest extent possible. If samples are permitted, the pharmacy should control these products to ensure proper storage, records, labeling, and product integrity.

Patient Care

Pharmaceutical care, defined as the responsible provision of drug therapy for the purpose of achieving definite outcomes that improve a patient's quality of life, has been adopted by much of the pharmacy profession.[23] The concept of pharmaceutical care is evolving into a more comprehensive, patient-focused model of pharmacist-provided care, sometimes termed *pharmacist patient care*. The principal elements of such care are the same: it is *medication related*; it is *care* that is *directly provided* to the patient; it is provided to produce *definite outcomes*; these outcomes are intended to improve the patient's *quality of life*; and the provider accepts personal *responsibility* for the outcomes.[23]

The mission of the pharmacist is to help people make the best use of medications. At a minimum, pharmacists are responsible for assessing the legal and clinical appropriateness of medication orders (or prescriptions), educating and counseling patients on the use of their medications, monitoring the effects of medication therapy, and maintaining patient profiles and other records. In the home infusion care setting, these responsibilities are best accomplished through the provision of pharmacist-provided patient care in which pharmacists are responsible for establishing relationships with patients and providers that will facilitate coordination and continuity of care, improve access to care, and improve patient outcomes.

Preadmission Assessment. The pharmacist, alone or in collaboration with other home infusion health care providers (e.g., nurses), should ensure that each patient referred for home infusion is assessed for appropriateness on the basis of admission criteria, including the following:

- The patient, family, and caregiver agree with provision of infusion services in the home.
- The patient or caregiver is willing and able to be educated about the correct administration of medications.
- The pharmacy can provide this education in a manner that the patient, family and caregiver can understand.
- The home environment is conducive to the provision of home infusion services (e.g., electricity and running water are present, and the home is clean and safe).
- The home infusion provider has reasonable geographic access to the patient.
- There is psychosocial and family support (e.g., caregiver requirements and financial concerns are manageable, and the family environment is suitable).
- There is ongoing prescriber involvement in the assessment and treatment of the patient.
- The medical condition and prescribed medication therapy are suitable for home infusion services, and there is a prognosis with clearly defined outcome goals.
- The indication, dosage, and route and method of administration of medications are appropriate.
- Appropriate laboratory tests are ordered for monitoring the patient's response to medications.

Using the information collected during the preadmission assessment, the pharmacist, in conjunction with the other health care providers involved in the patient's care and the patient or caregiver, will determine the patient's appropriateness for home infusion services. The conclusions of the assessment should be communicated to all parties and appropriately documented.

Initial Patient Database and Assessment. The complete patient database should be documented in the patient's home infusion record in a timely manner. This database should include, at a minimum, the following:

- The patient's name, address, telephone number, and date of birth
- The person to contact in the event of an emergency, including the legal guardian or representative, if applicable
- Information on the existence, content, and intent of an advance directive, if applicable
- The patient's height, weight, and gender

- All diagnoses
- The location and type of termination site of the vascular access device and internal and external catheter lengths, if applicable
- Pertinent laboratory test results
- Pertinent medical history and physical findings
- Nutrition screening test results
- An accurate history of allergies
- Initial and ongoing pharmaceutical assessments
- A detailed medication profile, including all medications (prescription and nonprescription), immunizations, home remedies, and investigational and nontraditional therapies
- The prescriber's name, address, and telephone number and any other pertinent information (e.g., Drug Enforcement Administration number, National Provider Identifier [NPI])
- Other agencies and individuals involved in the patient's care and directions for contacting them
- A history of medication use
- A care plan and a list of drug-related problems, if any

To obtain this information, the pharmacist could use the medical record; laboratory test results; direct communication with the patient, caregiver, nurse, and prescriber; and direct observation. When the pharmacist cannot directly observe the patient, the patient's home infusion nurse or other appropriate health care provider could provide the results of direct observation and physical assessment. If a shared-service agreement exists among multiple providers, the pharmacist should ensure that this agreement specifies the responsibilities of each provider for obtaining and sharing pertinent patient information.

Medication Reconciliation. Pharmacists should prepare or have access to comprehensive medication histories for each patient, including prescription drugs, nonprescription drugs, and alternative therapies. A pharmacist-conducted medication history for each patient is desirable; however, another appropriate health care provider (e.g., home infusion nurse, pharmacy technician) may obtain and maintain current medication histories, provided this information is accessible to the pharmacist and other health care providers.

Development of Care Plans. The pharmacist, in collaboration with the patient or caregiver and other health care providers, is responsible for developing an appropriate and individualized care plan for each patient. The pharmacist's contribution to the care plan should be based on information obtained from the initial pharmacy assessment and other relevant information obtained from the nurse, prescriber, patient, and caregivers. At a minimum, the pharmacist's contribution to the care plan should include the following:

- A description of actual or potential drug therapy problems and their proposed solutions
- A description of desired outcomes of the drug therapy provided
- A proposal for patient education and counseling
- A plan specifying proactive objective and subjective monitoring (e.g., vital signs, laboratory tests, physical findings, patient response, toxicity, adverse reactions, and noncompliance) and the frequency with which monitoring is to occur

The care plan should be developed at the start of therapy and regularly reviewed and updated; the degree of detail of the plan should be based on the complexity of drug therapy and the patient's condition. Updates or changes to the plan, as they occur, should be communicated to other health care providers involved in the patient's care, to the patient, and to caregivers. The care plan and updates should be a part of the patient's record.

Clinical Monitoring. The pharmacist is responsible, in collaboration with other health care providers, for ongoing clinical monitoring of the patient's drug therapy according to the care plan and for appropriately documenting and communicating the results of all pertinent monitoring activities to other health care providers involved in the patient's care. The pharmacist is also responsible for ensuring that relevant information is obtained from the patient, the caregiver, and other health care providers and for documenting this information in the patient's home infusion record.

Pharmacists may, in collaboration with prescribers and others, wish to develop clinical monitoring protocols for various therapies that could be individualized in specific care plans. Pharmacists may receive laboratory test results before other health care providers. In such cases, the pharmacist is responsible for communicating the test results to the prescriber and other health care providers. The pharmacist should provide an interpretive analysis of the information and recommendations for dosage adjustments and for continuation or discontinuation of drug therapy. The pharmacist should ensure that sufficient laboratory test results are readily available for monitoring the patient's therapy. In shared-service arrangements, clinical monitoring responsibilities should be delineated.

The patient, the family, the caregiver, and all health care providers involved in the patient's care should have access to a pharmacist 24 hours a day. The pharmacist is responsible for providing a summary of all relevant clinical information to another pharmacist providing coverage for that patient (e.g., an on-call pharmacist) before transferring patient care responsibilities.

Patient Consultation and Education. Home infusion pharmacists will primarily consult patients or caregivers over the telephone. Home visits should be considered for enhancing compliance or simplifying complex drug-related patient issues.

The home infusion pharmacist, or the home infusion nurse as the agent, should ensure that the patient, caregiver, and other health care providers understand the proper use and administration of medications provided, including vascular access and infusion devices, as required. The home infusion pharmacist, or the nurse as the agent, should explain to the patient or the patient's agent the directions for use and any additional information.

The pharmacist is responsible for ensuring that the patient or caregiver receives appropriate education and counseling about the patient's medication therapy.[24] The pharmacist should verify that the patient or caregiver understands the therapy. Other health care providers may be involved in the education and counseling. A home infusion pharmacist should be readily accessible if questions or problems arise.

Supplementary written information should be provided to reinforce oral communications. Contingencies should be available to provide education, counseling, and written materials to patients whose understanding of English may be compromised. Depending on the need, this might require access to interpreters or bilingual pharmacists. Patients who have hearing and sight impairments will potentially need other support or communication resources.

Professional judgment is required to determine what information should be included in patient education and counseling. The following should be considered:

- A description of medication therapy, including drug, dose, route of administration, dosage interval, and duration of therapy
- The goals of medication therapy and indicators of progress toward those goals
- Self-assessment techniques for monitoring the effectiveness of therapy
- The importance of following the therapeutic plan
- Proper aseptic technique
- Hand hygiene
- Proper care of the vascular-access device and site, if applicable
- Precautions and directions for administering medications
- Inspection of medications, containers, and supplies prior to use
- Equipment use, maintenance, and troubleshooting
- Home inventory management and procedures for securing additional supplies and medications when needed
- Potential adverse effects, drug–drug interactions, drug–nutrient interactions, contraindications, adverse reactions, and the management of those events
- Special precautions and directions for the preparation, storage, handling, and disposal of drugs, supplies, and biomedical waste
- Information on contacting health care providers involved in the patient's care
- Examples of situations that should be brought to the attention of the pharmacist or other health care providers involved in the patient's care (e.g., missed doses, doses not given at the proper time, and low supplies)
- Emergency procedures

Patient counseling and education should be performed in accordance with applicable state regulations and documented in the patient's home infusion record.

Communication with Patients and Caregivers. Effective communication among pharmacists, patients, and caregivers is also essential to ensuring high-quality care. The pharmacist providing home infusion services should establish free and open channels of communication with patients and caregivers. The pharmacist should contact the patient or the caregiver, as appropriate, to

- Obtain information needed for the initial pharmacy assessment.
- Provide supplemental patient education and counseling as needed.
- Assess compliance with drug therapy.
- Assess progress toward the goal of therapy.
- Inform the patient how to contact the pharmacist when needed.
- Assess drug therapy problems (e.g., failure to respond to therapy and adverse drug events).

All contacts with the patient should be documented in the patient's home infusion record.

Communication with Physicians, Prescribers, Nurses, and Other Health Care Providers. Effective communication among pharmacists and other health care providers is essential to ensuring continuous, coordinated care. The pharmacist should ensure that effective channels of communication about care are in place, including shared-service arrangements (e.g., regarding pain assessments and laboratory test data). Oral and written communication methods can be used for communicating patient information. All relevant clinical communication should be documented in the patient's home infusion record. The pharmacist is responsible for protecting the patient's privacy and confidentiality while communicating this information to other health care providers. Personnel involved in the care of the patient should meet regularly to discuss the clinical status of the patient and any operational issues related to the patient's care.

Medication Administration. Policies and procedures on the administration of medications should be available. Only personnel who are authorized by the home infusion organization and are appropriately trained and licensed should be permitted to administer medications to a patient. Pharmacists, where legally permitted, may be authorized to administer medications after receiving appropriate training.

Emergency Medical Care. The home infusion pharmacist should participate in decisions about the emergency care of patients at home, including the development of protocols for using emergency drugs in the home. Policies and procedures should exist within the organization for providing appropriate levels of patient care during emergency situations 24 hours a day, including access to the pharmacist responsible for the care, when appropriate. Appropriately trained pharmacists should have an authorized role in responding to medical emergencies. The pharmacy should participate in the development of policies and procedures to ensure availability of, access to, and security of emergency medications.

Discharge from Home Infusion. When patients have completed therapy as ordered, they should be discharged from service. Items that should be documented in the medical record upon discharge include the patient's response to therapy and status at discharge.

Transfer to Another Care Setting. The pharmacist should ensure continuity of pharmacist care to and from the home and other patient-care settings. The pharmacist should routinely contribute to processes ensuring that each patient receives pharmacist care regardless of transitions that occur across different health care settings (for example, among different components of a health system and different types of home infusion services). When home infusion patients are admitted to a hospital, the home infusion pharmacy should inform the hospital about (1) the medications the patient is currently receiving from the home infusion pharmacy and (2) known allergies. The home infusion pharmacy should recognize hospital policy when considering whether properly stored medications and medical equipment from the home can be used during the home infusion patient's hospitalization.

Documentation in the Home Infusion Medical Record. Clinical actions and recommendations by pharmacists that are intended to ensure safe and effective use of medications and that have a potential effect on patient outcomes should be documented in patients' home infusion medical records. Pharmacists should provide oral or written consultations to other health professionals regarding medication therapy selection and management. Consultations should be documented in the patient's home infusion medical record. The pharmacy should have an ongoing process for consistent documentation (and reporting to physicians, administrators, and others) of pharmacist care and patient outcomes resulting from medication therapy and other pharmacy actions. Patient privacy and confidentiality should be protected at all times.

A home infusion record should be developed and used for documenting the home infusion services provided to each patient. Written organizational policies and procedures should address the security of home infusion records and specify personnel authorized to review patient records and to make entries. The need to maintain confidentiality of patient information should be stressed to all personnel. The pharmacist is responsible for documenting all pharmacy clinical activities in the patient's record in a timely manner. General clinician-oriented forms are preferred over specific nursing, pharmacy, and other health care professional forms to minimize duplication of information. It may be advisable for organizations that provide multiple home infusion services (e.g., pharmacy, nursing, respiratory therapy, dieticians) to use a single home infusion record for documenting all clinical information regarding each patient. The patient's record should be accessible at all times to authorized personnel involved in the care of the patient, but confidentiality should be maintained.

Selection of Products, Devices, and Ancillary Supplies. The pharmacist, in collaboration with other health care providers and the patient, is responsible for selecting infusion devices, ancillary drugs (e.g., heparin lock flush solution, 0.9% sodium chloride flush), and ancillary supplies (e.g., dressing kits, syringes, and administration sets). Pharmacists should be thoroughly trained and knowledgeable in the selection, proper use, and maintenance of these devices, drugs, and supplies. Factors involved in the selection of devices and ancillary supplies may include the following:

- The stability and compatibility of prescribed medications in infusion device reservoirs
- The ability of an infusion device to accommodate the appropriate volume of medication and diluent, and to deliver the prescribed dose at the appropriate rate
- The ability of the patient or caregiver to learn to operate an infusion device
- The potential for patient complications and noncompliance
- Patient preference
- Nursing or caregiver experience with therapies and selected devices
- Prescriber preferences
- Cost considerations
- The safety features of infusion devices

Patient's Own Medications. Drug products and related devices not dispensed by the home infusion pharmacy that are to be used during the patient's course of therapy should be documented in the patient's home infusion medical record. When home infusion patients are known to be admitted to a hospital or other extended care facility, the home infusion pharmacy should inform the hospital about the medications the patient is currently receiving from the home infusion pharmacy and about any known allergies. The home infusion pharmacy should recognize hospital policy when considering whether properly stored medications and medical equipment from the home can be used during the home infusion patient's hospitalization.

Emergency Medications. The home infusion pharmacist, in consultation with the prescriber, should determine when emergency medications and supplies (e.g., anaphylaxis "kits") should be dispensed to home infusion patients. When standing orders for ancillary drugs or supplies or standardized treatment protocols are used, the pharmacist should review each protocol to determine its appropriateness for the patient.

Performance Improvement Activities

The home infusion pharmacy should have an ongoing, systematic program for assessing pharmacist patient care, and pharmacists should be active participants in performance improvement activities. A performance improvement program for home infusion should monitor patient satisfaction and outcomes, and the program should also include appropriate quality control measures for compounding sterile preparations and other activities. Performance improvement activities based on assessments should be integrated with the health system's overall performance improvement activities, as applicable. The performance improvement team should work with frontline staff to implement systems that include proper checks and balances focused on protecting against human error. Performance improvement initiatives should be focused on error reporting trends and high-risk functions such as dispensing high-alert medications.

Benchmarking. As part of the performance improvement program, operational and outcomes data should be benchmarked with those of other home infusion pharmacy services of similar size and scope. The results, including follow-up actions for improvement, should be documented and provided to the organization's managers, the frontline staff using the system, and others as appropriate.

Clinical Outcomes. Most accrediting bodies and some regulatory agencies require the home infusion pharmacy to monitor clinical patient outcomes. Common measures that are tracked routinely by home infusion companies include the rate of catheter-related infections, adverse drug reactions, medication errors, warehouse/delivery errors, equipment malfunctions, and unplanned hospitalizations. In addition, the organization should have an infection control program in which both staff and patient infection (communicable diseases) rates are monitored. The organization may also select outcomes that are monitored over a short time as a specific process is improved.

Medication Error Reporting. Medication error monitoring and prevention should be part of every pharmacy's performance improvement program. Information about strategies to prevent medication errors is available from several sources, including ISMP, which produces regular newsletters on this topic.

All pharmacies should have processes in place that are designed to prevent and detect medication errors before they leave the pharmacy. If an error does occur, the pharmacy director and staff should determine how and why the error happened, and what can be done to prevent similar errors from occurring. Medication errors should be reported to voluntary national reporting systems and, as required, to accrediting organizations or regulatory agencies. Reports should be documented, analyzed, trended and reviewed consistent with National Coordinating Council for Medication Error Reporting and Prevention (NCC-MERP) standards.

Patient Satisfaction. Most accrediting bodies require the home infusion pharmacy to measure patient satisfaction with treatment and services. This function can be performed in-house by mailing questionnaires to the patient, or it can be outsourced to a contractor. Patient satisfaction surveys that are returned should be reviewed for both positive and negative comments so that corrective action can be targeted to service issues.

Medication-Use Evaluation. An ongoing program of monitoring drug utilization and costs should be in place to ensure that medications are used appropriately, safely, and effectively, and to increase the probability of desired outcomes within defined populations of patients. The medication-use policy committee should define specific parameters for evaluation (e.g., disease state, pharmacologic category, high-use/high-cost drug products, high-alert medications) as appropriate for the organization. Through this ongoing evaluation, areas in need of improvement in medication prescribing and management can be identified and targeted for intervention.

Adverse Drug Event Reporting. The home infusion pharmacist should take a leadership role in the development of a program for reporting and monitoring all adverse drug events and device-related events, including adverse drug reactions and medication errors. The pharmacist should ensure that the prescriber is notified promptly of any suspected adverse drug events. Adverse drug events should serve as outcome indicators of quality, and the monitoring of adverse drug events should be a part of the organization's ongoing performance improvement program. Relevant trends should be integrated into staff development and in-service education programs for pharmacists and nurses to improve the quality of care and patient outcomes. Serious adverse drug reactions and device-related problems should be reported promptly to the manufacturer and to the Food and Drug Administration's MedWatch program.[25]

Operations

Hours of Operation. Home infusion pharmacy services shall be available 24 hours a day, seven days a week. A pharmacist should be available for consultation or dispensing after hours. Home infusion pharmacy staff may be supplemented by knowledgeable and experienced part-time or on-call personnel to extend pharmacy services coverage.

Pharmacy Security and After-Hours Access. Only authorized pharmacy personnel should have access to the pharmacy area. Other home infusion organization personnel may be in the pharmacy area only when an authorized pharmacist is present, in accordance with the home infusion organization's policies or as required by laws and regulations. In an emergency situation in which a pharmacist is not present, such as a fire or security alarm, policies and procedures should guide safe access to the pharmacy area and provide for notification of the pharmacist in charge or a designee.

Emergency Preparedness and Business Continuity Planning. Policies and procedures should be available that include a plan for providing pharmacy services in case of an area-wide disaster affecting the home infusion pharmacy or patients' home infusion settings. Appropriately trained pharmacists and representatives from the pharmacy team should be members of emergency preparedness teams and participate in drills. Patients should be informed about what to do to safely continue needed home therapies in the event of a disaster. The health system's business continuity plan should address the provision of pharmacy services in non-emergency situations, such as information system failures or disruptions of the drug procurement process.[19,26]

Communications. Staff meetings should be conducted on a regular basis for various purposes, which may include:

- Brief daily meeting to review on-call issues, upcoming referrals, and current daily plan
- Hand-off communications to and from evening staff or on-call personnel
- In-services regarding updates to policies or procedures, law, regulation, or services
- Review of new medications
- Analysis of sales and marketing efforts
- Performance improvement functions
- Team building among the staff
- Interdisciplinary meetings or case conferences to communicate the pharmacist's care plan for a patient (with patients, caregivers, physicians, prescribers, or other health professionals)

Equipment Management. Equipment may be owned, leased, or rented by the infusion pharmacy. It is usually most cost-effective to lease-purchase infusion pumps that are used in high volume. Pumps with specialized uses (e.g., micro-infusers) may be used less frequently and may be rented as needed. Equipment may be purchased or rented from a properly qualified vendor. Routine maintenance (i.e., basic safety checks, alarm testing, and accuracy validation) is performed between patient use, and preventive maintenance for medical equipment is defined by the manufacturer for each specific device. The manufacturer's preventive maintenance recommendations should be followed, and all equipment should be maintained so that the preventive maintenance is not overdue during patient use. Technical repair of medical equipment should be done by a properly qualified service technician. Home infusion pharmacies typically do not have the capacity to employ staff on site with the technical certification required for equipment preventive maintenance or repair. Outsourcing these functions is usually the most efficient and cost-effective way to maintain equipment in good working order.

Records Storage and Maintenance. Adequate space should be available for maintaining and storing records, including medication profiles and other patient information, management information, equipment maintenance sheets, controlled-substances inventory sheets, and MSDSes, among others, to ensure compliance with laws, regulations, accreditation requirements, and sound management practices. Patient records shall be secure. Records shall be retained according to applicable laws and regulations, which may vary by state and by Centers for Medicare & Medicaid Services (CMS) participation guidelines. There may be additional record retention requirements for specific patient population (e.g., pediatric patients) medical records in some states and according to accreditation standards.

Information Technology. Computer resources should be used to maintain patient medication profiles, perform necessary patient billing procedures, manage drug product inventories, and interface with other available computerized systems to obtain patient-specific clinical information for drug therapy monitoring and other clinical functions and to facilitate the continuity of care after patients transfer to and from other care settings.

Home Infusion Medical Record Systems. A patient medication profile should be maintained by all home infusion pharmacies regardless of where the dispensing of medications takes place. The home infusion medical record should include assessment and care planning documents, progress notes, laboratory test results, and other patient information related to determining the appropriateness of medications and monitoring their effects. The system should provide safeguards against the improper manipulation or alteration of records and provide an audit trail.

An automated information system is preferred, but the system may be manual, automated, or a combination of the two. If an automated information system is used, an auxiliary record-keeping procedure should be available for documenting medication information in case the automated system is inoperative, and a daily data backup system should be in place.

Hazardous Waste Management and Disposal. There are many ways to dispose of hazardous waste generated by the pharmacy. In addition to the established waste management companies, there are also mail-back services. For the traditional services, it is important to follow the company's requirements. Since much of the waste eventually is sent to dump sites, waste that needs to be incinerated should be discarded separately. The companies that provide mail-back service also incinerate all the waste they receive, so it is not necessary to separate the waste. It is also important that the pharmacist understand the OSHA and RCRA requirements regarding management and disposal of hazardous substances. There should be a designated area for hazardous waste, including sharps. Spill kits should be readily available in locations where hazardous substances are handled, and all personnel who handle these agents should be trained on using these kits.[4,22]

Facilities

To ensure optimal operational performance and quality patient care, adequate space, equipment, and supplies should be available for all professional and administrative functions related to medication use. These resources should be located in areas that facilitate the provision of services to patients, nurses, prescribers, and other health care providers and should be integrated with the home infusion organization's communications, delivery, or transportation systems. Facilities should be constructed, arranged, and equipped to promote safe and efficient work and to avoid damage to or deterioration of drug products.

Ambulatory Infusion Center or Infusion Suite. Pharmacies that have an on-site (ambulatory) infusion suite must include appropriate access to the facility (e.g., handicapped parking, sidewalk ramp) and other internal design features (e.g., restroom grab bar) according to the Americans with Disabilities Act. Local building code regulations may also apply. Accreditation standards for home care organizations typically include a section on infusion suites and cover such items as patient access, facility safety checks, nursing procedures, and room sanitation. State and local authorities may have additional regulations for ambulatory treatment centers; these should be researched before planning to offer ambulatory treatment services.

Home Infusion Pharmacies. Designated space and equipment for compounding and packaging sterile preparations should be available.[7,8] The compounding environment should be monitored and maintained on an ongoing basis. Appropriate facility space, equipment, and supplies for compounding hazardous preparations should be available.[7,8,22] Adequate facilities and equipment should be established for decontaminating, cleaning, and maintaining infusion devices, including durable medical equipment.

General Work Area. The pharmacy work area should allow pharmacists to observe work being done by support staff (telephone calls to patients, computer data entry, compounding, etc.). Pharmacies should consider having an area dedicated to the function of checking compounded preparations and other prescriptions that is out of the main traffic pattern and where the checking pharmacist is not distracted by noise, telephones, or conversation.

Stockroom and Storage Areas. Facilities should be available for storing and preparing medications in the home infusion pharmacy under proper conditions of sanitation, temperature, light, moisture, ventilation, segregation, and security to ensure medication integrity and personnel safety and to prevent drug diversion.[27] Adequate refrigeration and freezer capacity should be provided within the secure pharmacy area.

Office and Meeting Space. Office and meeting areas should be available for administrative, clinical, technical, and reimbursement staff. Ideally, interdisciplinary team members from pharmacy, nursing, and reimbursement are located within a proximate space.

Cleanroom and Anteroom (Compounding Area). The home infusion pharmacy should follow all applicable federal, state, and local requirements, including USP Chapter 797,[8] for building and maintaining the pharmacy's compounding facilities. Options for building out a cleanroom include purchase of a modular prefabricated unit or building out an existing space with only those materials needed to bring the facility into compliance with laws, regulation, and guidance. Design and organization of the cleanroom should allow for the pharmacist's view of compounding activities through a large window or clear wall and efficient flow of materials and compounding documents into the cleanroom for processing and out of the cleanroom for the checking/verification step.

Sterile medications shall be compounded within a primary engineering control such as a laminar flow hood or a compounding aseptic containment isolator. Compounding facilities shall be cleaned and maintained following federal, state, and local laws or regulations as well as applicable guidance (e.g., ASHP guidelines, *USP* Chapter 797).[7,8] Environmental monitoring of the compounding facilities shall be ongoing and should include all elements required by federal, state, and local laws or regulations as well as applicable guidance (e.g., ASHP guidelines, USP 797).[7,8]

References

1. Health Insurance Portability and Accountability Act of 1996. Pub. L. No. 104-191. www.cms.hhs.gov/HIPAAGenInfo/Downloads/HIPAALaw.pdf (accessed 12 February 2011).
2. U.S. Department of Health and Human Services Office of Inspector General Exclusions Program. http://oig.hhs.gov/fraud/exclusions.asp (accessed 12 January 2011).
3. American Society of Hospital Pharmacists. ASHP statement on continuing education. *Am J Hosp Pharm.* 1990; 47:1855.
4. United States Department of Labor Occupational Safety & Health Administration. http://osha.gov/SLTC/bloodbornepathogens/index.html (accessed 12 February 2011).
5. National Institute of Occupational Safety and Health. NIOSH List of Antineoplastic and Other Hazardous Drugs in Healthcare Settings 2010. www.cdc.gov/niosh/docs/2010-167/pdfs/2010-167.pdf (accessed 12 February 2011).
6. United States Department of Labor Occupations Safety & Health Administration, Hazard Communication: Foundation of Workplace Chemical Safety Program. www.osha.gov/dsg/hazcom/index.html (accessed 12 February 2011).
7. American Society of Health-System Pharmacists. ASHP guidelines on quality assurance for pharmacy-prepared sterile products. *Am J Health-Syst Pharm.* 2000; 57:1150–69.
8. Pharmaceutical compounding—sterile preparations (general information chapter 797). In: The United States pharmacopeia, 34th rev., and The national formulary, 29th ed. Rockville, MD: The United States Pharmacopeial Convention; 2011: 336–73.
9. American Society of Health-System Pharmacists. ASHP guidelines on the pharmacy and therapeutics committee and the formulary system. *Am J Health-Syst Pharm.* 2008; 65:1272–83.
10. American Society of Health-System Pharmacists. ASHP guidelines on clinical drug research. *Am J Health-Syst Pharm.* 1998; 55:369–76.
11. American Society of Hospital Pharmacists. ASHP guidelines for pharmaceutical research in organized health-care settings. *Am J Hosp Pharm.* 1989; 46:129–30.
12. American Society of Health-System Pharmacists. ASHP guidelines on the safe use of automated dispensing devices. *Am J Health-Syst Pharm.* 2010; 67:483–90.
13. American Society of Health-System Pharmacists. ASHP statement on the pharmacist's role in substance abuse prevention, education, and assistance. *Am J Health-Syst Pharm.* 2014; 71:243–6.
14. American Society of Health-System Pharmacists. ASHP guidelines on the pharmacist's role in the development, implementation, and assessment of critical pathways. *Am J Health-Syst Pharm.* 2004; 61:939–45.
15. American Society of Hospital Pharmacists. ASHP guidelines for selecting pharmaceutical manufacturers and suppliers. *Am J Hosp Pharm.* 1991; 48:523–4.
16. American Society of Health-System Pharmacists. ASHP guidelines on medication cost management strategies for hospitals and health systems. *Am J Health-Syst Pharm.* 2008; 65:1368–84.
17. American Society of Health-System Pharmacists (ASHP). ASHP Drug Shortages Resource Center. www.ashp.org/shortages (accessed 21 Mar 2013).
18. U.S. Food and Drug Administration. Drug shortages. www.fda.gov/cder/drug/shortages/ (accessed 21 Mar 2013).
19. American Society of Health-System Pharmacists. ASHP guidelines on managing drug product shortages in hospitals and health systems. *Am J Health-Syst Pharm.* 2009; 66:1399–406.
20. Institute for Safe Medication Practices (ISMP). ISMP's List of High-Alert Medications. www.ismp.org/tools/highalertmedications.pdf (accessed 21 Mar 2013).
21. American Society of Health-System Pharmacists. ASHP guidelines on outsourcing sterile compounding services. *Am J Health-Syst Pharm.* 2010; 67:757–65.
22. American Society of Health-System Pharmacists. ASHP guidelines on handling hazardous drugs. *Am J Health-Syst Pharm.* 2006; 63:1172–93.
23. Hepler CD, Strand LM. Opportunities and responsibilities in pharmaceutical care. *Am J Hosp Pharm.* 1990;47:533–43.
24. American Society of Health-System Pharmacists. ASHP guidelines on pharmacist-conducted patient education and counseling. *Am J Health-Syst Pharm.* 1997; 54:431–4.

25. American Society of Health-System Pharmacists. ASHP guidelines on adverse drug reaction monitoring and reporting. *Am J Health-Syst Pharm.* 1995; 52:417–9.
26. American Society of Health-System Pharmacists. ASHP statement on the role of health-system pharmacists in emergency preparedness. *Am J Health-Syst Pharm.* 2003; 60:1993–5.
27. American Society of Hospital Pharmacists. ASHP technical assistance bulletin on hospital drug distribution and control. *Am J Hosp Pharm.* 1980; 37:1097–103.

Approved by the ASHP Board of Directors on June 28, 2013. Developed through the ASHP Section of Ambulatory Care Practitioners Section Advisory Group on Home Infusion. These guidelines supersede the ASHP Guidelines on the Pharmacist's Role in Home Care dated April 27, 2000, and the ASHP Guidelines: Minimum Standard for Home Care Pharmacies dated November 14, 1998.

Barbara J. Petroff, M.S., FASHP; Donald Filibeck, Pharm.D., M.B.A.; Anna Nowobilski-Vasilios, Pharm.D., M.B.A., CNSC, BCNSP, FASHP; R. Stephen Olsen, Pharm.D.; Carol J. Rollins, Pharm.D., M.S., RD, BCNSP; and Cathy Johnson, B.S.Pharm., are gratefully acknowledged for authoring these guidelines.

ASHP gratefully acknowledges the contributions of the following individuals to these guidelines: Mitra Gavgani, Pharm.D.; Brian G. Swift, Pharm.D., M.B.A.; Lisa Linn Siefert, B.S.Pharm., ASQ-CQM, FASHP; Kelly Rogers, B.S.Pharm.; and Caryn M. Bing, M.S., FASHP.

ASHP also gratefully acknowledges the following organizations and individuals for reviewing these guidelines (review does not imply endorsement): Academy of Managed Care Pharmacy (AMCP); American Academy of Ambulatory Care Nursing (AAACN); American Society for Parenteral and Enteral Nutrition (ASPEN); Infusion Nurses Society; Rhode Island Society of Health-System Pharmacists; Jeanette Spain Adams, Ph.D., RN, ACNS, BC, CRNI; Mary Alexander, M.A., RN, CRNI, CAE, FAAN; Dominick A. Caselnova III, B.S.Pharm., M.H.A., FASHP; Toby Clark, M.Sc., FASHP; Sharon M. Durfee, B.S.Pharm., BCNSP; Michael Edwards, Pharm.D., M.B.A., BCOP, FASHP; Allen Flynn, Pharm.D., CPHIMS, CHS; Peggi Guenter, Ph.D., RN, CNSN (ASPEN); Kathleen M. Gura, Pharm.D., BCNSP, FASHP, FPPAG; Richelle Hamblin, RN, M.S.N., CRNI (AAACN); John Hertig, Pharm.D., M.S.; Tim Lanese, M.B.A., FASHP; Jay Lewandowski, Pharm.D.; Mary R. Monk-Tutor, Ph.D., FASHP; Richard D. Paoletti, M.B.A., FASHP; Susan M. Paschke, M.S.N., RN-BC, NEA-BC (AAACN); Stephanie Peshek, Pharm.D., M.B.A., FASHP; Nicole Pilch, Pharm.D., MSCR, BCPS; James A. Ponto, M.S., BCNP, FASHP; Tony Powers, Pharm.D.; Curt W. Quap, M.S., FASHP; Armando Riggi, Pharm.D.; Jean S. Rutledge, Ph.D.; Elizabeth Sampsel, Pharm.D., M.B.A., BCPS (AMCP); Robert A. Smaglia, B.S.Pharm.; Nancy R. Smestad, M.S.; Rex Speerhas, CDE, BCNSP; Melisa Tong, Pharm.D.; and Kristine Widboom.

Copyright © 2014, American Society of Health-System Pharmacists, Inc. All rights reserved. Contact ASHP for reprint and permissions requests. This content may not be used for commercial purposes without the express written consent of ASHP.

The bibliographic citation for this document is as follows: American Society of Health-System Pharmacists. ASHP Guidelines on Home Infusion Pharmacy Services. *Am J Health-Syst Pharm.* 2014; 71:325–41.

ASHP Guidelines: Minimum Standard for Ambulatory Care Pharmacy Practice

In recent years, there has been an increasing emphasis in health systems on the provision of ambulatory care services. Payers have created incentives to decrease hospitalization rates and length of stay, making way for a new shift toward pay-for-performance, outcomes-based reimbursement, and accountable care. There is also an increasing focus in medicine on preventive health, patient education, and care transitions. Yet, the number of patients with multiple chronic medical conditions that require longitudinal and integrated care management across a continuum of care settings is growing. Appropriate medication therapy in the ambulatory care setting is often the most common and most cost-effective form of treatment, yet the consequences of adverse drug events (ADEs) and the inappropriate use of medications in this setting can be catastrophic.[1] Ambulatory care pharmacy services are therefore an essential component of any comprehensive healthcare delivery system.

Pharmacists have become integral members of healthcare teams in a variety of settings, such as patient-centered medical homes, community health centers, long-term care facilities, hospital outpatient departments, and freestanding pharmacies, among others; the care they provide has enabled patients, other providers, and payers to achieve their clinical, humanistic, and economic goals.[2,3] There is growing recognition and understanding that ambulatory care pharmacy services extend far beyond the dispensing of medications and include direct patient care and the design and management of complex medication regimens and care delivery systems. Current evidence demonstrates that the inclusion of pharmacists practicing in ambulatory care settings on the healthcare team improves quality of care, enhances patient outcomes, and contributes to cost avoidance.[4] Most states now allow pharmacists to provide direct patient care services under a physician–pharmacist collaborative agreement, further supporting the expansion of ambulatory care pharmacy services.

The primary purpose of these guidelines is to outline the minimum requirements for the operation and management of services for patients in this rapidly evolving ambulatory care setting. The elements of service that are critical to optimal, safe, and effective medication use in the ambulatory setting include (1) leadership and practice management, (2) patient care, (3) drug distribution and control, and (4) facilities, equipment, and other resources. Although the scope of pharmacy services will vary from site to site, depending on the needs of the patients served and the resources available, these elements are directly linked to improved patient, population, and health-system outcomes. Specific attention to each element is essential to delivering patient care of the highest quality. As providers of care to patients in ambulatory care settings, pharmacists should be concerned with and take responsibility for the outcomes of their services in addition to the provision of these services. Care should also extend into and be coordinated with care providers in other settings; therefore, these guidelines should be used, as applicable, in conjunction with minimum standards for other practice settings. Rather than including detailed advice in this document, readers should refer to other referenced documents that address many of the outlined topics for additional information and guidance. Aspects of these guidelines may not be applicable in some settings due to differences in settings and organizational arrangements and complexity. Pharmacists practicing in ambulatory care settings should use their professional judgment in assessing and adapting these guidelines to meet the needs of their own practice settings.

These guidelines are intended to be a comprehensive overview of current minimum requirements for the operation and management of services for patients in the ambulatory care setting. These guidelines are complemented by the ASHP/ASHP Foundation Ambulatory Conference and Summit consensus recommendations,[5] which provide a long-term vision for aspirational and forward-thinking pharmacy practice models that will ensure that pharmacists participate as members of the ambulatory healthcare team who are responsible and accountable for patient and population outcomes.

Standard I. Practice Management

Effective leadership and practice management skills are necessary for the delivery of pharmacy services in a manner consistent with the health system's and the patient's needs. Such leadership should foster continuous improvement in patient care outcomes. The management of ambulatory care pharmacy services should focus on the pharmacist's value and responsibilities as a patient care provider and leader of the pharmacy enterprise through the development of organizational structures that support this mission. Development of such structures will require communication and collaboration with other departments and services throughout the health system that support ambulatory care, which every member of the pharmacy team should cultivate at every opportunity.

A. Pharmacy and Pharmacist Services

Pharmacy Mission, Goals, and Scope of Services. Ambula-tory care pharmacy services should have a written mission statement that, at a minimum, reflects both pharmacy patient care and service responsibilities. The mission should be consistent with the mission of the health system. The development and prioritization of goals, objectives, and work should be consistent with the mission statement. The mission statement may also incorporate consensus-based national goals, such as those expressed in the recommendations from the ASHP Pharmacy Practice Model Initiative.[6]

Ambulatory care pharmacy services should also maintain a written document describing the scope of pharmacy services. These services should be consistent with the health system's scope of services and should be applied in all practice sites. The mission, goals, and scope of services should be clearly communicated to everyone involved in the provision of pharmacy services.

DOI 10.37573/9781585287048.100

Practice Standards and Guidelines. The standards and regulations of all relevant government bodies (e.g., state boards of pharmacy, departments of health) shall be met. The practice standards and guidelines of the American Society of Health-System Pharmacists, the Joint Commission, the National Committee for Quality Assurance, and other appropriate accrediting bodies should be assessed and adapted, as applicable. Guidelines set forth by other independent organizations such as the Institute for Safe Medication Practices (ISMP) should be assessed and adapted as applicable. The health system and the pharmacy should strive to meet these standards, regardless of the particular financial and organizational arrangements by which pharmacy services are provided to the health system and its patients. Pharmacists practicing in ambulatory care settings should play a critical role in ensuring that the health system adheres to medication-related national quality indicators and evidence-based practice guidelines.

B. Laws and Regulations

Compliance with local, state, and federal laws and regulations applicable to the ambulatory care pharmacy shall be required. The pharmacy shall maintain relevant documentation of compliance with requirements concerning procurement, distribution, and disposal of drug products; security of patient information; and workplace safety from the state board of pharmacy, Food and Drug Administration (FDA), Drug Enforcement Administration (DEA), Centers for Medicare and Medicaid Services (CMS), Occupational Safety and Health Administration, and others. Ambulatory care pharmacies dispensing medications across state boundaries shall comply with out-of-state licensure requirements as well as other state and federal interstate laws and regulations. Pharmacists practicing in ambulatory care settings may enter into prescriptive authority and collaborative practice agreements that are state specific in scope. Finally, pharmacists practicing in ambulatory care settings should be knowledgeable about reimbursement rules and compliance and billing requirements.

C. Policies and Procedures

Policies and Procedures Manual. A policy and procedures manual governing the scope of the ambulatory care pharmacy services being provided (e.g., administrative, operational, and clinical) should be available and consistent with current department processes. The manual should be reviewed and revised on a regular basis to reflect changes in policies and procedures, the scope of services, organizational arrangements, objectives, or practices. All personnel should be familiar with and adhere to the contents of the manual. Appropriate mechanisms should be established to ensure compliance with all policies and procedures.

Personnel Safety. Ambulatory care pharmacy personnel should be involved in the health system's plans for emergency response, infection prevention and control, management of hazardous substances and waste, and incident reporting. All pharmacy staff shall be familiar with these plans.

Emergency Preparedness. Policies and procedures should exist for providing pharmacy services during facility, local, or areawide disasters affecting the organization's patients. Appropriately trained pharmacists and representatives from the pharmacy team should be members of emergency preparedness teams and participate in drills. Patients should be informed about what to do to safely continue medication therapy in the event of a disaster.[7]

The health system's business continuity plan should consider the provision of pharmacist patient care services in emergency situations. Factors to consider should include system failures and breakdowns in the drug procurement process.

Medical Emergencies. Policies and procedures should exist within the organization for providing appropriate levels of patient care during emergency situations 24 hours a day, including access to the pharmacist responsible for patient care, when appropriate. Pharmacists in the ambulatory care setting are an essential part of both rapid-response teams and resuscitation teams. Appropriately trained pharmacists should have an authorized role in responding to medical emergencies. The pharmacy should participate in the development of policies and procedures to ensure the availability of, access to, and security of emergency medications, including antidotes.

Preventive and Postexposure Immunization Programs. If appropriate, the pharmacy team should participate in the development of policies and procedures concerning preventive and wellness programs and postexposure programs for infectious diseases (e.g., human immunodeficiency virus, tuberculosis, hepatitis) for patients and employees. As appropriate, pharmacists should promote the use of immunizations and, when legally allowed, participate as active immunizers.[8]

Substance Abuse Programs. If appropriate, the pharmacy team should assist in the development of and participate in the health system's substance abuse education, prevention, identification, and organization-sponsored programs for staff and patients.[9]

D. Human Resources

Position Descriptions. Areas of responsibility within the scope of pharmacy services shall be clearly defined. The responsibilities and related competencies of pharmacy personnel shall be clearly defined in written position descriptions. Pharmacists should be responsible for the provision of patient care and for the supervision and management of support staff. Sufficient support staff (pharmacy technicians, clerical) should be employed to facilitate the provision of care. Technicians should be responsible for aspects of drug procurement, dialogue with third-party payers, support of pharmacists' patient care activities, and preparation of prescription orders for a pharmacist's clinical review.

Director of Ambulatory Care Pharmacy Services. These guidelines use the term *director of ambulatory care pharmacy services* (or, more simply, *director*) to indicate the person responsible for managing these services. Depending on the health system's organizational structure and other factors, designations such as manager or pharmacist-in-charge may also be used. Ambulatory care pharmacy services shall be managed by a professionally competent, legally qualified pharmacist. The director should be knowledgeable about and have experience in all aspects of pharmacy care for ambulatory care patients. Completion of an advanced management degree (e.g., M.B.A., M.H.A., M.S., M.P.H.), a residency, or both is desirable. Completion of an ASHP-accredited postgraduate year 1 (PGY1) residency should be considered a minimum competency, while completion of an ASHP-accredited postgraduate year 2 (PGY2) residency would be optimal.

The director of ambulatory care pharmacy services shall be responsible for

- Establishing the mission, vision, goals, and scope of services of the ambulatory care pharmacy practice setting on the basis of the needs of the patients served, the needs of the health system, and developments and trends in healthcare and pharmacy practice.
- Developing, implementing, evaluating, and updating plans and activities to fulfill the mission, vision, goals, and scope of services.
- Actively working with health-system leadership to develop and implement policies and procedures that provide safe and effective medication use for all patients served by the organization.
- Ensuring the development and implementation of policies and procedures that provide safe and effective medication use for the patients served by the organization.
- Mobilizing and managing the resources, both human and financial, necessary for the optimal provision of pharmacy services.
- Ensuring that patient care services provided by pharmacists and other pharmacy personnel are delivered in compliance with applicable state and federal laws and regulations as well as national practice standards.

A part-time director shall have the same obligations and responsibilities as a full-time director.[10,11]

The ambulatory care pharmacy team should be a cross-functional group whose skills set includes operations management, clinical care, financial management, process improvement, and informatics. Depending on the size and scope of the setting, these functional responsibilities may be assigned to a single person or a team. It is the responsibility of the director to monitor the status of the goals set forth in the vision, provide feedback to the pharmacy team as necessary, and support the team's implementation of the core functions of the pharmacy practice.

Pharmacist Licensure and Certification. All pharmacists must possess a current state license to practice pharmacy. Functional responsibilities may mandate additional degrees (M.S., M.B.A., M.H.A., M.P.H.), certificates, or credentials (e.g., Board of Pharmacy Specialties certification). Pharmacists who provide direct patient care and drug therapy management should be certified through the most appropriate Board of Pharmacy Specialties certification process. As appropriate, these pharmacists should also be privileged and credentialed by the health system.

Technician Requirements. The ambulatory care setting shall adhere to all state guidelines regarding pharmacy technician registration, certification, and licensure, as applicable. All pharmacy technicians should successfully complete a training course approved by the ambulatory care site that includes education on at least the following topics: the prescription-dispensing process, patient service skills, patient and employee safety, and pharmacy technician duties and responsibilities as defined by the board of pharmacy for that state. Pharmacy technicians should have completed an ASHP-accredited pharmacy technician training program and be certified by the Pharmacy Technician Certification Board (PTCB). The pharmacy should hire pharmacy technician trainees without those qualifications only if those individuals (1) are required to both successfully complete an ASHP-accredited pharmacy technician training program and successfully complete PTCB certification within 24 months of employment and (2) are limited to positions with lesser responsibilities until they successfully complete such training and certification. The pharmacy should require ongoing PTCB certification as a condition of continued employment.

Education and Training. All personnel should possess the education and training needed to fulfill their job responsibilities. All personnel should participate in relevant continuing-education programs, staff development programs, and other activities as necessary to maintain or enhance their competence. Both the ambulatory care pharmacy department and the health system should make available to personnel, as appropriate, training and education on new processes, procedures, and methods of patient care.[12] For pharmacists, ASHP-accredited PGY1 residency should be considered a minimum competency, while completion of an ASHP-accredited PGY2 residency would be optimal.

Recruitment, Selection, and Retention of Personnel. Qualities to consider in recruitment include completion of one or two years of postgraduate residency training, board certification, previous participation in a collaborative practice environment, and other credentials and privileges as appropriate. An ASHP-accredited PGY1 residency should be considered a minimum competency, while completion of an ASHP-accredited PGY2 residency would be optimal. Personnel should be recruited and selected on the basis of requirements in established position descriptions. Criteria used in the selection process should include the candidate's performance of similar job-specific duties, education history relevant to job-specific duties, and willingness to contribute to achieving the mission of the department and the health system. The director should assist in identifying the professional and technical requirements that a candidate must meet to qualify for the position. Clinical specialist positions are a necessary part of any health system in order to advance practice, education, and research activities. An employee retention plan is desirable.[13]

Orientation of Personnel. Personnel who are new to either a specific position or the organization should be oriented to their position through an established and structured procedure. During the orientation process, personnel should be trained in their new job functions by an employee knowledgeable in the work assigned. During the orientation period, the trainer's normal workload should be reduced in order to provide dedicated instruction time to the person being oriented, particularly in distributive settings. The orientation period of new personnel should be tailored to both the new employee's needs and the functions of the employee's position. Evaluation of the effectiveness of orientation programs should be done in conjunction with the competency assessment required before a new hire can assume full responsibility for the new position.

Work Schedules and Assignments. Assignments of pharmacists and pharmacy technicians should be clearly defined to allow the optimal use of personnel and resources. Work schedules should take into account peak demand times for pharmacist-provided patient care. Sufficient personnel should be available to ensure the safe and timely delivery of pharmacy services. Hours of operation should be designed to meet the needs of the patient population given the available resources of the health system.

Performance Evaluation and Job-Specific Competencies. Scheduled periodic evaluations of performance should occur for all pharmacy personnel. Performance should be evaluated on the basis of position description requirements and expected competencies, and the evaluation format should be consistent with that used by the health system. Evaluations should include comments from professional and technical staff as well as other members of the healthcare team. Pharmacy staff should meet the expectations defined in their position descriptions for adequate performance of their duties. The director should ensure that an ongoing competency assessment program is in place for all staff, and each staff member should have a continuous professional development plan.

E. Facilities, Equipment, and Other Resources

Pharmacy. To ensure optimal performance and quality patient care, adequate space, equipment, and other resources should be available for all professional, administrative, distributive, and direct patient care functions. Patient care areas, which include the pharmacy counter, counseling rooms, and clinic offices or examination rooms where direct patient care is provided, should ensure proper patient confidentiality, promote safe and efficient patient care, and contain all tools and supplies necessary for the provision of such care. Pharmacy services operations shall be located in areas that facilitate the provision of services to patients and healthcare providers. Distributive areas should be constructed, arranged, and equipped to promote safe and efficient workflow for staff and patients and to ensure medication integrity. All facilities shall be designed to comply with applicable state and federal guidelines.

Medication Storage and Preparation Areas. Facilities should exist for the preparation and storage of drug products and medications under proper conditions of sanitation, temperature, light, moisture, ventilation, segregation, and security throughout the pharmacy and other patient care areas. Monitored, adequate refrigerator and freezer capacity should be available within the secure pharmacy area and, as necessary, in nonpharmacy areas.

Compounding and Packaging Areas. There shall be suitable facilities to enable the compounding, preparation, packaging, and labeling of sterile and nonsterile drug products, including hazardous drug products, in accordance with established quality-assurance procedures. The work environment should promote orderliness and efficiency and minimize the potential for medication errors and contamination of products.[14–19]

Patient Care and Counseling Areas. A designated area should be available for private patient care and counseling by pharmacists to enhance patients' knowledge and understanding of and adherence to prescribed medication therapy regimens and monitoring plans, to provide disease state management and patient care services, and to foster continuity of care. Space should accommodate the pharmacist and patient and, as appropriate, parents, caregivers, or chaperones. These areas should be stocked with relevant supplies and equipment, including computers, drug references, monitoring equipment, and other necessary tools.[20]

Office and Meeting Areas. Adequate office and meeting areas should be available for administrative, educational, and training activities. These areas should be stocked with relevant supplies and equipment, including computers, drug references, and other necessary tools.

Automated Systems. Automated mechanical systems and software can promote safe, accurate, and efficient medication ordering and preparation, drug distribution, and clinical monitoring. Barcode technology that is associated with any of these systems provides an additional level of safety. The potential for medication errors with any of these systems should be thoroughly understood, evaluated, and eliminated to the greatest extent possible. Organizations should have policies and procedures for the evaluation, selection, use, calibration, monitoring, and maintenance of all automated pharmacy systems.[21,22] The greatest benefits to safety and productivity are seen with robust functionality, proper system maintenance, and the prevention of workarounds.

Automated systems and devices should interface with pharmacy-based systems and support and augment the medication-use process. The replenishment of dispensing equipment should be overseen by pharmacists or by technicians who have been certified as part of a technician-checking program, depending on specific state board requirements. Calibration, maintenance, and certification as required by applicable standards, laws, and regulations should be continual and documented. All automated systems shall include adequate safeguards to maintain the confidentiality and security of patient records, and there shall be procedures to provide essential patient care services in case of equipment failure or downtime.

Health Information Technology. A comprehensive pharmacy computer system shall be employed and should be integrated to the fullest extent possible with other health-system information systems and software. Computer resources should be used to support clerical functions, maintain patient medication profile records, provide clinical decision support, perform necessary patient-billing procedures, manage drug product inventories, provide drug information, access the patient medical record, manage electronic prescribing, and interface with other computerized systems to obtain patient-specific clinical information for medication therapy monitoring and other clinical functions and to facilitate the continuity and transitions of care to and from other care settings.

Pharmacy-based systems experts who act as resources and consultants in maintaining current systems, planning for implementations and upgrades, and assisting in performance improvement and evaluation are critical to the success of informatics implementation and use.

Record and Equipment Maintenance. Adequate space should exist for maintaining and storing records (e.g., prescription records, equipment maintenance, controlled substances inventory) to ensure compliance with laws, regulations, accreditation requirements, and sound management practices. Appropriate licenses, permits, tax stamps, and other documents shall be on display or on file as required by law or regulation. All equipment shall be adequately maintained and certified in accordance with applicable standards, laws, and regulations. Equipment maintenance and certification shall be documented.

F. Managing Financial Resources

Budget Management. The pharmacy shall have a budget that is consistent with the health system's financial management process and supports the scope of and demand for pharmacy services. Oversight of workload and financial performance should be managed in accordance with the health system's requirements. Management should provide for the determination and analysis of pharmacy service costs, capital equipment costs, and new project growth.

The ambulatory care pharmacy budget processes should enable the analysis of pharmacy services by unit of service and other parameters appropriate to the organization (e.g., organizationwide costs by medication therapy, clinical service, specific disease management categories, and patient third-party enrollment). The director should have an integral part in the organization's financial management process.

Health-System Integration. Other functional units within the health system should factor the cost of pharmacy services being provided by the ambulatory care pharmacy into the departmental budget when appropriate.

Third-Party Contract Review. In conjunction with the organization's legal or contracting department, the pharmacy director's team should review third-party payer contracts to ensure that reimbursement is appropriate for services being rendered (including dispensing, patient care, and disease state management services) and the terms of the contract are in the best interest of the patient and the health system. The organization, pharmacy, or pharmacist should contract with third-party payers that are relevant to the ambulatory care pharmacy's patient population.

Revenue, Reimbursement, and Compensation. The director should be knowledgeable about revenues for pharmacy services, including reimbursement for medication dispensing, patient care, and disease state and drug therapy management services. Processes should exist for the routine verification of payment from third-party payers.

Drug Expenditures. Specific policies and procedures for managing drug expenditures should address such methods as utilization review programs, inventory management, and cost-effective care for patients with limited income and resources. The pharmacy department should use practices such as competitive bidding, group purchasing, and specialized pricing (e.g., 340B Drug Pricing Program) when applicable to develop a responsible drug purchasing model.

G. Committee Involvement

A pharmacist representative from the ambulatory care pharmacy team shall be a member of and actively participate on committees responsible for establishing and implementing medication-related policies and procedures, ambulatory care leadership, the provision of patient care, informatics, and performance improvement, as appropriate. Members of the pharmacy team should take part in staff recognition, patient service programs, and other programs as identified in the ambulatory care pharmacy service. Members of the pharmacy team should participate in the activities of similar committees of the health system, as applicable

Standard II. Managing the Medication-Use Process

A. Medication-Use Policy Development

Medication-use policy decisions should be founded on the evidence-based clinical, ethical, legal, social, philosophical, quality-of-life, safety, and economic factors that result in optimal patient care. Committees within the organization that make decisions concerning medication use (e.g., pharmacy and therapeutics, infection control) should include the active and direct involvement of physicians, pharmacists, other appropriate healthcare professionals, and patients, where appropriate. Pharmacists practicing in ambulatory care settings should actively participate on committees whose decisions could affect the quality, safety, effectiveness, or cost of pharmacy services or the medication-use process. Institutional and health-system pharmacists and pharmacy technicians shall be members of an interprofessional team accountable and responsible for medication reconciliation, patient counseling, and medication-related outcomes by establishing a medication-related continuity-of-care process for all patients. Pharmacists practicing in ambulatory care settings should be actively involved in the development, maintenance, and updating of medication-use policies, including tracking and trending of health-system antibiotic resistance patterns.

B. Formulary Management and Integration

Both the patients' diseases and the medications authorized for use by patients' third-party prescription drug programs should be taken into account when determining the ambulatory care pharmacy's inventory. The pharmacy should have access to specialty medications distributed through closed-network systems when needed to support consistent delivery of patient care and medication reconciliation.

Health systems should maintain a formulary that is efficacious and cost-effective. This formulary should be developed with feedback from professional healthcare providers (pharmacists, physicians, social workers, case managers). When possible, charity programs (patient assistance programs, copayment foundations) should be accessed to help patients with limited income and resources to procure their medications.

C. Clinical Care Plans and Disease State Management

Pharmacists in their scope of practice should be involved as part of an interprofessional team in the development and implementation of clinical care plans with prescriptive authority in the healthcare setting (clinical practice guidelines, critical pathways) and disease state management programs involving collaborative drug therapy management (CDTM) agreements and treatment protocols. In addition, medication therapy management (MTM) services should be developed to assist with collaborative patient care. Emphasis should be placed on clinical care plans, primary care, and medication treatment protocols that cover dosage calculations and limits and medications frequently associated with adverse (potential and actual) events, including medication errors.[23,24] Primary care protocols should consider whole-patient needs for health promotion and disease prevention measures as well as appropriate patient assessments, comprehensive management of chronic disease states, management of medication-related care problems, and referrals for acute medical care. The targeting of diseases should consider the prevalence of the disease in the population served by the organization and the potential impact on clinical and economic outcomes.[25]

D. Drug Information

Policies and procedures should be in place for reviewing responses to requests for drug information for the purpose of performance improvement, safety, and education. Pharmacists should provide accurate, comprehensive, and patient-specific drug information to patients, caregivers, other pharmacists, physicians, nurses, and other healthcare providers as appropriate, both proactively and in response to requests associated with the delivery of pharmacist-provided patient care, educational programs, and publications. Expertise in evaluating literature on drugs should be considered essential to the provision of drug therapy management.

Drug information sources should include current professional and scientific periodicals, Web-based research tools (e.g., AHFS-DI, MicroMedex, Lexicomp Online), and the latest editions of reference books in appropriate pharmaceutical and biomedical subject areas that can be easily accessed. Available sources should support research on patient care issues, facilitate the provision of patient care, and promote safety in the medication-use process. When possible, a pharmacist should play a role in addressing complex drug information questions presented by professional staff within the health system (e.g., pharmacists, nurses, physicians).

E. Development of Patient Care Services

Pharmacists who practice in ambulatory care settings should be involved in the development, implementation, and evaluation of new or changing patient care services and drug therapy management services within the organization, such as the development of new clinic or office sites, medical homes, or accountable care organizations. In reviewing the potential for new services, both the value added to patient care by the new service and the financial and logistical implications of the new service should be considered. These efforts should promote the continuity of pharmacist-provided patient care across the continuum of care, practice settings, and geographically dispersed facilities, particularly for newly discharged patients. New services should be developed when opportunities arise for earlier involvement in medication therapy decisions (e.g., clinic rounds) and for continuity between patient encounters for the purpose of assessing therapy success, tolerance, toxicity, and adherence.

Standard III. Drug Product Procurement and Inventory Management

The pharmacy or contracted network pharmacies should be responsible for the procurement, distribution, and control of all drug products used in the treatment of the organization's patients. The pharmacy is responsible for the development of policies and procedures governing medication distribution and control. Policies and procedures should be developed in collaboration with other appropriate professionals, departments, and interprofessional committees of the organization.[26]

A. Purchasing and Maintaining the Availability of Drug Products

Drug Product Acquisition and Availability. Drug products approved for routine use should be purchased, stored, and available in sufficient quantities to meet the needs of ambulatory care patients. Drug products not approved for routine use but necessary to meet the needs of specific patients or categories of patients should be obtained in response to orders, according to established policies and procedures.

Pharmaceutical Manufacturers and Suppliers. Criteria for selecting pharmaceutical manufacturers and suppliers shall be established to ensure that patients receive pharmaceuticals and related supplies of the highest quality and at the lowest cost.[27] Although these duties may be delegated in part to a group purchasing organization, the pharmacy maintains sole responsibility for ensuring the quality of drug products used in the hospital.[27,28]

Pharmaceutical Manufacturers' Representatives. Policies and procedures should be developed governing the activities of manufacturers' representatives or vendors of drug products (including related supplies and devices) within the pharmacy, ambulatory care setting, and organization.[29] Representatives should not be permitted access to patient care areas and should be provided with written guidance on permissible activities. All promotional materials and activities shall be reviewed and approved by the pharmacy.[29–31]

B. Managing Inventory

Medication Storage. Medication storage areas must have proper environmental controls (i.e., proper temperature, light, humidity, conditions of sanitation, ventilation, and segregation), be secure, and be constructed so that drugs are accessible only to authorized personnel.[32] Adequate inventory controls must be maintained to allow proper inventory levels of medications based on utilization.

Drug Shortages. There should be policies and procedures for managing drug shortages, and pharmacy staff should monitor reliable sources of information regarding drug product shortages (e.g., drug shortages Web resource centers of ASHP[33] and FDA[34]). The pharmacy should develop strategies for identifying alternative therapies, working with suppliers, collaborating with physicians and other healthcare providers, and conducting an awareness campaign in the event of a drug shortage.[35]

Samples. The use of drug product samples should be prohibited to the extent possible.[32] However, if samples are permitted under certain circumstances, policies and procedures for their storage, control, and distribution should be in place. The pharmacy should oversee procurement, storage, and distribution of these products to ensure proper storage, record-keeping maintenance, product integrity, and compliance with all applicable packaging and labeling laws, regulations, standards, and patient education requirements. Pharmacists should be involved in the organization's efforts to secure safe and effective low-cost medications for low-income patients.[32,36]

Patient Care Area Stock. Inventory of drug products held in nonpharmacy areas (e.g., nursing station, clinic, physicians' offices) for direct administration to ambulatory care patients should be minimal. To the extent possible, medications administered to patients in nonpharmacy areas should be prepared by the pharmacy. If this is not possible, automated medication dispensing machines should be used to dispense medications to patients. The list of medications to be accessible and the policies and procedures regarding their use shall be developed by an interprofessional committee of physicians, pharmacists, and nurses.[36] Access to medications should be limited to cases in which the committee determines that an urgent clinical need for the medication outweighs the potential patient safety risks of making the medication accessible. A separate assessment should occur for every location where a medication may be stocked.

Controlled Substances. Policies and procedures should ensure the distribution of controlled substances and other medications with the potential for abuse. Policies and procedures should be consistent with applicable laws and regulations and should include methods for preventing and detecting diversion.[33]

Emergency Medications and Devices. The pharmacy should ensure the availability, access, and security of emergency medications, including antidotes. The telephone number of the local poison information center should be posted at or near all telephones for staff access. Pharmacists should have an authorized role in responding to medical emergencies.

All emergency medications should be stored in sealed containers that enable the staff to readily determine that the contents are complete and have not expired. All emergency medications should be available, controlled, and secured in the patient procedure areas.

Patient's Own Medications. Drug products and related devices brought into the organization by patients shall be identified by the pharmacy and documented on the patient's medical record if the medications are to be used. These medications shall be administered only pursuant to a prescriber's order and according to policies and procedures, which should ensure the pharmacist's identification and validation of the integrity as well as the secure and appropriate storage and management of such medications.

C. Drug Product Storage Area Inspections

All stocks of drug products, whether located within or outside the pharmacy area, should be inspected routinely and managed by pharmacy and location staff to ensure the absence of outdated, unusable, recalled, or mislabeled products. Storage conditions that would foster medication deterioration, storage arrangements that might contribute to medication errors, and other safety issues shall be assessed, documented, and corrected.[33]

D. Drug Recall and New Prescribing Information

Written procedures should exist for the timely intervention and dissemination of information regarding drug recalls. Procedures should include an established process for removing from use any drugs or devices subjected to a recall, notifying appropriate healthcare professionals, identifying any patients who may have been exposed to the recalled medication, and, if necessary, communicating available alternative therapies to prescribers. The pharmacy shall be notified of any defective drug products or related supplies and equipment encountered by nursing or medical staff. All drug product defects should be reported to FDA's MedWatch program.[33]

Standard IV. Patient Care

Pharmacists play an integral role in the provision of pharmaceutical care, which is defined as the responsible provision of drug therapy for the purpose of achieving definite outcomes that improve a patient's quality of life.[37] The concept of pharmaceutical care has evolved into a comprehensive, patient-focused model of pharmacist-provided care. The principal elements of pharmaceutical care are that it is medication related, is directly provided to the patient, and is provided to produce definite outcomes; these outcomes are intended to improve the patient's quality of life, and the provider must accept personal responsibility for the outcomes.[37] In 2008, a joint working group consisting of members and leadership from the American College of Clinical Pharmacy, the American Pharmacists Association, and the American Society of Health-System Pharmacists created a definition of ambulatory care practice as part of a petition to the Board of Pharmacy Specialties requesting recognition of ambulatory care pharmacy practice as a specialty. The definition described ambulatory care pharmacy practice as a specialty in medication use for preventive and chronic care:

> Ambulatory care pharmacy practice is the provision of integrated, accessible healthcare services by pharmacists who are accountable for addressing medication needs, developing sustained partnerships with patients, and practicing in the context of family and community. This is accomplished through direct patient care and medication management for ambulatory patients, long-term relationships, coordination of care, patient advocacy, wellness and health promotion, triage and referral, and patient education and self-management.[38–40]

The mission of the pharmacist is to help people make the best use of medications. At a minimum, pharmacists are responsible for assessing the legal and clinical appropriateness of medication orders (or prescriptions), educating and counseling patients on the use of their medications, monitoring the effects of medication therapy, and maintaining patient profiles and other records. In the ambulatory care setting, these responsibilities are best accomplished through the provision of pharmacist-provided patient care, whether in the context of collaborative agreements with physicians or independent of such agreements. Pharmacists are responsible for establishing relationships with patients and providers who will facilitate the coordination and continuity of care, improve access to care, and improve patient outcomes.

Providing Comprehensive Patient Care. The addition of clinical pharmacy services to healthcare teams has produced significant cost savings to the healthcare system and improved patient satisfaction, medication safety, and therapy outcomes.[4] Clinical pharmacy services are designed to improve patients' access to care, provide disease management, and focus on quality-related outcomes.

Recommendation B9 from the ASHP Pharmacy Practice Model Initiative specifically states that "for hospitals and health systems that provide ambulatory care services, drug-therapy management should be available from a pharmacist for each outpatient."[6] Furthermore, many of the PPMI recommendations support the comprehensive care of patients by pharmacists practicing in ambulatory care settings through transitions of care; quality, safety, and financial outcomes; and facilitating continuity of care and medication reconciliation.

Interprofessional care models are accepted and promoted by the medical community. The American College of Physicians and the American Society of Internal Medicine have stated that "collaborative drug therapy is one of the best examples of how pharmacists work with physicians. It is designed to maximize the patient's health-related quality of life, reduce the frequency of avoidable drug-related problems, and improve the societal benefits of pharmaceuticals."[41] In addition, governmental agencies support the work of pharmacists in the provision of direct patient care. The Medicare Modernization Act of 2003[42] mandated that MTM services be offered by prescription drug plans to Medicare beneficiaries at high risk for ADEs.[43] While neither the legislation nor the final CMS regulation provided guidance on the design or reimbursement structure for MTM services, CMS stated that these programs should be "patient-focused services aimed at improving therapeutic outcomes that are developed in conjunction with practicing pharmacists."[42] The Centers for Disease Control and Prevention endorsed pharmacists as integral members of the interprofessional healthcare team and supports the pharmacist's role in providing MTM services to improve patient outcomes.[44] The strongest statement about pharmacist-delivered direct patient care to date was presented in a report to the U.S. Surgeon General.[4] This report described how innovative models of care that include pharmacists as members of the healthcare team can help to improve safety, access, quality, and cost while improving outcomes. Lastly, as the Patient Protection and Affordable Care Act is fully implemented, the involvement of pharmacists practicing in ambulatory care settings will be critical in the establishment of accountable care organizations. These integrated systems of care will heavily rely on the expertise of pharmacists to support safe and appropriate medication use.

Patient Care and Disease State Management Services. The purpose of a direct patient care or disease state management service is to optimize therapeutic outcomes for patients. Such services may include elements designed to promote enhanced patient understanding, increase patient adherence, and detect ADEs. Possible services may include performing a comprehensive medication review (comprehensive or targeted) to identify, resolve, and prevent medication-related problems (including ADEs); performing patient health status assessments; formulating medication treatment plans; selecting, initiating, modifying, discontinuing, or administering medication therapy; managing high-cost and specialty medications; administering antibiotic stewardship programs; evaluating and monitoring patient response to drug therapy; documenting the care delivered for and communicating essential information to the patient's other primary care providers; providing education and training designed to enhance patient understanding and appropriate use of his or her medications; providing information, support services, and resources designed to enhance patient adherence with his or her therapeutic regimens; coordinating and integrating MTM services within the broader healthcare management services being provided to the patient; and selecting, initiating, modifying, discontinuing, or administering medication therapy under state-approved CDTM agreements.

Relationships with Patients. Successful disease state and medication management begins with the relationship between the patient and the pharmacist. Pharmacists practicing in ambulatory care settings who provide direct patient care should develop and maintain a rapport with and the trust of the patient and the caregiver. The pharmacist should coordinate all aspects of the individual's pharmacist-provided patient care, serve as a patient advocate, and encourage patients to take responsibility for their health. The pharmacist should be flexible and adapt to patient-specific variables such as the patient's perception of how an illness or symptoms affect his or her life and the patient's readiness for change.

Relationships with Providers: CDTM Agreements. Almost every state has amended its pharmacy practice act to allow for the expansion of pharmacists' scope of practice. Pharmacists should actively participate in medication therapy decision-making and management through collaboration with patients, caregivers, physicians, and other healthcare providers. By participating in CDTM, the pharmacist takes an active role in the initiation, management, and monitoring of medication therapy based on pharmacokinetic parameters, genetic characteristics of the patient, serum concentrations of medications, laboratory values, and other patient-related health and social factors in order to take responsibility and have authority for achieving desired therapeutic outcomes. PPMI recommendation B14 states that, when possible through credentialing and privileging processes, pharmacists should include in their scope of practice prescribing as part of the collaborative practice team.[6] A collaborative care agreement between the pharmacist and physician or other healthcare provider must comply with applicable laws and regulations and the organization's policies and procedures.

Patient History and Medication Reconciliation. Upon patient presentation for ambulatory care services, a pharmacist should obtain a patient and medication history and update and validate the patient's current medication list. Pharmacists should be integral in identifying, developing, reviewing, and approving new medications by conducting a patient-specific medication review before first-dose administration and evaluating patient response to therapy. The history should include pertinent demographic information; known health problems and diseases; applicable measurements and laboratory values; known drug allergies and ADEs; behavioral, lifestyle, and socioeconomic influences on healthcare; and a comprehensive list of prescription and nonprescription medications and related medical devices currently being used. The current medication list should be maintained and updated during subsequent patient encounters in both the inpatient and ambulatory care settings.

Pharmacists should routinely contribute to processes that ensure that each patient's care is maintained, regardless of transitions across the continuum of care and practice settings (e.g., between inpatient and community pharmacies or home care services). Moreover, pharmacists are uniquely positioned to aid in establishing a patient medication complexity index, which includes severity of illness, number of medications, and comorbidities.

Medication Therapy Assessment. Pharmacists practicing in ambulatory care settings must ensure safe and effective medication therapy. The assessment should include the appropriateness of the prescribed medication for the patient's diagnosis and history, identification of medication-related problems, and interventions for resolution. In addition, the assessment should produce a plan for monitoring patient adherence, therapeutic and adverse effects, and patient outcomes.

Medication Therapy Monitoring. The pharmacist should monitor patients' understanding of and adherence to the medication therapy plan as well as its effects and outcomes. During subsequent encounters, pharmacists should obtain appropriate information from patients, assess their progress, and identify and resolve problems. All interventions and assessments of the care plan should be documented and made available to all providers participating in the patient's care.

Documentation of Care Plan and Coordination of Care. Pharmacists should maintain a comprehensive care plan, preferably as a component of an interprofessional CDTM agreement. The care plan should be documented in the patient's medical record and be accessible to other healthcare professionals involved in patient care. The pharmacist is responsible for communicating the plan to the patient and other healthcare providers. The care plan should document the patient's medical and medication history, medication therapy assessment, and medication therapy regimen, including drug name, strength, and route of administration, indication for therapy, goal of therapy, monitoring parameters, and proposed length of therapy.

Pharmacist Skills and Competency. Pharmacists participating in direct patient care activities should demonstrate competency in the areas of care provided. Postdoctoral residency training, board certification, and continuing-education certification programs should be completed by all pharmacists and documented in a retrievable format. PPMI recommendation B10 states that pharmacists who provide drug therapy management should be certified through the most appropriate Board of Pharmacy Specialties certification process.[6] Examples of minimum requirements include demonstration of proficient communication skills, basic physical assessment, laboratory interpretation, and disease- and age-specific competencies. Minimum requirements for level of education, experience, or postgraduate training may be established for specific responsibilities or positions. Pharmacists in frontline practice should not be limited to competency in drug distribution and reactive order processing, and pharmacists engaged specifically in drug therapy management must have an understanding of and responsibility for the medication-use and delivery systems. Individual pharmacists must maintain competence in and accept responsibility for both the clinical and distributive activities of the pharmacy department. A model for ongoing evaluation, which may include peer review, should be developed to ensure that pharmacists remain competent.

Outcomes. Outcome measurements used to quantify the impact of the interventions of pharmacists practicing in ambulatory care settings can be divided into three categories: clinical, economic, and humanistic. Clinical outcomes may include rates of medication adherence, ADEs, and achievement and maintenance of evidence-based therapeutic goals. Examples of economic outcomes include hospitalization rates, emergency room visits, census growth, and revenue generation. Humanistic outcomes may include provider satisfaction, patient satisfaction, and measurements of impact on patient quality of life and personal productivity.

Patient Confidentiality. Policies and procedures for access to and dissemination of confidential patient information must meet all applicable legal and regulatory requirements, including those of the Health Insurance Portability and Accountability Act,[45] and be made readily available.

Standard V. Preparing, Packaging, and Labeling Medications

A. Preparing Medications

Preparation. The pharmacist should prepare or supervise the preparation of, in a timely and accurate manner, drug formulations, strengths, dosage forms, and packages prescribed.

Extemporaneous Compounding. Drug formulations, dosage forms, strengths, and packaging that are not available commercially but are deemed necessary for patient care should be prepared by appropriately trained personnel in accordance with applicable standards and regulations (e.g., FDA, United States Pharmacopeia [USP], state boards of pharmacy). Adequate quality-control and quality-assurance procedures should exist for these operations. Written master formulas and batch records (including product test results, as appropriate) shall be maintained, and a lot number or other method to identify each finished product with its production and control history shall be assigned to each batch. Commercially available products should be used to the maximum extent possible.[14,15,17,18,46–48]

Compounded Sterile Preparations. Sterile compounding is regulated by various state and federal agencies and shall meet all applicable laws and regulations. When possible, manufactured sterile preparations should be preferred to compounding in the pharmacy. Whenever compounded sterile preparations are prepared, properly-trained staff shall use appropriate techniques to avoid contamination and assure quality; this includes but is not limited to the following: (1) using aseptic technique; (2) maintaining clean, uncluttered, and functionally separate areas for product preparation to minimize the possibility of contamination; (3) using a primary engineering control that provides an International Organization for Standardization class 5 environment while preparing any intravenous admixture, any sterile preparation made from nonsterile ingredients, or any sterile preparation that will not be used within 1 hour; and (4) visually inspecting the integrity of the medications. *USP* Chapter 797[18] and the ASHP Guidelines on Quality Assurance for Pharmacy-Prepared Sterile Products[14] further define the compounding of sterile preparations and should be consulted by those responsible for this area of practice.

All sterile medications for use in the ambulatory care facility or for use by patients in the home should be prepared in a suitable environment by appropriately trained personnel and labeled appropriately for the user. Quality-control and quality-assurance procedures for the preparation of sterile products should exist, including annual competency assessment of the preparer's aseptic technique. For additional guidance regarding therapy in the patient home, refer to ASHP Guidelines on Home Infusion Pharmacy Services.[49]

Hazardous Drug Products. All hazardous drug products for use in the ambulatory care facility or for use by patients in the home should be prepared in a suitable environment by appropriately trained personnel and labeled appropriately for the user.[16] Special precautions, equipment, supplies (spill and eyewash kits), and training for storage, handling, and disposal of hazardous drug products should be in place to ensure the safety of personnel, patients, visitors, the community, and the environment. Quality-control and quality-assurance procedures for the preparation of hazardous products should be in place. Institutional policy should address the risk to personnel handling hazardous drug products, including periodic monitoring of personnel for adverse effects.[16]

B. Packaging and Labeling Medications

Packaging. Medications dispensed to ambulatory care patients should be packaged and labeled in compliance with applicable federal and state laws and regulations and with USP and other standards. When feasible, dispensing in unopened manufacturers' containers and in tamper-evident packaging is desirable. Packaging materials should be selected that preserve the integrity, cleanliness, and potency of compounded and commercially available drug products. Containers, including unit dose packages, for patients' home use shall comply with the Poison Prevention Packaging Act.[50]

Labeling. At a minimum, labels for patient home use of medications shall comply with applicable federal and state laws and regulations. Generally, labels contain the name, address, and telephone number of the pharmacy; date of dispensing; serial number of the prescription; patient's full name; name, strength, and dosage form of the medication; directions to the patient for use of the medication; name of the prescriber; precautionary information; authorized refills; and initials (or name) of the responsible pharmacist. Other information may be required by individual state laws and regulations.

Standard VI. Medication Delivery

A. Dispensing Medications

Prescribing. Policies and procedures should be available to ensure that healthcare providers have applicable state and federal licensure and, if required, organizational authorization for prescribing medications. Medications should be administered and dispensed to ambulatory care patients only after receiving the spoken, written, faxed, or electronic prescription of an authorized prescriber. Spoken orders should be limited to nonroutine and emergency situations and should be strongly discouraged for drug products and regimens prone to medication errors and other ADEs. A pharmacist should, as soon as possible, reduce spoken orders to writing and verify them using the Joint Commission read-back procedure.

Pharmacists practicing in ambulatory care settings should advocate and foster healthcare provider conformance with the formulary, clinical care plans, disease state management programs, and standardized Joint Commission–approved terminology and abbreviations. Pharmacists practicing in ambulatory care settings should advocate the development and use of electronic prescribing systems (direct order entry by the prescriber).

Therapeutic Purpose. Before dispensing any medication, the pharmacist should substantiate the indication for which the medication was prescribed. Prescribers should be encouraged to routinely communicate the condition being treated or the therapeutic purpose with all medication orders.

Medication Orders. Medication orders (or prescriptions) shall contain at a minimum the following information: patient name and address; medication name, dose, frequency, route, and quantity or duration; prescriber name, address, and telephone number; and prescriber DEA number for controlled substances. All medication orders shall be reviewed for legality and clinical appropriateness by a pharmacist before being dispensed. Any questions should be resolved with the prescriber, and any approved changes to the prescription shall be documented in a written notation on the face of the prescription. Information concerning changes should be appropriately communicated to the patient, caregiver, and other involved healthcare providers.

Drug Delivery Systems and Administration Devices. Pharmacists should provide leadership and advice in organizational and clinical decision-making regarding drug delivery systems and administration devices and should participate in the evaluation, use, and monitoring of these systems and devices. The potential for medication errors associated with such systems and devices should be thoroughly evaluated. Follow-up and education of staff should occur after systems errors are discovered to prevent future systems errors.

Mail Distribution. The pharmacy may mail medications to patients, preferably as part of a comprehensive pharmaceutical care program that gives patients access to a pharmacist. Mailed medications shall conform to all federal and state laws and regulations. Outer mailing packages and medication containers should protect the medication from heat, humidity, and other environmental conditions that can affect stability.[51] A toll-free telephone service that is answered during normal business hours should be provided to enable communication between a patient or the patient's physician and a pharmacist with access to the patient's records. The pharmacy should have procedures for investigating, replacing, and reporting, as required, medications lost during delivery. Special requirements for mailing controlled substances vary according to state laws and regulations.

Standard VII. Evaluating the Effectiveness of the Medication-Use System

A. Assessing Pharmacy Services and Practices

Documentation and Measurement of Patient Care, Interventions, and Outcomes. An ongoing process should be in place for consistent documentation and measurement (and reporting to medical staff, administrators, and others) of pharmacist interventions, patient outcomes from MTM (including patient satisfaction with the care provided and quality of life), and pharmacists' contributions to patient care.[52] Documenting pharmacy plans and recommendations in the patient's medical record is important for providing continuity of care between healthcare providers, communicating care plans, and underscoring the professional and legal responsibility a pharmacist assumes when making patient-specific recommendations and modifications in medication regimens. Participating in this program is an essential part of the role of every pharmacist practicing in ambulatory care settings. An electronic medical record should be used for documentation and measurement whenever possible, and the record should be designed to align pharmacists' documentation outlining care provided as well as a method to trace and ensure the quality of care provided with signed recommendations and follow-up notes in the patient's medical record.

Performance Improvement. The ambulatory care pharmacy service should have an ongoing, systematic program for assessing pharmacist-provided patient care.[53] Performance improvement activities based on assessments should be integrated with the health system's overall performance improvement activities, as applicable. The performance improvement team should work with frontline staff to implement systems that include proper checks and balances focused on protecting against human error. Performance improvement initiatives should be focused on error reporting trends and high-risk functions such as dispensing high-alert medications.

As part of the performance improvement program, operational and outcomes data should be benchmarked with those of other ambulatory care pharmacy services of similar size and scope. The results, including follow-up actions for improvement, should be documented and provided to the organization's managers, the frontline staff using the system, and others as appropriate.

B. Improving the Medication-Use Process

Medication-Use Evaluation. An ongoing program of both prospective and retrospective monitoring of drug utilization and costs should be in place to ensure that medications are used appropriately, safely, and effectively and to increase the probability of desired outcomes within defined populations of patients. Proactive and continuous quality-improvement strategies aid in risk mitigation of medication-use systems. Pharmacists practicing in ambulatory care settings should play an integral role in this program. The medication-use policy committee should define specific variables for evaluation (disease state, pharmacologic category, high-use/high-cost drug products, high-alert medications, high-risk therapies, problem-prone regimens) as appropriate for the organization. Through this ongoing evaluation, areas in need of improvement in medication prescribing and management can be identified and targeted for intervention.

Medication Safety. Ambulatory care pharmacy services should be part of the health system's program for preventing medication errors and ADEs. The health system's medication safety team should be a cross-functional group of employees (e.g., pharmacists, physicians, nurses) and patients, when applicable. Pharmacists who practice in ambulatory care settings are an essential part of this medication safety team. The medication safety program should foster a just culture for error reporting. The medication safety team should

- Use a systems-based approach to review errors.
- Review near-miss medication errors (i.e., errors that did not cause patient harm but, if repeated, could cause patient harm).
- Analyze the root cause of medication errors.
- Work with frontline staff to implement systems that include proper checks and balances focused on protecting against human error and mitigating risk.

The occurrence of medication errors should be reported to voluntary national reporting systems (e.g., USP Medication Errors Reporting Program, ISMP, and FDA MedWatch) to help prevent similar errors from occurring in other practice settings. Serious medication errors that result in temporary or permanent harm, disability, or death should be reported to the appropriate regulatory agency or accrediting body.

Patient Safety. Ambulatory care pharmacy services should be part of a health system's program to encourage patients' participation in and accountability for their care. Patient education should be sensitive to the individual patient's health literacy. To maximize the benefits of medication therapy and reduce the potential for errors, the program should encourage patients to ask questions about their medications and should emphasize adherence to their therapy plan. Pharmacist–patient dialogue, pamphlets, and videos should be used to teach patients how to ask questions about their medications. This process is particularly important for recently discharged patients.

Antimicrobial Stewardship and Infection Prevention and Control. There shall be policies and procedures to promote the optimal use of antimicrobial agents, reduce the transmission of infections, and educate health professionals, patients, and the public about these topics. Pharmacists should participate in antimicrobial stewardship and infection prevention and control efforts through clinical endeavors focused on proper antimicrobial utilization and membership on relevant interprofessional work groups and committees within the health system.

Pharmacists should monitor patients' laboratory reports of microbial sensitivities or applicable diagnostic markers and advise prescribers if microbial resistance is suspected, evaluate trends in microbial prescribing relative to changes in microbial resistance patterns, and assist in developing prescribing patterns to help minimize the development of drug resistance.[54]

Integration of Population-Based and Patient-Specific Activities. A mechanism should be in place for ensuring that the clinical and economic findings of population-based activities are appropriately incorporated into daily patient-specific practice. Population-based activities provide insight and guidance for the treatment of the average patient; however, all variables identified in the patient-specific encounter should be considered in therapeutic decision-making for individual patients.[55]

Standard VIII. Research

The pharmacist should initiate, participate in, and support clinical and practice-related research appropriate to the goals, objectives, and resources of the specific health system.

Policies and Procedures. The pharmacist shall ensure that policies and procedures for the safe and proper use of investigational drugs and medication-related devices are established and followed and that these policies and procedures meet all applicable laws and regulations. There shall be a procedure to ensure that informed consent is obtained from the patient before the first dose of the study drug is administered.[56,57]

Procurement, Distribution, and Control of Investigational Drugs. The pharmacy shall be responsible for overseeing the procurement, distribution, and control of all investigational drugs. Investigational drugs shall be approved for use by an institutional review board and shall be dispensed and administered to consenting patients according to an approved protocol.[38,56,57]

Institutional Review Board. A pharmacist shall be a member of the hospital's institutional review board (or equivalent body), if one exists.[56]

Drugs Not Approved by FDA. The pharmacy should seek and obtain documented authorization from appropriate committees (e.g., pharmacy and therapeutics committee) for the pharmacologic use of any chemical substance that has not received FDA approval for use as a drug. Documentation should exist to ensure that appropriate risk-management measures (e.g., obtaining informed consent) have been taken.

Information Regarding Investigational Drugs. The pharmacy shall have access to information on all investigational studies and similar research projects involving medications and medication-related devices used in the hospital. The pharmacy shall provide pertinent written information (to the extent known) about the safe and proper use of investigational drugs, including possible adverse effects and adverse drug reactions, to nurses, pharmacists, physicians, and other healthcare professionals called on to prescribe, dispense, and administer these medications.[56,57]

References

1. Johnson JA, Bootman JL. Drug-related morbidity and mortality, a cost-of-illness model. *Arch Intern Med.* 1995; 155:1949–56.
2. Lewis RK, Carter BL, Glover DG, et al. Comprehensive services in an ambulatory care pharmacy. *Am J Health-Syst Pharm.* 1995; 52:1793–7.
3. Segarra-Newnham M, Soisson KT. Provision of pharmaceutical care through comprehensive pharmacotherapy clinics. *Hosp Pharm.* 1997; 32:845–50.
4. Giberson S, Yoder S, Lee MP. Improving patient and health system outcomes through advanced pharmacy practice. A report to the U.S. Surgeon General (December 2011). www.usphs.gov/corpslinks/pharmacy/documents/2011AdvancedPharmacyPracticeReporttotheUSSG.pdf (accessed 2013 Mar 18).
5. American Society of Health-System Pharmacists. ASHP/ASHP Foundation Ambulatory Conference and Summit: consensus recommendations (March 4, 2014). www.ashpmedia.org/amcare14/docs/preliminary_recommendations_2014-03-04.pdf (accessed 2014 Jul 8).
6. The consensus of the Pharmacy Practice Model Summit. *Am J Health-Syst Pharm.* 2011; 68:1148–52.
7. American Society of Health-System Pharmacists. ASHP statement on the role of health-system pharmacists in emergency preparedness. *Am J Health-Syst Pharm.* 2003; 60:1993–5.
8. American Society of Health-System Pharmacists. ASHP guidelines on the pharmacist's role in immunization. *Am J Health-Syst Pharm.* 2003; 60:1371–7.
9. American Society of Health-System Pharmacists. ASHP statement on the pharmacist's role in substance abuse prevention, education, and assistance (2013). www.ashp.org/DocLibrary/BestPractices/SpecificStSubstance.aspx (accessed 2013 Jul 29).
10. Crane VS, Hatwig CA, Hayman JN, et al. Developing a management planning and control system for ambulatory pharmacy resources. *Pharm Pract Manag Q.* 1998; 18:52–71.
11. Rosum RW. Planning for an ambulatory care service. *Am J Health-Syst Pharm.* 1997; 54:1584–7.
12. American Society of Hospital Pharmacists. ASHP statement on continuing education. *Am J Hosp Pharm.* 1990; 47:1855.
13. American Society of Health-System Pharmacists. ASHP guidelines on the recruitment, selection, and retention of pharmacy personnel. *Am J Health-Syst Pharm.* 2003; 60:587–93.
14. American Society of Health-System Pharmacists. ASHP guidelines on quality assurance for pharmacy-prepared sterile products. *Am J Health-Syst Pharm.* 2000; 57:1150–69.
15. American Society of Hospital Pharmacists. ASHP technical assistance bulletin on compounding nonsterile products in pharmacies. *Am J Hosp Pharm.* 1994; 51:1441–8.
16. American Society of Health-System Pharmacists. ASHP guidelines on handling hazardous drugs. *Am J Health-Syst Pharm.* 2006; 63:1172–93.
17. American Society of Hospital Pharmacists. ASHP guidelines for repackaging oral solids and liquids in single unit and unit dose packages. *Am J Hosp Pharm.* 1983; 40:451–2.
18. Pharmaceutical compounding—sterile preparations (general information chapter 797). In: The United States pharmacopeia, 34th rev., and The national formulary, 29th ed. Rockville, MD: United States Pharmacopeial Convention; 2011: 336–73.

19. Pharmaceutical compounding—nonsterile preparations (general information chapter 795. In: The United States pharmacopeia, 34th rev., and The national formulary, 29th ed. Rockville, MD: United States Pharmacopeial Convention; 2011:330–6.
20. American Society of Health-System Pharmacists. ASHP guidelines on pharmacist-conducted patient education and counseling. *Am J Health-Syst Pharm.* 1997; 54:431–4.
21. American Society of Health-System Pharmacists. ASHP guidelines on the safe use of automated dispensing devices. *Am J Health-Syst Pharm.* 2010; 67:483–90.
22. Glover DG. Automated medication dispensing devices. *J Am Pharm Assoc.* 1997; NS37:353–60.
23. Kernodle SJ. Improving health care with clinical practice guidelines and critical pathways: implications for pharmacists in ambulatory practice. *Pharm Pract Manag Q.* 1997; 17:76–89.
24. LaCalamita S. Role of the pharmacist in developing critical pathways with warfarin therapy. *J Pharm Pract.* 1997; 10:398–410.
25. Curtiss FR. Lessons learned from projects in disease management in ambulatory care. *Am J Health-Syst Pharm.* 1997; 54:2217–29.
26. American Society of Health-System Pharmacists. ASHP statement on the pharmacist's responsibility for distribution and control of drug products. In: Hawkins BH, ed. Best practices for hospital and health-system pharmacy, 2013–2014 edition. Bethesda, MD: American Society of Health-System Pharmacists; 2013:125.
27. American Society of Hospital Pharmacists. ASHP guidelines for selecting pharmaceutical manufacturers and suppliers. *Am J Hosp Pharm.* 1991; 48:523–4.
28. American Society of Health-System Pharmacists. ASHP guidelines on medication cost management strategies for hospitals and health systems. *Am J Health-Syst Pharm.* 2008; 65:1368–84.
29. American Society of Hospital Pharmacists. ASHP guidelines for pharmacists on the activities of vendors' representatives in organized health care systems. *Am J Hosp Pharm.* 1994; 51:520–1.
30. American Society of Hospital Pharmacists. ASHP guidelines on pharmacists' relationships with industry. *Am J Hosp Pharm.* 1992; 49:154.
31. PhRMA code on interactions with healthcare professionals. Washington, DC: Pharmaceutical Research and Manufacturers of America; 2004 Jan.
32. American Society of Hospital Pharmacists. ASHP guidelines on hospital drug and distribution control. *Am J Hosp Pharm.* 1980; 37:1097–103.
33. American Society of Health-System Pharmacists. ASHP Drug Shortages Resource Center. www.ashp.org/shortages (accessed 2013 Jul 17).
34. Food and Drug Administration. Drug shortages. www.fda.gov/cder/drug/shortages (accessed 2013 Apr 3).
35. American Society of Health-System Pharmacists. ASHP guidelines on managing drug product shortages in hospitals and health systems. *Am J Health-Syst Pharm.* 2009; 66:1399–406.
36. American Society of Health-System Pharmacists. ASHP guidelines on the pharmacy and therapeutics committee and the formulary system. *Am J Health-Syst Pharm.* 2008; 65:1272–83.
37. American Society of Hospital Pharmacists. ASHP statement on pharmaceutical care. *Am J Hosp Pharm.* 1993; 50:1720–3.
38. Lewis RK, Lasack NL, Lambert BL, et al. Patient counseling—a focus on maintenance therapy. *Am J Health-Syst Pharm.* 1997; 54:2084–98.
39. Hepler CD, Strand LM. Opportunities and responsibilities in pharmaceutical care. *Am J Hosp Pharm.* 1990; 47:533–43.
40. Brennan C, Goode JV, Haines ST, et al. A petition to the Board of Pharmaceutical Specialties requesting recognition of ambulatory care pharmacy practice as a specialty (November 2008). www.accp.com/docs/positions/petitions/BPS_Ambulatory_Care_Petition.pdf (accessed 2015 Mar 19).
41. Keely JL, for the American College of Physicians–American Society of Internal Medicine. Pharmacist scope of practice. *Ann Intern Med.* 2002; 136:79–85.
42. Medicare Prescription Drug, Modernization, and Improvement Act of 2003, Pub. L. No. 108–173 (2003).
43. Academy of Managed Care Pharmacy. Sound medication therapy management programs: 2006 consensus document. www.pharmacist.com/sites/default/files/files/mtm_sound_programs_2006.pdf (accessed 2013 Jul 17).
44. Centers for Disease Control and Prevention. A program guide for public health: partnering with pharmacists in the prevention and control of chronic diseases. www.cdc.gov/dhdsp/programs/spha/docs/pharmacist_guide.pdf (accessed 2015 Mar 19).
45. Health Insurance Portability and Accountability Act of 1996. Pub. L. No. 104-191. www.cms.hhs.gov/HIPAAGenInfo/Downloads/HIPAALaw.pdf (accessed 2013 Jul 17).
46. American Society of Health-System Pharmacists. ASHP guidelines: minimum standard for pharmacies in hospitals (2012). www.ashp.org/DocLibrary/Best-Practices/SettingsGdlMinHosp.aspx (accessed 2013 Jul 17).
47. American Society of Hospital Pharmacists. ASHP technical assistance bulletin on single unit and unit dose packages of drugs. *Am J Hosp Pharm.* 1985; 42:378–9.
48. Pharmaceutical compounding—nonsterile preparations (general information chapter 795). In: The United States pharmacopeia, 35th rev., and The national formulary, 30th ed. Rockville, MD: United States Pharmacopeial Convention; 2011:344–50.
49. American Society of Health-System Pharmacists. ASHP guidelines on home infusion pharmacy services. *Am J Health-Syst Pharm.* 2014; 71:325–41.
50. Poison Prevention Packaging Act, 15 U.S.C. 1471–6.
51. General notices and requirements—preservation, packaging, storage, and labeling. In: The United States pharmacopeia, 30th rev., and The national formulary, 25th ed. Rockville, MD: United States Pharmacopeial Convention; 2007:9–12.

52. Borgsdorf LR, Mian JS, Knapp KK. Pharmacist-managed medication review in a managed care system. *Am J Hosp Pharm.* 1994; 51:772–7.
53. MacKinnon N. Performance measures in ambulatory pharmacy. *Pharm Pract Manage Q.* 1997; 17:52–62.
54. American Society of Health-System Pharmacists. ASHP statement on the pharmacist's role in antimicrobial stewardship and infection prevention and control. *Am J Health-Syst Pharm.* 2010; 67:575–7.
55. Mutnick AH, Sterba KJ, Szymusiak-Mutnick BA. Integration of quality assessment and a patient-specific intervention/outcomes program. *Pharm Pract Manage Q.* 1998; 17:25–36.
56. American Society of Health-System Pharmacists. ASHP guidelines on clinical drug research. *Am J Health-Syst Pharm.* 1998; 55:369–75.
57. American Society of Hospital Pharmacists. ASHP guidelines for pharmaceutical research in organized health-care settings. *Am J Hosp Pharm.* 1989; 46:129–30.

Developed through the ASHP Section of Ambulatory Care Practitioners and approved by the ASHP Board of Directors on September 19, 2014. These guidelines supersede the ASHP Guidelines: Minimum Standard for Pharmaceutical Services in Ambulatory Care dated April 21, 1999.

Jennifer Askew Buxton, Pharm.D., CPP, is Deputy Director, Pharmacy Services, Cape Fear Clinic, Wilmington, NC; at the time of writing she was Manager of Outpatient/Employee Pharmacy Services, New Hanover Regional Medical Center, Wilmington. Rose-Marie Babbitt, B.S.Pharm., M.A., is Vice President, Federal Contracts and Grants, American Pharmacists Association, Washington, DC; at the time of writing she was Associate Director, Pharmacy Services, Parkland Health and Hospital System, Dallas, TX. Cyndy A. Clegg, B.S.Pharm., M.H.A., is Director, Retail and Home Care Pharmacy, Swedish Medical Center, Edmonds, WA; at the time of writing she was Assistant Director, Ambulatory Pharmacy Services, Harborview Medical Center, Seattle, WA, and Clinical Associate Professor, University of Washington School of Pharmacy, Seattle. Sandra F. Durley, Pharm.D., is Associate Director, Ambulatory Care Pharmacy Department, and Clinical Assistant Professor, University of Illinois at Chicago (UIC), Chicago. Kelly T. Epplen, Pharm.D., BCACP, FASHP, is Associate Professor of Clinical Pharmacy Practice, James L. Winkle College of Pharmacy, University of Cincinnati, Cincinnati, OH; at the time of writing she was Clinical Coordinator, Ambulatory Pharmacy Services, Health Alliance, Greater Cincinnati, Florence, KY. Laurel M. Marsden, B.S.Pharm., M.S.H.A., is Assistant Director of Pharmacy, Virginia Commonwealth University Health System, Richmond. Bridgette A. Thomas, Pharm.D., is Clinical Applications Manager, Johns Hopkins Outpatient Pharmacy, Baltimore, MD. Nathan S. Thompson, B.S.Pharm., M.B.A., is Director, Outpatient Pharmacy, Johns Hopkins Home Care Group, Baltimore.

The contributions of the Section of Ambulatory Care Practitioners Executive Committee (Seena L. Haines, Pharm.D., FASHP, FAPhA, BCACP, BC-ADM, CDE; Gloria P. Sachdev, Pharm.D.; Jennifer Askew Buxton, Pharm.D., CPP; Melanie A. Dodd, Pharm.D., Ph.C., BCPS; Sandra Leal, Pharm.D., FAPhA, CDE; Steven M. Riddle, Pharm.D., BCPS, FASHP; and Justine Coffey, J.D., LL.M.) to this document are gratefully acknowledged.

The following organizations and individuals are acknowledged for reviewing draft versions of these Guidelines (review does not imply endorsement): Academy of Managed Care Pharmacy (AMCP); American Association of Critical-Care Nurses (AACN); American College of Clinical Pharmacy (ACCP); American Geriatric Society; Joint Commission; Cindi Brennan, Pharm.D., M.H.A.; Mark N. Brueckl, M.B.A. (AMCP); Anne Burns, Pharm.D.; Frank P. Castronovo, Jr., Ph.D.; Sharon Connor, Pharm.D.; Paul F. Davis, B.S.Pharm.; Ernest Dole, Pharm.D., FASHP; Melanie A. Dodd, Pharm.D., Ph.C., BCPS; Scott R. Drab, Pharm.D., CDE, BC-ADM; Sarah K. Ford, Pharm.D., BCPS, CPP; Seena L. Haines, Pharm.D., FASHP, FAPhA, BCACP, BC-ADM, CDE; Deanne L. Hall, Pharm.D., CDE; Philip E. Johnson, M.S., FASHP; Tom Kaye, M.B.A., FASHP; Sandra Leal, Pharm.D., FAPhA, CDE; Jeff Little, Pharm.D., M.P.H., BCPS; Jimmy R. Mitchell, M.S., M.P.H.; Bruce A. Nelson, M.S.; Colleen O'Malley, M.S., B.S.Pharm.; James A. Ponto, M.S., BCNP; Matt Ransom, Pharm.D., BCACP; Steven M. Riddle, Pharm.D., BCPS, FASHP; Christine Ruby, Pharm.D., BCPS; Gloria P. Sachdev, Pharm.D.; Paul M. Schyve, M.D. (Joint Commission); Pamela Shellner, B.S.N., M.A., RN (AACN); Melissa Somma-McGivney, Pharm.D., CDE; Richard L. Stambaugh, M.S., Pharm.D., BCPS; Marc H. Stranz, Pharm.D.; Megan Wagner, Pharm.D.; C. Edwin Webb, Pharm.D., M.P.H. (ACCP); and Jody Jacobson Wedret, B.S.Pharm., FASHP, FCSHP.

Copyright © 2015, American Society of Health-System Pharmacists, Inc. All rights reserved. Contact ASHP for reprint and permissions requests. This content may not be used for commercial purposes without the express written consent of ASHP.

The bibliographic citation for this document is as follows: American Society of Health-System Pharmacists. ASHP Guidelines: minimum standard for ambulatory care pharmacy practice. *Am J Health-Syst Pharm.* 2015; 72:1221–36.

ASHP Guidelines: Minimum Standard for Pharmacies in Hospitals

Purpose

The following minimum standard guidelines are intended to serve as a basic guide for the provision of pharmacy services in hospitals. These guidelines outline a minimum level of services that most hospital pharmacy departments should consistently provide. The reader is strongly encouraged to review the American Society of Health-System Pharmacy (ASHP) guidance documents referenced throughout these guidelines for more detailed descriptions. Certain elements of these guidelines may be applicable to other health care settings or may be useful in evaluating the scope and quality of pharmacy services.

Elements of Care

The mission of pharmacists is to help people make the best use of medications.[1] Therefore, pharmacists shall be concerned with not only the provision but the outcomes of pharmacy services. The elements of pharmacy services that are critical to safe, effective, and cost-conscious medication use in a hospital include (1) practice management, (2) medication-use policy development, (3) optimizing medication therapy, (4) drug product procurement and inventory management, (5) preparing, packaging, and labeling medications, (6) medication delivery, (7) monitoring medication use, (8) evaluating the effectiveness of the medication-use system, and (9) research. Although the scope of pharmacy services will vary from site to site, depending upon the needs of patients and the hospital as well as the resources available, these core elements are inextricably linked to successful outcomes. Failure to provide any of these services may compromise the quality of patient care.

Terminology

In these guidelines, the term "shall" is used to indicate a minimum standard of practice set forth in this document, in other ASHP policies, or in requirements established by laws, regulations, accrediting bodies, or other binding authorities. The term "should" is used to indicate a best practice that is strongly encouraged by ASHP but which may not be applicable to all institutions or in all circumstances.

Standard I. Practice Management

Effective leadership and practice management skills are necessary for the delivery of pharmacy services in a manner consistent with the hospital's and patients' needs. Such leadership should foster continuous improvement in patient care outcomes. The management of pharmacy services should focus on the pharmacist's responsibilities as a patient care provider and leader of the pharmacy enterprise through the development of organizational structures that support that mission. Development of such structures will require communication and collaboration with other departments and services throughout the hospital, which every member of the pharmacy team should cultivate at every opportunity.

A. Pharmacy and Pharmacist Services

Pharmacy Mission, Goals, and Scope of Services. The pharmacy shall have a written mission statement that reflects both patient care and operational responsibilities. Other aspects of the pharmacy's mission may require definition as well (e.g., educational and research responsibilities). The mission statement shall be consistent with the mission of the hospital and, if applicable, aligned with the health system of which the hospital is a component. The development, prioritization, and implementation of the pharmacy's goals should be consistent with the mission statement. Determination of short- and long-term goals and the undertaking of implementation activities should be performed in collaboration with institutional leadership and other hospital staff (e.g., pharmacy, nursing, and medical staff), and these should be integrated with the goals of the hospital. The mission statement may also incorporate consensus-based national goals, such as those expressed in the recommendations from the ASHP Pharmacy Practice Model Initiative.[2]

The pharmacy shall also maintain a written document describing the scope of pharmacy services. These services should be consistent with the hospital's scope of services and should be applied throughout the hospital in all practice sites.

The mission, goals, and scope of services shall be clearly communicated to everyone involved in the provision of pharmacy services, including pharmacists, residents, students, technicians, and support staff.

24-Hour Pharmacy Services. Adequate hours of operation for the provision of needed pharmacy services shall be maintained; 24-hour pharmacy services should be provided when possible. Twenty-four hour pharmacy services should be employed in all hospitals with clinical programs that require intensive medication therapy (e.g., transplant programs, open-heart surgery programs, neonatal intensive care units, and trauma centers). When 24-hour pharmacy services are not feasible, a pharmacist shall be available on an on-call basis. Remote medication order processing may be employed (to the extent permitted by law and regulation) to help provide pharmacy services but is not a substitute for an on-call pharmacist.[3] Automated drug dispensing equipment and computer databases are also not a substitute for the skills and knowledge of a pharmacist and should not be considered alternatives to 24-hour pharmacy services.[4]

After-Hours Pharmacy Access. In the absence of 24-hour pharmacy services, access to a limited supply of medications shall only be available to authorized, licensed health care professionals for use in carrying out urgent medication orders. Access to such medications shall be carefully monitored and documented, and after-hours access shall be reviewed regularly to ensure appropriate use. The list of medications to be accessible and the policies and procedures to be used (including subsequent review of all activity by a pharmacist)

DOI 10.37573/9781585287048.101

shall be developed by a multidisciplinary committee of physicians, pharmacists, and nurses (e.g., by the pharmacy and therapeutics [P&T] committee or its equivalent).[5] Access to medications should be limited to cases in which the P&T committee (or its equivalent) determines that the urgent clinical need for the medication outweighs the potential risks of making the medication accessible. The potential safety risks of medications should be considered in the decision to make them accessible, and medications, quantities, dosage forms, and container sizes that might endanger patients should be limited whenever possible.

Routine after-hours access to the pharmacy by nonpharmacists for access to medications shall not be permitted. The use of well-designed night cabinets, after-hours medication carts, automated dispensing devices,[6] and other methods precludes the need for nonpharmacists to enter the pharmacy.[4]

Practice Standards and Guidelines. The standards and regulations of all relevant government bodies (e.g., state boards of pharmacy, departments of health) shall be met. The practice standards and guidelines of ASHP, appropriate accrediting bodies (e.g., Joint Commission, American Osteopathic Association Healthcare Facilities Accreditation Program, Det Norske Veritas), and the Centers for Medicare and Medicaid Services shall be viewed as applicable, and the hospital should strive to meet all applicable standards.

B. Laws and Regulations

Applicable local, state, and federal laws and regulations shall be met, and relevant documentation of compliance shall be maintained.

C. Policies and Procedures

Policy and Procedures Manual. There shall be a policy and procedures manual governing pharmacy functions (e.g., administrative, operational, and clinical), and all pharmacy personnel shall follow those policies and procedures. The manual may include a statement of the pharmacy's mission, philosophy, or values (e.g., the pharmacy's mission or vision statement), but it should concentrate on operational policies and procedures to guide and direct all pharmacy services. The pharmacy's policies and procedures should be consistent with the hospital's policies and procedures, and the manual should be reviewed by a designated medical staff committee for potential conflicts and other medical issues. The manual shall be reviewed by pharmacy staff on a regular basis and revised as necessary to reflect changes in procedures, organization, objectives, or practices. The manual shall be accessible to pharmacy department personnel as well as other hospital employees (e.g., through the hospital's intranet), and all pharmacy personnel should be familiar with its contents. Appropriate mechanisms to ensure compliance with the policies and procedures should be established.

Personnel Safety. Pharmacy employees should be involved in the development of the hospital's plans for emergency response, infection prevention and control, management of hazardous substances and waste, and incident reporting, and all pharmacy staff shall receive education about those plans.

Emergency Preparedness. Facility emergency preparedness plans shall describe the role of pharmacy staff in emergency response (including evacuation), and the facility's business continuity plan shall include procedures for providing safe and efficient pharmacy services in case of emergencies. Appropriately trained pharmacists should be members of emergency preparedness teams and participate in applicable preparations and drills.[7] The pharmacy shall establish, in conjunction with the hospitalwide emergency plan, policies and procedures for the safe and orderly evacuation of pharmacy personnel in the event of an emergency in the hospital.

Medical Emergencies. The pharmacy shall participate in hospital decisions about the contents of code carts, emergency medication kits and trays, and the role of pharmacists in medical emergencies. Pharmacists should serve on cardiopulmonary resuscitation teams, and such pharmacists should receive appropriate training and maintain appropriate certifications (e.g., Basic Life Support, Advanced Cardiopulmonary Life Support, Pediatric Acute Life Support).

Immunization Programs. The pharmacy shall participate in the development of hospital policies and procedures concerning preventive and postexposure immunization programs for patients and hospital employees.[8] When practical, pharmacists should participate as active immunizers for hospital and health-system-based preventive immunization programs (e.g., influenza).

Substance Abuse Programs. The pharmacy shall assist in the development of and participate in hospital substance abuse education, prevention, identification, treatment, and employee assistance programs.[9]

D. Human Resources

Position Descriptions. Areas of responsibility within the scope of pharmacy services shall be clearly defined. The responsibilities and related competencies of professional and supportive personnel shall be clearly defined in written position descriptions. These position descriptions shall be reviewed and revised as required by the hospital's policies. Position descriptions should reflect more general aspects of performance (e.g., communication, motivation, teamwork) in addition to specific responsibilities and competencies.

Director of Pharmacy. The pharmacy shall be managed by a professionally competent, legally qualified pharmacist. The director of pharmacy should be thoroughly knowledgeable about and have experience in hospital pharmacy practice and management. An advanced management degree (e.g., M.B.A., M.H.A., or M.S.) or an administrative specialty residency[10] is desirable.

The director of pharmacy shall be responsible for

- Establishing the mission, vision, goals, and scope of services of the pharmacy based on the needs of the patients served, the needs of the hospital (and any health system of which the hospital may be a component), and developments and trends in health care and hospital pharmacy practice.
- Developing, implementing, evaluating, and updating plans and activities to fulfill the mission, vision, goals, and scope of services of the pharmacy.
- Actively working with or as a part of hospital or health-system leadership to develop and implement policies and procedures that provide safe and effective medication use for the patients served by the institution.

- Mobilizing and managing the resources, both human and financial, necessary for the optimal provision of pharmacy services.
- Ensuring that patient care services provided by pharmacists and other pharmacy personnel are delivered in adherence to applicable state and federal laws and regulations, hospital privileging requirements, and national practice standards.

A part-time director of pharmacy shall have the same obligations and responsibilities as a full-time director.

Pharmacists. The pharmacy shall employ an adequate number of competent, legally qualified pharmacists to meet the specific medication-use needs of the hospital's patients. Pharmacists hired on a temporary or contract basis shall meet the same requirements as those employed by the hospital.

Support Personnel. Sufficient support personnel (e.g., pharmacy technicians and clerical or secretarial personnel) shall be employed to facilitate pharmacy services. Support positions shall have a written job description that includes a statement of the competencies required for that position. Support staff shall be properly trained and supervised, and professional development programs for them are desirable. Pharmacy technicians should have completed an ASHP-accredited pharmacy technician training program, should be certified by the Pharmacy Technician Certification Board, and shall meet the requirements of applicable laws and regulations. Pharmacy technicians working in advanced roles should have additional training and demonstrate competencies specific to the tasks to be performed.

Education and Training. All personnel shall possess the education and training required to fulfill their responsibilities and shall participate in relevant continuing-education programs and activities as necessary to maintain or enhance their competence.[11]

Recruitment, Selection, and Retention of Personnel. Personnel should be recruited and selected by the pharmacy director on the basis of job-related qualifications and prior performance. An employee retention plan is desirable.[12]

Orientation of Personnel. There shall be an established, structured procedure for orienting new personnel to the pharmacy, the hospital, and their respective positions.[9] Evaluation of the effectiveness of orientation programs should be done in conjunction with the competency assessment required before a new hire can assume full responsibility for the new position.

Work Schedules and Assignments. The director of pharmacy shall ensure that work schedules, procedures, and assignments optimize the use of personnel and resources. There shall be a written departmental staffing plan that addresses how patients' needs will be met during periods of staff shortages and fluctuation in workload and/or patient acuity. Remote medication order processing may be employed to help address staff shortages or workload fluctuations.[3]

Performance Evaluation. There shall be procedures for regularly scheduled evaluation of the performance of pharmacy personnel. The evaluation format should be consistent with that used by the hospital. The competencies of the position shall be well defined in the position description, short- and long-term goals should be established for each employee, and the employee's competency shall be assessed regularly. The pharmacy director shall ensure that an ongoing competency assessment program is in place for all staff, and each staff member should have a continuous professional development plan.

Effective Communication. There should be established methods for communicating important information to staff in a timely manner (e.g., electronic communications, staff meetings, newsletters, bulletin boards). The pharmacy should establish appropriate mechanisms to regularly assess the effectiveness of such communications.

Ethical Conduct. Standards of ethical conduct shall be established, and there shall be procedures for educating all pharmacy staff regarding these standards. The institution's conflict-of-interest and ethical conduct policies shall be clearly communicated to all staff, with appropriate staff acknowledgement of conformance with these policies.[13]

E. Facilities

Pharmacy. Adequate space, equipment, and supplies shall be available for all professional and administrative functions relating to pharmacy services. These resources shall meet all applicable laws and regulations; shall be located in areas that facilitate the provision of services to patients, nurses, prescribers, and other health care providers; and shall be integrated with the hospital's communication and delivery or transportation systems.

Medication Storage and Preparation Areas. There shall be suitable facilities to enable the receipt, storage, and preparation of medications under proper conditions of sanitation, temperature, light, moisture, ventilation, segregation, and security to ensure medication integrity and personnel safety throughout the hospital.[4]

Compounding Areas. There shall be suitable facilities to enable the compounding, preparation, and labeling of sterile and nonsterile products, including hazardous drug products, in accordance with established quality-assurance procedures. The work environment should promote orderliness and efficiency and minimize the potential for medication errors and contamination of products.[14–20]

Patient Assessment and Consultation Area. In outpatient settings, a private area for pharmacist–patient consultations shall be available to confidentially enhance patients' knowledge of and adherence to prescribed medication regimens.[21]

Office and Meeting Space. Adequate office and meeting areas shall be available for administrative, educational, and training activities.

Automated Systems. There shall be policies and procedures for the evaluation, selection, use, calibration, monitoring, and maintenance of all automated pharmacy systems. Automated mechanical systems and software can promote safe, accurate, and efficient medication ordering and preparation, drug distribution, and clinical monitoring. Use of such systems and software shall be structured so as to not hinder the pharmacist's review of (and opportunity to intervene in) medication orders before the administration of first doses. The maintenance, calibration, and certification of all automated systems shall be performed and documented as required by all applicable laws, regulations, and standards.[6,22,23] All automated systems shall include adequate safeguards to maintain the confidentiality and security of patient records, and there shall be procedures to provide essential patient care services in case of equipment failure or downtime.

Information Technology. A comprehensive pharmacy computer system shall be employed and should be integrated to the fullest extent possible with other hospital information systems and software, including computerized provider-order-entry, medication administration, electronic health record, and patient billing systems. Computer resources should be used to support clerical functions, maintain patient medication profile records, provide clinical decision support, perform necessary patient billing procedures, manage drug product inventories, provide drug information, access the patient medical record, manage electronic prescribing, and interface with other computerized systems to obtain patient-specific clinical information for medication therapy monitoring and other clinical functions and to facilitate the continuity of care to and from other care settings. Pharmacists should be involved in the development and maintenance of order sets, templates, and dose ranges used in computerized provider-order-entry and clinical decision-support systems. Pharmacy computer systems should be integrated with the hospital's clinical, financial, and administrative information systems. All computer systems shall include adequate safeguards to maintain the confidentiality and security of patient records, and a backup system should be available to continue essential computerized functions (e.g., those that support patient care) during equipment failure.

Drug Information. Adequate space, current resources, and information-handling and communication technology shall be available to facilitate the provision of drug information. The department of pharmacy shall select its drug information resources, and pharmacists shall play a leadership role in the selection of drug information resources used by other health care providers in the hospital. Up-to-date, objective drug information shall be available, including current print or electronic periodicals, newsletters, best-practices guidelines, and recent editions of reference books in appropriate pharmaceutical and biomedical subject areas. Electronic drug information databases are preferred because they are frequently updated and can be made available to all health care professionals, but sufficient access to print information shall be available in case of equipment failure or downtime. Electronic and print drug information may be supplemented with medical libraries and other available resources. Appropriate drug information resources shall be readily accessible to pharmacists located in patient care areas.

Electronic databases and convenient methods of data dissemination (e.g., e-mail and handheld devices) are desirable. If such tools are employed, they should be made available to all health care practitioners who require access to the data.

Record Maintenance. All records shall be maintained in accordance with applicable laws, regulations, and institutional policies. Adequate space shall exist for maintaining and storing records (e.g., equipment maintenance, controlled substances inventory, and material safety data sheets) to ensure compliance with laws, regulations, accreditation requirements, and sound management practices. Appropriate licenses and permits shall be on display or on file as required by law or regulation. Equipment shall be adequately maintained and certified in accordance with applicable practice standards, laws, and regulations. There shall be documentation of equipment maintenance and certification.

F. Committee Involvement

A pharmacist shall be a member of and actively participate in hospital and health-system committees responsible for establishing and implementing medication-related policies and procedures as well as those committees responsible for the provision of patient care, including the P&T, infection-prevention and control, patient care, medication-use evaluation, medication safety, nutrition, and pain management committees (or their equivalents), as well as the institutional review board, quality-improvement, and information technology committees (or their equivalents).[5,24–26]

Standard II. Medication-Use Policy Development

A. Policy Development

All committees that make decisions concerning medication management and use shall have at least one pharmacist as a member. This includes the P&T, infection-control, patient care, medication-use evaluation, medication safety, nutrition, pain management, and information technology committees, as well as the institutional review board (or their equivalents).[5,24–26] Pharmacists shall be involved in the development, implementation, and assessment of care plans (protocols, critical pathways, disease statement management programs, or clinical practice guidelines), standing orders, and order sets that involve medication therapy.[27]

B. Formulary Management

Formulary. A well-controlled formulary of approved medications shall be maintained and regularly updated by the P&T committee (or its equivalent). The impact of and compliance with the formulary should be periodically reviewed (e.g., through drug-utilization reviews), and the P&T committee should regularly review the formulary for safety information. The P&T committee shall be responsible for developing and maintaining written criteria for drug product selection, which shall address formulary requests for medications intended for use in special populations (e.g., pediatric or geriatric populations). The P&T committee shall be responsible for developing and maintaining adequate product specifications to aid in the purchase of medications and related supplies. The pharmacy shall disseminate the formulary by electronic (preferred) or other means to meet the needs of all health care professionals.

There shall be policies and procedures that address the use of dietary supplements and other alternative therapies.

There shall be policies and procedures for the procurement, control, and use of nonformulary medications required for patient care.[5]

Medication Therapy Monographs. Medication therapy monographs for medications under consideration for formulary addition or deletion shall be made available to the

P&T committee for use in the decision-making process. These monographs should be based on evidence gathered through review and evaluation of the pertinent literature. Each monograph shall include a comparative therapeutic, economic, and risk assessment (inclusive of black-box warnings) of each medication. The risk assessment should address the likelihood of an error occurring and the risk of injury should that error occur.[5]

Nondrug Substances. There shall be policies and procedures that describe how the pharmacy shall seek and obtain documented authorization from appropriate medical staff and hospital committees prior to the medical use of any chemical substance that has not received Food and Drug Administration (FDA) approval for use as a drug or medical nutrition therapy. All chemical or biological substances whose administration is intended for pharmacological or medical effect or as a substitute for or complement to approved drugs shall be under the control of the pharmacy. Documentation shall exist to ensure that appropriate risk management measures (e.g., obtaining informed consent) have been taken.

C. Drug Information

Drug Information Requests. The pharmacist shall provide patient-specific drug information and accurate and comprehensive information about drugs and drug therapy to health professionals, patients, and patients' caregivers as appropriate. Responses to general and patient-specific drug information requests shall be provided in an accurate and timely manner by a pharmacist, and there should be a process for assessing and ensuring the quality of responses.[28]

Dissemination of Drug Information. Pharmacists shall keep the hospital's staff and health care providers informed about the use of medications on an ongoing basis through appropriate publications, presentations, and programs. Pharmacists shall ensure timely dissemination of drug product information (e.g., recall notices, labeling changes, and changes in product availability). Electronic communications (e.g., websites, email newsletters, intranet postings) are preferred because of their timeliness and accessibility.[28]

Standard III. Optimizing Medication Therapy

An important responsibility of the pharmacist is optimizing medication use. Pharmacists, in collaboration with medical and nursing staff, shall develop policies and procedures based on demonstrated best practices for ensuring the quality of medication therapy. Clinical imperatives should be the primary determinants of medication-use decisions.

A. Creating a Relationship with the Patient

Pharmacist Role in Direct Patient Care. Hospital and pharmacy department policies should encourage pharmacists to provide direct patient care to the greatest extent possible in both inpatient and outpatient settings. Hospital and pharmacy department policies should encourage pharmacists to engage in medication therapy management,[29] collaborative drug therapy management, immunization, medication ordering and administration, and other patient care activities to the extent permitted by law, regulation, and hospital requirements.

Continuity of Care. Pharmacists should assume responsibility for continuity of care for patients' medication therapy. Pharmacists and pharmacy departments should take a leadership role in developing and implementing policies and procedures for admissions, discharges, and transfers so that patients' medication therapy is well managed regardless of patient transitions across care settings (e.g., among different components of a health system or between inpatient and community pharmacies or home care services).

Patient Confidentiality. Systems shall be in place to ensure that patient confidentiality is maintained in accordance with applicable laws and regulations. All pharmacy personnel shall respect and protect patient confidentiality by safeguarding access to all patient information. Patient information shall be shared only with authorized health professionals and others authorized within the hospital or health system as needed for the care of patients.[30] Pharmacy personnel should periodically receive training in how to comply with patient confidentiality laws and regulations.

B. Acquiring Essential Patient Data

Pharmacists should obtain, prepare, or have immediate access to comprehensive medication histories for each patient, from the patient's medical record or other databases (e.g., a medication profile), or both. A pharmacist-conducted medication history for each patient is desirable. Electronic medical records should be constructed so that medication histories and other data required for medication management, including medication reconciliation, are available to all health professionals caring for a patient.

C. Consulting With Other Health Professionals About Medication Therapy

Pharmacist's Consultations. Pharmacists should provide oral and written consultations to other health professionals regarding medication therapy selection and management.[30]

Medical Record Documentation. There shall be policies and procedures for pharmacist review of and documentation in patients' medical records. Recommendations made by the pharmacist and actions taken in response to those recommendations should be documented in the patient's medical record so that other health care providers have access to that information.[30]

Medication Therapy Decisions. The pharmacist's prerogatives to initiate, monitor, and modify medication therapy for individual patients, and to order laboratory tests to exercise those responsibilities, consistent with laws, regulations, and hospital policy, shall be clearly delineated and approved by the appropriate committee (e.g., P&T, patient care, or medical executive committee).

Standard IV. Drug Product Procurement and Inventory Management

The pharmacy shall be responsible for the procurement, distribution, and control of all drug products used in the hospital for inpatient and ambulatory patients. Policies and procedures governing these functions shall be developed by the pharmacy with input from other appropriate hospital staff and committees.[4]

A. Selecting Sources of Pharmaceutical Products

Medication Acquisition. There shall be policies and procedures for managing medication acquisition. These policies and procedures should address such issues as formulary development (including initial evaluation for formulary consideration, medication-utilization review programs, and therapeutic interchange), competitive bidding, group purchasing, best practices, medication shortages, outsourcing, and cost-effective patient services. Benchmarking of medication costs should be performed to determine whether medication expenses and the change in medication expenses over time are consistent with industry standards.[4,31,32]

Pharmaceutical Manufacturers and Suppliers. Criteria for selecting drug product manufacturers and suppliers shall be established by the pharmacy to ensure the highest quality of and the best price for drug products. Although these duties may be delegated in part to a group purchasing organization, the pharmacy maintains the sole responsibility for ensuring the quality of drug products used in the hospital.[31,32]

Pharmaceutical Manufacturers' Representatives. There shall be written policies governing the activities of manufacturers' representatives or vendors of drug products (including related supplies and devices) within the hospital. Representatives should not be permitted access to patient care areas and should be provided with written guidance on permissible activities within the hospital. All promotional materials and activities shall be reviewed and approved by the pharmacy.[33]

B. Managing Inventory

Medication Storage. Medications shall be received, stored, and prepared under proper conditions of sanitation, temperature, light, moisture, ventilation, segregation, and security to ensure medication integrity and personnel safety.[4]

Drug Shortages. There shall be policies and procedures for managing drug product shortages. The pharmacy's inventory management system should be designed to detect subminimum inventory levels and alert the pharmacy to potential shortages, and pharmacy staff should monitor reliable sources of information regarding drug product shortages (e.g., the ASHP[34] and FDA[35] drug shortages web resource centers). The pharmacy should develop strategies for identifying alternative therapies, working with suppliers, collaborating with physicians and other health care providers, and conducting an awareness campaign in the event of a drug product shortage.[36]

Samples. The use of medication samples shall be eliminated to the extent possible. Medication samples shall never be used for inpatient treatment. If use of samples is otherwise permitted, there shall be policies and procedures to ensure their safe use. The pharmacy shall oversee the procurement, storage, and distribution of these products to ensure proper storage, maintenance of records, product integrity, and compliance with all applicable packaging and labeling laws, regulations, standards, and patient education requirements. Pharmacists should be involved in hospital efforts to secure safe and effective low-cost medications for low-income patients (e.g., through manufacturer patient assistance programs).[4,5,33]

Patient Care Area Stock. The proper use of automated dispensing devices reduces the need for medications to be stored in nonpharmacy areas.[6] Storage of medications in nonpharmacy areas (e.g., patient care and procedural areas) shall to the extent possible be limited to medications for emergency use and routinely used personal care items (e.g., mouthwash and antiseptic solutions). The list of medications to be accessible and the policies and procedures regarding their use shall be developed by a multidisciplinary committee of physicians, pharmacists, and nurses (e.g., the P&T committee).[5] Access to medications should be limited to cases in which the committee determines that the urgent clinical need for the medication outweighs the potential patient-safety risks of making the medication accessible. A separate assessment should occur for every location where a medication may be stocked.

Controlled Substances. There shall be policies and procedures to ensure control of the distribution and use of controlled substances and other medications with a potential for abuse. These policies and procedures shall be consistent with applicable laws and regulations and shall include methods for preventing and detecting diversion.[4]

Patient's Own Medications. Drug products and related devices brought into the hospital by patients shall be identified by pharmacy and documented in the patient's medical record if the medications are to be used during hospitalization. They shall be administered only pursuant to a prescriber's order and according to hospital policies and procedures, which should ensure the pharmacist's identification and validation of medication integrity as well as the secure and appropriate storage and management of such medications.

C. Inspecting Storage Areas and Inventory Items

All stocks of medications shall be inspected routinely to ensure the absence of outdated, unusable, recalled, or mislabeled products. Storage conditions that would foster medication deterioration, storage arrangements that might contribute to medication errors, and other safety issues shall be assessed, documented, and corrected.[4]

D. Returning Recalled, Expired, and Other Unusable Items

There shall be a written procedure for the timely handling and documentation of a drug product recall. These procedures should include an established process for removing from use any drugs or devices subjected to a recall, notifying appropriate health care professionals, identifying patients who may have been exposed to the recalled medication, and, if necessary, communicating available alternative therapies to prescribers. The pharmacy shall be notified of any defective drug products or related supplies and equipment encountered by the nursing or medical staffs. All drug product defects should be reported to the FDA's MedWatch reporting program.[4]

Standard V. Preparing, Packaging, and Labeling Medications

A. Preparing Medications

Compounding. Drug formulations, dosage forms, strengths, and packaging that are not available commercially but are needed for patient care shall be prepared by appropriately trained personnel in accordance with applicable practice standards and regulations. The pharmacy shall provide adequate quality-assurance procedures for these operations. Written master formulas and batch records (including product test results, as appropriate) shall be maintained, and a lot number or other method to identify each finished product with its production and control history shall be assigned to each batch.[14–20]

Sterile Preparations. When possible, manufactured sterile preparations should be preferred to compounding in the pharmacy. All sterile medications shall be prepared and labeled in a suitable environment by appropriately trained personnel in accordance with established quality-assurance and expiration dating procedures.[14,19] The use of sterile medications compounded outside the pharmacy should be avoided to the extent possible; when they are used, there shall be procedures for aseptic preparation, quality assurance, expiration dating, and ongoing competency evaluations for compounding personnel.[14,19,37] Sterile compounding outside the pharmacy or satellite pharmacies (e.g., on nursing units) should be minimized and occur only in emergency situations.[14,19]

Hazardous Drug Products. There shall be policies and procedures that describe special precautions, equipment, and training for preparation, handling, storage, and disposal of hazardous drug products and products used in their preparation. These policies and procedures shall be consistent with applicable laws and regulations and should be adequate to ensure the safety of staff, patients, visitors, the community, and the environment.[17]

B. Packaging Medications

Unit Dose Packaging. Whenever possible, medications shall be available for inpatient use in single-unit packages and in a ready-to-administer form. Manipulation of medications before administration (e.g., withdrawal of doses from containers, reconstitution of powdered drug products, labeling of containers, and splitting of tablets) by final users should be minimized.[15]

Bar-Coding of Unit Dose Packaging and Point of Care Administration. Unit dose packages should contain a bar code and that code should be used in inventory management, dose preparation and packaging, dispensing, and administration. It is the responsibility of the pharmacy department to ensure the quality of all aspects of bar-code medication administration, including scanability of bar codes and database management.[38,39]

Standard VI. Medication Dispensing and Delivery

A. Medication Dispensing

Prescribing. Medications shall be prescribed by individuals who have been granted appropriate clinical privileges in the hospital and are legally permitted to order medications. The pharmacy shall advocate and foster practitioners' conformance with standardized, approved, and safe terminology and abbreviations to be used throughout the hospital when prescribing medications and discourage use of nonstandard and unapproved terminology and abbreviations.[4]

Diagnostic or Therapeutic Purpose. Pharmacists should have immediate access to the patient's diagnosis or the intended therapeutic or medical purpose of medications.

Medication Orders. All patient medication orders shall be contained in the patient's medical record. A direct copy of the prescriber's order, either hard copy (including facsimile) or prescriber-entered electronic transmission (preferred method), shall be received by the pharmacist. Oral orders should be avoided to the extent possible. When oral orders are necessary, they shall follow the organization's established procedures for their use and documentation. Order transmittal safeguards should be used to ensure the security of the prescriber's order. Appropriate records of each medication order and its processing in the pharmacy shall be maintained in accordance with applicable laws and regulations.

A system shall exist to ensure that medication orders are not inappropriately continued.[4]

Review of Medication Orders. All medication orders shall be prospectively reviewed by a pharmacist and assessed in relation to pertinent patient and clinical information before the first dose is administered or made available in an automated dispensing device, except in emergent situations in which the treatment of the patient would be significantly compromised by the delay that would result from pharmacist review of the order. There shall be a procedure for retrospective review of these orders.

Any questions regarding an order shall be resolved with the prescriber prior to administration, and any action taken as a result of this intervention should be documented in the patient's medical record. Information concerning changes shall be communicated to the appropriate health professionals caring for the patient.[4]

B. Medication Delivery and Administration

Drug Delivery Systems, Administration Devices, and Automated Distribution Devices. The pharmacy shall have responsibility for developing policies, procedures, and quality-assurance programs regarding drug delivery systems, administration devices, and automated distribution devices that ensure safety, accuracy, security, and patient confidentiality. The potential for medication errors associated with such systems and devices should be thoroughly evaluated.[4,6] Pharmacy personnel shall supervise the stocking and documentation of medications in automated dispensing devices.[6] Whenever possible, automated dispensing cabinets should employ profile-based technology integrated with remote medication order-entry capabilities.

Medication Administration. Only personnel who are authorized by the hospital in accordance with applicable laws and regulations and appropriately trained shall be permitted to administer medications to a patient. All administered, refused, or omitted medication doses should be recorded in the patient's medical record according to an established procedure, and all medications that have not been administered should be returned to the pharmacy. No medication should be administered to a patient unless medical and nursing personnel have been provided with adequate information about, and are familiar with, its therapeutic use, method of administration, potential adverse effects, and dosage.

Standard VII. Monitoring Medication Use

A. Reviewing Patient Responses to Medication Therapy

Medication therapy monitoring shall be conducted by pharmacists. Medication therapy monitoring includes a proactive assessment of patient problems and an assessment of

a. The therapeutic appropriateness of the patient's medication regimen.
b. Therapeutic duplication or omissions in the patient's medication regimen.
c. The appropriateness of the dose of the medication, as well as the route, method, and frequency of administration of the medication.
d. Patient adherence to the prescribed medication regimen.
e. Medication–medication, medication–food, medication–dietary supplement, medication–laboratory test, and medication–disease interactions.
f. Adverse drug reactions and other undesired effects.[40]
g. Patient medication allergies and sensitivities.
h. Clinical and pharmacokinetic laboratory data to evaluate the efficacy and safety of medication therapy and to anticipate toxicity and adverse effects.
i. Physical signs and clinical symptoms relevant to the patient's medication therapy.
j. Assessment of the effectiveness of the patient's medication therapy.

B. Educating and Counseling Patients and Family

Pharmacists shall be available to participate in patient education. Pharmacists should help to ensure that all patients are given adequate information about the medications they receive in order to help patients participate in their own health care decisions and encourage adherence to medication regimens. Patient education activities shall be coordinated with the nursing, medical, and other clinical staff as needed. Medication-related material developed by other services and departments as well as commercial sources should be reviewed by the pharmacy staff for accuracy, currency, literacy appropriateness, and completeness. If necessary, interpretative language services (written or oral) should be made available to patients.[21]

Standard VIII. Evaluating the Effectiveness of the Medication-Use System

There shall be an ongoing, systematic program for quality assessment and improvement of pharmacy services and the medication-use system. The program should include routinely evaluating the literature for new technologies or successful practices that have been demonstrated to enhance safety in other organizations to determine if such technologies or practices can improve the hospital's medication-use system. This program should be integrated with the hospital's or health system's quality assessment and quality improvement activities. Quality-improvement activities related to the selection, prescription, procurement, storage, preparation, dispensing, distribution, administration, documentation, monitoring, and use of medications shall be routinely performed in cooperation with other health care providers. Feedback to appropriate individuals or entities about the quality achieved shall be provided.

A. Assessing Pharmacy Services and Practices

Documentation of Pharmacist-Provided Patient Care Services and Medication Therapy Outcomes. The pharmacy shall have an ongoing process for consistent documentation of the patient care services provided by pharmacists and patient outcomes from medication therapy.[30]

Workload and Financial Performance. A process shall exist to routinely monitor and document workload and financial performance. Metrics should encompass the full scope of patient care services provided by pharmacists and the pharmacy enterprise. This process should provide for the determination and analysis of hospital and systemwide costs of medication therapy. A pharmacist should be an integral part of the hospital's leadership teams (e.g., administrative, financial).

B. Improving the Medication-Use Process

Medication-Use Evaluation. There shall be an ongoing program for monitoring drug utilization and costs to ensure that medications are used appropriately, safely, and effectively and to increase the probability of desired patient outcomes. The P&T committee (or its equivalent) should define specific parameters for evaluation (e.g., disease state, pharmacological category, or high-use/high-cost drug products) as appropriate for the organization. Through the ongoing evaluation of medication use, areas in need of improvement in medication prescribing and management can be identified and targeted for intervention.[32,41]

Medication Safety. Pharmacists should provide leadership to and participate in collaborative, multidisciplinary efforts to prevent, detect, and resolve drug-related problems that can result in patient harm. Pharmacists and other appropriate hospital personnel shall establish and regularly revise policies and procedures regarding medication error and adverse event prevention and reporting. Monitoring, detecting, review, and analysis of the hospital and health system's medication errors and near-misses should be an ongoing process in a just culture environment,[42] and corresponding corrective actions should be documented. An ongoing program for preventing, monitoring, resolving, and reporting adverse drug events shall be developed.[40] A pharmacist shall participate in appropriate organizational committees and work with physicians, nurses, administrators, and others to examine and improve systems to ensure that medication-use processes are safe.[41]

Antimicrobial Stewardship and Infection Prevention and Control. There shall be policies and procedures to promote the optimal use of antimicrobial agents, reduce the transmission of infections, and educate health professionals, patients, and the public about these topics. Pharmacists should participate in antimicrobial stewardship and infection-prevention and control efforts through clinical endeavors focused on proper antimicrobial utilization and membership on relevant multidisciplinary work groups and committees within the health system.

Pharmacists should monitor patients' laboratory reports of microbial sensitivities or applicable diagnostic markers and advise prescribers if microbial resistance is suspected, evaluate trends in microbial prescribing relative to changes in microbial resistance patterns, and assist in developing prescribing patterns to help minimize the development of drug resistance.[24]

Standard IX. Research

The pharmacist should initiate, participate in, and support clinical and practice-related research appropriate to the goals, objectives, and resources of the specific hospital.

Policies and Procedures. The pharmacist shall ensure that policies and procedures for the safe and proper use of investigational drugs and medication-related devices are established and followed and that these policies and procedures meet all applicable laws and regulations. There shall be a procedure to assure that informed consent is obtained from the patient before the first dose of the study drug is administered.[5,44,45]

Procurement, Distribution, and Control of Investigational Drugs. The pharmacy shall be responsible for overseeing the procurement, distribution, and control of all investigational drugs. Investigational drugs shall be approved for use by an institutional review board and shall be dispensed and administered to consenting patients according to an approved protocol.[5,44,45]

Institutional Review Board. A pharmacist shall be a member of the hospital's institutional review board (or equivalent body), if one exists.[44]

Information Regarding Investigational Drugs. The pharmacy shall have access to information on all investigational studies and similar research projects involving medications and medication-related devices used in the hospital. The pharmacy shall provide pertinent written information (to the extent known) about the safe and proper use of investigational drugs, including possible adverse effects and adverse drug reactions, to nurses, pharmacists, physicians, and other health care professionals called upon to prescribe, dispense, and administer these medications.[44,45]

References

1. American Society of Health-System Pharmacists. Mission statement of the American Society of Health-System Pharmacists. *Am J Health-Syst Pharm.* 2001; 58:1524.
2. American Society of Health-System Pharmacists. The consensus of the Pharmacy Practice Model Summit. *Am J Health-Syst Pharm.* 2011; 68:1148–52.
3. American Society of Health-System Pharmacists. ASHP guidelines on remote medication order processing. *Am J Health-Syst Pharm.* 2010; 67:672–7.
4. American Society of Hospital Pharmacists. ASHP technical assistance bulletin on hospital drug distribution and control. *Am J Hosp Pharm.* 1980; 37:1097–103.
5. American Society of Health-System Pharmacists. ASHP guidelines on the pharmacy and therapeutics committee and the formulary system. *Am J Health-Syst Pharm.* 2008; 65:1272–83.
6. American Society of Health-System Pharmacists. ASHP guidelines on the safe use of automated dispensing devices. *Am J Health-Syst Pharm.* 2010; 67:483–90.
7. American Society of Health-System Pharmacists. ASHP statement on the role of health-system pharmacists in emergency preparedness. *Am J Health-Syst Pharm.* 2003; 60:1993–5.
8. American Society of Health-System Pharmacists. ASHP guidelines on the pharmacist's role in immunization. *Am J Health-Syst Pharm.* 2003; 60:1371–7.
9. American Society of Health-System Pharmacists. ASHP statement on the pharmacist's role in substance abuse prevention, education, and assistance. *Am J Health-Syst Pharm.* 2003; 60:1995–8.
10. American Society of Health-System Pharmacists. ASHP residency accreditation. www.ashp.org/menu/Accreditation/ResidencyAccreditation.aspx (accessed 2012 Jan 10).
11. American Society of Hospital Pharmacists. ASHP statement on continuing education. *Am J Hosp Pharm.* 1990; 47:1855.
12. American Society of Health-System Pharmacists. ASHP guidelines on the recruitment, selection, and retention of pharmacy personnel. *Am J Health-Syst Pharm.* 2003; 60:587–93.
13. American Pharmacists Association. Code of Ethics for Pharmacists. www.pharmacist.com/AM/Template.cfm?Section=Search1&template=/CM/HTMLDisplay.cfm&ContentID=2903 (accessed 2012 Jan 10).
14. American Society of Health-System Pharmacists. ASHP guidelines on quality assurance for pharmacy-prepared sterile products. *Am J Health-Syst Pharm.* 2000; 57:1150–69.
15. American Society of Hospital Pharmacists. ASHP technical assistance bulletin on single unit and unit dose packages of drugs. *Am J Hosp Pharm.* 1985; 42:378–9.
16. American Society of Hospital Pharmacists. ASHP technical assistance bulletin on compounding nonsterile products in pharmacies. *Am J Hosp Pharm.* 1994; 51:1441–8.
17. American Society of Health-System Pharmacists. ASHP guidelines on handling hazardous drugs. *Am J Health-Syst Pharm.* 2006; 63:1172–93.
18. American Society of Hospital Pharmacists. ASHP technical assistance bulletin on repackaging oral solids and liquids in single unit and unit dose packages. *Am J Hosp Pharm.* 1983; 40:451–2.
19. Pharmaceutical compounding—sterile preparations (general information chapter 797). In: The United States pharmacopeia, 34th rev., and The national formulary, 29th ed. Rockville, MD: United States Pharmacopeial Convention; 2011:336–73.
20. Pharmaceutical compounding—nonsterile preparations (general information chapter 795). In: The United States pharmacopeia, 34th rev., and The national formulary, 29th ed. Rockville, MD: United States Pharmacopeial Convention; 2011:330–6.
21. American Society of Health-System Pharmacists. ASHP guidelines on pharmacist-conducted patient

education and counseling. *Am J Health-Syst Pharm.* 1997; 54:431–4.

22. American Society of Health-System Pharmacists. ASHP guidelines on the safe use of automated compounding devices for the preparation of parenteral nutrition admixtures. *Am J Health-Syst Pharm.* 2000; 57:1343–8.
23. American Society of Health-System Pharmacists. ASHP guidelines on pharmacy planning for implementation of computerized provider order entry systems in hospitals and health systems. *Am J Health-Syst Pharm.* 2011; 68:e9–e31.
24. American Society of Health-System Pharmacists. ASHP statement on the pharmacist's role in antimicrobial stewardship and infection prevention and control. *Am J Health-Syst Pharm.* 2010; 67:575–7.
25. American Society of Health-System Pharmacists. ASHP statement on the pharmacist's role in informatics. *Am J Health-Syst Pharm.* 2007; 64:200–3.
26. American Society of Health-System Pharmacists. ASHP statement on the roles and responsibilities of the pharmacy executive. *Am J Health-Syst Pharm.* 2009; 66:499–502.
27. American Society of Health-System Pharmacists. ASHP guidelines on the pharmacist's role in the development, implementation, and assessment of critical pathways. *Am J Health-Syst Pharm.* 2004; 61:939–45.
28. American Society of Health-System Pharmacists. ASHP guidelines on the provision of medication information by pharmacists. *Am J Health-Syst Pharm.* 1996; 53:1843–5.
29. Office of the Law Revision Counsel, United States House of Representatives. USC*prelim*. 42 U.S.C. Sec. 299b-35(c), MTM services to eligible individuals. http://uscode.house.gov/lawrevisioncounsel.shtml (accessed 2012 Apr 24).
30. American Society of Health-System Pharmacists. ASHP guidelines on documenting pharmaceutical care in patient medical records. *Am J Health-Syst Pharm.* 2003; 60:705–7.
31. American Society of Hospital Pharmacists. ASHP guidelines for selecting pharmaceutical manufacturers and suppliers. *Am J Hosp Pharm.* 1991; 48:523–4.
32. American Society of Health-System Pharmacists. ASHP guidelines on medication cost management strategies for hospitals and health systems. *Am J Health-Syst Pharm.* 2008; 65:1368–84.
33. American Society of Hospital Pharmacists. ASHP guidelines for pharmacists on the activities of vendors' representatives in organized health care systems. *Am J Hosp Pharm.* 1994; 51:520–1.
34. American Society of Health-System Pharmacists. ASHP Drug Shortages Resource Center. www.ashp.org/shortages (accessed 2012 Jan 11).
35. Food and Drug Administration. Drug shortages. www.fda.gov/cder/drug/shortages/ (accessed 2012 Jan 11).
36. American Society of Health-System Pharmacists. ASHP guidelines on managing drug product shortages in hospitals and health systems. *Am J Health-Syst Pharm.* 2009; 66:1399–406.
37. American Society of Health-System Pharmacists. ASHP guidelines on outsourcing sterile compounding services. *Am J Health-Syst Pharm.* 2010; 67:757–65.
38. American Society of Health-System Pharmacists. ASHP statement on bar-code-enabled medication administration technology. *Am J Health-Syst Pharm.* 2009; 66:588–90.
39. American Society of Health-System Pharmacists. ASHP statement on bar-code verification during inventory, preparation, and dispensing of medications. *Am J Health-Syst Pharm.* 2011; 68:442–5.
40. American Society of Health-System Pharmacists. ASHP guidelines on adverse drug reaction monitoring and reporting. *Am J Health-Syst Pharm.* 1995; 52:417–9.
41. American Society of Health-System Pharmacists. ASHP guidelines on medication-use evaluation. *Am J Health-Syst Pharm.* 1996; 53:1953–5.
42. Khatri N, Brown GD, Hicks LL. From a blame culture to a just culture in health care. *Health Care Manage Rev.* 2009; 34(4):312–22.
43. American Society of Hospital Pharmacists. ASHP guidelines on preventing medication errors in hospitals. *Am J Hosp Pharm.* 1993; 50:305–14.
44. American Society of Health-System Pharmacists. ASHP guidelines on clinical drug research. *Am J Health-Syst Pharm.* 1998; 55:369–76.
45. American Society of Hospital Pharmacists. ASHP guidelines for pharmaceutical research in organized health-care settings. *Am J Hosp Pharm.* 1989; 46:129–30.

Developed through the ASHP Council on Pharmacy Practice and approved by the ASHP Board of Directors on April 13, 2012.

This document supersedes a previous version approved by the ASHP Board of Directors on September 22, 1995.

ASHP gratefully acknowledges the contributions made by the following individuals to various drafts of these guidelines: Thomas S. Brenner, B.S.Pharm., FASHP; Harold N. Godwin, M.S., FASHP, FAPhA; William A. Gouveia, M.S., FASHP; Brian D. Hodgkins, Pharm.D., FCSHP, FASHP; Stanley S. Kent, M.S., FASHP; Patricia C. Kienle, M.P.A., FASHP; Harold J. Kornfuhrer, B.S.Pharm., FASHP; Emory S. Martin III, Pharm.D., BCPS; J. Russell May, Pharm.D., FASHP; Gerald E. Meyer, Pharm.D., M.B.A., FASHP; Thomas E. O'Brien, Pharm.D., M.S., FASHP; Sherri L. Ramsey, D.Ph., BCPS; Frank G. Saya, Pharm.D., FCSHP, FASHP; Donna L. Soflin, B.S.Pharm., FASHP; David K. Solomon, Pharm.D., FASHP; Kasey K. Thompson, Pharm.D., M.S.; and Billy W. Woodward, B.S.Pharm.

ASHP also gratefully acknowledges the following organizations and individuals for reviewing drafts of these guidelines (review does not imply endorsement): American Nurses Association (ANA); Institute for Safe Medication Practices (ISMP); Rhode Island Society of Health-System Pharmacists (RISHP); South Carolina Society of Health-System Pharmacists (SCSHP); Wyoming Society of Health-System Pharmacy (WSHP); Tuesday Adams, RN-C, WCC; John A. Armitstead, M.S., FASHP; Phil Ayers, Pharm.D., BCNSP; Ronald Barnes, M.S.; Paul J. Barrett, Pharm.D., BCPS; Carol J. Bickford, Ph.D., RN-BC, CPHIMS (ANA); P. Justin Boyd, Pharm.D., BCPS, CDM; Tim Brown, Pharm.D., BCACP; Margaret Chrymko, Pharm.D.; Toby Clark, M.Sc., FASHP; Wayne F. Conrad, Pharm.D., FASHP; Gayle A. Cotchen, Pharm.D., M.B.A.; Debra Lynn Painter

Cowan, Pharm.D., FASHP; Arash Dabestani, Pharm.D., M.H.A., FASHP, FABC; Denise F. Daly, Pharm.D., BCPS; Tina H. Denetclaw, Pharm.D., BCPS; Deanna Dossey, Pharm.D.; William L. Fritz, M.S., FASHP; Daphne Hsu Galang, RPhT, CPhT, B.S., M.H.A.; Michael A. Gillette, Pharm.D., BCPS, BCACP; Kathleen M. Gura, Pharm.D., BCNSP, FASHP, FPPAG; Reginald L. Hain, B.S.Pharm.; Thomas G. Hall, Pharm.D.; George Hatfield, Pharm.D.; Jesse Hogue, Pharm.D.; Andrew Jarrell, Pharm.D.; Jack G. Kitrenos, Pharm.D., FASHP; Jamie Kuo, Pharm.D.; Jim Lile, Pharm.D.; Charles "Kurt" Mahan, Pharm.D., Ph.C.; Linda Gore Martin, Pharm.D., M.B.A., BCPS (WSHP); Justine Medina, M.S., RN; Dayna Mitchell, Pharm.D., BCPS; Holly Monatt, Pharm.D., BCPS; Selma Morrison; Robert J. Moura, M.S.; Jonathan M. Mundy, M.B.A. (RISHP); Bruce A. Nelson, M.S.; Beth Norman, M.S., RN, CNS, ACNS-BC; Robert S. Oakley, M.S.; Fred J. Pane, B.S.Pharm., FASHP; Shreya Parekh, Pharm.D.; Jennifer Phillips, Pharm.D.; James Ponto, BCNP, FASHP; Curt W. Quap, M.S., FASHP; Todd Rowland, Pharm.D.; Renee B. Sager, Pharm.D.; Joseph Sceppa, M.S., M.B.A.; Nicole Shumiloff, Pharm.D.; Nancy R. Smestad, M.S.; Carolyn M. Smith, Pharm.D., M.B.A., BCPS (SCSHP); William E. Smith, Pharm.D., M.P.H., Ph.D., FASHP; Richard L. Stambaugh, Pharm.D., M.S., BCPS; Therese Staublin, Pharm.D.; Marc Stranz, Pharm.D.; Timothy P. Stratton, Ph.D.; Pamela Swarny, Pharm.D., J.D.; Jane Tennis, B.S.Pharm., M.B.A.; Sherry Umhoefer, M.B.A.; Allen J. Vaida, Pharm.D., FASHP (ISMP); Jody Jacobson Wedret, FASHP, FCSHP; Roger Woolf, Pharm.D.; and Kevin Zak, Pharm.D.

Copyright © 2013, American Society of Health-System Pharmacists, Inc. All rights reserved. Contact ASHP for reprint and permissions requests. This content may not be used for commercial purposes without the express written consent of ASHP.

The bibliographic citation for this document is as follows: American Society of Health-System Pharmacists. ASHP guidelines: minimum standard for pharmacies in hospitals. *Am J Health-Syst Pharm.* 2013; 70:1619–30.

ASHP Guidelines on Pharmacy Services in Correctional Facilities

Correctional facilities include county, state, and federal jails, prisons, and detention centers whose populations may be adult or juvenile, U.S. citizen or noncitizen, sentenced inmates or detainees awaiting judicial proceedings. They may be managed directly by the relevant jurisdiction, run by a private company providing services under contract, or a combination of the two. Case law and historical precedent have established the inmate-patient's right to healthcare, notably in *Estelle* v. *Gamble*[1] and more recently in *Brown* v. *Plata*.[2] (Incarcerated individuals served by correctional pharmacists are referred to as *inmate-patients* in these guidelines; some jurisdictions may prefer other terms.) Correctional facilities should provide, at a minimum, a basic, humane, and appropriate level of healthcare services, consistent with community standards of care and made available to inmate-patients 24 hours a day, as needed. An important component of this basic provision is safe and effective pharmacist-provided patient care. As such, it is recommended that all correctional facilities obtain the services of a pharmacist.[3]

The size and scope of individual correctional facilities vary greatly. The concepts, principles, and recommendations contained in this document are intended to be generally applicable. In settings that may not have the ability to obtain the services of one or more full-time pharmacists, part-time, contract, or consultant pharmacists maintain the same basic obligations and responsibilities as their full-time counterparts in larger settings.

Correctional pharmacy practice, defined herein, encompasses many aspects of community, hospital, and consultant pharmacy practice while remaining a unique and distinct field of pharmacy practice. These guidelines are intended to address aspects unique to correctional pharmacy practice and detail the valuable clinical services and leadership provided by pharmacists in this arena.

Pharmacists who practice in correctional settings are responsible for maintaining familiarity with community standards of care, as well as the *Standards for Health Services* promulgated by the National Commission on Correctional Health Care[4,5] and the standards of the American Correctional Association.[6,7] Other pertinent guidelines of ASHP, the National Commission on Correctional Health Care, and the American Correctional Association should be reviewed as well as regulations and laws set by applicable federal, state, and local jurisdictions. Pharmacists who practice in correctional settings must also be familiar with the current literature, laws, and regulations governing confidentiality, consent, and other aspects of correctional healthcare that may differ from standard pharmacy practice.

The pharmacy director, in conjunction with the medical director or other responsible health authority and the correctional institution's administrators, should develop policies and procedures that complement these guidelines and add institution-specific details.

The Pharmacy Director

A licensed pharmacist in good standing with a state board of pharmacy recognized by the National Association of Boards of Pharmacy should be appointed the pharmacy director of the facility. He or she should be available, at a minimum, on a consulting basis. Pharmacist staffing should be proportionate to the healthcare needs of the facility.[8]

If the only pharmacy services provided are those of a consultant pharmacist, the consultant pharmacist must assume the role of the pharmacy director. If the correctional facility contracts with a vendor who provides pharmacy services, the vendor should designate and provide support for a pharmacist to assume the role of pharmacy director of the institution, with the associated responsibilities.[9]

The pharmacy director assumes responsibility for pharmacy operations and application of policy as approved by the responsible health authority and administration of the correctional facility and/or pharmacy vendor.

Therapeutic and Clinical Policies

Commensurate with the expanding role of clinical pharmacists, correctional pharmacists are well positioned to serve in an active role on the inmate-patient's medical team and provide direct patient care to improve health outcomes and minimize the risk of harm. Pharmacists can provide a plethora of services to correctional facilities and information on topics including but not limited to drug interactions, nutrition counseling and drug–nutrient interactions, food and drug allergies, drug abuse and withdrawal treatment, prenatal pharmaceutical care for pregnant women, disaster planning and response, emergency medications, proper antidotes for overdoses or poisonings, screening for and management of chronic diseases, mental health, anticoagulation, transitions of care, and medical devices and supplies. Correctional pharmacists should be involved in the administration of the annual influenza vaccine and other indicated vaccines to staff and inmate-patients. A pharmacist should be involved in the care of all inmate-patients with chronic infectious disease, especially tuberculosis, human immunodeficiency virus (HIV) infection, and viral hepatitis, to ensure proper drug therapy management of these complex conditions common to the correctional environment. Improper pharmaceutical management of these patients can contribute to disease outbreaks and the development of lifelong drug resistance.

The pharmacy director or a pharmacist designee should be a member of the institutional pharmacy and therapeutics (P&T) committee or its equivalent. A formulary should exist in accordance with the ASHP Statement on the Pharmacy and Therapeutics Committee and the Formulary System and the ASHP Guidelines on the Pharmacy and Therapeutics Committee and the Formulary System.[10,11]

Drug products selected for formulary inclusion should serve the needs of the inmate-patient population,

DOI 10.37573/9781585287048.102

be consistent with national clinical guidelines, and be as cost-effective as possible.[12] Institutional safety and security should also be considered when analyzing formulary options and restricted-use criteria. The correctional pharmacist must be aware that certain medications and delivery devices can be sold, bartered, abused, or modified into weapons or paraphernalia for drug use. The therapeutic benefits must be weighed against the risk of harm in cooperation with correctional services staff. Dosage forms such as liquids and injections should be considered for drugs identified as having abuse potential. However, pharmacists should advocate that cost and potential safety risks are not the sole determinants for drug product selection. Procedures should exist for the provision of nonformulary medications when medically appropriate.

For correctional institutions that offer a commissary or general store that sells medications or drug products, a pharmacist should be permitted to provide input into which nonprescription medications are made available for purchase. To prevent possible overdose, purchase quantity limits should be considered. The pharmacy director may determine which (if any) nonprescription medications are available from the pharmacy for inmate-patients who cannot afford them. The pharmacy director should also be involved in ensuring that the nonprescription medications are appropriately stored, and he or she should inspect any areas where medications are kept at regular intervals to ensure the integrity of these medications.

Regular consultation with the facility's medical, nursing, and mental health staff and leadership should occur, especially for maintaining policies and procedures for the use of psychotropic medications, medications for the treatment of infectious and communicable diseases, and other diseases or medical conditions common to the specific inmate-patient population, as necessary.[13] Pharmacists should provide input into antibiotic stewardship and infection-control policies and procedures pertinent to medication use and contact with medical supplies. Pharmacists should also be utilized appropriately in clinical decision-making, quality and safety improvement, policy and procedure development, drug regimen review, medication-use evaluation,[14] and direct patient care, in accordance with their skills and qualifications.[15]

Personnel

The pharmacy director should oversee pharmacy personnel and retain appropriate supervisory controls for support personnel, ensuring that pharmacy services are available commensurate with the needs of the facility. A pharmacist should visit and inspect the medication areas in the facility as required by policy but no less than quarterly.

Sufficient support personnel should be available to maximize the use of pharmacists in tasks requiring professional judgment.[16] Pharmacy technicians used as support personnel must meet jurisdictional requirements. Pharmacy technicians should have completed a pharmacy technician training program accredited by ASHP and the Accreditation Council for Pharmacy Education, obtained Pharmacy Technician Certification Board certification, and be in good standing with the state board of pharmacy.[17] When faced with a shortage of qualified pharmacy technicians, the health authority may need to consider the use of other legally qualified personnel with appropriate training and credentials to support pharmacy and departmental operations.

All personnel involved in the pharmaceutical distribution process should possess comparable education, training, licensure, and certifications to those of their community counterparts. The competencies, credentials, and licensure of all pharmacy staff should be maintained, inspected, and developed through ASHP-accredited residencies, relevant continuing-education activities, and advanced clinical training. Eligible pharmacists are encouraged to pursue board certification and credentialing as a certified correctional health professional through the National Commission on Correctional Health Care.[4,5] Pharmacists in correctional settings are encouraged to instruct or precept student pharmacists and pharmacy residents, as resources permit, to expose students and residents to correctional pharmacy as a potential career path.

Fiscal Resources

The pharmacy director or his or her designee should be involved in the appropriate administrative committee or board that establishes the budget for pharmacy department operations. Pharmacists serving correctional institutions should strive to provide high-quality care to inmate-patients while managing expenses. The ASHP Guidelines on Medication Cost Management Strategies for Hospitals and Health Systems provides a framework for cost-effectiveness decisions.[12]

The annual pharmacy budget can be forecast by weekly average utilization multiplied by 52 weeks. It should account for the total inmate capacity, average daily inmate population, demographics and health status of the inmate population, regional variability of disease burden, unforeseen needs, drug shortages, variability in drug pricing, and the disproportionate number or severity of patients with chronic or communicable diseases at the institution.[18]

Medication Purchasing and Control

Control of medications as they enter and move within the institution is an essential element of pharmacy operations in the correctional setting. Adequate methods to ensure that the appropriately trained staff members are involved in meeting these responsibilities should be established.

A pharmacist should be responsible for purchasing and controlling all prescription drug products. The responsibility, if any, for the ordering, issuance, accountability, and monitoring of other products that may be dispensed by or stored in the pharmacy should be made clear in policy. These items may include nonprescription medications, diagnostic and drug-related devices, needles, syringes, batteries, eyeglasses, contact lenses, and medical or surgical devices such as supplies for wound or ostomy care, suture and surgical kits, dental equipment, prosthetics, shoe inserts, compression garments, splints, and similar items. Accountability may include electronic controls, physical counts, and perpetual inventories.

The pharmacy director is responsible for selecting reputable and appropriate sources from which to obtain drug products and for ensuring that all drug products meet applicable legal requirements. Additional guidance on the obligations of drug product suppliers and purchasers appears in the ASHP Guidelines for Selecting Pharmaceutical Manufacturers and Suppliers.[19] Pharmacists must use professional judgment and prudence when considering the practice of redispensing unused medications or determining whether to allow inmate-patients to use medications brought in from outside the facility. These practices are not generally recommended, as the medications may have been adulterated or stored under improper conditions.

Drug Product Distribution

Inmate workers should not be utilized at any point in the distribution process. An ideal drug product distribution system will vary from one institution to another but should include as many of the following components as possible.[20] The drug distribution system will

- Be safe and cost-effective.
- Foster drug control and active drug-use monitoring by utilizing medication administration records to reduce medication errors and adverse drug reactions.
- Provide ongoing processes for the monitoring and reporting of adverse drug reactions and the detection and prevention of medication errors.
- Implement a unit dose or unit-of-use drug distribution and control system for all drug products used in directly observed therapy; to the extent practical, these items should be purchased or packaged in single-unit or unit dose packages or manually unit dosed with appropriate labeling.[21] Blister packaging, often called blister cards or bingo cards, may also be used for this purpose, provided they are appropriately labeled.
- Allow for the recovery of larger quantities of medications dispensed to inmate-patients to self-carry or keep on their person, after the discontinuance of orders or in compliance with automatic stop orders.
- Monitor and prevent the dispensing of unusually large quantities of medications, especially sufficient doses to potentially enable suicide attempts; individuals who are determined to be at high risk for suicide should be identified to the appropriate medical providers, including pharmacists.
- Provide opportunities for population-based reporting and analysis.
- Utilize modern, secure, and functional electronic hardware and software for data management and automated drug dispensing in accordance with the ASHP Guidelines on the Safe Use of Automated Dispensing Devices.[22]
- Allow access to patient medication records only to authorized personnel with a need for access.
- Protect patient confidentiality throughout the distribution process, especially for patients receiving medications for sensitive conditions (e.g., sexually transmitted infections, HIV).[23]
- Grant pharmacists full access to review and enter clinical interventions and documentation into the inmate-patient's medical record to ensure patient safety and the appropriateness of medication orders.[24]
- Require that the pharmacist review all medication orders before the first dose is dispensed, with the exception of emergency situations.
- Document refills and chain of custody from receiving to dispensing to the end user or destruction in accordance with state and federal laws and regulations.
- Detect and document patterns of inmate-patient medication behavior (e.g., use, misuse, refusal to use) in the patient's medical record.
- Allow for continuity of care both outside and within different areas of an institution.
- Minimize or eliminate the ability of inmate-patients to transfer, barter, trade, or share medications.
- Minimize unauthorized use of medications by anyone other than the intended patient, including pilferage by other inmates and staff. Multiuse containers and devices must not be shared among multiple inmate-patients.
- Deter the act of cheeking (pretending to but not actually swallowing a medication) through the use of injectable, immediate-release, or liquid medications; by crushing tablets and floating them in water (if appropriate); and by performing visual mouth checks.
- Have mechanisms to replace medication that is confiscated by staff or lost and alert the pharmacist to provide appropriate counseling for inappropriate medication behaviors such as stockpiling and cheeking.
- Account for situations unique to or made more complex by the nature of the correctional environment, such as an institutional lockdown, disease outbreaks, utility outages, and floods.

Medication Administration

In correctional settings, the responsibility of medication administration is sometimes assigned to appropriately trained nonhealthcare personnel if traditional administration by nurses is impracticable. The Standards of the National Commission on Correctional Health Care address this issue in greater detail.[4,5]

The pharmacy director should participate in the development of medication administration forms and ensure that all relevant information is incorporated into the forms, including medications administered, doses, frequency of administration, start and stop dates, and medication allergies. These forms should be stored electronically or kept in an area inaccessible to inmates.

The pharmacy director is responsible for creating policies and procedures for how medication will be administered to inmate-patients assigned to work details or work-release programs; being transported or escorted to a court hearing or other proceeding; or assigned to special housing units, segregation from the general population, or other special settings. Procedures should also be in place to ensure continuity of medication therapy upon transfer or release, within the capacity and limitations of the institution. For example, upon release, inmate-patients could either be issued an actual supply of medications proportionate to the anticipated time that they will need to reestablish care in the community or have their discharge prescriptions transmitted to a community pharmacy, compliant with the laws and regulations of both the transmitting and receiving state with the approval of the prescribing medical provider.

Education

Pharmacists in correctional settings are encouraged to take an active role in training facility and fellow healthcare staff on issues of pharmacist-provided patient care and pharmacy policies and procedures within the institution. Staff educational programs should include information on indications, administration, and the proper use of medications stocked for emergency use; monitoring for adverse events and allergic reactions; documentation; accountability; confidentiality; drug information; and the importance of adherence to medication regimens. The important role of correctional facility officers and their expectations as first responders in medical emergencies should be emphasized.

Pharmacists should also provide appropriate counseling to inmate-patients through the provision of language- and age-appropriate educational materials, direct counseling, small-group meetings, or other technological means (e.g., videoconferencing, telehealth) as available.[25] Poor health literacy is common among inmates, and efforts should be made to address and improve their understanding of their health and well-being while incarcerated. Inmate-patients should have reasonable access to drug information or pharmacist consultation upon request and within an acceptable time period to allow them to make informed choices regarding their own care. Pharmacists with the qualifications necessary to administer direct patient care services or medication therapy management should be authorized to do so, assuming that legal requirements are met and necessary collaborative practice agreements are in place.

Research

Performance of prospective and retrospective research is needed to advance the practice of correctional pharmacy and provide evidence-based rationales for clinical decisions and programs. However, inmates are federally protected as subjects in medical research as a result of the inherent loss of autonomy associated with incarceration and historical abuses.[26] The responsibility for ethical research begins with the professionalism of the primary investigators, including research pharmacists. All research with the potential to impact patient care must include provisions for informed consent and be approved by the institutional review board or its equivalent at all institutions involved, with special attention to medicolegal issues, ethics, criminology, and the endemic patient population.[27]

Adherence to federal regulations on medical research in correctional facilities is essential.[28] Extreme care should be taken to prevent situations in which inmates are or may appear to be coerced, rewarded, or penalized for their participation or nonparticipation in research. A common principle is that the inmate population should not bear the actual or possible risk burden of the research if it is unequal to the actual or possible benefits that this population stands to gain from the research.[29] All correctional research that involves medications should be conducted in consultation with a pharmacist, at a minimum.

Facilities

Several models of onsite and remote pharmacy facilities exist in the correctional environment and provide effective pharmacist patient care services. Pharmacy services may be provided in the absence of an onsite pharmacy. The definition of a pharmacy in the context of a correctional facility may or may not match the legal definition of a pharmacy for state or federal regulatory purposes, and associated registration requirements may differ. If the pharmacy is located onsite, it should be located within or in an area contiguous to the space provided for other healthcare services in order to accommodate interdisciplinary cooperation in patient care and facilitate inmate-patient perception of the pharmacy as a provider of healthcare services. Facilities and equipment should be adequate to accommodate appropriate security of all drug products, especially controlled substances. Only pharmacists designated by the pharmacy director should have access to the pharmacy. These pharmacists may possess keys, combinations, or trackable, secured electronic entry to the pharmacy and controlled substance safes. If state law allows, an authorized administrator may also possess these items. However, emergency access to the pharmacy for medical reasons should be minimized or eliminated through night stock medication availability or an emergency medication cart or locker maintained by a pharmacist. If urgent entry to the pharmacy must occur for nonmedical situations, such entries must be documented and reviewed by the pharmacy director.

Adequate and secure networked computers and electronic systems should be present with appropriate access to software to include electronic medical records, drug information resources, and programs necessary for the pharmacist to complete assigned tasks and duties.[30]

The safety and physical security of pharmacy staff should be priorities. All pharmacy staff should be appropriately equipped and trained to use communication devices, correctional tools, and self-defense techniques in accordance with institutional policy. Institutional correctional staff should ensure that all safety and security equipment is functional and well maintained. Pharmacy staff should not be asked to perform correctional duties outside their abilities or scope of training, except in emergencies, and should be trained and included in emergency drills and contingency planning. Procedures to address safety concerns to administrators should be in place.

Drug Storage

The pharmacy director is responsible for ensuring that medications are securely stored in every location in which they are kept in order to deter misuse and abuse. All drug products must be stored in accordance with the manufacturer's and/or *United States Pharmacopeia* requirements. Expired drug products must be segregated from those that remain in drug storage areas and must never be dispensed to inmate-patients. Refrigeration, freezers, and warmers should be adequate and functional, with appropriate monitoring and record keeping.

The number of areas where medications are stored should be kept to a minimum, and access to these areas should be off-limits to inmates and accessible only by approved and appropriately trained staff. The designated pharmacy personnel should inspect these areas on a consistent basis as determined by the pharmacy director. Controlled substances must be processed and stored in a manner consistent with the *Pharmacist's Manual* released by the Drug Enforcement Administration.[31] Theft and losses, especially suspected diversion, must be promptly reported to the appropriate regulatory agencies and to management of the correctional facility.

Reporting and Documentation

The pharmacy director should provide and explain reports of pharmacy activities to administration, other medical staff, and other stakeholders at regular intervals, depending on the level of pharmacy services provided. The pharmacy director is also responsible for maintaining and reviewing documentation for accuracy, especially medication administration records. Reports should be stored securely in hard copy or secure electronic format and for an appropriate period of time.

Basic reporting and documentation include

- The quantity and costs of drugs and services furnished
- Destruction of unusable or outdated medications
- Inventory value and quantities
- Records of meetings with administrators, physicians, midlevel providers, nurses, and other staff, as well as changes implemented as a result of those meetings
- Minutes of P&T committee (or equivalent) meetings[11]
- Medication administration records
- Actions taken on drug recalls or shortages
- Results of quality-control and quality-improvement activities, such as drug-use evaluations and chart reviews
- Reports generated as required by applicable state and federal laws regulating the practice of pharmacy, unless otherwise exempt or inapplicable
- All forms required by the Drug Enforcement Administration

Policies and Procedures

Following policies and procedures closely ensures safe, fair, consistent, and equitable distribution of pharmacist-provided patient care and ensures accountability. A written policies and procedures manual should be created to address specific aspects of pharmacy practice in each correctional facility or complex, including but not limited to the areas detailed in these guidelines. This manual should be reviewed and updated by the pharmacy director at least annually and signed by the administrator of the correctional facility and medical director or other responsible health authority. The manual should also address

- Transportation and storage of inmate-patients' medications within and among facilities and units.
- Security of drug products, especially controlled substances and drug-related items with needles and syringes.
- Contingency plans for maintaining accessibility of medications and services in the event of a lockdown, disaster, riot, or other emergency.
- The use of emergency kits of medications in life-threatening situations. The maintenance of such items should be the responsibility of a pharmacist, and their use should always be reported to the pharmacy director as soon as practical.
- Procedures in place to protect patient privacy. Correctional institutions must comply with the Health Insurance Portability and Accountability Act, though there are some minor differences regarding the sharing of health information and notification of privacy practices for inmate-patients.[32]
- Destruction procedures for expired, unused, or wasted drugs and controlled substances in accordance with the environmental regulations of the state or jurisdiction.
- The use of investigational drugs within the facility.[33]

ASHP acknowledges that individuals make personal moral decisions about capital punishment but opposes pharmacists' participation in capital punishment and affirms that pharmacists have a right to decline to participate in capital punishment without retribution.[34] Correctional pharmacists are committed to helping inmate-patients achieve optimal health outcomes.

Conclusion

High-quality pharmacist-provided patient care in correctional institutions contributes to the overall correctional mission of jails and prisons and to improving public health and reducing health disparities.[35–37] The pharmacy director and pharmacy staff should attempt to build and maintain positive relationships with other healthcare staff and institution administration to facilitate open and productive lines of communication. Adherence to detailed policies and procedures, together with ongoing surveillance and quality improvement, will create an environment that is conducive to safe and effective inmate-patient care. Improvements in health status and health behavior that occur due to the interventions of a pharmacist can begin a cascade of lasting benefits for inmate-patients and prepare them to return to their communities and to society.

References

1. *Estelle v. Gamble*, 429 U.S. 97 (1976).
2. *Brown v. Plata*, 131 S.Ct. 1910 (2011).
3. American Society of Health-System Pharmacists. ASHP guidelines: minimum standard for pharmacies in hospitals. *Am J Health-Syst Pharm.* 2013; 70:1619–30.
4. Standards for health services in jails: 2014. Chicago: National Commission on Correctional Health Care; 2014.
5. Standards for health services in prisons: 2014. Chicago: National Commission on Correctional Health Care; 2014.
6. Adult correctional institutions. 4th ed. Alexandria, VA: American Correctional Association; 2014.
7. American Correctional Association. Performance-based standards for correctional health care in adult correctional facilities. 1st ed. Alexandria, VA: American Correctional Association; 2014.

8. American Society of Health-System Pharmacists. ASHP statement on the roles and responsibilities of the pharmacy executive. *Am J Health-Syst Pharm.* 2009; 66:499–502.
9. American Society of Health-System Pharmacists. ASHP guidelines on remote medication order processing. *Am J Health-Syst Pharm.* 2010; 67:672–7.
10. American Society of Health-System Pharmacists. ASHP statement on the pharmacy and therapeutics committee and the formulary system. *Am J Health-Syst Pharm.* 2008; 65:2384–6.
11. American Society of Health-System Pharmacists. ASHP guidelines on the pharmacy and therapeutics committee and the formulary system. *Am J Health-Syst Pharm.* 2008; 65:1272–83.
12. American Society of Health-System Pharmacists. ASHP guidelines on medication cost management strategies for hospitals and health systems. *Am J Health-Syst Pharm.* 2008; 65:1368–84.
13. American Society of Health-System Pharmacists. ASHP statement on the pharmacist's role in antimicrobial stewardship and infection prevention and control. *Am J Health-Syst Pharm.* 2010; 67:575–7.
14. American Society of Health-System Pharmacists. ASHP guidelines on medication-use evaluation. *Am J Health-Syst Pharm.* 1996; 53:1953–5.
15. American Society of Health-System Pharmacists. ASHP guidelines on pharmacist-conducted patient education and counseling. *Am J Health- Syst Pharm.* 1997; 54:431–4.
16. American Society of Health-System Pharmacists. ASHP guidelines on the recruitment, selection, and retention of pharmacy personnel. *Am J Health-Syst Pharm.* 2003; 60:587–93.
17. American Society of Health-System Pharmacists. ASHP policy position 1519: pharmacy technician and certification. www.ashp.org/DocLibrary/BestPractices/EducationPositions.aspx (accessed 2015 Nov 9).
18. Schafer JJ, Gill TK, Sherman EM, McNicholl IR. ASHP guidelines on pharmacist involvement in HIV care. *Am J Health-Syst Pharm.* 2016; 73:468–94.
19. American Society of Hospital Pharmacists. ASHP guidelines for selecting pharmaceutical manufacturers and suppliers. *Am J Hosp Pharm.* 1991; 48:523–4.
20. American Society of Hospital Pharmacists. ASHP technical assistance bulletin on hospital drug distribution and control. *Am J Hosp Pharm.* 1980; 37:1097–103.
21. American Society of Hospital Pharmacists. ASHP technical assistance bulletin on single unit and unit dose packages of drugs. *Am J Hosp Pharm.* 1985; 42:378–9.
22. American Society of Health-System Pharmacists. ASHP guidelines on the safe use of automated dispensing devices. *Am J Health-Syst Pharm.* 2010; 67:483–90.
23. American Society of Health-System Pharmacists. ASHP statement on confidentiality of patient health care information. *Am J Health-Syst Pharm.* 2009; 66:411–2.
24. American Society of Health-System Pharmacists. ASHP guidelines on documenting pharmaceutical care in patient medical records. *Am J Health-Syst Pharm.* 2003; 60:705–7.
25. Thompson B, Conrad G, Gum MO et al. ASHP guidelines on remote medication order processing. *Am J Health-Syst Pharm.* 2010; 67:672–7.
26. Hornblum AM. They were cheap and available: prisoners as research subjects in twentieth century America. *BMJ.* 1997; 315:1437–41.
27. American Society of Hospital Pharmacists. ASHP guidelines for pharmaceutical research in organized health-care settings. *Am J Hosp Pharm.* 1989; 46:129–30.
28. 45 C.F.R. 4. www.hhs.gov/ohrp/policy/ohrpregulations.pdf (accessed 2015 Jun 2).
29. U.S. Department of Health and Human Services. The Belmont report: ethical principles and guidelines for the protection of human subjects of research (April 1979). www.hhs.gov/ohrp/policy/belmont.html (accessed 2015 Jul 2).
30. American Society of Health-System Pharmacists. ASHP statement on the pharmacist's role in clinical informatics. *Am J Health-Syst Pharm.* 2016; 73:410–3.
31. Leonhart M. Pharmacist's manual: an informational outline of the Controlled Substances Act of 1970. Washington, DC: Drug Enforcement Administration; 2010.
32. 45 C.F.R. 160, 164.
33. American Society of Health-System Pharmacists. ASHP guidelines on clinical drug research. *Am J Health-Syst Pharm.* 1998; 55:369–76.
34. American Society of Health-System Pharmacists. ASHP policy position 1531: pharmacist role in capital punishment. www.ashp.org/DocLibrary/BestPractices/EthicsPositions.aspx (accessed 2015 Sep 1).
35. American Society of Health-System Pharmacists. ASHP statement on the role of health-system pharmacists in public health. *Am J Health-Syst Pharm.* 2008; 65:462–7.
36. American Society of Health-System Pharmacists. ASHP statement on racial and ethnic disparities in health care. *Am J Health-Syst Pharm.* 2008; 65:728–33.
37. Bina C. Correctional pharmacy: public health challenges and opportunities. In: Truong H, Bressette J, Sellers J, eds. The pharmacist in public health, education, applications and opportunities. Washington, DC: American Pharmacists Association; 2010.

Approved by the ASHP Board of Directors on February 12, 2016, and developed through the Council on Pharmacy Practice. These guidelines supersede the ASHP Guidelines on Pharmacy Services in Correctional Facilities dated April 26, 1995.

The author has declared no potential conflicts of interest.

Quinn D. Bott, Pharm.D., CCHP, U.S. Public Health Service, United States Penitentiary/FPC Leavenworth, Leavenworth, KS.

ASHP gratefully acknowledges the following organizations and individuals for reviewing these guidelines (review does not imply endorsement): American Association of Pharmacy Technicians; American Pharmacists Association; Melissa Badowski, Pharm.D., BCPS, AAHIVP; Amanda Barner, Pharm.D., BCPS; Carol J. Bickford,

Ph.D., RN-BC, CPHIMS, FAAN; Timothy R. Brown, Pharm.D., BCACP, FASHP; Juliana Chan, Pharm.D., FCCP, BCACP; Steven J. Davis, Pharm.D., M.S.; Kathleen M. Gura, Pharm.D., BCNSP, FASHP; Matthew Keith, B.S.Pharm., BCPS, FASHP; Patricia C. Kienle, M.P.A., FASHP; Peter Lee, Pharm.D.; Robert C. Macky, Pharm.D.; Karen E. Malcolm, Pharm.D., BCACP, FASHP; Peggy Malovrh, Pharm.D.; Linda Gore Martin, Pharm.D., M.B.A., BCPS, FASHP; Ezra P. Mell, Pharm.D., MSE, BCPS; Julie A. Nelson, B.S., M.S., J.D.; Denise Nesbitt; B.S.Pharm.; Kathleen Pawlicki, B.S., M.S., FASHP; Barbara Petroff, M.S., FASHP; James Ponto, M.S., FASHP; James R. Rinehart, M.S., FASHP; Donald P. Rogers, Pharm.D., BCPS; Richard I. Sakai, Pharm.D., FASHP, FCSHP; Randy Vogenberg, Ph.D., FASHP; and Yvon Yeo, Pharm.D.

Copyright © 2016, American Society of Health-System Pharmacists, Inc. All rights reserved. Contact ASHP for reprint and permissions requests. This content may not be used for commercial purposes without the express written consent of ASHP.

The bibliographic citation for this document is as follows: American Society of Health-System Pharmacists. ASHP guidelines on pharmacy services in correctional facilities. *Am J Health-Syst Pharm.* 2016; 73:1784–90.

Research

DOI 10.37573/9781585287048

Research

2207

INSTITUTIONAL REVIEW BOARD AND INVESTIGATIONAL USE OF DRUGS

Source: Council on Pharmacy Practice

To support mandatory education and training on human subject protections and research bioethics for members of institutional review boards (IRBs), principal investigators, and all others involved in clinical research; further,

To advocate that principal investigators discuss their proposed clinical drug research with representatives of the pharmacy department before submitting a proposal to the IRB; further,

To advocate for the pharmacist's roles in ethical clinical research, including but not limited to serving as a principal investigator, developing protocols, executing research, determining rational-use decisions for the off-label use of drug products, and publishing research findings, and for adequately resourced, sustainable models for filling those roles; further,

To advocate that IRBs include pharmacists as voting members; further,

To advocate that IRBs inform pharmacy of all approved clinical research involving drugs within the hospital or health system; further,

To advocate that pharmacists act as liaisons between IRBs and pharmacy and therapeutics committees in the management and conduct of clinical drug research studies; further,

To support pharmacists' management of drug products used in clinical research.

This policy supersedes ASHP policy 0711.

Rationale

The Food and Drug Administration (FDA), under its regulations, defines an institutional review board (IRB) as a group of people that have been formally designated to review and monitor biomedical research involving human subjects. In accordance with FDA regulations, an IRB has the authority to approve, require modifications in (to secure approval), or disapprove research.

Human subjects research is codified in 45 CFR Section 46, and 45 CFR Section 46.102(e)(1) states that a human subject is:

a living individual about whom an investigator (whether professional or student) conducting research:

i. Obtains information or biospecimens through intervention or interaction with the individual, and uses, studies, or analyzes the information or biospecimens; or

ii. Obtains, uses, studies, analyzes, or generates identifiable private information or identifiable biospecimens.

Evidence-based healthcare decisions are highly dependent on sound principles of research and investigation. ASHP believes the healthcare workforce needs to be competent in understanding the research process and the protection of human subjects involved in research trials. In addition, hospitals and health systems are home to investigational drug services that support the conduct of clinical trials involving medication use. Pharmacists are critical to the successful management of these trials and therefore need to be engaged in decisions related to developing, conducting, and evaluating research within their institutions.

2243

ENROLLMENT OF UNDERREPRESENTED POPULATIONS IN CLINICAL TRIALS

Source: Council on Therapeutics

To support the enrollment of underrepresented populations in clinical trials; further,

To advocate that drug product manufacturers and researchers conduct and report outcomes of pharmacokinetic, pharmacodynamic, and pharmacogenomic research in underrepresented populations to facilitate safe and effective dosing of medications in these patient populations; further,

To advocate that if such research considers age, sex, gender, ethnicity, or race, the reason for such consideration be based on validated ethical or scientific reasons and be specified in the research protocol; further,

To foster the use and development of postmarketing research strategies to support the safe and effective use of drug products for approved and off-label indications in underrepresented populations; further,

To advocate that pharmacists should be involved in the design of clinical trials to provide guidance on drug dosing, administration, and monitoring in all patient populations.

This policy supersedes ASHP policy 1723.

Rationale

Pregnant patients, fetuses, neonates, children, members of racial or ethnic minority groups, the elderly, and transgender individuals are populations in which the pharmacokinetic, pharmacodynamic, and pharmacogenomic properties of medications may differ from those of people typically enrolled in clinical trials. These differences can dramatically alter the behavior of drugs, producing supra- or subtherapeutic levels, which may result in adverse effects. While there has been legislation that provides incentives for drug manufacturers to study these effects, many drugs already approved by the FDA do not have such information or robust outcomes reporting for these at-risk populations. The need for this guidance is supported by the complexity of dosing for these patients, which varies based on medication- and patient-specific characteristics. There is a paucity of research in these patient populations, which is similar to the lack of preapproval studies in obese patients. ASHP also encourages independent clinical and practice-based research in which pharmacists are involved in the study design to further define clinical use of medications in the treatment of these patients, as well as clinician reporting of patient experience via published articles and clinical registries.

1920

RESEARCH ON DRUG USE IN OBESE PATIENTS

Source: Council on Therapeutics

To encourage drug product manufacturers to conduct and publish pharmacokinetic and pharmacodynamic research in obese patients to facilitate safe and effective dosing of

DOI 10.37573/9781585287048.103

medications in this patient population, especially for medications most likely to be affected by obesity; further,

To encourage manufacturers to include in the Food and Drug Administration (FDA)–approved labeling detailed information on characteristics of individuals enrolled in drug dosing studies; further,

To advocate that the FDA develop guidance for the design and reporting of studies that support dosing recommendations in obese patients; further,

To advocate for increased enrollment and outcomes reporting of obese patients in clinical trials of medications; further,

To encourage independent research on the clinical significance of obesity on drug use, as well as the reporting and dissemination of this information via published literature, patient registries, and other mechanisms; further,

To recognize that pharmacists are medication therapy experts who should provide guidance on appropriate drug dosing for obese patients.

This policy supersedes ASHP policy 1515.

Rationale

Given the growing rate of obesity in the United States, ASHP is concerned about the uncertainty surrounding how obesity affects drug dosing, effectiveness, and safety, especially for medications most likely to be affected by obesity (defined as body mass index of >30 kg/m^2). The FDA does not require that studies of obese patient populations be performed, despite the growing proportion of obese patients in the United States. Obese patients are subject to variable pharmacokinetic effects of oral, parenteral, and topical therapeutic agents.

Drug product manufacturers should be encouraged to complete pharmacokinetic and pharmacodynamic dosing studies of obese patients, especially for drugs for which obesity is expected to have a significant clinical impact (e.g., antimicrobials, highly lipophilic drugs). If these voluntary studies are not completed, then manufacturers should include in the FDA-approved labeling complete information on the population enrolled in dosing studies and the methods used to determine dosing so that clinicians can assess the extent to which that population reflects patients being treated.

ASHP advocates that the FDA develop guidance for voluntary drug dosing studies of obese patients that would define study design and reporting with the intent of standardizing this research to the extent possible. The need for this guidance is supported by the complexity of drug dosing for obese patients, which varies based on drug and patient characteristics. A paucity of research in this population is noted, similar to the lack of preapproval studies in geriatric and pediatric patients. Such studies could help standardize research methods and promote comparative effectiveness research.

ASHP also encourages independent clinical and practice-based research to further define clinical use of drugs in the treatment of obese patients, as well as clinician reporting of patient experience in articles and clinical registries. ASHP also believes that pharmacists are uniquely positioned to review and apply this literature to make dosing recommendations based the most appropriate weight classification for obese patients, including ideal body weight, adjusted body weight, or total body weight.

1804

DRUG DOSING IN CONDITIONS THAT MODIFY PHARMACOKINETICS OR PHARMACODYNAMICS

Source: Council on Therapeutics

To encourage research on the pharmacokinetics and pharmacodynamics of drugs in acute and chronic conditions; further,

To advocate healthcare provider education and training that facilitate optimal patient-specific dosing in populations of patients with altered pharmacokinetics and pharmacodynamics; further,

To support development and use of standardized models, laboratory assessment, genomic testing, utilization biomarkers, and electronic health record documentation of pharmacokinetic and pharmacodynamic changes in acute and chronic conditions; further,

To collaborate with stakeholders in enhancing aggregation and publication of and access to data on the effects of such pharmacokinetic and pharmacodynamic changes on drug dosing within these patient populations.

This policy supersedes ASHP policy 1720.

This policy was reviewed in 2023 by the Council on Therapeutics and by the Board of Directors and was found to still be appropriate.

Rationale

The pharmacokinetic and pharmacodynamic properties of drugs found in drug information monographs are based on the drug's absorption, distribution, metabolism, and excretion in healthy, adult patients during Phase I of a drug's clinical trials. Many patients receiving drug therapy do not fit this profile, and many have compromised organ function. The medical community has long recognized the need for a standardized approach to evaluating organ system dysfunction. Although there are methods to determine organ function (e.g., the Cockcroft-Gault equation for renal function or the Child-Turcotte-Pugh Classification for Severity of Cirrhosis), there is debate as to whether these methods are true indicators of organ function, as the components that comprise these equations may fluctuate based on severity and patient status. Traditional laboratory values used to evaluate organ dysfunction can be bidirectional and conflicting as well.

In addition, with the exception of adjustments for renal dysfunction, there is not much information regarding dosage adjustment for specific drugs. Many organ systems are involved in a drug's absorption, distribution, metabolism, and excretion. Hepatic effects, for example, are a risk area, as those effects are slower to be seen and have not been the subject of much research, and the number of drugs affected are smaller in number than renally excreted drugs. Both acute and chronic aspects of patient conditions may require monitoring and adjustment, including sepsis, encephalopathies, pregnancy, heart failure exacerbations, and cystic fibrosis. Certain protocols, such as therapeutic hypothermia, can also have clinically significant impact on a drug's pharmacokinetic and pharmacodynamic behavior. There is also need to promote research and utilization of biomarkers into practice, as these may reflect organ function and may provide pharmacists with a more complete clinical picture.

Given the complex dose adjustments and variety of conditions, education of pharmacists and other healthcare professionals is critically important to appropriately treat patients.

ASHP Statement on Pharmaceutical Research in Organized Health-Care Settings

Pharmacy practice is grounded in the physicochemical, biological, and socioeconomic sciences. Hence, the continued and future success and self-esteem of the profession are dependent on the expanded knowledge base that can be produced through dynamic and rigorous scientific research and development. This research, to be meaningful and productive in terms of pharmacy's needs and goals in organized health-care settings, must include the participation of pharmacists practicing in those settings.

Pharmacists in organized health-care settings function in cooperation with other health-care professionals. They contribute a unique expertise to the drug-related aspects of patient care and take personal professional responsibility for the outcomes from the pharmaceutical care they provide to patients. Improvements in drug therapy depend on new knowledge generated by scientific research. Thus, pharmacists in organized health-care settings have a professional obligation to participate actively in and increase pharmacy-related and drug-related research efforts.[1,2]

Reflecting the collaborative nature of contemporary health care, this research should be multidisciplinary to be most beneficial. Thus, ASHP encourages pharmacists with a researchable idea or problem to seek the advice and active participation of people and organizations with scientific expertise such as

- College faculty (especially college of pharmacy faculty).
- Other staff and departments within the setting.
- Staff and departments in other health-care organizations.
- Industrial research personnel and laboratories.

It also is appropriate for pharmacists to function as principal investigators in research projects.

ASHP encourages pharmacists to increase their involvement in the following kinds of scientific research and development:

- Pharmaceutical research, including the development and testing of new drug dosage forms and drug preparation and administration methods and systems.
- Clinical research, such as the therapeutic characterization, evaluation, comparison, and outcomes of drug therapy and drug treatment regimens.
- Health services research and development, including behavioral and socioeconomic research such as research on cost–benefit issues in pharmaceutical care.
- Operations research, such as time and motion studies and evaluation of new and existing pharmacy programs and services.

This research will be a critical contribution of pharmacy to health care and must be fostered by all facets of the profession.

References

1. American Society of Hospital Pharmacists. ASHP guidelines for pharmaceutical research in organized healthcare settings. *Am J Hosp Pharm.* 1989; 46:129–30.
2. American Society of Hospital Pharmacists. ASHP guidelines for the use of investigational drugs in organized healthcare settings. *Am J Hosp Pharm.* 1991; 48:315–9.

Approved by the ASHP Board of Directors, November 14, 1990, and the ASHP House of Delegates, June 3, 1991. Revised by the ASHP Council on Professional Affairs. Supersedes a previous statement, "ASHP Statement on Institutional Pharmacy Research," approved by the ASHP House of Delegates on June 3, 1985, and the ASHP Board of Directors on November 14–15, 1984.

Copyright © 1991, American Society of Hospital Pharmacists, Inc. All rights reserved. Contact ASHP for reprint and permissions requests. This content may not be used for commercial purposes without the express written consent of ASHP.

The bibliographic citation for this document is as follows: American Society of Hospital Pharmacists. ASHP statement on pharmaceutical research in organized health-care settings. *Am J Hosp Pharm.* 1991; 48:1781.

DOI 10.37573/9781585287048.104

ASHP Guidelines on Clinical Drug Research

Purpose

The use of drug products to manage diseases and improve patients' quality of life is increasing as more effective and safer agents become available. Research to develop these agents is occurring in health system practice settings throughout the world. The credibility of this research and the protection of human subjects is a major responsibility of all health professionals involved.

ASHP believes pharmacists should play a pivotal role in the management of drugs used in the conduct of clinical research.[1-3] Pharmacists have become essential components of health system infrastructures supporting clinical research with both approved drugs and investigational drugs.[a,b] Pharmacists' roles in clinical research generally fall into one of two categories: (1) drug storage, preparation, and record keeping, frequently through an investigational drug service, and (2) serving as a principal investigator or a subinvestigator, manager, or coordinator within a research team that may include other health care professionals, research sponsors, monitors, contract research organizations, institutional review boards (IRBs), and institutional administrators.

The purposes of this document are to (1) outline the principles of clinical research, (2) describe the roles of participants in clinical research, (3) define pharmacists' roles in the use of drugs in clinical research, and (4) provide guidance to pharmacists and others responsible for the medication management component of clinical research. ASHP believes these guidelines are applicable to clinical research conducted in any health-system practice setting. These guidelines are an interpretation of federal laws, regulations, and standards for pharmacy practice in health systems. They should be used in conjunction with the applicable federal and state laws and regulations, not as a substitute for them. This document uses the term *shall* when the content is based on law or regulation and the term *should* for advice based on other guidelines, professional judgment, or expert opinion.

Background

The United States has benefited from a system for researching and marketing drug products that is codified in federal and state laws and regulations. The federal Food, Drug, and Cosmetic Act and its amendments[4] regulate drug product quality, safety, and effectiveness. The Food and Drug Administration (FDA) is the federal agency charged with enforcing the act and promulgating regulations for its implementation. FDA regulations concerning the conduct of clinical research with drug products of particular relevance for health-system pharmacists include Title 21 Code of Federal Regulations (CFR) Part 50, Protection of Human Subjects; Title 21 CFR Part 56, Institutional Review Boards; and Title 21 CFR Part 312, Investigational New Drug Application. Also applicable are the Department of Health and Human Services regulations in Title 45 CFR Part 46, Protection of Human Subjects. Requirements for and guidance on compliance with regulations are provided in FDA Information Sheets.

FDA has also published the Good Clinical Practice Consolidated Guideline[5] that was prepared under the auspices of the International Conference on Harmonisation of Technical Requirements for Registration of Pharmaceuticals for Human Use. The guideline offers a unified standard for designing, conducting, recording, and reporting trials that involve the participation of human subjects in the United States, Japan, and the European Union. In particular, the guideline provides a clearer understanding of behavioral and compliance standards for regulated drug research.

Basic Principles

The institutional components and practice settings of health systems participating in clinical drug research shall develop mechanisms, generally in the form of policies and procedures, for the approval, planning, and implementation of protocols. Good clinical practices, consistent with national and international standards, are the cornerstone of drug research in humans. Principles consistent with good clinical practices include the following:

1. An organization participating in human drug research studies shall ensure that such studies contain adequate safeguards for human subjects, its staff, and the scientific integrity of the study. There shall be written policies and procedures for the approval, management, and control of research involving investigational (not FDA-approved) drugs and post-marketing studies of FDA-approved drugs used in a research protocol. All research team members shall be fully informed about and comply with these policies and procedures.
2. The clinical trial shall have adequate prior information to justify use of human subjects, have a clearly defined protocol, and have received IRB approval before implementation.
3. All drug studies shall meet accepted ethical, legal, and scientific standards and be conducted by appropriately qualified investigators. Investigator qualifications, such as prior training and experience in research and with certain disease states, are required to be reviewed by IRBs, study sponsors, and FDA if the research will be submitted under an investigational new drug application (IND).
4. Every member of the research team shall be qualified by experience or training to perform his or her respective role.
5. All subjects must freely provide informed consent (documented in writing) before treatment with study drugs is begun. Accurate and complete information about the study's objectives, risks, and benefits must be provided before consent is obtained from the subject or his or her legally authorized representative. No unreasonable inducements (i.e., coercion or undue influence) shall be offered to subjects to encourage their participation in the study.
6. All clinical trial data shall be recorded and the records stored in such a way that the subject's rights of privacy and confidentiality are protected. All records shall be

DOI 10.37573/9781585287048.105

managed in a way that permits accurate reporting, verification, and retrieval after archiving.

7. Qualified pharmacists and other nonphysicians may serve as principal investigators as long as medical decisions made for the subjects are always the responsibility of a qualified physician or dentist.

Health-System Organization and Oversight

The health system should have processes for the administration of research that ensure that the aforementioned principles are upheld and the following responsibilities are met.

1. The health system shall be able to review and approve a protocol in the context of federal, state, and local laws and regulations. The health system should consider whether its own sponsored research or intellectual property development of drugs requires an IND for drugs not commercially available and approved drugs for unlabeled uses. An IND may be required if proposed research on the use of a marketed drug is intended to support the sponsor's change in drug labeling, advertising, or indications for use; a significant increase in risk; or a change in dosage level or route of administration. The health system should consult FDA for guidance.
2. The health system should have a mechanism for review and approval of the financial aspects of drug research, whether the study is sponsored by government agencies, foundations, or the pharmaceutical industry or is not sponsored.[6] Financial aspects may include contractual agreements stipulating cost recovery for resources, intellectual property agreements, insurance provisions, indemnification terms, and conflict-of-interest statements. Cost identification, allocation, and recovery mechanisms are imperative items for review and approval.
3. As required by federal regulation, clinical research shall be reviewed and approved by an IRB or equivalent committee (21 CFR 56.109). This committee shall evaluate each proposed clinical research study in terms of human subject protections and compliance with recognized ethical, legal, and scientific standards. No clinical study may be initiated unless approved in writing by the committee. Spoken IRB approval may be granted in emergency situations for a single subject's access to an investigational drug, but emergency use shall be reported to the IRB within five days; subsequent use requires full IRB review. Studies on the use of drugs in emergency or critical care settings do not in themselves qualify for single-subject approval and emergency exemption. Specific regulations govern research in the emergency setting and should be consulted in preparing protocols, IRB submissions, and consent procedures.[c,7]

   Treatment IND protocols are also subject to IRB review and approval. These protocols permit patient access to investigational drugs through a special program established by a sponsor. The physician and patient must agree that use of the agent may be in the patient's best interest and must document this agreement on a consent form.

   The IRB shall monitor approved studies to ensure that they are carried out appropriately and that the protocols are reassessed at least annually. Health system policies and procedures shall provide guidance on the conversion of human subjects to other therapies in the event that approval of an existing protocol is withdrawn by the IRB. The investigational-drug pharmacist, pharmacy director, or pharmacy director's designee should be a member of the IRB and should be consulted by the committee whenever drug studies are reviewed.
4. Investigational drugs shall be used only under the supervision of the principal investigator or authorized subinvestigators, all of whom shall be members of the professional staff. The determination of qualifications for investigators is the responsibility of the sponsor, IRB, and FDA when appropriate. Properly qualified pharmacists with experience and training in research may serve as principal investigators or subinvestigators.
5. The principal investigator or designee is responsible for obtaining informed consent from each subject who is eligible for participation in the study (i.e., meets inclusion and exclusion criteria).[c] The informed consent process shall conform to current federal and state regulations. IRB approval of the consent form (and assent form for minors) is required. Review by legal counsel may be desirable. The following points shall be included in the consent document and in an accompanying oral explanation by the investigator:
   a. That the trial involves research.
   b. The nature and purpose of the study and its expected benefits and foreseeable risks or discomforts. The name and telephone number of the principal investigator and persons to contact for questions about the study or drug.
   c. A balanced description of the alternative treatments available, including their respective risks and benefits.
   d. A general description of the study procedures, identification of any procedures that are experimental, expected length of therapy with the drug, and the subject's responsibilities. The name(s) of the investigational drug(s), including brand and generic names of commercial products.
   e. A statement that (1) participation is voluntary, (2) the subject may withdraw from the study at any time, (3) refusal to participate in or withdrawal from the study will involve no penalty or loss of benefits to which the subject is otherwise entitled, and (4) the principal investigator may remove the subject from the study if circumstances warrant. The investigator shall supply any new information that may affect a subject's desire to continue in a study.
   f. The name and signature of the subject (or his or her legally authorized representative), the name and signature of the principal investigator or subinvestigator, and the name and signature of the person presenting the consent form, with lines for each to personally date the signature.
   g. A statement of who will have access to any study records that contain subject identifiers, including monitoring personnel from the study sponsor or FDA who may inspect the records to assess

compliance with the study protocol and all regulations, or institutional personnel auditing the quality of clinical research or financial transactions.

h. Compensation or treatment available for a research-related injury.

i. Anticipated payments to subjects, pro rata terms, or expenses subjects may incur. Any costs for which the subject will be responsible.

The consent form shall be as detailed as is practical, with the goal of minimizing the amount of in-formation that must be presented orally yet enabling comprehension by most persons reading the form. For non-English-speaking subjects the consent form shall be in the subject's own language when feasible, or adequate interpretation shall be provided. For children able to read, an assent form shall be used to document their participation in the research process. The subject (or his or her representative) must have adequate time to read the consent form before signing it and shall receive a copy of the signed and dated form, along with any amendments to it. The subject shall retain a copy of the consent form. Additional copies of the consent form shall be kept on file as required by the sponsor, the IRB, the individual health system, and the medical records department.

Under certain protocols, patient drug or medical information may be collected from existing medical or pharmacy records. Pharmacists and investigators should consult the IRB to determine protocol-review and informed-consent requirements for any proposed studies.

6. The principal investigator is responsible for the proper maintenance of case report forms and all other study records required by the health system, the sponsor, and FDA.

7. The health system's medication-use system shall contain the following elements concerning drugs used in clinical research:

   a. Drugs shall be properly packaged in accordance with all applicable federal and state laws, regulations, and standards (e.g., FDA, *The United States Pharmacopeia and The National Formulary* [*USP–NF*], and the Poison Prevention Packaging Act).

   b. Drugs shall be labeled properly to ensure their safe use by the research and institutional staff and the subject.

   c. There shall be a mechanism to ensure that sufficient supplies of the drugs will be always available for the duration of the study.

   d. A mechanism shall be in place to allow the pharmacist or other designated health care provider, in a medical emergency during a randomized and blinded trial, to break the blinding code and reveal the identity of the study drug to other health care professionals. A reason to break the blind might be the need for a treatment decision that can be made only with knowledge of drug assignment.

   e. Nurses, pharmacists, physicians, and other health care practitioners (e.g., respiratory therapists, physician assistants) called on to administer or dispense investigational drugs should have adequate written information about (1) pharmacology (particularly adverse effects), (2) storage requirements, (3) method of dose preparation and administration, (4) disposal of unused drug, (5) precautions to be taken, including handling recommendations, (6) authorized prescribers, (7) human subject safety monitoring guidelines, and (8) any other material pertinent to safe and proper use of investigational drugs. These health care providers should be informed about the overall study objectives and procedures and shall have available a complete copy of the protocol for reference. Under all circumstances, investigational drugs shall be safely controlled, administered, and destroyed.

   f. Bulk supplies of the investigational drug shall be properly stored and adequately secured. When practical, all bulk supplies shall be stored in the pharmacy to ensure that storage, dispensing, accountability, and security are in compliance with federal and state laws and regulations and with standards used by the pharmacy department.

   g. There shall be a method for ensuring that only an authorized practitioner or designee prescribes the investigational drug.

   h. Records of the amount of investigational drug received from the sponsor and of its disposition (e.g., amounts dispensed to subjects or returned to sponsor) shall be maintained. These records shall be retained as required by regulation. Generally, records shall be maintained for at least two years after the date of an approved new-drug application (NDA) for the indication that is being investigated or, if the application is not approved or no application is filed, for at least two years after the investigation is discontinued and FDA is notified. Institutions should consider retaining records indefinitely. For studies involving international sites, records shall be maintained for 15 years after study closure. The sponsor may also request that records be stored longer than the minimum required time.

   i. If the subject is to receive the investigational drug at another facility, suitable arrangements shall be made for transfer of the drug. Sufficient information for safe use of the investigational drug, including copies of the subject's signed consent form, the study protocol, and the IRB approval letter, shall accompany the drug. The responsibilities of the facility to which the drug is transferred are based on whether that facility is providing care incidental to or as a participant in the research protocol.[8]

   j. The institution's records on investigational-drug studies should be designed so that various descriptive reports (e.g., names of all drugs under study, names of subjects who have received a given drug) can be generated conveniently and expeditiously. Once a study is closed, a copy of all pharmacy-related records should be provided to the principal investi-gator for storage. For its own records, the pharmacy should have a mechanism for long-term storage. The drug control responsibilities previously described shall be assigned to a pharmacist. If a pharmacist is not available, the investigator shall make arrangements to comply with these standards.

Pharmaceutical Services

A pharmacist should be responsible for ensuring that procedures for the control of drugs used in clinical research are developed and implemented. Each health system should develop a structure and procedures specific to its own needs and organization.

1. A copy of the IRB-approved research protocol and investigator's brochure or drug data sheet (see item 2 below), or both, and all amendments should be kept by a pharmacist.
2. Using the protocol and additional information (if needed) supplied by the principal investigator and sponsor, the pharmacist should prepare an investigational-drug data sheet that concisely summarizes for the medical, nursing, and pharmacy staffs information pertinent to use of the drug. This communication should contain, at a minimum
   a. Drug designation and common synonyms.
   b. Dosage forms and strengths.
   c. Usual dosage range, including dosage schedule and route of administration.
   d. Indications pursued in this study.
   e. Expected therapeutic effect to be studied.
   f. Expected and potential adverse effects, including symptoms of toxicity and their treatment.
   g. Drug–drug and drug–food interactions.
   h. Contraindications.
   i. Storage requirements.
   j. Instructions for dosage preparation and administration, including stability and handling guidelines.
   k. Instructions for disposition of unused doses.
   l. Names and telephone numbers of principal and authorized subinvestigators and study coordinators.

   Confidential copies should be distributed to the appropriate pharmacy staff and all areas within the health system where the investigational drug will be administered and the subjects monitored. Through the pharmacy or health-system computer system, this information can be made available to all staff members who need it. It is staff members' responsibility to become familiar with the information in these data sheets and to not share the information with persons who do not need it.
3. When it is practical, investigational-drug supplies should be stored in a pharmacy. When the drug is stored outside a pharmacy (e.g., small quantities in the investigator's office or in clinics where the drug is administered), methods used by the investigator responsible for the drug shall be audited by a pharmacist to ensure that storage, dispensing, accountability, and security comply with federal and state laws and regulations and with institutional policy.
4. The pharmacist shall maintain a perpetual inventory record for investigational drugs stored in the pharmacy. This record shall contain the drug's name, dosage form and strength, lot number, and expiration date; the name, address, and telephone number of the sponsor; the protocol number; and any other information needed for ordering the drug. Space shall be provided for recording data on the disposition of the drug (amounts received, transferred, wasted, or dispensed, with dates; the names of or codes for persons receiving the drug; and the names of prescribers), the amount currently on hand, the minimum reorder level, and the recorder's initials. The inventory record shall reflect drug doses that were dispensed but not administered and were returned to the pharmacist. These records are commonly audited by the sponsor, the sponsor's representatives, or FDA.[9,10]
5. The dispensing of investigational drugs should be integrated with the rest of the medication-use system, including, but not limited to, order review, profile maintenance, packaging, labeling, delivery, and quality-assurance procedures. However, prescription labels for investigational drugs shall be marked "investigational drug" or otherwise distinguished from other labels. The label should also include an alert to any possible hazards. There shall be a method for verifying that a valid, signed consent has been obtained. The investigational drug shall be dispensed only on the order of an authorized investigator or designee.
6. Educating patients and monitoring therapy (including adverse drug reaction monitoring) are two clinical functions that are particularly important and applicable to investigational drugs. The protocol should specify the provision of these functions by the pharmacists, the authorized investigator(s), and other members of the research team.
7. At the conclusion of the study, the pharmacist shall return, transfer, or dispose of all unused investigational drugs according to the specific instructions provided by the sponsor and in accordance with applicable regulations.
8. The pharmacist should prepare an annual or semiannual descriptive summary of investigational-drug use for the pharmacy director and pharmacy and therapeutics committee. This summary should include the number of studies in progress, a list of all drugs studied during the previous period, and a financial statement.
9. Drug costs and other expenses associated with drug studies (e.g., costs of record keeping and drug administration) should be properly allocated and reimbursed. Policies and procedures should address the role pharmacists play in billing sponsors, subjects, and third-party payers for services and goods related to research. In general, sponsors and health systems cannot charge subjects for an investigational drug. Sponsors may petition FDA for an exception. Health systems may charge subjects for drug preparation and other services necessary to deliver a final product, as is customary for delivery of services within the practice setting and when sponsors do not reimburse for this service. The anticipated costs of research should be described in

the consent form. Subjects must be advised that they or their third-party payers are responsible for these charges and that a third-party payer may refuse to pay for charges related to research.

10. The investigational drugs shall be stored under appropriate environmental control in a limited-access area separate from routine drug stocks and shall be inventoried on a regular basis.
11. Pharmacists may be confronted with circumstances related to a patient who is receiving an investigational drug provided by an investigator at a nonaffiliated practice setting and is admitted to their own practice setting for care incidental to the research protocol. Pharmacists should have a policy for managing investigational drugs under those circumstances that meets FDA guidelines.[8]
12. Pharmacists must ensure the scientific integrity of drug studies by managing access to treatment-assignment records in blinded studies and by ensuring that the correct drug was dispensed. The pharmacist, investigator, and sponsor must agree on a procedure for unblinding treatment assignment in emergencies.
13. Pharmacists who are assigned to manage investigational drugs may at times have to delegate certain dispensing activities to other pharmacists within the health system. To ensure continuity of quality dispensing services, the responsible pharmacist should design and implement procedures for educating other members of the pharmacy staff about the protocol and dispensing requirements. Often this can be accomplished by personal instruction and by preparing written directives and references for use by other pharmacists when they are called upon to dispense an investigational drug.
14. Pharmacists managing investigational drugs are in a unique position to monitor patient adherence to medication regimens. Because of the requirement that medication dispensed and returned be accounted for, pharmacists can readily surmise whether study pa-tients are consuming the medication in the prescribed man ner. At a minimum, pharmacists should counsel the investigator's research staff with regard to patient adherence. Pharmacists' skills in patient counseling should be used to support the investigators' efforts to encourage patients to adhere to their protocols.

Pharmaceutical Research Sponsors, Monitors, and Contract Research Organizations

The pharmaceutical company, or any study sponsor, that supports the use of investigational drugs in health systems should receive reliable and valid data. The following recommendations will serve as a guide to the pharmaceutical industry or other study sponsors to ensure that investigational drug use is managed appropriately and that studies are conducted effectively, efficiently, and safely.

1. Drugs shall be properly packaged in accordance with all applicable federal and state laws, regulations, and standards (e.g., FDA, *USP–NF*, and the Poison Prevention Packaging Act).
2. Drugs shall be properly labeled in accordance with applicable laws, regulations, and standards. If possible, ample space shall be left on the drug product container for further labeling by the pharmacist. Expiration dates and lot numbers should also be noted on the label.
3. A 24-hour telephone number should be available to study personnel, including the principal investigator and the pharmacy department. In the event of an emergency, information should be available pertaining to (1) adverse effects and their treatment, (2) emergency protocol management and dosing and administration guidelines, (3) the ability to break a "blinded code" to determine the treatment regimen, and (4) the mechanism for procuring a supply of medication under an emergency-use protocol.
4. Company representatives should be designated to handle routine requests, such as those for additional forms and resupply of investigational drugs. If possible, direct telephone or fax access should be available to expedite requests.
5. Investigational drugs should be shipped to the principal investigator in care of a pharmacist. The following information about procurement should also be supplied to the pharmacist:
   a. Name and telephone number of the sponsor's study monitor or field representative responsible for drug ordering.
   b. Estimated time for fulfillment of orders.
   c. Limits on quantities that can be ordered.
   d. Special ordering instructions.
   e. How the order is to be shipped (e.g., specific package-shipping firms).
   f. Disposition of invoice or drug receipt form once the drug is received.
6. The following information should be supplied by a sponsor or investigator to the pharmacist, preferably in an investigator's brochure, as applicable:
   a. Storage conditions required before and after preparation.
   b. Amounts and types of diluents for reconstitution and administration and the resulting final concentration of active drug.
   c. Stability of the prepared (i.e., ready-to-administer, reconstituted, or diluted) product and compatibility with drug delivery systems, diluents or i.v. fluids, containers, i.v. tubing, and filters.
   d. Known compatibility or incompatibility with other products.
   e. Light sensitivity.
   f. Filtration needs.
   g. Expiration dates or retest dates.
   h. Special instructions for preparation and admin-istration.
   i. Acceptable and recommended routes and methods of administration, including rates of infusion for injectable products.
   j. Known adverse effects during or after administration (e.g., pain, phlebitis, and nausea) and how to avoid and treat them.
   k. Usual dosage regimens and highest dose tested for specific disease states, including dosage

expressions for prescribing and labeling that could minimize misreading and misinterpretation.

- **l.** Contraindications.
- **m.** Drug interactions.
- **n.** Special precautions for storage, handling, and disposal of the drugs, including cytotoxic and hazardous drugs. For all hazardous drugs, the pharmacy department must be supplied with material safety data sheets.
- **o.** Pharmacology, including mechanism of action.
- **p.** Pharmacokinetic characteristics.

7. If all unused drugs are to be returned to the sponsor, information regarding storage and return procedures should be provided to the pharmacist. Drugs that are contaminated, outdated, or otherwise unsuitable should be returned to the sponsor or destroyed according to the institution's policies and procedures and applicable laws and regulations. These options should be agreed on beforehand by the sponsor and the pharmacist.

8. A complete current copy of the research protocol and investigator's brochure should be supplied to the pharmacist. Additional educational materials for use in informing pharmacists, physicians, and nurses about the investigational drug and research protocol should also be provided.

9. An appropriate allotment of research funds should be designated as reimbursement for

- **a.** Personnel.
- **b.** Storage facilities.
- **c.** Equipment.
- **d.** Ancillary products, such as diluents, syringes, and needles.
- **e.** Forms and miscellaneous clerical materials.
- **f.** Computer and other data-processing costs.
- **g.** Other expenses attributable to the pharmacist's involvement in the study.
- **h.** Apportioned pharmacy overhead costs.

10. Sponsors should respond to requests for information from pharmacists involved in treating patients without formal research approval at that institution. This may occur, for example, when a patient is hospitalized (e.g., in an emergency) at a facility other than his or her usual care site.

11. When seeking marketing approval for an investigational drug, sponsors should consult pharmacists, physicians, and others involved in their investigational-drug studies for information. Because of their experience with the drug, these practitioners can supply valuable suggestions for labeling, packaging, palatability, routes of administration, and other dosage form characteristics, as well as information regarding patient monitoring and education.

12. The sponsor of an investigational drug study should provide final closure details within six months of trial completion. This includes prompt notification of closure, directions for drug disposition, and final audits of all study records.

13. These recommendations should also apply to the post-marketing approval of drugs under study for new indications or diseases.

References

1. Stolar MH, ed. Pharmacy-coordinated investigational drug services. Revised ed. Bethesda, MD: American Society of Hospital Pharmacists; 1986.
2. American Society of Health-System Pharmacists. ASHP guidelines: minimum standard for pharmacies in hospitals. *Am J Health-Syst Pharm.* 1995; 52:2711–7.
3. American Society of Hospital Pharmacists. ASHP statement on the use of medications for unlabeled uses. *Am J Hosp Pharm.* 1992; 49:2006–8.
4. Federal Food, Drug, and Cosmetic Act (21 U.S.C. 301 et seq.) 1938, as amended.
5. Food and Drug Administration, Department of Health and Human Services. International conference on harmonisation; good clinical practice consolidated guideline. *Fed Regist.* 1997; 62:25692–709.
6. Wermeling DP, Piecoro LT, Foster TS. Financial impact of clinical research on a health system. *Am J Health-Syst Pharm.* 1997; 54:1742–51.
7. Bailey EM, Habowski SR. How to apply for emergency use of an investigational agent. *Am J Health-Syst Pharm.* 1996; 53:208–10.
8. Food and Drug Administration. Use of investigational products when subjects enter a second institution. IRB operations and clinical investigation information sheet. http://www.fda.gov/oc/oha/useofinv.html (accessed August 25, 1997).
9. Food and Drug Administration. Institutional review board inspections. IRB operations and clinical investigation information sheet. http://ww.fda.gov/oc/oha/institut.html (accessed August 25, 1997).
10. Food and Drug Administration. Inspections of clinical investigators. IRB operations and clinical investigation information sheet. http://ww.fda.gov/oc/oha/inspect.html (accessed August 25, 1997).

Suggested Internet Source

Food and Drug Administration information for clinical investigators. http://www.fda.gov/cder/about/smallbiz/clinical_investigator.htm.

Glossary[d]

Adverse drug reaction (ADR): In preapproval clinical experience with a new medicinal product or its new usages, particularly since the therapeutic dose(s) may not be established, all noxious and unintended responses to a medicinal product related to any dose should be considered adverse drug reactions. "Responses to a medicinal product" means that a causal relationship between a medicinal product and an adverse event is at least a reasonable possibility (i.e., that the relationship cannot be ruled out).

An ADR to a marketed medicinal product is a response to a drug that is noxious and unintended and that occurs at doses normally used in humans for prophylaxis, diagnosis, or therapy of diseases or for modification of physiological function.

Adverse event (AE): An AE is any untoward medical event that occurs in a patient or clinical investigation subject administered a pharmaceutical product and that does not necessarily have a causal relationship to this treatment. An AE can therefore be any unfavorable and unintended sign (including an abnormal laboratory finding), symptom, or disease temporally associated with the use of a medicinal (investigational) product, whether or not related to the medicinal (investigational) product.

Audit: A systematic and independent examination of trial-related activities and documents to determine whether the evaluated trial-related activities were conducted and the data were recorded, analyzed, and accurately reported according to the protocol, sponsor's standard operating procedures, good clinical practice, and the applicable regulatory requirements.

Audit report: A written evaluation by the sponsor's auditor of the results of the audit.

Case report form: A printed, optical, or electronic document designed to record all of the protocol-required information to be reported to the sponsor on each trial subject.

Clinical trial or study: Any investigation in human subjects that is intended to discover or verify the clinical, pharmacologic, or other pharmacodynamic effects of an investigational product, to identify any adverse reactions to an investigational product, or to study absorption, distribution, metabolism, and excretion of an investigational product with the object of ascertaining its safety, efficacy, or both. (The terms clinical trial and clinical study are synonymous.)

Clinical trial/study report: A written description of a trial or study of any therapeutic, prophylactic, or diagnostic agent conducted in humans, in which the clinical and statistical description, presentations, and analyses are fully integrated into a single report.

Contract research organization: A person or organization (commercial, academic, or other) contracted by the sponsor to perform one or more of a sponsor's trial-related duties and functions.

Direct access: Permission to examine, analyze, verify, and reproduce any records and reports that are important in the evaluation of a clinical trial. Any party (e.g., domestic and foreign regulatory authorities, sponsors, monitors, and auditors) with direct access should take all reasonable precautions within the constraints of the applicable regulatory requirements to maintain the confidentiality of subjects' identities and sponsors' proprietary information.

Documentation: All records, in any form (including but not limited to written, electronic, magnetic, and optical records and scans, roentgenograms, and electrocardiograms) that describe or record the methods, conduct, or results of a trial, the factors affecting a trial, and the actions taken.

Essential documents: Documents that individually and collectively permit evaluation of the conduct of a study and the quality of the data produced.

Good clinical practice: A standard for the design, conduct, performance, monitoring, auditing, recording, analysis, and reporting of clinical trials that provides assurance that the data and reported results are credible and accurate and that the rights, integrity, and confidentiality of trial subjects are protected.

Independent ethics committee: An independent body (institutional, regional, national, or supranational review board or committee), constituted of medical or scientific professionals and nonmedical or nonscientific members, whose responsibility it is to ensure the protection of the rights, safety, and well-being of human subjects involved in a trial and to provide public assurance of that protection by, among other things, reviewing and approving or providing favorable opinion on the trial protocol and the suitability of the investigators, the facilities, and the methods and material to be used in obtaining and documenting informed consent of the trial subjects.

Informed consent: A process by which a subject voluntarily confirms his or her willingness to participate in a particular trial, after having been informed of all aspects of the trial that are relevant to the decision to participate. Informed consent is documented by means of a written, signed, and dated form.

Investigator's brochure: A compilation of clinical and nonclinical data on an investigational product that are relevant to the study of the product in human subjects.

Monitoring: Overseeing the progress of a clinical trial and ensuring that it is conducted, recorded, and reported in accordance with the protocol, standard operating procedures, good clinical practice, and the applicable regulatory requirements.

Monitoring report: A written report from the monitor to the sponsor after each site visit or other trial-related communication, according to the sponsor's standard operating procedures.

Protocol: A document that describes the objectives, design, methods, statistical considerations, and organization of a trial. The protocol usually also gives the background and rationale for the trial, but these could be provided in other protocol-referenced documents. (Throughout the ICH GCP Guideline, the term protocol refers to protocol and protocol amendments.)

Serious adverse event or serious adverse drug reaction: Any untoward medical event that occurs in a patient or subject receiving a drug at any dose and results in death, is life-threatening, requires inpatient hospitalization or prolongation of existing hospitalization, results in persistent or significant disability or incapacity, or is a congenital anomaly or birth defect.

Source data: All information in original records and certified copies of original records of clinical findings, observations, or other activities in a clinical trial that is necessary for the reconstruction and evaluation of the trial. Source data are contained in source documents (original records or certified copies).

Source documents: Original documents, data, and records (e.g., hospital records, clinical and office charts, laboratory notes, memoranda, subjects' diaries or evaluation checklists, pharmacy dispensing records, recorded data from automated instruments, copies or transcriptions certified after verification as being accurate and complete, microfiches, photographic negatives, microfilm or magnetic media, roentgenograms, and subject files and records kept at the pharmacy, the laboratories, and the medicotechnical departments involved in the clinical trial).

Sponsor: An individual, a company, an institution, or an organization that takes responsibility for the initiation, management, or financing of a clinical trial.

Sponsor–investigator: An individual who both initiates and conducts, alone or with others, a clinical trial, and under whose immediate direction the investigational product is administered to, dispensed to, or used by a subject. The term does not include any person other than an individual (e.g., it does not include a corporation or an agency). The obligations of a sponsor-investigator include both those of a sponsor and those of an investigator.

---

[a]In this document investigational drugs are defined as those that are being considered for but have not yet received marketing approval by FDA for human use and those that have FDA approval for at least one indication but are being studied for new indications, new routes of administration, or new dosage forms.

[b]The principles and procedures described here are applicable to all clinical drug studies, not just those involving investigational drugs.

[c]In certain emergency situations, prior consent may be waived (21 CFR 50.24).

[d]Definitions selected from reference 5.

These guidelines were reviewed in 2003 by the Council on Professional Affairs and by the Board of Directors and were found to still be appropriate.

Approved by the ASHP Board of Directors, November 15, 1997. Developed by the ASHP Council on Professional Affairs. Supersedes the ASHP Guidelines for the Use of Investigational Drugs in Organized Health-Care Settings, dated November 14, 1990.

Copyright © 1998, American Society of Health-System Pharmacists, Inc. All rights reserved. Contact ASHP for reprint and permissions requests. This content may not be used for commercial purposes without the express written consent of ASHP.

The bibliographic citation for this document is as follows: American Society of Health-System Pharmacists. ASHP guidelines on clinical drug research. *Am J Health-Syst Pharm.* 1998; 55:369–76.

ASHP Guidelines for the Management of Investigational Drug Products

Purpose

The purpose of these guidelines is to describe a standardized approach for the management of investigational drug products by the clinical research pharmacy, pharmaceutical industry, and cooperative and research network groups. The scope of these guidelines includes the receipt, accountability, storage, handling, preparation, dispensing, and final disposition of investigational drug products to ensure inspection readiness and compliance with regulations as provided in the Code of Federal Regulations (CFR), 21 CFR, Part 312,[1] as well as International Conference on Harmonisation of Technical Requirements for Registration of Pharmaceuticals for Human Use (ICH) E6 Good Clinical Practice[2] (GCP) (described in 21 CFR Part 312, section 120) and Good Manufacturing Practice[3] (GMP) (described in 21 CFR Part 211), and the approved clinical study protocols. These guidelines will facilitate the adoption of best practices by new and established clinical research pharmacies (e.g., investigational drug service [IDS]) in collaboration with the pharmaceutical industry for the optimal management of investigational drug products. The ultimate goals of standardizing the management of investigational drug products are to improve patient safety, improve efficiency, and provide robust clinical data that allow new and innovative medications to reach the patients who need them.

Value of a Clinical Research Pharmacy

Since 1962, the Kefauver-Harris Amendments[4] to the Federal Food, Drug and Cosmetic Act have required drug manufacturers to prove that new drugs are safe and effective. This requirement is the foundation for clinical studies as they are known today. The pharmaceutical industry spends billions of dollars each year to test investigational drug products for safety and efficacy, and it may take a decade or more for a drug product to obtain market approval.[5] Thousands of subjects have been asked to consent and take part in the clinical research study process.

The current practice of the biopharmaceutical industry is to manufacture, distribute, and monitor investigational drug products for clinical research use while utilizing the expertise of healthcare providers, especially pharmacists, who manage the products at clinical study sites. It is imperative that pharmacists participating in these studies have the expertise to manage investigational drug products appropriately. The clinical research pharmacist is a critical member of the clinical study site team and has the expertise to understand the special handling requirements of investigational drug products.[6] Clinical research pharmacists understand the importance of managing and properly documenting investigational product receipt, storage, dispensing, returns, and final disposition. Failure to accurately document investigational product accountability can undermine the validity of clinical study data, which could spur sponsors to halt a site's participation in current or future studies and result in a loss of local patients' access to clinical studies.

Clinical research pharmacy is a specialized area of pharmacy practice that has evolved to meet the needs of the clinical study sites, help ensure research participants' safety, and protect the integrity of clinical study data. Clinical research pharmacists possess an expert working knowledge of the clinical research study process, human subject protection, and national and local regulations governing drug research. They are responsible for providing information to the appropriate healthcare team members, including pharmacy staff, who may be unfamiliar with the investigational drug product, enabling them to correctly dispense it as described in the clinical protocol and ensure its safe use.

Clinical Research Pharmacy Models

A clinical research pharmacy may be as simple as a part-time pharmacist or as complex as a team of dedicated clinical research pharmacists, technicians, and coordinators. It most commonly is part of the larger pharmacy organization (e.g., the hospital pharmacy). In rare cases, it may be a freestanding entity. As the complexity and volume of clinical studies at an institution increases, the decision to create a dedicated clinical research pharmacy with highly trained and specialized personnel and management can be made.

When establishing a clinical research pharmacy, the appropriate institutional metrics (e.g., staffing-to-order volume ratios)[6,7] should be used to determine the appropriate staffing, facility, and storage requirements needed to manage investigational drug products. A comprehensive approach will allow institutional leadership to fully support the creation of a clinical research pharmacy and should include a review of the types and therapeutic areas of studies that will be handled.

Each institution must also establish a funding model to support the clinical research pharmacy. This model may include (1) direct cost recovery from the sponsor–investigator, (2) indirect funding (e.g., based on institutional overhead such as grants to conduct research), (3) foundation underwriting of the research, or (4) institutions absorbing the cost of the clinical research. Clinical research pharmacy fees should be included at an early stage during the negotiation of each clinical study budget. Investigational drug products provided by sponsors at no cost to the clinical study site for use in clinical studies must not be charged to study participants.

Within the organization, pharmacy leadership, the clinical research pharmacist, institutional research leadership, and investigators should establish the locations where research participants will receive their care with the appropriate pharmacy support. A review of pharmacy activities and workflow for investigational drug product handling should be performed for the following locations, as appropriate: (1) inpatient units, (2) clinical research unit, (3) ambulatory care or outpatient clinic setting, and (4) a combination of inpatient and outpatient areas. The organization should develop a mechanism to handle participants being treated at multiple locations and facilities.

DOI 10.37573/9781585287048.106

A dedicated team should be identified as the clinical research pharmacy staff. In institutions with a large volume of clinical studies, the clinical research pharmacy staff may form an IDS with the appropriate management structure depending on the practice environment. Members of the clinical research pharmacy staff must have knowledge and documented training on ICH GCP,[2] the Health Insurance Portability and Accountability Act,[8] institutional review board (IRB) review and protection of human subjects,[9] the *Belmont Report*,[10] and all other competencies and policies required by the institution or the pharmacy.

Facilities, Security, and Limited Staff Access

According to GCP guidelines, the investigational drug product should be stored in a secure location as specified by the sponsor and in accordance with all applicable regulatory requirements.[2] Some institutions may have separate rooms for the storage of investigational drug products; others may have a separate storage area within the pharmacy department. In either case, the area should be secured (e.g., by key or electronic lock), with entry restricted to clinical research pharmacy or delegated staff.

Each institution must evaluate its ability to provide secure, limited access to investigational drug products. A clinical research pharmacy that does not have continuous (24-hour/365-day) support to provide access to investigational drug products may mitigate the need for access by utilizing regular pharmacy staff and considering on-call support by the clinical research pharmacists to supplement this staff.

Temperature Control and Monitoring

Control and monitoring of investigational drug product storage conditions are important for maintaining the integrity of the products and for the safety of the research participants. Documentation that proper storage conditions in the pharmacy have been maintained must be available. The sponsor shall determine and communicate acceptable storage temperatures, storage conditions (e.g., protection from light), and storage times for the products.[11] The clinical research pharmacist must be able to document the temperature storage conditions of the investigational drug products at all times while managed by the pharmacy. Each pharmacy location where investigational drug products are stored must be monitored to ensure that proper temperature storage conditions have been maintained.

Clinical research pharmacy and the pharmaceutical industry shall follow *United States Pharmacopeia* standards for controlled temperature storage.[12] Before the start of activities at the clinical study site, the sponsor should establish and communicate known allowable out-of-range temperatures and the maximum allowable deviation time (i.e., acceptable time out of range) for the investigational drug product. This information will enable the clinical research pharmacy to make independent decisions without quarantining the investigational drug product supply for acceptable excursions. An investigational drug product that does not meet the allowable excursion parameters must be quarantined under the proper storage conditions by the clinical research pharmacy, and the sponsor and principal investigator (PI) must be notified. Prompt direction from the sponsor regarding how to handle the quarantined product must be adequately documented and kept in the site study file.

If the investigational drug product is sensitive to humidity, the sponsor must work directly with the clinical research pharmacy regarding monitoring requirements for relative humidity.

All locations, including refrigerator, freezer, and room-temperature areas, storing the investigational drug product must have a temperature monitoring device or system. In addition, the temperature monitoring system should be calibrated at least annually to meet National Institute of Standards and Technology standards.[13] Documentation of the calibration of each device must be maintained and available for inspection. If an electronic temperature monitoring system is not available, a calibrated manual thermometer with the ability to capture daily maximum and minimum temperatures should be used. A daily record of the maximum and minimum temperatures should be maintained.

Equipment used to store investigational drug product should be connected to a backup power supply in the event of power failure. All refrigerators and freezers shall have preventive maintenance completed annually. All calibration and maintenance records should be archived per institutional policy.

Site Qualification

The site qualification by the sponsor determines whether the site meets the potential protocol requirements.[11] A pharmacy assessment should be part of the sponsor's site qualification. Ideally, the sponsor's agent should review the site's policies and procedures and applicable sponsor site qualification requirements with the clinical research pharmacy staff. If the sponsor provides a written report of the site qualification to the site PI, a copy should also be forwarded to the clinical research pharmacy. This report serves as the minutes of the visit and agreement of the scope and services the clinical research pharmacy may provide. If a report is not provided, informal notes or minutes may be taken by clinical research pharmacy personnel and kept on file.

Clinical Research Pharmacy Staff Responsibilities

The clinical research pharmacy should be included in the pre-IRB review for new clinical protocols. During this pre-IRB review, the clinical research pharmacy should determine the safety and feasibility of conducting the clinical research study at the institution with respect to its policies, pharmacy services, and the fees that will be charged for the services provided. For this review, the clinical research pharmacist should compile the following documents and information from the clinical study site team and sponsor:

- Clinical trial protocol, including the following:
  - Research participant location (inpatient, outpatient, or both)
  - Number of research participants expected to be enrolled at the site and number of dispensing visits
  - Duration of the study, including recruitment and treatment periods
  - Randomization method (i.e., how participants are randomized in the clinical trial)

    - Blinding (e.g., open label, single blind, double blind, third-party blinding by clinical research pharmacy)
- Investigator's brochure (known investigational drug product information including safety data, any relevant animal and human data, and the doses previously studied; provided by sponsor)
- Investigational drug product handling manual (pharmacy manual), if available, which should include the following:
    - Interactive response technology (IRT) (e.g., interactive voice or Web response systems [IVRS/IWRS]) instructions, if applicable
    - Description of investigational drug product (e.g., dosage forms, strength, packaging)
    - Investigational drug product and ancillary supply sourcing (e.g., provided by sponsor, sourced locally by clinical research pharmacy)
    - Ancillary supplies required (e.g., filters, bags, tubing, bag covers)
    - Supply of concomitant medications required (e.g., adjunctive therapies, premedications)
        - A discussion should be raised during the study setup to determine which concomitant medications will be reimbursed and which will be considered standard of care
    - Investigational drug product storage conditions (e.g., temperature, humidity)
    - Special handling precautions (e.g., protect from light, hazardous handling precautions)
    - Investigational drug product preparation or dispensing information (e.g., diluents, stability of reconstituted vial and solution for administration, dispensing in original container or repackaging)
    - Handling of containers used in preparing dose
    - Handling of participant investigational drug product returns
- Administration of investigational drug product (e.g., flushing of infusion line, order of investigational drug product administration in relation to other drugs administered at the same visit, drug and food interactions)

Pharmacist Listing on Statement of Investigator

The decision whether to list a pharmacist on the Statement of Investigator (Form FDA 1572) depends on the contribution the individual makes to the study.[14] If the individual will make a direct and significant contribution to the data or is directly involved in the treatment or evaluation of participants, he or she should be listed. If the individual will provide ancillary or intermittent contributions, he or she should not be listed. A pharmacist who prepares investigational drug product doses and maintains drug accountability for multiple clinical studies that are conducted at an institution would not be making a direct and significant contribution to the data for a particular study; therefore, it would not be necessary to list the pharmacist as a subinvestigator. However, the pharmacist should be listed in the investigator's study records as an individual to whom specific responsibilities have been delegated.

Delegation of Authority to Technicians and Pharmacy Support Staff

Many sites utilize individuals who are not pharmacists to perform some of the functions of the clinical research pharmacy under the direction of a licensed pharmacist. Certified pharmacy technicians or pharmacy coordinators may be delegated tasks, according to institutional policy, that do not require a pharmacist license. The clinical research pharmacist is responsible for ensuring compliance with laws, rules, and regulations regarding technician responsibilities. In many states, a technician may only perform certain duties under the direct supervision of a pharmacist, and the pharmacist is ultimately responsible for the work performed by the technician; therefore, only the clinical research pharmacist should sign the sponsor's Delegation of Authority log.

Clinical Research Pharmacy Staff Training

The clinical research pharmacist must be a participant in the sponsor's site initiation visit or the internal site initiation meeting (for sponsor–investigator or cooperative group studies). The clinical research pharmacist must participate in the pharmacy-specific training session and have the opportunity to discuss the investigational drug product dispensing logistics with the sponsor and clinical site study team. The clinical research pharmacist should provide the sponsor with key policies and procedures and standard operating procedures (SOPs) for review and approval, if not provided at the site qualification visit. These may include but are not limited to SOPs on training and delegation of tasks assigned to pharmacy personnel regarding investigational drug product handling, temperature monitoring, onsite investigational drug product destruction, essential document retention, and monitoring visit guidelines. Occasionally, sponsors conduct the site initiation remotely via telephone or Internet conference. The clinical research pharmacist must be invited and should participate in the pharmacy-specific training session.

At the site initiation visit, the pharmacy responsibilities are determined and the Delegation of Authority form is completed and signed by the clinical research pharmacist and PI. Specific tasks need to be determined at study initiation by the clinical research pharmacy and the clinical study site team (e.g., which team member is accessing the IRT for randomization, kit/bottle assignment). The clinical research pharmacist should determine which qualified pharmacy staff member will perform the delegated roles. The clinical research pharmacist should also determine which pharmacy staff will require electronic signatures (user name and passwords) for protocol systems such as IRT and coordinate with the sponsor to obtain them.

All pharmacy staff who may dispense investigational drug products should be trained in the proper dispensing process and in GCP[2] as it relates to PI-delegated roles. Training should be completed upon hire, and the information should be reviewed periodically. Records of training must be maintained and made available for inspection by regulatory agencies and sponsors.

Clinical research pharmacists and staff are required to follow all relevant pharmacy practice standards, institution policies and procedures, state and federal laws, and Joint Commission or other accreditation standards, as well as GCP guidance.[2] Clinical research pharmacy staff should maintain all certifications and competencies specified by the pharmacy department and the institution related to this requirement.

Formal sponsor training for every pharmacy staff member for each protocol and all protocol amendments is often not practical. Pharmacy staff should be trained to refer to the most recent version of the study-specific dispensing guidelines every time a delegated responsibility is performed. This practice ensures that the most recent procedures are used each time the investigational drug product is prepared and dispensed. Therefore, study-specific training by the sponsor is not indicated for all pharmacy staff. A pharmacy signature log with staff initials should be maintained and archived centrally by the pharmacy department for the purpose of verifying study-related records.

Sponsors frequently request the curriculum vitae (CV) of all pharmacy staff handling investigational drug product. However, since the institution maintains licensure and credentialing information, it is appropriate for clinical research pharmacy staff to only provide CVs to the sponsor if the pharmacist is listed on Form FDA 1571 (Investigational New Drug Application) or Form FDA 1572 (Statement of Investigator).[1]

The clinical research pharmacist should determine whether interested parties can confirm pharmacist licensing information at the individual state licensing office and, if so, provide the sponsor with access information. It is not necessary to provide proof of pharmacy technician certification.

Clinical Research Pharmacy Study Setup

The process of opening a new clinical research study should include preparing dispensing guidelines, a model physician order (prescription template), and a template of the dispensing label. The process should also include creating a protocol-specific study drug entry and order set in the electronic medical record as well as setting up a clinical research pharmacy study file.

Dispensing guidelines should be prepared by the clinical research pharmacist using the clinical protocol and any other relevant information provided to the clinical research pharmacy by the sponsor (e.g., investigational drug product handling manual, site initiation visit materials, investigator's brochure). It is the responsibility of the PI to ensure that the research pharmacy has the most up-to-date versions of all study documents. Dispensing guidelines describe the protocol-specific functions that the clinical research pharmacy staff must perform in order to adhere to the protocol and complete all responsibilities delegated to the pharmacy by the PI.[14] The dispensing guidelines are intended to operationalize the management of investigational drug products for a specific protocol within the institution and are used as a training tool by the pharmacy staff involved in the preparation and dispensing of the investigational drug product. A sample of dispensing guidelines has been previously published.[15] A draft version of the dispensing guidelines should be prepared before the site initiation visit to allow the clinical research pharmacist to identify the information that needs to be obtained at the meeting and to ensure that the clinical site will have all of the information needed before enrolling the first participant into the study.

Dispensing guidelines should be revised as appropriate after IRB approval of protocol amendments or other changes to study procedures. The clinical research pharmacist should maintain a system to document version control. Dispensing guidelines should be available (in print or electronic formats) to any pharmacy staff responsible for participant care.

The physician order template for the investigational drug product should be prepared by the clinical research pharmacist using the clinical protocol and other relevant information provided by the sponsor.[5] In institutions that use computerized provider order entry, the clinical research pharmacist should ensure that an order set is available in the system.

The investigational drug product should be entered into the pharmacy computer dispensing systems, if available. A dispensing label template should be created to ensure that information required by the clinical protocol is included on the label and that the administration instructions are consistent with the clinical protocol.

The dispensing label for the investigational drug product must comply with all state and federal rules and regulations as well as protocol requirements. The information on the label should be consistent with the information and instructions on the physician's order as well as the original drug container. The institution's contact information should be included on the label to aid in coordination of the participant's care by an outside institution. Special instructions should be included on the dispensing label or provided as auxiliary labels (e.g., food intake recommendations, storage conditions).

If the clinical research pharmacy repackages the investigational drug product, the Federal Investigational Drug Caution Statement—"Caution: New Drug—Limited by Federal (or United States) law to investigational use"—should be on the clinical site pharmacy label.[16] All labeling must also comply with applicable local and state regulations. In addition, the clinical research pharmacist should ensure that any required medication counseling (e.g., for psychiatric or teratogenic medications) is to be provided by the clinical research pharmacist or an appropriate member of the clinical site study team.

Considerations for Blinded Studies

When preparing dispensing guidelines for blinded studies in which the clinical research pharmacy staff are unblinded, the clinical research pharmacist should be cognizant that there are clinical site personnel with direct patient care responsibilities who are blinded to the research participant's treatment assignment, and the dispensing guidelines should be designed accordingly. Ideally, unblinded clinical site personnel should not be involved in direct patient care for study participants. Interactions between blinded and unblinded personnel should be minimized, and care should be taken to avoid communication that could inadvertently reveal a participant's treatment assignment. Any pharmacy staff member who is unblinded must use extreme care when communicating with blinded staff regarding any patient care information in order to avoid revealing the participant's blinded treatment assignment.

Active and placebo investigational drug products must be identical in appearance, labeling, preparation time, expiration date and time, and supplies used. Considerations when preparing blinded investigational drug products include

- Ensuring that the preparation times for the active drug and the placebo dose are the same.
- Providing the identical information on the active drug and placebo labels, including the expiration date and time; if the active drug and placebo products have different expiration dates and times, the shorter of the 2 times should be used.
- Making the port on intravenous bags look the same (i.e., if a commercial bag of diluent is used as the placebo, insert a needle into the port using aseptic technique to give the appearance that a drug has been added; if additive port covers are used, ensure matching covers).
- Using the same type of needle and tubing for administration of the active drug and the placebo dose.

An unblinding process must be established that allows the blinded treatment assignment to be determined. Examples of events that require unblinding include a research participant experiencing a severe adverse reaction and an unauthorized person ingesting or being administered the investigational drug product. An unblinding process that allows for immediate determination of the participant's treatment assignment or access to the sponsor's medical monitor should be developed. In order to allow continuous access to the unblinding process in the event of an emergent need to determine a participant's treatment assignment, a clinical site-specific plan should be developed that is not dependent solely on the PI.

When labeling a blinded study medication, the clinical research pharmacy must label it such that the blinding is protected and that clinical site study staff are not able to determine the actual contents of the container. The product should be labeled as "drug name or placebo." The protocol acronym should not be used solely in place of the product name; if a research participant presents at an emergency department, the treating physician should be able to identify the potential contents of the container so that treatment is not delayed.

Barcoding of Investigational Drug Products

Improved patient safety with barcoding has been well documented.[17] Although barcoding is desirable, the lack of a standard system limits its ability to be implemented with investigational drug products. Development of a standardized barcode lexicon that will facilitate the implementation of a global barcoding system is necessary. ASHP has urged the Food and Drug Administration (FDA) and other regulatory agencies, standard-setting bodies, contracting entities, health systems, and pharmaceutical manufacturers to develop and implement a universal symbology (e.g., barcodes, radio frequency identifiers) that are readily deciphered by commonly used scanning equipment to code for the National Drug Code, lot number, and expiration date on all unit dose, unit-of-use, and injectable drug packaging.[18]

Investigational Drug Product Accountability and Documentation

Detailed records, required to be kept by the sponsor, must identify the investigator to whom the investigational drug product is shipped as well as the date, quantity, and batch or code mark of such shipment.[19] The clinical site is required to maintain records detailing the participant to whom the investigational drug product was dispensed, the date, the quantity, and the batch or code mark dispensed. Incomplete or inaccurate drug accountability is a deficiency frequently cited in Form FDA 483 Inspectional Observations notices.[20] U.S. law does not require the use of an expiration date, use-by date, or retest date on product labels. In many cases, the date may be found on the packing slip; however, the clinical research pharmacy may reach out to the sponsor to request documentation of the retest or expiration date.

Routine inventory counts (e.g., monthly) should be performed for each investigational drug product in order to ensure that the physical quantity on hand corresponds to the quantities recorded on the drug accountability record form (DARF) and to manage investigational drug product with limited use dates. Any discrepancy should be reviewed and resolved for each investigational drug product.

According to the CFR and GCP guidelines,[1,2] investigational drug product receipt, dispensing, participant returns, and disposition are required transactions that must be documented. Sponsors may provide investigational drug product accountability records, or individual clinical research pharmacies may have their own accountability records. Frequently, sponsor-provided DARFs do not contain sections to document all of the required transactions. For clinical research pharmacies with multiple ongoing clinical studies, DARFs from different sponsors requiring inconsistent information can cause confusion. Use of standardized DARFs containing sections for the required transactions would ensure consistency and compliance with applicable regulations. **Figure 1** displays a template for a DARF, which can be customized for different clinical protocols and sites but maintains a standard appearance that will allow clinical research pharmacy personnel to complete the forms correctly and provide sponsors with the required documentation. The form allows the site to document the receipt and dispensing of individual bottles, vials, or kits, and the header of the form can be customized for the specific needs of the protocol. If a hard copy of the DARF is required by sponsors and an electronic dispensing/accountability system is used, it must have the capability of printing a hard copy of the DARF that shows the required transactions. At a minimum, the items on the form should be adhered to, ensuring site and sponsor compliance with regulatory agencies. The clinical research pharmacy DARF may be customized to include additional information requested by sponsors, such as the time of dose preparation or investigational drug product container numbers.

When the investigational drug product is transferred from the clinical research pharmacy to a satellite pharmacy or dispensing location, a separate DARF must be maintained with the investigational drug product. The DARF in the clinical research pharmacy should reflect the transfer of investigational drug product to the satellite location, and the satellite location's DARF should reflect receipt of the investigational drug product from the clinical research pharmacy. The satellite location's DARF should reflect all dispensing activity at that location. Any remaining investigational drug product must be returned to the clinical research pharmacy and documented in both DARFs accordingly.

The DARF is an official record, and, as such, any corrections that are made must be performed by making a line through the original entry, accompanied by the recorder's initials and date. The original entry may not be obscured.[21]

FIGURE 1. Template of a drug accountability record form. PI = principal investigator, CRA = clinical research associate.

(site name) Clinical Research Pharmacy
Drug Accountability Record Form (DARF)

Protocol Title:			Internal Protocol #:
PI:	Source:		Lot:
Study Drug Name:	Synonym:	Drug Location:	Kit:
Strength:		Drug Storage:	Exp/Retest:
Dosage Form:	Units Per Container:	Room Temp ___ Refrig # ___ Other ___	

Receipt Or Dispense Date dd/mmm/yyyy	Rx# or Pt Care Unit	Patient Initials FML or F - L	Patient Study #	Dose/ Frequency	Quantity Received or Dispensed	Balance	Staff Init	CRA Verify Init	Patient Returns			Disposition			CRA Verify Init
									# Returned	Date Returned	Staff Init	Return to Sponsor or Destroy	Date	Staff Init	

Comments: ____________________ Page ___ of ___

Investigational Drug Product Receipt

The clinical protocol or investigational drug product handling manual will indicate how to obtain the investigational drug product once a study site is approved to receive the product from the sponsor. The study site may need to enroll the first research participant before the product is shipped, or a study site may be allowed to have the investigational drug product onsite in anticipation of participant enrollment. When the product is shipped, the sponsor must ensure it is appropriately labeled so that it is easily identified as an investigational drug product for a specific clinical protocol. The immediate packaging container for the investigational drug product is required to bear the statement "Caution: New Drug—Limited by Federal (or United States) law to investigational use."[16]

In addition, it is strongly recommended that the sponsor's investigational drug product label contain the following information[22]:

- Investigational drug product name
  - ▸ Investigational drug product name may be the generic name, company molecule name, or compound name but must match the name used in the clinical protocol; the sole use of protocol acronyms should be avoided.
  - ▸ If the investigational drug product used in the clinical research study is blinded and placebo controlled, the label must indicate "[Investigational Drug Product Name] or Placebo."
- Investigational drug product strength or concentration unless this aspect of the trial is blinded
- Investigational drug product quantity (e.g., number of tablets, volume)
- Investigational drug product lot number and/or container or kit number
  - ▸ Lot number(s) should be referenced in the packing slip or receipt document, and terminology should be consistent with the clinical research study-related documentation (i.e., if the lot number is labeled as "Lot Number" on the package, it should not be referred to as "Batch Number" in supporting documentation).
  - ▸ Investigational drug products may also contain a unique container or kit number that will be used to identify the contents or to assign specific container or kit to a participant; in that case, the container or kit number may appear in place of the lot number, but the container or kit number must be cross-referenced with the packing slip.
- Expiration or retest date (period of use) of the investigational drug product
  - ▸ While it is preferred to be on the investigational drug product label, this information may be provided on the packing slip or via a memo included with the shipment to the clinical study site.
- Sponsor or manufacturer name and address
- Clinical research protocol number
  - ▸ When a sponsor is working on clinical studies using the same investigational drug product in parallel protocols for different indications, it may be difficult for a clinical site to determine which protocol the product belongs to unless this information is provided on the container.

- The sponsor may provide pooled supplies of investigational drug products to be used for multiple clinical research studies at the same clinical study site. The investigational drug product may be labeled with multiple clinical research protocol numbers, or the clinical research pharmacy may be required to assign each individual unit to a specific clinical research study at the time of dispensing. The assignment process must be clearly explained in the investigational drug product handling manual or the clinical protocol and be communicated clearly to the clinical research pharmacies.

- Oral medication intended to be dispensed to a participant for self-administration at home must comply with the Federal Poison Prevention Packaging Act[23] and be packaged in a child-resistant container. If the disease indicated in the clinical protocol is not conducive to this type of packaging, a statement must be included in the consent form alerting the potential participant that there is a risk to children in the home due to the lack of child-resistant packaging.

The investigational drug product shipment must be accompanied by a packing slip. Clinical research pharmacy staff are responsible for verifying the contents against the packing slip and assessing the condition of the package. Proof of receipt should be provided to the sponsor or supplier; this should be clearly outlined in the protocol or investigational drug product handling manual or on the packing slip. Any discrepancies (e.g., broken vials, missing product, temperature excursions) must be reported immediately, and the resolution of discrepancies must be appropriately documented. Sponsors may request that the product be quarantined in the interim; quarantined product must be maintained under the specified storage conditions. Sponsors should be prompt in responding to discrepancies or temperature excursions. The packing slip, shipment temperature records, and any other documents received with the investigational product shipment shall be stored in the pharmacy study-specific file. All investigational drug products received must be documented on a DARF.

Investigational Drug Product Dose Preparation and Dispensing

When preparing and dispensing an investigational drug product, the clinical research pharmacy should utilize site-developed, study-specific dispensing guidelines to ensure the investigational drug product handling requirements in the protocol are met. The clinical research pharmacy may store partial or empty vials of nonhazardous investigational drug product in a limited-access, secure area until returned or destroyed per the sponsor's direction. Sponsors should be diligent in the reconciliation and disposition of the used materials. Used and partial vials of hazardous investigational drug product should be destroyed according to the institutional policies and procedures immediately after dose preparation.

Remote Site or Clinic Dispensing

Remote site or clinic dispensing within a health system may be considered when clinical research pharmacy involvement may present a hardship for research participants or adversely affect the conduct of the clinical research study, especially in situations where timely access to the investigational drug product may be a challenge.

The clinical research pharmacy should review studies that may require remote site or clinic dispensing before IRB review to assist in determining how the investigational drug product should be managed at the remote site or clinic and in determining the best dispensing option. In situations in which pharmacist dispensing is not practical, physician dispensing may be an option. State laws and regulations should be reviewed to determine whether physician dispensing is permitted. If physician dispensing is allowed, all applicable state and federal laws and regulations with respect to handling investigational drug products (e.g., secure storage conditions, labeling requirements for outpatient use) as well as those regulating accountability and dispensing must be followed. The clinical research pharmacy should provide guidance on the applicable state laws and regulations that apply.

In such cases, the PI must maintain appropriate study-specific accountability records. These records should document the investigational drug product received and dispensed to participants enrolled in the clinical research study. Investigational drug product returned from participants and final disposition of investigational drug product must also be recorded.

The clinical research pharmacy should also perform periodic audits and inspections of storage facilities and drug accountability procedures that are managed by the PI.[24]

Investigational Drug Product Returned from Participants

Per GCP, the PI is responsible for ensuring and assessing clinical research protocol adherence.[2] This may include receiving, counting, and documenting investigational drug product returned from participants in the case report form or the electronic medication administration record, if required, in the protocol. This function may be delegated by the PI to the clinical research pharmacy; in such cases, the unused supply and empty investigational drug product containers should be returned to the clinical research pharmacy for documentation of the unused investigational drug product returns from participants and its final disposition. The clinical research pharmacy should record on the DARF the date and the quantity of investigational drug product returned, as directed in the investigational drug product handling manual. On occasion, the date of the investigational drug product count may differ from the actual date of participant return because the clinical research pharmacy may not be able to process the return immediately. Returned investigational drug product should be deemed not usable and should be stored in an area separate from the investigational drug product that is available for dispensing to research participants.

Used or partially used nonhazardous investigational drug product returns should be stored by the clinical research pharmacy in a limited-access, secure area until directed by the sponsor to return or destroy the product. The clinical research pharmacy should determine storage space availability and notify the sponsors in advance of any space limitations. The sponsor should visit the clinical research pharmacy at appropriate intervals based on study activity to return or destroy used investigational drug product. If such visits do not occur, the clinical research pharmacy should contact the sponsor to obtain permission to destroy or return the product.

Hazardous investigational drug product returns and returns of investigational drug product supplied by the National Cancer Institute should not be stored onsite. These products should be destroyed under the appropriate institutional hazardous drug disposal procedures immediately after counting and documentation on the DARF; exceptions should require approval by the clinical research pharmacist and the PI and should be stated in the dispensing guidelines. Each site should refer to its specific institutional policies regarding the destruction of hazardous drug products.

Investigational Drug Product Final Disposition

For investigational drug product returned to the sponsor or destroyed onsite, the return or destruction must be documented on the DARF by the clinical research pharmacy. If required by the sponsor, a separate return or destruction form may be used to document return or destruction of the investigational drug product. If the return of unused investigational drug product to the sponsor is required per the clinical research protocol, instructions on the return procedure should be provided to the clinical research pharmacy staff by the sponsor. If destruction of investigational drug product by the clinical research pharmacy is approved by the sponsor, the product should be destroyed per institutional policy. If the sponsor requests return of a hazardous investigational drug product, the shipper must comply with U.S. Department of Transportation regulations for shipping hazardous material.[25] Investigational drug products that are controlled substances should be returned to the sponsor for final disposition or destroyed per institutional policy; returns of such drug products must adhere to Drug Enforcement Administration regulations for shipping controlled substances.[26]

Clinical Research Pharmacy Study File

The clinical research pharmacy should create a study-specific pharmacy file using selected essential documents that are deemed necessary by the clinical research pharmacist for the routine management of investigational drug products. Original documents (e.g., DARFs, investigational drug product physician orders, packing slips) that are part of the clinical research study-specific pharmacy file are considered source documentation. These essential clinical research pharmacy documents will be retained throughout the study and must be readily available for inspection by the sponsor (or designee), PI (or designee), and regulatory agencies (e.g., FDA). Copies of temperature monitoring logs and policies do not need to be filed in individual clinical research-specific files but should be available on request.

Documents in the pharmacy file may be stored in hard copy or electronic format and should include sponsor-provided and site-prepared documents. Sponsor-provided documents should include the following:

- IRB-approved clinical research protocol and associated amendments
- Investigator's brochure and associated amendments
- Investigational drug product handling manual (version controlled) and associated amendments
- Investigational drug product ordering instructions and forms
- IRT (IVRS/IWRS) manuals (instructions and forms)
- Investigational drug product shipment documentation (e.g., packing slips, other drug receipt documents)
- Supporting investigational drug product information (e.g., package insert, safety data sheet, certificate of analysis, as applicable)
- Expiration and retest correspondence (period of use)
- Temperature excursion forms (if required)
- Correspondence (e.g., communication sheet, letters, e-mails)
- Investigational drug product disposition information and forms
- Miscellaneous documents (e.g., worksheets, sponsor-specific forms)

Site-prepared documents should include the following:

- IRB approval letter
- Access to IRB-approved consent (to establish documentation of research participant-specific medication training disclosure)
- Pharmacy-prepared dispensing guidelines
- Pharmacy fee sheet with billing information
- Pharmacy computer system entry information
- Investigational drug product physician order or prescription template(s)
- List of authorized prescribers for the clinical trial
- Research participant list and treatment assignment (if applicable)
- Clinical research pharmacy and pharmacy satellite DARFs (if applicable)
- Monitoring visit and audit forms
- Notes to file

If an investigational drug product is not dispensed from the clinical research pharmacy, a satellite-specific file should be created that includes a research participant list, dispensing guidelines, DARFs, and other study-specific documents (e.g., investigational drug product dose calculation worksheets); the file should be kept in the satellite pharmacy where the investigational drug product is being dispensed.

Monitoring Visits or Audits of the Clinical Research Pharmacy

It is the responsibility of the sponsor to monitor the progress of the clinical research study to ensure data integrity and participant safety.[1] If the clinical research study is an investigator-initiated protocol (sponsor–investigator), it is the responsibility of the local PI to meet all of the requirements of the sponsor, including monitoring and safety-reporting regulations.

The sponsor may delegate the monitoring and auditing responsibilities to a contract research organization. Clinical research associates who are employees of the sponsor or their agents from a contract research organization will be sent to monitor the clinical site. Sponsor audits at clinical sites may be conducted by representatives of the sponsor or independent auditors as well as inspectors from regulatory authorities. Communication regarding clinical site monitoring expectations will occur during the site initiation visit.

The clinical research associate (monitor) will visit the clinical study site to review the records and verify the accuracy of the documentation with the source documents onsite. Source documents include any original documents, data, and records, including (but not limited to) patient medical records, visit notes, protocol data collection forms, laboratory notes, participant drug administration diaries, and the clinical research pharmacy DARFs and associated records. The monitor must have access to the source documents; in some cases, this may require access to electronic medical records. Access to these systems should be provided in accordance with institutional policies.

The monitor should communicate with the clinical study site to determine a mutually agreeable time to meet with study staff and reserve a space to work. The clinical site should accommodate these visits whenever possible. The clinical study site should have a dedicated space in the same area as the protocol records where the monitor can work. The PI must be available for questions and discussion at some time during the visit. Some research protocols will allow remote monitoring activities in lieu of a visit to the site, and monitors may send queries to the clinical site for clarification. Depending on the time required by the clinical research pharmacy staff to respond to information requests, an additional charge may be imposed to accommodate these remote visits.

The monitor will need to visit the clinical research pharmacy to review pharmacy documentation. If the clinical research protocol is a blinded study and the clinical research pharmacist is unblinded, there should be a separate unblinded monitor specifically for clinical research pharmacy review. The unblinded contact(s) should be clearly stated in the pharmacy records. All others should be considered blinded and communications handled accordingly. An appointment should be made for each clinical research pharmacy visit to allow the staff to adequately prepare.[27] The clinical research pharmacy staff should meet with the monitor and provide access to pharmacy source documents for review. The monitor should confirm drug accountability and storage conditions and review a participant's returned investigational drug product. The monitor may return investigational drug product to the sponsor or authorize its destruction. All personal health information of the participants should be removed from investigational product labels and forms before being returned to the sponsor or should be destroyed.

Monitoring Visit Logs

The clinical research pharmacy staff should document monitoring visits and the reason for the meeting. Information documenting the identity of the monitor, company affiliation, study reviewed, and the duration of the visit to the clinical research pharmacy is useful to the sponsor and the pharmacy department. **Figure 2** provides an IDS monitor/visitor log template to capture such information.

At the end of a monitoring visit, the clinical research pharmacy staff or the sponsor should document any outstanding requests or issues that need to be completed before the next visit. A template of a study monitor exit summary report that can be used to capture issues for follow-up appears in **Figure 3**. Both the clinical research pharmacist

FIGURE 2. Template of an investigatioinal drug service monitor/visitor log.

Clinical Research Pharmacy Monitor/Visitor Log Month ________ Page ________

DATE	Internal Protocol #	DRUG/STUDY	NAME	TIME IN	TIME OUT	REASON FOR VISIT

FIGURE 3. Study monitor exit summary report template. CRP = clinical research pharmacy.

> **Clinical Research Pharmacy**
> **Study Monitor Exit Summary Report**
>
> **Internal Protocol#__________**
>
> ☐ **No Clinical Research Pharmacy action required**
>
> ☐ **Follow-up Clinical Research Pharmacy action required**
>
> **Study Monitor/Date** | **CRP Staff/Date (R.Ph. required for follow-up)**
>
> **Contact Information:**

and the monitor should sign the form to document their understanding of requests.

Study Close and Archiving of the Clinical Research Pharmacy Study Files

A site is required to retain all records for at least 2 years after the marketing application is approved for the indication being investigated. If the drug is not approved or if no application is filed, then records must be retained for 2 years after the investigation is discontinued.[26] Many institutions have retention policies that exceed these requirements. Trials taking place in other countries may also be subject to longer retention periods. Sponsors should indicate when this is the case and follow retention requirements where applicable. It is the responsibility of the sponsor to notify the clinical site and the clinical research pharmacy of these requirements. Each site must be familiar with state, local, and institutional policies and regulations regarding record retention. The clinical research pharmacy should provide written notice to the sponsor of impending document destruction.

Upon termination of a study, the clinical research pharmacy should work with the PI to determine who will maintain the following pharmacy-related documents:

- Drug accountability records and documentation of investigational drug product destruction
    - Investigational drug product shipment documentation
        - Proof of receipt and/or packing list
        - Certificates of analysis
        - Safety data sheets
    - Participant enrollment log
    - Participant identification code list
    - Participant-specific preparation records (batch control records for compounded items) and worksheets
        - Certain pharmacy documents, such as filled prescriptions or medication orders, must remain with the clinical research pharmacy in accordance with state board of pharmacy rules and regulations.
        - IRT-related documents
- Instructions for handling investigational drug product
    - Site-specific dispensing guidelines
- Signature sheet and pharmacy delegation log
- Sponsor investigational drug product and pharmacy-related correspondence

Nonessential pharmacy documents (e.g., protocols, amendments, investigator's brochure, IRB correspondence) shall be stored by the PI in the investigator study file. The clinical research pharmacy does not need to maintain copies of these documents.

The clinical research pharmacy files for terminated studies that are not returned to the PI should be maintained onsite, as space allows, and then moved to offsite, long-term storage as needed and if available. The clinical research pharmacy should maintain an onsite record of location for retrieval from long-term storage. Records must be readily retrievable in the event of an audit.

Clinical Research Pharmacists as IRB Members

IRB members must disclose any actual and perceived conflicts of interest throughout their membership term and must file a financial disclosure with the IRB office. This information should be considered during assignment of IRB submissions for review to avoid conflicts of interest.

An IRB member may be involved in the conduct of a research study that solely involves the provision of a service to a study (e.g., a pharmacist from the clinical research pharmacy who prepares and dispenses study medications, a radiologist who performs diagnostic imaging that is part of the research). In these cases, the IRB should not consider this a conflict of interest with regard to reviewing an IRB submission, provided the member's role in the study is limited to the provision of a service to the PI and he or she is not otherwise engaged in the study. Under these circumstances, the clinical research pharmacist serving on an IRB should not be listed on the Statement of Investigator (Form FDA 1572).

Summary

Clinical study sites that handle a significant volume of clinical studies should establish a formal IDS pharmacy utilizing these best practices as a foundation. Standardizing the processes for managing investigational drug products used by clinical research pharmacies will improve patient safety and protect study data integrity while maintaining regulatory compliance. Standardization will also provide guidance for clinical study sites that are new to handling investigational drug products. Adopting these best practices will enable clinical research pharmacies to enhance their collaboration with sponsors and the biopharmaceutical industry by aligning processes and systems to improve clinical study execution. Ultimately, these best practices will support the development of new and innovative medications for the patients who need them most.

References

1. Investigational New Drug Application, 21 CFR 312. www.ecfr.gov/cgi-bin/text-idx?SID=0261b7eecf94bade1f78efd3b22ee7f6&mc=true&node=pt21.5.312&rgn=div5 (accessed 2017 Jun 19).
2. International Conference on Harmonisation of Technical Requirements for Registration of Pharmaceuticals for Human Use. ICH harmonized tripartite guideline: guideline for good clinical practice. *J Postgrad Med.* 2001; 47:45–50.
3. Current Good Manufacturing Practice for Finished Pharmaceuticals (21 CFR 211). www.ecfr.gov/cgi-bin/text-idx?SID=0261b7eecf94bade1f78efd3b22ee7f6&mc=true&node=pt21.4.211&rgn=div5 (accessed 2017 Jun 19).
4. Drug Amendments of 1962. Pub. L. 87-781, Oct. 10, 1962, 76 Stat. 780 (21 U.S.C. 301). http://uscode.house.gov/table3/87_781.htm (accessed 2017 Jun 19).
5. DiMasi JA, Grabowski HG, Hansen RW. Cost of developing a new drug (November 2014). http://csdd.tufts.edu/files/uploads/Tufts_CSDD_briefing_on_RD_cost_study_-_Nov_18,_2014..pdf (accessed 2017 Jun 19).
6. Rough SS, McDaniel M, Rinehart JR. Effective use of workload and productivity monitoring tools in health-system pharmacy, part 1. *Am J Health-Syst Pharm.* 2010; 67:300–11.
7. Rough SS, McDaniel M, Rinehart JR. Effective use of workload and productivity monitoring tools in health-system pharmacy, part 2. *Am J Health-Syst Pharm.* 2010; 67:380–8.
8. Health Insurance Portability and Accountability Act of 1996 (Pub. L. 104-191). http://uscode.house.gov/table3/104_191.htm (accessed 2017 Jun 19).
9. Protection of Human Research Subjects (45 CFR 46). www.hhs.gov/ohrp/regulations-and-policy/regulations/45-cfr-46/index.html (accessed 2017 Jun 19).
10. National Commission for the Protection of Human Subjects of Biomedical and Behavioral Research. Ethical principles and guidelines for the protection of human subjects of research (April 18, 1979). www.hhs.gov/ohrp/regulations-and-policy/belmont-report/index.html (accessed 2017 Jun 19).
11. General responsibilities of sponsors (21 CFR 312.50). www.ecfr.gov/cgi-bin/text-idx?SID=10f9559cb05469f95eb97b446651b615&mc=true&node=se21.5.312_150&rgn=div8 (accessed 2017 Jun 20).
12. The United States pharmacopeia, 36th rev., and The national formulary, 31st ed. Rockville, MD: United States Pharmacopeial Convention; 2013:11.
13. National Institute of Standards and Technology. Good measurement practice for assignment and adjustment of calibration intervals for laboratory standards (January 2016). www.nist.gov/sites/default/files/documents/pml/wmd/labmetrology/GMP_11_20160121.pdf (accessed 2017 Jun 19).
14. Food and Drug Administration. Information sheet guidance for sponsors, clinical investigators, and IRBs: frequently asked questions—statement of investigator, Form FDA 1572 (May 2010). www.fda.gov/downloads/RegulatoryInformation/Guidances/UCM214282 (accessed 2017 Jun 19).
15. Siden R, Tamer HR, Skyles AJ et al. Pharmacist-prepared dispensing guidelines for drugs used in clinical research. *Am J Health-Syst Pharm.* 2012; 69:1021–6.
16. General responsibilities of investigators (21 CFR 312.60). www.ecfr.gov/cgi-bin/text-idx?SID=10f9559cb05469f95eb97b446651b615&mc=true&node=se21.5.312_160&rgn=div8 (accessed 2017 Jun 19).
17. Poon EG, Keohane CA, Yoon CS, et al. Effect of barcode technology on the safety of medication administration. *N Engl J Med.* 2010; 362:1698–707.
18. American Society of Health-System Pharmacists. ASHP statement on barcode-enabled medication administration technology. *Am J Health-Syst Pharm.* 2009; 66:588–90.
19. Recordkeeping and record retention (21 CFR 312.57). www.ecfr.gov/cgi-bin/text-idx?SID=10f9559cb05469f95eb97b446651b615&mc=true&node=se21.5.312_157&rgn=div8 (accessed 2017 Jun 19).
20. Office of Scientific Investigations. OSI metrics. www.fda.gov/AboutFDA/CentersOffices/OfficeofMedicalProductsandTobacco/CDER/ucm256374.htm (accessed 2017 Jun 19).
21. National Cancer Institute. Pharmaceutical management branch investigational drug accountability series. Drug accountability record form (DARF) basics. http://ctep.cancer.gov/branches/pmb/drug_training_videos/DARF_Basics_Handout.pdf (accessed 2017 Jun 19).
22. Institute for Safe Medication Practices. Product-related issues make error potential enormous with investigational drugs (November 1, 2007). www.ismp.org/newsletters/acutecare/articles/20071101.asp (accessed 2017 Jun 19).
23. Poison Prevention Packaging Act of 1970 (15 U.S.C. 1471–17; Pub. L. 91-601, 84 Stat. 16). www.cpsc.gov/s3fs-public/pppa.pdf (accessed 2017 Jun 19).
24. Shehab N, Tamer HR. Investigational drugs not dispensed by pharmacy: regulatory issues and the role of the investigational drug service. *Am J Health-Syst Pharm.* 2004; 61:1882–4.
25. Shippers—general requirements for shipments and packagings (49 CFR 173). www.ecfr.gov/cgi-bin/text-idx?SID=5b920076cbe059040feb2b85e9951775&mc=true&tpl=/ecfrbrowse/Title49/49CIsubchapC.tpl (accessed 2016 Jul 19).

26. Ultimate user delivery for the purpose of recall or investigational use of drugs (21 CFR Part 1317.85). www.ecfr.gov/cgi-bin/text-idx?SID=26cb45a08d172513244d104e129e0caf&mc=true&node=se21.9.1317_185&rgn=div8 (accessed 2017 Jun 19).
27. Siden R, Tankanow RM, Tamar HR. Understanding and preparing for clinical drug trial audits. *Am J Health-Syst Pharm.* 2002; 59:2301–8.

These guidelines were developed through the ASHP Section of Inpatient Practitioners and approved by the ASHP Board of Directors on November 8, 2017.

Stephen C. Kay, B.S.Pharm., Clinical Research Pharmacy, Pfizer, Andover, MA.

Darlette G. Luke, B.S.Pharm., Investigational Drug Service, Fairview Health Services, University of Minnesota Medical Center, Minneapolis, MN.

Helen R. Tamer, Pharm.D., Research Pharmacy, Michigan Medicine (University of Michigan), Ann Arbor, MI.

ASHP gratefully acknowledges the following individuals for reviewing these guidelines (review does not imply endorsement): Uzma Afzal, Pharm.D.; Beth McLendon Arvik, Pharm.D.; Molly A. Camis, Pharm.D., BCPS; Scott Fields, Pharm.D.; Mark G. Klang, Ph.D., M.S., BCNSP; Eimeira Padilla-Tolentino, Pharm.D.; Michele Page, M.B.A.; John Petrich, M.S.; Marjorie Shaw Phillips, M.S., FASHP; Kenneth Rockwell Jr., Pharm.D., M.S.; Erika L. Thomas, M.B.A., B.S. Pharm.; and John Vetrano, Pharm.D.

The authors have declared no potential conflicts of interest.

Copyright © 2018, American Society of Health-System Pharmacists, Inc. All rights reserved. Contact ASHP for reprint and permissions requests. This content may not be used for commercial purposes without the express written consent of ASHP.

The bibliographic citation for this document is as follows: American Society of Health-System Pharmacists. ASHP guidelines for the management of investigational drug products. *Am J Health-Syst Pharm.* 2018; 75:561–73.

ASHP Guidelines for Pharmaceutical Research in Organized Health-Care Settings

The promotion of research in the health and pharmaceutical sciences and in pharmaceutical services is a purpose of the American Society of Hospital Pharmacists, as stated in its Charter.[1] In keeping with this purpose, pharmacists in organized health-care settings should understand the (1) basic need for research and systematic problem solving in pharmacy practice; (2) fundamental scientific approach; (3) basic components of a research plan; (4) process of documenting and reporting findings; and (5) responsibilities of investigators with respect to patients, employers, grantors, and science in general.

In its purest form, scientific research is the systematic, controlled, empirical, and critical investigation of hypothetical propositions (theories) about presumed relationships among natural phenomena.[2] Aspects of the research process (e.g., problem definition, systematic data gathering, interpretation, and reporting), however, are also applicable to resolving specific practice problems. Independent, intraprofessional, and interdisciplinary collaborative research and problem solving are encouraged.

Need

Since pharmacy is based on the theories of the pharmaceutical, medical, and social sciences, pharmacy's advancement is linked to advancement in those sciences. Scientific inquiry, through formal research and systematic problem solving, leads to an expansion of knowledge and thus to advancement. Both research and systematic problem solving in organized health-care settings are needed for developing knowledge in pharmaceutics and drug therapy and for evaluation, modification, and justification of specific practices. Therefore, an understanding of the research process is important to pharmacists in such settings.

Primary areas for research by pharmacists in organized health-care settings are those in which pharmacists possess special expertise or unique knowledge. These areas include drug therapy, pharmaceutics, bioavailability, pharmacy practice administration, sociobehavioral aspects of pharmaceutical service systems, and application of information handling and computer technology to pharmacy practice.

The Scientific Approach

Aspects of the scientific approach may be applied to formal research and systematic problem solving. The scientific approach consists of four basic steps:

1. ***Problem—Obstacle—Idea.***[3] The scientist experiences an obstacle to understanding or curiosity as to why something is as it is. The scientist's first step is to express the idea in some reasonably manageable form, even if it is ill defined and tentative.
2. ***Hypothesis.*** The scientist looks back on experience for possible solutions—personal experience, the literature, and contacts with other scientists. A tentative proposition (hypothesis) is formulated about the relationship between two or more variables in the problem; for example, "If such and such occurs, then so and so results."
3. ***Reasoning—Deduction.*** The scientist deduces the consequences of the formulated hypothesis. The scientist may find that the deductions reveal a new problem that is quite different from the original one. On the other hand, deductions may lead to the conclusion that the problem cannot be solved with existing techni-cal tools. Such reasoning can help lead to wider, more basic, and more significant problems as well as to more narrow (testable) implications of the original hypothesis.
4. ***Observation—Test—Experiment.*** If the problem has been well stated, the hypotheses have been adequately formulated, and the implications of the hypotheses have been carefully deduced, the next step is to test the relationships expressed by the hypotheses, that is, the relationships among the variables. All testing is for one purpose: putting the relationships among the variables to an empirical test. It is not the hypotheses that are tested but the deduced implications of the hypotheses. On the basis of the research evidence, each hypothesis is either accepted or rejected.

Components of a Research Plan

Formal research frequently requires the development of a written plan (protocol or proposal). In funded research, the plan may take the form of a grant application. A typical plan might include

1. A problem statement.
2. A review of available literature on the subject.
3. The objectives for the project, including the hypotheses and the to-be-tested relationships among variables.
4. A description of the methodology to be used.
5. A description of statistical analyses to be applied to the data collected.
6. A budget and time frame for the project (where applicable).
7. The expected applicability of the research findings.

Documentation and Reporting

The structure of a research report is similar to the structure of a research plan. A typical outline is as follows:

1. Problem.
   a. Theories, hypotheses, and definitions.
   b. Previous research: the literature.
2. Methodology.
   a. Sample and sampling method.
   b. Experimental procedures and instrumentation.
   c. Measurement of variables.
   d. Statistical methods of analysis.
   e. Pretesting and pilot studies.
3. Results, interpretation, and conclusions.

DOI 10.37573/9781585287048.107

The statement of the problem sets the general stage for the reader and may be in question form. A common practice is to state the broader, general problem and then to state the hypotheses, both general and specific. All important variables should be defined, both in general and in operational terms, giving a justification for the definitions used, if needed.

The general and research literature related to the problem is discussed to explain the theoretical rationale of the problem, to tell the reader what research has and has not been carried out on the problem, and to show that this particular investigation has not been conducted before (except in the case of validating research).

The methodology section should meticulously describe what was done so as to enable another investigator to reproduce the research, reanalyze the data, and arrive at unambiguous conclusions about the adequacy of the methods. This section should tell what samples were used, how they were selected, and why they were selected. The means of measurement of the variables should be described. The data analysis methods should be outlined and justified. Where pilot studies and pretesting were used, they should be described.

Results and data should be condensed and expressed in concise form. Limitations and weaknesses of the study should be discussed. The question of whether the data support the hypotheses must be foremost in the mind of the report writer. Everything written should relate the results and data to the problem and the hypotheses.

Investigators' Responsibilities

Investigators bear a general responsibility to be scientifically objective in their research inquiries, conclusions, and reports. They bear a responsibility for being methodical and meticulous in the gathering of research data. They also bear both a fiduciary and a reporting responsibility to employers and grantors. In general, employee investigators are at least partially responsible to their employer organizations in the choice of research topics. Research funded from sources outside an investigator's organization may impose additional contractual obligations on the investigator and the organization.

In research involving patients, investigators are responsible for protecting patients from harm while the patients are participating in the research. All research involving patients should be reviewed and approved, before initiation, by an institutional review board. Written, informed consent should be obtained from every patient participating in each research project.[4] Meticulous recordkeeping is required regarding the clinical experience of patients participating in research projects.

Employee investigators bear responsibility for helping their organizations differentiate true, objective research from product marketing trials and promotions that may purport to be research projects. Grants for bona fide research typically bear a direct cost-recovery relationship to projects and typically involve the direct transfer of grant funds from grantors to the employee investigator's employer organization. Specific institutional policies vary widely, but employee investigators can generally better fulfill their fiduciary responsibilities when funds are not distributed directly from grantors to investigators. In keeping with their fiduciary responsibilities and their responsibility to be scientifically objective, investigators should be wary of arrangements in which prospective grantors offer inducements of value (gifts, trips, experiences, publicity, publications, etc.) to investigators, institutions, or patients before, during, or after the completion of proposed projects.

Investigators should make legitimate efforts to document publicly the findings of research in scientific, objectively refereed publications.

References

1. American Society of Hospital Pharmacists. Governing documents of the American Society of Hospital Pharmacists. Bethesda, MD: American Society of Hospital Pharmacists; 1984.
2. Kerlinger F. Foundations of behavioral research. New York: Holt, Rinehart and Winston; 1964:13.
3. Dewey J. How we think. Boston: Heath; 1933:106–18, as adapted to the scientific framework by Kerlinger, op cit., p 13–5.
4. American Society of Hospital Pharmacists. ASHP guidelines for the use of investigational drugs in institutions. *Am J Hosp Pharm.* 1983; 40:449–51.

Approved by the ASHP Board of Directors, September 30, 1988. Developed by the Council on Professional Affairs. Supersedes the "ASHP Guidelines for Scientific Research in Institutional Pharmacy" approved on November 15, 1977.

Copyright © 1989, American Society of Hospital Pharmacists, Inc. All rights reserved. Contact ASHP for reprint and permissions requests. This content may not be used for commercial purposes without the express written consent of ASHP.

The bibliographic citation for this document is as follows: American Society of Hospital Pharmacists. ASHP guidelines for pharmaceutical research in organized health-care settings. *Am J Hosp Pharm.* 1989; 46:129–30.

ASHP
Therapeutic Position Statements

DOI 10.37573/9781585287048

ASHP Therapeutic Position Statement on the Cessation of Tobacco Use

Position

The American Society of Health-System Pharmacists (ASHP) discourages all use of tobacco products and supports evidence-based tobacco-control policies and activities that reduce the prevalence of tobacco use. ASHP strongly encourages health care providers to take an active role in promoting the health of their patients by systematically integrating into routine patient care (a) the identification of tobacco users and (b) the delivery of evidence-based tobacco-cessation interventions. ASHP recommends behavioral and pharmacologic therapies for cessation, advocates their use for all patients attempting to quit smoking (except when medically contraindicated or in specific populations for which there is insufficient evidence of effectiveness), and advises that these therapeutic interventions be reimbursed under health insurance plans.

To enable more effective and consistent identification of tobacco use and drug interactions with smoking, ASHP urges that all patient records, including those in electronic medical records and pharmacy information technology systems, include a designated field for the collection of tobacco-use data and that this field be integrated within the system such that clinically significant drug interactions with tobacco products are identified. Schools that offer health professional degree programs are encouraged to integrate comprehensive tobacco-cessation training as part of their core curricula, and licensed clinicians are advised to participate in continuing-education programs as necessary to acquire and maintain tobacco-cessation counseling skills. Given the established dangers of secondhand smoke exposure, ASHP supports legislation promoting smoke-free environments for the employees and patrons of all workplaces and public venues. Furthermore, because the sale of tobacco products contradicts the clinician's role in promoting health, ASHP strongly opposes the sale or distribution of tobacco products in all establishments where health care services are rendered.

Epidemiology of Tobacco Use

As the former U.S. Surgeon General C. Everett Koop stated in 1982, "Cigarette smoking is the chief single, avoidable cause of death in our society and the most important public health issue of our time."[1] This statement remains true today, nearly three decades later. The Centers for Disease Control and Prevention (CDC) estimates that nearly 438,000 Americans die each year from smoking,[2] and approximately 50,000 persons die annually due to involuntary exposure to tobacco smoke.[3] Cigarettes are the only marketed consumable product that, when used as intended, will contribute to the death of half or more of its users.[4]

While cigarettes are, by far, the most frequently used form of tobacco in the United States, other forms of smoked tobacco (e.g., cigars, clove cigarettes [kreteks], pipe tobacco, bidis, hookah) and smokeless tobacco (e.g., chewing tobacco, snuff) can also lead to dependence and should be addressed by clinicians. Despite the proven negative health consequences of tobacco use and the fact that approximately 70% of smokers want to quit,[5] 20.8% of the U.S. adult population continues to smoke either every day (16.7%) or some days (4.1%).[6] In 2006, more men (23.9%) than women (18.0%) were smokers.[6] The prevalence of smoking also varied by race or ethnicity (non-Hispanic American Indian/Alaska Native, 32.4%; non-Hispanic white, 21.9%; non-Hispanic black, 23.0%; Hispanic, 15.2%; non-Hispanic Asian, 10.4%), education level (higher education is associated with a lower prevalence), and poverty level (20.4% of individuals living at or above the federal poverty level; 30.6% of individuals living below the poverty level).[6] An estimated 44.3% of cigarettes smoked in the United States are by persons with mental illness.[7]

Smoking prevalence varies across the nation. In 2006, the highest median prevalence of smoking was evident in Kentucky (28.6%) and the lowest was in Utah (9.8%).[8] Because most teens who smoke at least monthly continue to smoke in adulthood,[9] tobacco-use trends among youth are viewed as a key indicator of future national health trends.[10] In 2007, an estimated 21.6% of 12th graders (23.1% of males and 19.6% of females) had smoked one or more cigarettes in the past 30 days.[11] The prevalence of smoking has declined among adolescents over the past decade; however, the downward trend has largely diminished among 12th graders in recent years.

In the past decade, the prevalence of cigarette smoking has decreased while the per-capita consumption of cigars has increased.[12] However, beginning in 2005, there has been a slight trend toward decreased cigar use. In 2007, the prevalence of cigar smoking (one or more cigars in the past month) among persons 12 years or older was 5.4%.[13] Cigar weight and nicotine content vary widely, with most cigars ranging in weight from 1 to 22 g. In comparison, a typical U.S. cigarette weighs <1 g. The nicotine content in 10 commercially available cigars studied in 1996 ranged from 10 to 444 mg.[14] Cigarette brands sold by major manufacturers in the United States have a lower and less-variable total nicotine content, ranging from 11.9 to 14.5 mg of nicotine per cigarette.[15] As such, it is possible for one large cigar to contain as much tobacco as an entire pack of cigarettes and to deliver enough nicotine to establish and maintain dependence.[14]

In 2007, an estimated 8.1 million Americans 12 years of age or older (3.2%) had used smokeless tobacco in the past month; men (6.3%) were more likely than were women (0.4%) to be users.[13] The prevalence of smokeless tobacco use is highest among individuals ages 18–25 years and is substantially higher among American Indians, Alaskan Natives, and residents of the southern United States and rural areas.[13,16] While sales of most forms of smokeless tobacco (e.g., looseleaf, plug, twist) have declined since the mid-1980s, moist snuff sales have increased steadily since the late 1980s.[12]

An enormous economic burden accompanies tobacco use. Each pack of cigarettes smoked costs society $7.18 ($3.45 for associated medical care and $3.73 for productivity losses), for a total of $157 billion in annual health-related economic losses.[17] The lifelong smoker (e.g., one pack per

DOI 10.37573/9781585287048.108

day for 50 years) spends more than $100,000 on his or her smoking habit in addition to the associated medical care costs of tobacco use.

Extensive evidence implicates tobacco as the primary known preventable cause of death in the United States. As such, ASHP strongly supports evidence-based tobacco-control initiatives that aim to reduce the prevalence of tobacco use by (a) preventing the initiation of tobacco use and (b) promoting and maintaining cessation. Tobacco-control initiatives (e.g., those described in each state's comprehensive cancer control plan) should comply with recommendations set forth by CDC as delineated in the "Best Practices for Comprehensive Tobacco Control Programs"[18] and the "Guide to Community Preventive Services: Tobacco Use Prevention and Control."[19]

Nicotine Pharmacology

Tobacco products are carefully engineered formulations that optimize the delivery of nicotine, a chemical that meets established criteria for an addictive substance.[20] Once absorbed, nicotine induces a variety of central nervous system, cardiovascular, and metabolic effects. Within seconds after inhalation, nicotine reaches the brain and stimulates the release of various neurotransmitters including dopamine, which induces nearly immediate feelings of pleasure and relieves nicotine-withdrawal symptoms. This rapid dose response reinforces the need to repeat the administration of nicotine, thereby perpetuating smoking behavior.[21] The short half-life ($t_{1/2}$ = 2 hours) of nicotine generally necessitates frequent dosing throughout the day, and tobacco users become adept at titrating nicotine intake to maintain pleasure and arousal, modulate mood, and avoid withdrawal symptoms.[21]

When nicotine is discontinued, the following withdrawal symptoms may develop: irritability, impatience, anxiety, difficulty concentrating, restlessness, hunger, depression, insomnia, and cravings.[22–24] Most physical withdrawal symptoms generally manifest within 24–48 hours after quitting and gradually dissipate over two to four weeks[23]; however, strong cravings for tobacco can persist for months or even years.[25] The nicotine levels generated by smokeless tobacco are similar to those of smoking, although their onset of action is less rapid. Upon quitting, smokeless tobacco users experience withdrawal symptoms similar to those of smokers.[26] Although nicotine is the dependence-causing component of tobacco, it is not directly responsible for the myriad of negative health consequences of tobacco use.

Health Consequences of Tobacco Use and Exposure to Secondhand Smoke

Smoking. According to the 2004 Surgeon General's report on the health consequences of smoking,[27] smoking harms nearly every organ of the body, is causally associated with numerous diseases (**Table 1**), and reduces the health of smokers in general. In addition to contributing to the development of disease, smoking also can lead to exacerbation or reduced control of existing conditions such as hypertension, diabetes mellitus, and asthma. On average, men and women lose 13.2 and 14.5 years of life because of smoking, respectively.[17] Between 1997 and 2001, an estimated 437,902 annual U.S. deaths were attributable to smoking. Of these deaths, 158,529 (36.2%) were due to cancer, 137,979 (31.5%) to cardiovascular disease, and 101,454 (23.2%) to respiratory disease.[2]

TABLE 1.
Diseases and Other Adverse Health Effects Caused by Smoking[27]

Cancers
- Acute myeloid leukemia
- Bladder
- Cervical
- Esophageal
- Gastric
- Kidney
- Laryngeal
- Lung
- Oral cavity and pharyngeal
- Pancreatic

Cardiovascular diseases
- Abdominal aortic aneurysm
- Coronary heart disease (angina pectoris, ischemic heart disease, myocardial infarction)
- Cerebrovascular disease (transient ischemic attacks, stroke)
- Peripheral arterial disease

Pulmonary diseases
- Acute respiratory illnesses
  - Upper respiratory tract (rhinitis, sinusitis, laryngitis, pharyngitis)
  - Lower respiratory tract (bronchitis, pneumonia)
- Chronic respiratory illnesses
  - Chronic obstructive pulmonary disease
  - Respiratory symptoms: cough, phlegm, wheezing, dyspnea
  - Poor asthma control
  - Reduced lung function in infants exposed in utero to maternal smoking

Reproductive effects
- Reduced fertility in women
- Pregnancy and pregnancy outcomes
  - Preterm or premature rupture of membranes
  - Placenta previa
  - Placental abruption
  - Preterm delivery
  - Low infant birth weight
- Infant mortality (sudden infant death syndrome)

Other effects
- Cataract
- Osteoporosis (reduced bone density in postmenopausal women, increased risk of hip fracture)
- Periodontitis
- Peptic ulcer disease (in patients who are infected with *Helicobacter pylori*)
- Adverse surgical outcomes
  - Poor wound healing
  - Respiratory complications

Smokeless Tobacco. Users of smokeless forms of tobacco are often under the mistaken impression that these formulations are a "safe" alternative to smoking cigarettes. In addition to cosmetic effects such as halitosis and staining of the teeth, smokeless tobacco use is associated with serious health effects, including cancer, soft tissue alterations (e.g., leukoplakia), and periodontal effects.[16] Smokeless tobacco contains high concentrations of carcinogens, which have direct contact with mucosal tissues over prolonged periods of time. The most serious consequence of smokeless tobacco use is an increased risk of developing oral and pharyngeal cancers, and the risk appears to be dose related, in that heavy, longtime users are more likely to develop oral cancer than are nonusers. The health effects of smokeless tobacco with regard to cardiovascular disease are not well understood, and published data are conflicting.[28–30] Although smokeless tobacco products do not confer many of the risks associated with the inhalation of combusted tobacco (e.g., pulmonary disease, lung cancer), these products do impose harm and should not be recommended as aids for smoking cessation, because safer, effective products (i.e., medications with FDA-approved labeling for use in smoking cessation) are available.[31]

Secondhand Smoke Exposure. Exposure to secondhand smoke results in an estimated 50,000 deaths annually, in addition to contributing to numerous diseases among nonsmoking children and adults.[3] Major conclusions of the Surgeon General's report "The Health Effects of Involuntary Exposure to Tobacco Smoke" included the following:

1. Many millions of Americans, both children and adults, are still exposed to secondhand smoke in their homes and workplaces despite substantial progress in tobacco control.
2. Secondhand smoke exposure causes disease and premature death in children and adults who do not smoke.
3. Children exposed to secondhand smoke are at an increased risk for sudden infant death syndrome (SIDS), acute respiratory infections, ear problems, and more severe asthma; smoking by parents causes respiratory symptoms and slows lung growth in their children.
4. Exposure of adults to secondhand smoke has immediate adverse effects on the cardiovascular system and causes coronary heart disease and lung cancer.
5. The scientific evidence indicates that there is no risk-free level of exposure to secondhand smoke.
6. Eliminating smoking in indoor spaces fully protects nonsmokers from exposure to secondhand smoke; separating smokers from nonsmokers, cleaning the air, and ventilating buildings cannot eliminate exposures of nonsmokers to secondhand smoke.

Supplementing the evidence presented in the Surgeon General's report,[3] the California Environmental Protection Agency in January 2006 designated secondhand smoke as a "toxic air contaminant" and, in addition to noting the tobacco-related diseases described in the Surgeon General's report, specified that exposure to smoke is associated with breast cancer in younger, primarily premenopausal women.[32]

Drug Interactions with Tobacco Smoke. Various substances in tobacco interact with several commonly prescribed drugs.[33,34] It is widely recognized that polycyclic aromatic hydrocarbons (PAHs), the products of the incomplete combustion of tobacco, are largely responsible for the majority of drug interactions with smoking. PAHs are found in appreciably large quantities in tobacco smoke and are potent inducers of hepatic microsomal (cytochrome P-450) enzymes CYP1A1, CYP1A2, and possibly CYP2E1. Although other substances in tobacco smoke such as acetone, pyridines, benzene, nicotine, carbon monoxide, and heavy metals (e.g., cadmium) might also interact with hepatic enzymes, their effects appear to be less significant.[34] To enable more effective screening for tobacco use and drug interactions with smoking, all patient records, including those stored and accessed via medical records and pharmacy information technology systems, should include a designated field for collection of tobacco-use data. This field should be integrated into the system so that relevant drug interactions with tobacco smoke can be identified.

Health Benefits of Smoking Cessation

Quitting smoking produces immediate as well as long-term benefits, reducing the risk of developing diseases caused by smoking and improving health in general.[35] Some benefits are incurred almost immediately—within the first 24 hours—after quitting. Within two weeks to three months after quitting, circulation improves, walking becomes easier, and lung function increases up to 30%. Within 1 year, the excess risk of coronary heart disease is decreased to half that of a smoker, and after 5–15 years, stroke risk is reduced to a rate similar to that of people who have never smoked. Ten years after quitting, an individual's chance of dying of lung cancer is approximately half that of continuing smokers. In addition, the risk for mouth, throat, esophagus, bladder, kidney, or pancreatic cancer is decreased. Fifteen years after quitting, an individual's risk of coronary heart disease is reduced to a rate similar to that of people who have never smoked. Quitting at ages 30, 40, 50, and 60 has been shown to be associated with 10, 9, 6, and 3 years of life gained, respectively.[4] Thus, the benefits of quitting the use of tobacco are significant. It is never too late to quit to incur health benefits, but there are clear advantages to quitting earlier.

Strategies for Promoting Tobacco Cessation

Because of the immense societal burden that smoking imposes, tobacco use and dependence should be addressed during each clinical encounter. Routine screening for tobacco-use status enables clinicians to prevent the initiation of tobacco use among nonusers, facilitate cessation among current users, and promote continued abstinence among former users.

For most smokers, the quitting process is characterized by a series of quit attempts and subsequent relapses. On average, former smokers report 10.8 quit attempts over a period of 18.6 years before achieving long-term cessation.[36] Most quit attempts are undertaken without assistance, and approximately 95% of attempts end in relapse.[37]

Given the decades of strong, consistent findings in support of the efficacy and cost-effectiveness of both behavioral and pharmacologic interventions to facilitate tobacco cessation, ASHP recommends the use of evidenced-based behavioral and pharmacologic strategies for all patients attempting to quit smoking (except when medically contraindicated or in specific populations for which there is insufficient evidence of effectiveness [e.g., pregnant women, smokeless tobacco users, light smokers, adolescents]). Treatment for tobacco dependence is highly cost-effective relative to other medical interventions (e.g., periodic mammography screening, treatment for hypertension and hyperlipidemia) and should be made available to all tobacco users.[37] In accordance with recommendations set forth in the 2008 clinical practice guideline, Treating Tobacco Use and Dependence,[37] ASHP recommends that (1) all insurance plans include counseling and evidence-based pharmacotherapy treatments as a reimbursable benefit and (2) clinicians be reimbursed for providing treatment for tobacco dependence, just as they are reimbursed for treatment of other chronic conditions.

Data consistently reveal that behavioral interventions (e.g., counseling from a health care provider) and pharmacotherapy, used either alone or in combination, increase patients' odds for quitting their use of tobacco.[37] In a meta-analysis of 29 studies, it was determined that patients who receive a tobacco-cessation intervention from a nonphysician clinician or a physician clinician are 1.7 and 2.2 times as likely to quit (for at least five months), respectively, compared with patients who do not receive an intervention from a clinician.[37] Estimates of the efficacy of various behavioral and pharmacotherapy treatment strategies are shown in **Table 2.**

As delineated in the clinical practice guideline, clinicians should routinely screen for tobacco use and apply appropriate interventions (**Figure 1**), addressing five key components for comprehensive tobacco-cessation counseling (the 5 A's): (1) asking patients about tobacco use, (2) advising tobacco users to quit, (3) assessing their willingness to make a quit attempt, (4) assisting patients with quitting, and (5) arranging follow-up care (**Appendix A**). To increase the odds for success, patients who are not ready to quit should receive tailored motivational interventions that address the 5 R's[37] (**Appendix B**). Patients who are ready to quit should be provided with a treatment plan that includes behavioral counseling plus pharmacotherapy (as appropriate) and follow-up counseling.

Clinicians should become familiar with local community-based resources for tobacco cessation, including group programs and telephone counseling.[37] When expertise, practice site logistics, or time constraints do not afford an opportunity to provide comprehensive tobacco-cessation counseling, clinicians should apply a truncated 5 A's model whereby they *ask* about tobacco use, *advise* tobacco users to quit, and then *refer* patients to appropriate cessation providers or programs. With the October 2004 introduction of a national toll-free quit line number (1-800-QUIT-NOW), all residents of the United States can receive tobacco-cessation counseling at no cost. In clinical trials, telephone counseling services for smoking cessation have been shown to be effective among the patients who use them.[37–39] These positive results have been shown to translate into real-world effectiveness,[40] as evidenced in several meta-analytic reviews.[37,38,41,42]

Even the busiest of clinicians can serve an important role by spending approximately one minute per patient to identify tobacco users and to provide referrals to the quit line for more comprehensive counseling. When patients indicate a willingness to set a quit date in the next month, clinicians should consider a proactive approach whereby they obtain

TABLE 2.
Efficacy of Treatment Methods for Tobacco Use and Dependence[a,b]

Treatment Method	Estimated Odds Ratio[c] (95% CI)	Estimated Abstinence[d] Rate (95% CI)
Behavioral interventions		
Advice to quit		
No advice to quit	1.0	7.9
Physician advice to quit	1.3 (1.1–1.6)	10.2 (8.5–12.0)
Clinician intervention		
No counseling by a clinician	1.0	10.2
Counseling by a nonphysician	1.7 (1.3–2.1)	15.8 (12.8–18.8)
Counseling by a physician	2.2 (1.5–3.2)	19.9 (13.7–26.2)
Format of smoking cessation counseling		
No format	1.0	10.8
Self-help	1.2 (1.0–1.3)	12.3 (10.9–13.6)
Proactive telephone counseling[e]	1.2 (1.1–1.4)	13.1 (11.4–14.8)
Group counseling	1.3 (1.1–1.6)	13.9 (11.6–16.1)
Individual counseling	1.7 (1.4–2.0)	16.8 (14.7–19.1)
Pharmacotherapy		
Placebo	1.0	13.8
First-line agents		
Bupropion SR	2.0 (1.8–2.2)	24.2 (22.2–26.4)
Nicotine gum (6–14 wk)	1.5 (1.2–1.7)	19.0 (16.5–21.9)
Nicotine inhaler	2.1 (1.5–2.9)	24.8 (19.1–31.6)
Nicotine lozenge (2 mg)	2.0 (1.4–2.8)	24.2[f]
Nicotine patch (6–14 wk)	1.9 (1.7–2.2)	23.4 (21.3–25.8)
Nicotine nasal spray	2.3 (1.7–3.0)	26.7 (21.5–32.7)
Varenicline (2 mg/day)	3.1 (2.5–3.8)	33.2 (28.9–37.8)
Second-line agents		
Clonidine	2.1 (1.2–3.7)	25.0 (15.7–37.3)
Nortriptyline	1.8 (1.3–2.6)	22.5 (16.8–29.4)
Combination therapy		
Patch (>14 weeks) + *ad lib* nicotine	3.6 (2.5–5.2)	36.5 (28.6–45.3)
Nicotine patch + bupropion SR	2.5 (1.9–3.4)	28.9 (23.5–35.1)
Nicotine patch + nortriptyline	2.3 (1.3–4.2)	27.3 (17.2–40.4)
Nicotine patch + nicotine inhaler	2.2 (1.2–3.6)	25.8 (17.4–36.5)

[a]Reprinted from reference 43, with permission.
[b]Data from reference 37.
[c]Estimated relative to referent group. CI = confidence interval.
[d]Abstinence percentages for specified treatment method.
[e]A quitline that responds to incoming calls and makes outbound follow-up calls. After an initial request by the smoker or via a fax-to-quit program, the clinician initiates telephone contact to counsel the patient.
[f]One qualifying randomized trial; 95% CI not reported.

FIGURE 1. Assessing readiness to quit.[38] Algorithm for treating tobacco use.

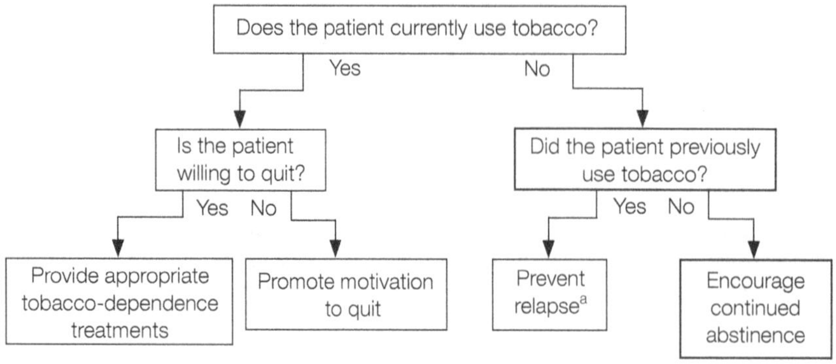

[a]Relapse-prevention interventions are not necessary for adults who have not used tobacco for many years.

the patient's permission to contact the quit line directly on the patient's behalf as opposed to their providing a passive referral (by simply offering the patient contact information for the quit line).[38]

Pharmacotherapy for Cessation. All patients attempting to quit using tobacco should be encouraged to use effective pharmacotherapies (**Table 3**) for smoking cessation,[43] except when medically contraindicated or in specific populations in which there is insufficient evidence of effectiveness (e.g., pregnant women, smokeless tobacco users, light smokers, adolescents).[37] Currently, the agents with approved FDA labeling for smoking cessation include five nicotine-replacement therapy (NRT) dosage forms, sustained-release bupropion, and varenicline. Pharmacologic agents that have not received FDA approval for use in smoking cessation but have demonstrated efficacy are clonidine and nortriptyline.[37]

NRT. Formulations of NRT products currently available in the United States include nicotine gum, lozenge, transdermal patch, nasal spray, and oral inhaler (Table 3). These agents improve quit rates by reducing the symptoms of nicotine withdrawal, enabling the patient to focus on behavior modification and coping with the psychological aspects of quitting. In addition, because the onset of action with NRT is not as rapid as that of nicotine obtained through tobacco (**Figure 2**), patients become less accustomed to the nearly immediate, reinforcing effects of tobacco. Patients using NRT are approximately two times as likely to quit smoking than are those receiving placebo.[37]

For selected patients with cardiovascular disease,[37] NRT should be used with caution, because nicotine can increase the heart rate and blood pressure and also act as a coronary vasoconstrictor.[44] Despite these effects, randomized, controlled trials have found no significant increase in the incidence of cardiovascular events or mortality among patients with cardiovascular disease receiving NRT when compared with that of patients receiving placebo.[45–47] However, because these studies specifically excluded patients with severe, underlying cardiac diseases, the clinical practice guideline[37] recommends that because of a lack of safety data in these higher-risk populations, NRT should be used with caution among patients who have experienced a myocardial infarction within the past two weeks and among those with serious arrhythmias or unstable angina.[37] A large observational study of more than 33,000 patients found that NRT use was not associated with an increased risk of myocardial infarction, stroke, or death.[48] Because the serum concentrations of nicotine achieved with the recommended dosages of NRT are generally much lower than those attained with smoking, most experts have concluded that the risks associated with NRT use in patients with cardiovascular disease are minimal relative to the risks of continued tobacco use.[44,49–52]

Other conditions for which NRT should be used with caution include active temporomandibular joint disease, pregnancy, and lactation. Patients with active temporomandibular joint disease should not use nicotine gum because doing so might exacerbate their condition. FDA classifies prescription formulations of nicotine as pregnancy category D, indicating that there is evidence of risk to the human fetus. Accordingly, none of the NRT formulations have received FDA approval for use during pregnancy. Although NRT may pose a risk to the developing fetus, it is arguably less than the risks associated with continued smoking.[53] However, because NRT has the potential to cause fetal harm and because of insufficient evidence supporting its efficacy in pregnant women, the 2008 clinical practice guideline does not recommend use during pregnancy.[37] Nicotine is secreted in breast milk[53] and, while the risk is slight, clinicians should be aware that the nursing infant is at risk for nicotine toxicity, especially if the mother concomitantly smokes and uses NRT.

Sustained-Release Bupropion. The first nonnicotine medication FDA approved for smoking cessation was sustained-release bupropion (Zyban, GlaxoSmithKline, Philadelphia). This agent, which was originally marketed as an antidepressant, is hypothesized to promote smoking cessation by inhibiting the reuptake of dopamine and norepinephrine in the central nervous system[54] and may function as a nicotinic acetylcholine-receptor antagonist.[55] The neurochemical effects are believed to modulate the dopamine reward pathway and reduce the cravings for nicotine and symptoms of withdrawal.[37] Bupropion is effective in smokers with or without a history of major depression,[56] suggesting that the mechanism of action is independent of the agent's antidepressant effects. Clinical trials involving almost 10,000 participants have confirmed the effectiveness of sustained-release bupropion as an aid to tobacco cessation; a recent meta-analysis of 31 trials concluded that the odds of tobacco abstinence at six or more months was 1.9 (sustained-release bupropion relative to placebo, 95% CI, 1.7–2.2).[57] Patients receiving sustained-release bupropion are approximately two times more likely to quit smoking than are patients receiving placebo.[44]

Bupropion is contraindicated in patients (1) with a seizure disorder, (2) with a history of anorexia or bulimia nervosa, (3) who are using another formulation of bupropion (Wellbutrin, Wellbutrin SR, Wellbutrin XL), (4) who have used a monoamine oxidase inhibitor within the past 14 days, and (5) who are undergoing abrupt discontinuation of alcohol or sedatives (including benzodiazepines).[58] In clinical trials for smoking cessation, the frequency of seizures with bupropion was <0.1% (seven seizures among 8000 bupropion-treated patients).[57] This frequency is comparable to the report rate of seizures (0.1%) when sustained-release bupropion was used in the treatment of depression.[59] For this reason, bupropion should be used with extreme caution in patients with a history of seizures, those who have experienced cranial trauma, and those receiving medications known to lower the seizure threshold or those with underlying severe hepatic cirrhosis. In addition, caution should be exercised in patients with certain depressive or psychiatric disorders. FDA has recently reclassified bupropion as a pregnancy category C drug, meaning that either (1) animal studies have demonstrated that the drug exerts animal-teratogenic or embryocidal effects, but there are no controlled studies in women, or (2) no studies are available in either animals or women. The pregnancy category reclassification resulted after the reanalysis of preclinical animal data demonstrated an increased incidence of fetal malformations and skeletal variations in rabbits receiving dosages approximately twofold higher than the maximum recommended human dose (on a milligram per square meter basis) of bupropion. The manufacturer continues to recommend that bupropion be used during pregnancy only if clearly needed.[58]

Varenicline. A partial agonist selective for the $\alpha_4\beta_2$ nicotinic acetylcholine receptor, varenicline (Chantix, Pfizer, Inc., New York, NY) was approved in May 2006 for use as an aid to smoking cessation. The drug's efficacy in smoking cessation is believed to be the result of low-level agonist activity at the receptor site combined with the competitive inhibition of nicotine binding. The partial agonist activity induces modest receptor stimulation that attenuates the symptoms of nicotine withdrawal. In addition, by blocking the ability of nicotine to activate $\alpha_4\beta_2$ nicotinic acetylcholine receptors, varenicline inhibits the surges of dopamine release that are believed to be responsible for the reinforcement and reward associated with smoking.[60]

Data from meta-analyses suggest that the use of varenicline significantly increases long-term smoking-abstinence rates relative to placebo and sustained-release bupropion.[37,61] FDA has classified varenicline as a pregnancy category C drug. The manufacturer recommends varenicline use during pregnancy only if the potential benefit justifies the potential risk to the fetus.[62]

In February 2008, FDA issued a public health advisory to alert health care providers about reports of serious neuropsychiatric symptoms in patients attempting to quit smoking while using varenicline, including changes in behavior, depressed mood, agitation, and suicidal ideation and behavior. The warnings and precautions sections of the drug's prescribing information have been updated, and FDA recommends that (1) patients tell their health care providers about any history of psychiatric illness before starting varenicline and (2) clinicians and patients monitor for changes in mood and behavior during treatment with varenicline.[63]

Second-Line Agents. Second-line agents that have not received an FDA indication for smoking cessation include the prescription medications clonidine and nortriptyline.[37] Controlled trials suggest that these agents are effective in treating tobacco dependence (Table 2), but they have a greater incidence of adverse effects and should be reserved for patients unable to quit with medications approved for smoking cessation.[37]

Combination Therapy. Certain combinations of medications have been shown to be effective smoking-cessation treatments. In the previous guideline, combination therapy was recommended only for patients unable to quit after monotherapy with a first-line agent. Based on data from eight clinical trials, the 2008 clinical practice guideline recommends that clinicians consider using combinations of first-line agents for patients who are willing to quit.[37] Combination NRT involves the use of a long-acting formulation (e.g., nicotine patch) along with a short-acting formulation (i.e., gum, lozenge, inhaler, or nasal spray). The long-acting formulation, which delivers nicotine at relatively constant levels, is used to prevent the onset of severe withdrawal symptoms; the short-acting formulation, which delivers nicotine at a more rapid rate, is used as needed to control the withdrawal symptoms that may occur during potential relapse situations (e.g., after meals, during times of stress, when around other smokers).

Controlled trials suggest that the nicotine patch in combination with short-acting NRT formulations (i.e., gum, nasal spray, or inhaler) significantly increases quit rates relative to placebo.[37] Similar results have been observed in trials using combination therapy with sustained-release bupropion and the nicotine patch. Results from an open-label trial suggest that a more-aggressive approach consisting of triple agent NRT (e.g., inhaler, patch, and nasal spray) with or without sustained-release bupropion is safe and effective among highly dependent smokers.[64] Clinicians should be aware that while the combination of the nicotine patch and sustained-release bupropion has been approved by FDA, the concurrent use of two NRT products is not FDA-approved for tobacco cessation. Furthermore, the optimal combinations, dosages, and duration of dual NRTs are currently unknown. The safety and effectiveness of varenicline used with sustained-release bupropion or NRT have not been established. Pilot data suggest that patients receiving both varenicline and the nicotine patch are more likely to experience adverse effects (nausea, headache, vomiting, dizziness, dyspepsia, and fatigue) than are those receiving the patch alone.[62]

Smoke-Free Environments

Smoking initiation and cessation result from the interplay of numerous factors, including but not limited to environmental influences.[21] Smokers in one's environment can both promote initiation and inhibit cessation.

Data on state-specific trends in smoke-free working environments indicate that 73.4% of employees who work indoors were covered by a smoke-free workplace policy, according to a survey of 14 states conducted in 2005.[65] Smoke-free workplaces have been shown to not only protect individuals from secondhand smoke but also to reduce the prevalence of smoking.[66] In a simulation study, smoke-free workplace policies were estimated to be approximately nine times more cost-effective per patient than are programs that provide NRT at no cost.[67]

TABLE 3.
Medications with FDA-Approved Indications for Smoking Cessation[43,a]

Product Name and Availability	Precautions	Dosing	Administration and Pt Information
Nicorette gum, generic, nonprescription, 2 or 4 mg	Pregnancy[c] (Category D), breastfeeding, recent (≤2 wk) MI, serious underlying arrhythmia, serious or worsening angina pectoris, TMJ disease	≥25 cigarettes/day: 4 mg, <25 cigarettes/day: 2 mg Wk 1–6: 1 piece every 1–2 hr, wk 7–9: 1 piece every 2–4 hr, wk 10–12: 1 piece every 4–8 hr Maximum, 24 pieces/day Duration, up to 12 wk	Chew each piece slowly, park between cheek and gum when peppery or tingling sensation appears (~15–30 chews), resume chewing when taste or tingle fades, repeat chew/park steps until most of the nicotine is gone (taste or tingle does not return; generally 30 min), park in different areas of mouth, no food or beverages 15 min before or during use
Commit lozenges, generic nonprescription, 2 or 4 mg	Pregnancy[c] (Category D), breastfeeding, recent (≤2 wk) MI, serious underlying arrhythmia, serious or worsening angina pectoris	First cigarette ≤30 min after waking: 4 mg, first cigarette >30 min after waking: 2 mg Wk 1–6: 1 lozenge every 1–2 hr, wk 7–9: 1 lozenge every 2–4 hr, wk 10–12: 1 lozenge every 4–8 hr Maximum, 20 lozenges/day Duration, up to 12 wk	Allow to dissolve slowly (20-30 min), nicotine release may cause a warm, tingling sensation, do not chew or swallow, occasionally rotate to different areas of the mouth, no food or beverages 15 min before or during use
Nicoderm CQ transdermal patch, nonprescription, 24-hr release; 7,14, or 21 mg	Pregnancy[c] (Category D), breastfeeding, recent (≤2 wk) MI, serious underlying arrhythmia, serious or worsening angina pectoris	>10 cigarettes/day: 21 mg/day × 6 wk, 14 mg/day × 2 wk, 7 mg/day × 2 wk ≤10 cigarettes/day: 14 mg/day × 6 wk, 7 mg/day × 2 wk Duration: 8–10 wk	May wear patch for 16 hr if pt has sleep disturbances (remove at bedtime)
Generic patch (formerly Habitrol), prescription or nonprescription, 24-hour release; 7,14, or 21 mg	Pregnancy[c] (Category D), breastfeeding, recent (≤2 wk) MI, serious underlying arrhythmia, serious or worsening angina pectoris	>10 cigarettes/day: 21 mg/day × 4 wk, 14 mg/day × 2 wk, 7 mg/day × 2 wk ≤10 cigarettes/day: 14 mg/day x 6 wk, 7 mg/day × 2 wk Duration: 8–10 wk	May wear patch for 16 hr if pt has sleep disturbances (remove at bedtime)
Nicotrol NS, metered spray, prescription 0.5 mg nicotine in 50 μL aqueous nicotine solution	Pregnancy[c] (Category D), breastfeeding, recent (≤2 wk) MI, serious underlying arrhythmia, serious or worsening angina pectoris, underlying chronic nasal disorders (rhinitis, nasal polyps, sinusitis), severe reactive airway disease	1–2 doses/hr (8–40 doses/day) 1 dose = 2 sprays (1 in each nostril); each spray delivers 0.5 mg of nicotine Maximum of 5 doses/hr or 40 doses/day Duration, 3–6 mo	For best results, initially use at least 8 doses/day; pts should not sniff, swallow, or inhale through nose as spray is administered

Adverse Effects	Advantages	Disadvantages	Cost/Day[b]
Mouth/jaw soreness, hiccups, dyspepsia, hypersalivation, effects associated with incorrect chewing technique (lightheadedness, nausea/ vomiting, throat and mouth irritation)	Might satisfy oral cravings, may delay weight gain; pts can adjust therapy to manage withdrawal symptoms; available in a variety of flavors	Gum chewing may not be socially acceptable, might be problematic for patients with significant dental work; pts must use proper chewing technique to minimize adverse effects	2 mg: \$3.28–\$6.58 (9 pieces), 4 mg: \$4.31–\$6.58 (9 pieces)
Nausea, hiccups, cough, heartburn, headache, flatulence, insomnia	Might satisfy oral cravings, might delay weight gain, easy to use and conceal; pts can adjust therapy to manage withdrawal symptoms; available in a variety of flavors	Adverse gastrointestinal effects (nausea, hiccups, heartburn) might be bothersome; need for frequent dosing can compromise adherence	2 mg or 4 mg: \$3.66–\$5.26 (9 pieces)
Local skin reactions (erythema, pruritus, burning), headache, sleep disturbances (insomnia), abnormal or vivid dreams (associated with nocturnal nicotine absorption)	Provides consistent nicotine levels over 24 hr; easy to use and conceal; once-daily administration associated with fewer adherence problems	Pts cannot adjust dosage; allergic reactions to adhesive might occur, pts with dermatological conditions should not use patch	\$1.90–\$3.89 (1 patch)
Local skin reactions (erythema, pruritus, burning), headache, sleep disturbances (insomnia), abnormal or vivid dreams (associated with nocturnal nicotine absorption)	Provides consistent nicotine levels over 24 hr; easy to use and conceal; once-daily administration associated with fewer adherence problems	Pts cannot adjust dosage; allergic reactions to adhesive might occur, pts with dermatological conditions should not use patch	\$1.90–\$3.89 (1 patch)
Nasal or throat irritation (hot, peppery, or burning sensation), rhinitis, tearing, sneezing, cough, headache	Pts can adjust therapy to manage withdrawal symptoms	Nasal or throat irritation may be bothersome; dependence can result; pts must wait 5 min before driving or operating heavy machinery; pts with chronic nasal disorders or severe reactive airway disease should not use spray; need for frequent dosing can compromise adherence	\$3.72 (8 doses)

Continued on next page

TABLE 3. (*Continued*)
Medications with FDA-Approved Indications for Smoking Cessation[43,a]

Product Name and Availability	Precautions	Dosing	Administration and Pt Information
Nicotrol inhaler, prescription, 10-mg cartridge delivers 4 mg inhaled nicotine vapor	Pregnancy[c] (Category D), breastfeeding, recent (≤2 wk) MI, serious underlying arrhythmia, serious or worsening angina pectoris, bronchospastic disease	6–16 cartridges/day for up to 6 mo, individualized dosing Duration, 3–6 mo	Initially, use at least 6 cartridges/day; best effects with continuous puffing for 20 min; nicotine in cartridge depleted after 20 min of active puffing; pt should inhale into back of throat or puff in short breaths; do not inhale into lungs (like a cigarette) but "puff" as if lighting a pipe; open cartridge retains potency for 24 hr
Zyban (bupropion SR), generic and prescription 150-mg sustained-release tablets	Pregnancy[c] (Category C), breastfeeding, concomitant therapy with medications or medical conditions known to lower the seizure threshold, severe hepatic cirrhosis *Contraindications:* Seizure disorder, concomitant bupropion (e.g., Wellbutrin) therapy, current or prior diagnosis of bulimia or anorexia nervosa, simultaneous abrupt discontinuation of alcohol or sedatives (including benzodiazepines), MAOI therapy in previous 14 days	150 mg p.o. every morning x 3 days, then increase to 150 mg p.o. twice daily; not to exceed 300 mg/day Duration: 7–12 wk, with maintenance up to 6 mo in selected patients	Treatment should be initiated while pt is still smoking; set quit date 1–2 wk after initiation of therapy; allow at least 8 hr between doses; avoid bedtime administration to minimize insomnia; dose tapering not necessary; can be used safely with NRT
Chantix (varenicline), prescription, 0.5- and 1-mg tablets	Pregnancy[c] (Category C), breastfeeding, severe renal impairment (dosage adjustment is necessary), safety and efficacy have not been established in patients with serious psychiatric illness	Days 1–3: 0.5 mg p.o. every morning, days 4–7: 0.5 mg p.o. twice daily, wk 2–12:1 mg p.o. twice daily Duration: 12 wks; an additional 12-wk course may be used in selected patients	Pts should begin therapy 1 wk before quit date; take dose after eating with full glass of water; dose tapering is not necessary; nausea and insomnia are side effects that are usually temporary

[a]Reprinted from reference 43, with permission. Copyright © 1999-2007 The Regents of the University of California, University of Southern California, and Western University of Health Sciences. All rights reserved. For complete prescribing information, please refer to the manufacturers' package inserts. FDA = Food and Drug Administration, MI = myocardial infarction, TMJ = temporomandibular joint, NRT = nicotine-replacement therapy, MAOI = monoamine oxidase inhibitor.

Over the past few years, numerous cities and states have adopted clean indoor air laws in workplaces.[68] Nationally, the effects of transitioning all workplaces to smoke-free environments would yield an estimated 4.5% decrease in the overall prevalence of smoking.[66] In its first year of implementation, a nationwide smoke-free workplace policy would produce an estimated 1.3 million new quitters, 1500 fewer myocardial infarctions, 350 fewer strokes, and a direct saving of nearly $60 million in medical costs.[69] Given this substantial impact on public health, ASHP supports the implementation of smoke-free policies for the employees and patrons of all workplaces and public venues, including but not limited to offices, restaurants, bars, bowling alleys, and casinos, and for establishments where health care services are rendered. ASHP also strongly supports smoke-free campuses for all health care institutions and facilities. In practice, clinicians should educate patients about the dangers of secondhand smoke and encourage patients who continue to smoke to do so outdoors.

The Clinician's Role

To ensure that all future clinicians have received adequate training for treating tobacco use and dependence, schools offering health-profession courses or degrees are advised to incorporate comprehensive tobacco-cessation training as part of the required curriculum for all students.[37] Licensed clinicians who have not received the formal training necessary to provide comprehensive tobacco-cessation counseling are encouraged to complete continuing-education programs. Furthermore, clinicians should systematically integrate the identification of tobacco users and the delivery of evidence-based tobacco-use cessation interventions into routine patient care. In the absence of time or expertise to provide comprehensive cessation counseling, clinicians should—at a minimum—ask patients about tobacco use, advise patients to quit, and refer these patients to external resources such as the toll-free quit line (1-800-QUIT-NOW)

Adverse Effects	Advantages	Disadvantages	Cost/Day[b]
Mouth or throat irritation, unpleasant taste, cough, headache, rhinitis, dyspepsia, hiccups	Pts can adjust therapy to manage withdrawal symptoms; mimics hand-to-mouth ritual of smoking	Initial throat or mouth irritation can be bothersome; cartridges should not be stored in very warm conditions or used in very cold conditions; pts with underlying bronchospastic disease must use inhaler with caution; need for frequent dosing can compromise adherence	$5.29 (6 cartridges)
Insomnia, dry mouth, nervousness/difficulty concentrating, rash, constipation, seizures (risk is 1/1,000 [0.1%])	Easy to use; oral formulation might be associated with fewer compliance problems; can be used with NRT; might be beneficial in patients with depression	Seizure risk is increased; several contraindications and precautions can preclude use	$3.62–$7.40 (2 tablets)
Nausea, sleep disturbances (insomnia, abnormal dreams), constipation, flatulence, vomiting, neuropsychiatric symptoms (behavior changes, agitation, depressed mood, suicidal ideation or behavior)	Easy to use; oral formulation might be associated with fewer compliance problems; offers new mechanism of action for pts who have not succeeded with other agents	May induce nausea in up to one third of pts; postmarketing surveillance data indicate potential for neuropsychiatric symptoms	$4.49–$4.75 (2 tablets)

[b]Average wholesale price from Medi-Span Electronic Drug File. Indianapolis, IN, Wolters Kluwer Health, September 2008.
[c]The U.S. clinical practice guideline states that pregnant smokers should be encouraged to quit without medication based on insufficient evidence and hypothetical concerns with safety. Pregnant smokers should be offered cessation counseling interventions that exceed minimal advice to quit.[37]

or a group program.[37] Because higher quit rates result when patients receive assistance from multiple health care providers,[37] clinicians are encouraged to work in tandem with other providers as part of a team approach to helping patients quit smoking. **Table 4** provides useful online links to assist clinicians in tobacco-control initiatives.

Given that the sale of tobacco contradicts both the clinician's role in promoting health and the pharmacist's code of ethics,[70] ASHP strongly opposes the sale or distribution of tobacco products in all establishments where health care services are rendered (e.g., hospitals, clinics, retail chain and community pharmacies).[71] For more than three decades, the pharmacy profession has repeatedly voiced opposition to the sale of tobacco products in pharmacies,[72] including formal resolutions from state and national organizations. Notably, few licensed pharmacists (estimated at <2%)[73] and pharmacy students (3.5%)[74] are in favor of tobacco sales in pharmacies. Given this overwhelming lack of support, members of the profession are advised to insist that tobacco sales no longer occur in the environments where pharmaceutical care is rendered. Furthermore, in accordance with a 2003 resolution set forth by the American Association of Colleges of Pharmacy, ASHP encourages colleges and schools of pharmacy to give preference as clerkship sites to those pharmacies that choose not to sell tobacco products.[74]

Conclusion

Given the extensive body of data implicating tobacco as the primary known preventable cause of death in the United States, ASHP strongly supports evidence-based tobacco-control initiatives that aim to reduce the prevalence of tobacco use. These efforts should address a continuum of services, activities, and policies ranging from the integration of tobacco-cessation counseling as a routine component of patient care to the adoption of clean indoor air laws. ASHP

FIGURE 2. Plasma nicotine concentrations for nicotine-containing products. Reprinted with permission from reference 43.

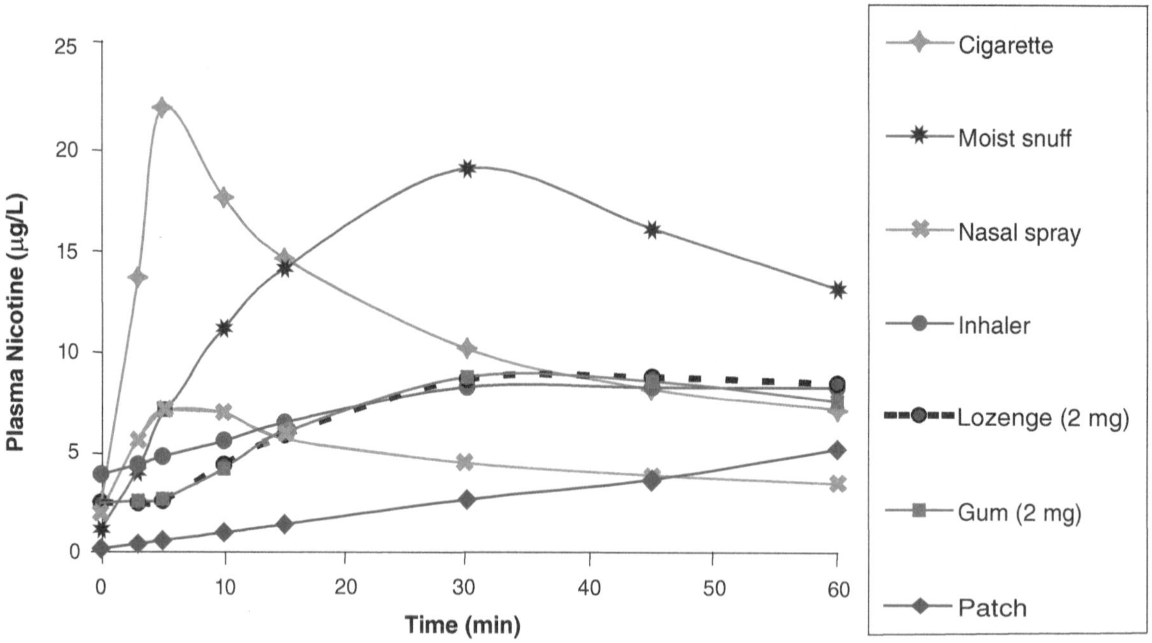

believes that the active involvement of health care providers is crucial to effective tobacco control at the population level and that the pharmacy profession—as a primary and accessible point of contact between the health care system and the public (including the medically underserved)—has a unique opportunity to serve as a cornerstone for the nation's tobacco-control efforts.

References

1. The health consequences of smoking: cancer. A report of the Surgeon General. http://profiles.nlm.nih.gov/NN/B/C/D/W/_/nnbcdw.pdf (accessed 2008 Jul 16).
2. Centers for Disease Control and Prevention. Annual smoking-attributable mortality, years of potential life lost, and productivity losses—United States, 1997-2001. *MMWR*. 2005; 54:625–8.
3. U.S. Department of Health and Human Services. 2006 Surgeon General's report: the health consequences of involuntary exposure to tobacco smoke. www.cdc.gov/tobacco/data_statistics/sgr/sgr_2006/index.htm (accessed 2008 Jul 16).
4. Doll R, Peto R, Boreham J, et al. Mortality in relation to smoking: 50 years' observations on male British doctors. *BMJ*. 2004; 328:1519.
5. Centers for Disease Control and Prevention. Cigarette smoking among adults—United States, 2000. *MMWR*. 2002; 51:642–5.
6. Centers for Disease Control and Prevention. Cigarette smoking among adults—United States, 2006. *MMWR*. 2007; 56:1157–61.
7. Lasser K, Boyd JW, Woolhandler S, et al. Smoking and mental illness: a population-based prevalence study. *JAMA*. 2000; 284:2606–10.
8. Centers for Disease Control and Prevention. State-specific prevalence of cigarette smoking among adults and quitting among persons aged 18-35 years—United States, 2006. *MMWR*. 2007; 56:993–6.
9. U.S. Department of Health and Human Services. 1994 Surgeon General's report—preventing tobacco use among young people. www.cdc.gov/tobacco/data_statistics/sgr/sgr_1994/index.htm (accessed 2008 Aug 13).
10. U.S. Department of Health and Human Services. Healthy People 2010. Vol. I and II. www.healthypeople.gov/publications/ (accessed 2008 Jul 16).
11. Johnston LD, O'Malley PM, Bachman JG, et al. Teen smoking resumes decline. www.monitoringthefuture.org/data/07data.html#2007data-cigs (accessed 2008 May 21).
12. U.S. Department of Agriculture. Tobacco outlook. Report TBS-263. http://usda.mannlib.cornell.edu/usda/ers/TBS//2000s/2007/TBS-10-24-2007.pdf (accessed 2008 Aug 13).
13. Substance Abuse and Mental Health Services Administration Offices of Applied Studies (2008). Results from the 2007 National Survey on Drug Use and Health: National findings (DHHS publication no. SMA 08-4343). Rockville, MD.
14. Henningfield JE, Fant RV, Radzius A, et al. Nicotine concentration, smoke pH and whole tobacco aqueous pH of some cigar brands and types popular in the United States. *Nicotine Tob Res*. 1999; 1:163–8.
15. Connolly GN, Alpert HR, Wayne GF, et al. Trends in nicotine yield in smoke and its relationship with design characteristics among popular US cigarette brands, 1997-2005. *Tob Control*. 2007; 16:e5.

TABLE 4.
Tobacco-Cessation Resources

Resource	Contact Information
Governmental agencies	
Centers for Disease Control and Prevention	www.cdc.gov
Environmental Protection Agency	www.epa.gov
Federal Trade Commission	www.ftc.gov
Office of the Surgeon General	www.surgeongeneral.gov
National Institutes of Health	www.nih.gov
National Cancer Institute	www.cancer.gov
National Heart, Lung, and Blood Institute	www.nhlbi.nih.gov
National Institute on Drug Abuse	www.nida.nih.gov
Organizations	
American Cancer Society	www.cancer.org
American Heart Association	www.americanheart.org
American Legacy Foundation	www.americanlegacy.org
American Lung Association	www.lungusa.org
American Society of Health-System Pharmacists	www.ashp.org/s_ashp/tobacco
Campaign for Tobacco-Free Kids	www.tobaccofreekids.org
Global Network of Pharmacists Against Tobacco	www.fip.org/pharmacistsagainsttobacco
North American Quitline Consortium	www.naquitline.org
Society for Research on Nicotine & Tobacco	www.srnt.org
University of California Smoking Cessation Leadership Center	smokingcessationleadership.ucsf.edu
University of California Tobacco-Related Disease Research Program	www.trdrp.org
World Health Organization	www.who.int
Documents	
Clinical Practice Guideline for Treating Tobacco Use and Dependence	www.surgeongeneral.gov/tobacco
Legacy Tobacco Industry Documents Archive	www.legacy.library.ucsf.edu
Pharmacologic aids for cessation—online support	
Committed Quitters Program	
Nicorette gum	www.nicorette.com
Nicoderm patch	www.nicodermcq.com
Commit lozenge	www.commitlozenge.com
GETQUIT Support Plan	
Chantix	www.chantix.com
Helping Hand Program	
Nicotrol nasal spray and inhaler	www.nicotrol.com
Smoke-Free Program	
Generic patch (formerly Habitrol)	www.habitrol.com
Nonpharmaceutical cessation support and programs	
QuitKey (handheld computer for scheduled gradual reduction of smoking)	www.quitkey.com
QuitNet (comprehensive online tobacco-cessation support program)	www.quitnet.com
Rx for Change: Clinician-Assisted Tobacco Cessation (evidence-based tobacco-cessation training materials for educating health professional students and licensed clinicians)	rxforchange.ucsf.edu
Tobacco-Free Nurses (national program focused on helping nurses and student nurses to stop smoking)	www.tobaccofreenurses.org
Toll-free quit lines (telephone counseling for cessation, available at no cost to all callers)	1-800-QUIT-NOW

16. Ebbert JO, Carr AB, Dale LC. Smokeless tobacco: an emerging addiction. *Med Clin North Am.* 2004; 88:1593–605.
17. Centers for Disease Control and Prevention. Annual smoking-attributable mortality, years of potential life lost, and economic costs—United States, 1995–1999. *MMWR.* 2002; 51:300–3.
18. Best practices for comprehensive tobacco control programs—2007. Atlanta: Centers for Disease Control and Prevention; 2007.
19. Task Force on Community Preventive Services. The guide to community preventive services: tobacco use prevention and control. *Am J Prev Med.* 2001; 20(suppl 2):1–88.
20. U.S. Department of Health and Human Services. The health consequences of smoking: nicotine addiction: a report of the Surgeon General. http://profiles.nlm.nih.gov/NN/B/B/Z/D/_/nnbbzd.pdf (accessed 2008 Jul 16).

21. Benowitz NL. Clinical pharmacology of nicotine: implications for understanding, preventing and treating tobacco addiction. *Clin Pharm Ther.* 2008; 83:531–41.
22. Hughes JR, Gust SW, Skoog K, et al. Symptoms of tobacco withdrawal: a replication and extension. *Arch Gen Psychiatry.* 1991; 48:52–9.
23. Hughes JR. Effects of abstinence from tobacco: valid symptoms and time course. *Nicotine Tob Res.* 2007; 9:315–327.
24. American Psychiatric Association. Diagnostic and statistical manual of mental disorders, 4th edition. Washington, DC: American Psychiatric Publishing; 1994.
25. Benowitz NL. Cigarette smoking and nicotine addiction. *Med Clin North Am.* 1992; 76:415–37.
26. Hatsukami DK, Gust SW, Keenan RM. Physiologic and subjective changes from smokeless tobacco withdrawal. *Clin Pharmacol Ther.* 1987; 41:103–7.
27. Centers for Disease Control and Prevention. U.S. 2004 Surgeon General's report—the health consequences of smoking. www.cdc.gov/tobacco/data_statistics/sgr/sgr_2004/index.htm (accessed 2008 Jul 16).
28. Henley SJ, Thun MJ, Connell C, et al. Two large prospective studies of mortality among men who use snuff or chewing tobacco (United States). *Cancer Causes Control.* 2005; 16:347–58.
29. Hergens MP, Ahlbom A, Andersson T, et al. Swedish moist snuff and myocardial infarction among men. *Epidemiology.* 2005; 16:12–16.
30. Gupta R, Gurm H, Bartholomew JR. Smokeless tobacco and cardiovascular risk. *Arch Intern Med.* 2004; 164:1845–9.
31. Henley SJ, Connell CJ, Richter P, et al. Tobacco-related disease mortality among men who switched from cigarettes to spit tobacco. *Tob Control.* 2007; 16:22–8.
32. California Environmental Protection Agency. Proposed identification of environmental tobacco smoke as a toxic air contaminant: executive summary. www.arb.ca.gov/regact/ets2006/ets2006.htm (accessed 2008 Oct 1).
33. Kroon LA. Drug interactions with smoking. *Am J Health-Syst Pharm.* 2007; 64:1917–21.
34. Zevin S, Benowitz NL. Drug interactions with tobacco smoking. *Clin Pharmacokinet.* 1999; 36:425–38.
35. U.S. Department of Health and Human Services. The benefits of smoking cessation. A report of the surgeon general (DHHS publication no. CDC 90-8416). U.S. Department of Health and Human Services, Public Health Service, Centers for Disease Control and Prevention and Health Promotion, Office on Smoking and Health. 1990.
36. Hazelden Foundation. Survey on current and former smokers—1998. www.hazelden.org/web/public/smokers 1998.page (accessed 2008 Aug 13.).
37. Fiore MC, Jaen CR, Baker TB, et al. Treating tobacco use and dependence—2008 update. Clinical practice guideline. www.surgeongeneral.gov/tobacco/treating_tobacco_use08.pdf (accessed 2008 Jul 16).
38. Stead L, Perera R, Lancaster T. Telephone counselling for smoking cessation. *Cochrane Database Syst Rev.* 2006; 3:CD002850.
39. Ossip-Klein DJ, McIntosh S. Quitlines in North America: evidence base and applications. *Am J Med Sci.* 2003; 326:201–5.
40. Zhu SH, Anderson CM, Tedeschi GJ, et al. Evidence of real-world effectiveness of a telephone quitline for smokers. *N Engl J Med.* 2002; 347:1087–93.
41. Lichtenstein E, Glasgow RE, Lando HA, et al. Telephone counseling for smoking cessation: rationales and meta-analytic review of evidence. *Health Educ Res.* 1996; 11:243–57.
42. Hopkins DP, Briss PA, Ricard CJ, et al. Reviews of evidence regarding interventions to reduce tobacco use and exposure to environmental tobacco smoke. *Am J Prev Med.* 2001; 20(2, suppl):16–66.
43. Rx for Change: clinician-assisted tobacco cessation. http://rxforchange.ucsf.edu (accessed 2008 Oct 1).
44. Benowitz NL. Cigarette smoking and cardiovascular disease: pathophysiology and implications for treatment. *Prog Cardiovasc Dis.* 2003; 46:91–111.
45. Working Group for the Study of Transdermal Nicotine in Patients with Coronary Artery Disease. Nicotine replacement therapy for patients with coronary artery disease. *Arch Intern Med.* 1994; 154:989–95.
46. Joseph AM, Norman SM, Ferry LH, et al. The safety of transdermal nicotine as an aid to smoking cessation in patients with cardiac disease. *N Engl J Med.* 1996; 335:1792–8.
47. Tzivoni D, Keren A, Meyler S, et al. Cardiovascular safety of transdermal nicotine patches in patients with coronary artery disease who try to quit smoking. *Cardiovasc Drugs Ther.* 1998; 12:239–44.
48. Hubbard R, Lewis S, Smith C, et al. Use of nicotine replacement therapy and the risk of acute myocardial infarction, stroke, and death. *Tob Control.* 2005; 14:416–21.
49. McRobbie H, Hajek P. Nicotine replacement therapy in patients with cardiovascular disease: guidelines for health professionals. *Addiction.* 2001; 96:1547–51.
50. Joseph AM, Fu SS. Safety issues in pharmacotherapy for smoking in patients with cardiovascular disease. *Prog Cardiovasc Dis.* 2003; 45:429–41.
51. Benowitz NL, Gourlay SG. Cardiovascular toxicity of nicotine: implications for nicotine replacement therapy. *J Am Coll Cardiol.* 1997; 29:1422–31.
52. Meine TJ, Patel MR, Washam JB, et al. Safety and effectiveness of transdermal nicotine patch in smokers admitted with acute coronary syndromes. *Am J Cardiol.* 2005; 95:976–8.
53. Benowitz NL, Dempsey DA. Pharmacotherapy for smoking cessation during pregnancy. *Nicotine Tob Res.* 2004;6(Suppl 2):S189–202.
54. Ascher JA, Cole JO, Colin J, et al. Bupropion: a review of its mechanism of antidepressant activity. *J Clin Psychiatry.* 1995; 56:395–401.
55. Slemmer JE, Martin BR, Damaj MI. Bupropion is a nicotinic antagonist. *J Pharmacol Exp Ther.* Oct 2000; 295:321–7.
56. Hayford KE, Patten CA, Rummans TA, et al. Efficacy of bupropion for smoking cessation in smokers with a former history of major depression or alcoholism. *Br J Psychiatry.* 1999; 174:173–8.

57. Hughes J, Stead L, Lancaster T. Antidepressants for smoking cessation. *Cochrane Database Syst Rev.* 2007(1):CD000031.
58. Zyban (bupropion hydrochloride) package insert. Research Triangle Park, NC: GlaxoSmithKline, Inc.; 2007 Aug.
59. Dunner DL, Zisook S, Billow AA, et al. A prospective safety surveillance study for bupropion sustained-release in the treatment of depression. *J Clin Psy-chiatry.* 1998; 59:366–73.
60. Foulds J. The neurobiological basis for partial agonist treatment of nicotine dependence: varenicline. *Int J Clin Pract.* May 2006; 60:571–6.
61. Cahill K, Stead LF, Lancaster T. Nicotine receptor partial agonists for smoking cessation. *Cochrane Database Syst Rev.* 2008(3):CD006103.
62. Chantix (varenicline) package insert. New York: Pfizer, Inc.; 2008 May.
63. Food and Drug Administration. Varenicline information. www.fda.gov/cder/drug/infopage/varenicline/default.htm (accessed 2008 May 22).
64. Bars MP, Banauch GI, Appel D, et al. Tobacco Free With FDNY: the New York City Fire Department World Trade Center Tobacco Cessation Study. *Chest.* 2006; 129:979–87.
65. State-specific prevalence of current cigarette smoking among adults and second hand smoke rules and policies in homes and workplaces, United States, 2005. *MMWR.* 2006; 55:1148–51.
66. Fichtenberg CM, Glantz SA. Effect of smoke-free workplaces on smoking behaviour: systematic review. *BMJ.* 2002; 325:188.
67. Ong MK, Glantz SA. Free nicotine replacement therapy programs vs implementing smoke-free workplaces: a cost-effectiveness comparison. *Am J Public Health.* 2005; 95:969–75.
68. American Nonsmokers' Rights Foundation. States, commonwealths, and municipalities with 100% smoke-free laws in workplaces, restaurants or bars. www.no-smoke.org/pdf/100ordlist.pdf (accessed 2008 Aug 13).
69. Ong MK, Glantz SA. Cardiovascular health and economic effects of smoke-free workplaces. *Am J Med.* 2004; 117:32–8.
70. American Pharmacists Association. Code of ethics for pharmacists. http://www.pharmacist.com/AM/Template.cfm?Section=Code_of_Ethics_for_Pharmacists&Template=/CM/HTMLDisplay.cfm&ContentID=5420 (accessed 2008 Aug 13).
71. American Society of Health-System Pharmacists. ASHP policy position 0713: tobacco and tobacco products. http://www.ashp.org/s_ashp/docs/files/BP07/HR_Positions.pdf (accessed 2008 Aug 13).
72. Davis RM. Tobacco sales in pharmacies: mixing good drugs and bad drugs. *Tob Control.* 1992; 1:84–96.
73. Hudmon KS, Prokhorov AV, Corelli RL. Tobacco cessation counseling: pharmacists' opinions and practices. *Patient Educ Couns.* 2006; 61:152–60.
74. Hudmon KS, Corelli RL, Fenlon CM, et al. Pharmacy student perceptions of tobacco sales in pharmacies and suggested methods for promoting tobacco-free experiential sites. *Am J Pharm Educ.* 2006; 70:75.

Appendix A—The 5 A's of Tobacco Cessation Counseling[37]

Step	Action	Strategies for Implementation
Ask—Systematically identify all tobacco users at every visit	Implement a system that ensures that, for every patient at every clinic visit, tobacco use status is queried and documented.[a]	Expand the vital signs to include tobacco use, or use an alternative universal identification system.[b] VITAL SIGNS Blood Pressure: _______ Pulse: ___ Weight: _____ Temperature: ______ Respiratory Rate: _______ Tobacco Use (circle one): Current Former Never
Advise—Strongly urge all tobacco users to quit	In a clear, strong, and personalized manner, urge every tobacco user to quit.	Advice should be: • Clear—"It is important that you quit smoking (or using chewing tobacco) now, and I can help you." "Cutting down while you are ill is not enough." "Occasional or light smoking is still dangerous." • Strong—"As your clinician, I need you to know that quitting smoking is the most important thing you can do to protect your health now and in the future. The clinic staff and I will help you." • Personalized—Tie tobacco use to current symptoms and health concerns, and/or its social and economic costs, and/or the impact of tobacco use on children and others in the household. "Continuing to smoke makes your asthma worse, and quitting may dramatically improve your health." "Quitting smoking may reduce the number of ear infections your child has."
Assess—Determine willingness to make a quit attempt	Assess every tobacco user's willingness to make a quit attempt at the time.	Assess patient's willingness to quit: "Are you willing to give quitting a try?" • If the patient is willing to make a quit attempt at the time, provide assistance. ό If the patient will participate in an intensive treatment, deliver such a treatment or link/refer to an intensive intervention. ό If the patient is a member of a special population (e.g., adolescent, pregnant smoker, racial/ethnic minority), consider providing additional information. • If the patient clearly states that he or she is unwilling to make a quit attempt at the time, provide an intervention shown to increase future quit attempts.
Assist—Aid the patient in quitting (provide counseling and medication)	Help the patient with a quit plan.	STAR: A patient's preparations for quitting: • **S**et a quit date. Ideally, the quit date should be within 2 weeks. • **T**ell family, friends, and coworkers about quitting, and request understanding and support. • **A**nticipate challenges to the upcoming quit attempt, particularly during the critical first few weeks. These include nicotine withdrawal symptoms. • **R**emove tobacco products from your environment. Prior to quitting, avoid smoking in places where you spend a lot of time (e.g., work, home, car). Make your home smoke-free.
	Recommend the use of approved medication, except when contraindicated or with specific populations for which there is insufficient evidence of effectiveness.	Recommend the use of medications found to be effective. Explain how these medications increase quitting success and reduce withdrawal symptoms. The first-line medications include: bupropion SR, nicotine gum, nicotine inhaler, nicotine lozenge, nicotine nasal spray, nicotine patch, and varenicline; second-line medications include: clonidine and nortriptyline. There is insufficient evidence to recommend medications for certain populations (e.g., pregnant women, smokeless tobacco users, light smokers, adolescents).
	Provide practical counseling (problem solving/skills training).	• Abstinence: Striving for total abstinence is essential. Not even a single puff after the quit date. • Past quit experience: Identify what helped and what hurt in previous quit attempts. Build on past success. • Anticipate triggers or challenges in the upcoming attempt. Discuss challenges/triggers and how the patient will successfully overcome them (e.g., avoid triggers, alter routines). • Alcohol: Because alcohol is associated with relapse, the patient should consider limiting/abstaining from alcohol while quitting. (Note that reducing alcohol intake could precipitate withdrawal in alcohol-dependent persons.) • Other smokers in the household: Quitting is more difficult when there is another smoker in the household. Patients should encourage housemates to quit with them or to not smoke in their presence.

Appendix A—The 5 A's of Tobacco Cessation Counseling[37] *(continued)*

Step	Action	Strategies for Implementation
	Provide intratreatment social support.	Provide a supportive clinical environment while encouraging the patient in his or her quit attempt. "My office staff and I are available to assist you." "I'm recommending treatment that can provide ongoing support."
	Provide supplementary materials, including information on quitlines.	• Sources: Federal agencies, nonprofit agencies, national quitline network (1-800-QUIT-NOW), or local/state/tribal health departments/quitlines. • Type: Culturally/racially/educationally/age-appropriate for the patient. • Location: Readily available at every clinician's workstation.
Arrange—Ensure follow-up contact	Arrange for follow-up contacts, either in person or via telephone.	• Timing: Follow-up contact should begin soon after the quit date, preferably during the first week. A second follow-up contact is recommended within the first month. Schedule further follow-up contacts as indicated. • Actions during followup contact: For all patients, identify problems already encountered and anticipate challenges in the immediate future. Assess medication use and problems. Remind patients of quitline support (1-800-QUIT-NOW). Address tobacco use at next clinical visit (treat tobacco use as a chronic disease). • For patients who are abstinent, congratulate them on their success. If tobacco use has occurred, review circumstances and elicit recommitment to total abstinence. Consider use of or link to more intensive treatment.

[a]Repeated assessment is not necessary in the case of the adult who has never used tobacco or has not used tobacco for many years and for whom this information is clearly documented in the medical record.

[b]Alternatives to expanding the vital signs include using tobacco use status stickers on all patient charts or indicating tobacco use status via electronic medical records or computerized reminder systems.

Appendix B—Enhancing Motivation to Quit: The 5 R's of Tobacco-Cessation Counseling[37]

Relevance

Encourage the patient to indicate why quitting is personally relevant, being as specific as possible. Motivational information has the greatest impact if it is relevant to a patient's disease status or risk, family or social situation (e.g., having children in the home), health concerns, age, gender, and other important patient characteristics (e.g., prior quitting experience, personal barriers to cessation).

Risks

The clinician should ask the patient to identify potential negative consequences of tobacco use. The clinician may suggest and highlight those that seem most relevant to the patient. The clinician should emphasize that smoking low-tar/low-nicotine cigarettes or use of other forms of tobacco (e.g., smokeless tobacco, cigars, and pipes) will not eliminate these risks. Examples of risks are:

- Acute risks: Shortness of breath, exacerbation of asthma, increased risk of respiratory infections, harm to pregnancy, impotence, infertility.
- Long-term risks: Heart attacks and strokes, lung and other cancers (e.g., larynx, oral cavity, pharynx, esophagus, pancreas, stomach, kidney, bladder, cervix, and acute myelocytic leukemia), chronic obstructive pulmonary diseases (chronic bronchitis and emphysema), osteoporosis, long-term disability, and need for extended care.
- Environmental risks: Increased risk of lung cancer and heart disease in spouses; increased risk for low birth-weight, sudden infant death syndrome (SIDS), asthma, middle ear disease, and respiratory infections in children of smokers.

Rewards

The clinician should ask the patient to identify potential benefits of stopping tobacco use. The clinician may suggest and highlight those that seem most relevant to the patient. Examples of rewards include:

- Improved health
- Food will taste better
- Improved sense of smell
- Saving money
- Feeling better about oneself
- Home, car, clothing, breath will smell better
- Setting a good example for children and decreasing the likelihood that they will smoke
- Having healthier babies and children
- Feeling better physically
- Performing better in physical activities
- Improved appearance, including reduced wrinkling/aging of skin and whiter teeth

Roadblocks

The clinician should ask the patient to identify barriers or impediments to quitting and provide treatment (problem solving counseling, medication) that could address barriers. Typical barriers might include:

- Withdrawal symptoms
- Fear of failure
- Weight gain
- Lack of support
- Depression
- Enjoyment of tobacco
- Being around other tobacco users
- Limited knowledge of effective treatment options

Repetition

The motivational intervention should be repeated every time an unmotivated patient visits the clinic setting. Tobacco users who have failed in previous quit attempts should be told that most people make repeated quit attempts before they are successful.

Developed by the ASHP Council on Therapeutics and approved by the ASHP Board of Directors on June 30, 2008.

Karen Suchanek Hudmon, Dr.P.H., M.S., and Robin L. Corelli, Pharm.D., are gratefully acknowledged for authoring this therapeutic position statement. Dr. Suchanek Hudmon is Associate Professor, Department of Pharmacy Practice, Purdue University School of Pharmacy and Pharmaceutical Sciencs, West Lafayette, IN. Dr. Corelli is Professor of Clinical Pharmacy, Department of Clinical Pharmacy, University of California San Francisco, San Francisco.

The following individuals are acknowledged for reviewing draft versions of this statement: John R. Hughes, M.D., Connie C. Revell, M.A., Mary H. Zimmerman, BCPS, CACP, Thomas P. Houston, M.D., FAAFP, FACPM, Candice Garwood, Pharm.D., BCPS, Karen Gunning, Pharm.D., BCPS, Carol Southard, R.N., M.S.N., Frank Vitale, M.A., Alan J. Zillich, Pharm.D., Laura B. Hanson, Pharm.D., Daniel A. Hussar, Ph.D., and the American Nurses Association.

Copyright © 2009, American Society of Health-System Pharmacists, Inc. All rights reserved. Contact ASHP for reprint and permissions requests. This content may not be used for commercial purposes without the express written consent of ASHP.

The bibliographic citation for this document is as follows: American Society of Health-System Pharmacists. ASHP therapeutic position statement on the cessation of tobacco use. *Am J Health-Syst Pharm.* 2009; 66:291–307.

ASHP Therapeutic Position Statement on the Institutional Use of 0.9% Sodium Chloride Injection to Maintain Patency of Peripheral Indwelling Intermittent Infusion Devices

Statement of Position

0.9% Sodium chloride injection is a safe and effective indwelling solution for maintaining catheter patency of peripheral indwelling intermittent infusion devices (PIIIDs) in adults and children age one year or older. ASHP supports the use of 0.9% sodium chloride injection in preference to heparin-containing flush solutions (heparin flush) in the institutional setting, on the basis of clinical evidence indicating that 0.9% sodium chloride injection (1) is as effective as heparin flush in maintaining the patency of PIIIDs when blood is not aspirated into the device, (2) is safer to use than heparin flush because of a lower potential for adverse effects, (3) avoids drug incompatibilities associated with heparin flush, and (4) is a cost-effective alternative to heparin flush. Because of limited and conflicting available scientific evidence to date, this recommendation is not applicable to children under the age of one year or patients in the home or other outpatient settings. This document is not applicable to catheters used for central venous or arterial access (including peripherally inserted central catheters and midline catheters) and the maintenance of patency in indwelling venipuncture devices used to obtain blood samples. Further research on PIIID patency in the aforementioned patient populations and settings is warranted.

Background

PIIIDs, often referred to as "saline locks" and frequently and inappropriately called "heparin locks," are used to provide convenient i.v. access in patients who require intermittent i.v. administration of medications without a continuous infusion of i.v. fluids. The advantages of PIIIDs include patient mobility and comfort and reduced fluid load.[1–4] PIIIDs most commonly consist of an intravenously inserted catheter attached to a short external cannula with a resealable injection port that is designed to facilitate multiple needle entries; thus, these devices eliminate the unnecessary trauma of multiple venipunctures.[4] A problem frequently encountered with PIIIDs is the loss of patency because of clot formation within the catheter. To prevent clot formation, catheters are commonly flushed after each administration of i.v. medication and every 8–12 hours when the device is not in use.[5] Because of heparin's anticoagulant effects, diluted solutions of heparin in 0.9% sodium chloride injection (e.g., 10 or 100 units/mL) have traditionally been used to periodically flush and fill these devices and prevent the formation of clots. Diluted heparin solutions are used to maintain patency while avoiding the systemic effects associated with therapeutic doses of heparin.[6]

However, due to the aforementioned concerns regarding heparin administration and the potential for medication dose error, many clinicians preferentially began using sodium chloride for flushes even before evidence was available that supported the use of sodium chloride instead of heparin.

Efficacy

Studies have indicated that 0.9% sodium chloride injection alone is as effective as heparin-containing solutions in maintaining PIIID patency.[7–16] In several randomized, double-blind studies in which PIIIDs composed principally of fluoroethylene propylene (Teflon) were used, 0.9% sodium chloride injection for flushing was associated with patency rates similar to those achieved with flush solutions containing heparin sodium 10 or 100 units/mL.[10–12] The frequency of phlebitis associated with the use of these solutions was also similar.[7,8,17–19] The type of solution used to maintain PIIID patency may not be as important as the positive pressure maintained in the i.v. line by the capped (sealed) injection device, which appears to prevent blood reflux and clot formation in the devices.[8,19] Several studies provide a scientific basis for using heparin flush,[6,20,21] but most published research supports 0.9% sodium chloride injection as an effective alternative to heparin flush in maintaining the patency of PIIIDs. However, 0.9% sodium chloride or heparin flush may not be the appropriate flush solution when flushing drugs that may not be compatible with 0.9% sodium chloride or heparin. Specific examples of such drugs include liposomal amphotericin B, doxorubicin, and i.v. immune globulin.[22] These drugs may need to be "preflushed" with another compatible solution such as 5% dextrose injection before and after administering the incompatible drug. In addition, the size of the i.v. catheter in pediatric patients appears to be a contributing factor in determining success with 0.9% sodium chloride for maintaining the patency of PIIIDs. Evidence supports the use of 0.9% sodium chloride flushes over heparin in pediatric patients,[23–27] and 0.9% sodium chloride injection is the preferred solution mentioned in the available nursing guidelines on infusion standards.[28]

One survey found that in neonates, it was common practice to flush catheter devices with heparin 1–2 units/mL,[29] and the literature supports the use of heparin 0.5 unit/mL added to continuous infusions through peripheral lines.[30] Concentrations of heparinized 0.9% sodium chloride injection 1–10 units/mL for flushing have been studied in neonatal patients, with no significant difference in catheter life or patency between 0.9% sodium chloride injection and heparinized 0.9% sodium chloride injection.[31–33] A limitation of these studies is small sample size, indicating low statistical power. Despite the lack of evidence-based literature supporting the superiority of heparin over 0.9% sodium chloride injection or vice versa for neonatal peripheral i.v. flushes, current guidelines published by the National Association of Neonatal Nurses state that heparinized 0.9% sodium chloride

DOI 10.37573/9781585287048.109

0.5 unit/mL should be used to flush peripheral i.v. catheters using 0.2–0.5 mL every three to four hours.[34] If using 0.9% sodium chloride injection in pediatric patients, avoid bacteriostatic 0.9% sodium chloride, especially in neonates.

One trial of pregnant women demonstrated significantly increased efficacy and decreased complication rates with heparin-infused catheters compared with those flushed with 0.9% sodium chloride.[35] A subsequent study of pregnant women found no significant differences in the number of patent catheters or in complications with catheters flushed with either heparin or 0.9% sodium chloride.[36] However, the authors from both studies noted that their sample sizes were small and not powered sufficiently to detect a significant difference in patency or complications, possibly affecting the true clinical significance of their results. While published data from pregnant patients are conflicting, common practice is to use 0.9% sodium chloride flushes for peripheral i.v. catheters in this patient population.

Adverse Effects of Heparin Flush

Heparin, even when used in small doses, may elicit adverse reactions in some patients. The potential for bleeding complications increases when patients receive multiple unmonitored heparin flushes.[37] Repeated injections of heparin, even in small doses, can alter activated partial thromboplastin time.[38] Allergic reactions are an inherent risk of using heparin. Although rare, heparin-flush-associated thrombocytopenia and hemorrhage have been reported.[37,39–41] The risks of these adverse effects may be avoided by using 0.9% sodium chloride injection instead of heparin flush. Heparin is incompatible with many anthracyclines, including daunorubicin and doxorubicin, as well as benzodiazepines such as diazepam and midazolam.[22]

Cost Implications

Enhanced quality of patient care should be the primary reason for deciding to use 0.9% sodium chloride injection for flushing. Secondarily, the choice of 0.9% sodium chloride injection may avoid substantial costs associated with drugs, related supplies, and staff time.[9]

Summary

Because current therapeutic evidence supports the efficacy of 0.9% sodium chloride injection in maintaining PIIID patency and due to the inherent risks associated with heparin, ASHP believes that the use of 0.9% sodium chloride injection is appropriate for maintaining the patency of PIIIDs in adults and children age one year or older in institutional settings. Because of limited and conflicting scientific evidence available to date, this recommendation is not applicable to neonates, patients in the home or other outpatient settings, catheters used for central venous or arterial access (including peripherally inserted central catheters and midline catheters), which was beyond the scope of this therapeutic position statement, and the maintenance of patency in indwelling venipuncture devices used to obtain blood samples.

References

1. Millam DA. Intermittent devices. *NITA*. 1981; 4:142–5.
2. Larkin M. Heparin locks. *NITA*. 1979; 2:18–9.
3. Thomas RB, Salter FJ. Heparin locks: their advantages and disadvantages. *Hosp Formul.* 1975; 10:536–8.
4. Deeb EN, Di Mattia PE. How much heparin in the lock? *Am J IV Ther.* 1976; 3:22–6.
5. Tuten SH, Gueldner SH. Efficacy of sodium chloride versus dilute heparin for maintenance of peripheral intermittent intravenous devices. *Appl Nurs Res.* 1991; 2:63–71.
6. Hanson RL, Grant AM, Majors KR. Heparin-lock maintenance with ten units of sodium heparin in one milliliter of normal saline solution. *Surg Gynecol Obstet.* 1976; 142:373–6.
7. Barrett PJ, Lester RL. Heparin versus saline flushing solutions in a small community hospital. *Hosp Pharm.* 1990; 25:115–8.
8. Dunn DL, Lenihan SF. The case for the saline flush. *Am J Nurs.* 1987; 87:798–9.
9. Fry B. Intermittent heparin flushing protocols. A standardization issue. *J Intraven Nurs.* 1992; 15:160–3.
10. Epperson EL. Efficacy of 0.9% sodium chloride injection with and without heparin for maintaining indwelling intermittent injection sites. *Clin Pharm.* 1984; 3:626–9.
11. Garrelts JC, LaRocca J, Ast D, et al. Comparison of heparin and 0.9% sodium chloride injection in the maintenance of indwelling intermittent i.v. devices. *Clin Pharm.* 1989; 8:34–9.
12. Hamilton RA, Plis JM, Clay C, et al. Heparin sodium versus 0.9% sodium chloride injection for maintaining patency of in-dwelling intermittent infusion devices. *Clin Pharm.* 1988; 7:439–43.
13. Shearer J. Normal saline versus dilute heparin flush: a study of peripheral intermittent i.v. devices. *NITA*. 1987; 10:425–7.
14. Miracle V, Fangman B, Kayrouz P, et al. Normal saline vs. heparin lock flush solution: one institution's findings. *Ky Nurse.* 1989; 37(Jul–Aug):1, 6–7.
15. Ashton J, Gibson V, Summers S. Effects of heparin versus saline solution on intermittent infusion device irrigation. *Heart Lung.* 1990; 19:608–12.
16. Hook ML, Ose P. Heparin vs. normal saline. *J Intraven Nurs.* 1990; 13:150–1. Letter.
17. Garrelts JC. White clot syndrome and thrombocytopenia: reasons to abandon heparin i.v. lock flush solution. *Clin Pharm.* 1992; 11:797–9.
18. Weber DR. Is heparin really necessary in the lock and, if so, how much? *DICP.* 1991; 25:399–407.
19. Goode CJ, Titler M, Rakel B, et al. A meta-analysis of effects of heparin flush and saline flush: quality and cost implications. *Nurs 2Res.* 1991; 40:324–30.
20. Cyganski JM, Donahue JM, Heaton JS. The case for the heparin flush. *Am J Nurs.* 1987; 87:796–7.
21. Holford NH, Vozeh S, Coates P, et al. More on heparin lock. *N Engl J Med.* 1977; 296:1300–1. Letter.

22. Trissel LA. Handbook on injectable drugs. 16th ed. Bethesda, MD: American Society of Health-System Pharmacists; 2011.
23. Mok E, Kwong TK, Chan MF. A randomized controlled trial for maintaining peripheral intravenous lock in children. *Int J Nurs Pract.* 2007; 13:33–45.
24. Hanrahan KS, Kleiber C, Fagan CL. Evaluation of saline for iv locks in children. *Pediatr Nurs.* 1994; 20:549–52.
25. Kleiber C, Hanrahan K, Fagan CL, et al. Heparin vs saline for peripheral i.v. locks in children. *Pediatr Nurs.* 1993; 19:405–9.
26. Danek G, Noris EM. Pediatric iv catheters: efficacy of saline flush. *Pediatr Nurs.* 1992; 18:111–3.
27. LeDuc K. Efficacy of normal saline solution versus heparin solution for maintaining patency of peripheral intravenous catheters in children. *J Emerg Nurs.* 1997; 23:306–9.
28. Intravenous Nurses Society. Infusion nursing standards of practice. *J Infus Nurs.* 2011; 34:37–72.
29. Romanowski GL, Zenk KE. Intravenous flush solutions for neonates. Paper presented at ASHP Midyear Clinical Meeting. New Orleans, LA; 1991 Dec 10.
30. Klenner AF, Fusch C, Rakow A, et al. Benefit and risk of heparin for maintaining peripheral venous catheters in neonates: a placebo-controlled trial. *J Pediatr.* 2003; 143:741–5.
31. Shah PS, Ng E, Sinha AK. Heparin for prolonging peripheral intravenous catheter use in neonates. *Cochrane Database Syst Rev.* 2005; 4:CD002774.
32. Goldberg M, Sankaran R, Givelichan L, et al. Maintaining patency of peripheral intermittent infusion devices with heparinized saline and saline. *Neonatal Intensive Care.* 1999; 12:18–22.
33. Heilskov J. A randomized trial of heparin and saline for maintaining intravenous locks in neonates. *J Soc Pediatr Nurs.* 1998; 3:111–6.
34. Altimier L, Brown B, Tedeschi L. NANN guidelines for neonatal nursing policies, procedures, competencies, and clinical pathways. 4th ed. Glenview, IL: National Association of Neonatal Nurses; 2006.
35. Meyer BA, Little CJ, Thorp JA, et al. Heparin versus normal saline as a peripheral line flush in maintenance of intermittent intravenous lines in obstetric patients. *Obstet Gynecol.* 1995; 85:433–6.
36. Niesen KM, Harris DY, Parkin LS, et al. The effects of heparin versus normal saline for maintenance of peripheral intravenous locks in pregnant women. *J Obstet Gynecol Neonatal Nurs.* 2003; 32:503–8.
37. Passannante A, Macik BG. The heparin flush syndrome: a cause of iatrogenic hemorrhage. *Am J Med Sci.* 1988; 296:71–3.
38. Heparin sodium monograph. In: McEvoy GK, ed. *AHFS Drug Information.* Bethesda, MD: American Society of Health-System Pharmacists; 2006:2616.
39. Heeger PS, Backstrom JT. Heparin flushes and thrombocytopenia. *Ann Intern Med.* 1986; 105:143. Letter.
40. Doty JR, Alving BM, McDonnell DE, et al. Heparin-associated thrombocytopenia in the neurosurgical patient. *Neurosurgery.* 1986; 19:69–72.
41. Cines DB, Tomaski A, Tannenbaum S. Immune endothelial-cell injury in heparin-associated thrombocytopenia. *N Engl J Med.* 1987; 316:581–9.

Approved by the ASHP Board of Directors on April 13, 2012. Developed through the Council on Therapeutics.

This document supersedes the ASHP therapeutic position statement on the institutional use of 0.9% sodium chloride injection to maintain patency of peripheral indwelling intermittent infusion devices approved by the ASHP Board of Directors on January 12, 2006.

Kim W. Benner, Pharm.D., BCPS, FASHP, and Amber J. Lucas, Pharm.D., BCPS, FASHP, are gratefully acknowledged for authoring this document.

Copyright © 2012, American Society of Health-System Pharmacists, Inc. All rights reserved. Contact ASHP for reprint and permissions requests. This content may not be used for commercial purposes without the express written consent of ASHP.

The bibliographic citation for this document is as follows: American Society of Health-System Pharmacists. ASHP therapeutic position statement on the institutional use of 0.9% sodium chloride injection to maintain patency of peripheral indwelling intermittent infusion devices. *Am J Health-Syst Pharm.* 2012; 69:1252–4.

ASHP Therapeutic Position Statement on the Role of Pharmacotherapy in Preventing Venous Thromboembolism in Hospitalized Patients

Position

Hospitals should develop formal policies, guidelines, practices, and procedures to address the appropriate prevention of venous thromboembolism (VTE). In addition, all hospitalized patients should be assessed for risk for both VTE and bleeding to determine if pharmacologic, mechanical, or combination VTE prophylaxis should be initiated. Patients should also be reassessed following any pertinent clinical changes. In at-risk patients without contraindications (i.e., risk for bleeding, active bleeding, or allergy), pharmacologic thromboprophylaxis should be initiated as soon as possible and within the first 24 hours of arrival at the hospital. Mechanical methods should be used when pharmacologic prophylaxis is contraindicated. Active interdisciplinary, multifaceted VTE prevention programs, in contrast to passive strategies, should be used to improve appropriate VTE prophylaxis within hospitals. These programs should incorporate provider, staff, and patient education; audits and feedback; hospital guidelines and policies; clinical decision-support software; monitoring for appropriate anticoagulant use; and provider reminders. Guidelines and policies need to be individualized at the hospital level, depending on the degree to which pharmacy, providers, nursing, and other staff are involved. The National Quality Forum (NQF) and the Joint Commission recommend creating policies and guidelines regarding anticoagulation. This is also a key recommendation of the American College of Chest Physicians (ACCP). Pharmacy professionals should actively participate in the development, implementation, and monitoring of anticoagulation and VTE prophylaxis programs. In addition, because pharmacologic prophylaxis is the primary method to prevent VTE, pharmacy professionals should take a leadership role in these hospital programs.

Background

Burden of Disease and Pharmacologic Prophylaxis. VTE comprises pulmonary embolism (PE) and deep vein thrombosis (DVT). Despite a wealth of information regarding the mortality and morbidity associated with VTE, hospitals worldwide continue to do poorly at preventing VTE events for at-risk patients. Between 60,000[1] and 300,000[2] deaths occur annually in the United States from PE, and as many as 200,000 of those deaths occur in U.S. hospitals.[3] Approximately 70% of fatal PEs are first detected postmortem.[4,5] Furthermore, up to 2,000,000 new DVTs occur annually within the United States.[1] VTE occurs in approximately 64.4% of surgical patients and 41.5% of medical patients.[6] PE is the most preventable cause of death among all causes for patients; therefore, VTE prevention is the best strategy for improving patient safety in U.S. hospitals.[7,8] In the absence of thromboprophylaxis, 1 in 10 hospital deaths is attributed to PE.[9] Recurrent VTE occurs in 7% of patients at six months,[10] increasing to up to 30% at 8–10 years[11,12] for patients despite treatment for the initial VTE. The risk of developing VTE rises sharply when the number of risk factors increases.[13] At 1 year after the initial VTE, the mortality rates associated with PE and DVT are particularly high in patients older than 65 years (39% and 21%, respectively).[14] The risk of recurrent VTE continues for up to 90 days after hospitalization.[15,16]

Approximately 60% of VTE events[17] and 75% of autopsy-confirmed fatal PE[18–21] occur in nonsurgical patients. More importantly, PE and proximal DVT are occurring more frequently in medical patients than in surgical patients.[22] This increase may be partially attributable to medical patients having historically lower rates of thromboprophylaxis compared with surgical patients. In addition, VTE prophylaxis for surgical patients has been studied for approximately 50 years, whereas well-designed studies for medical patients began surfacing in the mid-1990s. In placebo-controlled studies, VTE events have been reduced by 50–65% in acutely ill patients when prophylaxis was used.[23–25] Examples of avoided morbidity associated with VTE are recurrent VTE, postthrombotic syndrome (PTS), congestive heart failure, and pulmonary hypertension. PTS is the term used to describe signs and symptoms that may occur as a long-term complication of DVT and includes swelling, pain, edema, venous ectasia, and skin induration of the affected limb.[26] In severe PTS, patients may have painful, intractable leg ulcers, which decrease mobility and require additional medical care.[26] PTS is associated with an annualized cost as high as $11,667[27] and can lead to loss of quality of life and functional status. After a symptomatic DVT, the overall incidence of PTS is 20–50%, and severe PTS occurs in 5–10% of patients.[28] Within 2 years after the development of PE, chronic thromboembolic pulmonary hypertension occurs in approximately 3.8% of patients.[29] Results from clinical trials have shown that when pharmacologic prophylaxis is administered at appropriate doses and durations in medical patients, the breakthrough occurrence of VTE is clinically uncommon (2.8–5.6%).[23–25] The use of thromboprophylaxis has been shown to reduce mortality in both primary studies and meta-analyses.[25,30,31] This position statement focuses on key issues and guideline recommendations for the prevention of VTE in hospitalized patients augmented by health-system pharmacists.

Current Hospital Performance and Barriers. Globally, 41.5% of surgical patients and 60.5% of medical patients at risk for VTE do not receive appropriate prophylaxis therapy.[6] The concept of "appropriate VTE prophylaxis" has recently emerged and denotes appropriate drug, dose, and duration of therapy. Recent studies have demonstrated appropriate prophylaxis rates of only 13–33% in hundreds of U.S. hospitals.[32–35]

Barriers to VTE prophylaxis include concerns about bleeding complications; underestimation of the VTE risk; gaps in provider knowledge of VTE prevention; lack of knowledge regarding recommendations and standards;

DOI 10.37573/9781585287048.110

heterogeneous patient populations; perceived difficulties in risk assessment; lack of familiarity, agreement, or confidence with guidelines; belief that implementing guidelines is ineffective in improving outcomes; resistance to changing established practice patterns; need for approval and funding to implement guidelines; and lack of clarity and ease of use of guidelines.[36–38]

National Impact and Readmissions. Currently, VTE has an estimated financial burden of $13.5 billion–$69.3 billion per year in the United States, with $4.5 billion–$39.3 billion of this being preventable with pharmacist-driven or other VTE prevention programs.[39,40] Because of the gravity of the problem and poor performance of U.S. hospitals, many of the leading U.S. organizations began to prioritize VTE as a top initiative for improvement within the last decade. Some of these organizations include NQF, the Agency for Healthcare Research and Quality, the Institute for Healthcare Improvement, the Joint Commission, the Centers for Disease Control and Prevention (CDC), and the Centers for Medicaid and Medicare Services (CMS).[41]

Interestingly, a 2007 study found that approximately 5.3% of patients previously hospitalized for a DVT or PE are readmitted within one year for VTE.[42] A clear trend of hospital readmission occurred within the first 30 days of the initial event for these patients, with 27.1% readmitted for a DVT and 44.3% readmitted for a PE.[42]

Guidelines and Quality Measures

Many national and international guidelines exist for appropriate, evidence-based treatment of VTE prophylaxis. These include the ACCP guidelines, which were last updated in 2012,[43–45] and the International Union of Angiology guidelines from June 2006.[46] Oncology-specific guidelines, such as those created by the American Society of Clinical Oncology (ASCO)[47] and the National Comprehensive Cancer Network (NCCN),[48] are also available and are very specific about contraindications for prophylaxis, which is helpful to the practicing clinician. ASCO and NCCN guidelines were updated in 2007 and 2011, respectively.

Both the Joint Commission and CMS have initiated quality measures to promote VTE prophylaxis in hospitalized patients. In 2008, the Joint Commission implemented a National Patient Safety Goal that focuses on anticoagulation management in the hospital setting for both medical and surgical patients.[49] CMS also added DVT and PE after total knee replacement (TKR) or total hip replacement (THR) procedures to a list of conditions whose associated costs will not be reimbursed if acquired during a hospital stay.[50] The Joint Commission collaborated with NQF on the development of these measures to promote VTE prophylaxis, which were piloted in U.S. hospitals and then endorsed by NQF in 2008.[51] In October 2009, the Joint Commission made available a core measure set for VTE (**Table 1**), focusing on prophylaxis, treatment, and one outcome measure of "preventable" VTE.[52] Hospitals may choose this VTE core measure set as one of four required core measure sets on which to report.[52] However, because these measures alone do not give detailed recommendations on VTE prophylaxis, hospitals should base their guidelines, policies, practices, and recommendations on the most recent edition of the ACCP guidelines. At this time, only 60 of approximately 5000 acute care hospitals are reporting on the VTE core measure set. Therefore, hospitals should also adopt the Joint Commission's VTE measure set for core measure reporting to aid in improving patient care and reduce health care costs.

Mechanical Methods of Prophylaxis in Hospitalized Patients. While the focus of this manuscript is pharmacologic prophylaxis, pharmacists should familiarize themselves with mechanical methods of prophylaxis to make appropriate recommendations for patients when a pharmacologic contraindication exists. Mechanical methods of prophylaxis may be dynamic, static, or a combination of the two. Dynamic methods include intermittent pneumatic compression (IPC) devices, sequential compression devices, and venous foot pumps. Static methods include graduated compression stockings, elastic stockings, and thromboembolic deterrent hose. Mechanical methods of prophylaxis have been shown to only reduce the rates of DVT, not PE or death, in contrast with pharmacologic prophylaxis.[8] A 2005 meta-analysis of IPC device use in surgical patients found a 60% risk reduction in DVT with no substantial reduction in PE risk, compared with no prophylaxis ($p < 0.001$).[53,54]

Inferior vena cava filters (IVCFs) are an alternative static method of mechanical prophylaxis. To date, IVCFs have been shown to reduce recurrent PE at the expense of an increased risk of DVT in the absence of anticoagulation.[55] Hospitals should use IVCFs for patients with confirmed

TABLE 1.
The Joint Commission Venous Thromboembolism (VTE) National Hospital Inpatient Quality Measures[a]

Set Measure ID #	Measure Short Name
VTE-1	Venous thromboembolism prophylaxis
VTE-2	Intensive care unit venous thromboembolism prophylaxis
VTE-3	Venous thromboembolism patients with anticoagulant overlap therapy
VTE-4	Venous thromboembolism patients receiving unfractionated heparin therapy with dosages/platelet count monitoring by protocol
VTE-5	Venous thromboembolism discharge instructions
VTE-6	Incidence of potentially preventable venous thromboembolism

[a]Reprinted from the *Specifications Manual for National Hospital Inpatient Quality Measures,* version 4.1, March 2012, a collaborative work of the Centers for Medicare and Medicaid Services and the Joint Commission. This manual is periodically updated, and users of the manual must update their software and associated documentation based on the published manual production timelines.

proximal DVT who have an absolute contraindication to full-dose anticoagulation (e.g., patients with active bleeding) or who have not responded to standard anticoagulant regimens (e.g., patients who developed recurrent thromboembolism despite full-dose anticoagulant therapy) or in high-risk patients who have major surgery planned in the very near future. Once the absolute contraindication to anticoagulation subsides or the major surgery is completed, treatment with an appropriate anticoagulant should be initiated or resumed, depending on the clinical scenario.[8]

The health care team should ensure patients' compliance with mechanical methods of VTE prophylaxis throughout their hospitalization, as compliance is the most important determinant of efficacy.[56] Most devices used for mechanical VTE prophylaxis should be used for a minimum of 20 hours per day to be effective. Because of these compliance issues, hospitals and physicians should attempt to use mobile, battery-powered IPC devices that have the ability to record and report the hours the devices are used.[8,43–45] Mechanical methods of prophylaxis should be reserved for patients who are actively bleeding or at high risk for bleeding, with inclusion of such documentation in the patient record, or possibly as an adjunct to pharmacologic methods of prophylaxis.[8] Studies have demonstrated greater reductions in VTE rates among certain groups of patients (i.e., trauma patients, patients with spinal cord injury, and high-risk patients undergoing TKR, THR, hip fracture surgery, neurosurgery, and elective spine surgery) receiving combination pharmacologic and mechanical VTE prophylaxis compared with pharmacologic prophylaxis alone.[8]

Health-system pharmacists should evaluate patients for potential contraindications to anticoagulation therapies. They should also familiarize themselves with the specific mechanical methods available at their institution, which could be used in patients with such contraindications.

Risk Stratification and Identification

Most hospitalized patients have at least one risk factor for VTE, and approximately 40% have multiple risk factors.[8] Common risk factors for VTE are listed in **Table 2**, and DVT rates among various patient groups are presented in **Table 3**.[57] Most critically ill patients have multiple risk factors for VTE. Risk factors that may precede admission to a critical care unit may include trauma, active infection (e.g., sepsis), recent surgery, active malignancy, stroke, advanced age, congestive heart failure, respiratory failure, history of VTE, and pregnancy. In addition, patients admitted to critical care units have an increased risk of developing VTE due to immobilization, placement of central venous lines, sepsis, pharmacologic paralysis, mechanical ventilation, vasopressor use, and the need for surgical procedures and dialysis.[8,58]

PE is the second most common cause of death in patients with cancer.[8] Patients with hematologic malignancies, lung cancer, and gastrointestinal cancer have the highest rates of VTE. Within the first three months after being diagnosed with cancer, patients have an approximate 50-fold increased risk of developing a VTE compared with patients with no cancer.[59] Even during therapeutic anticoagulation after a VTE, fatal PE outnumbers fatal bleeding events in an approximate 3:1 ratio.[60] Certain cancer treatments, including chemotherapy, hormonal manipulation, erythropoiesis, and the presence of a central venous catheter, are also risk factors for VTE.[8] Chemotherapy is associated with an approximate sixfold increased risk of VTE,[61–63] with specific drugs contributing to higher VTE rates, including tamoxifen, anastrozole, letrozole, exemestane, bevacizumab, thalidomide, and lenalidomide.[64–73] Tamoxifen is associated with a higher rate of VTE than the aromatase inhibitors anastrozole, letrozole, and exemestane.[74–77]

TABLE 2.
Venous Thromboembolism (VTE) Risk Factors[8,57]

Risk Factor Category	Risk Factors
Common general risk factors	Previous VTE; surgery; trauma; thrombophilia; obesity (body mass index of >25 kg/m^2); acute hospitalization for medical illness; immobility or lower-extremity paresis; active or occult malignancy; cancer therapy, such as radiotherapy, hormonal therapy, chemotherapy, or angiogenesis inhibitors; venous compression from sources such as tumor, hematoma, or arterial abnormality; increasing age; pregnancy and the postpartum period; estrogen-containing oral contraceptives or hormone-replacement therapy; selective estrogen-receptor modulators; erythropoiesis-stimulating agents; inflammatory bowel disease; nephrotic syndrome; myeloproliferative disorders; paroxysmal nocturnal hemoglobinuria; central venous catheterization
Specific medical risk factors	
High risk	History of deep venous thrombosis or pulmonary embolism, family history of thrombosis, acute infection, active malignancy, age >75 yr, stroke, myocardial infarction, congestive heart failure, prolonged immobility (≥4 days), pregnancy or postpartum period, acute or chronic lung disease, acute inflammatory disease, inflammatory bowel disease, shock
Probable risk	High-dose estrogen therapy, obesity (body mass index of >25 kg/m^2), varicose veins, heparin-induced thrombocytopenia, congenital or acquired thrombophilia, antithrombin deficiency, positive lupus anticoagulant, antiphospholipid antibodies, protein S or C deficiency, positive factor V Leiden, elevated anticardiolipin antibodies, positive prothrombin gene mutation 20210A
Possible risk	Paraproteinemia, Behçet's disease, disorders of plasminogen and plasminogen activation, nephrotic syndrome, polycythemia, elevated serum homocysteine levels, dysfibrinogenemia, myeloproliferative disorders, age ≥ 41 yr, sepsis (<1 mo)

TABLE 3.

Frequency of DVT Associated with Various Patients Groups and Conditions in the Absence of Prophylaxis[8,57,a]

Patient Group or Condition	Frequency of DVT, %
General medical patients	10–26
Myocardial infarction	17–34
Stroke	11–75
Congestive heart failure	20–40
Medical intensive care	25–42
Critical care patients	10–80
General surgical patients	15–40
Major gynecological surgery	15–40
Major urologic surgery	15–40
Neurosurgery	15–40
Major orthopedic surgery of the hip or knee[b]	40–60
Trauma	40–80
Spinal cord injury	60–80

[a]DVT = deep venous thrombosis.
[b]Total knee or hip replacement or hip fracture surgery.

Furthermore, surgical patients with cancer have at least twice the risk of developing a postoperative DVT and three times the risk of developing a fatal PE as compared with patients with no cancer undergoing the same surgeries.[8] VTE recurrence rates are high both during anticoagulation and after anticoagulation has been discontinued.[78–81] Patients with cancer who develop a VTE have a substantial reduction in survival compared with cancer patients who do not develop a VTE.[82–84]

Research into other risk factors for VTE continues,[85–87] though validation of these risk factors will be needed. Risk-assessment models (RAMs) have been developed for the hospitalized patient and have proved useful in identifying patients at risk for VTE and bleeding.[8] The health-system pharmacist should take initiative and lead the collaborative implementation of RAMs within the hospital.

Several methods of risk assessment to reduce hospital-acquired VTE exist. Some methods may use one process or form for all patients being evaluated, while others may use specific processes or forms for specific patient groups. Both methods can be computerized (i.e., using electronic alerts) or completed manually. RAMs could also be based on a scoring system (i.e., positive points for specific risk factors and negative points for contraindications) or they could assess risk factors by patient groups based on guideline recommendations.[8]

Several RAMs have been proposed for hospitalized patients, incorporating both predisposing and exposing risk factors (e.g., major surgery, acute medical illness).[88–92] For example, Caprini et al.[88] developed a RAM for both hospitalized surgical and medical patients, with the surgical RAM being validated in 2009,[90] and Cohen et al.[90] developed an algorithm-based RAM for medical patients. Another recent, predictive, evidence-based, weighted-risk scoring system was developed from the large International Medical Prevention Registry on Venous Thromboembolism (IMPROVE) database for medical patients.[92] The risk scores were derived from the hazard ratios of seven independent clinical risk factors for VTE. The Padua prediction score is another RAM that uses 11 risk factors to determine VTE risk in the medical patient and categorizes a patient's VTE risk as low or high.[93] For all patients, the risk of bleeding should be determined using a group-appropriate RAM or guideline-delineated risk factors. A clear advantage of the IMPROVE RAM is that its derivation is evidence based, whereas the Padua prediction score is not.[91] Collectively, these RAMs further validate the concept of weighted scoring, demonstrating that all VTE risk factors are not equally associated with VTE risk.

Because risk factors are not weighted equally, clinicians should carefully examine risk factors to determine the individual care needed for each patient. Furthermore, efforts should be made to maximize the number of risk factors assessed with the RAM, as this will capture a greater number of patients at risk for VTE and maximize the sensitivity of the model.[94]

Although a review of all risk-assessment programs to reduce VTE is beyond the scope of this position statement, several reviews reiterate key characteristics that are essential to such programs.[94–97] Risk-assessment programs should be multifaceted, and those involved in such programs should provide active interventions instead of merely handing out guidelines or placing incomplete risk-assessment forms in patient charts. These programs should also educate and remind health care providers about the need for VTE prophylaxis, educate patients, use audit and feedback for the program itself and for individuals ignoring alerts (i.e., alert fatigue), monitor for inappropriate use of thromboprophylaxis, and use clinical decision-support software, either electronically or manually.

Pharmacist-driven VTE programs have helped improve the care received by hospitalized patients.[39,98–102] The implementation of one such program led to a significant increase in appropriate type, dose, and duration of prophylaxis while also significantly reducing "preventable" VTE events (relative risk reduction = 74%, $p = 0.0006$).[39] Another pharmacist-driven program significantly increased optimal VTE prophylaxis among hospitalized nonsurgical patients from 11% to 44% ($p < 0.001$). The program consisted of presentations, newsletters, and VTE prophylaxis recommendations made during clinical pharmacy rounds.[98] In addition, a multidisciplinary program that included pharmacists in the surgical intensive care unit achieved substantial reductions in both hospital-acquired and preventable VTE.[103] Lastly, the use of a simple, nonscoring, three-tiered (low, moderate, or high) VTE RAM led to an 86% reduction in preventable hospital-acquired VTE over three years.[104] This RAM was modular and embedded into computerized provider-order-entry (CPOE) order sets but was not a pharmacist-driven program.

Efficacy of Antithrombotic Prophylaxis and Recommendations

Heparins and Fondaparinux. Three prospective, randomized, placebo-controlled studies have been conducted to evaluate the efficacy of low-molecular-weight heparins (LMWHs) and fondaparinux for VTE prophylaxis in medical patients. These include the MEDENOX[23] (enoxaparin),

PREVENT[24] (dalteparin), and ARTEMIS[25] (fondaparinux) trials. The number needed to treat to avoid a VTE ranged from 11 to 45 in these studies. Major bleeding rates were 1.7%, 0.49%, and 0.2% in the MEDENOX, PREVENT, and ARTEMIS trials, respectively. The three studies demonstrated significant relative risk reductions of 63%, 55%, and 49.5% for VTE, respectively, with no significant differences in major bleeding rates. In the United States, enoxaparin and dalteparin have Food and Drug Administration (FDA)-approved indications for VTE prophylaxis in acutely ill medical patients; fondaparinux does not. Fondaparinux does carry this indication in certain European Union countries. In the recent PROTECT trial, investigators randomized critical care patients to dalteparin 5000 units daily or unfractionated heparin (UFH) 5000 units twice daily and found no significant difference in the rate of proximal DVT, major bleeding, or inhospital death. However, there was a significant reduction in the occurrence of PE with dalteparin as compared with UFH.[105]

According to a recent systematic review conducted by the American College of Physicians (ACP), the use of heparin in medical patients to prevent VTE decreases the rate of pulmonary embolism but does not decrease mortality and leads to more bleeding complications.[106,107] No differences in risks or benefits were found between the types of heparin used, though there was a nonsignificant difference favoring LMWH over UFH for PE (odds ratio, 0.67; confidence interval [CI], 0.45–1.00; $p = 0.053$; $I^2 = 0\%$). The use of mechanical devices led to adverse outcomes and did not demonstrate any benefit. Therefore, in medical and stroke patients, ACP currently recommends assessing the risks of VTE and bleeding before starting VTE prevention and only using pharmacologic prophylaxis if the risk of VTE is greater than the risk of bleeding. In addition, ACP recommends against using mechanical devices to prevent VTE.[106–108] These recommendations are similar to those of ACCP, which recommends an LMWH, a UFH two or three times daily, or fondaparinux for patients not at risk of bleeding but at risk of VTE. However, ACCP does recommend mechanical means of prophylaxis, such as IPC devices and graduated compression stockings for patients at risk of bleeding and VTE. ACCP analyses did not note any substantial difference in bleeding, VTE, or heparin-induced thrombocytopenia between UFH two and three times daily.[43] Because ACCP guidelines are in their ninth edition and ACP guidelines are newly released, we recommend using ACCP guidelines. Key guideline recommendations for the medical patient are listed in **Table 4**.

Warfarin versus LMWHs and Fondaparinux. Because of its slow onset of action, variable responses among patients, drug–drug and drug–food interactions, lower efficacy compared with LMWHs, need for frequent monitoring, and complexity of both inhospital and postdischarge supervision, warfarin has largely been abandoned as thromboprophylaxis in Europe. Similarly, the ACCP guidelines concluded that LMWHs, and likely fondaparinux by indirect comparison, are more effective than warfarin in preventing inhospital VTE and should be preferred.[8] Health-system pharmacists should continue to educate themselves on emerging evidence on the use of thromboprophylactic agents. They should also familiarize themselves with the risks, benefits, and duration of use in relation to transitions among levels of care.

Optimal Duration for Thromboprophylaxis

With the average length of stay in U.S. hospitals being approximately 5 days,[109] the recommended duration of prophylaxis in studies and within drug labeling is often not reached. Studies have suggested that the inappropriate duration of therapy is a major cause for failure to receive appropriate thromboprophylaxis among hospitalized patients.[15,33] ACCP guidelines advocate extended thromboprophylaxis of up to 35 days with an LMWH in patients undergoing major orthopedic surgery (especially hip fracture repair and hip replacement) and up to 28 days in patients with active cancer undergoing surgery for their cancer.[8] Recent results from the EXCLAIM study suggest that there is a high-risk subgroup of hospitalized medical patients (namely, women, patients with advanced age, or patients with complete immobility) who may benefit from extended outpatient thromboprophylaxis.[110] Results from two recent trials evaluating the use of rivaroxaban and apixaban in VTE prophylaxis did not demonstrate additional benefits with either drug when used for approximately one month.[111,112] Further studies are needed to determine whether the use of thromboprophylaxis for the duration recommended in the drug labeling is safe and improves outcomes in medical patients. The VTE Discharge Alert Trial is currently assessing if a human alert to physicians within 48 hours of planned patient discharge has any effect on increasing postdischarge prophylaxis or reducing VTE within 90 days of hospital admission in the medical patient. Major bleeding events within 30 days of hospital admission are also being monitored.[113] At a minimum, for the majority of at-risk patients, the optimal duration of prophylaxis is the length of the hospital stay if exposing risk factors are still present while considering the primary diagnosis and predisposing risk factors. Importantly, no studies evaluating the impact of ambulation on VTE have been conducted. A recent study found that despite timely ambulation, medical patients were still at risk of VTE, and this risk was substantially reduced with enoxaparin prophylaxis.[114] Therefore, patient ambulation or mobility should not be used as a reason to discontinue, or restrict, prophylaxis during hospitalization. Currently, ACCP guidelines recommend against extending the duration of thromboprophylaxis beyond the hospital stay or period of patient immobilization in the medical patient.[43]

Safety of Antithrombotic Prophylaxis

One of the major adverse events that can occur with the use of heparin is heparin-induced thrombocytopenia (HIT). HIT is an antibody-mediated adverse effect of heparin that is strongly associated with venous and arterial thrombosis. HIT is diagnosed when any of the following events occurs in association with the presence of HIT antibodies: an otherwise unexplained decrease in platelet count, venous or arterial thrombosis, skin lesions at heparin injection sites, and acute systemic reactions (fever or chills, tachycardia, hypertension, dyspnea, cardiopulmonary arrest) that occur after i.v. heparin bolus administration.[115] Although HIT can occur with a prophylactic dose of both LMWH and UFH, it happens about threefold more frequently with UFH than with LMWH and incurs approximately $41,133 of additional costs per case.[116,117] Because the occurrence of HIT

TABLE 4.

Existing Guideline Recommendations for Thromboprophylaxis of Hospitalized Medical and Critical Care Patients[a]

Group and Recommendations	Modality and Grade of Recommendation(s)
American College of Chest Physicians (2012)	
Acutely ill hospitalized medical patients at low risk of thrombosis: Do not use pharmacologic prophylaxis or mechanical prophylaxis.	No thromboprophylaxis
Acutely ill hospitalized medical patients at increased risk of thrombosis: Provide anticoagulant thromboprophylaxis with LMWH, low-dose UFH twice or three times daily, or fondaparinux and suggests against extending the duration of thromboprophylaxis beyond the period of patient immobilization or acute hospital stay.	Grade 1B[b]
Acutely ill hospitalized medical patients at increased risk of thrombosis who are bleeding or are at high risk for major bleeding: Use mechanical thromboprophylaxis using GCSs or IPC.	Grade 2C
Critically ill patients: Use LMWH or low-dose UFH for thromboprophylaxis.	Grade 2C
Critically ill patients who are bleeding or are at high risk for major bleeding: Use mechanical thromboprophylaxis with GCSs and/or IPC at least until the bleeding risk decreases.	Grade 2C
American College of Physicians (2011)	
Recommends assessment of the risk for thromboembolism and bleeding in medical (including stroke) patients before initiation of prophylaxis of VTE	Grade: strong recommendation; moderate-quality evidence
Recommends pharmacologic prophylaxis with heparin or a related drug for VTE in medical (including stroke) patients unless the assessed risk for bleeding outweighs the likely benefits	Grade: strong recommendation; moderate-quality evidence
Recommends against the use of mechanical prophylaxis with GCSs for prevention of VTE	Grade: strong recommendation; moderate-quality evidence
Policy implication: The American College of Physicians does not support the application of performance measures in medical (including stroke) patients that promote universal VTE prophylaxis regardless of risk.	
International Union of Angiology (2006)	
Acutely ill medical patients (patients older than 40 years with acute medical illness and/or reduced mobility with one of the following morbidities: acute heart failure NYHA class III/IV, respiratory disease [respiratory failure with or without ventilation or exacerbation of respiratory disease], active cancer requiring therapy, acute infective disease including severe infection and sepsis, rheumatic disease, ischemic stroke, or acute myocardial infarction) should be considered for prophylaxis. Patients with acute medical illness with reduced mobility and one of the following risk factors—history of VTE, malignant disease, or older than 75 years—should also be considered for prophylaxis.	UFH 5000 units three times daily (grade A), enoxaparin 40 mg once daily (grade A), dalteparin 5000 units once daily (grade A), fondaparinux 2.5 mg once daily (grade B)
National Comprehensive Cancer Network (2011) Cancer patients	LMWH, UFH 5000 units three times daily
American Society of Clinical Oncology (2007) Hospitalized medical patients	LMWH, UFH 5000 units three times daily

[a]LMWH = low-molecular-weight heparin, UFH = unfractionated heparin, GCSs = graduated compression stockings, IPC = intermittent pneumatic compression, NYHA = New York Heart Association, VTE = venous thromboembolism.
[b]Fondaparinux is not approved by the Food and Drug Administration for medical prophylaxis in the United States.

is more frequent with UFH, overall costs are likely reduced by using LMWH over UFH. Taking into consideration that HIT may be a serious, limb-threatening and life-threatening complication, LMWH may be favored over UFH. Only a limited number of case reports of fondaparinux-induced thrombocytopenia have been reported, and this may be an advantage of fondaparinux over LMWH and UFH. The new oral agents will likely also have an advantage over UFH and LMWH with regard to HIT and may be a useful alternative in patients with a history of HIT.

Major and minor bleeding can also occur with the use of prophylactic LMWH, warfarin, fondaparinux, and UFH. Overall, pharmacologic means of VTE prophylaxis carry a slightly higher risk of bleeding than placebo or mechanical means, but major bleeding rates are negligible with prophylactic doses in well-controlled clinical trials.[23–25,118–121] In studies evaluating the safety and efficacy of VTE prophylaxis in medical and surgical patients, the rate of major bleeding was between 0.2% and 2.7% among patients given pharmacologic prophylaxis. One recent meta-analysis in medical patients demonstrated no difference in major bleeding between pharmacologic prophylaxis and placebo and also showed a reduction in fatal PE with pharmacologic prophylaxis versus placebo.[122] Another meta-analysis concluded that the use of UFH was associated with substantially higher rates of major bleeding than LMWH.[123] A meta-analysis and two primary studies have also demonstrated lower rates of injection-site hematoma with LMWH than UFH.[124,125] Bleeding rates with fondaparinux appear comparable to those with LMWHs for both the medical and surgical patient.[40,116]

Patient groups at high risk for bleeding include those with serious comorbid diseases, especially active malignancy or cerebrovascular, kidney, heart, and liver disease; older patients; those receiving concurrent antithrombotic medications, including antiplatelets and fibrinolytics; patients with thrombocytopenia (<100,000 mm^3), a hemoglobin concentration of <13 g/dL (in surgical patients), severe renal insufficiency (creatinine clearance [CLcr] of <30 mL/min), active or recent peptic ulcer disease, recent gastrointestinal or major bleeding, uncontrolled arterial hypertension (systolic blood pressure of >200 mm Hg, diastolic blood pressure of >120 mm Hg, or both), or bacterial endocarditis; and those who have undergone spinal tap or epidural anesthesia within 12 hours.[43–45,126]

A bleeding RAM from the IMPROVE registry was developed and can be accessed at **http://omnifik.com/dev/improve/bleeding/**.[127] Risk factors for bleeding continue to be discovered and are individualized by patient group. Contraindications to VTE prophylaxis should be agreed on at the institution and pharmacy levels.

The overall avoidance of a substantial number of VTE events and their subsequent morbidity is what makes VTE prophylaxis so persuasive and important. A recent review concluded that mortality rates associated with PE were substantially higher than those associated with major bleeding from the use of anticoagulants, further supporting the focus on the prevention of the initial PE.[128] The initial cost of prophylaxis reduces overall costs by avoiding VTE and its associated morbidity. By and large, there is strong evidence that appropriately dosed thromboprophylaxis has an advantageous and favorable risk:benefit ratio.[8,46]

Recommendations

Most hospitalized patients have multiple risk factors for VTE. Patients at high risk include those in critical care, as well as burn, trauma, surgical, and cancer patients. All hospitalized patients, including patients in critical care or with burns, should be assessed for the risk of VTE using a RAM. Importantly, patients should be reassessed every 24-48 hours, or with pertinent clinical changes, for new or resolved VTE, bleeding risk factors, and contraindications to prophylaxis. According to these risks, patients should be given an LMWH, a UFH, or fondaparinux prophylactically. However, if there is a contraindication to pharmacologic prophylaxis (e.g., active bleeding, high risk of bleeding, allergy [including HIT within 100 days]), with inclusion of such documentation in the patient records, mechanical methods should be used for prophylaxis. Providers should refer to current ACCP guidelines and NCCN/ASCO guidelines for detailed recommendations for VTE prophylaxis for hospitalized patients. Special considerations for trauma, surgical, and cancer patients as well as for obese patients, patients with renal impairment, or pregnant patients are discussed below.

Major Trauma Patients. Trauma patients, including those with acute spinal cord injury, are among those with the highest risk of developing VTE. Recommendations are to administer thromboprophylaxis to all trauma patients.[55] One meta-analysis concluded that UFH alone as thromboprophylaxis in trauma patients was not any more effective than not using thromboprophylaxis.[129] Therefore, according to ACCP guidelines, LMWH is preferred over UFH in trauma patients. One trial demonstrated that UFH combined with mechanical ankle flexion devices was superior to UFH alone in orthopedic trauma patients.[130] Therefore, if used in this patient population, UFH should be combined with mechanical methods and not used alone. For patients undergoing rehabilitation, prophylaxis is recommended to continue with LMWH or warfarin (target International Normalized Ratio [INR] of 2.5 [range, 2–3]) until the risk of VTE subsides, until full ambulation, or for up to three months in trauma patients with spinal cord injury.[8,46]

Patients with Cancer. VTE prevention in this group is particularly important, not only because patients with cancer have a higher risk of VTE but because VTE is often more difficult to diagnose and treat in this population.[8] Patients who are confined to a bed and with an active malignancy should receive prophylaxis with an LMWH, a UFH, or fondaparinux.[8,46] If there is a contraindication to pharmacologic prophylaxis, graduated compression stockings or an IPC device should be used, with strong attention paid to compliance.[8] Although patients with cancer have a particularly increased risk of developing VTE, they continue to have the lowest rates of appropriate VTE prophylaxis.[32–35,131]

VTE prophylaxis should be initiated in cancer patients with solid tumors and additional VTE risk factors, including previous venous thrombosis, immobilization, and the use of hormonal therapy, angiogenesis inhibitors, thalidomide, and lenalidomide.[43] Agents of choice include UFH and LMWH. Additional studies are needed to evaluate anticoagulants in patients with cancer who do not have a traditional indication for thromboprophylaxis, such as those with recent cancer now in remission or undergoing outpatient chemotherapy.[8,46] Agreement on contraindications differs between key organizations and international experts, with some suggesting that pharmacologic prophylaxis be used with platelet counts as low as 5,000 per microliter and others suggesting a low of 50,000.[47] For more information on when to administer prophylaxis to cancer patients, refer to ACCP, NCCN, and ASCO guidelines.

Surgical Patients. An abundance of trials involving surgical patients have demonstrated substantial reductions in VTE with UFH, LMWH, fondaparinux, and warfarin over placebo or equivalence or noninferiority to other effective anticoagulants.[8,44–46] Because the number of surgical studies is so expansive and recommendations vary by patient group, readers are referred to the 2012 ACCP guidelines for specific details. ACCP guidelines include recommendations and background on

- General, vascular, laparoscopic, gynecological, urologic, bariatric, thoracic, and coronary bypass surgery; abdominal–pelvic surgery (including gastrointestinal); major trauma

- THR, TKR, knee arthroscopy, hip fracture surgery, timing of thromboprophylaxis initiation, screening for DVT before hospital discharge, and duration of thromboprophylaxis for the aforementioned major orthopedic surgeries
- Isolated lower-extremity injuries distal to the knee
- Craniotomy and spinal surgery

The following key points should be considered when initiating thromboprophylaxis for surgical patients:

1. Aspirin and warfarin, with a target INR of 2.5, may be used for the orthopedic population.
2. Select mechanical methods may be used alone for THR; TKR; hip fracture surgery; gynecologic, urologic, laparoscopic, or coronary artery bypass surgical groups; elective spine surgery; and neurosurgery.[8]
3. LMWH, fondaparinux, and three times daily UFH are typically options for surgical patients with multiple VTE risk factors (i.e., high risk), with LMWH and fondaparinux being preferred over three times daily UFH in many high-risk surgical groups.[8]
4. LMWH, fondaparinux, and twice-daily UFH are options in most moderate-risk surgical groups.[8]
5. The combination of IPC with pharmacologic prophylaxis typically conveys a 60% further risk reduction in VTE events.[8]
6. LMWH is the preferred agent in THR, TKR, and hip fracture surgery if patients do not have an increased risk of bleeding.

Obese Patients. Although more studies are needed, evidence supports the use of weight-based prophylactic dosing of LMWHs in obese patients (i.e., body mass index of >30 kg/m^2). Studies assessing anti-Xa levels at both treatment and prophylactic dosages demonstrated appropriate anti-Xa levels and no accumulation of drug. Appropriate anti-Xa levels have been reported in obese patients receiving enoxaparin, tinzaparin, and dalteparin dosed based on total body weights of up to 144, 165, and 190 kg, respectively.[132–136] One meta-analysis verified that major bleeding rates were not increased in obese patients who received weight-based LMWH when compared with non-obese individuals.[137]

Nadroparin and enoxaparin have been studied in prospective studies of obese patients undergoing bariatric surgery and orthopedic surgery.[138–142] Of note, nadroparin is not available in the United States. The usual recommended prophylactic doses of these agents may be inadequate for VTE prophylaxis in obese patients. For LMWHs, ACCP guidelines recommend using weight-based dosing for obese patients.[8] For enoxaparin, the specific dosing that appeared to be more favorable in bariatric surgery was 40 mg twice daily, though this may still be inadequate in some patients, and higher dosing may be more beneficial.[142] Although dosing suggestions are not yet well-defined in the literature, enoxaparin 0.5 mg/kg every 12–24 hours (e.g., depending on the level of obesity, with every-12-hour administration used for patients with higher body mass indexes) has been used successfully for prophylaxis at some centers.[143–145] Dosage increases of up to 30% have also been suggested.[145]

Patients with Renal Impairment. Several studies have assessed the effects of LMWHs in patients with renal impairment. Tinzaparin and dalteparin offer the most convincing data that these drugs may not accumulate in patients with severe renal impairment in both prophylactic and treatment doses.[147–154] However, one recent study comparing tinzaparin with UFH for the treatment of VTE in elderly patients with renal insufficiency found increased mortality in the tinzaparin group.[155] The trial was stopped early because of these interim results, though the increased mortality was not related to increased bleeding or VTE. There were nonsignificant trends for tinzaparin-treated patients having higher rates of VTE than those receiving UFH[155]; thus, more data are needed. Of note, tinzaparin production was recently discontinued in the United States.[156]

The recent Dalteparin's Influence on Renally Compromised anti-Ten-A (DIRECT) trial was a prospective study of 120 critically ill patients with a CLcr of <30 mL/min, who had at least one trough anti-Xa level measured.[150] The investigators analyzed the safety of prophylactic dosages of dalteparin and found no bioaccumulation of the drug in the patients. Interestingly, 62% of patients had acute renal failure at some point during their prophylactic regimen. These data suggest that in critically ill patients with severe renal insufficiency, VTE prophylaxis with dalteparin is unlikely to contribute to bleeding and is not associated with an excessive anticoagulant effect due to bioaccumulation.[150] Enoxaparin, however, has shown accumulation when used at treatment dosages.[157–161]

Because there is conflicting evidence regarding the accumulation of LMWHs in renally impaired patients, further studies are needed. At this time, ACCP recommends using an alternative agent or dosage-adjusted LMWH in patients who are renally impaired (CLcr of <30 mL/min). Because laboratory results are not immediately available on admission, it is important for pharmacists to review patients' history to determine if their LMWH dose needs to be adjusted or if they should be switched to another agent. Twice-daily UFH 5000 units is an appropriate option in both hemodialysis patients and patients with severe renal impairment in the absence of contraindications. A recent review with recommendations by Nutescu and colleagues[146] addressed LMWH use in both renal impairment and obesity across a wide array of patients.

Pregnant Patients. Pregnancy itself is a risk factor for the development of VTE. VTE in this patient population is complicated, and a thorough clinical history and risk assessment should be sought to determine antepartum and postpartum prophylaxis needs. In general, an LMWH is preferred over a UFH for the prevention and treatment of VTE because of UFH's increased risks of HIT and osteoporosis. At-risk pregnant patients should receive appropriate VTE prophylaxis per ACCP guidelines. For women undergoing cesarean delivery with at least one major or two minor risk factors, LMWH should be used or mechanical prophylaxis for patients with contraindications to LMWH. For women undergoing cesarean delivery with multiple additional risk factors, LMWH should be combined with mechanical methods until discharge. For selected high-risk patients, extended prophylaxis should be considered. Readers are referred to the ACCP guidelines for recommendations regarding the prevention of VTE in pregnant patients.[162]

Emerging Anticoagulant Options

At present, dabigatran, rivaroxaban, and warfarin are the only oral anticoagulants available, though dabigatran and rivaroxaban have only recently gained approval for stroke prevention in nonvalvular atrial fibrillation.[163–166] Dabigatran does not have other indications at this time, and its efficacy is based on the recently published RELY trial, which demonstrated that dabigatran was superior to warfarin with a similar rate of bleeding at a dosage of 150 mg twice daily.[165] Although warfarin has been the only oral anticoagulant available for more than five decades, it has several disadvantages when used for VTE prophylaxis in hospitalized patients, as discussed above. The development of new anticoagulants has focused on finding new oral formulations, specifically targeting single procoagulant complexes critical to the coagulation process, including blocking the initiation of coagulation, preventing the propagation of coagulation, and inhibiting thrombin.[167,168] There are several types of monotargeted oral anticoagulants: direct inhibitors of activated factors IXa and Xa, which are involved in the propagation of coagulation, and direct inhibitors of thrombin activity, which target factor IIa. Rivaroxaban and dabigatran have recently been approved by FDA. The approval of apixaban, however, has been delayed due to FDA's request for additional information.

Rivaroxaban. Rivaroxaban is an oral, reversible, once-daily factor Xa inhibitor that has an oral bioavailability of 80% and a half-life of 7–11 hours; it is 67% renally cleared.[164] Rivaroxaban is a substrate for P-glycoprotein 1 transporter, located in the gut and kidneys, and is also metabolized via cytochrome P-450 isoenzyme 3A4 (CYP3A4), so the use of strong inducers or inhibitors of this isoenzyme should be avoided in patients receiving rivaroxaban. The safety and efficacy of rivaroxaban for VTE prevention after TKR and THR have been evaluated in four Phase III studies (RECORD trials) in Europe and the United States.[169–172] The RECORD 1 and 2 trials were conducted in patients undergoing TKR; the RECORD 3 and 4 trials were conducted in those undergoing THR. Rivaroxaban was found to be superior to enoxaparin for preventing VTE and all-cause mortality with similar bleeding rates. In two of the four RECORD trials, rivaroxaban was superior to enoxaparin in the prevention of symptomatic VTE. The agent is approved for these indications in Europe and Canada and has recently gained FDA approval for the same indications within the United States.[164] In the Phase III MAGELLAN study, the safety and efficacy of extended prophylaxis with oral rivaroxaban (10 mg daily for 31–39 days) were compared to short-term prophylaxis with subcutaneous enoxaparin (40 mg daily for 6–14 days) for the prevention of VTE in medical patients. The results of this study indicate the superiority of rivaroxaban over enoxaparin at day 35 for the composite endpoint of asymptomatic proximal DVT, symptomatic DVT, symptomatic nonfatal PE, and VTE-related death. However, this came at the cost of substantially more major bleeding events.[109] The relative risk of bleeding compared with enoxaparin at 10 and 35 days was 2.3 ($p < 0.001$) and 2.5 ($p < 0.001$), respectively. Because of these safety results, the risk:benefit ratio of rivaroxaban in medical patients is questionable. In the ROCKET-AF study, based on the primary endpoint of stroke or systemic embolism in patients with nonvalvular atrial fibrillation, rivaroxaban was found to be noninferior to warfarin (hazard ratio, 0.88; 95% CI, 0.74–1.03; $p < 0.001$) ($p = 0.12$ for superiority). Rivaroxaban received FDA approval for VTE prevention in TKR, THR, and atrial fibrillation in 2011. However, because of the safety data and higher rates of clinically relevant bleeding, its use in medical patients cannot be recommended at this time.

Apixaban. Apixaban is a new, reversible, direct-acting oral pyrazole-based factor Xa inhibitor that is 25% renally cleared, is 60% bioavailable, and has a half-life of 9–14 hours. The drug is also cleared via the CYP3A4 isoenzyme system; therefore, strong inducers and inhibitors will need to be avoided. Apixaban is currently in advanced stages of testing for the prevention and treatment of thrombotic disorders. It binds to the active site of factor Xa without requiring antithrombin.[167,168]

Currently, there are several multinational Phase III studies of apixaban being conducted for the prevention of thrombotic events, including DVT and PE, in patients undergoing knee or hip replacement surgery. The results for one of these trials (ADVANCE-1) showed that the primary endpoint (symptomatic or asymptomatic DVT, PE, or death from any cause) occurred in 9.0% of apixaban recipients (2.5 mg twice daily), compared with 8.9% of those treated with enoxaparin (30 mg twice daily) in TKR.[173,174] Despite being numerically similar, these figures did not meet the statistical criteria for apixaban noninferiority. The ADVANCE-2 trial was conducted in patients undergoing TKR. The results demonstrated that apixaban (2.5 mg twice daily) was superior to enoxaparin 40 mg subcutaneously once daily for VTE prevention without increased bleeding. The ADVANCE-3 trial was conducted in patients undergoing THR, and its results demonstrated that apixaban was superior to enoxaparin for VTE prevention at 35 days postsurgery with a similar rate of bleeding. In the ADOPT study of apixaban for VTE prevention in medical patients, apixaban showed substantially increased major bleeding at 30 days without demonstrating superiority on the primary composite VTE efficacy endpoint.[168] These results are similar to those of the MAGELLAN trial mentioned above. The agent is also in Phase II clinical testing in patients with metastatic cancer.[174]

Dabigatran. Dabigatran is a potent, competitive, reversible direct thrombin (factor IIa) inhibitor with 80% renal excretion, a 14 to 17-hour half-life, and 6% oral bioavailability.[163] Dabigatran inhibits free thrombin, fibrin-bound thrombin, and thrombin-induced platelet aggregation. It is also a substrate of Pgp1; therefore, strong inducers and inhibitors should be avoided.[167,168] Dabigatran has completed Phase III clinical trials in Europe and the United States to evaluate its potential in thromboembolic disorders. It was approved for marketing by FDA in October 2010 for the prevention of stroke and systemic embolism in patients with nonvalvular atrial fibrillation. It has also been approved by the European Medicines Agency for primary prevention of VTE in adult patients who have undergone elective hip or knee replacement and has been subsequently launched in the United Kingdom and Germany.[168]

Three Phase III trials (RE-MODEL, RE-NOVATE, RE-MOBILIZE) have been undertaken to study dabigatran versus enoxaparin in the prevention of major VTE and VTE-related mortality after both knee and hip replacement surgery. The RE-MODEL (TKR) and RE-NOVATE (THR) met noninferiority criteria versus enoxaparin 40 mg daily, but the RE-MOBILIZE (TKR) failed to meet noninferiority criteria against enoxaparin 30 mg twice daily. Rates of major bleeding were comparable between the treatment groups.[173,174]

Potential Benefits and Limitations of Emerging Agents. The new oral anticoagulants are considered to be more convenient and simpler to use than vitamin K antagonists, because routine measuring of anticoagulant effects and dose adjustment are not required. Their oral route of administration as compared with injectables is favorable and may improve adherence and simplify postdischarge prophylaxis. Ecarin clotting time, thrombin time, activated partial thromboplastin time, and activated clotting time have theoretical potential to be used for measures of anticoagulant effect of dabigatran, whereas factor Xa levels and prothrombin time have the potential to measure the anticoagulant effect of apixaban and rivaroxaban. In addition, direct thrombin inhibitor measurement assays and reversal agents are under development for dabigatran. Most of these agents undergo renal clearance, which could lead to drug accumulation in patients with renal impairment.

Currently, there are no antidotes for rivaroxaban, apixaban, or dabigatran to rapidly reverse drug effects if required. This is also a current limitation shared by fondaparinux. LMWH can be partially reversed by protamine, whereas UFH can be fully reversed with protamine. Because these novel oral anticoagulants have longer half-lives than UFH and LMWH, any adverse effects caused by direct inhibition of thrombin or factor Xa will continue for several hours or days after the cessation of therapy.

Cost-Effectiveness of Antithrombotic Prophylaxis

For the initial hospital admission, the costs of DVT and PE are $9,805 and $14,146, respectively, and readmission costs for the same events are $11,862 (DVT cost significantly higher, $p = 0.006$) and $14,722, respectively.[42] With the cost of prophylaxis for approximately 10 days being $20–$250 for most pharmacologic agents, cost efficacy for pharmacologic prophylaxis is well established. A median of 10 days is a common duration of therapy for prophylaxis used in many medical and surgical trials not requiring an extended duration of therapy. A minimum duration of 10 days is also recommended for THR, TKR, and hip fracture surgery patients. Length of hospitalization and hospital costs have also been found to be substantially increased for patients who develop VTE.[175,176] One retrospective analysis demonstrated that total costs were not different for patients who were given prophylaxis with LMWH versus UFH, though VTE rates were substantially lower with LMWH versus UFH.[177] Two other studies found lower total costs of LMWH versus UFH[178,179] and cost-effectiveness of primary prophylaxis to prevent VTE over no prophylaxis.[111] With the introduction of generic enoxaparin and future agents—including a generic fondaparinux, dabigatran, apixaban, and rivaroxaban—the cost of VTE prophylaxis will likely continue to decrease.

Monitoring Antithrombotic Prophylaxis

Although the incidence of HIT with LMWH and UFH varies by patient group, HIT occurs much more frequently (i.e., threefold) with the use of UFH compared with LMWH. Postoperative orthopedic, cardiac, and vascular surgery patients receiving UFH for one to two weeks for thromboprophylaxis have the highest risk of HIT, ranging from 1% to 5%.[115] In this patient group, platelet count should be monitored at least every other day between postoperative days 4 and 14 or until UFH is stopped (if before day 14), whichever occurs first.[115] The risk of HIT is lower (0.1–1%) among postoperative patients receiving an LMWH or intravascular catheter UFH flushes and medical or obstetric patients receiving LMWH after previously receiving UFH. For these patients, platelet monitoring should occur at least every two or three days from day 4 to 14, or until the UFH or LMWH is stopped (if before day 14), whichever comes first.[115] When the estimated risk of HIT is less than 0.1%, the risk is described as "rare." Patients in this group include medical and obstetric patients receiving only LMWH or medical patients receiving only intravascular catheter UFH flushes, and platelet monitoring is not recommended.

Because LMWH and fondaparinux are cleared renally, pharmacists play an integral role in monitoring the safety and efficacy of therapy. They should pay close attention to patients' renal function and make appropriate dosage changes or modify prophylaxis to other appropriate regimens in collaborative environments. This may be accomplished by measuring anti-Xa levels.

Summary

Despite decades of evidence showing that pharmacologic and mechanical means can help prevent VTE in hospitalized at-risk patients, current national and international prevention strategies remain suboptimal. National organization positions are shifting to include omission of appropriate care as an adverse event or adverse drug event. Therefore, omission of VTE prophylaxis in a patient who develops a VTE is considered an adverse drug event if pharmacologic prophylaxis was indicated or as an adverse event if mechanical prophylaxis was indicated. To date, no adverse-drug-event studies are including "omission" of VTE prophylaxis as an adverse drug event. Inclusion of this adverse drug event will substantially increase the financial implications of adverse drug events nationally.

Future studies are needed in VTE prevention, including elicitation of the optimal duration of thromboprophylaxis (especially after hospital discharge because of the short lengths of stay in U.S. hospitals), the optimal use of currently approved agents for prophylaxis, the impact of preventable VTE as an adverse event or adverse drug event, and validation of individual scoring methods, especially in hospitalized settings. Hospital pharmacy leadership and proactive engagement are driving forces to ensure appropriate prophylactic management of VTE in hospitalized patients.

Recent data revealed that inhospital, pharmacy-driven VTE prevention programs can increase the use of appropriate thromboprophylaxis and reduce VTE events. VTE prophylaxis programs and anticoagulation management, especially in hospitalized settings, are opportunities that pharmacists can take advantage of in their respective health care settings to reduce unnecessary morbidity and mortality from this disease. Because of their expertise in pharmacotherapy, pharmacists are poised to take a leadership role in VTE prevention programs to positively affect patient care within hospitals and beyond.

References

1. Hirsh J, Hoak J. Management of deep vein thrombosis and pulmonary embolism. *Circulation.* 1996; 93:2212–45.
2. Heit JA, Cohen AT, Anderson FA Jr, on behalf of the VTE Impact Assessment Group. Estimated annual number of incident and recurrent, non-fatal and fatal venous thromboembolism (VTE) events in the US. *Blood.* 2005; 106:11. Abstract.
3. Cohen AT, Agnelli G, Anderson FA, et al. Venous thromboembolism (VTE) in Europe. The number of VTE events and associated morbidity and mortality. *Thromb Haemost.* 2007; 98:756–64.
4. Sandler DA, Martin JF. Autopsy proven pulmonary embolism in hospital patients: are we detecting enough deep vein thrombosis? *J R Soc Med.* 1989; 82:203–5.
5. Stein PD, Henry JW. Prevalence of acute pulmonary embolism among patients in a general hospital and at autopsy. *Chest.* 1995; 108:978–81.
6. Cohen AT, Tapson VF, Bergmann J, et al. Venous thromboembolism risk and prophylaxis in the acute hospital care setting (ENDORSE study): a multinational cross-sectional study. *Lancet.* 2008; 371:387–94.
7. Shojania KG, Duncan BW, McDonald KM, et al. Making health care safer: a critical analysis of patient safety practices. AHRQ Publication No. 01-E058. Rockville, MD: Agency for Healthcare Research and Quality; 2001.
8. Geerts WH, Bergqvist D, Pineo GF, et al. Prevention of venous thromboembolism. *Chest.* 2008; 133(suppl): 381S–453S.
9. Anderson FA Jr, Wheeler HB, Goldberg RJ, et al. A population-based perspective of the hospital incidence and case fatality rates of deep vein thrombosis and pulmonary embolism. The Worcester DVT Study. *Arch Intern Med.* 1991; 151:933–8.
10. White RH. The epidemiology of venous thromboembolism. *Circulation.* 2003; 107:14–8.
11. Prandoni P, Lensing AW, Cogo A, et al. The long-term clinical course of acute deep venous thrombosis. *Ann Intern Med.* 1996; 125:1–7.
12. Heit JA, Mohr DN, Silverstein MD, et al. Predictors of recurrence after deep vein thrombosis and pulmonary embolism: a population-based cohort study. *Arch Intern Med.* 2000; 160:761–8.
13. Anderson FA Jr, Spencer FA. Risk factors for venous thromboembolism. *Circulation.* 2003; 107:I9–16.
14. Kniffin WD Jr, Baron JA, Barrett J, et al. The epidemiology of diagnosed pulmonary embolism and deep venous thrombosis in the elderly. *Arch Intern Med.* 1994; 154:861–6.
15. Spencer FA, Gore KM, Lessard D, et al. Patient outcomes after deep vein thrombosis and pulmonary embolism: the Worcester Venous Thromboembolism Study. *Arch Intern Med.* 2008; 168:425–30.
16. Edelsberg J, Hagiwara M, Taneja C, et al. Risk of venous thromboembolism among hospitalized medically ill patients. *Am J Health-Syst Pharm.* 2006; 63(suppl 6):S16–22.
17. Goldhaber SZ, Tapson VF. A prospective registry of 5,451 patients with ultrasound-confirmed deep vein thrombosis. *Am J Cardiol.* 2004; 93:259–62.
18. Nielsen HK, Bechgaard P, Nielsen FP, et al. 178 fatal cases of pulmonary embolism in a medical department. *Acta Med Scand.* 1981; 209:351–5.
19. Hauch O, Jorgensen LN, Khattar SC, et al. Fatal pulmonary embolism associated with surgery: an autopsy study. *Acta Chir Scand.* 1990; 156:747–9.
20. Sperry KL, Key CR, Anderson RE. Toward a population-based assessment of death due to pulmonary embolism in New Mexico. *Hum Pathol.* 1990; 21:159–65.
21. Cohen AT, Edmondson RA, Phillips MJ, et al. The changing pattern of venous thromboembolic disease. *Haemostasis.* 1996; 26:65–71.
22. Piazza G, Seddighzadeh A, Goldhaber SZ. Double trouble for 2,609 hospitalized medical patients who developed deep vein thrombosis: prophylaxis omitted more often and pulmonary embolism more frequent. *Chest.* 2007; 132:554–61.
23. Samama MM, Cohen AT, Darmon JY, et al. A comparison of enoxaparin with placebo for the prevention of venous thromboembolism in acutely ill medical patients. *N Engl J Med.* 1999; 341:793–800.
24. Leizorovicz A, Cohen AT, Turpie AG, et al. Randomized, placebo-controlled trial of dalteparin for the prevention of venous thromboembolism in acutely ill medical patients. *Circulation.* 2004; 110:874–9.
25. Cohen AT, Davidson BL, Gallus AS, et al. Efficacy and safety of fondaparinux for the prevention of venous thromboembolism in older acute medical patients: randomised placebo controlled trial. *BMJ.* 2006; 332:325–9.
26. Ashrani AA, Heit JA. Incidence and cost burden of post-thrombotic syndrome. *J Thromb Thrombolysis.* 2009; 28:465–76.
27. MacDougall DA, Feliu AL, Boccuzzi SJ, et al. Economic burden of deep-vein thrombosis, pulmonary embolism, and post-thrombotic syndrome. *Am J Health-Syst Pharm.* 2006; 63(suppl 6):S5–15.
28. Kahn S, Ginsberg JS. Relationship between deep venous thrombosis and the postthrombotic syndrome. *Arch Intern Med.* 2004; 164:17–26.
29. Pengo V, Lensing AW, Prins MH, et al. Incidence of chronic thromboembolic pulmonary hypertension after pulmonary embolism. *N Engl J Med.* 2004; 350:2257–64.
30. Sagar S, Massey J, Sanderson JM. Low-dose heparin prophylaxis against fatal pulmonary embolism. *Br Med J.* 1975; 4:257–9.
31. Burleigh E, Wang C, Foster D, et al. Thromboprophylaxis in medically ill patients at risk for venous thromboembolism. *Am J Health-Syst Pharm.* 2006; 63(suppl 6):S23–9.
32. Yu HT, Dylan ML, Lin J, et al. Hospitals' compliance with prophylaxis guidelines for venous thromboembolism. *Am J Health-Syst Pharm.* 2007; 64:69–76.
33. Amin A, Stemkowski S, Lin J, et al. Thromboprophylaxis rates in US medical centers: success or failure? *J Thromb Haemost.* 2007; 5:1610–6.
34. Amin A, Stemkowski S, Lin J, et al. Appropriate thromboprophylaxis in hospitalized cancer patients. *Clin Adv Hematol Oncol.* 2008; 6:910–20.

35. Amin A, Spyropoulos AC, Dobesh P, et al. Are hospitals delivering appropriate VTE prevention? The venous thromboembolism study to assess the rate of thromboprophylaxis (VTE start). *J Thromb Thrombolysis.* 2010; 29:326–39.
36. Geerts WH, Pineo GF, Heit JA, et al. Prevention of venous thromboembolism: the Seventh ACCP Conference on Antithrombotic and Thrombolytic Therapy. *Chest.* 2004; 126(suppl):338S–400S.
37. Khorana AA. The NCCN clinical practice guidelines on venous thromboembolic disease: strategies for improving VTE prophylaxis in hospitalized cancer patients. *Oncologist.* 2007; 12:1361–70.
38. Cabana MD, Rand CS, Powe NR, et al. Why don't physicians follow clinical practice guidelines? A framework for improvement. *JAMA.* 1999; 282:1458–65.
39. Mahan CE, Hussein MA, Amin AN, et al. Venous thromboembolism pharmacy intervention management program with an active, multifaceted approach reduces preventable venous thromboembolism and increases appropriate prophylaxis. *Clin Appl Thromb Hemost.* 2012; 18:45–58.
40. Mahan CE, Borrego ME, Woersching AL, et al. Venous thromboembolism: annualised United States models for total, hospital-acquired and preventable costs utilising long-term attack rates. *Thromb Haemost.* 2012; 108:291–302.
41. Centers for Disease Control and Prevention. National Center on Birth Defects and Developmental Disabilities strategic plan 2011–2015. www.cdc.gov/NCBDDD/AboutUs/documents/NCBDDD_StrategicPlan_2-10-11.pdf (accessed 2012 Feb 27).
42. Spyropoulos AC, Lin J. Direct medical costs of venous thromboembolism and subsequent hospital readmission rates: an administrative claims analysis from 30 managed care organizations. *J Manag Care Pharm.* 2007; 13:475–86.
43. Kahn SR, Lim W, Dunn AS, et al. Prevention of venous thromboembolism in non-surgical patients. *Chest.* 2012; 141(suppl 2):e195s–226s.
44. Gould MK, Garcia DA, Wren SM, et al. Prevention of venous thromboembolism in nonorthopedic surgical patients. *Chest.* 2012; 141(suppl 2):e227s–77s.
45. Falck-Ytter Y, Francis CW, Johanson NA, et al. Prevention of venous thromboembolism in orthopedic surgery patients. *Chest.* 2012; 141(suppl 2):e278s–325s.
46. Cardiovascular Disease Educational and Research Trust, Cyprus Cardiovascular Disease Educational and Research Trust, European Venous Forum, et al. Prevention and treatment of venous thromboembolism. International consensus statement (guidelines according to scientific evidence). *Int Angiol.* 2006; 25:101–61.
47. Lyman GH, Khorana AA, Falanga A, et al. American Society of Clinical Oncology guideline: recommendations for venous thromboembolism prophylaxis and treatment in patients with cancer. *J Clin Oncol.* 2007; 25:5490–505.
48. National Comprehensive Cancer Network. NCCN clinical practice guidelines in oncology. Venous thromboembolic disease, version 2.2011. www.nccn.org/professionals/physician_gls/PDF/vte.pdf (accessed 2012 Feb 27).
49. Joint Commission. National Patient Safety Goals effective January 1, 2012. www.jointcommission.org/standards_information/npsgs.aspx (accessed 2012 Feb 27).
50. Centers for Medicare and Medicaid Services. Fact sheet: Medicare takes new steps to help make your hospital stay safer. www.cms.hhs.gov/apps/media/press/factsheet.asp?Counter=3227&intNumPerPage=10&checkDate=&checkKey=&srchType=1&numDays=3500&srchOpt=0&srchData=&keywordType=All&chkNewsType=6&intPage=&showAll=&pYear=&year=&desc=&cboOrder=date (accessed 2008 Aug 4).
51. National Quality Forum. National voluntary consensus standards for prevention and care of venous thromboembolism: policy, preferred practices and performance measures. www.qualityforum.org/Projects/s-z/VTE_Phase_I/Venous_Thromboembolism_%28VTE%29_I.aspx (accessed 2012 Feb 27).
52. Joint Commission. Performance measurement initiatives. Specifications manual for national hospital inpatient quality measures. www.jointcommission.org/specifications_manual_for_national_hospital_inpatient_quality_measures.aspx (accessed 2012 Feb 27).
53. Urbankova J, Quiroz R, Kucher N, et al. Intermittent pneumatic compression and deep vein thrombosis prevention. *Thromb Haemost.* 2005; 94:1181–5.
54. Lacut K, Bressollette L, Le Gal G, et al. Prevention of venous thrombosis in patients with acute intracerebral hemorrhage. *Neurology.* 2005; 65:865–9.
55. Mismetti P, Rivron-Guillot K, Quenet S, et al. A prospective long-term study of 220 patients with a retrievable vena cava filter for secondary prevention of venous thromboembolism. *Chest.* 2007; 131:223–9.
56. Morris R, Woodcock JP. Evidence-based compression prevention of stasis and deep vein thrombosis. *Ann Surg.* 2004; 239:162–71.
57. Spyropoulos AC, Mahan CE. Prevention of venous thromboembolism in medical patients. In: Fang MC, ed. Inpatient anticoagulation. Hoboken, NJ: Wiley-Blackwell; 2011.
58. Cook D, Crowther M, Meade M, et al. Deep venous thrombosis in medical-surgical critically ill patients: prevalence, incidence, and risk factors. *Crit Care Med.* 2005; 33:1565–71.
59. Blom JW, Doggen CJ, Osanto S, et al. Malignancies, prothrombotic mutations, and the risk of venous thrombosis. *JAMA.* 2005; 293:715–22.
60. Monreal M, Falgá C, Valdés M, et al. Fatal pulmonary embolism and fatal bleeding in cancer patients with venous thromboembolism: findings from the RIETE registry. *J Thromb Haemost.* 2006; 4:1950–6.
61. Heit JA, Silverstein MD, Mohr DN, et al. Risk factors for deep vein thrombosis and pulmonary embolism: a population-based case-control study. *Arch Intern Med.* 2000; 160:809–15.
62. Haddad TC, Greeno EW. Chemotherapy-induced thrombosis. *Thromb Res.* 2006; 118:555–68.
63. Khorana AA, Francis CW, Culakova E, et al. Risk factors for chemotherapy-associated venous thromboembolism in a prospective observational study. *Cancer.* 2005; 104:2822–9.

64. Hussein MA. Thromboembolism risk reduction in multiple myeloma patients treated with immunomodulatory drug combinations. *Thromb Haemost.* 2006; 95:924–30.

65. Johnson DH, Fehrenbacher L, Novotny WF, et al. Randomized phase II trial comparing bevacizumab plus carboplatin and paclitaxel with carboplatin and paclitaxel alone in previously untreated locally advanced or metastatic non-small cell lung cancer. *J Clin Oncol.* 2004; 22:2184–91.

66. Zangari M, Barlogie B, Anaissie E, et al. Deep vein thrombosis in patients with multiple myeloma treated with thalidomide and chemotherapy: effects of prophylactic and therapeutic anticoagulation. *Br J Haematol.* 2004; 126:715–21.

67. Barlogie B, Tricot G, Anaissie E, et al. Thalidomide and hematopoietic-cell transplantation for multiple myeloma. *N Engl J Med.* 2006; 354:1021–30.

68. El Accaoui RN, Shamseddeen WA, Taher AT. Thalidomide and thrombosis: a meta-analysis. *Thromb Haemost.* 2007; 97:1031–6.

69. Fisher B, Costantino J, Redmond C, et al. A randomized clinical trial evaluating tamoxifen in the treatment of patients with mode-negative breast cancer who have estrogen receptor-positive tumors. *N Engl J Med.* 1989; 320:479–84.

70. Fisher B, Costantino JP, Wickerham DL, et al. Tamoxifen for prevention of breast cancer: report of the National Surgical Adjuvant Breast and Bowel Project P-1 study. *J Natl Cancer Inst.* 1998; 90:1371–88.

71. Fisher B, Costantino JP, Wickerham DL, et al. Tamoxifen for the prevention of breast cancer: current status of the National Surgical Adjuvant Breast and Bowel Project P-1 study. *J Natl Cancer Inst.* 2005; 97:1652–62.

72. Lee AY, Levine MN. Venous thromboembolism and cancer: risks and outcomes. *Circulation.* 2003; 107:I-17–21.

73. Saphner T, Tormey DC, Gray R. Venous and arterial thrombosis in patients who received adjuvant therapy for breast cancer. *J Clin Oncol.* 1991; 9:286–94.

74. Thürlimann B, Keshaviah A, Coates AS, et al. A comparison of letrozole and tamoxifen in postmenopausal women with early breast cancer. *N Engl J Med.* 2005; 353:2747–57.

75. Baum M, Budzar AU, Cuzick J, et al. Anastrozole alone or in combination with tamoxifen versus tamoxifen alone for adjuvant treatment of postmenopausal women with early breast cancer: first results of the ATAC randomised trial. *Lancet.* 2002; 359:2131–9.

76. Bonnetere J, Buzdar A, Nabholtz JM, et al. Anastrozole is superior to tamoxifen as first-line therapy in hormone receptor positive advanced breast carcinoma: results of two randomized trials designed for combined analysis. *Cancer.* 2001; 92:2247–58.

77. Coombes RC, Hall E, Gibson LJ, et al. A randomized trial of exemestane after two to three years of tamoxifen therapy in postmenopausal women with primary breast cancer. *N Engl J Med.* 2004; 350:1081–92.

78. Prandoni P, Lensing AW, Piccioli A, et al. Recurrent venous thromboembolism and bleeding complications during anticoagulant treatment in patients with cancer and venous thrombosis. *Blood.* 2002; 100:3484–8.

79. Elting LS, Escalante CP, Cooksley C, et al. Outcomes and cost of deep venous thrombosis among patients with cancer. *Arch Intern Med.* 2004; 164:1653–61.

80. Blom JW, Vanderschoot JP, Oostindier MJ, et al. Incidence of venous thrombosis in a large cohort of 66,329 cancer patients: results of a record linkage study. *J Thromb Haemost.* 2006; 4:529–35.

81. Descourt R, Le Gal G, Couturaud F, et al. Recurrent venous thromboembolism under anticoagulant therapy: a high risk in adenocarcinoma? *Thromb Haemost.* 2006; 95:912–3.

82. Chew HK, Wun T, Harvey D, et al. Incidence of venous thromboembolism and its effect on survival among patients with common cancers. *Arch Intern Med.* 2006; 166:458–64.

83. Sorensen HT, Mellemkjaer L, Olsen JH, et al. Prognosis of cancers associated with venous thromboembolism. *N Engl J Med.* 2000; 343:1846–50.

84. Alcalay A, Wun T, Khatri V, et al. Venous thromboembolism in patients with colorectal cancer: incidence and effect on survival. *J Clin Oncol.* 2006; 24:1112–8.

85. Ageno W, Prandoni P, Romualdi E, et al. The metabolic syndrome and the risk of venous thrombosis: a case-control study. *J Thromb Haemost.* 2006; 4:1914–8.

86. Ageno W, Becattini C, Brighton T, et al. Cardiovascular risk factors and venous thromboembolism: a meta-analysis. *Circulation.* 2008; 117:93–102.

87. Masopust J, Maly R, Andrys C, et al. Markers of thrombogenesis are activated in unmedicated patients with acute psychosis: a matched case control study. *BMC Psychiatry.* 2011; 11:2.

88. Lutz L, Haas S, Hach-Wunderle V, et al. [Venous thromboembolism in internal medicine: risk assessment and pharmaceutical prophylaxis: publication for the specialist forum.] *Med Welt.* 2002; 53:231–4. In German.

89. Caprini JA, Arcelus JI, Reyna JJ. Effective risk stratification of surgical and nonsurgical patients for venous thromboembolic disease. *Semin Hematol.* 2001; 38(suppl 5):12–9.

90. Bahl V, Hu HM, Henke PK, et al. A validation study of a retrospective venous thromboembolism risk scoring method. *Ann Surg.* 2010; 251:344–50.

91. Cohen AT, Alikhan R, Arcelus JI, et al. Assessment of venous thromboembolism risk and the benefit of thromboprophylaxis in medical patients. *Thromb Haemost.* 2005; 94:750–9.

92. Spyropoulos AC, Anderson FA Jr, Fitzgerald G, et al. Predictive and associative models to identify hospitalized medical patients at risk for venous thromboembolism. *Chest.* 2011; 140:706–14.

93. Barbar S, Noventa F, Rossetto V, et al. A risk assessment model for the identification of hospitalized medical patients at risk for venous thromboembolism: the Padua Prediction Score. *J Thromb Haemost.* 2010; 8:2450–7.

94. Mahan CE, Spyropoulos AC. Venous thromboembolism prevention: a systematic review of methods to

increase prophylaxis and decrease events in the hospitalized patient. *Hosp Pract.* 2010; 38:97–108.

95. Tooher R, Middleton P, Pham C, et al. A systematic review of strategies to improve prophylaxis for venous thromboembolism in hospitals. *Ann Surg.* 2005; 241:397–415.
96. Michota FA. Bridging the gap between evidence and practice in venous thromboembolism prophylaxis: the quality improvement process. *J Gen Intern Med.* 2007; 22:1762–70.
97. Cohn SL. Prophylaxis of venous thromboembolism in the US: improving hospital performance. *J Thromb Haemost.* 2009; 7:1437–45.
98. Dobesh PP, Stacy ZA. Effect of a clinical pharmacy education program on improvement in the quantity and quality of venous thromboembolism prophylaxis for medically ill patients. *J Manag Care Pharm.* 2005; 11:755–62.
99. Bauer JB, Chun DS, Karpinski TA. Pharmacist-led program to improve venous thromboembolism prophylaxis in a community hospital. *Am J Health-Syst Pharm.* 2008; 65:1643–7.
100. Sobieraj DM. Development and implementation of a program to assess medical patients' need for venous thromboembolism prophylaxis. *Am J Health-Syst Pharm.* 2008; 65:1755–60.
101. Cronin M, Hill T, Reich DA, et al. Implementation of a multidisciplinary, pharmacy-led, thromboprophylaxis program in total-joint arthroplasty patients. *Am J Health-Syst Pharm.* 2009; 66:171–5.
102. Galanter WL, Thambi M, Rosencranz H, et al. Effects of clinical decision support on venous thromboembolism risk assessment, prophylaxis, and prevention at a university teaching hospital. *Am J Health-Syst Pharm.* 2010; 67:1265–73.
103. Stein J, Chesson M, Killian A, et al. Combined effect of multidisciplinary bedside rounding and real-time visualization of prophylaxis status on hospital acquired VTE in a surgical intensive care unit. Paper presented at 2011 Southern Hospital Medicine Annual Meeting. Grapevine, TX; 2011 May 11.
104. Maynard GA, Morris TA, Jenkins IH. Optimizing prevention of hospital-acquired venous thromboembolism (VTE): prospective validation of a VTE risk assessment model. *J Hosp Med.* 2010; 5:8–10.
105. Cook D, Meade M, Guyatt G, et al. Dalteparin vs unfractionated heparin in critically ill patients. *N Engl J Med.* 2011; 364:1305–14.
106. Lederle FA. Venous thromboembolism prophylaxis in hospitalized medical patients and those with stroke: a background review for an American College of Physicians clinical practice guideline. *Ann Intern Med.* 2011; 155:602–15.
107. Baker DW, Qaseem A. Evidence-based performance measures: preventing unintended consequences of quality measurement. *Ann Intern Med.* 2011; 155:625–32.
108. Qaseem A. Chou R, Humphrey L, et al. Venous thromboembolism prophylaxis in hospitalized patients: a clinical practice guideline from the American College of Physicians. *Ann Intern Med.* 2011; 155:625–32.
109. Centers for Disease Control and Prevention. Quick stats: average length of hospital stay, by diagnostic category—United States, 2003. *MMWR.* 2005; 54:680.
110. Hull RD, Schellong SM, Tapson VF, et al. Extended-duration venous thromboembolism (VTE) prophylaxis in acutely ill medical patients with recent reduced morbidity: the EXCLAIM study. *Ann Intern Med.* 2010; 153:8–18.
111. Goldhaber SZ. Apixaban versus enoxaparin for thromboprophylaxis in medically ill patients. *N Engl J Med.* 2011; 365:2167–77.
112. American College of Cardiology. Rivaroxaban compares favorably with enoxaparin in preventing venous thromboembolism in acutely ill patients without showing a net clinical benefit. www.cardiosource.org/News-Media/Media-Center/News-Releases/2011/04/MAGELLAN.aspx (accessed 2012 Feb 27).
113. ClinicalTrials.gov. VTE Discharge Alert Trial.: http://clinicaltrials.gov/ct2/show/NCT00853463 (accessed 2012 Feb 27).
114. Amin AN, Girard F, Samama MM. Does ambulation modify venous thromboembolism risk in acutely ill medical patients? *Thromb Haemost.* 2010; 104:955–61.
115. Warkentin TE, Greinacher A, Koster A, et al. Treatment and prevention of heparin-induced thrombocytopenia. *Chest.* 2008; 133:340–80.
116. Hirsh J, Bauer KA, Donati MB, et al. Parenteral anticoagulants: American College of Chest Physicians evidence-based clinical practice guidelines (8th edition). *Chest.* 2008; 133(suppl):141S–159S.
117. Creekmore FM, Oderda GM, Pendleton RC, et al. Incidence and economic implications of heparin-induced thrombocytopenia in medical patients receiving prophylaxis for venous thromboembolism. *Pharmacotherapy.* 2006; 26:1438–45.
118. Mcleod RS, Geerts WH, Sniderman KW, et al. Subcutaneous heparin versus low-molecular-weight heparin as thromboprophylaxis in patients undergoing colorectal surgery: results of the Canadian colorectal DVT prophylaxis trial: a randomized, double-blind trial. *Ann Surg.* 2001; 233:438–44.
119. Colwell CW Jr, Collis DK, Paulson R, et al. Comparison of enoxaparin and warfarin for the prevention of venous thromboembolic disease after total hip arthroplasty: evaluation during hospitalization and three months after discharge. *J Bone Joint Surg Am.* 1999; 81:932–40.
120. Leclerc JR, Geerts WH, Desjardins L, et al. Prevention of venous thromboembolism after knee arthroplasty: a randomized, double-blind trial comparing enoxaparin with warfarin. *Ann Intern Med.* 1996; 124:619–26.
121. Turpie AG, Bauer KA, Eriksson BI, et al. Fondaparinux vs enoxaparin for the prevention of venous thromboembolism in major orthopedic surgery: a meta-analysis of 4 randomized double-blind studies. *Arch Intern Med.* 2002; 162:1833–40.
122. Dentali F, Douketis JD, Gianni M, et al. Meta-analysis: anticoagulant prophylaxis to prevent symptomatic venous thromboembolism in hospitalized medical patients. *Ann Intern Med.* 2007; 146:278–88.
123. Mismetti P, Laporte-Simitsidis S, Tardy B, et al. Prevention of venous thromboembolism in internal

medicine with unfractionated or low-molecular-weight heparins: a meta-analysis of randomised clinical trials. *Thromb Haemost.* 2000; 83:14–9.

124. Kleber FX, Witt C, Vogel G, et al Randomized comparison of enoxaparin with unfractionated heparin for the prevention of venous thromboembolism in medical patients with heart failure or severe respiratory disease. *Am Heart J.* 2003; 145:614–21.
125. Lechler E, Schramm W, Flosbach CW. The venous thrombotic risk in non-surgical patients: epidemiological data and efficacy/safety profile of a low-molecular-weight heparin (enoxaparin). *Haemostasis.* 1996; 26(suppl 2):49–56.
126. Cheer SM, Dunn CJ, Foster R. Tinzaparin sodium: a review of its pharmacology and clinical use in the prophylaxis and treatment of thromboembolic disease. *Drugs.* 2004; 64:1479–502.
127. Decousus H, Tapson VF, Vergmann JF, et al. Factors at admission associated with bleeding risk in medical patients: findings from IMPROVE. *Chest.* 2011; 139:69–79.
128. Mahan CE, Spyropoulos AC. Venous thromboembolism prophylaxis with unfractionated heparin in the hospitalized medical patient: the case for thrice daily over twice daily dosing. *Intern Emerg Med.* 2010; 5:299–306.
129. Velmahos GC, Kern J, Chan LS, et al. Prevention of venous thromboembolism after injury: an evidence-based report; part I. Analysis of risk factors and evaluation of the role of vena caval filters. *J Trauma.* 2000; 49:132–9.
130. Fuchs S, Heyse T, Rudofsky G, et al. Continuous passive motion in the prevention of deep-vein thrombosis: a randomised comparison in trauma patients. *J Bone Joint Surg Br.* 2005; 87:1117–22.
131. Tapson VF, Decousus H, Pini M, et al. Venous thromboembolism prophylaxis in acutely ill hospitalized medical patients: findings from the International Medical Prevention Registry on Venous Thromboembolism. *Chest.* 2007; 132:936–45.
132. Sanderink G, Liboux A, Jariwala N, et al. The pharmacokinetics and pharmacodynamics of enoxaparin in obese volunteers. *Clin Pharmacol Ther.* 2002; 72:308–18.
133. Wilson S, Wilbur K, Burton E, et al. Effect of patient weight on the anticoagulant response to adjusted therapeutic dosage of low-molecular-weight heparin for the treatment of venous thromboembolism. *Haemostasis.* 2001; 31:42–8.
134. Smith J, Canton E. Weight-based administration of dalteparin in obese patients. *Am J Health-Syst Pharm.* 2003; 60:683–7.
135. Al-Yaseen E, Wells PS, Anderson J, et al. The safety of dosing dalteparin based on actual body weight for the treatment of acute venous thromboembolism in obese patients. *J Thromb Haemost.* 2005; 3:100–2.
136. Hainer J, Barrett J, Assaid C, et al. Dosing in heavy-weight/obese patients with the LMWH tinzaparin: a pharmacodynamic study. *Thromb Haemost.* 2002; 87:817–23.
137. Spinler S, Inverso S, Cohen M, et al. Safety and efficacy of unfractionated heparin versus enoxaparin in patients who are obese and patients with severe renal impairment: analysis from the ESSENCE and TIMI 11B studies. *Am Heart J.* 2003; 146:33–41.
138. Samama M, Verhill C, Carchy L. Relation between weight, obesity, and frequency of deep venous thrombosis after enoxaparin in orthopedic surgery. *Thromb Haemost.* 1995; 73:977.
139. Frederiksen S, Hedenbro J, Norgren L. Enoxaparin effect depends on body-weight and current doses may be inadequate in obese patients. *Br J Surg.* 2003; 90:547–8.
140. Heizmann M, Baerlocher G, Steinmann F, et al. Anti-Xa activity in obese patients after double standard dose of nadroparin for prophylaxis. *Thromb Res.* 2002; 106:179–81.
141. Kalfarentzos F, Stavropoulou F, Yarmenitis S, et al. Prophylaxis of venous thromboembolism using two different doses of low-molecular-weight heparin (nadroparin) in bariatric surgery: a prospective randomized trial. *Obes Surg.* 2001; 11:670–6.
142. Scholten D, Hoedema R, Scholten S. A comparison of two different prophylactic dose regimens of low molecular weight heparin in bariatric surgery. *Obes Surg.* 2002; 12:19–24.
143. Freeman A, Horner T, Pendleton RC, et al. Prospective comparison of three enoxaparin dosing regimens to achieve target anti-factor Xa levels in hospitalized, medically ill patients with extreme obesity. *Am J Hematol.* 2012; 87:740–3.
144. Rondina MT, Wheeler M, Rodgers GM, et al. Weight-based dosing of enoxaparin for VTE prophylaxis in morbidly obese, medically ill patients. *Thromb Res.* 2010; 125:220–3.
145. Ludwig KP, Simons HJ, Mone M, et al. Implementation of an enoxaparin protocol for venous thromboembolism prophylaxis in obese surgical intensive care unit patients. *Ann Pharmacother.* 2011; 45:1356–62.
146. Nutescu EA, Spinler SA, Wittkowsky A, et al. Low-molecular-weight heparins in renal impairment and obesity: available evidence and clinical practice recommendations across medical and surgical settings. *Ann Pharmacother.* 2009; 43:1064–83.
147. Siguret V, Pautas E, Fevrier M, et al. Elderly patients treated with tinzaparin administered once daily (175 anti-Xa IU/kg): anti-Xa and anti-IIa activities over 10 days. *Thromb Haemost.* 2000; 84:800–4.
148. Rabbat CG, Cook DJ, Crowther MA, et al. Dalteparin thromboprophylaxis for critically ill medical-surgical patients with renal insufficiency. *J Crit Care.* 2005; 20:357–63.
149. Tincani E, Mannucci C, Casolari B, et al. Safety of dalteparin for the prophylaxis of venous thromboembolism in elderly medical patients with renal insufficiency: a pilot study. *Haematologica.* 2006; 91:976–9.
150. Douketis JD, Cook D, Meade M, et al. Prophylaxis against deep vein thrombosis in critically ill patients with severe renal insufficiency with the low-molecular-weight heparin dalteparin—an assessment of safety and pharmacodynamics: the DIRECT study. *J Arch Intern Med.* 2008; 168:1805–12.
151. Shprecher AR, Cheng-Lai A, Madsen EM, et al. Peak antifactor Xa activity produced by

dalteparin treatment in patients with renal impairment compared with controls. *Pharmacotherapy.* 2005; 25:817–22.

152. Mahe I, Aghassarian M, Drouet L, et al. Tinzaparin and enoxaparin given at prophylactic dose for eight days in medical elderly patients with impaired renal function. *Thromb Haemost.* 2007; 97:581–6.
153. Lim W, Dentali F, Eikelboom W, et al. Meta-analysis: low-molecular-weight heparin and bleeding in patients with severe renal insufficiency. *Ann Intern Med.* 2006; 144:673–84.
154. Cestac P, Bagheri H, Lapeyre-Mestre M, et al. Utilisation and safety of low molecular weight heparins: prospective observational study in medical inpatients. *Drug Saf.* 2003; 26:197–207.
155. Tinzaparin: excess mortality in elderly patients with renal failure. Unfractionated heparin is best in this setting. *Prescrire Int.* 2009; 18:216.
156. American Society of Health-System Pharmacists. Tinzaparin sodium injection. www.ashp.org/DrugShortages/NotAvailable/bulletin.aspx?id=749 (accessed 2012 Oct 12).
157. Brophy D, Wazny L, Behr T, et al. The pharmacokinetics of subcutaneous enoxaparin in end-stage renal disease. *Pharmacotherapy.* 2001; 21:169–74.
158. Becker R, Spencer F, Gibson M, et al. Influence of patient characteristics and renal function on factor Xa inhibition pharmacokinetics and pharmacodynamics after enoxaparin administration in non-ST-segment elevation acute coronary syndromes. *Am Heart J.* 2002; 143:753–9.
159. Chow S, Zammit K, West K, et al. Correlation of antifactor Xa concentrations with renal function in patients on enoxaparin. *J Clin Pharmacol.* 2003; 43:586–90.
160. Sanderink G, Guimart C, Ozoux ML, et al. Pharmacokinetics and pharmacodynamics of the prophylactic dose of enoxaparin once daily over 4 days in patients with renal impairment. *Thromb Res.* 2002; 105:225–31.
161. Gerlach A, Pickworth K, Seth S, et al. Enoxaparin and bleeding complications: a review in patients with and without renal insufficiency. *Pharmacotherapy.* 2000; 20:771–5.
162. Bates SM, Greer IA, Pabinger I, et al. Venous thromboembolism, thrombophilia, antithrombotic therapy, and pregnancy: American College of Chest Physicians Evidence-Based Clinical Practice Guidelines (8th edition). *Chest.* 2008; 133(suppl):844S–886S.
163. Boehringer Ingelheim. Pradaxa (dabigatran etexilate) prescribing information. www.pradaxa.com (accessed 2012 Oct 2).
164. Janssen Pharmaceuticals. Xarelto (rivaroxaban) prescribing information. www.xarelto-us.com (accessed 2012 Oct 2).
165. Connelly S, Ezekowitz MD, Yusuf S, et al. Dabigatran versus warfarin in patients with atrial fibrillation. *N Engl J Med.* 2009; 361:1139–51.
166. Patel MR, Mahaffey KW, Garg J, et al. Rivaroxaban versus warfarin in nonvalvular atrial fibrillation. *N Engl J Med.* 2011; 365:883–91.
167. Mahan CE, Fanikos J. New antithrombotics: the impact on global health care. *Thromb Res.* 2011; 127:518–24.
168. Weitz JI, Eikelboom JW, Samama MM. New antithrombotic drugs: Antithrombotic Therapy and Prevention of Thrombosis, 9th edition: American College of Chest Physicians Evidence-Based Clinical Practice Guidelines. *Chest.* 2012; 141(suppl):e120S–51S.
169. Eriksson BI, Borris LC, Friedman RJ, et al. Rivaroxaban versus enoxaparin for thromboprophylaxis after hip arthroplasty. *N Engl J Med.* 2008; 358:2765–75.
170. Kakkar AK, Brenner B, Dahl OE, et al. Extended duration rivaroxaban versus short-term enoxaparin for the prevention of venous thromboembolism after total hip arthroplasty: a double-blind, randomised controlled trial. *Lancet.* 2008; 372:31–9.
171. Lassen MR, Ageno W, Borris LC, et al. Rivaroxaban versus enoxaparin for thromboprophylaxis after total knee arthroplasty. *N Engl J Med.* 2008; 358:2776–86.
172. Turpie AG, Lassen MR, Davidson BL, et al. Rivaroxaban versus enoxaparin for thromboprophylaxis after total knee arthroplasty (RECORD 4): a randomised trial. *Lancet.* 2009; 373:1673–80.
173. Merli G, Spyropoulos A, Caprini J. Use of emerging oral anticoagulants in clinical practice. *Ann Surg.* 2009; 250:219–28.
174. Gomez-Outes A, Lecumberri R, Pozo C, et al. New anticoagulants: focus on venous thromboembolism. *Curr Vasc Pharmacol.* 2009; 7:309–29.
175. Ollendorf DA, Vera-Llonch M, Oster G. Cost of venous thromboembolism following major orthopedic surgery in hospitalized patients. *Am J Health-Syst Pharm.* 2002; 59:1750–4.
176. Mcgarry LJ, Stokes ME, Thompson D. Outcomes of thromboprophylaxis with enoxaparin vs. unfractionated heparin in medical inpatients: a retrospective database analysis. *Thromb J.* 2006; 4:17.
177. Weinberg R, Lichtig LK, Caprini JA, et al. Cost implications of using unfractionated heparin or enoxaparin in medical patients at risk for venous thromboembolic events. *P&T.* 2006; 31:322–3.
178. Deitelzweig SB, Becker R, Lin J, et al. Comparison of the two-year outcomes and costs of prophylaxis in medical patients at risk of venous thromboembolism. *Thromb Haemost.* 2008; 100:810–20.

Approved by the ASHP Board of Directors on April 13, 2012. Developed through the ASHP Council on Therapeutics.

The following individuals are acknowledged for reviewing draft versions of this statement: Kathleen Achor, Jill Bates, Pharm.D., M.S., BCOP; Tim Brown, Pharm.D.; Debra Cowan, Pharm.D.; Michele Danish, Pharm.D., FASHP; Jean B. Douglas Pharm.D., FASHP; Stuart T. Haines, Pharm.D., BCPS, FASHP; Jody Jacobson Wedret, B.S.Pharm., FASHP, FCSHP; Patrick McDonnell, Pharm.D.; Nicole L. McMaster-Baxter, Pharm.D., M.S., BCPS; Fred Meister, Pharm.D.; Charles D. Ponte, Pharm.D., DPNAP, FCCP, FAPhA, FASHP; James A. Ponto, M.S., B.S.Pharm., FASHP; and Kay Ryan, M.S., M.B.A.

Charles E. Mahan, Pharm.D., Ph.C., is Director of Outcomes Research, New Mexico Heart Institute, Albuquerque, NM. Alex C. Spyropoulos, M.D., FACP, FCCP, FRCPC, is Associate Professor of

Medicine, Division of Hematology/Oncology, James P. Wilmot Cancer Center, University of Rochester Medical Center, Rochester, NY.

Dr. Mahan is a participant in the Traveling Fellowship Program for the North American Thrombosis Forum. Dr. Spyropoulos serves on the advisory board of Johnson and Johnson, Pfizer, and Bristol-Myers Squibb and on the steering committee of Bayer and Eisai. He also serves on the data safety monitoring board of Portola.

Copyright © 2012, American Society of Health-System Pharmacists, Inc. All rights reserved. Contact ASHP for reprint and permissions requests. This content may not be used for commercial purposes without the express written consent of ASHP.

The bibliographic citation for this document is as follows: American Society of Health-System Pharmacists. ASHP therapeutic position statement on the role of pharmacotherapy in preventing venous thromboembolism in hospitalized patients. *Am J Health-Syst Pharm.* 2012; 69:2174–90.

ASHP Therapeutic Position Statement on Strategies for Identifying and Preventing Pneumococcal Resistance

Position

The American Society of Health-System Pharmacists (ASHP) supports the establishment of state and national surveillance systems to track the prevalence of drug-resistant *Streptococcus pneumoniae* so that appropriate antimicrobial regimens can be used to treat infections caused by this common community-acquired pathogen.

ASHP supports continued educational efforts to promote the rational use of antimicrobials as a strategy for preventing the development of drug-resistant bacteria.

ASHP supports pharmacist leadership and involvement on antimicrobial stewardship teams and the addition of antimicrobial stewardship as a core component of pharmacy services.

ASHP supports the pharmacist in administration of vaccines for all persons at risk for acquiring pneumococcal disease. ASHP encourages the development of pharmacy-based programs to increase pneumonia vaccination rates of at-risk patients. Use of pneumococcal vaccines is a reliable strategy to decrease the morbidity and mortality associated with invasive infections due to *S. pneumoniae*.

Background

S. pneumoniae, also known as pneumococcus, is the most common cause of community-acquired, bacterial, respiratory-tract infections. It is a frequent cause of meningitis, otitis media, and community-acquired pneumonia. Infections caused by *S. pneumoniae* have been associated with increased morbidity and mortality, especially in children under two years of age and elderly adults. Infections caused by *S. pneumoniae* have historically been successfully treated with a variety of antimicrobials, including penicillin, cephalosporins, and erythromycin. In the early 1990s, the first reports of penicillin-nonsusceptible *S. pneumoniae* (PNSP) began to appear in the United States; these strains include both intermediately resistant and resistant strains of *S. pneumoniae*. To date, reports of increasing resistance of *S. pneumoniae* to penicillin and cephalosporins continue. In the late 1990s, reports of increasing resistance to trimethoprim–sulfamethoxazole, macrolides, and fluoroquinolones began to appear. Many isolates developed resistance to multiple classes of drugs and became known as multidrug-resistant *S. pneumoniae* (MDRSP). The increasing prevalence of MDRSP has created a challenge for health care providers in treating this common community-acquired pathogen.

The clinical significance of drug-resistant *S. pneumoniae* on treatment outcomes is unclear. Most of the available data on clinical outcomes are from retrospective reviews, case–control studies, and case reports. There is evidence that meningitis due to PNSP does not respond to treatment with either penicillin or standard doses of cephalosporins, leading to poor clinical outcomes.[1] In contrast, there does not appear to be a significant difference in clinical outcome, primarily mortality, when pneumonia or other nonmeningeal infections due to PNSP are treated with penicillin or cephalosporins. On the contrary, macrolides and fluoroquinolones with poor in vitro activity against *S. pneumoniae* have been associated with poor clinical outcomes and even treatment failures. It is likely that clinical outcomes are dependent on the mechanism and degree of resistance, the site of infection, and the pharmacokinetic and pharmacodynamic characteristics of the antimicrobial agents used in treatment.

Definitions. The Clinical and Laboratory Standards Institute (CLSI), previously known as the National Committee for Clinical Laboratory Standards, revised the definitions of *S. pneumoniae* susceptibility to several antimicrobials in its 2002 standards. Since that time, there have been two sets of interpretive criteria for *S. pneumoniae* isolates for i.v. penicillin and i.v. cephalosporins, depending on whether meningeal disease is present. *S. pneumoniae* resistant to penicillin is defined in terms of the minimum inhibitory concentration (MIC) of penicillin. Strains in a patient with meningeal disease may be distinguished as susceptible (MIC < 0.06 μg/mL) or resistant (MIC ≥ 0.12 μg/mL). Strains in a patient with nonmeningeal disease may be characterized as susceptible (MIC ≤ 2 μg/mL), intermediately resistant (MIC = 4 μg/mL), or highly resistant (MIC ≥ 8 μg/mL).[2] CLSI accounted for the pharmacokinetic and pharmacodynamic factors of a drug in redefining susceptibility breakpoints. The definition of MDRSP is a strain resistant to three or more classes of antibacterials (where those antibacterials may have activity).

Epidemiology. Numerous national and international surveillance studies have been conducted to determine the prevalence of *S. pneumoniae* resistance.[3–7] Although many of these surveillance studies have discontinued the annual collection of data, the Active Bacterial Core Surveillance, known as the ABCs, remains active in the United States.[8] These networks used similar methodologies and specimens: clinical isolates of *S. pneumoniae* from sterile body sites or the respiratory tract, with susceptibility testing in accordance with CLSI standards. Although these studies showed differing resistance rates to the antimicrobials tested, some common trends emerged. The incidence of strains highly resistant to penicillin has surpassed that of intermediately resistant strains. The rates of resistance to non-β-lactams have also increased: the prevalence of macrolide resistance is 20–30%, and trimethoprim–sulfamethoxazole resistance ranges between 24% and 38%. *S. pneumoniae* resistance to levofloxacin is hovering around less than 1%. ABCs personnel evaluate the incidence and susceptibility of invasive *S. pneumoniae* infections in the United States.[8] This surveillance group does not distinguish resistance based on location of disease (i.e., meningeal versus nonmeningeal). For the 2010 isolates, the rates of strains intermediately resistant and highly resistant to penicillin were similar (5.5% and 5.1%, respectively).[8] Resistance to macrolides was 25.7%, which greatly surpassed

DOI 10.37573/9781585287048.111

the intermediately resistant strains (0.5%), leaving 73.8% of strains susceptible. Trimethoprim–sulfamethoxazole susceptibility was slightly higher than the macrolides, at 77.6%, and tetracycline susceptibility was higher at 84.9%. Fluoroquinolone (levofloxacin specifically) resistance remained low at 0.3%, and vancomycin remained universally susceptible (100%). Previously, there were reports from Canada[9] and the Centers for Disease Control and Prevention (CDC)[10] of increasing resistance of *S. pneumoniae* to fluoroquinolones. Most fluoroquinolone-resistant isolates are resistant to other antimicrobials. Fluoroquinolone-resistant organisms are more likely to be found in persons over age 65 years, as this population has the highest usage rate of fluoroquinolones.

Persons at Risk. The greatest risk factor for becoming infected with a drug-resistant strain of *S. pneumoniae* is prior antimicrobial use. Other risk factors include carriage of *S. pneumoniae*, daycare attendance, exposure to children who attend daycare, severe medical comorbidities, immunosuppression, and high alcohol intake.[1] Smoking has been identified as a risk factor for developing invasive *S. pneumoniae* infections.[11] The risk of invasive *S. pneumoniae* infections is 4-fold if the patient is a smoker and 2.5-fold if the patient is exposed to secondhand smoke.[11] The risk of invasive disease declines over time for persons who have stopped smoking.

Mechanisms of Resistance. Resistance of *S. pneumoniae* to β-lactams is due to genetic mutations leading to alterations in three or four of the five high-molecular-weight penicillin-binding proteins (PBPs).[12] The degree of *S. pneumoniae* resistance is dependent on which PBPs are involved and the affinity of the β-lactam agent to the PBP. The differences in expression of these PBPs explain the differences in susceptibility to a variety of β-lactams.

S. pneumoniae resistance to macrolides occurs primarily through two mechanisms: active drug efflux (M phenotype) or ribosomal modification (MLS_{β} phenotype).[13] Active drug efflux confers resistance to all macrolide agents, whereas ribosomal modification confers resistance not only to the macrolides but also to lincosamides (e.g., clindamycin) and streptogramins. Almost 100% of macrolide-resistant *S. pneumoniae* found in the United States is attributable to ribosomal modification via methylation.[13]

Resistance of *S. pneumoniae* to fluoroquinolones is primarily a result of the mutations of the *parC* and *gyrA* genes, though efflux pumps may also play a role.[14] Alterations in the *parC* subunit of topoisomerase IV result in the reduced susceptibility of *S. pneumoniae* to gatifloxacin, levofloxacin, and moxifloxacin. This single-step mutation is difficult to detect clinically because isolates with a *parC* mutation are reported as susceptible using standard laboratory testing. This is concerning because isolates with single-step mutations are the progenitors for fully drug-resistant strains of *S. pneumoniae*, which have additional mutations in the *gyrA* subunit of DNA gyrase.

Establishment of Surveillance Systems

Surveillance systems are an integral component of combating bacterial resistance. The data gathered from surveillance systems can be used for many purposes, including identifying and tracking global outbreaks, identifying new strains and resistance profiles, setting public health policy, heightening awareness of health care providers to local resistance patterns that may affect the routine care of patients, and determining appropriate treatment for infections.

Health systems should develop a mechanism for the local surveillance of bacterial resistance and participate in state and national surveillance programs when available. Ideally, the surveillance system should identify trends in bacterial susceptibility patterns and correlate them with antimicrobial use in both health systems and communities.[15] The clinical microbiology laboratory, pharmacy, infection prevention, and information technology departments play important roles in maintaining an active surveillance system.

At a national level, data acquired through surveillance systems such as those used by CDC and the World Health Organization (WHO) can aid in the research and development of policies and treatment guidelines for pneumococcal disease. State and local surveillance is also essential, as national trends may not reflect trends within specific regions. On a local level, surveillance programs can help raise provider and public awareness of drug-resistant *S. pneumoniae* and direct patient care on an institutional level and potentially on the unit level. Institutional antibiograms should be updated annually, and microbiological data used for diagnosis should be stored in a way that will facilitate resistance surveillance.[16,17] Surveillance data may also be useful for tracking the impact of interventions, such as formulary changes and antimicrobial stewardship interventions, targeting the inappropriate or unnecessary use of antibiotics.

Rational Use of Antimicrobials

There is an abundance of literature showing the relationship between antimicrobial-use patterns and the development of bacterial resistance.[18–21] However, the bulk of this literature thus far has been generated from hospital or institutional studies and has little bearing on PNSP. Since *S. pneumoniae* is primarily a community-acquired pathogen, antimicrobial use in the outpatient setting has the greatest influence on its susceptibility profile. Few studies have shown a relationship between outpatient prescription use or antimicrobial stewardship interventions and *S. pneumoniae* susceptibility patterns. In the United States, Diekema and colleagues[22] found a positive correlation between high usage rates of outpatient β-lactam agents and the decreased penicillin susceptibility of *S. pneumoniae*. No correlation was found between the use of other antimicrobial classes (e.g., macrolides, tetracyclines, fluoroquinolones) and the decreased penicillin susceptibility of *S. pneumoniae*. More recently, Hicks et al.[23] reviewed outpatient antimicrobial prescription data (penicillins, cephalosporins, macrolides, and trimethoprim–sulfamethoxazole) and found a consistent relationship between higher prescription rates and increased rates of *S. pneumoniae* nonsusceptibility to the respective antimicrobial class. This study also found that when comparing sites with high versus low antimicrobial prescription rates for the same class of antimicrobials, macrolide and cephalosporin prescriptions were both associated with serotype 19A, despite yearly decreases in outpatient antimicrobial prescribing rates. Both of these studies were large, retrospective database studies and did not account for patient adherence to antimicrobial regimens. However, these studies demonstrated that antimicrobial use in the community is substantial and plays a role in the development of microbial resistance.

Approximately 50% of prescriptions for antimicrobials are unnecessary or inappropriate.[24] These agents are usually prescribed for treatment of the common cold, upper-respiratory-tract infections, acute rhinosinusitis, and bronchitis, ailments often caused by viruses that do not respond to antibacterials. Recent clinical practice guidelines from the Infectious Diseases Society of America for acute bacterial rhinosinusitis in children and adults acknowledged the difficulty in distinguishing between viral and bacterial etiologies. To decrease inappropriate antibacterial use, the guidelines recommend initiating antibacterials only if the patient has symptoms that are persistent and not improving (duration of ≥10 days), severe (≥3–4 days), or worsening or "double sickening" (subsequent worsening of symptoms or additional symptoms after earlier improvement). Prescribers for patients who do not yet meet the criteria for antibacterial treatment of rhinosinusitis will occasionally give a prescription for antibacterials with the instructions to fill and take the medication if symptoms are persistent. Pharmacists can assist patients in making appropriate decisions on antimicrobial use by counseling patients on the appropriate timing of initiating antibacterials as well as the importance of completing the prescribed treatment course. In addition, empirical antibacterial selection should not include amoxicillin, macrolides, trimethoprim–sulfamethoxazole, or monotherapy with second- or third-generation cephalosporins due to high rates of resistance in *S. pneumoniae*. Finally, a shorter course of antibacterial treatment (5–7 days) is recommended for adults, compared with the 10–14 days recommended for children. Several national organizations,[15,24] CDC, and WHO have advocated antimicrobial stewardship as a mechanism to limit the development of bacterial resistance.[25,26] One of the cornerstones of antimicrobial stewardship is the appropriate use of antimicrobials. Pharmacists should take active roles in antimicrobial stewardship programs, and the infectious diseases pharmacist is considered a core member of the antimicrobial stewardship team.[24,27]

In 1995, CDC launched the National Campaign for Appropriate Antibiotic Use in the Community, which, in 2003, was renamed Get Smart: Know When Antibiotics Work campaign.[28] This campaign was launched in response to growing antimicrobial resistance with respiratory pathogens and aims to reduce the rise of antimicrobial resistance through the promotion of appropriate prescribing, decrease the demand for antimicrobials to treat viral respiratory infections, and increase patient adherence with antimicrobials prescribed for upper-respiratory-tract infections. This program provides a wealth of information for the antimicrobial stewards and the public to help increase awareness at their facilities and includes promotional material for inpatient, outpatient, and long-term-care settings.

Vaccination

Pneumococcal infection has been associated with 2.4 million days of hospitalization and approximately 5000 deaths annually in the United States.[29] As vaccination may contribute to a reduction in these numbers and because hospitalization is an underutilized opportunity for vaccination, the Joint Commission (in collaboration with the Centers for Medicare and Medicaid Services) in January 2012 expanded the pneumococcal vaccination process measure to include all patients regardless of diagnosis. This measure evaluates if, before hospital discharge, patients age 6 years or older were screened for pneumococcal vaccine status and received the pneumococcal vaccine if appropriate. Infections caused by *S. pneumoniae* continue to cause significant morbidity and mortality despite the availability of effective vaccines.

The 23-valent pneumococcal polysaccharide vaccine (PPSV23), the 13-valent pneumococcal conjugate vaccine (PCV13), and the 7-valent pneumococcal conjugate vaccine (PCV7) have been shown to be highly effective in providing protection against the most commonly isolated pneumococcal serotypes that cause human disease, including those serotypes known to be antimicrobial resistant. While the use of these vaccines will not prevent the development of drug-resistant *S. pneumoniae*, they will likely prevent invasive infection caused by a drug-resistant organism. PPSV23 is recommended for all adults age 65 years or older and other adults with certain comorbid conditions.[30]

TABLE 1.
Patients Who Should Receive the 13-Valent Pneumococcal Conjugate Vaccine (PCV13)

Risk Group	Underlying Medical Condition
Immunocompetent persons	Cerebrospinal fluid leak Cochlear implant
Immunocompromised persons	Congenital or acquired immune deficiency Human immunodeficiency virus infection Chronic renal failure Nephrotic syndrome Leukemia Lymphoma Hodgkin disease Generalized malignancy Iatrogenic immunosuppression (diseases requiring treatment with immunosuppressive drugs, including long-term systemic corticosteroids and radiation therapy) Solid organ transplant Multiple myeloma
Persons with functional or anatomical asplenia	Sickle cell disease or other hemaglobinopathy Congenital or acquired asplenia

It may also be given to select groups of high-risk patients over 2 years of age (such as those with cochlear implants) as long as it is administered at least eight weeks after administration of the last dose of PCV7 or PCV13. This PPSV23 vaccine does not produce an adequate immunologic response in children under 2 years old and should not be used in that population. PCV7 was added to the standard recommended pediatric vaccines in October 2000.[31] PCV13 was added in 2010. The PCV series should be given to all children beginning at age 2 months. A single supplemental dose of PCV13 is recommended for all children age 14–59 months and for children age 60–71 months with certain underlying medical conditions who have already received an age-appropriate PCV7 series.[32] The CDC National Immunization Program has established recommendations for pneumococcal vaccine administration.[30,32]

PPSV23 was licensed in the early 1980s and has demonstrated good immunogenicity in both young and older adults; however, an individual will not develop an immune response to all 23 pneumococcal serotypes.[33] The reason for this is unclear. Despite the vaccine's long-standing availability and documented effectiveness, approximately 64% of eligible persons actually receive it.[34] One of the Healthy People 2020 goals is for 90% of eligible adults to receive the

TABLE 2.

Medical Conditions or Other Indications for Administration of 13-Valent Pneumococcal Conjugate Vaccine (PCV13), and Indications for 23-Valent Pneumococcal Polysaccharide Vaccine (PPSV23) Administration and Revaccination for Adults Age 19 Years or Older[24,a]

	PCV13	PPSV23	
Risk Group and Underlying Medical Condition	Recommended	Recommended	Revaccination 5 Years After First Dose
Immunocompetent persons			
Chronic heart disease[b]		X	
Chronic lung disease[c]		X	
Diabetes mellitus		X	
Cerebrospinal fluid leak	X	X	
Cochlear implant	X	X	
Alcoholism		X	
Chronic liver disease, cirrhosis		X	
Cigarette smoking		X	
Persons with functional or anatomic asplenia			
Sickle cell disease or other hemaglobinopathy	X	X	X
Congenital or acquired asplenia	X	X	X
Immunocompromised persons			
Congenital or acquired immunodeficiency[d]	X	X	X
Human immunodeficiency virus infection	X	X	X
Chronic renal failure	X	X	X
Nephrotic syndrome	X	X	X
Leukemia	X	X	X
Lymphoma	X	X	X
Hodgkin disease	X	X	X
Generalized malignancy	X	X	X
Iatrogenic immunosuppression[e]	X	X	X
Solid organ transplant	X	X	X
Multiple myeloma	X	X	X

[a]All adults age ≥65 years should receive a dose of PPSV23, regardless of previous history of vaccination with pneumococcal vaccine.
[b]Including congestive heart failure and cardiomyopathies, excluding hypertension.
[c]Including chronic obstructive pulmonary disease, emphysema, and asthma.
[d]Includes B- (humoral) or T-lymphocyte deficiency, complement deficiencies (particularly C1, C2, C3, and C4 deficiencies), and phagocytic disorders (excluding chronic granulomatous disease).
[e]Diseases requiring treatment with immunosuppressive drugs, including long-term systemic corticosteroids and radiation therapy.

pneumococcal vaccine.[35] This is an excellent opportunity for pharmacists to improve the vaccination rate of older adult patients and help promote national health care goals.

Revaccination with PPSV23 is recommended for adults over age 65 years if the first dose was administered when they were under 65 years old at the time of vaccination and at least 5 years has elapsed since the first dose.[30] In addition, persons younger than 65 years with immunocompromising conditions may receive a one-time revaccination if 5 years has elapsed since the first dose of PPSV23. Revaccination with PPSV23 results in a somewhat blunted immune response and is associated with increased injection-site reactions.[33]

PCV7 for children has been available since February 2000. Use of this vaccine has been shown to decrease the carriage rate of *S. pneumoniae* and the incidence of invasive pneumococcal disease, acute otitis media, and pneumonia in vaccinated populations.[36,37] The rate of vaccine-specific serotype *S. pneumoniae* carriage in vaccinated children remains below the rate for nonvaccinated children over prolonged periods of time. Widespread vaccination of children with PCV7 has shown a "herd effect" in decreasing the carriage rate of *S. pneumoniae* in children, who are an important vector for the transmission of *S. pneumoniae* to other children and adults.[36] This is similar to what was seen with widespread use of the *Haemophilus influenzae* type B vaccine and the marked decrease in *H. influenzae*-related infections.

PCV13 for children and adults has been available since February 2010 and has taken the place of the discontinued PCV7. All children age 2–59 months should have routine immunization with PCV13.[32] CDC has established routine and catch-up schedules for vaccination. Recommendations by the CDC Advisory Committee on Immunization Practices for the use of PCV13 in adults were established in 2012.[30] Patients who have immunocompromising conditions should receive PCV13 in addition to PPSV23 (**Tables 1 and 2**). Screening and vaccination should occur in all appropriate adult patients. Timing of PCV13 and PPSV23 administration is important to ensure maximal immune response. If the person has never received a dose of PCV13 or PPSV23, he or she should receive a dose of PCV13 followed by a dose of PPSV23 at least eight weeks later. If the patient has received one or more doses of PPSV23, the patient should receive one dose of PCV13 at least one year after the last dose of PPSV23.

Health care institutions should develop robust programs to increase pneumococcal vaccination rates as pneumococcal disease continues to contribute to a significant amount of morbidity and mortaility in the United States. More than 65% of patients with severe pneumococcal disease have been hospitalized in the preceding—three to five years, but few have received vaccine.[34] Most people who succumb to preventable infections have visited a health care provider in the preceding year but were not vaccinated.[38–42] Clinicians should ensure that patients receive proper immunizations,[43,44] and pharmacists can promote vaccination efforts by serving as educators, facilitators, and vaccinators. Currently, all 50 states allow pharmacists to administer vaccines, and 49 states allow pharmacists to administer pneumococcal vaccines.[45] Variability exists among the states regarding patient age limitations and pharmacist-administered vaccines, with 13 states authorizing pharmacists to vaccinate patients of any age.[46] Although vaccinations are typically administered in the ambulatory care setting, clinicians must also seize opportunities to vaccinate hospitalized patients (**Figure 1**). Pharmacists have demonstrated that they can increase the number of persons receiving needed vaccines in both inpatient and ambulatory care settings.[47]

Summary

The incidence of MDRSP continues to increase, causing significant morbidity and mortality. Health care providers should seize the opportunity to promote the judicious use of antimicrobials and vaccinate patients with the pneumococcal vaccines as a means to lessen this significant health problem. Pharmacists are poised to play a key role in patient care by assessing for the need and administering vaccines in compliance with the current guidelines. A pharmacist should have a key role on the antimicrobial stewardship team.

References

1. Pallares R, Fenoll A, Liñares J, for the Spanish Pneumococcal Infection Study Network. The epidemiology of antibiotic resistance in *Streptococcus pneumoniae* and the clinical relevance of resistance to cephalosporins, macrolides and fluoroquinolones. *Int J Antimicrob Agents.* 2003; 22(suppl 1):S15–24.
2. Performance standards for antimicrobial susceptibility testing; 23rd informational supplement. Wayne, PA: Clinical and Laboratory Standards Institute; 2013.
3. Centers for Disease Control and Prevention. ABCs report: *Streptococcus pneumoniae,* 2001. www.cdc.gov/abcs/reports-findings/survreports/spneu01.html (accessed 2013 Nov 20).
4. Jacobs MR, Felmingham D, Appelbaum PC, et al. The Alexander Project 1998–2000: susceptibility of pathogens isolated from community-acquired respiratory tract infection to commonly used antimicrobial agents. *J Antimicrob Chemother.* 2003; 52:229–46.
5. Doern G, Rybak MJ. Activity of telithromycin against *Streptococcus pneumoniae* resistant to penicillin, macrolides and fluoroquinolones isolated from respiratory tract infections: PROTEK US year 2 (2001–2002). Presented at 43rd Annual Interscience Conference on Antimicrobial Agents and Chemotherapy. Chicago, IL; 2003 Sep.
6. Doern GV, Heilmann KP, Huynh HK, et al. Antimicrobial resistance among clinical isolates of *Streptococcus pneumoniae* in the United Stated during 1999–2000, including a comparison of resistance rates since 1994–1995. *Antimicrob Agents Chemother.* 2001; 45:1721–9.
7. Karlowsky JA, Thornsberry C, Jones ME, et al. Factors associated with relative rates of antimicrobial resistance among *Streptococcus pneumoniae* in the United States: results from the TRUST surveillance program (1998–2002). *Clin Infect Dis.* 2003; 36:963–70.
8. Centers for Disease Control and Prevention. ABCs report: *Streptococcus pneumoniae,* 2010. www.cdc.gov/abcs/reports-findings/survreports/spneu10.html (accessed 2013 Nov 20).

FIGURE 1. Example pneumococcal vaccine administration pathway with notification for adult patients. PCV13 = 13-valent pneumococcal conjugate vaccine, PPSV23 = 23-valent pneumococcal polysaccharide vaccine, CDC = Centers for Disease Control and Prevention.

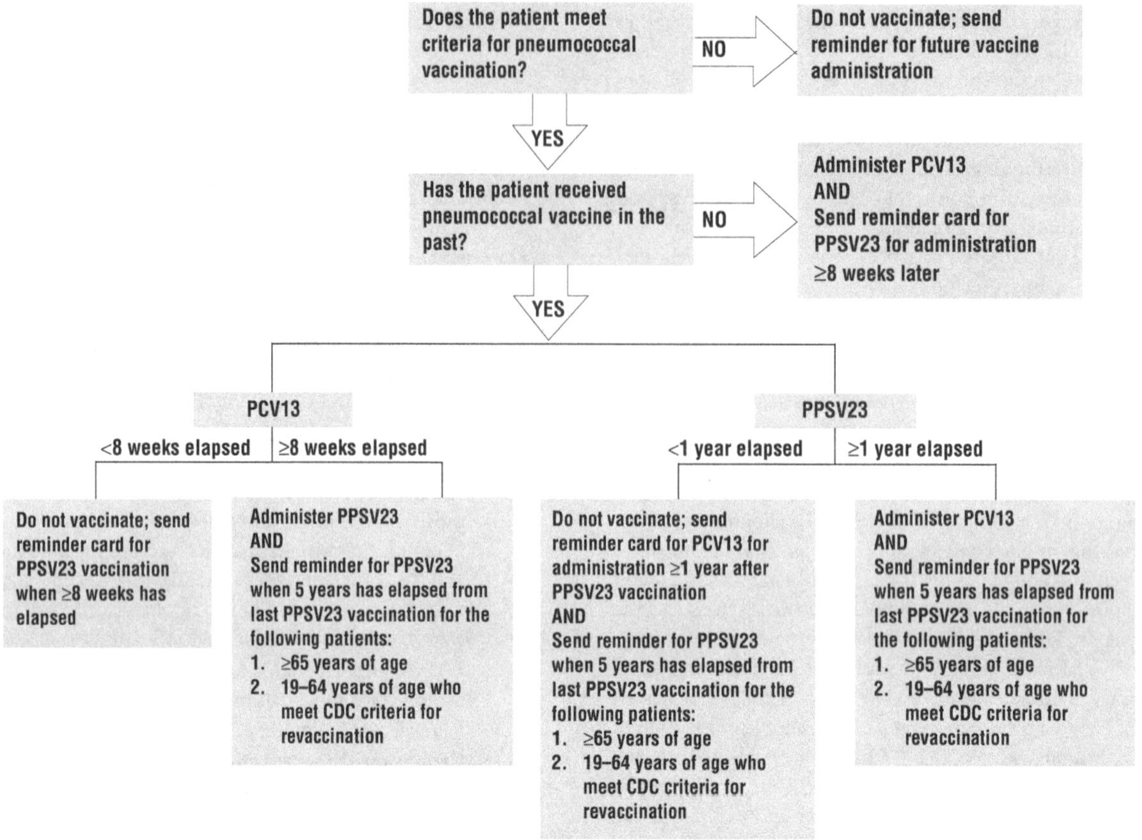

9. Chen DK, McGeer A, de Azavedo JC, et al. Decreased susceptibility of *Streptococcus pneumoniae* to fluoroquinolones in Canada. *N Engl J Med.* 1999; 341:233–9.
10. Centers for Disease Control and Prevention. Resistance of *Streptococcus pneumoniae* to fluoroquinolones—United States, 1995–1999. *MMWR.* 2001; 50:800–4.
11. Nuorti JP, Butler JC, Farley MM, et al. Cigarette smoking and invasive pneumococcal disease. *N Engl J Med.* 2000; 342:681–9.
12. Appelbaum PC. Resistance among *Streptococcus pneumoniae*: implications for drug selection. *Clin Infect Dis.* 2002; 34:1613–20.
13. Lynch JP, Martinez FJ. Clinical relevance of macrolide-resistant *Streptococcus pneumoniae* for community-acquired pneumonia. *Clin Infect Dis.* 2002; 34(suppl 1):S27–46.
14. Hooper DC. Fluoroquinolone resistance among gram-positive cocci. *Lancet Infect Dis.* 2002; 2:530–8.
15. Shales DM, Gerding DN, John JF. et al. Society for Healthcare Epidemiology of America and Infectious Diseases Society of America Joint Committee on Prevention of Antimicrobial Resistance: guidelines for the prevention of antimicrobial resistance in hospitals. *Clin Infect Dis.* 1997; 25:584–99.
16. Analysis and presentation of cumulative antimicrobial susceptibility test data; approved guideline, third edition. CLSI document M39-A3. Wayne, PA: Clinical and Laboratory Standards Institute; 2009.
17. World Health Organization. Surveillance standards for antimicrobial resistance. http://whqlibdoc.who.int/hq/2002/WHO_CDS_CSR_DRS_2001.5.pdf (accessed 2013 Nov 20).
18. Davies J, Davies D. Origins and evolution of antibiotic resistance. *Microbiol Mol Biol Rev.* 2010; 74:417–33.
19. Freire-Moran L, Aronsson B, Manz C, et al. Critical shortage of new antibiotics in development against multidrug-resistant bacteria-Time to react is now. *Drug Resist Updat.* 2011; 14:118–24.
20. Peleg AY, Hooper DC. Hospital-acquired infections due to gram-negative bacteria. *N Engl J Med.* 2010; 362:1804–13.
21. Meyer E, Schwab F, Schroeren-Boersch B, et al. Dramatic increase of third-generation cephalosporin-resistant E. coli in German intensive care units: secular trends in antibiotic drug use and bacterial resistance, 2001 to 2008. *Crit Care.* 2010; 14:R113.
22. Diekema DJ, Brueggemann AB, Doern GV. Antimicrobial-drug use and changes in resistance in *Streptococcus pneumoniae. Emerg Infect Dis.* 2000; 6:552–6.
23. Hicks LA, Chien YW, Taylor TH Jr, et al. Outpatient antibiotic prescribing and nonsusceptible *Streptococcus pneumoniae* in the United States, 1996–2003. *Clin Infect Dis.* 2011; 53:631–9.

24. Dellit TH, Owens RC, McGowan JE Jr, et al. Infectious Diseases Society of America and the Society for Healthcare Epidemiology of America guidelines for developing an institutional program to enhance antimicrobial stewardship. *Clin Infect Dis.* 2007; 44:159–77.
25. Centers for Disease Control and Prevention. Public health action plan to combat antimicrobial resistance. www.cdc.gov/drugresistance/actionplan/introduction_overview.html (accessed 2014 Jan 23).
26. Leung E, Weil DE, Raviglione M, et al. The WHO policy package to combat antimicrobial resistance. *Bull World Health Organ.* 2011; 89:390–2.
27. ASHP statement on the pharmacist's role in antimicrobial stewardship and infection prevention and control. *Am J Health-Syst Pharm.* 2010; 67:575–7.
28. Centers for Disease Control and Prevention. About the Get Smart campaign. www.cdc.gov/getsmart/campaign-materials/about-campaign.html (accessed 2013 Nov 20).
29. Specifications manual for national hospital inpatient quality measures discharges 07-01-12 (3Q12) through 12-31-12 (4Q12). Oakbrook Terrace, IL: Joint Commission; 2011.
30. Centers for Disease Control and Prevention. Recommended adult immunization schedule—United States, 2013. www.cdc.gov/vaccines/schedules/downloads/adult/adult-schedule.pdf (accessed 2013 Nov 20).
31. Centers for Disease Control and Prevention. Preventing pneumococcal disease among infants and young children: recommendations of the Advisory Committee on Immunization Practices (ACIP). *MMWR.* 2000; 49(RR-9):1–35.
32. Centers for Disease Control and Prevention. Birth—18 years and "catch-up" immunization schedules; Uniteed States, 2013. www.cdc.gov/vaccines/schedules/hcp/child-adolescent.html (accessed 2013 Nov 21).
33. Artz AS, Ershler WB, Longo DL. Pneumococcal vaccination and revaccination of older adults. *Clin Microbiol Rev.* 2003; 16:308–18.
34. Centers for Disease Control and Prevention. Epidemiology and prevention of vaccine-preventable diseases. The pink book: course textbook. www.cdc.gov/vaccines/pubs/pinkbook/pneumo.html#vaccines (accessed 2013 Nov 20).
35. Department of Health and Human Services. Healthy People 2020. www.healthypeople.gov (accessed 2012 Sep 27).
36. Dagan R, Fraser D. Conjugate pneumococcal vaccine and antibiotic-resistant *Streptococcus pneumoniae*: herd immunity and reduction of otitis morbidity. *Pediatr Infect Dis J.* 2000; 19(suppl):S79–88.
37. Whitney CG, Farley MM, Hadler J, et al. Decline in invasive pneumococcal disease after the introduction of protein-polysaccharide conjugate vaccine. *N Engl J Med.* 2003; 348:1737–46.
38. Williams WW, Hickson MA, Kane MA, et al. Immunization policies and vaccine coverage among adults. The risk for missed opportunites. *Ann Intern Med.* 1988; 108:616–25.
39. Fedson DS, Hickson MA, Kane MA, et al. Hospital-based pneumococcal immunization. Epidemiologic rationale from the Shenandoah study. *JAMA.* 1990; 264:1117–22.
40. Fedson DS. Influenza and pneumococcal immunization strategies for physicians. *Chest.* 1987; 91:436–43.
41. Magnussen CR, Valenti WM, Mushlin AI. Pneumococcal vaccine strategy. Feasibility of a vaccination program directed at hospitalized and ambulatory patients. *Arch Intern Med.* 1984; 144:1755–7.
42. Vondracek TG, Pham TP, Huycke MM. A hospital-based pharmacy interventions program for pneumococcal vaccination. *Arch Intern Med.* 1998; 158:1543–7.
43. American Society of Health-System Pharmacists. ASHP guidelines on the pharmacist's role in immunization. *Am J Health-Syst Pharm.* 2003; 60:1371–7.
44. Grabenstein JD, Bonasso J. Health-system pharmacists' role in immunizing adults against pneumococcal disease and influenza. *Am J Health-Syst Pharm.* 1999; 56(suppl 2):S2–24.
45. Immunization Action Coalition. States authorizing pharmacists to vaccinate. www.immunize.org/laws/pharm.asp (accessed 2012 Dec 27).
46. American Pharmacists Association. Pharmacist administered vaccines. www.pharmacist.com/sites/default/files/files/PharmacistIMZAuthority_June18_2012%20%5BRead-Only%5D.pdf (accessed 2012 Dec 27).
47. Noped JC, Schomberg R. Implementing an inpatient pharmacy-based pneumococcal vaccination program. *Am J Health-Syst Pharm.* 2001; 58:1852–5.

Kimberly A. Couch, Pharm.D., M.A., FIDSA, FASHP, is President, Infectious Diseases Pharmacy Associates, Stevensville, MD, and Clinical Pharmacist, Complete Rx, Seaford, DE. Teresa Geide, Pharm.D., BCPS, CGP, is Clinical Pharmacy Specialist, Infectious Diseases, Orlando Veterans Affairs Medical Center, Orlando, FL.

Developed through the ASHP Council on Therapeutics and approved by the ASHP Board of Directors on August 2, 2013.

The following individuals are acknowledged for reviewing draft versions of this statement: Arthur Chaput; Steven Dzierba, Pharm.D., M.S., FASHP; Kathleen M. Gura, Pharm.D., BCNSP, FASHP, FPPAG; Mojdeh Heavner, Pharm.D., BCPS; Jody Jacobson Wedret, B.S.Pharm., FASHP, FCSHP; Kristi Kuper, Pharm.D., BCPS; Fred Meister, Pharm.D., FASHP; Robert J. Moura, B.S.Pharm., M.S.; Michael Postelnick, B.S.Pharm, BCPS-AQ Infectious Diseases; and Michael Powell, B.S.P., M.S.P., FASHP.

The authors have declared no potential conflicts of interest.

This document supersedes the ASHP therapeutic position statement for identifying and preventing pneumococcal resistance approved by the ASHP Board of Directors on April 15, 2004.

Copyright © 2014, American Society of Health-System Pharmacists, Inc. All rights reserved. Contact ASHP for reprint and permissions requests. This content may not be used for commercial purposes without the express written consent of ASHP.

The bibliographic citation for this document is as follows: American Society of Health-System Pharmacists. ASHP therapeutic position statement on strategies for identifying and preventing pneumococcal resistance. *Am J Health-Syst Pharm.* 2014; 71:417–24.

ASHP Therapeutic Position Statement on the Use of Antipsychotic Medications in the Treatment of Adults with Schizophrenia and Schizoaffective Disorder

Position

The American Society of Health-System Pharmacists (ASHP) recognizes that schizophrenia and schizoaffective disorder are serious mental illnesses that can significantly affect an individual's perceptual, behavioral, affective, and cognitive functions. These conditions are usually chronic and recurrent, necessitating continuous treatment over the patient's lifetime. Individuals with these disorders frequently require lengthy and expensive hospitalizations, as well as a variety of ongoing rehabilitative and supportive services that can impose a significant burden on society.[1] In addition, high rates of suicidal behavior and completed suicides have been observed in patients with schizophrenia or schizoaffective disorder.[2] The management of the psychotic symptoms associated with these disorders typically requires long-term treatment with antipsychotic medications, the use of adjunctive pharmacologic treatments, and ongoing psychosocial and supportive interventions to reduce morbidity and mortality.

For the pharmacologic management of psychosis associated with schizophrenia and schizoaffective disorder, ASHP encourages health professionals to select either a first-generation antipsychotic agent (FGA) or a second-generation antipsychotic (SGA) based upon the adverse effect profile of the drug and the individual characteristics of the patient. Antipsychotics, both first- and second-generation agents, have similar efficacy and are the treatment of choice in individuals with schizophrenia or schizoaffective disorder with psychosis.

All antipsychotics have limitations and, in the usual dosage range doses, FGAs are generally equivalent in tolerability to SGAs.[3] Patients have different reasons for not tolerating a particular agent, and antipsychotic selection should be individualized to the patient. Upon selection of an effective treatment, clinicians must monitor therapy on an ongoing basis to ensure tolerability and adherence in order to optimize treatment outcomes.

The goal of this therapeutic position statement (TPS) is to provide a summary of FGAs and SGAs and provide recommendations for the clinician to consider when selecting an appropriate agent to treat psychosis in the adult patient with schizophrenia and schizoaffective disorder.

Background

Schizophrenia and schizoaffective disorder are serious, chronic mental illnesses that affect perceptual, behavioral, affective, and cognitive functioning. Individuals with schizophrenia generally exhibit a mixture of positive, negative, and cognitive symptoms with varying intensity throughout the course of the illness The DSM-5 (*Diagnostic and Statistical Manual of Mental Health Disorders, Fifth Edition*) diagnostic criteria for schizophrenia states that at least 2 out of 5 symptoms must be present for at least 1 month, and at least one of those one of those symptoms must be delusions, hallucinations, or disorganized speech (**Table 1**).[4] The symptoms of schizophrenia must be continuous for at least 6 months. Schizoaffective disorder differs from schizophrenia in that delusions or hallucinations only have to occur for a minimum of 2 weeks without signs of a mood disturbance sometime during the course of the illness. Symptoms of mania or depression are present during the majority of the longitudinal course of the illness.[4] Unlike in schizophrenia, social and occupational dysfunction need not occur for diagnosis of schizoaffective disorder according to DSM-5 criteria (Table 1).[4] The worldwide lifetime prevalence of schizophrenia and schizoaffective disorder is about 1.2%.[5,6] Schizophrenia and schizoaffective disorders have been studied together in many clinical trials and will be considered together for the purpose of this document.

First episode psychosis (FEP) refers to the first acute episode of psychosis following a prodromal period. The prodromal period is defined as a period of time in which an individual begins to experience behavioral changes (eg, anxiety, sleep disturbances, social withdrawal, and irritability, a reduction in concentration and motivation and/or suspiciousness) prior to the onset of the first episode of psychosis. As many as 100,000 teens and young adults in the United States experience FEP each year, with the peak onset occurring between 15 and 25 years of age.[7] It is important to recognize and treat FEP because the duration of untreated psychosis, defined as the time between the first psychotic symptoms and initiation of antipsychotic treatment, plays a major role in clinical patient outcomes.[8] The longer an individual goes untreated, the worse their long-term behavioral and cognitive symptoms, morbidity and mortality, quality of life, and functional capacity.[8] Patients with FEP tend to present late for medical attention; on average, the duration between the first symptoms and adequate treatment is 7 to 10 years.[8] In addition, as many as 80% of individuals with FEP will experience a relapse of symptoms requiring inpatient care and adding to the total cost of care.[9] The highest risk of suicide in individuals with psychosis occurs during the first 5 years of the illness, deemed the critical period.[10] A recent study assessed the 12-month mortality for patients with FEP as being 24 times higher than the general US population.[11]

Childhood-onset schizophrenia resembles the essential features seen in schizophrenia. Prodromal symptoms of psychosis occurring in children and adolescents (eg, apathy, social withdrawal) may be present before the first psychotic break, but the full symptoms of these disorders are rare in this population. In children, delusions and auditory and visual hallucinations are common but may be less sophisticated than those symptoms seen in adults. It is important to differentiate between childhood-onset schizophrenia and other diagnoses seen in children, such as autism spectrum disorder and attention deficit hyperactivity disorder, post-traumatic stress disorder, as well as normal fantasy play. Childhood-onset schizophrenia includes significant negative symptoms and typically has a poor outcome, including

DOI 10.37573/9781585287048.112

TABLE 1.
DSM-5 Criteria for Schizophrenia and Schizoaffective Disorder[4]

Schizophrenia Criteria	Schizoaffective Disorder Criteria
A. Two (or more) of the following symptoms, each present for the greater part of a one- month period (or less if treated successfully). At least one of these must be 1, 2, or 3 below. 1. Delusions 2. Hallucinations 3. Disorganized speech (eg, frequent derailment or incoherence). 4. Grossly disorganized or catatonic behavior 5. Negative symptoms (ie, diminished emotional expression or avolition) B. Level of function in a major area (personal or occupational functioning) must be less than prior to the onset of symptoms. C. There must be continuous signs of the illness for at least 6 months. During this 6- month time frame there must be a least 1 month of symptoms from A. above, and may include prodromal, residual or negative symptoms. D. Schizoaffective, depressive or bipolar disorder has been ruled out. E. The disturbance is not due to the effects of a substance (medication or drug of abuse) or a medical condition. F. If there is a history of autism spectrum or a communication disorder or childhood, a diagnosis of schizophrenia is only made if hallucinations or delusions are prominent.	A. An uninterrupted period of illness during which there is a major mood episode (major depressive or manic) concurrent with Criterion A of schizophrenia. (Note: The major depressive episode must include Criterion A1: Depressed mood.) B. Delusions or hallucinations for 2 or more weeks in the absence of a major mood episode (depressive or manic) during the lifetime duration of the illness. C. Symptoms that meet criteria for a major mood episode are present for the majority of the total duration of the active as well as the residual portions of the illness. D. The disturbance is not the result of a substance (medication or drug of abuse) or a medical condition. E. The following specifiers are based on the presentation of the mood episode: • Bipolar type: includes episodes of mania and sometimes depression • Depressive type: only major depressive episodes

significant, progressive impairment in the social, occupational, and academic functioning of affected individuals.[12]

Late-onset schizophrenia, occurring after 40 years of age, may have an otherwise similar course to typical adult-onset schizophrenia. Often individuals with late-onset illness will maintain affect and social functioning; often they will be or have been married during their life. Often the symptoms of psychosis, such as hallucinations and delusions, may not be as severe as they appear in those with an earlier onset of the illness.[13] Very late onset of schizophrenia is diagnosed if the first appearance of the illness occurs after the age of 65. This occurs more frequently in women and in those with general medical conditions like dementia.[13]

Pathophysiology of Schizophrenia

The effectiveness of FGAs, whose primary mechanism of action is blockade of dopamine in the brain, led to the initial hypothesis regarding dopamine's role in schizophrenia.[14] While it is apparent that increased dopamine in the mesolimbic pathway is responsible for the positive symptoms of schizophrenia, it is now understood that psychosis frequently involves numerous neurochemical abnormalities.[14,15] Psychosis has been observed in individuals with idiopathic and drug-induced hypofunction of the glutamate system.[16,17] In addition, the high rate of nicotine dependence in individuals with schizophrenia—up to 88% in one study—led to the identification of alpha 7 nicotinic acetylcholine-receptor abnormalities in the pathophysiology of schizophrenia.[18,19]

Pharmacologic Characteristics of Antipsychotic Drugs

The FGAs primarily exert their therapeutic effects by antagonizing postsynaptic dopamine2 receptors in the cortical and nigrostriatal pathway. However, these drugs are not selective in their activity. Each of the FGAs has effects on other receptors to varying degrees, including serotonin 2A, alpha 1, muscarinic, and histaminic receptors. The level of receptor binding correlates to the specific antipsychotic adverse effect profile. Low potency agents, dosed in the 100s of milligrams (eg, chlorpromazine, thioridazine), have a greater propensity to causing orthostatic hypotension, QT interval prolongation, anticholinergic effects, and sedation. High potency agents, dosed in the 10's of milligrams (eg, haloperidol, fluphenazine, loxapine, perphenazine, thiothixene, trifluoperazine), are more likely to cause extrapyramidal side effects (eg, dystonias, parkinsonism, akathisia) and tardive dyskinesia (**Table 2**).[20] FGAs are also associated with hematologic (eg, agranulocytosis), endocrine (eg, prolactin elevation, menstrual irregularities, sexual dysfunction), dermatologic (eg, blue-gray skin coloration, photosensitivity, allergic reactions) and ophthalmologic (eg, pigmentary retinopathy, corneal and lenticular deposits leading to cataracts, and rare cases of photophobia, and difficulty with visual accommodation). Other adverse effects include seizures, difficulty regulating body temperature and increased incidence of falls.[20]

The SGAs share the common pharmacologic action of dual serotonin-dopamine antagonism (**Table 3**). Aripiprazole, brexpiprazole and cariprazine differ slightly in that they function as partial agonists at dopamine receptors, reducing dopamine activity in the mesolimbic pathway.[21,22] In addition to antagonism at serotonin 2A and D2 receptors, SGAs interact with a multitude of other receptors including muscarinic, histaminic and alpha adrenergic receptors. Like FGAs some of the SGAs block D2 in the hypothalamic pituitary region causing hyperprolactinemia. Other SGAs block dopamine in the nigrostriatal area causing extrapyramidal motor effects. Some of the SGAs may alter insulin resistance and increase fasting cholesterol levels secondary to actions at receptors that are not currently well understood. None of

TABLE 2.
First-Generation Antipsychotics Currently Available in the United States

Drug (Trade Name)	Usual Therapeutic Doses	Year Approved
Chlorpromazine (Thorazine)	300–1,000 mg (maximum, 1,000 mg/day)	1953
Fluphenazine (Prolixin)	5–20 mg (maximum, 40 mg/day)	1959
Haloperidol (Haldol)	2–20 mg (maximum, 100 mg/day)	1967
Loxapine (Loxitane/Adasuve)	50–150 mg (maximum, 250 mg/day or 10 mg/day [inhalation])	1975
Perphenazine (Trilafon)	16–64 mg (maximum, 64 mg/day)	1957
Pimozide (Orap)	2–10 mg (maximum, 10 mg/day)	1985
Thioridazine (Mellaril)	100–800 mg (maximum, 800 mg/day)	1958
Thiothixene (Navane)	4–50 mg (maximum, 60 mg)	1967
Trifluoperazine (Stelazine)	5–40 mg (maximum, 40 mg/day)	1959

TABLE 3.
Second-Generation Antipsychotics Currently Available in the United States

Drug (Trade Name)	Usual Therapeutic Doses	Year Approved
Aripiprazole (Abilify)	15–30 mg/day	2002
Asenapine (Saphris)	10–20 mg/day	2009
Brexpiprazole (Rexulti)	2–4 mg/day	2015
Cariprazine (Vraylar)	1.5–6 mg/day	2015
Clozapine (Clozaril)	100–800 mg/day (maximum 900 mg)	1989
Iloperidone (Fanapt)	6–24 mg/day	2009
Lurasidone (Latuda)	40–120 mg/day	2010
Olanzapine (Zyprexa)	10–20 mg/day	1996
Paliperidone (Invega)	3–12 mg/day	2006
Quetiapine (Seroquel)	300–800 mg/day	1997
Risperidone (Risperdal)	2–8 mg/day	1993
Ziprasidone (Geodon)	80–160 mg/day	2001

the SGAs have identical neurotransmitter binding profiles, which gives each of them a unique clinical profile.

Efficacy for Negative Symptoms

Negative symptoms are considered to be the core deficit in schizophrenia.[23] Primary negative symptoms include flattened or blunted affect, avolition, asociality, amotivation, alogia and apathy.[24] Individuals diagnosed with schizophrenia typically experience a prodromal period, characterized by negative symptoms, in their late teens to mid-twenties. The prodromal period precedes the onset of psychotic or positive symptoms. Based upon DSM-5 criteria, positive symptoms such as delusions and hallucinations have to last for at least 1 month (untreated), but often last for 3 to 6 months prior to resolution.[4,24] After the resolution of positive symptoms the period of chronicity is called residual schizophrenia. This period is marked by continued negative symptoms which are a source of poor outcomes for many individuals.[24,25] Because of the difficulty in treating a deficit syndrome, greater effort has been given to treating positive symptoms of schizophrenia with antipsychotics, but it has been suggested that antipsychotics aggravate negative symptoms.[26,27] Some references divide negative symptoms into primary negative symptoms (disease related) and secondary negative symptoms (due to side effects of medications, substance abuse, and environmental issues).[28] For the purposes of this TPS, we will focus on primary negative symptoms.

Negative symptoms have been difficult to treat. Antidepressants, stimulants and antipsychotics are among the treatment strategies that have been studied for negative symptoms.[29] There was initial excitement with the use of SGAs because many of them appeared to demonstrate efficacy for both positive and negative symptoms in initial registration studies.[30] Clozapine, olanzapine, quetiapine, risperidone, asenapine, paliperidone and lurasidone all demonstrated effectiveness for negative symptoms in these studies.[25] Unfortunately, these studies suffered from small sample sizes, inconsistent diagnoses or stage of illness, and length of trial (typically 6-12 weeks).[25] Improvement of negative symptoms was measured during the active phase of the illness, and it is difficult to differentiate what improvements are from changes in the positive symptoms versus the negative symptoms.[25] Larger studies, such as the CUtLASS trial, did not show a significant difference between FGAs and SGAs in the treatment of negative symptoms.[3] The 2009 Patient Outcomes Research

Team (PORT) guidelines state that "the level of evidence is currently insufficient to support a treatment recommendation for any pharmacological treatment of negative symptoms in schizophrenia."[31]

Efficacy for Positive Symptoms

Positive symptoms are typically seen during exacerbations of schizophrenia. Positive symptoms include hallucinations, delusions, thought disorders, and disorganized speech. Finding medications to treat these symptoms has led positive symptoms to be the primary focus in the treatment of schizophrenia.[10] First- and second-generation antipsychotic agents have been demonstrated to be equally effective in the treatment of positive symptoms of schizophrenia when used in therapeutic doses.[3]

Neurocognitive Effects

Impaired cognitive functioning has long been observed as a core feature of schizophrenia. Longitudinal studies have shown that patients with schizophrenia have progressive brain tissue loss after onset of illness. These impairments are relatively stable over the natural course of the illness, regardless of the frequency of acute exacerbations of psychotic symptoms.[32] Furthermore, cognitive impairment may have a greater impact on psychosocial functioning than any other feature of schizophrenia.[33,34]

Many domains of cognition, including attention, short-term memory, and executive function, are affected by schizophrenia.[35] Treatment with antipsychotic drugs, while relieving positive symptoms of psychosis, do little to improve cognitive functioning. The concomitant use of anticholinergic drugs intended to prevent or treat EPS that accompany antipsychotic therapy may actually worsen some cognitive functions.[36]

Early studies of SGAs suggested that they might have a role in the treatment of cognition and psychosocial function in schizophrenia.[37–41] More recent studies have not established a significant effect of SGAs over FGAs on cognition, and there is a suggestion on review of previous studies that differences in results may be due to practice or placebo effect.[42–57]

First-Episode Psychosis

Patients with FEP are more responsive to treatment than patients with multiple psychotic episodes, but can also be more sensitive to the side effects of antipsychotics.[58] The majority of patients with FEP are responsive to treatment with more than 70% achieving full remission of signs and symptoms of psychosis within 3 to 4 months, and 83% achieving stable remission by the end of 1 year.[1,59]

Studies have shown that patients with FEP often respond well to low-dose antipsychotic medication.[58–60] Selection of an antipsychotic should be based upon patient preference, side effect profile, route of administration, presence of co-morbid medical conditions, and potential interactions with other prescribed medications, and cost. Patients with FEP initiated on an antipsychotic should be monitored closely to evaluate treatment response.[60] Adherence to treatment is crucial and can minimize the emotional distress and disruption of the patient's life.[60] Patients with a first episode of psychosis should continue treatment for at least 12 months after remission.[31,58] As many as 83% of patients with FEP will experience a relapse in symptoms within 5 years.[61]

Multi-Episode Schizophrenia

Multi-episode schizophrenia or relapse is part of the natural continuum of psychotic illness. The most common causes of relapse include stress, nonadherence, and substance use.[58] It is important to recognize that it is not uncommon to have a relapse in psychotic symptoms even while maintaining adherence.[58] The average rate of relapse is between 15% and 37% after 1 year of maintenance antipsychotic therapy, while the rate of relapse for patients on placebo is between 60% and 80%.[31,58,62–63]

When relapse occurs it is important to determine the reasons behind it, and to re-establish treatment as quickly as possible with the same or another medication.[58] The antipsychotic chosen should be based on the patient's previous response, side effects, route of administration, co-morbid medical conditions, potential drug interactions and the patient's preference.[58] Once an antipsychotic agent has been chosen, the dose should be initiated at an appropriate starting dose and titrated to a therapeutic dose. Titrating the dose too rapidly or using a dose above the therapeutic range may be associated with nonadherence and intolerance. Improvement in symptoms may take between 6 to 12 weeks.[58] If no symptom improvement is seen in 2 weeks at therapeutic doses, consider switching medications.[58] If a partial response is seen within 12 weeks, consider increasing the dose to the highest therapeutic dose as long as the patient is not experiencing side effects.[58] If the patient continues to experience only a partial response to this dose, consider augmentation with a different agent or switching to another antipsychotic agent. While evidence supporting augmentation is based upon limited and sometimes mixed results, it may benefit individuals who have a partial response versus initiating a new antipsychotic. Lifetime treatment with the lowest effective dose of an antipsychotic is recommended in individuals who have experienced multiple relapses.[58]

Treatment-Resistant Schizophrenia

Treatment-resistant schizophrenia is defined as inadequate improvement in target symptoms despite treatment with 2 or more antipsychotics (at least 1 of those should be a SGA) from differing chemical classes given at therapeutic doses for a minimum of 2 to 8 weeks per agent.[1,58,64–66]

A trial of clozapine is generally warranted for patients who demonstrate a suboptimal response to 2 or more trials with first- and second-line antipsychotic agents, and it is considered to be the third-line agent for all guidelines.[58] In addition, the adjunctive use of antidepressants, mood stabilizers, or anxiolytics may be beneficial in select patients.[58] The combined use of more than 1 antipsychotic drug is a controversial and costly practice.[67] Very little published evidence supports the use of multiple oral antipsychotics, except when attempting to transition a patient from one agent to another.[68] In the case of non-response or inability to tolerate clozapine other treatment strategies include treatment with other SGAs, augmentation, antipsychotic combinations, and electroconvulsive therapy, although there is limited evidence for these strategies.[69]

Clozapine, the first SGA introduced in the United States, has an established level of efficacy for use in individuals with psychosis resistant to treatment with other antipsychotics. Kane et al conducted the landmark trial that demonstrated the superior efficacy of clozapine in individuals with treatment resistant psychosis.[65] This trial enrolled only patients whose psychosis was treatment resistant, defined as not responding to at least 3 periods of treatment in the preceding 5 years with antipsychotics from 2 different chemical classes at dosages equivalent to 1,000 mg/day of chlorpromazine for 6 weeks. The previous antipsychotic trials must have failed to provide periods of good functioning or significant symptomatic relief.

A 6-week trial of haloperidol (mean dosage, 61 mg/day) and benztropine followed to confirm lack of drug response. Participants whose psychosis did not respond to haloperidol were randomized to receive clozapine (up to 900 mg/day) or chlorpromazine (up to 1,800 mg/day) with benztropine. Using a priori criteria, response rates were 30% for patients treated with clozapine versus 4% for the chlorpromazine group. The authors found that improvements in the Brief Psychiatric Rating Scale (BPRS) total scores and Clinical Global Impression (CGI) scale were 3 times greater in the patients treated with clozapine. These results were confirmed in large pragmatic trials and meta-analyses in which clozapine was compared to SGAs in treatment resistant patients resulting in symptom improvement and median time to discontinuation.[70,71]

Adverse Effects

Since the efficacy between FGAs and SGAs in treating psychosis is equivalent, the decision for choosing a particular agent often rests on the individual person with psychosis and the adverse effect profile of a specific antipsychotic. SGAs were originally marketed as having fewer adverse effects, especially fewer neurologic and motor symptoms and increased tolerability compared to FGAs. Much of this information came from short-term, industry-sponsored trials with carefully selected patient populations, and non-inferiority comparisons of symptom ratings.[72,73] Sponsored rigorously randomized studies designed to match real-world treatment scenarios have provided information that demonstrates first- and second-generation agents have nearly equal limitations; this supports the widely held notion that selection of an antipsychotic drug should be an individualized process.[3,69]

Motor Symptoms. Treatment with FGAs has long been associated with both acute and chronic motor adverse effects. Acute extrapyramidal symptoms (EPS)—dystonia, pseudoparkinsonism, and akathisia (a syndrome of subjective anxiety and restlessness)—are thought to be related to drug-induced blockade of dopamine receptors in the nigrostriatal pathway in the brain.

Improved tolerability with SGAs has given this class of medications some advantage over the first generation agents; however experience has shown that all of the SGAs excluding clozapine, quetiapine and iloperidone, have the propensity to cause some degree of EPS.[74] Recent trials have shown that there is no advantage to SGA agents in improving tolerability and effectiveness over FGAs. Akathisia is estimated to occur in 25% of patients taking a FGA while it is estimated to occur with SGAs at an incidence of 7% to 30% depending on the SGA used.[3,75–84]

Tardive dyskinesia, a potentially irreversible chronic motor disorder caused by long-term exposure to dopamine antagonists, has been another serious concern with FGAs. The average rate of tardive dyskinesia with the FGAs is between 24% to 30%.[85,86] SGAs were initially thought to have a lower risk of treatment emergent tardive dyskinesia with maintenance treatment. Studies suggest that the risk of tardive dyskinesia with SGAs (excluding clozapine) is more than half of that with FGAs, or more than two-thirds of the risk with clozapine.[87] A meta-analysis of 203 studies from 2017 reported that the prevalence of tardive dyskinesia with SGAs (20.7%) is slightly lower than with treatment using FGAs (30%).[87] The data suggest that the risk of tardive dyskinesia may be slightly lower with SGAs, but not eliminated.[88]

The first step in treating tardive dyskinesia is to discontinue the antipsychotic that is thought to have caused the adverse effect.[89] If discontinued too quickly the patient may experience withdrawal dyskinesia, so a slow taper is recommended.[89] A risk benefit analysis regarding discontinuing the offending agent may find that the individual will continue to need an antipsychotic agent.[89] In this case, switching to an agent with a lower risk of tardive dyskinesia, such as clozapine is recommended.

Clozapine appears to have an especially favorable profile for the prevention and management of antipsychotic-induced movement disorders. In comparative trials, clozapine exhibited little to no evidence of inducing treatment emergent EPS.[65,90,91] The risk of tardive dyskinesia associated with clozapine treatment also appears to be minimal.[92,93] In fact, clozapine has been used to successfully treat preexisting tardive dyskinesia. Remission of symptoms has been reported in some, but not all, cases of preexisting tardive dyskinesia treated with clozapine.[58,65,66] In addition, withdrawal of clozapine in patients with tardive dyskinesia has resulted in either maintenance of reduced movements or worsening of dyskinesias.[94] The inconsistent nature of tardive dyskinesia treatment makes prevention of this syndrome a very important consideration in the pharmacotherapy of schizophrenia and schizoaffective disorder.[95]

Valbenazine, a VMAT2 (vesicular monoamine transporter 2) inhibitor, has been FDA approved for the treatment of tardive dyskinesia.[96,97] There is some evidence for two other VMAT2 inhibitors as well, tetrabenazine and deutetrabenazine, both FDA approved for the treatment of Huntington's chorea. Tetrabenazine is currently in phase III trials for schizophrenia and schizoaffective disorders.[98,99] Deutetrabenazine was approved for tardive dyskinesia in August, 2017.[100]

Studies have noted modest benefit for the use of adjunctive vitamin E in low doses to protect against worsening symptoms of tardive dyskinesia.[101,102] There is limited evidence for the efficacy of clonazepam, amantadine, zonisamide, levetiracetam, essential fatty acids, melatonin, piracetam, propranolol, reservatol, ginkgo biloba and vitamin B6 for use in treatment.[93,103–106] Branched chain amino acids (BCAAs) have been FDA approved for use in treating tardive dyskinesia in men only.[107]

Prolactin Elevation. Dopamine antagonists may elevate serum prolactin levels by decreasing the prolactin inhibitory effects of dopamine in the hypothalamus. Prolactin elevation has been reported to cause an irregular or suppressed menstrual cycle, galactorrhea, gynecomastia, and sexual dysfunction in the short-term.[108–110] With long-term elevation of plasma prolactin levels, suppression of estrogen and testosterone may occur. These effects may lead to a decrease in bone mineral density and to osteoporosis.[111]

The degree of prolactin elevation that an antipsychotic agent may exert appears to be related to its dopamine- and serotonin-binding properties. Significant prolactin elevation and its associated adverse effects can occur with moderate-to-high doses of the FGAs, paliperidone, and risperidone. [111] Risperidone has been consistently associated with the greatest degree of prolactin elevation among both the SGAs and the FGAs.[112,113] Clozapine causes the least prolactin elevation (<5%), while olanzapine, quetiapine, ziprasidone, asenapine, lurasidone, and brexpiprazole cause low to moderate hyperprolactinemia (10% to 40%).[114–116] Cariprazine does not appear to affect prolactin levels.[117] Aripiprazole causes hypoprolactinemia and may be used adjunctively to decrease prolactin level elevations occurring with other antipsychotics.[118–120]

Weight Gain. The metabolic effects of antipsychotic drug therapy have become a source of concern for clinicians and patients. Schizophrenia and antipsychotic drug treatments have long been associated with comorbid obesity and its related conditions: type 2 diabetes mellitus and cardiovascular disease.[121–125] In addition, drug treatments and lifestyle changes aimed at weight reduction may be ineffective or difficult to implement in this population.[126–128]

In multiple published analyses, clozapine and olanzapine have been associated with the greatest degree of weight gain among the antipsychotics (**Table 4**).[129,130] For example, in an analysis of data from registration trials, Allison et al found that at 10 weeks of treatment, olanzapine-treated patients gained an average of 4.15 kg, while clozapine-treated patients gained 4.45 kg.[129] Weight changes with clozapine and olanzapine are known to continue for up to 1 year or more.[131,132]

Drugs associated with a moderate degree of treatment-emergent weight gain include SGAs iloperidone, quetiapine, and risperidone and the FGA chlorpromazine. These agents typically produce weight gain of about 2 to3 kg in the first 10 to 12 weeks of treatment.[129,133] A lower degree of weight gain is seen with higher potency FGAs, such as haloperidol and fluphenazine, and SGAs aripiprazole, asenapine, lurasidone, and ziprasidone. Mean observed weight gain with these agents in 10- to 12-week clinical studies has been 2 kg or less. [118,122]

TABLE 4.
Mean Body Weight Changes at 10–12 Weeks in Patients Receiving Antipsychotics[129,131,133]

Treatment	Weight Change (kg)
Placebo	−0.75
Molindone	−0.39
Ziprasidone	0.04
Fluphenazine	0.43
Lurasidone	0.59
Paliperidone	1.03
Haloperidol	1.08
Asenapine	1.24
Risperidone	2.10
Iloperidone	2.16
Chlorpromazine	2.58
Thioridazine	3.19
Mesoridazine	3.19
Olanzapine	4.15
Clozapine	4.45

Diabetes Mellitus. Individuals with a prodromal and first episode schizophrenia have an increased incidence of developing diabetes regardless of treatment with antipsychotics.[121,134] In addition, new-onset hyperglycemia and diabetes mellitus have been observed with antipsychotic treatment. In some instances, the initial presentation consists of life-threatening diabetic ketoacidosis or hyperosmolar coma.[135] Frequently, clinically significant weight gain does not occur before the diagnosis of diabetes.[136]

In an analysis of public health registries and commercial databases carried out by Hirsch et al, the most consistent associations of type 2 diabetes mellitus diagnosis were found with olanzapine and clozapine treatment.[137] Other antipsychotics, including aripiprazole, quetiapine, risperidone, and ziprasidone, demonstrated statistically significant associations with type 2 diabetes.[138]

Dyslipidemia. Hyperlipidemia is another significant cardiac risk associated with 40% of antipsychotic naïve individuals diagnosed with schizophrenia as well as some antipsychotic treatments.[139,140] While risk factors for hyperlipidemia typically include glucose intolerance, dietary changes and weight gain, increases in serum triglycerides and low-density lipoproteins with SGAs have not always correlated with significant weight gain.[141,142] Antipsychotic medications may have an effect on adipose tissue leading to increased lipogenesis, insulin resistance, and decreased lipolysis.[142]

Of the antipsychotics, haloperidol and aripiprazole are considered to be lipid neutral, with ziprasidone, risperidone, and other high potency antipsychotics potentially causing mild to no risk of dyslipidemia. Low potency phenothiazines (chlorpromazine and thioridazine), clozapine, olanzapine, and quetiapine cause a significant increase in serum cholesterol and triglycerides.[143–146]

A 2004 consensus panel that included experts from the American Diabetes Association, American Psychiatric Association, American Association of Clinical Endocrinologists, and the North American Association for the Study of Obesity was convened. Using data collected during a comprehensive literature review and presentations from representatives from the pharmaceutical industry and FDA, the consensus panel developed a statement outlining the metabolic risks of treatment with SGAs.[147] The panel recommended careful consideration of metabolic risks whenever SGAs are initiated, especially in high-risk patients. The panel also recommended considering switching antipsychotics in patients who gain more than 7% of their initial weight, experience worsening hyperglycemia, or develop worsening hyperlipidemia. The most recent American Diabetes Association Standards of Care Guideline recommends that individuals taking atypical antipsychotics should be screened annually for prediabetes or diabetes.[148] Adolescents and adults with changes in their weight glycemic control and lipid levels should be monitored.[148] The British Association of Psychopharmacology recently published guidelines similar to the ADA guidelines with the exception of adding a review of the ratio of total cholesterol to high-density lipoprotein at 12 weeks, 6 months, and annually.[149]

Cardiovascular Risk. Antipsychotic medications can cause cardiovascular effects such as arrhythmia, elevations in blood pressure, orthostatic hypotension, and more rarely, congestive heart failure, myocarditis and sudden death.[150] Antipsychotic naïve individuals with schizophrenia are at a higher risk of mortality due to cardiovascular factors than the general population, so the use of antipsychotics in these individuals increases patient risk factors.[150] Certain antipsychotic medications have been associated with clinically significant prolongation of the corrected QT (QTc) interval, which may lead to torsades de pointes, a fatal ventricular arrhythmia. The risk of cardiac mortality associated with psychotropic drug treatment is particularly troublesome because of its spontaneous and unpredictable nature.

The FGAs thioridazine, pimozide, and droperidol have been implicated in numerous cases of sudden unexpected death.[151] Electrocardiographic data have revealed that patients receiving droperidol and thioridazine are more likely to have an abnormally long QTc interval.[152] Numerous reports of patient fatalities and the availability of safer alternatives have prompted the FDA to recommend that thioridazine, pimozide, and droperidol only be used as alternative agents with extreme caution.[153]

Although regulatory scrutiny for cardiac assessment heightened during the development of SGAs, these agents are generally associated with a low risk of electrocardiologic abnormalities. Ziprasidone was found to be associated with modest QTc prolongation during its premarketing studies. A comparative study that sought to determine the extent of QTc prolongation seen with the target therapeutic dosages of haloperidol, risperidone, olanzapine, quetiapine, and ziprasidone was later presented to the FDA.[153] Thioridazine was associated with an average QTc interval increase of 35.8 milliseconds. Of the second-generation agents included in the study, ziprasidone was associated with the greatest mean increase in the QTc interval (20.6 milliseconds). Haloperidol-treated subjects had an average QTc interval increase of 4.7 milliseconds, the smallest change observed in this study.[154] Coadministration of other interacting drugs (eg, cytochrome P-450 isoenzyme inhibitors) did not lead to significant changes in QTc measurement. Ziprasidone's labeling warned of its greater potential of QTc interval prolongation and discouraged use in patients with electrolyte abnormalities, cardiac comorbidity, or concomitant use of metabolic inhibitors.[155] Since this study was completed several new antipsychotics have come to market and several of those have QTc ranges that have been measured in clinical trials. Of those agents, iloperidone appears to have a QTc of 9 milliseconds, but when combined with CYP-450 inhibitors its QTc can increase to 19 milliseconds.[156] It is important to recognize that most of the SGA's do cause QTc prolongation, but currently there is not enough data to stratify agents by potential to cause QT prolongation, so drug choice should be made keeping the cardiovascular risk factors and the QTc of the patient in mind.[157]

Clozapine has been associated with treatment-emergent myocarditis and cardiomyopathy. Myocarditis associated with clozapine treatment presents as an acute inflammation of the myocardium, which may lead to congestive heart failure.[158] The incidence has been estimated between 0.7 and 3%.[159–161] The greatest risk of fatal events appears to exist during the first month of therapy. Cardiomyopathy associated with clozapine is an insidious process characterized by ventricular dilatation, impaired contraction, and symptoms of congestive heart failure.[158]

Cerebrovascular Events. The use of antipsychotics for the treatment for dementia-related agitation and psychosis in elderly patients is an unlabeled use that is generally supported by efficacy data in published controlled clinical trials.[162] However, post hoc analyses of the safety data for these trials revealed an elevated risk of cerebrovascular adverse events (CVAEs), including stroke and transient ischemic attacks, among patients treated with antipsychotics.[163–166] In 2003, the FDA requested that manufacturers of antipsychotic agents place a black box warning describing this treatment risk on the labeling of these products.[167] A closer look at the applicable safety data reveals that the patients in the dementia trials were often at elevated risk for CVAEs because of advanced age, poor control of chronic cardiovascular disease, and the underlying etiology of the dementia.[168] Cases of CVAEs included nonspecific events, such as hypotensive episodes, periods of unresponsiveness, and slurred speech. For example, the pooled results of 6 placebo-controlled randomized studies of risperidone for the treatment of behavioral disturbances in patients with dementia revealed 33 CVAEs (3.3%) in 1,009 subjects receiving the drug. The frequency of CVAEs was 1.1% (8 of 712) among placebo-treated patients ($P = 0.004$). However, serious CVAEs (fatal events, life-threatening events, or CVAEs associated with hospitalization or disability) occurred in 15 (1.5%) of 1,009 patients treated with risperidone and 4 (0.6%) of 712 patients treated with placebo, a difference that failed to reach statistical significance. Furthermore, most patients experiencing stroke had risk factors, including hypertension, atrial fibrillation, and previous strokes.[168]

The nature of this type of safety data makes it difficult to determine causality. It has been postulated that the adverse effects of sedation, hypotension, pseudoparkinsonism, and enhanced platelet aggregation may contribute to the observed increase in CVAEs.[168] In addition; these findings have not been widely observed among patients with schizophrenia and schizoaffective disorder. It would therefore be advisable to monitor high risk elderly patients on antipsychotics for symptoms of stroke.

Hematologic Toxicity. Transient cases of agranulocytosis can occur in 0.01% of patients receiving FGAs during the first 8 weeks of therapy. The greatest incidence of agranulocytosis in the FGAs occurs with thioridazine and chlorpromazine. Among the SGA's the greatest incidence of neutropenia occurs with clozapine and olanzapine.[169]

Despite its superior efficacy for treatment-resistant schizophrenia, clozapine has remained underutilized due to concerns about its minor risk of agranulocytosis.[170–172] Agranulocytosis has been estimated to occur in 0.38% of patients treated with clozapine.[173] Episodes tend to occur between 2 and 6 months after initiation of treatment.[174] Fatal infectious complications may occur as a result of reduced white blood cell count.[175] Clozapine-induced agranulocytosis can be reversed with the prompt discontinuation of treatment.[176]

In 2015, the FDA established a new Risk Evaluation and Mitigation Strategy (REMS) program that transitioned the oversight of hematologic monitoring from the use of multiple manufacturer-based registries to a centralized program.[177] As with prior manufacturer-based registries, the Clozapine REMS Program requires coordination between prescribers and pharmacies to ensure regular blood monitoring of patients in order to initiate or continue treatment with clozapine. The new REMS program differs from the guidelines used in the previous registry programs in that the primary basis for treatment recommendations is now the patient's absolute neutrophil count (ANC), regardless of total white blood cell (WBC) counts.

The REMS program also provides separate guidelines for patients with benign ethnic neutropenia (BEN), a hereditary condition seen in 10% to 30% of individuals of African and Middle Eastern descent who have no history of repeated infections despite maintaining lower baseline WBC and ANC levels.[178,179] Individuals with BEN do not have a greater risk of clozapine-induced agranulocytosis, and are therefore not considered neutropenic within the ANC range of 1,000-1,500 cells/μL.[180]

Respiratory Depression. Respiratory depression is more common with clozapine and olanzapine than with other antipsychotics. Respiratory collapse has been associated with rapid dosage adjustment, alcohol, and concomitant benzodiazepine use.[181] It is therefore recommended that clozapine dosage be gradually adjusted from the starting dose if the patient is new to clozapine treatment or if 2 or more days have elapsed since the last dose. It is recommended to avoid the combination of clozapine and olanzapine with benzodiazepines if possible, and if used together, monitor the patient for respiratory depression.[182,183]

Seizure Threshold Changes. Most FGAs and SGAs lower the seizure threshold, with the greatest risk in patients with risk factors for seizures including epilepsy, traumatic brain injury, hyponatremia, rapid titration of antipsychotic agent, and higher drug serum levels. Risk of seizures is highest (>1%) for chlorpromazine at doses >1,000 mg/day and clozapine at doses >300 mg/day.[152] There is an intermediate risk of seizures for chlorpromazine doses <1,000 mg/day, clozapine 300 mg/day, olanzapine, quetiapine, and thioridazine.[184] A low risk of seizures (<0.5%) is associated with the high-potency antipsychotics, aripiprazole, ziprasidone, risperidone and paliperidone.[185–187] Precautions should be taken for patients with seizure disorders receiving antipsychotic treatment, potentially including the concurrent use of an antiseizure medication, such as lamotrigine or levetiracetam.[188]

Drug Selection and Dosing Considerations

With the notable exception of clozapine, the principal differences among the available antipsychotics lie in their adverse-effect profiles and dosage forms. Selection of an initial treatment for a patient whose psychosis is not considered to be treatment resistant should be individualized based on the patient's specific tolerability concerns.[189,190] For example, individuals with a known sensitivity to EPS may benefit from quetiapine. Patients with preexisting metabolic disorders or those at risk for developing metabolic disorder may benefit from high-potency FGAs or SGAs, such as aripiprazole, lurasidone, and ziprasidone, that have a lower propensity for causing metabolic adverse effects.

The availability of orally disintegrating tablets, sublingual tablets, oral liquid formulations, and long-acting injectable formulations of several antipsychotics provide options for patients who have difficulty taking standard oral tablets or capsules, those with a history of poor treatment adherence, or those with an expressed interest for these dosage forms.[191–193] Loxapine is also available as a powder for oral inhalation that has been FDA approved for treatment of acute agitation associated with schizophrenia or bipolar disorder. Its use is restricted by an FDA-approved REMS program which requires that it be given in a healthcare facility due to the risk of bronchospasm, pulmonary distress, and pulmonary arrest.

Dosing. The dosage ranges of antipsychotic drugs used for symptom remission in acute schizophrenia have been established in registration trials and in some post-marketing analyses.[194–196] The target doses of FGAs and SGAs for acute treatment are listed in Tables 2 and 3.

Maintenance therapy can frequently be achieved with lower dosages, thereby reducing toxicity. Special populations, such as the elderly or individuals with hepatic impairment, may require lower doses due to increased sensitivity to adverse effects. In some individuals with a history of suboptimal response to antipsychotic treatment, additional benefit has been gained using SGAs with doses higher than the maximum recommended in the product labeling.[206]

Long-Acting Injectable Formulations. The development and use of long-acting injectable (LAI) antipsychotic formulations have sought to reduce some barriers to treatment adherence and provide more convenient options for patients.[191,192,198] LAI agents are administered in intervals ranging from 2 to 12 weeks between doses, reducing the need to administer oral drug on a daily basis.

The available LAI antipsychotics are described on **Table 5**. The first generation agents, fluphenazine decanoate and haloperidol decanoate are oil-based formulations that are released gradually from muscle tissue after injection and hydrolysis to the active drug.[198] The newer second generation LAIs are water-based products that use a variety of delivery technologies to release the active drug over time.

While LAI antipsychotics have consistently demonstrated symptomatic efficacy and reduced relapse frequency compared to placebo, it has been more difficult to establish these outcomes in head-to-head studies with oral antipsychotics due to methodologic limitations.[200] Adverse effect

TABLE 5.
Long-Acting Injectable Antipsychotics Available in the United States

Drug	Starting Dose	Oral Supplementation	Maintenance Dose	Dosing Interval	Notes
Fluphenazine decanoate	12.5–25 mg	None	12.5–100 mg	2–3 weeks	
Haloperidol decanoate	100 mg	None	100–300 mg	4 weeks	
Risperidone microspheres (Risperdal Consta)	25 mg	3 weeks	25–50 mg	2 weeks	
Olanzapine pamoate (Zyprexa Relprevv)	210–405 mg	None	150–405 mg	2–4 weeks	Requires postinjection observation for 3 hours after each dose due to risk of post-injection delirium sedation syndrome. Because of this risk, it is available only through a restricted distribution program called Zyprexa Relprevv Patient Care Program and requires prescriber, healthcare facility, patient, and pharmacy enrollment.
Paliperidone palmitate (Invega Sustenna)	234 mg, then 156 mg	None	78–234 mg	Monthly	Loading doses given as two doses 3-11 days apart
Paliperidone palmitate (Invega Trinza)	273–819 mg	None	273–819 mg	Every 3 months	To be initiated only in patients stabilized on Invega Sustenna
Aripiprazole monohydrate (Abilify Maintena)	400 mg	2 weeks	300–400 mg	Monthly	
Aripiprazole lauroxil (Aristada)	441–882 mg	3 weeks	441–882 mg	4–6 weeks	
	1,064 mg			8 weeks	

profiles of LAI antipsychotics are generally comparable to those of the corresponding oral drug. However, due to their extended duration of action, any untoward effects from LAI treatment are not easily reversible.

The LAI formulations should be considered in patients with a stated preference for their use or in individuals with a previous history of poor adherence. They may be initiated after patients have achieved a degree of clinical stability with the corresponding oral medication.

Patient Monitoring

Frequent and continuous monitoring is necessary for individuals treated with antipsychotics in order to assess for therapeutic response and adverse effects. An evaluation of efficacy is warranted after week 2 of treatment, as it has been shown that nonresponse at this point predicts a low likelihood of response.[201] A longer trial is generally warranted for clozapine. Gradual reductions in the severity of psychotic symptoms (eg, suspiciousness, hallucinations) are expected with adequate treatment.

Monitoring for metabolic adverse effects of antipsychotic therapy should consist of regular assessments of body weight, glucose levels, and lipid values (**Table 6**).[149,202] Treatment with clozapine requires weekly assessment of complete blood count and absolute neutrophil count for the first 6 months. If no evidence of neutropenia or granulocytopenia is found, the monitoring frequency can be reduced to every two weeks for the next 6 months and then every 4 weeks thereafter.

Despite the lower propensity for causing adverse motor effects, all patients receiving SGAs, in addition to patients receiving FGAs, should be monitored for symptoms of dystonia, parkinsonism, akathisia, and tardive dyskinesia.[203] Patients should be evaluated for acute EPS weekly until two weeks after dose stabilization, from when antipsychotics are initiated or adjusted. Assessments for tardive dyskinesia should be conducted at least once yearly for individuals receiving continuous treatment with antipsychotics.[204]

Measurement of antipsychotic plasma levels is not clinically indicated, except to assess for treatment adherence or suspected drug interactions. However, a minimum plasma clozapine concentration of 350 ng/mL has been correlated with treatment response among patients whose psychosis has been identified as treatment resistant.[203–205] In maintenance treatment, a clozapine serum level of at least 200 ng/mL optimally correlated with low risk of relapse.[206]

Pharmacogenomics

Schizophrenia is a complex illness with an etiology involving environmental factors and approximately 80% heritability.[197] Studies have shown that there is a higher incidence of synaptic pruning in the brains of those individuals diagnosed with schizophrenia versus those in the general population.[207] Genome wide association studies have shown multiple

TABLE 6.
Monitoring Guidelines for Patients Treated with Second-Generation Antipsychotics

Assessment	Monitoring Frequency
Fasting blood glucose	All drugs: at baseline, then monthly for the first 3 months and every 6 months thereafter; more frequent assessments are indicated for individuals noted to be gaining weight
Weight assessment	All drugs: at baseline and monthly thereafter (self-monitoring of weight should be encouraged)
Electrocardiogram	Clozapine and ziprasidone: at baseline and annually thereafter; more frequent assessments may be indicated in patients over age 50 years and in patients with a history of cardiac arrhythmias
Complete blood count with differential	Clozapine: weekly for the first 6 months, every other week for the next 6 months, and every 4 weeks thereafter if no abnormalities are noted
Fasting total cholesterol, low- and high-density lipoproteins,	All drugs: at baseline and every 2 years thereafter if no abnormalities are noted; every 6 months for individuals noted to have hyperlipidemia or receiving lipid-lowering therapy

susceptibility loci for schizophrenia, yet these studies have been difficult to replicate.[208]

Treatment of schizophrenia can be difficult due to lack of an empirical approach to choosing appropriate medications. Individuals with schizophrenia are typically treated based on a "trial and error" basis which can lead to nonadherence and adverse effects.[209] As many as 30% to 40% of individuals taking an antipsychotic will not respond to an individual agent, even though other individuals taking the same medication at the same dose for the same amount of time will exhibit response and even remission.[210] Variability in treatment response is also complex. Environmental factors—such as cigarette smoking, alcohol consumption, and dietary choices—can impact drug response. Comorbid psychiatric diagnoses, concurrent medications, and demographic factors, including gender, age, and ethnicity play a role in medication response as well. Pharmacogenomic factors help account for the wide variability of treatment responses seen across the population.

The Clinical Pharmacogenetics Implementation Consortium and Dutch Pharmacogenetics Working Group provide valuable analyses and guidance related to pharmacogenomic considerations for select medications, including medications used in schizophrenia and schizoaffective disorder. Pharmacogenomic research on antipsychotics has focused on metabolic enzymes (cytochrome P450), neurotransmitters (dopamine, serotonin), and drug transporters (p-glycoprotein). A very large number of potential genes involved in efficacy and adverse effects of antipsychotics have been identified. For example, over 90 variants of the CYP2D6 gene have been recognized.[211] However, many of these pharmacogenomic studies have been difficult to replicate or are limited to in vitro studies.

Pharmacogenomic testing has become commercially available for clinical use, but standardized guidelines for their use predicting antipsychotic treatment response have not yet been established.[212] Analysis of polymorphisms across the neurotransmitters, metabolic enzymes, and drug transporters need to be systematically analyzed in large enough sample sizes to develop enough sensitivity and specificity to provide clinicians with adequate guidance to predict individual response to antipsychotics.

Despite the current limitations in utility of pharmacogenomic application in schizophrenia treatment, some antipsychotics carry FDA labelling indicating that they have potentially applicable biomarkers.[213] This pharmacogenomic information is primarily useful for initiating and targeting doses that might result in drug interactions (**Table 7**). Guidance to clinicians on who should receive this testing is still unclear. Improvements in testing options continue to grow. Not all companies that test genetic variants test for the same medications, so it is important to ascertain whether the test used for an individual will give the results that the clinician is seeking.[213]

Treatment Outcomes

Schizophrenia and related disorders are characterized by chronic courses and periodic exacerbations. Exacerbations in the positive symptoms of schizophrenia may precipitate costly hospitalizations and may result in encounters with the legal system. However, negative and cognitive symptoms may have the greatest impact on patients' functional status.[214] Among the domains of functioning affected include activities of daily living, employment, treatment adherence, socialization, and quality of life.[215,216] A variety of evidence-based psychosocial treatments have been demonstrated to have a positive impact on functional outcomes.[217]

Studies addressing the effect of antipsychotics on hospitalization have repeatedly found that these agents reduce the length of stay and readmission rate compared with placebo.[62] Rabinowitz, et al calculated a two-year rehospitalization rate of 31% to 33% for patients discharged from inpatient psychiatric hospitalization receiving olanzapine or risperidone, compared with a 48% rate for patients discharged on conventional antipsychotics ($P = 0.02$).[218] In a landmark double-blind trial of risperidone versus haloperidol, Csernansky et al measured relapse by examining rehospitalization, signs of clinical decompensation, and increasing requirements for supervision.[219] They found significantly lower relapse rates at 1 year and longer times to relapse with risperidone treatment. FDA accepted this trial as sufficient evidence to allow the manufacturer to indicate in the product labeling the drug's efficacy in delaying relapse. Kishimoto and colleagues in a

TABLE 7.
Pharmacogenomic Considerations with Use of Antipsychotic Medications[211–213,222–228]

Antipsychotic[a]	FDA Labeling Information
Aripiprazole[b]	In CYP2D6 PM and individuals receiving aripiprazole in addition to a strong CYP2D6 or CYP3A4 inhibitor, decrease dose of aripiprazole by half (50%) In individuals taking a strong CYP2D6 or CYP3A4 inhibitor in addition to aripiprazole, decreased the dose of aripiprazole to a quarter of the dose (25%) The mean elimination half-lives are about 75 hours and 146 hours for aripiprazole in NMs and PMs, respectively
Aripiprazole, extended-release injectable suspension	CYP2D6 PMs, adjust 300-mg dose to 200 mg In individuals taking 400 mg receiving a strong CYP2D6 and CYP3A4 inhibitor, decrease dose to 300 mg In those individuals taking 300 mg, decrease dose to 200 mg in strong CYP2D6 and CYP3A4 inhibitors and decrease the dose to 160 mg in those taking a combination of CYP2D6 and CYP3A4 inhibitors Do not use in CYP3A4 inducers concomitantly with aripiprazole extended-release
Clozapine	May have higher plasma levels in CYP1A2/3A4/2C19 PMs Use 33% of clozapine dose if given with CYP1A2 inhibitors Do not use clozapine with strong CYP3A4 inducers
Iloperidone	Reduce dose 50% in CYP2D6 and CYP3A4 PM
Perphenazine	CYP2D6 PMs will have higher concentrations than NMs
Risperidone	CYP2D6 NMs convert risperidone rapidly into 9- hydroxyrisperidone; CYP2D6 PMs convert it more slowly. CYP2D6 NMs have lower risperidone and higher 9-hydroxyrisperidone concentration than PMs. Given that 9-hydroxyrisperidone is an active metabolite, no changes in dose need to be made
Thioridazine	Thioridazine is contraindicated in CYP2D6 PMs. Reduced CYP2D6 activity in individuals taking thioridazine may cause prolongation of QTc inverval and may lead to cardiac arrhythmias (torsades de pointes)

CYP, cytochrome P-450; PM, poor metabolizer; NM, normal metabolizer (previously called extensive metabolizer).
[a]Clinical Pharmacogenetics Implementation Consortium make no recommendations for dose changes in patients receiving antipsychotic agents.
[b]Dutch Pharmacogenomics Working Group recommends using no more than 10 mg of aripiprazole in CYP2D6 PMs.[229]

meta-analysis showed no difference between FGAs and SGAs in regards to relapse unless you pool all of the SGAs.[62] If all SGA agents studied are pooled, results do show some superiority for relapse, treatment failure, hospitalization and tolerability over FGAs.

Suicide is a leading cause of death in this patient population, with a lifetime suicide mortality rate estimated at 4% to 6%.[220] Risk factors of suicidality in schizophrenia include depressed mood, history of previous suicide attempts, male gender, number of psychiatric hospitalizations and young age. In addition to having favorable effects on mood symptoms, there are indications that SGAs may also reduce suicide rates in some populations, with clozapine demonstrating a particular benefit in this regard.[221] In a study of 980 patients with schizophrenia or schizoaffective disorder at high risk for suicide, treatment with clozapine was associated with a significantly lower rate of suicide attempts and hospitalizations compared with olanzapine (20.8% versus 28.8%, $P < 0.005$).[2]

Summary

Schizophrenia and schizoaffective disorder are chronic illnesses that can present with a broad range of symptoms and can affect many domains of functioning. The currently available antipsychotic drugs, while not curative, can have a dramatic effect on the acute symptoms of psychosis and the overall trajectory of schizophrenia and schizoaffective disorder. Clozapine has demonstrated a unique level of efficacy for individuals with treatment-resistant schizophrenia and for individuals at high risk for suicide and is very valuable in these subgroups, despite the additional adverse hematologic and cardiovascular effects.

Metabolic adverse effects, including weight gain, glucose abnormalities, and hyperlipidemias, cause significant concern for patients receiving SGAs and must be managed proactively by clinicians. Extrapyramidal effects, including dystonic reactions, parkinsonism, and akathisia affect the tolerability of antipsychotics and should be monitored throughout the treatment course. Pharmacists and health care professionals in all settings should play an active role in assisting in the selection of an appropriate antipsychotic agent, ensuring appropriate monitoring, and providing counseling to help achieve optimal outcomes with treatment.

References

1. Lehman AF, Lieberman JA, Dixon LB, et al. Practice guidelines for the treatment of patients with schizophrenia, second edition. *Am J Psychiatry.* 2010;161(2)(suppl):1–56.
2. Meltzer HY. Alphs L, Green AI. Clozapine treatment for suicidality in schizophrenia. International Suicide Prevention Trial (InterSePT). *Arch Gen Psychiatry.* 2003;60(1):82–91.

3. Jones PB, Barnes TR, Davies L, et al. Randomized controlled trial of the effect on quality of life of second- vs first-generation antipsychotic drugs in schizophrenia: cost utility of the latest antipsychotic drugs in schizophrenia (CUtLASS 1). *Arch Gen Psychiatry.* 2006;63(10):1079–1087.
4. Schizophrenia spectrum and other psychotic disorders. In: American Psychiatric Association. *DSM-5: Diagnostic and Statistical Manual of Mental Disorders, 5th Edition.* Washington, DC: American Psychiatric Press; 2013.
5. Ross CA. Problems with the psychosis section of DSM-5. *Psychosis.* 2014;6:3, 235–241.
6. Peraia J. Lifetime prevalence of psychotic and bipolar I disorders in a general population. *Arch Gen Psychiatry.* 2007; 64(1):19–28.
7. Heinssen RK, Goldstein AB, Azrin ST; for National Institute for Mental Health. Evidence-based treatments for first episode psychosis: components of coordinated specialty care. RAISE website. https://www.nimh.nih.gov/health/topics/schizophrenia/raise/nimh-white-paper-csc-for-fep_147096.pdf. Published April 14, 2014. Accessed August 7, 2018.
8. Addington J, Heinssen RK, Robinson DG, et al. Duration of untreated psychosis in community treatment settings in the United States. *Psychiatric Serv.* 2015;66(7):753–756.
9. Nicholl D, Akhras KS, Diels J, Schadrack J. Burden of schizophrenia in recently diagnosed patients: healthcare utilization and cost perspective. *Curr Med Res Opin.* 2010;26(4):943–955.
10. Byrne P. Managing the acute psychotic episode. *BMJ.* 2007;334:686–692.
11. Schoenbaum M, Sutherland JM, Chappel A, et al. Twelve-month health care use and mortality in commercially insured young people with incident psychosis in the United States. *Schizophrenia Bull.* 2017;43(6):1962–1972.
12. Driver DI, Gogtay N, Rapoport JL. Childhood onset schizophrenia and early onset schizophrenia spectrum disorders. *Child Adolesc Psychiatr Clin N Am.* 2013;22(4):539–555.
13. Folsom DP, Lebowitz BD, Lindamer LA, et al. Schizophrenia in late life: emerging issues. *Dialogues Clin Neurosci.* 2016;8(1):45–52.
14. Howes OD, Kapur S. The dopamine hypothesis of schizophrenia: version III—the final common pathway. *Schizophrenia Bull.* 2009;35(3)549–562.
15. Brisch R, Saniotis A, Wolk R, et al. The role of dopamine in schizophrenia from a neurobiological and evolutionary perspective: old fashioned, but still in vogue. *Front Psychiatry.* 2014:5:110.
16. Javitt DC. Glutamatergic theories of schizophrenia. *J Psych Relat Sci.* 2010;47(1):4–16.
17. Javitt DC, Zukin SR, Heresco-Levy U, Umbricht D. Has an angel shown the way? Etiological and therapist implications of the PCP/NMDA model of schizophrenia. *Schizophrenia Bull.* 2012;38(5)958–966.
18. Hughes JR, Hatsukami DK, Mitchell JE, et al. Prevalence of smoking among psychiatric outpatients. *Am J Psychiatry.* 1986;143:993–997.
19. Brunzell D, McIntosh JM. Alpha 7 nicotinic acetylcholine receptors modulate motivation to self-administer nicotine: implications for smoking and schizophrenia. *Neuropsychopharmacology.* 2012;37:1134–1143.
20. Jibson MD, Marder S, Hermann R. First-generation antipsychotic medications: pharmacology, administration, and comparative side effects. UpToDate [database online]. Waltham, MA: Wolters Kluwer Health. https://www.uptodate.com/contents/first-generationantipsychotic-medications-pharmacologyadministration-and-comparative-sideeffects. Accessed March 6, 2017.
21. Stahl SM. Dopamine system stabilizers, aripiprazole, and the next generation of antipsychotics, part I: "Goldilocks" actions at dopamine receptors. *J Clin Psychiatry.* 2001; 62:841–842.
22. Stahl SM. Dopamine system stabilizers, aripiprazole, and the next generation of antipsychotics, part II: illustrating their mechanism of action. *J Clin Psychiatry.* 2001; 62:923–924.
23. Möller H. The relevance of negative symptoms in schizophrenia and how to treat them with psychopharmaceuticals? *Psychiatria Danubina.* 2016;28(4):435–440.
24. Dollfus S, Lyne J. Negative symptoms: history of the concept and their position in diagnosis of schizophrenia. *Schizophr Res.* 2017;186:3–7.
25. Mitra S, Mahintamani T, Kavoor AR, Nizamie SH. Negative symptoms in schizophrenia. *Ind Psychiatry J.* 2016;25(2):135–144.
26. Kantrowicz JT. Managing negative symptoms of schizophrenia: how far have we come? *CNS Drugs.* 2017;31:373–388.
27. Aleman A, Lincoln TM, Bruggeman R, et al. Treatment of negative symptoms: where do we stand and where do we go. *Schizophr Res.* 2017;186:55–62.
28. Kirschner M, Aleman A, Kaiser S. Secondary negative symptoms—a review of mechanisms, assessment and treatment. *Schizophr Res.* 2017;186:29–38.
29. Remington G, Foussias G, Fervaha G, et al. Treating negative symptoms in schizophrenia: an update. *Curr Treat Options Psychiatry.* 2016;3:133–150.
30. Leucht S, Cipriani A, Spineli L. Comparative efficacy and tolerability of 15 antipsychotic drugs in schizophrenia: a multiple-treatments meta-analysis. *Lancet.* 2013;382:951–962.
31. Buchanan RW, Kreyenbuhl J, Kelly DL, et al. The 2009 schizophrenia PORT psychopharmacological treatment recommendations and summary statements. *Schizophr Bull.* 2010;36:71–93.
32. Andreasen NC, Liu D, Ziebell S, et al. Relapse duration, treatment intensity, and brain tissue loss in schizophrenia: a prospective longitudinal MRI study. *Am J Psychiatry.* 2013;170:609–615.
33. Green MF. What are the functional consequences of neurocognitive deficits of schizophrenia? *Am J Psychiatry.* 1996;153:321–330.
34. Liddle PF. Cognitive impairment in schizophrenia: its impact on social functioning. *Acta Psychiatr Scand Suppl.* 2000;400:11–6.
35. Sharma T, Antonova L. Cognitive function in schizophrenia: deficits, functional consequences, and future treatment. *Psychiatr Clin North Am.* 2003;26:25–40.

36. Spohn HE, Strauss ME. Relation of neuroleptic and anticholinergic medication to cognitive functions in schizophrenia. *J Abnorm Psychol.* 1989;98:367–380.
37. Bilder RM, Goldman RS, Volavka J, et al. Neurocognitive effects of clozapine, olanzapine, risperidone and haloperidol in patients with chronic schizophrenia or schizoaffective disorder. *Am J Psychiatry.* 2002;159:11018–11028.
38. Hagger C, Buckley P, Kenny JT, et al. Improvement in cognitive functions and psychiatric symptoms in treatment-refractory schizophrenic patients receiving clozapine. *Biol Psychiatry.* 1993;34:702–712.
39. Grace J, Bellus SB, Raulin ML, et al. Long-term impact of clozapine and psychosocial treatment on psychiatric symptoms and cognitive functioning. *Psychiatr Serv.* 1996;47:41–45.
40. Buchanan RW, Holstein C, Breier A. The comparative efficacy and long-term effect of clozapine on neuropsychological test performance. *Biol Psychiatry.* 1994;36:717–725.
41. Cornblatt B, Kern RS, Carson WH, et al. Neurocognitive effects of aripiprazole versus olanzapine in stable psychosis. Presented at 23rd Collegium Internationale Neuropsychopharmacologicum Congress; June 2002; Montreal, Canada.
42. Davidson M, Galderisi S, Weiser M, et al. Cognitive effects of antipsychotic drugs in first-episode schizophrenia and schizophreniform disorder: a randomized, open-label clinical trial (EUFEST). *Am J Psychiatry.* 2009;166(6):675–682.
43. Keefe RS, Bilder RM, Davis SM, et al. Neurocognitive effects of antipsychotic medications in patients with chronic schizophrenia in the CATIE trial. *Arch Gen Psychiatry.* 2007;64:633–647.
44. Goldberg TE, Goldman RS, Burdick KE, et al. Cognitive improvements after treatment with SGAs in first episode schizophrenia: is it a practice effect? *Arch Gen Psychiatry.* 2007; 64:1115–1122.
45. Albus M, Hubmann W, Mohr F, et al. Neurocognitive functioning in patients with first-episode schizophrenia. *Eur Arch Psychiatry Clin Neurol.* 2006;256:442–451.
46. Hill SK, Shuepback D, Herbener ES, Keshavan MS, Sweeney JA. Pretreatment and longitudinal studies of neuropsychological deficits in antipsychotic-naïve patients with schizophrenia. *Schizophr Res.* 2004; 68:49–63.
47. Hoff AL, Sakuma M, Wieneke M, Horon R, Kushner M, DeLisi LE. Longitudinal neuropsychological follow-up study of patients with first-episode schizophrenia. *Am J Psychiatry.* 1999;156:1336–1341.
48. Keefe RS, Perkins DO, Gu H, Zipursky RB, Christensen BK, Lieberman JA. A longitudinal study of neurocognitive function in individuals at-risk for psychosis. *Schizophr Res.* 88:26–35.
49. Crespo-Facorro B, Rodriguez-Sanchez JM, Perez-Inglesias R, et al. Neurocognitive effectiveness of haloperidol, risperidone, and olanzapine in first episode psychosis: a randomized, controlled 1-year follow-up comparison. *J Clin Psychiatry.* 70:717–729.
50. Keefe RS, Malhotra AK, Meltzer H, et al. Efficacy and safety of donepezil in patients with schizophrenia or schizoaffective disorder: significant placebo/practice effects in a 12 week, randomized, double-blind, placebo-controlled trial. *Neuropsychopharmacology.* 2008;33:1217–1228.
51. Hill SK, Bishop JR, Palumbo D, Sweeney JA. Effect of second-generation antipsychotics on cognition: current issues and future challenges. *Expert Rev Neurother.* 2010;10(1):43–57.
52. Andersen R, Fagerlund B, Rasmussen H, et al. Cognitive effects of six months of treatment with quetiapine in antipsychotic-naïve first-episode schizophrenia. *Psychiatry Res.* 2011;187 (1-2):49–54.
53. Suzuki H, Gen K, Inoue Y. An unblended comparison of the clinical and cognitive effects of switching from first-generation antipsychotics to aripiprazole, perospirone or olanzapine in patients with chronic schizophrenia. *Prog Neuropsychopharmacology Biological Psychiatry.* 2011;35(1):161–168.
54. Cuesta MJ, Jalon EG, Campos MS, Peralta V. Cognitive effectiveness of olanzapine and risperidone in first-episode psychosis. *Br J Psychiatry.* 2009;194:439–445.
55. Guo X, Zhai J, Wei Q, et al. Neurocognitive effects of first- and second-generation antipsychotic drugs in early-stage schizophrenia: a naturalistic 12-month follow-up study. *Neuroscience Lett.* 2011;503(2):141–146.
56. Robles O, Zabala A, Bombin I, et al. Cognitive efficacy of quetiapine and olanzapine in early-onset first-episode psychosis. *Schizophrenia Bull.* 2011;37(2):405–415.
57. Frazier JA, Giuiano AJ, Johnson JL, et al. Neurocognitive outcomes in the treatment of early-onset schizophrenia spectrum disorders study. *J Am Acad Child Adolesc Psychiatry.* 2012;51(5):496–505.
58. Hasan A, Falkai P, Wobrock T, et al. World Federation of Societies of Biological Psychiatry (WFSBP) guidelines for the biological treatment of schizophrenia, part 1: update 2012 on the acute treatment of schizophrenia and the management of treatment resistance. *World J Biol Psychiatry.* 2012;13:318–378.
59. Gardner KN, Nasrallah HA. Managing first-episode psychosis: an early state of schizophrenia with distinct treatment needs. *Curr Psychiatr.* 2015;14(5):32–42.
60. Rosenheck R, Leslie D, Sint K, et al. Cost effectiveness of comprehensive, integrated care for first episode psychosis in the NIMH RAISE early treatment program. *Schizophrenia Bull.* 2016;42(4):896–906.
61. Zipursky RB, Menezes NM, Streiner DL. Risk of symptom recurrence with medication discontinuation in first-episode psychosis: a systematic review. *Schizophrenia Res.* 2014;152:408–414.
62. Kishimoto T, Agarwal V, Kishi T, Leucht S, Kane JM, Correll CY. Relapse prevention in schizophrenia: a systematic review and meta-analysis of second-generation antipsychotics versus first generation antipsychotics. *Mol Psychiatry.* 2013;18:53–66.
63. Leucht S, Tardy M, Komossa K, et al. Antipsychotic drugs versus placebo for relapse prevention in schizophrenia: a systematic review and meta-analysis. *Lancet.* 2012;379:2063–2071.
64. National Collaborating Centre for Mental Health. *The NICE guideline on core interventions in the treatment and management of schizophrenia in adults in primary*

and secondary care (updated edition). London, UK: British Psychological Society; 2010.
65. Kane J, Honigfeld G, Singer J, et al. Clozapine for the treatment-resistant schizophrenic, a double-blind comparison with chlorpromazine. *Arch Gen Psychiatry*. 1994;152:20–26.
66. McIlwain ME, Harrison J, Wheeler AJ, Russell BR. Pharmacotherapy for treatment-resistant schizophrenia. *Neuropsychiatr Dis Treat*. 2011;7:135–149.
67. Stahl SM. Antipsychotic polypharmacy: squandering precious resources? *J Clin Psychiatry*. 2002;63:93–94.
68. Newcomer JW, Weiden PJ, Buchanan RW. Switching antipsychotic medications to reduce adverse event burden in schizophrenia: establishing evidence-based practice. *J Clin Psychiatry*. 2013;74(11):1108–1120.
69. Lieberman JA, Stroup TS, McEvoy JP, et al. Effectiveness of antipsychotic drugs in patients with chronic schizophrenia. *N Engl J Med*. 2005;353:1209–1223.
70. Siskind D, McCartney L, Goldschlager R, Kisely S. Clozapine v. first- and second-generation antipsychotics in treatment-refractory schizophrenia: systematic review and meta-analysis. *Br J Psychiatry*. 2016;209(5):382–392.
71. Siskind D, McCartney L, Goldschlager R, Kisely S. Systematic review and meta-analysis of clozapine for treatment refractory schizophrenia. *Aust N Z J Psychiatry*. 2015;49:73–74.
72. Heres S, Davis J, Maino K, et al. Why olanzapine beats risperidone, risperidone beats quetiapine, and quetiapine beats olanzapine: an exploratory analysis of head-to-head comparison studies of second-generation antipsychotics. *Am J Psychiatry*. 2006;163:185–194.
73. Lewis S, Lieberman J. CATIE and CUtLASS: can we handle the truth? *Br J Psychiatry*. 2008; 192:161–163.
74. Farah A. Atypicality of atypical antipsychotics revisited. *Curr Psychiatry Rev*. 2013;9(4):316–324.
75. Weiden PJ. EPS profiles: the atypical antipsychotics are not all the same. *J Psychiatry Pract*. 2007;(13)(1):13–24.
76. Casey DE. Implications of the CATIE trial on treatment: extrapyramidal symptoms. *CNS Spectr*. 2006;11(7):25–31.
77. Tandon R. Antipsychotics in the treatment of schizophrenia: an overview. *J Clin Psychiatry*. 2011;72(1):4–8.
78. Fischer-Barnicol D, Lanquillon S, Haen E, et al. Typical and atypical antipsychotics-the misleading dichotomy: results from the working group "Drugs in Psychiatry (AGATE)," *Neuropsychobiology*. 2008;57:80–87.
79. Shirzadi AA, Ghaemi SN. Side effects of atypical antipsychotics: extrapyramidal symptoms and the metabolic syndrome. *Harv Rev Psychiatry*. 2006;14(3):152–164.
80. Jesic MP, Jesic A, Filipovic JB, et al. Extrapyramidal syndromes caused by antipsychotics. *Medicinski Pregled*. 2012;65:521–526.
81. Kumar R, Sachdev PS. Akathisia and second-generation antipsychotic drugs. *Curr Opin Psychiatry*. 2009;293–299.
82. Miller DD, Caroff SN, Davis SM, et al. Extrapyramidal side-effects of antipsychotics in a randomized trial. *Br J Psychiatry*. 2008;193(4):279–288.
83. Kane JM, Fleischhacker WW, Hansen L, Perlis R, Pikalov A, Talbott SA. Akathisia: an updated review focusing on second-generation antipsychotics. *J Clin Psychiatry*. 2009;70(5):629–643.
84. Thomas JE, Cabellero J, Arrington CA. The incidence of akathisia in the treatment of schizophrenia with aripiprazole, asenapine, and lurasidone: a meta analysis. *Curr Neuropharmacology*. 2015;13:681–691.
85. Casey DE. Tardive dyskinesia and atypical antipsychotic drugs. *Schizophr Res*. 1999;35:S61-S66.
86. Llorca P, Chereau I, Bayle F, Lancon C. Tardive dyskinesia and antipsychotics: a review. *Eur Psychiatry*. 2002; 17(3):129–138.
87. Carbon M, Hsied CH, Kane JM, Correll CU. Tardive dyskinesia prevalence in the period of second-generation antipsychotic use: a meta-analysis. *J Clin Psychiatry*. 2017;78(3):e278. doi;10.4888/JCP.16r10832
88. Correll CU, Leucht S, Kane JM. Lower risk for tardive dyskinesia associated with second- generation antipsychotics: a systematic review of 1-year studies. *Am J Psychiatry*. 2004; 161:414–425.
89. Vijayakumar D, Jankovic J. Drug-induced dyskinesia, part 2: treatment of tardive dyskinesia. *Drugs*. 2016;76:779–787.
90. Povlssen UJ, Noring U, Fog R, et al. Tolerability and therapeutic effect of clozapine: a retrospective investigation of 216 patients treated with clozapine for up to 12 years. *Acta Psychiatr Scand*. 1985;71:176–185.
91. Kurz M, Hummer M, Oberbauer H, et al. Extrapyramidal side effects of clozapine and haloperidol. *Psychopharmacology*. 1995;118:52–56.
92. Casey DE. Clozapine: neuroleptic-induced EPS and tardive dyskinesia. *Psychopharmacology*. 1989;99:S47-S53.
93. Lerner PP, Miodownik C, Lerner V. Tardive dyskinesia (syndrome): current concept and modern approaches to its management. *Psychiatry Clin Neurosci*. 2015;69(6):321–334.
94. Hazari N, Kate N, Grover S. Clozapine and tardive movement disorders: a review. *Asian J Psychiatr*. 2013;6(6):439–451.
95. Ahmed S, Chengappa KN, Naidu VR, et al. Clozapine withdrawal-emergent dystonias and dyskinesias: a case series. *J Clin Psychiatry*. 1998;59:472–477.
96. O'Brien CD, Jimenez R, Hauser RA, et al. NBI-98854, a selective monoamine transport inhibitor for the treatment of tardive dyskinesia: a randomized, double-blind, placebo-controlled study. *Mov Disord*. 2015;30:1681–1687.
97. Hauser RA, Factor SA, Marder SR, et al. KINECT 3: a phase 3 randomized, double-blind, placebo-controlled trial of valbenzapine for tardive dyskinesia. *Am J Psychiatry*. 2017;174:476–484.
98. Kaur N, Kumar P, Jamwal S, et al. Tetrabenazine: spotlight on drug review. *Ann Neurosci*. 2016;23:176–185.
99. Fernandez HH, Factor SA, Hauser RA, et al. Randomized controlled trial of deutetrabenzaine for tardive dyskinesia: the ARM-TD study. *Neurology*. 2017;88:2003–2010.
100. Brooks M. FDA OKs deutetrabenazine (Austedo) for tardive dyskinesia. Medscape Medical News.

www.medscape.com/viewarticle/885051. Accessed August 7, 2018.

101. Barak Y, Swartz M, Shamir E, et al. Vitamin E (alpha-tocopheol) in the treatment of tardive dyskinesia: a statistical meta-analysis. *Ann Clin Psychiatry.* 1998;10:101–105.
102. Soares-Weiser K, Maayan N, McGrath J. Vitamin E for neuropetic-induced tardive dyskinesia. *Cochrance Database Syst Rev.* 2011;2:CD000209.
103. Thaker GK, Nguyen JA, Strauss ME, Jacobson R, Kaup BA, Tamminga CA. Clonazepam treatment of tardive dyskinesia: a practical GABAmimetic strategy. *Am J Psychiatry.* 1990;147:445–451.
104. Pappa S, Tsouli S, Apostolou G, Mavreas V, Konitsiotis S. Effects of amantadine on tardive dyskinesia: a randomized, double-blind, placebo-controlled study. *Clin Neuropharmacol.* 2010;33:271–275.
105. Zheng W, Xiang YQ, Ng CH, et al. Extract of Gingko biloba for tardive dyskinesia: meta-analysis of randomized controlled trials. *Pharmacopsychiatry.* 2016;49:107–111.
106. Adelufosi AO, Abayomi O, Ojo TM. Pyridoxal 5 phosphate for neuroleptic-induced tardive dyskinesia. *Cochrane Database Syst Rev.* 2015;4:CDO01501.
107. Richardson MA, Bevans ML, Read LL, et al. Efficacy of the branched-chain amino acids in the treatment of tardive dyskinesia in men. *Am J Psychiatry.* 2003;160;1117–1124.
108. Dickson RA, Seeman MV, Corenblum B. Hormonal side effects in women: typical versus atypical antipsychotic treatment. *J Clin Psychiatry.* 2000;61(suppl 3):10–15.
109. Windgassen K, Wesselman W, Schulze-Monking H. Galactorreha and hyperprolactineia in schizophrenic patients on neuroleptics: frequency and etiology. *Neuropsychobiology.* 1996; 33:142–146.
110. Arana GW. An overview of side effects caused by typical antipsychotics. *J Clin Psychiatry.* 2000;61 (suppl 8):5–11.
111. Petty RG. Prolactin and antipsychotic medications: mechanisms of action. *Schizophr Res.* 1999;35(suppl): S67–73.
112. David SR, Taylor CC, Kinon BJ, et al. The effects of olanzapine, risperidone, and haloperidol on plasma prolactin levels in patients with schizophrenia. *Clin Ther.* 2000;22:1085–1096.
113. Bunker MT, Marken PA, Schneiderhan ME, et al. Attenuation of antipsychotic-induced hyperprolactinemia with clozapine. *J Child Adolesc Psychopharmacol.* 1997;7:65–69.
114. Inder WJ, Castle D. Antipsychotic-induced hyperprolactinemia. *Aust NZ J Psychiatry.* 2011;45:830–837.
115. Melkersson K. Differences in prolactin elevation and related symptoms of atypical antipsychotics in schizophrenic patients. *J Clin Psychiatry.* 2005;66:761–767.
116. Bruijnzeel D, Tandon R. Spotlight on brexpiprazole and its potential in the treatment of schizophrenia and as adjunctive therapy for the treatment of major depression. *Drug Des Devel Ther.* 2016:10;1641–1647.
117. Mattingly G, Anderson R. Cariprazine for schizophrenia and bipolar I disorder. *Curr Psychiatry.* 2016;15(1):e1-e6.
118. Sogawa R, Shimomura Y, Minami C. Aripiprazole-associated hypoprolactinemia in the clinical setting. *J Clin Psychiatry.* 2016;36(4)385–387.
119. Chen JX, Su YA, Bian QT, Wei LH, Zhang RZ. Adjunctive aripiprazole in the treatment of risperidone-induced hyperprolactinemia: a randomized, double-blind, placebo-controlled, dose response study. *Psychoneuroendocrinology.* 2015;58:130–140.
120. Qiao Y, Yang F, Guo Q, Wen H, Zhu S, et al. Add-on effects of a low-dose aripiprazole in resolving hyperprolactinemia induced by risperidone or paliperidone. *J Child Adolesc Psychopharmacol.* 2016;26(5):490–491.
121. Cordes J, Bechdolk A, Engelke C, et al. Prevalence of metabolic syndrome in female and male patients at risk of psychosis. *Schizophr Res.* 2017;179:57–63.
122. Allison DB, Fontaine KR, Heo M, et al. The distribution of body mass index among individuals with and without schizophrenia. *J Clin Psychiatry.* 1999;60:215–220.
123. Mukherjee S, Decina P, Bocola V, et al. Diabetes mellitus in schizophrenic patients. *Compr Psychiatry.* 1996;37:68–73.
124. Brambilla F, Guastalla A, Guerrini A, et al. Glucose-insulin metabolism in chronic schizophrenia. *Dis Nerv Syst.* 1976;37:98–103.
125. Tsuang MT, Perkins K, Simpson JC. Physical diseases in schizophrenia and affective disorder. *J Clin Psychiatry.* 1983;44:42–46.
126. Borovicka MC, Fuller MA, Konicki PE, et al. Phenylpropanolamine appears not to promote weight loss in patients with schizophrenia who have gained weight during clozapine treatment. *J Clin Psychiatry.* 2002;63:345–348.
127. Ball MP, Coons VB, Buchanan RW. A program for treating olanzapine-related weight gain. *Psychiatr Serv.* 2001;52:967–969.
128. Green AI, Patel JK, Goisman RM, et al. Weight gain from novel antipsychotic drugs: need for action. *Gen Hosp Psychiatry.* 2000;22:224–235.
129. Allison DB, Mentore JL, Heo M, et al. Antipsychotic-induced weight gain: a comprehensive research synthesis. *Am J Psychiatry.* 1999;156:1686–1696.
130. Leucht S, Cipriani A, SpineliL. Comparative efficacy and tolerability of 15 antipsychotic drugs in schizophrenia: a multiple-treatments meta-analysis. *Lancet.* 2013;382:951–962.
131. Bak M, Fransen A, Jansen J, van Os J, Drukker M. Almost all antipsychotics result in weight gain: a meta-analysis. *Plos One.* 2014;9(4):e94112.
132. Lu ML, Wang TN, Lin TY, et al. Differential effects of olanzapine and clozapine on plasma levels of adipocytokines and total ghrelin. *Prog Neuropsychopharmacol Biol Psychiatry.* 2015;58(3)47–50.
133. De Hert M, Yu W, Detraux J, et al. Body weight and metabolic adverse effects of asenapine, iloperidone, lurasidone and paliperidone in the treatment of schizophrenia and bipolar disorder: a systematic review and exploratory meta-analysis. *CNS Drugs.* 2012;26(9):733–759.
134. Greenhalgh AM, Gonzalez-Blanco L, Garcia-Rizo C, et al. Meta-analysis of glucose tolerance,

insulin, and insulin resistance in antipsychotic-naïve patients with non-affective psychosis. *Schizophr Res.* 2017;179:57–63.

135. Muench J, Carey M. Diabetes mellitus associated with second-generation antipsychotic medications: new case report and review of the literature. *J Am Board Fam Pract.* 2001; 14:278–282.
136. Jin H, Meyer JM, Jeste DV. Phenomenology of and risk factors for new onset diabetes mellitus associated with second-generation antipsychotics: an analysis of 45 published cases. *Ann Clin Psychiatry.* 2002;14:59–64.
137. Hirsch L, Yang J, Bresee L, et al. Second-generation antipsychotics and metabolic side effects: a systematic review of population-based studies. *Drug Saf.* 2017. doi: 10.1007/s40264-017-0543-0. Accessed August 7, 2018.
138. Falissar B, Mauro M, Shaw K, et al. The METEOR study: frequency of metabolic disorders in patients with schizophrenia. Focus on first and second generation and level of risk of antipsychotic drugs. *Int Clin Psychopharmacol.* 2011;26(6):291–302.
139. Mitchell AJ, Vancamptfort D, Sweers K, van Winkel R, Yu W, De Hert M. Prevalence of metabolic syndrome and metabolic abnormalities in schizophrenia and related disorders—a systematic review and meta-analysis. *Schizophr Bull.* 2013;39(2):304–318.
140. Misiak B, Stanczykiewicz B, Lacmanski L, Frydecka D. Lipid profile disturbances in antipsychotic naïve patietns with first-episode non-affective psychosis: a systematic review and meta-analysis. *Schizophr Res.* 2017. http://dx.doi.org/10.1016/j.schres.2017.03.031. Accessed August 7, 2018.
141. Meyer JM. Novel antipsychotics and severe hyperlipidemia. *J Clin Psychopharmacol.* 2001; 21:369–374.
142. Gonclaves P, Araujo JR, Martel F. Antipsychotic-induced metabolic alterations: focus on adipose tissue and molecular mechanisms. *Eur Neuropsychopharmacology.* 2015;25:1–16.
143. Olfson M, Marcus SC, Corey-Lisle P, Tuomari AV, Hines P, L'Italien GJ. Hyperlipidemia following treatment with antipsychotic medications. *Am J Psychiatry.* 2006;163(10):1821–1825.
144. Clark M, Dubowski K, Colmore J. The effect of chlorpromazine on serum cholesterol in chronic schizophrenic patients. *Clin Pharmacol Ther.* 1970;11(6):883–889.
145. Meyer JM, Koro CE. The effects of antipsychotic therapy on serum lipids: a comprehensive review. *Schizophrenia Res.* 2004;70(1):1–17.
146. Koro CE, Meyer JM. Atypical antipsychotic treatment and hyperlipidemia: a review. *Essn Psychopharm.* 2005;6(3):148–157.
147. American Diabetes Association, American Psychiatric Association, American Association of Clinical Endocrinologists et al. Consensus development conference on antipsychotic drugs and obesity and diabetes. *Diabetes Care.* 2004;27:596–601.
148. American Diabetes Association. Standards of medical care in diabetes—2017. *Diabetes Care.* 2017;4(suppl 1): S1-S134.
149. Cooper SJ, Reynolds GP. The BAP guidelines on the management of weight gain, metabolic disturbances, and cardiovascular risk associated with psychosis and antipsychotic drug treatment. *J Psychopharmacol.* 2016;30(8):717–748.
150. Khasawneh FT, Shankar GS. Minimizing cardiovascular adverse effects of atypical antipsychotic drugs in patients with schizophrenia. *Cardiol Res Pract.* 2014. http://dx.doi.org/10.1155/2014/273060. Accessed August 7, 2018.
151. Mehtonen OP, Aranko K, Malkonen L, et al. A survey of sudden death associated with the use of antipsychotic or antidepressant drugs: 49 cases in Finland. *Acta Psychiatr Scand.* 1991; 84:58–64.
152. Reilly JG, Ayis SA, Ferrier IN, et al. QTc-interval abnormalities and psychotropic drug therapy in psychiatric patients. *Lancet.* 2000;355:1048–1052.
153. Food and Drug Administration. *Psychopharmacological Drugs Advisory Committee. Briefing document for Zeldox capsules (ziprasidone HCl).* https://www.fda.gov/AdvisoryCommittees/CommitteesMeetingMaterials/Drugs/PsychopharmacologicDrugsAdvisoryCommittee/ucm535446.htm. Accessed August 7, 2018.
154. Laughren T, Gordon M. *FDA background on Zeldox (ziprasidone hydrochloride capsules) Pfizer, Inc.* Psychopharmacological Drugs Advisory Committee. July 19, 2000.
155. Geodon [prescribing information]. New York, NY: Pfizer Inc.; November 2006.
156. Iloperidone [package insert]. Washington, DC: Vanda Pharmaceuticals; May 2016.
157. Hasnain M, Vieweg WV. QTc interval prolongation and torsade de pointes associated with second-generation antipsychotics and antidepressants: a comprehensive review. *CNS Drugs.* 2014;28(10):887–920.
158. Merrill DB, Dec GW, Goff DC. Adverse cardiac effects associated with clozapine. *J Clin Psychopharmacol.* 2005;25:32–41.
159. Ronaldson KJ, Fitzgerald PB, McNeil JJ. Clozapine-induced myocarditis, a widely overlooked adverse reaction. *Acta Psychiatr Scand.* 2015;132(4):231–240.
160. Karjalainen J, Heikkila J. Incidence of three presentations of acute myocarditis in young men in military service. A 20-year experience. *Eur Heart J.* 1999;20:1120–1125.
161. Haas SJ, Hill R, Krum H, et al. Clozapine-associated myocarditis: a review of 116 cases of suspected myocarditis associated with the use of clozapine in Australia during 1993-2003. *Drug Saf.* 2007;30:47–57.
162. Sink KM, Holden KF, Yaffe K. Pharmacological treatment of neuropsychiatric symptoms of dementia: a review of the evidence. *JAMA.* 2005;293:596–608.
163. Hsu WT, Esmaily-Fard A, Lai CC, et al. Antipsychotics and the risk of cerebrovascular accident: a systematic review and meta-analysis of observational studies. *J Am Med Dir Assoc.* 2017;18 (8):692–699.
164. Wang PS, Schneeweiss S, Avorn J, et al. Risk of death in elderly users of conventional vs. atypical antipsychotic medications. *N Engl J Med.* 2005;353:2335–2341.

165. Chen WY, Chen LY, Liu HC, et al. Antipsychotic medications and stroke in schizophrenia: a case-crossover study. *PLoS One.* 2017;12(6):e0179424.
166. Hsieh PH, Hsiao FY, Gau CS. Use of antipsychotics and risk of cerebrovascular events in schizophrenic patients: a nested case-control study. *J Clin Psychopharmacol.* 2013;33:299–305.
167. Food and Drug Administration. FDA public health advisory: deaths with antipsychotics in elderly patients with behavioral disturbances. http://psychrights.org/Drugs/FDAatypicalswarning4elderly.pdf. Accessed August 7, 2018.
168. Herrmann N, Lanctot KL. Do atypical antipsychotics cause stroke? *CNS Drugs.* 2005;19:91–103.
169. Hasan A, Falkai P, Wobrock T, et al. World Federation of Societies of Biological Psychiatry (WFSBP) guidelines for biological treatment of schizophrenia, part 2: update 2012 on the long-term treatment of schizophrenia and management of antipsychotic induced side-effects. *World J Biol Psychiatry.* 2013;14:2–44.
170. Bogers JPAM, Schulte PFJ, Van Dijk D. Clozapine underutilization in the treatment of schizophrenia: how can clozapine prescription rates be improved? *J Clin Psychopharmacology.* 2016;36(2):109–111.
171. Sanders K, McLean AJ, Adair DK, Hepburn B, Sims B. Clozapine underutilization: addressing the barriers 2016. https://www.nasmhpd.org/sites/default/files/Assessment%201_Clozapine%20Underutilization.pdf. Accessed August 7, 2018.
172. Stanton RJ, Paxos C, Geldenhuys WJ, Boss JL. Clozapine underutilization in treatment-resistant schizophrenia. *Ment Health Clin.* 2015;5(2)63–67.
173. Hill M, Freudenreich O. Clozapine: key discussion points for prescribers. *Clin Schizophr Relat Psychoses.* 2013;6(4):177–185.
174. Alvir JJ, Lieberman JA, Safferman AZ, et al. Clozapine-induced agranulocytosis-incidence and risk factors in the United States. *N Engl J Med.* 1993;329:162–167.
175. Lally J, Flanagan RJ. Severe neutropenia and agranulocytosis. In: *Life-Threatening Effects of Antipsychotic Drugs.* Cambridge, MA: Academic Press; 2016:105.
176. Raja M, Raja S. Clozapine safety, 40 years later. *Curr Drug Saf.* 2014;9:163–195.
177. Food and Drug Administration. FDA drug safety communication: FDA modifies monitoring for neutropenia associated with schizophrenia medicine clozapine; approves new shared REMS program for all clozapine medicines. http://www.fda.gov/Drugs/DrugSafety/ucm461853.htm. Accessed August 7, 2018.
178. Haddy TB, Rana SR, Castro O. Benign ethnic neutropenia: what is a normal absolute neutrophil count? *J Lab Clin Med.* 1999;133:15–22.
179. Thobakgale CF, Ndung'u T. Neutrophil counts in persons of African origin. *Curr Opin Hematol.* 2014;21:50–57.
180. Manu P, Sarvaiya N, Rogozea LM, Kane JM, Correll CU. Benign ethnic neutropenia and clozapine use: a systematic review of the evidence and treatment recommendations. *J Clin Psychiatry.* 2016;77:e909-e916.
181. Wilson MP, Chen N, Vilke GM, Castillo EM, MacDonald KS, Minassian A. Olanzapine in ED patients: differential effects on oxygenation in patients with alcohol intoxication. *Am J Emerg Med.* 2012;30:1196–1202.
182. Bitter R, Bemler TL, Opler L. Safety evaluation of the concomitant use of clozapine and benzodiazepines: a retrospective, cross-sectional chart review. *J Psych Pract.* 2008;14:265–270.
183. Wilson MP, MacDonald K, Vilke GM, Feifel D. Potential complications of combining intramuscular olanzapine with benzodiazepines in emergency department patients. *J Emerg Med.* 2012;43:889–896.
184. Williams AM, Park SH. Seizure associated with clozapine: incidence, etiology, and management. *CNS Drugs.* 2015;62:345–354.
185. Alper K, Schwartz KA, Kolts RL, Khan A. Seizure incidence in psychopharmacological clinical trials: an analysis of Food and Drug Administration (FDA) summary basis of approval reports. *Biol Psychiatry.* 2007;62:345–354.
186. Marks RC, Luchins DJ. Antipsychotic medications and seizures. *Psychol Med.* 1991;9(1):37–52.
187. Pisani F, Oteri G, Costa C, DiRaimondo G, DiPerri R. Effects of psychotropic drugs on the seizure threshold. *Drug Saf.* 2002;25(2):91–110.
188. Citrome L, McEvoy JP, Saklad SR. A guide to the management of clozapine-related tolerability and safety concerns. *Clin Schizophr Relat Psychoses.* 2016;10:163–177.
189. Sprague DA, Loewen PS, Raymond CB. Selection of atypical antipsychotics for the management of schizophrenia. *Ann Pharmacother.* 2004;38:313–319.
190. Correll CU, Canas F, Larmo I, et al. Individualizing antipsychotic treatment selection in schizophrenia: characteristics of empirically derived patient subgroups. *Eur Psychiatry.* 2011;26:3–16.
191. Heres SI, Schmitz FS, Leucht S. The attitude of patients towards antipsychotic depot treatment. *Int Clin Psychopharmacol.* 2007;22(5):275–282.
192. Patel MX, De Zoysa N, Bernadt M, David A. Depot and oral antipsychotics: patient preferences and attitudes are not the same thing. *J Psychopharmacol.* 2009;23:789–796.
193. San L, Casillas M, Ciudad A, Gilaberte I. Olanzapine orally disintegrating tablet: a review of efficacy and compliance. *CNS Neurosci Ther.* 2008;14:203–214.
194. Love RC, Conley RR, Kelly DL, et al. A dose-outcome analysis of risperidone. *J Clin Psychiatry.* 1999;60: 771–775.
195. Citrome L, Jaffe A, Levine J, Lindenmayer JP. Dosing of quetiapine in schizophrenia: how clinical practice differs from registration studies. *J Clin Psychiatry.* 2005;66:1512–1516.
196. Citrome L, Jaffe A, Levine J. How dosing of ziprasidone in a state hospital system differs from product labeling. *J Clin Psychiatry.* 2009;70:975–982.
197. Gejman PV, Sanders AR, Duan J. The role of genetics in the etiology of schizophrenia. *Psychiatr Clin North Am.* 2016;33:35–66.
198. Marcus SC, Zummo J, Pettit AR, et al. Antipsychotic adherence and rehospitalization in schizophrenia patients receiving oral versus long-acting injectable

antipsychotics following hospital discharge. *J Manag Care Spec Pharm.* 2015;21:754–768.

199. Beresford R, Ward A. Haloperidol decanoate: a preliminary review of its pharmacodynamic and pharmacokinetic properties and therapeutic use in psychosis. *Drugs.* 1987:33;31–49.
200. Correll CU, Citrome L, Haddad PM, et al. The use of long-acting injectable antipsychotics in schizophrenia: evaluating the evidence. *J Clin Psychiatry.* 2016;77(suppl 3):1–24.
201. Samara MT, Leucht C, Leeflang MM, et al. Early improvement as a predictor of later response to antipsychotics in schizophrenia: a diagnostic test review. *Am J Psychiatry.* 2015;172:617–629.
202. Marder SR, Essock SM, Miller AL, et al. Physical health monitoring of patients with schizophrenia. *Am J Psychiatry.* 2004;161:1334–1349.
203. Spina E, Avenoso A, Facciola G, et al. Relationship between plasma concentrations of clozapine and norclozapine and therapeutic response in patients with schizophrenia resistant to conventional neuroleptics. *Psychopharmacol (Berl).* 2000;148:83–89.
204. Kronig MH, Munne RA, Szymanski S, et al. Plasma clozapine levels and clinical response for treatment refractory schizophrenic patients. *Am J Psychiatry.* 1995;152:179–182.
205. Gaertner I. Gaertner HJ, Vonthein R, et al. Therapeutic drug monitoring of clozapine in relapse prevention: a five-year prospective study. *J Clin Psychopharmacol.* 2001;21:305–310.
206. Xiang YQ, Zhang, ZJ, Weng YZ, et al. Serum concentrations of clozapine and norclozapine in the prediction of relapse of patients with schizophrenia. *Schizophr Res.* 2006;83:201–210.
207. Miller BJ, Culpepper N, Rapaport MH, Buckley P. Prenatal inflammation and neurodevelopment in schizophrenia: a review of human studies. *Prog Neuropsychopharmacol Biol Psychiatry.* 2013;42:92 100.
208. Lee KW, Woon PS, Teo YY, Sim K. Genome wide studies (GWAS) and copy number variation (CNV) studies of the major psychoses: what have we learnt? *Neurosci Biobehav Rev.* 2012:36:556–571.
209. Xu Q, Wu X, Xiong Y, Xing Q, He L, Qin S. Pharmacogenomics can improve antipsychotic treatment in schizophrenia. *Front Med.* 2013;7(2):180–190.
210. Meltzer HY. Treatment resistant schizophrenia-the role of clozapine. *Curr Med Res Opin.* 1999;14(1)1–20.
211. Kirchheiner J, Nickchen K, Bauer M, et al. Pharmacogenetics of antidepressants and antipsychotics: the contribution of allelic variations to the phenotype of drug response. *Mol Psychiatry.* 2004;9(5):442–473.
212. Eum S, Lee Am, Bishop JR. Pharmacogenetic tests for antipsychotic medications: clinical implications and considerations. *Dialogues Clin Neurosci.* 2016;18:323–337.
213. Drozda K, Muller DJ, Bishop JR. Pharmacogenomic testing for neuropsychiatric drugs: current status of drug labeling, guidelines for using genetic information, and test options. *Pharmacotherapy.* 2014;34(2):166–184.
214. Carbon M, Correll CU. Thinking and acting beyond the positive: the role of the cognitive and negative symptoms in schizophrenia. *CNS Spectr.* 2004;19(suppl S1):38–52.
215. Kitchen H, Rofail D, Heron L, Sacco P. Cognitive impairment associated with schizophrenia: a review of the humanistic burden. *Adv Ther.* 2012;29:148–162.
216. Foussias G, Agid O, Fervaha G, Remington G. Negative symptoms of schizophrenia: clinical features, relevance to real world functioning and specificity versus other CNS disorders. *Eur Neuropsychopharmacol.* 2014;24:693–709.
217. Mueser KT, Deavers F, Penn DL, Cassisi JE. Psychosocial treatments for schizophrenia. *Ann Rev Clin Psychol.* 2013;9:465–497.
218. Rabinowirz J, Lichtenberg P, Kaplan Z, et al. Rehospitalization rates of chronically ill schizophrenic patients discharged on a regimen of risperidone, olanzapine, or conventional antipsychotics. *Am J Psychiatry.* 2001;158: 266–269.
219. Csernansky JG, Mahmoud R, Brenner R. A comparison of risperidone and haloperidol for the prevention of relapse in patients with schizophrenia. *N Engl J Med.* 2002;346:16–22.
220. Palmer BA, Pankratz VS, Bostwick JM. The lifetime risk of suicide in schizophrenia: a reexamination. *Arch Gen Psychiatry.* 2005;62:247–253.
221. Meltzer HY, Okayli G. Reduction of suicidality during clozapine treatment of neuroleptic- resistant schizophrenia: impact on risk-benefit assessment. *Am J Psychiatry.* 1995; 152:183–190.
222. Relling MV, Klein TE. CPIC: Clinical Pharmacogenetics Implementation Consortium of the Pharmacogenomics Research Network. *Clin Pharmacol Ther.* 2011;89:464–471.
223. Bank PCD, Caudle KE, Swen JJ, et al. Comparison of the guidelines of the Clinical Pharmacogenetics Implementation Consortium and the Dutch Pharmacogenomics Working Group. *Clin Pharmacol Ther.* 2018;103:595–618.
224. Abilify [prescribing information]. Princeton, NJ: Otsuka Pharmaceutical Co; 2014.
225. Abilify Maintena [prescribing information]. Princeton, NJ: Otsuka Pharmaceutical Co; 2013.
226. Clozaril [prescribing information]. Rosemount, PA; HLS Therapeutics; 2017.
227. Fanapt [prescribing information]. Rockville, MD; Vanda Pharmaceuticals; 2009.
228. Risperidal [prescribing information]. Titusville, NJ; Janssen Pharmaceuticals; 2003.
229. Dutch Pharmacogenomics Working Group. PharmGKB search engine. https://www.pharmgkb.org/. Accessed August 7, 2018.

Developed through the ASHP Council on Therapeutics and approved by the ASHP Board of Directors on September 27, 2018. This document supersedes the ASHP therapeutic position statement on the use of second-generation antipsychotic medications in the treatment of adults with psychotic disorders approved by the ASHP Board of Directors on June 24, 2006.

The following organizations and individuals are acknowledged for reviewing draft versions of this statement: Candis M. Morello, PharmD, CDE, FASHP; Roberta J Wong, PharmD, FASHP, FCSHP; Randy Kuiper, PharmD, BCPS, FASHP; Ian R. McGrane, PharmD, BCPS, BCPP; Amy Werremeyer, PharmD, BCPP; Charles A.

Reynolds, PharmD, BCPP; Jarvin Enosh T. Tan, RPh; Stepan Uhlyar, PharmD; Austin De La Cruz, PharmD, BCPP; Jody Jacobson Wedret, RPh, FASHP, FCSHP; James Rinehart, RPh, MS, FASHP; Brittany Finocchio, PharmD, BCPP; Edna Patatanian, PharmD; Christopher W. Ellison, PharmD, BCPS; Erika Tillery, PharmD, BCPP, BCGP; American Pharmacists Association; and Academy of Managed Care Pharmacy.

Jason M. Noel, PharmD, BCPP, University of Maryland School of Pharmacy, Baltimore, MD.

Cherry W. Jackson, PharmD, BCPP, FASHP, FCCP, Auburn University Harrison School of Pharmacy, Auburn, AL, and Department of Psychiatry and Behavioral Neurobiology, University of Alabama, Birmingham, School of Medicine, Birmingham, AL.

Copyright © 2020, American Society of Health-System Pharmacists, Inc. All rights reserved. Contact ASHP for reprint and permissions requests. This content may not be used for commercial purposes without the express written consent of ASHP.

The bibliographic citation for this document is as follows: American Society of Health-System Pharmacists. ASHP therapeutic position statement on the use of antipsychotic medications in the treatment of adults with schizophrenia and schizoaffective disorder. *Am J Health-Syst Pharm.* 2020;77:2114–2132.

ASHP
Therapeutic Guidelines

DOI 10.37573/9781585287048

Clinical Practice Guidelines for Antimicrobial Prophylaxis in Surgery

These guidelines were developed jointly by the American Society of Health-System Pharmacists (ASHP), the Infectious Diseases Society of America (IDSA), the Surgical Infection Society (SIS), and the Society for Healthcare Epidemiology of America (SHEA). This work represents an update to the previously published ASHP Therapeutic Guidelines on Antimicrobial Prophylaxis in Surgery,[1] as well as guidelines from IDSA and SIS.[2,3] The guidelines are intended to provide practitioners with a standardized approach to the rational, safe, and effective use of antimicrobial agents for the prevention of surgical-site infections (SSIs) based on currently available clinical evidence and emerging issues.

Prophylaxis refers to the prevention of an infection and can be characterized as primary prophylaxis, secondary prophylaxis, or eradication. Primary prophylaxis refers to the prevention of an initial infection. Secondary prophylaxis refers to the prevention of recurrence or reactivation of a preexisting infection. Eradication refers to the elimination of a colonized organism to prevent the development of an infection. These guidelines focus on primary perioperative prophylaxis.

Guidelines Development and Use

Members of ASHP, IDSA, SIS, and SHEA were appointed to serve on an expert panel established to ensure the validity, reliability, and utility of the revised guidelines. The work of the panel was facilitated by faculty of the University of Pittsburgh School of Pharmacy and University of Pittsburgh Medical Center Drug Use and Disease State Management Program who served as contract researchers and writers for the project. Panel members and contractors were required to disclose any possible conflicts of interest before their appointment and throughout the guideline development process. Drafted documents for each surgical procedural section were reviewed by the expert panel and, once revised, were available for public comment on the ASHP website. After additional revisions were made to address reviewer comments, the final document was approved by the expert panel and the boards of directors of the above-named organizations.

Strength of Evidence and Grading of Recommendations. The primary literature from the previous ASHP Therapeutic Guidelines on Antimicrobial Prophylaxis in Surgery[1] was reviewed together with the primary literature published between the date of the previous guidelines, 1999, and June 2010, identified by searches of MEDLINE, EMBASE, and the Cochrane Database of Systematic Reviews. Particular attention was paid to study design, with greatest credence given to randomized, controlled, double-blind studies. There is a limited number of adequately powered randomized controlled trials evaluating the efficacy of antimicrobial prophylaxis in surgical procedures. Guidelines development included consideration of the following characteristics: validity, reliability, clinical applicability, flexibility, clarity, and a multidisciplinary nature as consistent with ASHP's philosophy on therapeutic guidelines.[4] The limitations of the evidence base are noted within each individual procedure section of the guidelines. Published guidelines with recommendations by experts in a procedure area (e.g., American College of Obstetricians and Gynecologists [ACOG]) and noted general guidelines (e.g., Centers for Disease Control and Prevention [CDC], Scottish Intercollegiate Guidelines Network, *Medical Letter*, SIS, SHEA/IDSA) were also considered.[2,3,5–11]

DOI 10.37573/9781585287048.113

Recommendations for the use of antimicrobial prophylaxis are graded according to the strength of evidence available. The strength of evidence represents only support for or against prophylaxis and does not apply to the antimicrobial agent, dose, or dosage regimen. Studies supporting the recommendations for the use of antimicrobial therapy were classified as follows:

- Level I (evidence from large, well-conducted, randomized, controlled clinical trials or a meta-analysis)
- Level II (evidence from small, well-conducted, randomized, controlled clinical trials)
- Level III (evidence from well-conducted cohort studies)
- Level IV (evidence from well-conducted case–control studies)
- Level V (evidence from uncontrolled studies that were not well conducted)
- Level VI (conflicting evidence that tends to favor the recommendation)
- Level VII (expert opinion or data extrapolated from evidence for general principles and other procedures)

This system has been used by the Agency for Healthcare Research and Quality, and ASHP, IDSA, SIS, and SHEA support it as an acceptable method for organizing strength of evidence for a variety of therapeutic or diagnostic recommendations.[4] Each recommendation was categorized according to the strength of evidence that supports the use or nonuse of antimicrobial prophylaxis as category A (levels I–III), category B (levels IV–VI), or category C (level VII).

When higher-level data are not available, a category C recommendation represents a consensus of expert panel members based on their clinical experience, extrapolation from other procedures with similar microbial or other clinical features, and available published literature. In these cases, the expert panel also extrapolated general principles and evidence from other procedures. Some recommendations include alternative approaches in situations in which panel member opinions were divided.

A major limitation of the available literature on antimicrobial prophylaxis is the difficulty in establishing significant differences in efficacy between prophylactic antimicrobial agents and controls (including placebo, no treatment, or other antimicrobial agents) due to study design and low SSI rates for most procedures. A small sample size increases the likelihood of a Type II error; therefore, there may be no apparent difference between the antimicrobial agent and placebo when in fact the antimicrobial has a beneficial effect.[12] A valid study is placebo controlled and randomized with a sufficient sample in each group to avoid a Type II error. Of note, prophylaxis is recommended in some cases due to the severity of complications of postoperative infection (e.g., an infected device that is not easily removable) necessitating precautionary measures despite the lack of statistical support.

Summary of Key Updates. These guidelines reflect substantial changes from the guidelines published in 1999.[1] Highlights of those changes are outlined here.

Preoperative-dose timing. The optimal time for administration of preoperative doses is within 60 minutes before surgical incision. This is a more-specific time frame than the previously recommended time, which was "at induction of anesthesia." Some agents, such as fluoroquinolones and vancomycin, require administration over one to two hours; therefore, the administration of these agents should begin within 120 minutes before surgical incision.

Selection and dosing. Information is included regarding the approach to weight-based dosing in obese patients and the need for repeat doses during prolonged procedures.[13–18] Obesity has been linked to an increased risk for SSI. The pharmacokinetics of drugs may be altered in obese patients, so dosage adjustments based on body weight may be warranted in these patients. For all patients, intraoperative redosing is needed to ensure adequate serum and tissue concentrations of the antimicrobial if the duration of the procedure exceeds two half-lives of the drug or there is excessive blood loss during the procedure (**Table 1**). Recommendations for selection of antimicrobial agents for specific surgical procedures and alternative agents (e.g., for patients with allergies to β-lactam antimicrobials) are provided in **Table 2**.

Duration of prophylaxis. New recommendations for a shortened postoperative course of antimicrobials involving a single dose or continuation for less than 24 hours are provided. Further clarity on the lack of need for postoperative antimicrobial prophylaxis based on the presence of indwelling drains and intravascular catheters is included.

Common principles. A section addressing concepts that apply to all types of surgical procedures has been added. Expanded and new recommendations are provided for plastic, urology, cardiac, and thoracic procedures, as well as clarity on prophylaxis when implantable devices are inserted. The latest information on the use of mupirocin and on the role of vancomycin in surgical prophylaxis is summarized in these updated guidelines.

Application of Guidelines to Clinical Practice. Recommendations are provided for adult (age 19 years or older) and pediatric (age 1–18 years) patients. These guidelines do not specifically address newborn (premature and full-term) infants. While the guidelines do not address all concerns for patients with renal or hepatic dysfunction, antimicrobial prophylaxis often does not need to be modified for these patients when given as a single preoperative dose before surgical incision.

The recommendations herein may not be appropriate for use in all clinical situations. Decisions to follow these recommendations must be based on the judgment of the clinician and consideration of individual patient circumstances and available resources.

These guidelines reflect current knowledge of antimicrobial prophylaxis in surgery. Given the dynamic nature of scientific information and technology, periodic review, updating, and revisions are to be expected.

Special Patient Populations. *Pediatric patients.* Pediatric patients undergo a number of procedures similar to adults that may warrant antimicrobial prophylaxis. Although pediatric-specific prophylaxis data are sparse, available data have been evaluated and are presented in some of the procedure-specific sections of these guidelines. Selection of antimicrobial prophylactic agents mirrors that in adult guidelines, with the agents of choice being first- and second-generation cephalosporins, reserving the use of vancomycin for patients with documented β-lactam allergies.[19,20] While the use of a penicillin with a β-lactamase inhibitor in combination with cefazolin or vancomycin and gentamicin has also been studied in pediatric patients, the number of patients included in these evaluations remains small.[20–23] As with adults, there is little evidence supporting the use of vancomycin, alone or in combination with other antimicrobials, for routine perioperative antimicrobial prophylaxis in institutions that have a high prevalence of methicillin-resistant *Staphylococcus aureus* (MRSA). Vancomycin may be considered in children known to be colonized with MRSA and, in one retrospective historical cohort study, was shown to decrease MRSA infections.[21] Mupirocin use has been studied in and is efficacious in children colonized with MRSA, but there are limited data supporting its use perioperatively.[24–30] However, there is little reason to think that the impact and effect would be any different in children, so its use may be justified. Additional studies in this setting are needed to establish firm guidelines.

Unless noted in specific sections, all recommendations for adults are the same for pediatric patients, except for dosing. In most cases, the data in pediatric patients are limited and have been extrapolated from adult data; therefore, nearly all pediatric recommendations are based on expert opinion. In some sections, pediatric efficacy data do not exist and thus are not addressed in these guidelines. Fluoroquinolones should not be routinely used for surgical prophylaxis in pediatric patients because of the potential for toxicity in this population. The same principle of preoperative dosing within 60 minutes before incision has been applied to pediatric patients.[20–23] Additional intraoperative dosing may be needed if the duration of the procedure exceeds two half-lives of the antimicrobial agent or there is excessive blood loss during the procedure.[19,21] As with adult patients, single-dose prophylaxis is usually sufficient. If antimicrobial prophylaxis is continued postoperatively, the duration should be less than 24 hours, regardless of the presence of intravascular catheters or indwelling drains.[19,22,23,31,32] There are sufficient pharmacokinetic studies of most agents to recommend pediatric dosages that provide adequate systemic exposure and, presumably, efficacy comparable to that demonstrated in adults. Therefore, the pediatric dosages provided in these guidelines are based largely on pharmacokinetic data and the extrapolation of adult efficacy data to pediatric patients. Because few clinical trials have been conducted in pediatric surgical patients, strength of evidence criteria have not been applied to these recommendations. With few exceptions (e.g., aminoglycoside dosages), pediatric dosages should not exceed the maximum adult recommended dosages. Generally, if dosages are calculated on a milligram-per-kilogram basis for children weighing more than 40 kg, the calculated dosage will exceed the maximum recommended dosage for adults; adult dosages should therefore be used.

TABLE 1.

Recommended Doses and Redosing Intervals for Commonly Used Antimicrobials for Surgical Prophylaxis

	Recommended Dose			
Antimicrobial	Adults[a]	Pediatrics[b]	Half-life in Adults With Normal Renal Function, hr[19]	Recommended Redosing Interval (From Initiation of Preoperative Dose), hr[c]
Ampicillin–sulbactam	3 g (ampicillin 2 g/ sulbactam 1 g)	50 mg/kg of the ampicillin component	0.8–1.3	2
Ampicillin	2 g	50 mg/kg	1–1.9	2
Aztreonam	2 g	30 mg/kg	1.3–2.4	4
Cefazolin	2 g, 3 g for pts weighing ≥120 kg	30 mg/kg	1.2–2.2	4
Cefuroxime	1.5 g	50 mg/kg	1–2	4
Cefotaxime	1 g[d]	50 mg/kg	0.9–1.7	3
Cefoxitin	2 g	40 mg/kg	0.7–1.1	2
Cefotetan	2 g	40 mg/kg	2.8–4.6	6
Ceftriaxone	2 g[e]	50–75 mg/kg	5.4–10.9	NA
Ciprofloxacin[f]	400 mg	10 mg/kg	3–7	NA
Clindamycin	900 mg	10 mg/kg	2–4	6
Ertapenem	1 g	15 mg/kg	3–5	NA
Fluconazole	400 mg	6 mg/kg	30	NA
Gentamicin[g]	5 mg/kg based on dosing weight (single dose)	2.5 mg/kg based on dosing weight	2–3	NA
Levofloxacin[f]	500 mg	10 mg/kg	6–8	NA
Metronidazole	500 mg	15 mg/kg Neonates weighing <1200 g should receive a single 7.5-mg/kg dose	6–8	NA
Moxifloxacin[f]	400 mg	10 mg/kg	8–15	NA
Piperacillin–tazobactam	3.375 g	Infants 2–9 mo: 80 mg/kg of the piperacillin component Children >9 mo and ≤40 kg: 100 mg/kg of the piperacillin component	0.7–1.2	2
Vancomycin	15 mg/kg	15 mg/kg	4–8	NA
Oral antibiotics for colorectal surgery prophylaxis (used in conjunction with a mechanical bowel preparation)				
Erythromycin base	1 g	20 mg/kg	0.8–3	NA
Metronidazole	1 g	15 mg/kg	6–10	NA
Neomycin	1 g	15 mg/kg	2–3 (3% absorbed under normal gastrointestinal conditions)	NA

[a]Adult doses are obtained from the studies cited in each section. When doses differed between studies, expert opinion used the most-often recommended dose.

[b]The maximum pediatric dose should not exceed the usual adult dose.

[c]For antimicrobials with a short half-life (e.g., cefazolin, cefoxitin) used before long procedures, redosing in the operating room is recommended at an interval of approximately two times the half-life of the agent in patients with normal renal function. Recommended redosing intervals marked as "not applicable" (NA) are based on typical case length; for unusually long procedures, redosing may be needed.

[d]Although FDA-approved package insert labeling indicates 1 g,14 experts recommend 2 g for obese patients.

[e]When used as a single dose in combination with metronidazole for colorectal procedures.

[f]While fluoroquinolones have been associated with an increased risk of tendinitis/tendon rupture in all ages, use of these agents for single-dose prophylaxis is generally safe.

[g]In general, gentamicin for surgical antibiotic prophylaxis should be limited to a single dose given preoperatively. Dosing is based on the patient's actual body weight. If the patient's actual weight is more than 20% above ideal body weight (IBW), the dosing weight (DW) can be determined as follows: DW = IBW + 0.4(actual weight – IBW).

TABLE 2.

Recommendations for Surgical Antimicrobial Prophylaxis

Type of Procedure	Recommended Agents[a,b]	Alternative Agents in Patients with β-Lactam Allergy	Strength of Evidence[c]
Cardiac			
Coronary artery bypass	Cefazolin, cefuroxime	Clindamycin,[d] vancomycin[d]	A
Cardiac device insertion procedures (e.g., pacemaker implantation)	Cefazolin, cefuroxime	Clindamycin, vancomycin	A
Ventricular assist devices	Cefazolin, cefuroxime	Clindamycin, vancomycin	C
Thoracic			
Noncardiac procedures, including lobectomy, pneumonectomy, lung resection, and thoracotomy	Cefazolin, ampicillin–sulbactam	Clindamycin,[d] vancomycin[d]	A
Video-assisted thoracoscopic surgery	Cefazolin, ampicillin–sulbactam	Clindamycin,[d] vancomycin[d]	C
Gastroduodenale			
Procedures involving entry into lumen of gastrointestinal tract (bariatric, pancreaticoduodenectomy[f])	Cefazolin	Clindamycin or vancomycin + aminoglycoside[g] or aztreonam or fluoroquinolone[h-j]	A
Procedures without entry into gastrointestinal tract (antireflux, highly selective vagotomy) for high-risk patients	Cefazolin	Clindamycin or vancomycin + aminoglycoside[g] or aztreonam or fluoroquinolone[h-j]	A
Biliary tract			
Open procedure	Cefazolin, cefoxitin, cefotetan, ceftriaxone,[k] ampicillin–sulbactam[h]	Clindamycin or vancomycin + aminoglycoside[g] or aztreonam or fluoroquinolone[h-j] Metronidazole + aminoglycoside[g] or fluoroquinolone[h-j]	A
Laparoscopic procedure			
Elective, low-risk[l]	None	None	A
Elective, high-risk[l]	Cefazolin, cefoxitin, cefotetan, ceftriaxone,[k] ampicillin–sulbactam[h]	Clindamycin or vancomycin + aminoglycoside[g] or aztreonam or fluoroquinolone[h-j] Metronidazole + aminoglycoside[g] or fluoroquinolone[h-j]	A
Appendectomy for uncomplicated appendicitis	Cefoxitin, cefotetan, cefazolin + metronidazole	Clindamycin + aminoglycoside[g] or aztreonam or fluoroquinolone[h-j] Metronidazole + aminoglycoside[g] or fluoroquinolone[h-j]	A
Small intestine			
Nonobstructed	Cefazolin	Clindamycin + aminoglycoside[g] or aztreonam or fluoroquinolone[h-j]	C
Obstructed	Cefazolin + metronidazole, cefoxitin, cefotetan	Metronidazole + aminoglycoside[g] or fluoroquinolone[h-j]	C
Hernia repair (hernioplasty and herniorrhaphy)	Cefazolin	Clindamycin, vancomycin	A

Continued on next page

TABLE 2. ***(continued)***

Type of Procedure	Recommended Agents[a,b]	Alternative Agents in Patients with β-Lactam Allergy	Strength of Evidence[c]
Colorectal[m]	Cefazolin + metronidazole, cefoxitin, cefotetan, ampicillin–sulbactam,[h] ceftriaxone + metronidazole,[n] ertapenem	Clindamycin + aminoglycoside[g] or aztreonam or fluoroquinolone[h-j] metronidazole + aminoglycoside[g] or fluoroquinolone[h-j]	A
Head and neck			
Clean	None	None	B
Clean with placement of prosthesis (excludes tympanostomy tubes)	Cefazolin, cefuroxime	Clindamycin[d]	C
Clean-contaminated cancer surgery	Cefazolin + metronidazole, cefuroxime + metronidazole, ampicillin–sulbactam	Clindamycin[d]	A
Other clean-contaminated procedures with the exception of tonsillectomy and functional endoscopic sinus procedures	Cefazolin + metronidazole, cefuroxime + metronidazole, ampicillin–sulbactam	Clindamycin[d]	B
Neurosurgery			
Elective craniotomy and cerebrospinal fluid-shunting procedures	Cefazolin	Clindamycin,[d] vancomycin[d]	A
Implantation of intrathecal pumps	Cefazolin	Clindamycin,[d] vancomycin[d]	C
Cesarean delivery	Cefazolin	Clindamycin + aminoglycoside[g]	A
Hysterectomy (vaginal or abdominal)	Cefazolin, cefotetan, cefoxitin, ampicillin–sulbactam[h]	Clindamycin or vancomycin + aminoglycoside[g] or aztreonam or fluoroquinolone[h-j] Metronidazole + aminoglycoside[g] or fluoroquinolone[h-j]	A
Ophthalmic	Topical neomycin–polymyxin B–gramicidin or fourth-generation topical fluoroquinolones (gatifloxacin or moxifloxacin) given as 1 drop every 5–15 min for 5 doses[o] Addition of cefazolin 100 mg by subconjunctival injection or intracameral cefazolin 1–2.5 mg or cefuroxime 1 mg at the end of procedure is optional	None	B
Orthopedic			
Clean operations involving hand, knee, or foot and not involving implantation of foreign materials	None	None	C
Spinal procedures with and without instrumentation	Cefazolin	Clindamycin,[d] vancomycin[d]	A
Hip fracture repair	Cefazolin	Clindamycin,[d] vancomycin[d]	A

TABLE 2. *(continued)*

Type of Procedure	Recommended Agents[a,b]	Alternative Agents in Patients with β-Lactam Allergy	Strength of Evidence[c]
Implantation of internal fixation devices (e.g., nails, screws, plates, wires)	Cefazolin	Clindamycin,[d] vancomycin[d]	C
Total joint replacement	Cefazolin	Clindamycin,[d] vancomycin[d]	A
Urologic			
Lower tract instrumentation with risk factors for infection (includes transrectal prostate biopsy)	Fluoroquinolone,[h-j] trimethoprim–sulfamethoxazole, cefazolin	Aminoglycoside[g] with or without clindamycin	A
Clean without entry into urinary tract	Cefazolin (the addition of a single dose of an aminoglycoside may be recommended for placement of prosthetic material [e.g., penile prosthesis])	Clindamycin,[d] vancomycin[d]	A
Involving implanted prosthesis	Cefazolin ± aminoglycoside, cefazolin ± aztreonam, ampicillin–sulbactam	Clindamycin ± aminoglycoside or aztreonam, vancomycin ± aminoglycoside or aztreonam	A
Clean with entry into urinary tract	Cefazolin (the addition of a single dose of an aminoglycoside may be recommended for placement of prosthetic material [e.g., penile prosthesis])	Fluoroquinolone,[h-j] aminoglycoside[g] with or without clindamycin	A
Clean-contaminated	Cefazolin + metronidazole, cefoxitin	Fluoroquinolone,[h-j] aminoglycoside[g] + metronidazole or clindamycin	A
Vascular[p]	Cefazolin	Clindamycin,[d] vancomycin[d]	A
Heart, lung, heart–lung transplantation[q]			
Heart transplantation[r]	Cefazolin	Clindamycin,[d] vancomycin[d]	A (based on cardiac procedures)
Lung and heart–lung transplantation[r,s]	Cefazolin	Clindamycin,[d] vancomycin[d]	A (based on cardiac procedures)
Liver transplantation[q,t]	Piperacillin–tazobactam, cefotaxime + ampicillin	Clindamycin or vancomycin + aminoglycoside[g] or aztreonam or fluoroquinolone[h-j]	B
Pancreas and pancreas–kidney transplantation[r]	Cefazolin, fluconazole (for patients at high risk of fungal infection [e.g., those with enteric drainage of the pancreas])	Clindamycin or vancomycin + aminoglycoside[g] or aztreonam or fluoroquinolone[h-j]	A

Continued on next page

TABLE 2. ***(continued)***

Type of Procedure	Recommended Agents[a,b]	Alternative Agents in Patients with β-Lactam Allergy	Strength of Evidence[c]
Plastic surgery	Cefazolin	Clindamycin or vancomycin + aminoglycoside[g] or aztreonam or fluoroquinolone[h-j]	A
Clean with risk factors or clean-contaminated	Cefazolin, ampicillin–sulbactam	Clindamycin,[d] vancomycin[d]	C

[a]The antimicrobial agent should be started within 60 minutes before surgical incision (120 minutes for vancomycin or fluoroquinolones). While single-dose prophylaxis is usually sufficient, the duration of prophylaxis for all procedures should be less than 24 hours. If an agent with a short half-life is used (e.g., cefazolin, cefoxitin), it should be readministered if the procedure duration exceeds the recommended redosing interval (from the time of initiation of the preoperative dose [see Table 1]). Readministration may also be warranted if prolonged or excessive bleeding occurs or if there are other factors that may shorten the half-life of the prophylactic agent (e.g., extensive burns). Readministration may not be warranted in patients in whom the half-life of the agent may be prolonged (e.g., patients with renal insufficiency or failure).

[b]For patients known to be colonized with methicillin-resistant *Staphylococcus aureus*, it is reasonable to add a single preoperative dose of vancomycin to the recommended agent(s).

[c]Strength of evidence that supports the use or nonuse of prophylaxis is classified as A (levels I–III), B (levels IV–VI), or C (level VII). Level I evidence is from large, well-conducted, randomized controlled clinical trials. Level II evidence is from small, well-conducted, randomized controlled clinical trials. Level III evidence is from well-conducted cohort studies. Level IV evidence is from well-conducted case–control studies. Level V evidence is from uncontrolled studies that were not well conducted. Level VI evidence is conflicting evidence that tends to favor the recommendation. Level VII evidence is expert opinion.

[d]For procedures in which pathogens other than staphylococci and streptococci are likely, an additional agent with activity against those pathogens could be considered. For example, if there are surveillance data showing that gram-negative organisms are a cause of surgical-site infections (SSIs) for the procedure, practitioners may consider combining clindamycin or vancomycin with another agent (cefazolin if the patient is not β-lactam allergic; aztreonam, gentamicin, or single-dose fluoroquinolone if the patient is β-lactam allergic).

[e]Prophylaxis should be considered for patients at highest risk for postoperative gastroduodenal infections, such as those with increased gastric pH (e.g., those receiving histamine H_2-receptor antagonists or proton-pump inhibitors), gastroduodenal perforation, decreased gastric motility, gastric outlet obstruction, gastric bleeding, morbid obesity, or cancer. Antimicrobial prophylaxis may not be needed when the lumen of the intestinal tract is not entered.

[f]Consider additional antimicrobial coverage with infected biliary tract. See the biliary tract procedures section of this article.

[g]Gentamicin or tobramycin.

[h]Due to increasing resistance of *Escherichia coli* to fluoroquinolones and ampicillin–sulbactam, local population susceptibility profiles should be reviewed prior to use.

[i]Ciprofloxacin or levofloxacin.

[j]Fluoroquinolones are associated with an increased risk of tendonitis and tendon rupture in all ages. However, this risk would be expected to be quite small with single-dose antibiotic prophylaxis. Although the use of fluoroquinolones may be necessary for surgical antibiotic prophylaxis in some children, they are not drugs of first choice in the pediatric population due to an increased incidence of adverse events as compared with controls in some clinical trials.

[k]Ceftriaxone use should be limited to patients requiring antimicrobial treatment for acute cholecystitis or acute biliary tract infections which may not be determined prior to incision, not patients undergoing cholecystectomy for noninfected biliary conditions, including biliary colic or dyskinesia without infection.

[l]Factors that indicate a high risk of infectious complications in laparoscopic cholecystectomy include emergency procedures, diabetes, long procedure duration, intraoperative gallbladder rupture, age of >70 years, conversion from laparoscopic to open cholecystectomy, American Society of Anesthesiologists classification of 3 or greater, episode of colic within 30 days before the procedure, reintervention in less than one month for noninfectious complication, acute cholecystitis, bile spillage, jaundice, pregnancy, nonfunctioning gallbladder, immunosuppression, and insertion of prosthetic device. Because a number of these risk factors are not possible to determine before surgical intervention, it may be reasonable to give a single dose of antimicrobial prophylaxis to all patients undergoing laparoscopic cholecystectomy.

[m]For most patients, a mechanical bowel preparation combined with oral neomycin sulfate plus oral erythromycin base or with oral neomycin sulfate plus oral metronidazole should be given in addition to i.v. prophylaxis.

[n]Where there is increasing resistance to first- and second-generation cephalosporins among gram-negative isolates from SSIs, a single dose of ceftriaxone plus metronidazole may be preferred over the routine use of carbapenems.

[o]The necessity of continuing topical antimicrobials postoperatively has not been established.

[p]Prophylaxis is not routinely indicated for brachiocephalic procedures. Although there are no data in support, patients undergoing brachiocephalic procedures involving vascular prostheses or patch implantation (e.g., carotid endarterectomy) may benefit from prophylaxis.

[q]These guidelines reflect recommendations for perioperative antibiotic prophylaxis to prevent SSIs and do not provide recommendations for prevention of opportunistic infections in immunosuppressed transplantation patients (e.g., for antifungal or antiviral medications).

[r]Patients who have left-ventricular assist devices as a bridge and who are chronically infected might also benefit from coverage of the infecting microorganism.

[s]The prophylactic regimen may need to be modified to provide coverage against any potential pathogens, including gram-negative (e.g., *Pseudomonas aeruginosa*) or fungal organisms, isolated from the donor lung or the recipient before transplantation. Patients undergoing lung transplantation with negative pretransplantation cultures should receive antimicrobial prophylaxis as appropriate for other types of cardiothoracic surgeries. Patients undergoing lung transplantation for cystic fibrosis should receive 7–14 days of treatment with antimicrobials selected according to pretransplantation culture and susceptibility results. This treatment may include additional antibacterial or antifungal agents.

[t]The prophylactic regimen may need to be modified to provide coverage against any potential pathogens, including vancomycin-resistant enterococci, isolated from the recipient before transplantation.

Patients with prosthetic implants. For patients with existing prosthetic implants who undergo an invasive procedure, there is no evidence that antimicrobial prophylaxis prevents infections of the implant. However, updated guidelines from the American Heart Association (AHA) suggest that prophylaxis may be justified in a limited subset of patients for the prevention of endocarditis.[11]

Common Principles and Procedure-Specific Guidelines. The Common Principles section has been developed to provide information common to many surgical procedures. These principles are general recommendations based on currently available data at the time of publication that may change over time; therefore, these principles need to be applied with careful attention to each clinical situation. Detailed information pertinent to specific surgical procedures is included in the procedure-specific sections of these guidelines.

In addition to patient- and procedure-specific considerations, several institution-specific factors must be considered by practitioners before instituting these guidelines. The availability of antimicrobial agents at the institution may be restricted by local antimicrobial-use policy or lack of approval for use by regulatory authorities. Medications that are no longer available or not approved for use by the Food and Drug Administration (FDA) are so noted. Local resistance patterns should also be considered in selecting antimicrobial agents and are discussed in the colonization and resistance patterns section of the Common Principles section.

Requirements for Effective Surgical Prophylaxis

Appendix A lists the wound classification criteria currently used by the CDC National Healthcare Safety Network (NHSN) and Healthcare Infection Control Practices Advisory Committee (HICPAC).[33–35]

Criteria for defining an SSI have also been established by NHSN (**Appendix B**).[8,36] These definitions assist in evaluating the importance of providing antimicrobial prophylaxis and the potential consequences of infection, including the need for treatment. Some criteria vary slightly by procedure.

Although antimicrobial prophylaxis plays an important role in reducing the rate of SSIs, other factors such as attention to basic infection-control strategies,[37] the surgeon's experience and technique, the duration of the procedure, hospital and operating-room environments, instrument-sterilization issues, preoperative preparation (e.g., surgical scrub, skin antisepsis, appropriate hair removal), perioperative management (temperature and glycemic control), and the underlying medical condition of the patient may have a strong impact on SSI rates.[5,8] These guidelines recognize the importance of these other factors but do not include a discussion of or any recommendations regarding these issues beyond the optimal use of prophylactic antimicrobial agents. Patient-related factors associated with an increased risk of SSI include extremes of age, nutritional status, obesity, diabetes mellitus, tobacco use, coexistent remote body-site infections, altered immune response, corticosteroid therapy, recent surgical procedure, length of preoperative hospitalization, and colonization with microorganisms. Antimicrobial prophylaxis may be justified for any procedure if the patient has an underlying medical condition associated with a high risk of SSI or if the patient is immunocompromised (e.g., malnourished, neutropenic, receiving immunosuppressive agents).

Antimicrobial prophylaxis may be beneficial in surgical procedures associated with a high rate of infection (i.e., clean-contaminated or contaminated procedures) and in certain clean procedures where there are severe consequences of infection (e.g., prosthetic implants), even if infection is unlikely. While prophylactic antimicrobials are not indicated for some clean surgical procedures,[8] available data suggest that the relative risk reduction of SSI from the use of antimicrobial prophylaxis is the same in clean and in higher-risk procedures.[38] The decision to use prophylaxis depends on the cost of treating and the morbidity associated with infection compared with the cost and morbidity associated with using prophylaxis. Antimicrobial prophylaxis is justified for most clean-contaminated procedures. The use of antimicrobial agents for dirty procedures (Appendix A) or established infections is classified as treatment of presumed infection, not prophylaxis. See the procedure-specific sections for detailed recommendations.

Quality-Improvement Efforts. National, state, local, and institutional groups have developed and implemented collaborative efforts to improve the appropriateness of surgical antimicrobial prophylaxis. Various process and outcomes measures are employed, and results are disseminated. Institutional epidemiology and infection-control programs, state-based quality-improvement campaigns (e.g., the Michigan Surgical Quality Collaborative, the Washington State Surgical Clinical Outcomes Assessment Program[39,40]), CDC, NHSN, the National Surgical Quality Improvement Program, the Joint Commission, and the National Quality Forum have been instrumental in developing programs to prevent SSIs.

Over the past decade or more, several organizations, payers, and government agencies, including the Centers for Medicare and Medicaid Services (CMS), have established national quality improvement initiatives to further improve the safety and outcomes of health care, including surgery.[41–47] One area of focus in these initiatives for patients undergoing surgical procedures is the prevention of SSIs. The performance measures used, data collection and reporting requirements, and financial implications vary among the initiatives. The Surgical Care Improvement Project (SCIP) began in 2002 as the Surgical Infection Prevention (SIP) project, focusing on the timing, selection, and duration of prophylactic antimicrobial agents.[41,42] The SIP project was expanded to SCIP to include additional process measures surrounding patient safety and care during surgical procedures, including glucose control, venous thromboembolism prophylaxis, hair removal, and temperature control. Similar measures have been adopted by the Joint Commission.[43] The Physicians Quality Reporting System was established in 2006 to provide financial incentives to physicians meeting performance standards for quality measures, including surgery-related measures similar to those reported for SCIP and the Joint Commission.[44] Data are required to be collected by institutions and reported to payers.[42,44,46] Data for CMS and the Physicians Quality Reporting System measures are displayed on public websites to allow consumers to compare performance among hospitals. Institutional data collection and reporting are required, with financial incentives tied to performance to varying degrees, including payment for reporting, payment increases for meeting or exceeding minimum levels of performance, payment reduction for poor performance, and lack of payment for the development of surgical complications, such as mediastinitis.

Quality-improvement initiatives and mandated performance reporting are subject to change, so readers of these guidelines are advised to consult their local or institutional quality-improvement departments for new developments in requirements for measures and data reporting that apply to their practice.

Cost Containment. Few pharmacoeconomic studies have addresed surgical antimicrobial prophylaxis; therefore, a cost-minimization approach was employed in developing these guidelines. The antimicrobial agent recommendations are based primarily on efficacy and safety. Individual institutions must consider their acquisition costs when implementing these guidelines.

Additional cost savings may be realized through collaborative management by pharmacists and surgeons to select the most cost-effective agent and minimize or eliminate postoperative dosing.[48–50] The use of standardized antimicrobial order sets, automatic stop-order programs, and educational initiatives has been shown to facilitate the adoption of guidelines for surgical antimicrobial prophylaxis.[51–58]

Common Principles

Ideally, an antimicrobial agent for surgical prophylaxis should (1) prevent SSI, (2) prevent SSI-related morbidity and mortality, (3) reduce the duration and cost of health care (when the costs associated with the management of SSI are considered, the cost-effectiveness of prophylaxis becomes evident),[51,52] (4) produce no adverse effects, and (5) have no adverse consequences for the microbial flora of the patient or the hospital.[53] To achieve these goals, an antimicrobial agent should be (1) active against the pathogens most likely to contaminate the surgical site, (2) given in an appropriate dosage and at a time that ensures adequate serum and tissue concentrations during the period of potential contamination, (3) safe, and (4) administered for the shortest effective period to minimize adverse effects, the development of resistance, and costs.[8,59,60]

The selection of an appropriate antimicrobial agent for a specific patient should take into account the characteristics of the ideal agent, the comparative efficacy of the antimicrobial agent for the procedure, the safety profile, and the patient's medication allergies. A full discussion of the safety profile, including adverse events, drug interactions, contraindications, and warnings, for each antimicrobial agent is beyond the scope of these guidelines. Readers of these guidelines should review the FDA-approved prescribing information and published data for specific antimicrobial agents before use. For most procedures, cefazolin is the drug of choice for prophylaxis because it is the most widely studied antimicrobial agent, with proven efficacy. It has a desirable duration of action, spectrum of activity against organisms commonly encountered in surgery, reasonable safety, and low cost. There is little evidence to suggest that broad-spectrum antimicrobial agents (i.e., agents with broad in vitro antibacterial activity) result in lower rates of postoperative SSI compared with older antimicrobial agents with a narrower spectrum of activity. However, comparative studies are limited by small sample sizes, resulting in difficulty detecting a significant difference between antimicrobial agents; therefore, antimicrobial selection is based on cost, safety profile, ease of administration, pharmacokinetic profile, and bactericidal activity.

Common Surgical Pathogens

The agent chosen should have activity against the most common surgical-site pathogens. The predominant organisms causing SSIs after clean procedures are skin flora, including *S. aureus* and coagulase-negative staphylococci (e.g., *Staphylococcus epidermidis*).[61] In clean-contaminated procedures, including abdominal procedures and heart, kidney, and liver transplantations, the predominant organisms include gram-negative rods and enterococci in addition to skin flora. Additional details on common organisms can be found in procedure-specific sections of these guidelines.

Recommendations for the selection of prophylactic antimicrobials for various surgical procedures are provided in Table 2. Adult and pediatric dosages are included in Table 1. Agents that are FDA-approved for use in surgical antimicrobial prophylaxis include cefazolin, cefuroxime, cefoxitin, cefotetan, ertapenem, and vancomycin.[62–67]

Trends in Microbiology. The causative pathogens associated with SSIs in U.S. hospitals have changed over the past two decades. Analysis of National Nosocomial Infections Surveillance (NNIS) System data found that the percentage of SSIs caused by gram-negative bacilli decreased from 56.5% in 1986 to 33.8% in 2003.[68] *S. aureus* was the most common pathogen, causing 22.5% of SSIs during this time period. NHSN data from 2006 to 2007 revealed that the proportion of SSIs caused by *S. aureus* increased to 30%, with MRSA comprising 49.2% of these isolates.[61] In a study of patients readmitted to U.S. hospitals between 2003 and 2007 with a culture-confirmed SSI, the proportion of infections caused by MRSA increased significantly from 16.1% to 20.6% ($p < 0.0001$).[69] MRSA infections were associated with higher mortality rates, longer hospital stays, and higher hospital costs compared with other infections.

Spectrum of Activity. Antimicrobial agents with the narrowest spectrum of activity required for efficacy in preventing infection are recommended in these guidelines. Alternative antimicrobial agents with documented efficacy are also listed herein. Individual health systems must consider local resistance patterns of organisms and overall SSI rates at their site when adopting these recommendations. Resistance patterns from organisms causing SSIs—in some cases procedure-specific resistance patterns—should take precedence over hospitalwide antibiograms.

Vancomycin. In 1999, HICPAC, an advisory committee to CDC and the Secretary of the Department of Health and Human Services, collaborated with other major organizations to develop recommendations for preventing and controlling vancomycin resistance.[70] The recommendations are echoed by these and other guidelines.[6,7,41,71] Routine use of vancomycin prophylaxis is not recommended for any procedure.[8] Vancomycin may be included in the regimen of choice when a cluster of MRSA cases (e.g., mediastinitis after cardiac procedures) or methicillin-resistant coagulase-negative staphylococci SSIs have been detected at an institution. Vancomycin prophylaxis should be considered for patients with known MRSA colonization or at high risk for MRSA colonization in the absence of surveillance data (e.g., patients with recent hospitalization, nursing-home residents, hemodialysis patients).[5,41,72] In institutions with SSIs attributable to community-associated MRSA, antimicrobial agents with known in vitro activity against this pathogen may be considered as an alternative to vancomycin.

Each institution is encouraged to develop guidelines for the proper use of vancomycin. Although vancomycin is commonly used when the risk for MRSA is high, data suggest that vancomycin is less effective than cefazolin for preventing SSIs caused by methicillin-susceptible *S. aureus* (MSSA).[73,74] For this reason, vancomycin is used in combination with cefazolin at some institutions with both MSSA and MRSA SSIs. For procedures in which pathogens other than staphylococci and streptococci are likely, an additional agent with activity against those pathogens should be considered. For example, if there are surveillance data showing that gram-negative organisms are a cause of SSIs for the procedure, practitioners may consider combining vancomycin with another agent (cefazolin if the patient does not have a β-lactam allergy; an aminoglycoside [gentamicin or tobramycin], aztreonam, or single-dose fluoroquinolone if the patient has a β-lactam allergy). The use of vancomycin for MRSA prophylaxis does not supplant the need for routine surgical prophylaxis appropriate for the type of procedure. When vancomycin is used, it can almost always be used as a single dose due to its long half-life.

Colonization and Resistance. A national survey determined that *S. aureus* nasal colonization in the general population decreased from 32.4% in 2001–02 to 28.6% in 2003–04 ($p < 0.01$), whereas the prevalence of colonization with MRSA increased from 0.8% to 1.5% ($p < 0.05$) during the same time periods.[75] Colonization with MRSA was independently associated with health care exposure among men, having been born in the United States, age of >60 years, diabetes, and poverty among women. Similarly, children are colonized with *S. aureus* and MRSA, but colonization varies by age. Children under 5 years of age have the highest rates, mirroring rates seen in patients over age 60 years.[76] The rates drop in children between 5 and 14 years of age and gradually increase to rates seen in the adult population. Lo et al.[77] reported that in a large cohort of children, 28.1% were colonized with *S. aureus* between 2004 and 2006. Between 2007 and 2009, 23.3% of children were colonized with *S. aureus*, but the proportion of children colonized with MRSA had increased from 8.1% in 2004 to 15.1% in 2009.

Surgical antimicrobial prophylaxis can alter individual and institutional bacterial flora, leading to changes in colonization rates and increased bacterial resistance.[78–84] Surgical prophylaxis can also predispose patients to *Clostridium difficile*-associated colitis.[81] Risk factors for development of *C. difficile*-associated colitis include longer duration of prophylaxis or therapy and use of multiple antimicrobial agents.[85] Limiting the duration of antimicrobial prophylaxis to a single preoperative dose can reduce the risk of *C. difficile* disease.

The question of what antimicrobial surgical prophylaxis to use for patients known to be colonized or recently infected with multidrug-resistant pathogens cannot be answered easily or in a manner that can be applied uniformly to all patient scenarios. Whether prophylaxis should be expanded to provide coverage for these pathogens depends on many factors, including the pathogen, its antimicrobial susceptibility profile, the host, the procedure to be performed, and the proximity of the likely reservoir of the pathogen to the incision and operative sites. While there is no evidence on the management of surgical antimicrobial prophylaxis in a patient with past infection or colonization with a resistant gram-negative pathogen, it is logical to provide prophylaxis with an agent active against MRSA for any patient known to be colonized with this gram-positive pathogen who will have a skin incision; specific prophylaxis for a resistant gram-negative pathogen in a patient with past infection or colonization with such a pathogen may not be necessary for a purely cutaneous procedure. Similarly, a patient colonized with vancomycin-resistant enterococci (VRE) should receive prophylaxis effective against VRE when undergoing liver transplantation but probably not when undergoing an umbilical hernia repair without mesh placement. Thus, patients must be treated on a case-by-case basis, taking into account multiple considerations.

Patients receiving therapeutic antimicrobials for a remote infection before surgery should also be given antimicrobial prophylaxis before surgery to ensure adequate serum and tissue levels of antimicrobials with activity against likely pathogens for the duration of the operation. If the agents used therapeutically are appropriate for surgical prophylaxis, administering an extra dose within 60 minutes before surgical incision is sufficient. Otherwise, the antimicrobial prophylaxis recommended for the planned procedure should be used. For patients with indwelling tubes or drains, consideration may be given to using prophylactic agents active against pathogens found in these devices before the procedure, even though therapeutic treatment for pathogens in drains is not indicated at other times. For patients with chronic renal failure receiving vancomycin, a preoperative dose of cefazolin should be considered instead of an extra dose of vancomycin, particularly if the probable pathogens associated with the procedure are gram-negative. In most circumstances, elective surgery should be postponed when the patient has an infection at a remote site.

Allergy to β-Lactam Antimicrobials. Allergy to β-lactam antimicrobials may be a consideration in the selection of surgical prophylaxis. The β-lactam antimicrobials, including cephalosporins, are the mainstay of surgical antimicrobial prophylaxis and are also the most commonly implicated drugs when allergic reactions occur. Because the predominant organisms in SSIs after clean procedures are gram-positive, the inclusion of vancomycin may be appropriate for a patient with a life-threatening allergy to β-lactam antimicrobials.

Although true Type 1 (immunoglobulin E [IgE]-mediated) cross-allergic reactions between penicillins, cephalosporins, and carbapenems are uncommon, cephalosporins and carbapenems should not be used for surgical prophylaxis in patients with documented or presumed IgE-mediated penicillin allergy. Confusion about the definition of true allergy among patients and practitioners leads to recommendations for alternative antimicrobial therapy with the potential for a lack of efficacy, increased costs, and adverse events.[86,87] Type 1 anaphylactic reactions to antimicrobials usually occur 30–60 minutes after administration. In patients receiving penicillins, this reaction is a life-threatening emergency that precludes subsequent use of penicillins.[88] Cephalosporins and carbapenems can safely be used in patients with an allergic reaction to penicillins that is not an IgE-mediated reaction (e.g., anaphylaxis, urticaria, bronchospasm) or exfoliative dermatitis (Stevens-Johnson syndrome, toxic epidermal necrolysis), a life-threatening hypersensitivity reaction that can be caused by β-lactam antimicrobials and other medications.[88,89] Patients should be carefully questioned about their history of antimicrobial allergies to determine whether a true allergy exists before selection of agents for prophylaxis. Patients with allergies to cephalosporins, penicillins, or both have been excluded from many clinical trials. Alternatives to β-lactam antimicrobials are provided in Table 2 based mainly on the antimicrobial activity profiles against predominant procedure-specific organisms and available clinical data.

Drug Administration

The preferred route of administration varies with the type of procedure, but for a majority of procedures, i.v. administration is ideal because it produces rapid, reliable, and predictable serum and tissue concentrations.

Timing of Initial Dose. Successful prophylaxis requires the delivery of the antimicrobial to the operative site before contamination occurs. Thus, the antimicrobial agent should be administered at such a time to provide serum and tissue concentrations exceeding the minimum inhibitory concentration (MIC) for the probable organisms associated with the procedure, at the time of incision, and for the duration of the procedure.[41,90] In 1985, DiPiro et al.[91] demonstrated that higher serum and tissue cephalosporin concentrations at the time of surgical incision and at the end of the procedure were achieved when the drugs were given intravenously at the time of anesthesia induction compared with administration in the operating room. The average interval between antimicrobial administration and incision was 17–22 minutes[91] (Dellinger EP, personal communication, 2011 May).

A prospective evaluation of 1708 surgical patients receiving antimicrobial prophylaxis found that preoperative administration of antimicrobials within 2 hours before surgical incision decreased the risk of SSI to 0.59%, compared with 3.8% for early administration (2–24 hours before surgical incision) and 3.3% for any postoperative administration (any time after incision).[92] In a study of 2048 patients undergoing coronary bypass graft or valve replacement surgery receiving vancomycin prophylaxis, the rate of SSI was lowest in those patients in whom an infusion was started 16–60 minutes before surgical incision.[93] This time interval (16–60 minutes before incision) was compared with four others, and the rates of SSIs were significantly lower when compared with infusions given 0–15 minutes before surgical incision ($p < 0.01$) and 121–180 minutes before incision ($p = 0.037$). The risk of infection was higher in patients receiving infusions 61–120 minutes before incision (odds ratio [OR], 2.3; 95% confidence interval [CI], 0.98–5.61) and for patients whose infusions were started more than 180 minutes before surgical incision (OR, 2.1; 95% CI, 0.82–5.62).[93]

In a large, prospective, multicenter study from the Trial to Reduce Antimicrobial Prophylaxis Errors (TRAPE) study group, the timing, duration, and intraoperative redosing of antimicrobial prophylaxis and risk of SSI were evaluated in 4472 patients undergoing cardiac surgery, hysterectomy, or hip or knee arthroplasty.[94] The majority of patients (90%) received antimicrobial prophylaxis per the SCIP guidelines.[41] Patients were assigned to one of four groups for analysis. Group 1 (n = 1844) received a cephalosporin (or other antimicrobial with a short infusion time) administered within 30 minutes before incision or vancomycin or a fluoroquinolone within one hour before incision. Group 2 (n = 1796) received a cephalosporin 31–60 minutes before incision or vancomycin 61–120 minutes before incision. Group 3 (n = 644) was given antimicrobials earlier than recommended, and group 4 (n = 188) received their initial antimicrobial doses after incision. The infection risk was lowest in group 1 (2.1%), followed by group 2 (2.4%) and group 3 (2.8%). The risk of infection was highest in group 4 (5.3%, $p = 0.02$ compared with group 1). When cephalosporins and other antimicrobials with short infusion times were analyzed separately (n = 3656), the infection rate with antimicrobials administered within 30 minutes before incision was 1.6% compared with 2.4% when antimicrobials were administered 31–60 minutes before incision ($p = 0.13$).

In a multicenter Dutch study of 1922 patients undergoing total hip arthroplasty, the lowest SSI rate was seen in patients who received the antimicrobial during the 30 minutes before incision.[95] The highest risk for infection was found in patients who received prophylaxis after the incision.

It seems intuitive that the entire antimicrobial dose should be infused before a tourniquet is inflated or before any other procedure that restricts blood flow to the surgical site is initiated; however, a study of total knee arthroplasties compared cefuroxime given 10–30 minutes before tourniquet inflation with cefuroxime given 10 minutes before tourniquet deflation and found no significant difference in SSI rates between the two groups.[96]

Overall, administration of the first dose of antimicrobial beginning within 60 minutes before surgical incision is recommended.[41,94,97] Administration of vancomycin and fluoroquinolones should begin within 120 minutes before surgical incision because of the prolonged infusion times required for these drugs. Because these drugs have long half-lives, this early administration should not compromise serum levels of these agents during most surgical procedures. Although the recent data summarized above suggest lower infection risk with antimicrobial administration beginning within 30 minutes before surgical incision, these data are not sufficiently robust to recommend narrowing the optimal window to begin infusion to 1–30 minutes before surgical incision. However, these data do suggest that antimicrobials can be administered too close to the time of incision. Although a few articles have suggested increased infection risk with administration too close to the time of incision,[93,96,97] the data presented are not convincing. In fact, all of these articles confirm the increased rate of SSI for antimicrobials given earlier than 60 minutes before incision. In one article, the infection rate for patients given an antimicrobial within 15 minutes of incision was lower than when antimicrobials were given 15–30 minutes before incision.[97] In another article, small numbers of patients were reported, and an assertion of high infection rates for infusion within 15 minutes of incision was made, but no numeric data or p values were provided.[98] In a third article, only 15 of over

2000 patients received antimicrobials within 15 minutes before incision.[93] Earlier studies found that giving antimicrobials within 20 minutes of incision and as close as 7 minutes before incision resulted in therapeutic levels in tissue at the time of incision.[41,90,91,94,97,98]

Dosing. To ensure that adequate serum and tissue concentrations of antimicrobial agents for prophylaxis of SSIs are achieved, antimicrobial-specific pharmacokinetic and pharmacodynamic properties and patient factors must be considered when selecting a dose. One of the earliest controlled studies of antimicrobial prophylaxis in cardiac surgery found a lower rate of infection in patients with detectable concentrations of the drug in serum at the end of surgery compared with patients in whom the drug was undetectable.[99] In another study, higher levels of antimicrobial in atrial tissue at the time of starting the pump for open-heart surgery were associated with fewer infections than were lower antimicrobial concentrations.[100] In patients undergoing colectomy, infection levels were inversely related to the serum gentamicin concentration at the time of surgical closure.[17] In general, it seems advisable to administer prophylactic agents in a manner that will ensure adequate levels of drug in serum and tissue for the interval during which the surgical site is open.

Weight-based dosing. The dosing of most antimicrobials in pediatric patients is based on body weight, but the dosing of many antimicrobials in adults is not based on body weight, because it is safe, effective, and convenient to use standardized doses for most of the adult patient population. Such standardized doses avoid the need for calculations and reduce the risk for medication errors. However, in obese patients, especially those who are morbidly obese, serum and tissue concentrations of some drugs may differ from those in normal-weight patients because of pharmacokinetic alterations that depend on the lipophilicity of the drug and other factors.[101] Limited data are available on the optimal approach to dosing of antimicrobial agents for obese patients.[102,103] If weight-based dosing is warranted for obese patients, it has not been determined whether the patient's ideal body weight or total (i.e., actual) body weight should be used. In theory, using the ideal body weight as the basis for dosing a lipophilic drug (e.g., vancomycin) could result in subtherapeutic concentrations in serum and tissue, and the use of actual body weight for dosing a hydrophilic drug (e.g., an aminoglycoside) could result in excessive concentrations in serum and tissue. Pediatric patients weighing more than 40 kg should receive weight-based doses unless the dose or daily dose exceeds the recommended adult dose.[104]

Conclusive recommendations for weight-based dosing for antimicrobial prophylaxis in obese patients cannot be made because data demonstrating clinically relevant decreases in SSI rates from the use of such dosing strategies instead of standard doses in obese patients are not available in the published literature.

In a small, nonrandomized, two-phase study of morbidly obese adults undergoing gastroplasty and normal-weight adults undergoing upper abdominal surgery, blood and tissue concentrations of cefazolin after the administration of a 1-g preoperative dose were consistently lower in morbidly obese patients than in the normal-weight patients.[101] The concentrations in morbidly obese patients also were lower than the MICs needed for prophylaxis against gram-positive cocci and gram-negative rods. In the second phase of the study, adequate blood and tissue cefazolin concentrations were achieved in morbidly obese patients receiving preoperative doses of cefazolin 2 g, and the rate of SSIs was significantly lower in these patients compared with morbidly obese patients receiving 1-g doses during the first phase of the study.

While the optimal cefazolin dose has not been established in obese patients, a few pharmacokinetic studies have investigated the cefazolin concentrations in serum and tissue during surgical procedures.[13,105] Two small pharmacokinetic studies found that administering 1- or 2-g doses of cefazolin may not be sufficient to produce serum and tissue concentrations exceeding the MIC for the most common pathogens. In a small, single-center study, 38 adults undergoing Roux-en-Y gastric bypass surgery were classified by body mass index (BMI) in one of three groups.[13] All patients were given cefazolin 2 g i.v. 30–60 minutes before the incision, followed by a second 2-g i.v. dose three hours later. The mean serum drug concentration before the second dose of cefazolin was lower than the resistance breakpoint in all three BMI groups. Serum drug concentrations were lower in patients with a high BMI than in patients with lower BMI values. Tissue drug concentrations were lower than a targeted concentration of 8 μg/mL at all measurement times, except the time of skin closure in the patients with the lowest BMIs. These results suggest that a 1-g dose of cefazolin may be inadequate for obese patients undergoing gastric bypass surgery. A weakness of the literature on drug dosing in morbidly obese patients is the practice of reporting results by BMI rather than weight.

Doubling the normal dose of cephalosporins or making fewer adjustments based on renal dysfunction may produce concentrations in obese patients similar to those achieved with standard doses in normal-weight patients.[103] Considering the low cost and favorable safety profile of cefazolin, increasing the dose to 2 g for patients weighing more than 80 kg and to 3 g for those weighing over 120 kg can easily be justified.[41] For simplification, some hospitals have standardized 2-g cefazolin doses for all adult patients.

Gentamicin doses have been compared for prophylaxis only in colorectal surgery, where a single dose of gentamicin 4.5 mg/kg in combination with metronidazole was more effective in SSI prevention than multiple doses of gentamicin 1.5 mg/kg every eight hours.[16,17] In obese patients who weigh 20% above their ideal body weight, the dose of gentamicin should be calculated using the ideal body weight plus 40% of the difference between the actual and ideal weights.[106] If gentamicin will be used in combination with a parenteral antimicrobial with activity against anaerobic agents for prophylaxis, it is probably advisable to use 4.5–5 mg/kg as a single dose.[16] This dose of gentamicin has been found safe and effective in a large body of literature examining the use of single daily doses of gentamicin for therapeutic indications.[106–113] When used as a single dose for prophylaxis, the risk of toxicity from gentamicin is very low.

Obese patients are often underrepresented in clinical trials and are not currently considered a special population for whom FDA requires separate pharmacokinetic studies during antimicrobial research and development by the drug manufacturer. Obesity has been recognized as a risk factor for SSI; therefore, optimal dosing of antimicrobial prophylaxis is needed in these patients.[114] While a BMI of >30 kg/m^2 is commonly used to define obesity, the body fat percentage (>25% in men and >31% in women) may better predict SSI risk, because the BMI may not reflect body composition. In a recent prospective cohort study of 590 patients undergoing elective surgery, there was no significant difference in SSI rates in nonobese and obese patients when the BMI was used to define obesity (12.3% versus 11.6%, respectively).[115] However, when the body fat percentage (determined by bioelectrical impedance analysis) was used as the basis for identifying obesity (>25% in men and >31% in women), obese patients had a fivefold-higher risk of SSI than did nonobese patients (OR, 5.3; 95% CI, 1.2–23.1; $p = 0.03$). These findings suggest that body fat percentage is a more sensitive and precise measurement of SSI risk than is the BMI.

Redosing. Intraoperative redosing is needed to ensure adequate serum and tissue concentrations of the antimicrobial if the duration of the procedure exceeds two half-lives of the antimicrobial or there is excessive blood loss (i.e., >1500 mL).[17,41,94,116–121] The redosing interval should be measured from the time of administration of the preoperative dose, not from the beginning of the procedure. Redosing may also be warranted if there are factors that shorten the half-life of the antimicrobial agent (e.g., extensive burns). Redosing may not be warranted in patients in whom the half-life of the antimicrobial agent is prolonged (e.g., patients with renal insufficiency or renal failure). See Table 1 for antimicrobial-specific redosing recommendations.

Duration. The shortest effective duration of antimicrobial administration for preventing SSI is not known; however, evidence is mounting that postoperative antimicrobial administration is not necessary for most procedures.[6,7,41,122–124] The duration of antimicrobial prophylaxis should be less than 24 hours for most procedures. Cardiothoracic procedures for which a prophylaxis duration of up to 48 hours has been accepted without evidence to support the practice is an area that remains controversial. The duration of cardiothoracic prophylaxis in these guidelines is based on expert panel consensus because the available data do not delineate the optimal duration of prophylaxis. In these procedures, prophylaxis for the duration of the procedure and certainly for less than 24 hours is appropriate.

A 1992 meta-analysis of studies comparing first-generation cephalosporins and antistaphylococcal antimicrobials (e.g., penicillins) with second-generation cephalosporins in patients undergoing cardiothoracic surgery found a reduction in the rate of SSI with second-generation cephalosporins but no benefit from continuing surgical prophylaxis beyond 48 hours.[125] Reports published in 1980,[126] 1993,[127] 1997,[128] and 2000[129] involving seven studies that compared single-dose prophylaxis or prophylaxis only during the operation with durations of one to four days failed to show any reduction in SSIs with the longer durations of prophylaxis. In a more-recent observational four-year cohort study of 2641 patients undergoing coronary artery bypass graft (CABG) surgery, the extended use of antimicrobial prophylaxis (>48 hours) instead of a shorter duration of prophylaxis (<48 hours) failed to reduce the risk of SSI (OR, 1.2; 95% CI, 0.8–1.6).[130] Moreover, prolonged prophylaxis was associated with an increased risk of acquired antimicrobial resistance (cephalosporin-resistant Enterobacteriaceae and VRE) compared with short-term prophylaxis (OR, 1.6; 95% CI, 1.1–2.6).

There are no data to support the continuation of antimicrobial prophylaxis until all indwelling drains and intravascular catheters are removed.[19,31,32,41,131–134]

Topical Administration of Irrigations, Pastes, and Washes

I.V. and oral antimicrobial administration are the main focus of these guidelines, and these routes of administration are used for most surgical procedures addressed by these guidelines, with the exception of ophthalmic procedures, for which topical administration is the primary route of administration. Limited high-quality data are available regarding the use of antimicrobial irrigations, pastes, and washes that are administered topically. Studies published in the early 1980s demonstrated that prophylactic topical administration of antimicrobials in the surgical incision during various non-ophthalmic procedures is superior to placebo but not superior to parenteral administration, and topical administration does not increase the efficacy of parenteral antimicrobials when used in combination for prophylaxis.[135–138] Additional high-quality data on the safety and efficacy of topical antimicrobial administration as an adjunct to i.v. administration are needed to determine the role of topical antimicrobial prophylaxis.

One area of interest for topical administration of antimicrobials, mainly gentamicin and vancomycin, is application to the sternum during cardiac procedures in combination with i.v. agents to prevent mediastinitis. This strategy has been evaluated in cohort and randomized controlled studies.[139–142] While the studies found a significantly lower rate of SSI with topical antimicrobials compared with standard prophylaxis,[140] placebo,[142] and a historical control,[139] a smaller, randomized, placebo-controlled study found no difference between groups.[141]

More recently, implantable gentamicin collagen sponges failed to show any efficacy in reducing SSIs in a large prospective study of patients undergoing cardiac surgery and resulted in an increased infection rate in patients undergoing colectomy.[143,144] The safety and efficacy of topical antimicrobials have not been clearly established; therefore, routine use of this route cannot be recommended in cardiac or other procedures.[145]

Preoperative Screening and Decolonization

S. aureus is the most common pathogen causing SSIs, accounting for 30% of SSIs in the United States. Colonization with *S. aureus*, primarily in the nares, occurs in roughly one in four persons and increases the risk of SSI by 2- to 14-fold.[146–152] A national survey assessing nasal colonization with *S. aureus* in the general population conducted from 2001 through 2004 found that while the rate of colonization with *S. aureus* decreased from 32.4% in 2001–02 to 28.6% in 2003–04 ($p < 0.01$), the rate of colonization with MRSA increased from 0.8% to 1.5% ($p < 0.05$).[75]

Preoperative screening for *S. aureus* carriage and decolonization strategies have been explored as means to reduce the rate of SSIs. Anterior nasal swab cultures are most commonly used for preoperative surveillance, but screening additional sites (pharynx, groin, wounds, rectum) can increase detection rates.[153] Such preoperative surveillance swabs that can be cultured on selective or nonselective media or sent for rapid polymerase chain reaction (PCR)-based screening can be used to identify colonized patients in the preoperative period. When properly used, all of these techniques can identify MSSA and MRSA. However, not all PCR-based systems will identify both MRSA and MSSA so verification with the laboratory is needed. While many studies have focused specifically on MRSA screening in high-risk hospitalized patients in an effort to prevent MRSA SSI and hospital-acquired infections, the risk of developing an SSI remains elevated for any *S. aureus* carrier. While some authors advocate screening for MRSA carriage in the general population, the data supporting universal screening in the surgical population are more controversial.[154,155] Screening has been advocated to both identify candidates for *S. aureus* decolonization and inform the selection of optimal prophylactic antimicrobials, such as the addition of vancomycin for those colonized with MRSA.

FDA has approved intranasal mupirocin to eradicate MRSA nasal colonization in adult patients and health care workers.[156] It is noted in the prescribing information that there are insufficient data to support use in prevention of autoinfection of high-risk patients from their own nasal colonization with *S. aureus*. However, additional data have demonstrated that the use of intranasal mupirocin in nasal carriers of *S. aureus* decreases the rate of *S. aureus* infections.[157,158] One meta-analysis of seven studies focused on surgical patients only[157]; the other meta-analysis of nine studies included high-quality studies in dialysis patients.[158]

Recent studies have confirmed that *S. aureus* decolonization of the anterior nares decreases SSI rates in many surgical patients.[159] The data are most compelling in cardiac and orthopedic surgery patients. There are fewer data in general surgery patients. A large, randomized controlled trial of general, cardiac, and neurosurgical patients (n = 3864) revealed that prophylactic intranasal application of mupirocin did not significantly reduce the overall rate of *S. aureus* SSIs (2.3% in the mupirocin group versus 2.4% in the control group) but did decrease the rate of *S. aureus* SSI among *S. aureus* carriers (3.7% in the mupirocin group versus 5.9% in the control group).[160]

Another randomized controlled trial found no significant difference in the rate of postoperative *S. aureus* SSIs among cardiac surgery patients receiving intranasal mupirocin and those receiving placebo, but the study was limited by the small numbers of patients (n = 257) and reported SSIs (n = 5).[161] Among elective orthopedic patients undergoing implantation and other procedures, a randomized clinical trial demonstrated a nonsignificant reduction in the rate of postoperative *S. aureus* SSIs in patients receiving mupirocin (n = 315, 3.8%) compared with those receiving placebo (n = 299, 4.7%).[150]

A recent randomized, double-blind, placebo-controlled, multicenter study conducted in the Netherlands found that the use of mupirocin nasal ointment and chlorhexidine baths in identified *S. aureus* carriers reduced the risk of hospital-associated *S. aureus* infections.[162] In the study, a real-time PCR assay was used to rapidly identify *S. aureus* nasal carriers; all of the *S. aureus* isolates were susceptible to methicillin. Deep SSIs occurred in 0.9% of the mupirocin–chlorhexidine-treated group (4 of 441 patients) versus 4.4% of the placebo group (16 of 367 patients) (relative risk, 0.21; 95% CI, 0.07–0.62). The reduction in superficial SSIs was less marked (1.6% versus 3.5%; relative risk, 0.45; 95% CI, 0.18–1.11). It is plausible that this approach would be beneficial in a setting of MRSA, but it has not been proven.

Most studies conclude that the use of preoperative intranasal mupirocin in colonized patients is safe and potentially beneficial as an adjuvant to i.v. antimicrobial prophylaxis to decrease the occurrence of SSIs. However, the optimal timing and duration of administration are not standardized. In most studies, mupirocin was used for five days before the operation. While *S. aureus* resistance to mupirocin has been detected,[148,162] raising concerns about the potential for widespread problems with resistance from routine use of this agent, resistance has only rarely been seen in the preoperative setting. Low-level resistance is associated with an increased rate of failure of decolonization and has been seen in institutions that use standardized mupirocin decolonization protocols.[163] Therefore, when decolonization therapy (e.g., mupirocin) is used as an adjunctive measure to prevent *S. aureus* SSI, surveillance of susceptibility of *S. aureus* isolated from SSIs to mupirocin is recommended.[164] While universal use of mupirocin is discouraged, specific recommendations for the drug's use can be found in the cardiac and orthopedic sections of these guidelines.

Future Research

Additional research is needed in several areas related to surgical antimicrobial prophylaxis. The risks and benefits of continuing antimicrobial prophylaxis after the conclusion of the operative procedure, including dosing and duration, need to be further evaluated. Insight is needed to make specific recommendations for intraoperative repeat dosing, weight-based dosing in obese patients, and timing of presurgical antimicrobials that must be administered over a prolonged period (e.g., vancomycin, fluoroquinolones). Additional clarification is needed regarding targeted antimicrobial concentrations and intraoperative monitoring of antimicrobial serum and tissue concentrations to optimize efficacy. The role of topical administration of antimicrobial agents as a substitute for or an adjunct to i.v. antimicrobial prophylaxis needs to be further evaluated. Additional data are needed to guide the selection of antimicrobial agents for prophylaxis, particularly combination regimens, for patients with allergies to β-lactam antimicrobials. Data are also needed to devise strategies to optimize antimicrobial prophylaxis in patients and facilities with a high risk or high prevalence of resistant organisms implicated in SSIs (e.g., MRSA). Optimal strategies for screening for *S. aureus* and decolonization for certain procedures need to be identified. Finally, outcomes studies are needed to assess the impact of using quality measures and pay-for-performance incentives designed to reduce surgical morbidity and mortality.

Cardiac Procedures

Background. Cardiac procedures include CABG procedures, valve repairs, and placement of temporary or permanent implantable cardiac devices, including ventricular assist devices (VADs). SSIs, including mediastinitis and sternal wound infection, are rare but serious complications after cardiac procedures. In patients undergoing CABG, the mean frequency of SSIs depending on NHSN SSI risk index category ranges from 0.35 to 8.49 per 100 operations when donor sites are included.[165] The mean frequency of SSIs depending on NHSN SSI risk index category for patients undergoing CABG with only chest incisions ranges from 0.23 to 5.67 per 100 operations.[165] Most of these infections are superficial in depth. Patient-related and procedure-related risk factors for SSIs after cardiac procedures have been identified from several single-center cohort and case–control studies.[117,128,166–176] These include diabetes,[166,169,171–175] hyperglycemia,[177–182] peripheral vascular disease,[171,172,174] chronic obstructive pulmonary disease,[166,174,175] obesity (BMI of >30 kg/m^2),[166–168,171,173–176] heart failure,[171,172] advanced age,[117,128,166,172] involvement of internal mammary artery,[168–172] reoperation,[169–171] increased number of grafts,[171] long duration of surgery,[117,166,167,176] and *S. aureus* nasal colonization.[146,160]

Patients requiring extracorporeal membrane oxygenation (ECMO) as a bridge to cardiac or lung transplantation should be treated with a similar approach. If there is no history of colonization or previous infection, the general recommendations for SSI antimicrobial prophylaxis for the specific procedure should be followed. For ECMO patients with a history of colonization or previous infection, changing the preoperative antimicrobial prophylaxis to cover these pathogens must be considered, weighing whether the pathogen is relevant to SSIs in the planned procedure.

Organisms. Almost two thirds of organisms isolated in both adult and pediatric patients undergoing cardiac procedures are gram-positive, including *S. aureus*, coagulase-negative *staphylococcus*, and, rarely, *Propionibacterium acnes*. Gram-negative organisms are less commonly isolated in these patients and include *Enterobacter* species, *Pseudomonas aeruginosa*, *Escherichia coli*, *Klebsiella pneumoniae*, *Proteus mirabilis*, and *Acinetobacter* species.[93,139,146,183–192]

Efficacy. The SSI rate in cardiac procedures is low, but there are potential consequences if infection occurs. Multiple studies have found that antimicrobial prophylaxis in cardiac procedures lowers the occurrence of postoperative SSI up to fivefold.[125]

Choice of agent. Cephalosporins have been the most studied antimicrobials for the prevention of SSIs in cardiac procedures. Both first-generation (cefazolin) and second-generation (cefamandole and cefuroxime) cephalosporins have been shown to be effective in reducing SSI in cardiac surgery; however, the superiority of one class over another has not been proven.[125,127,193–199]

A meta-analysis comparing cephalosporins with glycopeptides (e.g., vancomycin) as antimicrobial prophylaxis regimens for cardiac procedures found a higher frequency of postoperative chest and deep-chest SSIs and a trend toward an increased risk of gram-positive SSI in the glycopeptide group but a lower frequency of SSIs caused by resistant gram-positive pathogens.[72] The routine use of vancomycin for the prevention of SSIs is not recommended, based on limited evidence of efficacy and concerns of increased glycopeptide resistance of microorganisms.[8,116] There is no clear evidence to support the use of vancomycin, alone or in combination with other antimicrobials, for routine antimicrobial prophylaxis in institutions that have a high prevalence of MRSA.[8,11,41,72,73,116,200] Vancomycin should be considered in patients who are colonized with MRSA.[41,116,201] The accepted alternative antimicrobial for β-lactam-allergic patients undergoing cardiac procedures is vancomycin or clindamycin for gram-positive coverage.[41,116,201,202] The addition of an aminoglycoside, aztreonam, or a fluoroquinolone may be prudent when gram-negative pathogens are a concern.[8,116]

Mupirocin. The proportion of infections related to *S. aureus* among patients undergoing cardiac surgery and the increase in MRSA as a cause of SSIs at some institutions have led to investigations of methods for preoperative eradication, particularly with intranasal mupirocin.[203] Readers are referred to the Common Principles section of these guidelines for discussion of the use of intranasal mupirocin. Of note, the data demonstrated a 45% reduction in *S. aureus* SSIs with the use of preoperative mupirocin among patients known to be colonized with *S. aureus* who undergo cardiac procedures.[157,193] Institutions should monitor for mupirocin resistance periodically.

Topical administration. Additional information on topical administration of antimicrobials can be found in the Common Principles section of these guidelines. Use of topical antimicrobials, mainly gentamicin or vancomycin, applied to the sternum during cardiac procedures in combination with i.v. agents to prevent mediastinitis has been evaluated in both cohort[139] and randomized controlled studies.[140–142] While the studies found a significantly lower rate of SSIs with topical antimicrobials compared with standard prophylaxis,[140] placebo,[142] and a historical control,[139] a smaller randomized, placebo-controlled study found no difference between groups.[141] More recent studies of gentamicin collagen sponges failed to show any efficacy in a large prospective study of cardiac surgery.[143] The safety and efficacy of topical antimicrobials have not been clearly established and therefore cannot be recommended for routine use in cardiac procedures.[139–142]

Cardiopulmonary bypass. Cardiopulmonary bypass (CPB) is a common surgical technique in cardiac procedures that alters the volume of distribution and bioavailability of medications administered during the procedure.[116,204,205] Several small cohort or comparative studies[128,204–213] have evaluated the serum and tissue concentrations of several routinely used antimicrobial prophylactic agents (i.e., cefazolin, cefuroxime, gentamicin, and vancomycin) in patients undergoing CPB during cardiac procedures. Until further clinical outcomes data and well-designed studies become available to inform alternative dosing strategies, routinely used doses of common antimicrobial agents should be used in patients undergoing CPB during cardiac procedures.

Duration. The optimal duration of antimicrobial prophylaxis for cardiac procedures continues to be evaluated. Data support a duration ranging from a single dose up to 24 hours postoperatively.[41,99,131,191,214–217] No significant differences were found in several small studies in patients undergoing cardiac procedures between these dosing strategies in patients primarily receiving first- or second-generation cephalosporins. Although a recent meta-analysis suggested the possibility of increased efficacy with cardiac surgical prophylaxis extending beyond 24 hours, the authors noted that the findings were limited by the heterogeneity of antimicrobial regimens used and the risk of bias in the published studies.[218] The comparisons of varying durations were performed with different antimicrobials with differing efficacy and do not support longer durations. Consequently, this meta-analysis does not provide evidence to support changing the currently accepted prophylaxis duration of less than 24 hours, particularly given the evidence from studies involving noncardiac operations. The currently accepted duration of prophylaxis for cardiac procedures is less than 24 hours, but prophylaxis should be continued for the duration of the procedure.[41,59,126–129,131,201]

Two small studies did not support the continuation of antimicrobial prophylaxis until intravascular catheters or intraaortic balloon pumps were removed, due to a lack of influence on infections or catheter colonization compared with short-course (24 hours) cefazolin or cefuroxime.[219,220] The practice of continuing antimicrobial prophylaxis until all invasive lines, drains, and indwelling catheters are removed cannot be supported due to concerns regarding the development of drug-resistant organisms, superinfections, and drug toxicity.[41,131]

Pediatric Efficacy. The rate of SSI in pediatric cardiac procedures is sometimes higher than in adult patients.[20,31,221] Significant risk factors in pediatric patients with a mediastinal SSI included the presence of other infections at the time of the procedure, young age (newborns and infants), small body size, the duration of the procedure (including CPB time), the need for an intraoperative blood transfusion, an open sternum postoperatively, the need for a reexploration procedure, the length of stay in the intensive care unit, an NNIS/NHSN risk score of 2, and the performance of emergency procedures.[20,31,221]

The organisms of concern in pediatric patients are the same as those in adult patients.[20,21,31,221] However, MRSA is rarely a concern in this population as a risk factor for SSI.[221] Pediatric patients considered at high risk for MRSA infection are those with preoperative MRSA colonization or a history of MRSA infection, neonates younger than one month of age, and neonates under three months of age who have been in the hospital since birth or have a complex cardiac disorder.[21] Strategies such as intranasal mupirocin and changes in antimicrobial prophylactic agent to vancomycin led to decreased rates of MRSA carriage and the absence of MRSA infections in one time-series evaluation; however, the overall clinical impact of these efforts is still unclear.[21,221]

No well-controlled studies have evaluated the efficacy of antimicrobial prophylaxis in pediatric patients undergoing cardiac procedures. Therefore, the efficacy of antimicrobial prophylaxis is extrapolated from adult studies and should be considered the standard of care for pediatric cardiac surgery patients.[19]

No well-designed studies or consensus has established the appropriate doses for common antimicrobial prophylactic agents for use in pediatric cardiac patients. Antibiotic doses have been extrapolated from guidelines for the prevention of bacterial endocarditis.[11] In recent evaluations, doses of cefazolin have ranged from 25 to 50 mg/kg,[19–21,31] and vancomycin doses have ranged from 10 to 20 mg/kg.[19–21,31,222–226] Gentamicin doses used in studies have included 2.5[20] and 5 mg/kg[22]; however, the study authors[22] felt that the higher dose was excessive. The expert panel recognizes that the usual total daily dose for pediatric patients older than six months can be 6.5–7.5 mg/kg and that dosing schedules for younger patients may be complicated.

Recommendations. For patients undergoing cardiac procedures, the recommended regimen is a single preincision dose of cefazolin or cefuroxime with appropriate intraoperative redosing (Table 2). Currently, there is no evidence to support continuing prophylaxis until all drains and indwelling catheters are removed. Clindamycin or vancomycin is an acceptable alternative in patients with a documented β-lactam allergy. Vancomycin should be used for prophylaxis in patients known to be colonized with MRSA. If organizational SSI surveillance shows that gram-negative organisms cause infections for patients undergoing these operations, practitioners should combine clindamycin or vancomycin with another agent (cefazolin if the patient is not β-lactam allergic; aztreonam, aminoglycoside, or single-dose fluoroquinolone if the patient is β-lactam allergic). Mupirocin should be given intranasally to all patients with documented *S. aureus* colonization. (Strength of evidence for prophylaxis = A.)

Cardiac Device Insertion Procedures

Background. Antimicrobial prophylaxis is the standard of care for patients undergoing cardiac implantable device insertion (e.g., pacemaker implantation).[227] Based on available data and perceived infection risk, antimicrobial prophylaxis is not routinely recommended for cardiac catheterization or transesophageal echocardiogram.[228]

NHSN has reported a mean SSI rate after pacemaker placement of 0.44 per 100 procedures.[165] This rate may underestimate the risk of late SSI and complications.[229] Risk factors for device-related infection after implantation of cardioverter–defibrillator systems or pacemakers identified in two large, prospective, multicenter cohort studies[230,231] and a large case–control study[232] included fever within 24 hours before implantation, temporary pacing before implantation, and early reintervention for hematoma or lead replacement[230]; corticosteroid use for more than one month during the preceding year and more than two leads in place compared with two leads[232]; and development of pocket hematoma.[231] In all of the evaluations, antimicrobial prophylaxis was found to be protective against device-related infection.[230–232] Limited data are available on the efficacy and optimal dose and duration of antimicrobial prophylaxis in patients undergoing implantation of a new pacemaker, pacing system, or other cardiac device.

A meta-analysis of 15 prospective, randomized, controlled, mainly open-label studies evaluated the effectiveness of systemic antimicrobial prophylaxis compared with controls (no antimicrobials) on infection rates after pacemaker implantation.[227] Antibiotics included penicillins or cephalosporins with a duration ranging from a single preoperative dose to four days postoperatively. A consistent and significant protective effect of antimicrobial prophylaxis was found and encouraged the routine use of antimicrobial prophylaxis in patients undergoing permanent pacemaker implantation. A prospective, single-center cohort study found a low rate (1.7%) of SSI complications with a single 2-g dose of cefazolin in patients undergoing implantation of a new pacemaker, pulse-generator replacement, or upgrading of a preexisting pacing system.[233] A notable limitation of the study was the exclusion of patients with temporary percutanous cardiac stimulators who are at high risk of infection.

A large, randomized, double-blind, placebo-controlled study found a significantly lower rate of SSI with a single 1-g dose of cefazolin (0.64%) compared with placebo (3.28%) ($p = 0.016$) given immediately before device implantation or generator replacement in a permanent pacemaker, implantable cardioverter defibrillator, or cardiac resynchronization device in a surgical operating room.[231] The expert panel noted that the cefazolin dose was not adjusted for patient weight. Recently, AHA produced evidence-based guidelines that recommend the use of a single dose of a preoperative antimicrobial.[229]

VADs are increasingly used to bridge patients to transplantation or to support individuals who do not respond to medical therapy for congestive heart failure. Very limited data exist on infection rates, and there are no published studies that demonstrate the effectiveness of preoperative antimicrobial therapy. Using 2006–08 data from the Interagency Registry for Mechanically Assisted Circulatory Support, Holman and colleagues[234] reported that most infections related to mechanical cardiac support devices were bacterial (87%), with the remainder associated with fungal (9%), viral (1%), protozoal (0.3%), or unknown (2%) causes. Driveline infections are primarily caused by staphylococcal species from the skin. Fungal organisms also play an important role in VAD infections, most notably *Candida* species, and carry a high risk of mortality. A recent survey of antimicrobial surgical prophylaxis with VADs illustrates the variability and lack of consensus with regimens, using anywhere from one to four drugs for a duration of 24–72 hours.[235] Immediate postoperative infections are caused by gram-positive organisms. Complications from long-term infections should not be confused with immediate postprocedure SSIs.[236] Based on the consensus of the expert panel, antimicrobial prophylaxis for replacement of a VAD due to ongoing or recent infection should incorporate coverage directed at the offending organism or organisms. While many centers use vancomycin plus ciprofloxacin plus fluconazole, this practice is not based on the published evidence.

Recommendation. A single dose of cefazolin or cefuroxime is recommended for device implantation or generator replacement in a permanent pacemaker, implantable cardioverter defibrillator, or cardiac resynchronization device. (Strength of evidence for prophylaxis = A.) There is limited evidence to make specific recommendations for VADs, and each practice should tailor protocols based on pathogen prevalence and local susceptibility profiles. Clindamycin or vancomycin is an acceptable alternative in patients with a documented β-lactam allergy. Vancomycin should be considered for prophylaxis in patients known to be colonized with MRSA.

Thoracic Procedures

Background. Noncardiac thoracic procedures include lobectomy, pneumonectomy, thoracoscopy, lung resection, and thoracotomy. In addition to SSIs, postoperative nosocomial pneumonia and empyema are of concern after thoracic procedures.[237]

NHSN has reported that the rate of infection associated with thoracic surgery ranges from 0.76% to 2.04%.[165] Studies have found that the reported rate of SSIs after thoracic procedures in patients receiving antimicrobial prophylaxis ranged from 0.42% to 4%.[238–241] One study found an SSI rate of 14% when prophylaxis was not used.[239] The reported rates of pneumonia and empyema with antimicrobial prophylaxis are 3–24% and 0–7%, respectively.[237,239–244]

Video-assisted thoracoscopic surgery (VATS) is commonly used for thoracic procedures. In some settings, VATS constitutes one third or more of all thoracic surgical procedures.[245] Since VATS uses small incisions, the rate of SSIs is lower compared with the rate associated with open thoracic surgical procedures.[246] A prospective cohort study (n = 346) confirmed a low rate of SSIs (1.7%) after minimally invasive VATS procedures.[240] An additional prospective study of 988 lung resection patients confirmed that the SSI rate was significantly lower (5.5%) in VATS patients than in open thoracotomy patients (14.3%).[247] Furthermore, SSI correlated with the duration of surgery, serum albumin, concurrent comorbidity, age, and forced expiratory volume in one second. Antimicrobial prophylaxis recommendations in this section refer to both open thoracotomy and VATS procedures. Based on available data and perceived infection risk, antimicrobial prophylaxis is not routinely recommended for chest tube insertion.

Results of a prospective cohort and case–control study revealed the following independent risk factors for pneumonia after thoracic procedures: extent of lung resection, intraoperative bronchial colonization, chronic obstructive pulmonary disease, BMI of >25 kg/m^2, induction therapy (chemotherapy, radiotherapy, or chemoradiotherapy), advanced age (≥75 years old), and stage III or IV cancer.[243,244]

Organisms. The organisms reported from SSIs in patients undergoing thoracic procedures were *S. aureus* and *S. epidermidis*.[237] Organisms isolated in patients with postoperative pneumonia included gram-positive (*Streptococcus* and *Staphylococcus* species), gram-negative (*Haemophilus influenzae*, *Enterobacter cloacae*, *K. pneumoniae*, *Acinetobacter* species, *P. aeruginosa*, and *Moraxella catarrhalis*), and fungal (*Candida* species) pathogens.[237,239–243]

Efficacy. Antimicrobial prophylaxis is the standard of care for patients undergoing noncardiac thoracic surgery, including pulmonary resection.[11,201,237] One randomized, double-blind, placebo-controlled, single-center study of patients in Spain undergoing pulmonary resection, persistent pneumothorax without thoracotomy tube before surgery, and nonpulmonary thoracic surgical procedures, excluding those involving the esophagus and exploratory thoracotomies, compared a single dose of cefazolin 1 g i.v. and placebo given 30 minutes before the procedure.[239] The study was stopped early due to the significant difference in SSI rates between groups (1.5% with cefazolin versus 14% with placebo, p < 0.01). No differences in the rates of pneumonia and empyema were seen between groups, but these were not endpoints of the study.

Choice of agent. There is no clear optimal choice for antimicrobial prophylaxis in thoracic procedures. The need to consider pneumonia and empyema as well as SSIs after thoracic procedures has been raised in the literature.[237,241–244] There are a limited number of small, single-center, randomized controlled or cohort studies that evaluated several antimicrobial agents. One small, randomized controlled study and one cohort study found that ampicillin–sulbactam was significantly better than cephalosporins (cefazolin and cefamandole) for preventing pneumonia.[242,243] No statistically significant difference was found between cefuroxime and cefepime in the rate of postoperative SSI, pneumonia, or empyema in a small, randomized controlled study in patients undergoing elective thoracotomy.[241] Lower rates of infections and susceptibility of all organisms were noted with cefuroxime compared with cefepime. Therefore, the study authors concluded that cefuroxime was marginally more effective and was more cost-effective than cefepime.

Duration. No clear consensus on the duration of antimicrobial prophylaxis has been established. Studies have evaluated different dosing strategies for cephalosporins or penicillins, with most studies using single doses given preoperatively within 60 minutes before surgical incision.[237,239,240,242,244] Studies found differing results when comparing agents given for 24 hours (cefepime, ampicillin-sulbactam) and 48 hours (cefuroxime, cefamandole); however, these findings may be attributable to the different antimicrobials tested.[241,243] Additional discussion on dosing is provided in the Common Principles section of these guidelines.

Recommendations. In patients undergoing thoracic procedures, a single dose of cefazolin or ampicillin–sulbactam is recommended (Appendix B). Clindamycin or vancomycin is an acceptable alternative in patients with a documented β-lactam allergy. Vancomycin should be used for prophylaxis in patients known to be colonized with MRSA. If organizational SSI surveillance shows that gram-negative organisms are associated with infections during these operations or if there is risk of gram-negative contamination of the surgical site, practitioners should combine clindamycin or vancomycin with another agent (cefazolin if the patient is not β-lactam allergic; aztreonam, aminoglycoside, or single-dose fluoroquinolone if the patient is β-lactam allergic). (Strength of evidence for prophylaxis for VATS = C; strength of evidence for prophylaxis for other thoracic procedures = A.)

Gastroduodenal Procedures

Background. The gastroduodenal procedures considered in these guidelines include resection with or without vagotomy for gastric or duodenal ulcers, resection for gastric carcinoma, revision required to repair strictures of the gastric outlet, percutaneous endoscopic gastrostomy (PEG) insertion, perforated ulcer procedures (i.e., Graham patch repair), pancreaticoduodenectomy (Whipple procedure), and bariatric surgical procedures (gastric bypass, gastric banding, gastroplasty, other restrictive procedures, biliopancreatic diversion). Studies specifically addressing antimicrobial prophylaxis for gastroesophageal reflux disease procedures (Nissen fundoplication) or highly selective vagotomy for ulcers (usually done laparoscopically) could not be identified. Antireflux procedures and highly selective vagotomy are clean procedures in contrast to essentially all other gastroduodenal procedures that are clean-contaminated. Other procedures that are generally performed using laparoscopic or endoscopic techniques (e.g., endoscopic retrograde cholangiopancreatography) are not specifically discussed in this document. Natural orifice transluminal endoscopic surgery (NOTES) is a developing operative technique using natural orifices (e.g., vagina, anus, mouth, stomach) for entry into the abdomen that leaves no visible scar.[248] No studies on antimicrobial prophylaxis using NOTES have been published. SSI rates reported in patients not receiving antimicrobial prophylaxis were 6% after vagotomy and drainage, 13% after gastric ulcer procedures, 6.8–17% after procedures for gastric cancer,[249–253] 8% for pancreaticoduodenectomy,[254] and 23.9–26% after PEG insertion.[255,256]

The stomach is an effective barrier to bacterial colonization; this is at least partially related to its acidity. The stomach and the duodenum typically contain small numbers of organisms (<10^4 colony-forming units [CFU]/mL), the most common of which are streptococci, lactobacilli, diphtheroids, and fungi.[257,258] Treatment with agents that increase gastric pH increases the concentration of gastric organisms.[259–261] Alterations in gastric and duodenal bacterial flora as a result of increases in gastric pH have the potential to increase the postoperative infection rate.[262,263]

The risk of postoperative infection in gastroduodenal procedures depends on a number of factors, including the gastroduodenal procedure performed. Patients who are at highest risk include those with achlorhydria, including those receiving pharmacotherapy with histamine H_2-receptor antagonists or proton-pump inhibitors,[264] gastroduodenal perforation, decreased gastric motility, gastric outlet obstruction, morbid obesity, gastric bleeding, or cancer.[265] Similar to other types of surgical procedures, risk factors for SSIs related to gastroduodenal procedures include long procedure duration,[252,266,267] performance of emergency procedures,[250,261] greater than normal blood loss,[251,252] American Society of Anesthesiologists (ASA) classification of ≥3, and late administration of antimicrobials.[268]

Organisms. The most common organisms cultured from SSIs after gastroduodenal procedures are coliforms (*E. coli*, *Proteus* species, *Klebsiella* species), *staphylococci*, *streptococci*, *enterococci*, and occasionally *Bacteroides* species.[101,269–276]

Efficacy. Randomized controlled trials have shown that prophylactic antimicrobials are effective in decreasing postoperative infection rates in high-risk patients after gastroduodenal procedures. The majority of available studies were conducted in single centers outside of the United States. Relative to other types of gastrointestinal tract procedures, the number of clinical trials evaluating antimicrobial prophylaxis for gastroduodenal procedures is limited. In placebo-controlled trials, infection rates ranged from 0% to 22% for patients receiving cephalosporins or penicillins and from 1.7% to 66% for patients receiving placebo.[270,271,273–275,277–284] The difference was significant in most studies.

Data support antimicrobial prophylaxis for patients undergoing PEG insertion.[264,285–287] A Cochrane review of systemic antimicrobial prophylaxis for PEG procedures that included 11 randomized controlled trials and 1196 patients found a statistically significant reduction in peristomal infections with antimicrobial prophylaxis (OR, 0.35; 95% CI, 0.23–0.48).[288] Two meta-analyses found statistically significant decreases in SSIs with antimicrobial prophylaxis compared with placebo or controls, from 23.9–26% to 6.4–8%, respectively.[255,256] Most well-designed, randomized controlled studies found a significant decrease in postoperative SSIs or peristomal infections with single i.v. doses of a cephalosporin or penicillin, ranging from 11% to 17%, compared with from 18% to 66% with placebo or no antimicrobials.[279–282,288] Conflicting results have been seen in studies evaluating the use of preoperative patient MRSA screening, decontamination washes and shampoos, five-day preoperative treatment with intranasal mupirocin, and single-dose teicoplanin preoperative prophylaxis to decrease postoperative MRSA infections during PEG insertion.[289,290]

While there have been no well-designed clinical trials of antimicrobial prophylaxis for patients undergoing bariatric surgical procedures, treatment guidelines support its use based on morbid obesity and additional comorbidities as risk factors for postoperative infections.[264,291] There is no consensus on the appropriate antimicrobial regimen; however, higher doses of antimicrobials may be needed for adequate serum and tissue concentrations in morbidly obese patients.[13,268,291]

A notable risk factor for SSIs after esophageal and gastroduodenal procedures is decreased gastric acidity and motility resulting from malignancy or acid-suppression therapy.[264,276] Therefore, antimicrobial prophylaxis is indicated for patients undergoing gastric cancer procedures (including gastrectomy) and gastroduodenal procedures related to gastric and duodenal ulcer disease or bariatric surgery or pancreaticoduodenectomy. Evaluations of practice for pancreaticoduodenectomy show that antimicrobials are typically given due to concerns of bile contamination. Prophylaxis for gastroduodenal procedures that do not enter the gastrointestinal tract, such as antireflux procedures, should be limited to high-risk patients due to lack of data supporting general use in all patients. Furthermore, laparoscopic antireflux procedures are associated with very low SSI rates (0.3%) compared with open antireflux procedures (1.4%), just as laparoscopic gastric bypass procedures are associated with lower rates than in open procedures (0.4% versus 1.2%).[292]

Choice of agent. The most frequently used agents for gastroduodenal procedures were first-generation[271,273,277,278,284,293–297] and second-generation[269,270,274,275,280,293,294,298] cephalosporins. No differences in efficacy between first- and second-generation cephalosporins were found. Amoxicillin–clavulanate[279,282,283,299] and ciprofloxacin[269,300] were also evaluated with similar results. Relatively few studies have compared the efficacy of different agents in reducing postoperative infection rates.

One meta-analysis recommended using a single dose of an i.v. broad-spectrum antimicrobial for SSI prophylaxis in these patients,[256] while another found no differences between penicillin- or cephalosporin-based regimens and three-dose or single-dose regimens.[255] In a comparative study, oral or i.v. ciprofloxacin and i.v. cefuroxime were similarly effective in upper gastrointestinal procedures, including gastrectomy, vagotomy, and fundoplication.[300] No differences in efficacy were seen between ceftriaxone and combination ceftriaxone and metronidazole for PEG insertion in pediatric patients.[301] An open-label study found a significant decrease in local peristomal and systemic infection (i.e., pneumonia) after PEG insertion after a single 1-g i.v. dose of ceftriaxone was given 30 minutes before surgery when compared with placebo (13.3% and 36.3%, respectively; $p < 0.05$).[281] No differences were noted between cefotaxime and piperacillin–tazobactam for PEG SSIs.[288] Ampicillin–sulbactam and cefazolin had equal efficacy in gastrectomy.[253] One study found that piperacillin–tazobactam in combination with ciprofloxacin or gentamicin was the most active regimen against bacteria recovered from bile in pancreatoduodenectomy patients.[302]

Duration. The majority of studies evaluated a single dose of cephalosporin or penicillin.[256,279–284,288,290,297] The available data indicate that single-dose and multiple-dose regimens are similarly effective. Three studies compared single- and multiple-dose regimens of cefamandole,[294] amoxicillin–cluvulanate,[299] and ampicillin–sulbactam and cefazolin.[253] There were no significant differences in SSI rates. Multiple-dose regimens of first-generation (cefazolin) or second-generation (cefotiam) cephalosporins of four days, operative day only, and three days in duration did not differ in overall SSI rates.[295]

Recommendations. Antimicrobial prophylaxis in gastroduodenal procedures should be considered for patients at highest risk for postoperative infections, including risk factors such as increased gastric pH (e.g., patients receiving acid-suppression therapy), gastroduodenal perforation, decreased gastric motility, gastric outlet obstruction, gastric bleeding, morbid obesity, ASA classification of ≥3, and cancer.

A single dose of cefazolin is recommended in procedures during which the lumen of the intestinal tract is entered (Table 2). (Strength of evidence for prophylaxis = A.) A single dose of cefazolin is recommended in clean procedures, such as highly selective vagotomy, and antireflux procedures only in patients at high risk of postoperative infection due to the presence of the above risk factors. (Strength of evidence for prophylaxis = C.) Alternative regimens for patients with β-lactam allergy include clindamycin or vancomycin plus gentamicin, aztreonam, or a fluoroquinolone. Higher doses of antimicrobials are uniformly recommended in morbidly obese patients undergoing bariatric procedures. Higher doses of antimicrobials should be considered in significantly overweight patients undergoing gastroduodenal and endoscopic procedures.

Biliary Tract Procedures

Background. Biliary tract procedures include cholecystectomy, exploration of the common bile duct, and choledochoenterostomy. These guidelines pertain only to patients undergoing biliary tract procedures with no evidence of acute biliary tract infection and to patients with community-acquired acute cholecystitis of mild-to-moderate severity. As noted in the Common Principles section, patients receiving therapeutic antimicrobials for an infection before surgery should be given additional antimicrobial prophylaxis before surgery.

These guidelines do not address patients requiring biliary tract procedures for more-severe infections, including community-acquired acute cholecystitis with severe physiological disturbance, advanced age, or immunocompromised state; acute cholangitis; and health-care-associated or nosocomial biliary infections. These biliary tract infections are treated as complicated intraabdominal infections.[303] All patients with a suspected biliary tract infection who undergo biliary tract surgery should receive preoperative i.v. antimicrobials.

The majority of published literature regarding SSIs in biliary tract procedures focuses on cholecystectomy. The overall reported rate of postoperative infection in open biliary tract procedures with antimicrobial prophylaxis is 1–19%.[292,304–311] Infection rates after laparoscopic cholecystectomy range from 0% to approximately 4% in patients without antimicrobial prophylaxis[308,312–320] and from 0% to 7% with prophylaxis.[292,304–323] Several studies found that laparoscopic cholecystectomy SSI rates were significantly lower than those associated with open cholecystectomy.[292,306–311]

Risk factors associated with postoperative SSIs after biliary procedures include performance of emergency procedures,[305] diabetes,[305,306,311,315,317] longer procedure duration (over 120 minutes),[305,317,324] intraoperative gallbladder rupture,[305] age of >70 years,[6,311,315,317,325] open cholecystectomy,[7,311] conversion of laparoscopic to open cholecystectomy,[7] higher ASA classification (≥3),[306,310,317] episode of biliary colic within 30 days before the procedure,[315,316] reintervention in less than a month for noninfectious complications,[310] acute cholecystitis,[6,7,306] bile spillage,[7] jaundice,[6,7,306] pregnancy,[7] nonfunctioning gallbladder,[6] and immunosuppression.[7]

The biliary tract is usually sterile. Patients with bacteria in the bile at the time of surgery may be at higher risk of postoperative infection[305,326,327]; however, some studies have found no association between the presence of bacteria in the bile and infection.[305,315,316,319,321] Obesity (a BMI of >30 kg/m^2) was found to be a risk factor in some studies[306] but not in others.[315,319] Laparoscopic cholecystectomy was associated with a significantly decreased risk for SSI.[292,310,324,325]

Organisms. The organisms most commonly associated with infection after biliary tract procedures include *E. coli, Klebsiella* species, and enterococci; less frequently, other gram-negative organisms, streptococci, and staphylococci are isolated.[305,306,312,315,316,318,319,321,326,328–338] Anaerobes are occasionally reported, most commonly *Clostridium* species.

Recent studies have documented increasing antimicrobial resistance in the causative pathogens in biliary tract infections and other intra-abdominal infections, with up to 40% of *E. coli* isolates resistant to ampicillin–sulbactam and fluoroquinolones.[339–341] Due to this increasing resistance of *E. coli* to fluoroquinolones and ampicillin–sulbactam, local population susceptibility profiles should be reviewed to determine the optimal antimicrobials for SSI prevention in biliary tract procedures.

Efficacy. Numerous studies have evaluated the use of prophylactic antimicrobials during biliary tract procedures, with a focus on laparoscopic cholecystectomy. Laparoscopic cholecystectomy has replaced open cholecystectomy as the standard of practice because of the reduction in recovery time and shorter hospital stay. The majority of studies of antimicrobial prophylaxis for laparoscopic cholecystectomy were underpowered and varied in control groups used (placebo, active, or no treatment), follow-up (from 30 to 60 days, while some studies did not clearly define length of time), and how SSIs were detected and reported.[308,312–316,318,319,321,322] Some studies included patients who were converted from laparoscopic to open cholecystectomy and others did not.

A large, multicenter, quality-assurance study in Germany assessed the effectiveness of antimicrobial prophylaxis in laparoscopic and open cholecystectomies.[308] This study included 4477 patients whose antimicrobial choice and dosage regimens were at the discretion of the medical center and surgeon. Antimicrobials used included first-, second-, and third-generation cephalosporins or penicillins alone or in combination with metronidazole, gentamicin, or both metronidazole and gentamicin. The most common cephalosporin used was ceftriaxone, allowing its data to be separated from data for other antimicrobials. Antimicrobial prophylaxis was administered to 2217 patients (ceftriaxone [n = 787 laparoscopic and n = 188 open] and other antimicrobials [n = 229 laparoscopic and n = 229 open]); none was given to 1328 laparoscopic and 932 open cholecystectomy patients. Significantly lower overall infectious complications occurred in patients receiving antimicrobial prophylaxis (0.8% ceftriaxone and 1.2% other antimicrobials), compared with 5% of those who received no prophylaxis ($p < 0.05$). The overall rates of infectious complications were 0.6%, 0.8%, and 3.3% in patients undergoing laparoscopic cholecystectomy receiving ceftriaxone, other antimicrobials, and no prophylaxis, respectively, and 1.6%, 3.9%, and 7.4%, respectively, for patients undergoing open cholecystectomy. Significantly lower rates of SSIs and postoperative pneumonia were noted in patients receiving antimicrobials compared with those who did not receive prophylaxis ($p < 0.05$). SSI rates were significantly decreased in laparoscopic cholecystectomy patients who received ceftriaxone (0.1%) or other antimicrobials (0.2%) compared with those who received no antimicrobial prophylaxis (1.6%). SSI rates were significantly decreased in open cholecystectomy patients who received ceftriaxone (1.0%) or other antimicrobials (2.6%) compared with those who received no antimicrobial prophylaxis (4.4%). The study authors concluded that antimicrobial prophylaxis should be administered to all patients undergoing cholecystectomy, regardless of approach. The study had several limitations, including lack of randomization, lack of adequate controls, and lack of clear definition of patient selection for the antimicrobial regimens. The statistical analysis was not clearly defined. The study appears to have compared only the use and lack of use of antimicrobials (with ceftriaxone and other antimicrobials combined for analysis) and did not specifically compare the laparoscopic and open approaches.

The findings of this study contrast with those of several other published studies. A meta-analysis of 15 randomized controlled studies evaluated the need for antimicrobial prophylaxis in elective laparoscopic cholecystectomy for patients at low risk of infection.[313] Low risk was defined as not having any of the following: acute cholecystitis, a history of acute cholecystitis, common bile duct calculi, jaundice, immune suppression, and prosthetic implants. A total of 2961 patients were enrolled in the studies, including 1494 who received antimicrobial prophylaxis, primarily with cephalosporins, vancomycin, fluoroquinolones, metronidazole, and amoxicillin–clavulanate, and 1467 controls receiving placebo or no treatment. No significant difference was found in the rates of infectious complications (2.07% in patients receiving antimicrobial prophylaxis versus 2.45% in controls) or SSIs (1.47% in patients receiving antimicrobial prophylaxis versus 1.77% in controls). The authors of the meta-analysis concluded that antimicrobial prophylaxis was not necessary for low-risk patients undergoing elective laparoscopic cholecystectomy. An additional meta-analysis of 9 randomized controlled trials (n = 1437) also concluded that prophylactic antimicrobials do not prevent infections in low-risk patients undergoing laparoscopic cholecystectomy.[342]

A small, prospective, nonrandomized study compared the use of cefotaxime 1 g i.v. during surgery with an additional two i.v. doses given eight hours apart after surgery (n = 80) with no antimicrobial prophylaxis (n = 86) in patients undergoing elective laparoscopic cholecystectomy with accidental or incidental gallbladder rupture and spillage of bile.[317] Patients who had spillage of gallstone calculi or whose operations were converted to open operations were excluded from the study. The rate of SSIs did not significantly differ between treatment groups (2.5% with antimicrobials versus 3.4% without antimicrobial prophylaxis). Based on results of multivariate analysis, routine antimicrobial prophylaxis was not recommended for these patients unless they were diabetic, were older than 60 years, or had an ASA classification of ≥3 or the duration of the procedure exceeded 70 minutes.

Current data do not support antimicrobial prophylaxis for low-risk patients undergoing elective laparoscopic cholecystectomies or those with incidental or accidental gallbladder rupture. Antimicrobial prophylaxis should be considered for patients at high risk of infection, including those undergoing open cholecystectomy, as described above, or who are considered to be at high risk for conversion to an open procedure.

Choice of agent. The data do not indicate a significant difference among first-, second-, and third-generation cephalosporins. First-generation,[307,308,312,315,319,323,330,336,338,343,344] second-generation,[308,314,315,318,323,327–329,331,332,335,344–352] and third-generation[308,309,315–317,321,322,332,333,338,349,353,354] cephalosporins have been studied more extensively than other antimicrobials. Limited data are available for ampicillin with gentamicin,[355] piperacillin,[356] amoxicillin–clavulanate,[305,338,351,354] ciprofloxacin,[320,333,352,357] and cephalosporins or penicillins alone or in combination with metronidazole, gentamicin, or both metronidazole and gentamicin.[308]

Several studies have compared first-generation cephalosporins with second- or third-generation age nts.[315,336,338,344–347,353,358] With one exception,[347] there was no significant difference in efficacy among agents. Other studies found no significant differences in efficacy between ampicillin and cefamandole,[335] ciprofloxacin and ceftriaxone,[333] amoxicillin–clavulanate and cefotaxime,[354] amoxicillin–clavulanate and cefamandole,[351] ceftriaxone and ceftazidime,[321] and oral and i.v. ciprofloxacin and i.v. cefuroxime.[352,357] One study found that i.v. ampicillin–sulbactam was associated with significantly lower rates of infection compared with cefuroxime[306] and that patients treated with oral ceftibuten had significantly lower infection rates than those who received amoxicillin–clavulanate.[338]

Duration. The effect of duration of prophylaxis on outcome has been evaluated. A single dose of a cephalosporin was compared with multiple doses in several studies; no significant differences in efficacy were found.[327,329,330,348,349,353,359] The largest study compared one dose of cefuroxime with three doses in 1004 patients with risk factors for infection who were undergoing biliary tract surgery.[327] There was no significant difference in the rates of minor or major SSIs between the single- and multiple-dose groups. In the majority of studies, one dose of an antimicrobial was administered at induction of anesthesia,[306,312,338,352,354] within 30 minutes before incision,[338] or 1[315,316,320,321] or 2[338] hours before incision. Additional doses were given as follows: one dose 12 hours after administration of the initial dose,[352] two doses 12 and 24 hours after administration of the initial dose,[338] two doses every 6[338] or 8[317,319] hours after surgery, and one dose 24 hours after surgery[315] and five days after surgery.[352] In one study, a second dose of amoxicillin–clavulanate or cefotaxime was administered for procedures lasting longer than 4 hours.[354]

Recommendations. A single dose of cefazolin should be administered in patients undergoing open biliary tract procedures (Table 2). (Strength of evidence for prophylaxis = A.) Alternatives include ampicillin–sulbactam and other cephalosporins (cefotetan, cefoxitin, and ceftriaxone). Alternative regimens for patients with β-lactam allergy include clindamycin or vancomycin plus gentamicin, aztreonam, or a fluoroquinolone; or metronidazole plus gentamicin or a fluoroquinolone.

Antimicrobial prophylaxis is not necessary in low-risk patients undergoing elective laparoscopic cholecystectomies. (Strength of evidence against prophylaxis for low-risk patients = A.) Antimicrobial prophylaxis is recommended in patients undergoing laparoscopic cholecystectomy who have an increased risk of infectious complications. Risk factors include performance of emergency procedures, diabetes, anticipated procedure duration exceeding 120 minutes, risk of intraoperative gallbladder rupture, age of >70 years, open cholecystectomy, risk of conversion of laparoscopic to open cholecystectomy, ASA classification of ≥3, episode of biliary colic within 30 days before the procedure, reintervention in less than a month for noninfectious complications of prior biliary operation, acute cholecystitis, anticipated bile spillage, jaundice, pregnancy, nonfunctioning gallbladder, and immunosuppression. Because some of these risk factors cannot be determined before the surgical intervention, it may be reasonable to give a single dose of antimicrobial prophylaxis to all patients undergoing laparoscopic cholecystectomy. (Strength of evidence for prophylaxis for high-risk patients = A.)

Appendectomy Procedures

Background. Cases of appendicitis can be described as complicated or uncomplicated on the basis of the pathology. Patients with uncomplicated appendicitis have an acutely inflamed appendix. Complicated appendicitis includes perforated or gangrenous appendicitis, including peritonitis or abscess formation. Because complicated appendicitis is treated as a complicated intra-abdominal infection,[303] it has not been addressed separately in these guidelines. All patients with a suspected clinical diagnosis of appendicitis, even those with an uncomplicated case, should receive appropriate preoperative i.v. antimicrobials for SSI prevention, which, due to the common microbiology encountered, requires similar antimicrobial choices to those used to treat complicated appendicitis.

Approximately 80% of patients with appendicitis have uncomplicated disease.[59] SSI has been reported in 9–30% of patients with uncomplicated appendicitis who do not receive prophylactic antimicrobials, though some reports suggest lower complication rates in children with uncomplicated appendicitis.[165,360–365] Mean SSI rates for appendectomy reported in the most recent NHSN report (2006–08) were 1.15% (60 of 5211) for NHSN risk index categories 0 and 1 versus 3.47% (23 of 663) for NHSN risk index categories 2 and 3.[165] Laparoscopic appendectomy has been reported to produce lower rates of incisional (superficial and deep) SSIs than open appendectomy in adults and children in multiple meta-analyses and several randomized clinical trials.[292,310,366–371] However, the rate of organ/space SSIs (i.e., intra-abdominal abscesses) was significantly increased with laparoscopic appendectomy.

Organisms. The most common microorganisms isolated from SSIs after appendectomy are anaerobic and aerobic gram-negative enteric organisms. *Bacteroides fragilis* is the most commonly cultured anaerobe, and *E. coli* is the most frequent aerobe, indicating that the bowel flora constitute a major source for pathogens.[59,372,373] Aerobic and anaerobic streptococci, *Staphylococcus* species, and *Enterococcus* species also have been reported. *P. aeruginosa* has been reported infrequently.

Efficacy. Antibiotic prophylaxis is generally recognized as effective in the prevention of postoperative SSIs in patients undergoing appendectomy when compared with placebo.[374]

Choice of agent. Randomized controlled trials have failed to identify an agent that is clearly superior to other agents in the prophylaxis of postappendectomy infectious complications. An appropriate choice for SSI prophylaxis in uncomplicated appendicitis would be any single agent or combination of agents that provides adequate gram-negative and anaerobic coverage. The second-generation cephalosporins with anaerobic activity and a first-generation cephalosporin plus metronidazole are the recommended agents on the basis of cost and tolerability. Given the relatively equivalent efficacy between agents, a cost-minimization approach is reasonable; the choice of agents should be based on local drug acquisition costs and antimicrobial sensitivity patterns.

A wide range of antimicrobials have been evaluated for prophylaxis in uncomplicated appendicitis. The most commonly used agents were cephalosporins. In general, a second-generation cephalosporin with anaerobic activity (cefoxitin or cefotetan) or third-generation cephalosporins with partial anaerobic activity (cefotaxime) were effective, with postoperative SSI rates of <5% in most studies.[364,375–381]

Piperacillin 2 g was comparable to cefoxitin 2 g in a well-controlled study.[381] Metronidazole used alone was less effective than cefotaxime, with infection rates above 10%.[376] However, when metronidazole was combined with cefazolin, ampicillin,[382] or gentamicin,[378,383] the post-operative SSI rates were 3–6%.

A double-blind, randomized, controlled trial was conducted at two hospitals to evaluate the effect of metronidazole, which is effective against most anaerobes, and cefazolin, which is effective against many aerobic organisms, singly and in combination, on the rate of sepsis after appendectomy.[384] Patients were randomized into one of four groups: metronidazole and placebo, cefazolin and placebo, metronidazole and cefazolin, or double placebo. Patients with generalized peritonitis were excluded for ethical reasons. Treatment was started before the procedure and continued every 8 hours for 24 hours. All patients in the trial were followed for about two weeks after discharge from the hospital, and their surgical sites were inspected. A total of 271 patients were assessed. Sepsis rates at the two hospitals were similar. Patients who received both cefazolin and metronidazole had a significantly lower infection rate compared with the other groups.[384] Consistent with the antibacterial spectrum of the agents, a prospective study of antimicrobial prophylaxis for colorectal procedures found that the combination of metronidazole with aztreonam did not show adequate coverage of gram-positive organisms.[385] The Common Principles section of these guidelines provides additional considerations for weight-based dosing.

Duration. In most of the studies of second- or third-generation cephalosporins or metronidazole combinations, a single dose[376–378,380,383] or two or three doses[364,379,382] were given. Although direct comparisons were not made, there was no discernible difference in postoperative SSI rates between single-dose and multidose administration in most studies. A randomized trial specifically comparing different durations of regimens found no statistical difference between a single preoperative dose, three doses (preoperative dose plus two additional doses), or a five-day regimen.[386] A large cohort study found that single doses of metronidazole and gentamicin in patients undergoing open appendectomy were effective and sufficient in decreasing the SSI rate.[387]

Pediatric Efficacy. In pediatric patients, as with adults, preoperative determination of complicated versus uncomplicated appendicitis is difficult. A comprehensive review is not provided here, but this topic has been addressed by SIS.[388]

Two pediatric studies demonstrated no difference in SSI rates between placebo and several antimicrobials. The first study compared metronidazole, penicillin plus tobramycin, and piperacillin.[389] The second study compared single-dose metronidazole and single-dose metronidazole plus cefuroxime.[390] A meta-analysis including both adult and pediatric studies found that for pediatric patients, antimicrobial prophylaxis trended toward being beneficial, but the results were not statistically significant.[374] A retrospective chart review questioned the routine need for antimicrobial prophylaxis in children with simple appendicitis, due to relatively low infection rates in children not receiving prophylaxis.[365] However, these and other study authors have suggested antimicrobial prophylaxis may be considered due to the morbidity associated with infectious complications (e.g., prolonged hospitalization, readmission, reoperation) and due to the inability to preoperatively identify appendicitis.

As a single agent, metronidazole was no more effective than placebo in two double-blind studies that included children 10 years of age or older[360] and 15 years of age or older.[363] In a randomized study that included pediatric patients, ceftizoxime and cefamandole were associated with significantly lower infection rates and duration of hospitalization than placebo.[391] Both cefoxitin and a combination of gentamicin and metronidazole were associated with a lower rate of postoperative infection in a randomized study that included pediatric patients younger than 16 years.[378] Second-generation cephalosporins with anaerobic activity (cefoxitin or cefotetan) and third-generation cephalosporins with anaerobic activity (cefotaxime) were effective, with post-operative infection rates of <5% in two studies that included pediatric patients younger than 12 years.[364,378,379] A single dose of gentamicin with clindamycin was found to be safe and effective in children with simple appendicitis.[392]

Recommendations. For uncomplicated appendicitis, the recommended regimen is a single dose of a cephalosporin with anaerobic activity (cefoxitin or cefotetan) or a single dose of a first-generation cephalosporin (cefazolin) plus metronidazole (Table 2). For β-lactam-allergic patients, alternative regimens include (1) clindamycin plus gentamicin, aztreonam, or a fluoroquinolone and (2) metronidazole plus gentamicin or a fluoroquinolone (ciprofloxacin or levofloxacin). (Strength of evidence for prophylaxis = A.)

Small Intestine Procedures

Background. Small intestine procedures, or small bowel surgery as defined by NHSN, include incision or resection of the small intestine, including enterectomy with or without intestinal anastomosis or enterostomy, intestinal bypass, and strictureoplasty; it does not include small-to-large bowel anastomosis.

The risk of SSI in small bowel surgery is variable. The Surgical Site Infection Surveillance Service in England (data collected by 168 hospitals in 13 categories of surgical procedures between 1997 and 2002) reported an SSI rate of 8.9% (94 of 1056).[393] Mean SSI rates for small bowel procedures reported in the most recent NHSN report (2006–08) were 3.44% for NHSN risk index category 0 versus 6.75% for NHSN risk index categories 1, 2, and 3. A study of 1472 patients undergoing bowel surgery (small bowel and colon) at 31 U.S. academic medical centers between September and December 2002 found an SSI rate of 8.7% for all wound categories. For patients with clean-contaminated wounds, the SSI rate was 7.9%; for those with contaminated or dirty-infected wounds, the SSI rates were 12.0% and 20.4%, respectively.[394]

In a study of 178 penetrating stomach and small bowel injuries, 94% of which were operated on within six hours of presentation, SSIs occurred in nearly 20% of cases. When associated colon injuries were excluded, SSIs occurred in 16% of gastric injuries and 13% of small bowel injuries. Although 74% of patients received antimicrobials, the specific timing of antimicrobial administration was not provided.[395] Other studies of small bowel injury confirm similar SSI rates.[396–400]

Antimicrobial prophylaxis is recommended for small bowel surgery, based on inferring effectiveness from other clean-contaminated procedures. No specific prospective randomized studies could be identified that addressed antimicrobial prophylaxis for small bowel surgery. Antimicrobial prophylaxis for small bowel surgical procedures related to a diagnosis of complicated intra-abdominal infection is not addressed separately in these guidelines, as antimicrobial therapy for established intraabdominal infection should be initiated preoperatively.

Organisms. The most common microorganisms isolated from SSIs after small bowel surgery are aerobic gram-negative enteric organisms. Among the species isolated from patients with SSI after small intestine surgery are gram-negative bacilli of gastrointestinal enteric origin (aerobic and anaerobic) and gram-positive species, such as streptococci, staphylococci, and enterococci, which is consistent with similar studies.[401] *E. coli* is the most frequently identified aerobe, indicating that the bowel flora constitute a major source of pathogens. Aerobic and anaerobic streptococci, *Staphylococcus* species, and *Enterococcus* species also have been reported.

The microbiology of 2280 SSIs after upper or lower abdominal surgery conducted from 1999 to 2006 was described in the Prevalence of Infections in Spanish Hospitals (EPINE) study.[402] The most frequent microorganisms isolated were *E. coli* (28%), *Enterococcus* species (15%), *Streptococcus* species (8%), *P. aeruginosa* (7%), and *S. aureus* (5%; resistant to methicillin, 2%). The microbiology of SSIs after upper abdominal tract surgery did not show any significant differences compared with SSIs of the lower tract, though there were relatively more staphylococci, *K. pneumoniae*, *Enterobacter* species, *Acinetobacter* species, and *Candida albicans* isolates and fewer *E. coli*, *B. fragilis*, and *Clostridium* species in the upper abdominal surgery group.[402]

Efficacy. Antibiotic prophylaxis is generally recognized as effective in the prevention of postoperative SSIs in patients undergoing small bowel surgery when compared with placebo. However, there are no prospective placebo-controlled trials to definitively establish the efficacy of prophylactic antimicrobials in this patient population.

Choice of agent. The antimicrobials selected for prophylaxis must cover the expected pathogens for the small intestine. The microbial ecology of the proximal small intestine (i.e., jejunum) is similar to that of the duodenum, whereas the microbial flora of the ileum are similar to those of the colon. In patients with small intestine obstruction, the microbial flora are similar to those of the colon.

No randomized controlled trials have confirmed that one antimicrobial agent is superior to other agents for SSI prophylaxis in small bowel surgery. An appropriate antimicrobial choice for SSI prophylaxis in small bowel surgery is any single agent or combination of agents that provides adequate coverage for the small intestinal microbes. In patients with small bowel obstruction, additional coverage of anaerobic bacteria is also desirable.

For small intestine procedures with no evidence of obstruction, a first-generation cephalosporin (cefazolin) is recommended. For patients with small intestine obstruction, a first-generation cephalosporin with metronidazole or a second-generation cephalosporin with anaerobic activity (cefoxitin or cefotetan) is the recommended agent. The choice of agents should be based on local drug acquisition costs and antimicrobial sensitivity patterns. The Common Principles section of these guidelines provides additional considerations for weight-based dosing.

Duration. Preoperative dosing of antimicrobials for SSI prevention, with additional intraoperative antimicrobial dosing dependent on the duration of the operation and no postoperative dosing, is recommended for patients undergoing small bowel surgery.

Pediatric Efficacy. In pediatric patients, as with adults, antimicrobial prophylaxis for SSI prevention in small bowel surgery is recommended.

Recommendations. For small bowel surgery without obstruction, the recommended regimen is a first-generation cephalosporin (cefazolin) (Table 2). For small bowel surgery with intestinal obstruction, the recommended regimen is a cephalosporin with anaerobic activity (cefoxitin or cefotetan) or the combination of a first-generation cephalosporin (cefazolin) plus metronidazole. For β-lactam-allergic patients, alternative regimens include (1) clindamycin plus gentamicin, aztreonam, or a fluoroquinolone and (2) metronidazole plus gentamicin or a fluoroquinolone (ciprofloxacin or levofloxacin). (Strength of evidence for prophylaxis = C.)

Hernia Repair Procedures (Hernioplasty and Herniorrhaphy)

Background. All patients who undergo hernioplasty (prosthetic mesh repair of hernia) or herniorrhaphy (suture repair of hernia) should receive appropriate preoperative i.v. antimicrobials for SSI prevention. The risk of SSIs is higher in hernioplasty compared with herniorrhaphy.[403] There is a significant risk of requiring prosthetic mesh removal in hernioplasty patients who develop an SSI, and determination of whether mesh placement will be required for hernia repair is not always possible in the preoperative period.

Mean SSI rates for herniorrhaphy reported in the most recent NHSN report (2006–08) were 0.74% (21 of 2852) for NHSN risk index category 0, 2.42% (81 of 3348) for NHSN risk index category 1, and 5.25% (67 of 1277) for NHSN risk index categories 2 and 3.[165]

A Cochrane meta-analysis of 17 randomized trials (n = 7843; 11 hernioplasty trials, 6 herniorrhaphy trials) in elective open inguinal hernia repair reported SSI rates of 3.1% versus 4.5% in the antimicrobial prophylaxis and control groups, respectively (OR, 0.64; 95% CI, 0.50–0.82).[404] The subgroup of patients with herniorrhaphy had SSI rates of 3.5% and 4.9% in the prophylaxis and control groups, respectively (OR, 0.71; 95% CI, 0.51–1.00). The subgroup of patients with hernioplasty had SSI rates of 2.4% and 4.2% in the prophylaxis and control groups, respectively (OR, 0.56; 95% CI, 0.38–0.81).

A meta-analysis of nine randomized trials of open hernioplasty for inguinal hernia documented SSI rates of 2.4% (39 of 1642) in the antimicrobial group and 4.2% (70 of 1676) in the control group. Antibiotics showed a protective effect in preventing SSI after mesh inguinal hernia repair (OR, 0.61; 95% CI, 0.40–0.92). Antibiotic prophylaxis did reduce the rate of SSI in hernia patients undergoing mesh hernioplasty.[405]

Based on the results of these two systematic reviews, preoperative antimicrobial prophylaxis for SSI prevention is recommended for both herniorrhaphy and hernioplasty. Compared with open hernia repair, laparoscopic hernia repair has been reported to produce lower rates of incisional (superficial and deep) SSIs in randomized clinical trials.[406–408] In a recent multicenter randomized trial of laparoscopic versus open ventral incisional hernia repair (n = 162), SSI was significantly less common in the laparoscopic group than in the open repair group (2.8% versus 21.9%; OR, 10.5; 95% CI, 2.3–48.2; p = 0.003).[409] A meta-analysis of eight randomized trials comparing laparoscopic and open incisional or ventral hernia repair with mesh revealed that laparoscopic hernia repair was associated with decreased SSI rates (relative risk, 0.22; 95% CI, 0.09–0.54) and a trend toward fewer infections requiring mesh removal.[410]

Organisms. The most common microorganisms isolated from SSIs after herniorrhaphy and hernioplasty are aerobic gram-positive organisms. Aerobic streptococci, *Staphylococcus* species, and *Enterococcus* species are common, and MRSA is commonly found in prosthetic mesh infections.[411]

Efficacy. Antibiotic prophylaxis is generally recognized as effective when compared with placebo in the prevention of postoperative SSIs in patients undergoing herniorrhaphy and hernioplasty.

Choice of agent. Randomized controlled trials have failed to identify an agent that is clearly superior to other agents for SSI prophylaxis in hernia repair. A first-generation cephalosporin is the recommended agent on the basis of cost and tolerability. The Common Principles section of these guidelines provides additional considerations for weight-based dosing.

Duration. Based on the evidence to date, a single preoperative dose of antimicrobial is recommended in hernioplasty and herniorrhaphy, with redosing as recommended in the Common Principles section of these guidelines (if the procedure duration exceeds the recommended redosing interval from the time of initiation of the preoperative dose or if there is prolonged or excessive bleeding).

Recommendations. For hernioplasty and herniorrhaphy, the recommended regimen is a single dose of a first-generation cephalosporin (cefazolin) (Table 2). For patients known to be colonized with MRSA, it is reasonable to add a single preoperative dose of vancomycin to the recommended agent. For β-lactam-allergic patients, alternative regimens include clindamycin and vancomycin. (Strength of evidence for prophylaxis = A.)

Colorectal Procedures

Background. SSIs have been reported to occur in approximately 4–10% of patients undergoing colon procedures, 3–7% in small bowel procedures, and 3–27% in patients after rectal procedures, based on the risk index.[165] However, when patients are followed carefully in clinical trials, rates tend to be considerably higher (17–26%).[412] Other septic complications, such as fecal fistula, intra-abdominal abscesses, peritonitis, and septicemia, are serious concerns but are much less common.[413] Infectious complication rates range from 30% to 60% without antimicrobial prophylaxis[59,414] and are <10% with appropriate antimicrobial prophylaxis. A pooled analysis of clinical trials of antimicrobial prophylaxis in colon procedures demonstrated that antimicrobial use significantly reduced mortality rates (11.2% for control versus 4.5% for treatment) and SSI rates.[415]

The type and duration of the procedure can affect the risk of infection. Rectal resection is associated with a higher risk of infection than is intraperitoneal colon resection.[416–418] Other risk factors include extended procedure duration (e.g., >3.5 hours),[59,412,418,419] impaired host defenses,[418] age of >60 years,[418] hypoalbuminemia,[419,420] bacterial or fecal contamination of the surgical site,[418,420] inadvertent perforation or spillage,[412,421] corticosteroid therapy,[419] perioperative transfusion of packed red blood cells,[394,418] hypothermia,[422] hyperglycemia,[423,424] and obesity.[412,418]

Organisms. The infecting organisms in colorectal procedures are derived from the bowel lumen, where there are high concentrations of organisms. *B. fragilis* and other obligate anaerobes are the most frequently isolated organisms from the bowel, with concentrations 1,000–10,000 times higher than those of aerobes.[425] *E. coli* is the most common aerobe. *B. fragilis* and *E. coli* comprise approximately 20–30% of the fecal mass. They are the most frequently isolated pathogens from infected surgical sites after colon procedures.

Efficacy. Results from randomized controlled trials and a Cochrane review of 182 studies of over 30,000 patients support the routine use of prophylactic antimicrobials in all patients undergoing colorectal procedures.[426]

Choice of agent. The agent chosen for antimicrobial prophylaxis in colorectal procedures should have activity against the anaerobic and aerobic floras of the bowel. The most appropriate regimen for antimicrobial prophylaxis for colorectal procedure (e.g., oral, i.v, oral–i.v. combination) and the optimal choice of antimicrobial agent have not been fully resolved.

Oral regimens. The efficacy of oral prophylactic antimicrobial agents has been established in studies only when used with mechanical bowel preparation (MBP). A variety of oral agents administered after MBP have been evaluated for prophylaxis for colorectal procedures. The most common combinations include an aminoglycoside (neomycin and, less often, kanamycin, which is only available in injectable form in the United States) plus a medication with anaerobic activity, usually erythromycin[427–434] or metronidazole.[432,433,435–439] In placebo-controlled studies, the oral combination was significantly more effective than placebo in reducing SSIs.[427,433,434,439,440] Postoperative SSI rates were 0–11% with neomycin plus erythromycin[427–432] and 2–13% with neomycin and metronidazole.[436–438] Combinations of neomycin and tetracycline,[440] neomycin and clindamycin,[436] and neomycin and tinidazole[441] have also been used successfully, with postoperative SSI rates of <10%. The use of metronidazole as a single agent appears to be less effective, with reported SSI rates of 12–15%.[442–444]

Oral antimicrobials have been compared with i.v. agents in a few studies. Oral neomycin plus oral erythromycin was similarly effective as i.v. cefoxitin in one study[429] but inferior in another[445] and was similarly effective as i.v. ceftriaxone plus i.v. metronidazole in patients undergoing elective colorectal procedures.[431] The addition of i.v. cefamandole to oral neomycin plus oral erythromycin did not improve efficacy.[430] In one of these studies, oral neomycin and erythromycin were more effective than i.v. cefoxitin for procedures lasting longer than 4 hours.[445] A randomized controlled study was stopped early due to the significantly higher rate of infection in the oral neomycin and erythromycin group (41%) compared with the single-dose i.v. metronidazole and ceftriaxone group (9.6%) ($p < 0.01$).[446] Similarly, a study of oral metronidazole and kanamycin compared with the same medications given intravenously found an increased rate of postoperative sepsis (36% versus 6.5%, respectively) ($p < 0.001$), greater numbers of *E. coli* resistant to kanamycin, more bacterial overgrowth, and antimicrobial-associated pseudomembranous colitis in the oral group.[447] However, the oral antimicrobials were not given on a schedule expected to be effective, as they were discontinued 36 hours before the procedure. The fact that oral antibiotics were given for three days rather than less than one day, as is the current practice, was suggested as a possible reason for the resistance and colitis observed.

I.V. regimens. A wide range of i.v. antimicrobials have been evaluated for prophylaxis in colorectal procedures. Cephalosporins are the most common agents, usually administered as a single agent. The majority of studies found that single-agent first-generation cephalosporins (cefazolin and cephalothin)[445,448–451] were ineffective, with postoperative SSI rates ranging from 12% to 39%.[448,449] The lack of efficacy is likely due to their lack of *B. fragilis* activity. The combination of cefazolin and metronidazole provides adequate coverage of pathogens and may be a cost-effective prophylaxis strategy.[6,41]

Second-generation cephalosporins with anaerobic activity, such as cefoxitin and cefotetan, have been widely evaluated. In single-agent therapy, SSI rates ranged from 0% to 17%[91,417,445,452–459]; however, more than half of the studies found SSI rates of >10%.

Third-generation agents, cefotaxime and ceftriaxone, have been evaluated in a few trials; postoperative SSI rates were 8–19% with single-agent use.[456,460,461] In some studies, second- or third-generation cephalosporins were combined with other i.v. agents, most commonly metronidazole.[452,459–462] However, in all but one of these studies, a combination of a second- or third-generation cephalosporin plus metronidazole was no more effective than the cephalosporin alone. The use of third- or fourth-generation cephalosporins for routine antimicrobial prophylaxis is not recommended as use may lead to development of resistant organisms.[6,41,444,463] However, in institutions where there is increasing gram-negative resistance from isolates to first- and second-generation cephalosporins, a single dose of ceftriaxone plus metronidazole may be preferred over routine use of carbapenems.

Three small studies, with under 200 patients each, found i.v. ampicillin–sulbactam or amoxicillin–clavulanate to be as effective as i.v. combinations of gentamicin and metronidazole,[464] gentamicin and clindamycin,[465] and cefotaxime and metronidazole for preventing SSIs in elective colorectal procedures.

A randomized controlled study of adult patients undergoing elective colon or rectal procedures evaluated the use of a single high dose of gentamicin 4.5 mg/kg i.v. plus metronidazole 500 mg i.v. in sequential order over 30 minutes compared with multiple standard doses of gentamicin 1.5 mg/kg plus metronidazole given preoperatively and every 8 hours for 24 hours postoperatively.[16] All patients underwent MBP before surgery. Patients with a serum creatinine concentration exceeding 1.7 mg/L were excluded from the study. No statistically significant differences were seen in deep and superficial incisional SSI rates between groups. Significantly fewer superficial SSIs were seen in the single-dose group compared with the multidose group in procedures lasting longer than 3.5 hours (22.2% versus 55%, $p = 0.021$). A pharmacodynamic study of these patients found the gentamicin concentration at the time of surgical-site closure as the strongest independent factor for infection.[17] Of note, the infection rate was 80% in 10 patients with gentamicin concentrations of <0.5 mg/L.

Other i.v. agents that have been evaluated either alone or in combination include aminoglycosides,[464,466–469] clindamycin,[466] ampicillin,[467,469–471] penicillins plus β-lactamase inhibitors,[464,465,468,472,473] doxycycline,[470,474–476] piperacillin,[91,473] imipenem,[462] and ciprofloxacin.[300]

Ertapenem, a broad-spectrum carbapenem, is approved by FDA for the prophylaxis of SSIs after elective colorectal procedures.[67] Cefotetan is also FDA approved for surgical prophylaxis in clean-contaminated procedures (e.g., gastrointestinal procedures) in adult patients undergoing elective colon or rectal procedures.[62] A large, multicenter, randomized controlled study compared a single 1-g i.v. dose of ertapenem with cefotetan 2 g i.v. infused within 60 minutes before surgical incision.[412] All patients received MBP preoperatively. SSI rates were significantly lower in the ertapenem group versus cefotetan in the per-protocol (18.1% and 31.1%, respectively) and the modified intent-to-treat (17.1% and 50.9%) populations. Ertapenem was found to be superior to cefotetan for SSI prevention. Although not statistically significant, higher rates of skin-related events (i.e., pruritis and rash), gastrointestinal events, and *C. difficile* infection were seen in the ertapenem group. The study authors concluded that ertapenem is an acceptable alternative to cefotetan and cefoxitin. Routine use of ertapenem for surgical prophylaxis remains controversial due to theoretical concerns regarding increases in resistant organisms and a potential increase in adverse events.[477]

Alternative agents for patients with a high likelihood of past serious adverse event or allergy to β-lactams include (1) clindamycin plus an aminoglycoside, aztreonam, or a fluoroquinolone and (2) metronidazole plus an aminoglycoside or a fluoroquinolone.[41]

Combination oral and i.v. regimens. Combinations of oral and i.v. antimicrobials have been used in an attempt to further reduce postoperative infection rates. Regimens include oral neomycin and erythromycin plus i.v. administration of a cephalosporin,[416,417,429,445,449,478,479] metronidazole,[480,481] and gentamicin plus clindamycin.[466] Postoperative SSI rates in these studies ranged from 0% to 7%. With one exception,[416] there was no significant difference between oral neomycin–erythromycin plus an i.v. antimicrobial and oral neomycin–erythromycin alone.[429,449,466,478] When combination oral and i.v. agents were compared with i.v. agents alone, combination therapy was favored in five of six studies[417,429,445,449,480,482]; the difference was significant in three.[417,449,482] The most recent Cochrane review found that the infection rate was significantly lower with the combination of oral plus i.v. prophylaxis when compared with i.v. alone (relative risk, 0.55; $p = 0.000084$) or with oral prophylaxis alone (relative risk, 0.34; $p = 0.024$).[426] A recent report of over 2000 patients recorded prospectively in the Michigan Surgical Quality Collaborative—Colectomy Best Practices Project and analyzed retrospectively revealed a significantly lower rate of postoperative infections when 370 colectomy patients received MBP and oral antimicrobial prophylaxis compared with propensity-matched patients receiving i.v. prophylaxis alone.[483]

A multicenter, randomized, controlled study of 491 patients who received MBP plus oral antimicrobials (kanamycin and erythromycin) with i.v. cefmetazole (not available in the United States but noted by the expert panel to have a similar spectrum of activity as cefotetan) or i.v. cefmetazole alone found no difference in SSI between groups for colon procedures.[484] However, the combination of oral and i.v. antimicrobials was significantly better than i.v. alone for rectal procedures, particularly abdominoperineal excision. Another study found the postoperative SSI rates after rectal resection were 23% and 11%, respectively, for patients receiving i.v. cefoxitin and cefoxitin plus oral neomycin and erythromycin.[417]

The safety and tolerability of oral antimicrobials have been investigated in two studies. One case–control study found an increased incidence of *C. difficile* colitis among patients with oral plus i.v. antimicrobials and MBP compared with i.v. antimicrobials and MBP alone.[485] However, another case–control study found a lower rate (not statistically significant) of *C. difficile* infection in patients who had received oral antimicrobials compared with those who had not (1.6% versus 2.9%, $p = 0.09$).[486] A randomized controlled study of 300 patients undergoing elective colorectal procedures found significantly higher rates of nausea and vomiting among patients receiving three doses of oral antimicrobials (neomycin and metronidazole, 44% and 31%, respectively) in combination with i.v. cefoxitin and MBP compared with regimens including one dose of oral antimicrobials (18% and 11%, respectively) and no oral antimicrobials (13% and 9%, respectively).[487] No difference was noted between groups for rates of abdominal pain, SSIs, or intraabdominal abscesses. An increased number of gastrointestinal adverse events was also reported in another comparative study in the combination oral and i.v. group (2.9%) compared with the i.v.-only group (2.1%), although the results were not statistically significant.[484] Overall, the evidence suggests that the combination of oral antimicrobials with MBP in addition to i.v. prophylactic antimicrobials reduces the rate of postoperative infections compared with i.v. antimicrobials alone without MBP, although the addition of oral antimicrobials increases gastrointestinal symptoms.

Duration. Single and multiple doses were compared in several studies.[454–456,461,471,475] However, only two of these studies compared single doses with multiple doses of the same antimicrobial.[471,475] There was no significant difference in infection rates between single-dose and multidose administration. One study found a single dose of cefotaxime plus metronidazole was significantly more effective than three doses of cefotaxime alone.[461] The most recent Cochrane review found no benefit to extending the duration of prophylaxis ($p = 0.58$).[426] Generally, antimicrobial prophylaxis should be continued for no more than 24 hours and can typically be stopped when the procedure is completed and the surgical site is closed.[6,41,444] No evidence supports greater efficacy for doses given after the completion of the procedure. Additional discussion on this topic is found in the Common Principles section of these guidelines.

Consideration should be given to an additional dose of the i.v. antimicrobial if an agent with a short half-life is used and the procedure duration exceeds the recommended redosing interval (starting from the time of initiation of the preoperative dose) and if intraoperative blood loss occurs.[6,41,120,418,444,445] No significant difference was seen in SSI rates with single-dose cefazolin, single-dose cefotetan, and cefazolin given as one preoperative dose and a second dose three hours later for procedures with a duration of less than three hours.[118] SSI rates were significantly higher with a single dose of cefazolin for procedures with a duration of greater than three hours. Using an agent with a longer half-life can decrease the necessity to redose the antimicrobial during long procedures.

Pediatric Efficacy. No well-controlled studies have evaluated the efficacy of antimicrobial prophylaxis in pediatric patients undergoing colorectal procedures. However, there is no reason to suspect that prophylaxis efficacy would be different. The safety, efficacy, tolerability, and cost-effectiveness of intestinal lavage have been demonstrated in two studies of 20 and 21 pediatric patients.[488,489]

Recommendations. A single dose of second-generation cephalosporin with both aerobic and anaerobic activities (cefoxitin or cefotetan) or cefazolin plus metronidazole is recommended for colon procedures (Table 2). In institutions where there is increasing resistance to first- and second-generation cephalosporins among gram-negative isolates from SSIs, the expert panel recommends a single dose of ceftriaxone plus metronidazole over routine use of carbapenems. An alternative regimen is ampicillin–sulbactam. In most patients, MBP combined with a combination of oral neomycin sulfate plus oral erythromycin base or oral neomycin sulfate plus oral metronidazole should be given in addition to i.v. prophylaxis. The oral antimicrobial should be given as three doses over approximately 10 hours the afternoon and evening before the operation and after the MBP. Alternative regimens for patients with β-lactam allergies include (1) clindamycin plus an aminoglycoside, aztreonam, or a fluoroquinolone and (2) metronidazole plus an aminoglycoside or a fluoroquinolone. Metronidazole plus aztreonam is not recommended as an alternative because this combination has no aerobic gram-positive activity.[385] (Strength of evidence for prophylaxis = A.)

Head and Neck Procedures

Background. Elective procedures of the head and neck are predominantly clean or clean-contaminated.[490] Clean procedures include thyroidectomy and lymph node excisions. Clean-contaminated procedures include all procedures involving an incision through the oral or pharyngeal mucosa, ranging from parotidectomy, submandibular gland excision, tonsillectomy, adenoidectomy, and rhinoplasty to complicated tumor-debulking and mandibular fracture repair procedures requiring reconstruction. The frequency of SSIs reported for clean procedures without antimicrobial prophylaxis is <1%.[491,492] In contrast, infection rates in patients undergoing complicated head and neck cancer surgery are quite high, with infection occurring in 24–87% of patients without antimicrobial prophylaxis.[493–497] While many of these head and neck cancer procedures are clean-contaminated, these procedures can fall into different wound classifications. Head and neck cancer patients often have many of the risk factors for infection mentioned below.[498]

Postoperative SSI rates are affected by age, nutritional status, and the presence of concomitant medical conditions such as diabetes mellitus, anemia, and peripheral vascular disease.[496,499–504] Use of tobacco,[498,505] alcohol,[505,506] or drugs of abuse[507] has also been associated with a higher risk of postoperative infection, particularly in patients with mandibular fracture. The hospital course, including length of hospitalization before operation, duration of antimicrobial use before operation, length of operation, presence of implants, and previous tracheotomy can also affect postoperative SSI rates.[496,497,501–504,508] In patients with cancer, preoperative radiation and chemotherapy as well as the stage of the malignancy may also affect infection risk.[497,498,502–504] Procedure-related risk factors for infection include radical or bilateral neck dissections[501,508] and reconstruction with myocutaneous flaps or microvascular-free flaps.[497–499,508]

Organisms. The normal floras of the mouth and the oropharynx are responsible for most infections that follow clean-contaminated head and neck procedures.[6,8,496,498,499,506,509–519] Anaerobic and aerobic bacteria are abundant in the oropharynx. As a result, postoperative SSIs are usually polymicrobial and involve both aerobic and anaerobic bacteria. The predominant oropharyngeal organisms include various streptococci (aerobic and anaerobic species), other oral anaerobes including *Bacteroides* species (but not *B. fragilis*), *Peptostreptococcus* species, *Prevotella* species, *Fusobacterium* species, *Veillonella* species, Enterobacteriaceae, and staphylococci. Nasal flora includes *Staphylococcus* species and *Streptococcus* species.

Efficacy. *Clean procedures.* Systemic administration of prophylactic antimicrobials has not been proven effective in reducing SSI rates in patients undergoing clean procedures of the head and neck and are not recommended for routine use.[6–8,497,520] One randomized, double-blind, multicenter study of 500 patients undergoing thyroid procedures for goiter or carcinoma found no difference in postoperative SSI rates in those who received antimicrobial prophylaxis (0.8%) and those who did not (0.4%).[491]

Clean-contaminated procedures. Based on the best available evidence, current guidelines and review articles recommend the use of antimicrobial prophylaxis for the majority of clean-contaminated procedures.[6–8,497,520,521] However, antimicrobial prophylaxis did not lower infection risk in randomized controlled trials of patients undergoing adenoidectomy, tonsillectomy,[522,523] and septoplasty,[524] and systematic reviews have not recommended prophylaxis for these procedures.[7,525,526]

The efficacy of antimicrobial prophylaxis is best established for head and neck cancer surgery. Several small randomized, controlled trials found high infection rates in placebo groups (24–78%) and markedly lower infection rates in the prophylaxis groups (5.8–38%) using a variety of regimens, including cefazolin, third-generation cephalosporins, and ampicillin plus cloxacillin. Although these studies were small, the results are concordant, and the high infection rates allowed the studies to reach statistical significance despite the small sample sizes. Similar results were reported in several additional small, uncontrolled studies.[500,527–529]

Choice of agent. Several randomized, single-center studies have compared antimicrobial regimens for clean-contaminated procedures. In one study, 189 patients undergoing head and neck cancer procedures were randomized to receive cefazolin 1 g (n = 92) or amoxicillin–clavulanate (n = 97), both given within one hour of incision and every eight hours postoperatively for three doses.[511] The postoperative SSI rates were 24% with cefazolin and 21% with amoxicillin–clavulanate; there was no statistically significant difference in infection rates in this underpowered study. Two studies have compared ampicillin–sulbactam to clindamycin and yielded discordant results. One study of 242 patients (169 evaluable) undergoing head and neck cancer procedures compared ampicillin–sulbactam 1.5 g (n = 119) and clindamycin 600 mg (n = 123) given within one to two hours of incision and every six hours postoperatively for a total of four doses.[510] No difference in SSIs was found, with 15 infections reported in each group (13% for the ampicillin–sulbactam group and 12% for the clindamycin group). There was no significant difference in adverse events between groups. There was a higher rate of *C. difficile*-positive patients in the clindamycin group (n = 7) than in the ampicillin–sulbactam group (n = 1), with no reported statistical analysis. Another study of 212 patients undergoing clean-contaminated head and neck oncology surgery found significantly fewer infections in the ampicillin–sulbactam group (13.3%) compared with the clindamycin group (27.1%) (p = 0.02).[530] A greater number of gram-negative pathogens were recovered from patients randomized to the clindamycin group. The combination of gentamicin and clindamycin was superior to cefazolin in one older clinical trial.[531]

Duration. Studies of clean-contaminated head and neck procedures found no difference in efficacy between regimens of 24 hours and longer regimens of three, five, or seven days.[499–501,505,507,512,524,531–534] Limited data exist on single-dose prophylaxis in these procedures.

One study of patients undergoing free-flap reconstruction after head and neck procedures found a significantly lower rate of acquisition and infection with MRSA in patients receiving short-term cefuroxime and metronidazole (one dose during induction of anesthesia and one dose eight hours postoperatively) compared with long-term therapy (same antimicrobials with additional doses every eight hours for up to five days) ($p = 0.005$ and $p = 0.01$, respectively, for acquisition and infection).[535]

Recommendations. *Clean procedures.* Antimicrobial prophylaxis is not required in patients undergoing clean surgical procedures of the head and neck. If there is placement of prosthetic material, a preoperative dose of cefazolin or cefuroxime is reasonable, though there are few data supporting the efficacy of prophylaxis in this setting (Table 2). A reasonable alternative for patients with β-lactam allergies is clindamycin. (Strength of evidence against prophylaxis without prosthesis placement = B; strength of evidence for prophylaxis with prosthesis placement = C.)

Clean-contaminated procedures. Antimicrobial prophylaxis has not been shown to benefit patients undergoing tonsillectomy or functional endoscopic sinus procedures. The preferred regimens for patients undergoing other clean-contaminated head and neck procedures are (1) cefazolin or cefuroxime plus metronidazole and (2) ampicillin–sulbactam. Clindamycin is a reasonable alternative in patients with a documented β-lactam allergy. The addition of an aminoglycoside to clindamycin may be appropriate when there is an increased likelihood of gram-negative contamination of the surgical site. (Strength of evidence for prophylaxis in cancer surgery patients = A; strength of evidence for prophylaxis for other clean-contaminated procedures except tonsillectomy and functional endoscopic sinus procedures = B.)

Neurosurgery Procedures

Background. Nosocomial central nervous system (CNS) infections do not often occur but have potentially serious consequences and poor outcomes, including death.[536] One of the greatest risks for these infections in children and adults is undergoing a neurosurgical procedure. A classification system for neurosurgery, validated by Narotam et al.,[537] divides procedures into five categories: clean, clean with foreign body, clean-contaminated, contaminated, and dirty. Risk factors for postoperative infections after neurological procedures include an ASA classification of ≥2,[538] postoperative monitoring of intracranial pressure[538,539] or ventricular drains[536,538] for five or more days, cerebrospinal fluid (CSF) leak,[539–541] procedure duration of more than two to four hours,[540,542–544] diabetes,[544] placement of foreign body,[536] repeat or additional neurosurgical procedures,[538,541–543] concurrent (remote, incision, or shunt) or previous shunt infection,[536,539,545,546] and emergency procedures.[542,545]

Organisms. Data from most published clinical trials indicate that SSIs are primarily associated with gram-positive bacteria, *S. aureus*, and coagulase-negative *staphylococci.*[6,8,537–545,547–554] Several cohort studies revealed high rates (up to 75–80% of isolates) of MRSA[540–543,548–552] and coagulase-negative staphylococci among patients undergoing a variety of neurosurgical procedures.[539,540,543,549] Other skin organisms such as *P. acnes* may be seen after CSF shunt placement, craniotomy, and other procedures.[536,555,556] Gram-negative bacteria have also been isolated as the sole cause of postoperative neurosurgical SSIs in approximately 5–8% of cases and have been isolated in polymicrobial infections.[537–539,541–545,547–550,552,553]

Efficacy. *Clean procedures.* Antimicrobial prophylaxis is recommended for adult and pediatric patients undergoing craniotomy and spinal procedures.[7,520] One meta-analysis of six studies found decreased odds of meningitis in patients undergoing craniotomy who received antimicrobial prophylaxis (1.1%) versus no prophylaxis (2.7%) ($p = 0.03$).[557] Two cohort studies[540,543] in patients undergoing craniotomy at the same institution found that antimicrobial prophylaxis with cloxacillin or amoxicillin–clavulanate, clindamycin for β-lactam-allergic patients, and other antimicrobials (not detailed) had a significantly lower infection rate (5.8%) than no prophylaxis (9.7%) ($p < 0.0001$).[543] A significantly lower infection rate of 4.6% was seen in low-risk patients (clean craniotomy, no implant) with antimicrobial prophylaxis compared with those without prophylaxis (4.6% versus 10%, $p < 0.0001$). A significantly lower rate of scalp infections, bone flap osteitis, and abscess or empyema was seen with antimicrobial prophylaxis compared with no prophylaxis. Antimicrobial prophylaxis demonstrated no difference in postoperative meningitis[540,543] and infection rates in high-risk patients (those undergoing emergency, clean-contaminated, and dirty procedures or reoperation or with operative times exceeding four hours).[543]

Prospective studies involving large numbers of patients have also demonstrated lower neurosurgical postoperative infection rates when antimicrobial prophylaxis is used.[558–561] One such study of patients undergoing craniotomy, spinal, or shunting procedures was stopped early because of an excessive number of SSIs in the placebo group.[562]

Choice of agent. Studies of clean neurosurgical procedures reported antimicrobial regimens including clindamycin,[540,543,557] vancomycin,[542,557] cefotiam (not marketed in the United States),[557] piperacillin,[557] cloxacillin,[540,543,557] oxacillin,[542,557] cefuroxime,[547] cefotaxime,[548] sulfamethoxazole–trimethoprim,[548] cefazolin,[542,544] penicillin G,[542] and amoxicillin–clavulanate.[540,542,543] A meta-analysis found no significant difference in the rates of postcraniotomy meningitis with various antimicrobial regimens (single-dose regimens of clindamycin, vancomycin, or cefotiam; three doses of piperacillin; four doses of cloxacillin; and six doses of oxacillin).[557]

A randomized, open-label, multicenter study of 613 adult patients undergoing elective craniotomy, shunt, or stereotactic procedures found no difference in single doses of cefotaxime and trimethoprim–sulfamethoxazole in postoperative abscess formation, SSIs, and shunt infections.[548]

Duration. The majority of studies included single doses of antimicrobials; therefore, the use of single-dose antimicrobial prophylaxis given within 60 minutes before surgical incision in patients undergoing neurosurgery is generally recommened.[6,7,520,540,543,547,548,557,563]

Efficacy for CSF-Shunting Procedures. Antimicrobial prophylaxis is recommended for adults undergoing placement of a CSF shunt.[7] Prophylaxis in patients undergoing ventriculostomy or intraventrical prophylaxis at the time of ventriculoperitoneal shunt insertion has shown some benefit in reducing infection but remains controversial due to limited evidence.[6,7]

Because CNS infections after shunting procedures are responsible for substantial mortality and morbidity, especially in children, the possible role of prophylactic antimicrobials in such procedures has been studied in numerous small, well-conducted, randomized controlled trials.[564–571] Meticulous surgical and aseptic techniques and short procedure times were determined to be important factors in lowering infection rates after shunt placement. Although the number of patients studied in each trial was small, two meta-analyses of these data demonstrated that antimicrobial prophylaxis use in CSF-shunting procedures reduced the risk of infection by approximately 50%.[572,573]

Intrathecal pump placement involves the implantation of a permanent intrathecal catheter to allow instillation of medication. CNS infections may occur after these procedures, which are performed in both pediatric and adult populations. Several retrospective series have reported infection rates of 4.5–9% after intrathecal baclofen pump placement.[574-576] There are minimal published trial data regarding appropriate prophylaxis for intrathecal pump procedures. It has been suggested that prophylaxis for intrathecal pump procedures be managed similarly to prophylaxis for CSF-shunting procedures.[577]

There is no consensus on the use of antimicrobial prophylaxis in patients with extraventricular drains (EVDs) or intracranial pressure monitors.[134] An international survey of neurosurgeons and critical care medicine and infectious diseases specialists illustrates the difference in practices. The majority of neurosurgeons used or recommended the use of antimicrobial prophylaxis with EVDs (73.5%) and other monitoring devices (59%), compared with rates of 46–59% for critical care medicine specialists and 35% for infectious diseases specialists. The majority of specialists did not recommend or use antimicrobial-coated EVD catheters.

Two randomized controlled studies comparing antimicrobial-impregnated shunts to standard, non-antimicrobial-impregnated shunts along with antimicrobial prophylaxis with i.v. cephalosporin found a decrease in rates of shunt infections[549] and a significant decrease in CSF infection with antimicrobial-impregnated shunts.[545] At this time, routine use of antimicrobial-impregnated devices is not recommended; additional well-designed studies are needed to establish their place in therapy.[7,578]

Choice of agent. In CSF-shunting procedures, no single antimicrobial agent has been demonstrated to have greater efficacy than others.[546,548,551–554,579] There is a lack of data on the necessity of antimicrobials with CNS penetration relating to prevention of infection in CNS shunting procedures.

Duration. The majority of studies support the use of single-dose prophylaxis regimens or regimens with a duration of 24–48 hours postoperatively.[6–8,520,539,546,549–552,579] There is a lack of data evaluating the continuation of EVDs with and without antimicrobial prophylaxis. The international survey mentioned above asked respondents to indicate their recommended duration for antimicrobial prophylaxis with EVDs as either periprocedural, for 24 hours, for the first three days, for the entire time the device is in place, or other.[135] The respondents from the specialties of neurosurgery, neurocritical care, and critical care had similar results, with 28–31% using or recommending periprocedural antimicrobials, 4–10% for 24 hours, 2–4% for the first three days, 43–64% for the entire time the device is in place, and 0–14% for other. The infectious diseases specialists reported rates of 62%, 19%, 4%, 12%, and 4%, respectively.

One retrospective single-center cohort study of 308 patients with EVDs placed for three days or more received antimicrobial prophylaxis for the duration of EVD use (n = 209) compared with patients receiving cefuroxime 1.5 g i.v. every eight hours for three doses or less frequently periprocedurally (timing not clearly defined in article) (n = 99).[580] The overall rate of bacterial ventriculitis was 3.9%, with 8 patients (3.8%) in the extended-use group and 4 patients (4%) in the short-term prophylaxis group, the difference of which was not significant. The study authors concluded that there was no benefit to the use of a prolonged duration of antimicrobial prophylaxis.

Pediatric Efficacy for CSF-Shunting Procedures. Antimicrobial prophylaxis is recommended for children undergoing a CSF-shunting procedure.[7] The efficacy of antimicrobial prophylaxis is extrapolated from adult studies.

A retrospective pediatric study of 384 CSF-shunting procedures found a lower infection rate in patients who received antimicrobials (2.1%) compared with those who did not (5.6%), but this difference failed to reach statistical significance.[581] Two randomized, prospective studies that included pediatric patients did not demonstrate a significant difference in infection rates between the control group and the groups that received cefotiam[571] (not available in the United States) or methicillin.[568] A randomized, double-blind, placebo-controlled study that included pediatric patients undergoing ventriculoperitoneal shunt surgeries failed to demonstrate that the use of perioperative sulfamethoxazole–trimethoprim reduced the frequency of shunt infection.[564]

Other studies have demonstrated efficacy for prophylactic antimicrobials.[566,582] A single-center, randomized, double-blind, placebo-controlled trial of perioperative rifampin plus trimethoprim was performed in pediatric patients.[582] Among patients receiving rifampin plus trimethoprim, the infection rate was 12%, compared with 19% in patients receiving placebo. The study was ended because of the high infection rates before significance could be achieved. Infection rates at the study institution had been 7.5% in the years before the study. An open-label randomized study, including pediatric patients, demonstrated a lower infection rate in a group receiving oxacillin (3.3%) than in a control group (20%).[566]

Recommendations. A single dose of cefazolin is recommended for patients undergoing clean neurosurgical procedures, CSF-shunting procedures, or intrathecal pump placement (Table 2). Clindamycin or vancomycin should be reserved as an alternative agent for patients with a documented β-lactam allergy (vancomycin for MRSA-colonized patients). (Strength of evidence for prophylaxis = A.)

Cesarean Delivery Procedures

Background. Approximately 1.2 million infants are born by cesarean delivery in the United States annually.[583] The infection rate after cesarean delivery has been reported to be 4–15%,[583] though recent NHSN data showed an infection rate of 2–4%.[165]

Postpartum infectious complications are common after cesarean delivery. Endometritis (infection of the uterine lining) is usually identified by fever, malaise, tachycardia, abdominal pain, uterine tenderness, and sometimes abnormal or foul-smelling lochia.[584] Fever may also be the only symptom of endometritis.

Endometritis has been reported to occur in up to 24% of patients in elective cesarean delivery and up to approximately 60% of patients undergoing nonelective or emergency section.[584,585] Risk factors for endometritis include cesarean delivery, prolonged rupture of membranes, prolonged labor with multiple vaginal examinations, intrapartum fever, and low socioeconomic status.[585,586] Patients with low socioeconomic status may have received inadequate prenatal care.

The factor most frequently associated with infectious morbidity in postcesarean delivery is prolonged labor in the presence of ruptured membranes. Intact chorioamniotic membranes serve as a protective barrier against bacterial infection. Rupture of the membrane exposes the uterine surface to bacteria from the birth canal. The vaginal fluid with bacterial flora is drawn into the uterus when it relaxes between contractions during labor. Women undergoing labor for more than six to eight hours in the presence of ruptured membranes should be considered at high risk for developing endometritis.[587] Other risk factors for SSIs after cesarean delivery include systemic illness, poor hygiene, obesity, and anemia.[587,588]

Organisms. The normal flora of the vagina include staphylococci, *streptococci*, *enterococci*, *lactobacilli*, diphtheroids, *E. coli*, anaerobic streptococci (*Peptococcus* species and *Peptostreptococcus* species), *Bacteroides* species (e.g., *Bacteroides bivius*, *B. fragilis*), and *Fusobacterium* species.[584,587,589–592] Endometritis infections are often polymicrobial and include aerobic streptococcus (particularly group B β-hemolytic streptococcus and enterococci), gram-negative aerobes (particularly *E. coli*), gram-negative anaerobic rods (particularly *B. bivius*), and anaerobic *cocci* (*Peptococcus* species and *Peptostreptococcus* species). *Ureaplasma urealyticum* has been commonly isolated from endometrial and surgical-site cultures. Additional commonly isolated organisms from SSIs include *Staphylococcus* species and enterococci.

Efficacy. While the use of antimicrobial prophylaxis in low-risk procedures (i.e., those with no active labor and no rupture of membranes) has been brought into question by the results of several randomized, placebo-controlled studies that found no reduction in infectious complications (fever, SSI, urinary tract infection, or endometritis) with the use of prophylaxis, the majority of these evaluations were underpowered and included administration of antimicrobial prophylaxis at cord clamping.[593–599] However, the efficacy of antimicrobial prophylaxis in cesarean delivery has been shown in several studies and two meta-analyses for both elective and nonelective procedures. Therefore, prophylaxis is recommended for all patients undergoing cesarean delivery.[584,592]

One meta-analysis that reviewed 7 placebo-controlled randomized trials in low-risk elective cesarean delivery found that prophylaxis was associated with a significant decrease in endometritis and fever.[592] A larger meta-analysis of 81 randomized trials with 11,937 women undergoing both elective and nonelective cesarean delivery found that antimicrobial prophylaxis was associated with a significant reduction in risk of fever, endometritis, SSI, urinary tract infection, and serious infection.[585] The relative risk for endometritis in elective cesarean section was 0.38 (95% CI, 0.22–0.64) in those receiving antimicrobial prophylaxis compared to those receiving no prophylaxis.

Choice of agent. Although several different antimicrobials used alone or in combination for antimicrobial prophylaxis during cesarean delivery have been evaluated, the use of first-generation cephalosporins (specifically cefazolin) has been advocated by ACOG and the American Academy of Pediatrics (AAP), based on their efficacy, narrow spectrum of activity, and low cost.[584] This recommendation is supported by a meta-analysis of 51 randomized controlled trials comparing at least two antimicrobial regimens that concluded that ampicillin and first-generation cephalosporins have similar efficacy.[600]

Newer prospective randomized controlled and cohort studies have evaluated the addition of metronidazole, azithromycin,[601–603] or doxycycline[601] to a first- or second-generation cephalosporin to extend the spectrum of activity against common organisms isolated from endometrial and surgical-site cultures, specifically *U. urealyticum* and *Mycoplasma* species. These studies found significantly lower rates of postoperative infections (including endometritis and SSI) and a shorter duration of hospital stay compared with prophylaxis with a first- or second-generation cephalosporin alone.[601–604] Antibiotic administration occurred either postoperatively or after cord clamping in these studies. Further study, particularly with preoperative antimicrobial administration, is needed to confirm these preliminary findings and establish a place in therapy for this practice.

Timing. Historically, administration of antimicrobials in cesarean delivery was delayed until after cord clamping.[600,605,606] The principal reasons were to avoid suppression of the neonate's normal bacterial flora that could promote the selection of resistant organisms and concern that the antimicrobials could potentially mask neonatal infection, complicating evaluation of neonatal sepsis. However, more contemporary data support the administration of antimicrobial prophylaxis before surgical incision to protect against bacterial contamination of the surgical site and decrease the risk of infection. The practice of antimicrobial prophylaxis administration before surgical incision is endorsed by ACOG and AAP.[584,607] See the Common Principles section of these guidelines for additional discussion on antimicrobial timing.

A meta-analysis of three randomized controlled trials and two nonrandomized controlled studies provided evidence that preoperative antimicrobial administration significantly decreased the rate of endometritis compared with administration after cord clamping (3.9% and 8.9%, respectively; $p = 0.012$).[605] A lower SSI rate was also seen with preoperative antimicrobial administration (3.2% versus 5.4%), though this difference was not significant. The overall rate of infection-related morbidity was also significantly lower. No differences between the groups were seen in neonatal outcomes, including sepsis, sepsis workups, and neonatal intensive care unit admissions. The largest study included in this meta-analysis was a prospective, randomized, controlled, double-blind, single-center, double-dummy study of 357 patients comparing cefazolin 1 g i.v. given preoperatively and after cord clamping, which had results consistent with the overall meta-analysis.[606]

In a recent randomized trial of more than 1100 women undergoing cesarean section between 2004 and 2010, Witt and colleagues[608] found no difference in SSI rates for patients having antimicrobial administration before surgical incision compared with those who received antimicrobial prophylaxis at the time of cord clamping. All patients received a single dose of cefazolin 2 g.

Duration. A meta-analysis of 51 studies found that multidose regimens provided no apparent benefit over single-dose regimens.[600] The use of single-dose prophylaxis is supported by ACOG and AAP for procedures lasting less than two hours.[584] Additional intraoperative doses may be warranted for patients with excessive blood loss or for whom the duration of the procedure is extended.

For additional discussion of dosing, see the Common Principles section of these guidelines.

Recommendation. The recommended regimen for all women undergoing cesarean delivery is a single dose of cefazolin administered before surgical incision (Table 2). (Strength of evidence for prophylaxis = A.) For patients with β-lactam allergies, an alternative regimen is clindamycin plus gentamicin.

Hysterectomy Procedures

Background. Hysterectomy is second only to cesarean delivery as the most frequently performed major gynecological procedure in the United States, with over 600,000 hysterectomies performed annually.[609] Uterine fibroid tumors account for 40% of all presurgical diagnoses leading to hysterectomy.[609] Other common diagnoses are dysfunctional uterine bleeding, genital prolapse, endometriosis, chronic pelvic pain, pelvic inflammatory disease, endometrial hyperplasia, and cancer.

Hysterectomy involves the removal of the uterus and, occasionally, one or two fallopian tubes, the ovaries, or a combination of ovaries and fallopian tubes.[610] Radical hysterectomy entails removal of the uterus, fallopian tubes, and ovaries and extensive stripping of the pelvic lymph nodes in patients with extension of their cancer. Hysterectomies are performed by a vaginal or abdominal approach using a laparoscopic- or robot-assisted method. During a vaginal hysterectomy, the procedure is completed through the vagina with no abdominal incision. Abdominal hysterectomy involves an abdominal incision. Laparoscopic and robotic methods involve small incisions and require additional equipment, increased operator experience, and increased length of procedures.[611,612] In the United States, between 2000 and 2004, the abdominal approach for hysterectomy was used in 67.9% of surgical procedures and the vaginal approach in 32.1%. Of hysterectomies performed via the vaginal approach, 32.4% also used laparoscopy.[609] The ACOG Committee on Gynecologic Practice recommends vaginal hysterectomy as the approach of choice for benign disease, based on evidence of better outcomes and fewer complications.[613] Laparoscopic abdominal hysterectomy is an alternative when the vaginal route is not indicated or feasible.[613,614] Of note, ACOG has stated that the supracervical approach—removal of the uterus with preservation of the cervix—should not be recommended as a superior technique for hysterectomy due to the lack of advantage in postoperative complications, urinary symptoms, or sexual function and the increased risk of future trachelectomy to remove the cervical stump.[615]

Infections after hysterectomy include superficial and organ/space (vaginal cuff infection, pelvic cellulitis, and pelvic abscess) SSIs.[589] The reported SSI rates between January 2006 and December 2008 in the United States, based on NNIS risk index category, were 0.73–1.16 per 100 procedures for vaginal hysterectomy and 1.10–4.05 per 100 procedures for abdominal hysterectomy.[165] A multicenter surveillance study found a mean infection rate of 2.53% associated with all types of hysterectomy and a significantly lower mean rate of infection with laparoscopic versus abdominal hysterectomies (1.15% versus 3.44%, respectively).[325]

Risk factors for infection after vaginal or abdominal hysterectomy include longer duration of surgery, young age, diabetes, obesity, peripheral vascular disease, collagen disease, anemia, transfusion, poor nutritional status, and previous history of postsurgical infection.[590,616–622] The depth of subcutaneous tissue is also a significant risk factor for infection after abdominal hysterectomy.[623] Additional risk factors for infection after radical hysterectomy for cervical cancer include the presence of malignancy, prior radiation therapy, and the presence of indwelling drainage catheters.[619,620]

Organisms. The vagina is normally colonized with a wide variety of bacteria, including gram-positive and gram-negative aerobes and anaerobes. The normal flora of the vagina includes staphylococci, streptococci, enterococci, lactobacilli, diphtheroids, *E. coli*, anaerobic streptococci, *Bacteroides* species, and *Fusobacterium* species.[589,624] Postoperative vaginal flora differs from preoperative flora; the amount of enterococci, gram-negative bacilli, and *Bacteroides* species increases postoperatively. Postoperative changes in flora may occur independently of prophylactic antimicrobial administration and are not by themselves predictive of postoperative infection.[589,625,626] Postoperative infections associated with vaginal hysterectomy are frequently polymicrobial, with enterococci, aerobic gram-negative bacilli, and *Bacteroides* species isolated most frequently. Postoperative SSIs after abdominal and radical hysterectomies are also polymicrobial; gram-positive cocci and enteric gram-negative bacilli predominate, and anaerobes are frequently isolated.[626,627]

Efficacy. A meta-analysis of 25 randomized controlled trials demonstrated the efficacy of antimicrobial prophylaxis, including first- and second-generation cephalosporins and metronidazole, in the prevention of infections after abdominal hysterectomy.[628] The infection rates were 21.1% with placebo or no prophylaxis and 9.0% with any antimicrobial. Another meta-analysis found that the rate of postoperative infection (surgical and pelvic sites) in women undergoing vaginal hysterectomy who received placebo or no prophylactic antimicrobial ranged from 14% to 57%, which was significantly higher than the 10% rate reported with antimicrobials.[629]

Malignant disease as the reason for hysterectomy is a common exclusion from studies of antimicrobial prophylaxis. Older, prospective, placebo-controlled studies found a lower rate of SSIs with antimicrobial prophylaxis after radical hysterectomy.[619,630–633] The applicability of these results is limited by small sample size and the inclusion of antimicrobials not available in the United States. Radical hysterectomy is primarily completed through an abdominal approach but can also be performed by a vaginal approach and using laparoscopic or robotic methods.[634] Therefore, antimicrobial prophylaxis would be warranted, regardless of approach. No placebo-controlled studies have been conducted to evaluate the efficacy of antimicrobial prophylaxis when used for laparoscopic hysterectomy.

Choice of agent. Cephalosporins are the most frequently used and studied antimicrobials for prophylaxis in vaginal and abdominal hysterectomies. Studies directly comparing different cephalosporins have found no significant differences in rates of infection in vaginal hysterectomy and have indicated that first-generation cephalosporins (primarily cefazolin) are equivalent to second- and third-generation agents.[635–644] In abdominal hysterectomy, no significant differences in the rates of serious infections were noted between second- and third-generation cephalosporin regimens.[641,645–649] Few comparisons have been made between second-generation cephalosporins and cefazolin. Cefazolin has been at least as effective in preventing infectious complications as second- and third-generation cephalosporins.[636,650–652] However, one double-blind controlled study of 511 women undergoing abdominal hysterectomy found that the risk of major SSIs requiring antimicrobial therapy was significantly higher in the group receiving preoperative cefazolin 1 g (11.6%; relative risk, 1.84; 95% CI, 1.03–3.29) than in those treated with cefotetan 1 g (6.3%).[617] A multicenter, randomized, double-blind, active- and placebo-controlled study compared single doses of ampicillin, cefazolin, and placebo administered to women undergoing elective total abdominal hysterectomy at two centers in Thailand.[653] The study found a significantly lower rate of infection, including superficial and deep SSIs, urinary tract infections, vaginal cuff infection, and pneumonia, with cefazolin (10.3%) compared with placebo (26.9%) and ampicillin (22.6%). No difference was seen between ampicillin and placebo. The study authors concluded that cefazolin was more effective than ampicillin for elective total abdominal hysterectomy.

A randomized controlled study of 511 patients undergoing laparoscopic gynecological procedures at one center in Italy compared single doses of amoxicillin–clavulanate 2.2 g and cefazolin 2 g i.v. administered 20–30 minutes before the procedure.[654] A second dose was given if the surgery lasted over three hours or there was extensive blood loss (>1500 mL). No significant differences in the rates of any postoperative infection, including SSIs, were found between groups. The statistical power of the study was not stated.

In light of the organisms encountered in the vaginal canal and comparative studies conducted among different classes of cephalosporins, cefazolin, cefotetan, cefoxitin, cefuroxime, and ampicillin–sulbactam have been supported as appropriate first-line choices for prophylaxis during vaginal or abdominal hysterectomy.[6,9,41] Alternative agents for patients with a history of immediate hypersensitivity to penicillin include either clindamycin or metronidazole plus an aminoglycoside or a fluoroquinolone (ciprofloxacin, levofloxacin, or moxifloxacin) or aztreonam (with clindamycin only).

Duration. Studies comparing single doses of one antimicrobial with multidose regimens of a different antimicrobial have shown the two regimens to be equally effective in reducing the postoperative infection rate in women undergoing vaginal and abdominal hysterectomies.[635–643,645–650,655–663] The limited comparative trials involving single-dose cefazolin[637,654,655,664] or ampicillin–sulbactam[654,663] indicate that a single dose of antimicrobial is sufficient prophylaxis for SSIs for vaginal hysterectomy. Single doses of cefotetan, ceftizoxime, or cefotaxime appear to be as effective as multiple doses of cefoxitin.[644–649,665] A second dose of antimicrobial is warranted when the procedure lasts three hours or longer or if blood loss exceeds 1500 mL.[9,654]

Recommendation. The recommended regimen for women undergoing vaginal or abdominal hysterectomy, using an open or laparoscopic approach, is a single dose of cefazolin (Table 2). Cefoxitin, cefotetan, or ampicillin–sulbactam may also be used. Alternative agents for patients with a β-lactam allergy include (1) either clindamycin or vancomycin plus an aminoglycoside, aztreonam, or a fluoroquinolone and (2) metronidazole plus an aminoglycoside or a fluoroquinolone. (Strength of evidence for prophylaxis = A.)

Ophthalmic Procedures

Background. Ophthalmic procedures include cataract extractions, vitrectomies, keratoplasties, intraocular lens implantation, glaucoma procedures, strabotomies, retinal detachment repair, laser in situ keratomileusis, and laser-assisted subepithelial keratectomy. Most of the available data regarding antimicrobial prophylaxis involve cataract procedures. The goal of prophylaxis is primarily to reduce acute postoperative endophthalmitis, defined as severe intraocular inflammation due to infection, which can lead to loss of vision if untreated.[666] Since 2000, the reported frequency of endophthalmitis after ophthalmic procedures is low worldwide, ranging from 0% to 0.63%.[667–680] The reported time from procedure to diagnosis of endophthalmitis ranges from one day to six weeks, with the majority of infections identified within one week.[666,669,671,673,674,681–683]

Potential risk factors for postoperative ophthalmic infections include preoperative factors such as diabetes,[666] active ocular infection or colonization,[666,684] lacrimal drainage system infection or obstruction, age of >85 years,[685] and immunodeficiency.[684] Procedure-related risk factors include clear corneal incisions (as opposed to scleral tunnel incisions),[680,686] any surgical complication, vitreous loss,[684] posterior capsule tear,[681,684,685] silicone intraocular lens implantation,[677,680] and the nonuse of facemasks in the operating theater.[681]

Organisms. Among organisms isolated from patients developing postoperative endophthalmitis after cataract procedure, approximately 25–60% were coagulase-negative *Staphylococcus* species, primarily *S. epidermidis.*[668,670,671,673,674,678,683,684,686] Other gram-positive organisms identified included *S. aureus*, *Streptococcus* species, *Enterococcus* species, *P. acnes*, and *Corynebacterium* species. Gram-negative organisms isolated included *Serratia* species, *Klebsiella* species, *P. mirabilis*, and *P. aeruginosa*. These organisms represent the normal flora isolated pre-operatively in a number of studies.[675,687–693]

Efficacy. Data on antimicrobial prophylaxis efficacy in ophthalmic procedures to prevent endophthalmitis are limited; however, prophylaxis is common.[684] The low rate of postoperative endophthalmitis makes it difficult to complete an adequately powered study to show efficacy of antimicrobial prophylaxis in ophthalmic procedures; therefore, surrogate markers of eradication of normal flora bacteria and reduction of bacterial count on the conjunctiva, lower and upper eyelids, eyelashes, and inner canthus (corner of the eye) preoperatively and postoperatively are used. Many of the available studies are flawed with retrospective or uncontrolled design, inadequate follow-up, variations in surgical techniques (including disinfection, antimicrobial prophylaxis strategies, and methods for performing procedures), and limited reporting of clinical outcomes.

The large, randomized, partially-masked, placebo-controlled, multinational, multicenter study conducted by the European Society of Cataract and Refractive Surgeons (ESCRS) compared the rate of postoperative endophthalmitis in over 16,600 patients undergoing routine cataract procedures at 24 centers in Europe randomized to one of four perioperative prophylaxis groups.[679,680,694] Patients received no antimicrobial prophylaxis, intracameral cefuroxime at the end of the procedure alone, perioperative levofloxacin 0.5% ophthalmic solution given within the hour before the procedure, or both intracameral cefuroxime and perioperative levofloxacin. All patients had the eye area disinfected with povidone–iodine 5% preoperatively and received topical levofloxacin postoperatively. The study was stopped after an interim analysis due to results of a multivariate analysis indicating that patients not receiving intracameral cefuroxime were approximately five times more likely to develop endophthalmitis. The study has been questioned for its high rate of endophthalmitis, selection of cefuroxime due to gaps in gram-negative coverage, unknown drug concentrations in the aqueous humor, risks of hypersensitivity, the lack of a commercially available preparation, the lack of a subconjunctival cefuroxime treatment group, selection of topical levofloxacin, and methods for statistical analysis.[695–697]

Two single-center, historical-controlled studies in hospitals in Spain reported decreases in acute postoperative endophthalmitis among patients undergoing cataract procedure with intracameral cefazolin added to the previous routine prophylaxis of preoperative eyelid cleansing with soap for three days[670] and povidone–iodine eye area preparation,[670,674] topical antimicrobial, and corticosteroid preparations given at the end of the procedure and postoperatively. One study found a significant decrease and a relative risk reduction of 88.7% in postoperative endophthalmitis with intracameral cefazolin.[670] The other found a decrease from 0.63% to 0.055% in postoperative endophthalmitis with intracameral cefazolin.[674] No statistical analysis was performed in this study.

A retrospective cohort study of patients undergoing cataract procedure at one center in Canada between 1994 and 1998 found no significant difference in the rate of postoperative endophthalmitis with preoperative topical antimicrobials compared with none.[668] A significant decrease in endophthalmitis was seen with subconjunctival administration of antimicrobials at the end of the procedure compared with no antimicrobials.

Several prospective studies have shown decreases in ocular flora, measured by bacterial isolate and CFU counts, with preoperative antimicrobial irrigation,[675] topical antimicrobials,[687,688,691,692,698–700] and intracameral antimicrobials.[682] These studies did not report rates of endophthalmitis, limiting the application of the results.

Choice of agent. Along with careful site preparation and disinfection, the ideal antimicrobial prophylaxis agent should be bactericidal against common pathogens of postoperative endophthalmitis and be used safely in the eye.[6,8,684] There is no consensus on the agent of choice for antimicrobial prophylaxis in ophthalmic procedures, and no agent is FDA-approved for this indication. There are limited studies evaluating the efficacy of a particular choice of antimicrobial prophylaxis for ophthalmic surgeries. The most efficacious antimicrobial cannot be determined from the available data due to study flaws and a lack of direct comparisons. Local ocular flora resistance patterns should be monitored to aid in the selection of appropriate agents for prophylaxis.[683,689,701]

Based on the available literature, use of povidone-iodine as a preoperative antiseptic agent is recommended to decrease ocular microbes and thereby prevent endophthalmitis.[6,684,702] Povidone–iodine 5% or 10% is instilled in the conjunctival sac and applied topically to the ocular skin surface.[703] The most effective protocol has not been established, as povidone–iodine is frequently used in combination with other antimicrobials.[670,674,675,678,687,704] Chlorhexidine has been used as an effective alternative to povidone–iodine, particularly in patients who are iodine allergic.[682,703]

Ophthalmic surgeons surveyed in the United Kingdom reported that commonly used antimicrobial prophylactic agents included cephalosporins, aminoglycosides, vancomycin, chloramphenicol, neomycin alone or in combination with polymyxin, and fluoroquinolones.[695,703] A similar survey of members of the American Society of Cataract and Refractive Surgery found that over 90% of respondents used fluoroquinolones (mainly fourth-generation agents), vancomycin, and cephalosporins.[697] These antimicrobials have been recommended in practice guidelines.[6]

Cephalosporins, specifically cefazolin, cefuroxime, and ceftazidime, have been shown to be safe and effective in decreasing postoperative endophthalmitis when added to regimens of povidone–iodine and topical antimicrobials.[670,674,677,679,680,699] Vancomycin has been shown to decrease cultures and reach adequate concentrations to prevent and treat most corneal pathogens.[675,705] Aminoglycosides alone[687] or in combination with an antiseptic agent (chlorhexidine)[682] showed no significant difference in the reduction of culture results compared with an antiseptic alone (povidone–iodine or chlorhexidine)[682,690] and no antimicrobial prophylaxis.

A randomized controlled study compared the antimicrobial activity and safety of trimethoprim 0.1%–polymyxin B sulfate 10,000 units/mL ophthalmic solution and tobramycin 0.3% ophthalmic solution in patients undergoing cataract procedures.[692] All patients received one drop and a subconjunctival injection of corticosteroids and gentamicin postoperatively followed by one drop of study medication four times daily for five to seven days. No significant differences were seen between groups for positive culture results from conjunctiva at baseline, at procedure, or at postoperative days 5–7 or in lid margin culture at baseline and postoperative days 5–7. A higher rate of positive cultures at procedure was seen in the trimethoprim–polymyxin group (37 of 59 cultures, 63%) compared with 13 (41%) of 32 cultures in the tobramycin group (p = 0.043). Both medications eradicated the majority of bacteria on the day of procedure and postoperative days 5–7. Aqueous humor concentrations did not achieve the MICs of *S. aureus* or *S. epidermidis* and were undetectable for polymyxin B sulfate. The adverse events of irritation and allergic reaction were experienced by three patients in the trimethoprim–polymyxin group. The study authors concluded that there was no difference between trimethoprim and tobramycin in ocular flora reduction.

A randomized controlled study compared conjunctiva and contact lens culture results after treatment with tobramycin 0.3% versus ofloxacin 0.3% ophthalmic solutions in patients undergoing photorefractive keratectomy.[693] No differences were seen among preoperative, postoperative, or contact lens cultures between treatment groups. Although not statistically significant, logistic regression found that cultures from patients treated with tobramycin were two times more likely to be positive than those treated with ofloxacin. The study had low power and did not compare baseline and posttreatment culture results for any treatment group.

Fluoroquinolones have been found in studies to significantly decrease the ocular culture results from baseline[667,673,691,698,700,706]; achieve aqueous humor, vitreal, and corneal tissue concentrations adequate to prevent and treat common ocular pathogens[705,707–710]; and result in improved ocular measurements (i.e., visual acuity, epithelial cell counts, and epithelial healing).[711–716] A retrospective multicenter case series of 20,013 patients who underwent uncomplicated cataract surgeries and received fourth-generation fluoroquinolones preoperatively and postoperatively reported the rates of postoperative endophthalmitis.[673] Endophthalmitis occurred in 9 (0.06%) of 16,209 surgeries in patients treated with gatifloxacin 0.3% ophthalmic solution (95% CI, 0.03–0.1%) and in 5 (0.1%) of 3,804 surgeries in patients treated with moxifloxacin 0.5% ophthalmic solution (95% CI, 0.05–0.3%). There were no significant differences in efficacy between agents.

In a retrospective cross-sectional study conducted over a 10-year period with third- and fourth-generation fluoroquinolones, significantly lower rates of endophthalmitis were reported for the fourth-generation agents moxifloxacin and gatifloxacin (0.56 per 1000 cataract surgeries) than for the third-generation agents ciprofloxacin and ofloxacin (1.97 per 1000 surgeries) ($p = 0.0011$).[671]

Route. There is no consensus on the most effective route of antimicrobial administration for the prevention of endophthalmitis. The routes of antimicrobial administration used in ophthalmic procedures include preoperative topical antimicrobial ophthalmic drops, addition of antimicrobials to the irrigation solution, instillation of antimicrobials intracamerally at the end of surgery, subconjunctival injection of antimicrobials, and postoperative topical application of antimicrobials.[6,684,702,717]

The ESCRS randomized controlled study mentioned above found that patients not receiving intracameral cefuroxime were approximately six times more likely to develop postoperative endophthalmitis.[679,680,694] Surveys of the impact of the ESCRS study findings found that there was an increase in the use of intracameral over subconjunctival cefuroxime based on preliminary study results.[703] For respondents who had not adopted this practice, the reported reasons for not using intracameral cefuroxime included the need for further study, concerns about risk and cost of therapy, the lack of a subconjunctival comparator group, the high rate of endophthalmitis in the control groups, concerns about statistical analysis, and questions regarding the selection of cefuroxime due to gaps in ophthalmic pathogen coverage.[695,697] There is no commercially available cefuroxime formulation for intracameral administration, which was reported as one of the main barriers to use of this route. Concerns regarding compounded intracameral antimicrobials expressed by survey respondents included inflammation, dilution errors, corneal endothelial injury, and the risk for bacterial contamination and infection.

A retrospective cohort study compared the efficacy of intracameral cefuroxime versus subconjunctival cefuroxime in reducing the rate of endophthalmitis after cataract procedures at one center in northeast England.[718] A total of 19,425 patients received antimicrobial prophylaxis with preoperative povidone–iodine 5% in the conjunctival sac and subconjunctival injection of cefuroxime 50 mg at the end of the procedure, and 17,318 patients received intracameral cefuroxime 1 mg at the end of the procedure. There were two groups of patients excluded from the analysis: protocol violators who received no prophylaxis and patients who were enrolled in the ESCRS study. The overall rate of endophthalmitis in analyzed patients was 35 cases in 36,743 procedures (0.95 per 1,000 cases). Of these, 27 occurred in the subconjunctival cefuroxime group (1.39 per 1,000 cases), and 8 occurred in the intracameral group (0.46 per 1,000 cases) (OR, 3.01; 95% CI, 1.37–6.63; $p = 0.0068$).

Several studies found a lower rate of endophthalmitis with the addition of intracameral cephalosporins (cefazolin and cefuroxime) at the end of the surgical procedure after routine perioperative and postoperative topical antimicrobial prophylaxis regimens.[670,674] A case–control study revealed a 5.7 times increased likelihood of developing postoperative endophthalmitis with topical antimicrobial prophylaxis only (including gentamicin 0.3% and chlorhexidine 0.05%) compared with the addition of intracameral cefuroxime 1 mg to the regimen in cataract procedure.[677] Both intracameral cephalosporins and moxifloxacin have been shown as safe, with no adverse events and no effects on visual acuity and endothelial cell counts.[670,674,699,715,716]

One study involving healthy adult volunteers found that orally administered levofloxacin and moxifloxacin achieved adequate aqueous humor concentrations to provide activity against gram-positive and most gram-negative ocular pathogens without adverse events.[707]

The addition of subconjunctival antimicrobials to existing topical antimicrobial prophylaxis regimens has also been shown to reduce the rate and risk of endophthalmitis in intraocular procedures compared with topical antimicrobials alone.[668,681,686] Topical antimicrobials have been shown to be safe and effective in lowering rates of endophthalmitis,[671,673] decreasing bacterial organisms and CFUs in conjunctiva,[667,675,691,692,698,700] and achieving adequate concentrations to be effective against most ocular pathogens,[705,706,708–710,719] with no notable adverse events.[711–714]

Duration and timing. There are a lack of clear evidence and no consensus on the appropriate duration and timing of antimicrobial prophylaxis in ophthalmic procedures.[6,684] Commonly reported times of antimicrobial prophylaxis include preoperatively, intraoperatively, at the end of the procedure, and postoperatively.[684] Few studies have investigated the differences between the timing and duration of antimicrobial prophylaxis regimens. Many of the regimens are used in combination, making it difficult to determine the optimal timing and duration. Preoperative antimicrobial timing reported in the literature has ranged from one to multiple drops within an hour preoperatively on the day of the procedure[671,673,679,680,692–694,698,703,709,710,716] or one to three days before the procedure.[667,698,700,703,708,710,712,714]

Two topical moxifloxacin regimens were compared for conjunctival bacterial flora and aqueous humor concentrations in a randomized controlled study of patients undergoing cataract procedures.[691,719] In one regimen, patients were administered moxifloxacin 0.5% four times a day beginning one day before the procedure plus one drop two hours before the procedure (total of five drops before the procedure); the other group received moxifloxacin 0.5% two hours before surgery and every 15 minutes for the first hour of the procedure (total of five drops). There were no cases of postoperative endophthalmitis up to six months after the procedure in any patient. Administration of moxifloxacin on the day of the procedure was found to result in a significant decrease in median CFU compared with baseline and was found (based on change in log CFU) to be more effective than antimicrobial administration on the day before the procedure. Mean aqueous humor concentrations of moxifloxacin at the beginning of the procedure were significantly higher in the group who received the drug on the day of the procedure.

A small, randomized controlled study compared aqueous humor concentrations of levofloxacin and ciprofloxacin in patients undergoing a cataract procedure with routine phacoemulsification given as (1) one or two drops four times daily for two days before the procedure, with the last dose given immediately before bedtime on the night before the procedure, (2) five doses (one or two drops) delivered every 10 minutes in the hour before the procedure, or (3) a combination of both dosing strategies.[706] Aqueous humor concentrations of levofloxacin were significantly higher than those of ciprofloxacin. Significantly higher doses of drug were delivered to the aqueous humor in the group receiving same-day prophylaxis than in patients receiving levofloxacin or ciprofloxacin two days before surgery. No cases of endophthalmitis or ocular or systemic toxicities were reported.

A randomized controlled study compared the effectiveness of topical ofloxacin in the reduction or elimination of conjunctival bacterial flora when given as one drop every five minutes for three applications one hour before the procedure alone (control group) or combined with ofloxacin one drop four times daily for three days (study group) before cataract procedures.[688] No differences in positive conjunctival cultures were seen between groups five days before topical antimicrobials or before the administration of ofloxacin on the day of the procedure. Significantly higher positive culture rates were seen in the control group than in the study group one hour after the administration of the preoperative antimicrobial and before povidone–iodine, immediately before the procedure, and at the conclusion of the procedure. Mean CFU counts did not significantly differ five days preoperatively and immediately before the procedure but were significantly higher in the control group at all other time points. Neither outcomes of endophthalmitis nor patient compliance with antimicrobial use was reported. The study's authors concluded that three days of topical ofloxacin was more effective than administration just one hour before the procedure in reducing the number of positive bacterial cultures at several time points perioperatively.

Numerous studies have evaluated the efficacy of intracameral and subconjunctival injections of antimicrobials given at the end of surgery.[6,674,677,679–682,697,699,703,716,718] The most commonly reported dose of intracameral cefuroxime was 1 mg,[677,679,680,682,699,718] and the most commonly reported subconjunctival dose was 50 mg.[718] Doses of 2.5 or 1 mg of intracameral cefazolin were studied,[670,674] as were 250- and 500-μg doses of intracameral moxifloxacin.[715,716] Postoperative dosing strategies reported in the literature include four times daily for 3–7 days[667,670,671,673–675,679,680,692,711,712,715] and for up to 15 days[713,714] or until the bottle was empty.[716]

Despite the lack of well-controlled trials, the consequences of bacterial endophthalmitis support the use of prophylactic antimicrobials. No definitive studies have clearly delineated superiority of antimicrobial route, timing, or duration.

Recommendation. Due to the lack of robust data from trials, specific recommendations cannot be made regarding choice, route, or duration of prophylaxis. As a general principle, the antimicrobial prophylaxis regimens used in ophthalmic procedures should provide coverage against common ocular pathogens, including *Staphylococcus* species and gram-negative organisms, particularly *Pseudomonas* species.

Preoperative antisepsis with povidone–iodine is recommended, based on available evidence. Appropriate topical antimicrobials include commercially available neomycin–polymyxin B–gramicidin solution or fluoroquinolones (particularly fourth-generation agents) given as one drop every 5–15 minutes for five doses within the hour before the start of the procedure (Table 2). The addition of subconjunctival cefazolin 100 mg or intracameral cefazolin 1–2.5 mg or cefuroxime 1 mg at the end of the procedure is optional. While some data have shown that intracameral antimicrobials may be more effective than subconjunctival antimicrobials, there are no commercially available antimicrobials approved for these routes of administration. (Strength of evidence for prophylaxis = B.)

Orthopedic Procedures

Background. Orthopedic procedures considered in these guidelines include clean orthopedic procedures (not involving replacement or implantations), spinal procedures with or without instrumentation, repair of hip fractures, implantation of internal fixation devices (screws, nails, plates, and pins), and total-joint-replacement procedures. Grade III open fractures (extensive soft tissue damage and crushing) are often associated with extensive surgical-site contamination and are routinely managed with empirical antimicrobial treatment and surgical debridement, for which guidelines have been published separately.[720] Available guidelines recommend that antimicrobial prophylaxis in grade I (clean wound with ≤1-cm laceration) and grade II (clean wound with >1-cm laceration without extensive soft tissue damage) open fractures be handled similarly to other clean orthopedic procedures.[721–724]

Between 2006 and 2008, SSIs were reported nationally, based on risk category, in approximately 0.7–4.15 per 100 procedures for patients undergoing spinal fusion, 0.72–2.3 per 100 procedures in patients undergoing laminectomy, 0.67–2.4 per 100 procedures in patients undergoing hip prosthesis, and 0.58–1.60 per 100 procedures in patients undergoing knee prosthesis.[165] Postoperative SSI is one of the most costly complications of orthopedic procedures due to hospital readmissions, extended hospital length of stay, the need for additional procedures (often removal and reimplantation of implanted hardware), convalescent or nursing home care between procedures, and significant increases in direct hospital costs (e.g., prolonged antimicrobial therapy).[725,726] Studies have found that the estimated economic impact of one deep SSI was $100,000 in hospital costs alone after hip arthroplasty and $60,000 after knee arthroplasty.[727–731]

In light of the serious consequences, antimicrobial prophylaxis is well accepted in procedures involving the implantation of foreign materials.[8,732] Prophylaxis is also indicated in spinal procedures without instrumentation, where an SSI would pose catastrophic risks.[726,733–738]

Organisms. Skin flora are the most frequent organisms involved in SSIs after orthopedic procedures. The most common pathogens in orthopedic procedures are *S. aureus*, gram-negative bacilli, coagulase-negative staphylococci (including *S. epidermidis*), and β-hemolytic streptococci.[739–743] Spinal procedures may be complicated by polymicrobial infection that includes gram-negative bacteria.[740]

A contributing factor to SSIs in arthroplasty is the formation of bacterial biofilm, particularly with *S. aureus* and *S. epidermidis*, on inert surfaces of orthopedic devices. Bacterial biofilm confers antimicrobial resistance and makes antimicrobial penetration difficult.[744–748]

There is increasing concern regarding the emergence of SSIs due to resistant microorganisms, specifically VRE and MRSA in surgical patients. Several studies have investigated MRSA colonization and SSIs and evaluated the effect of decolonization, including the use of topical mupirocin, in orthopedic procedures.[150,157,741,749–753] Mupirocin decolonization protocols as an adjunct to i.v. cephalosporin prophylaxis in orthopedic patients resulted in significant decreases in nasal MRSA carriage[150,751] and overall SSIs.[157,750–752] Preoperative decolonization with intranasal mupirocin may have utility in patients undergoing elective orthopedic procedures who are known to be colonized or infected with either MRSA or MSSA.[150,151,157,741,749–755] Readers are referred to additional discussion in the Common Principles section of these guidelines.

Clean Orthopedic Procedures Not Involving Implantation of Foreign Materials

Background. In clean orthopedic procedures, such as knee, hand, and foot procedures, and those not involving the implantation of foreign materials, the need for antimicrobial prophylaxis is not well established.[738,749,756] Antimicrobial prophylaxis in patients undergoing diagnostic and operative arthroscopic procedures is controversial.[6,757–760] The risks of SSI and long-term sequelae are low for procedures not involving implantation.

Efficacy. The efficacy of antimicrobial prophylaxis in clean orthopedic procedures was first investigated in the middle part of the 20th century. A number of these studies and reviews have since been found to be flawed, as patients were not randomized to treatment groups and the timing and duration of antimicrobial prophylaxis were not studied.[761,762] Further, patients were administered prophylactic antimicrobials after the surgical procedure, which may have led to invalid results. The low rate of infection and absence of serious morbidity failed to justify the expense or potential for toxicity and resistance associated with routine use of antimicrobial prophylaxis in the setting of clean orthopedic procedures.

Recommendations. Antimicrobial prophylaxis is not recommended for patients undergoing clean orthopedic procedures, including knee, hand, and foot procedures, arthroscopy, and other procedures without instrumentation or implantation of foreign materials. (Strength of evidence against prophylaxis = C.) If the potential for implantation of foreign materials is unknown, the procedure should be treated as with implantation.

Spinal Procedures with and without Instrumentation

Background. Data support the use of antimicrobial prophylaxis for orthopedic spinal procedures with and without instrumentation, including fusions, laminectomies, and minimally invasive disk procedures, to decrease the rate of postoperative spinal infection.[8,543,563,732,733,739,763–766] SSIs after orthopedic spinal procedures, including minimally invasive disk procedures, are associated with high morbidity. Invasion of the epidural space in organ/space SSIs is of particular concern after spinal procedures.[8,145,767]

SSI rates vary with the complexity of the procedure. One retrospective, multicenter study of 1274 adult patients found an overall SSI rate of 0.22% with antimicrobial prophylaxis after minimally invasive spinal procedures (i.e., any spinal procedures performed through a tubular retractor-type system).[768] Procedures included simple decompressive procedures (such as microscopic or endoscopic discectomy or foraminotomy or decompression of stenosis), minimally invasive arthrodeses with percutaneous instrumentation, and minimally invasive intradural procedures. The SSI rate in patients receiving antimicrobial prophylaxis undergoing spinal procedures with instrumentation has ranged from 2.8% to 9.7%.[165,764,765,769,770] Monosegmental instrumentation has a reported SSI rate of <2%, compared with 6.7% for instrumentation at multiple levels.[771]

Several case–control studies of adults undergoing spinal procedures with and without instrumentation have found the following notable patient-related risk factors for SSI: prolonged preoperative hospitalization,[771] diabetes,[767,772–775] elevated serum glucose concentration (>125 mg/dL preoperatively [within 30 days] or >200 mg/dL postoperatively),[773] older age,[767,776] smoking and alcohol abuse,[776] previous procedure complicated by infection,[774–776] and obesity.[770–775,777] Procedure-related risk factors include extended duration of procedure (defined in studies as two to five hours or greater than five hours,[775] greater than three hours,[771] and greater than five hours[776]), excessive blood loss (>1 L),[771,775] staged procedure,[776] multilevel fusions,[777] foreign-body placement (e.g., screw, rod, plate),[767] combined anterior and posterior fusion,[776] and suboptimal antimicrobial timing (>60 minutes before or after incision).[773] A significant decrease in SSIs was seen with procedures at the cervical spine level[772,773] or with an anterior surgical approach.[775]

Efficacy. Despite the lack of comparative studies evaluating prophylaxis for spinal procedures with and without instrumentation (implantation of internal fixation devices), antimicrobial prophylaxis is recommended due to the associated morbidity and assumed costs of SSIs.[771] A meta-analysis of six studies with 843 patients undergoing spinal procedures (types of procedures were not differentiated in the analysis) demonstrated an overall effectiveness of antimicrobial prophylaxis.[732] Antimicrobials studied included single-dose or multidose regimens of <24 hours' duration of cephaloridine (a first-generation cephalosporin no longer available in the United States), vancomycin and gentamicin, cefazolin with and without gentamicin, piperacillin, and oxacillin. The pooled SSI rate with antimicrobial prophylaxis was 2.2%, compared with 5.9% in controls (OR, 0.37; 95% CI, 0.17–0.78; $p < 0.01$). One randomized controlled study of 1237 adult patients undergoing spinal procedures to repair a herniated disk (hemilaminectomy, laminectomy, flavectomy, spondylosyndesis) found no significant difference in the rate of SSIs between single-dose cefuroxime 1.5 g i.v. (1.3%) and placebo (2.9%) given within 60 minutes before surgical incision. No significant difference was seen between treatment groups for incisional SSIs (0.98% and 1.12%, respectively) or deep SSIs (0.33% and 0.32%, respectively), but the difference in organ/space infections was significant between groups (0% and 1.44%, respectively; $p < 0.01$).[778]

Choice of agent. There is no clearly superior antimicrobial agent or regimen for spinal procedures.[563,769] The antimicrobials most often studied for prophylaxis in orthopedic procedures are first-generation cephalosporins, particularly cefazolin. Cefazolin has been noted as a suitable agent for spinal procedures with its spectrum of activity (e.g., against *Staphylococcus* species and gram-negative bacilli such as *E. coli*) and adequate tissue[121] and disk concentrations.[779,780]

Second- and third-generation cephalosporins offer no major advantages over first-generation agents. Their routine use is not recommended due to their higher cost and potential to promote resistance, particularly among healthcare-associated gram-negative bacilli.[8] Broader coverage may be considered for instrumented fusion due to the risk of poly-microbial infections, including those caused by gram-negative bacteria.[563,769]

Clindamycin and vancomycin have adequate activity against the most common pathogens involved in orthopedic procedures and would be acceptable alternatives under certain circumstances, such as prophylaxis for patients with a β-lactam allergy. Vancomycin should be included with cefazolin or used as an alternative agent for routine antimicrobial prophylaxis for patients who are known to be colonized with MRSA.[6,8,41,733,781]

Duration. The majority of available studies of antimicrobial prophylaxis in spinal procedures have used single doses or regimens of <24 hours' duration.[732] There is no high-quality evidence supporting a duration of >24 hours,[782] and some sources recommend only a single preoperative dose.[8,769,778]

Pediatric Efficacy. While no studies have evaluated the efficacy of antimicrobial prophylaxis in pediatric patients undergoing spinal procedures with or without instrumentation, the incidence and risk factors for SSIs in this population have been reported. The frequencies of SSIs in pediatric patients undergoing spinal fusion were 3.5% (<18 years old),[783] 3.8% (<19 years old),[784] 4.4% (ages 1–22 years old), and 5.2% (<17 years old)[764] for varying conditions, including Scheuermann's kyphosis,[784] myelodysplasia,[764] idiopathic scoliosis,[783,785] neuromuscular scoliosis,[785] kyphosis,[783] and spondylolisthesis.[783] The majority of patients in studies reporting antimicrobial prophylaxis received cefazolin, vancomycin, or clindamycin.[764,783,785]

Risk factors for SSIs after spinal procedures with instrumentation in a pediatric population include myelodysplasia,[764] procedure at the sacral spine, obesity,[785] ASA classification of >2, a complex medical condition (including spinal bifida, cerebral palsy, Marfan syndrome, achondroplasia, osteogenesis imperfecta, other unspecified genetic disease, muscular dystrophy, spinal muscular atrophy, or other debilitating myopathies),[783] and previous spinal procedures. One study found a decreased risk of infection with hypothermia (core body temperature of <35.5 °C for the duration of the procedure).[785]

Two studies found suboptimal antimicrobial prophylaxis as a risk factor for SSIs in spinal procedures.[764,783] Optimal antimicrobial prophylaxis was defined as cefazolin 20 mg/kg (up to 2 g) given within 30 minutes[764] or 60 minutes[783] before surgical incision, vancomycin 10 mg/kg (up to 1 g) given within 60 minutes[783] or 150 minutes[764] before surgical incision, or clindamycin 10 mg/kg (up to 600 mg) given within 60 minutes before surgical incision.[783] Intraoperative redosing was defined as appropriate for cefazolin if administered for procedures lasting more than four hours and for vancomycin or clindamycin for procedures lasting more than six hours in one study[783] and for cefazolin administered every eight hours in the other study.[764] A third study found that use of clindamycin as the perioperative antimicrobial increased the risk of SSI.[785]

Recommendations. Antimicrobial prophylaxis is recommended for orthopedic spinal procedures with and without instrumentation. The recommended regimen is cefazolin (Table 2). (Strength of evidence for prophylaxis in orthopedic spinal procedures = A.) Clindamycin and vancomycin should be reserved as alternative agents as described in the Common Principles section. If there are surveillance data showing that gram-negative organisms are a cause of SSIs for the procedure, practitioners may consider combining clindamycin or vancomycin with another agent (cefazolin if the patient is not β-lactam allergic; aztreonam, gentamicin, or single-dose fluoroquinolone if the patient is β-lactam allergic). Mupirocin should be given intranasally to all patients known to be colonized with *S. aureus*.

Hip Fracture Repair

Background. Data support the use of antimicrobial prophylaxis for hip fracture repair to reduce the rate of SSIs, particularly in procedures that involve internal fixation (e.g., nails, screws, plates, wires). SSIs after hip fracture repair can result in extensive morbidity, including prolonged and repeated hospitalization, sepsis, persistent pain, device replacement, and possible death.[726,739,786–790]

Efficacy. The efficacy of antimicrobial prophylaxis in hip fracture repair has been illustrated in two meta-analyses.[787,788] One meta-analysis of 15 hip fracture procedure trials (the majority of procedures involved closed, proximal femoral, or trochanteric fractures with internal fixation) demonstrated that any dose and duration of prophylaxis are superior to no prophylaxis with respect to preventing SSIs (deep and superficial SSIs were analyzed together).[787] The rate of SSIs was 10.4% in controls versus 5.39% in treatment groups. A second meta-analysis of 22 studies reiterated the efficacy of antimicrobial prophylaxis in fracture procedures.[788] The analysis included the same hip fracture studies examined in the first meta-analysis, with additional studies of long-bone fracture repair (i.e., closed ankle fracture and other closed fractures, some noted with internal fixation). This second meta-analysis reviewed 10 studies of 1896 patients receiving a preoperative and two or more postoperative doses of a parenteral antimicrobial compared with a placebo or with no treatment. The authors found a relative risk of deep SSIs of 0.36 (95% CI, 0.21–0.65) and a relative risk of superficial SSIs of 0.48 (95% CI, 0.28–0.81) associated with antimicrobial use.

Choice of agent. The antimicrobials most often studied for prophylaxis in orthopedic procedures are first-generation cephalosporins due to their ease of administration, low cost, and safety profile.[787,788,791] Second- and third-generation cephalosporins have not been shown to offer clear advantages over first-generation agents. These agents are not recommended for routine use due to their higher cost, potential to promote resistance, and association with adverse events (e.g., *C. difficile*-associated diarrhea).[8,790,792]

Alternative regimens may be needed for institutions with highly resistant organisms, such as MRSA or *C. difficile*. Success in decreasing rates of *C. difficile*-associated disease and mortality was seen in a single-center study with the antimicrobial prophylaxis regimen change from three doses of cefuroxime[790,792] to a single preoperative dose of cefuroxime plus gentamicin.[792] In another study, *C. difficile*-associated disease decreased after the prophylaxis regimen was changed from cefuroxime to amoxicillin–clavulanate.[790]

Clindamycin and vancomycin have adequate activity against the most common pathogens involved in orthopedic procedures and would be acceptable alternatives under certain circumstances, such as prophylaxis for patients with a β-lactam allergy. Vancomycin should be included with cefazolin or used as an alternative agent for routine antimicrobial prophylaxis for patients who are known to be colonized with MRSA.[6,8,41,733,781]

Duration. For effective prophylaxis, the MIC of the antimicrobial needs to be exceeded at the target site from the moment of incision until surgical-site closure.[788] Two meta-analyses demonstrating the efficacy of antimicrobial prophylaxis in long-bone and hip fracture procedures also showed that multiple perioperative doses did not offer an advantage over a single preoperative dose.[787,788] These studies support a duration of antimicrobial prophylaxis of ≤24 hours.

Recommendations. The recommended regimen in hip fracture repair or other orthopedic procedures involving internal fixation is cefazolin. Clindamycin and vancomycin should be reserved as alternative agents, as described in the Common Principles section. If there are surveillance data showing that gram-negative organisms are a cause of SSIs for the procedure, practitioners may consider combining clindamycin or vancomycin with another agent (cefazolin if the patient is not β-lactam allergic; aztreonam, gentamicin, or single-dose fluoroquinolone if the patient is β-lactam allergic). Mupirocin should be given intranasally to all patients with documented colonization with *S. aureus*. (Strength of evidence for prophylaxis = A.)

Total Joint Replacement

Background. In 2005, more than 750,000 hip or knee replacements were performed in the United States.[793] The reported frequency of SSIs complicating hip, knee, elbow, ankle, or shoulder replacement ranges from 0.6% to 12%.[743,786,794–797] SSI rates as high as 11% after hip replacement and 12% after elbow replacement have been reported.[786,797] However, for hip and knee replacements, the most common joint arthroplasties, infection rates are typically less than 2%.[165]

The introduction of antimicrobial prophylaxis, stringent infection-control protocols, and the use of ultraclean operating rooms has led to a substantial reduction in SSI rates (to ≤1%).[734,786,796,798,799] Postoperative prosthetic joint infection is an organ/space SSI that occurs early (within 3 months postoperatively), is delayed (3–12 months postoperatively), or occurs late (>12 months after surgery).[748] These infections frequently require removal of the prosthesis, a prolonged course of antimicrobials, and one- or two-stage reimplantation of the prosthesis and may result in permanent disability.[796,800] Studies have shown an estimated economic impact of one deep SSI of $100,000 in hospital costs alone after hip arthroplasty and $60,000 after knee arthroplasty.[727–731]

Common risk factors for prosthetic joint infection[748] include advanced age; obesity; diabetes mellitus; corticosteroid use; malignancy; rheumatoid arthritis; previous arthroplasty on the same joint; arthroplasty undertaken to treat a fracture; type of joint replaced (e.g., risk is greater for the knee than the hip); perioperative surgical-site complications, including superficial SSI; hematoma; and persistent surgical-site drainage. Operative risk factors include ASA classification of ≥3, duration of procedure exceeding the 75th percentile for the procedure or exceeding three hours, surgical site classified as contaminated or dirty, and no systemic antimicrobial prophylaxis. Excluding the presence of a systemic antimicrobial, patients with these operative risk factors are at the greatest risk of developing an SSI.

A contributing factor to SSIs in arthroplasty is the formation of bacterial biofilm, particularly with *S. aureus* and *S. epidermidis*, on inert surfaces of orthopedic devices to confer antimicrobial resistance and difficulty in antimicrobial penetration.[744–748]

Efficacy. The majority of studies that have evaluated antimicrobial prophylaxis in joint replacements have been conducted in patients undergoing total hip or total knee arthroplasty.[801] There is a lack of efficacy data involving elbow, shoulder, and ankle arthroplasty; however, the same antimicrobial prophylaxis principles can be applied. In light of the serious potential consequences, antimicrobial prophylaxis is well accepted in procedures involving the implantation of foreign materials.[8,543,732,733]

A meta-analysis supports the use of antimicrobial prophylaxis for SSI reduction in patients undergoing total joint replacement.[801] Of the 26 randomized controlled studies examined, 24 included patients undergoing total hip or total knee arthroplasty. The meta-analysis noted that the studies did not clearly state if the arthroplasties were primary or revision. The SSIs were defined as visible purulent exudates at the surgical site (deep or superficial) in the included studies. Seven studies (n = 3065 patients) pooled to compare antimicrobial prophylaxis with placebo found a relative risk reduction of SSIs of 81%.

Choice of agent. There are no data supporting superiority of one class of antimicrobials over another for antimicrobial prophylaxis in total joint replacement. A meta-analysis of studies, mainly in total hip or total knee replacement, found no difference in SSIs between cephalosporins with teicoplanin (not available in the United States) in five studies with 2625 patients, cephalosporins and penicillin derivatives in three studies of 386 patients, and first- and second-generation cephalosporins in eight studies of 2879 patients.[801] Selection should be based on cost, availability, and local resistance patterns. First-generation cephalosporins are the agents most commonly studied and used for antimicrobial prophylaxis in joint replacement procedures.

Clindamycin and vancomycin have adequate activity against the most common pathogens involved in orthopedic procedures and would be acceptable alternatives under certain circumstances, such as prophylaxis for patients with a β-lactam allergy. Vancomycin should be included with cefazolin or used as an alternative agent for routine antimicrobial prophylaxis in institutions that have a high prevalence of MRSA SSIs and for patients who are known to be colonized with MRSA.[6,8,41,733,781] Readers are referred to the section on implantation of internal fixation devices for further discussion of antimicrobial prophylaxis choice.

Antimicrobial-laden bone cement. The use of antimicrobial-laden bone cement in conjunction with i.v. antimicrobial prophylaxis is common worldwide, particularly for the prevention of infection in primary hip and knee arthroplasties.[802–806] FDA has approved premixed aminoglycoside (i.e., gentamicin and tobramycin) in bone cement products for use in hip, knee, or other joints in second-stage revision of total joint arthroplasty.[807] The products are not approved for prophylaxis in primary joint replacement procedures. While antimicrobial bone cement has not been shown to be superior to i.v. antimicrobials,[808,809] there is evidence that supports the combination of using antimicrobial-laden bone cement together with systemic antimicrobial prophylaxis.

Although the evidence for the prophylactic use of antimicrobial-laden bone cement in primary joint arthroplasty looks favorable, a recent multicenter evaluation of risk factors for SSI in patients undergoing total hip arthroplasty did not find that use of antimicrobial-laden bone cement reduced the risk for infection.[95] In addition, questions remain regarding the risk for antimicrobial resistance and allergy, as well as the increased cost.[41,802–807,810–813] Readers are referred to reviews of this topic for additional information about tissue penetration, clinical application, and safety.[805,810–815]

Duration. The duration of prophylaxis in joint replacement procedures has been controversial. More recent data and clinical practice guidelines do not support prophylaxis beyond 24 hours.[6,41,133,723] Studies involving total hip replacement have used antimicrobials for 12 hours to 14 days postoperatively.[726,734–737,816] A duration of 24 hours was supported in a randomized trial of 358 patients undergoing total hip arthroplasty, total knee arthroplasty, or hip fracture repair that compared prophylaxis that lasted 24 hours versus 7 days of either nafcillin or cefazolin started 20 minutes before the procedure.[816] The difference in SSI rates between groups was not significant. There is no evidence of benefit of antimicrobial administration until all drains or catheters are removed.[32,41,133]

Recommendations. The recommended regimen for patients undergoing total hip, elbow, knee, ankle, or shoulder replacement is cefazolin. Clindamycin and vancomycin should be reserved as alternative agents, as described in the Common Principles section. If there are any surveillance data showing that gram-negative organisms are a cause of SSIs for the procedure, practitioners may consider combining clindamycin or vancomycin with another agent (cefazolin if the patient is not β-lactam allergic; aztreonam, gentamicin, or a single-dose fluoroquinolone if the patient is β-lactam allergic). Mupirocin should be given intranasally to all patients with documented colonization with *S. aureus*. (Strength of evidence for prophylaxis = A.)

Urologic Procedures

Background. The goals of antimicrobial prophylaxis in urologic procedures are the prevention of bacteremia and SSIs and the prevention of postoperative bacteriuria.[59] Postoperative urinary tract infections (UTIs) are the main concern for morbidity in patients after urologic procedures.[817,818] Bacteriuria, defined as $>10^3$ or $>10^4$ CFU/mL in symptomatic UTI and $>10^5$ CFU/mL in asymptomatic bacteriuria, within 30 days postoperatively is a frequent primary outcome in urologic procedure studies.[819–825] The benefits of preventing postoperative bacteriuria are not clearly known.[825]

In addition to general risk factors discussed in the Common Principles section of these guidelines, urologic-specific risk factors include anatomic anomalies of the urinary tract,[818] urinary obstruction,[826] urinary stone,[817,825,826] and indwelling or externalized catheters.[817,818,822,826] Preoperative UTI, particularly if recurrent, is recognized as a high-risk factor for postoperative infection, which is typically treated before procedures and is a common exclusion criterion from studies of efficacy of antimicrobial prophylaxis in urologic procedures.[817,826–828] Additional urologic operation-specific risk factors include length of post-operative catheterization,[829] mode of irrigation (closed versus open), and postoperative pyuria.[821]

Organisms. *E. coli* is the organism most commonly isolated in patients with postoperative bacteriuria; however, other gram-negative bacilli and enterococci may also cause infection.[818,821,827,830–839] Organisms such as *S. aureus*, coagulase-negative *Staphylococcus* species, and group A *Streptococcus* species are also a concern in procedures entering the skin with or without entering the urinary tract.[818,827,830–832,838,840,841] There is also some concern with biofilm-forming bacteria (*S. epidermidis* and *P. aeruginosa*) in patients with prosthesis implantation.[842]

Efficacy. The efficacy of antimicrobial prophylaxis in select urologic procedures has been investigated in several clinical trials. Of note, many of these placebo-controlled studies have excluded patients with risk factors for infection, those requiring antimicrobial prophylaxis for another indication (e.g., infective endocarditis), and those with preoperative UTI or bacteriuria.

The efficacy of antimicrobial prophylaxis in clean procedures among patients at low risk of complications has been variable. One randomized, placebo-controlled study of oral antimicrobials in 2083 patients undergoing flexible cystoscopy found a positive urine culture (bacteriuria with $>10^5$ CFU/mL) in 9.1% of patients receiving placebo, 4.6% of patients receiving trimethoprim, and 2.8% of patients receiving ciprofloxacin.[839] The rates of bacteriuria compared with baseline were significantly higher with placebo and significantly lower with use of antimicrobials compared with placebo. A randomized, placebo-controlled study of 517 patients undergoing prostate brachytherapy found no significant difference in postimplantation epididymitis with or without antimicrobial prophylaxis (0.4% and 1.5%, respectively).[843] A meta-analysis of eight randomized, placebo-controlled or no-treatment-controlled studies with 995 patients undergoing urodynamic studies found a decrease in bacteriuria with antimicrobial prophylaxis (OR, 0.39; 95% CI, 0.24–0.61).[820] The number needed to treat was 13 to prevent one episode of asymptomatic bacteriuria using a pooled rate of 13.7% for bacteriuria. One study found that not using antimicrobial prophylaxis was a significant risk factor for bacteriuria caused by urinary dynamic studies.[821]

Antimicrobial prophylaxis has been studied in urologic procedures involving entry into the gastrointestinal tract, with the majority of the literature on transurethral resection of the prostate (TURP) and prostate biopsy. Two large meta-analyses have suggested prophylactic antimicrobials may be effective in all patients undergoing TURP, including low-risk patients and those with preoperatively sterile urine.[844,845] One meta-analysis of 32 trials with 4260 patients found that prophylactic antimicrobials decreased the combined bacteriuria (>10^5 CFU/mL) event rate from 26% to 9.1%, for a relative risk reduction of 65% (95% CI, –55 to –72), and the combined clinical septicemia episode rate from 4.4% to 0.7% in TURP patients, including low-risk patients.[846] Another meta-analysis of 28 trials that included a total of 4694 patients found prophylactic antimicrobials decreased the post-TURP rate of bacteriuria, fever, and bacteremia, as well as the need for additional postoperative antimicrobials.[847] An additional multicenter, open-label, randomized, active- and placebo-controlled trial in patients with sterile urine undergoing TURP found a decreased rate of bacteriuria (≥5 CFU/mL) with antimicrobial prophylaxis (21% with levofloxacin and 20% with sulfamethoxazole–trimethoprim) compared with placebo (30%) ($p = 0.009$).[822]

Three randomized, placebo-controlled studies of patients undergoing transrectal needle biopsy of the prostate found significant differences in infectious complications (including bacteriuria, positive urine cultures, and UTI) in patients treated with single doses of oral antimicrobial prophylaxis compared with placebo.[819,837,838] These three studies support the routine use of antimicrobial prophylaxis in all patients undergoing transrectal needle biopsy of the prostate. Of note, all patients undergoing transrectal needle biopsy of the prostate received a cleansing enema before the procedure.[819,837,838] Use of MBP has been reported in urologic procedures that involve entering the gastrointestinal tract (e.g., urinary diversion).[844,846]

The use of antimicrobial prophylaxis in patients undergoing extracorporeal shock wave lithotripsy (ESWL) and ureterorenoscopy is supported by the results of a meta-analysis[847] and a small randomized controlled trial.[848] The meta-analysis included eight randomized controlled trials with 885 patients and six clinical case series involving 597 patients undergoing ESWL.[845] The overall rate of UTI in the randomized controlled trials ranged from 0% to 7.7% with antimicrobial prophylaxis and from 0% to 28% in the control groups (relative risk, 0.45; 95% CI, 0.22–0.93). A randomized, placebo-controlled study of 113 patients undergoing ureterorenoscopy found a rate of postoperative bacteriuria of 1.8% with antimicrobial prophylaxis and 12.5% without ($p = 0.0026$).[848] No patients had symptomatic UTI or inflammation complications of the urogenital tract postoperatively.

There are no studies of antimicrobial prophylaxis in major open or laparoscopic procedures (cystectomy, radical prostatectomy, and nephrectomy); therefore, data have been extrapolated from other major intraabdominal procedures.

Choice of agent. No single antimicrobial regimen appears superior for urologic procedures. A wide range of antimicrobial regimens, including cephalosporins,[658,835,836,843,849–855] aminoglycosides,[856,857] piperacillin–tazobactam,[849,858,859] trimethoprim–sulfamethoxazole,[822,838,860] trimethoprim,[839] nitrofurantoin,[861] and fluoroquino-lones,[819,821,822,824,831,835–837,839,840,843,848,851,853–855,862,863] have been evaluated in urologic procedures. The efficacy of fluoroquinolones for antimicrobial prophylaxis in urologic surgical procedures has been well established. One study found better reduction of bacteriuria with either ciprofloxacin or trimethoprim compared with placebo,[839] while other studies found no difference in efficacy between a fluoroquinolone and sulfamethoxazole–trimethoprim, both of which were better than placebo.[822,838] No differences were found in studies between oral or i.v. fluoroquinolones (ciprofloxacin or ofloxacin) compared with i.v. or intramuscular cephalosporins (ceftriaxone, cefotaxime, or cefazolin) and intramuscular penicillin (piperacillin–tazobactam) in various urologic procedures.[835,836,851,854,855,858] In several studies, fluoroquinolones were administered orally, which appears to be feasible in patients undergoing procedures not involving opening the urinary or gastrointestinal tract, when the i.v. route would be preferred.[822,836,838,851,855,858] Recently, resistance to fluoroquinolones has been emerging; the fact that most of the literature was published before resistance became prevalent should be considered, since resistance may decrease the relevance of these studies.[836,846,847,858,864] Local resistance patterns to fluoroquinolones, particularly with *E. coli*, should be evaluated to help guide antimicrobial selection.

Broad-spectrum antimicrobials, such as third-generation cephalosporins and carbapenems, are no more effective than first- or second-generation cephalosporins, aminoglycosides, or oral agents (trimethoprim–sulfamethoxazole, nitrofurantoin, or fluoroquinolones) and should be reserved for patients with active infection or who require additional coverage for intestinal organisms.[6,826,827] Their routine use is not recommended due to their higher cost and potential to promote resistance, particularly among health-care-associated gram-negative bacilli.[8]

Duration. While longer durations of postoperative prophylaxis (up to three weeks) have been studied,[856,858,860,861] more-recent data support the use of shorter durations (i.e., a single dose or less than 24 hours' duration) in urologic procedures.[658,817,818,823,824,826,831,832,834,836,846,853,857,859,862,865,866] Based on bioavailability, oral antimicrobial prophylaxis should be administered 1–2 hours before surgical incision or start of the procedure.[817,819–822,824,826,836,838,840,848,851,855]

Pediatric Efficacy. Limited data on antimicrobial prophylaxis are available for pediatric patients undergoing urologic procedures. One prospective, open-label, nonrandomized study of boys undergoing hypospadias repair with tabularized incision plate urethroplasty allocated patients to receive cefonicid (no longer available in the United States) with one i.v. dose before the procedure only or the addition of oral cephalexin three times daily starting on postoperative day 1 until 2 days after catheter removal (median, 8.3 days).[833] More patients in the single-dose group had bacteriuria and complications (urethrocutaneous fistula and meatal stenosis); however, the rate of infection and infection-related complications did not significantly differ between groups.

Recommendations. No antimicrobial prophylaxis is recommended for clean urologic procedures in patients without risk factors for postoperative infections. Patients with preoperative bacteriuria or UTI should be treated before the procedure, when possible, to reduce the risk of postoperative infection. For patients undergoing lower urinary tract instrumentation with risk factors for infection, the use of a fluoroquinolone or trimethoprim–sulfamethoxazole (oral or i.v.) or cefazolin (i.v. or intramuscular) is recommended (Table 2). For patients undergoing clean urologic procedures without entry into the urinary tract, cefazolin is recommended, with vancomycin or clindamycin as an alternative for those patients allergic to β-lactam antimicrobials. For patients undergoing clean urologic procedures with entry into the urinary tract, cefazolin is recommended, with alternative antimicrobials to include a fluoroquinolone, the combination of an aminoglycoside plus metronidazole, or an aminoglycoside plus clindamycin. For clean-contaminated procedures of the urinary tract (often entering the gastrointestinal tract), antimicrobials as recommended for elective colorectal surgery are recommended. This would generally include the combination of cefazolin with or without metronidazole, cefoxitin, or, for patients with β-lactam allergy, a combination of either a fluoroquinolone or aminoglycoside given with either metronidazole or clindamycin. The medical literature does not support continuing antimicrobial prophylaxis until urinary catheters have been removed. See the colorectal procedures section of these guidelines for recommendations pertaining to procedures entering the gastrointestinal tract. (Strength of evidence for prophylaxis = A.)

Vascular Procedures

Background. Infection after vascular procedures occurs with low frequency but can be associated with extensive morbidity and mortality.[867,868] Postoperative infections involving vascular graft material can result in limb loss and life-threatening conditions.[868] As a result, antimicrobial prophylaxis is widely used in procedures that involve implantation of prosthetic material and procedures for which there is greater risk of infection, such as aneurysm repair, thromboendarterectomy, and vein bypass.[6,41,867,869] Patients undergoing brachiocephalic procedures (e.g., carotid endarterectomy, brachial artery repair) without implantation of prosthetic graft material do not appear to benefit from routine antimicrobial prophylaxis.[6,41,867,870]

Risk factors for postoperative SSI in patients undergoing vascular procedures include lower-extremity sites, delayed procedures after hospitalization, diabetes mellitus, and a history of vascular or aortocoronary bypass procedures.[871,872] Currently, prospective data from well-designed studies on prophylaxis for endovascular stenting do not exist. However, if prophylaxis is desired, the same antimicrobials and short duration of therapy used for open vascular procedures should be given. Risk factors that warrant consideration of prophylaxis in patients undergoing endovascular stenting include prolonged procedures (more than two hours), reintervention at the surgical site within seven days, vascular stent placement in the groin through a hematoma or sheath, procedures in immunosuppressed patients, and the presence of another intravascular prosthesis.[873–877]

Organisms. The predominant organisms involved include *S. aureus*, *S. epidermidis*, and enteric gram-negative bacilli. MRSA is an emerging organism of concern.

Several studies evaluated the rate of colonization, carriage, and infection with MRSA in patients undergoing various vascular procedures.[878–884] Independent risk factors for MRSA infection included MRSA colonization, open abdominal aortic aneurysm, tissue loss, and lower-limb bypass.[878] Patients who have or develop MRSA infections before vascular procedures have increased risk of inhospital death, intensive care unit admission, repeat surgeries, increased length of stay, and delayed wound healing, compared with patients without infections.[880–883]

Efficacy. Prophylactic antimicrobials decrease the rate of infection after procedures involving the lower abdominal vasculature and procedures required to establish dialysis access. The follow-up time for patients with late surgical-site complications was at least once after hospital discharge (not further defined) for most studies,[829,865,871,885–887] at one month,[869,871,888,889] at six months,[872] and at three years.[138]

A meta-analysis of 10 randomized controlled trials in patients undergoing peripheral arterial reconstruction with biological or prosthetic graft procedures found an overall consistent reduction in SSIs with systemic antimicrobial prophylaxis compared with placebo (relative risk, 0.25; 95% CI, 0.17–0.38; $p < 0.00001$).[890] An overall reduction was found among 5 studies evaluating early graft infection (relative risk, 0.31; 95% CI, 0.11–0.85; $p = 0.02$), though no individual study found a significant reduction in SSIs.

The largest study included in the meta-analysis above was a randomized, prospective, double-blind, placebo-controlled study of patients undergoing peripheral vascular procedures ($n = 462$). The infection rate was significantly lower with cefazolin than with placebo (0.9% and 6.8%, respectively).[885] Four deep graft infections were observed in the placebo group; none occurred in the patients who received cefazolin. No infections were observed in patients who underwent brachiocephalic ($n = 103$), femoral artery ($n = 56$), or popliteal ($n = 14$) procedures.

Patients undergoing vascular access procedures for hemodialysis may benefit from the administration of antistaphylococcal antimicrobials. A placebo-controlled study of 408 patients undergoing permanent vascular access placement demonstrated an upper-extremity prosthetic polytetrafluoroethylene graft infection rate of 6% with placebo compared with 1% with vancomycin ($p = 0.006$).[869]

Choice of agent. Cefazolin remains the preferred and most cost-effective prophylactic agent for use in vascular procedures.[6,8,41,872,886,887] There was no significant difference in infection rates between cefazolin and cefuroxime in patients undergoing abdominal aortic and lower-extremity peripheral vascular procedures,[886] between cefazolin and cefamandole (no longer available in the United States) in patients undergoing aortic or infrainguinal arterial procedures,[887] or between cefazolin and ceftriaxone in patients undergoing arterial reconstruction involving infraclavicular sites.[872]

A multicenter, randomized, double-blind, prospective trial of 580 patients undergoing arterial procedures involving the groin who received either two doses of ciprofloxacin 750 mg orally or three doses of cefuroxime 1.5 g i.v. on the day of the procedure found an SSI rate of 9.2% (27 patients) and 9.1% (26 patients), respectively, within 30 days of the procedure.[889] Although oral ciprofloxacin was shown to be as effective as i.v. cefuroxime, this study did not address concerns about resistance with routine use of fluoroquinolones.[891] Therefore, i.v. cefazolin remains the first-line agent for this indication. The efficacy of oral agents for prophylaxis needs to be further evaluated.

There are limited data regarding the choice of an antimicrobial for β-lactam-allergic patients undergoing vascular procedures. The main alternative agents are vancomycin and clindamycin, since prophylaxis is largely directed against gram-positive cocci. Vancomycin can also be used for prophylaxis in institutions with MRSA or methicillin-resistant *S. epidermidis* (MRSE) clusters or in patients with β-lactam allergy.[6,8,41] Clindamycin may be an acceptable alternative to vancomycin, though local antimicrobial resistance patterns should be taken into account.

An aminoglycoside may be added to vancomycin for the addition of aerobic gram-negative bacilli coverage if the procedure involves the abdominal aorta or a groin incision, due to the potential for gastrointestinal flora. See the Common Principles section of these guidelines for further discussion of the use of vancomycin. Alternative antimicrobials for β-lactam-allergic patients receiving vancomycin may include a fluoroquinolone or aztreonam.[6]

Duration. A meta-analysis of three randomized controlled studies involving vascular procedures, including lower-limb reconstruction and open arterial procedures, found no additional benefit of continuing prophylactic antimicrobials for over 24 hours postoperatively compared with no more than 24 hours (relative risk, 1.28; 95% CI, 0.82–1.98).[890]

A randomized, double-blind study compared infection rates of a one-day and a three-day course of cefuroxime with placebo in 187 patients undergoing peripheral vascular procedures.[888] The infection rates were 16.7%, 3.8%, and 4.3% in the placebo, one-day, and three-day groups, respectively. The difference in the infection rates between the one- and three-day groups was not significant.

A randomized controlled study compared one day and five days of amoxicillin–clavulanate 1.2 g in 100 patients undergoing 108 lower-limb reconstruction procedures.[892] No difference was seen in the postoperative SSI rate between groups (9 patients [16%] and 12 patients [23%], respectively). The study authors selected the agent based on extended spectrum of activity and good tissue penetration. However, they concluded that due to the high rate of infection observed, the use of antimicrobial prophylaxis might not be as effective as once thought.

A randomized controlled study compared ticarcillin-clavulanate 3.1 g given as a single dose at induction of anesthesia with multiple doses given at induction and every 6 hours postoperatively until venous access lines were removed or a maximum of 20 doses (total of five days) in patients undergoing open arterial procedures.[893] Significantly more SSIs occurred in the single-dose group (28 [18%] of 153 patients) compared with the multidose group (15 [10%] of 149 patients) (relative risk, 2; 95% CI, −1.02 to 3.92; $p = 0.041$). Ticarcillin–clavulanate has a short duration of action and is not recommended as a routine agent for antimicrobial prophylaxis. Practice guidelines recommend single-dose prophylaxis in vascular procedures or a maximum duration of therapy of 24 hours postoperatively, regardless of the presence of invasive drains.[6,41]

Recommendations. The recommended regimen for patients undergoing vascular procedures associated with a higher risk of infection, including implantation of prosthetic material, is cefazolin (Table 2). (Strength of evidence for prophylaxis = A.) Clindamycin and vancomycin should be reserved as alternative agents as described in the Common Principles section of these guidelines. If there are surveillance data showing that gram-negative organisms are a cause of SSIs for the procedure, practitioners may consider combining clindamycin or vancomycin with another agent (cefazolin if the patient is not β-lactam allergic; aztreonam, gentamicin, or single-dose fluoroquinolone if the patient is β-lactam allergic), due to the potential for gastrointestinal flora exposure.

Heart, Lung, and Heart–Lung Transplantation

Background. Solid-organ transplant recipients are at high risk for infections due to the complexity of the surgical procedures, donor- or recipient-derived infections, reactivation of recipient-associated latent infections, preoperative recipient colonization, exposure to community pathogens, and opportunistic infections due to immunosuppression.[894–897] Infections occur more frequently in the first year after transplantation, due to aggressive immunosuppression. Transplant recipients with infections are commonly asymptomatic or have nonspecific symptoms or sequelae of infection, which makes detection and diagnosis of infections difficult.[855,857,894] Postoperative infections caused by bacterial, viral, and fungal pathogens, including SSIs, UTIs, bloodstream infections, and pneumonia, are of greater concern within the first month after transplantation.[895–897] Opportunistic infections that result from immunosuppression typically occur after the first month of transplantation. It is routine for transplant recipients to receive antimicrobial prophylaxis to prevent opportunistic infections.[894–897] A discussion of the prophylactic strategies for prevention of cytomegalovirus (CMV) infection, herpes simplex virus infection, pneumocystis, UTI in kidney transplant recipients, *Aspergillus* infection in lung transplant recipients, and other opportunistic infections outside of the immediate posttransplantation period is beyond the scope of these guidelines.

Few well-designed, prospective, comparative studies of antimicrobial prophylaxis have been conducted with patients undergoing solid-organ transplantation, and no formal recommendations are available from expert consensus panels or professional organizations; however, there are reviews that provide guidance.[8,41,894]

The recommendations given for each of the solid-organ transplant procedures are intended to provide guidelines for safe and effective surgical prophylaxis based on the best available literature. Antimicrobial surgical prophylaxis practice will vary considerably among transplantation centers throughout the United States, based on the organ involved, preexisting recipient and donor infections, and local antimicrobial susceptibilities.[894–897]

Heart Transplantation. *Background.* Heart transplantation is an option for selected patients with end-stage cardiac disease. In 2007, the United Network for Organ Sharing (UNOS) reported that 2209 heart transplants were performed in the United States, including 327 in children (<18 years of age).[898] The mean graft survival rate 10 years after heart transplantation is approximately 49%. Infection continues to be an important cause of morbidity and mortality after heart transplantation and is a primary cause of death in approximately 14% of patients within the first year after transplantation.[899]

Despite the large number of heart transplantation procedures performed, few studies have specifically examined postoperative SSI rates in this population. General cardiothoracic procedures have been associated with SSI rates ranging from 9% to 55% in the absence of antimicrobial prophylaxis.[214,900,901] Studies of general cardiothoracic procedures, including heart transplantation, found SSIs, particularly mediastinitis, in 3–6% of patients who received antimicrobial prophylaxis.[170,902] The frequency was highest in heart transplant recipients. The SSI rates reported in patients undergoing heart transplantation who received antimicrobial prophylaxis ranged from 5.8% to 8.8%, including mediastinitis in 3–7% of patients.[903,904]

Several independent risk factors for SSIs after cardiac and thoracic procedures have been identified (see the cardiac and thoracic sections of this article). Heart transplantation has been identified as an independent risk factor for SSIs.[170] Other independent risk factors for SSIs in heart transplantation include age,[905] receipt of ciprofloxacin alone for prophylaxis,[906] positive wire cultures,[907] a BMI of >30 kg/m^2, female sex,[908] previous cardiac procedures, previous left VAD placement, and hemodynamic instability requiring inotropic support.[903,904] Unfavorable functional outcomes were seen in patients who developed infections within the first year after heart transplantation associated with lung, bloodstream, and CMV infections.[909] Independent predictors of mortality in heart transplant recipients included serum creatinine levels, amyloid etiology, history of hypertension, pulmonary infection, and CNS infection. Additional predisposing factors for infection in heart transplantation include exposure to pathogens from the donor or transplant recipient, the time from organ recovery to reperfusion, and the immunosuppressive regimens used.[897,904,910] Similar risk factors for infection are noted in pediatric transplant recipients, with the addition of a naive immune system to several pathogens, most notably viruses, as well as incomplete primary immunization series.[897]

Patients with an indwelling VAD at the time of heart transplantation have additional prophylaxis concerns. Recipients who do not have a driveline infection and have no history of either colonization or infection should receive prophylaxis as described for recipients without a VAD in place. Patients with a history of colonization or previous infection should have the antimicrobial sensitivities of that organism considered when choosing the SSI prophylactic regimen administered, though the duration should still be less than 24 hours. Heart transplant recipients with an active VAD driveline infection at the time of heart transplantation should be given appropriate antimicrobials specifically for the treatment of that infection. This intervention will usually determine the actual perioperative prophylaxis regimen as well as the duration of therapy beyond the period of prophylaxis.

Patients requiring ECMO as a bridge to heart transplantation should be treated with a similar approach. If there is no history of colonization or previous infection, then the general recommendations for SSI antimicrobial prophylaxis for the specific procedure should be followed. In ECMO patients with a history of colonization or previous infection, changing the preoperative antimicrobial prophylaxis to cover these pathogens must be considered, weighing whether the pathogen is relevant to SSIs in the planned procedure.

Because heart transplantation is similar to other cardiac and thoracic procedures, similar considerations regarding the need for antimicrobial prophylaxis apply (see the cardiac and thoracic sections).[911] These guidelines do not address antimicrobial prophylaxis for infective endocarditis. Readers are referred to the current guidelines for prevention of infective endocarditis from AHA.[11,228]

Organisms. As with other types of cardiothoracic procedures, gram-positive organisms, mainly *Staphylococcus* species, are the primary pathogens that cause SSI after heart transplantation.[902,905–907,912,913] MRSA was reported in 12–21% of SSIs in several cohort studies.[903,905,906] Vancomycin-resistant *Enterococcus faecalis* was noted in 15% of infections in one cohort study.[903] Other gram-positive pathogens (e.g., coagulase-negative staphylococci, *Enterococcus* species)[903,905–907,913] and gram-negative organisms (e.g., Enterobacteriaceae, *P. aeruginosa*, *Stenotrophomonas maltophilia*) are also a concern for SSIs in heart transplant recipients, as are *Candida* species.[903,906]

Efficacy. Despite the paucity of literature on antimicrobial prophylaxis for the prevention of SSIs in heart transplantation, the efficacy noted in other cardiac surgical procedures has made it the standard of practice during transplantation.[896]

No randomized controlled trials have specifically addressed the use of antimicrobial prophylaxis in heart transplantation. In an open-label noncomparative study, the SSI rate was 4.5% among 96 patients administered cefotaxime plus floxacillin preoperatively and for 72 hours after cardiac procedures.[912] This rate of infection was similar to that seen in other cardiothoracic, nonheart transplantation procedures in which antimicrobial prophylaxis was used.

Choice of agent. Antimicrobial prophylaxis for heart transplantation should be similar to that used for other types of cardiothoracic procedures.[911] First- and second-generation cephalosporins are considered to be equally efficacious and are the preferred agents. There appear to be no significant differences in efficacy among prophylactic regimens using agents such as cefazolin and cefuroxime.[914] The use of antistaphylococcal penicillins, either alone or in combination with aminoglycosides or cephalosporins, failed to demonstrate superior efficacy to that of cephalosporin monotherapy (see the cardiac and thoracic sections) in other cardiothoracic procedures.

Several cohort studies examined antimicrobial prophylactic agents used for patients undergoing heart transplantation but did not evaluate efficacy.[902,903,905,906] Ciprofloxacin alone was found to be an independent risk factor for incisional SSIs.[906]

Duration. There is no consensus on the optimal duration of antimicrobial prophylaxis in cardiothoracic procedures, including heart transplantation. Cohort evaluations of patients undergoing heart transplantation reported durations of antimicrobial prophylaxis with cefazolin or vancomycin of 24 or 48 hours postoperatively.[902,903,905] Data from cardiothoracic procedures also support a range of prophylaxis durations, from a single dose to 24 or 48 hours postoperatively.[41,131] The currently accepted duration for these procedures, which do not include transplantation, is 24–48 hours postoperatively.[41,59,131,201] The duration of antimicrobial prophylaxis for patients who do not have their chest primarily closed is unclear; most centers continue prophylaxis until the chest is closed, but there is no evidence to support this practice.

Pediatric efficacy. No randomized controlled studies have specifically addressed antimicrobial prophylaxis for heart transplantation in pediatric patients. Infants are at risk for mediastinitis caused by gram-negative as well as gram-positive organisms. Pediatric patients undergoing heart transplantation should be treated according to recommendations for other types of cardiothoracic procedures. The recommended regimen for pediatric patients undergoing cardiothoracic procedures is cefazolin 25–50 mg/kg i.v. within 60 minutes before surgical incision and every 8 hours for up to 48 hours. Cefuroxime 50 mg/kg i.v. within 60 minutes before surgical incision and every 8 hours for up to 48 hours is an acceptable alternative. Vancomycin 10–20 mg/kg i.v. over 60–120 minutes, with or without gentamicin 2 mg/kg i.v., should be reserved as an alternative on the basis of guidelines from HICPAC for routine antimicrobial prophylaxis in institutions that have a high prevalence of MRSA, for patients who are colonized with MRSA, or for patients with a true β-lactam allergy.[8] Additional doses may be needed intraoperatively for procedures >4 hours in duration, for patients with major blood loss, or for extended use of CPB depending on the half-life of the prophylactic antimicrobial. Fluoroquinolones are not routinely recommended in pediatric patients.

Recommendations. Based on data for other types of cardiothoracic procedures, antimicrobial prophylaxis is indicated for all patients undergoing heart transplantation (see cardiac and thoracic sections). The recommended regimen is a single dose of cefazolin (Table 2). There is no evidence to support continuing prophylaxis until chest and mediastinal drainage tubes are removed. Alternatives include vancomycin or clindamycin with or without gentamicin, aztreonam, or a single fluoroquinolone dose. (Strength of evidence for prophylaxis = A.) The optimal duration of antimicrobial prophylaxis for patients who do not have their chest primarily closed is unclear. No recommendation is made for these patients. Patients who have left VADs as a bridge and who are chronically infected might also benefit from coverage of the infecting microorganism.

Lung and Heart–Lung Transplantation. *Background.* Lung transplantation is an accepted option for a variety of end-stage, irreversible lung diseases. The most common diseases for which lung transplantation is performed are idiopathic pulmonary fibrosis, chronic obstructive pulmonary disease, emphysema, cystic fibrosis, α-1-antitrypsin deficiency, and idiopathic pulmonary arterial hypertension.[915,916] UNOS reported that in the United States in 2007, 1468 lung transplantations and 31 heart–lung transplantations were conducted in adults, and 52 lung transplantations and 3 heart–lung transplantations were performed in children.[898,917] Ten-year survival rates were reported as 29.7% of double-lung, 17.5% of single-lung, and 25.8% of heart–lung transplant recipients.[899] The reported three-year survival rate for pediatric lung transplant recipients was 57%.[89]

Infections are the most common complications after lung and heart–lung transplantations.[899,915,918,919] In an analysis of UNOS data over an 18-year period, infection was the number one cause of death within the first year of transplantation, occurring in 24.8% of lung and 18.3% of heart–lung transplant recipients.[899] Among the top 10 primary causes of death within the first year after lung and heart–lung transplantations were sepsis, pneumonia, fungal infection (lung only), and CMV infection.[899] A study of two cohorts of patients undergoing heart, lung, and heart–lung transplantations who received antimicrobial prophylaxis evaluated the rate of SSIs and mediastinitis.[904,908] The rate of SSI among all transplant recipients was 12.98%, with the majority of infections (72%) being organ/space infections, followed by deep incisional infections (17%) and superficial incisional infections (10%).[908] The overall rate of mediastinitis in a similar cohort was 2.7%, with rates of 5.2% in heart–lung transplant recipients and 3.2% in bilateral lung transplant recipients.[904] Pneumonia was reported in 26.4% of transplantation patients overall, with rates of 20.7% in lung transplant recipients and 40% in heart–lung transplant recipients.[908] A cohort of lung transplant recipients reported a rate of 2.2 episodes of pneumonia per patient during a median follow-up period of 412 days (range, 1–1328 days).[920]

Bronchial anastomotic infections, especially fungal infections, can be serious and are potentially fatal in lung transplant recipients.[921,922] The lung allocation score (LAS) is a rating system adopted by the Organ Procurement and Transplant Network and UNOS in 2005 to improve organ allocation and transplantation outcomes. The LAS is based on the risk of death while on the waiting list for transplantation and the expected 1-year survival after transplantation. Patients with a low LAS are unlikely to undergo transplantation. A study of lung transplant recipients age 12 years or older revealed a higher rate of infection and other morbidities and a lower 1-year survival rate in patients with a high LAS at the time of transplantation than in patients with a low LAS at the time of transplantation.[923] Thus, the potential for bronchial anastomotic infection and a poor posttransplantation outcome needs to be considered in patients undergoing lung transplantation. Among lung transplantation patients, risk factors for nosocomial infections included α-1-antitrypsin deficiency and repeat transplantation. Risk factors for pneumonia included colonized or infected donor bronchus and perfusate and preoperative colonization with gram-negative rods. Risk factors for mortality among the transplant recipients were cystic fibrosis, nosocomial infection, and ventilation before transplantation.[908] Risk factors for mediastinitis after heart, lung, and heart–lung transplantation were degree of immunosuppression, impaired renal function, previous sternotomy, and reexploration due to bleeding.[904] There was a positive association between pretransplantation colonizing microorganisms from suppurative lung disease patients and pneumonia after transplantation.[920] Transplantation alters the physiological function of lungs, including the impairment of mucociliary clearance and interruption of the cough reflex, leading to a higher risk of pulmonary infections.[896]

In patients requiring ECMO as a bridge to lung transplantation who have no history of colonization or previous infection, the general recommendations for SSI antimicrobial prophylaxis for the procedure should be followed. In

ECMO patients with a history of colonization or previous infection, changing the preoperative antimicrobial prophylaxis to cover these pathogens must be considered, weighing whether the pathogen is relevant to SSIs in the planned procedure.

Organisms. While gram-positive and gram-negative organisms are of concern in heart transplantation, there is increased concern regarding gram-negative and fungal pathogens in mediastinitis and pneumonia in patients undergoing lung transplantation.[894,904,908] The most frequent organisms found in SSIs or mediastinitis in two cohort studies were *P. aeruginosa*,[904,908] *Candida* species, *S. aureus* (including MRSA),[908] enterococci, coagulase-negative staphylococci (e.g., *S. epidermidis*), *Burkholderia cepacia*,[904] *E. coli*, and *Klebsiella* species.

Patients undergoing lung transplantation are also at risk for bacterial or fungal pneumonia due to colonization or infection of the lower and upper airways of the donor, recipient, or both.[915] Organisms reported to cause pneumonia in lung transplantation patients include *P. aeruginosa*,[894,896,904,908,920] *S. aureus* (including MRSA),[894,896,904,908] *B. cepacia*,[896,904,908] *Enterobacter* species,[908] *S. maltophilia*, *Klebsiella* species,[904,908] *S. epidermidis*,[904] *E. coli*, *Aspergillus* species,[920] and VRE.[894] Similarly, organisms frequently seen in pediatric lung infections are nonfermenting gram-negative bacteria, such as *Pseudomonas* species, *Stenotrophomonas* species, *Alcaligenes* species, and fungi, including *Aspergillus* species.[897]

The donor lung appears to be a major route of transmission of pathogens; 75–90% of bronchial washings from donor organs are positive for at least one bacterial organism.[920,924,925] Organ recipients may also be the source of infection of the transplanted organ. This is particularly true in patients with cystic fibrosis because of the frequent presence of *P. aeruginosa* in the upper airways and sinuses before transplantation.[896,919] These pathogens are often multidrug resistant, likely due, in large part, to frequent administration of broad-spectrum antimicrobials during the course of the disease. Multidrug-resistant strains of *B. cepacia* and *S. maltophilia* may be a problem in cystic fibrosis patients in some transplantation centers.[919,926]

Efficacy. Although much has been published about general infectious complications associated with lung transplantation, no randomized controlled trials regarding antimicrobial prophylaxis for lung or heart–lung transplantation have been published; however, antimicrobial prophylaxis is considered standard practice in these patients.[896] Antimicrobial prophylaxis is routinely administered to patients undergoing lung or heart–lung transplantation, with the aim of preventing pneumonia as well as SSIs. The rate of pneumonia within the first two weeks postoperatively has reportedly been decreased from 35% to approximately 10% by routine antimicrobial prophylaxis.[927–929] Improvements in surgical technique and postoperative patient care are also important factors in the apparently lower rates of pneumonia after lung transplantation.

Choice of agent. No formal studies have addressed optimal prophylaxis for patients undergoing lung transplantation. Antimicrobial prophylaxis for lung and heart–lung transplantation should generally be similar to that used for other cardiothoracic procedures (see the cardiac and thoracic sections). First- and second-generation cephalosporins are considered equally efficacious and are the preferred agents for these procedures. However, prophylactic regimens should be modified to include coverage for any potential bacterial pathogens, including gram-negative and fungal organisms, that have been isolated from the recipient's airways or the donor lung through preoperative cultures.[894,896,904,908,915,920] Patients with end-stage cystic fibrosis should receive antimicrobials on the basis of the known susceptibilities of pretransplant isolates, particularly *P. aeruginosa*, *B. cepacia* complex, and *Aspergillus* species.

Antimicrobial prophylaxis regimens reported in cohort evaluations of thoracic transplantation, including lungs, have varied.[904,908,920] One study used ceftazidime, floxacillin, tobramycin, and itraconazole in these patients.[908] In addition, all patients received nebulized amphotericin B and oral itraconazole as antifungal prophylaxis. Another cohort study used cefepime for lung transplant recipients without known colonization; for those with known colonization, the selection of agents was based on organism susceptibility.[920] A third cohort reported use of metronidazole and aztreonam as prophylaxis for patients with a septic lung (positive sputum culture).[904]

Antifungal prophylaxis should be considered, especially when pretransplantation cultures reveal fungi in the donor lung[915] or the recipient's airway. There is no consensus on the appropriate antifungal agent for lung transplant recipients.[894,896,930] Selection is recommended based on patient risk factors for infection (e.g., cystic fibrosis) and colonization, pretransplantation and posttransplantation cultures, and local fungus epidemiology.[894,896,897,930] Because of the serious nature of fungal infections in the early posttransplantation period and the availability of antifungal agents, prophylaxis should be considered when *Candida* or *Aspergillus* species are isolated from the donor lung[915] or recipient's airway.

Duration. No well-conducted studies have addressed the optimal duration of antimicrobial prophylaxis for lung or heart–lung transplantation. In the absence of positive cultures from the donor or the recipient, prophylactic regimens of 48–72 hours and no longer than 7 days have been reported.[896,904,905,931] In patients with positive pretransplantation cultures from donor or recipient organs or patients with positive cultures after transplantation, postoperative antimicrobial treatment for 7–14 days or longer has been reported, particularly for patients with cystic fibrosis and previous *P. aeruginosa* and multidrug-resistant infections.[896,915,919] Such antimicrobial administration is viewed as treatment and not as surgical prophylaxis. Treatment may include additional antibacterial agents or antifungal agents.

Recommendations. Based on data from other types of cardiothoracic procedures, all adult patients undergoing lung transplantation should receive antimicrobial prophylaxis, because of the high risk of infection. Patients with negative pretransplantation cultures should receive antimicrobial prophylaxis as appropriate for other types of cardiothoracic procedures.

The recommended regimen is a single dose of cefazolin (Table 2). There is no evidence to support continuing prophylaxis until chest and mediastinal drainage tubes are removed. Alternatives include vancomycin with or without gentamicin, aztreonam, and a single fluoroquinolone dose. (Strength of evidence for prophylaxis = A.) The optimal duration of antimicrobial prophylaxis for patients who do not have their chest primarily closed is unclear. No recommendation is made for these patients.

The prophylactic regimen should be modified to provide coverage against any potential pathogens, including gram-negative (e.g., *P. aeruginosa*) and fungal organisms, isolated from the donor lung or the recipient pretransplantation. The prophylactic regimen may also include antifungal agents for *Candida* and *Aspergillus* species based on patient risk factors for infection (e.g., cystic fibrosis) and colonization, pretransplantation and posttransplantation cultures, and local fungus epidemiology. Patients undergoing lung transplantation for cystic fibrosis should receive treatment for at least seven days with antimicrobials selected according to pretransplantation culture and susceptibility results. (Strength of evidence for prophylaxis = B.)

Liver Transplantation

Background. Liver transplantation is a lifesaving procedure for many patients with end-stage hepatic disease for whom there are no other medical or surgical options.[932,933] In 2007, UNOS reported that 6494 liver transplantations were performed in the United States, 96% of which had a cadaveric donor and 4% had a living-related donor source.[934] These liver transplantations were performed in 5889 adults and 605 pediatric (<18 years old) patients. Reported 1-year patient survival rates for adults ranged from 76.9% to 95%[932,935–938] and from 80% to 91.7% for pediatric patients.[934,939–942] Survival at 3 and 5 years ranged from 68.5% to 80.9%[934] and from 61.6% to 76.5%[932,933] in adult patients, respectively. In pediatric patients, 3- and 5-year survival ranged from 73.2% to 86%[897,934,941] and from 69.2% to 80.1%,[934] respectively. One-year graft survival rates ranged from 74.2% to 94% in adults[934–936,938] and from 72.1% to 86.1% in pediatric patients.[934,941,942] Graft survival at 3 and 5 years ranged from 58.9% to 75.5% and from 51.6% to 70.5%, respectively, in adults and from 62.5% to 77.6% and from 68.4% to 71.4%, respectively, in pediatric patients.[934,941] No significant differences were noted in graft or patient survival between cadaveric and living-related donors in adult and pediatric liver transplant recipients.[934] Infection remains a major cause of morbidity and mortality in liver transplant recipients. Infections may occur in 31–83% of patients within three months of transplantation and are the cause of death in 4–53% of patients.[934,936,940,943–950] These rates are highly variable and do not seem to have changed despite advances in surgical technique and medical management. SSIs within 30 days after transplantation ranged from 4% to 48% with antimicrobial prophylaxis in several cohort and controlled studies.[935–938,941,942,948,949,951–964] Superficial SSIs are seen most often within the first two to three weeks postoperatively, whereas organ/space infections and deep infections are seen after three to four weeks.

Liver transplantation is often considered to be the most technically difficult of the solid-organ transplantation procedures. Surgical procedures lasting longer than 8–12 hours have been consistently identified as one of the most important risk factors for early infectious complications, including SSIs, intraabdominal infections, and biliary tract infections.[896,938,939,945,947,957] Other important risk factors for infectious complications related to liver transplantation surgery include previous hepatobiliary surgery,[896,939,945,947,952,963] previous liver or kidney transplantation,[937,951,952,965] and surgical complications such as anastomotic leakage.[896,938,939,945,947,951,952] Patient-related risk factors for infection after liver transplantation include antimicrobial use within three to four months before transplantation,[935,954] low pretransplantation serum albumin concentration,[938,958,963] high pretransplantation serum bilirubin concentration,[939,945,947] ascites,[938] obesity,[963] diabetes, and hemochromatosis.[966] Procedure-related risk factors for infection include transfusion of >4 units of red blood cells,[896,951] bacterial contamination due to entry into the gastrointestinal tract,[963] surgical incision method,[963] and use of muromonab-CD3 within the first week after transplantation.[938]

Organisms. The pathogens most commonly associated with early SSIs and intraabdominal infections are those derived from the normal flora of the intestinal lumen and the skin. Aerobic gram-negative bacilli, including *E. coli*,[935,937,939,940,942,945,947–949,951,967,968] *Klebsiella* species,[933,936,937,939,940,945,947–949,967–969] *Enterobacter* species,[936,939,940,942,945,947,952,959,964,967,968] *Acinetobacter baumannii*,[935–937,942,951] and *Citrobacter* species,[939,940,945,947,952,959,967,968] are common causes of SSIs and intraabdominal infections and account for up to 65% of all bacterial pathogens. Infections due to *P. aeruginosa* may also occur but are much less common in the early postoperative period.[936,937,939,940,942,945,947,948,952,959,969] Enterococci are particularly common pathogens and may be responsible for 20–46% of SSIs and intraabdominal infections.[894,933,935,937,938,940,943,945–947,951,952,955,964,965,969] *S. aureus* (frequently MRSA) and coagulase-negative staphylococci are also common causes of postoperative SSIs.[936–938,940,942,943,945–949,955,957–961,964,965,970,971] *Candida* species commonly cause both early and late postoperative infections.[933,936,937,940,942,943,945–947,949,951,969]

Several studies have noted increasing concern about antimicrobial resistance based on detection of resistant organisms, including *E. coli*,[935,937] *Enterococcus* species,[933,937,964,965] *Enterobacter* species,[964] *Klebsiella* species,[933,937] coagulase-negative staphylococci,[937,964] and *S. aureus*.[937,948,957–961,970] General information on antimicrobial resistance is provided in the Common Principles section of these guidelines. Of specific concern to the transplantation community is the emergence of multidrug-resistant *A. baumannii*,[972] carbapenem-resistant Enterobacteriaceae,[973,974] *K. pneumoniae* carbapenemase-producing organisms,[975] and *C. difficile*.[976–978]

Efficacy. Although there remains a high rate of infection directly related to the liver transplantation procedure, there are few well-controlled studies concerning optimal antimicrobial prophylaxis. In evaluating the efficacy of prophylactic regimens, it is important to differentiate between early infections (occurring within 14–30 days after surgery) and late infections (occurring more than 30 days after surgery). Infections occurring in the early postoperative period are most commonly associated with biliary, vascular, and abdominal surgeries involved in the transplantation procedure itself and are thus most preventable with prophylactic antimicrobial regimens.[939,940,943,945] The frequency of these infections varies from 10% to 55% despite antimicrobial prophylaxis.[939,940,943,945,979] It is difficult to assess the efficacy of prophylactic regimens in reducing the rate of infection, because prophylaxis has been routinely used in light of the complexity of the surgical procedure; therefore, reliable rates of infection in the absence of prophylaxis are not available. No controlled studies have compared prophylaxis with no prophylaxis.

Choice of agent. Antimicrobial prophylaxis should be directed against the pathogens most commonly isolated from early infections (i.e., gram-negative aerobic bacilli, staphylococci, and enterococci). Traditional prophylactic regimens have therefore consisted of a third-generation cephalosporin (usually cefotaxime, because of its antistaphylococcal activity) plus ampicillin.[936,937,943,944,946–948,951,952,954,962,965,967,979] The use of cefoxitin and ampicillin–sulbactam, cefotaxime and ampicillin–sulbactam and gentamicin,[957–959] cefuroxime and metronidazole,[971] ceftriaxone and metronidazole,[980] cefotaxime and metronidazole,[953] ceftriaxone and ampicillin,[949] ceftizoxime alone,[955] cefotaxime and tobramycin,[956] cefoxitin alone,[960,961] cefazolin alone,[951] amoxicillin–clavulanate and gentamicin,[970] amoxicillin–clavulanate alone,[951] glycopeptides and antipseudomonal penicillin,[951] quinolone and amoxicillin–clavulanate or glycopeptide,[951] vancomycin and aztreonam,[951,981] and piperacillin–tazobactam[964,970] has also been reported. Alternative prophylaxis regimens for β-lactam-allergic patients have included cefuroxime and metronidazole,[970] clindamycin and gentamicin or aztreonam,[948,960–962] ciprofloxacin and metronidazole,[970] and vancomycin or ciprofloxacin.[936] Imipenem alone was used in one study for patients with renal failure.[956] The efficacy of these regimens compared with cefotaxime plus ampicillin is difficult to assess due to different definitions of infection used in the available studies and variability of study design (many single-center cohort studies) in different countries. One prospective nonrandomized study found no difference in the frequency of SSIs in orthotopic liver transplant recipients with cefazolin alone and amoxicillin–clavulanate alone, both given one hour before surgical incision, with a second dose given in cases of significant bleeding or surgery lasting over six hours, as antimicrobial prophylaxis.[935] The study did find a significantly higher rate of *A. baumannii* in the cefazolin group than the amoxicillin–clavulanate group. The routine use of vancomycin as antimicrobial prophylaxis is not recommended because of the risk of developing vancomycin-resistant organisms,[8,950] but vancomycin may be reserved for centers with an MRSA or MRSE cluster.[8,950,957–959] No randomized controlled studies have been conducted to compare the efficacy of other antimicrobial prophylactic regimens in the prevention of early postoperative infections. For patients known to be colonized with MRSA, VRE, or resistant gram-negative pathogens, it is reasonable to consider prophylaxis specifically targeted at these organisms. See the Common Principles section for further discussion.

Postoperative infections with *Candida* species after liver transplantation are common, particularly in the abdomen, and are frequently considered organ/space SSIs. For this reason, the use of antifungal prophylaxis in the perioperative period has become common. Efficacy has been demonstrated for fluconazole,[964–984] lipid complex amphotericin B,[985–987] and caspofungin.[988] Finally, one meta-analysis found a decreased risk of fungal infection and death associated with fungal infection, though not overall mortality, among patients given antifungal prophylaxis.[989] Universal antifungal prophylaxis is probably not necessary, since the risk of invasive candidiasis is low in uncomplicated cases. Instead, prophylaxis is generally reserved for patients with two or more of the following risk factors: need for reoperation, retransplantation, renal failure, choledochojejunostomy, and known colonization with *Candida* species.[15] Risk is also increased with prolonged initial procedure or transfusion of >40 units of cellular blood products, but this cannot be predicted before the procedure.

Selective bowel decontamination to eliminate aerobic gram-negative bacilli and yeast from the bowel before the transplantation procedure has been evaluated in several studies and a meta-analysis.[936,943,949,955,956,967,968,980,990,991] These studies used combinations of nonabsorbable antibacterials (aminoglycosides, polymyxin B or E), antifungals (nystatin, amphotericin B), and other antimicrobials (cefuroxime in suspension) administered orally and applied to the oropharyngeal cavity in combination with systemically administered antimicrobials. Results are conflicting, with no differences in patient outcomes (e.g., infection rates, mortality) or cost and concerns of increasing gram-positive infections with potential resistance in several studies[939,955,956,980,991] and others with positive results.[936,949] Two randomized controlled studies found significantly fewer bacterial infections with early enteral nutrition plus lactobacillus and fibers.[971,980] Based on currently available data, the routine use of selective bowel decontamination or lactic acid bacteria and fibers in patients undergoing liver transplantation is not recommended.

Duration. No studies have assessed the optimal duration of antimicrobial prophylaxis in liver transplantation. Although antimicrobials have been administered in studies for five days[937,944,946,949,957–959] and seven days,[964] the majority of recent studies have limited the duration of prophylaxis to 72 hours,[981] 48 hours,[936,943,945,952,955,956,960,961,967,970,979,980,991] 36 hours,[981] 24 hours,[935,948,962,970] and a single dose,[963] with no apparent differences in early infection rates. A prospective, nonrandomized, controlled study found no difference in bacterial infections within the first three months after liver transplantation in patients receiving cefotaxime and ampicillin as short-term antimicrobial prophylaxis for two to three days, compared with long-term prophylaxis for five to seven days.[954] Of note, 5 of the 11 patients in the long-term prophylaxis group had detectable *C. difficile* toxin B in the feces and developed enteritis. No patients in the short-term group had detectable *C. difficile*. Two recent review articles noted that antimicrobial prophylaxis duration should be less than three days.[896,950]

Pediatric Efficacy. There are few data specifically concerning antimicrobial prophylaxis in liver transplantation in pediatric patients. The combination of cefotaxime plus ampicillin has been reportedly used in children undergoing living-related donor liver transplantation; the efficacy of this regimen appeared to be favorable.[946] A small, retrospective, single-center cohort study reported outcomes of children undergoing liver, heart, small bowel, or lung transplantation receiving piperacillin–tazobactam 120–150 mg/kg/day beginning before surgical incision and continuing for 48 hours postoperatively and found favorable results, with a superficial SSI rate of 8% and no deep SSIs.[992]

Recommendations. The recommended agents for patients undergoing liver transplantation are (1) piperacillin–tazobactam and (2) cefotaxime plus ampicillin (Table 2). (Strength of evidence for prophylaxis = B.) For patients who are allergic to β-lactam antimicrobials, clindamycin or vancomycin given in combination with gentamicin, aztreonam, or a fluoroquinolone is a reasonable alternative. The duration of prophylaxis should be restricted to 24 hours or less.

For patients at high risk of *Candida* infection, fluconazole adjusted for renal function may be considered. (Strength of evidence for prophylaxis = B.)

Pancreas and Pancreas–Kidney Transplantation

Background. Pancreas transplantation is an accepted therapeutic intervention for type 1 diabetes mellitus; it is the only therapy that consistently achieves euglycemia without dependence on exogenous insulin.[993–997] Simultaneous pancreas–kidney (SPK) transplantation is an accepted procedure for patients with type 1 diabetes and severe diabetic nephropathy. In 2007, UNOS reported that 469 pancreas transplantations and 862 SPK transplantations were performed in the United States, of which 60 and 4 patients, respectively, were under age 18 years.[998] Pancreas graft 1-year survival rates ranged from 70.2% to 89%, and the 3-year rates ranged from 48% to 85.8%.[998–1002] Patient survival with pancreas transplantation has been reported between 75% and 97% at 1 year and between 54% and 92.5% at 3 years.[998] Allograft survival is higher in recipients of SPK transplantations, with allograft survival rates of 86.1–95.1% at 1 year and 54.2–92.5% at 3 years. Reported patient survival rates in SPK are 91.7–97.6% at 1 year and 84.4–94.1% at 3 years. During pancreas transplantation, surgical complications with portal-hepatic drainage significantly decreased the 1-year and 3-year survival rates to 48% and 44%, respectively, in one cohort study.[999]

Infectious complications are a major source of morbidity and mortality in patients undergoing pancreas or SPK transplantation; the frequency of SSI is 7–50% with antimicrobial prophylaxis.[993–997,1000–1009] The majority of SSIs occurred within the first 30 days to three months after transplantation.[1000–1002,1005,1008,1009] UTIs are also a significant concern during the same time frame, with rates ranging from 10.6% to 49% in pancreas transplant recipients who received antimicrobial prophylaxis, and are much more common in recipients with bladder drainage compared with enteric drainage.[1000–1008]

Pancreas and SPK transplantation patients may be at increased risk of SSIs and other infections because of the combined immunosuppressive effects of diabetes mellitus and the immunosuppressive drugs used to prevent graft rejection.[995,1000] Other factors associated with increased SSI rates include prolonged operating and ischemic times (>4 hours), organ donor age of >55 years, and enteric rather than bladder drainage of pancreatic duct secretions.[895,995,1000] Prolonged organ preservation time (>20 hours) was shown to increase the risk of complications, including duodenal leaks and decreased graft survival in cadaveric pancreas transplant recipients.[1003] Risk factors for UTI are reviewed in the kidney transplant section.

Organisms. A majority of superficial SSIs after pancreas or SPK transplantation are caused by *Staphylococcus* species (both coagulase-positive and coagulase-negative) and gram-negative bacilli (particularly *E. coli* and *Klebsiella* species).[993–997,1000–1002,1004–1006,1009–1011] Deep SSIs also are frequently associated with gram-positive (*Enterococcus* species, *Streptococcus* species, and *Peptostreptococcus* species) and gram-negative organisms (*Enterobacter* species, *Morganella* species, and *B. fragilis*), as well as *Candida* species.[993–997,1000–1002,1004–1006,1009–1011] Although anaerobes are occasionally isolated, the necessity for specific treatment of anaerobes in SSIs after pancreas transplantation remains unclear.

Efficacy. Although no placebo-controlled studies have been conducted, several open-label, noncomparative, single-center studies have suggested that antimicrobial prophylaxis substantially decreases the rate of superficial and deep SSIs after pancreas or SPK transplantation. SSI rates were 7–33% with various prophylactic regimens,[995,1000–1002,1004,1005] compared with 7–50% for historical controls in the absence of prophylaxis.[1009,1010] The reason for the wide disparity in infection rates observed with prophylaxis is not readily apparent but may include variations in SSI definitions, variations in antimicrobial prophylaxis, immunosuppression protocols, and variations in surgical techniques.[999–1002,1005,1007,1008]

Choice of agent. Because of the broad range of potential pathogens, several studies have used multidrug prophylactic regimens, including imipenem–cilastatin plus vancomycin[995]; tobramycin, vancomycin, and fluconazole[1010]; cefotaxime, metronidazole, and vancomycin[1012]; cefotaxime, vancomycin, and fluconazole[1008]; ampicillin and cefotaxime[1007]; and piperacillin–tazobactam and fluconazole.[1006]

HICPAC recommendations for SSI prevention include limiting the use of vancomycin unless there is an MRSA or MRSE cluster or as an alternative for β-lactam-allergic patients, though transplantation procedures were not specifically covered in the guidelines.[8] Limited data are available on the use of vancomycin as antimicrobial prophylaxis in kidney or pancreas transplantation, or both. A small, randomized, active-controlled, single-center study evaluated the impact of vancomycin-containing antimicrobial prophylaxis regimens in kidney and pancreas (alone or SPK) transplant recipients on the frequency of gram-positive infections.[1004] Renal transplantation patients received either vancomycin and ceftriaxone or cefazolin, and pancreas transplantation patients received either vancomycin and gentamicin or cefazolin and gentamicin. There was no statistically significant difference in the risk of developing gram-positive infections between antimicrobial prophylaxis regimens with and without vancomycin. The study was not powered to detect a difference in efficacy between the antimicrobial regimens. For patients known to be colonized with MRSA, VRE, or resistant gram-negative pathogens, it is reasonable to consider prophylaxis targeted specifically for these organisms. See the Common Principles section for further discussion.

An evaluation of the surgical complications of pancreas transplant recipients with portal-enteric drainage found an intraabdominal infection rate of 12% in the 65 patients undergoing SPK transplantation and no cases in those undergoing pancreas transplantation alone.[999] All patients received either cefazolin 1 g i.v. every eight hours for one to three days, or vancomycin if the patient had a β-lactam allergy.

One study evaluated SSI rates in SPK transplantation after single-agent, single-dose prophylaxis with cefazolin 1 g i.v. to donors and recipients, as well as cefazolin 1-g/L bladder and intraabdominal irrigation in the recipient.[1009] Superficial SSIs developed in 2 patients (5%), and deep SSIs associated with bladder anastomotic leaks or transplant pancreatitis occurred in 4 additional patients (11%). This study reported similar SSI rates as with multidrug, multidose regimens.

Based on the regularity of isolation of *Candida* species from SSIs after pancreas transplantation and the frequent colonization of the duodenum with yeast, fluconazole is commonly added to prophylactic regimens. Although never studied in a randomized trial, a lower fungal infection rate was found in one large case series with the use of fluconazole (6%) compared with no prophylaxis (10%).[1013] Although enteric drainage of the pancreas has been identified as a risk factor for postoperative fungal infections, many institutions use fluconazole for prophylaxis with bladder-drained organs as well. In settings with a high prevalence of non-*albicans Candida* species, a lipid-based formulation of amphotericin B has been recommended in infectious diseases guidelines from the American Society of Transplantation and the American Society of Transplant Surgeons.[15]

Duration. Studies evaluating the use of antimicrobial prophylaxis regimens in pancreas and SPK transplantation, summarized above, ranged from a single preoperative dose of cefazolin to multidrug regimens of 2–5 days' duration.[995,1005,1009,1010,1012] More recent studies reported monotherapy regimens with cefazolin or vancomycin,[999] amoxicillin–clavulanate,[1001,1002] and piperacillin–tazobactam[1000–1002] 1–7 days in duration, with the majority using the regimen 48–72 hours after transplantation. The duration of fluconazole ranged from 7 to 28 days.[1002]

Recommendations. The recommended regimen for patients undergoing pancreas or SPK transplantation is cefazolin (Table 2). (Strength of evidence for prophylaxis = A.) For patients who are allergic to β-lactam antimicrobials, clindamycin or vancomycin given in combination with gentamicin, aztreonam, or a fluoroquinolone is a reasonable alternative. The duration of prophylaxis should be restricted to 24 hours or less. The use of aminoglycosides in combination with other nephrotoxic drugs may result in renal dysfunction and should be avoided unless alternatives are contraindicated. (Strength of evidence for prophylaxis = C.) For patients at high risk of *Candida* infection, fluconazole adjusted for renal function may be considered.

Kidney Transplantation

Background. In 2007, UNOS reported that 16,628 kidney transplantations were performed in the United States; of these, 796 patients were younger than 18 years.[998] The rate of postoperative infection after this procedure has been reported to range from 10% to 56%, with the two most common infections being UTIs and SSIs.[1004,1014–1024] Graft loss due to infection occurs in up to 33% of cases.[1017,1023] One study of adult and pediatric kidney transplant recipients (both living-related and cadaveric donor sources) found patient survival rates at 7 years after transplantation of 88.9% and 75.5%, respectively, and graft survival of 75% and 55.5%, respectively.[1025] No patients developed an SSI. Mortality associated with postoperative infections is substantial and ranges from approximately 5% to 30%.[1015,1017,1019,1022,1026,1027]

The frequency of SSIs in kidney transplant recipients has ranged from 0% to 11% with antimicrobial prophylaxis[1023–1025,1028,1029] to 2% to 7.5% without systemic prophylaxis.[1030,1031] The majority of these infections were superficial in nature and were detected within 30 days after transplantation.[1023,1028–1030] Risk factors for SSI after kidney transplantation include contamination of organ perfusate[1027]; pretransplantation patient-specific factors, such as diabetes,[1029,1030] chronic glomerulonephritis,[1030] and obesity[1027,1030,1032]; procedure-related factors, such as ureteral leakage and hematoma formation[1027]; immunosuppressive therapy[1024,1027,1029]; and postoperative complications, such as acute graft rejection, reoperation, and delayed graft function.[1030] In one study, the frequency of SSI was 12% in patients receiving immunosuppression with azathioprine plus prednisone but only 1.7% in patients receiving cyclosporine plus prednisone.[1033] A significant difference in SSI rates was noted after kidney transplantation between immunosuppression regimens including mycophenolate mofetil (45 [3.9%] of 1150 patients) versus sirolimus (11 [7.4%] of 144 patients).[1029] Sirolimus-containing immunosuppression was found to be an independent risk factor for SSIs. These recommendations refer to kidney transplant recipients; recommendations for living kidney donors can be found in the discussion of nephrectomy in the urologic section.

Organisms. Postoperative SSIs in kidney transplant recipients are caused by gram-positive organisms, particularly *Staphylococcus* species (including *S. aureus* and *S. epidermidis*) and *Enterococcus* species, gram-negative organisms, *E. coli*, *Enterobacter* species, *Klebsiella* species, *P. aeruginosa*, and yeast with *Candida* species.[1004,1014–1021,1023,1024,1026,1028,1030,1034] One study site in Brazil reported a high level of antimicrobial resistance.[1030] Organisms recovered from infections included MRSA (77%), methicillin-resistant coagulase-negative *Staphylococcus* (53.5%), extended-spectrum β-lactamase-producing *K. pneumoniae* (80%), and carbapenem-resistant *P. aeruginosa* (33.3%). Another center in Brazil reported a significant difference in resistance to broad-spectrum antimicrobials in pathogens isolated in UTIs from cadaveric kidney transplant recipients (n = 21, 19.1%) compared with living-related donor kidney transplant recipients (n = 2, 3.7%) (p = 0.008).[1024] One center in the United States reported 94% susceptibility to vancomycin of *Enterococcus* species within the first month after transplantation, while *E. coli*, cultured most commonly more than six months after transplantation, was 63% resistant to sulfamethoxazole–trimethoprim.[1023] This resistance may be related to the routine use of sulfamethoxazole–trimethoprim in prophylaxis of *Pneumocystis carinii* pneumonia and UTI.

Efficacy. A number of studies have clearly demonstrated that antimicrobial prophylaxis significantly decreases postoperative infection rates in patients undergoing kidney transplantation. These have included at least one randomized controlled trial[1014] and many prospective and retrospective studies comparing infection rates with prophylaxis and historical infection rates at specific transplantation centers.[1015–1018,1021,1033–1035] Based on the available literature, the routine use of systemic antimicrobial prophylaxis is justified in patients undergoing kidney transplantation.

Two studies that evaluated a triple-drug regimen consisting of an aminoglycoside, an antistaphylococcal penicillin, and ampicillin found infection rates of <2%, compared with 10–25% with no antimicrobial prophylaxis.[1018,1019] More specifically, infection rates in patients without antimicrobial prophylaxis (45 cadaveric and 44 living-related donors) were 10.1% in total (8.9% and 11.4%, respectively), compared with 1.5% in total (1.5% and 0%, respectively) with antimicrobial prophylaxis.[1018] Infection rates were as high as 33%

in living-related patients with no antimicrobial prophylaxis and 0–1% in both cadaveric and living-related transplant recipients with antimicrobial prophylaxis.[1021] Piperacillin plus cefuroxime was also shown to be efficacious; infection rates were 3.7%, compared with 19% in cadaveric transplant recipients not receiving prophylaxis.[1018] Several studies have shown that single-agent prophylaxis with an antistaphylococcal penicillin,[1029,1034] a first-generation cephalosporin,[1016,1017,1023,1024,1029] a second-generation cephalosporin,[1028,1035,1036] or a third-generation cephalosporin (e.g., cefoperazone, cefotaxime, ceftriaxone)[1024,1029,1033,1037] can reduce postoperative infection rates to 0–8.4%. All studies included cadaveric transplant recipients, whereas living-related transplant recipients were also included in select studies.[1017,1024,1028,1036] Where compared directly, infection rates between cadaveric and living-related transplant recipients receiving antimicrobial prophylaxis were not statistically different.[1024]

Choice of agent. The available data do not indicate a significant difference between single-drug and multidrug antimicrobial regimens.[1014,1018,1021] In addition, there appears to be no significant differences between single-agent regimens employing antistaphylococcal penicillins and first-, second-, or third-generation cephalosporins.[1016,1017,1033–1035,1037] Studies have directly compared antimicrobial regimens in a prospective, controlled fashion. Single-agent prophylaxis with both cefazolin and ceftriaxone has been reported to result in SSI rates of 0%.[1016,1024,1037]

A survey of 101 kidney transplant centers in 39 countries reported that 65% of the centers used single antimicrobial prophylaxis regimens, 20.8% used two-drug regimens, and 3% used three drugs; no prophylaxis was used in 11% of centers.[1036] Cephalosporins were used in 68 centers (55 alone, 7 in combination with penicillin, and 6 with other antimicrobials). Penicillins were used by 28 centers (13 alone, 7 with cephalosporin, and 8 with other antimicrobials). Other antimicrobials (specifics were not reported) were used in 2 centers as the single agent.

As noted above, HICPAC recommendations for SSI prevention include limiting the use of vancomycin to situations in which there is an MRSA or MRSE cluster or as an alternative for β-lactam-allergic patients.[8] Transplantation procedures were not specifically covered in the guidelines.

Duration. Studies have used various prophylactic regimens, ranging from a single-drug cephalosporin regimen, administered as a single preoperative dose or for up to 24 hours postoperatively, to multidrug regimens of two to five days' duration.[981,1004,1014–1018,1021,1023,1024,1028,1029,1033,1036,1038] Cefazolin for 24 hours was equivalent to seven days of surgical prophylaxis in living-related kidney transplant donors.[1039] There appear to be no significant differences in SSI rates between single-dose, 24-hour, and multidose regimens; therefore, the duration of antimicrobial should be restricted to 24 hours.

Pediatric Efficacy. Although pediatric patients were included in studies demonstrating the efficacy of antimicrobial prophylaxis, there are few data specific to pediatric patients.

One cohort of 96 pediatric patients who underwent 104 renal transplants (63% cadaveric and 37% living-related donors) ranged in age from six months to 18 years (mean age, 8.2 ± 5.5 years).[1040] Antimicrobial prophylaxis included one dose of cefotaxime 30-mg/kg i.v. bolus at the start of the procedure and cefotaxime 90 mg/kg/day in three divided doses during the intensive care unit stay, which averaged one to two days. No SSIs were reported.

Recommendations. The recommended agent for patients undergoing kidney transplantation is cefazolin (Table 2). (Strength of evidence for prophylaxis = A.) For patients who are allergic to β-lactam antimicrobials, clindamycin or vancomycin given in combination with gentamicin, aztreonam, or a fluoroquinolone is a reasonable alternative. The duration of prophylaxis should be restricted to 24 hours or less. The use of aminoglycosides in combination with other nephrotoxic drugs may result in renal dysfunction and should be avoided unless alternatives are contraindicated. (Strength of evidence for prophylaxis = C.) For patients at high risk of *Candida* infection, fluconazole adjusted for renal function may be considered.

Plastic Surgery and Breast Procedures

Background. Plastic surgery encompasses a broad range of procedures focused on reconstructive, dermatological, and cosmetic procedures.[1041] The primary goal of these procedures is to restore function to the affected area, with a secondary goal of improving appearance. The scope of procedures ranges from simple primary surgical-site closure, skin grafts, and skin flaps to composite tissue transplantations. Composite tissue transplantation for tissue reconstruction of the knee joint, larynx, uterus, abdominal wall, hand, face, and penis has been performed in a small number of patients.[1042,1043]

Most dermatological, breast (reduction and reconstructive), clean head and neck, and facial procedures have an associated SSI rate of <5%.[1044–1053] Oral procedures, such as wedge excision of lip or ear, flaps on the nose,[1046,1054] and head and neck flaps, have SSI rates of approximately 5–10%.[1053,1055–1060] In addition to general risk factors as described in the Common Principles section, factors that increase the risk of postoperative infectious complications for plastic surgery procedures include implants,[1061] skin irradiation before the procedure, and procedures below the waist.[1062,1063]

Organisms. The most common organisms in SSIs after plastic surgery procedures are *S. aureus*,[1045,1049,1050,1053,1054,1056,1063–1068] other staphylococci, and streptococci.[1045,1054,1064,1066,1067] Procedures involving macerated, moist environments (e.g., under a panus or axilla of an obese individual), below the waist, or in patients with diabetes are associated with a higher rate of infection with gram-negative organisms such as *P. aeruginosa*,[1068] *Serratia marcescens*, or Enterobacteriaceae, including *E. coli*,[1065,1068] *Klebsiella* species,[1068] and *P. mirabilis*.[1065]

Efficacy. The efficacy of antimicrobial prophylaxis in select plastic surgery procedures has been investigated in several clinical trials and cohort studies.

Most placebo-controlled and retrospective studies for many clean plastic surgery procedures have found that antimicrobial prophylaxis does not significantly decrease the risk of infection. These studies have evaluated head and neck procedures (facial bone fracture, tumor excision and reconstruction, radical neck dissection, rhinoplasty),[1049] flexor tendon injury repairs,[1051] augmentation mammoplasty using periareolar submuscular technique,[1052] carpal tunnel,[1069] and breast procedures (reduction mammoplasty, lumpectomy, mastectomy, axillary node dissection).[1056,1058,1070,1071]

However, a Cochrane review of seven randomized, placebo-controlled trials of 1984 patients undergoing breast cancer procedures (axillary lymph node dissection and primary nonreconstructive surgery) evaluated the effectiveness of preoperative or perioperative antimicrobial prophylaxis ($n = 995$) compared with placebo or no treatment ($n = 989$) in reducing the rate of postoperative infections.[1072] Pooled study results revealed a significant difference in SSI rates with antimicrobial prophylaxis (80 [8%] of 995), compared with 10.5% (104 of 989) for no antimicrobial prophylaxis (relative risk, 0.72; 95% CI, 0.53–0.97). Review authors concluded that antimicrobial prophylaxis is warranted to decrease the risk of SSIs in nonreconstructive breast cancer procedures.

Guidelines also support no antimicrobial prophylaxis in patients undergoing clean facial or nasal procedures without an implant.[7] For patients undergoing facial or nasal procedures with an implant, antimicrobial prophylaxis should be considered.[7]

A randomized, double-blind, controlled trial of 207 patients evaluated the use of three antimicrobial prophylaxis regimens in patients undergoing abdominoplasty procedures.[1066] The reported SSI rates were 13% for patients receiving no antimicrobial prophylaxis, 4.3% for those receiving preoperative antimicrobials only, and 8.7% for those receiving one preoperative dose and three days of postoperative antimicrobials. There was a significantly lower infection rate in the group receiving preoperative antimicrobials only compared with the placebo group ($p < 0.05$). The infection rate was slightly but not significantly higher in patients who received postoperative antimicrobials.

Choice of agent. There is no consensus on the appropriate antimicrobial agent to use for prophylaxis in plastic surgery procedures.[1055,1073] Agents with good gram-positive coverage and, depending on the site of surgery, activity against common gram-negative organisms are recommended for patients undergoing clean plastic surgery procedures with risk factors (listed in the Common Principles section and the background discussion of this section) or clean-contaminated procedures. Cefazolin or ampicillin–sulbactam is sufficient in most cases, with clindamycin and vancomycin as alternatives for patients with β-lactam allergy. There are no studies assessing the impact of MRSA on patients undergoing plastic surgery procedures or regarding the need to alter prophylaxis regimens in patients without known colonization with MRSA. When vancomycin or clindamycin is used and if a gram-negative organism is highly suspected, practitioners should consider adding cefazolin if the patient is not β-lactam allergic; if the patient is β-lactam allergic, the addition of aztreonam, gentamicin, or single-dose fluoroquinolone should be considered. If the surgical site involves the ear, an antipseudomonal fluoroquinolone may be considered to cover *Pseudomonas* species.[1045]

Although oral agents such as cephalexin, amoxicillin, clindamycin, and azithromycin have been recommended in reviews of antimicrobial prophylaxis in clean dermatological surgery, there is no evidence that supports their use.[13,1045,1046,1054]

Duration. Antimicrobial prophylaxis should be limited to the shortest duration possible to prevent SSIs (even if a drain or a catheter is left in place or an implant is inserted), limit adverse events, and prevent antimicrobial resistance.[8,512,1047,1048,1054,1056]

Multiple studies have found no significant differences in SSI rates after breast surgery with single-dose preoperative cephalosporin compared with extended-duration regimens that last from one to five days postoperatively.[1048,1054,1056]

A randomized, single-blind, controlled trial of 74 patients undergoing surgical ablation of head and neck malignancies with immediate free-flap reconstruction found no significant differences in SSI rate between clindamycin 900 mg i.v. every eight hours for 3 doses compared with 15 doses.[1057] Both groups were given clindamycin 900 mg i.v. immediately preoperatively, in addition to the postoperative regimens.

In a controlled study, 200 patients undergoing septorhinoplasty were randomized to a single preoperative dose of amoxicillin–clavulanate 2.2 g i.v. administered 30 minutes before surgical incision only ($n = 100$) or in combination with postoperative oral amoxicillin–clavulanate 1000 mg twice daily for seven days.[533] There was no significant difference in infection rates between the group receiving only a preoperative dose (0%) and the combination group (3%). There was a higher rate of adverse events (nausea, diarrhea, skin rash, and pruritus) among the combination group compared with the group receiving only a preoperative dose ($p = 0.03$). The study authors recommended the use of a single preoperative i.v. dose of amoxicillin–clavulanate for endonasal septorhinoplasty.

Pediatric Efficacy. Limited data on antimicrobial prophylaxis are available for pediatric patients undergoing plastic surgery procedures. There is no consensus among surgeons regarding the use of antimicrobial prophylaxis in the repair of cleft lip and palate.[1074] The occurrence of postoperative infections after these procedures is 1.3%.[1075] No controlled trials have evaluated the use of antimicrobial prophylaxis in these procedures.

Recommendations. Antimicrobial prophylaxis is not recommended for most clean procedures in patients without additional postoperative infection risk factors as listed in the Common Principles section of these guidelines and the background discussion of this section. Although no studies have demonstrated antimicrobial efficacy in these procedures, expert opinion recommends that patients with risk factors undergoing clean plastic procedures receive antimicrobial prophylaxis. The recommendation for clean-contaminated procedures, breast cancer procedures, and clean procedures with other risk factors is a single dose of cefazolin or ampicillin–sulbactam (Table 2). (Strength of evidence for prophylaxis = C.) Alternative agents for patients with β-lactam allergy include clindamycin and vancomycin. If there are surveillance data showing that gram-negative organisms cause SSIs for the procedure, the practitioner may consider combining clindamycin or vancomycin with another agent (cefazolin if the patient is not β-lactam allergic; aztreonam, gentamicin, or single-dose fluoroquinolone if the patient is β-lactam allergic). Postoperative duration of antimicrobial prophylaxis should be limited to less than 24 hours, regardless of the presence of indwelling catheters or drains.

References

1. American Society of Health-System Pharmacists. ASHP therapeutic guidelines on antimicrobial prophylaxis in surgery. *Am J Health-Syst Pharm.* 1999; 56:1839–88.
2. Dellinger EP, Gross PA, Barrett TL, et al. Quality standard for antimicrobial prophylaxis in surgical procedures. *Clin Infect Dis.* 1994; 18:422–7.
3. Page CP, Bohnen JM, Fletcher JR, et al. Antimicrobial prophylaxis for surgical wounds: guidelines for clinical care. *Arch Surg.* 1993; 128:79–88.
4. Dotson LR, Witmer DR. Development of ASHP therapeutic guidelines. *Am J Health-Syst Pharm.* 1995; 52:254–5.
5. Anderson DJ, Kaye KS, Classen D, et al. Strategies to prevent surgical site infections in acute care hospitals. *Infect Control Hosp Epidemiol.* 2008; 29(suppl 1):S51–61.
6. Antimicrobial prophylaxis for surgery. *Treat Guidel Med Lett.* 2009; 7:47–52.
7. Scottish Intercollegiate Guidelines Network. Antibiotic prophylaxis in surgery. www.sign.ac.uk/pdf/sign104.pdf (accessed 2009 Jul 30).
8. Mangram AJ, Horan TC, Pearson ML, et al. Guideline for prevention of surgical site infection. *Infect Control Hosp Epidemiol.* 1999; 20:250–78.
9. American College of Obstetricians and Gynecologists. Antibiotic prophylaxis for gynecologic procedures. ACOG practice bulletin no. 104. *Obstet Gynecol.* 2009; 113:1180–9.
10. AAP Comittee on Fetus and Newborn, ACOG Committee on Obstetric Practice, eds. Guidelines for perinatal care. 6th ed. Elk Grove Village, IL: American Academy of Pediatrics and American College of Obstetricians and Gynecologists; 2008.
11. Wilson W, Taubert KA, Gewitz M, et al. Prevention of infective endocarditis: guidelines from the American Heart Association: a guideline from the American Heart Association Rheumatic Fever, Endocarditis, and Kawasaki Disease Committee, Council on Cardiovascular Disease in the Young, and the Council on Clinical Cardiology, Council on Cardiovascular Surgery and Anesthesia, and the Quality of Care and Outcomes Research Interdisciplinary Working Group. *Circulation.* 2007; 116:1736–54.
12. Freiman JA, Chalmers TC, Smith H, et al. The importance of beta, the type II error and sample size in the design and interpretation of the randomized control trial. *N Engl J Med.* 1978; 299:690–4.
13. Edmiston CE, Krepel C, Kelly H, et al. Perioperative antibiotic prophylaxis in the gastric bypass patient: do we achieve therapeutic levels? *Surgery.* 2004; 136:738–47.
14. Claforan (cefotaxime sodium) for injection package insert. Bridgewater, NJ: Sanofi Aventis; 2009 Jul.
15. Pappas PG, Silveira FP. *Candida* in solid organ transplant recipients. *Am J Transplant.* 2009; 9(suppl 4):S173–9.
16. Zelenitsky SA, Silverman RE, Duckworth H, et al. A prospective, randomized, double-blind study of single high dose versus multiple standard dose gentamicin both in combination with metronidazole for colorectal surgical prophylaxis. *J Hosp Infect.* 2000; 46:135–40.
17. Zelenitsky SA, Ariano RE, Harding GK, et al. Antibiotic pharmacodynamics in surgical prophylaxis: an association between intraoperative antibiotic concentrations and efficacy. *Antimicrob Agents Chemother.* 2002; 46:3026–30.
18. Rybak MJ, Lomaestro BM, Rotschafer JC, et al. Vancomycin therapeutic guidelines: a summary of consensus recommendations from the Infectious Diseases Society of America, the American Society of Health-System Pharmacists, and the Society of Infectious Diseases Pharmacists. *Clin Infect Dis.* 2009; 49:325–7.
19. Alphonso N, Anagnostopoulos PV, Scarpace S, et al. Perioperative antibiotic prophylaxis in paediatric cardiac surgery. *Cardiol Young.* 2007; 17:12–25.
20. Maher KO, VanDerElzen K, Bove EL, et al. A retrospective review of three antibiotic prophylaxis regimens for pediatric cardiac surgical patients. *Ann Thorac Surg.* 2002; 74:1195–200.
21. Kato Y, Shime N, Hashimoto S, et al. Effects of controlled perioperative antimicrobial prophylaxis on infectious outcomes in pediatric cardiac surgery. *Crit Care Med.* 2007; 35:1763–8.
22. Haessler D, Reverdy ME, Neidecker J, et al. Antibiotic prophylaxis with cefazolin and gentamicin in cardiac surgery for children less than ten kilograms. *J Cardiothorac Vasc Anesth.* 2003; 17:221–5.
23. Vargas MR, Danton MH, Javaid SM, et al. Pharmacokinetics of intravenous flucloxacillin and amoxicillin in neonatal and infant cardiopulmonary bypass surgery. *Eur J Cardiothorac Surg.* 2004; 25:256–60.
24. Milstone AM, Budd A, Shepard JW, et al. Role of decolonization in a comprehensive strategy to reduce methicillin-resistant *Staphylococcus aureus* infections in the neonatal intensive care unit: an observational cohort study. *Infect Control Hosp Epidemiol.* 2010; 31:558–60.
25. Chua AN, Goldstein SL, Bell D, et al. Topical mupirocin/sodium hypochlorite reduces peritonitis and exit-site infection rates in children. *Clin J Am Soc Nephrol.* 2009; 4:1939–43.
26. Paglialonga F, Esposito S, Edefonti A, et al. Catheter-related infections in children treated with hemodialysis. *Pediatr Nephrol.* 2004; 19:1324–33.
27. Shiojima T, Ohki Y, Nako Y, et al. Immediate control of a methicillin-resistant *Staphylococcus aureus* outbreak in a neonatal intensive care unit. *J Infect Chemother.* 2003; 9:243–7.
28. Romance L, Nicolle L, Ross J, et al. An outbreak of methicillin-resistant *Staphylococcus aureus* in a pediatric hospital—how it got away and how we caught it. *Can J Infect Control.* 1991; 6:11–3.
29. Hayakawa T, Hayashidera T, Katsura S, et al. Nasal mupirocin treatment of pharynx-colonized methicillin resistant *Staphylococcus aureus*: preliminary study with 10 carrier infants. *Pediatr Int.* 2000; 42:67–70.
30. Liu CC, Hor LI, Wu YH, et al. Investigation and elimination of epidemic methicillin-resistant *Staphylococcus aureus* in a neonatal intensive care unit. *Min Kuo Hsiao Erh Ko I Hsueh Hui Tsa Chih.* (Chinese Medical Journal) 1993; 34:285–93.

31. Nateghian A, Taylor G, Robinson JL. Risk factors for surgical site infections following open-heart surgery in a Canadian pediatric population. *Am J Infect Control.* 2004; 32:397–401.
32. Bratzler DW, Houck PM, Richards C, et al. Use of antimicrobial prophylaxis for major surgery: baseline results from the National Surgical Infection Prevention Project. *Arch Surg.* 2005; 140:174–82.
33. National Healthcare Safety Network. Patient safety component manual: surgical site infection (SSI) event. www.cdc.gov/nhsn/PDFs/pscManual/9pscSSIcurrent.pdf (accessed 2011 Apr 5).
34. Horan TC, Gayness RP, Martone WJ, et al. CDC definitions of nosocomial surgical site infections, 1992: a modification of CDC definitions of surgical wound infections. *Infect Control Hosp Epidemiol.* 1992; 13:606–8.
35. National Healthcare Safety Network. Patient safety component manual: key terms. www.cdc.gov/nhsn/PDFs/pscManual/16pscKeyTerms_current.pdf (accessed 2012 Oct 23).
36. Horan TC, Andrus M, Dudeck MA. CDC/NHSN surveillance definition of health care-associated infection and criteria for specific types of infections in the acute care setting. *Am J Infect Control.* 2008; 36:309–32.
37. Ehrenkranz NJ, Pfaff SJ. Mediastinitis complicating cardiac operations: evidence of postoperative causation. *Rev Infect Dis.* 1991; 13:803–14.
38. Bowater RJ, Stirling SA, Lilford RJ. Is antibiotic prophylaxis in surgery a generally effective intervention? Testing a generic hypothesis over a set of meta-analyses. *Ann Surg.* 2009; 249:551–6.
39. Englesbe MJ, Dimick JB, Sonnenday CJ, et al. The Michigan Surgical Quality Collaborative: will a statewide quality improvement initiative pay for itself? *Ann Surg.* 2007; 246:1100–3.
40. Flum DR, Fisher N, Thompson J, et al. Washington state's approach to variability in surgical processes/outcomes: Surgical Clinical Outcomes Assessment Program (SCOAP). *Surgery.* 2005; 138:821–8.
41. Bratzler DW, Houck PM, for the Surgical Infection Prevention Guidelines Writers Workgroup. Antimicrobial prophylaxis for surgery: an advisory statement from the national surgical infection prevention project. *Clin Infect Dis.* 2004; 38:1706–15.
42. Fry DE. Surgical site infections and the Surgical Care Improvement Project (SCIP): evolution of national quality measures. *Surg Infect.* 2008; 9:579–84.
43. Watson DS. National patient safety goals and implementation. *AORN J.* 2009; 90:123–7.
44. Myles JL, Shamanski F, Witte D. The Physicians Quality Reporting Initiative: measure, development, implementation and current procedural terminology coding. *Adv Anat Pathol.* 2010; 17:49–52.
45. Callcut RA, Breslin TM. Shaping the future of surgery: the role of private regulation in determining quality standards. *Ann Surg.* 2006; 243:304–12.
46. Bratzler DW. The Surgical Infection Prevention and Surgical Care Improvement Projects: promises and pitfalls. *Am Surg.* 2006; 72:1010–6.
47. DePalma RG. Surgical quality programs in the Veterans Health Administration. *Am Surg.* 2006; 72:999–1004.
48. Gómez MI, Acosta-Gnass SI, Mosqueda-Barboza L, et al. Reduction in surgical antibiotic prophylaxis expenditure and the rate of surgical site infection by means of a protocol that controls the use of prophylaxis. *Infect Control Hosp Epidemiol.* 2006; 27:1358–65.
49. Bond CA, Raehl CL. Clinical and economic outcomes of pharmacist-managed antimicrobial prophylaxis in surgical patients. *Am J Health-Syst Pharm.* 2007; 64:1935–42.
50. Hermsen ED, Smith Shull S, Puumala SE, et al. Improvement in prescribing habits and economic outcomes associated with the introduction of a standardized approach for surgical antimicrobial prophylaxis. *Infect Control Hosp Epidemiol.* 2008; 29:457–61.
51. Alerany C, Campany D, Monterde J, et al. Impact of local guidelines and an integrated dispensing system on antibiotic prophylaxis quality in a surgical centre. *J Hosp Infect.* 2005; 60:111–7.
52. Allerberger F, Gareis R, Jindrák V, et al. Antibiotic stewardship implementation in the EU: the way forward. *Expert Rev Anti Infect Ther.* 2009; 7:1175–83.
53. Voit SB, Todd JK, Nelson B, et al. Electronic surveillance system for monitoring surgical antimicrobial prophylaxis. *Pediatrics.* 2005; 116:1317–22.
54. Kritchevsky SB, Braun BI, Bush AJ, et al. The effect of a quality improvement collaborative to improve antimicrobial prophylaxis in surgical patients: a randomized trial. *Ann Intern Med.* 2008; 149:472–80.
55. Potenza B, Deligencia M, Estigoy B, et al. Lessons learned from the institution of the Surgical Care Improvement Project at a teaching medical center. *Am J Surg.* 2009; 198:881–8.
56. Parker BM, Henderson JM, Vitagliano S, et al. Six sigma methodology can be used to improve adherence for antibiotic prophylaxis in patients undergoing noncardiac surgery. *Anesth Analg.* 2007; 104:140–6.
57. Rosenberg AD, Wambold D, Kraemer L, et al. Ensuring appropriate timing of antimicrobial prophylaxis. *J Bone Joint Surg Am.* 2008; 90:226–32.
58. Manniën J, Van Kasteren ME, Nagelkerke NJ, et al. Effect of optimized antibiotic prophylaxis on the incidence of surgical site infection. *Infect Control Hosp Epidemiol.* 2006; 27:1340–6.
59. Gorbach SL, Condon RE, Conte JE Jr, et al. Evaluation of new anti-infective drugs for surgical prophylaxis. *Clin Infect Dis.* 1992; 15(suppl 1):S313–38.
60. Källman J, Friberg Ö. Antibiotic prophylaxis in cardiac surgery—general principles. *APMIS.* 2007; 115:1012–5.
61. Hidron AI, Edwards JR, Patel J, et al., for the National Healthcare Safety Network Team and participating National Healthcare Safety Network facilities. Antimicrobial-resistant pathogens associated with healthcare-associated infections: annual summary of data reported to the National Healthcare Safety Network at the Centers for Disease Control and Prevention, 2006–2007. *Infect Control Hosp Epidemiol.* 2008; 29:996–1011.
62. Cefotetan package insert. Shaumburg, IL: Abraxis Pharmaceutical Products; 2007 Jul.

63. Cefazolin package insert. Shaumburg, IL: Abraxis Pharmaceutical Products; 2006 Jul.
64. Cefoxitin package insert. Shaumburg, IL: APP Pharmaceuticals, LLC; 2008 Feb.
65. Sterile vancomycin package insert. Shaumburg, IL: APP Pharmaceuticals, LLC; 2008 Apr.
66. Cefuroxime package insert. Shaumburg, IL: APP Pharmaceuticals; 2008 Nov.
67. Invanz (ertapenem injection) package insert. Whitehouse Station, NJ: Merck; 2010 Mar.
68. Gaynes R, Edwards JR. National Nosocomial Infections Surveillance System: overview of nosocomial infections caused by gram-negative bacilli. *Clin Infect Dis.* 2005; 41:848–54.
69. Weigelt JA, Lipsky BA, Tabak UP, et al. Surgical site infections: causative pathogens and associated outcomes. *Am J Infect Control.* 2010; 38:112–20.
70. Centers for Disease Control and Prevention. Recommendations for preventing the spread of vancomycin resistance. Recommendations of the Hospital Infection Control Practices Advisory Committee (HICPAC). www.cdc.gov/mmwr/PDF/RR/RR4412.PDF (accessed 2012 Dec 9).
71. Gould FK, Brindle R, Chadwick PR, et al. Guidelines (2008) for the prophylaxis and treatment of methicillin-resistant *Staphylococcus aureus* (MRSA) infections in the United Kingdom. *J Antimicrob Chemother.* 2009; 63:849–61.
72. Bolon MK, Morlote M, Weber SG, et al. Glycopeptides are no more effective than β-lactam agents for prevention of surgical site infection after cardiac surgery: a meta-analysis. *Clin Infect Dis.* 2004; 38:1357–63.
73. Finkelstein R, Rabino G, Mashiah T, et al. Vancomycin versus cefazolin prophylaxis for cardiac surgery in the setting of a high prevalence of methicillin-resistant staphylococcal infections. *J Thorac Cardiovasc Surg.* 2002; 123:326–32.
74. Bull AL, Worth LJ, Richards MJ. Impact of vancomycin surgical prophylaxis on the development of methicillin-sensitive *Staphylococcus aureus* surgical site infections: report from Australian surveillance data (VICNISS). *Ann Surg.* Epub ahead of print. 2012 Jul 20 (DOI 10.1097/SLA.0b013e31825fa398).
75. Gorwitz RJ, Kruszon-Moran D, McAllister SK, et al. Changes in the prevalence of nasal colonization with *Staphylococcus aureus* in the United States, 2001–2004. *J Infect Dis.* 2008; 197:1226–34.
76. Milstone AM, Carroll KC, Ross T, et al. Community-associated methicillin-resistant *Staphylococcus aureus* strains in pediatric intensive care unit. *Emerg Infect Dis.* 2010; 16:647–55.
77. Lo WT, Wang CC, Lin WJ, et al. Changes in the nasal colonization with methicillin-resistant *Staphylococcus aureus* in children: 2004–2009. *PLoS One.* 2010; 5:e15791.
78. Roberts NJ, Douglas RG. Gentamicin use and *Pseudomonas* and *Serratia* resistance: effect of a surgical prophylaxis regimen. *Antimicrob Agents Chemother.* 1978; 13:214–20.
79. Kriesel D, Savel TG, Silver AL, et al. Surgical antibiotic prophylaxis and *Clostridium difficile* toxin positivity. *Arch Surg.* 1995; 130:989–93.
80. Privitera G, Scarpellini P, Ortisi G, et al. Prospective study of *Clostridium difficile* intestinal colonization and disease following single-dose antibiotic prophylaxis surgery. *Antimicrob Agents Chemother.* 1991; 35:208–10.
81. Jobe BA, Grasley A, Deveney KE, et al. *Clostridium difficile* colitis: an increasing hospital-acquired illness. *Am J Surg.* 1995; 169:480–3.
82. Morris JG, Shay DK, Hebden JN. Enterococci resistant to multiple antimicrobial agents, including vancomycin: establishment of endemicity in a university medical center. *Ann Intern Med.* 1995; 123:250–9.
83. Sastry V, Brennan PJ, Levy MM. Vancomycin-resistant enterococci: an emerging problem in immunosuppressed transplant recipients. *Transplant Proc.* 1995; 27:954–5.
84. Rhinehart E, Smith NE, Wennersten C. Rapid dissemination of beta-lactamase producing aminoglycoside resistant *Enterococcus faecium* among patients and staff on an infant-toddler surgical ward. *N Engl J Med.* 1990; 323:1814–8.
85. Cohen SH, Gerding DN, Johnson S, et al. Clinical practice guidelines for *Clostridium difficile* infection in adults: 2010 update by the Society for Healthcare Epidemiology of America (SHEA) and the Infectious Diseases Society of America (IDSA). *Infect Control Hosp Epidemiol.* 2010; 31:431–55.
86. Salkind AR, Cuddy PG, Foxworth JW. Is this patient allergic to penicillin? An evidence-based analysis of the likelihood of penicillin allergy. *JAMA.* 2001; 285:2498–505.
87. Frumin J, Gallagher JC. Allergic cross-sensitivity between penicillin, carbapenem, and monobactam antibiotics: what are the chances? *Ann Pharmacother.* 2009; 43:304–15.
88. Cunha BA. Antibiotic selection in the penicillin-allergic patient. *Med Clin North Am.* 2006; 90:1257–64.
89. Pichichero ME. Use of selected cephalosporins in penicillin-allergic patients: a paradigm shift. *Diagn Microbiol Infect Dis.* 2007; 57:13s–18s.
90. Galandiuk S, Polk HC Jr, Jagelman DG, et al. Re-emphasis of priorities in surgical antibiotic prophylaxis. *Surg Gynecol Obstet.* 1989; 169:218–22.
91. DiPiro JT, Vallner JJ, Bowden TA, et al. Intraoperative serum and tissue activity of cefazolin and cefoxitin. *Arch Surg.* 1985; 120:829–32.
92. Classen DC, Evans RS, Pestotnik SL, et al. The timing of prophylactic administration of antibiotics and the risk of surgical-wound infection. *N Engl J Med.* 1992; 326:281–6.
93. Garey KW, Dao T, Chen H, et al. Timing of vancomycin prophylaxis for cardiac surgery patients and the risk of surgical site infections. *J Antimicrob Chemother.* 2006; 58:645–50.
94. Steinberg JP, Braun BI, Hellinger WC, et al. Timing of antimicrobial prophylaxis and the risk of surgical site infection: results from the Trial to Reduce Antimicrobial Prophylaxis Errors. *Ann Surg.* 2009; 250:10–6.
95. Van Kasteren ME, Mannien J, Ott A, et al. Antibiotic prophylaxis and the risk of surgical site infections following total hip arthroplasty: timely administration

is the most important factor. *Clin Infect Dis.* 2007; 44:921–7.

96. Soriano A, Bori G, Garcia-Ramiro S, et al. Timing of antibiotic prophylaxis for primary total knee arthroplasty performed during ischemia. *Clin Infect Dis.* 2008; 46:1009–14.
97. Weber WP, Marti WR, Zwahlen M, et al. The timing of surgical antimicrobial prophylaxis. *Ann Surg.* 2008; 247:918–26.
98. Dellinger EP. What is the ideal time for administration of antimicrobial prophylaxis for a surgical procedure? *Ann Surg.* 2008; 247:927–8.
99. Goldman DA, Hopkins CC, Karchmer AW, et al. Cephalothin prophylaxis in cardiac valve surgery. A prospective, double-blind comparison of two-day and six-day regimens. *J Thorac Cardiovasc Surg.* 1977; 73:470–9.
100. Platt R, Munoz A, Stella J, et al. Antibiotic prophylaxis for cardiovascular surgery. Efficacy with coronary artery bypass. *Ann Intern Med.* 1984; 101:770–4.
101. Forse RA, Karam B, MacLean LD, et al. Antibiotic prophylaxis for surgery in morbidly obese patients. *Surgery.* 1989; 106:750–6.
102. Falagas ME, Karageorgopoulos DE. Adjustment of dosing of antimicrobial agents for bodyweight in adults. *Lancet.* 2010; 375:248–51.
103. Pai MP, Bearden DT. Antimicrobial dosing considerations in obese adult patients. Insights from the Society of Infectious Diseases Pharmacists. *Pharmacotherapy.* 2007; 27:1081–91.
104. Johnson PN, Miller JL, Boucher EA, for the Pediatric Pharmacy Advisory Group Advocacy Committee. Medication dosing in overweight and obese children. www.ppag.org/obesedose (accessed 2010 Nov 22).
105. Koopman E, Nix DE, Erstad BL, et al. End-of-procedure cefazolin concentrations after administration for prevention of surgical-site infection. *Am J Health-Syst Pharm.* 2007; 64:1927–34.
106. Bauer LA, Edwards WA, Dellinger EP, et al. Influence of weight on aminoglycoside pharmacokinetics in normal weight and morbidly obese patients. *Eur J Clin Pharmacol.* 1983; 24:643–7.
107. Bailey TC, Little JR, Littenberg B, et al. A meta-analysis of extended-interval dosing versus multiple daily dosing of aminoglycosides. *Clin Infect Dis.* 1997; 24:786–95.
108. Barza M, Ioannidis JP, Cappelleri JC, et al. Single or multiple daily doses of aminoglycosides: a meta-analysis. *BMJ.* 1996; 312:338–45.
109. Blaser J, Konig C. Once-daily dosing of aminoglycosides. *Eur J Clin Microbiol Infect Dis.* 1995; 14:1029–38.
110. Murry KR, McKinnon PS, Mitrzyk B, et al. Pharmacodynamic characterization of nephrotoxicity associated with once-daily aminoglycoside. *Pharmacotherapy.* 1999; 19:1252–60.
111. Nicolau DP, Freeman CD, Belliveau PP, et al. Experience with a once-daily aminoglycoside program administered to 2,184 adult patients. *Antimicrob Agents Chemother.* 1995; 39:650–5.
112. Rao SC, Ahmed M, Hagan R. One dose per day compared to multiple doses per day of gentamicin for treatment of suspected or proven sepsis in neonates. *Cochrane Database Syst Rev.* 2006; 1:CD005091.
113. Zhanel GG, Ariano RE. Once daily aminoglycoside dosing: maintained efficacy with reduced nephrotoxicity? *Ren Fail.* 1992; 14:1–9.
114. Anaya DA, Dellinger EP. The obese surgical patient: a susceptible host for infection. *Surg Infect.* 2006; 7:473–80.
115. Waisbren E, Rosen H, Bader AM, et al. Percent body fat and prediction of surgical site infection. *J Am Coll Surg.* 2010; 210:381–9.
116. Engelman R, Shahian D, Shemin R, et al. The Society of Thoracic Surgeons practice guideline series: antibiotic prophylaxis in cardiac surgery, part II: antibiotic choice. *Ann Thorac Surg.* 2007; 83:1569–76.
117. Zanetti G, Giardina R, Platt R. Intraoperative redosing of cefazolin and risk for surgical site infection in cardiac surgery. *Emerg Infect Dis.* 2001; 7:828–31.
118. Scher KS. Studies on the duration of antibiotic administration for surgical prophylaxis. *Am Surg.* 1997; 63:59–62.
119. Markantonis SL, Kostopanagiotou G, Panidis D, et al. Effects of blood loss and fluid volume replacement on serum and tissue gentamicin concentrations during colorectal surgery. *Clin Ther.* 2004; 26:271–81.
120. Morita S, Nishisho I, Nomura T, et al. The significance of the intraoperative repeated dosing of antimicrobials for preventing surgical wound infection in colorectal surgery. *Surg Today.* 2005; 35:732–8.
121. Swoboda SM, Merz C, Kostuik J, et al. Does intraoperative blood loss affect antibiotic serum and tissue concentrations? *Arch Surg.* 1996; 131:1165–72.
122. DiPiro JT, Cheung RP, Bowden TA, et al. Single-dose systemic antibiotic prophylaxis of surgical wound infections. *Am J Surg.* 1986; 152:552–9.
123. Fonseca SN, Kunzle SR, Junqueira MJ, et al. Implementing 1-dose antibiotic prophylaxis for prevention of surgical site infection. *Arch Surg.* 2006; 141:1109–13.
124. McDonald M, Grabsch E, Marshall C, et al. Single-versus multiple-dose antimicrobial prophylaxis for major surgery: a systematic review. *Aust N Z J Surg.* 1998; 68:388–96.
125. Kreter B, Woods M. Antibiotic prophylaxis for cardiothoracic operations. Meta-analysis of thirty years of clinical trials. *J Thorac Cardiovasc Surg.* 1992; 104:590–9.
126. Austin TW, Coles JC, Burnett R, et al. Aortocoronary bypass procedures and sternotomy infections: a study of antistaphylococcal prophylaxis. *Can J Surg.* 1980; 23:483–5.
127. Galbraith U, Schilling J, Von Segesser LK, et al. Antibiotic prophylaxis in cardiovascular surgery: a prospective, randomized, comparative trial of one-day cefazolin vs single-dose cefuroxime. *Drugs Exp Clin Res.* 1993; 19:229–34.
128. Kriaras I, Michalopoulos A, Michalis A, et al. Antibiotic prophylaxis in cardiac surgery. *J Cardiovasc Surg.* 1997; 38:605–10.
129. Kriaras I, Michalopoulos A, Turina M, et al. Evolution of antimicrobial prophylaxis in cardiovascular surgery. *Eur J Cardiothorac Surg.* 2000; 18:440–6.

130. Harbarth S, Samore MH, Lichtenberg D, et al. Prolonged antibiotic prophylaxis after cardiovascular surgery and its effect on surgical site infections and antimicrobial resistance. *Circulation.* 2000; 101:2916–21.
131. Edwards FH, Engelman R, Houck P, et al. The Society of Thoracic Surgeons practice guideline series: antibiotic prophylaxis in cardiac surgery, part I: duration. *Ann Thorac Surg.* 2006; 81:397–404.
132. Lee KR, Ring JC, Leggiadro RJ. Prophylactic antibiotic use in pediatric cardiovascular surgery: a surgery of current practice. *Pediatr Infect Dis J.* 1995; 14:267–9.
133. American Academy of Orthopaedic Surgeons. Information statement: recommendations for the use of intravenous antibiotic prophylaxis in primary total joint arthroplasty. www.aaos.org/about/papers/advistmt/1027.asp (accessed 2008 May 13).
134. McCarthy PJ, Patil S, Conrad SA, et al. International and specialty trends in the use of prophylactic antibiotics to prevent infectious complications after insertion of external ventricular drainage devices. *Neurocrit Care.* 2010; 12:220–4.
135. Hares MM, Hegarty MA, Warlow J, et al. A controlled trial to compare systemic and intra-incisional cefuroxime prophylaxis in high risk gastric surgery. *Br J Surg.* 1981; 68:276–80.
136. Moesgaard F, Lykkegaard Nielsen M. Failure of topically applied antibiotics, added to systemic prophylaxis, to reduce perineal wound infection in abdominoperineal excision of the rectum. *Acta Chir Scand.* 1988; 154:589–92.
137. Pitt HA, Postier RG, Gadacz TR, et al. The role of topical antibiotics in "high-risk" biliary surgery. *Surgery.* 1982; 91:518–24.
138. Pitt HA, Postier RG, Mcgowan WA, et al. Prophylactic antibiotics in vascular surgery. Topical, systemic, or both. *Ann Surg.* 1980; 192:356–64.
139. Schersten H. Modified prophylaxis for preventing deep sternal wound infection after cardiac surgery. *APMIS.* 2007; 115:1023–6.
140. Friberg Ö, Svedjeholm R, Söderquist B, et al. Local gentamicin reduces sternal wound infections after cardiac surgery: a randomized controlled trial. *Ann Thorac Surg.* 2005; 79:153–62.
141. Eklund AM, Valtonen M, Werkkala KA. Prophylaxis of sternal wound infections with gentamicin-collagen implant: randomized controlled study in cardiac surgery. *J Hosp Infect.* 2005; 59:108–12.
142. Vander Salm TJ, Okike ON, Pasque MK, et al. Reduction of sternal infection by application of topical vancomycin. *J Thorac Cardiovasc Surg.* 1989; 98:618–22.
143. Bennett-Guerrero E, Ferguson TB Jr, Lin M, et al. Effect of an implantable gentamicin-collagen sponge on sternal wound infections following cardiac surgery: a randomized trial. *JAMA.* 2010; 304:755–62.
144. Bennett-Guerrero E, Pappas TN, Koltun WA, et al. Gentamicin-collagen sponge for infection prophylaxis in colorectal surgery. *N Engl J Med.* 2010; 363:1038–49.
145. McHugh SM, Collins CJ, Corrigan MA, et al. The role of topical antibiotics used as prophylaxis in surgical site infection prevention. *J Antimicrob Chemother.* 2011; 66:693–701.
146. Goodman J, Schaffner W, Collins H, et al. Infection after cardiovascular surgery. *N Engl J Med.* 1968; 278:117–23.
147. Perl TM. Prevention of *Staphylococcus aureus* infections among surgical patients: beyond traditional perioperative prophylaxis. *Surgery.* 2003; 134:s10–7.
148. Kluytmans JA, Mouton JW, Ijzerman EP, et al. Nasal carriage of *Staphylococcus aureus* as a major risk factor for wound infections after cardiac surgery. *J Infect Dis.* 1995; 171:216–9.
149. Kluytmans JA, Mouton JW, Vanden-Bergh MF, et al. Reduction of surgical-site infections in cardiothoracic surgery by elimination of nasal carriage of *Staphylococcus aureus*. *Infect Control Hosp Epidemiol.* 1996; 17:780–5.
150. Kalmeijer MD, Coertjens H, Van Nieuwland-Bollen PM, et al. Surgical site infections in orthopedic surgery: the effect of mupirocin nasal ointment in a double-blind, randomized, placebo-controlled study. *Clin Infect Dis.* 2002; 35:353–8.
151. Hacek DM, Robb WJ, Paule SM, et al. *Staphylococcus aureus* nasal decolonization in joint replacement surgery reduces infection. *Clin Orthop Relat Res.* 2008; 466:1349–55.
152. White A, Smith J. Nasal reservoir as the source of extranasal staphylococci. *Antimicrob Agents Chemother.* 1963; 161:679–83.
153. Lauderdale TL, Wang JT, Lee WS, et al. Carriage rates of methicillin-resistant *Staphylococcus aureus* (MRSA) depend on anatomic location, the number of sites cultured, culture methods, and the distribution of clonotypes. *Eur J Clin Microbiol Infect Dis.* 2010; 29:1553–9.
154. Jain R, Kralovic SM, Evans ME. Veterans Affairs initiative to prevent *Staphylococcus aureus* infections. *N Engl J Med.* 2011; 364:1419–30.
155. Harbarth S, Fankhauser C, Schrenzel J, et al. Universal screening for methicillin-resistant *Staphylococcus aureus* at hospital admission and nosocomial infection in surgical patients. *JAMA.* 2008; 299:1149–57.
156. Bactroban (mupirocin calcium ointment, 2%) nasal package insert. Research Triangle Park, NC: GlaxoSmithKline; 2009 Apr.
157. Kallen AJ, Wilson CT, Larson RJ. Perioperative intranasal mupirocin for the prevention of surgical-site infections: systematic review of the literature and meta-analysis. *Infect Control Hosp Epidemiol.* 2005; 26:916–22.
158. Van Rijen M, Bonten M, Wenzel R, et al. Mupirocin ointment for preventing *Staphylococcus aureus* infections in nasal carriers. *Cochrane Database Syst Rev.* 2008; 4:CD006216.
159. Hebert C, Robicsek A. Decolonization therapy in infection control. *Curr Opin Infect Dis.* 2010; 23:340–5.
160. Perl TM, Cullen JJ, Wenzel RP, et al. Intranasal mupirocin to prevent postoperative *Staphylococcus aureus* infections. *N Engl J Med.* 2002; 346:1871–7.
161. Konvalinka A, Errett L, Fong IW. Impact of treating *Staphylococcus aureus* nasal carriers on wound

infections in cardiac surgery. *J Hosp Infect.* 2006; 64:162–8.

162. Bode LG, Kluytmans JA, Wertheim HF, et al. Preventing surgical-site infections in nasal carriers of *Staphylococcus aureus*. *N Engl J Med.* 2010; 362:9–17.
163. Lee AS, Macedo-Vinas M, Francois P, et al. Impact of combined low-level mupirocin and genotypic chlorhexidine resistance on persistent methicillin-resistant *Staphylococcus aureus* carriage after decolonization therapy: a case-control study. *Clin Infect Dis.* 2011; 52:1422–30.
164. Muto CA, Jernigan JA, Ostrowsky BE, et al. SHEA guideline for preventing nosocomial transmission of multidrug-resistant strains of *Staphylococcus aureus* and *Enterococcus*. *Infect Control Hosp Epidemiol.* 2003; 24:362–86.
165. Edwards JR, Peterson KD, Mu Y, et al. National Healthcare Safety Network (NHSN) report: data summary for 2006 through 2008. *Am J Infect Control.* 2009; 37:783–805.
166. Kutsal A, Ibrisim E, Catav Z, et al. Mediastinitis after open heart surgery. Analysis of risk factors and management. *J Cardiovasc Surg.* 1991; 32:38–41.
167. Abboud CS, Way SB, Baltar VT. Risk factors for mediastinitis after cardiac surgery. *Ann Thorac Surg.* 2004; 77:676–83.
168. Crabtree TD, Codd JE, Fraser VJ, et al. Multivariate analysis of risk factors for deep and superficial sternal infection after coronary artery bypass grafting at a tertiary care medical center. *Semin Thorac Cardiovasc Surg.* 2004; 16:53–61.
169. Kohli M, Yuan L, Escobar M, et al. A risk index for sternal surgical wound infection after cardiovascular surgery. *Infect Control Hosp Epidemiol.* 2003; 24:17–25.
170. Lepelletier D, Perron S, Bizouarn P, et al. Surgical-site infection after cardiac surgery: incidence, microbiology and risk factors. *Infect Control Hosp Epidemiol.* 2005; 26:466–72.
171. Lu JC, Grayson AD, Jha P, et al. Risk factors for sternal wound infection and mid-term survival following coronary artery bypass surgery. *Eur J Cardiothorac Surg.* 2003; 23:943–9.
172. Tang GH, Maganti M, Weisel RD, et al. Prevention and management of deep sternal wound infection. *Semin Thorac Cardiovasc Surg.* 2004; 16:62–9.
173. Jakob HG, Borneff-Lipp M, Bach A, et al. The endogenous pathway is a major route for deep sternal wound infection. *Eur J Cardiothorac Surg.* 2000; 17:154–60.
174. Rahmanian PB, Adams DH, Castillo JG, et al. Impact of body mass index on early outcome and late survival in patients undergoing coronary artery bypass grafting or valve surgery or both. *Am J Cardiol.* 2007; 100:1702–8.
175. Vuorisalo S, Haukipuro K, Pokela R, et al. Risk features for surgical-site infections in coronary artery bypass surgery. *Infect Control Hosp Epidemiol.* 1998; 19:240–7.
176. Segers P, De Jong AP, Kloek JJ, et al. Risk control of surgical site infection after cardiothoracic surgery. *J Hosp Infect.* 2006; 62:437–45.
177. Zerr KJ, Furnary AP, Grunkemeier GL, et al. Glucose control lowers the risk of wound infection in diabetics after open heart operations. *Ann Thorac Surg.* 1997; 63:356–61.
178. Furnary AP, Zerr KJ, Grunkemeier GL, et al. Continuous intravenous insulin infusion reduces the incidence of deep sternal wound infection in diabetic patients after cardiac surgical procedures. *Ann Thorac Surg.* 1999; 67:352–62.
179. Dellinger EP. Preventing surgical-site infections: the importance of timing and glucose control. *Infect Control Hosp Epidemiol.* 2001; 22:604–6.
180. Latham R, Lancaster AD, Covington JF, et al. The association of diabetes and glucose control with surgical-site infections among cardiothoracic surgery patients. *Infect Control Hosp Epidemiol.* 2001; 22:607–12.
181. Furnary AP, Gao G, Grunkemeier GL, et al. Continuous insulin infusion reduces mortality in patients with diabetes undergoing coronary artery bypass grafting. *J Thorac Cardiovasc Surg.* 2003; 125:1007–21.
182. Gandhi GY, Nuttall GA, Abel MD, et al. Intraoperative hyperglycemia and perioperative outcomes in cardiac surgery patients. *Mayo Clin Proc.* 2005; 80:862–6.
183. Dohmen PM. Influence of skin flora and preventive measures on surgical site infection during cardiac surgery. *Surg Infect.* 2006; 7:S13–7.
184. Kittle C, Reed W. Antibiotics and extracorporeal circulation. *J Thorac Cardiovasc Surg.* 1961; 41:34–48.
185. Slonim R, Litwak R, Gadboys H, et al. Antibiotic prophylaxis of infection complicating open-heart operations. *Antimicrob Agents Chemother.* 1963; 3:731–5.
186. Garey KW, Amrutkar P, Dao-Tran TK, et al. Economic benefit of appropriate timing of vancomycin prophylaxis in patients undergoing cardiovascular surgery. *Pharmacotherapy.* 2008; 28:699–706.
187. Garey KW, Lai D, Dao-Tran TK, et al. Interrupted time series analysis of vancomycin compared to cefuroxime for surgical prophylaxis in patients undergoing cardiac surgery. *Antimicrob Agents Chemother.* 2008; 52:446–51.
188. Cimochowski GE, Harostock MD, Brown R, et al. Intranasal mupirocin reduces sternal wound infection after open heart surgery in diabetics and nondiabetics. *Ann Thorac Surg.* 2001; 71:1572–9.
189. Zangrillo A, Landoni G, Fumagalli L, et al. Methicillin-resistant *Staphylococcus* species in a cardiac surgical intensive care unit: a 5-year experience. *J Cardiothorac Vasc Anesth.* 2006; 20:31–7.
190. Fekety F, Cluff L, Sabiston D, et al. A study of antibiotic prophylaxis in cardiac surgery. *J Thorac Cardiovasc Surg.* 1969; 57:757–63
191. Conte J, Cohen S, Roe B, et al. Antibiotic prophylaxis and cardiac surgery: a prospective double-blind comparison of single-dose versus multi-dose regimens. *Ann Intern Med.* 1972; 76:943–9.
192. Firor W. Infection following open-heart surgery, with special reference to the role of prophylactic antibiotics. *J Thorac Cardiovasc Surg.* 1967; 53:371–8.
193. Slama T, Sklar S, Misinski J, et al. Randomized comparison of cefamandole, cefazolin and cefuroxime

prophylaxis in open-heart surgery. *Antimicrob Agents Chemother.* 1986; 29:744–7.

194. Kaiser A, Petracek M, Lea J, et al. Efficacy of cefazolin, cefamandole, and gentamicin as prophylactic agents in cardiac surgery. *Ann Surg.* 1987; 206:791–7.
195. Conklin C, Gray R, Neilson D, et al. Determinants of wound infection incidence after isolated coronary artery bypass surgery in patients randomized to receive prophylactic cefuroxime or cefazolin. *Ann Thorac Surg.* 1988; 46:172–7.
196. Wellens F, Pirlet M, Larbuisson R, et al. Prophylaxis in cardiac surgery: a controlled, randomized comparison between cefazolin and cefuroxime. *Eur J Cardiothorac Surg.* 1995; 9:325–9.
197. Townsend TR, Reitz BA, Bilker WB, et al. Clinical trial of cefamandole, cefazolin, and cefuroxime for antibiotic prophylaxis in cardiac operations. *J Thorac Cardiovasc Surg.* 1993; 106:664–70.
198. Curtis JJ, Boley TM, Walls JT, et al. Randomized, prospective comparison of first- and second-generation cephalosporins as infection prophylaxis for cardiac surgery. *Am J Surg.* 1993; 166:734–7.
199. Doebbeling BN, Pfaller MA, Kuhns KR, et al. Cardiovascular surgery prophylaxis: a randomized, controlled comparison of cefazolin and cefuroxime. *J Thorac Cardiovasc Surg.* 1990; 99:981–9.
200. Vuorisalo S, Pokela R, Syrjälä H. Comparison of vancomycin and cefuroxime for infection prophylaxis in coronary artery bypass surgery. *Infect Control Hosp Epidemiol.* 1998; 19:234–9.
201. Baddour LM, Bettmann MA, Bolger AF, et al. Nonvalvular cardiovascular device-related infections. *Circulation.* 2003; 108:2015–31.
202. Chamber CE, Eisenhauer MD, McNicol LB, et al. Infection control guidelines for the cardiac catheterization laboratory: society guidelines revisited. *Catheter Cardiovasc Interv.* 2006; 67:78–86.
203. Van Rijen M, Bonten M, Wenzel R, et al. Mupirocin ointment for preventing *Staphylococcus aureus* infections in nasal carriers. *Cochrane Database Syst Rev.* 2008; 4:CD006216.
204. Ortega GM, Martí-Bonmatí E, Guevara SJ, et al. Alteration of vancomycin pharmacokinetics during cardiopulmonary bypass in patients undergoing cardiac surgery. *Am J Health-Syst Pharm.* 2003; 60:260–5.
205. Nascimento JW, Carmona MJ, Strabelli TM, et al. Systemic availability of prophylactic cefuroxime in patients submitted to coronary artery bypass grafting with cardiopulmonary bypass. *J Hosp Infect.* 2005; 59:299–303.
206. Vuorisalo S, Pokela R, Syrjälä H. Is single-dose antibiotic prophylaxis sufficient for coronary artery bypass surgery? An analysis of peri- and postoperative serum cefuroxime and vancomycin levels. *J Hosp Infect.* 1997; 37:237–47.
207. Fellinger EK, Leavitt BJ, Hebert JC. Serum levels of prophylactic cefazolin during cardiopulmonary bypass surgery. *Ann Thorac Surg.* 2002; 74:1187–90.
208. Caffarelli AD, Holden JP, Baron EJ, et al. Plasma cefazolin levels during cardiovascular surgery: effects of cardiopulmonary bypass and profound hypothermic circulatory arrest. *J Thorac Cardiovasc Surg.* 2006; 131:1338–43.
209. Hutschala D, Skhirtladze K, Kinstner C, et al. In vivo microdialysis to measure antibiotic penetration into soft tissue during cardiac surgery. *Ann Thorac Surg.* 2007; 84:1605–10.
210. Waltrip T, Lewis R, Young V, et al. A pilot study to determine the feasibility of continuous cefazolin infusion. *Surg Infect.* 2002; 3:5–9.
211. Nascimento JW, Carmona MJ, Strabelli TM, et al. Perioperative cefuroxime pharmacokinetics in cardiac surgery. *Clinics.* 2007; 62:257–60.
212. Lewis DR, Longman TJ, Wisheart JD, et al. The pharmacokinetics of a single dose of gentamicin (4 mg/kg) as prophylaxis in cardiac surgery requiring cardiopulmonary bypass. *Cardiovasc Surg.* 1999; 7:398–401.
213. Kitzes-Cohen R, Farin D, Piva G, et al. Pharmacokinetics of vancomycin administered as prophylaxis before cardiac surgery. *Ther Drug Monit.* 2000; 22:661–7.
214. Austin T, Coles J, McKenzie P, et al. Cephalothin prophylaxis and valve replacement. *Ann Thorac Surg.* 1977; 23:333–6.
215. Sisto T, Laurikka J, Tarkka MR. Ceftriaxone vs cefuroxime for infection prophylaxis in coronary bypass surgery. *Scand J Thorac Cardiovasc Surg.* 1994; 28:143–8.
216. Nooyen SM, Overbeek BP, Brutel De La Riviere A, et al. Prospective randomised comparison of single-dose versus multiple-dose cefuroxime for prophylaxis in coronary artery bypass grafting. *Eur J Clin Microbiol Infect Dis.* 1994; 13:1033–7.
217. Tamayo E, Gualis J, Flórez S, et al. Comparative study of single-dose and 24-hour multiple-dose antibiotic prophylaxis for cardiac surgery. *J Thorac Cardiovasc Surg.* 2008; 136:1522–7.
218. Mertz D, Johnstone J, Loeb M. Does duration of perioperative antibiotic prophylaxis matter in cardiac surgery? A systematic review and meta-analysis. *Ann Surg.* 2011; 254:48–54.
219. Sandoe JA, Kumar B, Stoddart B, et al. Effect of extended perioperative antibiotic prophylaxis on intravascular catheter colonization and infection in cardiothoracic surgery patients. *J Antimicrob Chemother.* 2003; 52:877–9.
220. Niederhäuser U, Vogt M, Vogt P, et al. Cardiac surgery in a high-risk group of patients: is prolonged postoperative antibiotic prophylaxis effective? *J Thorac Cardiovasc Surg.* 1997; 114:162–8.
221. Huddleston CB. Mediastinal wound infections following pediatric cardiac surgery. *Semin Thorac Cardiovasc Surg.* 2004; 16:108–12.
222. McEvoy GK, Snow EK, Miller J, et al., eds. AHFS drug information. Bethesda, MD: American Society of Health-System Pharmacists; 2011.
223. Johns Hopkins Hospital, Arcara K, Tschudy M, Lee CK, eds. Harriet Lane handbook, 19th edition. Philadelphia: Elsevier, Inc.; 2012.
224. Lance LL, Lacey CF, Goldman MP, et al., eds. Quick-look drug book, 18th edition. Baltimore, MD: Lippincott Williams & Wilkins; 2011.

225. Lexi-Comp Online. Hudson, OH: Lexi-Comp, Inc.; 2011.
226. Smith KM, Riche DM, Henyan NN, eds. Handbook of clinical drug data. 11th ed. New York: McGrawHill; 2010.
227. Da Costa A, Kirkorian G, Cucherat M, et al. Antibiotic prophylaxis for permanent pacemaker implantation: a meta-analysis. *Circulation.* 1998; 97:1796–801.
228. Nishimura RA, Carabello BA, Faxon DP, et al. ACC/AHA 2008 guideline update on valvular heart disease: focused update on infective endocarditis: a report of the American College of Cardiology/American Heart Association Task Force on Practice Guidelines. *Circulation.* 2008; 118:887–96.
229. Baddour LM, Epstein AE, Erickson CC, et al. American Heart Association Rheumatic Fever, Endocarditis, and Kawasaki Disease Committee; Council on Cardiovascular Disease in Young; Council on Cardiovascular Surgery and Anesthesia; Council on Cardiovascular Nursing; Council on Clinical Cardiology; Interdisciplinary Council on Quality of Care; American Heart Association. Update on cardiovascular implantable electronic device infections and their management: a scientific statement from the American Heart Association. *Circulation.* 2010; 121:458–77.
230. Klug D, Balde M, Pavin D, et al. Risk factors related to infections of implanted pacemakers and cardioverter-defibrillators: results of a large prospective study. *Circulation.* 2007; 116:1349–55.
231. De Oliveira JC, Martinelli M, Nishioka SA, et al. Efficacy of antibiotic prophylaxis before the implantation of pacemakers and cardioverter-defibrillators: results of a large, prospective, randomized, double-blinded, placebo-controlled trial. *Circ Arrhythm Electrophysiol.* 2009; 2:29–34.
232. Sohail MR, Uslan DZ, Khan AH, et al. Risk factor analysis of permanent pacemaker infection. *Clin Infect Dis.* 2007; 45:166–73.
233. Bertaglia E, Zerbo F, Zardo S, et al. Antibiotic prophylaxis with a single dose of cefazolin during pacemaker implantation: incidence of long-term infective complications. *PACE.* 2006; 29:29–33.
234. Holman WL, Pae WE, Teutenberg JJ, et al. INTERMACS: interval analysis of registry data. *J Am Coll Cardiol.* 2009; 208:755–61.
235. Walker PC, DePrestel DD, Miles NA, et al. Surgical infection prophylaxis for left ventricular assist device implantation. *J Card Surg.* 2011; 26:440–3.
236. Califano S, Pagani FD, Malani PN. Left ventricular assist device-associated infections. *Infect Dis Clin North Am.* 2012; 26:77–87.
237. Radu DM, Jauréguy F, Seguin A, et al. Postoperative pneumonia after major pulmonary resections: an unsolved problem in thoracic surgery. *Ann Thorac Surg.* 2007; 84:1669–74.
238. Cardo D, Horan T, Andres M, et al. National Nosocomial Infections Surveillance (NNIS) system report: data summary from January 1992 through June 2004. *Am J Infect Control.* 2004; 32:470–85.
239. Aznar R, Mateu M, Miró JM, et al. Antibiotic prophylaxis in non-cardiac thoracic surgery: cefazolin versus placebo. *Eur J Cardiothorac Surg.* 1991; 5:515–8.
240. Rovera F, Imperatori A, Militello P, et al. Infections in 346 consecutive video-assisted thoracoscopic procedures. *Surg Infect.* 2003; 4:45–51.
241. Turna A, Kutlu CA, Ozalp T, et al. Antibiotic prophylaxis in elective thoracic surgery: cefuroxime versus cefepime. *Thorac Cardiov Surg.* 2003; 51:84–8.
242. Boldt J, Piper S, Uphus D, et al. Preoperative microbiologic screening and antibiotic prophylaxis in pulmonary resection operations. *Ann Thorac Surg.* 1999; 68:208–11.
243. Schussler O, Dermine H, Alifano M, et al. Should we change antibiotic prophylaxis for lung surgery? Postoperative pneumonia is the critical issue. *Ann Thorac Surg.* 2008; 86:1727–34.
244. Shiono S, Yoshida J, Nishimura M, et al. Risk factors of postoperative respiratory infections in lung cancer surgery. *J Thorac Oncol.* 2007; 2:34–8.
245. Imperatori A, Rotolo N, Gatti M, et al. Peri-operative complications of video-assisted thoracoscopic surgery (VATS). *Int J Surg.* 2008; 6:S78–81.
246. Solaini L, Prusciano F, Bagioni P, et al. Video-assisted thoracic surgery (VATS) of the lung: analysis of intraoperative and postoperative complications over 15 years and review of the literature. *Surg Endosc.* 2008; 22:298–310.
247. Imperatori A, Rovera F, Rotolo N, et al. Prospective study of infection risk factors in 988 lung resections. *Surg Infect.* 2006; 7:S57–60.
248. Chamberlain RS, Sakpal SV. A comprehensive review of single-incision laparoscopic surgery (SILS) and natural orifice transluminal endoscopic surgery (NOTES) techniques for chelecystectomy. *J Gastrointest Surg.* 2009; 13:1733–40.
249. Cruse PJ, Foord R. The epidemiology of wound infection: a ten-year prospective study of 62,939 wounds. *Surg Clin North Am.* 1980; 60:27–40.
250. Petrosillo N, Drapeau CM, Nicastri E, et al. Surgical site infections in Italian hospitals: a prospective multicenter study. *BMC Infect Dis.* 2008; 8:34.
251. Watanabe A, Kohnoe S, Shimabukuro R, et al. Risk factors associated with surgical site infection in upper and lower gastrointestinal surgery. *Surg Today.* 2008; 38:404–12.
252. Yasuda K, Shiraishi N, Adachi Y, et al. Risk factors for complications following resection of large gastric cancer. *Br J Surg.* 2001; 88:873–7.
253. Mohri Y, Tonouchi H, Kobayashi M, et al. Randomized clinical trial of single- versus multiple-dose antimicrobial prophylaxis in gastric cancer surgery. *Br J Surg.* 2007; 94:683–8.
254. Yeo CJ, Cameron JL, Sohn TA, et al. Pancreaticoduodenectomy with or without extended retroperitoneal lymphadenectomy for periampullary adenocarcinoma: comparison of morbidity and mortality and short-term outcome. *Ann Surg.* 1999; 229:613–24.
255. Jafri NS, Mahid SS, Minor KS, et al. Meta-analysis: antibiotic prophylaxis to prevent peristomal infection following percutaneous endoscopic gastrostomy. *Aliment Pharmacol Ther.* 2007; 25:647–56.
256. Sharma VK, Howden CW. Meta-analysis of randomized, controlled trials of antibiotic prophylaxis before

percutaneous endoscopic gastrostomy. *Am J Gastroenterol.* 2000; 95:3133–6.

257. Gorbach SL, Plaut AG, Nahas L, et al. Studies of intestinal microflora: II. Microorganisms of the small intestine and their relations to oral fecal flora. *Gastroenterology.* 1967; 53:856–67.
258. Gorbach SL. Intestinal microflora. *Gastroenterology.* 1971; 60:1110–29.
259. Ruddell WS, Axon AT, Findlay JM, et al. Effect of cimetidine on the gastric bacterial flora. *Lancet.* 1980; 1:672–4.
260. Driks MR, Craven DE, Bartolome RC, et al. Nosocomial pneumonia in intubated patients given sucralfate as compared with antacids or histamine type 2 blockers. *N Engl J Med.* 1987; 317:1376–82.
261. Long J, Desantis S, State D, et al. The effect of antisecretagogues on gastric microflora. *Arch Surg.* 1983; 118:1413–5.
262. Sjostedt S, Levin P, Malmborg AS, et al. Septic complications in relation to factors influencing the gastric microflora in patients undergoing gastric surgery. *J Hosp Infect.* 1989; 12:191–7.
263. Feretis CB, Contou CT, Papoutsis GG, et al. The effect of preoperative treatment with cimetidine on postoperative wound sepsis. *Am Surg.* 1984; 50:594–8.
264. Antimicrobial prophylaxis in surgery. *Treat Guidel Med Lett.* 2006; 4:83–8.
265. LoCiero J, Nichols RL. Sepsis after gastroduodenal operations; relationship to gastric acid, motility, and endogenous microflora. *South Med J.* 1980; 73:878–80.
266. Pessaux P, Msika S, Atalla D, et al. Risk factors for postoperative infectious complications in noncolorectal abdominal surgery: a multivariate analysis based on a prospective multicenter study of 4718 patients. *Arch Surg.* 2003; 138:314–24.
267. Imai E, Ueda M, Kanao K, et al. Surgical site infection surveillance after open gastrectomy and risk factors for surgical site infection. *J Infect Chemother.* 2005; 11:141–5.
268. Christou NV, Jarand J, Sylvestre JL, et al. Analysis of the incidence and risk factors for wound infections in open bariatric surgery. *Obes Surg.* 2004; 14:16–22.
269. McArdle CS, Morran CG, Pettit L, et al. Value of oral antibiotic prophylaxis in colorectal surgery. *Br J Surg.* 1995; 82:1046–8.
270. Nichols RL, Webb WR, Jones JW, et al. Efficacy of antibiotic prophylaxis in high risk gastroduodenal operations. *Am J Surg.* 1982; 143:94–8.
271. Stone HH. Gastric surgery. *South Med J.* 1977; 70:S35–7.
272. Morris DL, Yound D, Burdon DW, et al. Prospective randomized trial of single-dose cefuroxime against mezlocillin in elective gastric surgery. *J Hosp Infect.* 1984; 5:200–4.
273. Lewis RT, Allan CM, Goodall RG, et al. Discriminate use of antibiotic prophylaxis in gastroduodenal surgery. *Am J Surg.* 1979; 138:640–3.
274. Lewis RT, Allan CM, Goodall RG, et al. Cefamandole in gastroduodenal surgery: a controlled prospective, randomized, double-blind study. *Can J Surg.* 1982; 25:561–3.
275. Mitchell NJ, Evans DS, Pollock D. Pre-operative, single-dose cefuroxime antimicrobial prophylaxis with and without metronidazole in elective gastrointestinal surgery. *J Antimicrob Chemother.* 1980; 6:393–9.
276. Uchiyama K, Takifuji K, Tani M, et al. Prevention of postoperative infections by administration of antimicrobial agents immediately before surgery for patients with gastrointestinal cancers. *Hepatogastroenterology.* 2007; 54:1487–93.
277. Pories WJ, Van Rij AM, Burlingham BT, et al. Prophylactic cefazolin in gastric bypass surgery. *Surgery.* 1981; 90:426–32.
278. Polk H, Lopez-Meyer J. Postoperative wound infection: a prospective study of determinant factors and prevention. *Surgery.* 1969; 66:97–103.
279. Saadeddin A, Freshwater DA, Fisher NC, et al. Antibiotic prophylaxis for percutaneous endoscopic gastrostomy for non-malignant conditions: a double-blind prospective randomized controlled trial. *Aliment Pharmacol Ther.* 2005; 22:565–70.
280. Ahmad I, Mouncher A, Abdoolah A, et al. Antibiotic prophylaxis for percutaneous endoscopic gastrostomy—a prospective, randomized, double-blind trial. *Aliment Pharmacol Ther.* 2003; 18:209–15.
281. Dormann AJ, Wigginghaus B, Risius H, et al. Antibiotic prophylaxis in percutaneous endoscopic gastrostomy (PEG)—results from a prospective randomized multicenter trial. *Z Gastroenterol.* 2000; 38:229–34.
282. Preclik G, Grune S, Leser HG, et al. Prospective, randomized, double blind trial of prophylaxis with single dose of co-amoxiclav before percutaneous endoscopic gastrostomy. *BMJ.* 1999; 319:881–4.
283. Panigrahi H, Shreeve DR, Tan WC, et al. Role of antibiotic prophylaxis for wound infection in percutaneous endoscopic gastrostomy (PEG): result of a prospective double-blind randomized trial. *J Hosp Infect.* 2002; 50:312–5.
284. Sturgis TM, Yancy W, Cole JC, et al. Antibiotic prophylaxis in percutaneous endoscopic gastrostomy. *Am J Gastroenterol.* 1996; 91:2301–4.
285. Banerjee S, Shen B, Baron TH, for the American Society for Gastrointestinal Endoscopy Standards of Practice Committee. Antibiotic prophylaxis for GI endoscopy. *Gastrointest Endosc.* 2008; 67:791–8.
286. Rey JR, Axone A, Budzynska A, et al. Guidelines of the European Society of Gastrointestinal Endoscopy (E.S.G.E.) antibiotic prophylaxis for gastrointestinal endoscopy. *Endoscopy.* 1998; 30:318–24.
287. Allison MC, Sandoe JA, Tighe R, et al., for the Endoscopy Committee of the British Society of Gastroenterology. Antibiotic prophylaxis in gastrointestinal endoscopy. *Gut.* 2009; 58:869–80.
288. Gossner L, Keymling J, Hahn EG, et al. Antibiotic prophylaxis in percutaneous endoscopic gastrostomy (PEG): a prospective randomized clinical trial. *Endoscopy.* 1999; 31:119–24.
289. Rao GG, Osman M, Johnson L, et al. Prevention of percutaneous endoscopic gastrostomy site infections caused by methicillin-resistant *Staphylococcus aureus.* *J Hosp Infect.* 2004; 58:81–3.

290. Thomas S, Cantrill S, Waghorn DJ, et al. The role of screening and antibiotic prophylaxis in the prevention of percutaneous gastrostomy site infection caused by methicillin-resistant *Staphylococcus aureus*. *Aliment Pharmacol Ther.* 2007; 25:593–7.
291. Sauerland S, Angrisani L, Belachew M, et al. Obesity surgery. Evidence-based guidelines of the European Association for Endoscopic Surgery (EAES). *Surg Endosc.* 2005; 19:200–21.
292. Varela JE, Wilson SE, Nguyen NT. Laparoscopic surgery significantly reduces surgical-site infections compared with open surgery. *Surg Endosc.* 2010; 24:270–6.
293. Ueno T, Yamamoto K, Kawaoka T, et al. Current antibiotic prophylaxis in pancreatoduodenectomy in Japan. *J Hepatobiliary Pancreat Surg.* 2005; 12:304–9.
294. Stone HH, Haney BH, Kolb LD, et al. Prophylactic and preventive antibiotic therapy. Timing, duration and economics. *Ann Surg.* 1979; 189:691–9.
295. Kusachi S, Sumiyama Y, Nagao J, et al. Prophylactic antibiotics given within 24 hours of surgery, compared with antibiotics given for 72 hours perioperatively, increased the rate of methicillin-resistant *Staphylococcus aureus* isolated from surgical site infections. *J Infect Chemother.* 2008; 14:44–50.
296. Imamura H, Furukawa H, Iijima S, et al. Multicenter phase II study of antimicrobial prophylaxis in low-risk patients undergoing distal gastrectomy for gastric cancer. *Gastric Cancer.* 2006; 9:32–5.
297. Alexander JW, Rahn R. Prevention of deep wound infection in morbidly obese patients by infusion of an antibiotic into the subcutaneous space at the time of wound closure. *Obes Surg.* 2004; 14:970–4.
298. Radhakrishnan NV, Shenoy AH, Cartmill I, et al. Addition of local antiseptic spray to parenteral antibiotic regimen reduces the incidence of stomal infection following percutaneous endoscopic gastrostomy: a randomized controlled trial. *Eur J Gastroenterol Hepatol.* 2006; 18:1279–84.
299. Bates T, Roberts JV, Smith K, et al. A randomized trial of one versus three doses of augmentin as wound prophylaxis in at-risk abdominal surgery. *Postgrad Med J.* 1992; 68:811–6.
300. McArdle CS, Morran CG, Anderson JR, et al. Oral ciprofloxacin as prophylaxis in gastroduodenal surgery. *J Hosp Infect.* 1995; 30:211–6.
301. Rawat D, Srivistava A, Thomson M. Antibody prophylaxis for children undergoing percutaneous endoscopic gastrostomy. *J Pediatr Gastroenterol Nutr.* 2005; 40:234–5.
302. Cortes A, Sauvanet A, Bert F, et al. Effect of bile contamination on immediate outcomes after pancreaticoduodenectomy for tumor. *J Am Coll Surg.* 2006; 202:93–9.
303. Solomkin JS, Mazuski JE, Bradley JS, et al. Diagnosis and management of complicated intra-abdominal infection in adults and children: guidelines by the Surgical Infection Society and the Infectious Diseases Society of America. *Surg Infect.* 2010; 11:79–109.
304. Meijer WS, Schmitz PI, Jeekel J. Meta-analysis of randomized, controlled clinical trials of antibiotic prophylaxis in biliary tract surgery. *Br J Surg.* 1990; 77:282–90.
305. Den Hoed PT, Boelhouwer RU, Veen HF, et al. Infections and bacteriological data after laparoscopic and open gallbladder surgery. *J Hosp Infect.* 1998; 39:27–37.
306. Dervisoglou A, Tsiodras S, Kanellakopoulou K, et al. The value of chemoprophylaxis against *Enterococcus* species in elective cholecystectomy: a randomized study of cefuroxime vs ampicillin/sulbactam. *Arch Surg.* 2006; 141:1162–7.
307. Cainzos M, Sayek I, Wacha H, et al. Septic complications after biliary tract stone surgery: a review and report of the European Prospective Study. *Hepatogastroenterology.* 1997; 44:959–67.
308. Lippert H, Gastinger J. Antimicrobial prophylaxis in laparoscopic and conventional cholecystectomy. *Chemotherapy.* 1998; 44:355–63.
309. Siddiqui K, Khan AF. Comparison of frequency of wound infection: open vs laparoscopic cholecystectomy. *J Ayub Med Coll Abbottabad.* 2006; 18:21–4.
310. Romy S, Eisenring MC, Bettschart V, et al. Laparoscope use and surgical site infections in digestive surgery. *Ann Surg.* 2008; 247:627–32.
311. Rotermann M. Infection after cholecystectomy, hysterectomy or appendectomy. *Health Rep.* 2004; 15:11–23.
312. Chang WT, Lee KT, Chuang SC, et al. The impact of prophylactic antibiotics on postoperative infection complication in elective laparoscopic cholecystectomy: a prospective randomized study. *Am J Surg.* 2006; 191:721–5.
313. Zhou H, Zhang J, Wang Q, et al. Meta-analysis: antibiotic prophylaxis in elective laparoscopic cholecystectomy. *Aliment Pharmacol Ther.* 2009; 29:1086–95.
314. Dobay KJ, Freier DT, Albear P. The absent role of prophylactic antibiotics in low-risk patients undergoing laparoscopic cholecystectomy. *Am Surg.* 1999; 65:226–8.
315. Higgins A, London J, Charland S, et al. Prophylactic antibiotics for elective laparoscopic cholecystectomy: are they necessary? *Arch Surg.* 1999; 134:611–4.
316. Tocchi A, Lepre L, Costa G, et al. The need for antibiotic prophylaxis in elective laparoscopic cholecystectomy: a prospective randomized study. *Arch Surg.* 2000; 135:67–70.
317. Guzmán-Valdivia G. Routine administration of antibiotics to patients suffering accidental gallbladder perforation during laparoscopic cholecystectomy is not necessary. *Surg Laparosc Endosc Percutan Tech.* 2008; 18:547–50.
318. Harling R, Moorjani N, Perry C, et al. A prospective, randomized trial of prophylactic antibiotics versus bag extraction in the prophylaxis of wound infection in laparoscopic cholecystectomy. *Ann R Coll Surg Engl.* 2000; 82:408–10.
319. Illig KA, Schmidt E, Cavanaugh J, et al. Are prophylactic antibiotics required for elective laparoscopic cholecystectomy? *J Am Coll Surg.* 1997; 184:353–6.
320. Zurbuchen U, Ritz JP, Lehmann KS, et al. Oral vs intravenous antibiotic prophylaxis in elective laparoscopic cholecystectomy—an exploratory trial. *Langenbecks Arch Surg.* 2008; 393:479–85.

321. Al-Abassi AA, Farghaly MM, Ahmed HL, et al. Infection after laparoscopic cholecystectomy: effect of infected bile and infected gallbladder wall. *Eur J Surg.* 2001; 167:268–73.
322. Farello GA, Cerofolini A. Antimicrobial prophylaxis with ceftriaxone in laparoscopic cholecystectomy: a 7-year clinical experience involving 3,603 patients. *J Chemother.* 2000; 12(suppl 3):17–22.
323. McGuckin M, Shea JA, Schwartz JS. Infection and antimicrobial use in laparoscopic cholecystectomy. *Infect Control Hosp Epidemiol.* 1999; 20:624–6.
324. Biscione FM, Couto RC, Pedrosa TM, et al. Comparison of the risk of surgical site infection after laparoscopic cholecystectomy and open cholecystectomy. *Infect Control Hosp Epidemiol.* 2007; 28:1103–6.
325. Brill A, Ghosh K, Gunnarsson C, et al. The effects of laparoscopic cholecystectomy, hysterectomy, and appendectomy on nosocomial infection risks. *Surg Endosc.* 2008; 22:1112–8.
326. Cainzos M, Potel J, Puente JL. Prospective, randomized, controlled study of prophylaxis with cefamandole in high-risk patients undergoing operations upon the biliary tract. *Surg Gynecol Obstet.* 1985; 160:27–32.
327. Meijer WS, Schmitz PI. Prophylactic use of cefuroxime in biliary tract surgery: randomized, controlled trial of single versus multiple dose in high-risk patients. *Br J Surg.* 1993; 80:917–21.
328. Grant MD, Jones RC, Wilson SE, et al. Single-dose cephalosporin prophylaxis in high-risk patients undergoing surgical treatment of the biliary tract. *Surg Gynecol Obstet.* 1992; 174:347–54.
329. Lapointe RW, Roy AF, Turgeon PL, et al. Comparison of single-dose cefotetan and multidose cefoxitin as intravenous prophylaxis in elective, open biliary tract surgery: a multicentre, double-blind, randomized study. *Can J Surg.* 1994; 37:313–8.
330. Strachan CJ, Black J, Powis SJ, et al. Prophylactic use of cephazolin against wound sepsis after cholecystectomy. *Br Med J.* 1977; 1:1254–6.
331. Berne TV, Yellin AE, Appleman MD, et al. Controlled comparison of cefmetazole with cefoxitin for prophylaxis in elective cholecystectomy. *Surg Gynecol Obstet.* 1990; 170:137–40.
332. Wilson SE, Hopkins JA, Williams RA. A comparison of cefotaxime versus cefamandole in prophylaxis for surgical treatment of the biliary tract. *Surg Gynecol Obstet.* 1987; 164:207–12.
333. Kujath P. Antibiotic prophylaxis in biliary tract surgery. Ciprofloxacin versus ceftriaxone. *Am J Med.* 1989; 87(5A):255S–257S.
334. Garibaldi RA, Skolnck D, Maglio S, et al. Postcholecystectomy wound infection. *Ann Surg.* 1986; 204:650–4.
335. Levi JU, Martinez OV, Hutson DG, et al. Ampicillin versus cefamandole in biliary tract surgery. *Am Surg.* 1984; 50:412–7.
336. Kellum JM, Duma RJ, Gorbach SL, et al. Single-dose antibiotic prophylaxis for biliary surgery. *Arch Surg.* 1987; 122:918–22.
337. Muller EL, Pitt HA, Thompson JE, et al. Antibiotics in infections of the biliary tract. *Surg Gynecol Obstet.* 1987; 165:285–92.
338. Jewesson PJ, Stiver G, Wai A, et al. Double-blind comparison of cefazolin and ceftizoxime for prophylaxis against infections following elective biliary tract surgery. *Antimicrob Agents Chemother.* 1996; 40:70–4.
339. Montravers P, Lepape A, Dubreuil L, et al. Clinical and microbiological profiles of community-acquired and nosocomial intra-abdominal infections: results of the French prospective, observational EBIIA study. *J Antimicrob Chemother.* 2009; 63:785–94.
340. Baquero F, Hsueh PR, Paterson DL, et al. In vitro susceptibilities of aerobic and facultatively anaerobic gram-negative bacilli isolated from patients with intra-abdominal infections worldwide: 2005 results from Study for Monitoring Antimicrobial Resistance Trends (SMART). *Surg Infect.* 2009; 10:99–104.
341. Chow JW, Satishchandran V, Snyder TA, et al. In vitro susceptibilities of aerobic and facultative gram-negative bacilli isolated from patients with intra-abdominal infections worldwide: the 2002 Study for Monitoring Antimicrobial Resistance Trends (SMART). *Surg Infect.* 2005; 6:439–48.
342. Choudhary A, Bechtold ML, Puli SR, et al. Role of prophylactic antibiotics in laparoscopic cholecystectomy: a meta-analysis. *J Gastrointest Surg.* 2008; 12:1847–53.
343. Stone HH, Hooper CA, Kolb LD, et al. Antibiotic prophylaxis in gastric, biliary and colonic surgery. *Ann Surg.* 1976; 184:443–52.
344. Sirinek KR, Schauer PR, Yellin AE, et al. Single-dose cefuroxime versus multiple-dose cefazolin as prophylactic therapy for high-risk cholecystectomy. *J Am Coll Surg.* 1994; 178:321–5.
345. Drumm J, Donovan IA, Wise R. A comparison of cefotetan and cefazolin for prophylaxis against wound infection after elective cholecystectomy. *J Hosp Infect.* 1985; 6:277–80.
346. Crenshaw CA, Glanges E, Webber CE, et al. A prospective, randomized, double blind study of preventive cefamandole therapy in patients at high risk for undergoing cholecystectomy. *Surg Gynecol Obstet.* 1981; 153:546–52.
347. Leaper DJ, Cooper MJ, Turner A. A comparison trial between cefotetan and cephazolin for wound sepsis prophylaxis during elective upper gastrointestinal surgery with an investigation of cefotetan penetration into the obstructed biliary tree. *J Hosp Infect.* 1986; 7:269–76.
348. Maki DG, Lammers JL, Aughey DR. Comparative studies of multiple-dose cefoxitin vs. single-dose cefonicid for surgical prophylaxis in patients undergoing biliary tract operations or hysterectomy. *Rev Infect Dis.* 1984; 6(suppl 4):S887–95.
349. Garcia-Rodriquez JA, Puig-LaCalle J, Arnau C, et al. Antibiotic prophylaxis with cefotaxime in gastroduodenal and biliary surgery. *Am J Surg.* 1989; 158:428–32.
350. Targarona EM, Garau J, Munoz-Ramos C, et al. Single-dose antibiotic prophylaxis in patients at high risk for infection in biliary surgery: a prospective and randomized study comparing cefonicid with mezlocillin. *Surgery.* 1990; 107:327–34.

351. Krige JE, Isaacs S, Stapleton GN, et al. Prospective, randomized study comparing amoxicillin-clavulanic acid and cefamandole for the prevention of wound infection in high-risk patients undergoing elective biliary surgery. *J Hosp Infect.* 1992; 22(suppl A):33–41.
352. Agrawal CS, Sehgal R, Singh RK, et al. Antibiotic prophylaxis in elective cholecystectomy: a randomized, double blind study comparing ciprofloxacin and cefuroxime. *Indian J Physiol Pharmacol.* 1999; 43:501–4.
353. Kellum JM, Gargano S, Gorbach SL, et al. Antibiotic prophylaxis in high-risk biliary operations: multicenter trial of single preoperative ceftriaxone versus multidose cefazolin. *Am J Surg.* 1984; 148:15–21.
354. Tonelli F, Mazzei T, Novelli A, et al. Amoxicillin/clavulanic acid versus cefotaxime for antimicrobial prophylaxis in abdominal surgery: a randomized trial. *J Chemother.* 2002; 14:366–72.
355. McLeish AR, Keighley MR, Bishop HM. Selecting patients requiring antibiotics in biliary surgery by immediate Gram stains of bile at surgery. *Surgery.* 1977; 81:473–7.
356. Krajden S, Yaman M, Fuksa M, et al. Piperacillin versus cefazolin given perioperatively to high-risk patients who undergo open cholecystectomy: a double-blind, randomized trial. *Can J Surg.* 1993; 36:245–50.
357. McArdle CS. Oral prophylaxis in biliary tract surgery. *J Antimicrob Chemother.* 1994; 33:200–2.
358. Plouffe JF, Perkins RL, Fass RJ, et al. Comparison of the effectiveness of moxalactam and cefazolin in the prevention of infection in patients undergoing abdominal operations. *Diagn Microbiol Infect Dis.* 1985; 3:25–31.
359. Katz S, Glicksman A, Levy Y, et al. Cefuroxime prophylaxis in biliary surgery: single versus triple dose. *Israel J Med Sci.* 1993; 29:673–6.
360. Ahmed ME, Ibrahim SZ, Arabi YE, et al. Metronidazole prophylaxis in acute mural appendicitis: failure of a single intra-operative infusion to reduce wound infection. *J Hosp Infect.* 1987; 10:260–4.
361. Donovan IA, Ellis D, Gatehouse D, et al. One-dose antibiotic prophylaxis against wound infection after appendectomy: a randomized trial of clindamycin, cefazolin sodium and a placebo. *Br J Surg.* 1979; 66:193–6.
362. Gilmore OJ, Martin TD. Aetiology and prevention of wound infection in appendectomy. *Br J Surg.* 1974; 62:567–72.
363. Keiser TA, Mackenzie RL, Feld LN. Prophylactic metronidazole in appendectomy: a double-blind controlled trial. *Surgery.* 1983; 93:201–3.
364. Winslow RE, Rem D, Harley JW. Acute nonperforating appendicitis: efficacy of brief antibiotic prophylaxis. *Arch Surg.* 1983; 118:651–5.
365. Tonz M, Schmid P, Kaiser G. Antibiotic prophylaxis for appendectomy in children: critical appraisal. *World J Surg.* 2000; 24:995–8.
366. Wilson AP. Antibiotic prophylaxis and infection control measures in minimally invasive surgery. *J Antimicrob Chemother.* 1995; 36:1–5.
367. Aziz O, Athanasiou T, Tekkis PP. Laparoscopic versus open appendectomy in children: a meta-analysis. *Ann Surg.* 2006; 243:17–27.
368. Khan MN, Fayyad T, Cecil TD, et al. Laparoscopic versus open appendectomy: the risk of postoperative infectious complications. *JSLS.* 2007; 11:363–7.
369. Hansen J, Smithers MB, Schache D, et al. Laparoscopic versus open appendectomy: prospective randomised trial. *World J Surg.* 1996; 20:17–21.
370. Sauerland S, Lefering R, Neugebauer EA. Laparoscopic versus open surgery for suspected appendicitis. *Cochrane Database Syst Rev.* 2004; 4:CD001546.
371. Hemmila MR, Birkmeyer NJ, Arbabi S, et al. Introduction to propensity scores: a case study on the comparative effectiveness of laparoscopic vs open appendectomy. *Arch Surg.* 2010; 145:939–45.
372. Stone HH. Bacterial flora of appendicitis in children. *J Pediatr Surg.* 1976; 11:37–42.
373. Keighley MR. Infection: prophylaxis. *Br Med Bull.* 1988; 44:374–402.
374. Andersen BR, Kallehave FL, Andersen HK. Antibiotics versus placebo for prevention of post-operative infection after appendicectomy. *Cochrane Database Syst Rev.* 2005; 3:CD001439.
375. Helmer KS, Robinson EK, Lally KP, et al. Standardized patient care guidelines reduce infectious morbidity in appendectomy patients. *Am J Surg.* 2002; 183:608–13.
376. Lau WY, Fan ST, Yiu TF, et al. Prophylaxis of post-appendectomy sepsis by metronidazole and cefotaxime: a randomized, prospective and double-blind trial. *Br J Surg.* 1983; 70:670–2.
377. Lau WY, Fan ST, Chu KW, et al. Randomized, prospective, and double-blind trial of new beta-lactams in the treatment of appendicitis. *Antimicrob Agents Chemother.* 1985; 28:639–42.
378. Lau WY, Fan ST, Chu KW, et al. Cefoxitin versus gentamicin and metronidazole in prevention of post-appendectomy sepsis: a randomized, prospective trial. *J Antimicrob Chemother.* 1986; 18:613–9.
379. O'Rourke MG, Wynne MJ, Morahan RJ, et al. Prophylactic antibiotics in appendectomy: a prospective, double-blind, randomized study. *Aust N Z J Surg.* 1984; 54:535–41.
380. Liberman MA, Greason KL, Frame S, et al. Single-dose cefotetan or cefoxitin versus multiple-dose cefoxitin as prophylaxis in patients undergoing appendectomy for acute nonperforated appendicitis. *J Am Coll Surg.* 1995; 180:77–80.
381. Salam IM, Abu Galala KH, el Ashaal YI, et al. A randomized prospective study of cefoxitin versus piperacillin in appendicectomy. *J Hosp Infect.* 1994; 26:133–6.
382. Lau WY, Fan ST, Yiu TF, et al. Prophylaxis of postappendectomy sepsis by metronidazole and ampicillin: a randomized, prospective and double-blind trial. *Br J Surg.* 1983; 70:155–7.
383. Al-Dhohayan A, Al-Sebayl M, Shibl A, et al. Comparative study of Augmentin versus metronidazole/gentamicin in the prevention of infections after appendectomy. *Eur Surg Res.* 1993; 25:60–4.
384. Morris WT, Innes DB, Richardson RA, et al. The prevention of post-appendicectomy sepsis by

metronidazole and cefazolin: a controlled double-blind trial. *Aust N Z J Surg.* 1980; 50:429–33.

385. Morris DL, Wilson SR, Pain J, et al. A comparison of aztreonam/metronidazole and cefotaxime/metronidazole in elective colorectal surgery: antimicrobial prophylaxis must include gram-positive cover. *J Antimicrob Chemother.* 1990; 25:673–8.
386. Mui LM, Ng CS, Wong SK, et al. Optimum duration of prophylactic antibiotics in acute non-perforated appendicitis. *Aust N Z J Surg.* 2005; 75; 425–8.
387. Kasatpibal N, Nørgaard M, Sørensen HT, et al. Risk of surgical site infection and efficacy of antibiotic prophylaxis: a cohort study of appendectomy patients in Thailand. *BMC Infect Dis.* 2006; 6:111.
388. Nadler EP, Gaines BA. The Surgical Infection Society guidelines on antimicrobial therapy for children with appendicitis. *Surg Infect.* 2008; 9:75–83.
389. Kizilcan F, Tanyel FC, Buyukpamukcu N, et al. The necessity of prophylactic antibiotics in uncomplicated appendicitis during childhood. *J Pediatr Surg.* 1992; 27:586–8.
390. Soderquist-Elinder C, Hirsch K, Bergdahl S, et al. Prophylactic antibiotics in uncomplicated appendicitis during childhood: a prospective randomized study. *Eur J Pediatr Surg.* 1995; 5:282–5.
391. Browder W, Smith JW, Vivoda LM, et al. Nonperforative appendicitis: a continuing surgical dilemma. *J Infect Dis.* 1989; 159:1088–94.
392. Emil S, Laberge JM, Mikhail P, et al. Appendicitis in children: a ten-year update of therapeutic recommendations. *J Pediatr Surg.* 2003; 38:236–42.
393. Leong G, Wilson J, Charlett A. Duration of operation as a risk factor for surgical site infection: comparison of English and US data. *J Hosp Infect.* 2006; 63:255–62.
394. Walz MJ, Paterson CA, Seligowski JM, et al. Surgical site infection following bowel surgery: a retrospective analysis of 1446 patients. *Arch Surg.* 2006; 141:1014–8.
395. Salim A, Teixeira PG, Inaba K, et al. Analysis of 178 penetrating stomach and small bowel injuries. *World J Surg.* 2008; 32:471–5.
396. Witzke JD, Kraatz JJ, Morken JM, et al. Stapled versus hand sewn anastomoses in patients with small bowel injury: a changing perspective. *J Trauma.* 2000; 49:660–6.
397. Kirkpatrick AW, Baxter KA, Simons RK, et al. Intraabdominal complications after surgical repair of small bowel injuries: an international review. *J Trauma.* 2003; 55:399–406.
398. Brundage SI, Jurkovich GJ, Hoyt DB, et al. Stapled versus sutured gastrointestinal anastomoses in the trauma patient: a multicenter trial. *J Trauma.* 2001; 51:1054–61.
399. Hackam DJ, Ali J, Jastaniah SS. Effects of other intraabdominal injuries on the diagnosis, management, and outcome of small bowel trauma. *J Trauma.* 2000; 49:606–10.
400. Guarino J, Hassett JM Jr, Luchette FA. Small bowel injuries: mechanisms, patterns, and outcome. *J Trauma.* 1995; 39:1076–80.
401. Schnuriger B, Inaba K, Eberle BM, et al. Microbiological profile and antimicrobial susceptibility in surgical site infections following hollow viscus injury. *J Gastrointest Surg.* 2010; 14:1304–10.
402. Múñez E, Ramos A, Espejo TÁ, et al. [Microbiology of surgical site infections in abdominal tract surgery patients]. *Cir Esp.* 2011; 89:606–12. In Spanish.
403. Den Hartog D, Dur AH, Tuinebreijer WE, et al. Open surgical procedures for incisional hernias. *Cochrane Database Syst Rev.* 2008; 3:CD006438.
404. Sanchez-Manuel FJ, Lozano-García J, Seco-Gil JL. Antibiotic prophylaxis for hernia repair. *Cochrane Database Syst Rev.* 2012; 2:CD003769.
405. Yin Y, Song T, Liao B, et al. Antibiotic prophylaxis in patients undergoing open mesh repair of inguinal hernia: a meta-analysis. *Am Surg.* 2012; 78:359–65.
406. Goodney PP, Birkmeyer CM, Birkmeyer JD. Short-term outcomes of laparoscopic and open ventral hernia repair: a meta-analysis. *Arch Surg.* 2002; 137:1161–5.
407. Sajid MS, Bokhari SA, Mallick AS, et al. Laparoscopic versus open repair of incisional/ventral hernia: a meta-analysis. *Am J Surg.* 2009; 197:64–72.
408. Kaafarani HM, Kaufman D, Reda D, et al. Predictors of surgical site infection in laparoscopic and open ventral incisional herniorrhaphy. *J Surg Res.* 2010; 163:229–34.
409. Itani KM, Hur K, Kim LT, et al. Comparison of laparoscopic and open repair with mesh for the treatment of ventral incisional hernia: a randomized trial. *Arch Surg.* 2010; 145:322–8.
410. Forbes SS, Eskicioglu C, McLeod RS, et al. Meta-analysis of randomized controlled trials comparing open and laparoscopic ventral and incisional hernia repair with mesh. *Br J Surg.* 2009; 96:851–8.
411. Sanchez VM, Abi-Haidar YE, Itani KM. Mesh infection in ventral incisional hernia repair: incidence, contributing factors, and treatment. *Surg Infect.* 2011; 12:205–9.
412. Itani KM, Wilson SE, Awad SS, et al. Ertapenem versus cefotetan prophylaxis in elective colorectal surgery. *N Engl J Med.* 2006; 335:2640–51.
413. Bartlett S, Burton R. Effects of prophylactic antibiotics on wound infection after elective colon and rectal surgery. *Am J Surg.* 1983; 145:300–9.
414. Burton RC. Postoperative wound infection in colon and rectal surgery. *Br J Surg.* 1973; 60:363–8.
415. Baum M, Anish D, Chalmers T, et al. A survey of clinical trials of antibiotic prophylaxis in colon surgery: evidence against further use of no treatment controls. *N Engl J Med.* 1981; 305:795–9.
416. Coppa G, Eng K, Gouge T, et al. Parenteral and oral antibiotics in elective colorectal surgery: a prospective randomized trial. *Am J Surg.* 1983; 145:62–5.
417. Coppa G, Eng K. Factors involved in antibiotic selection in elective colon and rectal surgery. *Surgery.* 1988; 104:853–8.
418. Glenny AM, Song F. Antimicrobial prophylaxis in colorectal surgery. *Qual Health Care.* 1999; 8:132–6.
419. Suding P, Jensen E, Abramson MA, et al. Definitive risk factors for anastomotic leaks in elective open colorectal resection. *Arch Surg.* 2008; 143:907–12.
420. Svensson LG. Prophylactic antimicrobial administration. *S Afr J Surg.* 1985; 23:55–62.

421. Hojer H, Wetterfors J. Systemic prophylaxis with doxycycline in surgery of the colon and rectum. *Ann Surg.* 1978; 187:362–8.

422. Kurz A, Sessler DI, Lenhardt R, for the Study of Wound Infection and Temperature Group. Perioperative normothermia to reduce the incidence of surgical-wound infection and shorten hospitalization. *N Engl J Med.* 1996; 334:1209–15.

423. Ata A, Lee J, Bestle SL, et al. Postoperative hyperglycemia and surgical site infection in general surgery patients. *Arch Surg.* 2010; 145:858–64.

424. McConnell YJ, Johnson PM, Porter GA. Surgical site infections following colorectal surgery in patients with diabetes: association with postoperative hyperglycemia. *J Gastrointest Surg.* 2009; 13:508–15.

425. Nichols RL. Prophylaxis for intraabdominal surgery. *Rev Infect Dis.* 1984; 6(suppl 1):S276–82.

426. Nelson RL, Glenny AM, Song F. Antimicrobial prophylaxis for colorectal surgery. *Cochrane Database Syst Rev.* 2009; 1:CD001181.

427. Clarke J, Condon R, Bartlett J, et al. Preoperative oral antibiotics reduce septic complications of colon operations: results of a prospective randomized, double-blind clinical study. *Ann Surg.* 1977; 186:251–9.

428. Nichols R, Broldo P, Condon P, et al. Effect of pre-operative neomycin-erythromycin intestinal preparation on the incidence of infectious complications following colon surgery. *Ann Surg.* 1973; 178:453–62.

429. Stellato T, Danziger L, Gordon N, et al. Antibiotics in elective colon surgery: a randomized trial of oral, systemic, and oral/systemic antibiotics for prophylaxis. *Am Surg.* 1990; 56:251–4.

430. Petrelli N, Contre DC, Herrera L, et al. A prospective randomized trial of perioperative prophylactic cefamandole in elective colorectal surgery for malignancy. *Dis Colon Rectum.* 1988; 31:427–9.

431. Kling PA, Dahlgren S. Oral prophylaxis with neomycin and erythromycin in colorectal surgery; more proof for efficacy than failure. *Arch Surg.* 1989; 124:705–7.

432. Lewis RT, Goodall RG, Marien B, et al. Is neomycin necessary for bowel preparation in surgery of the colon? Oral neomycin plus erythromycin versus erythromycin–metronidazole. *Dis Colon Rectum.* 1989; 32:265–70.

433. Wapnick S, Gunito R, Leveen HH, et al. Reduction of postoperative infection in elective colorectal surgery with preoperative administration of kanamycin and erythromycin. *Surgery.* 1979; 85:317–21.

434. Bartlett J, Condon R, Gorbach S, et al. Veterans Administration Cooperative Study on bowel preparation for elective colorectal operations: impact of oral antibiotic regimen on colonic flora, wound irrigation cultures and bacteriology of septic complications. *Ann Surg.* 1978; 188:249–54.

435. Wolff B, Beart R, Dozios R, et al. A new bowel preparation for elective colon and rectal surgery: a prospective, randomized clinical trial. *Arch Surg.* 1988; 123:895–900.

436. Gahhos FN, Richards GK, Hinchey EJ, et al. Elective colon surgery: clindamycin versus metronidazole prophylaxis. *Can J Surg.* 1982; 25:613–6.

437. Dion YM, Richards GK, Prentis JJ, et al. The influence of oral metronidazole versus parenteral pre-operative metronidazole on sepsis following colon surgery. *Ann Surg.* 1980; 192:221–6.

438. Beggs FD, Jobanputra RS, Holmes JT. A comparison of intravenous and oral metronidazole as prophylactic in colorectal surgery. *Br J Surg.* 1982; 69:226–7.

439. Goldring J, McNaught W, Scott A, et al. Prophylactic oral antimicrobial agents in elective colonic surgery: a controlled trial. *Lancet.* 1975; 2:997–9.

440. Washington J, Dearing W, Judd E, et al. Effect of preoperative antibiotic regimen on development of infection after intestinal surgery. *Ann Surg.* 1974; 180:567–72.

441. Peruzzo L, Savio S, De Lalla F. Systemic versus systemic plus oral chemoprophylaxis in elective colorectal surgery. *Chemioterapia.* 1987; 6:601–3.

442. Willis A, Fergunson I, Jones P, et al. Metronidazole in prevention and treatment of *Bacteroides* infections in elective colonic surgery. *Br Med J.* 1977; 1:607–10.

443. Hagen TB, Bergan T, Liavag I. Prophylactic metronidazole in elective colorectal surgery. *Acta Chir Scand.* 1980; 146:71–5.

444. Song F, Glenny AM. Antimicrobial prophylaxis in colorectal surgery: a systematic review of randomized controlled trials. *Br J Surg.* 1998; 85:1232–41.

445. Kaiser A, Herrington J, Jacobs J, et al. Cefoxitin vs erythromycin, neomycin and cefazolin in colorectal surgery: importance of the duration of the operative procedure. *Ann Surg.* 1983; 198:525–30.

446. Weaver M, Burdon DW, Youngs DJ, et al. Oral neomycin and erythromycin compared with single-dose systemic metronidazole and ceftriaxone prophylaxis in elective colorectal surgery. *Am J Surg.* 1986; 151:437–42.

447. Keighley MR, Arabi Y, Alexander-Williams J, et al. Comparison between systemic and oral antimicrobial prophylaxis in colorectal surgery. *Lancet.* 1979; 1:894–7.

448. Lewis RT, Allan CM, Goodall RG, et al. Are first-generation cephalosporins effective for antibiotic prophylaxis in elective surgery of the colon? *Can J Surg.* 1983; 26:504–7.

449. Condon RE, Bartlett JG, Nichols RL, et al. Preoperative prophylactic cephalothin fails to control septic complications of colorectal operations: results of a controlled clinical trial. *Am J Surg.* 1979; 137:68–74.

450. McDermott F, Polyglase A, Johnson W, et al. Prevention of wound infection in colorectal resections by preoperative cephazolin with and without metronidazole. *Aust N Z J Surg.* 1981; 51:351–3.

451. Jones RN, Wojeski W, Bakke J, et al. Antibiotic prophylaxis to 1,036 patients undergoing elective surgical procedures. A prospective randomized comparative trial of cefazolin, cefoxitin, and cefotaxime in a prepaid medical practice. *Am J Surg.* 1987; 153:341–6.

452. Morton A, Taylor E, Wells G. A multicenter study to compare cefotetan alone with cefotetan and

metronidazole as prophylaxis against infection in elective colorectal operations. *Surg Gynecol Obstet.* 1989; 169:41–5.

453. Hoffman C, McDonald P, Watts J. Use of perioperative cefoxitin to prevent infection after colonic and rectal surgery. *Ann Surg.* 1981; 193:353–6.
454. Periti P, Mazzei T, Tonelli F. Single-dose cefotetan vs multiple dose cefoxitin. *Rectum.* 1989; 32:121–7.
455. Jagelman D, Fabian T, Nichols R, et al. Single-dose cefotetan versus multiple dose cefoxitin as prophylaxis in colorectal surgery. *Am J Surg.* 1988; 155:71–6.
456. Shatney CH. Antibiotic prophylaxis in elective gastro-intestinal tract surgery: a comparison of single-dose preoperative cefotaxime and multiple-dose cefoxitin. *J Antimicrob Chemother.* 1984; 14(suppl B):241–5.
457. Arnaud JP, Bellissant E, Boissel P, et al. Single-dose amoxycillin-clavulanic acid vs cefotetan for prophylaxis in elective colorectal surgery: a multicentre, prospective, randomized study. *J Hosp Infect.* 1992; 22(suppl A):23–32.
458. Periti P, Tonelli F, Mazzei T, et al. Antimicrobial chemoimmunoprophylaxis in colorectal surgery with cefotetan and thymostimulin: prospective, controlled, multicenter study. *J Chemother.* 1993; 5:37–42.
459. Skipper D, Karran SJ. A randomized, prospective study to compare cefotetan with cefuroxime plus metronidazole as prophylaxis in elective colorectal surgery. *J Hosp Infect.* 1992; 21:73–7.
460. Lumley JW, Siu SK, Pillay SP, et al. Single-dose ceftriaxone as prophylaxis for sepsis in colorectal surgery. *Aust N Z J Surg.* 1992; 62:292–6.
461. Hakansson T, Raahave D, Hansen OH, et al. Effectiveness of single-dose prophylaxis with cefotaxime and metronidazole compared with three doses of cefotaxime alone in elective colorectal surgery. *Eur J Surg.* 1993; 159:177–80.
462. Karran SJ, Sutton G, Gartell P, et al. Imipenem prophylaxis in elective colorectal surgery. *Br J Surg.* 1993; 80:1196–8.
463. Fukatsu K, Saito H, Matsuda T, et al. Influences of type and duration of antimicrobial prophylaxis on an outbreak of methicillin-resistant *Staphylococcus aureus* and on the incidence of wound infection. *Arch Surg.* 1997; 132:1320–5.
464. AhChong K, Yip AW, Lee FC, et al. Comparison of prophylactic ampicillin/sulbactam with gentamicin and metronidazole in elective colorectal surgery: a randomized clinical study. *J Hosp Infect.* 1994; 27:149–54.
465. Kwok SP, Lau WY, Leung KL, et al. Amoxicillin and clavulanic acid versus cefotaxime and metronidazole as antibiotic prophylaxis in elective colorectal resectional surgery. *Chemotherapy.* 1993; 39:135–9.
466. Barbar MS, Hirxberg BC, Rice C, et al. Parenteral antibiotics in elective colon surgery? A prospective, controlled clinical study. *Surgery.* 1979; 86:23–9.
467. Madsen M, Toftgaard C, Gaversen H, et al. Cefoxitin for one day vs ampicillin and metronidazole for three days in elective colorectal surgery: a prospective, randomized, multicenter study. *Dis Colon Rectum.* 1988; 31:774–7.
468. Blair J, McLeod R, Cohen Z, et al. Ticarcillin/clavulanic acid (Timentin) compared to metronidazole/netilmicin in preventing postoperative infection after elective colorectal surgery. *Can J Surg.* 1987; 30:120–2.
469. Mendes Da Costa P, Kaufman L. Amikacin once daily plus metronidazole versus amikacin twice daily plus metronidazole in colorectal surgery. *Hepatogastroenterology.* 1992; 39:350–4.
470. Roland M. Prophylactic regimens in colorectal surgery: an open randomized consecutive trial of metronidazole used alone or in combination with ampicillin or doxycycline. *World J Surg.* 1986; 10:1003–8.
471. Juul PZ, Klaaborg KE, Kronborg O. Single or multiple doses of metronidazole and ampicillin in elective colorectal surgery: a randomized trial. *Dis Colon Rectum.* 1987; 30:526–8.
472. University of Melbourne Colorectal Group. A comparison of single-dose Timentin with mezlocillin for prophylaxis of wound infection in elective colorectal surgery. *Dis Colon Rectum.* 1989; 32:940–3.
473. Stewart M, Taylor EW, Lindsay G. Infection after colorectal surgery: a randomized trial of prophylaxis with piperacillin versus sulbactam/piperacillin. *J Hosp Infect.* 1995; 29:135–42.
474. Bergman L, Solhaug JH. Single-dose chemoprophylaxis in elective colorectal surgery. *Ann Surg.* 1987; 205:77–81.
475. Goransson G, Nilsson-Ehle I, Olsson S, et al. Single-versus multiple-dose doxycycline prophylaxis in elective colorectal surgery. *Acta Chir Scand.* 1984; 150:245–9.
476. Andaker L, Burman LG, Eklund A, et al. Fosfomycin/metronidazole compared with doxycycline/metronidazole for the prophylaxis of infection after elective colorectal surgery: a randomized, double-blind, multicentre trial in 517 patients. *Eur J Surg.* 1992; 158:181–5.
477. Sexton DJ. Carbapenems for surgical prophylaxis? *N Engl J Med.* 2006; 355:2693–5.
478. Condon RE, Bartlett J, Greenlee H, et al. Efficacy of oral and systemic antibiotic prophylaxis in colorectal operations. *Arch Surg.* 1983; 118:496–502.
479. Condon RE. Preoperative antibiotic bowel preparation. *Drug Ther.* 1983; 83:29–37.
480. Hinchey E, Richards G, Lewis R, et al. Moxalactam as single agent prophylaxis in the prevention of wound infection following colon surgery. *Surgery.* 1987; 101:15–9.
481. Jagelman DG, Fazio VW, Lavery IC, et al. A prospective, randomized, double-blind study of 10% mannitol mechanical bowel preparation combined with oral neomycin and short-term, perioperative, intravenous Flagyl as prophylaxis in elective colorectal resections. *Surgery.* 1985; 98:861–5.
482. Lewis RT. Oral versus systemic antibiotic prophylaxis in elective colon surgery: a randomized study and meta-analysis send a message from the 1990s. *Can J Surg.* 2002; 45:173–80.
483. Englesbe MJ, Brooks L, Kubus J, et al. A statewide assessment of surgical site infection following colectomy: the role of oral antibiotics. *Ann Surg.* 2010; 252:514–20.

484. Kobayashi M, Mohri Y, Tonouchi H, et al. Randomized clinical trial comparing intravenous antimicrobial prophylaxis alone with oral and intravenous antimicrobial prophylaxis for the prevention of a surgical site infection in colorectal cancer surgery. *Surg Today.* 2007; 37:383–8.
485. Wren SM, Ahmed N, Jamal A, et al. Preoperative oral antibiotics in colorectal surgery increase the rate of *Clostridium difficile* colitis. *Arch Surg.* 2005; 140:752–6.
486. Krapohl GL, Phillips LR, Campbell DA, et al. Bowel preparation for colectomy and risk of *Clostridium difficile* infection. *Dis Colon Rectum.* 2011; 54:810–7.
487. Espin-Basany E, Sanchez-Garcia JL, Lopez-Cano M, et al. Prospective, randomised study on antibiotic prophylaxis in colorectal surgery. Is it really necessary to use oral antibiotics? *Int J Colorectal Dis.* 2005; 20:542–6.
488. Sondheimer JM, Sokol RJ, Taylor S, et al. Safety, efficacy, and tolerance of intestinal lavage in pediatric patients undergoing diagnostic colonoscopy. *J Pediatr.* 1991; 119:148–52.
489. Tuggle DW, Hoelzer DJ, Tunell WP, et al. The safety and cost-effectiveness of polyethylene glycol electrolyte solution bowel preparation in infants and children. *J Pediatr Surg.* 1987; 22:513–5.
490. Weber RS, Callender DL. Antibiotic prophylaxis in clean-contaminated head and neck oncologic surgery. *Ann Otol Rhinol Laryngol.* 1992; 101:16–20.
491. Avenia N, Sanguinetti A, Cirocchi R, et al. Antibiotic prophylaxis in thyroid surgery: a preliminary multicentric Italian experience. *Ann Surg Innov Res.* 2009; 3:10.
492. Johnson JT, Wagner RL. Infection following uncontaminated head and neck surgery. *Arch Otolaryngol Head Neck Surg.* 1987; 113:368–9.
493. Saginur R, Odell PF, Poliquin JF. Antibiotic prophylaxis in head and neck cancer surgery. *J Otolaryngol.* 1988; 17:78–80.
494. Mandell-Brown M, Johnson JT, Wagner RL. Cost-effectiveness of prophylactic antibiotics in head and neck surgery. *Otolaryngol Head Neck Surg.* 1984; 92:520–3.
495. Johnson JT, Yu VL, Myers EN, et al. Efficacy of two third-generation cephalosporins in prophylaxis for head and neck surgery. *Arch Otolaryngol.* 1984; 110:224–7.
496. Callender DL. Antibiotic prophylaxis in head and neck oncologic surgery: the role of gram-negative coverage. *Int J Antimicrob Agents.* 1999; 12(suppl 1):s21–7.
497. Simo R, French G. The use of prophylactic antibiotics in head and neck oncological surgery. *Curr Opin Otolaryngol Head Neck Surg.* 2006; 14:55–61.
498. Lotfi CJ, Cavalcanti Rde C, Costa e Silva AM, et al. Risk factors for surgical-site infections in head and neck cancer surgery. *Otolaryngol Head Neck Surg.* 2008; 138:74–80.
499. Liu SA, Tung KC, Shiao JY, et al. Preliminary report of associated factors in surgical site infection after major head and neck neoplasm operations—does the duration of prophylactic antibiotic matter? *J Laryngol Otol.* 2008; 122:403–8.
500. Sepehr A, Santos BJ, Chou C, et al. Antibiotics in head and neck surgery in the setting of malnutrition, tracheotomy, and diabetes. *Laryngoscope.* 2009; 119:549–53.
501. Coskun H, Erisen L, Basut O. Factors affecting wound infection rates in head and neck surgery. *Otolaryngol Head Neck Surg.* 2000; 123:328–33.
502. Robbins KT, Favrot S, Hanna D, et al. Risk of surgical site infection in patients with head and neck cancer. *Head Neck.* 1990; 12:143–8.
503. Tabet JC, Johnson JT. Wound infection in head and neck surgery: prophylaxis, etiology and management. *J Otolaryngol.* 1990; 19:197–200.
504. Girod DA, McCulloch TM, Tsue TT, et al. Risk factors for complications in clean-contaminated head and neck surgical procedures. *Head Neck.* 1995; 17:7–13.
505. Miles BA, Potter JK, Ellis E III. The efficacy of post-operative antibiotic regimens in the open treatment of mandibular fractures: a prospective randomized trial. *J Oral Maxillofac Surg.* 2006; 64:576–82.
506. Penel N, Fournier C, Roussel-Delvallez M, et al. Prognostic significance of surgical site infections following major head and neck cancer surgery: an open non-comparative prospective study. *Support Care Cancer.* 2004; 12:634–9.
507. Lovato C, Wagner JD. Infection rates following perioperative prophylactic antibiotics versus postoperative extended regimen prophylactic antibiotics in surgical management of mandibular fractures. *J Oral Maxillofac Surg.* 2009; 67:827–32.
508. Strauss M, Saccogna PW, Allphin AL. Cephazolin and metronidazole prophylaxis in head and neck surgery. *J Laryngol Otol.* 1997; 111:631–4.
509. Simons JP, Johnson JT, Yu VL, et al. The role of topical antibiotic prophylaxis in patients undergoing contaminated head and neck surgery with flap reconstruction. *Laryngoscope.* 2001; 111:329–35.
510. Johnson JT, Kachman K, Wagner RL, et al. Comparison of ampicillin/sulbactam versus clindamycin in the prevention of infection in patients undergoing head and neck surgery. *Head Neck.* 1997; 19:367–71.
511. Skitarelić N, Morović M, Manestar D. Antibiotic prophylaxis in clean-contaminated head and neck oncological surgery. *J Craniomaxillofac Surg.* 2007; 35:15–20.
512. Andrews PJ, East CA, Jayaraj SM, et al. Prophylactic vs. postoperative antibiotic use in complex septorhinoplasty surgery: a prospective, randomized, single-blind trial comparing efficacy. *Arch Facial Plast Surg.* 2006; 8:84–7.
513. Becker GD, Welch WD. Quantitative bacteriology of closed-suction wound drainage in contaminated surgery. *Laryngoscope.* 1990; 100:403–6.
514. Johnson JT, Yu VL. Role of aerobic gram-negative rods, anaerobes, and fungi in surgical site infection after head and neck surgery: implications for antibiotic prophylaxis. *Head Neck.* 1989; 11:27–9.
515. Rubin J, Johnson JT, Wagner RL, et al. Bacteriologic analysis of surgical site infection following major head

and neck surgery. *Arch Otolaryngol Head Neck Surg.* 1988; 114:969–72.

516. Brown BM, Johnson JT, Wagner RL. Etiologic factors in head and neck surgical site infections. *Laryngoscope.* 1987; 97:587–90.
517. Penel N, Fournier C, Lefebvre D, et al. Multivariate analysis of risk factors for surgical site infection in head and neck squamous cell carcinoma surgery with opening of mucosa. Study of 260 surgical procedures. *Oral Oncol.* 2005; 41:294–303.
518. Brook I. Microbiology and management of post-surgical wounds infection in children. *Pediatr Rehabil.* 2002; 5:171–6.
519. Brook I. Microbiology and principles of antimicrobial therapy for head and neck infections. *Infect Dis Clin N Am.* 2007; 21:355–91.
520. National Institute for Health and Clinical Excellence. Surgical site infection (clinical guideline 74) 2008. www.nice.org.uk/CG74 (accessed 2012 Dec 9).
521. Andreasen JO, Jensen SS, Schwartz O, et al. A systematic review of prophylactic antibiotics in the surgical treatment of maxillofacial fractures. *J Oral Maxillofac Surg.* 2006; 64:1664–8.
522. O'Reilly BJ, Black S, Fernandes J, et al. Is the routine use of antibiotics justified in adult tonsillectomy? *J Laryngol Otol.* 2003; 117:382–5.
523. Lee WC, Duignan MC, Walsh RM, et al. An audit of prophylactic antibiotic treatment following tonsillectomy in children. *J Laryngol Otol.* 1996; 110:357–9.
524. Caniello M, Passerotti GH, Goto EY, et al. Antibiotics in septoplasty: is it necessary? *Braz J Otorhinolaryngol.* 2005; 71:734–8.
525. Dhiwakar M, Eng CY, Selvaraj S, et al. Antibiotics to improve recovery following tonsillectomy: a systematic review. *Otolaryngol Head Neck Surg.* 2006; 134:357–64.
526. Dhiwakar M, Clement WA, Supriya M, et al. Antibiotics to reduce post-tonsillectomy morbidity. *Cochrane Database Syst Rev.* 2008; 2:CD005607.
527. Fennessy BG, Harney M, O'Sullivan MJ, et al. Antimicrobial prophylaxis in otorhinolaryngology/head and neck surgery. *Clin Otolaryngol.* 2007; 32:204–7.
528. Seven H, Sayin I, Turgut S. Antibiotic prophylaxis in clean neck dissections. *J Laryngol Otol.* 2004; 118:213–6.
529. Slattery WH III, Stringer SP, Cassisi NJ. Prophylactic antibiotic use in clean, uncontaminated neck dissection. *Laryngoscope.* 1995; 105:244–6.
530. Weber RS, Raad I, Frankenthaler R, et al. Ampicillin-sulbactam vs clindamycin in head and neck oncologic surgery. The need for gram-negative coverage. *Arch Otolaryngol Head Neck Surg.* 1992; 118:1159–63.
531. Johnson JT, Myers EN, Thearle PB, et al. Antimicrobial prophylaxis for contaminated head and neck surgery. *Laryngoscope.* 1984; 94:46–51.
532. Righi M, Manfredi R, Farneti G, et al. Short-term versus long-term antimicrobial prophylaxis in oncologic head and neck surgery. *Head Neck.* 1996; 18:399–404.
533. Rajan GP, Fergie N, Fischer U, et al. Antibiotic prophylaxis in septorhinoplasty? A prospective, randomized study. *Plast Reconstr Surg.* 2005; 116:1995–8.
534. Abubaker AO, Rollert MK. Postoperative antibiotic prophylaxis in mandibular fractures: a preliminary randomized, double-blind, and placebo-controlled clinical study. *J Oral Maxillofac Surg.* 2001; 59:1415–9.
535. Avery CM, Ameerally P, Castling B, et al. Infection of surgical wounds in the maxillofacial region and free flap donor sites with methicillin-resistant *Staphylococcus aureus. Br J Oral Maxillofac Surg.* 2006; 44:217–21.
536. Gantz NM. Nosocomial central nervous system infections. In: Mayhall CG, ed. Hospital epidemiology and infection control. 3rd ed. Philadelphia: Lippincott Williams and Wilkins; 2004.
537. Narotam PK, van Dellen JR, du Trevou MD, et al. Operative sepsis in neurosurgery: a method of classifying surgical case. *Neurosurgery.* 1994; 34:409–16.
538. Kourbeti IS, Jacobs AV, Koslow M, et al. Risk factors associated with postcraniotomy meningitis. *Neurosurgery.* 2007; 60:317–26.
539. Rebuck JA, Murry KR, Rhoney DH, et al. Infection related to intracranial pressure monitors in adults: analysis of risk factor and antibiotic prophylaxis. *J Neurol Neurosurg Psychiatry.* 2000; 69:381–4.
540. Korinek AM, Baugnon T, Golmard JL, et al. Risk factors for adult nosocomial meningitis after craniotomy: role of antibiotic prophylaxis. *Neurosurgery.* 2006; 58:126–33.
541. Lietard C, Thébaud V, Besson G, et al. Risk factors for neurosurgical site infections: an 18-month prospective survey. *J Neurosurg.* 2008; 109:729–34.
542. Korinek AM, for the French Study Group of Neurosurgical Infections SEHP C-CLIN Paris-Nord. Risk factors for neurosurgical site infections after craniotomy: a prospective multicenter study of 2944 patients. *Neurosurgery.* 1997; 41:1073–81.
543. Korinek AM, Golmard JL, Elcheick A, et al. Risk factors for neurosurgical site infections after craniotomy: a critical reappraisal of antibiotic prophylaxis on 4578 patients. *Br J Neurosurg.* 2005; 19:155–62.
544. Valentini LG, Casali C, Chatenoud L, et al. Surgical site infections after elective neurosurgery: a survey of 1747 patients. *Neurosurgery.* 2007; 61:88–96.
545. Zabramski JM, Whiting D, Darouiche RO, et al. Efficacy of antimicrobial-impregnated external ventricular drain catheters: a prospective, randomized controlled trial. *J Neurosurg.* 2003; 98:725–30.
546. Biyani N, Grisaru-Soen G, Steinbok P, et al. Prophylactic antibiotics in pediatric shunt surgery. *Childs Nerv Syst.* 2006; 22:1465–71.
547. Holloway KL, Smith KW, Wilberger JE, et al. Antibiotic prophylaxis during clean neurosurgery: a large, multicenter study using cefuroxime. *Clin Ther.* 1996; 18:84–94.
548. Whitby M, Johnson BC, Atkinson RL, et al. The comparative efficacy of intravenous cefotaxime and trimethoprim/sulfamethoxazole in preventing infection after neurosurgery: a prospective, randomized study. *Br J Neurosurg.* 2000; 14:13–18.
549. Govender ST, Nathoo N, van Dellen JR. Evaluation of an antibiotic-impregnated shunt system for the treatment of hydrocephalus. *J Neurosurg.* 2003; 99:831–9.

550. Tacconelli E, Cataldo MA, Albanese A, et al. Vancomycin versus cefazolin prophylaxis for cerebrospinal shunt placement in a hospital with a high prevalence of methicillin-resistant *Staphylococcus aureus*. *J Hosp Infect.* 2008; 69:337–44.
551. Wong GK, Poon WS, Lyon D, et al. Cefepime vs ampicillin/sulbactam and aztreonam as antibiotic prophylaxis in neurosurgical patients with external ventricular drain: result of a prospective randomized controlled clinical trial. *J Clin Pharm Ther.* 2006; 31:231–5.
552. Ragal BT, Browd SR, Schmidt RH. Surgical shunt infection: significant reduction when using intraventricular and systemic antibiotic agents. *J Neurosurg.* 2006; 105:242–7.
553. Sarguna P, Lakshmi V. Ventriculoperitoneal shunt infections. *Indian J Med Microbiol.* 2006; 24:52–4.
554. Langley JM, Gravel D, Moore D, et al. Study of cerebrospinal fluid shunt-associated infections in the first year following placement, by the Canadian Nosocomial Infection Surveillance Program. *Infect Control Hosp Epidemiol.* 2009; 30:285–8.
555. Nisbet M, Briggs S, Ellis-Pegler R, et al. *Propionibacterium acnes*: an under-appreciated cause of post-neurosurgical infection. *J Antimicrob Chemother.* 2007; 60:1097–103.
556. Conen A, Walti LN, Merlo A, et al. Characteristics and treatment outcome of cerebrospinal fluid shunt-associated infections in adults: a retrospective analysis over an 11-year period. *Clin Infect Dis.* 2008; 47:73–82.
557. Barker FG II. Efficacy of prophylactic antibiotics against meningitis after craniotomy: a meta-analysis. *Neurosurgery.* 2007; 60:887–94.
558. Haines SJ, Goodman ML. Antibiotic prophylaxis of postoperative neurosurgical wound infection. *J Neurosurg.* 1982; 56:103–5.
559. Quartey GR, Polyzoidis K. Intraoperative antibiotic prophylaxis in neurosurgery: a clinical study. *Neurosurgery.* 1981; 8:669–71.
560. Savitz MH, Katz SS. Prevention of primary wound infection in neurosurgical patients: a 10-year study. *Neurosurgery.* 1986; 18:685–8.
561. Blomstedt GC, Kytta J. Results of a randomized trial of vancomycin prophylaxis in craniotomy. *J Neurosurg.* 1988; 69:216–20.
562. Shapiro M, Wald U, Simchen E, et al. Randomized clinical trial of intraoperative antimicrobial prophylaxis of infection after neurosurgical procedures. *J Hosp Infect.* 1986; 8:283–95.
563. Watters WC III, Baisden J, Bono CM, et al. Antibiotic prophylaxis in spine surgery: an evidence-based clinical guideline for the use of prophylactic antibiotics in spine surgery. *Spine J.* 2009; 9:142–6.
564. Wang EL, Prober CG, Hendrick BE. Prophylactic sulfamethoxazole and trimethoprim in ventriculoperitoneal shunt surgery. A double-blind, randomized, placebo-controlled trial. *JAMA.* 1984; 251:1174–7.
565. Blomstedt GC. Results in trimethoprim-sulfamethoxazole prophylaxis in ventriculostomy and shunting procedures. *J Neurosurg.* 1985; 62:694–7.
566. Djindjian M, Fevrier MJ, Ottervbein G, et al. Oxacillin prophylaxis in cerebrospinal fluid shunt procedures: results of a randomized, open study in 60 hydrocephalic patients. *Surg Neurol.* 1986; 24:178–80.
567. Blum J, Schwarz M, Voth D. Antibiotic single-dose prophylaxis of shunt infections. *Neurosurg Rev.* 1989; 12:239–44.
568. Schmidt K, Gjerris F, Osgaard O, et al. Antibiotic prophylaxis in cerebrospinal fluid shunting: a prospective randomized trial in 152 hydrocephalic patients. *Neurosurgery.* 1985; 17:1–5.
569. Griebel R, Khan M, Tan L. CSF shunt complications: an analysis of contributory factors. *Childs Nerv Syst.* 1985; 1:77–80.
570. Lambert M, MacKinnon AE, Vaishnav A. Comparison of two methods of prophylaxis against CSF shunt infection. *Z Kinderchir.* 1984; 39(suppl):109–10.
571. Zentner J, Gilsbach J, Felder T. Antibiotic prophylaxis in cerebrospinal fluid shunting: a prospective randomized trial in 129 patients. *Neurosurg Rev.* 1995; 18:169–72.
572. Haines SJ, Walters BC. Antibiotic prophylaxis for cerebrospinal fluid shunts: a meta-analysis. *Neurosurgery.* 1994; 34:87–92.
573. Langley JM, LeBlanc JC, Drake J, et al. Efficacy of antimicrobial prophylaxis in placement of cerebrospinal fluid shunts: meta-analysis. *Clin Infect Dis.* 1993; 17:98–103.
574. Borowski A, Littleton AG, Borkhuu B, et al. Complications of intrathecal baclofen pump therapy in pediatric patients. *J Pediatr Orthop.* 2010; 30:76–81.
575. Motta F, Buonaguro V, Stignani C. The use of intrathecal baclofen pump implants in children and adolescents: safety and complications in 200 consecutive cases. *J Neurosurg.* 2007; 107(suppl):32–5.
576. Fjelstad AB, Hommelstad J, Sorteberg A. Infections related to intrathecal baclofen therapy in children and adults: frequency and risk factors. *J Neurosurg Pediatr.* 2009; 4:487–93.
577. Follett KA, Boortz-Marx RL, Drake JM, et al. Prevention and management of intrathecal drug delivery and spinal cord stimulation system infections. *Anesthesiology.* 2004; 100:1582–94.
578. Ratilal BO, Costa J, Sampaio C. Antibiotic prophylaxis for surgical introduction of intracranial ventricular shunts. *Cochrane Database Syst Rev.* 2006; 3:CD005365.
579. Arnaboldi L. Antimicrobial prophylaxis with ceftriaxone in neurosurgical procedures: a prospective study of 100 patients undergoing shunt operations. *Chemotherapy.* 1996; 42:384–90.
580. Alleyne CH, Hassan M, Zabramski JM. The efficacy and cost of prophylactic and periprocedural antibiotics in patients with external ventricular drains. *Neurosurgery.* 2000; 47:1124–9.
581. Shurtleff DB, Stuntz JT, Hayden PW. Experience with 1201 cerebrospinal fluid shunt procedures. *Pediatr Neurosci.* 1985–1986; 12:49–57.
582. Walters BC, Goumnerova L, Hoffman HJ, et al. A randomized, controlled trial of perioperative rifampin/trimethoprim in cerebrospinal fluid shunt surgery. *Childs Nerv Syst.* 1992; 8:253–7.

583. Martin JA, Hamilton BE, Sutton PD, et al. Births: final data for 2006. *Natl Vital Stat Rep.* 2009; 57:1–104.

584. Obstetric and medical complications. In: American Academy of Pediatrics and American College of Obstetricians and Gynecologists. Guidelines for perinatal care. 6th ed. Elk Grove Village, IL: American Academy of Pediatrics; 2008:175–204.

585. Hofmeyr GJ, Smaill F. Antibiotic prophylaxis for cesarean section. *Cochrane Database Syst Rev.* 2002; 3:CD000933.

586. Killian C, Graffunder EM, Vinciguerra T, et al. Risk factors for surgical-site infections following cesarean section. *Infect Control Hosp Epidemiol.* 2001; 22:613–7.

587. Faro S. Infectious disease relations to cesarean section. *Obstet Gynecol Clin North Am.* 1989; 16:363–71.

588. Olsen MA, Butler AM, Willers DM, et al. Risk factors for surgical site infection after low transverse cesarean section. *Infect Control Hosp Epidemiol.* 2008; 29:477–84.

589. Hemsell DL. Infections after gynecologic surgery. *Obstet Gynecol Clin North Am.* 1989; 16:381–400.

590. Faro S. Antibiotic prophylaxis. *Obstet Gynecol Clin North Am.* 1989; 16:279–89.

591. Tita AT, Rouse DJ, Blackwell S, et al. Emerging concepts in antibiotic prophylaxis for cesarean delivery: a systematic review. *Obstet Gynecol.* 2009; 113:675–82.

592. Chelmow D, Ruehli MS, Huang E. Prophylactic use of antibiotics for nonlaboring patients undergoing cesarean delivery with intact membranes: a meta-analysis. *Am J Obstet Gynecol.* 2001; 184:656–61.

593. Duff P, Smith PN, Keiser JF. Antibiotic prophylaxis in low-risk cesarean section. *J Reprod Med.* 1982; 27:133–8.

594. Apuzzio JJ, Reyelt C, Pelosi MA, et al. Prophylactic antibiotics for cesarean section: comparison of high- and low-risk patients for endometritis. *Obstet Gynecol.* 1982; 59:693–8.

595. Duff P. Prophylactic antibiotics for cesarean delivery: a simple cost-effective strategy for prevention of postoperative morbidity. *Am J Obstet Gynecol.* 1987; 157:794–8.

596. Jakobi P, Weissman A, Sigler E, et al. Post-cesarean section febrile morbidity. Antibiotic prophylaxis in low-risk patients. *J Reprod Med.* 1994; 39:707–10.

597. Rizk DE, Nsanze H, Mabrouk MH, et al. Systemic antibiotic prophylaxis in elective cesarean delivery. *Int J Gynaecol Obstet.* 1998; 61:245–51.

598. Rouzi AA, Khalifa F, Ba'aqeel H, et al. The routine use of cefazolin in cesarean section. *Int J Gynecol Obstet.* 2000; 69:107–12.

599. Bagratee JS, Moodley J, Kleinschmidt I, et al. A randomized controlled trial of antibiotic prophylaxis in elective caesarean delivery. *Br J Obstet Gynaecol.* 2001; 108:143–8.

600. Hopkins L, Smaill F. Antibiotic prophylaxis regimens and drugs for cesarean section. *Cochrane Database Syst Rev.* 1999; 2:CD001136.

601. Andrews WW, Hauth JC, Cliver SP, et al. Randomized clinical trial of extended spectrum antibiotic prophylaxis with coverage for *Ureaplasma urealyticum* to reduce post-cesarean delivery endometritis. *Obstet Gynecol.* 2003; 101:1183–9.

602. Tita AT, Hauth JC, Grimes A, et al. Decreasing incidence of postcesarean endometritis with extended-spectrum antibiotic prophylaxis. *Obstet Gynecol.* 2008; 111:51–6.

603. Tita AT, Owen J, Stamm A, et al. Impact of extended-spectrum antibiotic prophylaxis on incidence of postcesarean surgical wound infection. *Am J Obstet Gynecol.* 2008; 199:303.e1–e3.

604. Meyer NL, Hosier KV, Scott K, et al. Cefazolin versus cefazolin plus metronidazole for antibiotic prophylaxis at cesarean section. *South Med J.* 2003; 96:992–5.

605. Costantine MM, Rahman M, Ghulmiyah L, et al. Timing of perioperative antibiotics for cesarean delivery: a metaanalysis. *Am J Obstet Gynecol.* 2008; 199:301.e1–e6.

606. Sullivan SA, Smith T, Chang E, et al. Administration of cefazolin prior to skin incision is superior to cefazolin at cord clamping in preventing postcesarean infectious morbidity: a randomized, controlled trial. *Am J Obstet Gynecol.* 2007; 196:455.e1–e5.

607. Committee Opinion No. 465: antimicrobial prophylaxis for cesarean delivery: timing of administration. *Obstet Gynecol.* 2010; 116:791–2.

608. Witt A, Döner M, Petricevic L, et al. Antibiotic prophylaxis before surgery vs after cord clamping in elective cesarean delivery: a double-blind, prospective, randomized, placebo-controlled trial. *Arch Surg.* 2011; 146:1404–9.

609. Whiteman MK, Hillis SD, Jamieson DJ, et al. Inpatient hysterectomy surveillance in the United States, 2000–2004. *Am J Obstet Gynecol.* 2008; 198:34.e1–e7.

610. Schorge JO, Schaffer JI, Halvorson LM, et al. Surgeries for benign gynecologic conditions. Chap. 41. In: Schorge JO, Schaffer JI, Halvorson LM, et al., eds. Williams gynecology. New York: McGraw-Hill Professional; 2008.

611. Drahonovsky J, Haakova L, Otcenasek M, et al. A prospective randomized comparison of vaginal hysterectomy, laparoscopically assisted vaginal hysterectomy, and total laparoscopic hysterectomy in women with benign uterine disease. *Eur J Obstet Gynecol.* 2009; 148:172–6.

612. Sokol AI, Green IC. Laparoscopic hysterectomy. *Clin Obstet Gynecol.* 2009; 52:304–12.

613. ACOG Committee Opinion No. 444: choosing the route of hysterectomy for benign disease. *Obstet Gynecol.* 2009; 114:1156–8.

614. Nieboer TE, Johnson N, Lethaby A, et al. Surgical approach to hysterectomy for benign gynaecological disease. *Cochrane Database Syst Rev.* 2009; 3:CD003677.

615. American College of Obstetricians and Gynecologists. ACOG Committee Opinion No. 388: supracervical hysterectomy. *Obstet Gynecol.* 2007; 110:1215–7.

616. Jennings RH. Prophylactic antibiotics in vaginal and abdominal hysterectomy. *South Med J.* 1978; 71:251–4.

617. Hemsell D, Johnson ER, Hemsell PG, et al. Cefazolin is inferior to cefotetan as single-dose prophylaxis for

women undergoing elective total abdominal hysterectomy. *Clin Infect Dis.* 1995; 20:677–84.

618. Goosenberg J, Emich JP Jr, Schwarz RH. Prophylactic antibiotics in vaginal hysterectomy. *Am J Obstet Gynecol.* 1969; 105:503–6.
619. Marsden DE, Cavanagh D, Wisniewski BJ, et al. Factors affecting the incidence of infectious morbidity after radical hysterectomy. *Am J Obstet Gynecol.* 1985; 152:817–21.
620. Mann W, Orr J, Shingleton H, et al. Perioperative influences on infectious morbidity in radical hysterectomy. *Gynecol Oncol.* 1981; 11:207–12.
621. Löfgren M, Poromaa IS, Stjerndahl JH, et al. Postoperative infections and antibiotic prophylaxis for hysterectomy in Sweden: a study by the Swedish National Register for Gynecologic Surgery. *Acta Obstet Gynecol Scand.* 2004; 83:1202–7.
622. Olsen MA, Higham-Kessler J, Yokoe DS, et al. Developing a risk stratification model for surgical site infection after abdominal hysterectomy. *Infect Control Hosp Epidemiol.* 2009; 30:1077–83.
623. Soper DE, Bump RC, Hurt GW. Wound infection after abdominal hysterectomy: effect of the depth of subcutaneous tissue. *Am J Obstet Gynecol.* 1995; 173:465–71.
624. Soper DE. Infections of the female pelvis. In: Mandell GL, Bennett JE, Dolin R, eds. Mandell, Douglas and Bennett's principles and practice of infectious diseases. 7th ed. New York: Churchill Livingstone; 2009:1514–6.
625. Ohm MJ, Galask RP. The effect of antibiotic prophylaxis on patients undergoing vaginal operations. II. Alterations of microbial flora. *Am J Obstet Gynecol.* 1975; 123:597–604.
626. Ohm MJ, Galask RP. The effect of antibiotic prophylaxis on patients undergoing total abdominal hysterectomy. II. Alterations of microbial flora. *Am J Obstet Gynecol.* 1976; 125:448–54.
627. Appelbaum P, Moodley J, Chatterton S, et al. Metronidazole in the prophylaxis and treatment of anaerobic infection. *S Afr Med J.* 1978; 1:703–6.
628. Mittendorf R, Aronson MP, Berry RE, et al. Avoiding serious infections associated with abdominal hysterectomy: a meta-analysis of antibiotic prophylaxis. *Am J Obstet Gynecol.* 1993; 169:1119–24.
629. Duff P. Antibiotic prophylaxis for abdominal hysterectomy. *Obstet Gynecol.* 1982; 60:25–9.
630. Miyazawa K, Hernandez E, Dillon MB. Prophylactic topical cefamandole in radical hysterectomy. *Int J Gynaecol Obstet.* 1987; 25:133–8.
631. Micha JP, Kucera PR, Birkett JP, et al. Prophylactic mezlocillin in radical hysterectomy. *Obstet Gynecol.* 1987; 69:251–4.
632. Sevin B, Ramos R, Lichtinger M, et al. Antibiotic prevention of infection complicating radical abdominal hysterectomy. *Obstet Gynecol.* 1984; 64:539–45.
633. Rosenshein NB, Ruth JC, Villar J, et al. A prospective randomized study of doxycycline as a prophylactic antibiotic in patients undergoing radical hysterectomy. *Gynecol Oncol.* 1983; 15:201–6.
634. Zakashansky K, Bradley WH, Nezhat FR. New techniques in radical hysterectomy. *Curr Opin Obstet Gynecol.* 2008; 20:14–9.
635. Hemsell D, Menon M, Friedman A. Ceftriaxone or cefazolin prophylaxis for the prevention of infection after vaginal hysterectomy. *Am J Surg.* 1984; 148:22–6.
636. Hemsell DL, Johnson ER, Bawdon RE, et al. Ceftriaxone and cefazolin prophylaxis for hysterectomy. *Surg Gynecol Obstet.* 1985; 161:197–203.
637. Soper D, Yarwood R. Single-dose antibiotic prophylaxis in women undergoing vaginal hysterectomy. *Obstet Gynecol.* 1987; 53:879–82.
638. Rapp RP, Connors E, Hager WD, et al. Comparison of single-dose moxalactam and a three-dose regimen of cefoxitin for prophylaxis in vaginal hysterectomy. *Clin Pharm.* 1986; 5:988–93.
639. Roy S, Wilkins J. Single-dose cefotaxime versus 3- to 5-dose cefoxitin for prophylaxis of vaginal or abdominal hysterectomy. *J Antimicrob Chemother.* 1984; 14(suppl B):217–21.
640. Roy S, Wilkins J, Hemsell DL, et al. Efficacy and safety of single-dose ceftizoxime vs. multiple-dose cefoxitin in preventing infection after vaginal hysterectomy. *J Reprod Med.* 1988; 33(suppl 1):149–53.
641. Roy S, Wilkins J, Galaif E, et al. Comparative efficacy and safety of cefmetazole or cefoxitin in the prevention of postoperative infection following vaginal and abdominal hysterectomy. *J Antimicrob Chemother.* 1989; 23(suppl D):109–17.
642. Mercer LJ, Murphy HJ, Ismail MA, et al. A comparison of cefonicid and cefoxitin for preventing infections after vaginal hysterectomy. *J Reprod Med.* 1988; 33:223–6.
643. Hemsell DL, Heard ML, Nobles BJ, et al. Single-dose cefoxitin prophylaxis for premenopausal women undergoing vaginal hysterectomy. *Obstet Gynecol.* 1984; 63:285–90.
644. McGregor JA, Phillips LE, Dunne JT, et al. Results of a double-blind, placebo controlled clinical trial program of single-dose ceftizoxime versus multiple-dose cefoxitin as prophylaxis for patients undergoing vaginal and abdominal hysterectomy. *J Am Coll Surg.* 1994; 178:12–31.
645. Orr JW Jr, Varner RE, Kilgore LC, et al. Cefotetan versus cefoxitin as prophylaxis in hysterectomy. *Am J Obstet Gynecol.* 1986; 154:960–3.
646. Orr JW Jr, Sisson PF, Barrett JM, et al. Single center study results of cefotetan and cefoxitin prophylaxis for abdominal or vaginal hysterectomy. *Am J Obstet.* 1988; 158(3 pt 2):714–6.
647. Berkeley AS, Orr JW, Cavanagh D, et al. Comparative effectiveness and safety of cefotetan and cefoxitin as prophylactic agents in patients undergoing abdominal or vaginal hysterectomy. *Am J Surg.* 1988; 155:81–5.
648. Berkeley AS, Freedman KS, Ledger WJ, et al. Comparison of cefotetan and cefoxitin prophylaxis for abdominal and vaginal hysterectomy. *Am J Obstet Gynecol.* 1988; 158:706–9.
649. Gordon SF. Results of a single center study of cefotetan prophylaxis in abdominal or vaginal hysterectomy. *Am J Obstet Gynecol.* 1988; 158:710–4. [Erratum, *Am J Obstet Gynecol.* 1989; 160:1025.]
650. Campillo F, Rubio JM. Comparative study of single-dose cefotaxime and multiple doses of cefoxitin and

cefazolin as prophylaxis in gynecologic surgery. *Am J Surg.* 1992; 164(suppl):12S–15S.
651. Berkeley AS, Haywork SD, Hirsch JC, et al. Controlled, comparative study of moxalactam and cefazolin for prophylaxis of abdominal hysterectomy. *Surg Gynecol Obstet.* 1985; 161:457–61.
652. Tuomala RE, Fischer SG, Munoz A, et al. A comparative trial of cefazolin and moxalactam as prophylaxis for preventing infection after abdominal hysterectomy. *Obstet Gynecol.* 1985; 66:372–6.
653. Chongsomchai C, Lumbiganon P, Thinkhamrop J, et al. Placebo-controlled, double-blind, randomized study of prophylactic antibiotics in elective abdominal hysterectomy. *J Hosp Infect.* 2002; 52:302–6.
654. Cormio G, Di Fazio F, Lorusso F, et al. Antimicrobial prophylaxis in laparotomic gynecologic surgery: a prospective randomized study comparing amoxicillin-clavulanic acid with cefazolin. *J Chemother.* 2002; 14:618–22.
655. Lett WJ, Ansbacher R, Davison BL, et al. Prophylactic antibiotics for women undergoing vaginal hysterectomy. *J Reprod Med.* 1977; 19:51–4.
656. Hamod KA, Spence MR, Roshenshein NB, et al. Single and multidose prophylaxis in vaginal hysterectomy: a comparison of sodium cephalothin and metronidazole. *Am J Obstet Gynecol.* 1980; 136:976–9.
657. Hemsell DL, Johnson ER, Heard MC, et al. Single dose piperacillin versus triple dose cefoxitin prophylaxis at vaginal and abdominal hysterectomy. *South Med J.* 1989; 82:438–42.
658. Turano A. New clinical data on the prophylaxis of infections in abdominal, gynecologic, and urologic surgery. *Am J Surg.* 1992; 164(suppl):16S–20S.
659. D'Addato F, Canestrelli M, Repinto A, et al. Perioperative prophylaxis in abdominal and vaginal hysterectomy. *Clin Exp Obstet Gynecol.* 1993; 20:95–101.
660. Gonen R, Hakin M, Samberg I, et al. Short-term prophylactic antibiotic for elective abdominal hysterectomy: how short? *Eur J Obstet Gynecol Reprod Biol.* 1985; 20:229–34.
661. Scarpignato C, Labruna C, Condemi V, et al. Comparative efficacy of two different regimens of antibiotic prophylaxis in total abdominal hysterectomy. *Pharmatherapeutica.* 1980; 2:450–5.
662. Hemsell DL, Hemsell PG, Heard ML, et al. Preoperative cefoxitin prophylaxis for elective abdominal hysterectomy. *Am J Obstet Gynecol.* 1985; 153:225–6.
663. Triolo O, Mancuso A, Pantano F. Amoxycillin/clavulanate prophylaxis in gynecologic surgery. *Int J Gynaecol Obstet.* 2004; 85:59–61.
664. Su HY, Ding DC, Chen DC, et al. Prospective randomized comparison of single-dose versus 1-day cefazolin for prophylaxis in gynecologic surgery. *Acta Obstet Gynecol Scand.* 2005; 84:384–9.
665. Tchabo JG, Cutting ME, Butler C. Prophylactic antibiotics in patients undergoing total vaginal or abdominal hysterectomy. *Int Surg.* 1985; 70:349–52.
666. Read RW. Endophthalmitis. In: Yanoff M, Duker JS, eds. Ophthalmology. 3rd ed. St. Louis: Mosby; 2009.
667. Bucci FA, Amico LM, Evans RE. Antimicrobial efficacy of prophylactic gatifloxacin 0.3% and moxifloxacin 0.5% in patients undergoing phacoemulsification surgery. *Eye Contact Lens.* 2008; 34:39–42.
668. Colleaux KM, Hamilton WK. Effect of prophylactic antibiotics and incision type on the incidence of endophthalmitis after cataract surgery. *Can J Ophthalmol.* 2000; 35:373–8.
669. Eifrig CW, Flynn HW Jr, Scott IU, et al. Acute-onset postoperative endophthalmitis: review of incidence and visual outcomes (1995–2001). *Ophthalmic Surg Lasers.* 2002; 33:373–8.
670. Garat M, Moser CL, Martín-Baranera M, et al. Prophylactic intracameral cefazolin after cataract surgery: endophthalmitis risk reduction and safety results in a 6-year study. *J Cataract Refract Surg.* 2009; 35:637–42.
671. Jensen MK, Fiscella RG, Moshirfar M, et al. Third- and fourth-generation fluoroquinolones: retrospective comparison of endophthalmitis after cataract surgery performed over 10 years. *J Cataract Refract Surg.* 2008; 34:1460–7.
672. Mollan SP, Mollan AJ, Konstantinos C, et al. Incidence of endophthalmitis following vitreoretinal surgery. *Int Ophthalmol.* 2009; 29:203–5.
673. Moshirfar M, Feiz V, Vitale AT, et al. Endophthalmitis after uncomplicated cataract surgery with the use of fourth-generation fluoroquinolones: a retrospective observational case series. *Ophthalmology.* 2007; 114:686–91.
674. Romero P, Méndez I, Salvat M, et al. Intracameral cefazolin as prophylaxis against endophthalmitis in cataract surgery. *J Cataract Refract Surg.* 2006; 32:438–41.
675. Soto AM, Mendívil MP. The effect of topical povidone-iodine, intraocular vancomycin, or both on aqueous humor cultures at the time of cataract surgery. *Am J Ophthalmol.* 2001; 131:293–300.
676. Taban M, Behrens A, Newcomb RL, et al. Incidence of acute endophthalmitis following penetrating kerato plasty. *Arch Ophthalmol.* 2005; 123:605–9.
677. Wejde G, Samolov B, Seregard S, et al. Risk factors for endophthalmitis following cataract surgery: a retrospective case-control study. *J Hosp Infect.* 2005; 61:251–6.
678. Wu PC, Li M, Chang SJ, et al. Risk of endophthalmitis after cataract surgery using different protocols for povidone-iodine preoperative disinfection. *J Ocul Pharmacol Ther.* 2006; 22:54–61.
679. Barry P, Seal DV, Gettinby G, et al. ESCRS study of prophylaxis of postoperative endophthalmitis after cataract surgery: preliminary report of principal results from a European multicenter study. *J Cataract Refract Surg.* 2006; 32:407–10.
680. ESCRS Endophthalmitis Study Group. Prophylaxis of postoperative endophthalmitis following cataract surgery: results of the ESCRS multicenter study and identification of risk factors. *J Cataract Refract Surg.* 2007; 33:978–88.
681. Kamalarajah S, Ling R, Silvestri G, et al. Presumed infectious endophthalmitis following cataract surgery in the UK: a case-control study of risk factors. *Eye.* 2007; 21:580–6.

682. Montan PG, Setterquist H, Marcusson E, et al. Preoperative gentamicin eye drops and chlorhexidine solution in cataract surgery: experimental and clinical results. *Eur J Ophthalmol.* 2000; 10:286–92.
683. Recchia FM, Busbee BG, Pearlman RB, et al. Changing trends in the microbiologic aspects of postcataract endophthalmitis. *Arch Ophthalmol.* 2005; 123:341–6.
684. American Academy of Ophthalmology. Cataract in the adult eye, preferred practice pattern. http://one.aao.org/CE/PracticeGuidelines/PPP_Content.aspx?cid=a80a87ce-9042-4677-85d7-4b876deed276 (accessed 2012 Dec 9).
685. Hatch WV, Cernat G, Wong D, et al. Risk factors for acute endophthalmitis after cataract surgery: a population-based study. *Ophthalmology.* 2009; 116:425–40.
686. Lertsumitkul S, Myers PC, O'Rourke MT, et al. Endophthalmitis in the western Sydney region: a case-control study. *Clin Experiment Ophthalmol.* 2001; 29:400–5.
687. De Kaspar HM, Chang RT, Singh K, et al. Prospective randomized comparison of 2 different methods of 5% povidone-iodine applications for anterior segment intraocular surgery. *Arch Ophthalmol.* 2005; 123:161–5.
688. Ta CN, Egbert PR, Singh K, et al. Prospective randomized comparison of 3-day versus 1-hour preoperative ofloxacin prophylaxis for cataract surgery. *Ophthalmology.* 2002; 109:2036–41.
689. Fernández-Rubio E, Urcelay JL, Cuesta-Rodriguez T. The antibiotic resistance pattern of conjunctival bacteria: a key for designing a cataract surgery prophylaxis. *Eye.* 2009; 23:1321–8.
690. Gelfand YA, Mezer E, Linn S, et al. Lack of effect of prophylactic gentamicin treatment on intraocular and extraocular fluid cultures after pars plana vitrectomy. *Ophthalmic Surg Lasers.* 1998; 29:497–501.
691. Vasavada AR, Gajjar D, Raj SM, et al. Comparison of 2 moxifloxacin regimens for preoperative prophylaxis: prospective randomized triple-masked trial. Part 2: residual conjunctival flora. *J Cataract Refract Surg.* 2008; 34:1383–8.
692. Osher RH, Amdahl LD, Cheetham JK. Antimicrobial efficacy and aqueous humor concentration of preoperative and postoperative topical trimethoprim/polymyxin B sulfate versus tobramycin. *J Cataract Refract Surg.* 1994; 20:3–8.
693. Barequet IS, Jabbur NS, Barron Y, et al. Perioperative microbiologic profile of the conjunctiva in photoreactive keratectomy. *J Refract Surg.* 2001; 17:55–62.
694. Seal DV, Barry P, Gettinby G, et al. ESCRS study of prophylaxis of postoperative endophthalmitis after cataract surgery: case for a European multicenter study. *J Cataract Refract Surg.* 2006; 32:396–406.
695. Gore DM, Anjunawela RI, Little BC. United Kingdom survey of antibiotic prophylaxis practice after publication of the ESCRS endophthalmitis study. *J Cataract Refract Surg.* 2009; 35:770–3.
696. O'Brien TP, Arshinoff SA, Mah FS. Perspective on antibiotics for postoperative endophthalmitis prophylaxis: potential role of moxifloxacin. *J Cataract Refract Surg.* 2007; 33:1790–800.
697. Chang DF, Braga-Mele R, Mamalis N, et al. Prophylaxis of postoperative endophthalmitis after cataract surgery: results of the 2007 ASCRS member survey. *J Cataract Refract Surg.* 2007; 33:1801–5.
698. De Kaspar HM, Kreutzer TC, Aguirre-Romo I, et al. A prospective randomized study to determine the efficacy of preoperative topical levofloxacin in reducing conjunctival bacterial flora. *Am J Ophthalmol.* 2008; 145:136–42.
699. Montan PG, Wejde G, Setterquist H, et al. Prophylactic intracameral cefuroxime: evaluation of safety and kinetics in cataract surgery. *J Cataract Refract Surg.* 2002; 28:982–7.
700. Chisari G, Cavallaro G, Reibaldi M, et al. Presurgical antimicrobial prophylaxis: effect on ocular flora in healthy patients. *Int J Clin Pharmacol Ther.* 2004; 42:35–8.
701. Park SH, Lim JA, Choi JS, et al. The resistance patterns of normal ocular bacterial flora to 4 fluoroquinolone antibiotics. *Cornea.* 2009; 28:68–72.
702. Ciulla TA, Starr MB, Masket S. Bacterial endophthalmitis prophylaxis for cataract surgery: an evidence-based update. *Ophthalmology.* 2002; 109:13–26.
703. Gordon-Bennett P, Karas A, Flanagan D, et al. A survey of measures used for the prevention of postoperative endophthalmitis after cataract surgery in the United Kingdom. *Eye.* 2008; 22:620–7.
704. Ta CN, Singh K, Egbert PR, et al. Prospective comparative evaluation of povidone-iodine (10% for 5 minutes versus 5% for 1 minute) as prophylaxis for ophthalmic surgery. *J Cataract Refract Surg.* 2008; 34:171–2.
705. Cahane M, Ben Simon GJ, Barequet IS, et al. Human corneal stromal tissue concentration after consecutive doses of topically applied 3.3% vancomycin. *Br J Ophthalmol.* 2004; 88:22–4.
706. Bucci FA. An in vivo study comparing the ocular absorption of levofloxacin and ciprofloxacin prior to phacoemulsification. *Am J Ophthalmol.* 2004; 137:308–12.
707. García-Sáenz MC, Arias-Puente A, Fresnadillo-Martinez MJ, et al. Human aqueous humor levels of oral ciprofloxacin, levofloxacin and moxifloxacin. *J Cataract Refract Surg.* 2001; 27:11969–74.
708. Hariprasad SM, Blinder KJ, Shah GK, et al. Penetration pharmacokinetics of topically administered 0.5% moxifloxacin ophthalmic solution in human aqueous and vitreous. *Arch Ophthalmol.* 2005; 123:39–44.
709. Holland EJ, McCarthy M, Holland S. The ocular penetration of levofloxacin 1.5% and gatifloxacin 0.3% ophthalmic solutions in subjects undergoing corneal transplant surgery. *Curr Med Res Opin.* 2007; 23:2955–60.
710. Costello P, Bakri SJ, Beer PM, et al. Vitreous penetration of topical moxifloxacin and gatifloxacin in humans. *Retina.* 2006; 26:191–5.
711. Burka JM, Bower KS, Vanroekel RC, et al. The effect of fourth-generation fluoroquinolones gatifloxacin and moxifloxacin on epithelial healing following photorefractive keratectomy. *Am J Ophthalmol.* 2005; 140:83–7.

712. Durrie DS, Trattler W. A comparison of therapeutic regimens containing moxifloxacin 0.5% ophthalmic solution and gatifloxacin 0.3% ophthalmic solution for surgical prophylaxis in patients undergoing LASIK or LASEK. *J Ocul Pharmacol Ther.* 2005; 21:236–41.
713. Campos M, Ávila M, Wallau A, et al. Efficacy and tolerability of a fixed-dose moxifloxacin-dexamethasone formulation for topical prophylaxis in LASIK: a comparative, double-masked clinical trial. *Clin Ophthalmol.* 2008; 2:331–8.
714. Freitas LL, Soriano E, Muccioli C, et al. Efficacy and tolerability of a combined moxifloxacin/dexamethasone formulation for topical prophylaxis and reduction of inflammation in phacoemulsification: a comparative, double masked clinical trial. *Curr Med Res Opin.* 2007; 23:3123–30.
715. Lane SS, Osher RH, Masket S, et al. Evaluation of the safety of prophylactic intracameral moxifloxacin in cataract surgery. *J Cataract Refract Surg.* 2008; 34:1451–9.
716. Espiritu CR, Caparas VL, Bolinao JG. Safety of prophylactic intracameral moxifloxacin 0.5% ophthalmic solution in cataract surgery patients. *J Cataract Refract Surg.* 2007; 33:63–8.
717. Olson RJ. Reducing the risk of postoperative endophthalmitis. *Surv Ophthalmol.* 2004; 49(suppl 2):s55–61.
718. Yu-Wai-Man P, Morgan SJ, Hildreth AJ, et al. Efficacy of intracameral and subconjunctival cefuroxime in preventing endophthalmitis after cataract surgery. *J Cataract Refract Surg.* 2008; 34:447–51.
719. Vasavada AR, Gajjar D, Raj SM, et al. Comparison of 2 moxifloxacin regimens for preoperative prophylaxis: prospective randomized triple-masked trial. Part 1: aqueous concentration of moxifloxacin. *J Cataract Refract Surg.* 2008; 34:1379–82.
720. Eron LJ. Prevention of infection following orthopedic surgery. *Antibiot Chemother.* 1985; 33:140–64.
721. Gosselin RA, Roberts I, Gillespie WJ. Antibiotics for preventing infection in open limb fractures. *Cochrane Database Syst Rev.* 2004; 1:CD003764.
722. Hauser CJ, Adams CA Jr, Eachempati SR, et al. Surgical Infection Society guideline: prophylactic antibiotic use in open fractures: an evidence-based guideline. *Surg Infect.* 2006; 7:379–405.
723. Jaeger M, Maier D, Kern WV, et al. Antibiotics in trauma and orthopedic surgery—a primer of evidence-based recommendations. *Injury.* 2006; 37:s74–80.
724. Luchette FA, Bone LB, Born CT, et al. Practice management guidelines for prophylactic antibiotic use in open fractures. www.east.org/tpg/openfrac.pdf (accessed 2008 May 26).
725. Whitehouse JD, Friedman ND, Kirkland KB, et al. The impact of surgical-site infections following orthopedic surgery at a community hospital and university hospital: adverse quality of life, excess length of stay and extra cost. *Infect Control Hosp Epidemiol.* 2002; 23:183–9.
726. Boyd RJ, Burke JF, Colton T. A double-blind clinical trial of prophylactic antibiotics in hip fractures. *J Bone Joint Surg.* 1973; 55:1251–8.
727. Sculco TP. The economic impact of infected joint arthroplasty. *Orthopaedics.* 1995; 18:871–3.
728. Kurtz SM, Lau E, Schmier J, et al. Infection burden for hip and knee arthroplasty in the United States. *J Arthroplasty.* 2008; 23:984–91.
729. Bozic KJ, Ries MD. The impact of infection after total hip arthroplasty on hospital and surgeon resource utilization. *J Bone Joint Surg Am.* 2005; 87:1746–51.
730. Hebert CK, Williams RE, Levy RS, et al. Cost of treating an infected total knee replacement. *Clin Orthop Related Res.* 1996; 331:140–5.
731. Anderson DJ, Kaye KS, Schmader KE, et al. Clinical and financial outcomes due to methicillin resistant *Staphylococcus aureus* surgical site infection: a multicenter matched outcomes study. *PLoS One.* 2009; 4:e8305.
732. Brown EM, Path FR, Pople IK, et al. Prevention of postoperative infection in patients undergoing spinal surgery. *Spine.* 2004; 29:938–45.
733. Barker FG II. Efficacy of prophylactic antibiotic therapy in spinal surgery: a meta-analysis. *Neurosurgery.* 2002; 51:391–401.
734. Ericson C, Lidgren L, Lindberg L. Cloxacillin in the prophylaxis of postoperative infections of the hip. *J Bone Joint Surg.* 1973; 55:808–13.
735. Pollard JP, Hughes SP, Scott JE, et al. Antibiotic prophylaxis in total hip replacement. *Br Med J.* 1979; 1:707–9.
736. Burnett JW, Gustilo RB, Williams DN, et al. Prophylactic antibiotics in hip fractures. *J Bone Joint Surg.* 1980; 62:457–62.
737. Tengve B, Kjellander J. Antibiotic prophylaxis in operations on trochanteric femoral fractures. *J Bone Joint Surg.* 1978; 60:97–9.
738. Pavel A, Smith RL, Ballard A, et al. Prophylactic antibiotics in clean orthopedic surgery. *J Bone Joint Surg.* 1974; 56:777–82.
739. Boxma H, Broekhuizen T, Patka P, et al. Randomised controlled trial of single-dose antibiotic prophylaxis in surgical treatment of closed fractures: the Dutch Trauma Trial. *Lancet.* 1996; 347:1133–7.
740. Weinstein MA, McCabe JP, Cammisa FP Jr. Postoperative spinal wound infection: a review of 2,391 consecutive index procedures. *J Spinal Disord.* 2000; 13:422–6.
741. Trampuz A, Zimmerli W. Antimicrobial agents in orthopedic surgery: prophylaxis and treatment. *Drugs.* 2006; 66:1089–105.
742. Yamaguchi K, Adams RA, Morrey BF. Infection after total elbow arthroplasty. *J Bone Joint Surg Am.* 1998; 80:481–91.
743. Bohsali KI, Wirth MA, Rockwood CA Jr. Complications of total shoulder arthroplasty. *J Bone Joint Surg Am.* 2006; 88:2279–92.
744. Meehan J, Jamali AA, Nguyen H. Prophylactic antibiotics in hip and knee arthroplasty. *J Bone Joint Surg Am.* 2009; 91:2480–90.
745. Costerton JW, Stewart PS, Greenberg EP. Bacterial biofilms: a common cause of persistent infections. *Science.* 1999; 284:1318–22.

746. Costerton JW. Biofilm theory can guide the treatment of device-related orthopaedic infections. *Clin Orthop Related Res.* 2005; 437:7–11.
747. Lewis K. Riddle of biofilm resistance. *Antimicrob Agents Chemother.* 2001; 45:999–1007.
748. Matthews PC, Berendt AR, McNally MA, et al. Diagnosis and management of prosthetic joint infection. *BMJ.* 2009; 338:1378–83.
749. Prokuski L. Prophylactic antibiotics in orthopaedic surgery. *J Am Acad Orthop Surg.* 2008; 16:283–93.
750. Gernaat-Van Der Sluis AJ, Hoogenboom-Verdegaal AM, Edixhoven PJ, et al. Prophylactic mupirocin could reduce orthopedic wound infections: 1044 patients treated with mupirocin compared with 1260 historical controls. *Acta Orthop Scand.* 1998; 69:412–4.
751. Wilcox MH, Hall J, Pike H, et al. Use of perioperative mupirocin to prevent methicillin resistant *Staphylococcus aureus* (MRSA) orthopedic surgical site infections. *J Hosp Infect.* 2003; 54:196–201.
752. Coskun D, Aytac J. Decrease in *Staphylococcus aureus* surgical-site infection rates after orthopaedic surgery after intranasal mupirocin ointment. *J Hosp Infect.* 2004; 58:90–1.
753. Van Rijen MM, Bonten M, Wenzel RP, et al. Intranasal mupirocin for reduction of *Staphylococcus aureus* infections in surgical patients with nasal carriage: a systematic review. *J Antimicrob Chemother.* 2008; 61:254–61.
754. Rao N, Cannella B, Crossett LS, et al. A preoperative decolonization protocol for *Staphylococcus aureus* prevents orthopaedic infections. *Clin Orthop Relat Res.* 2008; 466:1343–8.
755. Kim DH, Spencer M, Davidson SM, et al. Institutional prescreening for detection and eradication of methicillin-resistant *Staphylococcus aureus* in patients undergoing elective orthopaedic surgery. *J Bone Joint Surg Am.* 2010; 92:1820–6.
756. Zgonis T, Jolly GP, Garbalosa JC. The efficacy of prophylactic intravenous antibiotics in elective foot and ankle surgery. *J Foot Ankle Surg.* 2004; 43:97–103.
757. Kurzweil PR. Antibiotic prophylaxis for arthroscopic surgery. *Arthroscopy.* 2006; 22:452–4.
758. Wieck JA, Jackson JK, O'Brien TJ, et al. Efficacy of prophylactic antibiotics in arthroscopic surgery. *Orthopedics.* 1997; 20:133–4.
759. Bert JM, Giannini D, Nace L. Antibiotic prophylaxis for arthroscopy of the knee: is it necessary? *Arthroscopy.* 2007; 23:4–6.
760. Babcock HM, Carroll C, Matava M, et al. Surgical site infections after arthroscopy: outbreak investigation and case control study. *Arthroscopy.* 2003; 19:172–81.
761. Olix ML, Klug TJ, Coleman CR, et al. Prophylactic antibiotics in elective operations on bones, joints, and tendons. *Surg Forum.* 1960; 10:818–9.
762. Tachdjian MO, Compere EL. Postoperative wound infections in orthopedic surgery: evaluation and prophylactic antibiotics. *J Int Coll Surg.* 1957; 28:797–805.
763. Beiner JM, Grauer J, Kwon BK, et al. Postoperative wound infections of the spine. *Neurosurg Focus.* 2003; 15:1–5.
764. Labbé AC, Demers AM, Rodrigues R, et al. Surgical-site infection following spinal fusion: a case-control study in a children's hospital. *J Infect Control Hosp Epidemiol.* 2003; 24:591–5.
765. Lonstein J, Winter R, Moe J, et al. Wound infection with Harrington instrumentation and spine fusion for scoliosis. *Clin Orthop Relat Res.* 1973; 96:222–33.
766. Dimick JB, Lipsett PA, Kostuik JP. Spine update: antimicrobial prophylaxis in spine surgery: basic principles and recent advances. *Spine.* 2000; 25:2544–8.
767. Kanafani ZA, Dakdouki GK, El-Dbouni O, et al. Surgical site infections following spinal surgery at a tertiary care center in Lebanon: incidence, microbiology, and risk factors. *Scand J Infect Dis.* 2006; 38:589–92.
768. O'Toole JE, Eichholz KM, Fessler RG. Surgical site infection rates after minimally invasive spinal surgery. *J Neurosurg Spine.* 2009; 11:471–6.
769. Hellbusch LC, Helzer-Julin M, Doran SE, et al. Single-dose vs multiple-dose antibiotic prophylaxis in instrumented lumbar fusion—a prospective study. *Surg Neurol.* 2008; 70:622–7.
770. Pull Ter Gunne AF, van Laarhoven CJ, Cohen DB. Incidence of surgical site infection following adult spinal deformity surgery: an analysis of patient risk. *Eur Spine J.* 2010; 19:982–8.
771. Wimmer C, Gluch H, Franzreb M, et al. Predisposing factors for infection in spine surgery: a survey of 850 spinal procedures. *J Spinal Disord.* 1998; 11:125–8.
772. Friedman ND, Sexton DJ, Connelly SM, et al. Risk factors for surgical site infection complicating laminectomy. *Infect Control Hosp Epidemiol.* 2007; 28:1060–5.
773. Olsen MA, Nepple JJ, Riew D, et al. Risk factors for surgical site infection following orthopaedic spinal operations. *J Bone Joint Surg Am.* 2008; 90:62–9.
774. Hollenbeak CS, Lave JR, Zeddies T, et al. Factors associated with risk of surgical wound infections. *Am J Med Qual.* 2006; 21(suppl):29S–34S.
775. Pull Ter Gunne AF, Cohen DB. Incidence, prevalance, and analysis of risk factors for surgical site infection following adult spinal surgery. *Spine.* 2009; 34:1422–8.
776. Fang A, Hu SS, Endres N, et al. Risk factors for infection after spinal surgery. *Spine.* 2005; 30:1460–5.
777. Patel N, Bagan B, Vadera S, et al. Obesity and spine surgery: relations to perioperative complications. *J Neurosurg Spine.* 2007; 6:291–7.
778. Petignat C, Francioli P, Harbarth S, et al. Cefuroxime prophylaxis is effective in noninstrumented spine surgery: a double-blind, placebo-controlled study. *Spine.* 2008; 33:1919–24.
779. Walters R, Moore R, Fraser R. Penetration of cefazolin in human lumbar intervertebral disk. *Spine.* 2006; 31:567–70.
780. Rimoldi RL, Haye W. The use of antibiotics for wound prophylaxis in spinal surgery. *Orthop Clin North Am.* 1996; 27:47–52.
781. American Academy of Orthopaedic Surgeons. Information statement: the use of prophylactic antibiotics in orthopaedic medicine and the emergence of vancomycin-resistant bacteria. www.aaos.org/about/papers/advistmt/1016.asp (accessed 2008 May 13).

782. Dobzyniak MA, Fischgrund JS, Hankins S, et al. Single versus multiple dose antibiotic prophylaxis in lumbar disc surgery. *Spine.* 2003; 28:453–5.
783. Milstone AM, Maragakis LL, Townsend T, et al. Timing of preoperative antibiotic prophylaxis: a modifiable risk factor for deep surgical site infections after pediatric spinal fusion. *Pediatr Infect Dis J.* 2008; 27:704–8.
784. Coe JD, Smithe JS, Berven S, et al. Complications of spinal fusion for Scheuermann kyphosis: a report of the Scoliosis Research Society Morbidity and Mortality Committee. *Spine.* 2010; 35:99–103.
785. Linam WM, Margolis PA, Staat MA, et al. Risk factors associated with surgical site infection after pediatric posterior spinal fusion procedure. *Infect Control Hosp Epidemiol.* 2009; 30:109–16.
786. Fitzgerald RH. Infections of hip prosthesis and artificial joints. *Infect Dis Clin North Am.* 1989; 3:329–38.
787. Southwell-Keely JP, Russo RR, App B, et al. Antibiotic prophylaxis in hip fracture surgery: a meta-analysis. *Clin Orthop Relat Res.* 2004; 410:179–84.
788. Gillespie WJ, Walenkamp G. Antibiotic prophylaxis for surgery for proximal femoral and other closed long bone fractures. *Cochrane Database Syst Rev.* 2001; 1:CD000244.
789. Hahnel J, Burdekin H, Anand S. Re-admissions following hip fracture surgery. *Ann R Coll Surg Engl.* 2009; 91:591–5.
790. Gulihar A, Nixon M, Jenkins D, et al. *Clostridium difficile* in hip fracture patients: prevention, treatment and associated mortality. *Injury.* 2009; 40:746–51.
791. Cunha BA, Gossling HR, Pasternak HS, et al. The penetration characteristics of cefazolin, cephalothin, and cephradine into bone in patients undergoing total hip replacement. *J Bone Joint Surg.* 1977; 59:856–9.
792. Starks I, Ayub G, Walley G, et al. Single-dose cefuroxime with gentamicin reduces *Clostridium difficile*-associated disease in hip-fracture patients. *J Hosp Infect.* 2008; 70:21–6.
793. DeFrances CJ, Hall MJ. 2005 National Hospital Discharge Survey. *Adv Data.* 2007; 385:1–19.
794. Glazebrook MA, Arsenault K, Dunbar M. Evidence-based classification of complications in total ankle arthroplasty. *Foot Ankle Int.* 2009; 30:945–9.
795. Gougoulias N, Khanna A, Maffulli N. How successful are current ankle replacements? A systematic review of the literature. *Clin Orthop Relat Res.* 2010; 468:199–208.
796. Blom AW, Brown J, Taylor AH, et al. Infection after total knee arthroplasty. *J Bone Joint Surg Br.* 2004; 86:688–91.
797. Kasten MD, Skinner HB. Total elbow arthroplasty. An 18-year experience. *Clin Orthop Relat Res.* 1993; 290:177–88.
798. Periti P, Stringa G, Mini E, et al. Comparative multicenter trial of teicoplanin versus cefazolin for antimicrobial prophylaxis in prosthetic joint implant surgery. *Eur J Clin Microbiol Infect Dis.* 1999; 18:113–9.
799. Minnema B, Vearncombe M, Augustin A, et al. Risk factors for surgical-site infection following primary total knee arthroplasty. *Infect Control Hosp Epidemiol.* 2004; 25:477–80.
800. Blom AW, Taylor AH, Pattison G, et al. Infection after total hip arthroplasty. *J Bone Joint Surg Br.* 2003; 85:956–9.
801. AlBuhairan B, Hind D, Hutchinson A. Antibiotic prophylaxis for wound infections in total joint arthroplasty. *J Bone Joint Surg Br.* 2008; 90:915–9.
802. Fish DN, Hoffman HM, Danziger LH. Antibiotic impregnated cement use in U.S. hospitals. *Am J Hosp Pharm.* 1992; 49:2469–74.
803. Malik MH, Gambhir AK, Bale L, et al. Primary total hip replacement: a comparison of a nationally agreed guide to practice and current surgical technique as determined by the North West Regional Arthroplasty Registry. *Ann R Coll Surg Engl.* 2004; 86:113–8.
804. Bourne RB. Prophylactic use of antibiotic bone cement: an emerging standard—in the affirmative. *J Arthroplasty.* 2004; 19(suppl 1):69–72.
805. Engesaeter LB, Lie SA, Espehaug B, et al. Antibiotic prophylaxis in total hip arthroplasty: effects of antibiotic prophylaxis systemically and in bone cement on the revision rate of 22,170 primary hip replacements followed 0 to 14 years in the Norwegian Arthroplasty Register. *Acta Orthop Scand.* 2003; 74:644–51.
806. Espehaug B, Engesaeter LB, Vollset SE, et al. Antibiotic prophylaxis in total hip arthroplasty: review of 10,905 primary cemented total hip replacements reported to the Norwegian Arthroplasty Register, 1987 to 1995. *J Bone Joint Surg Br.* 1997; 79:590–5.
807. Jiranek WA, Hanssen AD, Greenwald AS. Antibiotic-loaded bone cement for infection prophylaxis in total joint replacement. *J Bone Joint Surg.* 2006; 88:2487–500.
808. McQueen MM, Hughes SP, May P, et al. Cefuroxime in total joint arthroplasty. Intravenous or in bone cement. *J Arthroplasty.* 1990; 5:169–72.
809. Josefsson G, Kolmert L. Prophylaxis with systematic antibiotics versus gentamicin bone cement in total hip arthroplasty. A ten-year survey of 1,688 hips. *Clin Orthop Relat Res.* 1993; 292:210–4.
810. Hanssen AD, Osmon DR. The use of prophylactic antimicrobial agents during and after hip arthroplasty. *Clin Orthop Relat Res.* 1999; 369:124–38.
811. Jiranek W. Antibiotic-loaded cement in total hip replacement: current indications, efficacy, and complications. *Orthopedics.* 2005; 28(suppl):s873–7.
812. Diefenbeck M, Mückley T, Hofman GO. Prophylaxis and treatment of implant-related infections by local application of antibiotics. *Injury.* 2006; 37(suppl 2):S95–104.
813. Hanssen AD. Prophylactic use of antibiotic bone cement: an emerging standard—in opposition. *J Arthroplasty.* 2004; 19(suppl 1):73–7.
814. Block JE, Stubbs HA. Reducing the risk of deep wound infection in primary joint arthroplasty with antibiotic bone cement. *Orthopedics.* 2005; 28:1334–45.
815. Wininger DA, Fass RJ. Antibiotic-impregnated cement and beads for orthopedic infections. *Antimicrob Chemother.* 1996; 40:2675–9.

816. Nelson CL, Green TG, Porter RA, et al. One day versus seven days of preventive antibiotic therapy in orthopedic surgery. *Clin Orthop Relat Res.* 1983; 176:258–63.
817. Matsumoto T, Kiyota H, Matsukawa M, et al. Japanese guidelines for prevention of perioperative infections in urological field. *Int J Urol.* 2007; 14:890–909.
818. Wolf JS Jr, Bennett CJ, Dmochowski RR, et al. Best practice policy statement on urologic surgery antimicrobial prophylaxis. *J Urol.* 2008; 179:1379–90.
819. Kapoor DA, Klimberg IW, Malek GH, et al. Single-dose oral ciprofloxacin versus placebo for prophylaxis during transrectal prostate biopsy. *Urology.* 1998; 52:552–8.
820. Latthe PM, Foon R, Toozs-Hobson P. Prophylactic antibiotics in urodynamics: a systematic review of effectiveness and safety. *Neurourol Urodyn.* 2008; 27:167–73.
821. Kartal ED, Yenilmez A, Kiremitci A, et al. Effectiveness of ciprofloxacin prophylaxis in preventing bacteriuria caused by urodynamic study: a blind, randomized study of 192 patients. *Urology.* 2006; 67:1149–53.
822. Wagenlehner FM, Wagenlehner C, Schinzel S, et al. Prospective, randomized, multicentric, open, comparative study on the efficacy of a prophylactic single dose of 500 mg levofloxacin versus 1920 mg trimethoprim/sulfamethoxazole versus a control group in patients undergoing TUR of the prostate. *Eur Urol.* 2005; 47:549–56.
823. Takeyama K, Takahashi S, Maeda T, et al. Comparison of 1-day, 2-day, and 3-day administration of antimicrobial prophylaxis in radical prostatectomy. *J Infect Chemother.* 2007; 13:320–3.
824. Briffaux R, Coloby P, Bruyere F, et al. One preoperative dose randomized against 3-day antibiotic prophylaxis for transrectal ultrasonography-guided prostate biopsy. *BJU Int.* 2008; 103:1069–73.
825. Bootsma AM, Pes MP, Geerlings SE, et al. Antibiotic prophylaxis in urologic procedures: a systematic review. *Eur Urol.* 2008; 54:1270–86.
826. Grabe M, Bishop MC, Bjerklund-Johansen TE, et al. Guidelines on urological infections. www.uroweb.org (accessed 2010 Mar 18).
827. Yamamoto S, Kanamaru S, Kunishima Y, et al. Perioperative antimicrobial prophylaxis in urology: a multi-center prospective study. *J Chemother.* 2005; 17:189–97.
828. Hamasuna R, Betsunoh H, Sueyoshi T, et al. Bacteria of preoperative urinary tract infections contaminate the surgical fields and develop surgical site infections in urologic operations. *Int J Urol.* 2004; 11:941–7.
829. Richter S, Lang R, Zur F, et al. Infected urine as a risk factor for postprostatectomy wound infection. *Infect Control Hosp Epidemiol.* 1991; 12:147–9.
830. Carson CC. Diagnosis, treatment and prevention of penile prosthesis infection. *Int J Impot Res.* 2003; 15(suppl 5):S139–46.
831. Schaeffer AJ, Montorsi F, Scattoni V, et al. Comparison of a 3-day with a 1-day regimen of an extended-release formulation of ciprofloxacin as antimicrobial prophylaxis for patients undergoing transrectal needle biopsy of the prostate. *BJU Int.* 2007; 100:51–7.
832. Hara N, Kitamura Y, Saito T, et al. Perioperative antibiotics in radical cystectomy with ileal conduit urinary diversion: efficacy and risk of antimicrobial prophylaxis on the operation day alone. *Int J Urol.* 2008; 15:511–5.
833. Meir DB, Livne PM. Is prophylactic antimicrobial treatment necessary after hypospadias repair? *J Urol.* 2004; 171:2621–2.
834. Doğan HS, Şahin A, Çetinkaya Y, et al. Antibiotic prophylaxis in percutaneous nephrolithotomy: prospective study in 81 patients. *J Endourol.* 2002; 16:649–53.
835. Cox CE. Comparison of intravenous ciprofloxacin and intravenous cefotaxime for antimicrobial prophylaxis in transurethral surgery. *Am J Med.* 1989; 87(suppl 5A):252S–254S.
836. Cam K, Kayikci A, Akman Y, et al. Prospective assessment of the efficacy of single dose versus traditional 3-day antimicrobial prophylaxis in 12-core transrectal prostate biopsy. *Int J Urol.* 2008; 18:997–1001.
837. Aron M, Rajeev TP, Gupta NP. Antibiotic prophylaxis for transrectal needle biopsy of the prostate: a randomized controlled study. *BJU Int.* 2000; 85:682–5.
838. Isen K, Küpeli B, Sinik Z, et al. Antibiotic prophylaxis for transrectal biopsy of the prostate: a prospective randomized study of the prophylactic use of single dose oral fluoroquinolone versus trimethoprim-sulfamethoxazole. *Int Urol Nephrol.* 1999; 31:491–5.
839. Johnson MI, Merrilees D, Robson WA, et al. Oral ciprofloxacin or trimethoprim reduces bacteriuria after flexible cystoscopy. *BJU Int.* 2007; 100:826–9.
840. Yokoyama M, Fujii Y, Yoshida S, et al. Discarding antimicrobial prophylaxis for transurethral resection of bladder tumor: a feasibility study. *Int J Urol.* 2009; 16:61–3.
841. Takeyama K, Matsukawa M, Kunishima Y, et al. Incidence of and risk factors for surgical site infections in patients with radical cystectomy with urinary diversion. *J Infect Chemother.* 2005; 11:177–81.
842. Gomelsky A, Dmochowski RR. Antibiotic prophylaxis in urologic prosthetic surgery. *Curr Pharm Des.* 2003; 9:989–96.
843. Hoffelt SC, Wallner K, Merrick G. Epididymitis after prostate brachytherapy. *Urology.* 2004; 63:293–6.
844. Ferguson KH, McNeil JJ, Morey AF. Mechanical and antibiotic bowel preparation for urinary diversion surgery. *J Urol.* 2002; 167:2352–6.
845. Pearle MS, Roehrborn CG. Antimicrobial prophylaxis prior to shock wave lithotripsy in patients with sterile urine before treatment: a meta-analysis and cost-effectiveness analysis. *Urology.* 1997; 49:679–86.
846. Berry A, Barratt A. Prophylactic antibiotic use in transurethral prostatic resection: a meta analysis. *J Urol.* 2002; 167:571–7.
847. Qiang W, Jianchen W, MacDonald R, et al. Antibiotic prophylaxis for transurethral prostatic resection in men with preoperative urine containing less than 100,000 bacteria per ml: a systematic review. *J Urol.* 2005; 173:1175–81.
848. Knopf HJ, Graff H, Schulze H. Perioperative antibiotic prophylaxis in ureteroscopic stone removal. *Eur Urol.* 2003; 44:115–8.

849. Brewster SF, MacGowan AP, Gingell JC. Antimicrobial prophylaxis for transrectal prostatic biopsy: a prospective, randomized trial of cefuroxime versus piperacillin/tazobactam. *Br J Urol.* 1995; 76:351–4.
850. DeBessonet DA, Merlin AS. Antibiotic prophylaxis in elective genitourinary tract surgery: a comparison of single-dose preoperative cefotaxime and multiple-dose cefoxitin. *J Antimicrob Chemother.* 1984; 14(suppl B):271–5.
851. Christiano AP, Hollowell CM, Kim H, et al. Double-blind randomized comparison of single-dose ciprofloxacin versus intravenous cefazolin in patients undergoing outpatient endourologic surgery. *Urology.* 2000; 55:182–5.
852. Bhatia NN, Karram MM, Bergman A. Role of antibiotic prophylaxis in retropubic surgery for stress urinary incontinence. *Obstet Gynecol.* 1989; 74:637–9.
853. Terai A, Ichioka K, Kohei N, et al. Antibiotic prophylaxis in radical prostatectomy: 1-day versus 4-day treatments. *Int J Urol.* 2006; 13:1488–93.
854. Gombert ME, DuBouchet L, Aulicino TM, et al. Brief report: intravenous ciprofloxacin versus cefotaxime prophylaxis during transurethral surgery. *Am J Med.* 1989; 87(suppl 5A): 250S–251S.
855. Klimberg IW, Malek GH, Cox CE. Single-dose oral ciprofloxacin compared with cefotaxime and placebo for prophylaxis during transurethral surgery. *J Antimicrob Chemother.* 1999; 43(suppl A):77–84.
856. Gibbons RP, Stark RA, Gorrea RJ, et al. The prophylactic use—or misuse—of antibiotics in transurethral prostatectomy. *J Urol.* 1978; 119:381–3.
857. Ramsey E, Sheth NK. Antibiotic prophylaxis in patients undergoing prostatectomy. *Urology.* 1983; 21:376–8.
858. Cormio L, Berardi B, Callea A, et al. Antimicrobial prophylaxis for transrectal prostatic biopsy: a prospective study of ciprofloxacin vs. piperacillin/tazobactam. *BJU Int.* 2002; 90:700–2.
859. Sakura M, Kawakami S, Yoshida S, et al. Prospective comparative study of single dose versus 3-day administration of antimicrobial prophylaxis in minimum incision endoscopic radical prostatectomy. *Int J Urol.* 2008; 15:328–31.
860. Hills NH, Bultitude MI, Eykyn S. Co-trimoxazole in prevention of bacteriuria after prostatectomy. *Br Med J.* 1976; 2:498–9.
861. Matthew AD, Gonzales R, Jeffords D, et al. Prevention of bacteriuria after transurethral prostatectomy with nitrofurantoin macrocrystals. *J Urol.* 1978; 120:442–3.
862. Hammarsten J, Lindqvist K. Norfloxacin as prophylaxis against urethral strictures following transurethral resection of the prostate: an open, prospective, randomized study. *J Urol.* 1993; 150:1722–4.
863. Siracusano S, Knez R, Tiberio A, et al. The usefulness of antibiotic prophylaxis in invasive urodynamics in postmenopausal female subjects. *Int Urogynecol J.* 2008; 19:939–42.
864. Patel U, Kirby R. Infections after prostate biopsy and antibiotic resistance. *BJU Int.* 2008; 101:1201–4.
865. Hall JC, Christiansen KJ, England P, et al. Antibiotic prophylaxis for patients undergoing transurethral resection of the prostate. *Urology.* 1996; 47:852–6.
866. Liu GG, Nguyen T, Nichol MB. An economic analysis of antimicrobial prophylaxis against urinary tract infection in patients undergoing transurethral resection of the prostate. *Clin Ther.* 1999; 21:1589–603.
867. Burnakis TG. Surgical antimicrobial prophylaxis: principles and guidelines. *Pharmacotherapy.* 1984; 4:248–71.
868. Homer-Vanniasinkam S. Surgical site and vascular infections: treatment and prophylaxis. *Int J Infect Dis.* 2007; 11:S17–22.
869. Zibari GB, Gadallah MF, Landreneau M, et al. Preoperative vancomycin prophylaxis decreases incidence of postoperative hemodialysis vascular access infections. *Am J Kidney Dis.* 1997; 30:343–8.
870. Naylor AR, Payne D, London NJ, et al. Prosthetic patch infection after carotid endarterectomy. *Eur J Vasc Endovasc Surg.* 2002; 23:11–6.
871. Richet HM, Chidiac C, Prat A, et al. Analysis of risk factors for surgical wound infections following vascular surgery. *Am J Med.* 1991; 91:171S–172S.
872. Ross CB, Wheeler WG II, Jones MJ, et al. Ceftriaxone versus cefazolin in peripheral arterial operations: a randomized, prospective trial. *South Med J.* 1997; 90:16–22.
873. Ryan JM, Ryan BM, Smith TP. Antibiotic prophylaxis in interventional radiology. *J Vasc Interv Radiol.* 2004; 15:547–56.
874. McDermott VG, Schuster MG, Smith TP. Antibiotic prophylaxis in vascular and interventional radiology. *Am J Roentgenol.* 1997; 169:31–8.
875. Beddy P, Ryan JM. Antibiotic prophylaxis in interventional radiology—anything new? *Tech Vasc Interv Radiol.* 2006; 9:69–76.
876. Malek AM, Higashida RT, Reilly LM, et al. Subclavian arteritis and pseudoaneurysm formation secondary to stent infection. *Cardiovasc Interv Radiol.* 2000; 23:57–60.
877. Venkatesan AM, Kundu S, Sacks D, et al. Practice guideline for adult antibiotic prophylaxis during vascular and interventional radiology procedures. *J Vasc Interv Radiol.* 2010; 21:1611–30.
878. Thompson M. An audit demonstrating a reduction in MRSA infection in a specialized vascular unit resulting from a change in infection control protocol. *Eur J Vasc Endovasc Surg.* 2006; 31:609–15.
879. Morange-Saussier V, Giraudeau B, van der Mee N, et al. Nasal carriage of methicillin-resistant *Staphylococcus aureus* in vascular surgery. *Ann Vasc Surg.* 2006; 20:767–72.
880. Taylor MD, Napolitano LM. Methicillin-resistant *Staphylococcus aureus* infections in vascular surgery: increasing prevalence. *Surg Infect.* 2004; 5:180–7.
881. Grimble SA, Magee TR, Galland RB. Methicillin resistant *Staphylococcus aureus* in patients undergoing major amputation. *Eur J Vasc Endovasc Surg.* 2001; 22:215–8.
882. Nasim A, Thompson MM, Naylor AR, et al. The impact of MRSA on vascular surgery. *Eur J Vasc Endovasc Surg.* 2001; 22:211–4.
883. Cowie SE, Ma I, Lee SK, et al. Nosocomial MRSA infection in vascular surgery patients: impact

on patient outcome. *Vasc Endovasc Surg.* 2005; 39:327–34.

884. Fawley WN, Parnell P, Hall J, et al. Surveillance for mupirocin resistance following introduction of routine peri-operative prophylaxis with nasal mupirocin. *J Hosp Infect.* 2006; 62:327–32.
885. Kaiser A, Clayton KR, Mulherin JL, et al. Antibiotic prophylaxis in vascular surgery. *Ann Surg.* 1978; 188:283–9.
886. Edwards WH, Kaiser AB, Kernodle DS, et al. Cefuroxime versus cefazolin as prophylaxis in vascular surgery. *J Vasc Surg.* 1992; 15:35–42.
887. Edwards WH Jr, Kaiser AB, Tapper S, et al. Cefamandole versus cefazolin in vascular surgical wound infection prophylaxis: cost-effectiveness and risk factors. *J Vasc Surg.* 1993; 18:470–5.
888. Hasselgren PO, Ivarson L, Risberg B, et al. Effects of prophylactic antibiotics in vascular surgery. A prospective, randomized, double-blind study. *Ann Surg.* 1984; 200:86–92.
889. Risberg B, Drott C, Dalman P, et al. Oral ciprofloxacin versus intravenous cefuroxime as prophylaxis against postoperative infection in vascular surgery: a randomized double-blind, prospective multicentre study. *Eur J Endovasc Surg.* 1995; 10:346–51.
890. Stewart AH, Eyers PS, Earnshaw JJ. Prevention of infection in peripheral arterial reconstruction: a systematic review and meta-analysis. *J Vasc Surg.* 2007; 46:148–55.
891. Murray BE. Problems and dilemmas of antimicrobial resistance. *Pharmacotherapy.* 1992; 12:86–93.
892. Earnshaw JJ, Slack RC, Hopkinson BR, et al. Risk factors in vascular surgical sepsis. *Ann R Coll Surg Engl.* 1988; 70:139–43.
893. Hall JC, Christiansen KJ, Goodman M, et al. Duration of antimicrobial prophylaxis in vascular surgery. *Am J Surg.* 1998; 175:87–90.
894. Fishman JA. Infection in solid-organ transplant recipients. *N Engl J Med.* 2007; 357:2601–14.
895. Fischer SA. Infections in the transplant recipient. *Med Health R I.* 2002; 85:125–7.
896. Soave R. Prophylaxis strategies for solid-organ transplantation. *Clin Infect Dis.* 2001; 33(suppl 1):s26–31.
897. Keough WL, Michaels MG. Infectious complications in pediatric solid organ transplantation. *Pediatr Clin North Am.* 2003; 50:1451–69.
898. United Network for Organ Sharing. Organ Procurement and Transplantation Network data (as of September 5, 2008). http://optn.transplant.hrsa.gov/data/ (accessed 2012 Dec 9).
899. Cai J. Thoracic transplantation in the United States: an analysis of UNOS registry data. *Clin Transplant.* 2006; 41–56.
900. Fong I, Baker C, McKee D. The value of prophylactic antibiotics in aorta-coronary bypass operations. *J Thorac Cardiovasc Surg.* 1979; 78:908–13.
901. Penketh A, Wansbrough-Jones M, Wright E, et al. Antibiotic prophylaxis for coronary artery bypass graft surgery. *Lancet.* 1985; 1:1500.
902. Muñoz P, Menasalvas A, Bernaldo de Quirós JC, et al. Postsurgical mediastinitis: a case-control study. *Clin Infect Dis.* 1997; 25:1060–4.
903. Filsoufi F, Rahmanian PB, Castillo JG, et al. Incidence, treatment strategies and outcome of deep sternal wound infection after orthotopic heart transplantation. *J Heart Lung Transplant.* 2007; 26:1084–90.
904. Abid Q, Nkere UU, Hasan A, et al. Mediastinitis in heart and lung transplantation: 15 years experience. *Ann Thorac Surg.* 2003; 75:1565–71.
905. Carrier M, Perrault LP, Pellerin M, et al. Sternal wound infection after heart transplantation: incidence and results with aggressive surgical treatment. *Ann Thorac Surg.* 2001; 72:719–24.
906. Ramos A, Asensio A, Muñoz E, et al. Incisional surgical infection in heart transplantation. *Transpl Infect Dis.* 2008; 10:298–302.
907. Sénéchal M, LePrince P, Tezenas du Montcel S, et al. Bacterial mediastinitis after heart transplantation: clinical presentation, risk factors and treatment. *J Heart Lung Transplant.* 2004; 23:165–70.
908. Mattner F, Fischer S, Weissbrodt H, et al. Post-operative nosocomial infections after lung and heart transplantation. *J Heart Lung Transplant.* 2007; 26:241–9.
909. Van De Beek D, Kremer WK, Del Pozo JL, et al. Effect of infectious diseases on outcome after heart transplant. *Mayo Clin Proc.* 2008; 83:304–8.
910. Keay S. Cardiac transplantation: pre-transplant infectious diseases evaluation and post-transplant prophylaxis. *Curr Infect Dis Rep.* 2002; 4:285–92.
911. Kaiser AB. Use of antibiotics in cardiac and thoracic surgery. In: Sabiston DC Jr, Spencer FC, eds. Surgery of the chest. 6th ed. Philadelphia: W. B. Saunders; 1995:98–116.
912. Khaghani A, Martin M, Fitzgerald M, et al. Cefotaxime and flucloxacillin as antibiotic prophylaxis in cardiac transplantation. *Drugs.* 1988; 35(suppl 2):124–6.
913. Montoya JG, Giraldo LF, Efron B, et al. Infectious complications among 620 consecutive heart transplant patients at Stanford University Medical Center. *Clin Infect Dis.* 2001; 33:629–40.
914. Petri WA Jr. Infections in heart transplant recipients. *Clin Infect Dis.* 1994; 18:141–8.
915. Trulock EP. Lung transplantation. *Am J Respir Crit Care Med.* 1997; 155:789–818.
916. U.S. Department of Health and Human Services. Organ Procurement and Transplantation Network/ Scientific Registry of Transplant Recipients annual report. Table 12.4. Transplant recipient characteristics, 1999 to 2008. Recipients of deceased donor lungs. 2009 May 4. http://optn.transplant.hrsa.gov/ar2009/1204_rec-dgn_lu.htm (accessed 2011 Mar 17).
917. Hosenpud JD, Novick RJ, Bennett LE, et al. The registry of the International Society for Heart and Lung Transplantation: thirteenth official report. *J Heart Lung Transplant.* 1996; 15:655–74.
918. Davis RD Jr, Pasque MK. Pulmonary transplantation. *Ann Surg.* 1995; 221:14–28.
919. Kotloff RM, Zuckerman JB. Lung transplantation for cystic fibrosis. Special considerations. *Chest.* 1996; 109:787–98.
920. Campos S, Caramori M, Teixeira R, et al. Bacterial and fungal pneumonia after lung transplantation. *Transplant Proc.* 2008; 40:822–4.

921. Krishnam MS, Suh RD, Tomasian A, et al. Postoperative complications of lung transplantation: radiologic findings along a time continuum. *Radiographics.* 2007; 27:957–74.

922. Helmi M, Love RB, Welter D, et al. *Aspergillus* infection in lung transplant recipients with cystic fibrosis: risk factors and outcomes comparison to other types of transplant recipients. *Chest.* 2003; 123:800–8.

923. Russo MJ, Iribarne A, Hong KN, et al. High lung allocation score is associated with increased morbidity and mortality following transplantation. *Chest.* 2010; 137:651–7.

924. Dowling RD, Zenati M, Yousem S, et al. Donor-transmitted pneumonia in experimental lung allografts. *J Thorac Cardiovasc Surg.* 1992; 103:767–72.

925. Low DE, Kaiser LR, Haydock DA, et al. The donor lung: infectious and pathologic factors affecting outcome in lung transplantation. *J Thorac Cardiovasc Surg.* 1993; 106:614–21.

926. Steinbach S, Sun L, Jiang RZ, et al. Transmissibility of *Pseudomonas cepacia* infection in clinic patients and lung-transplant recipients with cystic fibrosis. *N Engl J Med.* 1994; 331:981–7.

927. Dauber JH, Paradis IL, Dummer JS. Infectious complications in pulmonary allograft recipients. *Clin Chest Med.* 1990; 11:291–308.

928. Deusch E, End A, Grimm M, et al. Early bacterial infections in lung transplant recipients. *Chest.* 1993; 104:1412–6.

929. Paradis IL, Williams P. Infection after lung transplantation. *Semin Respir Infect.* 1993; 8:207–15.

930. Husain S, Zaldonis D, Kusne S, et al. Variation in antifungal prophylaxis strategies in lung transplantation. *Transpl Infect Dis.* 2006; 8:213–8.

931. Noyes BE, Kurland G, Orenstein DM. Lung and heart-lung transplantation in children. *Pediatr Pulmonol.* 1997; 23:39–48.

932. Moreno R, Berenguer M. Post-liver transplantation medical complications. *Ann Hepatol.* 2006; 5:77–85.

933. Muiesan P, Vergani D, Mieli-Vergani G. Liver transplantation in children. *J Hepatol.* 2007; 46:340–8.

934. United Network for Organ Sharing. Organ Procurement and Transplantation Network: data. **http://optn.transplant.hrsa.gov/data/**. Based on OPTN data as of September 26, 2008.

935. García Prado ME, Matia EC, Ciuro FP, et al. Surgical site infection in liver transplant recipients: impact of the type of perioperative prophylaxis. *Transplantation.* 2008; 85:1849–54.

936. Kuo PC, Bartlett ST, Lim JW, et al. Selective bowel decontamination in hospitalized patients awaiting liver transplantation. *Am J Surg.* 1997; 174:745–9.

937. Kim YJ, Kim SI, Wie SH, et al. Infectious complications in living-donor liver transplant recipients: a 9-year single-center experience. *Transplant Infect Dis.* 2008; 10:316–24.

938. Hollenbeak CS, Alfrey EJ, Souba WW. The effect of surgical site infections on outcomes and resource utilization after liver transplantation. *Surgery.* 2001; 130:388–95.

939. Kibbler CC. Infections in liver transplantation: risk factors and strategies for prevention. *J Hosp Infect.* 1995; 30(suppl):209–17.

940. Wade JJ, Rolando N, Hayllar K, et al. Bacterial and fungal infections after liver transplantation: an analysis of 284 patients. *Hepatology.* 1995; 21:1328–36.

941. Shepherd RW, Turmelle Y, Nadler M, et al. Risk factors for rejection and infection in pediatric liver transplantation. *Am J Transplant.* 2008; 8:396–403.

942. Hollenbeak CS, Alfrey EJ, Sheridan K, et al. Surgical site infections following pediatric liver transplantation: risks and costs. *Transpl Infect Dis.* 2003; 5:72–8.

943. Arnow PM, Carandang GC, Zabner R, et al. Randomized controlled trial of selective bowel decontamination for prevention of infections following liver transplantation. *Clin Infect Dis.* 1996; 22:997–1003.

944. Colonna JO II, Drew WJ, Brill JE, et al. Infectious complications in liver transplantation. *Arch Surg.* 1988; 123:360–4.

945. George DL, Arnow PM, Fox AS, et al. Bacterial infection as a complication of liver transplantation: epidemiology and risk factors. *Rev Infect Dis.* 1991; 13:387–96.

946. Uemoto S, Tanaka K, Fujita S, et al. Infectious complications in living related liver transplantation. *J Pediatr Surg.* 1994; 29:514–7.

947. Kusne S, Dummer JS, Singh N, et al. Infections after liver transplantation. An analysis of 101 consecutive cases. *Medicine.* 1988; 67:132–43.

948. Singh N, Paterson DL, Gayowski T, et al. Predicting bacteremia and bacteremic mortality in liver transplant recipients. *Liver Transpl.* 2000; 6:54–61.

949. Hjortrup A, Rasmussen A, Hansen BA, et al. Early bacterial and fungal infections in liver transplantation after oral selective bowel decontamination. *Transplant Proc.* 1997; 29:3106–10.

950. Villacian JS, Paya CV. Prevention of infections in solid organ transplant recipients. *Transpl Infect Dis.* 1999; 1:50–64.

951. Asensio A, Ramos A, Cuervas-Mons V, et al. Effect of antibiotic prophylaxis on the risk of surgical site infection in orthotopic liver transplant. *Liver Transpl.* 2008; 14:799–805.

952. Arnow PM, Zachary KC, Thistlethwaite JR, et al. Pathogenesis of early operative site infections after orthotopic liver transplantation. *Transplantation.* 1998; 65:1500–3.

953. Mattner F, Kola A, Fischer S, et al. Impact of bacterial and fungal donor organ contamination in lung, heart-lung, heart and liver transplantation. *Infection.* 2008; 36:207–12.

954. Barkholt LM, Andersson J, Ericzon BG, et al. Stool cultures obtained before liver transplantation are useful for choice of perioperative antibiotic prophylaxis. *Transplant Int.* 1997; 10:432–8.

955. Hellinger WC, Yao JD, Alvarez S, et al. A randomized, prospective, double-blinded evaluation of selective bowel decontamination in liver transplantation. *Transplantation.* 2002; 73:1904–9.

956. Zwaveling JH, Maring JK, Klompmaker IJ, et al. Selective decontamination of the digestive tract to prevent

postoperative infection: a randomized placebo-controlled trial in liver transplant patients. *Crit Care Med.* 2002; 30:1204–9.

957. Hashimoto M, Sugawara Y, Tamura S, et al. Impact of new methicillin-resistant *Staphylococcus aureus* carriage postoperatively after living donor liver transplantation. *Transplant Proc.* 2007; 39:3271–5.
958. Hashimoto M, Sugawara Y, Tamura S, et al. Bloodstream infection after living donor liver transplantation. *Scand J Infect Dis.* 2008; 40:509–16.
959. Hashimoto M, Sugawara Y, Tamura S, et al. *Pseudomonas aeruginosa* infection after living-donor liver transplantation in adults. *Transpl Infect Dis.* 2009; 11:11–9.
960. Bert F, Galdbart JO, Zarrouk V, et al. Association between nasal carriage of *Staphylococcus aureus* and infection in liver transplant recipients. *Clin Infect Dis.* 2000; 31:1295–9.
961. Bert F, Bellier C, Lassel L, et al. Risk factors for *Staphylococcus aureus* infection in liver transplant recipients. *Liver Transpl.* 2005; 11:1093–9.
962. Chang FY, Singh N, Gayowski T, et al. *Staphylococcus aureus* nasal colonization and association with infections in liver transplant recipients. *Transplantation.* 1998; 65:1169–72.
963. Mehrabi A, Fonouni H, Wente M, et al. Wound complications following kidney and liver transplantation. *Clin Transplant.* 2006; 20(suppl 17):97–110.
964. Kawecki D, Chmura A, Pacholczyk M, et al. Surgical site infections in liver recipients in the early posttransplantation period: etiological agents and susceptibility profiles. *Transplant Proc.* 2007; 39:2800–6.
965. Bedini A, Codeluppi M, Cocchi S, et al. Gram-positive bloodstream infections in liver transplant recipients: incidence, risk factors, and impact on survival. *Transplant Proc.* 2007; 39:1947–9.
966. Dar FS, Faraj W, Zaman MB, et al. Outcome of liver transplantation in hereditary hemochromatosis. *Transplant Int.* 2009; 22:717–24.
967. Arnow PM, Furmaga K, Flaherty JP, et al. Microbiological efficacy and pharmacokinetics of prophylactic antibiotics in liver transplant patients. *Antimicrob Agents Chemother.* 1992; 36:2125–30.
968. Gorensek MJ, Carey WD, Washington JA II, et al. Selective bowel decontamination with quinolones and nystatin reduces gram-negative and fungal infections in orthotopic liver transplant recipients. *Cleve Clin J Med.* 1993; 60:139–44.
969. Piselli P, Zanfi C, Corazza V, et al. Incidence and timing of infections after liver transplant in Italy. *Transplant Proc.* 2007; 39:1950–2.
970. Desai D, Desai N, Nightingale P, et al. Carriage of methicillin-resistant *Staphylococcus aureus* is associated with an increased risk of infection after liver transplantation. *Liver Transpl.* 2003; 9:754–9.
971. Rayes N, Seehofer D, Theruvath T, et al. Supply of pre- and probiotics reduces bacterial infection rates after liver transplantation—a randomized, double-blind trial. *Am J Transplant.* 2005; 5:125–30.
972. Reid GE, Grim SA, Aldeza CA, et al. Rapid development of *Acinetobacter baumannii* resistance to tigecycline. *Pharmacotherapy.* 2007; 27:1198–201.
973. Chen H, Zhang Y, Chen YG, et al. Sepsis resulting from *Enterobacter aerogenes* resistant to carbapenems after liver transplantation. *Hepatobiliary Pancreat Dis Int.* 2009; 8:320–2.
974. Chen YG, Zhang Y, Yu YS, et al. In vivo development of carbapenem resistance in clinical isolates of *Enterobacter aerogenes* producing multiple ß-lactamases. *Int J Antimicrob Agents.* 2008; 32:302–7.
975. Bennett JW, Herrera ML, Lewis JS II, et al. KPC-2-producing *Enterobacter cloacae* and *Pseudomonas putida* coinfection in a liver transplant recipient. *Antimicrob Agents Chemother.* 2009; 53:292–4.
976. Carignan A, Allard C, Pépin J, et al. Risk of *Clostridium difficile* infection after perioperative antibacterial prophylaxis before and during an outbreak of infection due to a hypervirulent strain. *Clin Infect Dis.* 2008; 46:1838–46.
977. Stelzmueller I, Goegele H, Biebl M, et al. *Clostridium difficile* in solid organ transplantation—a single-center experience. *Dig Dis Sci.* 2007; 52:3231–6.
978. Hashimoto M, Sugawara Y, Tamura S, et al. *Clostridium difficile*-associated diarrhea after living donor liver transplantation. *World J Gastroenterol.* 2007; 13:2072–6.
979. Bion JF, Badger I, Crosby HA, et al. Selective decontamination of the digestive tract reduces gram-negative pulmonary colonization but not systemic endotoxemia in patients undergoing elective liver transplantation. *Crit Care Med.* 1994; 22:40–9.
980. Rayes N, Seehofer D, Hansen S, et al. Early enteral supply of lactobacillus and fiber versus selective bowel decontamination: a controlled trial in liver transplant recipients. *Transplantation.* 2002; 74:123–8.
981. González-Segura C, Pascual M, Garcia Huete L, et al. Donors with positive blood culture: could they transmit infections to the recipients? *Transplant Proc.* 2005; 37:3664–6.
982. Lumbreras C, Cuervas-Mons V, Jara P, et al. Randomized trial of fluconazole versus nystatin for the prophylaxis of *Candida* infection following liver transplantation. *J Infect Dis.* 1996; 174:583–8.
983. Winston DJ, Pakrasi A, Busuttil RW. Prophylactic fluconazole in liver transplant recipients. A randomized, double-blind, placebo-controlled trial. *Ann Intern Med.* 1999; 131:729–37.
984. Sharpe MD, Ghent C, Grant D, et al. Efficacy and safety of itraconazole prophylaxis for fungal infections after orthotopic liver transplantation: a prospective, randomized, double-blind study. *Transplantation.* 2003; 76:977–83.
985. Castroagudin JF, Ponton C, Bustamante M, et al. Prospective interventional study to evaluate the efficacy and safety of liposomal amphotericin B as prophylaxis of fungal infections in high-risk liver transplant recipients. *Transplant Proc.* 2005; 37:3965–7.
986. Lorf T, Braun F, Ruchel R, et al. Systemic mycoses during prophylactical use of liposomal amphotericin B (Ambisome) after liver transplantation. *Mycoses.* 1999; 42:47–53.
987. Tollemar J, Hockerstedt K, Ericzon BG, et al. Liposomal amphotericin B prevents invasive fungal infections in liver transplant recipients. A randomized,

placebo-controlled study. *Transplantation.* 1995; 59:45–50.

988. Fortun J, Martin-Davila P, Montejo M, et al. Prophylaxis with caspofungin for invasive fungal infections in high-risk liver transplant recipients. *Transplantation.* 2009; 87:424–35.

989. Cruciani M, Mengoli C, Malena M, et al. Antifungal prophylaxis in liver transplant patients: a systematic review and meta-analysis. *Liver Transpl.* 2006; 12:850–8.

990. Weisner RH, Hermans PE, Rakela J, et al. Selective bowel decontamination to decrease gram-negative aerobic bacterial and candidal colonization and prevent infection after orthotopic liver transplantation. *Transplantation.* 1988; 45:570–4.

991. Safdar N, Said A, Lucey MR. The role of selective digestive decontamination for reducing infection in patients undergoing liver transplantation: a systematic review and meta-analysis. *Liver Transpl.* 2004; 10:817–27.

992. Wiesmayr S, Stelzmueller I, Mark W, et al. Experience with the use of piperacillin-tazobactam in pediatric non-renal solid organ transplantation. *Pediatr Transplant.* 2007; 11:38–48.

993. Barker RJ, Mayes JT, Schulak JA. Wound abscesses following retroperitoneal pancreas transplantation. *Clin Transplant.* 1991; 5:403–7.

994. Douzdjian V, Abecassis MM, Cooper JL, et al. Incidence, management, and significance of surgical complications after pancreas-kidney transplantation. *Surg Gynecol Obstet.* 1993; 177:451–6.

995. Everett JE, Wahoff DC, Statz C, et al. Characterization and impact of wound infection after pancreas transplantation. *Arch Surg.* 1994; 129:1310–7.

996. Ozaki CF, Stratta RJ, Taylor RJ, et al. Surgical complications in solitary pancreas and combined pancreas-kidney transplantations. *Am J Surg.* 1992; 164:546–51.

997. Sollinger HW, Ploeg RJ, Eckhoff DE, et al. Two hundred consecutive simultaneous pancreas-kidney transplants with bladder drainage. *Surgery.* 1993; 114:736–44.

998. United Network for Organ Sharing. Organ Procurement and Transplantation Network: data. **http://optn.transplant.hrsa.gov/data/**. Based on OPTN data as of October 2, 2008.

999. Reddy KS, Stratta RJ, Shokouh-Amiri MH, et al. Surgical complications after pancreas transplantation with portal-enteric drainage. *J Am Coll Surg.* 1999; 189:305–13.

1000. Berger N, Wirmsberger R, Kafka R, et al. Infectious complications following 72 consecutive enteric-drained pancreas transplants. *Transpl Int.* 2006; 19:549–57.

1001. Bonatti H, Berger N, Kafka R, et al. Experience with ATG short course high dose induction therapy in a series of 112 enteric drained pancreatic transplants. *Ann Transplant.* 2002; 7:22–7.

1002. Berger N, Guggenbichler S, Steurer W, et al. Bloodstream infection following 217 consecutive systemic-enteric drained pancreas transplants. *BMC Infect Dis.* 2006; 6:127.

1003. Humar A, Kandawamy R, Drangstveit MB, et al. Prolonged preservation increases surgical complications after pancreas transplants. *Surgery.* 2000; 127:545–51.

1004. Pfundstein J, Roghmann MC, Schwalbe RS, et al. A randomized trial of surgical antimicrobial prophylaxis with and without vancomycin in organ transplant patients. *Clin Transplant.* 1999; 13:245–52.

1005. Smets YF, van der Pijl JW, van Dissel JT, et al. Infectious disease complications of simultaneous pancreas-kidney transplantation. *Nephrol Dial Transplant.* 1997; 12:764–71.

1006. Michalak G, Kwiatkowski A, Bieniasz M, et al. Infectious complications after simultaneous pancreas-kidney transplantation. *Transplant Proc.* 2005; 37:3560–3.

1007. Linhares MM, Gonzalez AM, Triviño T, et al. Simultaneous pancreas-kidney transplantation: infectious complications and microbiological aspects. *Transplant Proc.* 2004; 36:980–1.

1008. Bassetti M, Salvalaggio PR, Topal J, et al. Incidence, timing and site of infections among pancreas transplant recipients. *J Hosp Infect.* 2004; 56:184–90.

1009. Barone GW, Hudec WA, Sailors DM, et al. Prophylactic wound antibiotics for combined kidney and pancreas transplants. *Clin Transplant.* 1996; 10:386–8.

1010. Freise CE, Stock PG, Roberts JP, et al. Low postoperative wound infection rates are possible following simultaneous pancreas-kidney transplantation. *Transplant Proc.* 1995; 27:3069–70.

1011. Smets YF, van der Pijl JW, van Dissel JT, et al. Major bacterial and fungal infections after 50 simultaneous pancreas-kidney transplantations. *Transplant Proc.* 1995; 27:3089–90.

1012. Douzdjian V, Gugliuzza KK. Wound complications after simultaneous pancreas-kidney transplants: midline versus transverse incision. *Transplant Proc.* 1995; 27:3130–2.

1013. Bartlett ST. Pancreatic transplantation after thirty years: still room for improvement. *J Am Coll Surg.* 1996; 183:408–10.

1014. Cohen J, Rees AJ, Williams G. A prospective randomized controlled trial of perioperative antibiotic prophylaxis in renal transplantation. *J Hosp Infect.* 1988; 11:357–63.

1015. Hoy WE, May AG, Freeman RB. Primary renal transplant wound infections. *N Y State J Med.* 1981; 81:1469–73.

1016. Kohlberg WI, Tellis VA, Bhat DJ, et al. Wound infections after transplant nephrectomy. *Arch Surg.* 1980; 115:645–6.

1017. Muakkassa WF, Goldman MH, Mendez-Picon G, et al. Wound infections in renal transplant patients. *J Urol.* 1983; 130:17–9.

1018. Novick AC. The value of intraoperative antibiotics in preventing renal transplant wound infections. *J Urol.* 1981; 125:151–2.

1019. Ramos E, Karmi S, Alongi SV, et al. Infectious complications in renal transplant recipients. *South Med J.* 1980; 73:752–4.

1020. Rubin RH, Wolfson JS, Cosimi AB, et al. Infection in the renal transplant recipient. *Am J Med.* 1981; 70:405–11.

1021. Tilney NL, Strom TB, Vineyard GC, et al. Factors contributing to the declining mortality rate in renal transplantation. *N Engl J Med.* 1978; 299:1321–5.

1022. Muñoz P. Management of urinary tract infections and lymphocele in renal transplant recipients. *Clin Infect Dis.* 2001; 33(suppl 1):S53–7.

1023. Alangaden GJ, Thyagarajan R, Gruber SA, et al. Infectious complications after kidney transplantation: current epidemiology and associated risk factors. *Clin Transplant.* 2006; 20:401–9.

1024. Dantas SP, Kuboyama RH, Mazzali M, et al. Nosocomial infections in renal transplant patients: risk factors and treatment implications associated with urinary tract and surgical site infections. *J Hosp Infect.* 2006; 63:117–23.

1025. Celik A, Sifil A, Cavdar C, et al. Outcome of renal transplantation: 7-year experience. *Transplant Proc.* 2001; 33:2657–9.

1026. Lai MK, Huang CC, Chu SH, et al. Surgical complications in renal transplantation. *Transplant Proc.* 1994; 26:2165–6.

1027. Schmaldienst S, Hoerl WH. Bacterial infections after renal transplantation. *Nephron.* 1997; 75:140–53.

1028. Maraha B, Bonten H, van Hooff H, et al. Infectious complications and antibiotic use in renal transplant recipients during a 1-year follow-up. *Clin Microbiol Infect.* 2001; 7:619–25.

1029. Ramos A, Asensio A, Muñoz E, et al. Incisional surgical site infection in kidney transplantation. *Urology.* 2008; 72:119–23.

1030. Menezes FG, Wey SB, Peres CA, et al. Risk factors for surgical site infection in kidney transplant recipients. *Infect Control Hosp Epidemiol.* 2008; 29:771–3.

1031. Stephan RN, Munschauer CE, Kumar MS. Surgical wound infection in renal transplantation. Outcome data in 102 consecutive patients without perioperative systemic antibiotic coverage. *Arch Surg.* 1997; 132:1315–9.

1032. Sawyer RG, Pelletier SJ, Pruett TL. Increased early morbidity and mortality with acceptable long-term function in severely obese patients undergoing liver transplantation. *Clin Transplant.* 1999; 13:126–30.

1033. Koyle MA, Glasscock RJ, Ward HJ, et al. Declining incidence of wound infection in cadaveric renal transplant recipient. *Urology.* 1988; 31:103–6.

1034. Judson RT. Wound infection following renal transplantation. *Aust N Z J Surg.* 1984; 54:223–4.

1035. Del Rio G, Dalet F, Chechile G. Antimicrobial prophylaxis in urologic surgery: does it give some benefit? *Eur Urol.* 1993; 24:305–12.

1036. Midtvedt K, Hartmann A, Midtvedt T, et al. Routine perioperative antibiotic prophylaxis in renal transplantation. *Nephrol Dial Transplant.* 1998; 13:1637–41.

1037. Capocasale E, Mazzoni MP, Tondo S, et al. Antimicrobial prophylaxis with ceftriaxone in renal transplantation. Prospective study of 170 patients. *Chemotherapy.* 1994; 40:435–40.

1038. Wakelin SJ, Casey J, Robertson A, et al. The incidence and importance of bacterial contaminants of cadaveric renal perfusion fluid. *Transplant Int.* 2005; 17:680–6.

1039. Zomorrodi A, Buhluli A. Is antibiotic usage necessary after donor nephrectomy? A single center experience. *Saudi J Kidney Dis Transpl.* 2008; 19:200–5.

1040. Pape L, Offner G, Ehrich JH, et al. A single center clinical experience in intensive care management of 104 pediatric renal transplantations between 1998 and 2002. *Pediatr Transplant.* 2004; 8:39–43.

1041. Thorne CH. Techniques and principles in plastic surgery. In: Thorne CH, Beasley RW, Aston SJ, et al., eds. Grabb and Smith's plastic surgery. 6th ed. Philadelphia: Lippincott Williams and Wilkins; 2007.

1042. Chełmoński A, Jabłecki J, Sycz Z. Composite allotransplantations of knee joint, larynx, uterus, abdominal wall, face and penis. *Ann Transplant.* 2007; 12:5–11.

1043. Bonatti H, Brandacher G, Margreiter R, et al. Infectious complications in three double hand recipients: experience from a single center. *Transplant Proc.* 2009; 41:517–20.

1044. Babcock MD, Grekin RC. Antibiotic use in dermatologic surgery. *Dermatol Clin.* 2003; 21:337–48.

1045. Messingham MJ, Arpey CJ. Updates on the use of antibiotics in cutaneous surgery. *Dermatol Surg.* 2005; 31:1068–78.

1046. Wright TI, Baddour LM, Berbari EF, et al. Antibiotic prophylaxis in dermatologic surgery: advisory statement 2008. *J Am Acad Dermatol.* 2008; 59:464–73.

1047. Throckmorton AD, Boughey JC, Boostrom SY, et al. Postoperative prophylactic antibiotics and surgical site infection rates in breast surgery patients. *Ann Surg Oncol.* 2009; 16:2464–9.

1048. Khan UD. Breast augmentation, antibiotic prophylaxis, and infection: comparative analysis of 1,628 primary augmentation mammoplasties assessing the role and efficacy of antibiotics prophylaxis duration. *Aesthetic Plast Surg.* 2010; 34:42–7.

1049. Baran CN, Sensöz Ö, Ulusoy MG. Prophylactic antibiotics in plastic and reconstructive surgery. *Plast Reconstr Surg.* 1999; 103:1561–6.

1050. Mekako AI, Chetter IC, Coughlin PA, et al., on behalf of the Hull Antibiotic pRophylaxis in varicose VEin Surgery Trialists (HARVEST). Randomized clinical trial of co-amoxiclav versus no antibiotic prophylaxis in varicose vein surgery. *Br J Surg.* 2010; 97:29–36.

1051. Stone JF, Davidson JS. The role of antibiotics and timing of repair in flexor tendon injuries of the hand. *Ann Plast Surg.* 1998; 40:7–13.

1052. LeRoy J, Given KS. Wound infection in breast augmentation: the role of prophylactic perioperative antibiotics. *Aesthetic Plast Surg.* 1991; 15:303–5.

1053. Stewart KJ, Stewart DA, Coghlan B, et al. Complications of 278 consecutive abdominoplasties. *J Plast Reconstr Aesth Surg.* 2006; 59:1152–5.

1054. Rosengren H, Dixon A. Antibacterial prophylaxis in dermatologic surgery: an evidence-based review. *Am J Clin Dermatol.* 2010; 11:35–44.

1055. Landes G, Harris PG, Lemaine V, et al. Prevention of surgical site infection and appropriateness of antibiotic prescribing habits in plastic surgery. *J Plast Reconstr Aesthet Surg.* 2008; 61:1347–56.

1056. Ahmadi AH, Cohen BE, Shayani P. A prospective study of antibiotic efficacy in preventing infection in reduction mammaplasty. *Plast Reconstr Surg.* 2005; 116:126–31.

1057. Carroll WR, Rosenstiel D, Fix JR, et al. Three-dose vs. extended-course clindamycin prophylaxis for free-flap reconstruction of the head and neck. *Arch Otolaryngol Head Neck Surg.* 2003; 129:771–4.
1058. Serletti JM, Davenport MS, Herrera HR, et al. Efficacy of prophylactic antibiotics in reduction mammoplasty. *Ann Plast Surg.* 1994; 33:476–80.
1059. Halpern AC, Leyden JJ, Dzubow LM, et al. The incidence of bacteremia in skin surgery of the head and neck. *J Am Acad Dermatol.* 1988; 19:112–6.
1060. Samra S, Sawh-Martinez R, Barry O, et al. Complication rates of lipoabdominoplasty versus traditional abdominoplasty in high-risk patients. *Plast Reconstr Surg.* 2010; 125:683–90.
1061. Olsen MA, Lefta M, Dietz JR, et al. Risk factors for surgical site infection after major breast operation. *J Am Coll Surg.* 2008; 207:326–35.
1062. Dixon AJ, Dixon MP, Dixon JB. Prospective study of skin surgery in patients with and without known diabetes. *Dermatol Surg.* 2009; 35:1035–40.
1063. Wahie S, Lawrence CM. Wound complications following diagnostic skin biopsies in dermatology inpatients. *Arch Dermatol.* 2007; 143:1267–71.
1064. Gravante G, Araco A, Sorge R, et al. Wound infections in post-bariatric patients undergoing body contouring abdominoplasty: the role of smoking. *Obes Surg.* 2007; 17:1325–31.
1065. Rey JE, Gardner SM, Cushing RD. Determinants of surgical site infection after breast biopsy. *Am J Infect Control.* 2005; 33:126–9.
1066. Sevin A, Senen D, Sevin K, et al. Antibiotic use in abdominoplasty: prospective analysis of 207 cases. *J Plast Reconstr Aesthet Surg.* 2007; 60:379–82.
1067. Gravante G, Caruso R, Araco A, et al. Infections after plastic procedures: incidences, etiologies, risk factors, and antibiotic prophylaxis. *Aesthetic Plast Surg.* 2008; 32:243–51.
1068. Bertin ML, Crowe J, Gordon SM. Determinants of surgical site infection after breast surgery. *Am J Infect Control.* 1998; 26:61–5.
1069. Harness NG, Inacio MC, Pfeil FF, et al. Rate of infection after carpal tunnel release surgery and effect of antibiotic prophylaxis. *J Hand Surg.* 2010; 35:189–96.
1070. Platt R, Zucker JR, Zaleznik DF, et al. Perioperative antibiotic prophylaxis and wound infection following breast surgery. *J Antimicrob Chemother.* 1993; 31(suppl B):43–8.
1071. Kompatscher P, von Planta A, Spicher I, et al. Comparison of the incidence and predicted risk of early surgical site infections after breast reduction. *Aesthetic Plast Surg.* 2003; 27:308–14.
1072. Bunn F, Cunningham ME, Handscomb K. Prophylactic antibiotics to prevent surgical site infection after breast cancer surgery. *Cochrane Database Syst Rev.* 2006; 2:CD005360.
1073. Perrotti JA, Castor SA, Perez PC, et al. Antibiotic use in aesthetic surgery: a national survey and literature review. *Plast Reconstr Surg.* 2002; 109:1685–93.
1074. Smyth AG, Knepil GJ. Prophylactic antibiotics and surgery for primary clefts. *Br J Oral Maxillofac Surg.* 2008; 46:107–9.
1075. Cocco JF, Antonetti JW, Burns JL, et al. Characterization of the nasal, sublingual and oropharyngeal mucosa microbiota in cleft lip and palate individuals before and after surgical repair. *Cleft Palate Craniofac J.* 2010; 47:151–5.

Appendix A—National Healthcare Safety Network Criteria for Classifying Wounds[35]

Clean: An uninfected operative wound in which no inflammation is encountered and the respiratory, alimentary, genital, or uninfected urinary tracts are not entered. In addition, clean wounds are primarily closed and, if necessary, drained with closed drainage. Operative incisional wounds that follow nonpenetrating (blunt) trauma should be included in this category if they meet the criteria.

Clean-contaminated: Operative wounds in which the respiratory, alimentary, genital, or urinary tracts are entered under controlled conditions and without unusual contamination. Specifically, operations involving the biliary tract, appendix, vagina, and oropharynx are included in this category, provided no evidence of infection or major break in technique is encountered.

Contaminated: Open, fresh, accidental wounds. In addition, operations with major breaks in sterile technique (e.g., open cardiac massage) or gross spillage from the gastrointestinal tract and incisions in which acute, nonpurulent inflammation is encountered are included in this category.

Dirty or infected: Includes old traumatic wounds with retained devitalized tissue and those that involve existing clinical infection or perforated viscera. This definition suggests that the organisms causing postoperative infection were present in the operative field before the operation.

Appendix B—National Healthcare Safety Network Criteria for Defining a Surgical-Site Infection (SSI)[8,36]

Superficial incisional SSI: Occurs within 30 days postoperatively and involves skin or subcutaneous tissue of the incision and at least one of the following: (1) purulent drainage from the superficial incision, (2) organisms isolated from an aseptically obtained culture of fluid or tissue from the superficial incision, (3) at least one of the following signs or symptoms of infection: pain or tenderness, localized swelling, redness, or heat, and superficial incision is deliberately opened by surgeon and is culture-positive or not cultured (a culture-negative finding does not meet this criterion), and (4) diagnosis of superficial incisional SSI by the surgeon or attending physician.

Deep incisional SSI: Occurs within 30 days after the operative procedure if no implant is left in place or within one year if implant is in place and the infection appears to be related to the operative procedure, involves deep soft tissues (e.g., fascial and muscle layers) of the incision, and the patient has at least one of the following: (1) purulent drainage from the deep incision but not from the organ/space component of the surgical site, (2) a deep incision spontaneously dehisces or is deliberately opened by a surgeon and is culture-positive or not cultured and the patient has at least one of the following signs or symptoms: fever (>38 °C) or localized pain or tenderness (a culture-negative finding does not meet this criterion), (3) an abscess or other evidence of infection involving the deep incision is found on direct examination, during reoperation, or by histopathologic or radiologic examination, and (4) diagnosis of a deep incisional SSI by a surgeon or attending physician.

Organ/space SSI: Involves any part of the body, excluding the skin incision, fascia, or muscle layers, that is opened or manipulated during the operative procedure. Specific sites are assigned to organ/space SSI to further identify the location of the infection (e.g., endocarditis, endometritis, mediastinitis, vaginal cuff, and osteomyelitis). Organ/space SSI must meet the following criteria: (1) infection occurs within 30 days after the operative procedure if no implant is in place or within 1 year if implant is in place and the infection appears to be related to the operative procedure, (2) infection involves any part of the body, excluding the skin incision, fascia, or muscle layers, that is opened or manipulated during the operative procedure, and (3) the patient has at least one of the following: (a) purulent drainage from a drain that is placed through a stab wound into the organ/space, (b) organisms isolated from an aseptically obtained culture of fluid or tissue in the organ/space, (c) an abscess or other evidence of infection involving the organ/space that is found on direct examination, during reoperation, or by histopathologic or radiologic examination, and (d) diagnosis of an organ/space SSI by a surgeon or attending physician.

The following individuals are acknowledged for their significant contributions to this manuscript: Sandra I. Berríos-Torres, M.D.; Rachel Bongiorno-Karcher, Pharm.D.; Colleen M. Culley, Pharm.D., BCPS; Susan R. Dombrowski, M.S., B.S.Pharm.; and Susan J. Skledar, B.S.Pharm., M.P.H., FASHP.

Financial support provided by Emory University, Johns Hopkins University, Northwestern University, Rush University, University of Colorado, University of Michigan, University of Oklahoma, University of Nebraska, University of Virginia, University of Washington, and West Virginia University.

Dr. Bratzler is a consultant for Telligen; Dr. Dellinger has received honoraria for participation on advisory boards and consultation for Merck, Baxter, Ortho-McNeil, Targanta, Schering-Plough, WebEx, Astellas, Durata, Pfizer, Applied Medical, Rib-X, 3M, the American Hospital Association, Premier Inc., Oklahoma Foundation for Medical Quality, and the Hospital Association of New York State; Dr. Perl serves on the advisory boards of Hospira and Pfizer and has received a grant from Merck; Dr. Auwaerter serves on the advisory panel of Genentech; Dr. Fish serves on the advisory board and speakers' bureau of Merck; and Dr. Sawyer serves as a consultant for Pfizer, Merck, Wyeth, 3M, and Ethicon and has received an R01 grant from the National Institute of General Medical Sciences and a T32 grant from the National Institute of Allergy and Infectious Diseases. Drs. Bolon, Napolitano, Olsen, Steinberg, Slain, and Weinstein have declared no potential conflicts of interest.

Copyright © 2013, American Society of Health-System Pharmacists, Inc. All rights reserved. Contact ASHP for reprint and permissions requests. This content may not be used for commercial purposes without the express written consent of ASHP.

The bibliographic citation for this article is as follows: Bratzler DW, Dellinger EP, Olsen KM, et al. Clinical practice guidelines for antimicrobial prophylaxis in surgery. *Am J Health-Syst Pharm.* 2013; 70:195–283.

Clinical Practice Guidelines for Sustained Neuromuscular Blockade in the Adult Critically Ill Patient

The decision to treat a patient in the intensive care unit (ICU) with neuromuscular blocking agents (NMBAs) (for reasons other than the placement of an endotracheal tube) is a difficult one that is guided more commonly by individual practitioner preference than by standards based on evidence-based medicine. Commonly cited reasons for the use of NMBAs in the ICU are to facilitate mechanical ventilation or different modes of mechanical ventilation and to manage patients with head trauma or tetanus. Independent of the reasons for using NMBAs, we emphasize that all other modalities to improve the clinical situation must be tried, using NMBAs only as a last resort.

In 1995 the American College of Critical Care Medicine (ACCM) of the Society of Critical Care Medicine (SCCM) published guidelines for the use of NMBAs in the ICU. The present document is the result of an attempt to reevaluate the literature that has appeared since the last guidelines were published and, based on that review, to update the recommendations for the use of NMBAs in the ICU. **Appendix A** summarizes our recommendations. Using methods previously described to evaluate the literature and grade the evidence, the task force reviewed the physiology of the neuromuscular receptor, the pharmacology of the NMBAs currently used in the ICU, the means to monitor the degree of blockade, the complications associated with NMBAs, and the economic factors to consider when choosing a drug.

Neuromuscular Junction in Health and Disease

The neuromuscular junction consists of a motor nerve terminus, the neurotransmitter acetylcholine, and the postsynaptic muscle endplate (**Figure 1**). The impulse of an action potential causes the release of acetylcholine from synaptic vesicles (each containing about 10,000 molecules of acetylcholine) diffusing across the 20-nm gap to the postsynaptic endplate. The motor endplate contains specialized ligand-gated, nicotinic acetylcholine receptors (nAChRs), which convert the chemical signal (i.e., binding of two acetylcholine molecules) into electrical signals (i.e., a transient permeability change and depolarization in the postsynaptic membrane of striated muscle).

There are depolarizing and nondepolarizing NMBAs. Depolarizing NMBAs physically resemble acetylcholine and, therefore, bind and activate acetylcholine receptors. Succinylcholine is currently the only available depolarizing NMBA and is not used for long-term use in ICUs.

Nondepolarizing NMBAs also bind acetylcholine receptors but do not activate them—they are competitive antagonists. The difference in the mechanism of action also accounts for different effects in certain diseases. If there is a long-term decrease in acetylcholine release, the number of acetylcholine receptors within the muscle increases. This upregulation causes an increased response to depolarizing NMBAs but a resistance to nondepolarizing NMBAs (i.e., more receptors must be blocked). Conditions in which there are fewer acetylcholine receptors (e.g., myasthenia gravis) lead to an increase in sensitivity to nondepolarizing NMBAs.

Adult skeletal muscle retains an ability to synthesize both the mature adult nAChR as well as an immature nAChR variant in which a gamma subunit is substituted for the normal epsilon subunit. Synthesis of immature (fetal) receptors may be triggered in the presence of certain diseases (e.g., Guillain-Barré syndrome, stroke) and other conditions producing loss of nerve function. These immature nAChRs are distinguished by three features. First, immature receptors are not localized to the muscle endplate but migrate across the entire membrane surface.[2] Second, the immature receptors are metabolically short-lived (<24 hours) and more ionically active, having a 2- to 10-fold longer channel "open time." Lastly, these immature receptors are more sensitive to the depolarizing effects of such drugs as succinylcholine and more resistant to the effects of competitive antagonists, such as pancuronium. This increase in the number of immature acetylcholine receptors may account for the tachyphylaxis seen with NMBAs and some of the complications associated with their use. For the remainder of this document, only nondepolarizing NMBAs will be discussed.

Pharmacology of Neuromuscular-Receptor Blockers

Aminosteroidal Compounds. The aminosteroidal compounds include pancuronium, pipecuronium, vecuronium, and rocuronium (**Tables 1 and 2**).[3–11]

Pancuronium. Pancuronium, one of the original NMBAs used in ICUs, is a long-acting, nondepolarizing compound that is effective after an intravenous bolus dose of 0.06–0.1 mg/kg for up to 90 minutes. Though it is commonly given as an i.v. bolus, it can be used as a continuous infusion[12] by adjusting the dose to the degree of neuromuscular blockade that is desired (Table 1). Pancuronium is vagolytic (more than 90% of ICU patients will have an increase in heart rate of ≥10 beats/min), which limits its use in patients who cannot tolerate an increase in heart rate.[12] In patients with renal failure or cirrhosis, pancuronium's neuromuscular blocking effects are prolonged because of its increased elimination half-life and the decreased clearance of its 3-hydroxypancuronium metabolite that has one-third to one-half the activity of pancuronium.

Pipecuronium. Pipecuronium is another long-acting NMBA with an elimination half-life of about two hours, similar to pancuronium's. Khuenl-Brady and colleagues[13] conducted an open-label evaluation of pipecuronium compared with pancuronium in 60 critically ill patients to determine the minimum doses required for ventilatory management. The administration of 8 mg of either drug followed by intermittent boluses of 4–6 mg when needed resulted in optimal paralysis. Patients were paralyzed for a mean duration of 62.6 hours (45–240 hours) and 61.5 hours (46–136 hours) with pancuronium and pipecuronium, respectively. No adverse effects were attributed to either drug. Perhaps because of this lack of difference and because there are no recent studies examining

DOI 10.37573/9781585287048.114

Figure 1. Neuromuscular Junction. Schematic model of the organization and structure of the neuromuscular junction, with focus and enlargement on the postsynaptic membrane. Agrin is the nerve-derived protein that triggers receptor clustering during synapse formation. Receptor aggregation appears to occur in distinct steps, however, initiated with acetylcholine receptors (AChR) localized together by rapsyn. Meanwhile, D-dystroglycan, the extracellular component of dystrophin-associated glycoprotein complex (DGC), is the agrin receptor which transduces final AChR clustering. This process utilizes the structural organization of additional proteins like utrophin, which stabilize the mature, immobile domains by interaction with the underlying cytoskeleton (actin). When completed, this process concentrates AChR density 1000-fold compared to typical muscle membrane. ACh = acetylcholine, MuSK = muscle-specific-receptor kirase, MASC = MuSK-accessory specificity component. (Reprinted with permission, from Wall MH, Prielipp RC. Monitoring the neuromuscular junction. In: Lake C, Blitt CD, Hines RL, eds. Clinical Monitoring: Practical Applications for Anesthesia and Critical Care. Philadelphia: W.B. Saunders, 2000, Figure 10-3.)

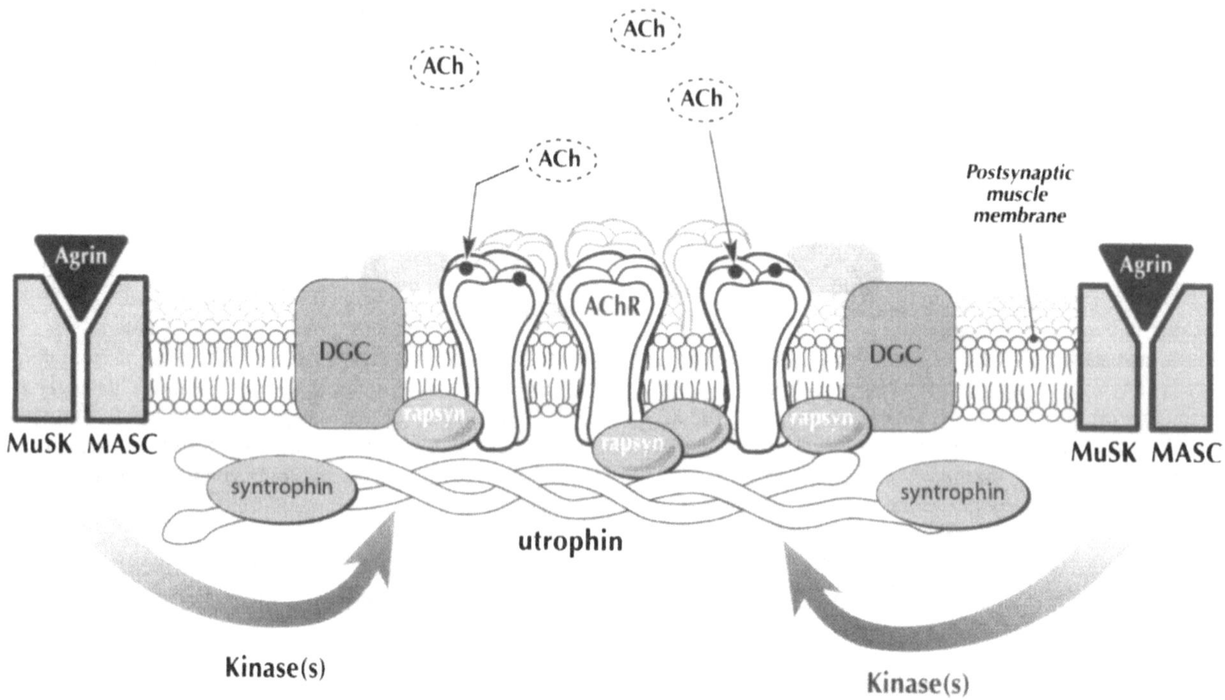

pipecuronium's use in the ICU, most clinicians continue to use the more familiar drug, pancuronium.

Vecuronium. Vecuronium is an intermediate-acting NMBA that is a structural analogue of pancuronium and is not vagolytic. An i.v. bolus dose of vecuronium 0.08–0.1 mg/kg, produces blockade within 60–90 seconds that typically lasts 25–30 minutes. After an i.v. bolus dose, vecuronium is given as a 0.8–1.2-μg/kg/min continuous infusion, adjusting the rate to the degree of blockade desired. Because up to 35% of a dose is renally excreted, patients with renal failure will have decreased drug requirements. Similarly, because up to 50% of an injected dose is excreted in bile, patients with hepatic insufficiency will also have decreased drug requirements to maintain adequate blockade. The 3-desacetylvecuronium metabolite has 50% of the pharmacologic activity of the parent compound, so patients with organ dysfunction may have increased plasma concentrations of both the parent compound and the active metabolite, which contributes to the prolongation of blockade if the dose is not adjusted. Vecuronium has been reported to be more commonly associated with prolonged blockade once discontinued, compared with other NMBAs[a]. Members of the task force believe that vecuronium is being used with decreased frequency in the ICU.

Vecuronium has been studied in open-label prospective trials.[14,15] In one of these studies, the mean infusion rate for vecuronium was 0.9 ± 0.1 μg/kg/min for a mean duration of 80 ± 7 hours. Recovery of a train-of-four (TOF) ratio of ≥0.7 was significantly longer than with cisatracurium.[15] Recovery time averaged 1–2 hours but ranged from ≤30 minutes to more than 48 hours.

Although Rudis, et al.[14] observed no difference in the incidence of prolonged blockade between patients receiving vecuronium with and without concomitant administration of corticosteroids, the opinion of the task force was that patients receiving vecuronium and corticosteroids were at increased risk of prolonged weakness once the drug was discontinued.

Rocuronium. Rocuronium is a newer nondepolarizing NMBA with a monoquaternary steroidal chemistry that has an intermediate duration of action and a very rapid onset. When given as a bolus dose of 0.6–1 mg/kg, blockade is almost always achieved within two minutes, with maximum blockade occurring within three minutes. Continuous infusions are begun at 10 μg/kg/min.[8] Rocuronium's metabolite, 17-des-acetylrocuronium, has only 5–10% activity compared with the parent compound.

Sparr, Khuenl-Brady, and colleagues[8,9] studied the dose requirements, recovery times, and pharmacokinetics of rocuronium in 32 critically ill patients, 27 of whom were given intermittent bolus doses, and 5 received a continuous infusion. The median duration of drug administration was 29 hours and 63.4 hours in the bolus dose and infusion groups, respectively. The mean dose of rocuronium required to maintain 80% blockade was 0.34 mg/kg, and the median infusion rate required to maintain one twitch of the TOF was

TABLE 1.

Selected Neuromuscular Blocking Agents[a] for ICU Use

Variable	Benzylisoquinolinium Drugs: D-Turbocurarine (Curare)	Cisatracurium (Nimbex)	Atracurium (Tracrium)	Doxacurium (Nuromax)	Mivacurium (Mivacron)
Introduced (yr)	1942	1995	1983	1991	1992
ED_{95}[b] dose (mg/kg)	0.51	0.05	0.25	0.025–0.03	0.075
Initial dose (mg/kg)	0.1–0.2	0.1–0.2	0.4–0.5	0.025–0.05	0.15–0.25
Duration (min)	80	45–60	25–35	120–150	10–20
Infusion described	. . .	Yes	Yes	Yes	Yes
Infusion dose (μg/kg/min)	. . .	2.5–3	4–12	0.3–0.5	9–10
Recovery (min)	80–180	90	40–60	120–180	10–20
% Renal excretion	40–45	Hofmann elimination	5–10 (uses Hofmann elimination)	70	Inactive metabolites
Renal failure	Increased duration	No change	No change	Increased duration	Increased duration
% Biliary excretion	10–40	Hofmann elimination	Minimal (uses Hofmann elimination)	Insufficient data	. . .
Hepatic failure	Minimal change to mild increased effect	Minimal to no change	Minimal to no change	. . .	Increased duration
Active metabolites	No	No	No, but can accumulate laudanosine	. . .	No
Histamine release hypotension	Marked	No	Minimal but dose dependent	No	Minimal but dose dependent
Vagal block tachycardia	Minimal	No	No	No	No
Ganglionic blockade hypotension	Marked	No	Minimal to none	No	No
Prolonged ICU block	. . .	Rare	Rare	Insufficient data	Insufficient data

Variable	Aminosteroidal Drugs: Pancuronium (Pavulon)	Vecuronium (Norcuron)	Pipecuronium (Arduan)	Rocuronium (Zemuron)
Introduced (yr)	1972	1984	1991	1994
ED_{95}[b] dose (mg/kg)	0.05	0.05	0.05	0.3
Initial dose (mg/kg)	0.06–0.1	0.08–0.1	0.085–0.1	0.6–1
Duration (min)	90–100	35–45	90–100	30
Infusion described	Yes	Yes	No	Yes
Infusion dose (μg/kg/min)	1–2	0.8–1.2	0.5–2	10–12
Recovery (min)	120–180	45–60	55–160	20–30
% Renal excretion	45–70	50	50+	33
Renal failure	Increased effect	Increased effect, especially metabolites	Increased duration	Minimal
% Biliary excretion	10–15	35–50	Minimal	<75
Hepatic failure	Mild increased effect	Variable, mild	Minimal	Moderate
Active metabolites	Yes, 3-OH and 17-OH-pancuronium	Yes, 3-desacetyl-vecuronium	Insufficient data	No
Histamine release hypotension	No	No	No	No
Vagal block tachycardia	Modest to marked	No	No	Some at higher doses
Ganglionic blockade hypotension	No	No	No	No
Prolonged ICU block	Yes	Yes	Insufficient data	Insufficient data

[a]Based on drugs for use in a 70-kg man. Modified with permission from Prielipp and Coursin. Reference 3.

[b]ED_{95} = effective dose for 95% of patients studied.

TABLE 2.
ICU Studies of Aminosteroidal Drugs[a]

Reference	Type of Study	Patients	Results	Level of Evidence
4	Prospective, observational, cohort	30	Median time to recovery with pancuronium was 3.5 hr in infusion group vs. 6.3 hr in the bolus dose group.	3
5	Prospective, open-label	25 PICU	Increased infusion requirements for pancuronium with anticonvulsants.	3
6	Prospective, open-label	6	Vecuronium clearance increased in 3 and decreased in 2 patients. V_D did not change.	3
7	Survey	...	Neuromuscular blockade monitored clinically with only 8.3% using TOF. All respondents indicated concomitant use of sedatives and/or opioids (75%).	5
8	Prospective, open-label	30 SICU	25 trauma patients received rocuronium 50-mg i.v. bolus dose followed by maintenance doses of 25 mg whenever TOF = 2, five patients were on continuous infusion at 25 mg/hr. Duration 1–5 days, recovery approximately 3 hr, and plasma clearance similar between groups.	3
9	Prospective, open-label	32	An initial dose of rocuronium 50 mg followed by maintenance doses of 25 mg with TOF = 2 (*n* = 27) or by continuous infusion to maintain TOF (*n* = 5). Pharmacokinetic data tabulated. Crossover with patients reported by Khuenl-Brady, et al.[8]	3
10	Prospective, randomized, controlled	20 CABG	Pancuronium (*n* = 10) was compared to rocuronium (*n* = 10). Incidence of residual block higher with pancuronium than rocuronium. No effect on time to extubation.	2
11	Prospective, open-label	12 ICU	12 patients, 4 with MODS. Patients given 0.6-mg/kg bolus dose of rocuronium followed by repeated bolus (*n* = 2) or continuous infusion (*n* = 10) started at 10–12 µg/kg/min and adjusted to TOF = 1–4. No evidence of prolonged blockade.	3

[a]PICU = pediatric intensive care unit, SICU = surgical intensive care unit, CABG = coronary artery bypass grafting, ICU = intensive care unit, TOF = train-of-four, V_D = volume of distribution, MODS = multiple organ dysfunction syndrome.

0.54 mg/kg/hr. The median time from the last bolus dose to the appearance of TOF response was 100 minutes; in the infusion group, the TOF response returned 60 minutes after the infusion was stopped.

Rapacuronium. Rapacuronium, a propionate analogue of vecuronium, was marketed as a nonde polarizing NMBA as an alternative to succinylcholine. It was withdrawn from the market on March 27, 2001, because of reports of morbidity (bronchospasm) and mortality associated with its use.

Benzylisoquinolinium Compounds. The benzylisoquinolinium compounds include D-tubocuranine, atracurium, cisatracurium, doxacurium, and mivacurium (**Tables 1 and 3**).[12,15,16,31]

D-Tubocurarine. Tubocurarine was the first nondepolarizing NMBA to gain acceptance and usage in the ICU. This long-acting benzylisoquinolinium agent is rarely used in ICUs because it induces histamine release and autonomic ganglionic blockade. Hypotension is rare, however, when the agent is administered slowly in appropriate dosages (e.g., 0.1–0.2 mg/kg). Metabolism and elimination are affected by both renal and hepatic dysfunction.

*Atracurium.*Atracurium is an intermediate-acting NMBA with minimal cardiovascular adverse effects and is associated with histamine release at higher doses. It is inactivated in plas-ma by ester hydrolysis and Hofmann elimination so that renal or hepatic dysfunction does not affect the duration of blockade.

Laudanosine is a breakdown product of Hofmann elimination of atracurium and has been associated with central nervous system excitation. This has led to concern about the possibility of precipitating seizures in patients who have received extremely high doses of atracurium or who are in hepatic failure (laudanosine is metabolized by the liver). There has been only one report of a surgical patient who had a seizure while receiving atracurium.[32]

Atracurium has been administered to various critically ill patient populations, including those with liver failure,[17] brain injury,[21] or multiple organ dysfunction syndrome (MODS), to facilitate mechanical ventilation. In these reports, atracurium infusion rates varied widely, but they typically ranged from 10 to 20 µg/kg/min with doses adjusted to clinical endpoints or by TOF monitoring. Infusion durations ranged from ≤24 hours to >200 hours. Recovery of normal neuromuscular activity usually occurred within one to two hours after stopping the infusions and was independent of organ function. Long-term infusions have been associated with the development of tolerance, necessitating significant dose increases or conversion to other NMBAs.[31,33] Atracurium has been associated with persistent neuromuscular weakness as have other NMBAs.[34–38]

Cisatracurium. Cisatracurium, an isomer of atracurium, is an intermediate-acting benzyliso-quinolinium NMBA that is increasingly used in lieu of atracurium. It produces few, if any, cardiovascular effects and has a lesser tendency to produce mast cell degranulation than atracurium. Bolus doses of 0.1–0.2 mg/kg result in paralysis in

TABLE 3.
ICU Studies of Benzylisoquinolinium Drugs[a]

Reference	Type of Study	Patients	Dose	Results	Level of Evidence
16	Review	. . .	. . .	Review of pharmacokinetics	5
17	Prospective, open-label, controlled	14 with hepatic failure vs. 11 controls	Cisatracurium 0.1-mg/kg i.v. bolus dose	V_D greater in liver patients but no differences in elimination $t_{1/2}$ or in duration of action	5
18	Prospective, randomized, single-blind	20 ICU	Cisatracurium (n = 12) 0.25 mg/kg/hr Atracurium (n = 8) 0.62 mg/kg/hr	Similar mean recovery time	2
19	Prospective, randomized	12 ICU	Cisatracurium 0.1-mg/kg bolus dose + 0.18-mg/ kg/hr infusion Atracurium: 0.5 mg/kg + 0.6-mg/kg/hr infusion	Measured V_D, Cl, $T_{1/2}$. Laudanosine concentration was lower in patients on cisatracurium	2
20	Randomized, open-label	61 ICU	Cisatracurium (n = 26) 0.1-mg/kg bolus, followed by an infusion of 3 μg/ kg/min; 14 pts infusion only Atracurium (n = 18) 0.5 mg/kg bolus followed by an infusion of 10 μg/kg/min; 3 pts infusion only Infusion adjusted to one twitch	118 ± 19 min recovery no change in HR, BP, and ICP with bolus	3
15	Prospective, randomized, double-blind, multicenter	58 ICU	Cisatracurium 2.5-μg/kg/min Vecuronium 1-μg/kg/min	Recovery profiles were significantly different with more prolonged recovery noted for vecuronium. TOF monitoring could not eliminate prolonged recovery and myopathy	1
21	Prospective, blinded, cross-over	14 with brain injury	Cisatracurium 0.15 mg/kg bolus Atracurium 0.75 mg/kg bolus	No change in ICP, CPP, CBF, MAP, $ETCO_2$, and HR and no histamine-related symptoms, with 3×ED_{95} cisatracurium. With 3×ED_{95} tracurium, ICP, CPP, CBF, and MAP decreased within 2–4 min. Five patients had typical histamine reaction; excluding these five patients, there was no difference in any variable compared with cisatracurium	2
22	Observational, prospective, open-label	24 with brain injury	0.1 or 0.2-mg/kg cisatracurium bolus dose	No change from baseline in ICP, CPP, MAP, $ETCO_2$, HR, and CBF velocity in both groups	5
23	Case	. . .	. . .	. . .	4
24	Case	. . .	. . .	. . .	4
25	Review	. . .	. . .	. . .	4
26	Editorial	. . .	. . .	. . .	4
27	Review	. . .	. . .	. . .	5
28	Review	. . .	. . .	. . .	5
12	Multicenter, prospective, double-blind, randomized	40 critically ill	Doxacurium 0.04-mg/kg bolus dose, 0.025-mg/kg maintenance; pancuronium: 0.07 mg/ kg bolus dose, 0.05-mg/kg maintenance	No difference in adverse reactions or onset of blockade; pancuronium had a more prolonged and variable recovery time	1
29	Prospective, open-label	8 mechanical ventilated ICU with HD monitoring and pHi <7.35	Doxacurium: 0.03-mg/kg load; 0.03-mg/kg/hr infusion	$DO_2 + VO_2$ decreased, pHi increased; VO_2 is decreased and pHi increased. NMBA causes redistribution of blood flow to splanchnic beds	5
30	Prospective, open-label study	8 ICU with traumatic head injury	Doxacurium 0.05 mg/kg then 0.25 μg/kg/min	No significant effect in HR, BP, ICP. No adverse effects	5
31	Case report	4 with atracurium tachyphylaxis	Doxacurium 0.25–0.75 μg/kg/min	No tachyphylaxis noted	5

[a]ICU = intensive care unit, TOF = train-of-four, V_D = volume of distribution, HR = heart rate, BP = blood pressure, ICP = intracranial pressure, CPP = cerebral perfusion pressure, CBF = cerebral blood flow, MAP = mean arterial pressure, NMBA = neuromuscular blocking agent, $ETCO_2$ = end tidal carbon dioxide, ED_{95} = effective dose for 95% of patients studied, HD = hemodynamic flow, pHi = gastric mucosal pH, DO_2 = oxygen delivery, VO_2 = oxygen consumption, CBF = cerebral blood flow.

an average of 2.5 minutes, and recovery begins at approximately 25 minutes; maintenance infusions should be started at 2.5–3 μg/kg/min. Cisatracurium is also metabolized by ester hydrolysis and Hofmann elimination, so the duration of blockade should not be affected by renal or hepatic dysfunction. Prolonged weakness has been reported following the use of cisatracurium.[38]

Cisatracurium has been compared with atracurium and vecuronium for facilitating mechanical ventilation in several open-label prospective trials.[15,18–21] Cisatracurium infusion rates ranged from 2 to 8 μg/kg/min and were adjusted to clinical endpoints or to TOF count. Infusion durations varied from 4 to 145 hours. Recovery of a TOF ratio >0.7 occurred within 34–85 minutes after drug discontinuation and was independent of organ function. These recovery times are similar to those seen with atracurium[18,21] and less than those observed with vecuronium.[15]

Doxacurium. Doxacurium, a long-acting benzylisoquinolinium agent, is the most potent NMBA currently available. Doxacurium is essentially free of hemodynamic adverse effects. Initial doses of doxacurium 0.05–0.1 mg/kg may be given with maintenance infusions of 0.3–0.5 μg/kg/min and adjusted to the degree of blockade desired. An initial bolus dose lasts an average of 60–80 minutes. Doxacurium is primarily eliminated by renal excretion. In elderly patients and patients with renal dysfunction, a significant prolongation of effect may occur.

Murray and colleagues[12] conducted a prospective, randomized, controlled, multicenter comparison of intermittent doses of doxacurium and pancuronium in 40 critically ill patients requiring neuromuscular blockade to optimize mechanical ventilation or to lower intracranial pressure (ICP). Patients were given another bolus dose based on TOF monitoring and were paralyzed for a mean duration of 2.6 days with doxacurium or 2.2 days with pancuronium. There was a clinically significant increase in heart rate after the initial bolus dose of pancuronium compared with baseline (120 ± 23 versus 109 ± 22 beats/min, respectively) without any differences after the initial dose of doxacurium (107 ± 21 versus 109 ± 21 beats/min, respectively). Once the drugs were discontinued, the pancuronium group had a more prolonged and variable recovery time (279 ± 229 min) than the doxacurium group (135 ± 46 min).

Mivacurium. Mivacurium is one of the shortest-acting NMBAs currently available. It consists of multiple stereoisomers and has a half-life of approximately two minutes, allowing for rapid reversal of the blockade. There are little data to support its use as a continuous infusion in the ICU.

Indications

NMBAs are indicated in a variety of situations (**Table 4**).[8,9,12–15,17–21,30,39,42] There have been no studies randomizing patients who are considered candidates for NMBAs to a placebo versus an NMBA. We therefore reviewed many studies comparing one NMBA to another to assess the clinical indications for enrolling patients in these studies. The most common indications for long-term administration of NMBAs included facilitation of mechanical ventilation, control of ICP, ablation of muscle spasms associated with tetanus, and decreasing oxygen consumption (**Figure 2**). NMBAs are often used to facilitate ventilation and ablate muscular activity in patients with elevated ICP or seizures but have no direct effect on either condition. Patients who are being treated for seizures who also take NMBAs should have electroencephalographic monitoring to ensure that they are not actively seizing while paralyzed.

With the exception of atracurium and cisatracurium, which need to be given continuously because of their short half-lives, bolus administration of NMBAs offers potential advantages for controlling tachyphylaxis; monitoring for accumulation, analgesia, and amnesia; and limiting complications related to prolonged or excessive blockade; and improving economics. However, in many ICUs, NMBAs are administered continuously, achieving adequate paralysis and faster recovery with TOF monitoring.

Facilitate Mechanical Ventilation. Numerous reports have described the use of NMBAs to facilitate mechanical ventilation. Most of the reports are limited to case studies, small prospective open-label trials, and small randomized open-label and double-blind trials enrolling a wide variety of critically ill patients to whom NMBAs were given to prevent respiratory dysynchrony, stop spontaneous respiratory efforts and muscle movement, improve gas exchange, and facilitate inverse ratio ventilation. However, none of these reports compared NMBAs to placebos.

Manage Increased ICP. The data supporting the use of NMBAs to control ICP are limited to a case report and an open-label trial. Prielipp[30] evaluated doxacurium use in eight patients with severe head injury in an open-label prospective study. NMBAs were given to facilitate ventilation or to manage brain injuries. Patients received an initial bolus injection of doxacurium 0.05 mg/kg followed by a continuous infusion of 0.25 μg/kg/min adjusted to maintain one twitch of the TOF. Doxacurium had no effect on ICP, heart rate, or blood pressure. Infusion rates were similar at the beginning (1 ± 0.1 mg/hr) and at the end (1.3 ± 0.2 mg/hr) of the study. TOF responses returned at 118 minutes; a TOF ratio of 0.7 was measured at 259 ± 24 minutes. No adverse events were reported.

McClelland, et al.[40] treated three patients with atracurium for four to six days to manage increased ICP. patients could undergo a neurologic examination within minutes after discontinuing atracurium. No adverse events were reported. There have been no controlled studies evaluating the role of NMBAs in the routine management of increased ICP.

Treat Muscle Spasms. Case studies describe the use of NMBAs in the treatment of muscle contractures associated with tetanus, drug overdoses, and seizures; many were published before 1994.

Anandaciva and Koay[41] administered a continuous rocuronium infusion to control muscle tone in patients with tetanus. Muscle spasms recurred at an infusion rate of 8 μg/kg/min, and neither administering a bolus dose of 0.9 mg/kg nor increasing the infusion rate to 10 μg/kg/min controlled the muscle contractures but did increase heart rate. Switching to a different NMBA could control the spasms.

Decrease Oxygen Consumption. Freebairn, et al.[42] evaluated the effects of vecuronium on oxygen delivery, oxygen consumption, oxygen extraction ratios, and gastric intramucosal pH in a randomized, placebo-controlled crossover trial in 18 critically ill patients with severe sepsis. Although the

TABLE 4.
Indications for the Long-Term Use of Neuromuscular Blocking Agents in Critically Ill Patients[a]

Indication	Agents (*n*)	Study Design	Underlying Diseases	Reference	Level of Evidence
Facilitate Mechanical Ventilation					
Facilitate management	Cisatracurium (40), atracurium (21)	Randomized, open-label	Hepatic failure, sepsis, cardiogenic shock, ARDS	20	2
Beneficial to management	Cisatracurium (12), atracurium (8)	Randomized, single-blind	Cardiac arrest, respiratory failure, postneurosurgery, trauma, multiorgan failure, asthma, cardiogenic shock	18	2
Facilitate management	Cisatracurium (6), atracurium (6)	Randomized, open-label	Multiple	19	2
Facilitate management	Cisatracurium (28), vecuronium (30)	Randomized, double-blind	Head trauma, intracranial hemorrhage, trauma, ARDS, sepsis, hepatic or renal failure, tetanus	15	2
Optimize mechanical ventilation, increase ICP	Doxacurium (19), pancuronium (21)	Prospective, randomized, double-blind	Not reported	12	2
Facilitate mechanical ventilation	Pipecuronium (30), pancuronium (30)	Prospective, open-label	Head injury, multiple trauma, sepsis, multiorgan failure	13	3
Facilitate mechanical ventilation; dose-finding pharmacokinetic study	Rocuronium (32)	Prospective, open-label	Respiratory failure, multiple trauma, blunt brain trauma	9	3
Facilitate mechanical ventilation; dose-finding pharmacokinetic study	Rocuronium (30)	Prospective, open-label	Multiple trauma and/or blunt brain trauma	8	3
Deterioration in gas exchange	Vecuronium and atracurium (1)	Case report	Respiratory failure in a kidney/pancreas transplant patient	39	5
Control ICP					
Facilitate mechanical ventilation and/or management of traumatic brain injury	Doxacurium (8)	Prospective, open-label	Severe head injury	30	3
Control ICP	Atracurium (4)	Case report	Severe head injury	40	5
Control Muscle Spasms					
Control tetanospasms	Rocuronium (1)	Case report	Tetanus	41	5
Decrease Oxygen Consumption					
Determine effect on oxygen delivery, consumption, and gastric intramucosal pH	Vecuronium (18)	Prospective, randomized, controlled, cross-over	Severe sepsis and septic shock	42	2

[a]ARDS = acute respiratory distress syndrome, ICP = intracranial pressure.

Figure 2. Use of neuromuscular blocking agents (NMBAs) in the ICU.

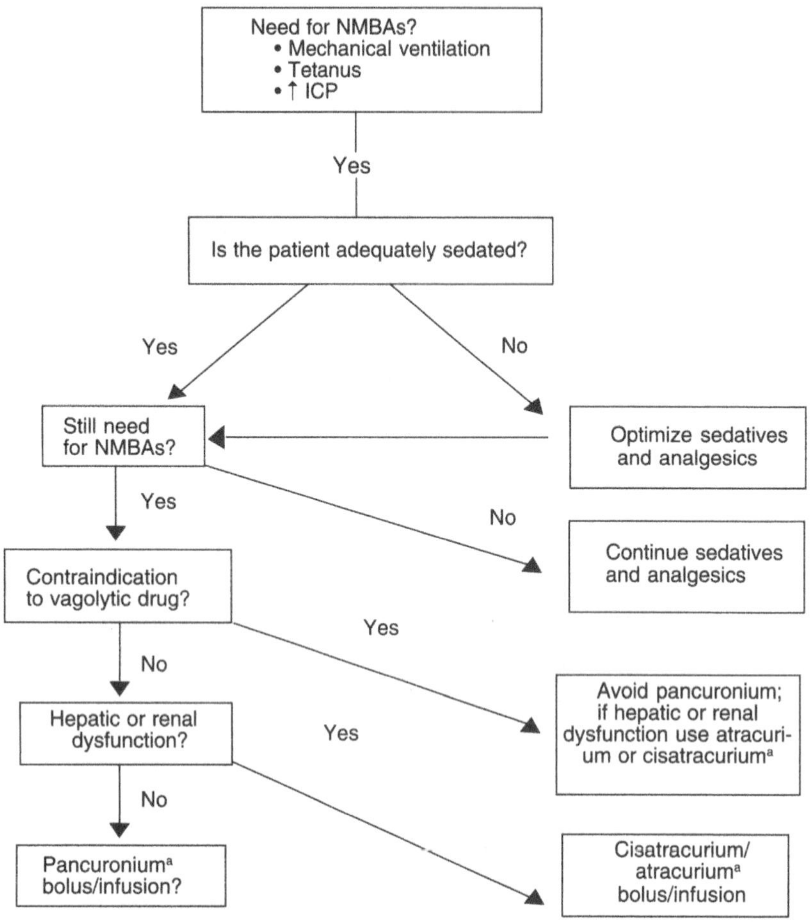

[a]Monitor train-of-four ratio, protect eyes, position patient to protect pressure points, and address deep venous thrombosis prophylaxis. Reassess every 12–24 hours for continued NMBA indication.

infusion of vecuronium achieved an adequate level of paralysis and improved respiratory compliance, it did not alter intramucosal pH, oxygen consumption, oxygen delivery, or oxygen extraction ratios.

Recommended Indications

There are no prospective, randomized, controlled trials assigning patients to an NMBA versus a placebo with a goal of documenting if such patients could be managed by means other than NMBA therapy.

> *Recommendation: NMBAs should be used for an adult patient in an ICU to manage ventilation, manage increased ICP, treat muscle spasms, and decrease oxygen consumption only when all other means have been tried without success. (Grade of recommendation = C)*

Recommended Drugs

There has, in essence, been no study since the last guidelines were published that questions the use of pancuronium for the majority of patients in an ICU. Those prospective, randomized, controlled trials (PRCTs) that have been conducted do not clearly show the benefits of using newer agents or any other agents instead of pancuronium.

There are no well-designed studies with sufficient power to make this a level A recommendation, but there is evidence in the literature that patients on pancuronium fare as well as or better than patients receiving any other NMBA.

The two adverse effects of pancuronium that are commented on frequently are vagolysis and an increase in heart rate. Therefore, patients who would not tolerate an increase in heart rate, i.e., those with cardiovascular disease, should probably receive an NMBA other than pancuronium. The indications for the use of an NMBA must outweigh the risk of tachycardia, and that is based on interpretation of the severity of the patient's underlying cardiovascular disease. For example, a patient with a history of atrial fibrillation now in sinus rhythm and otherwise hemodynamically stable might better tolerate pancuronium than a patient who is hospitalized with cardiogenic pulmonary edema and managed with mechanical ventilation. The clinician should choose an NMBA on the basis of other patient characteristics. Any benzylisoquinolinium compound or aminosteroidal compound could be substituted for pancuronium in these circumstances.

There are no ideal PRCTs that support this recommendation, but there are data suggesting that patients recover more quickly following administration of cisatracurium or atracurium compared with patients receiving other NMBAs if they have evidence of hepatic or renal disease.

> *Recommendations: The majority of patients in an ICU who are pre-scribed an NMBA can be managed effectively with pancuronium. (Grade of recommendation = B)*
>
> *For patients for whom vagolysis is contraindicated (e.g., those with cardiovascular disease), NMBAs other than pancuronium may be used. (Grade of recommendation = C)*
>
> *Because of their unique metabolism, cisatracurium or atracurium is recommended for patients with significant hepatic or renal disease. (Grade of recommendation = B)*

Monitoring

Monitoring neuromuscular blockade is recommended (**Table 5**).[12,14,43–55] Monitoring the depth of neuromuscular blockade may allow use of the lowest NMBA dose and may minimize adverse events. No PRCT has reported that reducing the dose of an NMBA can prevent persistent weakness. Despite this lack of evidence and the lack of a standardized

TABLE 5.
Monitoring the Degree of Neuromuscular Blockade[a]

Monitoring Method	Study Design	Reference	Level of Evidence
TOF vs. clinical assessment to guide dosing	Prospective, randomized, single-blind	14	2
TOF vs. clinical assessment to compare depth of neuromuscular blockade	Prospective, nonrandomized	43	4
Complications with various monitoring methods	Retrospective, nonrandomized cohort	44	4
Use of TOF in comparing NMBAs	Multicenter, double-blind, PRCT	12	2
Methods of monitoring NMBAs	Editorial	45	6
Methods of monitoring NMBAs	Review	46	6
Comparison of common NMBAs/pharmacology	Review	25	6
Frequency of NMBA monitoring methods	Nonrandomized, historic, descriptive	47	4
Comparison of NMBA monitoring methods	Editorial	48	6
Comparison of NMBA monitoring methods	Expert opinion	49	6
Comparison of NMBA monitoring methods	Expert opinion	50	6
Technical aspects and problems in NMBA monitoring	Review	51	6
Technical problems with NMBAs monitoring	Review	52	6
Technical problems with NMBA monitoring	Review	53	5
Methods of assessing depth of NMBA	Prospective, randomized, blinded	54	2
Patient assessment during NMBA use	Review	55	6

[a]TOF = train-of-four, NMBA = neuromuscular blocking agent, PRCT = prospective, randomized, controlled trial.

method of monitoring, assessment of the depth of neuromuscular blockade in ICU patients is recommended.[43]

Visual, tactile, or electronic assessment of the patient's muscle tone or some combination of these three is commonly used to monitor the depth of neuromuscular blockade. Observation of skeletal muscle movement and respiratory effort forms the foundation of clinical assessment; electronic methods include the use of ventilator software allowing plethysmographic recording of pulmonary function to detect spontaneous ventilatory efforts and "twitch monitoring," i.e., the assessment of the muscular response by visual, tactile, or electronic means to a transcutaneous delivery of electric current meant to induce peripheral nerve stimulation (PNS).

Since the last practice guidelines were published, only two studies have examined the best method of monitoring the depth of neuromuscular blockade, and none have compared the efficacy or accuracy of specific techniques. The first study was a prospective, randomized, single-blinded trial of 77 patients in a medical ICU who were administered vecuronium based on either clinical parameters (patient breathed above the preset ventilatory rate) or TOF monitoring, with a goal of one of four twitches.[44] PNS resulted in a significantly lower total dose and lower mean infusion rate of NMBA as well as a faster time to recovery of neuromuscular function and spontaneous ventilation.

A second study sought to compare the depth of blockade induced by atracurium either by "best clinical assessment" (i.e., maintenance of patient-ventilator synchrony and prevention of patient movement) or TOF monitoring (with a goal of three of four twitches). Analysis of the 36 medical ICU patients in this prospective, nonrandomized trial revealed no difference in the total dose, mean dose, or the mean time to clinical recovery.[43] This may have been due to sample size or study design.

An additional study examining the results of the implementation of a protocol using PNS to monitor the level of blockade in patients receiving a variety of NMBAs found a reduction in the incidence of persistent neuromuscular weakness.[49]

Other methods of electronic monitoring of the depth of blockade are fraught with difficulties; TOF monitoring of PNS remains the easiest and most reliable method available,[43,44,46–50] despite its shortcomings and technical pitfalls.[51–53] Currently, there is no universal standard for twitch monitoring. The choice of the number of twitches necessary for "optimal" blockade is influenced by the patient's overall condition and level of sedation. The choice of the "best" nerve for monitoring may be influenced by site accessibility, risk of false positives, considerations for the effect of stimulation on patient visitors, and whether faint twitches should be included in the assessment of blockade.[54–56] Despite these gaps in research-generated knowledge, evidence-based practice appears to be influencing the increasing frequency with which PNS is utilized.[47] The low correlation of blockade measured peripherally compared with that of the phrenic nerve and diaphragm underscores the importance of three issues: (1) more than one method of monitoring should be utilized, (2) poor technique in using any device will invariably produce inaccurate results, and (3) more clinical studies are necessary to determine the best techniques.

Recommendations for Monitoring Degree of Blockade

Even though the patient may appear quiet and "comfortable," experienced clinicians understand the indications and therapeutic limits of NMBAs. Despite multiple admonitions that NMBAs have no analgesic or amnestic effects, it is not uncommon to find a patient's degree of sedation or comfort significantly overestimated or even ignored. It is difficult to assess pain and sedation in the patient receiving NMBAs, but patients must be medicated for pain and anxiety, despite the lack of obvious symptoms or signs. In common practice, sedative and analgesic drugs are adjusted until the patient does not appear to be conscious and then NMBAs are administered. There have been no studies of the use of electrophysiologic monitoring in assessing adequacy of sedation or analgesia.

In a phenomenological study of 11 critically ill adult trauma patients who required therapeutic NMBA, patients compared their feelings of vagueness to dreaming.[56] Few patients recalled pain or painful procedures. Family members understood the rationale for the use of the drugs and remembered being encouraged to touch and talk with patients. The use of effective pain and sedation protocols and a liberalized visiting policy may have affected the findings.

Recommendations: Patients receiving NMBAs should be assessed both clinically and by TOF monitoring (Grade of recommendation = B), with a goal of adjusting the degree of neuromuscular blockade to achieve one or two twitches. (Grade of recommendation = C)

Before initiating neuromuscular blockade, patients should be medicated with sedative and analgesic drugs to provide adequate sedation and analgesia in accordance with the physician's clinical judgment to optimize therapy. (Grade of recommendation = C)

Complications

Skeletal muscle weakness in ICU patients is multifactorial, producing a confusing list of names and syndromes, including acute quadriplegic myopathy syndrome (AQMS), floppy man syndrome, critical illness polyneuropathy (CIP), acute myopathy of intensive care, rapidly evolving myopathy, acute myopathy with selective lysis of myosin filaments, acute steroid myopathy, and prolonged neurogenic weakness (**Table 6**).[57,58]

There are probably two adverse events related to prolonged paralysis following discontinuation of NMBAs. We define the first, "prolonged recovery from NMBAs," as an increase (after cessation of NMBA therapy) in the time to recovery of 50–100% longer than predicted by pharmacologic parameters. This is primarily due to the accumulation of NMBAs or metabolites. By comparison, the second, AQMS, presents with a clinical triad of acute paresis, myonecrosis with increased creatine phosphokinase (CPK) concentration, and abnormal electromyography (EMG). The latter is characterized by severely reduced compound motor action potential (CMAP) amplitudes and evidence of acute denervation. In the beginning, these syndromes are characterized by neuronal dysfunction; later (days or weeks), muscle atrophy and necrosis may develop.[59]

TABLE 6.
Weakness in ICU Patients: Etiologies and Syndromes[a]

1. Prolonged recovery from NMBAs (secondary to parent drug, drug metabolite, or drug-drug interaction)
2. Myasthenia gravis
3. Lambert-Eaton syndrome
4. Muscular dystrophy
5. Guillain-Barré syndrome
6. Central nervous system injury or lesion
7. Spinal cord injury
8. Steroid myopathy
9. Mitochondrial myopathy
10. HIV-related myopathy
11. Acute myopathy of intensive care
12. Disuse atrophy
13. Critical illness polyneuropathy
14. Severe electrolyte toxicity (e.g., hypermagnesemia)
15. Severe electrolyte deficiency (e.g., hypophosphatemia)

[a]ICU = intensive care unit, NMBAs = neuromuscular blocking agents, HIV = human immunodeficiency virus.

Prolonged Recovery from NMBAs. The steroid-based NMBAs are associated with reports of prolonged recovery and myopathy.[57,60] This association may reflect an increased risk inferred by these NMBAs or may reflect past practice patterns in which these drugs may have been more commonly used.[61] Steroid-based NMBAs undergo extensive hepatic metabolism, producing active drug metabolites. For instance, vecuronium produces three metabolites: 3-des-, 17-des-, and 3,17-desacetyl vecuronium.[62] The 3-desacetyl metabolite is estimated to be 80% as potent as the parent compound. The 3-desacetyl vecuronium metabolite is poorly dialyzed, minimally ultrafiltrated, and accumulates in patients with renal failure because hepatic elimination is decreased in patients with uremia. Thus, the accumulation of both 3- desacetyl vecuronium and its parent compound, vecuronium, in patients with renal failure contributes to a prolonged recovery by this ICU subpopulation. Other explanations have been proposed. One suggests that the basement membrane of the neuromuscular junction acts as a reservoir of NMBAs, maintaining NMBAs at the nAChRs long after the drug has disappeared from the plasma.[63]

Drug–drug interactions that potentiate the depth of motor blockade (**Table 7**) may also prolong recovery. The specific interaction of NMBAs and exogenous corticosteroids is discussed later.[57,62–65]

Physiologic changes of the nAChRs are enhanced when patients are immobilized or denervated secondary to spinal cord injury, and perhaps during prolonged NMBA drug-induced paralysis. The nAChRs may be triggered to revert to a fetal-variant structure (**Figure 3**), characterized by an increase in total number, frequent extrajunctional proliferation, and resistance to nondepolarizing NMBAs. The proliferation and distribution of these altered receptors across the myomembrane may account for tachyphylaxis and the neuromuscular blocking effects of these drugs.

AQMS. AQMS, also referred to as postparalytic quadriparesis, is one of the most devastating complications of NMBA therapy and one of the reasons that indiscriminate use of NMBAs is discouraged (**Table 8**).[65,66] This entity must be differentiated from other neuromuscular pathologies (Table 6) seen in an ICU and requires extensive testing. Reports of AQMS in patients receiving NMBAs alone are quite limited; no experimental model has been able to produce the histopathology of this syndrome by administering NMBAs. Afflicted patients demonstrate diffuse weakness that persists long after the NMBA is discontinued and the drug and its active metabolites are eliminated. Neurologic examination reveals a global motor deficit affecting muscles in both the upper and lower

TABLE 7.
Drug-Drug Interactions of Neuromuscular Blocking Agents (NMBAs)

Drugs that Potentiate the Action of Nondepolarizing NMBAs	Drugs that Antagonize the Actions of Nondepolarizing NMBAs
Local anesthetics	Phenytoin
Lidocaine	Carbamazepine
Antimicrobials (aminoglycosides, polymyxin B, clindamycin, tetracycline)	Theophylline
Antiarrhythmics (procainamide, quinidine)	Ranitidine
Magnesium	
Calcium channel blockers	
β-Adrenergic blockers	
Immunosuppresive agents (cyclophosphamide, cyclosporine)	
Dantrolene	
Diuretics	
Lithium carbonate	

Figure 3. Acetylcholine Receptor. The mature nicotinic acetylcholine receptor (AChR) (left) with its glycoprotein subunits arranged around the central cation core. Two molecules of acetylcholine bind simultaneously to the two alpha subunits to convert the channel to an open state. The immature, or fetal-variant, receptor is shown on the right, with a single subunit substitution which follows major stress such as burns or denervation. These immature receptors are characterized by 10-fold greater ionic activity, rapid metabolic turnover, and extrajunctional proliferation. (Reprinted, with permission, from Martyn JAJ, White DA, Gronert GA, et al. Up-and-down regulation of skeletal muscle acetylcholine receptors. *Anesthesiology.* 1992; 76:825.)

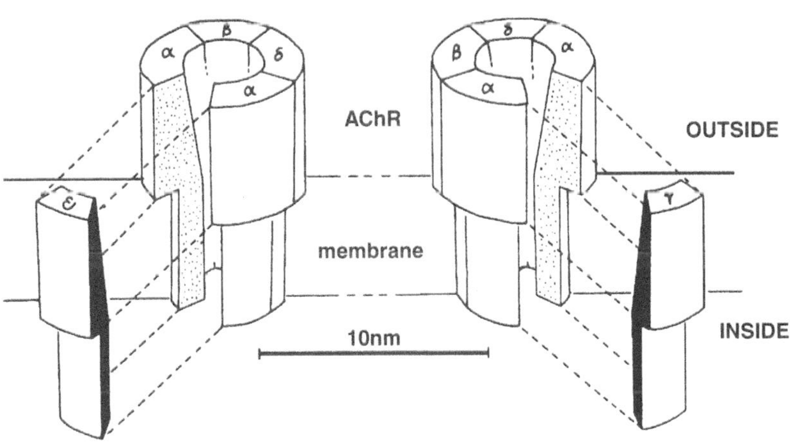

extremities and decreased motor reflexes. However, extraocular muscle function is usually preserved. This myopathy is characterized by low-amplitude CMAPs, and muscle fibrillations but normal (or nearly normal) sensory nerve conduction studies.[63,67] Muscle biopsy shows prominent vacuolization of muscle fibers without inflammatory infiltrate, patchy type 2 muscle fiber atrophy, and sporadic myofiber necrosis.[64] Modest CPK increases (0 to 15-fold above normal range) are noted in approximately 50% of patients and are probably dependent on the timing of enzyme measurements and the initiation of the myopathic process. Thus, there may be some justification in screening patients with serial CPK determinations during infusion of NMBAs, particularly if the patients are concurrently treated with corticosteroids. Also, since AQMS develops after prolonged exposure to NMBAs, there may be some rationale to daily "drug holidays" (i.e., stopping the drugs for a few to several hours and restarting them only when necessary). However, no one has demonstrated that drug holidays decrease the frequency of AQMS. Other factors that may contribute to the development of the syndrome include nutritional deficiencies, concurrent drug administration with aminoglycosides or cyclosporine, hyperglycemia, renal and hepatic dysfunction, fever, and severe metabolic or electrolyte disorders.

Evidence supports, but occasionally refutes,[14] the association of concurrent administration of NMBAs and corticosteroids with AQMS.[59,63,68,69] The incidence of myopathy may be as high as 30% in patients who receive corticosteroids and NMBAs. While no period of paralysis is risk free, NMBA administration beyond one or two days increases the risk of myopathy in this setting.[63] Similarly, there is an inconsistent correlation with the dose of corticosteroids, but total doses in excess of 1 g of methylprednisolone (or equivalent) probably increase the risk. Afflicted patients manifest an acute, diffuse, flaccid weakness and an inability to wean from mechanical ventilation. Sensory function is generally preserved.[63] Muscle biopsy shows extensive type 2 fiber atrophy, myonecrosis, disarray of sarcomere architecture, and an extensive, selective loss of myosin. Experimental evidence in animals shows that denervation for ≥24 hours induces profound negative nitrogen balance and increases expression of steroid receptors in muscle. Such denervation sensitizes muscle to even normal cortico steroid concentrations, and evidence suggests that the combination of denervation and high-dose corticosteroids precipitates myosinolysis.

Acute myopathy in ICU patients is also reported after administration of the benzylisoquinolinium NMBAs (i.e., atracurium, cisatracurium, doxacurium).[24,34,69] Common to all these reports is the coadministration of benzylisoquinolinium NMBAs and large doses of corticosteroids, aminoglycosides, or other drugs that affect neuromuscular transmission.

Recommendations: For patients receiving NMBAs and corticosteroids, every effort should be made to discontinue NMBAs as soon as possible. (Grade of recommendation = C)

Drug holidays (i.e., stopping NMBAs daily until forced to restart them based on the patient's condition) may decrease the incidence of AQMS. (Grade of recommendation = C)

Other nerve and muscle disorders have been recognized in the last decade in ICU patients (Table 6). For instance, CIP is a sensory and motor polyneuropathy identified in elderly, septic patients or those with MODS.[58,66,70] EMG testing reveals decreased CMAP, fibrillation potentials,

TABLE 8.
Potential Complications of Neuromuscular Blockade Use in the ICU[a]

Complications and Contraindications of Succinylcholine in the ICU	General Complications Associated with NMBAs in the ICU
Loss of airway	Awake, paralyzed patient-anxiety and panic
Hyperkalemia	Risk of ventilator disconnect or airway mishap
Plasma pseudocholinesterase deficiency	Autonomic and cardiovascular effects (i.e., vagolytic)
	Decreased lymphatic flow
	Risk of generalized deconditioning
	Skin breakdown
	Peripheral nerve injury
	Corneal abrasion, conjunctivitis
	Myositis ossificans
	Risk of prolonged muscle weakness, AQMS
	Potential central nervous system toxicity

[a]NMBA = neuromuscular blocking agent, AQMS = acute quadriplegic myopathy syndrome.

and positive sharp waves.[60,63,64] CIP is primarily an axonopathy and may be related to microvascular ischemia of the nerve but is not directly related to the use of NMBAs. Recovery from ICU myopathy requires a protracted (weeks or months) hospitalization. One economic analysis of 10 patients who developed AQMS showed the median additional hospital charge to be $66,000 per patient.[65] As for any critically ill patient, particularly immobilized patients, deep venous thrombosis (DVT) prophylaxis and physical therapy to maintain joint mobility are important.

Patients receiving NMBAs are also at risk of developing keratitis and corneal abrasion. Prophylactic eye care is highly variable and recommendations may include methylcellulose drops, ophthalmic ointment, taping the eyelids shut to ensure complete closure, or eye patches. In a study of 69 paralyzed or heavily sedated patients by Lenart and Garrity,[71] there was strong evidence that the use of an artificial tear ointment prevented corneal exposure. In this randomized study, patients served as their own controls.

Myositis Ossificans (Heterotopic Ossification). Myositis ossificans can develop in patients who are paralyzed for long periods of time, but inflammation is not characteristic of the ailment. The name is misleading because the process involves connective tissue (not muscle). The name originates from the ossification that occurs within the connective tissue of muscle but may also be seen in ligaments, tendons, fascia, aponeuroses, and joint capsules. The acquired form of the disease may occur at any age in either sex, especially around the elbows, thighs, and buttocks. The basic defect is the inappropriate differentiation of fibroblasts into osteoblasts and is usually triggered by trauma and muscle injury, paraplegia or quadriplegia, tetanus, and burns. Treatment consists of promoting an active range of motion around the affected joint and surgery when necessary.

Tachyphylaxis. For reasons mentioned earlier, tachyphylaxis to NMBAs can and does develop.

Coursin and colleagues[31] administered doxacurium to four patients who developed tolerance to atracurium infusions (range, 16 to 40 µg/kg/min). Patients were successfully blocked with infusion rates of doxacurium 0.25–0.75 µg/kg/min.

Tschida, et al.[72] described a patient whose atracurium requirement escalated from 5 to 30 µg/kg/min over 10 days. The patient was successfully blocked with a pancuronium infusion of 10–50 µg/kg/min for a period of five days.

Fish and Singletary[33] describe a patient who was inadequately blocked with a 60-µg/kg/min infusion of atracurium but adequately paralyzed for seven days with 2.3-mg/kg/hr infusion of vecuronium. Tachyphylaxis then developed to vecuronium which prompted discontinuation of NMBAs. Two days later, 50–µg/kg/min atracurium infusions were required with high-dose midazolam and fentanyl infusions to achieve adequate oxygenation and acceptable airway pressures.

Recommendations: Patients receiving NMBAs should have prophylactic eye care (Grade of recommendation = B), physical therapy (Grade of recommendation = C), and DVT prophylaxis. (Grade of recommendation = C)

Patients who develop tachyphylaxis to one NMBA should try another drug if neuromuscular blockade is still required. (Grade of recommendation = C)

Economics

There have been few formal pharmacoeconomic evaluations of NMBAs. In one of these economic evaluations, medication-related cost savings were found when voluntary prescribing guidelines for NMBAs were initiated in the operating room of a university hospital.[73] In another study that involved randomization to one of three NMBAs, there were no significant cost differences between atracurium, vecuronium, and rocuronium for surgeries lasting two hours or less, but vecuronium and rocuronium were economically advantageous if the duration of surgery was two to four hours.[74] In a third retrospective study, long-acting NMBAs (e.g., D-tubocurarine and pancuronium) were associated with prolonged postoperative recovery compared with shorter-acting agents (e.g., atracurium, mivacurium, and vecuronium). The authors noted in the discussion section of the paper that based on intrainstitutional recovery room costs, delays in recovery times seen with the longer-acting agents offset the expected savings in drug costs.[75] For patients transferred to the ICU, this may not be a major problem.

Two pharmacoeconomic investigations involving NMBAs in the ICU evaluated the costs associated with prolonged recovery following discontinuation of nondepolarizing NMBAs. In one study, overall costs were lower when TOF monitoring was employed.[76] In another study, patients who had prolonged motor weakness after discontinuing NMBAs were compared with a control group[77]; ICU and hospital costs were substantially higher in the patients with prolonged weakness.

A study involving 40 academic medical centers with patients undergoing coronary artery bypass graft surgery found no significant differences in duration of intubation or duration of ICU or hospital stay among patients who received pancuronium ($n = 732$), vecuronium ($n = 130$), or both ($n = 242$) agents.[78] It is unknown if these results pertain to subgroups of patients, such as those with renal or hepatic dysfunction. If the results of this study are confirmed, the choice of agent could be based solely on cost minimization using medication purchase cost information and equipotent dosage regimens.

A prospective, randomized trial comparing TOF to standard clinical assessment showed decreased NMBA usage and faster return of spontaneous ventilation with TOF monitoring.[14] TOF has the potential to decrease costs associated with NMBA use in ICUs.

Appendix B describes the basic steps involved in conducting a cost-effectiveness analysis of the NMBAs. Consequently, intrainstitutional data and assumptions can be used to perform the analysis along with local value judgments involved in selecting the appropriate agent(s).

Recommendations: Institutions should perform an economic analysis using their own data when choosing NMBAs for use in an ICU. (Grade of recommendation = C)

References

1. Society of Critical Care Medicine and American Society of Health-System Pharmacists. Sedation, analgesia, and neuromuscular blockade of the critically ill adult: revised clinical practice guidelines for 2002. *Am J Health-Syst Pharm.* 2002; 59:147–9.
2. Coakley JH, Nagendran K, Yarwood GD, et al. Patterns of neurophysiological abnormality in prolonged critical illness. *Intensive Care Med.* 1998; 24:801–7.
3. Prielipp RC, Coursin DB. Applied pharmacology of common neuromuscular blocking agents in critical care. *New Horizons.* 1994; 2:34–47.
4. De Lemos JM, Carr RR, Shalansky KF, et al. Paralysis in the critically ill: intermittent bolus pancuronium compared with continuous infusion. *Crit Care Med.* 1999; 27:2648–55.
5. Tobias JD, Lynch A, McDuffee A, et al. Pancuronium infusion for neuromuscular block in children in the pediatric intensive care unit. *Anesth Analg.* 1995; 81:13–6.
6. Segredo V, Caldwell JE, Wright PM, et al. Do the pharmacokinetics of vecuronium change during prolonged administration in critically ill patients? *Br J Anaesth.* 1998; 80:715–9.
7. Appadu BL, Greiff JM, Thompson JP. Postal survey on the long-term use of neuromuscular block in the intensive care unit. *Intensive Care Med.* 1996; 22:862–6.
8. Khuenl-Brady KS, Sparr H, Pühringer F, et al. Rocuronium bromide in the ICU: dose finding and pharmacokinetics. *Eur J Anaesthesiol Suppl.* 1995; 11:79–80.
9. Sparr HJ, Wierda JMKH, Proost JH, et al. Pharmacodynamics and pharmacokinetics of rocuronium in intensive care patients. *Br J Anaesth.* 1997; 78:267–73.
10. McEwin L, Merrick PM, Bevan DR. Residual neuromuscular blockade after cardiac surgery: pancuronium vs rocuronium. *Can J Anaesth.* 1997; 44:891–5.
11. Stene J, Murray M, de Ruyter M, et al. Selective rocuronium pharmacodynamics and kinetics during ICU infusion. *Anesthesiology.* 1998; 89:A477. Abstract.
12. Murray MJ, Coursin DB, Scuderi PE, et al. Double-blind, randomized, multicenter study of doxacurium vs. pancuronium in intensive care unit patients who require neuromuscular-blocking agents. *Crit Care Med.* 1995; 23:450–8.
13. Khuenl-Brady KS, Reitstatter B, Schlager A, et al. Long-term administration of pancuronium and pipecuronium in the intensive care unit. *Anesth Analg.* 1994; 78:1082–6.
14. Rudis MI, Sikora CP, Angus E, et al. A prospective, randomized, controlled evaluation of peripheral nerve stimulation versus standard clinical dosing of neuromuscular blocking agents in critically ill patients. *Crit Care Med.* 1997; 25:575–83.
15. Prielipp RC, Coursin DB, Scuderi PB, et al. Comparison of the infusion requirements and recovery profiles of vecuronium and cisatracurium 51W89 in intensive care unit patients. *Anesth Analg.* 1995; 81:3–12.
16. Hull CJ. Pharmacokinetics and pharmacodynamics of the benzylisoquinolinium muscle relaxants. *Acta Anaesthesiol Scand Suppl.* 1995; 106:13–7.
17. De Wolf AM, Freeman JA, Scott VL, et al. Pharmacokinetics and pharmacodynamics of cisatracurium in patients with end-stage liver disease undergoing liver transplantation. *Br J Anaesth.* 1996; 76:624–8.
18. Pearson AJ, Harper NJ, Pollard BJ. The infusion requirements and recovery characteristics of cisatracurium or atracurium in intensive care patients. *Intensive Care Med.* 1996; 22:694–8.
19. Boyd AH, Eastwood NB, Parker CJ, et al. Comparison of the pharmacodynamics and pharmacokinetics of an infusion of cisatracurium (51W89) or atracurium in critically ill patients undergoing mechanical ventilation in an intensive therapy unit. *Br J Anaesth.* 1996; 76:382–8.
20. Newman PJ, Quinn AC, Grounds RM, et al. A comparison of cisatracurium (51W89) and atracurium by infusion in critically ill patients. *Crit Care Med.* 1997; 25:1139–42.
21. Schramm WM, Papousek A, Michalek-Sauberer A, et al. The cerebral and cardiovascular effects of cisatracurium and atracurium in neurosurgical patients. *Anesth Analg.* 1998; 86:123–7.
22. Schramm WM, Jesenko R, Bartuneka A, et al. Effects of cisatracurium on cerebral and cardiovascular hemo-dynamics in patients with severe brain injury. *Acta Anaesthesiol Scand.* 1997; 41:1319–23.
23. Grigore AM, Brusco LJr, Kuroda M, et al. Laudanosine and atracurium concentrations in a patient receiving long-term atracurium infusion. *Crit Care Med.* 1998; 26:180–3.
24. Davis NA, Rodgers JE, Gonzalez ER, et al. Prolonged weakness after cisatracurium infusion: a case report. *Crit Care Med.* 1998; 26:1290–2.
25. Reeves ST, Turcasso NM. Nondepolarizing neuromuscular blocking drugs in the intensive care unit: a clinical review. *South Med J.* 1997; 90:769–74.

26. Miller RD. Use of neuromuscular blocking drugs in intensive care unit patients. *Anesth Analg.* 1995; 81:1–2.
27. Bion J, Prielipp RC, Bihari D, et al. Cisatracurium in intensive care. *Curr Opin Anesthesiol.* 1996; 9:S47–51.
28. Werba A, Schultz AM, Hetz H, et al. Benzylisochinoline muscle relaxants in clinical practice. *Acta Anaesthesiol Scan Suppl.* 1997; 111:109–10.
29. Marik PE, Kaufman D. The effects of neuromuscular paralysis on systemic and splanchnic oxygen utilization in mechanically ventilated patients. *Chest.* 1996; 109:1038–42.
30. Prielipp RC, Robinson JC, Wilson JA, et al. Dose response, recovery, and cost of doxacurium as a continuous infusion in neurosurgical intensive care unit patients. *Crit Care Med.* 1997; 25:1236–41.
31. Coursin DB, Meyer DA, Prielipp RC. Doxacurium infusion in critically ill patients with atracurium tachyphylaxis. *Am J Health Syst-Pharm.* 1995; 52:635–9.
32. Manthous CA, Chatila W. Atracurium and status epilepticus. *Crit Care Med.* 1995; 23:1440–2.
33. Fish DN, Singletary TJ. Cross-resistance to both atracurium- and vecuronium-induced neuromuscular blockade in a critically ill patient. *Pharmacotherapy.* 1997; 17:1322–7.
34. Meyer KC, Prielipp RC, Grossman JE, et al. Prolonged weakness after infusion of atracurium in two intensive care unit patients. *Anesth Analg.* 1994; 78:772–4.
35. Manthous CA, Chatila W. Prolonged weakness after the withdrawal of atracurium. *Am J Resp Crit Care Med.* 1994; 150:1441–3.
36. Branney SW, Haenal JB, Moore FA, et al. Prolonged paralysis with atracurium infusion: a case report. *Crit Care Med.* 1994; 22:1699–701.
37. Rubjo ER, Seelig CB. Persistent paralysis after prolonged use of atracurium in the absence of corticosteroids. *South Med J.* 1996; 89:624–6.
38. Hoey LL, Joslin SM, Nahum A, et al. Prolonged neuromuscular blockade in two critically ill patients treated with atracurium. *Pharmacotherapy.* 1995; 15:254–9.
39. Prielipp RC, Jackson MJ, Coursin DB. Comparison of neuromuscular recovery after paralysis with atracurium versus vecuronium in an ICU patient with renal insufficiency. *Anesth Analg.* 1994; 78:775–8.
40. McClelland M, Woster P, Sweasey T, et al. Continuous midazolam/atracurium infusions for the management of increased intracranial pressure. *J Neurosci Nurs.* 1995; 27:96–101.
41. Anandaciva S, Koay CW. Tetanus and rocuronium in the intensive care unit. *Anaesthesia.* 1996; 51:505–6.
42. Freebairn RC, Derrick J, Gomersall CD, et al. Oxygen delivery, oxygen consumption, and gastric intramucosal pH are not improved by a computer-controlled, closed-loop, vecuronium infusion in severe sepsis. *Crit Care Med.* 1997; 25:72–7.
43. Strange C, Vaughan L, Franklin C, et al. Comparison of train-of-four and best clinical assessment during continuous paralysis. *Am J Resp Crit Care Med.* 1997; 156:1556–61.
44. Frankel H, Jeng J, Tilly E, et al. The impact of implementation of neuromuscular blockade monitoring standards in a surgical intensive care unit. *Am Surg.* 1996; 62:503–6.
45. Sladen RN. Neuromuscular blocking agents in the intensive care unit: a two-edged sword. *Crit Care Med.* 1995; 23:423–8.
46. Ford EV. Monitoring neuromuscular blockade in the adult ICU. *Am J Crit Care.* 1995; 4:122–30.
47. Kleinpell R, Bedrosian C, McCormick L. Use of peripheral nerve stimulators to monitor patients with neuromuscular blockade in the ICU. *Am J Crit Care.* 1996; 5:449–54.
48. Murray MJ. Monitoring of peripheral nerve stimulation versus standard clinical assessment for dosing of neuromuscular blocking agents. *Crit Care Med.* 1997; 25:561–2.
49. Tavernier B, Rannou JJ, Vallet B. Peripheral nerve stimulation and clinical assessment for dosing of neuromuscular blocking agents in critically ill patients. *Crit Care Med.* 1998; 26:804–5.
50. Barnette RE, Fish DJ. Monitoring neuromuscular blockade in the critically ill. *Crit Care Med.* 1995; 23:1790–1.
51. Rudis M, Guslits B, Zarowitz B. Technical and interpretative problems of peripheral nerve stimulation in monitoring neuromuscular blockade in the intensive care unit. *Ann Pharmacother.* 1996; 30:165–72.
52. Tschida SJ, Loey LL, Bryan KV. Inconsistency with train-of-four monitoring in a critically ill paralyzed patient. *Pharmacotherapy.* 1995; 15:540–5.
53. Tschida SJ, Loey LL, Mather D. Train-of-four: to use or not to use. *Pharmacotherapy.* 1995; 15:546–50.
54. Martin R, Bourdua I, Theriault S, et al. Neuromuscular monitoring: does it make a difference? *Can J Anesth.* 1996; 43:585–8.
55. Luer JM. Sedation and chemical relaxation in critical pulmonary illness: suggestions for patient assessment and drug monitoring. *AACN Clin Issues.* 1995; 6:333–43.
56. Johnson KL, Cheung RB, Johnson SB, et al. Therapeutic paralysis of critically ill trauma patients: perceptions of patients and their family members. *Am J Crit Care.* 1999; 8:490–8.
57. Watling SM, Dasta JF. Prolonged paralysis in intensive care unit patients after the use of neuromuscular blocking agents: a review of the literature. *Crit Care Med.* 1994; 22:884–93.
58. Nates J, Cooper D, Day B, et al. Acute weakness syndromes in critically ill patients—a reappraisal. *Anaesth Intensive Care.* 1997; 25:502–13.
59. Road J, Mackie G, Jiang T, et al. Reversible paralysis with status asthmaticus, steroids, and pancuronium: clinical electrophysiological correlates. *Muscle Nerve.* 1997; 20:1587–90.
60. Lacomis D, Giuliani MJ, Van Cott A, et al. Acute myopathy of intensive care: clinical, electromyographic, and pathological aspects. *Ann Neurol.* 1996; 40:645–54.
61. Elliot J, Bion J. The use of neuromuscular blocking drugs in intensive care practice. *Acta Anaesthesiol Scand Suppl.* 1995; 106:70–82.

62. Leatherman J, Fluegel W, David W, et al. Muscle weakness in mechanically ventilated patients with severe asthma. *Am J Resp Crit Care Med.* 1996; 153:1686–90.
63. David W, Roehr C, Leatherman J. EMG findings in acute myopathy with status asthmaticus, steroids and paralytics: clinical and electrophysiologic correlation. *Electromyogr Clin Neurophysiol.* 1998; 38:371–6.
64. Faragher MW, Day BJ, Dennett X. Critical care myopathy: an electrophysiological and histological study. *Muscle Nerve.* 1996; 19:516–8.
65. Latronico N, Fenzi F, Recupero D, et al. Critical illness myopathy and neuropathy. *Lancet.* 1996; 347:1579–82.
66. Bolton CF. Muscle weakness and difficulty in weaning from the ventilator in the critical care unit. *Chest.* 1994; 106:1–2.
67. Barohn RJ, Jackson CE, Rogers SJ, et al. Prolonged paralysis due to nondepolarizing neuromuscular blocking agents and corticosteroids. *Muscle Nerve.* 1994; 17:647–54.
68. Zochodne DW, Ramsay DA, Shelley S. Acute necrotizing myopathy of intensive care: electrophysiologic studies. *Muscle Nerve.* 1994; 17:285–92.
69. Marik PE. Doxacurium-corticosteroid acute myopathy: another piece to the puzzle. *Crit Care Med.* 1996; 24:1266–7.
70. Hund E, Fogel W, Krieger D, et al. Critical illness polyneuropathy: clinical findings and outcomes of a frequent cause of neuromuscular weaning failure. *Crit Care Med.* 1996; 24:1328–33.
71. Lenart SG, Garrity J. Eye care for the mechanically ventilated patient receiving neuromuscular blockade or propofol. *Am J Crit Care.* 2000; 9:188–91.
72. Tschida SJ, Hoey LL, Nahum A, et al. Atracurium resistance in a critically ill patient. *Pharmacotherapy.* 1995; 15:533–9.
73. Gora-Harper ML, Hessel E, Shadick D. Effect of prescribing guidelines on the use of neuromuscular blocking agents. *Am J Health-Syst Pharm.* 1995; 52:1900–4.
74. Loughlin KA, Weingarten CM, Nagelhout J, et al. A pharmacoeconomic analysis of neuromuscular blocking agents in the operating room. *Pharmacotherapy.* 1996; 16:942–50.
75. Ballantyne JC, Chang Y. The impact of choice of muscle relaxant on postoperative recovery time: a retrospective study. *Anesth Analg.* 1997; 85:476–82.
76. Zarowitz BJ, Rudis MI, Lai K, et al. Retrospective pharmacoeconomic evaluation of dosing vecuronium by peripheral nerve stimulation versus standard clinical assessment in critically ill patients. *Pharmacotherapy.* 1997; 17:327–32.
77. Rudis MI, Guslits BJ, Peterson EL, et al. Economic impact of prolonged motor weakness complicating neuromuscular blockade in the intensive care unit. *Crit Care Med.* 1996; 24:1749–56.
78. Butterworth J, James R, Prielipp RC, et al. Do shorter-acting neuromuscular blocking drugs or opioids associate with reduced intensive care unit or hospital length of stay after coronary artery bypass grafting? *Anesthesiology.* 1998; 88:1437–46.

Appendix A—Summary of Recommendations

1. NMBAs should be used for an adult patient in an ICU to manage ventilation, manage increased ICP, treat muscle spasms, and decrease oxygen consumption only when all other means have been tried without success.[1] (Grade of recommendation = C)
2. The majority of patients in an ICU who are prescribed an NMBA can be managed effectively with pancuronium. (Grade of recommendation = B)
3. For patients for whom vagolysis is contraindicated (e.g., those with cardiovascular disease), NMBAs other than pancuronium may be used. (Grade of recommendation = C)
4. Because of their unique metabolism, cisatracurium or atracurium is recommended for patients with significant hepatic or renal disease. (Grade of recommendation = B)
5. Patients receiving NMBAs should be assessed both clinically and by TOF monitoring (Grade of recommendation = B), with a goal of adjusting the degree of neuromuscular blockade to achieve one or two twitches. (Grade of recommendation = C)
6. Before initiating neuromuscular blockade, patients should be medicated with sedative and analgesic drugs to provide adequate sedation and analgesia in accordance with the physician's clinical judgment to optimize therapy. (Grade of recommendation = C)
7. For patients receiving NMBAs and corticosteroids, every effort should be made to discontinue NMBAs as soon as possible. (Grade of recommendation = C)
8. Drug holidays (i.e., stopping NMBAs daily until forced to restart them based on the patient's condition) may decrease the incidence of AQMS. (Grade of recommendation = C)
9. Patients receiving NMBAs should have prophylactic eye care (Grade of recommendation = B), physical therapy (Grade of recommendation = C), and DVT prophylaxis. (Grade of recommendation = C)
10. Patients who develop tachyphylaxis to one NMBA should try another drug if neuromuscular blockade is still required. (Grade of recommendation = C)
11. Institutions should perform an economic analysis using their own data when choosing NMBAs for use in an ICU. (Grade of recommendation = C)

Appendix B—Determination of Cost Effectiveness Using Intrainstitutional Data[a]

1. For each adverse effect (e.g., prolonged recovery) of any given neuromuscular blocking agent (NMBA), add all associated costs together and multiply this figure by the probability of the occurrence of the adverse effect. If adverse effects A, B, and C are associated with an NMBA, then

   (Drug cost + cost A1) (probability of occurrence expressed as a decimal) = \$U
   (Drug cost + cost B1) (probability of occurrence expressed as a decimal) = \$V
   (Drug cost + cost C1) (probability of occurrence expressed as a decimal) = \$W

2. Calculate the product of the drug cost multiplied by the probability of occurrence of no adverse effects expressed as a decimal; add this product to the cost multiplied by the probability factor for each adverse effect calculated in step 1.

   (Drug cost) (probability of occurrence of no adverse effects) + $U + $V + $W = average cost of all pathways for agent

   Note: The probabilities of all adverse effects plus the probability of no adverse effects associated with the NMBA must add up to 1.

3. Determine the cost effectiveness of the agent by dividing the total costs associated with the agent by the probability of occurrence of no adverse effects expressed as a decimal.

   Example using pancuronium:

   a. [$224 (drug cost for 4 days of therapy) + $1000 (estimated cost of 1 extra day of ICU stay due to prolonged paralysis resulting from renal dysfunction)] [0.07 (estimated probability of renal dysfunction)] = $85.68 [$224 (drug cost for 4 days of therapy) + $1000 (estimated cost of 1 extra day of ICU (intensive care unit) stay due to prolonged paralysis resulting from hepatic dysfunction)] [0.04 (estimated probability of hepatic dysfunction)] = $48.96

   b. [$224 (drug cost for 4 days of therapy, assuming no adverse effects) × 0.89 (estimated probability of no adverse effects)] + $85.68 + $48.96 = $334.00

   c. Cost effectiveness of pancuronium = 334.00/0.89 (probability of no adverse effects) = $375.28

---

[a]Note that the term "adverse effects" includes problems such as prolonged paralysis resulting from decreased medication elimination due to impaired organ function. If a neuromuscular blocking agent is eliminated by more than one organ (e.g., kidney and liver), prolonged paralysis may result from impaired elimination due to a combination of organ problems. For example, one adverse effect may be prolonged paralysis associated with renal dysfunction, while another adverse effect may be prolonged paralysis associated with hepatic dysfunction, while a third adverse effect may be prolonged paralysis associated with combined renal and hepatic dysfunction.

Developed through the Task Force of the American College of Critical Care Medicine (ACCM) of the Society of Critical Care Medicine (SCCM), in collaboration with the American Society of Health-System Pharmacists (ASHP), and in alliance with the American College of Chest Physicians; and approved by the Board of Regents of ACCM and the Council of SCCM on November 15, 2001 and the ASHP Board of Directors on November 17, 2001.

Members of the 2001–2002 Commission on Therapeutics are William L. Greene, Pharm.D., BCPS, FASHP, *Chair;* Mary Lea Gora-Harper, Pharm.D., BCPS, *Vice Chair;* Kate Farthing, Pharm.D.; Charles W. Ham, Pharm.D., M.B.A.; Rita K. Jew, Pharm.D.; Rex S. Lott, Pharm.D.; Keith M. Olsen, Pharm.D., FCCP; Joseph J. Saseen, Pharm.D., BCPS; Beth A. Vanderheyden, Pharm.D., BCPS; Amy M. Blachere, R.Ph., *Student Member;* Jill E. Martin, Pharm.D., FASHP, *Board Liaison*; Dennis Williams, Pharm.D., FASHP, FCCP, FAPHA, BCPS, *Liaison Section of Clinical Specialist;* and Cynthia L. LaCivita, Pharm.D., *Secretary.*

Members of the Neuromuscular Blockade Task Force are Michael J. Murray, M.D., Ph.D., FCCM, *Chair,* Professor and Chair of Anesthesiology, and Dean, Mayo School of Health Sciences, Mayo Clinic Jacksonville, FL; Stanley Nasraway, Jr., M.D., FCCM, *Executive Director of Task Force,* Associate Professor, Surgery, Medicine, and anesthesia, Tufts-New England Medical Center, Boston, MA; Jay Cowen, M.D., Director, Medical Intensive Care Unit, LeHigh Valley Hospital, Allentown, PA; Heidi F. DeBlock, M.D., Department of Surgery, Albany Medical Center, Albany, NY; Brian L. Erstad, Pharm.D., FCCM, Department of Pharmacy Practice & Science, College of Pharmacy, University of Arizona, Tucson, AZ; Anthony W. Gray, Jr., M.D., FCCM, Section of Pulmonary and Critical Care, Medicine and Surgical Critical Care, Lahey Clinic Medical Center, Burlington, MA; Judith Jacobi, Pharm.D., FCCM, BCPS, Critical Care Pharmacy Specialist, Methodist Hospital–Clarian Health Partners, Indianapolis, IN; Philip D. Lumb, M.B., B.S., FCCM, Professor and Chairman, Department of Anesthesiology, Keck School of Medicine of USC, Los Angeles, CA; William T. McGee, M.D., M.H.A., Critical Care Division, Departments of Medicine & Surgery, Baystate Medical Center, Springfield, MA; William T. Peruzzi, M.D., FCCM, Associate Professor of Anesthesiology, Northwestern University School of Medicine, Chief, Section of Critical Care Medicine, Northwestern Memorial Hospital, Chicago, IL; Richard C. Prielipp, M.D., FCCM, Section Head, Critical Care and Department of Anesthesiology, Wake Forest University School of Medicine, Medical Center Boulevard, Winston-Salem, NC; Greg Susla, Pharm.D., FCCM, Clinical Center Pharmacy Department, National Institutes of Health, Bethesda, MD; Ann N. Tescher, R.N., Clinical Nurse Specialist, Mayo Clinic, Rochester, MN; Cynthia L. LaCivita, Pharm.D., Clinical Affairs Associate, *ASHP Staff Liaison*; Deborah L. McBride, Director of Publications, *SCCM Staff Liaison.*

Reviewers: American College of Chest Physicians; American Academy of Neurology; American Association of Critical Care Nurses; American Nurses Association; American Pharmaceutical Association; American College of Clinical Pharmacy; Joe Dasta, Pharm.D.; Doug Fish, Pharm.D.; Erkan Hassan, Pharm.D.; H. Mathilda Horst, M.D.; Carlayne E. Jackson, M.D.; Karen Kaiser, R.N.; Kathleen M. Kelly, M.D.; Carl Schoenberger, M.D.; Lori Schoonover, R.N.; and Gayle Takaniski, Pharm.D.

The recommendations in this document do not indicate an exclusive course of treatment to be followed. Variations, taking into account individual circumstances, may be appropriate.

Copyright © 2002, American Society of Health-System Pharmacists, Inc. and the Society of Critical Care Medicine. All rights reserved. Contact ASHP for reprint and permissions requests. This content may not be used for commercial purposes without the express written consent of ASHP.

The bibliographic citation is as follows: Society of Critical Care Medicine and American Society of Health-System Pharmacists. Clinical practice guidelines for sustained neuromuscular blockade in the adult critically ill patient. *Am J Health Syst Pharm.* 2002; 59:179–95.

Therapeutic Monitoring of Vancomycin for Serious Methicillin-resistant *Staphylococcus Aureus* Infections

A Revised Consensus Guideline and Review by the American Society of Health-System Pharmacists, the Infectious Diseases Society of America, the Pediatric Infectious Diseases Society, and the Society of Infectious Diseases Pharmacists

The first consensus guideline for therapeutic monitoring of vancomycin in adult patients was published in 2009. A committee representing 3 organizations (the American Society of Health-System Pharmacists [ASHP], Infectious Diseases Society of America [IDSA], and Society for Infectious Diseases Pharmacists [SIDP]) searched and reviewed all relevant peer-reviewed data on vancomycin as it related to in vitro and in vivo pharmacokinetic and pharmacodynamics (PK/PD) characteristics, including information on clinical efficacy, toxicity, and vancomycin resistance in relation to serum drug concentration and monitoring. The data were summarized, and specific dosing and monitoring recommendations were made. The primary recommendations consisted of eliminating routine monitoring of serum peak concentrations, emphasizing a ratio of area under the curve over 24 hours to minimum inhibitory concentration (AUC/MIC) of ≥400 as the primary PK/PD predictor of vancomycin activity, and promoting serum trough concentrations of 15 to 20 mg/L as a surrogate marker for the optimal vancomycin AUC/MIC if the MIC was ≤1 mg/L in patients with normal renal function. The guideline also recommended, albeit with limited data support, that actual body weight be used to determine the vancomycin dosage and loading doses for severe infections in patients who were seriously ill.[1]

Since those recommendations were generated, a number of publications have evaluated the impact of the 2009 guidelines on clinical efficacy and toxicity in patients receiving vancomycin for the treatment of methicillin-resistant *Staphylococcus aureus* (MRSA) infections. It should be noted, however, that when the recommendations were originally published, there were important issues not addressed and gaps in knowledge that could not be covered adequately because of insufficient data. In fact, adequate data were not available to make recommendations in the original guideline for specific dosing and monitoring for pediatric patients outside of the neonatal age group; specific recommendations for vancomycin dosage adjustment and monitoring in the morbidly obese patient population and patients with renal failure, including specific dialysis dosage adjustments; recommendations for the use of prolonged or continuous infusion (CI) vancomycin therapy; and safety data on the use of dosages that exceed 3 g per day. In addition, there were minimal to no data on the safety and efficacy of targeted trough concentrations of 15 to 20 mg/L.

This consensus revision evaluates the current scientific data and controversies associated with vancomycin dosing and serum concentration monitoring for serious MRSA infections (including but not limited to bacteremia, sepsis, infective endocarditis, pneumonia, osteomyelitis, and meningitis) and provides new recommendations based on recent available evidence. Due to a lack of data to guide appropriate targets, the development of this guideline excluded evaluation of vancomycin for methicillin-susceptible *S. aureus* (MSSA) strains, coagulase-negative staphylococci, and other pathogens; thus, the extrapolation of guideline recommendations to these pathogens should be viewed with extreme caution. Furthermore, serious invasive MRSA infections exclude nonbacteremic skin and skin structure and urinary tract infections. Since this guideline focuses on optimization of vancomycin dosing and monitoring, recommendations on the appropriateness of vancomycin use, combination or alternative antibiotic therapy, and multiple medical interventions that may be necessary for successful treatment of invasive MRSA infections are beyond the scope of this guideline and will not be presented.

DOI 10.37573/9781585287048.115

Methods

These are the consensus statements and guideline of ASHP, IDSA, the Pediatric Infectious Diseases Society (PIDS), and SIDP. Guideline panel composition consisted of physicians, pharmacists, and a clinical pharmacologist with expertise in clinical practice and/or research with vancomycin. Committee members were assigned key topics regarding vancomycin dosing and monitoring. A draft document addressing these specific areas was reviewed by all committee members and made available for public comments for 30 days through ASHP, IDSA, PIDS, and SIDP. The committee then met to review and revise the document based on the submitted comments, suggestions, and recommendations. After careful discussion and consideration, the document was revised and circulated among the committee and supporting organizations prior to final approval and publication. A search of PubMed and Embase was conducted using the following search terms: *vancomycin, pharmacokinetics, pharmacodynamics, efficacy, resistance, toxicity, obesity,* and *pediatrics*. All relevant and available peer-reviewed studies in the English-language literature published from 1958 through 2019 were considered. Studies were rated by their quality of evidence, and the subsequent recommendations were graded using the classification schemata described in **Table 1**.

Potential limitations of this review included the fact that there are few published randomized clinical trials of vancomycin dosing and monitoring available in the literature. Most published studies evaluating vancomycin dosing, dosage adjustment, and monitoring were retrospective PK or PD clinical assessments or retrospective observational studies in patients with MRSA infections.

PK/PD Efficacy Targets. To optimize the dosing of any antimicrobial agent, a firm understanding of the drug's exposure-effect and exposure-toxicity links are required. While a variety of PD indices for vancomycin have been suggested, an AUC/MIC ratio of ≥400 (with the MIC determined by

TABLE 1.
Grading System for Recommendations Based on Quality of Evidence[a]

Category and Grade	Definition
Strength of recommendation	
A	Good evidence to support a recommendation for or against use
B	Moderate evidence to support a recommendation for or against use
C	Poor evidence to support a recommendation
Quality of evidence	
I	Evidence from 1 or more properly randomized controlled trials
II	Evidence from 1 or more well-designed clinical trials, without randomization; from cohort or case controlled analytic studies (preferably from more than 1 center); from multiple time-series; or from dramatic results from uncontrolled experiments
III	Evidence from opinions of respected authorities, based on clinical experience, descriptive studies, or reports of expert committees

[a]Adapted from the Canadian Task Force on the Periodic Health Examination.[2]

broth microdilution [BMD]) is the current accepted critical PK/PD index in light of our limited experience and studies evaluating AUC/MIC values of <400.[1,3–7] In vitro and in vivo assessments of PK/PD models applicable to human MRSA infection have found that bactericidal activity (ie, a 1- to 2-log reduction in bacterial inoculum in the animal model) is achieved when the vancomycin AUC/MIC_{BMD} ratio approximates or exceeds 400. Furthermore, in vitro data suggest that an AUC of <400 potentiates the emergence of MRSA resistance and vancomycin-intermediate *S. aureus* strains.[8,9] There are also mounting clinical data, albeit mostly retrospective in nature, in support of this PK/PD target for vancomycin.[10–18] A summary of these investigations and their findings can be found in Table 1.[10–17,19–23]

Clinical PK/PD Data: Adults

While an AUC/MIC_{BMD} ratio of ≥400 is currently considered the optimal PK/PD "efficacy" target, it is important to recognize that this target has been largely derived from retrospective, single-center, observational studies of patients with MRSA bloodstream infections.[11–17] It is also important to recognize that most of the landmark clinical studies that established the contemporary PK/PD efficacy target relied on simple vancomycin clearance (CL) formulas based on daily vancomycin dose and estimated renal function to determine AUC values.[10,11,13] Current evaluation of these data demonstrates that these CL formulas provide imprecise estimates of the AUC.[24–26] This finding is not surprising, as there is considerable interpatient variability in vancomycin exposure profiles in clinical practice, and it is not possible to generate valid estimates of exposure variables in a given individual based on CL formulas that are derived from glomerular filtration rate estimation equations alone.[10,11,13] In most cases, the formula-based approach will overestimate vancomycin CL by approximately 40% to 50%.[16]

While it has been cumbersome to estimate AUC in the clinical setting in the past, Neely and colleagues[24] recently demonstrated that Bayesian software programs (refer to Therapeutic Monitoring section) can be used to generate accurate and reliable estimates of the daily AUC values with trough-only PK sampling. However, the accuracy of AUC estimation is higher with peak and trough measurements compared to trough-only PK sampling.[24] Using this validated Bayesian method to estimate the daily AUC in a single-center, retrospective study of patients with MRSA bloodstream infections, Lodise and colleagues[16] found that outcomes were maximized when day 1 and day 2 AUC/MIC_{BMD} ratios exceeded 521 and 650, respectively. Employing the same Bayesian approach to estimate daily AUC values, Casapao and colleagues[17] also noted that the risk of vancomycin treatment failure among patients with MRSA infective endocarditis was greatest among those with an AUC/MIC_{BMD} ratio of ≤600 and that this exposure-failure relationship persisted after adjusting for factors such as intensive care unit (ICU) admission, presence of heteroresistant vancomycin-intermediate *S. aureus*, and other comorbidities. In contrast to the studies by Lodise et al and Casapao et al, several small-scale, retrospective clinical evaluations of vancomycin exposure-response reported lower Bayesian-derived thresholds for AUC/MIC since the AUC was measured at steady-state conditions and indexed to the MIC, as determined by the Etest (bioMérieux USA, Hazelwood, MO) method, to arrive at an AUC/MIC_{Etest} value.[12,14,15] The MIC_{Etest} value tends to be 1.5- to 2-fold higher than the MIC_{BMD} value; therefore, it is likely that the AUC threshold needed for response from these 3 studies,[12,14,15] if calculated using the MIC_{BMD}, would align with the studies by Lodise et al[16] and Casapao et al.[17]

In an effort to surmount the limitations-associated with previous single-center, retrospective vancomycin exposure response clinical analyses, a multicenter, observational prospective study was performed to evaluate the relationship between the prespecified day 2 AUC/MIC ratios (ie, AUC/MIC_{Etest} of ≥320 and AUC/MIC_{BMD} of ≥650) and outcomes in adult patients (n = 265) with MRSA bacteremia. In the multivariate analyses, treatment failure rates were not significantly different between the prespecified day 2 AUC/MIC groups. Post hoc global outcomes analyses suggested that patients in the 2 lowest AUC exposure quintiles (ie, those with an AUC of ≤515 mg · h/L) experienced the best global outcome (defined as absence of both treatment failure and acute kidney injury [AKI]). While global outcomes were similar in the 2 lowest AUC-exposure quintiles, only 20% of the study population (n = 54) had an AUC of ≤400 mg · h/L, and it is unclear if efficacy outcomes are maintained at an AUC less than this threshold of 400 mg · h/L.[23] Notably, the higher AUC value cited above (515 mg · h/L) provides a new index that incorporates both efficacy and AKI that is still within the recommended AUC range of 400 to 600 mg · h/L (assuming a MIC of 1 mg/L).

Collectively, recent studies highlight the importance of generating valid estimates of the AUC values through Bayesian modeling techniques when conducting vancomycin exposure-outcomes analyses in patients. Current vancomycin exposure-effectiveness data originated largely from studies of MRSA bacteremia, with some studies for pneumonia and infective endocarditis and none for osteomyelitis and meningitis. Furthermore, outcomes data for a MIC of 2 mg/L are limited, suggesting the need for more studies to ascertain the optimal AUC/MIC target for this MIC value or consideration for the use of alternative antibiotics. The currently available data also highlight the critical need for large-scale, multicenter, randomized, vancomycin dose–optimized clinical outcomes trials. As data from future prospective, multicenter clinical studies emerge, it is important that clinicians recognize that our current understanding of the PK/PD target associated with maximal effect and toxicity is subject to change, and this may ultimately alter the current way we dose vancomycin to optimize effect and minimize toxicity.

Toxicodynamics: AKI

A major concern with vancomycin use is the occurrence of AKI. While multiple definitions of vancomycin-associated AKI have been employed in the literature, most studies defined it as an increase in the serum creatinine (SCr) level of ≥0.5 mg/dL, or a 50% increase from baseline in consecutive daily readings, or a decrease in calculated creatinine CL (CL_{cr}) of 50% from baseline on 2 consecutive days in the absence of an alternative explanation.[1] Recently, it has been proposed that a more sensitive threshold (ie, an increase in SCr of ≥0.3 mg/dL over a 48-hour period) may be considered as an indicator of vancomycin-associated AKI. This threshold was adopted from the Acute Kidney Injury Network (AKIN) and the Kidney Disease: Improving Global Outcomes (KDIGO) criteria.[27–29] The incidence of vancomycin-associated AKI has varied across published studies. In a meta-analysis by van Hal and colleagues,[29] the prevalence of vancomycin-associated AKI varied from 5% to 43%. Similarly, a recent meta-analysis of 13 studies by Sinha Ray et al[30] reported that the relative risk of AKI with vancomycin was 2.45 (95% confidence interval, 1.69–3.55), with an attributable risk of 59%. Most episodes of AKI developed between 4 and 17 days after initiation of therapy. Many patients, especially those who are critically ill, do not fully recover renal function after AKI,[31] and even mild AKI can significantly decrease long-term survival rates, increase morbidity, prolong hospitalizations, and escalate healthcare costs.[22,32]

With any drug, an understanding of its toxicodynamic profile is required for optimal dosing. Several studies, largely retrospective in nature, have attempted to quantify the relationship between vancomycin exposure and probability of AKI.[33,34] Although data are limited, the collective literature suggests that the risk of AKI increases as a function of the trough concentration, especially when maintained above 15 to 20 mg/L.[29] Similarly, there are recent data to suggest that the risk of AKI increases along the vancomycin AUC continuum, especially when the daily AUC exceeds 650 to 1,300 mg · h/L.[24,33–35] Furthermore, animal studies corroborate the finding that increased AUC rather than trough concentration is a strong predictor of AKI.[36,37]

Suzuki et al[33] evaluated the mean vancomycin AUC in relation to AKI. Most patients who developed AKI had AUC values between 600 and 800 mg · h/L, compared with 400 to 600 mg · h/L in those without AKI (P = 0.014). Furthermore, Lodise and colleagues[34] showed that the probability of AKI increased 2.5-fold among patients with AUC values above 1,300 mg · h/L compared with patients with lower values (30.8% vs 13.1%, P = 0.02). Although AUC values above 1,300 mg · h/L were associated with a substantial increase in AKI, an AUC exposure-response relationship appeared to exist, and the probability of a nephrotoxic event increased as a function of the daily AUC and patient's body weight.[38] A study by Zasowski et al[21] also reported a similar relationship between Bayesian-estimated vancomycin AUC thresholds and AKI in 323 patients; AUC values of ≥1,218 mg · h/L for 0 to 48 hours, ≥677 for 0 to 24 hours, and ≥683 for 24 to 48 hours or troughs of ≥18.2 mg/L were associated with a 3- to 4-fold increased risk of nephrotoxicity. Similarly, the aforementioned multicenter, prospective study of patients with MRSA bloodstream infections found that AKI increased along the day 2 AUC continuum in a stepwise manner and that patients with day 2 AUC values of ≥793 mg · h/L were at the greatest risk for AKI.[23]

Given the understanding about potential toxic concentrations, there are also data to suggest that AUC-guided vancomycin dosing may reduce the occurrence of vancomycin-associated AKI. In a retrospective, quasi-experimental study of 1,280 hospitalized patients, Finch et al[20] compared the incidence of nephrotoxicity in patients monitored by individualized AUC vs trough concentration. AUC-guided dosing was found to be independently associated with a significant decrease in AKI (odds ratio [OR], 0.52; 95% CI, 0.34-0.80; P = 0.003).[20] Median Bayesian-estimated AUC was significantly lower with AUC-guided dosing vs trough monitoring (474 [SD, 360-611] mg · h/L vs. 705 [SD, 540-883] mg · h/L; P < 0.001). In the prospective study by Neely et al,[22] 252 patients were monitored via troughs of 10 to 20 mg/L in year 1 vs Bayesian-estimated AUC values of ≥400 mg · h/L in years 2 and 3 of the investigation. Nephrotoxicity occurred in 8% of subjects in year 1 and in 0% and 2% of subjects in years 2 and 3, respectively (P = 0.01). The median trough concentration and AUC values associated with AKI were 15.7 mg/L and 625 mg · h/L, as compared with values of 8.7 mg/L and 423 mg · h/L in subjects without AKI (P = 0.02).[22]

Collectively, the published clinical exposure-response analyses suggest that a daily AUC of ≥400 is the driver of effectiveness and that the risk of AKI is related to AUC and trough values. More importantly, these data provide the foundation for the current understanding of the therapeutic window for vancomycin. When evaluating the toxicodynamics of vancomycin, it is important to recognize other factors that may complicate or exacerbate the risk of AKI. Host-related factors associated with nephrotoxicity include increased weight, pre-existing renal dysfunction, and critical illness. Concurrent administration of nephrotoxic agents such as aminoglycosides, loop diuretics, amphotericin B, intravenous (i.v.) contrast dye, and vasopressors has been shown to increase the risk of nephrotoxicity. Recently, piperacillin/tazobactam and flucloxacillin have been reported to increase the risk for AKI in patients receiving vancomycin.[39–44] It is unclear if the threshold for vancomycin-induced AKI varies according to these covariates, but clinicians should be mindful of the potential for additional risk when prescribing vancomycin to patients when these conditions are present.[34,40–50]

Based on the current best available evidence, daily vancomycin AUC values (assuming a MIC of 1 mg/L) should be maintained between 400 and 600 mg · h/L to minimize the likelihood of nephrotoxicity and maximize efficacy for suspected or definitive serious invasive MRSA infections. Once culture results or the clinical presentation rule out invasive MRSA infection, the empiric use of vancomycin at guideline-recommended exposures should be de-escalated, either by a decrease in vancomycin exposure or initiation of alternative antibiotics. Extrapolation of guideline recommendations to noninvasive MRSA and other pathogens should be viewed with extreme caution.

Therapeutic Monitoring

Therapeutic monitoring has centered on maintaining trough concentrations between 15 and 20 mg/L for serious infections due to MRSA. Previous expert guidelines recommended monitoring trough concentrations as a surrogate marker for the AUC/MIC ratio based on the historical difficulty in estimating the AUC in clinical practice.[1,5] In the past, calculation of AUC in clinical practice involved collection of multiple vancomycin serum concentrations during the same dosing interval, with subsequent use of PK software that was not readily available at all institutions. As such, the guideline viewed trough-directed dosing as a more practical alternative to AUC/MIC-guided dosing in clinical practice.

Although the recommendation to maintain trough values between 15 and 20 mg/L for serious infections due to MRSA has been well integrated into practice, the clinical benefits of maintaining higher vancomycin trough values have not been well documented.[38,51–55] From a PK/PD perspective, it is not surprising that there are limited clinical data to support the range of 15 to 20 mg/L. Recent studies have demonstrated that trough values may not be an optimal surrogate for AUC values.[26,56,57] While trough attainment ensures achievement of a minimum cumulative exposure, a wide range of concentration-time profiles can result in an identical trough value. Patel et al[26] reported a wide range of AUC values from several different dosing regimens yielding similar trough values. The therapeutic discordance between trough and AUC values is not surprising, as the AUC is the integrated quantity of cumulative drug exposure (ie, the serum drug concentration–time curve over a defined interval). In contrast, the trough represents a single exposure point at the end of the dosing interval. In clinical practice, monitoring of trough concentrations will translate into achievement of one specific minimum daily AUC value, whereas the 24-hour AUC (AUC_{24}) largely represents the average concentration during that time period [AUC_{24} (mg · h/L) = average concentration (mg/L) x 24 (hours)]. For troughs of 15 to 20 mg/L, this typically equates to a daily AUC in excess of 400 mg · h/L. However, there is considerable variability in the upper range of AUC values associated with a given trough value. Although trough-only monitoring is practical, the potential limitations surrounding the practice suggest that trough monitoring may be insufficient to guide vancomycin dosing in all patients.

Although the AUC/MIC ratio is considered the PK/PD driver of efficacy for vancomycin, clinicians trying to optimize vancomycin treatment for patients with serious MRSA infections may be best advised to use AUC-guided dosing and assume a MIC_{BMD} of 1 mg/L (unless it is known, through BMD, to be greater or less than 1 mg/L). The MIC value is of less importance for several reasons. First, the range of vancomycin MIC values among contemporary MRSA isolates is narrow, and the BMD MIC_{90} in most institutions is 1 mg/L or less.[58–62] Second, measurement of MIC values is imprecise, with dilution of $\pm 1 \log_2$ and variation of 10% to 20% considered acceptable; therefore, the variability of reported MIC values encountered in routine clinical practice is likely to reflect measurement error.[63] Third, there is a high degree of variability between commercially available MIC testing methods relative to the BMD method (see Vancomycin Susceptibility Testing section). Last, MIC results are typically not available within the first 72 hours of index culture collection, yet current data indicate that the vancomycin AUC/MIC ratio needs to be optimized early in the course of infection.

Daily AUC values (assuming a MIC_{BMD} of 1 mg/L) should be maintained between 400 and 600 mg · h/L to maximize efficacy and minimize the likelihood of AKI. In the past, AUC monitoring required the collection of multiple concentrations over the same dosing interval. With these data, a clinician would calculate the AUC using the linear-trapezoid rule. This approach required precise collection of vancomycin concentrations, making it largely impractical outside of a research setting. However, this is no longer the case. It is now possible to accurately estimate the AUC with limited PK sampling. One such approach involves the use of Bayesian software programs to estimate the vancomycin AUC value with minimal PK sampling (ie, 1 or 2 vancomycin concentrations) and provide AUC-guided dosing recommendations in real time. An alternative approach involves use of 2 concentrations (peak and trough) and simple analytic PK equations to estimate AUC values.[57,64]

Bayesian-Derived AUC Monitoring. Bayesian-guided dosing is based in part on Bayes' Theorem, as it quantifies the sequential relationship between the estimated probability distribution of an individual patient's PK parameter values (eg, volume [V_d] or CL) prior to administering the drug based on the way the drug behaved in a population of prior patients (the Bayesian prior) and the revised probability distribution of a specific patient's PK parameter values using exact dosing and drug concentration data (the Bayesian conditional posterior). In short, Bayesian dose optimization software uses a well-developed vancomycin population PK model as the Bayesian prior, together with the individual patient's observed drug concentrations in the data file, to calculate a Bayesian posterior parameter value distribution for that patient. The dose optimization software then calculates the optimal dosing regimen based on the specific patient's profile.[65–67]

An advantage of the Bayesian approach is that vancomycin concentrations can be collected within the first 24 to 48 hours rather than at steady-state conditions (after the third or fourth dose), and this information can be used to inform subsequent dosing (adaptive feedback control). As part of their output, Bayesian dosing programs provide innovative treatment schemes, such as front-loading doses with subsequent transition to a lower maintenance dosing regimen, to rapidly achieve target concentrations within the first 24 to 48 hours among critically ill patients. The Bayesian approach also provides the ability to integrate covariates, such as CL_{cr}, in the structural PK models (the Bayesian prior density file) that account for the pathophysiological changes that readily occur in critically ill patients. Incorporation of covariates that account for these "dynamic" changes serves as a way to identify dosing schemes that optimize effect and predict future dosing in a patient who has an evolving PK profile.[67]

Bayesian dose-optimizing software programs are now readily available and can be used in real time to identify the optimal vancomycin dosage that readily achieves the AUC target (assuming a MIC_{BMD} of 1 mg/L).[66,68] Bayesian programs offer numerous advantages over the traditional first order equation software programs. Using richly sampled vancomycin PK data from 3 studies comprising 47 adults with varying renal function, Neely and colleagues[24] demonstrated that Bayesian software programs, embedded with a PK model based on richly sampled vancomycin data as the Bayesian prior, can be used to generate accurate and reliable estimates of the daily AUC values with trough-only PK sampling. Of note, there was limited inclusion of special populations in this study, and it is unclear if this trough-only Bayesian AUC estimation approach can be applied to obese patients, critically ill patients, pediatric patients, and patients with unstable renal function. A randomized controlled study of 65 subjects by Al-Sulaiti et al[69] showed that estimating AUC using both peak and trough concentrations (vs trough only estimates) may improve vancomycin-associated therapeutic cure. Until more data are available, it is preferred to estimate the Bayesian AUC using 2 vancomycin concentrations (peak and trough).

First-Order PK Analytic Equations. Alternatively, the AUC can be accurately estimated based on the collection of 2 timed steady-state serum vancomycin concentrations and the use of first-order PK equations.[57] The equations used to compute AUC from 2 samples are based in part on an original approach proposed by Begg, Barclay, and Duffull[70] for aminoglycosides and modified by Pai and Rodvold.[57] It is preferred that a near steady-state, postdistributional peak (1 to 2 hours after end of infusion) and trough concentrations within the same dosing interval (if possible) are used when estimating the AUC with the equation-based methods.

The major advantage of this approach is that it is simpler and relies on fewer assumptions than the Bayesian approach. The first-order PK equations used to estimate the AUC are also familiar to most clinicians, facilitating ease of use in practice. Once the AUC_{24} is estimated, the clinician simply revises the total daily dose to achieve the desired AUC_{24}, as alterations of total daily dose will provide proportional changes in observed AUC_{24}.[6,71–73] The major limitation of this approach is that it is not adaptive like the Bayesian approach, as it can only provide a snapshot of the AUC for the sampling period. As such, this AUC calculation will not be correct if a physiologic change such as renal dysfunction occurs during or after the sampling period. Furthermore, it is extremely difficult to estimate the vancomycin AUC_{24} with the equation-based method in patients who receive multiple dosing regimens within a 24-hour period. If the vancomycin dosing interval is more frequent than once a day, the AUC_{24} will be a function of the number of identical doses administered during that interval (eg, AUC must be multiplied by 2 for a 12-hour dosing interval to calculate the true AUC_{24}). It is also highly preferred that concentrations are collected near steady-state conditions.

Despite its drawbacks, this estimate of AUC is a clear step above trough-only or peak-only concentration interpretation and is familiar to most clinicians. Several large medical centers within the United States have already adopted this approach of acquiring 2 postdose serum concentration estimates of the AUC to perform routine vancomycin dosing and monitoring and have demonstrated a considerable improvement in safety over the current trough-only concentration monitoring method.[37,64]

PK Sampling Time. Timing of achievement of targeted AUC values (assuming a MIC_{BMD} of 1 mg/L) remains unclear. The early AUC/MIC target ratios derived in animal models were based on the AUC value from 0 to 24 hours.[3,4] More recent clinical assessments that identified a link between AUC/MIC ratio and outcomes also assessed the AUC values achieved early in the course of therapy.[1,3,5–7,10,13,20–22] The 2009 vancomycin guideline stated that the trough should be assessed prior to steady-state conditions (ie, prior to the fourth dose).[1,5] In fact, steady-state conditions are difficult to determine in clinical practice, and the timing of the fourth dose is more dependent on the dosing interval (ie, 12 vs 24 hours) than steady-state conditions. Given the importance of early, appropriate therapy,[74] targeted AUC exposures should be achieved early during the course of therapy, preferably within the first 24 to 48 hours. If monitoring is initiated after the first dose, the contribution of the loading dose to the actual AUC may vary depending on the magnitude of the loading dose vs maintenance doses. The decision to delay therapeutic monitoring beyond 48 hours should be based on severity of infection and clinical judgment.

Summary and Recommendations

1. In patients with suspected or definitive serious MRSA infections, an individualized target of the AUC/MIC_{BMD} ratio of 400 to 600 (assuming a vancomycin MIC_{BMD} of 1 mg/L) should be advocated to achieve clinical efficacy while improving patient safety (A-II). Doses of 15 to 20 mg/kg (based on actual body weight) administered every 8 to 12 hours as an intermittent infusion are recommended for most patients with normal renal function when assuming a MIC_{BMD} of 1 mg/L (A-II). In patients with normal renal function, these doses may not achieve the therapeutic AUC/MIC target when the MIC is 2 mg/L.
2. Given the narrow vancomycin AUC range for therapeutic effect and minimal AKI risk, the most accurate and optimal way to manage vancomycin dosing should be through AUC-guided dosing and monitoring (A-II). We recommend to accomplish this in one of two ways.
   a. One approach relies on the collection of 2 concentrations (obtained near steady-state, postdistributional peak concentration [C_{max}] at 1 to 2 hours after infusion and trough concentration [C_{min}] at the end of the dosing interval), preferably but not required during the same dosing interval (if possible) and utilizing first-order PK equations to estimate the AUC (A-II).

b. The preferred approach to monitor AUC involves the use of Bayesian software programs, embedded with a PK model based on richly sampled vancomycin data as the Bayesian prior, to optimize the delivery of vancomycin based on the collection of 1 or 2 vancomycin concentrations, with at least 1 trough. It is preferred to obtain 2 PK samples (ie, at 1 to 2 hours post infusion and at end of the dosing interval) to estimate the AUC with the Bayesian approach (A-II). A trough concentration alone may be sufficient to estimate the AUC with the Bayesian approach in some patients, but more data are needed across different patient populations to confirm the viability of using trough-only data (B-II).

3. When transitioning to AUC/MIC monitoring, clinicians should conservatively target AUC values for patients with suspected or documented serious infections due to MRSA assuming a vancomycin MIC_{BMD} of 1 mg/L or less at most institutions. Given the importance of early, appropriate therapy, vancomycin targeted exposure should be achieved early during the course of therapy, preferably within the first 24 to 48 hours (A-II). As such, the use of Bayesian-derived AUC monitoring may be prudent in these cases since it does not require steady-state serum vancomycin concentrations to allow for early assessment of AUC target attainment.
4. Trough-only monitoring, with a target of 15 to 20 mg/L, is no longer recommended based on efficacy and nephrotoxicity data in patients with serious infections due to MRSA (A-II). There is insufficient evidence to provide recommendations on whether trough-only or AUC-guided vancomycin monitoring should be used among patients with noninvasive MRSA or other infections.
5. Vancomycin monitoring is recommended for patients receiving vancomycin for serious MRSA infections to achieve sustained targeted AUC values (assuming a MIC_{BMD} of 1 mg/L unless it is known to be greater or less than 1 mg/L by BMD). Independent of MRSA infection, vancomycin monitoring is also recommended for all patients at high risk for nephrotoxicity (eg, critically ill patients receiving concurrent nephrotoxins), patients with unstable (ie, deteriorating or significantly improving) renal function, and those receiving prolonged courses of therapy (more than 3 to 5 days). We suggest the frequency of monitoring be based on clinical judgment; frequent or daily monitoring may be prudent for hemodynamically unstable patients (eg, those with end-stage renal disease), with once-weekly monitoring for hemodynamically stable patients (B-II).

Vancomycin Susceptibility Testing

With the MIC being a component of the vancomycin AUC/MIC targeted surrogate for efficacy, it is important to be aware of local and national vancomycin susceptibility patterns for MRSA. Although in some centers there has been a steady increase in the average vancomycin MIC over several decades, recent national and international studies that have evaluated MRSA susceptibility to glycopeptides, lipopeptides, and beta-lactams have demonstrated that vancomycin MICs have remained constant over time, with a MIC of ≤1 mg/L demonstrated for more than 90% of isolates.[58–62] A meta-analysis of 29,234 MRSA strains from 55 studies revealed that the MIC determinations performed by BMD, Etest, and automated systems were predominately 1 mg/L and that there was no evidence of a MIC creep phenomenon.[75] Furthermore, a global surveillance program reported that 95% of 57,319 MRSA isolates had MICs of 1 mg/L, with no signs of MIC creep over 20 years.[76] While there does not seem to be a large number of organisms with a vancomycin MIC of ≥2 mg/L when reference methods are used, there is considerable variability in MIC results between the susceptibility testing methods. The challenge is that, according to the Clinical Laboratory Standards Institute (CLSI), acceptable variability for MIC measurement methods is within ±1 doubling dilution (essential agreement), such that current susceptibility testing methods are unable, with high reproducibility, to distinguish MICs of 1 mg/L from MICs of 0.5 mg/L or 2 mg/L. Most institutions routinely perform MIC testing using automated systems: BD Phoenix (BD, Franklin Lakes, NJ), MicroScan WalkAway (Beckman Coulter, Brea, CA), or Vitek 2 (bioMérieux), and in some cases the Etest methodology (bioMérieux). In a study of 161 MRSA blood isolates, when using the essential agreement definition of ±1 $\log_2$ dilution error, Vitek 2 and MicroScan WalkAway demonstrated a 96.3% agreement with BMD, whereas BD Phoenix demonstrated an 88.8% agreement.[77] The Etest method had the lowest agreement with BMD, at 76.4% (results were consistently higher by 1 to 2 dilutions). The Etest will likely produce a higher value (0.5 to 2 dilutions higher) than BMD. In another study, 92% of the strains were demonstrated to have a vancomycin MIC of 1 mg/L by BMD; corresponding figures were 70% for MicroScan WalkAway and Etest and 41% for Vitek 1.[78]

Rybak et al[79] compared MicroScan WalkAway, Vitek 2, BD Phoenix, and Etest to BMD methods among 200 MRSA strains. In contrast to previous studies, these investigators used an absolute agreement definition of ±0 $\log_2$ dilution error to better characterize the precision. Using this definition, results with BD Phoenix and MicroScan WalkAway had the highest agreement with BMD (66.2% and 61.8%, respectively), followed by Vitek 2 (54.3%). As noted above, Etest tended to produce results that were 1 to 2 dilutions higher (agreement with BMD was 36.7%). However, when compared to BMD, Etest identified a MIC of 2 mg/L 80% of the time. When compared to BMD, MicroScan WalkAway (prompt method) over-called MIC values of 1 mg/L by 74.1%, and BD Phoenix and Vitek 2 undercalled MIC values of 2 mg/L by 76% and 20%, respectively.

The high variability of MIC results among the 4 systems compared to BMD clearly poses a challenge to the clinician making treatment decisions based on MIC and poses questions as to the most relevant MIC method.[79] This variability between MIC values and testing methods routinely performed at most institutions further supports the use of AUC (assuming a MIC_{BMD} of 1 mg/L) to guide vancomycin empiric dosing. For nonserious infections, this variability may be inconsequential. In a critically ill patient infected by MRSA, who may require prompt achievement of the target AUC/MIC, it is imperative to verify the MIC by a standardized method (preferably BMD, as Etest may result in a higher MIC than BMD) as soon as possible to avoid a delay in effective therapy. An AUC/MIC_{BMD} of 400 to 600 is approximately equivalent to an AUC/MIC_{Etest} of 200 to 400, reflecting values that are 1 to 2 dilutions higher than those yielded by Etest. Furthermore, there are no data to support decreasing the dose to achieve the targeted AUC/MIC of 400 to 600 if the MIC is less than 1 mg/L.

Summary and Recommendations

6. Based on current national vancomycin susceptibility surveillance data, under most circumstances of empiric dosing, the vancomycin MIC should be assumed to be 1 mg/L. When the MIC_{BMD} is >1 mg/L, the probability of achieving an AUC/MIC target of ≥400 is low with conventional dosing; higher doses may risk unnecessary toxicity, and the decision to change therapy should be based on clinical judgment. In addition, when the MIC_{BMD} is <1 mg/L, we do not recommend decreasing the dose to achieve the AUC/MIC target. It is important to note the limitations in automated susceptibility testing methods, including the lack of precision and variability in MIC results depending on method used (B-II).

Continuous Infusion vs Intermittent Infusion

Administration of vancomycin by continuous infusion (CI) has been evaluated as an alternative to intermittent infusion (II) with potential advantages of earlier target attainment, less variability in serum concentrations, ease of drug level monitoring (less dependence on sampling time or multiple concentrations to calculate AUC), and lower the potential risk of AKI.

Comparative Studies. Published studies that compared intermittent to continuous administration primarily focused on 2 distinct populations, adult critically ill patients in the ICU with suspected or documented infections and those receiving outpatient antimicrobial therapy (OPAT) for bone and joint infections.[80-89] Most studies compared CI to II for the risk of AKI and attainment of target serum concentrations; only 4 studies included other outcome endpoints such as treatment failure and mortality.[80,84,87,89] Measures of vancomycin drug exposure reported in clinical trials include trough and average steady-state concentrations and AUC_{24}. One challenge when comparing clinical outcomes between CI and II is the lack of consistent reporting of exposure parameters between groups treated using the 2 dosing strategies. For CI, the most commonly reported drug exposure parameter was the steady-state concentration, while for II it was the trough concentration. For future investigations it would be beneficial to report AUC and/or average steady state concentration for both CI and II groups to enable direct comparison of drug exposure between groups and correlate with efficacy and safety endpoints.

Critically Ill Patients. A total of 7 studies compared CI vs II of vancomycin in critically ill patients.[81-87] Only one study, by Wysocki et al,[80] evaluated both efficacy and safety in a prospective randomized trial comparing vancomycin CI (n = 61) and II (n = 58) in 119 patients. Most patients had pneumonia or bacteremia, mostly due to MRSA. Mean serum steady-state and trough concentrations attained were 24 mg/L and 15 mg/L, respectively, for both the CI and II groups. AUC_{24} values were comparable between the CI and II groups, with significantly less variability in the CI group (P = 0.026). Clinical failure rates were similar in the CI and II groups on day 10 (21% vs 26%) and at end of treatment (21% vs 19%), although the mean AUC_{24} was shown to be lower in the CI group than in the II group (596 [SD, 159] mg · h/L vs 685 [SD, 260] mg · h/L, $P < 0.05$). Nephrotoxicity occurred in 18% of patients overall, with similar rates in the CI and II groups (16% vs 19%). However, dialysis was required more often in those who received CI vs II (6 of 10 patients vs 3 of 11 patients). Risk factors for nephrotoxicity such as diabetes and concomitant diuretic, aminoglycoside, and iodine use were similar between groups. It is notable that the study only had 23% power to detect a difference in clinical outcomes between groups.[1]

Another study compared mortality among critically ill burn patients receiving CI (n = 90) or II (n = 81).[84] Mortality rates in the hospital and on days 14 and 28 were numerically higher for those receiving CI, but the differences did not reach statistical significance (10% vs 6.2%, 18.9% vs 11%, and 32% vs 21%, respectively). However, when mortality was compared by treatment indications, those who received CI for non-gram-positive sepsis had significantly higher mortality (70% vs 16.7%, P = 0.001); nearly half of this subgroup had gram-negative bacteremia or candidemia. It is possible that the difference in outcome may be attributed to differences in the management of those infections and not directly related to vancomycin administration. Nephrotoxicity occurred numerically less frequently in the CI group than in the II group (percentage of patients with increase in Scr of 0.5 mg/dL at end of therapy, 6.7% vs 14.8%). While higher mean vancomycin concentrations were noted in the CI group relative to the II group (20 [SD, 3.8] mg/L vs 14.8 [SD, 4.4] mg/L, $P < 0.001$), which would be expected when comparing steady-state and trough concentrations, AUC_{24} was not reported, thereby precluding comparison of drug exposure between the CI and II groups.

Five other studies compared serum drug concentrations achieved and the risk of nephrotoxicity between CI and II in critically ill patients.[81-83,85,86] As expected, the ranges of measured vancomycin concentrations from the studies were significantly higher in the CI groups than in the II groups (steady state concentrations of 20-25 mg/L vs troughs of 10-15 mg/L, respectively). Another study showed that a higher percentage of patients attained a vancomycin concentration of >20 mg/L at least once during the treatment course with CI vs II administration (63.2% vs 44.9%, P = 0.065).[82] One study reported lower mean AUC_{24} with CI vs II (529 [SD, 98] mg · h/L vs 612 [SD, 213] mg · h/L, P value not stated), and increased steady state concentration compared with trough (25 ± 4 vs 17 ± 4.7 mg/L, respectively, P = 0.42) with CI vs. II.[83] The discordance observed in the relationship of trough concentration and AUC_{24} underscores the importance of measuring AUC_{24} to compare relative drug exposure with CI vs II in future studies.

In general, the rate of nephrotoxicity was reported to be similar or numerically lower with CI vs II administration (range, 4%-16% vs 11%-19%); the same trend but higher rates were reported in studies that applied the AKIN criteria for nephrotoxicity (26%-28% vs 35%-37%).[81-83,85,86] In addition, Saugel et al[85] noted significantly less frequent need for renal replacement therapy (RRT) during vancomycin treatment for patients in the CI group than for those in the II group (7% [7 of 94 patients] vs 23% [12 of 52 patients] required RRT; P = 0.007). Of interest, in the largest retrospective study comparing CI and II, conducted in 1,430 ICU patients, Hanrahan et al[86] reported a higher rate of nephrotoxicity in those receiving CI vs II (25% [161 of 653 patients] vs 20% [77 of 390 patients]; $P = 0.001$); bivariate analysis indicated that every 1-mg/L increase in serum concentration was associated with an 11% increase in the risk of nephrotoxicity, with lower odds in those receiving II. However, logistic regression analysis indicated the contrary in that II was associated with an 8-fold higher odds of nephrotoxicity (95% confidence interval, 2.87-23.41). The lack of information provided on confounding variables such as receipt of concomitant nephrotoxins and relative AUCs between treatment groups preclude drawing a definitive conclusion regarding the safety of CI, especially in light of the disparate results of bivariate and logistic regression analyses.

Patients Receiving OPAT. To date there have been 2 studies comparing the efficacy of vancomycin administration by CI vs II in patients whose therapy was initiated in the hospital and continued as OPAT. Duration of therapy ranged from 30 days to 14 weeks.[87,89] Most patients were treated for bone and joint and skin structure–related infections. In a small prospective study, rates of osteomyelitis cure, defined as remaining asymptomatic 12 months after completion of therapy, did not differ significantly between groups (94% vs 78%, $P = 0.3$), but only 27 patients were evaluable.[87]

Another study retrospectively evaluated the efficacy of vancomycin in patients with MRSA infections; most had bone and joint and skin structure–related infections, while 10% had bloodstream infections or endocarditis.[89] Rates of clinical failure were similar in the CI and II groups (19% [25 of 133 patients] vs 25% [9 of 36], $P = 0.41$) after excluding 29% of study patients who had subtherapeutic serum vancomycin concentrations for more than 1 week. However, it is not clear how frequent serum concentrations were monitored, if inhospital treatment duration before OPAT differed between groups, and whether treatment success rates differed by type of infection.

In studies that evaluated the safety of CI vancomycin as OPAT, treatment duration ranged from 4 to 14 weeks, with a reported average mean steady-state serum concentration of 13 to 30 mg/L.[87,88] In a retrospective matched cohort study of 80 patients, a trend towards less frequent occurrence of nephrotoxicity was observed in the CI group vs the II group (10% vs 25%, $P = 0.139$), and when nephrotoxicity did occur it had a later onset in the CI group ($P = 0.036$).[88] Patients were matched by age, comorbid conditions, gender, baseline Scr, and receipt of concurrent nephrotoxins; those who had an Scr of ≥1.5 mg/dL at baseline, developed nephrotoxicity as inpatients prior to OPAT, or experienced hypotension resulting in renal dysfunction were excluded. In another retrospective study,[90] the same investigators identified a steady-state average concentration of 28 mg/L as the threshold breakpoint for the development of nephrotoxicity using CART (classification and regression tree) analysis: Nephrotoxicity occurred in 71.4% (5 of 7) and 11.6% (11 of 95) patients with steady-state concentrations of ≥28 mg/L and <28 mg/L, respectively. In one prospective study of an elderly cohort (mean age, 70 years) receiving high-dose vancomycin therapy by CI, with targeting of a steady-state concentration of 30 to 40 mg/L for a median duration of 6 weeks, nephrotoxicity occurred in 32% of patients. Additionally, 4 patients in that study developed leukopenia.[91]

Dosing and Other Considerations for Use of CI. Most published studies of critically ill patients receiving vancomycin CI employed a loading dose of 15 to 20 mg/kg followed by daily maintenance infusions at doses of 30 to 40 mg/kg (up to 60 mg/kg) to achieve a target steady-state concentration of 20 to 25 mg/L. By simply multiplying the steady-state concentration by 24, a target steady-state concentration of 20 to 25 mg/L would equate to an AUC_{24}/MIC of 480 to 600 (assuming a MIC of 1 mg/L). Of note, the PK/PD target for CI has not been validated. All of the PK/PD data supporting an AUC_{24}/MIC ratio of >400 as the best correlate for clinical outcomes were derived from patients who received II vancomycin dosing.

Rapid attainment of target serum concentrations has been cited as a potential advantage of CI over II when treating acute infections, particularly in ICU patients early during the course of infection. In 2 comparative studies, target steady-state concentrations of 20 to 25 mg/L were achieved more rapidly with use of CI vs II: in a mean time of 36 (SD, 31) hours vs 51 (SD, 39) hours ($P = 0.03$) in one study and 16 (SD, 8) hours vs 50 (SD, 21) hours ($P < 0.001$) in the other.[81,83] Importantly, less variability in the steady-state concentration and fewer blood samples (a single steady-state concentration vs both peak and trough concentrations) are required to calculate AUC_{24} among patients receiving CI vs II. Timing of blood sampling for trough determinations is critical during II, whereas steady-state concentration can be measured any time after steady state has been reached during CI. In addition, vancomycin administration by CI in patients receiving OPAT has the theoretical advantage of a need for less frequent access to the i.v. catheter and thus less complications resulting from thrombus formation or infections. On the other hand, incompatibility of vancomycin with certain drugs (particularly at high concentrations), that are commonly administered in the critical care setting is a notable challenge of vancomycin CI.[92,93] The use of proper concentration, alternative agents, independent lines, or multiple catheters may be warranted if vancomycin is to be administered by CI.

Summary and Recommendations

7. The pharmacokinetics of CI suggest that such regimens may be a reasonable alternative to conventional II dosing when the AUC target cannot be achieved (B-II). Based on currently available data, a loading dose of 15 to 20 mg/kg, followed by daily maintenance CI of 30 to 40 mg/kg (up to 60 mg/kg) to achieve a target steady state concentration of 20 to 25 mg/L may be considered for critically ill patients (B-II). AUC_{24} can be simply calculated by multiplying the steady-state concentration (ie, the desired therapeutic range of 20 to 25 mg/L throughout the entire dosing interval) by a factor of 24. Attaining the desired drug exposure may be more readily accomplished given the ease of sampling time and dosage adjustment by changing the rate of infusion, which is a highly desirable feature in critically ill patients (B-II).
8. The risk of developing nephrotoxicity with CI appears to be similar or lower than that with intermittent dosing when targeting a steady-state concentration of 15 to 25 mg/L and a trough concentration of 10 to 20 mg/L (BII). Definitive studies are needed to compare drug exposure based on measured AUC_{24} and factors that predispose to

development of nephrotoxicity, such as receipt of concomitant nephrotoxins, diuretics, and/or vasopressor therapy in patients receiving CI vs II of vancomycin.

9. Incompatibility of vancomycin with other drugs commonly coadministered in the ICU requires the use of independent lines or multiple catheters when vancomycin is being considered for CI (A-III).

Loading Doses

Loading doses of vancomycin have been evaluated in several studies during the past decade.[94–109] Providing loading doses of 20 to 35 mg/kg based on actual body weight rapidly achieves targeted ranges of serum vancomycin concentrations and decreases the risk of subtherapeutic concentrations during the first days of therapy. Loading doses are recommended in patients who are critically ill or in the ICU,[95–102] require dialysis or renal replacement therapy,[102–106] or are receiving vancomycin CI therapy.[94–98,105,108] While this approach is not currently supported by evidence from large randomized clinical trials, vancomycin loading doses can be considered in the treatment of serious MRSA infections. Vancomycin should be administered in a dilute solution (eg, concentrations of no more than 5 mg/mL) and infused over a period of not less than 60 minutes or at a rate of 10 to 15 mg/min (≥1 hour per 1,000 mg) to minimize infusion-related adverse events. An infusion rate of 10 mg/min or less is associated with fewer infusion-related events. Loading doses of 25 to 35 mg/kg will require infusion times of at least 2 to 3 hours.[99] After administration of the loading dose, the initiation of the maintenance dose should occur at the next dosing interval (eg, an interval of every 6 hours indicates initiating the maintenance dose 6 hours after the start of the loading dose).

In most studies that have employed loading doses, vancomycin dosing was based on actual body weight. While this practice is commonplace, dosing by actual body weight assumes there is a linear relationship between key population PK parameters (ie, V_d and clearance) and the body size descriptor employed. While a wide variety of actual weight–based estimates of V_d (for example, 0.4 to 1 L/kg) have been reported in the literature,[6] mounting data suggest that it is not entirely accurate to describe vancomycin V_d as being proportional to body weight, particularly among obese patients (refer to Dosing in Obesity section). As noted in several recent articles discussing vancomycin PK in obesity, as weight increases the coefficient used to calculate V_d decreases.[48,110,111] At this point, dosing should be based on actual body weight, with doses capped at 3,000 mg (refer to Dosing in Obesity section).[112] More intensive therapeutic monitoring should also be performed in obese patients.

Summary and Recommendations

10. In order to achieve rapid attainment of targeted concentrations in critically ill patients with suspected or documented serious MRSA infections, a loading dose of 20 to 35 mg/kg can be considered for intermittent infusion administration of vancomycin (B-II).[1]

11. Loading doses should be based on actual body weight and not exceed 3,000 mg (refer to Dosing in Obesity section). More intensive and early therapeutic monitoring should also be performed in obese patients (BII).

Dosing in Obesity

The original vancomycin dosing strategies predate our current definitions of obesity and understanding of drug pharmacokinetics in obesity. Obesity is defined as a body mass index (BMI) of ≥30 kg/m^2 and is currently divided into 3 tiers: class I obesity (30.0–34.9 kg/m^2), class II obesity (35.0–39.9 kg/m^2), and class III, or morbid, obesity (≥40 kg/m^2).[113] The prevalence of obesity increased from approximately 10% in the 1950s to 39.8% in 2015-2016, and the average US adult weighs approximately 83 kg, compared to the historical standard of 70 kg.[114,115] This shift in the distribution of body size is relevant to the calculation of vancomycin doses based on patient body weight. Obesity may be associated with an increased risk of vancomycin-induced nephrotoxicity, in part due to supratherapeutic exposure resulting from maintenance doses calculated using actual body weight.[45,116]

The selection of vancomycin loading dose is dependent on the estimated V_d. Pharmacokinetic studies have repeatedly demonstrated that the vancomycin V_d increases with actual body weight; however, this PK parameter does not increase with actual body weight in a proportionate manner and is not reliably predictable in obese individuals.[111,117–121] Blouin and colleagues[111] demonstrated a statistically significant difference in weight-indexed V_d between obese and nonobese patients. Similarly, using data from 704 patients, Ducharme and colleagues[118] found that mean weight-indexed vancomycin V_d decreased with increasing body size. The average weight-indexed V_d in a study by Bauer and colleagues[119] was much lower in 24 morbidly obese patients (0.32 L/kg) than in 24 patients of normal weight (0.68 L/kg, $P < 0.001$). Recent studies in obese adults corroborate these findings and suggest that lower V_d estimates of approximately 0.5 L/kg or weight-independent central tendency estimates approaching 75 L are observed in obese adults.[112,120,121] The nonlinear relationship between vancomycin V_d and body weight can be resolved with piecewise functions of alternate weight descriptors, allometric scaling, use of lower mg/kg doses with increasing body size, or capping the dose at a threshold.[118,122] The underlying rationale for a loading dose is rapid attainment of therapeutic concentrations. Therefore, using actual body weight–based loading doses of 20 to 25 mg/kg (doses lower than previously recommended), with consideration of capping doses at 3,000 mg, is the most practical strategy in obese patients with serious infections.[112] For example, this strategy would result in calculated loading doses of 1,500 to 2,500 mg in patients weighing 80 to 99 kg, 2,000 to 3,000 mg in those weighing 100 to 119 kg, and 2,500 to 3,000 mg in patients with a weight of ≥120 kg (doses rounded to the nearest 250 mg). The decision of whether or not to employ a loading dose, as well as the magnitude of this dose, should be driven by the severity of infection and the urgency to achieve a therapeutic concentration rather than by body size alone.

Empiric maintenance dosing of vancomycin is reliant on estimated CL. Vancomycin CL is predicted by kidney function, which is most commonly estimated as CL_{cr} with the Cockcroft-Gault equation using patient age, sex, Scr, and body size.[123] There is considerable controversy regarding the optimal body size metric for this calculation in obese patients.[124] The Cockcroft-Gault equation predates the global standardization of Scr measurement traceable to isotopic dilution mass spectrometry (IDMS) standards advocated to reduce intralaboratory and interlaboratory measurement variability.[124] A recent population PK study by Crass and colleagues[112] of obese patients (n = 346) with BMI values of 30.1 to 85.7 kg/m^2 and body weights of 70 to 294 kg provided an equation to estimate vancomycin CL based on age, sex, Scr (IDMS traceable), and allometrically scaled body weight. This model or similar approaches to estimating vancomycin CL, such as that defined by Rodvold and colleagues,[125] can be used to estimate the total daily maintenance dose. The population model–estimated vancomycin CL multiplied by the target AUC estimates the initial daily maintenance dose.[112,120,122] For example, studies report an average vancomycin CL of approximately 6 L/h in obese patients that equates to achieving an AUC of approximately 500 mg · h/L with a daily dose of 3,000 mg. Empiric vancomycin maintenance dosages above 4,500 mg/day are not expected in obese adults, because vancomycin CL rarely exceeds 9 L/h.[112,120,121]

Population PK models of vancomycin cannot account for more than 50% of the interindividual variability, which supports therapeutic drug monitoring (TDM) in this population.[117,118,120,122] A reliable estimate of vancomycin V_d is necessary for AUC estimation when AUC is based solely on a trough concentration measurement.[24,121,126,127] This bias is addressed and precision is improved by measurement of both a peak (collected at least 1 hour after the end of infusion) and a trough concentration to estimate AUC accurately in obese patients.[126] Once a reliable PK estimate of vancomycin elimination is determined by using these 2 concentration measurements, subsequent vancomycin AUC estimation is achievable with trough-only measurements by Bayesian methods in physiologically stable patients.[57] For critically ill obese patients with unstable physiology, additional work to design adaptive feedback models to tailor doses is needed.

Summary and Recommendations

12. A vancomycin loading dose of 20 to 25 mg/kg using actual body weight, with a maximum dose of 3,000 mg, may be considered in obese adult patients with serious infections (B-II). Initial maintenance doses of vancomycin can be computed using a population PK estimate of vancomycin clearance and the target AUC in obese patients. Empiric maintenance doses for most obese patients usually do not exceed 4,500 mg/day, depending on their renal function (B-II). Early and frequent monitoring of AUC exposure is recommended for dose adjustment, especially when empiric doses exceed 4,000 mg/day (A-II). Measurement of peak and trough concentrations is recommended to improve the accuracy of vancomycin AUC estimation and maintenance dose optimization in obese patients, aligning with recommendations 2 and 5 for nonobese adults.

Renal Disease and Renal Replacement Therapies

Intermittent Hemodialysis. Despite the common use of vancomycin in patients receiving hemodialysis, there are few published outcome studies that provide guidance on the optimal PK/PD targets in this population. Previously published drug dosing recommendations generally targeted a predialysis serum concentration, even though other PD targets may be more appropriate. Predialysis vancomycin concentration to MRSA MIC ratios of >18.6 have been associated with improved bacteremic patient outcomes, suggesting that serum concentration monitoring is essential throughout the course of therapy.[128] Dosing to achieve predialysis vancomycin concentrations of 10 to 20 mg/L, as has been done clinically,[129] results in mean AUC_{24} values ranging from 250 to 450 mg · h/L, with some values below the AUC/MIC goals recommended in other populations.[130] Outcome studies validating the AUC_{24h} goal of 400 to 600 mg · h/L used in other patient populations have not been conducted in the hemodialysis population. Nonetheless, the maintenance doses recommended in this section aim to reach this AUC_{24} target (ie, 400-600 mg · h/L), as recommended throughout this document.

Many dialysis-related factors affect the degree of vancomycin exposure in these patients. These considerations include the amount of time between vancomycin dose administration and the scheduled time of the next dialysis session,[104] whether the dose is given during dialysis or after hemodialysis has ended, and the dialyzer's permeability if the dose is administered intradialytically.[131] Dialysis frequency also plays a role in dosing decisions. For non–critically ill patients receiving hemodialysis, 2 or 3 days is the most common interdialytic period. Some critically ill patients with severe catabolism and AKI may require more than thrice weekly hemodialysis for optimal metabolic control, and their maintenance vancomycin doses should be based on serum concentration monitoring.[132]

Vancomycin dosing in patients with acute or chronic kidney failure has transformed over time due to the changes in dialysis technology and techniques.[133] Older (pre-1990s) hemodialyzers were not very permeable to large molecules. Vancomycin (with a molecular weight of 1,450 Da) was not considered "dialyzable" because it poorly crossed the hemodialysis membranes of the era. Indeed, even today's vancomycin package insert, based on PK studies conducted in the 1980s, states that "vancomycin is poorly removed by dialysis."[134] As hemodialysis membrane technology has improved, dialyzers have become far more permeable. Vancomycin is cleared substantially by contemporary high-permeability hemodialyzers[135,136]; consequently, vancomycin dosing strategies have changed substantially as well. For example, in spite of the package insert statement "In anuria, a dose of 1000 mg every 7 to 10 days has been recommended" and the statement that "vancomycin is poorly removed by dialysis,"[134] far more frequent doses are needed to maintain therapeutic serum concentrations in patients receiving hemodialysis. The extent of vancomycin removal by dialysis is dependent on the permeability of the hemodialyzer used[131]; consequently, investigators have developed and published a wide variety of vancomycin dosing protocols in an attempt to compensate for the increase in vancomycin dialytic CL caused by increases in dialyzer permeability.

An added complication of appropriate vancomycin dosing in patients receiving hemodialysis is the prevailing practice of administering the drug during the final hours of the hemodialysis process, thus resulting in some of the infused drug being removed immediately by the hemodialyzer. This practice started back when low-permeability dialyzers were used and little vancomycin was eliminated by hemodialysis. The practice has persisted at most dialysis units because most dialysis units treat 3 shifts of patients per day, and holding a dialysis chair for 60 to 90 additional minutes while vancomycin infuses into a patient is not cost-effective. Indeed, it is more cost-effective to infuse "extra" vancomycin during the hemodialysis session to compensate for intradialytic loss than it is to keep a dialysis unit open later to allow vancomycin infusions. Intradialytically infused vancomycin results in reduced delivery of drug to the patient, similar to a first-pass phenomenon. The extent of intradialytic drug removal is variable and depends on patient and dialysis system factors, the most important of which is dialyzer membrane permeability.[135,137–139] Approximately 20% to 40% of an intradialytically administered vancomycin dose is removed by the simultaneous hemodialysis, with the highly permeable dialyzers tending to the higher end of this range.[137,140,141]

Maintenance dosing strategies that do not provide a dose with every hemodialysis session (eg, a maintenance dose is given with every second or third hemodialysis session) have been studied,[102,142,143] but none have been found to meet vancomycin exposure goals in the last day of the dosing interval without giving massive doses that result in very high peak concentrations. Consequently, maintenance vancomycin doses are recommended to be administered with each hemodialysis session to ensure therapeutic serum concentrations throughout the dosing interval. In the typical thrice-weekly hemodialysis schedule, 25% larger doses are needed for the 3-day interdialytic period (eg, Friday to Monday) to maintain sufficient vancomycin exposure on the third day.[130,144]

Dosing that is weight based appears to be superior to standard dosing schemes that do not account for patient size. Further, doses should be based on actual body weight rather than a calculated body weight (see Dosing in Obesity section for considerations on how to dose morbidly obese patients). Because vancomycin is water soluble, vancomycin dosing in fluid overloaded patients should also be based on actual body weight at the time of dosing rather than on some calculated adjusted weight.[102–105]

Serum concentration monitoring is a valuable tool to guide vancomycin dosing in patients receiving dialysis, provided that serum concentrations are obtained and interpreted correctly. For example, blood sampling for assessment of vancomycin concentrations should not occur during or for at least 2 hours after a hemodialysis treatment. These samples will not be reflective of the true vancomycin body load because of the dialytic removal of vancomycin. Vancomycin serum concentrations will be low immediately following a dialysis treatment but will rebound substantially as drug redistributes from the tissues back to the blood over the next few hours.[131,142,145] Dosing decisions based on serum concentrations obtained during or soon after hemodialysis will be inherently incorrect and could result in administration of doses higher than necessary.[145] Serum concentration monitoring performed with blood samples obtained prior to the hemodialysis treatment is recommended to guide dosing, although other serum concentration monitoring techniques have been suggested.[146]

Dosing to achieve predialysis vancomycin concentrations of 10 to 20 mg/L, as has been conducted clinically,[129] results in mean AUC_{24} values ranging from 250 to 450 mg · h/L, often below the AUC/MIC goals recommended in other populations.[130] Outcome studies validating the AUC target of 400 to 600 mg · h/L used in other patient populations have not been conducted in the hemodialysis population. While determination of AUC/MIC attainment is recommended, limited serum concentration monitoring is possible in patients receiving hemodialysis in the outpatient setting for 2 reasons. The first reason is that frequent phlebotomy must be avoided in order to preserve future hemodialysis vascular access needs; the second is that it is impractical to obtain blood samples aside from the predialysis sample that is obtained from the blood catheter inserted for use in the dialysis process. Patients leave the dialysis unit after hemodialysis and do not return until the next dialysis session days later. Consequently, since data are unavailable for an optimal AUC target in these patients, and no data are available to demonstrate efficacy below an AUC threshold value of 400, the goal should be to attain the AUC target of 400 to 600 mg · h/L used in other patient populations. It is most practical to continue monitoring based on predialysis concentrations and extrapolate these values to estimate AUC. Maintaining predialysis concentrations between 15 and 20 mg/L is likely to attain the AUC target of 400 to 600 mg · h/L in the previous 24 hours, with higher AUC/MIC values occurring on days prior.

Summary and Recommendations

13. The following tabulation outlines recommended vancomycin loading and maintenance doses for patients receiving hemodialysis, with accounting for permeability of the dialyzer and whether the dose is administered intradialytically or after dialysis ends (B-II).

Timing and Dialyzer Permeability	Vancomycin Dose, mg/kg[a]
After dialysis ends	
Low permeability	Loading: 25 Maint.: 7.5[b]
High permeability	Loading: 25 Maint.: 10[b]
Intradialytic	
Low permeability	Loading: 30 Maint.: 7.5-10[b]
High permeability	Loading: 35 Maint.: 10-15[b]

[a]From references 104, 129, 130, 137, 138, 140, and 147.

[b]Thrice-weekly dose administration.

14. Since efficacy data are unavailable for AUC values of <400 mg · h/L, monitoring based on predialysis serum concentrations and extrapolating these values to estimate AUC is most practical. Maintaining predialysis concentrations between 15 and 20 mg/L is likely to achieve the AUC of 400 to 600 mg · h/L in the previous 24 hours (C-III). Predialysis serum concentration monitoring should be performed not less than weekly and should drive subsequent dosing, as opposed to a strict weight-based recommendation, although these recommended doses provide a useful starting point until serum concentrations have been determined (BII).

Hybrid Hemodialysis Therapies. Contemporary renal replacement therapies used to treat kidney disease have expanded well beyond thrice-weekly, 3- to 4-hour hemodialysis sessions. In the outpatient setting, shorter, more frequent home hemodialysis treatments are used in a growing number of patients. In the inpatient setting, various types of "hybrid" hemodialysis therapies are employed. These hybrid treatments go by many names, including prolonged intermittent renal replacement therapy (PIRRT) and slow-low efficiency dialysis (SLED). Essentially these hybrid therapies use standard hemodialysis machines that run at slower blood and dialysate flow rates and for longer durations (usually 6 to 12 hours per day). Even hemodialysis itself differs in the inpatient and outpatient settings, as patients with AKI are often hemodynamically unstable and lack sufficient vascular access for robust blood flow through the dialysis vascular access. All these hybrid dialysis therapies clear vancomycin to a different extent than standard intermittent hemodialysis.[148,149] The timing of the vancomycin dose in relation to the hybrid hemodialysis session is essential in determining a dosing regimen. If hybrid hemodialysis is started soon after the dose is administered, much of the dose will be removed, whereas the same vancomycin dose given after the dialysis session ends will yield a much larger AUC_{24} and much higher average serum concentrations. As is the case with any hemodialysis therapy, serum concentrations obtained during or within 2 hours from the end of hemodialysis will be artificially low because dialysis will have efficiently removed vancomycin from the blood, and vancomycin located in the tissues will not have had time to redistribute back into the bloodstream. Calculation of maintenance doses based on an intra- or postdialytic vancomycin serum concentration may result in doses that are too high. Caution is recommended in basing any maintenance dosing on these serum concentration values.

Little has been published on the patient outcomes achieved when vancomycin is used in patients receiving hybrid dialysis. Authors of one small case series of 27 courses of vancomycin given to patients receiving a hybrid hemodialysis therapy reported that prescribers have tried a wide variety of dosing schemes.[150] By these authors' criteria, 89% of the prescribed vancomycin doses in their institution were too low. Given the absence of outcome data in patients receiving these therapies, it seems prudent to use the same vancomycin AUC goal recommended throughout this document (400 to 600 mg · h/L assuming a MIC of 1 mg/L).

Summary and Recommendations

15. Loading doses of 20 to 25 mg/kg actual body weight should be used, recognizing that these hybrid dialysis therapies efficiently remove vancomycin (B-III). Initial doses should not be delayed to wait for a dialysis treatment to end. Maintenance doses of 15 mg/kg should be given after hybrid hemodialysis ends or during the final 60 to 90 minutes of dialysis, as is done with standard hemodialysis (B-III).[130] Concentration monitoring should guide further maintenance doses.

Continuous Renal Replacement Therapies. The use of continuous renal replacement therapy (CRRT) modalities like continuous venovenous hemofiltration (CVVH), continuous venovenous hemodialysis (CVVHD), and continuous venovenous hemodiafiltration (CVVHDF) has grown in popularity in critically ill patients with AKI because of their superior ability to provide fluid and solute balance. Provided these therapies operate in an uninterrupted fashion, vancomycin CL is relatively constant over the dosing interval, although CL may decline as the hemodiafilter clogs over time.[151] Vancomycin is removed by CRRT and its CL is related closely to the rate of ultrafiltrate/dialysate flow,[105] with hemodiafilter type being of lesser importance, because contemporary hemodiafilters are all very permeable to the drug.

In patients on CRRT, serum concentration attainment goals often are not met with conventional dosing.[84,152] Although outcomes studies specific to patients receiving CRRT have not been conducted, it seems prudent to apply the same vancomycin AUC/MIC target (ie, 400-600) in these critically ill patients as is recommended throughout this document.

Summary and Recommendations

16. Loading doses of 20 to 25 mg/kg by actual body weight should be used in patients receiving CRRT at conventional, KDIGO-recommended effluent rates of 20 to 25 mL/kg/h (B-II).[153] Initial maintenance dosing for CRRT with effluent rates of 20 to 25 mL/kg/h should be 7.5 to 10 mg/kg every 12 hours (B-II). Maintenance dose and dosing interval should be based on serum concentration monitoring, which should be conducted within the first 24 hours to ensure AUC/MIC targets are met.[154] In fluid overloaded patients, doses may be reduced as patients become euvolemic and drug V_d decreases. The use of CI of vancomycin in patients receiving CRRT appears to be growing,[84,105] and this method could be used in place of intermittent vancomycin dosing, especially when high CRRT ultrafiltrate/dialysate flow rates are employed (B-II).

Pediatric Patients

In 2011, prior to the availability of alternative agents for MRSA in pediatrics, vancomycin was recommended as the drug of choice for invasive MRSA infections in children.[5] Although there are limited prospective, comparative data on the value of vancomycin therapeutic monitoring in adults with respect to improving outcomes and decreasing toxicity, virtually no prospectively collected data on outcomes of MRSA infection in newborns, infants and children exist. Further, for newborns (particularly premature infants) compared with older infants, immature renal elimination mechanisms and a relative increase in V_d by body weight further complicate dosing guidelines during the first several weeks of life. Additional complexity for dosing strategies during early childhood is based on a continual maturation of glomerular filtration, which is directly related to vancomycin CL. The glomerular filtration rate increases through the first years of life to rates in school-aged children that are greater than those in adults, with subsequent decline during the teen years to adult normal rates. Such a diversity of PK parameter values based on developmental pharmacology from neonates to adolescents provides a challenge to develop generalized vancomycin dosing. However, this has improved with the application of population-based PK models using allometric scaling and renal maturation covariates. In a population-based PK study by Colin and colleagues[155] that evaluated vancomycin PK throughout the entire age continuum from infancy to geriatric years using pooled data from 14 studies, age, weight, and kidney function were important factors in estimating clearance. Careful monitoring in the pediatric population is prudent, especially with the evident dynamic changes in renal function in this population. As with adults, comorbidities and concurrent medications can influence vancomycin tissue distribution, elimination, and toxicity.

Limitation of Outcomes Data. Recent retrospective studies on bacteremic *S. aureus* infections (both MRSA and MSSA strains) in children treated with vancomycin suggest that trough concentrations of >15 mg/L were not associated with improved outcomes, yet an increase in AKI was observed.[156–158] Furthermore, another retrospective pediatric study evaluating outcomes of MRSA bacteremia as a function of an AUC/MIC_{BMD} of ≥400 did not show improved outcomes.[159] Similarly, vancomycin trough concentrations of <10 mg/L, as compared with concentrations of >10 mg/L, were not associated with increased 30-day mortality and recurrent bacteremia in children, although the lower concentrations were associated with prolonged bacteremia.[160]

In the absence of prospective, comparative outcomes data in children regarding unique AUC/MIC exposures necessary for clinical and microbiologic success in treating serious MRSA infections in different neonatal and pediatric populations to validate the observations reported in adults (see Clinical PK/PD Data: Adults section), dosing in children should be designed to achieve an AUC of 400 mg · h/L and potentially up to 600 mg · h/L (assuming a MIC of 1 mg/L). This PD target range, specifically a range closer to an AUC/MIC of 400 rather than 600, has been widely used by investigators to model pediatric dosing and therapeutic monitoring. With inadequate PK studies and outcomes data to support the higher end of the AUC target range in pediatrics, it is prudent to aim for an AUC/MIC of 400 in pediatrics to limit the development of exposure-related AKI. Furthermore, in pediatrics, an AUC/MIC target of 400 is more readily achievable than it is in adults and correlates to trough concentrations of 7 to 10 mg/L rather than concentrations of 15 to 20 mg/L as are reported in adults. This wide variability in trough concentrations between these populations with regard to achieving an AUC/MIC of 400 corroborates the need for an AUC-guided approach to dosing and monitoring. It is possible that in otherwise healthy children with fewer comorbidities than are typically seen in adults, a lower target may yield outcomes equivalent to an AUC of 400 to 600 mg · hr/L. The decision to retain or increase AUC target exposure should be based on clinical judgment in the management of these patients.

With use of currently recommended vancomycin dosages of 45 to 60 mg/kg/day, widespread treatment failures in children have not been reported in the literature, which may be reflective of a younger host with a more robust systemic and immunologic response to infection, a different management approach (surgical and antibiotic) to invasive MRSA infection, lack of associated comorbidities, or publication bias. Prospective comparative clinical trials involving children with documented infections treated with different vancomycin dosages or exposures have not been published.

Empiric Maintenance Regimen. Published retrospective PK/PD data in children suggest that current vancomycin dosing of 45 to 60 mg/kg/day (in divided doses administered every 6 to 8 hours) may be insufficient to achieve currently recommended targets for adults of an AUC of 400 to 600 mg · h/L (assuming a MIC of 1 mg/L).[1] In fact, higher dosages, ranging from 60 to 80 mg/kg/day and given in divided doses every 6 hours, may be needed to achieve these targets for MRSA strains with a vancomycin MIC of 1 mg/L or less, presumably as a result of greater vancomycin CL than is seen in adults.[1,161–164] For children infected by MRSA pathogens with a MIC of >1 mg/L, it is unlikely that the target exposure can be reliably achieved with previously investigated dosages of vancomycin in children.

Le and colleagues[164] utilized population-based PK modeling to analyze 1,660 vancomycin serum concentrations obtained at 2 institutions from 2003 to 2011 among 702 children older than 3 months of age with varying comorbidities. They demonstrated that 4 important factors (age, weight, renal function as assessed by SCr, and MIC) contributed to vancomycin exposure. Monte Carlo simulations were created using population-based PK modeling with Bayesian estimation and MICs of clinical isolates as determined by Etest, with 85% of clinical isolates demonstrated to have a MIC_{Etest} of 1 mg/L or less. To achieve an AUC/MIC_{Etest} of ≥400 in 90% of subjects, a dosage of 80 mg/kg/day was necessary, particularly in those less than 12 years of age with normal renal function. At a dosage of 80 mg/kg/day, the median AUC and median trough concentration were 675 mg · h/L and 16 mg/L, respectively. As expected, subjects 12 years of age or older achieved similar exposure at lower dosages of 60 to 70 mg/kg/day. At a dosage of 60 to 70 mg/kg/day (divided doses administered every 6 hours), an AUC of 400 mg · h/L correlated to a mean trough of 8 to 9 mg/L.[164] The clinical applicability of this PK model for vancomyin CL estimation to determine AUC exposure was validated in a small study by Ploessl et al.[165]

Other studies corroborated Le and colleagues' findings regarding the need to use higher dosages, ranging from 60 to 80 mg/kg/day, depending on age and renal function.[162,164,166,167] Using the literature for vancomyin CL published in or before 2000 and Bayesian estimation for one 25-kg base subject, Frymoyer et al[163] evaluated the relationship between AUC and trough concentrations, showing that a dosage of 60 mg/kg/day achieved trough concentrations of 7 to 10 mg/L and an AUC/MIC of ≥400 in 90% of children for MRSA pathogens with a MIC of 1 mg/L. However, their finding may not be extrapolatable to the entire pediatric population given the variable ages and renal function. In a second study, these investigators demonstrated that a dosage of 60 mg/kg/day achieved AUC/MIC_{BMD} values between 386 and 583 (assuming a MIC_{BMD} of 1 mg/L) in children 2 to 12 years of age, indicating that some younger children may require higher doses to achieve target AUC/MIC_{BMD}.[162] The probability of target attainment was not provided, and dosages above 60 mg/kg/day were not evaluated in this study.

Two retrospective studies that utilized non-Bayesian methods evaluated trough concentration targets of 10 to 20 mg/L (a higher range than that used by Le et al[164] and Frymoyer et al[163], who also assessed AUC) in children 1 month to 18 years of age. An interesting finding of the study of Madigan et al[166] was that a dosage of 60 mg/kg/day achieved the target trough concentration in only 17% of preschool-aged children 2 to 5 years old, which was the lowest attainment for any pediatric age group. Eiland and colleagues[161] showed that dosages of 70 to 80 mg/kg/day were necessary to achieve trough concentrations of 10 to 20 mg/L. Another study, by Abdel et al,[168] demonstrated that dosages higher than 60 mg/kg/day were necessary to achieve an AUC/MIC of ≥400 in children with cancer. The mean age in this study cohort was 6 (SD, 2.5) years; it is possible that young age with greater CL may have been a contributing factor for the need for an increased dose, an observation uncovered in studies by Le et al[164] and Madigan et al.[166]

As a drug that demonstrates renal elimination, vancomycin requires dosage adjustment in children with acute or chronic renal insufficiency. Le and colleagues[169] conducted a population based PK analysis with Bayesian methods that evaluated 63 case control pairs (matched by age and weight) with 319 vancomycin serum concentrations. The mean age of this study cohort was 13 (SD, 6) years. The investigators reported that a vancomycin dosage of 45 mg/kg/day (ie, 15 mg/kg every 8 hours) in renally impaired children achieved AUC exposure similar to that achieved with a dosage of 60 mg/kg/day in children with normal renal function. Notably, they showed that in 87% of children with initial renal impairment, vancomycin CL improved (with a lag in the recovery of renal function as assessed by SCr) within the first 5 days of therapy, indicating some degree of renal function recovery, a finding that provides support for ongoing vancomycin TDM. In addition, vancomycin CL does not always correlate well with renal function (as assessed by creatinine CL) in children, particularly in those who are acutely ill in the ICU setting and have varying degrees of renal dysfunction. Rapid return of renal function may occur over the first few days after ICU admission. As such, therapeutic monitoring of both serum concentrations and renal function should be conducted during vancomycin therapy.[170,171]

Loading Doses. Loading doses of 25 to 30 mg/kg for critically ill adults have been suggested to achieve steady-state concentrations more quickly, but preliminary data on pediatric patients suggest that the benefit of a loading dose of 30 mg/kg is quickly lost if the maintenance dose is insufficient to provide adequate ongoing exposure.[167] However, the concept of a loading dose accompanied by a daily maintenance dose sufficient to achieve the target exposure and initiated at a specified time after the loading dose should be investigated.

Minimizing AKI Risk. Similar to the literature on adults, the literature in pediatrics suggests, in aggregate, that the risk of AKI increases as a function of vancomycin exposure, especially when the trough concentration exceeds 15 to 20 mg/L. In fact, Fiorito and colleagues[158] reported in a recent metaanalysis of 10 pediatric studies that troughs of ≥15 mg/L increased the OR for AKI by 2.7-fold (95% confidence interval, 1.82–4.05) and that AKI was further correlated with a stay in the pediatric ICU. McKamy and colleagues[172] published results of the first study that uncovered the association between vancomycin trough concentrations greater than 15 to 20 mg/L and AKI in pediatric patients. In addition, they showed that children who received concurrent nephrotoxic drugs (particularly furosemide) and stayed in the pediatric ICU were also more likely to experience AKI. Four studies published later corroborated these findings, indicating that the interplay of multiple factors in addition to vancomycin exposure contributed to AKI.[173-176] Interestingly, Sinclair et al[174] reported that a 5-mg/kg dose augmentation or each additional day of vancomycin use increased the risk of AKI. Knoderer and colleagues[173] evaluated late-onset AKI (defined as occurring after 7 days of vancomycin therapy) and observed that young age (<1 year) was independently associated with late AKI.

One pediatric study evaluated the relationship of AKI with vancomycin AUC and trough concentrations, both derived by Bayesian estimation. Le and colleagues[19] conducted a large population-based PK analysis using 1,576 serum concentrations collected from 680 pediatric subjects. A continuous exposure-response relationship was observed, with 10%, 33%, and 57% of patients who respectively achieved AUC values of ≥400, 800, and 1,000 mg · h/L experiencing AKI. Even after adjusting for ICU stay and concomitant use of nephrotoxic drugs, an AUC of ≥800 mg · h/L and trough concentrations of ≥15 mg/L were independently associated with a greater than 2.5-fold increased risk of AKI. The linkage of AUC to AKI, along with the strong correlation between AUC and trough concentrations (Spearman's coefficient, 0.963; $P < 0.001$), reinforces AUC as a plausible PK/PD parameter for therapeutic monitoring that encompasses both therapeutic and toxic responses. Vancomycin exposure should be maintained at an AUC of <800 mg · h/L to minimize AKI risk. As such, vancomycin dosages of ≥100 mg/kg/day should be avoided given that the projected median AUC and trough values are 843 mg · h/L and 21 mg/L, respectively, at a dosage of 100 mg/kg/day.[164] However, enhanced renal clearance of vancomycin may transiently occur in specific situations in children, in which case the dose of vancomycin may need to be higher than is usually prescribed to achieve an AUC of 400 mg · h/L, highlighting the need for therapeutic monitoring.

Therapeutic Monitoring. Recent literature on vancomycin in pediatrics has focused primarily on PK analysis to support optimal dosing. Le and colleagues[177] conducted a population-based PK analysis in 138 pediatric subjects who were more than 3 months of age, evaluating 712 serum vancomycin concentrations (collected mostly after the third or fourth dose). They showed that both accuracy and precision for estimating AUC_{24} (calculated by total daily dose over vancomycin CL, with the integration of Bayesian estimation) were improved using 2 concentrations (peak and trough), compared with trough-only monitoring. Furthermore, the 2-concentration approach improved the prediction of future AUC exposure in patients.[177] Another study, by Stockmann et al,[178] evaluated AUC-based vancomycin monitoring in 23 pediatric patients with cystic fibrosis. The researchers demonstrated that 2 concentrations calculated using a standard PK equation and a trough concentration calculated using a Bayesian population-based PK model produced similar AUC estimations. Despite the availability of limited studies on vancomycin monitoring in pediatrics, the findings appear congruent with adult data supporting AUC-guided therapeutic monitoring that incorporates the Bayesian method, especially if only a single trough concentration is available. Furthermore, this AUC-guided monitoring approach also appears prudent in order to predict toxicity in light of AKI data in pediatrics.

Overall, there are limited pediatric outcomes data to support the AUC target correlated with drug effectiveness in adults. Some of the differences found between adults and children treated for MRSA infections with vancomycin include the complexity of vancomycin CL in the various pediatric age groups, and the differences in tissue site-of-infection drug exposure (eg, common occurrence of multifocal complicated osteomyelitis in children requiring therapeutic bone concentrations, with rare occurrence of MRSA endocarditis) suggest that further studies in children that incorporate prospective assessment of clinical outcomes and large sample size are needed to identify the optimal dosing strategies for MRSA infections in pediatrics. Until additional data are available, the AUC target used in adults (ie, from 400 up to 600 mg · h/L [assuming a MIC of 1 mg/L]) appears to be the most appropriate initial target for vancomycin exposures in all pediatric age groups. For most children across the pediatric age groups, assuming a vancomycin MIC of 1 mg/L, published data suggest that a dosage of 60 to 80 mg/kg/day (given in divided doses every 6 hours) is required to achieve an AUC target of 400 to 600 mg · h/L.

Summary and Recommendations

17. Based on an AUC target of 400 mg · h/L (but potentially up to 600 mg · hr/L, assuming a vancomycin MIC of ≤1 mg/L for MRSA) from adult data, the initial recommended vancomycin dosage for children with normal renal function and suspected serious MRSA infections (including pneumonia, pyomyositis, multifocal osteomyelitis, complicated bacteremia, and necrotizing fasciitis) is:

- 60 to 80 mg/kg/day, in divided doses given every 6 hours, for children ages 3 months to less than 12 years or
- 60 to 70 mg/kg/day, in divided doses given every 6 to 8 hours, for those ≥12 years old (A-II).

The maximum empiric daily dose is usually 3,600 mg in children with adequate renal function (C-III). Most children generally should not require more than 3,000 mg/day, and doses should be adjusted based on observed concentrations to achieve the AUC/MIC target. Early monitoring of observed concentrations is recommended when doses exceed 2,000 to 3,000 mg/day (A-III). Furthermore, close monitoring of observed concentrations and renal function is prudent in patients with poor or augmented renal clearance, as resolution of their renal function abnormalities may occur within the first 5 days of therapy.

18. AUC-guided therapeutic monitoring for vancomycin, preferably with Bayesian estimation, is suggested for all pediatric age groups, based on developmental changes of vancomycin CL documented from the newborn to the adolescent. Based on current available data, the suggestion for AUC-guided monitoring in pediatrics aligns with the approach for adults, including the application of Bayesian estimation for 1 trough concentration or first-order PK equations with 2 concentrations (B-II). The Bayesian AUC-guided dosing strategy may be an optimal approach to individualize vancomycin therapy in pediatrics since it can incorporate varying ages, weights, and renal function. Both serum concentrations of vancomycin and renal function should be monitored since vancomycin CL and CL_{cr} are not always well correlated in pediatrics. Furthermore, aggressive dosing to maintain target AUC exposure and decrease the risk of potential AKI in treatment of MRSA infection necessitates drug monitoring.

19. Therapeutic monitoring may begin within 24 to 48 hours of vancomycin therapy for serious MRSA infections in children, as in adults (B-III). Any delay in therapeutic monitoring should be based on severity of infection and clinical judgment. Dosing adjustment should be made for those with renal insufficiency, those with obesity (see Pediatric Obesity), and those receiving concurrent nephrotoxic drug therapy. Following the initial dose, dosing adjustment is important for those with acute renal insufficiency, but subsequent adjustment (particularly within the first 5 days of therapy) may be necessary for those experiencing recovery of renal function. Sustained or subsequent decreases in dosage may be needed, particularly for those with chronic renal insufficiency and those receiving concurrent nephrotoxic drug therapy (B-III).

20. Vancomycin exposure may be optimally maintained below the thresholds for AUC of 800 mg · h/L and for trough concentrations of 15 mg/L to minimize AKI (BII). The safety of vancomycin dosages above 80 mg/kg/day has not been prospectively evaluated. Avoiding vancomycin dosages of ≥100 mg/kg/day is suggested since they are likely to surpass these thresholds (B-III).

21. Insufficient data exist on which to base a recommendation for a loading dose among the nonobese pediatric population. Loading doses from adult studies may be considered, but further studies are needed to elucidate the appropriate dose for the various pediatric populations from the neonate to adolescent (C-III).

Pediatric Obesity. Vancomycin is a large glycopeptide molecule that is hydrophilic, suggesting that distribution into tissues with high lipid concentrations, such as adipose tissue, is decreased, as noted above for adults (see Dosing in Obesity section). When vancomycin dosing is based on total body weight (mg/kg) for both obese and nonobese children, serum concentrations have been documented to be higher in obese children, assuming that renal CL is similar between the 2 populations.[179] Moffett retrospectively compared vancomycin pharmacokinetics in 24 obese children who were matched with 24 nonobese control children.[180] Vancomycin dose administration per child was slightly higher in the obese children, which resulted in increased trough concentrations. Similarly, 2 retrospective non-Bayesian studies by Heble et al[181] and Miller et al[182] documented higher vancomycin trough concentrations in overweight and obese children, as compared to normal-weight children, with dosing based on total body weight. No increase in AKI was noted in the overweight children.[182]

Collectively, non-Bayesian studies of obese children have evaluated maintenance regimens ranging from 40 to 80 mg/kg/day (calculated using total body weight), with some instituting maximum doses of 1 to 2 g over 1 to 2 hours.[180,181,183,184] As an alternative to total body weight, one study recommended the use of body surface area to dose vancomycin, which necessitates establishing a different dosing regimen and obtaining height measurements that may not always be readily available in clinical practice.[185] Body surface area is not typically used for dosing medications in children, except for chemotherapeutic agents.[186]

Using a Bayesian population-based PK analysis of 389 vancomycin serum concentrations collected from 87 pairs of obese and nonobese children (matched by age and baseline SCr), Le and colleagues[187] showed that the V_d was strongly correlated with actual or total body weight and that CL correlated with allometric weight (ie, weight x 0.75) and body surface area. Using this PK model, Nguyen and colleagues[164,166] concluded, using Monte Carlo simulations with Bayesian estimation, that vancomycin 60 mg/kg/day dosed by total body weight, as compared with other weight measures, resulted in the highest rate of achievement of the target AUC/MIC of ≥400 in obese children (ie, the target was achieved in 76% when vancomycin was given by total body weight, in 66% when given by adjusted body weight, and in 31% when given by allometric weight). Furthermore, when given dosages of vancomycin of 60 mg/kg/day by total body weight, fewer obese children of <12 vs ≥12 years of age achieved an AUC/MIC of ≥400 (70% and 84%, respectively), an age-based observation also identified in nonobese children.[164,166] Interestingly, the use of a 20-mg/kg loading dose based on total body weight in obese children increased achievement of an AUC/MIC of ≥400, especially within the first 12 hours of therapy. In addition, 1 of every 5 obese children had an AUC of ≥ 800 mg · h/L, indicating that routine therapeutic and safety monitoring is prudent.[188]

Summary and Recommendations

22. Data suggest that obese children are likely to have vancomycin exposures that may be statistically greater than those in normal-weight children when doses are calculated on a mg/kg basis, but these differences are not known to be of sufficient clinical importance to suggest different mg/kg empiric vancomycin dosages in obese children at this time. Similar to nonobese children, obese children < 12 years old, compared with those ≥ 12 years, may require a higher mg/kg dose (B-II).

23. Therapeutic monitoring is likely to be of particular value in obese children, both for therapeutic response and the risk of AKI. The specific recommendations for therapeutic monitoring in nonobese children may also apply for obese children (B-II).

24. A loading dose of 20 mg/kg by total body weight is recommended in obese children (A-III).

Neonates. Vancomycin therapeutic monitoring is important in neonates, based on developmental considerations of prominent increasing renal function that occurs over the first several weeks of life.[189] Models to predict vancomycin dosing have variously incorporated weight-based dosing, chronologic age–based dosing, postmenstrual age–based dosing, SCr-based dosing (except for the first week of life, when transplacental maternal creatinine in the neonatal circulation renders neonatal SCr values inaccurate in estimating renal function), or combinations of these strategies. Regardless of which model is used, therapeutic monitoring in the neonate is essential due to the rapid maturation of renal function over the first weeks of life.

Mehrotra et al[190] compared 4 models for predicting vancomycin serum concentrations, based on their population PK model, using a standard weight-based dose, a postmenstrual age–based dose, a postmenstrual and postnatal age–based dose, and a SCr-based dose. Serum creatinine–based dosing predicted trough concentrations with the smallest variability in both term and preterm neonates. However, for those who wish to achieve a target exposure based on high trough concentrations within a narrow range of 15 to 20 mg/L, it should be noted that only 13% to 21% of neonates were within this range across the 4 dosing regimens. Marqués-Miñana et al[191] also developed a population PK model and proposed dosing based on postmenstrual age. SCr-based rather than postmenstrual or postconceptional age–based dosing has been supported by Irikura et al[192] and Capparelli et al.[193] However, when evaluating published neonatal PK models, no consensus on an optimal dosing regimen was achieved by experts on neonatal vancomycin, Zhao et al reported.[194] After evaluating the predictive performance of 6 models, Zhao et al concluded the importance of evaluating analytical techniques for SCr and vancomycin concentrations best explained the variability of predictions between the models. Zhao et al found that the Jaffé method overestimated SCr concentrations when compared to the enzymatic method and that for vancomycin concentrations, the fluorescence polarization immunoassay method and enzyme-multiplied immunoassay method assays showed different predictive performances as well.[194]

With the knowledge that AUC, as compared with trough concentrations, is a more achievable target in pediatrics, Frymoyer and colleagues[195] evaluated the association between AUC and trough concentrations in neonates. Using 1,702 vancomycin concentrations (measured by the homogenous particle-enhanced turbidimetric inhibition immunoassay) collected from 249 neonates up to 3 months of age, population PK analysis was conducted to create a model for vancomycin CL that was based on weight, postmenstrual age, and SCr (measured by a modified kinetic Jaffé reaction). Monte Carlo simulations with Bayesian estimation demonstrated that trough concentrations ranging from 7 to 11 mg/L were highly predictive of an AUC_{24} of >400 mg · h/L in at least 90% of neonates. Dosages to achieve this PK/PD target ranged from 15 to 20 mg/kg every 8 to 12 hours, depending on postmenstrual age and SCr.[194] Stockmann et al[196] later supported the predictive performance and generalizability of this model in their study of 243 neonates with 734 vancomycin concentrations. While a trough concentration of 11 mg/L predicted the attainment of an AUC of ≥400 mg · h/L in 93% of neonates, Stockmann and colleagues noted that a trough concentration alone did not precisely predict AUC and concluded that Bayesian approaches to support vancomycin dosing decisions for neonates in the clinical setting are needed.[196] Furthermore, Cies et al[197] reported differences in vancomycin pharmacokinetics, in particular rapid vancomycin CL, in neonates with extracorporeal oxygenation life support, reiterating the need for Bayesian-derived dosing decision support in this vulnerable population. Lastly, Leroux et al[198] demonstrated the success of the clinical integration of a model-based vancomycin dosing calculator, developed from a population PK study, that was successful in improving the rate of attainment of a serum concentration of 15 to 25 mg/L from 41% to 72% without any cases of AKI.

As an alternative to intermittent administration, CI of vancomycin has been evaluated in infants. In a multicenter, randomized controlled trial involving 111 infants less than 90 days of age, Gwee et al[199] showed that the use of CI resulted in fewer dose adjustments and a lower mean daily dose than intermittent administration. The target trough

TABLE 2.
Primary Recommendations for Vancomycin Dosing and Therapeutic Drug Monitoring

A. ADULTS AND PEDIATRIC PATIENTS
1. In patients with suspected or definitive serious MRSA infections, an individualized target AUC/MIC_{BMD} ratio of 400 to 600 (assuming a vancomycin MIC_{BMD} of 1 mg/L) should be advocated to achieve clinical efficacy while improving patient safety (A-II).
2. When transitioning to AUC/MIC monitoring, clinicians should conservatively target AUCs for patients with suspected or documented serious infections due to MRSA, assuming a vancomycin MIC_{BMD} of 1 mg/L or less at most institutions. Given the importance of early, appropriate therapy, vancomycin targeted exposure should be achieved early during the course of therapy, preferably within the first 24 to 48 hours (A-II). As such, the use of Bayesian-derived AUC monitoring may be prudent in these cases since it does not require steady-state serum vancomycin concentrations to allow for early assessment of AUC target attainment.
3. Trough-only monitoring, with a target of 15 to 20 mg/L, is no longer recommended, based on efficacy and nephrotoxicity data in patients with serious infections due to MRSA (A-II). There is insufficient evidence to provide recommendations on whether trough-only or AUC-guided vancomycin monitoring should be used among patients with noninvasive MRSA or other infections.
4. Vancomycin monitoring is recommended for patients receiving vancomycin for serious MRSA infections to achieve a sustained targeted AUC (assuming a MIC_{BMD} of 1 mg/L unless it is known to be greater or less than 1 mg/L by BMD). Independent of MRSA infection, vancomycin monitoring is also recommended for all patients at high risk for nephrotoxicity (eg, critically ill patients receiving concurrent nephrotoxins), patients with unstable (ie, deteriorating or significantly improving) renal function, and those receiving prolonged courses of therapy (more than 3 to 5 days). We suggest the frequency of monitoring be based on clinical judgment; frequent or daily monitoring may be prudent for hemodynamically unstable patients (eg, those with end-stage renal disease), with once-weekly monitoring for hemodynamically stable patients (B-II).
5. Based on current national vancomycin susceptibility surveillance data, under most circumstances for empiric dosing, the vancomycin MIC should be assumed to be 1 mg/L. When the MIC_{BMD} is greater than 1 mg/L, the probability of achieving an AUC/MIC target of ≥400 is low with conventional dosing; higher doses may risk unnecessary toxicity, and the decision to change therapy should be based on clinical judgment. In addition, when the MIC_{BMD} is less than 1 mg/L, we do not recommend decreasing the dose to achieve the AUC/MIC target. It is important to note the limitations in automated susceptibility testing methods, including the lack of precision and variability in MIC results depending on the method used (B-II).
6. The pharmacokinetics of continuous infusion suggest that such regimens may be a reasonable alternative to conventional intermittent infusion dosing when the AUC target cannot be achieved (B-II).
7. Incompatibility of vancomycin with other drugs commonly coadministered in the ICU requires the use of independent lines or multiple catheters when vancomycin is being considered for continuous infusion (A-III).
B. ADULTS
8. Given the narrow vancomycin AUC range for therapeutic effect and minimal associated risk of acute kidney injury (AKI), the most accurate and optimal way to manage vancomycin dosing should be through AUC-guided dosing and monitoring (A-II). We recommend to accomplish this in one of two ways: a. One approach relies on the collection of 2 concentrations (obtained near the steady state, post-distributional peak concentration at 1 to 2 hours after infusion and trough at end of dosing interval), preferably but not required during the same dosing interval (if possible) and utilizing first-order pharmacokinetic (PK) equations to estimate the AUC (A-II). b. The preferred approach to monitor AUC involves the use of Bayesian software programs, embedded with a PK model based on richly sampled vancomycin data as the Bayesian prior, to optimize the delivery of vancomycin based on the collection of 1 or 2 vancomycin concentrations, with at least 1 trough. It is preferred to obtain 2 PK samples (ie, 1 to 2 hours post infusion and at the end of the dosing interval) to estimate the AUC with the Bayesian approach (A-II). A trough concentration alone may be sufficient to estimate the AUC with the Bayesian approach in some patients, but more data across different patient populations are needed to confirm the viability of using trough-only data (B-II).
9. Doses of 15 to 20 mg/kg (based on actual body weight) administered every 8 to 12 hours as an intermittent infusion are recommended for most patients with normal renal function when assuming a MIC_{BMD} of 1 mg/L (A-II). In patients with normal renal function, these doses may not achieve therapeutic AUC/MIC targets when the MIC is 2 mg/L.
10. *Continuous Infusion:* Based on current available data, a loading dose of 15 to 20 mg/kg, followed by daily maintenance CI of 30 to 40 mg/kg (up to 60 mg/kg), to achieve a target steady-state concentration of 20 to 25 mg/L may be considered for critically ill patients (B-II). AUC_{24} can be simply calculated when multiplying the steady-state concentration (ie, desired therapeutic range of 20 to 25 mg/L throughout the entire dosing interval) by a factor of 24 (B-II). Attaining the desired drug exposure may be more readily accomplished, given the ease of sampling time and dosage adjustment, by changing the rate of infusion, which is a highly desirable feature in critically ill patients (B-II).
11. The risk of developing nephrotoxicity with CI appears to be similar or lower compared to intermittent dosing when targeting a steady-state concentration of 15 to 25 mg/L and a trough concentration of 10 to 20 mg/L, respectively (B-II). Definitive studies are needed to compare drug exposure based on measured AUC_{24} and factors that predispose to development of nephrotoxicity, such as receipt of concomitant nephrotoxins, diuretics, and/or vasopressor therapy in patients receiving continuous vs intermittent infusion of vancomycin.
12. In order to achieve rapid attainment of targeted concentrations in critically ill patients with suspected or documented serious MRSA infections, a loading dose of 20 to 35 mg/kg can be considered for intermittent administration of vancomycin (B-II). Loading doses should be based on actual body weight and not exceed 3,000 mg. More intensive and early therapeutic monitoring should also be performed in obese patients (B-II).

Continued on next page

TABLE 2. *(continued)*
Primary Recommendations for Vancomycin Dosing and Therapeutic Drug Monitoring

B. ADULTS
13. *Adult Obesity:* A vancomycin loading dose of 20 to 25 mg/kg using actual body weight, with a maximum of 3,000 mg, may be considered in obese adult patients with serious infections (B-II). Empiric maintenance doses for most obese patients usually do not exceed 4,500 mg/day, depending on their renal function (B-II). Early and frequent monitoring of AUC exposure is recommended for dose adjustment, especially when empiric doses exceed 4,000 mg/day (A-II).
14. *Intermittent Hemodialysis:* Since efficacy data are unavailable for an AUC of <400 mg · h/L, monitoring based on predialysis serum concentrations and extrapolating these values to estimate AUC is most practical. Maintaining predialysis concentrations between 15 and 20 mg/L is likely to achieve the AUC of 400 to 600 mg · h/L in the previous 24 hours (C-III). Predialysis serum concentration monitoring should be performed not less than weekly and should drive subsequent dosing rather than a strict weight-based recommendation, although these recommended doses provide a useful starting point until serum concentrations have been determined (B-II).
15. *Hybrid Dialysis Therapies (eg, Slow-Low Efficiency Dialysis [SLED]):* Loading doses of 20 to 25 mg/kg actual body weight should be used, recognizing that these hybrid dialysis therapies efficiently remove vancomycin (B-III). Initial doses should not be delayed to wait for a dialysis treatment to end. Maintenance doses of 15 mg/kg should be given after hybrid hemodialysis ends or during the final 60 to 90 minutes of dialysis, as is done with standard hemodialysis (B-III). Concentration monitoring should guide further maintenance doses.
16. *Continuous Renal Replacement Therapy (CRRT):* Loading doses of 20 to 25 mg/kg by actual body weight should be used in patients receiving CRRT at conventional, KDIGO-recommended effluent rates of 20 to 25 mL/kg/h (B-II). Initial maintenance dosing for CRRT with effluent rates of 20 to 25 mL/kg/h should be 7.5 to 10 mg/kg every 12 hours (B-II). Maintenance dose and dosing interval should be based on serum concentration monitoring, which should be conducted within the first 24 hours to ensure AUC/MIC targets are met. In fluid overloaded patients, doses may be reduced as patients become euvolemic and drug V_d decreases. The use of CI vancomycin in patients receiving CRRT appears to be growing, and this method could be used in place of intermittent vancomycin dosing, especially when high CRRT ultrafiltrate/dialysate flow rates are employed (B-II).
C. PEDIATRIC PATIENTS
17. Based on an AUC target of 400 mg · h/L (but potentially up to 600 mg · hr/L assuming a MIC of ≤1 mg/L) from adult data, the initial recommended vancomycin dosage for children with normal renal function and suspected serious MRSA infections is 60 to 80 mg/kg/day, divided every 6 to 8 hours, for children ages 3 months and older (A-II).
18. The maximum empiric daily dose is usually 3,600 mg/day in children with adequate renal function (C-III). Most children generally should not require more than 3,000 mg/day, and doses should be adjusted based on observed concentrations to achieve the AUC/MIC target. Early monitoring of observed concentrations is recommended when doses exceed 2,000 to 3,000 mg/day (A-III). Furthermore, close monitoring of observed concentrations and renal function is prudent in patients with poor or augmented renal clearance as resolution of their renal function may occur within the first 5 days of therapy.
19. AUC-guided therapeutic monitoring for vancomycin, preferably with Bayesian estimation, is suggested for all pediatric age groups, based on developmental changes of vancomycin CL documented from the newborn to the adolescent. Based on current available data, the suggestion for AUC-guided monitoring in pediatrics aligns with the approach for adults, including the application of Bayesian estimation for 1 trough concentration, or first-order PK equations with 2 concentrations (B-II). The Bayesian AUC-guided dosing strategy may be an optimal approach to individualize vancomycin therapy in pediatrics since it can incorporate varying ages, weights, and renal function. Both serum concentrations of vancomycin and renal function should be monitored since vancomycin CL and creatinine CL are not always well correlated in pediatrics. Furthermore, aggressive dosing to maintain target AUC exposure and decrease the risk of potential AKI in treatment of MRSA infection necessitates drug monitoring.
20. Therapeutic monitoring may begin within 24 to 48 hours of vancomycin therapy for serious MRSA infections in children, as in adults (B-III). Any delay in therapeutic monitoring should be based on severity of infection and clinical judgment. Dosing adjustment should be made for those with renal insufficiency, or those with obesity, or for those receiving concurrent nephrotoxic drug therapy. Following the initial dose, dosing adjustment is important for those with acute renal insufficiency, but subsequent adjustment (particularly within the first 5 days of therapy) may be necessary for those experiencing recovery of renal function. Sustained or subsequent decreases in dosage may be needed, particularly for those with chronic renal insufficiency and those receiving concurrent nephrotoxic drug therapy (B-III).
21. Vancomycin exposure may be optimally maintained below the thresholds for AUC of 800 mg · h/L and for trough concentrations of 15 mg/L to minimize AKI (B-II). The safety of vancomycin above 80 mg/kg/day has not been prospectively evaluated. Avoiding vancomycin dosages of ≥100 mg/kg/day is suggested since they are likely to surpass these thresholds (B-III).
22. Insufficient data exist on which to base a recommendation for a loading dose among the nonobese pediatric population. Loading doses from adult studies may be considered, but further studies are needed to elucidate the appropriate dose for the various pediatric populations, from neonates to adolescents (C-III).
23. *Pediatric Obesity:* Data suggest that obese children are likely to have vancomycin exposures that may be statistically greater than in normal-weight children when doses are calculated on a mg/kg basis, but these differences are not known to be of sufficient clinical importance to suggest different mg/kg empiric vancomycin dosages in obese children at this time. Similar to nonobese children, obese children < 12 years old, compared with those ≥ 12 years, may require higher mg/kg doses (B-II).
24. *Pediatric Obesity:* Therapeutic monitoring is likely to be of particular value in obese children, both for therapeutic response and to minimize the risk of AKI. The specific recommendations for therapeutic monitoring in nonobese children may also apply for obese children (B-II). A loading dose of 20 mg/kg by total body weight is recommended in obese children (A-III).
25. *Neonates:* Dosages recommended to achieve an AUC of 400 mg · hr/L (assuming a MIC of 1 mg/L) in neonates and infants up to 3 months old range from 10 to 20 mg/kg every 8 to 48 hours depending on postmenstrual age, weight, and SCr (A-II).

Abbreviations (not defined in body of table): AUC, area under the curve; BMD, broth micodilution; CL, clearance; ICU, intensive care unit; KDIGO, Kidney Disease: Improving Global Outcomes; MIC, minimum inhibitory concentration; MRSA, methicillin-resistant *Staphylococcus aureus*; SCr, serum creatinine; V_d, volume of distribution.

concentrations were 10 to 20 mg/L for II, and the steady-state concentrations were 15 to 25 mg/L for CI. The AUC and clinical outcomes, including nephrotoxicity, could not be evaluated rigorously in this study due to the small sample size. Overall, the clinical utility of CI in neonates requires further evaluation, as the most common pathogen causing late-onset sepsis requiring vancomycin therapy is *Staphylococcus epidermidis*, with limited cases of *S. aureus* sepsis. While the optimal AUC/MIC target for *S. epidermidis* is not well studied, a lower target may be reasonable, but further data to support this recommendation are needed.

The incidence of vancomycin-associated AKI reported in neonates has been low, ranging from 1% to 9%.[200] Nonetheless, a positive correlation between increasing vancomycin trough concentrations and AKI has been reported by Bhargava et al.[201] Furthermore, in a large, retrospective, multicenter, propensity score–matched cohort study of 533 neonates receiving vancomycin and gentamicin and 533 receiving gentamicin alone, Constance et al[202] concluded that AKI was not associated with vancomycin alone but may occur in the presence of other recognized risk factors, including patent ductus arteriosus, concomitant nonsteroidal anti-inflammatory drug use, 1 or more positive blood cultures, low birth weight, and higher scores for severity of illness and risk of mortality.

Summary and Recommendations

25. Doses recommended to achieve an AUC of 400 mg · h/L (assuming a MIC of 1 mg/L) in neonates and infants up to 3 months old range from 10 to 20 mg/kg every 8 to 48 hours, depending on postmenstrual age, weight, and SCr (A-II). AUC-guided therapeutic dosing and monitoring, preferably with Bayesian estimation, can best achieve the target vancomycin exposure likely to be required for a successful outcome of treatment for a MRSA infection for all neonates, regardless of gestational and chronologic age. The specific recommendations for AUC-guided therapeutic monitoring in children should also apply for neonates (see recommendation 18, A-III).

Conclusion

To optimize vancomycin use for the treatment of serious infections caused by MRSA, we recommend targeting an AUC/MIC_{BMD} ratio of 400 to 600 (assuming an MIC_{BMD} of 1 mg/L) for empiric dosing in both adult and pediatric patients to maximize clinical efficacy and minimize AKI risk. Furthermore, the AUC should be therapeutically monitored using 1 or 2 postdose concentrations (ie, a peak concentration measured after the early vancomycin tissue distribution phase and a trough level measured prior to the next dose), preferably integrating the Bayesian approach. The primary recommendations are summarized in **Table 2**. The successful use of these guideline recommendations to positively impact patient outcomes may require multifaceted interventions, including educational meetings, guideline implementation, and dissemination of educational material on vancomycin dosing, monitoring, and nephrotoxicity.[203,204] While valuable literature pertaining to adults, children, and neonates has emerged since the last vancomycin guideline, future studies in all patient populations are necessary to address existing gaps, including (1) efficacy data to support vancomycin use in specific patient populations (including neonates and pediatric patients and patients with renal disease and obesity) and for other types of infections; (2) efficacy data for specific pathogens, including coagulase-negative staphylococcus and *Streptococcus* species; (3) robust pediatric efficacy data for MRSA and other gram-positive pathogens causing different types of serious infections; (4) optimal loading and maintenance dosing regimens for patients with obesity and renal insufficiency; (5) efficacy benefit and the need for a dosing algorithm (specifically incorporating a loading dose followed by maintenance infusion); and (6) toxicodynamics of vancomycin CI in critically ill patients.

References

1. Rybak MJ, Lomaestro BM, Rotschafer JC, et al. Therapeutic monitoring of vancomycin in adult patients: a consensus review of the American Society of Health-System Pharmacists, the Infectious Diseases Society of America, and the Society of Infectious Diseases Pharmacists. *Am J Health-Syst Pharm.* 2009; 66(1):82–98.
2. The periodic health examination. Canadian Task Force on the Periodic Health Examination. *Can Med Assoc J.* 1979; 121(9):1193–1254.
3. Craig WA. Basic pharmacodynamics of antibacterials with clinical applications to the use of beta-lactams, glycopeptides, and linezolid. *Infect Dis Clin North Am.* 2003; 17(3):479–501.
4. Drusano GL. Antimicrobial pharmacodynamics: critical interactions of 'bug and drug'. *Nat Rev Microbiol.* 2004; 2(4):289–300.
5. Liu C, Bayer A, Cosgrove SE, Daum RS et al. Clinical practice guidelines by The Infectious Diseases Society of America for the treatment of methicillin-resistant *Staphylococcus aureus* infections in adults and children: executive summary. *Clin Infect Dis.* 2011; 52(3):285–292.
6. Rybak MJ. The pharmacokinetic and pharmacodynamics properties of vancomycin. *Clin Infect Dis.* 2006; 42(Suppl 1):S35-S39.
7. Kullar R, Leonard SN, Davis SL et al. Validation of the effectiveness of a vancomycin nomogram in achieving target trough concentrations of 15-20 mg/L suggested by the vancomycin consensus guidelines. *Pharmacotherapy.* 2011; 31(5):441–448.
8. Singh NB, Yim J, Jahanbakhsh S, Sakoulas G, Rybak MJ. Impact of cefazolin co-administration with vancomycin to reduce development of vancomycin-intermediate *Staphylococcus aureus. Diagn Microbiol Infect Dis.* 2018; 91(4):363–370.
9. Vidaillac C, Gardete S, Tewhey R et al. Alternative mutational pathways to intermediate resistance to vancomycin in methicillin-resistant *Staphylococcus aureus. J Infect Dis.* 2013; 208(1):67–74.
10. Moise-Broder PA, Forrest A, Birmingham MC, Schentag JJ. Pharmacodynamics of vancomycin and other antimicrobials in patients with *Staphylococcus aureus* lower respiratory tract infections. *Clin Pharmacokinet.* 2004; 43(13):925–942.
11. Kullar R, Davis SL, Levine DP, Rybak MJ. Impact of vancomycin exposure on outcomes in patients with

methicillin-resistant *Staphylococcus aureus* bacteremia: support for consensus guidelines suggested targets. *Clin Infect Dis.* 2011; 52(8):975–981.

12. Brown J, Brown K, Forrest A. Vancomycin AUC_{24}/MIC ratio in patients with complicated bacteremia and infective endocarditis due to methicillin-resistant *Staphylococcus aureus* and its association with attributable mortality during hospitalization. *Antimicrob Agents Chemother.* 2012; 56(2):634–638.
13. Holmes NE, Turnidge JD, Munckhof WJ et al. Vancomycin AUC/MIC ratio and 30-day mortality in patients with *Staphylococcus aureus* bacteremia. *Antimicrob Chemother.* 2013; 57(4):1654–1663.
14. Gawronski KM, Goff DA, Brown J, Khadem TM, Bauer KA. A stewardship program's retrospective evaluation of vancomycin AUC_{24}/MIC and time to microbiological clearance in patients with methicillinresistant *Staphylococcus aureus* bacteremia and osteomyelitis. *Clin Ther.* 2013; 35(6):772–779.
15. Jung Y, Song KH, Cho Je et al. Area under the concentration-time curve to minimum inhibitory concentration ratio as a predictor of vancomycin treatment outcome in methicillin-resistant *Staphylococcus aureus* bacteraemia. *Int J Antimicrob Agents.* 2014; 43(2):179–183.
16. Lodise TP, Drusano GL, Zasowski E et al. Vancomycin exposure in patients with methicillin-resistant *Staphylococcus aureus* bloodstream infections: how much is enough? *Clin Infect Dis.* 2014; 59(5):666–675.
17. Casapao AM, Lodise TP, Davis SL et al. Association between vancomycin day 1 exposure profile and outcomes among patients with methicillin-resistant *Staphylococcus aureus* infective endocarditis. *Antimicrob Agents Chemother.* 2015; 59(6):2978–2985.
18. Mogle BT, Steele JM, Seabury RW, Dang UJ, Kufel WD. Implementation of a two-point pharmacokinetic AUC-based vancomycin therapeutic drug monitoring approach in patients with methicillin-resistant *Staphylococcus aureus* bacteraemia. *Int J Antimicrob Agents.* 2018; 52(6):805–810.
19. Le J, Ny P, Capparelli E et al. Pharmacodynamic characteristics of nephrotoxicity associated with vancomycin use in children. *J Pediatric Infect Dis Soc.* 2015; 4(4):e109-e116.
20. Finch NA, Zasowski EJ, Murray KP et al. A quasi-experiment to study the impact of vancomycin area under the concentration-time curve-guided dosing on vancomycin-associated nephrotoxicity. *Antimicrob Agents Chemother.* 2017; 61(12):e01293–17.
21. Zasowski EJ, Murray KP, Trinh TD et al. Identification of vancomycin exposure-toxicity thresholds in hospitalized patients receiving intravenous vancomycin. *Antimicrob Agents Chemother.* 2018; 62(1):e01684–17.
22. Neely MN, Kato L, Youn G et al. Prospective trial on the use of trough concentration versus area under the curve to determine therapeutic vancomycin dosing. *Antimicrob Agents Chemother.* 2018; 62(2):e02042–17.
23. Lodise TP, Rosenkranz SL, Finnemeyer M et al. The emperor's new clothes: prospective observational evaluation of the association between initial vancomycin exposure and failure rates among adult hospitalized patients with MRSA bloodstream infections (PROVIDE) [published online ahead of print June 3, 2019]. *Clin Infect Dis.* doi.10.1093/cid/ciz460.
24. Neely MN, Youn G, Jones B et al. Are vancomycin trough concentrations adequate for optimal dosing? *Antimicrob Agents Chemother.* 2014; 58(1):309–316.
25. Lesar TS, Rotschafer JC, Strand LM, Zolem LD, Zaske DE. Gentamicin dosing errors with four commonly used nomograms. *JAMA.* 1982; 248(10):1190–1193.
26. Patel N, Pai MP, Rodvold KA, Lomaestro B, Drusano GL, Lodise TP. Vancomycin: we can't get there from here. *Clin Infect Dis.* 2011; 52(8):969–974.
27. Mehta RL, Kellum JA, Shah SV et al.; Acute Kidney Injury Network. Acute Kidney Injury Network: report of an initiative to improve outcomes in acute kidney injury. *Crit Care.* 2007; 11(2):R31.
28. Roy AK, Mc Gorrian C, Treacy C et al. A comparison of traditional and novel definitions (RIFLE, AKIN, and KDIGO) of acute kidney injury for the prediction of outcomes in acute decompensated heart failure. *Cardiorenal Med.* 2013; 3(1):26–37.
29. van Hal SJ, Paterson DL, Lodise TP. Systematic review and meta-analysis of vancomycin-induced nephrotoxicity associated with dosing schedules that maintain troughs between 15 and 20 milligrams per liter. *Antimicrob Agents Chemother.* 2013; 57(2):734–744.
30. Sinha Ray A, Haikal A, Hammoud KA, Yu AS. Vancomycin and the risk of AKI: a systematic review and meta-analysis. *Clin J Am Soc Nephrol.* 2016; 11(12):2132–2140.
31. Singbartl K, Kellum JA. AKI in the ICU: definition, epidemiology, risk stratification, and outcomes. *Kidney Int.* 2012; 81(9):819–825.
32. Linder A, Fjell C, Levin A, Walley KR, Russell JA, Boyd JH. Small acute increases in serum creatinine are associated with decreased long-term survival in the critically ill. *Am J Respir Crit Care Med.* 2014; 189(9):1075–81.
33. Suzuki Y, Kawasaki K, Sato Y et al. Is peak concentration needed in therapeutic drug monitoring of vancomycin? A pharmacokinetic-pharmacodynamic analysis in patients with methicillin-resistant *Staphylococcus aureus* pneumonia. *Chemotherapy.* 2012; 58(4):308–312.
34. Lodise TP, Patel N, Lomaestro BM, Rodvold KA, Drusano GL. Relationship between initial vancomycin concentration-time profile and nephrotoxicity among hospitalized patients. *Clin Infect Dis.* 2009; 49(4):507–514.
35. Aljefri DM, Avedissian SN, Rhodes NJ, Postelnick MJ, Nguyen K, Scheetz MH. Vancomycin area under the curve and acute kidney injury: a meta-analysis. *Clin Infect Dis.* 2019; 69(11):1881–1887.
36. Avedissian SN, Pais GM, O'Donnell JN et al. Twenty-four hour pharmacokinetic relationships for intravenous vancomycin and novel urinary biomarkers of acute kidney injury in a rat model. *J Antimicrob Chemother.* 2019; 74(8):2326–2334.
37. Rhodes NJ, Prozialeck WC, Lodise TP et al. Evaluation of vancomycin exposures associated with elevations in novel urinary biomarkers of acute kidney injury in vancomycin-treated rats. *Antimicrob Agents Chemother.* 2016; 60(10):5742–5751.

38. Lodise TP, Graves J, Evans A et al. Relationship between vancomycin MIC and failure among patients with methicillin-resistant *Staphylococcus aureus* bacteremia treated with vancomycin. *Antimicrob Agents Chemother.* 2008; 52(9):3315–3320.
39. Tong SYC, Lye DC, Yahav D, et al; for Australasian Society for Infectious Diseases Clinical Research Network. Effect of vancomycin or daptomycin with vs without an antistaphylococcal β-lactam on mortality, bacteremia, relapse, or treatment failure in patients with MRSA bacteremia: a randomized clinical trial. *JAMA.* 2020; 323(6):527–537.
40. Moenster RP, Linneman TW, Finnegan PM, Hand S, Thomas Z, McDonald JR. Acute renal failure associated with vancomycin and beta-lactams for the treatment of osteomyelitis in diabetics: piperacillin-tazobactam as compared with cefepime. *Clin Microbiol Infect.* 2014; 20(6):O384-O389.
41. Gomes DM, Smotherman C, Birch A et al. Comparison of acute kidney injury during treatment with vancomycin in combination with piperacillin-tazobactam or cefepime. *Pharmacotherapy.* 2014; 34(7):662–669.
42. Burgess LD, Drew RH. Comparison of the incidence of vancomycin-induced nephrotoxicity in hospitalized patients with and without concomitant piperacillin-tazobactam. *Pharmacotherapy.* 2014; 34(7):670–676.
43. Navalkele B, Pogue JM, Karino S et al. Risk of acute kidney injury in patients on concomitant vancomycin and piperacillin-tazobactam compared to those on vancomycin and cefepime. *Clin Infect Dis.* 2017; 64(2):116–123.
44. Karino S, Kaye KS, Navalkele B et al. Epidemiology of acute kidney injury among patients receiving concomitant vancomycin and piperacillin-tazobactam: opportunities for antimicrobial stewardship. *Antimicrob Agents Chemother.* 2016; 60(6):3743–3750.
45. Lodise TP, Lomaestro B, Graves J, Drusano GL. Larger vancomycin doses (at least four grams per day) are associated with an increased incidence of nephrotoxicity. *Antimicrob Agents Chemother.* 2008; 52(4):1330–1336.
46. Minejima E, Choi J, Beringer P, Lou M, Tse E, Wong-Beringer A. Applying new diagnostic criteria for acute kidney injury to facilitate early identification of nephrotoxicity in vancomycin-treated patients. *Antimicrob Agents Chemother.* 2011; 55(7):3278–3283.
47. Cano EL, Haque NZ, Welch VL, et al. Incidence of nephrotoxicity and association with vancomycin use in intensive care unit patients with pneumonia: retrospective analysis of the IMPACT-HAP Database. *Clin Ther.* 2012; 34(1):149–157.
48. Vance-Bryan K, Rotschafer JC, Gilliland SS, Rodvold KA, Fitzgerald CM, Guay DR. A comparative assessment of vancomycin-associated nephrotoxicity in the young versus the elderly hospitalized patient. *J Antimicrob Chemother.* 1994; 33(4):811–821.
49. Jeffres MN, Isakow W, Doherty JA, Micek ST, Kollef MH. A retrospective analysis of possible renal toxicity associated with vancomycin in patients with health care-associated methicillin-resistant *Staphylococcus aureus* pneumonia. *Clin Ther.* 2007; 29(6):1107–1115.
50. Fullmer A, McCue D, Feng C. Retrospective review of vancomycin-induced nephrotoxicity in patients with leukemia. *J Oncol Pharm Pract.* 2014; 20(6):403–408.
51. Chung J, Oh JM, Cho EM et al. Optimal dose of vancomycin for treating methicillin-resistant *Staphylococcus aureus* pneumonia in critically ill patients. *Anaesth Intensive Care.* 2011; 39(6):1030–1037.
52. Hermsen ED, Hanson M, Sankaranarayanan J, Stoner JA, Florescu MC, Rupp ME. Clinical outcomes and nephrotoxicity associated with vancomycin trough concentrations during treatment of deep-seated infections. *Expert Opin Drug Saf.* 2010; 9(1):9–14.
53. Hidayat LK, Hsu DI, Quist R, Shriner KA, Wong-Beringer A. High-dose vancomycin therapy for methicillin-resistant *Staphylococcus aureus* infections: efficacy and toxicity. *Arch Intern Med.* 2006; 166(19):2138–2144.
54. Kralovicová K, Spanik S, Halko J et al. Do vancomycin serum levels predict failures of vancomycin therapy or nephrotoxicity in cancer patients? *J Chemother.* 1997; 9(6):420–426.
55. Zimmermann AE, Katona BG, Plaisance KI. Association of vancomycin serum concentrations with outcomes in patients with gram-positive bacteremia. *Pharmacotherapy.* 1995; 15(1):85–91.
56. Mohr JF, Murray BE. Point: vancomycin is not obsolete for the treatment of infection caused by methicillin-resistant *Staphylococcus aureus*. *Clin Infect Dis.* 2007; 44(12):1536–1542.
57. Pai MP, Neely M, Rodvold KA, Lodise TP. Innovative approaches to optimizing the delivery of vancomycin in individual patients. *Adv Drug Deliv Rev.* 2014; 77:50–57.
58. Diaz R, Afreixo V, Ramalheira E, Rodrigues C, Gago B. Evaluation of vancomycin MIC creep in methicillin resistant *Staphylococcus aureus* infections—a systematic review and meta-analysis. *Clin Microbiol Infect.* 2017; 24(2):97–104.
59. Diaz R, Ramalheira E, Afreixo V, Gago B. Evaluation of vancomycin MIC creep in *Staphylococcus aureus* infections. *J Glob Antimicrob Resist.* 2017; 10:281–284.
60. Sader HS, Farrell DJ, Flamm RK, Jones RN. Activity of ceftaroline and comparator agents tested against *Staphylococcus aureus* from patients with bloodstream infections in US medical centres (2009-13). *J Antimicrob Chemother.* 2015; 70(7):2053–2056.
61. Pfaller MA, Sader HS, Flamm RK, Castanheira M, Smart JI, Mendes RE. In vitro activity of telavancin against clinically important gram-positive pathogens from 69 U.S. medical centers (2015): potency analysis by U.S. Census Divisions. *Microb Drug Resist.* 2017; 23(6):718–726.
62. Duncan LR, Sader HS, Smart JI, Flamm RK, Mendes RE. Telavancin activity in vitro tested against a worldwide collection of gram-positive clinical isolates (2014). *J Glob Antimicrob Resist.* 2017; 10:271–276.
63. Mouton JW, Meletiadis J, Voss A, Turnidge J. Variation of MIC measurements: the contribution of strain and laboratory variability to measurement precision. *J Antimicrob Chemother.* 2018; 73(9):2374–2379.
64. Heil EL, Claeys KC, Mynatt RP et al. Making the change to area under the curve-based

vancomycin dosing. *Am J Health-Syst Pharm.* 2018; 75(24):1986–1995.

65. Jelliffe RW, Schumitzky A. Modeling, adaptive control, and optimal drug therapy. *Med Prog Technol.* 1990; 16(1-2):95–110.
66. Bayard DS, Jelliffe RW. A Bayesian approach to tracking patients having changing pharmacokinetic parameters. *J Pharmacokinet Pharmacodyn.* 2004; 31(1):75–107.
67. Fuchs A, Csajka C, Thoma Y, Buclin T, Widmer N. Benchmarking therapeutic drug monitoring software: a review of available computer tools. *Clin Pharmacokinet.* 2013; 52(1):9–22.
68. Turner RB, Kojiro K, Shephard EA et al. Review and validation of Bayesian dose-optimizing software and equations for calculation of the vancomycin area under the curve in critically ill patients. *Pharmacotherapy.* 2018; 38(12):1174–1183.
69. Al-Sulaiti FK, Nader AM, Saad MO et al. Clinical and pharmacokinetic outcomes of peak-trough-based versus trough-based vancomycin therapeutic drug monitoring approaches: a pragmatic randomized controlled trial. *Eur J Drug Metab Pharmacokinet.* 2019; 44(5):639–652.
70. Begg EJ, Barclay ML, Duffull SB. A suggested approach to once-daily aminoglycoside dosing. *Br J Clin Pharmacol.* 1995; 39(6):605–609.
71. Bauer LA. *Applied Clinical Pharmacokinetics.* 2nd ed. New York, NY: McGraw-Hill Medical; 2008.
72. Beringer P. *Winter's Basic Clinical Pharmacokinetics.* 6th ed. Philadelphia, PA: Wolters Kluwer Health; 2018.
73. Marsot A, Boulamery A, Bruguerolle B, Simon N. Vancomycin: a review of population pharmacokinetic analyses. *Clin Pharmacokinet.* 2012; 51(1):1–13.
74. Lodise TP, McKinnon PS, Swiderski L, Rybak MJ. Outcomes analysis of delayed antibiotic treatment for hospital-acquired *Staphylococcus aureus* bacteremia. *Clin Infect Dis.* 2003; 36(11):1418–1423.
75. Diaz R, Afreixo V, Ramalheira E, Rodrigues C, Gago B. Evaluation of vancomycin MIC creep in methicillin-resistant *Staphylococcus aureus* infections—a systematic review and meta-analysis. *Clin Microbiol Infect.* 2018; 24(2):97–104.
76. Diekema DJ, Pfaller MA, Shortridge D, Zervos M, Jones RN. Twenty-year trends in antimicrobial susceptibilities among *Staphylococcus aureus* from the SENTRY antimicrobial surveillance program. *Open Forum Infect Dis.* 2019; 6(suppl 1):S47-S53.
77. Kruzel MC, Lewis CT, Welsh KJ et al. Determination of vancomycin and daptomycin MICs by different testing methods for methicillin-resistant *Staphylococcus aureus. J Clin Microbiol.* 2011; 49(6):2272–2273.
78. Hsu DI, Hidayat LK, Quist R et al. Comparison of method-specific vancomycin minimum inhibitory concentration values and their predictability for treatment outcome of meticillin-resistant *Staphylococcus aureus* (MRSA) infections. *Int J Antimicrob Agents.* 2008; 32(5):378–385.
79. Rybak MJ, Vidaillac C, Sader HS et al. Evaluation of vancomycin susceptibility testing for methicillin-resistant *Staphylococcus aureus*: comparison of etest and three automated testing methods. *J Clin Microbiol.* 2013; 51(7):2077–2081.
80. Wysocki M, Delatour F, Faurisson F et al. Continuous versus intermittent infusion of vancomycin in severe staphylococcal infections: prospective multicenter randomized study. *Antimicrob Agents Chemother.* 2001; 45(9):2460–2467.
81. Schmelzer TM, Christmas AB, Norton HJ, Heniford BT, Sing RF. Vancomycin intermittent dosing versus continuous infusion for treatment of ventilator-associated pneumonia in trauma patients. *Am Surg.* 2013; 79(11):1185–1190.
82. Tafelski S, Nachtigall I, Troeger U, et al. Observational clinical study on the effects of different dosing regimens on vancomycin target levels in critically ill patients: continuous versus intermittent application. *J Infect Public Health.* 2015; 8(4):355–363.
83. Hutschala D, Kinstner C, Skhirdladze K, Thalhammer F, Muller M, Tschernko E. Influence of vancomycin on renal function in critically ill patients after cardiac surgery: continuous versus intermittent infusion. *Anesthesiology.* 2009; 111(2):356–365.
84. Akers KS, Cota JM, Chung KK, Renz EM, Mende K, Murray CK. Serum vancomycin levels resulting from continuous or intermittent infusion in critically ill burn patients with or without continuous renal replacement therapy. *J Burn Care Res.* 2012; 33(6):e254-e262.
85. Saugel B, Nowack MC, Hapfelmeier A et al. Continuous intravenous administration of vancomycin in medical intensive care unit patients. *J Crit Care.* 2013; 28(1):9–13.
86. Hanrahan TP, Harlow G, Hutchinson J et al. Vancomycin-associated nephrotoxicity in the critically ill: a retrospective multivariate regression analysis*. *Crit Care Med.* 2014; 42(12):2527–2536.
87. Vuagnat A, Stern R, Lotthe A et al. High dose vancomycin for osteomyelitis: continuous vs. intermittent infusion. *J Clin Pharm Ther.* 2004; 29(4):351–357.
88. Ingram PR, Lye DC, Fisher DA, Goh WP, Tam VH. Nephrotoxicity of continuous versus intermittent infusion of vancomycin in outpatient parenteral antimicrobial therapy. *Int J Antimicrob Agents.* 2009; 34(6):570–574.
89. Verrall AJ, Llorin R, Tam VH et al. Efficacy of continuous infusion of vancomycin for the outpatient treatment of methicillin-resistant *Staphylococcus aureus* infections. *J Antimicrob Chemother.* 2012; 67(12):2970–2973.
90. Ingram PR, Lye DC, Tambyah PA, Goh WP, Tam VH, Fisher DA. Risk factors for nephrotoxicity associated with continuous vancomycin infusion in outpatient parenteral antibiotic therapy. *J Antimicrob Chemother.* 2008; 62(1):168–171.
91. Dubée V, Zeller V, Lhotellier L et al. Continuous highdose vancomycin combination therapy for methicillin-resistant staphylococcal prosthetic hip infection: a prospective cohort study. *Clin Microbiol Infect.* 2013; 19(2):E98-E105.
92. Raverdy V, Ampe E, Hecq JD, Tulkens PM. Stability and compatibility of vancomycin for administration

by continuous infusion. *J Antimicrob Chemother.* 2013; 68(5):1179–1182.

93. Wade J, Cooper M, Ragan R. Simulated Y-site compatibility of vancomycin and piperacillin-tazobactam. *Hosp Pharm.* 2015; 50(5):376–379.
94. de Waele JJ, Danneels I, Depuydt P, Decruyenaere J, Bourgeois M, Hoste E. Factors associated with inadequate early vancomycin levels in critically ill patients treated with continuous infusion. *Int J Antimicrob Agents.* 2013; 41(5):434–438.
95. Ocampos-Martinez E, Penaccini L, Scolletta S et al. Determinants of early inadequate vancomycin concentrations during continuous infusion in septic patients. *Int J Antimicrob Agents.* 2012; 39(4):332–337.
96. Mohammedi I, Descloux E, Argaud L, Le Scanff J, Robert D. Loading dose of vancomycin in critically ill patients: 15 mg/kg is a better choice than 500 mg. *Int J Antimicrob Agents.* 2006; 27(3):259–262.
97. Li J, Udy AA, Kirkpatrick CM, Lipman J, Roberts JA. Improving vancomycin prescription in critical illness through a drug use evaluation process: a weight-based dosing intervention study. *Int J Antimicrob Agents.* 2012; 39(1):69–72.
98. Pea F, Furlanut M, Negri C et al. Prospectively validated dosing nomograms for maximizing the pharmacodynamics of vancomycin administered by continuous infusion in critically ill patients. *Antimicrob Agents Chemother.* 2009; 53(5):1863–1867.
99. Roberts JA, Taccone FS, Udy AA, Vincent JL, Jacobs F, Lipman J. Vancomycin dosing in critically ill patients: robust methods for improved continuous-infusion regimens. *Antimicrob Agents Chemother.* 2011; 55(6):2704–2709.
100. Truong J, Levkovich BJ, Padiglione AA. Simple approach to improving vancomycin dosing in intensive care: a standardised loading dose results in earlier therapeutic levels. *Intern Med J.* 2012; 42(1):23–29.
101. Wang JT, Fang CT, Chen YC, Chang SC. Necessity of a loading dose when using vancomycin in critically ill patients. *J Antimicrob Chemother.* 2001; 47(2):246.
102. Barth RH, DeVincenzo N. Use of vancomycin in high-flux hemodialysis: experience with 130 courses of therapy. *Kidney Int.* 1996; 50(3):929–936.
103. Brown M, Polisetty R, Gracely EJ, Cuhaci B, Schlecht HP. Weight-based loading of vancomycin in patients on hemodialysis. *Clin Infect Dis.* 2011; 53(2):164–166.
104. Vandecasteele SJ, de Bacquer D, de Vriese AS. Implementation of a dose calculator for vancomycin to achieve target trough levels of 15-20 microg/mL in persons undergoing hemodialysis. *Clin Infect Dis.* 2011; 53(2):124–129.
105. Covajes C, Scolletta S, Penaccini L et al. Continuous infusion of vancomycin in septic patients receiving continuous renal replacement therapy. *Int J Antimicrob Agents.* 2013; 41(3):261–266.
106. Decker BS, Kays MB, Chambers M, Kraus MA, Moe SM, Sowinski KM. Vancomycin pharmacokinetics and pharmacodynamics during short daily hemodialysis. *Clin J Am Soc Nephrol.* 2010; 5(11):1981–1987.
107. Alfandari S, Levent T, Descamps D et al. Evaluation of glycopeptide use in nine French hospitals. *Med Mal Infect.* 2010; 40(4):232–237.
108. Hochart C, Berthon C, Corm S et al. Vancomycin serum concentration during febrile neutropenia in patients with acute myeloid leukemia. *Med Mal Infect.* 2011; 41(12):652–656.
109. Lemaire X, Loiez C, Valette M et al. Comparison of vancomycin and teicoplanin trough serum levels in patients with infected orthopedic devices: new data for old therapies. *J Infect Chemother.* 2011; 17(3):370–374.
110. Grace E. Altered vancomycin pharmacokinetics in obese and morbidly obese patients: what we have learned over the past 30 years. *J Antimicrob Chemother.* 2012; 67(6):1305–1310.
111. Blouin RA, Bauer LA, Miller DD, Record KE, Griffen WO Jr. Vancomycin pharmacokinetics in normal and morbidly obese subjects. *Antimicrob Agents Chemother.* 1982; 21(4):575–580.
112. Crass RL, Dunn R, Hong J, Krop LC, Pai MP. Dosing vancomycin in the super obese: less is more. *J Antimicrob Chemother.* 2018; 73(11):3081–3086.
113. Clinical guidelines on the identification, evaluation, and treatment of overweight and obesity in adults: executive summary. Expert Panel on the Identification, Evaluation, and Treatment of Overweight in Adults. *Am J Clin Nutr.* 1998; 68(4):899–917.
114. Pastor PN, Reuben C, Xia H. *Chartbook on Trends in the Health of Americans.* Hyattsville, MD: National Center for Health Statistics; 2002.
115. Hales CM, Carroll MD, Fryar CD, Ogden CL. Prevalence of obesity among adults and youth: United States, 2015–2016. *NCHS Data Brief.* 2017; (288):1–8.
116. Choi YC, Saw S, Soliman D et al. Intravenous vancomycin associated with the development of nephrotoxicity in patients with class III obesity. *Ann Pharmacother.* 2017; 51(11):937–944.
117. Vance-Bryan K, Guay DR, Gilliland SS, Rodvold KA, Rotschafer JC. Effect of obesity on vancomycin pharmacokinetic parameters as determined by using a Bayesian forecasting technique. *Antimicrob Agents Chemother.* 1993; 37(3):436–440.
118. Ducharme MP, Slaughter RL, Edwards DJ. Vancomycin pharmacokinetics in a patient population: effect of age, gender, and body weight. *Ther Drug Monit.* 1994; 16(5):513–518.
119. Bauer LA, Black DJ, Lill JS. Vancomycin dosing in morbidly obese patients. *Eur J Clin Pharmacol.* 1998; 54(8):621–625.
120. Adane ED, Herald M, Koura F. Pharmacokinetics of vancomycin in extremely obese patients with suspected or confirmed *Staphylococcus aureus* infections. *Pharmacotherapy.* 2015; 35(2):127–139.
121. Hong J, Krop LC, Johns T, Pai MP. Individualized vancomycin dosing in obese patients: a two-sample measurement approach improves target attainment. *Pharmacotherapy.* 2015; 35(5):455–463.
122. Pai MP. Drug dosing based on weight and body surface area: mathematical assumptions and limitations in obese adults. *Pharmacotherapy.* 2012; 32(9):856–868.
123. Cockcroft DW, Gault MH. Prediction of creatinine clearance from serum creatinine. *Nephron.* 1976; 16(1):31–41.

124. Matzke GR, Aronoff GR, Atkinson AJ Jr et al. Drug dosing consideration in patients with acute and chronic kidney disease-a clinical update from Kidney Disease Improving Global Outcomes (KDIGO). *Kidney Int.* 2011; 80(11):1122–1137.
125. Rodvold KA, Blum RA, Fischer JH et al. Vancomycin pharmacokinetics in patients with various degrees of renal function. *Antimicrob Agents Chemother.* 1988; 32(6):848–852.
126. Pai MP, Hong J, Krop L. Peak measurement for vancomycin AUC estimation in obese adults improves precision and lowers bias. *Antimicrob Agents Chemother.* 2017; 61(4):e02490–16.
127. Carreno JJ, Lomaestro B, Tietjan J, Lodise TP. Pilot study of a Bayesian approach to estimate vancomycin exposure in obese patients with limited pharmacokinetic sampling. *Antimicrob Agents Chemother.* 2017; 61(5):e02478–16.
128. Fu CF, Huang JD, Wang JT, Lin SW, Wu CC. The ratio of pre-dialysis vancomycin trough serum concentration to minimum inhibitory concentration is associated with treatment outcomes in methicillin-resistant *Staphylococcus aureus* bacteremia. *PLoS One.* 2018; 13(3):e0193585.
129. Zelenitsky SA, Ariano RE, McCrae ML, Vercaigne LM. Initial vancomycin dosing protocol to achieve therapeutic serum concentrations in patients undergoing hemodialysis. *Clin Infect Dis.* 2012; 55(4):527–533.
130. Lewis SJ, Mueller BA. Contemporary vancomycin dosing in chronic hemodialysis patients does not meet AUC targets: development of a new dosing model using Monte Carlo simulation. Presentation at: Infectious Diseases Week; 2016; New Orleans LA.
131. Scott MK, Mueller BA, Clark WR. Vancomycin mass transfer characteristics of high-flux cellulosic dialysers. *Nephrol Dial Transplant.* 1997; 12(12):2647–2653.
132. Clark WR, Mueller BA, Kraus MA, Macias WL. Extracorporeal therapy requirements for patients with acute renal failure. *J Am Soc Nephrol.* 1997; 8(5):804–812.
133. Mueller BA, Smoyer WE. Challenges in developing evidence-based drug dosing guidelines for adults and children receiving renal replacement therapy. *Clin Pharmacol Ther.* 2009; 86(5):479–482.
134. Vancomycin hydrochloride for injection [package insert]. Lake Forest, IL: Hospira, Inc.; March 2017.
135. Lanese DM, Alfrey PS, Molitoris BA. Markedly increased clearance of vancomycin during hemodialysis using polysulfone dialyzers. *Kidney Int.* 1989; 35(6):1409–1412.
136. Quale JM, O'Halloran JJ, DeVincenzo N, Barth RH. Removal of vancomycin by high-flux hemodialysis membranes. *Antimicrob Agents Chemother.* 1992; 36(7):1424–1426.
137. Scott MK, Macias WL, Kraus MA, Clark WR, Carfagna MA, Mueller BA. Effects of dialysis membrane on intradialytic vancomycin administration. *Pharmacotherapy.* 1997; 17(2):256–262.
138. Mason NA, Neudeck BL, Welage LS, Patel JA, Swartz RD. Comparison of 3 vancomycin dosage regimens during hemodialysis with cellulose triacetate dialyzers: post-dialysis versus intradialytic administration. *Clin Nephrol.* 2003; 60(2):96–104.
139. Ariano RE, Fine A, Sitar DS, Rexrode S, Zelenitsky SA. Adequacy of a vancomycin dosing regimen in patients receiving high-flux hemodialysis. *Am J Kidney Dis.* 2005; 46(4):681–687.
140. Lucksiri A, Scott MK, Mueller BA, Hamburger RJ, Sowinski KM. CAHP-210 dialyzer influence on intradialytic vancomycin removal. *Nephrol Dial Transplant.* 2002; 17(9):1649–1654.
141. Nyman HA, Agarwal A, Senekjian HO, Leypoldt JK, Cheung AK. Removal of vancomycin administered during dialysis by a high-flux dialyzer. *Hemodial Int.* 2018; 22(3):383–387.
142. Pollard TA, Lampasona V, Akkerman S et al. Vancomycin redistribution: dosing recommendations following high-flux hemodialysis. *Kidney Int.* 1994; 45(1):232–237.
143. Crawford BS, Largen RF, Walton T, Doran JJ. Once-weekly vancomycin for patients receiving high-flux hemodialysis. *Am J Health-Syst Pharm.* 2008; 65(13):1248–1253.
144. El Nekidy WS, El-Masri MM, Umstead GS, Dehoorne-Smith M. Predicting maintenance doses of vancomycin for hospitalized patients undergoing hemodialysis. *Can J Hosp Pharm.* 2016; 69(5):341–347.
145. Pallotta KE, Manley HJ. Vancomycin use in patients requiring hemodialysis: a literature review. *Semin Dial.* 2008; 21(1):63–70.
146. Pai AB, Pai MP. Vancomycin dosing in high flux hemodialysis: a limited-sampling algorithm. *Am J Health-Syst Pharm.* 2004; 61(17):1812–1816.
147. Maxson R, Pate J, Starr J. Evaluation of weight-based vancomycin dosing for hospitalized hemodialysis patients. *Ren Fail.* 2016; 38(10):1677–1682.
148. Kielstein JT, Czock D, Schöpke T et al. Pharmacokinetics and total elimination of meropenem and vancomycin in intensive care unit patients undergoing extended daily dialysis. *Crit Care Med.* 2006; 34(1):51–56.
149. Scoville BA, Mueller BA. Medication dosing in critically ill patients with acute kidney injury treated with renal replacement therapy. *Am J Kidney Dis.* 2013; 61(3):490–500.
150. Harris LE, Reaves AB, Krauss AG, Griner J, Hudson JQ. Evaluation of antibiotic prescribing patterns in patients receiving sustained low-efficiency dialysis: opportunities for pharmacists. *Int J Pharm Pract.* 2013; 21(1):55–61.
151. Pasko DA, Churchwell MD, Salama NN, Mueller BA. Longitudinal hemodiafilter performance in modeled continuous renal replacement therapy. *Blood Purif.* 2011; 32(2):82–88.
152. Frazee EN, Kuper PJ, Schramm GE et al. Effect of continuous venovenous hemofiltration dose on achievement of adequate vancomycin trough concentrations. *Antimicrob Agents Chemother.* 2012; 56(12):6181–6185.
153. Kidney Disease: Improving Global Outcomes Acute Kidney Injury Work Group. KDIGO clinical practice

guideline for acute kidney injury. *Kidney Int Suppl.* 2012(2):S1-S138.

154. Chaijamorn W, Jitsurong A, Wiwattanawongsa K, Wanakamanee U, Dandecha P. Vancomycin clearance during continuous venovenous haemofiltration in critically ill patients. *Int J Antimicrob Agents.* 2011; 38(2):152–156.
155. Colin PJ, Allegaert K, Thomson AH et al. Vancomycin pharmacokinetics throughout life: results from a pooled population analysis and evaluation of current dosing recommendations. *Clin Pharmacokinet.* 2019; 58(6):767–780.
156. McNeil JC, Kok EY, Forbes AR et al. Healthcare-associated Staphylococcus aureus bacteremia in children: evidence for reverse vancomycin creep and impact of vancomycin trough values on outcome. *Pediatr Infect Dis J.* 2016; 35(3):263–268.
157. McNeil JC, Kaplan SL, Vallejo JG. The influence of the route of antibiotic administration, methicillin susceptibility, vancomycin duration and serum trough concentration on outcomes of pediatric *Staphylococcus aureus* bacteremic osteoarticular infection. *Pediatr Infect Dis J.* 2017; 36(6):572–577.
158. Fiorito TM, Luther MK, Dennehy PH, LaPlante KL, Matson KL. Nephrotoxicity with vancomycin in the pediatric population: a systematic review and meta-analysis. *Pediatr Infect Dis J.* 2018; 37(7):654–661.
159. Hahn A, Frenck RW Jr, Allen-Staat M, Zou Y, Vinks AA. Evaluation of target attainment of vancomycin area under the curve in children with methicillin-resistant *Staphylococcus aureus* bacteremia. *Ther Drug Monit.* 2015; 37(5):619–625.
160. Yoo RN, Kim SH, Lee J. Impact of initial vancomycin trough concentration on clinical and microbiological outcomes of methicillin-resistant *Staphylococcus aureus* bacteremia in children. *J Korean Med Sci.* 2017; 32(1):22–28.
161. Eiland LS, English TM, Eiland EH 3rd. Assessment of vancomycin dosing and subsequent serum concentrations in pediatric patients. *Ann Pharmacother.* 2011; 45(5):582–589.
162. Frymoyer A, Hersh AL, Benet LZ, Guglielmo BJ. Current recommended dosing of vancomycin for children with invasive methicillin-resistant *Staphylococcus aureus* infections is inadequate. *Pediatr Infect Dis J.* 2009; 28(5):398–402.
163. Frymoyer A, Guglielmo BJ, Hersh AL. Desired vancomycin trough serum concentration for treating invasive methicillin-resistant staphylococcal infections. *Pediatr Infect Dis J.* 2013; 32(10):1077–1079.
164. Le J, Bradley JS, Murray W et al. Improved vancomycin dosing in children using area under the curve exposure. *Pediatr Infect Dis J.* 2013; 32(4):e155-e163.
165. Ploessl C, White C, Manasco K. Correlation of a vancomycin pharmacokinetic model and trough serum concentrations in pediatric patients. *Pediatr Infect Dis J.* 2015; 34(10):e244-e247.
166. Madigan T, Sieve RM, Graner KK, Banerjee R. The effect of age and weight on vancomycin serum trough concentrations in pediatric patients. *Pharmacotherapy.* 2013; 33(12):1264–1272.
167. Demirjian A, Finkelstein Y, Nava-Ocampo A et al. A randomized controlled trial of a vancomycin loading dose in children. *Pediatr Infect Dis J.* 2013; 32(11):1217–1223.
168. Abdel Hadi O, Al Omar S, Nazer LH, Mubarak S, Le J. Vancomycin pharmacokinetics and predicted dosage requirements in pediatric cancer patients. *J Oncol Pharm Pract.* 2016; 22(3):448–453.
169. Le J, Vaida F, Nguyen E et al. Population-based pharmacokinetic modeling of vancomycin in children with renal insufficiency. *J Pharmacol Clin Toxicol.* 2014; 2(1):1017–1026.
170. Avedissian SN, Bradley E, Zhang D et al. Augmented renal clearance using population-based pharmacokinetic modeling in critically ill pediatric patients. *Pediatr Crit Care Med.* 2017; 18(9):e388-e394.
171. Zhang H, Wang Y, Gao P et al. Pharmacokinetic characteristics and clinical outcomes of vancomycin in young children with various degrees of renal function. *J Clin Pharmacol.* 2016; 56(6):740–748.
172. McKamy S, Hernandez E, Jahng M, Moriwaki T, Deveikis A, Le J. Incidence and risk factors influencing the development of vancomycin nephrotoxicity in children. *J Pediatr.* 2011; 158(3):422–426.
173. Knoderer CA, Gritzman AL, Nichols KR, Wilson AC. Late-occurring vancomycin-associated acute kidney injury in children receiving prolonged therapy. *Ann Pharmacother.* 2015; 49(10):1113–1119.
174. Sinclair EA, Yenokyan G, McMunn A, Fadrowski JJ, Milstone AM, Lee CK. Factors associated with acute kidney injury in children receiving vancomycin. *Ann Pharmacother.* 2014; 48(12):1555–1562.
175. Matson KL, Shaffer CL, Beck GL, Simonsen KA. Assessment of initial serum vancomycin trough concentrations and their association with initial empirical weight-based vancomycin dosing and development of nephrotoxicity in children: a multicenter retrospective study. *Pharmacotherapy.* 2015; 35(3):337–343.
176. Ragab AR, Al-Mazroua MK, Al-Harony MA. Incidence and predisposing factors of vancomycin-induced nephrotoxicity in children. *Infect Dis Ther.* 2013; 2(1):37–46.
177. Le J, Ngu B, Bradley JS et al. Vancomycin monitoring in children using Bayesian estimation. *Ther Drug Monit.* 2014; 36(4):510–518.
178. Stockmann C, Olson J, Rashid J et al. An evaluation of vancomycin area under the curve estimation methods for children treated for acute pulmonary exacerbations of cystic fibrosis due to methicillin-resistant *Staphylococcus aureus*. *J Clin Pharmacol.* 2019; 59(2):198–205.
179. Kendrick JG, Carr RR, Ensom MH. Pharmacokinetics and drug dosing in obese children. *J Pediatr Pharmacol Ther.* 2010; 15(2):94–109.
180. Moffett BS, Kim S, Edwards MS. Vancomycin dosing in obese pediatric patients. *Clin Pediatr (Phila).* 2011; 50(5):442–446.
181. Heble DE Jr, McPherson C, Nelson MP, Hunstad DA. Vancomycin trough concentrations in overweight or obese pediatric patients. *Pharmacotherapy.* 2013; 33(12):1273–1277.

182. Miller M, Miller JL, Hagemann TM, Harrison D, Chavez-Bueno S, Johnson PN. Vancomycin dosage in overweight and obese children. *Am J Health-Syst Pharm.* 2011; 68(21):2062–2068.
183. Nassar L, Hadad S, Gefen A et al. Prospective evaluation of the dosing regimen of vancomycin in children of different weight categories. *Curr Drug Saf.* 2012; 7(5):375–381.
184. Eiland LS, Sonawane KB. Vancomycin dosing in healthy-weight, overweight, and obese pediatric patients. *J Pediatr Pharmacol Ther.* 2014; 19(3):182–188.
185. Camaione L, Elliott K, Mitchell-Van Steele A, Lomaestro B, Pai MP. Vancomycin dosing in children and young adults: back to the drawing board. *Pharmacotherapy.* 2013; 33(12):1278–1287.
186. Natale S, Bradley J, Nguyen WH et al. Pediatric obesity: pharmacokinetic alterations and effects on antimicrobial dosing. *Pharmacotherapy.* 2017; 37(3):361–378.
187. Le J, Capparelli EV, Wahid U et al. Bayesian estimation of vancomycin pharmacokinetics in obese children: matched case-control study. *Clin Ther.* 2015; 37(6):1340–1351.
188. Nguyen WN, Bradley JS, Capparelli EV et al. Optimal weight-based vancomycin dosing in obese children using Bayesian estimation. Presentation at: Interscience Conference on Antimicroial Agents and Chemotherapy; September 21, 2015; San Diego, CA.
189. Rhodin MM, Anderson BJ, Peters AM et al. Human renal function maturation: a quantitative description using weight and postmenstrual age. *Pediatr Nephrol.* 2009; 24(1):67–76.
190. Mehrotra N, Tang L, Phelps SJ, Meibohm B. Evaluation of vancomycin dosing regimens in preterm and term neonates using Monte Carlo simulations. *Pharmacotherapy.* 2012; 32(5):408–419.
191. Marqués-Miñana MR, Saadeddin A, Peris JE. Population pharmacokinetic analysis of vancomycin in neonates. A new proposal of initial dosage guideline. *Br J Clin Pharmacol.* 2010; 70(5):713–720.
192. Irikura M, Fujiyama A, Saita F et al. Evaluation of the vancomycin dosage regimen based on serum creatinine used in the neonatal intensive care unit. *Pediatr Int.* 2011; 53(6):1038–1044.
193. Capparelli EV, Lane JR, Romanowski GL et al. The influences of renal function and maturation on vancomycin elimination in newborns and infants. *J Clin Pharmacol.* 2001; 41(9):927–934.
194. Zhao W, Lopez E, Biran V, Durrmeyer X, Fakhoury M, Jacqz-Aigrain E. Vancomycin continuous infusion in neonates: dosing optimisation and therapeutic drug monitoring. *Arch Dis Child.* 2013; 98(6):449–453.
195. Frymoyer A, Hersh AL, El-Komy MH et al. Association between vancomycin trough concentration and area under the concentration-time curve in neonates. *Antimicrob Agents Chemother.* 2014; 58(11):6454–6461.
196. Stockmann C, Hersh AL, Roberts JK et al. Predictive performance of a vancomycin population pharmacokinetic model in neonates. *Infect Dis Ther.* 2015; 4(2):187–198.
197. Cies JJ, Moore WS 2nd, Nichols K, Knoderer CA, Carella DM, Chopra A. Population pharmacokinetics and pharmacodynamic target attainment of vancomycin in neonates on extracorporeal life support. *Pediatr Crit Care Med.* 2017; 18(10):977–985.
198. Leroux S, Jacqz-Aigrain E, Biran V et al. Clinical utility and safety of a model-based patient-tailored dose of vancomycin in neonates. *Antimicrob Agents Chemother.* 2016; 60(4):2039–2042.
199. Gwee A, Cranswick N, McMullan B et al. Continuous versus intermittent vancomycin infusions in infants: a randomized controlled trial. *Pediatrics.* 2019; 143(2), pii:e20182179.
200. Lestner JM, Hill LF, Heath PT, Sharland M. Vancomycin toxicity in neonates: a review of the evidence. *Curr Opin Infect Dis.* 2016; 29(3):237–247.
201. Bhargava V, Malloy M, Fonseca R. The association between vancomycin trough concentrations and acute kidney injury in the neonatal intensive care unit. *BMC Pediatr.* 2017; 17(1):50.
202. Constance JE, Balch AH, Stockmann C et al. A propensity-matched cohort study of vancomycinassociated nephrotoxicity in neonates. *Arch Dis Child Fetal Neonatal Ed.* 2016; 101(3):F236-F243.
203. Phillips CJ, Wisdom AJ, McKinnon RA, Woodman RJ, Gordon DL. Interventions targeting the prescribing and monitoring of vancomycin for hospitalized patients: a systematic review with meta-analysis. *Infect Drug Resist.* 2018; 11:2081–2094.
204. Phillips CJ, McKinnon RA, Woodman RJ, Gordon DL. Sustained improvement in vancomycin dosing and monitoring post-implementation of guidelines: results of a three-year follow-up after a multifaceted intervention in an Australian teaching hospital. *J Infect Chemother.* 2018; 24(2):103–109.

Michael J. Rybak, PharmD, MPH, PhD, FCCP, FIDP, FIDSA, Anti-Infective Research Laboratory, Department of Pharmacy Practice, Eugene Applebaum College of Pharmacy & Health Sciences, Wayne State University, Detroit, MI, School of Medicine, Wayne State University, Detroit, MI, and Detroit Receiving Hospital, Detroit, MI.

Jennifer Le, PharmD, MAS, FIDSA, FCCP, FCSHP, BCPSAQ ID, Skaggs School of Pharmacy and Pharmaceutical Sciences, University of California San Diego, La Jolla, CA.

Thomas P. Lodise, PharmD, PhD, Albany College of Pharmacy and Health Sciences, Albany, NY, and Stratton VA Medical Center, Albany, NY.

Donald P. Levine, MD, FACP, FIDSA, School of Medicine, Wayne State University, Detroit, MI, and Detroit Receiving Hospital, Detroit, MI.

John S. Bradley, MD, JSB, FIDSA, FAAP, FPIDS, Department of Pediatrics, Division of Infectious Diseases, University of California at San Diego, La Jolla, CA, and Rady Children's Hospital San Diego, San Diego, CA.

Catherine Liu, MD, FIDSA, Division of Allergy and Infectious Diseases, University of Washington, Seattle, WA, and Vaccine and Infectious Disease Division, Fred Hutchinson Cancer Research Center, Seattle, WA.

Bruce A. Mueller, PharmD, FCCP, FASN, FNKF, University of Michigan College of Pharmacy, Ann Arbor, MI.

Manjunath P. Pai, PharmD, FCCP, University of Michigan College of Pharmacy, Ann Arbor, MI.

Annie Wong-Beringer, PharmD, FCCP, FIDSA, University of Southern California School of Pharmacy, Los Angeles, CA.

John C. Rotschafer, PharmD, FCCP, University of Minnesota College of Pharmacy, Minneapolis, MN.

Keith A. Rodvold, PharmD, FCCP, FIDSA, University of Illinois College of Pharmacy, Chicago, IL.

Holly D. Maples, PharmD, University of Arkansas for Medical Sciences College of Pharmacy & Arkansas Children's Hospital, Little Rock, AR.

Benjamin M. Lomaestro, PharmD, Albany Medical Center Hospital, Albany, NY.

Dr. Wong-Beringer received a grant from Merck & Co. and consulted for Rempex Pharmaceuticals, INSMED, Merck & Co., Nabriva Therapeutics, GlaxoSmithKline, Paratek Pharmaceuticals, Achaogen, Inc., Bayer HealthCare, and SIGA Technologies. Dr. Bradley served on a planning committee for the US Food and Drug Administration and European Medicines Agency at the American College of Clinical Pharmacy's annual meeting; participated in the design of a pediatric clinical trial; served on an executive committee for the United States Committee on Antimicrobial Susceptibility Testing; and consulted for Achaogen, Allergan, ContraFect, GlaxoSmithKline, Janssen, Melinta, Merck, Nabrive, Pfizer, Theravance, and Zavante. Dr. Liu received a research grant from Nohla Therapeutics and was a member of an Independent Efficacy Adjudication Committee with Theravance. Dr. Le received research awards from the Sternfels Prize for Drug Safety Innovation, Duke University, the National Institutes of Health (NIH) and National Institute of Child Health and Human Development, and JMI Laboratories; was an invited advisory board member for FDA, the Asian Pacific Health Foundation, and *Infectious Diseases and Therapy* journal. Dr. Levine served on the data safety monitoring board for Contrafect and served on an adjudication panel for Novartis. Dr. Lodise received grants from the Antibiotic Resistance Leadership Group (ARLG), Merck & Co, and Motif Bio PLC; served as a health outcomes project consultant for Paratek Pharmaceuticals, Allergan, Merck & Co., and Melinta Therapeutics; served on advisory boards for Paratek Pharmaceuticals, Motif Bio PLC, Achaogen, Nabriva, and Tetraphase; served as a consultant to Paratek Pharmaceuticals, ARLG, Allergan, Merck & Co., Melinta Therapeutics, Motif Bio PLC, Achaogen, Nabriva, and Tetraphase; and was a speaker for Melinta Therapeutics, Tetraphase, and Sunovion. Dr. Maples served as an international working group member for the European Cystic Fibrosis Society and North American Cystic Fibrosis Society, served on an advisory panel for the Centers for Disease Control and Prevention and Pew Charitable Trust, and was on a committee for the Arkansas Health Department. Dr. Mueller received research grants from Merck & Co. and Hope Pharmaceutical and served on an advisory board for NxStage and Baxter. Dr. Pai received a grant from Merck, Inc., served on an advisory board for Shinogi and Paratek Pharmaceuticals, and served on the meet the professor program for Merck. Dr. Rodvold received a grant from Theravance Biopharm, NIH, ARLG, and Allergan; consulted for BLC, Entasis, Merck, Paratek Pharmaceuticals, Shionogi, Tetraphase, and Wockhardt; was a speaker at the American Society for Microbiology and European Society for Clinical Microbiology and Infectious Diseases ASM/ESCMID conference; served on the 2015–2019 Program Committee and was 2016–2018 Program Co-Chairperson for the American Microbiology Society; and was a member of the 2017–2019 Antimicrobial Resistance Committee for IDSA. Dr. Rybak received research grants from Bayer Pharmaceuticals, the NIH Research Project Grant (RO1) Program, Merck, Allergan, the Michigan Department of Health and Human Services, Accelerate Diagnostics, Inc., NIH, Contrafect, Motif Biosciences, and the Michigan Translational Research and Commercialization Program; and served as a grant review panel member for NIH. The other authors have declared no potential conflicts of interest.

Copyright © 2020, American Society of Health-System Pharmacists, Inc. All rights reserved. Contact ASHP for reprint and permissions requests. This content may not be used for commercial purposes without the express written consent of ASHP.

The bibliographic citation for this document is as follows: Rybak MJ, Le J, Lodise TP, et al. Therapeutic monitoring of vancomycin for serious methicillin-resistant *Staphylococcus aureus* infections: A revised consensus guideline and review by the American Society of Health-System Pharmacists, the Infectious Diseases Society of America, the Pediatric Infectious Diseases Society, and the Society of Infectious Diseases Pharmacists. *Am J Health-Syst Pharm.* 2020; 77(11):835–864. https://doi.org/10.1093/ajhp/zxaa036